CHAPTER 32: Acute Gingival and Periodontal Conditions, Lesions of Endodontic Origin, and Avulsed Teeth

Procedure 32-1 Emergency Management of the Avulsed Tooth

CHAPTER 33: Caries Management: Fluoride and Nonfluoride Caries-Preventive Agents

Procedure 33-1 Professionally Applied Topical Fluoride Using the Tray Technique for In-Office Fluoride Treatment (Gel or Foam)
Procedure 33-2 Professionally Applied Sodium Fluoride Varnish Using the Paint-On Technique

CHAPTER 34: Pit and Fissure Sealants

Procedure 34-1 Applying Light-Cured (Photopolymerized) Sealants
Procedure 34-2 Applying Self-Cured (Autopolymerizing) Sealants

CHAPTER 35: Nutritional Counseling

Procedure 35-1 Food Record Instructions for Dental Patients

CHAPTER 37: Impressions, Study Casts, and Oral Appliances

Procedure 37-1 Selecting the Correct Tray Size and Preparing It for Use
Procedure 37-2 Mixing Alginate
Procedure 37-3 Making a Mandibular Preliminary Impression
Procedure 37-4 Making a Maxillary Preliminary Impression
Procedure 37-5 Making a Wax-Bite Registration
Procedure 37-6 Pouring the Cast and the Base
Procedure 37-7 Constructing a Custom-Made Oral Appliance (A Single-Layer Mouth Guard, a Fluoride Tray, or a Tooth-Whitening Tray)

CHAPTER 38: Restorative Therapy

Procedure 38-1 Applying a Rubber Dam
Procedure 38-2 Removing a Rubber Dam
Procedure 38-3 Placing a Tofflemire Matrix System
Procedure 38-4 Placing an Amalgam Restoration
Procedure 38-5 Finishing and Polishing Amalgam Restorations
Procedure 38-6 Placing and Finishing a Class III Composite Restoration
Procedure 38-7 Placing and Finishing a Class II Composite Restoration
Procedure 38-8 Placing a Resin-Modified Glass Ionomer (RMGI) Restoration of Class V Abrasion Lesions
Procedure 38-9 Placing a Stainless Steel Crown
Procedure 38-10 Placing Retraction Cord
Procedure 38-11 Preparing Reinforced Zinc Oxide Eugenol Temporary Restorations (Class II Cavity Preparation)

CHAPTER 39: Dentinal Hypersensitivity Management

Procedure 39-1 Administration of Desensitizing Agents

CHAPTER 40: Local Anesthesia

Procedure 40-1 Oraqix Topical Anesthetic Application for Use During Scaling and Root Planing
Procedure 40-2 Loading the Metallic or Plastic Cartridge-Type Syringe
Procedure 40-3 Unloading the Breech-Loading Metallic or Plastic Cartridge-Type Syringe
Procedure 40-4 Basic Techniques for a Successful Injection

CHAPTER 41: Nitrous Oxide–Oxygen Analgesia

Procedure 41-1 Administration of Nitrous Oxide–Oxygen Analgesic Using the Constant Liter Flow Technique

CHAPTER 42: Persons with Disabilities

Procedure 42-1 Transferring Client from Wheelchair to Dental Chair Using a One-Person Lift
Procedure 42-2 Transferring Client from Wheelchair to Dental Chair Using a Two-Person Lift

CHAPTER 46: Human Immunodeficiency Virus Infection

Procedure 46-1 Dental Hygiene Care for the Patient with Human Immunodeficiency Virus

CHAPTER 48: Persons with Autoimmune Diseases

Procedure 48-1 Implementation of a Stress Reduction Protocol

CHAPTER 50: Respiratory Diseases

Procedure 50-1 Management of an Acute Asthmatic Episode

CHAPTER 56: Persons with Fixed and Removable Dental Prostheses

Procedure 56-1 Professional Care for Clients with Removable Dental Prostheses
Procedure 56-2 Daily Oral and Denture Hygiene Care for Individuals with Removable Prostheses
Procedure 56-3 Daily Oral Care for Individuals with Fixed Dental Prostheses

ELSEVIER evolve

YOU'VE JUST PURCHASED MORE THAN A TEXTBOOK!*

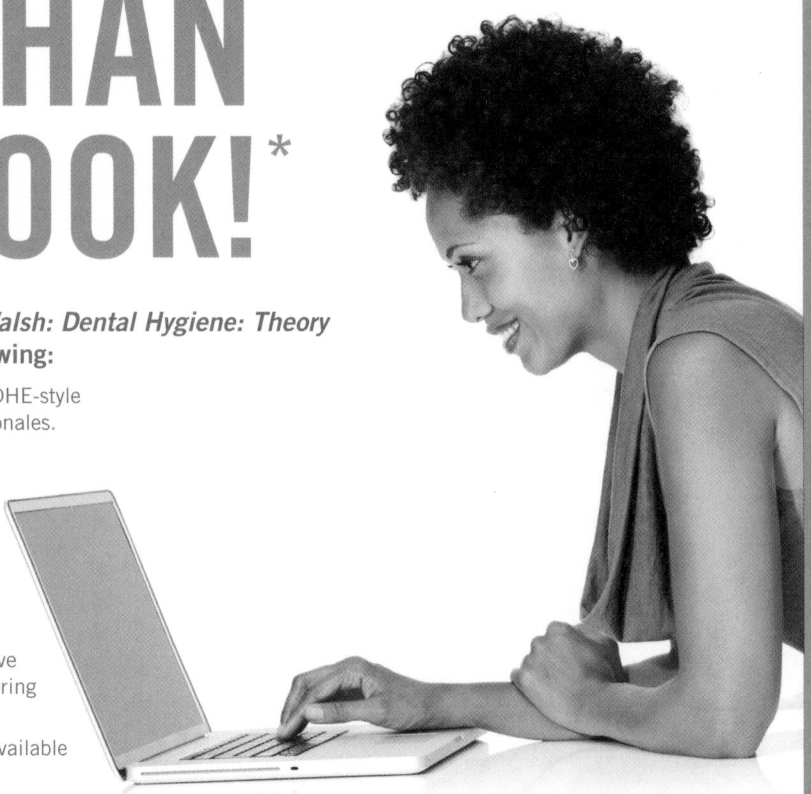

Evolve Student Resources for *Darby and Walsh: Dental Hygiene: Theory and Practice, 4th Edition* include the following:

- NEW! Practice Quizzes: Approximately 1300 NBDHE-style questions with instant-feedback answers and rationales.
- NEW! Flashcards: Text-only, interactive, and separated by chapter to help you master key terminology.
- Competency Evaluation Forms: Procedural assessments that can be completed and stored in a portfolio to demonstrate clinical competence.
- NEW! Procedure Sequencing Exercises: Interactive tool to allow students to practice the correct ordering of steps in key clinical procedures.
- Suggested Readings: Expanded print resources available on selected topics.
- Supplemental Material: Additional tables, figures, and boxes available for a select number of chapters.
- Web Resources: Hyperlinked suggested websites for further research.

To access your student resources, visit:

http://evolve.elsevier.com/Darby/hygiene

Fourth Edition

Dental Hygiene

THEORY AND PRACTICE

Michele Leonardi Darby, BSDH, MS
Professor Emeritus
Gene W. Hirschfeld School of Dental Hygiene
Old Dominion University
Norfolk, Virginia

Margaret M. Walsh, RDH, MS, EdD
Professor
Department of Preventative and Restorative Dental Sciences
School of Dentistry
University of California–San Francisco
San Francisco, California

Consulting Editor
Denise M. Bowen, RDH, MS
Professor Emeritus
Department of Dental Hygiene
Idaho State University
Pocatello, Idaho

ELSEVIER

ELSEVIER
SAUNDERS

3251 Riverport Lane
St. Louis, Missouri 63043

DENTAL HYGIENE: THEORY AND PRACTICE, FOURTH EDITION ISBN: 978-1-4557-4548-7

ISBN: 978-1-4557-4548-7

Vice President and Publisher: Linda Duncan
Executive Content Strategist: Kathy Falk
Content Strategist: Kristin Wilhelm
Content Development Specialist: Joslyn Dumas
Publishing Services Manager: Catherine Jackson
Project Manager: Carol O'Connell
Design Direction: Maggie Reid

Printed in the United States of America

Last digit is the print number: 9 8 7 6 5 4 3 2

To my parents, for their unwavering focus on what really matters in life.
To my husband, Dennis, and our children, Devan and Blake, for making everything worthwhile.

MLD

To my family, especially TJ and Rachel Langer and Martha and Ray Pfeiffer, and to my friends and colleagues, especially Babs, Denise, Jana, Catherine, Kirsten, Jane, JoAnn, and Ann for their love and support during my recent illness, and for the joy they always bring to my life.

MMW

CONTRIBUTORS

Gary C. Armitage, DDS, MS
Professor
Department of Orofacial Sciences
University of California–San Francisco
San Francisco, California
Chapter 20: *Potential Impact of Periodontal Infections on Overall General Health*

Joanna Asadoorian, RDH, PhD
Director and Associate Professor
School of Dental Hygiene
Faculty of Dentistry
University of Manitoba
Winnipeg, Manitoba, Canada
Chapter 31: *Chemotherapy for Control of Periodontal Disease*

Curtis Aumiller, MS, MBA RRT-NPS, RPFT
Associate Professor/Director of Clinical Education
Respiratory Therapist Program
Harrisburg Area Community College
Harrisburg, Pennsylvania
Chapter 50: *Respiratory Diseases*

Deborah Blythe Bauman, BSDH, MS
Assistant Dean, Associate Professor
College of Health Sciences
Old Dominion University
Norfolk, Virginia
Chapter 44: *Diabetes Mellitus*

Helene S. Bednarsh, BS, RDH, MPH
Director HIV Dental
HIV/AIDS Services Division
Boston Public Health Commission
Boston, Massachusetts
Chapter 9: *Infection Control*

Louise Bourassa, DH, BA, MA
Professor
Dental Hygiene Program
Cégep Garneau
Québec, Québec, Canada
Chapter 25: *Dentifrices*

Denise M. Bowen, RDH, MS
Professor Emeritus
Department of Dental Hygiene
Idaho State University
Pocatello, Idaho
Chapter 1: *The Dental Hygiene Profession*
Chapter 10: *Medical Emergencies*
Chapter 23: *Toothbrushing*
Chapter 24: *Mechanical Oral Biofilm Control: Interdental and Supplemental Self-Care Devices*
Chapter 59: *Orthodontic Care*

Jennifer L. Brame, BS, MS
Clinical Assistant Professor
Dental Ecology
UNC-Chapel Hill
Chapel Hill, North Carolina
Chapter 63: *Career Planning and Job Searching*

Lynn Bergstrom Bryan, BSDH, MEd
Associate Clinical Professor
Surgical Sciences–Periodontics
Marquette University School of Dentistry
Milwaukee, Wisconsin
Chapter 28: *Root Morphology and Instrumentation Implications*

Sue Camardese RDH, MS
Chase Brexton Health Services
Dental Department
Columbia, Maryland
President and Co-founder
Mid Atlantic Prevent Abuse and Neglect through Dental Awareness (PANDA) Coalition
Chapter 60: *Abuse and Neglect*

Denise Michelle Claiborne, BS, BSDH, MSDH
Lecturer
Dental Hygiene
Old Dominion University
Norfolk, Virginia
Chapter 8: *The Dental Hygiene Care Environment*

Brigette R. Cooper, RDH, BA, MS
Associate Professor
Dental Hygiene
Minnesota State University, Mankato
Mankato, Minnesota
Chapter 38: *Restorative Therapy*

Elizabeth T. Couch, RDH, MS
Research Analyst
Department of Preventive and Restorative Dental Sciences
School of Dentistry
University of California–San Francisco
San Francisco, California;
Clinical Supervisor
Dental Assisting Program
Foothill College
Los Altos, California
Chapter 61: *Palliative Oral Care*

Eve Cuny, BA, MS
Associate Professor
Dental Practice
University of the Pacific, Arthur A. Dugoni School of Dentistry
San Francisco, California
Chapter 9: *Infection Control*

Devan Leonardi Darby, MD, MPH
Chapter 6: Cultural Competence
Chapter 46: Human Immunodeficiency Virus Infection

Joan M. Davis, RDH, PhD
Professor
Dental Hygiene
Southern Illinois University
Carbondale, Illinois
Chapter 45: Cancer

Leeann R. Donnelly, Dip DH, BDSc(DH), MSc, PhD
Assistant Professor
Oral Biological and Medical Sciences
University of British Columbia
Vancouver, British Columbia, Canada
Chapter 56: Persons with Fixed and Removable Dental Prostheses

Catherine Kelly Draper, RDH, MS
Adjunct Faculty
Dental Hygiene
Foothill College
Los Altos Hills, California
Chapter 7: Professional Portfolios

Lori J. Drummer, RDH, MEd, EdM
Professor
Dental Hygiene
Health and Sciences Division
College of DuPage
Glen Ellyn, Illinois
Chapter 11: Ergonomics

Nadia Dubreuil, DH
Professor
Dental Hygiene
College Francois-Xavier-Garneau
Québec, Québec, Canada
Chapter 25: Dentifrices

Donna Eastabrooks, CDA, RDH, MA, PhD
Professor and Clinic Coordinator
Dental Hygiene Program
Manor College
Jenkintown, Pennsylvania
Chapter 17: Oral Hygiene Assessment: Soft and Hard Deposits

Kathy J. Eklund, RDH, MHP
Director of Occupational Health and Safety
The Forsyth Institute
Cambridge, Massachusetts;
Adjunct Faculty
Dental Hygiene
Massachusetts College of Pharmacy and Health Sciences
Boston, Massachusetts;
Adjunct Faculty
Dental Hygiene
Mount Ida College
Newton, Massachusetts
Chapter 9: Infection Control

Joan Gugino Ellison, RDH, BS, MS
Adjunct Faculty
Dental Hygiene and Allied Health
Harrisburg Area Community College
Harrisburg, Pennsylvania
Chapter 50: Respiratory Diseases

Maureen E. Fannon, RDH, MS
Lecturer/Clinical Instructor
Dental Hygiene
Kennedy King College
Chicago, Illinois
Chapter 34: Pit and Fissure Sealants

John D.B. Featherstone, MSc, PhD
Professor and Dean
Director Biomaterials, Biophysical Sciences, and Engineering Program
University of California–San Francisco
School of Dentistry
Department of Preventive and Restorative Dental Sciences
University of California San Francisco
San Francisco, California
Chapter 18: Dental Caries Management by Risk Assessment

Margaret J. Fehrenbach, RDH, MS
Dental Hygiene Educational Consultant
Dental Science Technical Writer
Seattle, Washington
Chapter 15: Extraoral and Intraoral Clinical Assessment

Jane L. Forrest, BSDH, MS, EdD
Professor of Clinical Dentistry
Dental Public Health and Pediatric Dentistry
Section Chair, Behavioral Science
University of Southern California
Los Angeles, California
Director, National Center for Dental Hygiene Research and Practice
Chapter 3: Evidence-Based Decision Making

Joan I. Gluch, RDH, PhD
Associate Dean, Academic Policies, Director of Community Health and Adjunct Associate Professor
Preventive and Restorative Sciences
University of Pennsylvania School of Dental Medicine
Philadelphia, Pennsylvania
Chapter 55: The Older Adult

JoAnn R. Gurenlian, RDH, PhD
Professor and Graduate Program Director
Idaho State University
Department of Dental Hygiene
Division of Health Sciences
Pocatello, Idaho
Chapter 48: Persons with Autoimmune Diseases

Joanna L. Harris-Worelds, RDH, MSDH
Instructor, SC-ADHA Advisor
Dental Hygiene
Clayton State University
Morrow, Georgia
Chapter 57: *Orofacial Clefts and Fractured Jaw*

Carol Dixon Hatrick, CDA, RDA, RDH, MS
Director
Dental Programs
Santa Rosa Junior College
Santa Rosa, California
Chapter 37: *Impressions, Study Casts, and Oral Appliances*

Kathleen O. Hodges, BSDH, MSDH
Professor
Dental Hygiene
Idaho Satae Univeristy, Office of Medical and Oral Health
Pocatello, Idaho
Chapter 27: *Ultrasonic Instrumentation*
Chapter 30: *Decision Making Related to Nonsurgical Periodontal Therapy*

Mehran Hossaini-Zadeh, DMD
Associate Clinical Professor
Oral and Maxillofacial Surgery
University of California–San Francisco
San Francisco, California
Chapter 58: *Osseointegrated Dental Implants*

Kirsten A. Jarvi, RDH, MS
Director of Professional Education
Interleukin Genetics, Inc
University of California–San Francisco
Guest lecturer
San Francisco, California
Chapter 36: *Tobacco Cessation*

Juliana J. Kim, BSDH, MS, MBA, PhD
Vice President, Scientific Affairs
Sunstar Americas, Inc.
Chicago, Illinois
Chapter 39: *Dentinal Hypersensitivity Management*

Ron J.M. Knevel, RDH, B Health, Med
Senior Lecturer, Course Coordinator Oral Health Science
Department of Dentistry and Oral Health
La Trobe University, La Trobe Rural Health School
Bendigo, Victoria, Australia
Chapter 6: *Cultural Competence*

Brenda S. Kunz, RDH, BA, MSET
Instructor
Department of Dental Hygiene
Carrington College California–Sacramento
Sacramento, California
Chapter 47: *Persons with Neurologic and Sensory Deficits*

Diana Lamoreux, RDH, BS, MEd
Retired Faculty
Cuyahoga Community College
Dental Hygiene Program;
Lorain County Community College
Dental Hygiene Program
Cleveland, Ohio
Private Practice
Chapter 33: *Caries Management: Fluoride and Nonfluoride Caries-Preventive Agents*

France Lavoie, HD, BA, MA, DU Posturology
Independent Practice
Professor
Cegep Trois-Rivieres
College Francois-Xavier-Garneau
Quebec, Quebec, Canada
Chapter 25: *Dentifrices*

Joan D. Leakey, DipDT, DipDH, DipPI, MEd
Clinical Associate Professor
Dental Hygiene Program
School of Dentistry
University of Alberta
Edmonton, Alberta, Canada
Chapter 16: *Dentition Assessment*

Margaret Lemaster, BSDH, MS
Assistant Professor
School of Dental Hygiene
Old Dominion University
Norfolk, Virgina
Chapter 52: *Alcohol and Substance Abuse Problems*

Laura Lee MacDonald, Dip DH, BScD(DH), MEd
Associate Professor and Faculty of Graduate Studies
School of Dental Hygiene
University of Manitoba
Winnipeg, Manitoba, Canada
Chapter 4: *Health and Health Promotion*
Chapter 53: *Eating Disorders*

Lisa F. Harper Mallonee, BSDH, MPH
Associate Professor
Dental Hygiene
Texas A&M Health Science Center
Baylor College of Dentistry
Dallas, Texas
Chapter 35: *Nutritional Counseling*

Leslie Ann Wilkerson Mallory, RDH, MS
Faculty
School of Dental Hygiene
College of Health Sciences
Old Dominion University
Norfolk, Virginia
Chapter 54: *Women's Health and the Health of Their Children*

Syrene A. Miller, BA
Director of Evidence Based Decision Making
The Center for Oral Health
Deer Park, Washington
Chapter 3: *Cultural Competence*

Cara M. Miyasaki, RDA, RDHEF, MS
Program Director
Dental Assisting Program
Foothill College;
Instructor
Dental Hygiene Department
Foothill College
Los Altos Hills, California
Chapter 13: *Vital Signs*

Laura Mueller-Joseph, BSDH, MS, EdD
Professor and Chair
Department of Dental Hygiene
State University of New York at Farmingdale
Farmingdale, New York
Chapter 43: *Cardiovascular Disease*

Kathleen B. Muzzin, RDH, MS
Associate Professor
Caruth School of Dental Hygiene
Baylor College of Dentistry
Texas A&M Health Science Center
Dallas, Texas
Chapter 42: *Persons with Disabilities*

Michaela Nguyen, RDH, MS
Clinical Associate Professor
Dental Hygiene
Ostrow School of Dentistry of USC
Los Angeles, California
Chapter 26: *Hand-Activated Instrumentation*

Elena Ortega, RDH, MS
Instructor
Dental Hygiene
Diablo Valley College
Pleasant Hill, California;
Instructor
Dental Hygiene
Chabot College
Hayward, California
Chapter 40: *Local Anesthesia*

Karen M. Palleschi, AS, BSDH, MS
Professor
Dental Hygiene
Hudson Valley Community College
Troy, New York
Chapter 22: *Dental Hygiene Care Plan, Evaluation, and Documentation*

Frieda Atherton Pickett, BS, MSDH
Adjunct Associate Professor
Graduate Dental Hygiene
Idaho State University
Pocatello, Idaho
Chapter 12: *The Health History*

Janice F.L. Pimlott, BScD, MSc
Professor Emeritus
Dentistry
University of Alberta
Edmonton, Alberta, Canada
Chapter 16: *Dentition Assessment*

Dorothy J. Rowe, RDH, MS, PhD
Associate Professor
Preventive and Restorative Dental Sciences
University of California–San Francisco
San Francisco, California
Chapter 47: *Persons with Neurologic and Sensory Deficits*

Kelly Marie Schulz, BSDH, MS
Adjunct Assistant Professor
Gene W. Hirschfeld School of Dental Hygiene
Old Dominion University
Norfolk, Virginia
Chapter 51: *Developmentally and Cognitively Challenged Persons*

Michelle Sirois, BSDH, MSDH
Assistant Professor
Dental Hygiene
Springfield Technical Community College
Springfield, Massachusetts
Chapter 62: *Practice Management*

Birgitta Söder, Dr, PhD, RDH
Professor Emeritus
Dental Medicine
Karolinska Institutet
Huddinge, Sweden
Chapter 32: *Acute Gingival and Periodontal Conditions, Lesions of Endodontic Origin, and Avulsed Teeth*

Ann Eshenaur Spolarich, RDH, PhD
Clinical Associate Professor
Division of Dental Public Health and Pediatric Dentistry
University of Southern California
Los Angeles, California;
Adjunct Associate Professor
Arizona School of Dentistry and Oral Health
A.T. Still University
Mesa, Arizona;
Clinical Instructor
Dean's Faculty
University of Maryland Dental School
Baltimore, Maryland
Chapter 14: *Pharmacologic History*
Chapter 48: *Persons with Autoimmune Diseases*

Phyllis Spragge, RDH, MA
Program Director
Dental Hygiene
Foothill College
Los Altos Hills, California
Chapter 7: *Professional Portfolios*

Joyce Y. Sumi, BSDH, MSDH
Associate Professor, Dental Hygiene
Co-Director, Advanced Dental Hygiene Sciences
Division of Periodontology, Diagnostic Sciences, and Dental Hygiene
Ostrow School of Dentistry
University of Southern California
Los Angeles, California
Chapter 26: *Hand-Activated Instrumentation*

Sheryl L. Ernest Syme, RDH, MS
Associate Professor
Division of Dental Hygiene
University of Maryland School of Dentistry;
Director, Degree Completion Program and Curriculum Management
Division of Dental Hygiene
University of Maryland School of Dentistry
Baltimore, Maryland
Chapter 60: *Abuse and Neglect*

Cheryl Thomas, RDH
Dentalinspirations, Inc.
Galveston, Texas
Chapter 49: *Renal Disease and Organ Transplantation*

Susan Lynn Tolle, BSDH, MS
Professor, University Professor, Director of Clinical Affairs
Dental Hygiene
Old Dominion University
Norfolk, Virginia
Chapter 19: *Periodontal and Risk Assessment*

Judy Yamamoto, RDH, MS
Professor
Dental Hygiene and Dental Assisting
Foothill College
Los Altos Hills, California
Chapter 34: *Pit and Fissure Sealants*

Pamela Zarkowski, JD, MPH, BSDH
Provost and Vice President for Academic Affairs
University of Detroit Mercy
McNichols Campus
Detroit, Michigan
Chapter 64: *Legal and Ethical Decision Making*

Evidence-Based Knowledge—The Foundation of Dental Hygiene

Dental Hygiene: Theory and Practice, Fourth Edition, is for students and professionals who are interested in the use of evidence-based knowledge to guide decision making in practice. Societal values and healthcare reforms forecast the need for dental hygienists who can assess situations, access information, make evidence-based decisions, and collaborate with dentists and other health professionals in providing quality, culturally appropriate healthcare. Research evidence provides a framework for making decisions, solving problems, explaining phenomena, and predicting outcomes that enables the practitioner to continually re-evaluate and advance service to society.

This book prepares dental hygienists to view their profession with pride, understand its scope, and influence its advancement. The book uses the process of care guided by a client's human needs to operationalize the roles of the dental hygienist as practitioner, client advocate, manager, researcher, and health promoter.

Dental Hygiene: Theory and Practice, Fourth Edition, is predicated on four key assumptions:

- Oral health and systemic health are inextricably linked; therefore collaboration with other healthcare professions is essential for quality client care.
- Theory, research, and client needs and values serve as the basis for decision making.
- Dental hygienists are responsible and accountable for the services they provide and for the professional judgments and decisions they render.
- Accountability requires a systematic approach to practice, and this approach is the dental hygiene process.

Given these assumptions, society has a right to access care from individuals who are competent in making dental hygiene assessments, diagnoses, and care plans; providing interventions; and evaluating clinical outcomes.

Human Needs Theory

Human needs theory serves as a unifying theme in this book. We have selected this theory for the following reasons: Dental hygiene promotes oral and systemic health through the fulfillment of human needs related to dental hygiene care. Human needs are universal, transcend all cultures, and are applicable to both individuals and groups. Human need fulfillment contributes to the quality of life of the individual, community, nation, and world. These facts were recognized by the World Health Organization when, in 1984, it redefined health as "the extent to which an individual or group is able, on the one hand, to realize aspirations and satisfy needs and, on the other hand, to change and cope with the environment."

Because dental hygiene care assists individuals in their attainment of human needs, it is an essential component of the healthcare system, it enhances quality of life, and it is valued in today's wellness-oriented society.

Terminology

An effort was made to use the most current terms (e.g., terms from the American Academy of Periodontology Classification of Periodontal Diseases and Conditions, American Dental Association insurance codes and definitions, diabetes mellitus type 1 and type 2, oral biofilm). Progressing through the book, the reader may quickly notice that the term *client* is used more frequently than *patient.* We are sensitive to the responses that the term *client* may evoke. In general, however, we deliberately use the term *client* because it is broader in scope than the term *patient*, and it can refer to a group as well as an individual. In addition, given that the focus of dental hygiene is to prevent oral disease and promote wellness, the term *client* recognizes that not all of those for whom we provide care are in need of "treatment" for a disease. Also, the term *client* acknowledges the autonomy of the recipient of care, because individuals who seek dental hygiene care generally choose to do so in partnership with the dental hygienist.

Textbook Format

Dental Hygiene: Theory and Practice, Fourth Edition, is organized into eight sections:

- Section I: Conceptual Foundations (7 chapters)
- Section II: Preparation for the Appointment (4 chapters)
- Section III: Assessments (9 chapters)
- Section IV: Critical Thinking in Dental Hygiene Practice (2 chapters)
- Section V: Implementation (16 chapters)
- Section VI: Pain and Anxiety Control (3 chapters)
- Section VII: Individuals with Special Needs (20 chapters)
- Section VIII: Management (3 chapters)

In terms of format, chapters include:

- **Competencies** to guide the teacher and the learner.
- **Evidence-based explanations** of the subject.
- **Procedures** with detailed steps and color illustrations to ensure that the learner attains clinical competence.
- **Client Education Tips** to remind the learner that there is more than just flossing and toothbrushing in educating a person about his or her oral and systemic health.
- **Legal, Ethical, and Safety Issues** that highlight areas in need of management to protect the health and welfare of both client and practitioner.
- **Key Concepts** that summarize the main points of the chapter at a glance.
- **Critical Thinking Exercises and Scenarios** that provide opportunities for independent thought, problem solving, reflection, and discussion.

Recognizing that this book may be used throughout North America, we have included, where appropriate, information that reflects the practice of dental hygiene in Canada.

Section I: Conceptual Foundations describes the evolving profession of dental hygiene, introduces human needs theory and the process of dental hygiene care, and provides the behavioral science and communication theory used by successful dental hygienists in human interactions. The dental hygiene process provides the framework for delivering quality care to all types of clients in a variety of settings and serves as the core of professional practice. Given dental hygiene's focus on oral disease prevention and health promotion, an entire chapter is devoted to evidence-based decision making. In addition, professional portfolios are introduced as a means of documenting the learner's progress in providing care and becoming a competent practitioner. Moreover, because we live in a global society and culture influences health, disease, behavior, beliefs, and lifestyle, a chapter on cultural competence is included in this section.

Section II: Preparation for the Appointment describes the dental hygiene care environment, guidelines for infection control, and strategies for adapting to guidelines as they change. One chapter is devoted to the management of medical emergencies, and another to the application of ergonomic principles to prevent occupational disabilities in practitioners.

Section III: Assessments includes chapters that delineate the competencies of the dental hygienist in assessment of a client's general, dental, and periodontal health and risk status. In addition, one chapter is devoted to the oral-systemic health connection.

Section IV: Critical Thinking in Dental Hygiene Practice explains the dental hygiene diagnosis and how a dental hygiene diagnosis is made. This section also details the value of including client goals in the care plan and demonstrates how evaluation is used to document outcomes of care. With evaluation and documentation, the dental hygienist is accountable for care provided and can be confident that interventions made a positive difference in the individual's systemic and oral health status.

Section V: Implementation presents numerous evidence-based interventions that comprise dental hygiene care. Specific clinical procedures, in table format, facilitate competency development in a variety of protocols within the context of total body health, including personal oral care, instrumentation and root morphology, stain management, nonsurgical periodontal therapy, periodontal chemotherapy, oral disease risk assessment and management, tobacco cessation, nutritional counseling, supportive diagnostic aids, and restorative therapy.

Section VI: Pain and Anxiety Control covers both the behavioral and pharmacologic management of the client via anxiety-reducing protocols and administration of desensitizing agents, intraoral local anesthetic agents, and nitrous oxide–oxygen analgesia. Pain and anxiety control is essential for quality dental hygiene care.

Section VII: Individuals with Special Needs recognizes that dental hygienists care for a growing number of individuals with diseases or disabilities that affect their daily living, self-care, and ability to access healthcare. Special needs clients that dental hygienists are likely to treat have been included to facilitate quality and access to care for all individuals.

Section VIII: Management provides the capstone for the dental hygienist who is interested in developing competencies in leadership, practice management, and legal and ethical decision making.

Glossary

At the end of the book, an abbreviated glossary defines essential terms. A fully comprehensive glossary is located on the Evolve companion website (see below).

New to This Edition

The Fourth Edition of *Dental Hygiene: Theory and Practice* includes the following three new chapters essential to helping the learner meet the challenge of contemporary dental hygiene practice:

Chapter 3: Evidence-Based Decision Making
Chapter 7: Professional Portfolios
Chapter 61: Palliative Oral Care

Evolve Companion Website

http://evolve.elsevier.com/Darby/Hygiene

A website found at http://evolve.elsevier.com/Darby/Hygiene has been revised to support the content of the book and to enhance the faculty's instructional repertoire and student learning. The website includes:

For Instructors

TEACH Instructor's Resources Manual

Detailed and customizable chapter support materials based on textbook learning objectives. The manual includes:

- Lesson Plans
- Lecture Outlines
- PowerPoint presentations
- Additional Activities

Test Question Bank

With the current emphasis on student and curricular learning outcomes, competence, and assessment, a bank of more than 1,650 test questions can easily become part of an educator's overall assessment plan. These questions available on the website can be used independently by students or integrated into benchmark examinations that verify student knowledge at various points throughout the curriculum. With so many questions available, along with supporting rationales for the correct answers, questions can be selected and integrated into an annual comprehensive exam to prepare students for the National Board Dental Hygiene Examination.

Image Collection

An electronic image collection can be downloaded for PowerPoint presentations, handouts, and examinations.

For Students

Practice Quizzes

Approximately 1,500 multiple-choice questions, separated by chapter, with instant-feedback answers, rationales, and page number references for remediation.

Competency-Based Evaluation Forms

Procedures from the textbook have been modified into Competency-Based Evaluation Forms and posted on the text website. These can be downloaded for use in laboratory, preclinical, or clinical settings. Once downloaded, these forms can be used for self-evaluation, peer evaluation, instructor evaluation, and/or re-evaluation.

Procedure Ordering Exercises

Drag-and-drop exercises take each procedure apart and encourage the student to correctly order the steps involved, providing valuable practice in mastering clinical functions.

Full Glossary

A comprehensive and searchable glossary defines terms efficiently for the busy reader and reflects contemporary usage of key words as found in current literature.

Web Resources

Website information and resources are posted on the website by chapter to connect users to Internet information on relevant and related topics. These are website resources that the dental hygienist will use to enhance knowledge and practice. These websites enrich the learning experience.

Suggested Readings

Suggested readings for some chapters can be accessed readily from the website. These relevant citations can be used to support evidence-based decisions or as a start to a search of the literature for a written paper, research project, oral presentation, or research poster/table clinic assignment or simply for those who need to know more.

Supplemental Material

Additional images, boxes, and tables are provided to supplement the core text content for certain chapters, as needed.

Procedure Videos

Several of the procedures in *Dental Hygiene: Theory and Practice*, Fourth Edition, contain the following logo:

Procedure 15-3 Conducting Cytology

This logo indicates that a video is available for that skill in Elsevier's new online video collection, *Dental Hygiene Procedures Videos*. These videos are sold separately and can be purchased through the online Evolve bookstore at http://evolve.elsevier.com.

ACKNOWLEDGMENTS

We would like to express our sincere appreciation to all the contributors who helped make *Dental Hygiene: Theory and Practice,* Fourth Edition, a reality, including all contributors to earlier editions. Special recognition is extended to our esteemed friend and colleague, Denise Bowen. Without her expertise and commitment, this project would not have been possible. Denise, you are the BEST!

Appreciation also is extended to the American Dental Hygienists' Association and the American Dental Association. We also acknowledge the authors and publishers who granted permission to use concepts, quotes, photographs, figures, and tables. Several individuals who contributed content reviews of selected areas and/or photographs and diagrams should be acknowledged:

Gail Bemis Stoops; Philips Oral Healthcare, Inc.; Gayle McCombs, RDH, MS; Caren Barnes, RDH, PhD, Director of Dental Research, University of Nebraska; Jane Eisen, DDS, ORALSCAN Laboratories, Inc.; Catherine Kavanagh; Joanna Hill; Mark Dellinges, DDS, University of California–San Francisco, School of Dentistry; Connie Drisko, RDH, DDS, University of North Carolina School of Dentistry; Thomas Flynn, DMD, University of Connecticut; Bruce Barker, DDS, University of Missouri–Kansas City School of Dentistry; James R. Clark, University of Washington School of Dentistry, Department of Orthodontics; Ann Gabrick, MSW, LSCSW, Eating Disorders Unit, Baptist Medical Center, Kansas City, Missouri; Robert Cowan, DDS, Advanced Education General Dentistry, University of Missouri–Kansas City School of Dentistry; Greg Mann; Theresa J. Kellerman; M.J. McDonald; M.A. Conover; Paul Hains, Down syndrome client, University of North Carolina School of Dentistry; Linda Ross Santiago, RDH, Diablo Valley College, Pleasant Hill, California; Kathleen Muzzin, Caruth School of Dental Hygiene, Baylor College of Dentistry, Texas A&M University System; Deborah Baldwin, Dr. Kenneth Marinak, and Dr. Frederick Ochave, Gene W. Hirschfeld School of Dental Hygiene, Old Dominion University, Norfolk, Virginia; Dr. Philip R. Melnick, University of California–Los Angeles, School of Dentistry; Dr. Christopher Wyatt and Dr. R.W. Priddy, Faculty of Dentistry, University of British Columbia, Vancouver, Canada; Dr. F.T. McIver, Department of Pediatric Dentistry, University of North Carolina School of Dentistry; Victoria Vick and Cindy Sensabaugh (formerly with Procter & Gamble), Professional and Scientific Relations; GlaxoSmithKline; Schick Technologies; Nordent, Inc.; A-dec, Inc.; LeeAnn Keefer (formerly with DENTSPLY International); Electro Medical Systems; Osprey Communications; Colgate Oral Pharmaceuticals; Premier Dental Products Company; Mary Littleton and Danielle A. Victoriano, Hu-Friedy Manufacturing Company, Inc.; Tony Riso Company; Florida Probe Corporation; Brasseler USA; American Eagle Instruments, Inc.; Miltex; Paradise Dental Technologies; LM-Instruments; Premier Dental Products Company; Hartzell & Son; Bausch and Lomb; DentalView, Inc.; Tech Poll Studios, Inc.; Singer Professional Services, Inc.; 3i-Implant Innovations; the QUE Corporation; GI America; Sunstar Americas, Inc.; and WaterPik, Inc.

Appreciation is extended to Musarrat Anjum Shah, Nakia Nate Howard, Grace H Kogi, and Claire Gwayi Chore for assistance in critical review, editing, and library research. Special thanks to Dr. Andrew Balas, Dean, College of Health Sciences, who provided some financial support to fund a student worker to help with this project.

Because the work of those who contributed to the first, second, and third editions remains central to this revision, we gratefully acknowledge Barbara Heckman, Renee Hannibrink, Christine Hovliaras, Margaret Tan, Ann Flynn Scarff, Glenn Gordon, Maria Perno-Goldie, Merry Greig Cosgrove, Mari-Anne L. Low, Pamela Parker Brangan, Deanne Shuman, Beth McKinney, Gerry J. Barker, Marilynn Beck, Kim Krust Bray, Joan Ellison, Ginger B. Mann, Cheryl A Cameron, Gwen Essex, Jacquelyn Fried, Ruth Hull, Sandra Kramer, Stacy Long, Richard B. McCoy, Jeanne Maloney, Anne Miller, Brenda Parton Maddox, Dorothy Perry, Sandra Rich, Michelle Sensat, Peggy Tsutsui, Lynn Utecht, Lee E. Wentworth, Karen Williams, Linda G. Kraemer, Dimitrias Karastathis, Brenda S. Kuunz, Irma LaCross, Kathleen M. Schlotthauer, Hope Oliver, Sandra Zagar, and Nancy Zinser.

Our special thanks to our Elsevier family, particularly Kristin Wilhelm, Content Strategist; Joslyn Dumas, Content Development Specialist; Sarah Vora, Editorial Assistant; and Carol O'Connell, Project Manager, for their incredible work, commitment, enthusiastic support, and encouragement as they shepherded the manuscript throughout the publication process. We also wish to express our sincere gratitude to Linda Duncan, Elsevier Vice President and Publisher; Kathy Falk, Executive Content Strategist; Catherine Jackson, Publishing Services Manager; and Maggie Reid, Design Direction, for their support, understanding and commitment during preparation of this textbook.

We also are indebted to Dr. Helen Yura Petro for her mentorship and generosity in sharing time and knowledge, without which the human needs conceptual model for dental hygiene would never have become a reality. Without the contributions of these outstanding individuals, the book would not have been possible.

As with any new text, we shall be grateful to readers who have suggestions for additions or revisions or who are interested in sharing their responses with us. This edition reflects our ever-evolving responses to feedback provided by our dental hygiene community.

Michele Leonardi Darby
Margaret M. Walsh

CONTENTS

CHAPTER 1

The Dental Hygiene Profession

Michele Leonardi Darby, Margaret M. Walsh, Denise M. Bowen

COMPETENCIES

1. Define the discipline of dental hygiene, the dental hygienist, and the dental hygiene process of care.
2. Explain the paradigm for the discipline of dental hygiene.
3. Describe the different dental hygiene conceptual models.
4. Describe the professional roles of the dental hygienist.
5. Explain professional regulation in dental hygiene, including the purpose of standards of practice, accreditation, practice acts, and licensure.
6. Explain the role and importance of professional dental hygiene associations.
7. Describe the different workforce models for dental hygienists.

What Is Dental Hygiene?

Dental hygiene is the science and practice of preventive oral healthcare, including the management of behaviors to prevent oral disease and to promote health.

Who Is the Dental Hygienist?

Dental hygienists are licensed preventive oral health professionals who have graduated from accredited dental hygiene programs in institutions of higher education.[1] Dental hygienists provide education, clinical services, and consultation to individuals and populations of all ages in many settings and capacities. The American Dental Hygienists' Association defines the professional roles of the dental hygienist as clinician, corporate, public health, researcher, educator, administrator, and entrepreneur.[2] Dental hygienists promote and maintain oral wellness and thereby contribute to overall health and quality of life. If an individual's oral health changes, the dental hygienist, within the scope of dental hygiene practice, provides the highest quality of dental hygiene care to guide the person back to oral wellness. If oral wellness cannot be achieved, dental hygiene care helps to attain the best possible degree of oral health. In addition, the dental hygienist assists individuals in seeking other healthcare services as needed.

What Is the Dental Hygiene Process of Care?

The dental hygiene process of care is a systematic approach to dental hygiene care that involves six key behaviors,[2] or steps, including the following:

- Assessment
- Diagnosis
- Planning
- Implementation
- Evaluation
- Documentation

Box 1-1 defines these six steps of the dental hygiene process. The dental hygienist conducts a thorough, individualized assessment of the client who may be with or at risk for oral disease or complications. The dental hygiene diagnosis[3] uses critical analysis of all assessment findings to identify existing or potential client needs and oral health problems. Goals for behavioral outcomes, oral health, and overall health are addressed by the dental hygienist while planning dental hygiene care, implementing specific interventions, evaluating their effectiveness, and documenting all related information. Throughout the dental hygiene process of care, the dental hygienist takes into account individual and environmental factors such as the following:

- The person's level of growth and maturity
- Psychomotor ability
- Age
- Gender
- Role
- Lifestyle
- Culture
- Attitudes
- Health beliefs and behaviors
- Level of knowledge

In addition to evaluating an individual's clinical circumstances, preferences, or values, the dental hygienist critically evaluates the scientific evidence and uses experience and judgment when providing care.

In this age of consumerism, wellness, and self-care, the preventive role of the dental hygienist has more value to the public than ever before. The consumer's role in healthcare is changing. The healthcare consumer is demanding greater rights in the healthcare process. Consumers expect to make healthcare decisions to prevent and control disease, have skeptical and questioning attitudes, view healthcare professionals as fallible, and challenge authority and the status quo.

The term *client* is used instead of *patient* with increasing frequency in some healthcare settings as a more accurate way to describe the contemporary healthcare consumer. This preference is based on the perspective that the term *patient* suggests a sick, dependent person who is in need of therapy, whereas *client* connotes wellness as well as illness and suggests a person who is an active participant in oral healthcare and who is responsible for personal choices and the consequences of those choices. Moreover, the term *patient* is limited in reference to an individual, whereas *client* is a broader term that may refer to an individual, family, group, community, or

BOX 1-1

Steps of the Dental Hygiene Process of Care[2]

STEPS	DEFINITION
Assessment	The systematic collection of data to identify oral and general health status based on client problems, needs, and strengths
Diagnosis	The use of critical decision-making skills to reach conclusions about the client's dental hygiene needs based on all available assessment data and evidence in the literature[3]
Planning	The establishment of realistic goals and outcomes based on client needs, expectations, values, and current scientific evidence to plan dental hygiene interventions to facilitate optimal oral health
Implementation	Delivery of dental hygiene services based on the dental hygiene care plan while minimizing risk and optimizing oral health
Evaluation	Review and assessment of the outcomes of dental hygiene care
Documentation	Complete and accurate recording of all collected data, interventions planned and provided, recommendations, and other information relevant to client care and treatment[2]

nation. Because of its versatility and meaning, *client* is used throughout this book to denote the recipient who is the central focus of the dental hygiene process of care.

The dental hygiene process of care is the foundation of professional dental hygiene practice and provides a framework for delivering high-quality dental hygiene care to all types of clients in any environment or professional role. This process requires decision making and assumes that dental hygienists are responsible for identifying and resolving client problems within the scope of dental hygiene practice.

Roles

Contemporary dental hygiene practice requires that dental hygienists possess a range of knowledge and skills in a variety of areas. In the past the principal services of dental hygienists were oral health education and professional removal of calculus, biofilm, and other exogenous accretions from the tooth surface. Changes in healthcare knowledge and practice have expanded the philosophy of dental hygiene to include the professional roles of clinician, corporate, public health, researcher, educator, administrator, and entrepreneur (Figure 1-1).[4] Dental hygienists in these seven roles share a common goal of improved oral health for society. Although most dental hygienists are clinical practitioners (Figure 1-2), others have pursued nonclinical careers by going into business for themselves (e.g., dental staff placement agencies, private continuing education companies, consulting firms, or independent oral healthcare providers in long-term care facilities), or working in public health, in private industry, in public schools or academia, or with government agencies.

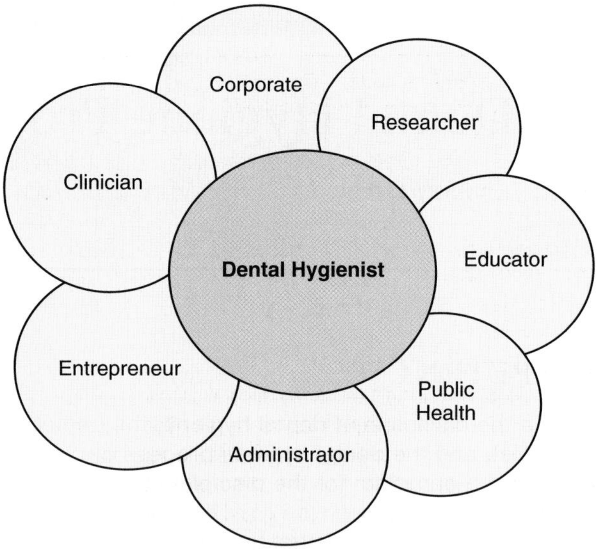

Figure 1-1. Seven professional roles of the dental hygienist identified by the American Dental Hygienists' Accociation.[4]

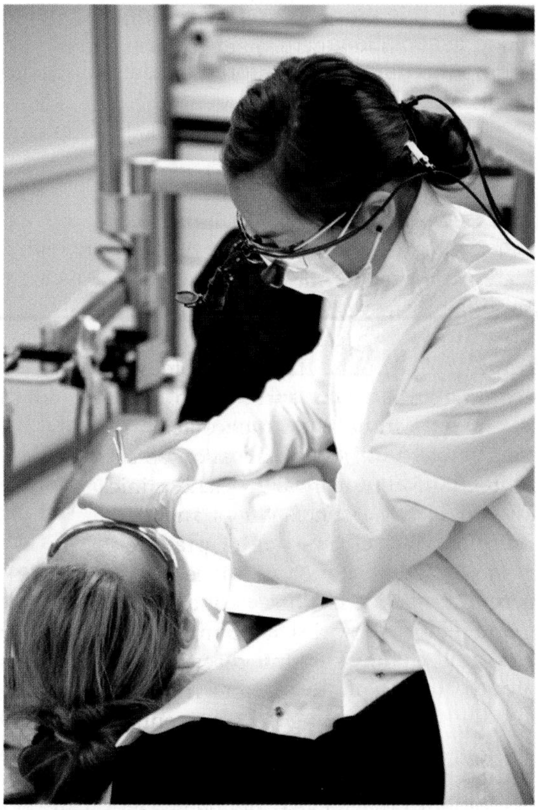

Figure 1-2. Dental hygiene clinician. (Courtesy Idaho State University Department of Dental Hygiene.)

Clinician

The role of the dental hygiene clinician includes assessing, diagnosing, planning, implementing, evaluating, and documenting treatment for prevention, intervention, and control of oral diseases, while practicing in collaboration with other health professionals.[4] The responsibilities of the dental hygiene clinician are summarized in Box 1-2 and include providing preventive, therapeutic, and educational services.

BOX 1-2

Responsibilities of the Dental Hygiene Clinician

Preventive
Methods employed to prevent oral disease and promote health (e.g., applying topical fluoride to teeth)

Therapeutic
Methods employed to arrest or control oral disease (e.g., scaling and root planing periodontally involved teeth)

Educational
Methods employed in both preventive and therapeutic aspects of clinical dental hygiene care to explain concepts regarding oral disease and health, to demonstrate self-care techniques, to reinforce learning, to evaluate understanding, and to determine ability to perform desired behaviors (e.g., teaching toothbrushing and flossing)

As a clinician the dental hygienist educates clients about their oral health and care options, helps them set oral health goals, and collaborates with them to meet those goals. The dental hygiene clinician makes decisions independently or in collaboration with the client and family, the dentist, or other healthcare professionals. The dental hygiene clinician also explains concepts regarding oral health and disease and their relationship to general health, explains and demonstrates oral self-care procedures, determines the client's understanding, motivates behavior change, reinforces learning or desired behavior, and evaluates the client's progress in learning.

The role of dental hygiene clinician involves effectively communicating with clients and with dentists and other healthcare professionals. This interprofessional role is critical in meeting the oral health and human needs of individuals, families, and communities. Practice acts in most legal jurisdictions specify oral health education as a responsibility of the dental hygienist. Dental hygiene clinicians work in a variety of clinical practice settings and deliver a variety of services (Table 1-1). The scope of practice for the clinician varies by country, state, or province. In general, however, dental hygiene clinicians assess and record findings from social and health histories including risk factors for oral disease (e.g., smoking, systemic disease); assess paraoral and intraoral hard and soft tissues and record findings; remove deposits on the teeth using debridement; apply preventive and therapeutic agents related to periodontal disease (e.g., subgingival controlled-release delivery systems containing chlorhexidine or antibiotics) and dental caries (e.g., topical fluoride, dental sealants); expose radiographs; educate clients about their oral health and its relationship to their general health; educate clients about self-care techniques and options for oral healthcare; refer clients to other health professionals for evaluation and care; evaluate outcomes of dental hygiene care; and document all related information. In many jurisdictions, dental hygiene clinicians administer local anesthetics and nitrous oxide–oxygen analgesia, make dental impressions, and place and/or remove periodontal sutures; in some, they place dental restorations.

Corporate Dental Hygienist

Corporate dental hygienists contribute their expertise regarding achieving and maintaining optimal oral and general health to companies that support the oral health and healthcare industry through the sale of products and services (see Table 1-1). They are employed as sales representatives and managers, product researchers, corporate educators, and corporate administrators. The industry values the clinical experience and understanding of oral healthcare delivery.

Public Health

Public health dental hygienists provide care to those who otherwise would not have access to oral healthcare.[2] They often design and deliver community health programs funded by government or nonprofit organizations.

Dental hygienists in public health departments develop oral health educational materials and protocols for service programs, such as fluoride rinse programs for elementary schoolchildren, dental screenings, and special programs for Native Americans or children served by Head Start. They may provide clinical services to these same clients or in urban and rural community clinics. Moreover, public health dental hygienists also provide classroom oral health education instruction to students, parents, and teachers (see Table 1-1).

Researcher

A dental hygiene **researcher** tests the assumptions of clinical practice and education and investigates dental hygiene problems to improve oral healthcare, the practice of dental hygiene, and educational approaches for teaching the theory and principles of dental hygiene. The entry-level information that students receive in school is not expected to sustain a lifelong career because knowledge and technology are forever evolving. Throughout a professional career the dental hygienist uses research-related skills to remain current in the art and science of dental hygiene and to make evidence-based decisions during clinical care; however, a dental hygiene researcher has a different role.

Many dental hygienists have chosen research as a primary focus of their dental hygiene careers. Such dedicated dental hygiene researchers are employed in academic settings; federal, state, or local health agencies; research institutions (e.g., National Institute of Dental and Craniofacial Research); and private industry. The minimal educational requirement for a career in research is a graduate degree in dental hygiene or a related field, with a doctoral degree preferred. (Visit the website at http://evolve.elsevier.com/Darby/hygiene for discussion of the different academic dental hygiene degrees available.)

Educator

Dental hygiene **educators** are in abundant demand.[2] Dental hygiene education programs are expanding in number and scope around the world. Colleges and universities require dental hygiene faculty who can apply educational theory and methodology to educate competent dental hygiene graduates. A faculty member in a school of dental hygiene prepares students for careers as professional dental hygienists. They may prepare dental hygiene students for all seven professional roles of the dental hygienist by teaching in programs and higher education institutions offering different degrees.

TABLE 1-1
Seven Roles of the Professional Dental Hygienist[4]

Roles	Sample Settings	Sample Responsibilities
Clinician	Clinical practice (e.g., private dental practices, community clinics, hospitals, prison facilities, independent practice, armed forces) Managed care programs Extended care facilities School-based programs	Uses the dental hygiene process of care (assesses, diagnoses, plans, implements, evaluates, and documents) to prevent, intervene in, and control oral diseases and to promote health Provides care to clients based on evidence-based decision making and skill with consideration of human needs Accepts clients as partners in their healthcare Collaborates with and refers to other healthcare professionals to promote client health and prevent disease Adheres to moral, ethical, and legal responsibilities
Corporate	Oral healthcare industry Product research industry Publishing industry	Applies educational and practice expertise to support the oral health industry in providing quality products, services, and information to the public and the profession
Public health	Public health clinics Indian Health Service settings Head Start programs State public health departments	Designs or participates in programs to address unmet needs of the underserved or groups with special needs Develops programs and delivers care in school-based or community-based settings Collaborates to include preventive oral health care delivered by dental hygienists in comprehensive public health programs Uses process of care to plan, conduct, and evaluate community oral health programs
Researcher	Clinical practice Research institutions Institutions of professional education Oral healthcare industry	Conducts needs assessment Develops clear statement of a specific problem, including environmental context, and dental hygiene roles and relationships Conducts and interprets a current literature review Develops an evidence-based strategic plan to address the problem with budget, expected outcomes, and evaluation procedures Implements research plan Interprets and evaluates research findings and applies findings to practice
Educator	Clinical practice settings Public health programs Public school programs Faculty in dental schools and dental hygiene schools Healthcare agencies Oral healthcare industry	Applies educational theory and the teaching-learning process (e.g., assessing the health knowledge and oral health status of individuals and groups; planning health education; transmitting current concepts of health promotion and disease prevention to individuals and groups; and evaluating educational outcomes) Promotes concepts of prevention in community-based programs designed for specific population groups Designs and produces instructional materials and media for the consumer Uses communication and interpersonal skills to meet learning needs of clients
Administrator	Community-based health-promotion and disease-prevention programs Educational institutions Clinical practice State dental health program administration Oral healthcare industry	Establishes short- and long-range goals Participates in strategic planning Formulates policies and procedures Coordinates human, material, and financial resources Motivates and evaluates staff, solves problems, makes decisions, resolves conflicts, and effects change Evaluates programs and modifies them based on evaluation outcomes
Entrepreneur	Practice management Business Oral healthcare industry Product development and sales industry Employment service centers Continuing education businesses Consulting businesses Nonprofit organizations	Initiate or finance new commercial enterprises Develops networking systems to bring available resources together to resolve problems or deliver professional services Monitors the quality of professional services Assists professionals in providing the best possible care using state-of-the-art knowledge, skills, and procedures Develops business opportunities to address healthcare needs of consumers and professional needs of providers Obtains resources to deliver needed services to clients served by nonprofit organizations

Dental hygiene educators work primarily as clinical and classroom instructors, academic faculty, program directors, and corporate educators.

Faculty members are responsible for teaching current dental hygiene theory and practice, advancing dental hygiene knowledge through research, and providing public service. Schools of dentistry often employ a dental hygienist to teach periodontal and preventive oral health concepts and skills to predoctoral dental students in classroom, laboratory, and clinical settings. Such dental hygiene educator positions require at least a baccalaureate degree and usually require a graduate degree in dental hygiene, public health, education, or some related basic or behavioral science discipline.

Administrator

In various settings in which dental hygiene care is provided, the dental hygienist acts as manager or administrator. An **administrator** is a person whose official position is to guide and direct the work of others. Responsibilities commonly associated with a manager include planning, assessing, decision making, organizing, staffing, and directing. Dental hygienists use organizational skills, communicate goals and objectives, identify and manage resources, and evaluate and change programs, primarily in health, education, and healthcare. The dental hygienist as administrator is knowledgeable about organizational structure and goals, the line of authority, responsibilities of various co-workers, and channels of communication; uses and contributes to organizational policies and procedures; and values human and material resources.

Dental hygiene administrators may serve as clinical directors, educational program directors or deans, executive directors of professional associations and nonprofit organizations, research administrators, or sales managers. These dental hygiene administrators also are employed in upper-level and middle management positions in federal, state, and local health departments, and in private companies that market oral healthcare products. The minimum educational requirement usually is a graduate degree in dental hygiene or a related field. Many academic administrative positions require that the dental hygienist have a doctoral degree.

Entrepreneur

The dental hygiene **entrepreneur** uses imagination and creativity to start or finance a new business or commercial endeavor.[4] Dental hygienists have been successful in a variety of enterprises and opportunities continue to expand (see Table 1-1). They have created businesses providing services related to practice management, employment, and consulting and have invented new products.

The term *entrepreneur* implies taking a risk to achieve this goal. Dental hygiene entrepreneurs must have skills and abilities in leadership, team building, negotiation, and consensus building. Training in business practices and finance also is an advantage.

Regardless of the roles selected by a dental hygienist during the span of a professional career, the focus of the dental hygienists' work remains prevention of oral disease and promoting oral wellness by working in collaboration with others involved in healthcare in a variety of settings for all populations.

Visit the website at http://evolve.elsevier.com/Darby/hygiene for additional resources regarding dental hygiene diagnosis and professional roles of the dental hygienist.

Dental Hygiene's Paradigm

A **paradigm** is a widely accepted worldview of a discipline that shapes the direction and methods of its practitioners, educators, administrators, and researchers.[5] A discipline's paradigm consists of the following:

- Major concepts selected for study by the discipline
- Statements about the major concepts that define them in a global manner

A paradigm specifies the unique perspective of each discipline and is the first level of distinction between disciplines.[5] In a discipline the body of knowledge progresses from a single paradigm to multiple conceptual models and multiple theories derived from each model[5] (Figure 1-3). The four major concepts of the paradigm for the discipline of dental

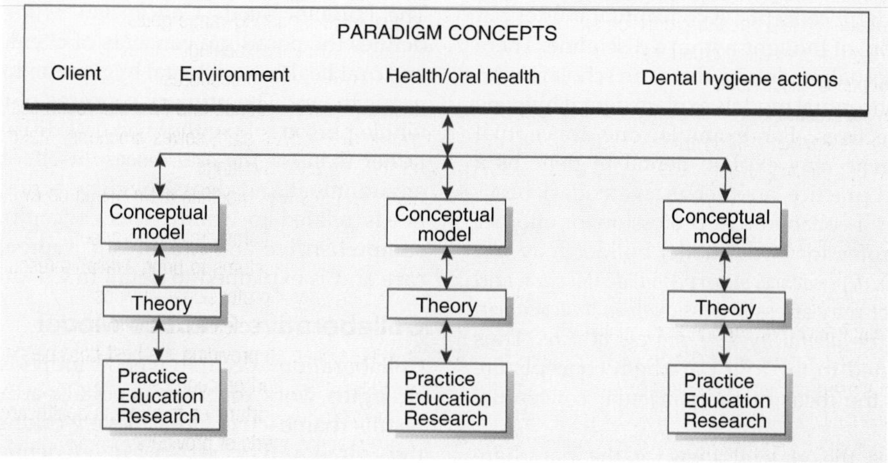

Figure 1-3. Dental hygiene theory development framework. (From American Dental Hygienists' Association: *Proceedings of the 69th Annual Session, House of Delegates*, Denver, June 1993.)

BOX 1-3

Four Major Concepts of the Dental Hygiene Paradigm

CONCEPTS	DEFINITION
Client	The recipient of dental hygiene care; includes persons, families, and groups and communities of people of all ages, genders, and sociocultural and economic states
Environment	Factors other than dental hygiene actions that affect the client's attainment of optimal oral health. These include economic, psychologic, cultural, physical, legal, educational, ethical, and geographic factors
Health and oral health	The client's state of being as it exists on a continuum from optimal wellness to illness and fluctuates over time as the result of biologic, psychologic, spiritual, and developmental factors. Oral health and overall health are interrelated because each influences the other.
Dental hygiene actions	Interventions that a dental hygienist can initiate to promote oral wellness and to prevent or control oral disease. These actions involve cognitive, affective, and psychomotor performances and may be provided in independent, interdependent, and collaborative relationships with the client and the healthcare team.

hygiene as defined by the American Dental Hygienists' Association (ADHA)[6] include the client, the environment, health and oral health, and dental hygiene actions. Definitions of these paradigm concepts are listed in Box 1-3. These four paradigm concepts are central to the discipline of dental hygiene. They are defined further and expanded in numerous ways by the development of conceptual models of dental hygiene.

Conceptual Models

Conceptual models are important for dental hygiene because they provide philosophic and practical perspectives about dental hygiene's paradigm concepts. A conceptual model can be thought of as a school of thought within a discipline. There can be as many conceptual models as there are scholars who can think them up. Conceptual models explain dental hygiene from different perspectives. For example, one conceptual model of dental hygiene may explain dental hygiene as a public health–oriented practice, another as an auxiliary occupation, still another as a collaborative profession, or another as an independent profession. One model builder may use terms such as *auxiliary, dependence, supervision, dental care,* and *duties,* whereas another may stress *professionalism, independent decision making,* and the *dental hygiene process of care.* Thus terms and beliefs related to the four paradigm concepts are defined according to the focus of the particular conceptual model.[5]

Table 1-2 describes the general view of the paradigm concept "dental hygiene actions" from the differing perspectives of the Occupational Model and the Professional Model of Dental Hygiene. These conceptual models as well as the Collaborative Practice Model and the Human Needs Conceptual Model are discussed in more detail in the following sections. (For information on additional conceptual models of Dental Hygiene, see http://evolve.elsevier.com/Darby/hygiene.)

Occupational Model versus the Professional Model

Table 1-2 compares some of the basic propositions related to dental hygiene actions of the Occupational Model of Dental Hygiene with those of the Professional Model of Dental Hygiene. The Occupational Model[5] presents the concept of dental hygiene actions as technically based. According to this model the dental hygienist is a dental auxiliary who implements treatment plans and carries out isolated duties as directed by the supervising dentist. This conceptual model emphasizes the provision of oral prophylaxis in the dental office (defined as oral hygiene instruction, thorough calculus removal, and coronal polishing) as the primary duty delegated to the dental hygienist by the dentist under direct supervision. Expertise, evaluation of the effect of dental hygiene care on oral health and disease, and decision making are not stressed.

In the Occupational Model the focus of assessment is to gather data for the dentist to use in determining the dental diagnosis and treatment plan, part of which will be implemented by the dental hygienist. This model conveys the idea that the dental hygienist, as an auxiliary person, is accountable to the supervising dentist, who is then accountable to the client.

In contrast, the Professional Model[5] perceives the paradigm concept of dental hygiene actions to be knowledge based. This model conveys the view that dental hygienists use a process of care to assess needs, diagnose dental hygiene problems, and plan, implement, evaluate, and document dental hygiene care. According to this model the dental hygienist is responsible for making decisions about dental hygiene care and is accountable to the client. Each of these conceptual models has a unique perspective on dental hygiene that guides dental hygiene education and clinical practice in different ways.

Human Needs Conceptual Model

The Human Needs Conceptual Model[7] of dental hygiene defines the paradigm concepts of client, environment, health and oral health, and dental hygiene actions in terms of human needs theory. The primary concerns of this model are for the whole person who either has oral disease or may develop it, rather than for the oral disease itself, and for the role of the environment and dental hygiene actions in meeting human needs related to health. This conceptual model provides a comprehensive and humanistic approach to dental hygiene care and is explained in detail in Chapter 2.

Collaborative Practice Model

Collaboration occurs when individuals with differing strengths work together as equal partners to achieve better results than each could achieve working alone. According to the Collaborative Practice Model[8] dentists and dental hygienists work together as colleagues, each offering professional expertise for the goal of providing optimum oral healthcare

TABLE 1-2

Sample Propositions About Dental Hygiene Actions from Two Conceptual Models of Dental Hygiene

Occupational Model	Professional Model
Dental hygienists implement preventive treatment plans developed by supervising dentist.	Dental hygienists implement self-generated preventive care regimens.
Dental hygienists are secondary care providers.	Dental hygienists are primary care providers.
Dental hygienists carry out isolated duties as indicated by supervising dentist.	Dental hygienists use a process of care to assess needs, plan and implement care, and evaluate outcomes.
Dental hygienists are auxiliaries of dentistry.	Dental hygienists are professionals who collaborate with the dentist and other health professionals.
Dental hygienists are responsible for less complex, easier oral healthcare services.	Dental hygienists are responsible for services that include some of the more difficult techniques to master in oral healthcare.
Dental hygiene care involves an oral prophylaxis every 6 months at a 30- to 45-min appointment.	Dental hygiene care involves multiple interventions that may require multiple appointments and appointment lengths.
Dentists are responsible for less valued services, leaving the dentist time for important services.	Dental hygienists are responsible for preventive and oral maintenance care, which is highly valued by today's wellness-oriented consumer.
Unsupervised dental hygiene practice reduces the quality of oral healthcare and increases client risks.	Unsupervised dental hygiene practice increases public access to oral hygiene care and lowers healthcare costs.
Dentists are responsible for making decisions about dental hygienists.	Dental hygienists are responsible for making decisions about dental hygienists.
Dentists are accountable to the dentist.	Dental hygienists are accountable to the client (consumer).
Dentists are responsible for the client's oral health.	Clients are responsible for their own oral health.
Dental hygienists fulfill their role through the function of a clinician.	Dental hygienists fulfill their role through functions of clinician, educator, administrator or manager, advocate, and researcher.
Dental hygiene actions are technically based.	Dental hygiene actions are knowledge based.

to the public. Although both professions can and should work together to improve the oral health status of the public, each has a specific role that complements and augments the effectiveness of the other. The collaborative practice model emphasizes the distinct roles of dental hygienist and dentist and their ability to enter into a collegial relationship as healthcare providers. In this model the dentist and the dental hygienist are in a co-therapist relationship. In a collaborative practice, dental hygienists are viewed as experts in their field, are consulted about appropriate dental hygiene interventions, are expected to make clinical dental hygiene decisions, and are given freedom in planning, implementing, and evaluating the dental hygiene component of the overall care plan.

The Dental Hygienist in Interprofessional Practice

Interprofessional collaboration, also known as interprofessional practice in healthcare, is defined as a team approach to comprehensive client-centered care by multiple health professionals with different backgrounds working together to provide quality care.[9] The term *practice* refers to clinical and nonclinical health-related services—for example, diagnosis, treatment, surveillance, and health communications. An interprofessional approach is important for improving client outcomes beyond what could be achieved by delivering care within one discipline because each profession brings complementary knowledge, skills, values, and attitudes to each client case.[10] For interprofessional healthcare workers to collaborate effectively and improve health outcomes, two or more professionals with different backgrounds must be given an opportunity to learn from one another and to learn about one another's discipline. This process of interprofessional education is becoming more common throughout the world to address rising demands and costs for healthcare.[9]

Dental hygienists work in interprofessional practice in a variety of settings with healthcare workers from multiple backgrounds. For example, dental hygienists work in clinics and medical practices with pediatricians, family physicians, and physician assistants completing pediatric oral assessments, applying fluoride varnish, and teaching parents about oral healthcare practices important to their child's oral health. Dental hygienists in long-term care facilities work with nurses' aides and registered nurses to monitor residents' oral health, care for dentures, provide preventive oral healthcare, and make dental care referrals. Clinical psychologists, dental hygienists, nutritionists, public health nurses, and social workers in Japan work collaboratively to deliver comprehensive healthcare services to pregnant women and young children.[9] The opportunities are expanding, and dental hygienists are being trained to work with healthcare providers in many disciplines. Dental hygienists are embracing these opportunities as well as their role as a primary healthcare provider to deliver comprehensive client services through interprofessional practice.[10]

Visit the website at http://evolve.elsevier.com/Darby/hygiene for additional information regarding interprofessional education and practice.

Professional Regulation

Accreditation

Accreditation is a formal, voluntary nongovernmental process that establishes a minimum set of national standards that promote and ensure quality in educational institutions and programs and serves as a mechanism to protect the public.[11] Accreditation documents include descriptions of all competencies and abilities that a beginning dental hygiene practitioner must consistently perform accurately and efficiently.

Standards of Dental Hygiene Practice

Standards in the United States

In 2008 the ADHA, building on the initial Standards developed in 1985, developed the *Standards for Clinical Dental Hygiene Practice.*[4] These updated Standards define and guide professional dental hygiene practice. The primary purpose of the *Standards for Clinical Dental Hygiene Practice* is to provide a resource for dental hygiene practitioners seeking to provide client-centered and evidence-based clinical care. In addition, dental hygienists functioning as educators, researchers, and administrators can use these *Standards* to guide implementation of collaborative, client-centered care in multidisciplinary teams of health professionals. Such collaborations occur in community-based settings such as community and public health centers, hospitals, schools, and long-term care programs. Although dental hygienists are individually accountable to the *Standards* set by the discipline, these *Standards* do not substitute for professional judgment. However, they do provide a framework that describes a competent level of dental hygiene care based on the dental hygiene process of care. These Standards likely will be modified based on new scientific evidence and federal and state regulations to ensure optimal, comprehensive client care.[4]

In addition to the *Standards for Clinical Dental Hygiene Practice,* the American Dental Education Association has developed statements of competencies for entry into the allied dental professions that include competencies for entry into the profession of dental hygiene.[12] These competencies describe the abilities of a dental hygienist entering the dental hygiene profession and inform dental hygiene accreditation bodies. The Standards, along with these competencies, serve the profession and society in the following ways:

- Define the activities of dental hygienists unique to dental hygiene.
- Provide consumers, employers, and colleagues with guidelines as to what constitutes high-quality dental hygiene care.
- Provide guidelines for establishing goals for clinical dental hygiene education.
- Serve as the foundation for competence assurance and continued professional development.

Standards in Canada

The current standards for dental hygiene practice in Canada, *Practice Competencies and Standards for Canadian Dental Hygienists,* was a collaborative project involving many stakeholders and released in 2010.[13] This document evolved from earlier versions of the standards originating in 1981 and defined a national perspective on the knowledge and abilities dental hygienists require to practice competently and responsibly.

The Canadian Dental Hygienists' Association (CDHA) combined competency statements and practice standards in the same document to be considered as a whole. The practice competencies are intended for use primarily by educators in curriculum development to define the outcomes of entry-level professional education. The practice standards specify a level to which entry-level dental hygienists must practice as outlined by the Federation of Dental Hygiene Regulatory Authorities. These standards also include the CDHA definition of dental hygiene and scope of practice. Some provincial professional associations have developed additional standards for practicing dental hygienists.

Practice Acts and Licensure

Dental practice acts are laws established in each state (United States) or province (Canada) to regulate the practice of dentistry and dental hygiene. Although the laws that regulate dental hygiene practice vary with each licensing jurisdiction, they have common elements. In general, the practice act does the following:

- Establishes criteria for dental hygiene education, licensure, and relicensure
- Defines the legal scope of dental hygiene practice
- Protects the public by making dental hygiene practice by uncredentialed and unlicensed persons illegal
- Creates a board empowered with legal authority to oversee the policies and procedures affecting the dental hygiene practice in that jurisdiction

The board in each jurisdiction is given legal authority to design and administer licensing examinations to graduates of approved schools of dental hygiene. Individuals who pass the licensing examination earn a license to practice dental hygiene as it is defined in that jurisdiction. The license can be denied, revoked, or suspended for a variety of reasons, such as incompetence, negligence, chemical dependency, illegal practice, and criminal misconduct. Realizing the limitation of single states requiring repeat licensing examinations for dental hygienists who are relocating, some state boards have established licensing by credential as an alternative. Licensing by credential recognizes the dental hygiene license received in other states when appropriate. Documents are provided for the board's approval in meeting licensure requirements so that the dental hygienist does not have to repeat a practical examination after relocating.

The Dental Hygiene National Board

To be eligible for regional and/or state clinical licensure examinations, after graduation from an accredited dental hygiene program, dental hygienists must also pass the written National Board Dental Hygiene Examination administered by the American Dental Association Joint Commission on National Dental Examinations. The purpose of the national examination is to assist state boards in determining qualifications of dental hygiene licensure applicants by assessing their ability to recall important information from basic biomedical, dental, and dental hygiene sciences, as well as their ability to apply such information in problem-solving situations. A case-based segment of the examination focuses on the ability to use knowledge related to clinical dental hygiene and the dental sciences in solving client problems and addressing client needs.

Visit the website at http://evolve.elsevier.com/Darby/hygiene for additional information on entry-level competencies and standards of dental hygiene practice in the United States and Canada.

Professional Dental Hygiene Organizations

Professional organizations collectively represent the views of a profession and influence resolution of issues relevant to education, practice, and research in that profession. Professional organizations have an enormous effect on dental hygiene because they address issues of professional growth, education, access to care, research and theory development, quality assurance, manpower, legislation, and collaboration with other professionals. Although many organizations exist, only the major ones are discussed in this chapter.

American Dental Hygienists' Association

The American Dental Hygienists' Association is a national organization of dental hygienists. To improve the total health of the public, ADHA's mission is to advance the art and science of dental hygiene.[14] ADHA works to achieve the following:

- Ensure access to quality oral healthcare.
- Increase awareness of the cost-effective benefits of prevention.
- Promote the highest standards of dental hygiene education, licensure, practice, and research.
- Represent and promote the interests of dental hygienists.

Founded in 1923, the ADHA has a tri-level structure by which individual members are automatically part of local (component), state (constituent), and national levels of governance. The official publications of the ADHA include the *Journal of Dental Hygiene and Access.* The House of Delegates is its legislative body, which is composed of voting members who proportionately represent each constituent. The Board of Trustees, presided over by the organization's elected president, consists of voting members (president, president-elect, vice president, treasurer, immediate past president, and 12 district trustees) and nonvoting, ex officio members (executive director and speaker of the House). The ADHA plays a major role in issues that deal with legislation, access to care, education, practice, research, public relations, and health policy. The ADHA offers a variety of tangible and intangible benefits. Membership and support by professional and student dental hygienists in the United States is important.

National Dental Hygienists' Association

In 1932 the National Dental Hygienists' Association (NDHA) was founded by African American dental hygienists to address the needs and special challenges of minority dental hygienists. The mission of the NDHA is to do the following[15]:

- Promote the highest standards of education and ethics for dental hygienists; create specific position statements on issues affecting the dental hygiene profession.
- Enhance recruitment efforts for communities of minority students in need.
- Assist in access to oral care for underserved communities in the United States.
- Provide public service as a means to enhance the Association's visibility.
- Provide a professional foundation for minority dental hygienists.
- Increase the number of minority dental hygienists.

The NDHA board includes five officers and five trustees elected by the growing general membership body.[12] NDHA has six component organizations functioning as official affiliated professional organizations. It holds an annual convention in conjunction with the National Dental Association and publishes a newsletter.

Canadian Dental Hygienists' Association

The Canadian Dental Hygienists' Association (CDHA), officially founded in 1965, is the national association for registered dental hygienists in Canada. The CDHA's purpose is to enable its members to provide quality preventive and therapeutic oral healthcare as well as health promotion for all members of the Canadian public.[16] As the collective voice of dental hygiene in Canada, the CDHA contributes to the health of the public by leading the development of national positions and encouraging standards related to dental hygiene practice, education, research, and regulation.

The CDHA Board's actions are directed toward attaining specific measurable outcomes, including the following[16]:

- Direct access to dental hygiene care
- Recognition by the Canadian public
- Supportive public policy and a strong national voice
- Interprofessional practice
- Professional identity and professional standards
- Knowledge and research
- Business success and workplace well-being
- Leadership development

With a structure similar to that of the ADHA, the CDHA has provincial organizations supported by local components. The CDHA publishes *The Canadian Journal of Dental Hygiene* as its official journal and has played a prominent role in developing continuing education, formal dental hygiene education, portability of licensure, and dental hygiene research and theory. The ADHA and CDHA have worked together to achieve many common goals.

International Federation of Dental Hygienists

In 1986 the International Federation of Dental Hygienists (IFDH) was formed in Oslo, Norway. The IFDH's purposes are as follows[17]:

- "Safeguard and defend the interests of the profession of dental hygiene, represent and advance the profession of dental hygiene.
- Promote professional alliances with its association members as well as with other associations, federations, and organizations whose objectives are similar.
- Promote and coordinate the exchange of knowledge and information about the profession, its education, and its practice.
- Promote access to quality preventive oral health services.
- Increase public awareness that oral disease can be prevented through proven regimens.

- Provide a forum for the understanding and discussion of issues pertaining to dental hygiene."

The IFDH recognizes that the need for dental hygiene is universal and that dental hygiene services should be unrestricted by consideration of nationality, sex, race, creed, color, politics, or social status. The IFDH provides a formal network by which dental hygienists worldwide can promote collegiality among nations, commitment to maintaining universal standards of dental hygiene care and education, and access to high-quality oral healthcare.

The IFDH is governed by its House of Delegates, which has two delegates from each country's association member. Normally this governing body meets every 3 years, in conjunction with the International Symposium on Dental Hygiene, hosted and organized by a selected member country. An executive council (president, president-elect, vice president, and treasurer) is elected by the House of Delegates to execute the goals established by the House of Delegates every 3 years.[17]

Workforce Model for Dental Hygienists

Dental hygienists work in various settings to deliver clinical oral healthcare and work under varying levels of supervision, depending on the state practice act and regulations. States progressively are recognizing the importance of increasing direct access to dental hygiene services. In 2012 dental hygienists were authorized in 35 states to work in community-based settings (e.g., public health or safety net clinics, schools, long-term care facilities) to provide preventive services without the presence of a dentist.[18] Expanding the professional practice settings of dental hygienists improves access to oral health services, use of oral health services, and oral health outcomes. ADHA, CDHA, NDHA, and others have called for new types of oral healthcare providers as well as increased options for delivery of dental hygiene care to the public.

Levels of Supervision

Dental hygienists work independently, with varying levels of supervision or in collaboration with dentists with the goal of comprehensive oral healthcare for each client. **Direct supervision** is defined as practicing with a dentist present in the facility where treatment is being rendered, commonly a private dental practice. **General supervision** requires a dentist to authorize services provided by a dental hygienist, but there is no need for the dentist to be present. General supervision also is common in private dental practices and often is extended to alternative practice settings in the community. **Public health supervision** allows dental hygienists to provide care without authorization of a dentist according to protocols established by state laws and regulations when the hygienist is delivering services in alternative settings. Examples of alternative settings include federally funded health centers and clinics; nursing homes; extended care facilities; home health; group homes for the elderly, disabled, and youth; schools; hospitals; migrant work facilities; and local and state public health facilities.

Direct access indicates that dental hygienists are able to provide services they determine appropriate without specific authorization. Laws and regulations in various states, provinces, and countries determine the level of supervision required, if any.

Some states allow for independent or collaborative practices and others provide for dental hygienists practicing as **registered dental hygienists in alternative practice (RDHAP)** or with **limited or extended access permits** (LAP or EAP). Such permits provide an opportunity for professionals with experience to specialize in treating clients with special needs. These clients may include patients with mental or physical disabilities, the elderly, and others whose health conditions limit their abilities to access quality dental care. Many of these dental hygienists deliver care to homebound clients, children in school or public health settings, and clients in residential care facilities and other institutions. In many states, dental hygienists are recognized and reimbursed as Medicaid providers. In some jurisdictions dental hygienists also may establish practices in communities that have been designated as dental health professional shortage areas. The workforce models are many, varied, and growing.

Independent Practitioner or Independent Contractor

An **independent dental hygiene practitioner** owns her own business, or independent practice, and provides preventive oral healthcare services to the public as a primary care provider where permitted by law. If supervision is required, the dental hygienist can contract with a dentist through a collaborative practice agreement or other means of satisfying supervision requirements while also addressing the dental treatment needs of the clients. Examples of businesses owned by a dental hygienist entrepreneur include a private dental hygiene practice, a community oral healthcare delivery service, or a provider of dental hygiene services in school settings. An **independent contractor** of dental hygiene care may own equipment and lease space in a dental office or clinic under a contractual arrangement, usually made with a dentist. Rather than being paid a salary and having the overhead costs paid by the dentist or other business owner, the dental hygienist is self-employed.

Dental hygienists who practice independently or provide direct access to dental hygiene care have a variety of backgrounds and diverse practice characteristics in the populations served and practice settings. The services provided were consistent with allowable services for unsupervised practice in states that allow it. Other states are expanding access to care by allowing for advanced dental hygiene practitioners.

The Advanced Dental Hygiene Practitioner

Historically in the United States, dental healthcare access has been limited by lack of dentists practicing in rural or inner-city areas and citizens victimized by education, economic, cultural, and health status disadvantages. Because of these barriers, some people suffer in pain or delay preventive care and treatment until the oral condition is severe and expensive to correct. When dental problems reach a crisis, some people seek dental care from hospital emergency rooms, where healthcare providers may alleviate pain temporarily but are not able to treat dental disease.

Following the *Surgeon General's National Call to Action to Promote Oral Health*[19] the American Dental Hygienists' Association developed a plan, model, and competencies for a new mid-level practitioner called the *advanced dental hygiene practitioner (ADHP)*.[20] The main role of this new mid-level practitioner is to increase societal access to primary oral healthcare cost effectively via assessment and evaluation, preventive, restorative, and therapeutic services. Unlike the dental hygienist who works primarily in private practice settings where people have a dental home, the ADHP works outside of the traditional private practice settings to provide services in nursing homes, schools, and community clinics closing the dental care gap for vulnerable populations. With advanced dental hygiene practitioners, more oral healthcare can be provided to underserved populations where they live, work, or play, resulting in improved oral health of the population at less cost. The concept is similar to other mid-level providers. Similar to other mid-level providers such as the advanced nurse practitioner, the occupational therapist, or the physical therapist, the ADHP requires graduate-level education. The Pew Center on the States reports that by 2014, with healthcare reform and the provision of dental insurance to millions of U.S. children, the demand for oral healthcare services will increase.[21] Another challenge is that a significant number of dentists are expected to retire from practice just as the need for dental care is expected to escalate. Given Pew's predictions, the ADHP will contribute significantly to closing the disparity gap between the number of people who need care and the number of providers able to meet the need.

The groundbreaking Master of Science in Advanced Dental Therapy (ADT) Program in Minnesota is the first to graduate dental hygienists as mid-level practitioners to work in collaboration with an authorizing dentist within the legal scope of practice.[22] Some advanced services include nonsurgical extractions of periodontally diseased permanent teeth with tooth mobility; dispensing analgesics, anti-inflammatories, and antibiotics; atraumatic restorative therapy; pulpotomies on primary teeth; cavity preparation and restoration of primary and permanent teeth; extraction of primary teeth; and preparation and placement of preformed crowns.

In 2012 four states considered legislation to establish new oral health providers that would allow some form of advanced practice for dental hygienists. The legislative proposals varied, but each would facilitate licensed dental hygienists pursuing additional education to administer an advanced clinical scope of services, including restorative care. The models are designed to extend the reach of the existing oral healthcare system to underserved populations.[19] Dental hygienists prepared as mid-level providers help the professions of dentistry and dental hygiene meet the oral healthcare needs of the community. The development of advanced dental hygiene practitioners, such as the ADTs or ADHPs, will result in cost-effective, quality, primary dental care and healthier citizens in the United States.

CLIENT EDUCATION TIPS

- The profession of dental hygiene emphasizes the prevention of oral disease and the client's role in controlling factors that cause disease.

LEGAL, ETHICAL, AND SAFETY ISSUES

Dental hygienists must be licensed in the jurisdiction in which they practice.

KEY CONCEPTS

- Dental hygiene is the study of preventive oral healthcare, including the management of behaviors to prevent oral disease and promote health.
- The dental hygienist is a licensed oral healthcare professional who assumes the professional roles of clinician, corporate, researcher, educator, public health, administrator, and entrepreneur to support total health through the prevention of oral disease and the promotion of health.
- The dental hygiene process includes assessment, diagnosis, planning, implementation, evaluation, and documentation. It is the foundation of professional dental hygiene practice and provides a model for organizing and providing dental hygiene care in a variety of settings.
- A paradigm specifies the unique perspective of each discipline and is the first level of distinction between disciplines.
- The paradigm for the discipline of dental hygiene consists of the following four major concepts: client, environment, health and oral health, and dental hygiene actions.
- A conceptual model can be thought of as a school of thought within a discipline. There can be as many conceptual models as there are scholars who can think them up.
- The occupational model presents dental hygiene as technically based. The professional model describes dental hygiene as knowledge based.
- The collaborative practice model assumes that dentists and dental hygienists work together as colleagues, each offering professional expertise for the goal of providing optimum oral healthcare to the public.
- The human needs conceptual model of dental hygiene defines the paradigm concepts of client, environment, health and oral health, and dental hygiene actions in terms of human needs theory.
- The dental hygiene clinician provides preventive, therapeutic, and educational services and makes decisions independently or in collaboration with the client and family, the dentist, or other healthcare professionals.
- The public health dental hygienist provides oral health information and services to those who otherwise would not have access to such care, usually in government or nonprofit programs, or community-based clinics, schools, and settings. The corporate dental hygienist works with the oral health and healthcare industries to improve oral health and total health-related products and services for the public. The dental hygiene researcher tests assumptions underlying dental hygiene practice and investigates dental hygiene problems to improve oral healthcare and the practice of dental hygiene.
- The entrepreneur initiates, owns, and operates a business providing oral health or total health-related goods and services, frequently with some risk of time, resources, and other such investments involved.
- Interprofessional collaboration or practice is an approach to provide comprehensive healthcare to clients through the teamwork of healthcare workers from more than one discipline.
- Standards of practice provide consumers, employers, and colleagues with guidelines as to what constitutes high-quality dental hygiene care.

- Licensure is the process by which a government agency certifies that individuals are minimally qualified to practice in its jurisdiction.
- Professional organizations represent collectively the views of a profession and influence resolution of issues relevant to that profession.
- Evidence-based decision making uses current best evidence in conjunction with clinical expertise and input from the client within the context of the client's clinical circumstances.
- Dental hygiene workforce models are expanding to meet the public's need for increased access to oral healthcare.
- The ADHP is a new member of the dental hygiene workforce that has the potential to increase access to care for those who otherwise do not have access to oral healthcare services.

CRITICAL THINKING EXERCISES

1. Select a conceptual model of dental hygiene and explain why you prefer it over all other models.
2. Interview two dental hygienists and determine which professional role(s) they assume as well as whether they are aware of dental hygienists who practice in all seven professional roles of the professional dental hygienist. Report to your classmates during a class session.

REFERENCES

1. American Dental Hygienists' Association (ADHA): *Educational standards position paper*, ADHA, 2011.
2. American Dental Hygienists' Association: *Standards of care for clinical dental hygiene practice*, 2008.
3. American Dental Hygienists' Association (ADHA): *Dental hygiene diagnosis: an ADHA position paper*, 2010.
4. American Dental Hygienists' Association (ADHA): Professional roles of the dental hygienist. *ADHA*, 2011.
5. Walsh M: Theory development in dental hygiene. *Probe* 25:12, 1991.
6. American Dental Hygienists' Association (ADHA): Policy statement. Theory Development/Paradigm Concepts 6-93. *ADHA*, 1993.
7. Darby M, Walsh M: Application of the human needs conceptual model to dental hygiene practice. *J Dent Hyg* 74:230, 2000.
8. Darby M: Collaborative practice model: the future of dental hygiene. *J Dent Educ* 47:589, 1983.
9. World Health Organization (WHO). (2010) Framework for Interprofessional Education and Collaborative Practice. Geneva, Switzerland. Available at www.who.int/hrh/nursing_midwifery/en/. Accessed on March 22, 2013.
10. Lawlor S: Interprofessional practice: enhancing the dental hygienists' role. *Can J Dent Hygiene* 47(1):11, 2013.
11. American Dental Association (ADA) Commission on Dental Accreditation: *Accreditation standards for dental hygiene education programs*, Chicago, 2007, revised 2013, ADA.
12. American Dental Education Association (ADEA): ADEA competencies for entry into the allied dental professions. *J Dent Educ* 75(7):949, 2011.
13. Canadian Dental Hygienists' Association. *Entry to practice competencies and standards for dental hygienists.* A collaborative project of the Canadian Dental Hygienists Association (CDHA), Federation of Dental Hygiene Regulatory Authorities (FDHRA), Commission on Dental Accreditation of Canada (CDAC), National Dental Hygiene Certification Board (NDHCB) and dental hygiene educators, 2010. Available at: www.cdha.ca/pdfs/Competencies_and_Standards.pdf. Accessed March 21, 2013.
14. American Dental Hygienists' Association (ADHA): ADHA website. Available at: www.adha.org. Accessed January 2013.
15. National Dental Hygienists' Association (NDHA): NDHA website. Available at: http://www.ndhaonline.org/index.html. Accessed March 21, 2013.
16. Canadian Dental Hygienists' Association (CDHA): CDHA website. Available at: www.cdha.ca. Accessed March 21, 2013.
17. International Federation of Dental Hygienists (IFDH): IFDH website. Available at: http://www.ifdh.org/about.html. Accessed January 2013.
18. American Dental Hygienists' Association. Facts about the dental hygiene workforce. October 2012. Available at http://www.adha.org/resources-docs/75118_Facts_About_the_Dental_Hygiene_Workforce.pdf. Accessed March 25, 2013.
19. U.S. Department of Health and Human Services. *National Call to Action to Promote Oral Health.* Rockville, MD: U.S. Department of Health and Human Services, Public Health Service, National Institutes of Health, National Institute of Dental and Craniofacial Research. NIH Publication No. 03-5303, Spring 2003.
20. American Dental Hygienists'Association. Competencies for the advanced dental hygiene practitioner. Available at: http://www.adha.org/resources-docs/72612_ADHP_Competencies.pdf. Accessed March 27, 2013.
21. The PEW Center on the States. Help wanted: *A policy makers guide to new dental providers.* Available at http://www.pewtrusts.org/uploadedFiles/wwwpewtrustsorg/Reports/State_policy/Dental_Report_final_Low%20Res.pdf. Accessed March 25, 2013.
22. Stolberg R, Brickle C, Darby M: Development and status of the advanced dental hygiene practitioner. *J Dent Hyg* 85(2):83, 2011.

EVOLVE RESOURCES

Please visit http://evolve.elsevier.com/Darby/hygiene for additional practice and study support tools.

Human Needs Theory and Dental Hygiene Care

CHAPTER 2

Margaret M. Walsh, Michele Leonardi Darby

COMPETENCIES

1. Explain why dental hygienists need to understand human needs theory.
2. Describe Maslow's hierarchy of needs.
3. Define the four paradigm concepts based on the dental hygiene Human Needs Conceptual Model.
4. Define the eight human needs related to dental hygiene care, including:
   - Explain a clinical example of each.
   - Identify at least one related deficit and plan a dental hygiene intervention to meet the unmet need.
5. Explain how to meet client needs simultaneously.

Background

Dental hygiene care promotes health and prevents oral disease over the human life span through the provision of educational, preventive, and therapeutic services.[1] To achieve this goal the dental hygienist is concerned with the whole person, applying specific knowledge about the client's emotions, values, family, culture, and environment, as well as general knowledge about the body systems. The dental hygienist views clients as being actively involved in their care, because ultimately clients must use self-care and seek professional care to obtain and maintain their oral wellness.

Human needs theory helps dental hygienists understand the relationship between human need fulfillment and human behavior. A **human need** is a tension within a person. This tension expresses itself in some goal-directed behavior that continues until the goal is reached. **Human needs theory** explains that need fulfillment dominates human activity, and behavior is organized in relation to unsatisfied needs.[2] The dental hygienist uses clients' unsatisfied human needs related to dental hygiene care as motivators to guide them toward disease prevention and optimal oral wellness.

Although many human need theorists have provided the theoretic substance for understanding human needs and the motivation inherent in meeting these needs, Maslow's work is highlighted here as a foundation for discussing dental hygiene human needs theory presented later in this chapter.

Maslow's Hierarchy of Needs

Abraham Maslow identified and assigned priorities to basic human needs. His theory maintains that certain human needs are more basic than others. As a result, some needs must be met before individuals turn their attention to meeting other needs.[2] Maslow prioritized human needs in a hierarchy of five categories based on their power and strength to motivate behavior (Figure 2-1). The hierarchy is arranged with the most imperative needs for survival at the bottom and the least imperative at the top. On the most basic, or first, level of human needs are **physiologic needs**, such as the need for food, fluids, sleep, and exercise. According to Maslow's theory, a person is dominated by physiologic needs; if these needs are not reasonably satisfied, all other categories of needs in the hierarchy may seem irrelevant or may be relegated to low priority.

On the second level are **safety needs**, including the need for physical and psychologic security. Safety needs include the need for stability, protection, structure, and freedom from fear and anxiety. In times of danger, the need to ensure safety and protection becomes paramount. Every other need becomes less important. Loss of parental protection, war, and being confronted with new tasks, strangers, or illness are threats to the need for safety.

On the third level are **love and belonging needs**. They include the need for affectionate relationships and the need for a place within one's culture, group, or family. Love and belonging needs are expressed in the desire for tenderness, affection, contact, intimacy, togetherness, and face-to-face encounters. Love needs involve giving and receiving love. Love and belonging needs also are expressed in the need to overcome feelings of alienation, aloneness, or strangeness brought on by the scattering of family, friends, and significant others.

On the fourth level of Maslow's hierarchy are **self-esteem needs**, such as feelings of confidence, usefulness, achievement, and self-worth. Esteem needs include the need for a stable, firmly based, wholesome self-evaluation; the need for respect and esteem of self as well as esteem from others; a desire for strength, mastery, and competitiveness; and a need for feeling confident, independent, and freed. Deprivation of these needs results in feelings of inferiority, helplessness, and discouragement. Fulfillment of esteem needs results in feelings of capability and a willingness to be a contributor to society.

The final level of the hierarchy is the need for what Maslow calls **self-actualization**, a state in which each person is fully achieving his or her potential and is able to solve problems and cope realistically with life's situations.

Maslow points out that those individuals in whom a certain need always has been met or satisfied are best equipped to withstand deprivation of that need at some future time. Individuals whose needs have not been met in the past respond differently to current need deprivation than do people who have never been deprived.

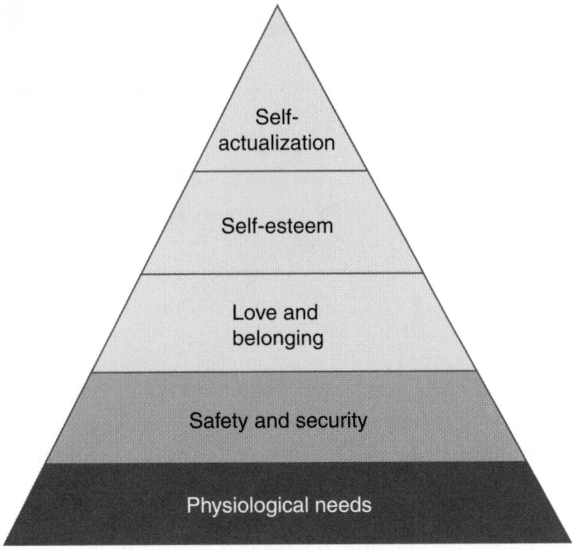

Figure 2-1. Maslow's hierarchy of needs. (Adapted from Potter PA, Perry AG: *Fundamentals of nursing*, ed 3, St Louis, 1993, Mosby.)

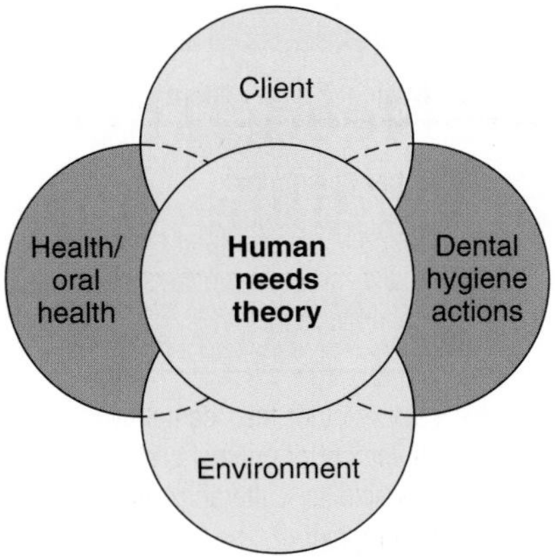

Figure 2-2. Dental hygiene's paradigm concepts are explained in terms of human needs theory in the Human Needs Conceptual Model. (Adapted from Yura H, Walsh M: *The nursing process*, ed 5, Norwalk, Conn, 1988, Appleton and Lange.)

Human Needs Conceptual Model of Dental Hygiene

Dental hygiene's Human Needs Conceptual Model is a theoretic framework for dental hygiene care.[3-6] This dental hygiene conceptual model, or school of thought, incorporates the dental hygiene process of care (assessment, diagnosis, planning, implementation, evaluation, and documentation) but defines the approach to dental hygiene care based on eight human needs especially related to oral disease prevention and health promotion. Human needs theory was selected as the conceptual framework for this model for the following reasons:

- Human needs transcend age, culture, gender, and nationality.
- Human needs connect the oral cavity with the total person.
- Human needs are recognized by the World Health Organization's definition of health as "the extent to which an individual or group is able, on the one hand, to realize aspirations and satisfy needs and, on the other hand, to change and cope with the environment."[7]
- Human needs fulfillment contributes to the quality of life of individuals, communities, and nations.
- Human needs fulfillment emphasizes a client-centered, humanistic approach to dental hygiene care.

The **Human Needs Conceptual Model** defines the four major concepts of the dental hygiene paradigm (client, environment, health and oral health, and dental hygiene actions) in terms of human needs theory (Figure 2-2) and provides a comprehensive and client-centered approach to the dental hygiene process. The manner in which human needs theory defines the paradigm concepts and the steps of the dental hygiene process is described in the following sections and compared with Global Paradigm definitions in Tables 2-1 and 2-2.

Concept 1: Client

In the Human Needs Conceptual Model, the **client** is a biologic, psychologic, spiritual, social, cultural, and intellectual human being who is an integrated, organized whole and whose behavior is motivated by human need fulfillment. Figure 2-3 illustrates this concept. Human need fulfillment restores a sense of wholeness as a human being. The client can be an individual, a family, or a group and is viewed as having eight human needs especially related to dental hygiene care.[2,3]

Concept 2: Environment

In the Human Needs Conceptual Model, the **environment** influences the manner, mode, and level of human need fulfillment for the person, family, and community. The concept of environment in the Human Needs Conceptual Model is defined as the milieu in which the client and dental hygienist find themselves. The environment affects the client and the dental hygienist, and the client and the dental hygienist also influence the environment. The concept of the environment is shown in Figure 2-4 and includes dimensions such as society, climate, geography, politics, economics, education, socioethnocultural factors, significant others, the family, the community, the state, the nation, and the world.

Concept 3: Health and Oral Health

The concept of **health and oral health** is defined as a state of well-being that exists on a continuum from maximal wellness to maximal illness (Figure 2-5). The higher the level of human need fulfillment, the higher the state of wellness for the individual. Maximal wellness is achieved with maximal fulfillment of human needs; maximal illness occurs with minimal or absent human need fulfillment. Along the health and oral health continuum, degrees of wellness and illness are associated with varying levels of human need fulfillment.

Concept 4: Dental Hygiene Actions

Dental hygiene actions are behaviors of the dental hygienist aimed at assisting clients in meeting their eight human needs related to optimal oral wellness and quality of life throughout the life cycle. Dental hygiene actions take into account such client and environmental factors as the individual's age, gender, roles, lifestyle, culture, attitudes, health beliefs, climate, and level of knowledge.

TABLE 2-1

Comparison of the Major Four Paradigm Concepts*

Paradigm Concepts	Global Definitions[8]	Human Needs Conceptual Model Definitions[3,4]
Client	The recipient of dental hygiene care; includes persons, families, groups, and communities of all ages, genders, and sociocultural and economic states	A biologic, psychologic, spiritual, social, cultural, and intellectual human being who is an integrated, organized whole and whose behavior is motivated by human need fulfillment; may be an individual, a family, or a group
Environment	Factors other than dental hygiene actions that affect the client's attainment of optimal oral health. These factors include economic, psychologic, cultural, physical, legal, educational, ethical, and geographic	The milieu in which the client and dental hygienist find themselves, which includes many dimensions (e.g., society, climate, geography, politics, economics) that influence the manner, mode, and level of human need fulfillment for the person, family, and community
Health and oral health	The client's state of well-being, which exists on a continuum from optimal wellness to illness and fluctuates over time as the result of biologic, psychologic, spiritual, and developmental factors. Oral health and overall health are interrelated because each influences the other	A state of well-being that exists on a continuum from maximum wellness to maximum illness. The higher the level of human need fulfillment, the higher the state of wellness for the client
Dental hygiene actions	Interventions that a dental hygienist can initiate to promote oral wellness and to prevent or control oral disease. These actions involve cognitive, affective, and psychomotor performances and may be provided in independent, interdependent, and collaborative relationships with the client and the healthcare team	Interventions that assist clients in meeting their human needs related to optimal oral wellness and quality of life throughout the life cycle

*Defined globally by dental hygiene's paradigm and further defined by the Human Needs Conceptual Model.

TABLE 2-2

Dental Hygiene Process*

Steps	Generic Definitions	Human Needs Conceptual Model
Assessment	Systematic collection and analysis of the following data to identify client needs and oral health problems: medical and dental histories; vital signs; extraoral and intraoral examination; periodontal and dental examination; radiographs; indices; and risk assessments (e.g., tobacco, systemic conditions, caries)[9]	Systematic data collection and evaluation of eight human needs as being met or unmet based on all available assessment data
Dental hygiene diagnosis	Use of critical decision-making skills to reach conclusions about the patient or client's dental hygiene needs based on all available assessment data[10]	Identification of unmet human needs among the eight related to dental hygiene care (i.e., human need deficit) and of the cause as evidenced by signs and symptoms
Planning	The establishment of realistic goals and treatment strategies to facilitate optimal oral health[9]	Establishment of goals for client behavior with time deadlines to meet identified unmet human needs
Implementation	Provision of treatment as identified in the assessment and planning phase[9]	The process of carrying out planned interventions targeting causes of unmet needs
Evaluation	Measurement of the extent to which goals identified in the treatment plan were achieved[9] The complete and accurate recording of all collected data, treatment planned and provided, recommendations, and other information relevant to client care	The outcome measurement of whether client goals have been met, partially met, or unmet The complete and accurate recording of human need deficits related to the client's 8 human needs, and dental hygiene diagnoses, goals, interventions, and evaluations based on human need theory

*Defined globally by the ADA Commission on Dental Hygiene Accreditation and/or by the American Dental Education Association and then further defined by the Human Needs Conceptual Model.

Inherent in the concept of dental hygiene actions is the dental hygiene process as shown in Figure 2-6. After initial collection of client histories, vital signs, and environmental, clinical, radiographic, and risk assessments, findings are evaluated to determine whether the eight human needs related to dental hygiene care are met (Box 2-1). These eight human needs relate to physical, emotional, intellectual, social, and cultural dimensions of the client and the environment that are relevant to dental hygiene care. Findings from the assessment of these human needs ensures a comprehensive

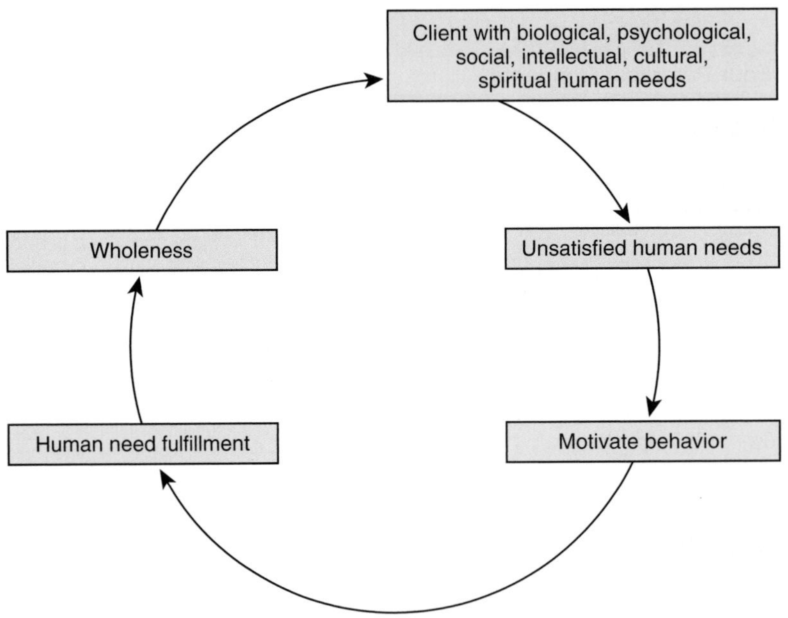

Figure 2-3. The concept of client in the Human Needs Conceptual Model of dental hygiene.

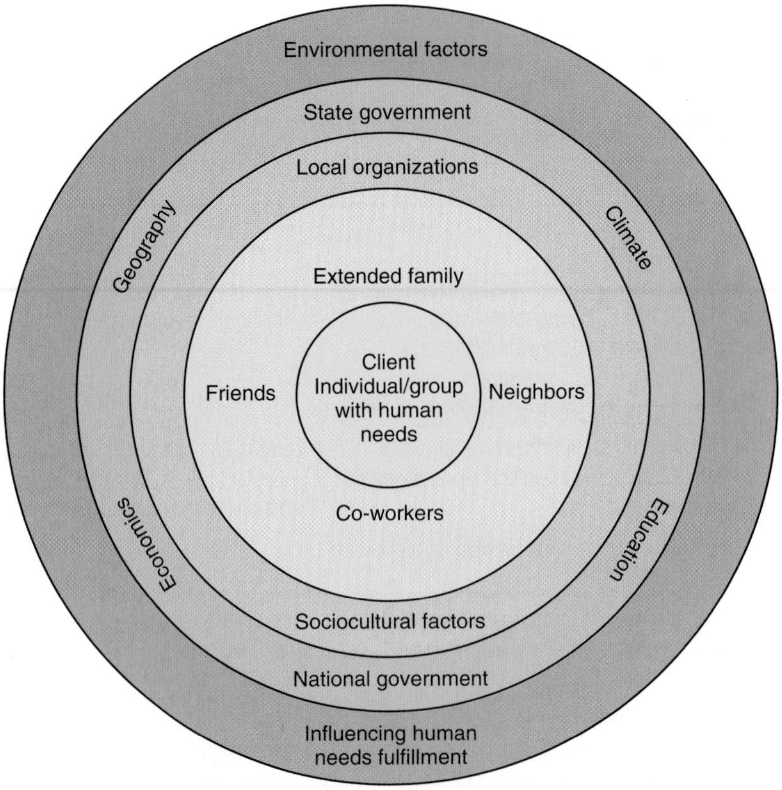

Figure 2-4. The concept of environment in the Human Needs Conceptual Model of dental hygiene.

and humanistic approach to care. Dental hygienists use these findings to make dental hygiene diagnoses based on *unmet* human needs (i.e., human need deficits) and then to plan (i.e., set goals, sequence appointments, select interventions), implement, and evaluate outcomes of dental hygiene care (i.e., goals met, partially met, or unmet). Figure 2-7 provides a sample clinical tool for use in assessing the eight human needs; making dental hygiene diagnoses; and planning, implementing, evaluating, and documenting dental hygiene interventions designed to meet the identified unmet human needs related to dental hygiene care. (Chapters 21 and 22 provide detailed explanations of how to apply the dental hygiene process in the context of the Dental Hygiene Human Needs Conceptual Model.)

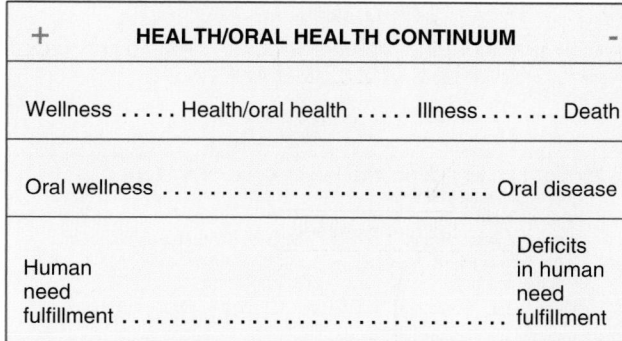

+ HEALTH/ORAL HEALTH CONTINUUM -
Wellness ..... Health/oral health ..... Illness....... Death
Oral wellness .... Oral disease
Human need fulfillment .... Deficits in human need fulfillment

Figure 2-5. The concept of health and oral health in the Human Needs Conceptual Model of dental hygiene. (Adapted from Yura H, Walsh M: *The nursing process,* ed 5, Norwalk, Conn, 1988, Appleton and Lange.)

BOX 2-1

Eight Human Needs Related to Dental Hygiene Care

- Protection from health risks
- Freedom from fear and stress
- Freedom from pain
- Wholesome facial image
- Skin and mucous membrane integrity of the head and neck
- Biologically sound and functional dentition
- Conceptualization and problem solving
- Responsibility for oral health

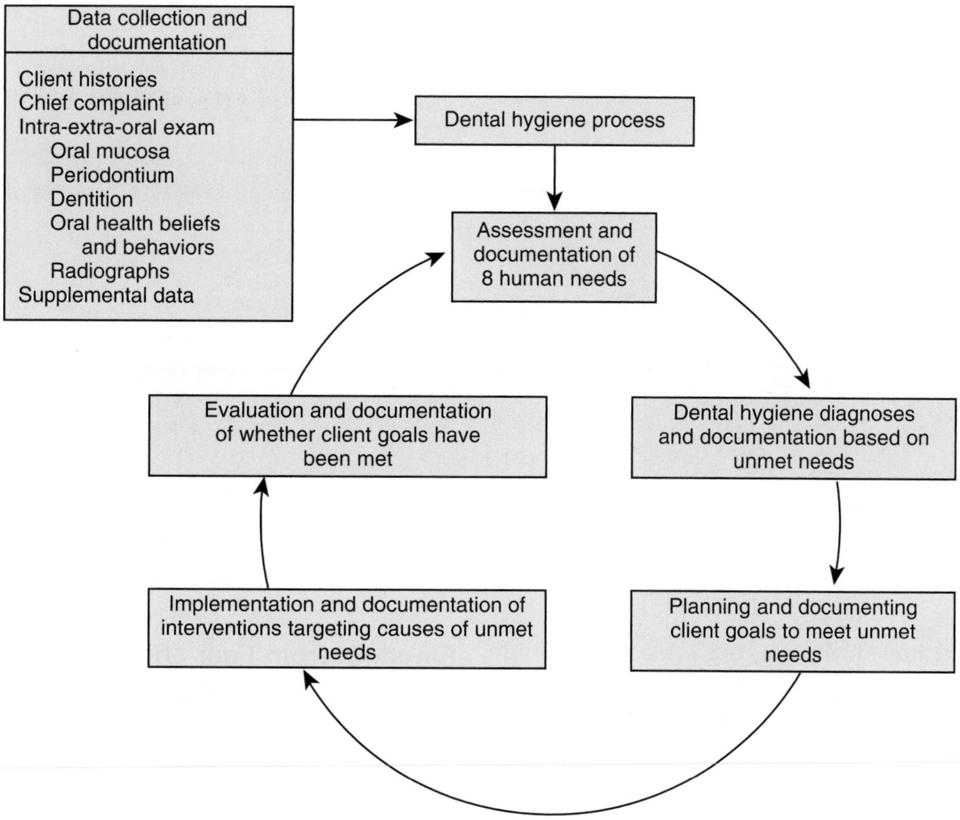

Figure 2-6. The concept of dental hygiene actions in the Human Needs Conceptual Model of dental hygiene as it relates to the dental hygiene process.

Dental Hygiene's Eight Human Needs

The eight human needs related to dental hygiene care are described in the following sections.

Protection from Health Risks

Protection from health risks is the need to avoid medical contraindications related to dental hygiene care and to be free from harm or danger involving the integrity of the body structure and environment around the person. This human need includes clients' need to be in a state of good general health through efficient functioning of body organs and systems, or under the active care of a physician in a controlled state of general health that provides for adequate function of body organs and systems.

Assessment

The dental hygienist obtains information related to the client's general health by careful evaluation of the client's verbal and nonverbal behavior during history taking, as well as by clinical, radiographic, and laboratory (if applicable) assessment. Indications that the client's need for protection from health risks is *unmet* include, but are not limited to, the following:

- Evidence from the client's health history of the need for immediate referral to, or consultation with, a physician

ASSESSMENT (circle signs & symptoms present)

1) **PROTECTION FROM HEALTH RISKS**
- vital signs outside of normal limits
- need for prophylactic antibiotics
- potential for injury
- other ______

2) **FREEDOM FROM FEAR AND STRESS**
* reports or displays:
- anxiety about proximity of clinician, confidentiality or previous dental experience
- oral habits
- substance abuse

* concern about:
- infection control, fluoride therapy, fluoridation, mercury toxicity

3) **FREEDOM FROM PAIN**
* extra-/intraoral pain or sensitivity
* other ______

4) **WHOLESOME FACIAL IMAGE**
* expresses dissatisfaction with appearance
- teeth - gingiva - facial profile - breath - other ______

5) **SKIN AND MUCOUS MEMBRANE INTEGRITY OF HEAD AND NECK**
- extra-/intraoral lesion
- swelling
- gingival inflammation
- BOP
- pockets > 4 mm
- attachment loss > 1 mm
- xerostomia
- other ______

6) **BIOLOGICALLY SOUND AND FUNCTIONAL DENTITION**
* reports difficulty in chewing
* presents with:
- defective restorations
- teeth with signs of disease
- missing teeth
- other ______
- ill fitting dentures, appliances
- abrasion erosion, abfraction
- active caries

7) **CONCEPTUALIZATION AND PROBLEM SOLVING**
* has questions about DH care and/or oral disease
* other ______

8) **RESPONSIBILITY FOR ORAL HEALTH**
* plaque and calculus present
* inadequate parental supervision of oral healthcare
* no dental exam within the last 2 years
* other ______

DENTAL HYGIENE DIAGNOSIS (List the unmet human need; then be specific about the etiology and about signs and symptoms evidencing a deficit)

(Unmet Human Need) due to (Etiology) as evidenced by (Signs and Symptoms)

CLIENT GOALS	**INTERVENTIONS** (target etiologies)	**EVALUATION** (goal met, partially met, or unmet)

APPOINTMENT SCHEDULE:

CONTINUED-CARE RECOMMENDATION:

Figure 2-7. Dental hygiene process of care form based on the Human Needs Conceptual Model.

regarding uncontrolled disease (e.g., blood pressure reading or blood glucose level outside of normal limits)
- Evidence of conditions that necessitate premedication with antibiotics to protect the client's health (e.g., complete hip replacement surgery within the past 2 years)
- Evidence of lifestyle practices that place the client at risk for oral injury (e.g., an athlete who plays contact sports without the benefit of an athletic mouth protector or guard) or for systemic or oral disease (e.g., a tobacco user)

Implications for Dental Hygiene Care

Dental hygienists with questions about a client's general health and its influence on dental hygiene care consult the client's physician before providing dental hygiene care. In general, clients with no physician of record are referred to one for examination. Obtaining initial information related to a client's general and oral health and updating it at each dental hygiene care appointment are essential to ensure that the client's need for protection from health risks is met. Box 2-2 provides an example of signs and symptoms of an actual or potential human need deficit related to this human need and suggested dental hygiene interventions.

Freedom from Fear and Stress

Freedom from fear and stress is the need to feel safe and to be free from emotional discomfort in the oral healthcare environment and to receive appreciation, attention, and respect from others.

Assessment

Fulfillment of this need can be assessed by evaluating the client's verbal and nonverbal behavior, as well as by careful examination of the face and oral cavity for signs of stress. Nonverbal behavior is evaluated by careful observation of the client on reception, during history taking, and throughout the provision of dental hygiene care. Indications that the client's need for freedom from fear and stress is unmet include but are not limited to the client's self-report or display of at least one of the following:
- Fear or anxiety about care to be provided
- Concern about the following:
  - Previous negative dental experiences
  - Cost of care
  - Infection control
  - Radiation exposure

BOX 2-2

Protection from Health Risks

SIGNS AND SYMPTOMS OF ACTUAL OR POTENTIAL DEFICIT

Client presents with potential deficit related to orofacial injury and concussion deterrence during participation in sports (Figure 2-8)

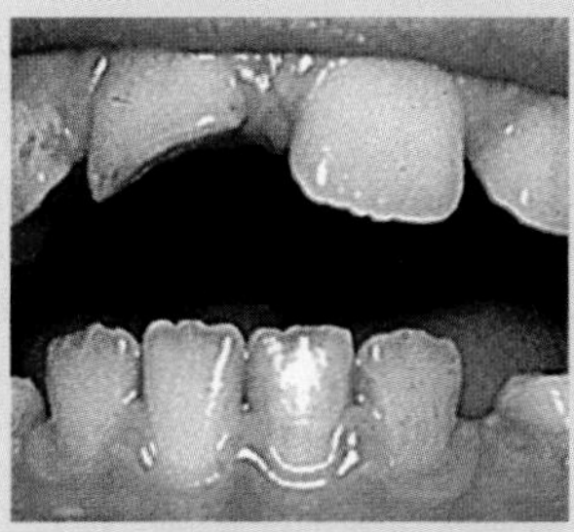

Figure 2-8. Fractured tooth from athletic injury. (Courtesy Dr. Margaret Walsh, University of California, San Francisco.)

INTERVENTION STRATEGIES

Recommend properly designed athletic mouthguard to protect against oral/facial injuries and concussion

Custom mouthguards (Figures 2-9 and 2-10): Recommended
- Designed by a health professional
- Proper fitting
- Good adaptation, retention, comfort, and stability
- No effect on breathing and communication
- Good concussion deterrence
- Long lasting

Pressure laminated mouthguard (Figure 2-11)
- Concussion deterrence
- Long lasting

Boil and bite mouthguard (Figure 2-12)
- Most commonly used
- Thermoplastic material
- Boiling water/formed in mouth
- Limited sizes
- Do not cover all posterior teeth
- Poor retention
- Gagging effects
- Bulky, interferes with speech and breathing
- Uncomfortable

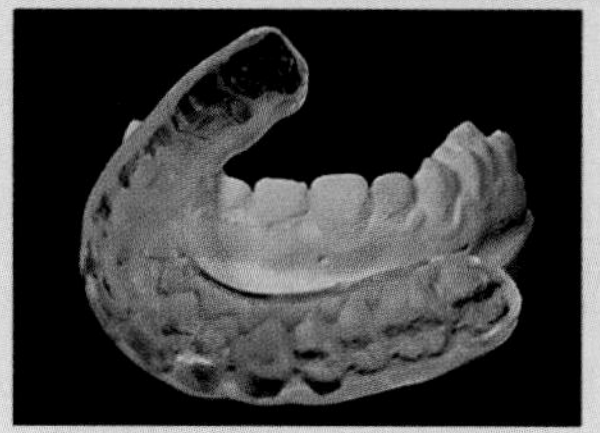

Figure 2-9. Custom mouth guard designed by a health professional.

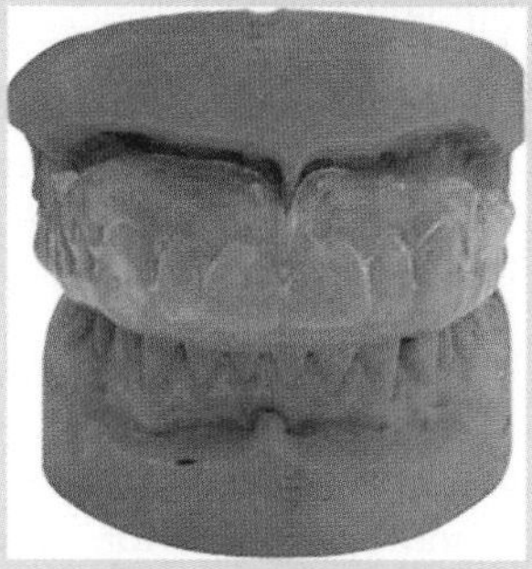

Figure 2-10. Custom mouthguard.

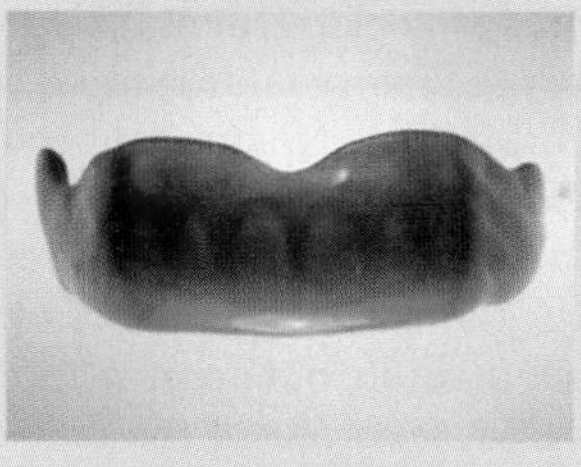

Figure 2-11. Pressure laminated mouthguard.

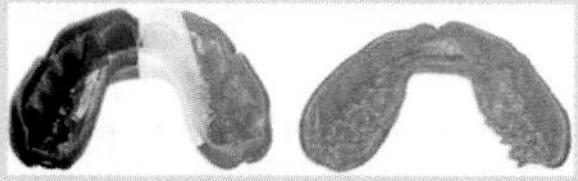

Figure 2-12. Over-the-counter boil and bite mouthguard.

  - Mercury toxicity
  - Fluoride toxicity
- Oral habits related to stress (e.g., bruxism, nailbiting, thumbsucking)
- Substance abuse (a maladaptive coping mechanism)
- Client's expression of dissatisfaction with the dental hygienist or dental hygiene care throughout any phase of the dental hygiene process of care
- Excessive perspiration (sweaty palms or beads of perspiration on forehead) or crying

Implications for Dental Hygiene Care

To some clients, the dental hygiene appointment itself may signal threat or danger and may trigger fear and stress. Being confronted with strangers, uncontrollable objects (e.g., dental hygiene instruments), loss of parental protection (for children), and the risk (however minute) of contracting an infectious or life-threatening disease such as acquired immunodeficiency syndrome (AIDS) are threats to the need for freedom from fear and stress.

If fear and stress are apparent at the beginning of, or during, the dental hygiene appointment, the dental hygienist initiates fear- or stress-control interventions immediately. Such interventions include reassuring the client that every effort will be made to provide care in as comfortable and safe a manner as possible; communicating with empathy; providing positive reinforcement of desired behavior; and answering all questions as completely as possible. For instance, clients may ask about safety factors associated with radiation, infection control, mercury-containing dental restorations (amalgam), water fluoridation, and fluoride therapy. The dental hygienist reassures about the safety of these procedures and provides evidence-based information about the rationales for their use. Box 2-3 provides an example of signs and symptoms of an actual or potential human need deficit related to this human need and suggested dental hygiene interventions.

At all times the dental hygienist demonstrates, through behavior, the unique worth of each client as a human being and ensures that the client's dignity is supported. It is particularly critical for the dental hygienist to be aware of and to exhibit respect for diversity in cultural and ethnic groups and the health beliefs, values, and behaviors associated with them. (See Chapter 6 on cultural competence and Chapter 41 on the use of nitrous oxide–oxygen analgesia for the apprehensive client. Moreover, on the website section associated with Chapter 41 is additional information on the behavioral management of pain and anxiety.)

Freedom from Pain

Freedom from pain is the need to be exempt from physical discomfort in the head and neck area. This human need is a strong motivator for clients to perform behavior that will lead to its fulfillment.

Assessment

Fulfillment of this need can be assessed by evaluating the client's verbal and nonverbal behavior, as well as by careful examination of the face and oral cavity for signs of physical discomfort. Verbal behavior is evaluated by inquiring about the client's reason for seeking dental hygiene care and by collecting data during history taking and during the intraoral and extraoral examinations. Nonverbal behavior is evaluated by careful observation of the client on reception, during history taking, and throughout the provision of dental hygiene care. Indications that the client's need for freedom from pain is unmet include, but are not limited to, client self-report or display of at least one of the following:

- Extraoral or intraoral pain or sensitivity
- Use of pain medication
- Difficulty with movement and/or tension in face, hands, and/or legs
- Discomfort or pain during dental hygiene care
- Speaking with hesitation or breaks in sentences
- Excessive perspiration (sweaty palms or beads of perspiration on forehead) and/or crying

Implications for Dental Hygiene Care

If pain is apparent at the beginning of or during the dental hygiene appointment, the dental hygienist initiates pain control interventions immediately, including client referral to the dentist for care. Ways in which the dental hygienist provides pain control for clients are discussed in Chapters 40 and 41. Because the mouth is very sensitive, dental hygienists perform instrumentation techniques as carefully and as gently as possible, especially when treating a client who is not anesthetized. Box 2-4 provides an example of signs and symptoms of an actual or potential human need deficit related to this human need and suggested dental hygiene interventions.

Wholesome Facial Image

Wholesome facial image is the need to feel satisfied with one's own oral-facial features and breath. Facial image is determined by individuals' perception of their physical characteristics and their interpretation of how that image is perceived by others. Facial image is influenced by normal and abnormal physical changes and by cultural and societal attitudes and values. For example, normal developmental changes such as growth and aging affect a person's facial image. Cultural values lead Surma women in Ethiopia to wear lip plates as a sign of physical beauty or Maori people to covet face tattoos that tell a story of a person's accomplishments and ancestry. In the United States, society emphasizes youth, beauty, and wholeness, a fact that is apparent in television programs, movies, and advertisements. These cultural attitudes and values affect how people perceive their physical bodies, because body image is a combination of the ideal and the real.[11]

People generally do not adapt quickly to changes in the physical body. For example, people who experience normal aging often report that they do not feel different, but when they look in the mirror they are surprised by their aged facial characteristics. Facial disfigurement resulting from disease, trauma, or surgery is an obvious stressor affecting body image. For example, tooth loss is a stressor that affects facial image through a change in personal appearance.

The importance of a change in appearance is determined partly by individual perceptions of the alteration and by personal estimations of how others perceive that alteration. For example, if someone associates possession of natural teeth with femininity or masculinity, loss of teeth may be a significant alteration, one that may threaten the person's sexuality or sense of self. Similarly, clients with dentures, a cleft lip, or facial disfigurement after surgical treatment of oral cancer may reduce social contacts out of fear of people's reactions to them. Such clients may feel isolated, excluded, stigmatized, or helpless. Their feelings of social isolation may be based in reality, because people may avoid contact with them for fear of causing embarrassment or offense. Thus body image stressors can negatively alter the client's body image, which in turn may alter negatively the client's self-concept and behavior.[11]

Indications that the client's need for a wholesome facial image is fulfilled include such evidence as the client's statement of satisfaction with his or her appearance, being neatly groomed, and making an effort to bring out the best of facial assets with careful makeup and attention to hairstyle.

Assessment

The dental hygienist assesses the client's need for a wholesome facial image based on information obtained from history taking, direct observation, and casual conversation with the client. For example, the client's satisfaction with the general appearance of the teeth, mouth, and facial profile can be determined by asking questions such as, "Does anything about your teeth bother you?" or "Is there anything about your mouth that concerns you?" Such questions may elicit responses indicating dissatisfaction with tooth stain, calculus, receding gums, bleeding gums, a discolored restoration, or malaligned teeth. Indications that the client's need for a wholesome facial image is unmet include but are not limited to clients' self-report of dissatisfaction with the following:

- Appearance of their teeth, gingivae, facial profile
- Their breath

BOX 2-3

Freedom from Fear and Stress

SIGNS AND SYMPTOMS OF ACTUAL OR POTENTIAL DEFICIT	INTERVENTION STRATEGIES
Client reports • Fear related to past negative dental experiences • Concern about cost of care • Concern about disease transmission • Concern about fluoride toxicity • Concern about care planned • Concern about mercury toxicity • Concern about radiation	• Communicate with empathy (Figure 2-13). • Answer all questions. • Provide music with headphones; use humor to establish rapport (Figure 2-14). • Offer and administer nitrous oxide analgesia if indicated (Figures 2-15 and 2-16).

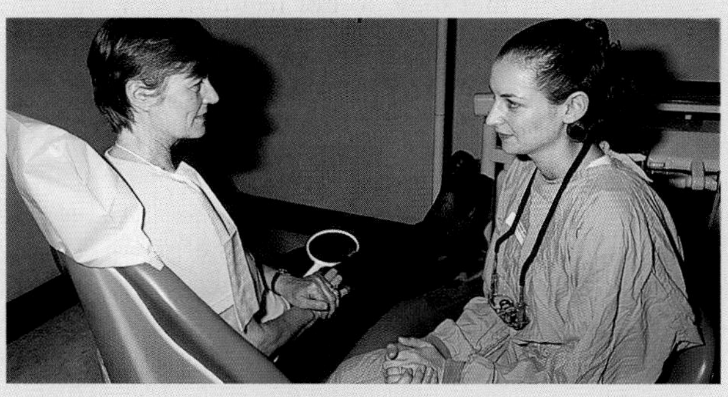

Figure 2-13. Dental hygienist actively listening to client.

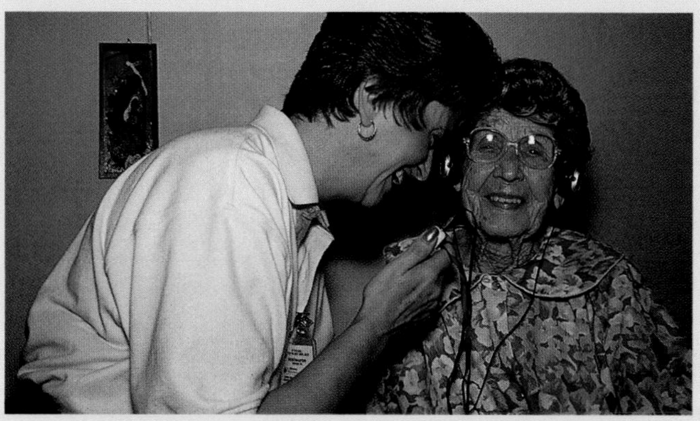

Figure 2-14. Dental hygienist sharing a joke with the client.

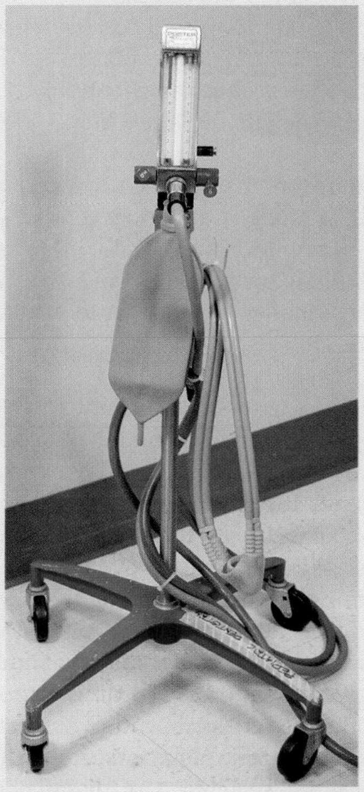

Figure 2-15. Portable nitrous oxide machine. (Courtesy Dr. Mark Dellinges and Cory Price.)

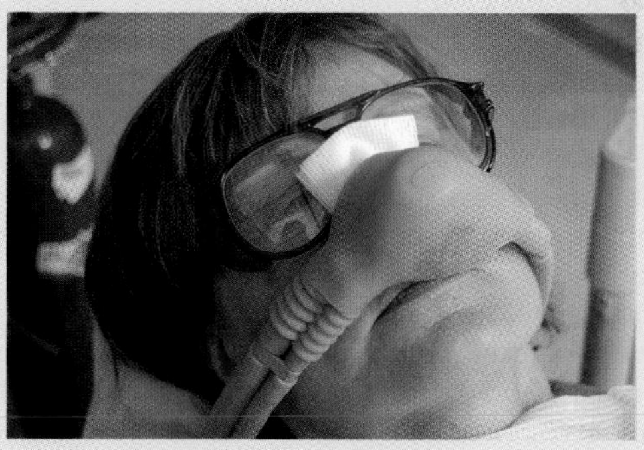

Figure 2-16. Client wearing nitrous oxide mask. (Courtesy Dr. Mark Dellinges and Cory Price.)

BOX 2-4

Freedom from Head and Neck Pain

SIGNS AND SYMPTOMS OF ACTUAL OR POTENTIAL DEFICITS	INTERVENTION STRATEGIES
Client reports • Extraoral or intraoral pain or sensitivity • Tenderness upon palpation • Discomfort during dental hygiene care	Initiate pain control interventions immediately (Figures 2-17 and 2-18).

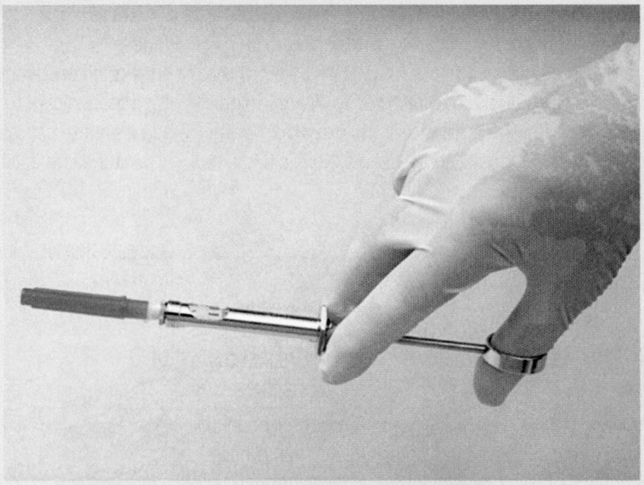

Figure 2-17. Intraoral syringe loaded with local anesthetic. (From Malamed SF: *Handbook of local anesthesia*, ed 6, St Louis, 2013, Mosby.)

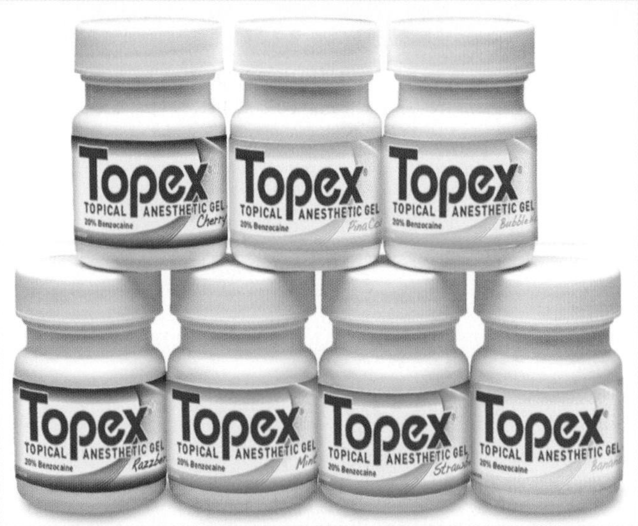

Figure 2-18. Topical local anesthetic. (Courtesy Beautlich LP, Pharmaceuticals, Waukegan, Illinois.)

Such unmet needs have implications for dental hygiene care, including referral to other health professionals (e.g., general dentist, periodontist, orthodontist) for additional care.

Implications for Dental Hygiene Care

Tooth loss, malaligned teeth, oral cancer, and facial disfigurement are examples of facial image stressors related to the face and oral cavity that dental hygiene clients may experience. The dental hygienist listens to client doubts about treatment outcomes related to these stressors and provides information, reassurance, and referrals as needed. Complimenting such clients on some aspect of their appearance assists them to focus on positive attributes and features. For some clients, encouragement to seek other support systems to share feelings about body changes may be helpful in assisting them to reinforce accomplishments, strengths, and positive attributes.[11]

Facial image stressors affect self-concept and motivate behavior, including oral health behavior. The dental hygienist's acceptance of a client with an altered self-concept because of facial image stressors may be the factor that stimulates positive rehabilitative results. For example, a client whose physical appearance has changed drastically from head and neck cancer surgery must adapt to a new facial image. For this client, being accepted by the dental hygienist as a human being with ideas, feelings, and values who is worthy and whole despite illness or physical alterations is important. This acceptance also can provide an example for the client and family members that affirms the client's self-worth.[11] The client's feelings of insecurity, fears of rejection, or loss of self-worth can be lessened through sensitive, knowledgeable dental hygiene care.

Dental hygienists must be in touch with their own feelings and expectations about clients undergoing such facial image stressors because the dental hygienist's reaction to a client's illness or physical alteration can have a significant impact on the client's self-concept and the outcome of care. Clients with low self-esteem because of altered facial image may be particularly sensitive to the way the dental hygienist involves them in their own care. A dental hygienist with mixed feelings about clients' physical alteration may be hesitant in making suggestions, thus inadvertently implying that they may be unable to follow suggestions. Alternatively, the hygienist may insist that such clients assume too much responsibility for their own care, thus causing anxiety and frustration. In either case, clients' self-esteem and facial image may be threatened additionally rather than strengthened. However, if the dental hygienist demonstrates confidence in a client's abilities and is confident in personal feelings about and expectations of the client, then the client's sense of wholesome facial image, as well as self-worth, will be reinforced.[11] Box 2-5 provides an example of signs and symptoms of an actual or potential human need deficit related to this human need and suggested dental hygiene interventions.

BOX 2-5

Wholesome Facial Image

SIGNS AND SYMPTOMS OF ACTUAL OR POTENTIAL DEFICIT	INTERVENTION STRATEGIES
Client reports • Dissatisfaction with facial profile, breath (Figure 2-19)	Refer to orthodontist. Review tooth brushing, flossing, and other aids for halitosis prevention.
• Dissatisfaction with esthetic appearance of teeth (Figure 2-20)	Provide oral prophylaxis with coronal polishing.
	Recommend tooth whitening using H_2O_2 to lighten teeth for a more esthetic smile, or recommend professionally dispensed whitening product (e.g., Crest Whitestrips Supreme) 14% H_2O_2 twice daily, 30 min for 3 weeks (Figure 2-21). Recommend professionally dispensed whitening product, e.g., Crest Whitestrips Supreme, 14% H_2O_2 twice daily, 30 min for 3 weeks.

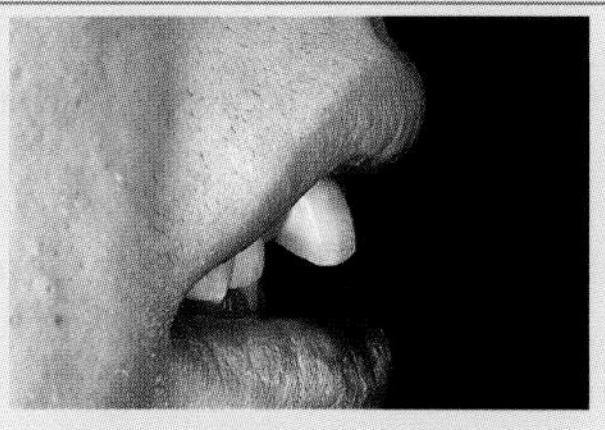

Figure 2-19. Malocclusion.

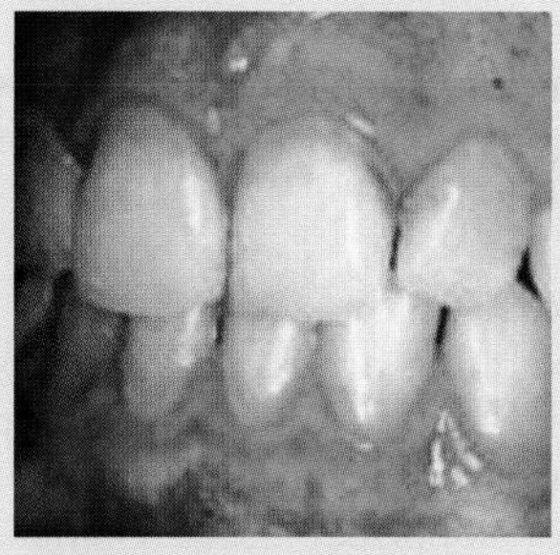

Figure 2-20. Green stain. (From Scully C, Welbury R, Flaitz C, Paes de Almeida O: *A color atlas of orofacial health and disease in children and adolescents*, ed 2, Oxford, England, 2002, Taylor and Francis.)

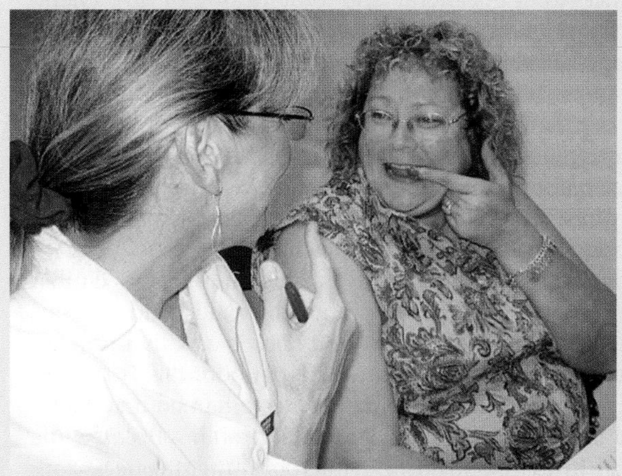

Figure 2-21. Dental hygienist talking with client. (Courtesy Michele Darby, BSDH, MS.)

Skin and Mucous Membrane Integrity of the Head and Neck

Skin and mucous membrane integrity of the head and neck is the need for an intact and functioning covering of the person's head and neck area, including the oral mucous membranes and periodontium. These intact tissues defend against harmful microbes, provide sensory information, resist injurious substances and trauma, and reflect adequate nutrition.

Assessment

Assessment of this human need occurs initially by careful observation of the client's face, head, and neck area as part of an overall client appraisal on reception and seating; and by careful examination of the oral cavity and adjacent structures and the periodontium before planning and implementing dental hygiene care (see Chapters 15, 19, and 32).

Indications that this human need is unmet include but are not limited to the presence of any of the following conditions:

- Extraoral and intraoral lesions, tenderness, or swelling
- Gingival inflammation
- Bleeding on probing (BOP)
- Probing depths or clinical attachment loss greater than 4 mm
- Xerostomia (dry mouth), with accompanying oral mucous membranes that are not uniform in color
- Extraoral or intraoral manifestations of nutritional deficiencies (see Chapter 35)
- Evidence of an eating disorder (e.g., trauma around the mouth from implements used to induce vomiting or enamel erosion) (see Chapter 53)

Implications for Dental Hygiene Care

The dental hygienist examines all skin and mucous membranes in and about the oral cavity, including the periodontium, documents findings, and informs the dentist and the client about evidence of abnormal tissue changes and/or disease. A variety of skin and oral mucosal lesions may be observed that may or may not be symptomatic. Recognition, treatment, and follow-up of specific lesions may be of great significance to the general and oral health of the client. Routine extraoral and intraoral examination of clients at the initial appointment and at each continued care appointment provides an excellent opportunity to control oral disease by early recognition and treatment. At least annually, clients are screened to detect potentially cancerous lesions. Moreover, a current appointment may be postponed because of a client's need for urgent medical consultation or because of evidence of infectious lesions, such as herpes labialis.

Because periodontal disease is epidemic in the United States and elsewhere, the human need for skin and mucous membrane integrity of the head and neck is usually unmet in clients seeking dental hygiene care. In periodontal disease the sulcular, or pocket, epithelium becomes inflamed and ulcerated and bleeds readily on periodontal probing. Because the epithelium is not intact, harmful microbes enter the periodontal tissues and the bloodstream. Under these circumstances, dental hygiene strategies to meet the human need for skin and mucous membrane integrity of the head and neck may include the following:

- Instruction on biofilm and related self-care techniques
- Scaling and root planing with or without extrinsic stain removal
- Subgingival placement of antimicrobial agents
- Referral to the general dentist or the periodontist for specialty care

Moreover, dental hygienists use their extraoral and intraoral examination and interviewing skills to identify nutritional problems and provide counseling or appropriate referral. Dental hygienists are in an excellent position to recognize signs of poor nutrition and to take steps to initiate change. Regular contact with continued-care clients at 3-, 4-, or 6-month intervals enables dental hygienists to make observations of clients' physical status, food intake, and response to dental hygiene care. The dental hygienist informs the dentist of observations that indicate a nutritional problem and incorporates approaches to solving the problem into the dental hygiene care plan. When malnutrition or a serious eating disorder such as anorexia nervosa or bulimia nervosa is suspected, client referral for medical evaluation is a priority (see Chapter 53). Box 2-6 provides an example of signs and symptoms of an actual or potential human need deficit related to this human need and suggested dental hygiene interventions.

Biologically Sound and Functional Dentition

Biologically sound and functional dentition refers to the need for intact teeth and restorations that defend against harmful microbes, provide for adequate functioning and esthetics, and reflect appropriate nutrition and diet.

Assessment

Assessment of this need is ongoing throughout the dental hygiene care appointment. However, initially it occurs while the hygienist is taking a careful dental history and carefully observing the client's dentition as part of a thorough examination of the oral cavity and adjacent structures preliminary to dental hygiene care. Indications that the client's need for a biologically sound dentition is unmet include but are not limited to client self-report or display of at least one of the following conditions:

- Difficulty in chewing
- Defective restorations
- Teeth with signs of dental caries, abrasion, abfraction, or erosion
- Missing teeth
- Ill-fitting prosthetic appliances
- Teeth with calculus, oral biofilm, or extrinsic stain
- Active caries
- High daily sugar intake
- Evidence of an eating disorder (e.g., erosion of teeth, particularly on the lingual and incisal surfaces of maxillary anterior teeth and the occlusal and palatal surfaces of maxillary molars)
- No examination by a dentist in the previous 2 years

Implications for Dental Hygiene Care

The dental hygienist documents existing conditions of the teeth, including restorations, deviations from normal, signs of caries, and missing teeth.

A bitewing radiographic survey may assist with evaluation and charting, especially between posterior teeth. All

BOX 2-6

Skin and Mucous Membrane Integrity of Head and Neck

SIGNS AND SYMPTOMS OF ACTUAL OR POTENTIAL DEFICITS	INTERVENTION STRATEGIES
Client presents with • Gingival inflammation • Bleeding on probing • Probing depths or attachment loss • Mucogingival problems • Oral manifestations of nutritional deficiencies	Scaling and root planing Referral to dentist/periodontist for further evaluation and possible surgical treatment (Figures 2-22, 2-23, 2-24) Nutritional assessment Referral to a physician when malnutrition or a serious eating disorder is suspected
• Extra and/or intraoral lesions (Figure 2-25)	Antifungal cream • Viaderm ointment 15 gram tube, apply thin coating 3×/day • Continue for a few more days after resolved Drooling: protect with water-based lip lubricant

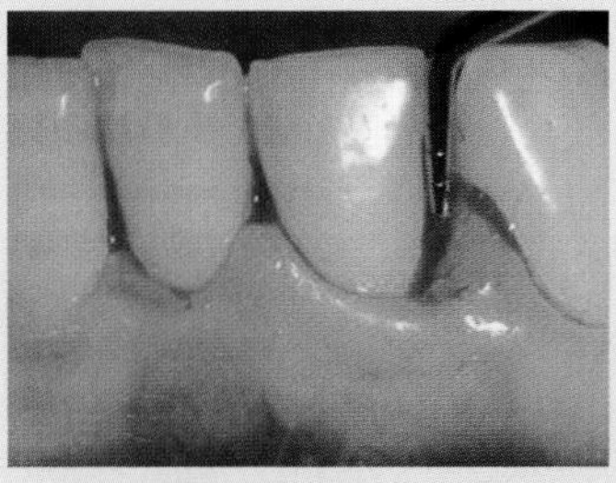

Figure 2-22. Gingival inflammation and bleeding on probing.

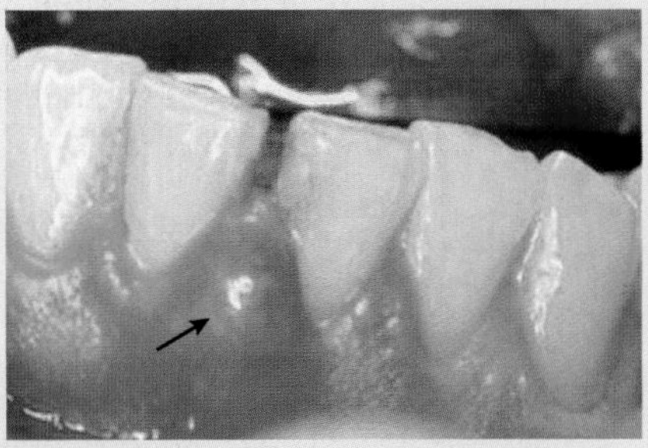

Figure 2-23. Inflamed and edematous interdental papilla.

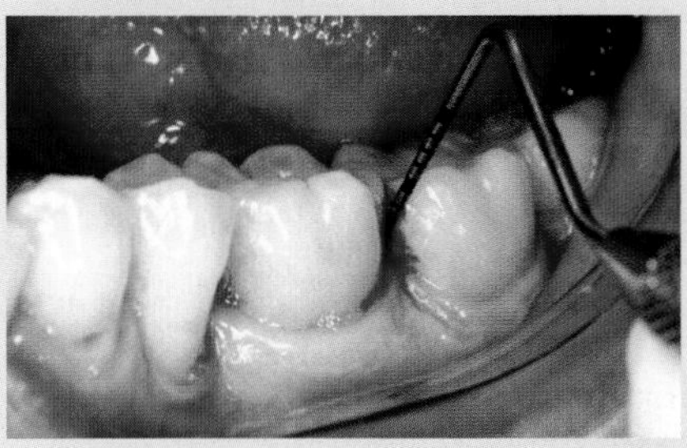

Figure 2-24. Bleeding on probing.

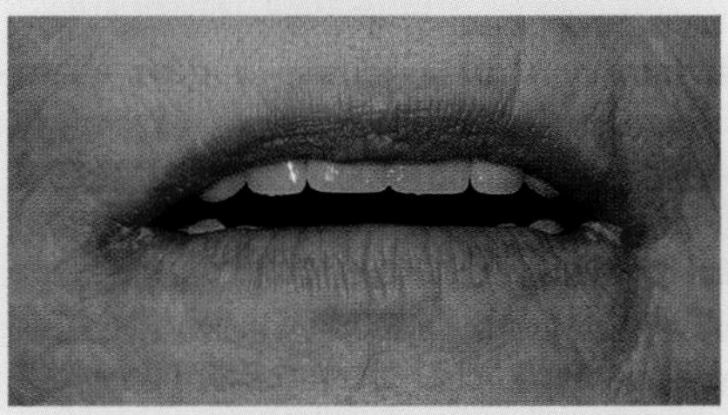

Figure 2-25. Angular cheilitus. (From Newman MG, Takei HH, Klokkevold PR, Carranza FA, eds: *Carranza's clinical periodontology,* ed 10, St Louis, 2012, Saunders.)

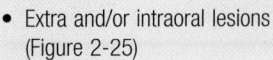

OTC, Over the counter.

teeth with signs of disease and/or functional problems should be called to the immediate attention of the dentist. Performing caries-risk assessment, exposing radiographs based on assessment data, providing fluoride therapy and sealants, recommending home fluoride therapy or xylitol use, and referring to the dentist for periodic oral examination are dental hygiene interventions most frequently used to meet the client's need for a biologically sound dentition.

Nutritional assessment also is particularly important for clients who may be at risk for nutritional problems related to tooth loss, ill-fitting dentures, dental caries, and periodontal diseases. A complete nutritional assessment includes collecting data from observation and a dietary history (see Chapter 35).

Conceptualization and Problem Solving

Conceptualization and problem solving involve the need to understand ideas and abstractions to make sound judgments about one's oral health (Box 2-7). This need is considered to be met if the client understands the rationale for recommended oral healthcare interventions; participates in setting goals for dental hygiene care; has no questions about professional dental hygiene care or dental treatment; and has no questions about the cause of the oral problem, its relationship to overall health, and the importance of the solution suggested to solve the problem.

Assessment

The dental hygienist assesses this need by listening to clients' questions and responses to the hygienist's answers.

BOX 2-7

Responsibility for Oral Health

SIGNS AND SYMPTOMS OF ACTUAL OR POTENTIAL DEFICIT	INTERVENTION STRATEGIES
Client presents with • Inadequate plaque biofilm control (Figures 2-26 and 2-27 • Inadequate caregiver supervision • No dental exam within 2 years	Oral hygiene education (Figures 2-28 and 2-29) Refer for dental examination Set goals for dental hygiene care in collaboration with the client
	Referral for dental exam (Figure 2-30)

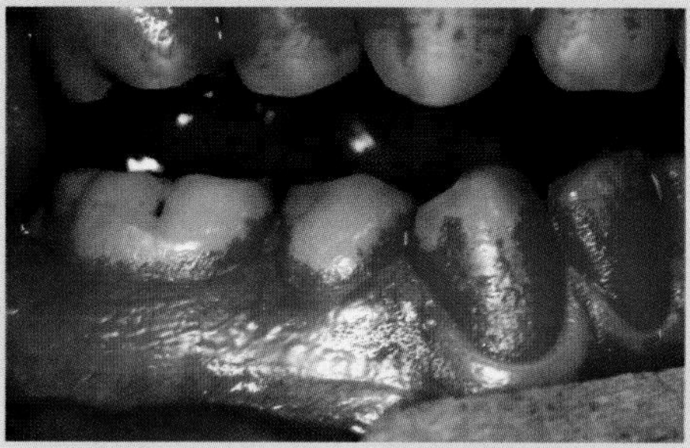

Figure 2-26. Disclosed plaque biofilm. (Courtesy Dr. George Blozis. From Ibsen OAC, Phelan JA: *Oral pathology for the dental hygienist*, ed 6, St Louis, 2013, Saunders.)

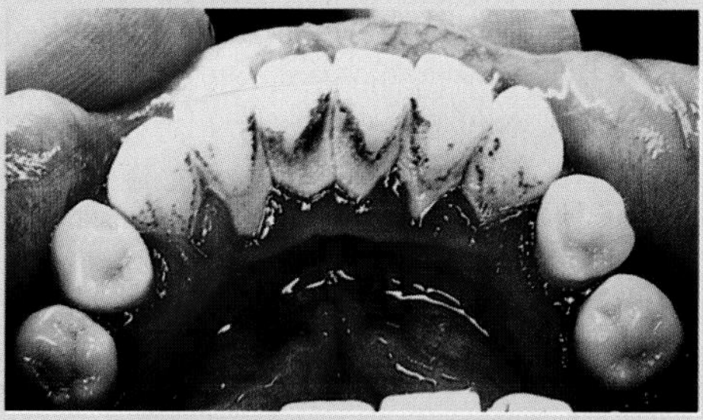

Figure 2-27. Supragingival calculus. (Courtesy Dr. Eli Whitney, Certified Specialist in Oral Medicine and Oral Pathology, Faculty of Dentistry, University of British Columbia, Vancouver, Canada.)

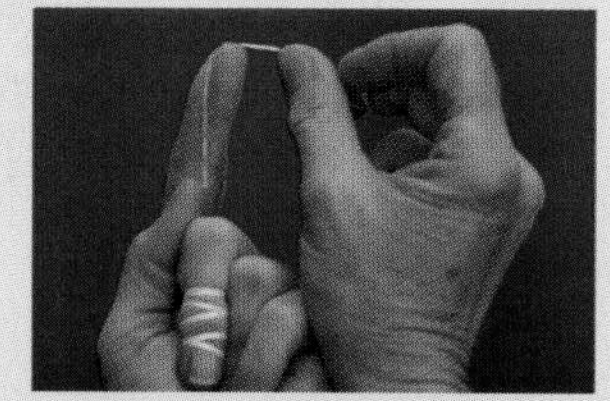

Figure 2-28. Flossing.

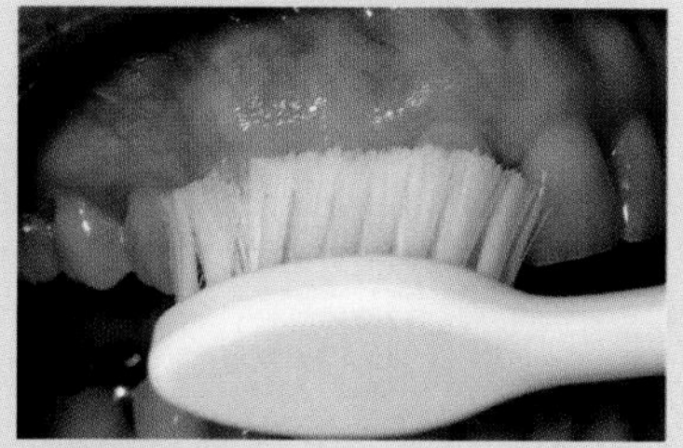

Figure 2-29. Toothbrushing.

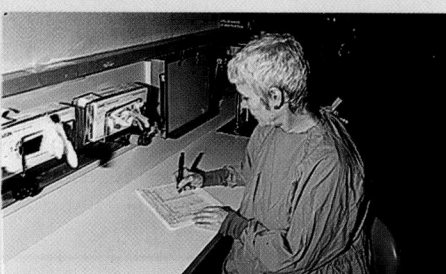

Figure 2-30. Dental hygienist documenting referral for dental exam.

Indications that this need is unmet include but are not limited to evidence that the client has questions, misconceptions, or a lack of knowledge about at least one of the following:
- Recommended dental or dental hygiene care
- Oral diseases, their causes, and their relation to general health
- Preventive self-care or professional procedures

Implications for Dental Hygiene Care

During client education, dental hygienists present the rationale and details of methods recommended for the prevention and control of oral diseases. In addition, they question clients to ensure understanding of concepts relevant to clients' oral health and recommended care and ask clients to demonstrate use of any explained home self-care device to clarify client understanding and evaluate ability to use the device. To ensure client understanding, the dental hygienist often augments verbal presentation with graphics and other types of visual aids. For example, to help a client conceptualize what biofilm is, where it is located, and its relationship to periodontal disease, the dental hygienist may do the following:
- Use a tablet or rinse to disclose the location of biofilm in a client's own mouth.
- Provide a mirror for clients to view the inflammatory response of their gingival tissues to biofilm.
- Demonstrate use of an oral self-care tool for biofilm removal in the client's own mouth (e.g., floss) while the client observes in a mirror; observe the client's use and provide feedback.
- Sketch on a pad of paper the location of biofilm on the cervical third of teeth and relate it graphically to periodontal destruction in the client's mouth.

Use commercially prepared materials to reinforce where biofilm accumulates and its effect on periodontal tissues, tooth structure, and oral malodor.

Box 2-8 provides an example of signs and symptoms of an actual or potential human need deficit related to this human need and suggested dental hygiene interventions.

Responsibility for Oral Health

Responsibility for oral health refers to the need for accountability for one's oral health as a result of interaction among

BOX 2-8

Conceptualization and Problem Solving

SIGNS AND SYMPTOMS OF ACTUAL OR POTENTIAL DEFICIT	INTERVENTION STRATEGIES
Client has questions or misconceptions associated with • Oral diseases • Rationale for daily self-care • DH care	Client education about oral health and disease and care needed (Figure 2-31)

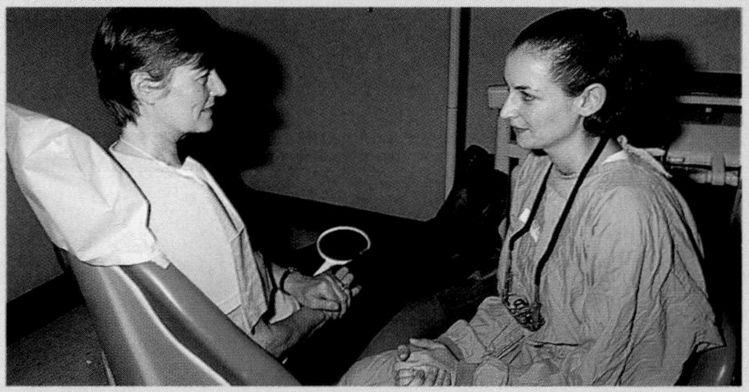

Figure 2-31. Dental hygienist providing client education.

one's motivation, physical and cognitive capability, and social environment.

Assessment

This need is assessed from data collected in the client's health, pharmacologic, dental, personal, and cultural histories and from direct observation of whether the client performs adequate daily oral self-care and seeks adequate professional care to prevent and control oral diseases. Indications that this need is unmet include but are not limited to the presence of any one of the following conditions:

- Inadequate oral self-care
- In the case of small children, inadequate parental caregiver supervision of daily oral hygiene care
- No dental examination within the last 2 years

Implications for Dental Hygiene Care

The dental hygienist assesses the client's oral health behaviors and suggests behaviors to the client (or to the parent/healthcare decision maker when the client is a child) that should be initiated to obtain and maintain oral wellness. In providing oral health education, the dental hygienist appeals to clients' sense of self-determination and empowerment to evoke the client's need for responsibility for oral health. The dental hygienist encourages the client to participate in setting goals for dental hygiene care, offers choices, and facilitates and reinforces client decision making. In addition, the hygienist addresses deficits in clients' psychomotor skill level and recommends strategies to enhance proper manipulation of the toothbrush, floss, or other oral self-care tools (e.g., use of lightweight power toothbrushes to compensate for psychomotor skill deficits that may be related to degenerative disabilities in arthritic clients).

A primary role of the dental hygienist is to motivate and empower clients to adopt and maintain positive oral health behaviors. In this effort the dental hygienist views the client as being actively involved in the process of care. Using information from the client's history, oral examination, radiographs, and all other data collected during the initial assessment, the dental hygienist in collaboration with the client establishes goals for dental hygiene care. These goals must be related realistically to the client's individual needs, values, and ability level. Because each client has personal requirements for self-care, clients must participate in setting goals and must commit personally to achieving them if oral disease control and prevention are to be successful over the life span. Box 2-9 provides an example of signs and symptoms of an actual or potential human need deficit related to this human need and suggested dental hygiene interventions.

Simultaneously Meeting Needs

Identification of the eight human needs related to dental hygiene care is a useful way for dental hygienists to evaluate and understand the needs of all clients and to achieve a client-centered practice. A client entering the oral care environment may have one or more unmet needs, and dental hygiene care delivered within a human needs conceptual framework addresses all of them simultaneously. The Human Needs Conceptual Model provides a holistic and humanistic perspective for dental hygiene care. The model addresses the client's needs in the physical, psychologic, emotional, intellectual, spiritual, and social dimensions and defines the territory for the practice of client-centered dental hygiene. Applying this model when interacting with clients, whether the client is an individual, a family, or a community, enhances the dental hygienist's relationship with the client and promotes the client's adoption of and adherence to the dental hygienist's professional recommendations.

Oral disease disrupts clients' ability to meet their human needs not only in the physical dimension but also in the emotional, intellectual, social, and cultural dimensions. Therefore the dental hygienist plans and provides interventions for clients with diverse needs. Using information from the client's histories, oral examination, radiographs, and all other data collected, the dental hygienist assesses clients for unmet needs and then considers how dental hygiene care can best help them meet those needs. After identifying which of

BOX 2-9

Biologically Sound and Functional Dentition

SIGN AND SYMPTOMS OF ACTUAL OR POTENTIAL DEFICIT	INTERVENTION STRATEGIES	
Client presents with • Missing or diseased teeth • Defective restorations • Abrasion, erosion, trauma • Ill-fitting dentures • Chewing difficulties Clinical signs of disease and/or functional problems	• Refer to dentist for restorative care • Establish homecare regimen: • Daily fluoride mouth rinsing (Figure 2-32) • Daily toothbrushing with fluoridated dentifrice and interproximal care • Chlorhexidine antimicrobial therapy daily for 1 week and monthly for 6 months until cariogenic bacteria controlled	Restorative care

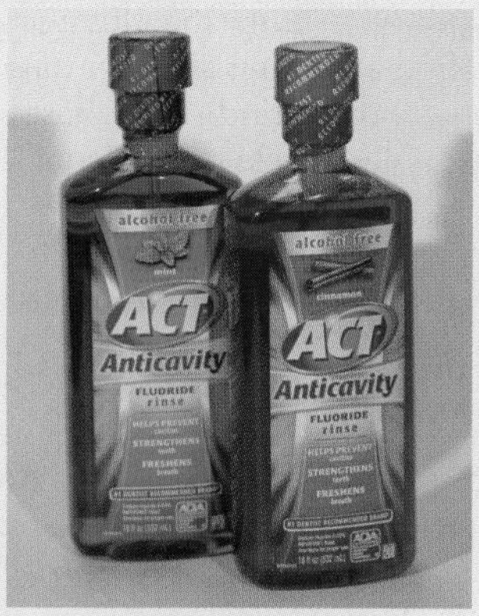

Figure 2-32. 0.05% sodium fluoride mouth rinse. (Courtesy Dr. Mark Dellinges.)

a client's human needs are unmet, the dental hygienist, in collaboration with the client, sets goals and establishes priorities for providing care to fulfill these needs. Setting goals and establishing priorities, however, does not mean that the dental hygienist provides care for only one need at a time. In emergency situations, of course, physiologic needs take precedence, but even then the dental hygienist is aware of the client's other psychosocial needs. For example, when providing care for a client with painful gingivitis, whose human needs for skin and mucous membrane integrity of the head and neck and for freedom from pain require immediate attention, the dental hygienist also takes into consideration the client's need for freedom from stress and wholesome facial image. Often one need may take priority and the dental hygienist must be concerned first with the highest-priority need (such as helping the client cope with a fear of having his or her teeth scaled before helping the client restore the integrity of the gingival tissues). However, frequently the dental hygienist simultaneously addresses needs such as assisting a client in meeting the need for responsibility for oral health while also helping the client achieve freedom from pain.

CLIENT EDUCATION TIPS

- Explain modification to care required because of medical conditions.
- Discuss client's previous negative experiences related to dental or dental hygiene care, and reassure that every effort will be made to provide care as comfortably and safely as possible.
- Listen to doubts about treatment outcomes expressed by clients undergoing treatment related to facial image stressors, and provides information and reassurance as needed.
- Present the rationale and details of methods recommended for the prevention and control of oral diseases, and ask questions to determine if the client needs clarification of concepts.
- Offer choices for self-care and professional care to evoke clients' need for responsibility for oral health.
- Encourage clients to participate in setting goals for dental hygiene care, and reinforce client decisions.

LEGAL, ETHICAL, AND SAFETY ISSUES

- Discuss all procedures with clients, obtain informed consent, and encourage their participation in the dental hygiene care plan.
- Postpone a current appointment because of a client's need for urgent medical consultation or because of evidence of infectious lesions such as herpes labialis or mucous patches.
- Address medical contraindications before performing any intraoral instrumentation associated with dental hygiene care.

KEY CONCEPTS

- Dental hygiene care focuses on the promotion of oral health and the prevention of oral disease over the life span.
- The dental hygienist is concerned with the whole person, applying specific knowledge about the client's emotions, values, family, culture, and environment as well as general knowledge about the body systems.
- Clients are viewed as active participants in the process of dental hygiene care because the ultimate responsibility to use self-care and seek professional care to obtain and maintain oral wellness is theirs.
- Dental hygiene's Human Needs Conceptual Model is a theoretic framework for dental hygiene care. This

conceptual model, or school of thought, defines an approach to dental hygiene care based on human needs theory.
- The Human Needs Conceptual Model defines the four major concepts of dental hygiene's paradigm (client, environment, health and oral health, and dental hygiene actions) in terms of human needs theory.
- Using information from the client's histories, oral examination, radiographs, and all other data collected, the dental hygienist uses these findings to assess whether or not the eight human needs related to dental hygiene are met.
- Assessment of the eight human needs ensures a comprehensive and humanistic approach to care. Dental hygienists use these findings to make dental hygiene diagnoses based on unmet human needs (i.e., human need deficits) and then to plan (i.e., set goals), implement, evaluate , and document outcomes of dental hygiene care (i.e., determining whether or not goals are met, partially met, or unmet).
- The Human Needs Conceptual Model provides a comprehensive and client-centered approach to the process of dental hygiene care.

CRITICAL THINKING EXERCISES

Given the following scenario, use the dental hygiene Human Needs Conceptual Model to list the human needs that are in deficit and to plan dental hygiene interventions to meet the identified human need deficits.

SCENARIO 2-1

Devan Sacks, age 12, is a new client in the dental practice and has been scheduled for dental hygiene care. Devan is in the seventh grade and is one of the star players on the girls' soccer team. She is accompanied by her mother, Margaret (age 32), and her sister, Bridget (age 10). After completing health, dental, and personal histories, the dental hygienist initiates the assessment phase of the dental hygiene process of care, including a baseline assessment of human needs related to dental hygiene care, a complete dental and periodontal assessment, and self-care and skill level assessment. Significant findings include 6-mm probing depths around teeth 19 and 30, and 4- to 5-mm pockets around teeth 22 to 27. Oral hygiene was generally poor. Client has a knowledge deficit regarding oral biofilm, periodontal disease process, and status of the oral cavity.

REFERENCES

1. American Dental Hygienists' Association: Dental hygiene: focus on advancing the profession, 2004-2005 (position paper). Available at: www.adha.org/downloads/ADHA_Focus_Report.pdf. Accessed September 26, 2008.
2. Maslow AH: *Motivation and personality*, ed 2, New York, 1970, Harper and Row.
3. Darby M, Walsh M: A human needs conceptual model for dental hygiene, Part I, *J Dent Hyg* 67:326, 1993.
4. Walsh M, Darby J: Application of the human needs conceptual model to the role of the clinician: Part II, *J Dent Hyg* 67:335, 1993.
5. Sato Y, Saito A, Nakamura-Miura A, et al: Application of the dental hygiene Human Needs Conceptual Model and the Oral Health–Related Quality of Life Model to the dental hygiene curriculum in Japan, *Int J Dent Hyg* 5:158, 2007.
6. Darby M, Walsh M: Application of the Human Needs Conceptual Model to dental hygiene practice, *J Dent Hyg* 74:230, 2000.
7. World Health Organization: Working for health: an introduction to the World Health Organization. Available at: www.who.int/about/brochure_en.pdf. Accessed February 4, 2008.
8. American Dental Hygienists' Association: Policy 18–96 Glossary, 1996.
9. American Dental Association Commission on Dental Accreditation: *Accreditation standards for dental hygiene education programs*, Chicago, 1998, American Dental Association. Available at: www.ada.org/prof/ed/accred/standards/dh.pdf. Accessed February 8, 2008.
10. American Dental Education Association: Exhibit 7: competencies for entry into the profession of dental hygiene. *J Dent Educ* 71(7):929, 2007. Available at: http://www.jdentaled.org/cgi/reprint/71/7/929.pdf. Accessed September 29, 2008.
11. Potter PA, Perry AG: *Fundamentals of nursing*, ed 7, St Louis, 2009, Mosby.

EVOLVE RESOURCES

Please visit http://evolve.elsevier.com/Darby/hygiene for additional practice and study support tools.

CHAPTER 3

Evidence-Based Decision Making

Jane L. Forrest, Syrene A. Miller

COMPETENCIES

1. **Explain evidence-based decision making and its importance in everyday practice.**
2. **Discuss the principles of EBDM.**
3. **Describe the steps and skills necessary to practice EBDM, including explain how EBDM can help you stay current in order to provide the most appropriate care for your clients.**

The desire to improve the oral health of clients must start with the hygienist's commitment to keeping current with important and useful scientific knowledge. The challenge, however, is finding relevant clinical evidence when needed to help make well-informed decisions and to answer client questions. Although dental hygienists may want to keep current, the increase in the number of published articles, new devices, products, and drugs has made it nearly impossible. However, as professionals, dental hygienists have an ethical responsibility to provide the most appropriate care to their clients. One approach to help clinicians bridge the gap between current research evidence and practice is through evidence-based decision making.[1]

For example, how would you respond to a client who watched a popular daytime talk show that discussed how an oral cancer screening is performed using different adjunctive devices and then questioned you about how thorough you were in performing an oral cancer screening because you did not use one of the devices? Would you know how to find the most current scientific information on this topic to determine if the evidence supports the procedure you performed, or what they learned on TV? Or, what about clients who refuse to have radiographs taken because of a report they saw on the evening news on a recent study associating dental x-rays with brain tumors (meningiomas)? Again, what would you say to them and would you know how to find the most current scientific information on this topic to be able to discuss it? Would you understand the level of evidence that was obtained in the study and how to present this to your clients?

The above two examples reinforce the importance of EBDM, which requires becoming a good consumer of the scientific literature so that clinicians understand what they are reading, the level of evidence it represents, and how much confidence can be put into the findings. In this regard, EBDM is client centered and supplements the traditional decision-making process by incorporating the most relevant scientific information.

What Is Evidence-Based Decision Making?

Evidence-based decision making (EBDM) is defined as "the integration of best research evidence with our clinical expertise and our patient's unique values and circumstances."[2] Thus optimal decisions are made when all components are considered (Figure 3-1). To practice EBDM, new online searching and evaluation skills are needed along with an understanding of research design. These skills and knowledge allow clinicians to access efficiently and appraise critically scientific articles to see if they are relevant to guiding their decision making or answering specific client questions. EBDM is not unique to medicine or any specific health discipline, which is why it is referred to here as EBDM rather than evidence-based dentistry or evidence-based dental hygiene.

Principles of Evidence-Based Decision Making

EBDM is about solving clinical problems, whether patient care issues, the client's clinical condition, or questions based on personal interest. In solving these problems, there are two fundamental principles of EBDM[3]:

1. Evidence alone is never sufficient to make a clinical decision: that is, clinical research is only one key component of the decision-making process and does not tell a practitioner what to do (see Figure 3-1).
2. Levels of evidence exist: a hierarchy of evidence is available to guide clinical decision making. As the term *hierarchy* implies, not all evidence is equal.
   - As you move up the hierarchy, the research designs allow more control so that intervention or treatment outcome differences are not due to chance.
   - As you move up the hierarchy, the number of published studies decreases, and yet these are more clinically relevant studies (Figure 3-2).[4]

Evidence Sources and Levels of Evidence

There are two categories of evidence sources: primary and secondary research. Understanding the distinction between these two helps with the search for evidence and critical analysis of it.

Primary research includes original research studies. These studies can be divided into two categories: experimental studies and nonexperimental, or observational, studies (see Figure 3-2).

1. In experimental research, the researcher is testing a hypothesis, most likely to establish cause and effect. To accomplish this goal:

- The researcher controls or manipulates the variables under investigation, such as in testing the effectiveness of a treatment.
- The researcher uses complex study designs that include randomized controlled trials and controlled clinical trials.

The **randomized controlled trial (RCT)** provides the strongest evidence for demonstrating cause and effect: that is, the treatment has caused the effect, rather than it happening by chance.

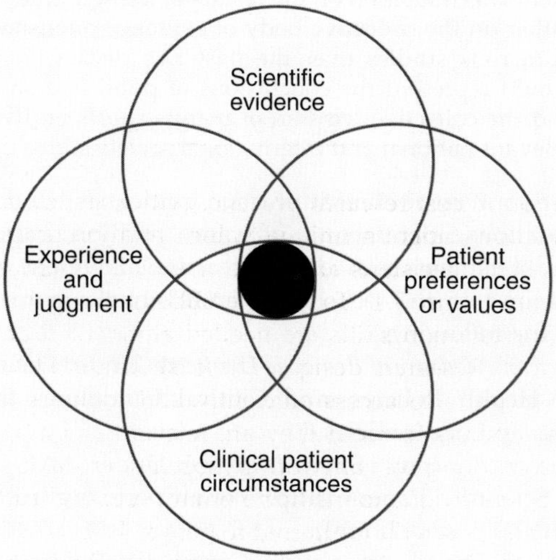

Figure 3-1. Evidence-based decision making. (Adapted from Forrest JL, Miller SA: Evidence-based decision making in dental hygiene education, practice, and research, *J Dent Hyg* 75:50, 2001.)

2. **Nonexperimental, or observational, research** includes studies in which the researcher *does not give a treatment, intervention, or provide an exposure*; that is, data are gathered without intervening to control variables.
   - This type of research includes cohort studies and case control studies.
   - **Cohort studies** and **case control studies** are used to describe and interpret conditions or relationships that already exist.
   - These studies are used when the possibility exists that testing a treatment or intervention has the potential to cause harm. For example, in a cohort study the investigator could not give tobacco to subjects to test if tobacco causes cancer but rather would recruit subjects who already are exposed to the risk (tobacco) and then follow them to see who develops cancer.
   - **Secondary research** sources include preappraised, or filtered research, that is research on already conducted individual studies. This category includes the following:
     - Evidence-based clinical practice guidelines
     - Meta-analyses (MAs)
     - Systematic reviews (SRs)
     - Evidence-based article reviews

In Figure 3-2, the hierarchy of evidence is shown. Sources regarded as providing level 1 evidence, the highest level of evidence, are within the category of secondary research. Also considered level 1 evidence is an individual RCT. This highest level of evidence is followed respectively by cohort studies (level 2), and case-control studies (level 3). Case reports, narrative reviews, and editorials (levels 4 and 5 evidence) do not involve a research design. Although animal and laboratory

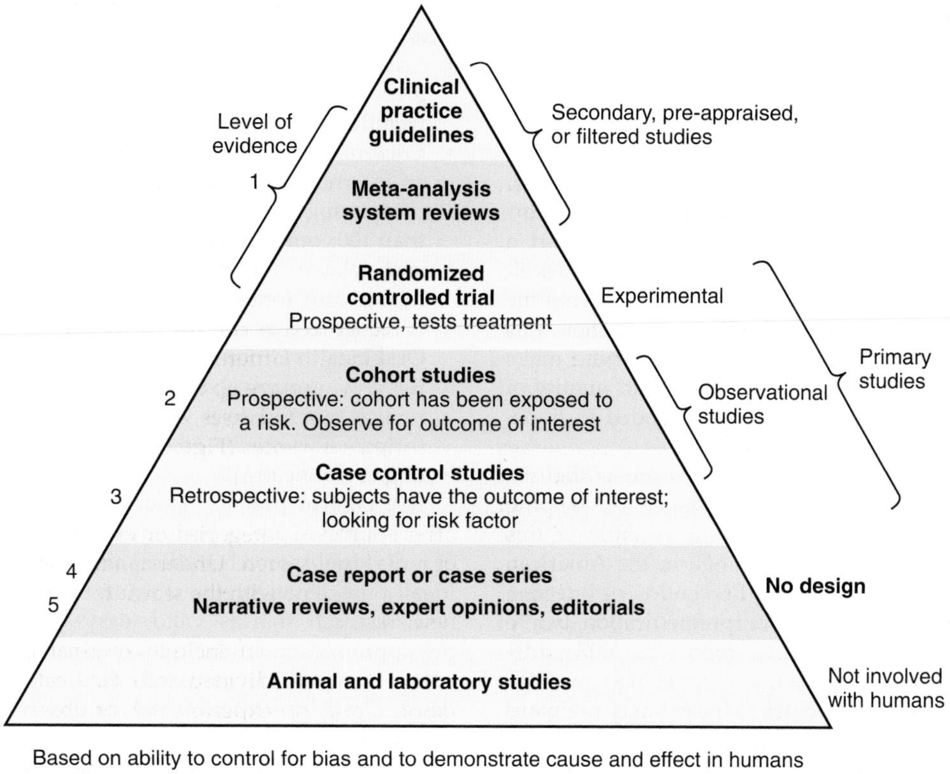

Figure 3-2. Hierarchy of research designs and levels of scientific evidence. (© 2012, JL Forrest, NCDHRP [National Center for Dental Hygiene Research & Practice].)

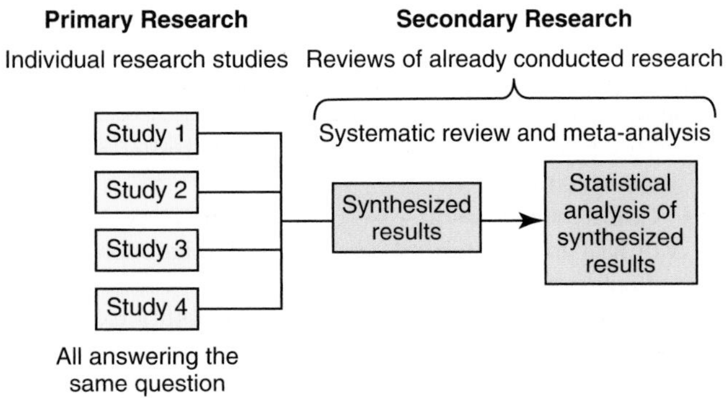

Figure 3-3. Primary vs. secondary research. (© 2008, JL Forrest & SA Miller, NCDHRP [National Center for Dental Hygiene Research & Practice].)

research studies are extremely important, they are at the bottom of the hierarchy because they do not involve human subjects, and evidence-based practice is all about how it works in people. An excellent short, graphic review of each of these research methods and designs can be found at the SUNY Downstate Medical Center, Evidence Based Medicine Course, "Guide to Research Methods—The Evidence Pyramid,"[5] which can be accessed at http://library.downstate.edu/EBM2/2100.htm.

Figure 3-3 illustrates the relationship between primary research, which includes individual studies (RCTs, cohort, and case-control studies), and secondary research, which is the synthesis of the findings from individual research studies that answer the same question (e.g., treatment, products, procedures, techniques, materials). A **systematic review (SR)** is the synthesis of the findings from individual studies on the same topic. When data from the individual studies that make up the SR can be combined, and an analysis conducted of this pooled data is known as a **meta-analysis**. The benefits of pooling the data are that the sample size and power usually increase and the combined effect can increase the precision of estimates of treatment effects and exposure risks.[6]

At the top of the hierarchy are **clinical practice guidelines**. A clinical practice guideline is secondary evidence that incorporates the best available scientific evidence to support a clinical practice. SRs and MAs support the process of developing clinical practice guidelines by putting together all the evidence known about a topic in an objective manner. This evidence then is analyzed by a panel of experts who make specific recommendations based on the level and quality of evidence. Clinical practice guidelines are intended to translate the research into practical applications.

Clinical practice guidelines change over time as the evidence evolves, underscoring the importance of keeping current with the scientific literature. One example of this evolving nature of evidence is the change in the American Heart Association Guidelines for the Prevention of Infective Endocarditis related to the need for premedication before dental and dental hygiene procedures.[7] Before the 2007 guidelines, the most recent premedication update was in 1997. Before 1997 there were eight updates to the primary regimens for dental procedures since the original guideline was first published in 1955. In the 2007 update, the rationale for revising the 1997 document was provided. Excerpts from their rationale include the following: (notice the references to types of studies, use of evidence, and experts in updating the guidelines)

> The rationale for prophylaxis was based largely on expert opinion and what seemed to be a rational and prudent attempt to prevent a life-threatening infection … Accordingly, the basis for recommendations for Infective Endocarditis (IE) prophylaxis was not well established, and the quality of evidence was limited to a few case-control studies or was based on expert opinion, clinical experience, and descriptive studies that utilized surrogate measures of risk … The present revised document was not based on the results of a single study but rather on the collective body of evidence published in numerous studies over the past two decades … and would represent the conclusions of published studies and the collective wisdom of many experts on IE and relevant national and international societies.[8]

Other sources of clinical practice guidelines, clinical recommendations, parameters of care, position papers, or academy statements related to clinical dental hygiene practice can be found on the websites of professional organizations, such as the following:

- *American Academy of Pediatric Dentistry:* Under Definitions, Oral Health Policies, and Clinical Guidelines (http://www.aapd.org/policies/)
- *American Academy of Periodontology:* Under AAP Clinical and Scientific Papers (http://www.perio.org/resources-products/posppr2.html)
- *American Dental Association:* Center for Evidence-based Dentistry website (http://ebd.ada.org) provides links to systematic reviews and critical summaries; clinical recommendations on fluorides, sealants, oral cancer screening along with chairside guides on many of these topics; and links to a variety of external resources, including PubMed and Cochrane
- *Centers for Disease Control and Prevention:* Under Guidelines and Recommendations (http://www.cdc.gov/OralHealth/guidelines.htm)
- ***Cochrane Collaboration:*** The Cochrane Collaboration is an international, independent, not-for-profit organization comprising more than 28,000 contributors from more than 100 countries dedicated to producing SRs as a reliable and relevant source of evidence about the effects of health care for making informed decisions. Their work is recognized as the gold standard for SRs. The Cochrane Oral Health Group is but one of 52 groups. All Cochrane Review groups have an obligation to update the review every 2 to 4 years to account for new evidence (http://www.cochrane.org [Oral Health Group, http://ohg.cochrane.org]).

If a clinical practice guideline does not exist, there are other sources of pre-appraised evidence (SRs, MAs, or reviews of individual research studies) available to help stay current. Ideally, the dental hygienist wants to be able to access quickly new research that is valid, easy to read, and has been pre-appraised, as in the two evidence-based dentistry journals. These evidence-based dentistry journals, *Evidence Based Dentistry* (http://www.nature.com/ebd/index.html) and the *Journal of Evidence-Based Dental Practice* (http://www.jebdp.com), specifically publish 1- to 2-page summaries of the SR or original research article with expert commentary including the clinical application. In addition, the

International Journal of Dental Hygiene and many of the general dentistry and specialty journals are publishing SRs and MAs that support the care provided in clinical dental hygiene practice.

EBDM Process and Skills: A Practical Application

The growth of "evidence-based" practice has been made possible through two factors. The first is the development of online scientific databases, such as **PubMed** (MEDLINE) and the Cochrane Library. The second factor is having access to computers and/or handheld devices that provide Internet access. This combination allows quick location of relevant clinical evidence so that there is no excuse for not doing so.

EBDM requires developing new skills. These **EBDM skills** consist of the abilities to find, critically appraise, and correctly apply current evidence from relevant research to clinical decisions made in practice so that the evidence known is reflected in the care provided. Translating these skills into action include the five steps outlined in Box 3-1.

These EBDM skills provide a structured process and, just as in learning technical clinical skills, these too require practice. Staying current is a not an option: it is a requirement for all professionals because the body of evidence is constantly evolving over time as individual research studies are conducted. What is learned in school during the first year may not be current by the time of graduation. Only by devoting time to this neverending process of updating current knowledge and skills will the dental hygienist be prepared to give clients the best evidence-based care.

How Is EBDM Used in Everyday Practice?

The following Clinical Scenario 3-1 is provided to illustrate the five steps and skills necessary to practice EBDM.

SCENARIO 3-1

Mrs. Sanchez is a 58-year-old woman who is concerned about her receding gums and whether she will begin to get cavities on the root surfaces. She knows her children have received fluoride treatments to prevent cavities on their teeth and asks you if she should be getting professionally applied fluoride treatments and what she should be doing at home.

Having recently read an article on the role of chlorhexidine varnish (CHx-V) for the prevention of adult caries you want to reread it and doublecheck to see if a fluoride regimen would be more effective, and if so, which fluoride(s). Because Mrs. Sanchez has a second appointment with you next week, you tell her you would like to look up the most current scientific information and discuss the findings with her at that appointment.

Step 1. Asking Good Questions: The PICO Process

Asking a good clinical question is a difficult skill to learn, but it is fundamental to EBDM. To help meet this challenge, the PICO process has been formulated.[2] The PICO process almost always begins with a client question or problem.

A "well-built" **PICO question** includes four parts beginning with the client problem or population (P); the intervention (I); the comparison (C), a second intervention and often the standard; and the outcome(s) (O). Once these four components are identified clearly, the following format is used to structure the following question:

> "For a client with _____ (P), will _____ (I) as compared to _____ (C) increase/decrease/provide better/be more effective in doing ___ (O)?"

The formality of using PICO to frame the question facilitates the computerized search by identifying key terms to use. Based on Mrs. Sanchez's clinical case, the PICO question would be,

> "For a client with gingival recession," will fluoride varnish (I) as compared to chlorhexidine varnish (C) be more effective in preventing root caries (O)?*

BOX 3-1

Skills Needed to Apply the EBDM Process[2]

- Convert information needs/problems into clinical questions so that they can be answered.
- Conduct a computerized search with maximum efficiency for finding the best external evidence with which to answer the question.
- Critically appraise the evidence for its validity and usefulness (clinical applicability).
- Apply the results of the appraisal, or evidence, in clinical practice.
- Evaluate the process and your performance.

Step 2. Conduct an Efficient Computerized Search

The second step in using EBDM is to conduct a computerized search to find the best external evidence for answering the question. Finding relevant evidence requires conducting a focused search of the peer-reviewed professional literature based on the appropriate research methodology.

PubMed is used to demonstrate finding the evidence because it provides free access to MEDLINE, the largest scientific database (PubMed, http://www.ncbi.nlm.nih.gov/pubmed/; Figure 3-4). Also, starting with PubMed may save time because many references found on other databases, including the ADA's Center for Evidence-Based Dentistry, directly link to PubMed.

Although it takes time to develop searching skills, the **PubMed Clinical Queries** feature can be used immediately (Figure 3-5). It provides specialized searches using evidence-based filters to retrieve articles. The built-in algorithms streamline the process of searching for clinically relevant articles, making it one of the most valuable features for busy professionals and students. Being able to search electronically

*For an in-depth review on EBDM and PICO, complete the course *Evidence-Based Decision Making: Introduction and Formulating Good Clinical Questions* on Dentalcare.com, under the Course Listings Topic of Electives, http://www.dentalcare.com/en-US/home.aspx.

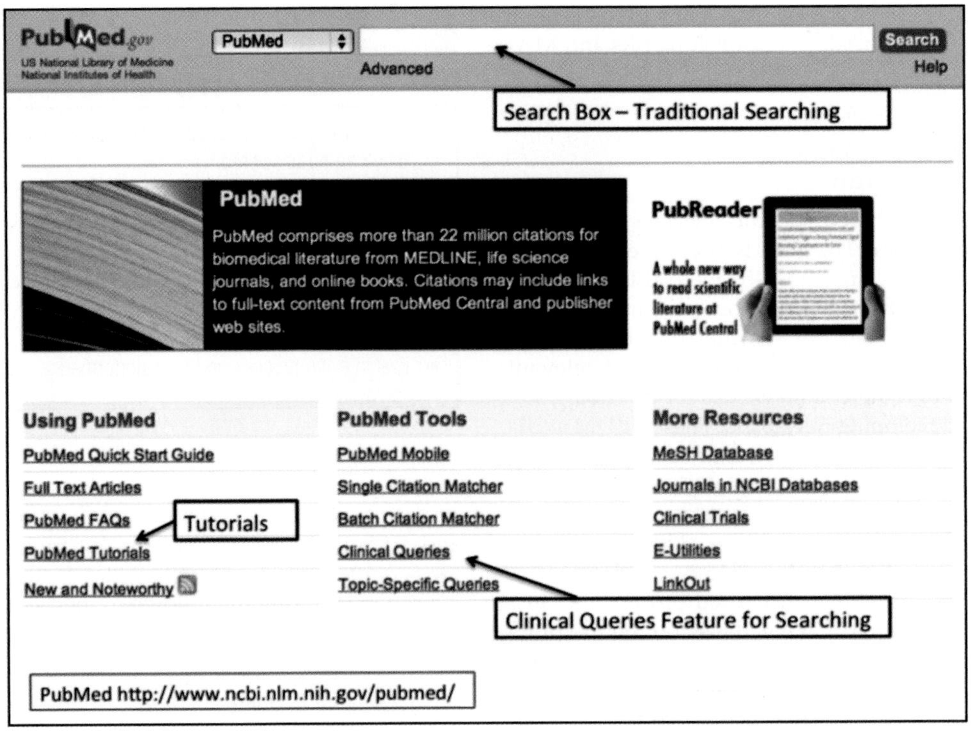

Figure 3-4. PubMed Homepage. Links to Clinical Queries and Other Key Features.

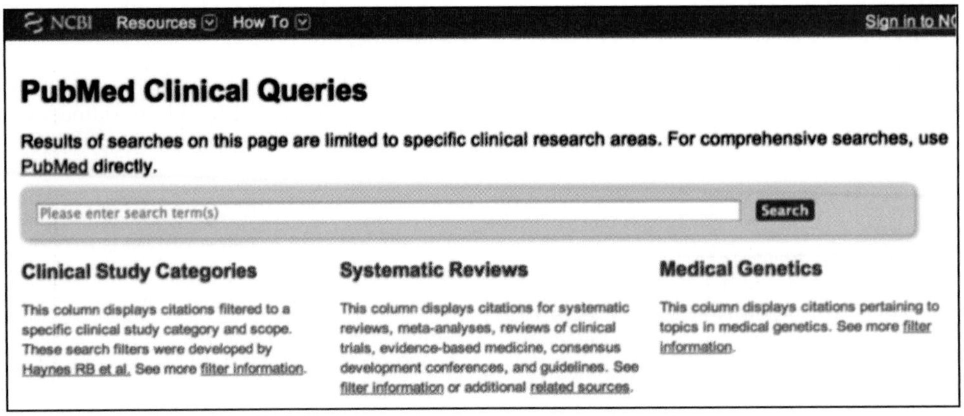

Figure 3-5. PubMed clinical queries.

across hundreds of journals at the same time for specific answers to client questions also overcomes the challenges of knowing which journals to subscribe to and to finding relevant clinical evidence when it is needed to help make well-informed decisions.

A link to the Clinical Queries feature is found on the PubMed homepage under PubMed Tools. The traditional search box and PubMed tutorials also are highlighted in Figure 3-4.

Of the three options on the Clinical Queries page, the primary focus is on using the first two options, the Clinical Study Categories and Systematic Reviews. Because the goal is to find quickly the highest level of evidence, the clinician should begin with reviewing the citations retrieved under Systematic Reviews. This option also finds citations for meta-analyses, reviews of clinical trials, evidence-based medicine, consensus development conferences, and guidelines. If there are none, or none that answer the question, the next option is to review the individual studies found under the Clinical Study Categories.

For the clinical scenario, the *Intervention* (fluoride varnish) and *Comparison* (chlorhexidine varnish) components of PICO are the primary search terms to use first. These are typed into the search box on the Clinical Queries page (Figure 3-6). Ideally, these two components retrieve SRs that compare the two and quickly assist in answering the question in one step.

In this case, six citations under Systematic Reviews and 70 individual studies were returned. In scanning through the abstracts, the most recent SRs and individual studies focus on the caries-preventive effectiveness of chlorhexidine (CHx) rather than comparing the two treatments.[9-11] However, reading the abstracts demonstrates that the evidence on using

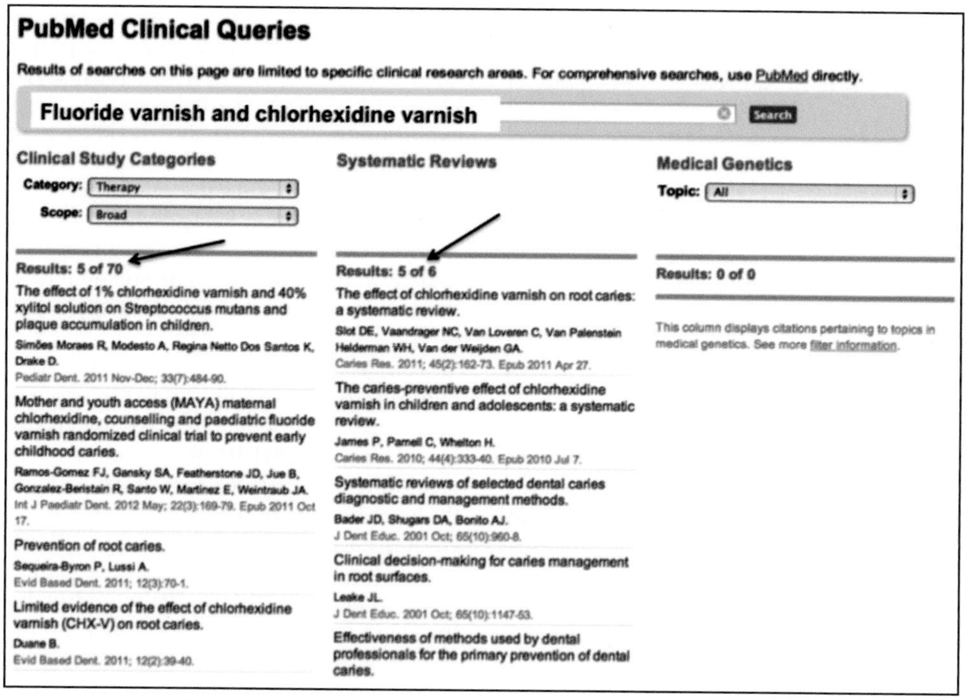

Figure 3-6. Fluoride varnish and chlorhexidine varnish search results.

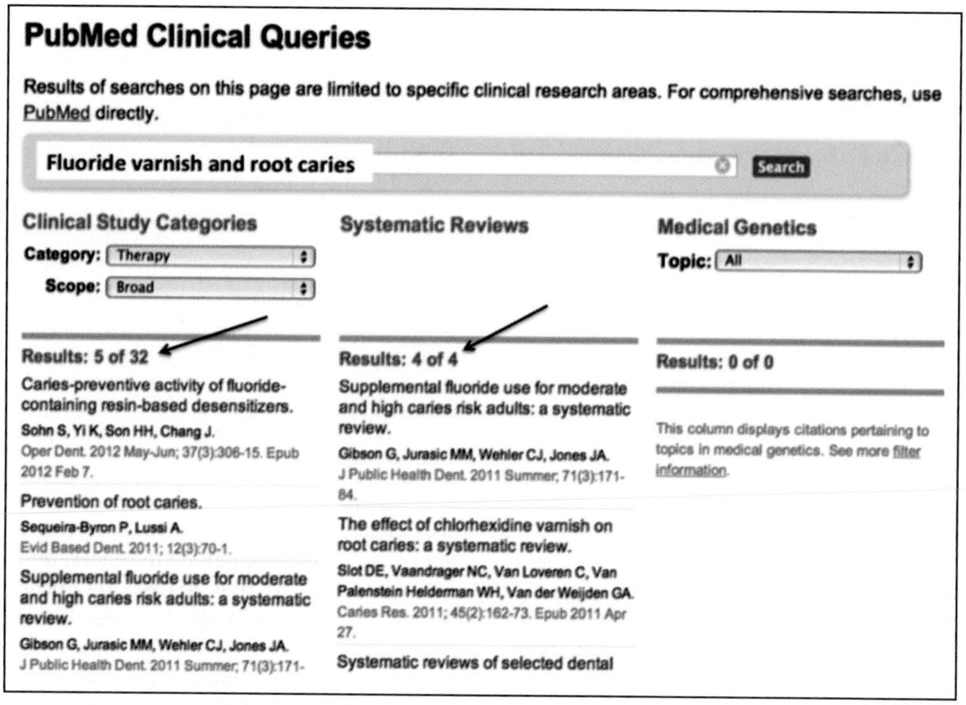

Figure 3-7. Fluoride varnish and root caries search results.

CHx varies from being weak at best[8] to inconclusive[9] or not recommending CHx at all.[11]

Subsequently, a second search is run for fluoride varnish and root caries (Figure 3-7). This search retrieves 4 SRs and 32 individual studies. Conclusions of the SR, *Supplemental fluoride use for moderate and high caries risk adults: a systematic review*,[12] found that 1.1% NaF pastes/gels and 5% NaF varnishes were moderately effective in higher-risk adults.

Because Mrs. Sanchez was interested in what she could do at home on a regular basis, the 32 individual studies also were scanned, and two promising studies were identified quickly. The first was a randomized trial comparing three different fluoride treatments to arrest initial root carious lesions (a chemo-mechanical technique and a 2.23% fluoride varnish, the 2.23% fluoride varnish alone, and a stannous fluoride solution [8%]).[13] The investigators concluded that the

BOX 3-2

Key Tips for Learning How to Search Using PubMed

- Keep the search simple.
- Limit the search terms to the key terms identified in the PICO question.
- Begin your search using the PubMed Clinical Queries feature.
- Complete the PubMed Tutorial to learn how to take full advantage of PubMed.
- Complete the courses on Dentalcare.com that are tailored to EBDM and Searching PubMed.

frequent topical application of fluoride could be a successful treatment for incipient root carious lesions, irrespective of the type of fluoride treatment used. In the second study, investigators hypothesized and found that a combination of professional applied acidulated phosphate fluoride (APF), and use of 1100-ppm-fluoride dentifrice would provide additional protection for dentin compared with 1100-ppm-fluoride dentifrice alone.[14]

Without knowing about the Clinical Queries feature or combining the Intervention and Comparison, the most common way of beginning a search is to type in the main search term in the search box on the homepage (see Figure 3-4). Typing in "fluoride varnish" garnered 705 citations. Someone not familiar with the PubMed filters feature or levels of evidence would spend considerable time reviewing the 705 titles and abstracts to determine which ones may be useful or become discouraged after reviewing the first 10 or 20 and stop.*

Key tips to keep in mind when beginning to learn how to search using PubMed are outlined in Box 3-2.

Step 3. Critically Appraise the Evidence for Its Validity and Usefulness (Clinical Applicability)

Once the most current evidence is located, the next step in the EBDM process is to understand it and its relevance to the client's problem and answering the PICO question. Three key questions guide the critical analysis process[2,15,16]:

1. Are the results of the study valid?
2. What are the results?
3. Will the results help in caring for my client?

The first question focuses the analysis on the research design, methods, and manner in which the study was conducted. This focus on results reinforces the importance of understanding research design and the corresponding level of evidence it provides. Little confidence can be placed in the results if the study was not conducted appropriately. Therefore answering the first question can help determine whether to continue reading that particular article. Fortunately, to assist with this process several evidence-based groups provide critical appraisal checklists of questions that can be downloaded to use.[15,16] These tools consist of a structured series of questions that help determine the study validity by exploring the strengths and weaknesses of how a study was conducted, or of how information was collected, and how useful and applicable the evidence is to the specific client problem or question being asked.

Once determined that the results are valid, the next step is to determine if the results or potential benefits (or harms) are important, and then whether to apply the evidence to client care.

The researchers' conclusions are specifically helpful as they discuss the implications for practice and research. As previously mentioned, the results related to CHx-V were inconclusive, either having weak or insufficient evidence to recommend CHx-V for root caries prevention. Had the same findings been true of fluoride varnish, or if all the fluoride studies had been conducted with children and adolescents, then the results would have to be extrapolated by the provider to decide if the results would be helpful in caring for the client. This situation would refer to the first fundamental principle of EBDM: the evidence alone is never sufficient to make a clinical decision, and the practitioner determines whether the level and quality of the evidence is useful and how much confidence can be placed on the findings. This principle helps practitioners decide which, if any, of the scientific evidence to incorporate with their experience and judgment, along with the clinical circumstances and client preferences or values.

Statistical vs. Clinical Significance

Another consideration in appraising the evidence is understanding the difference between statistical significance and clinical significance. **Statistical significance** refers to the likelihood that the results were unlikely to have occurred by chance at a specified probability level and that the differences would still exist each time the experiment was repeated. Therefore statistical significance is reported as the probability related to chance, or "p" level. Levels of statistical significance are set at thresholds at the point where the null hypothesis (the statement of no difference between groups) will be rejected, such as at $p < 0.05$, which means that the probability is less than 5 in 100 that the difference occurred by chance.

Clinical significance is used to distinguish the importance and meaning of the results reported in a study and is not based on a comparison of numbers, as is statistical significance. A study can have statistical significance without being clinically significant and vice versa. Statistical significance does not determine the practical or clinical implications of the data. For example, small differences may be statistically significant, a difference of 0.05 to 1.0 mm in levels of attachment; however, this difference may not be clinically significant because this small a difference could be due to measurement error and/or chance. On the other hand, analysis of the results of a study may find no statistically significant difference between two treatments, which may mean that a new treatment was as effective (no better or no worse) as the gold standard treatment. This finding could be clinically significant, especially if the new treatment is easier to apply/less technique sensitive, takes less time/fewer visits, and/or is less costly.

*For a comprehensive step-by-step guide on how to conduct a search using both Clinical Queries and the Traditional/Comprehensive PubMed mechanism, complete the course, *Strategies for Searching the Literature Using PubMed*, on Dentalcare.com, under the Course Listings Topic of Electives, http://www.dentalcare.com/en-US/home.aspx.

Step 4. Apply the Results of the Appraisal, or Evidence, in Clinical Practice

After completing the review of the evidence, the next step is to discuss findings with Mrs. Sanchez. For example, it appears that the results of the SR and individual studies demonstrate statistical and clinical significance for providing a fluoride treatment using either 1.1% NaF paste or gel, or a 5% NaF varnish,[13] or acidulated phosphate fluoride (APF) during her visit, and then having her follow up at home with use of a 1100-ppm fluoride dentifrice.[13] Other factors to consider are the frequency of professional applications, because the effectiveness of the fluoride treatments may have to be based on the same intervals used in the research studies as well as which of the investigated treatment regimens/types of professional fluoride treatment products are used in the office. Cost also may be a consideration because the 1100-ppm fluoride dentifrice is a prescription item.

Because the original case scenario focused on the comparison of CHx-V and Fluoride varnish, a second PICO question to investigate would be as follows:

> For a client with gingival recession and receiving a professional fluoride treatment, will an OTC ADA accepted fluoride dentifrice and mouthrinse (I) as compared with an OTC ADA accepted fluoride dentifrice alone (C) be as effective as a homecare regimen in preventing root caries (O)?

Step 5. Evaluate the Process and Your Performance

The final step in EBDM is evaluation of the effectiveness of the process. This step includes evaluating two aspects: the outcomes of the care provided and the application of the EBDM skills. Mastering the skills of EBDM takes time, practice, and reflection, and a clinician who is new to the steps should not be discouraged by early difficulties. Self-evaluation of developing skills is a most critical aspect in mastery of EBDM. Following the five skills/steps in the EBDM process, questions that can be used to evaluate performance are outlined in Box 3-3.

The path for development of expertise in any skill involves learning the basic steps followed by practice in applying the skills; however, practice without reflection on how to improve is trial-and-error learning rather than following a systematic process. Reflective practitioners are continually self-assessing results of their actions to enhance their abilities and development of expertise. This self-assessment also is the case with development of skills in EBDM. The practitioner who makes time to apply *and* evaluate the results of EBDM develops expertise and quickly and conveniently stays current with scientific findings on topics that are important to practice.

BOX 3-3

Questions for Evaluating the Evidence-Based Decision-Making Process

- Were my questions focused and answerable?
- Did I use the PICO components to find high levels of evidence quickly and efficiently?
- Did I appraise the evidence effectively?
- Was I able to integrate the appraisal with my own expertise and the unique features of the situation to present the findings in an unbiased and understandable manner to my client?
- Did I evaluate the outcome of care provided to my client?
- Did I make improvements based on feedback and past experiences?

Conclusion

EBDM provides a strategy for improving the efficiency of integrating new evidence into client care decisions. Being able to search electronically across hundreds of journals at the same time for specific answers to client questions overcomes the challenge of finding relevant clinical evidence when it is needed to help make well-informed decisions. As EBDM becomes standard practice, dental hygienists must be knowledgeable of what constitutes the evidence and how it is reported. Understanding research designs and levels of evidence allows the clinician to judge better the validity and relevance of reported findings. By integrating good science with clinical judgment and patient preferences, clinicians enhance their decision-making ability and maximize the potential for successful client care outcomes.

CLIENT EDUCATION TIPS

- Evidence-based decision making allows the clinician to discuss the rationale for new therapies and new approaches based on the evolving science so that clients can participate in making informed decisions.
- Evidence-based decision making allows the clinician to discuss the rationale for changing or eliminating previous procedures that now, through sound research, have been found not to be effective.

LEGAL, ETHICAL, AND SAFETY ISSUES

- Dental hygienists have an ethical responsibility to keep current to provide the most appropriate, evidence-based care for their clients.
- Treatment planning options and the care/interventions provided must be documented in the client's record.

KEY CONCEPTS

- The desire to improve the oral health of clients must start with the hygienist's commitment to keeping current with important and useful scientific knowledge. Although the increase in the number of published articles, new devices, products, and drugs has made it nearly impossible to keep up to date, dental hygienists have an ethical responsibility to provide the most appropriate care to their clients.
- EBDM skills and knowledge allow clinicians to access efficiently and appraise critically scientific articles to see if they are relevant to guiding their decision making or answering specific client questions.
- Evidence alone is never sufficient to make a clinical decision: that is, clinical research is only one key component of the decision making process and does not tell a practitioner what to do.
- A hierarchy of evidence exists to guide clinical decision making, and as a hierarchy implies, not all evidence is equal.

- There are two categories of evidence sources: primary and secondary research. Understanding the distinction between these two helps in searching for evidence and critically analyzing it.
- Evidence changes over time as more and more research is conducted, underscoring the importance of keeping current with the scientific literature.
- Multiple sources provide clinical practice guidelines, clinical recommendations, parameters of care, position papers or academy statements that support clinical dental hygiene practice.
- EBDM requires developing new skills, such as the abilities to find, critically appraise, and correctly apply current evidence from relevant research to decisions made in practice so that what is known is reflected in the care provided.
- Being able to search electronically across hundreds of journals at the same time for specific answers to client questions overcomes the challenges of knowing which journals to subscribe to and to finding relevant clinical evidence when it is needed to help make well-informed decisions. The PubMed Clinical Queries feature provides a starting place for finding relevant evidence since it uses evidence-based filters to retrieve articles.

CRITICAL THINKING EXERCISES

Kevin is a 27-year-old bartender who has used chewing tobacco for 13 years. He is a frequent user who chews almost 5 hours a day. He has just learned from his oral healthcare provider that he has developed precancerous lesions in the vestibular area where he holds the tobacco plug. This new information has motivated him to quit.

Kevin knows he cannot quit by willpower alone because he has tried in the past. He wants to know if Zyban, a non-nicotine aid, or if the nicotine patch is more effective in helping chewing tobacco users permanently quit.

1. Identify the PICO components and write out the PICO question.
2. Once you have the PICO question, conduct a PubMed search.
3. After finding citations, critically analyze them to determine which are helpful in answering your question.
4. Discuss how you would incorporate the evidence into your clinical decision making, including how you would discuss your findings with Kevin.
5. Evaluate your strengths and weaknesses in using the EBDM process.
6. Explain why evidence alone is never sufficient to make a clinical decision.
7. Explain why an RCT is not always the appropriate research design to use.
8. Discuss how EBDM influences dental hygiene practice today.
9. Once you have completed the EBDM process, discuss how you can use these skills to provide better care for your patients.

REFERENCES

1. Committee on Quality of Health Care in America, IOM. Crossing the Quality Chasm: *A New Health System for the 21st Century*, Washington, DC, 2000, The National Academy of Sciences.
2. Straus SE, Glasziou P, Richardson WS, et al: *Evidence-based medicine: how to practice and teach it*, ed 4, London, England, 2011, Churchill Livingstone Elsevier.
3. Evidence-Based Medicine Working Group: *Users' Guides to the Medical Literature, A Manual for EB Clinical Practice*, ed 2, Chicago, 2008, AMA.
4. McKibbon A, Eady A, Marks S: *PDQ, evidence-based principles and practice*, Hamilton, Ontario, 1999, B.C. Decker.
5. SUNY Downstate Medical Center, Evidence Based Medicine Course, Guide to Research Methods – The Evidence Pyramid. Available at: http://library.downstate.edu/EBM2/2100.htm. Accessed December 16, 2012.
6. Mulrow C: Rationale for systematic reviews. In Chalmers I, Altman DG, editors: *Systematic reviews*, London, England, 1995, BMJ Publishing Group, p 1.
7. Wilson W, Taubert KA, Gewitz M, et al: Prevention of infective endocarditis, guidelines from the American Heart Association: a guideline from the American Heart Association Rheumatic Fever, Endocarditis, and Kawasaki Disease Committee, Council on Cardiovascular Disease in the Young, and the Council on Clinical Cardiology, Council on Cardiovascular Surgery and Anesthesia, and the Quality of Care and Outcomes Research Interdisciplinary Working Group. *Circulation*, 1736-1754, 2007. Available at: http://circ.ahajournals.org/content/116/15/1736.full.pdf+html?sid=ada268bd-1f10-4496-bae4-b91806aaf341. Accessed December 16, 2012.
8. Wilson W, Taubert KA, Gewitz M, et al: Prevention of infective endocarditis. *Circulation* 116:1736, 2007.
9. Slot DE, Vaandrager NC, Van Loveren C, et al: The effect of chlorhexidine varnish on root caries: a systematic review. *Caries Res* 45(2):162, 2011.
10. James P, Parnell C, Whelton H: The caries-preventive effect of chlorhexidine varnish in children and adolescents: a systematic review. *Caries Res* 44(4):333, 2010.
11. Autio-Gold J: The role of chlorhexidine in caries prevention. *Oper Dent* 33(6):710, 2008.
12. Gibson G, Jurasic MM, Wehler CH, et al: Supplemental fluoride use for moderate and high caries risk adults: a systematic review. *J Public Health Dent* 71(3):171, 2011.
13. Fure S, Lingstrom P: Evaluation of different fluoride treatments of initial root carious lesions in vivo. *Oral Health Prev Dent* 7(2):147, 2009.
14. Vale GC, Tabchoury CP, Del Bel Cury AA, et al: APF and dentifrice effect on root dentin demineralization and biofilm. *J Dent Res* 90(1):77, 2011.
15. Centre for Evidence-Based Medicine, Critical Appraisal Tools. Available at: http://www.cebm.net/index.aspx?o=1157. Accessed December 16, 2012.
16. Critical Appraisal Skills Programme, Making sense of the evidence. CASP Critical Appraisal Checklists. Available at: http://www.casp-uk.net. Accessed December 16, 2012.

EVOLVE RESOURCES

Please visit http://evolve.elsevier.com/Darby/hygiene for additional practice and study support tools.

CHAPTER 4

Health and Health Promotion

Laura Lee MacDonald

COMPETENCIES

1. Explain the health continuum and dental hygiene care, including:
   - Explain how oral health can be viewed as an investment.
   - Describe a dental hygiene intervention for the three levels of prevention—primary, secondary, and tertiary.
   - Differentiate among disease treatment, disease prevention, and health promotion.
2. Describe health-promotion strategies the dental hygienist might employ to facilitate client oral health: oral health marketing, health education, collaboration, use of mass media, community organization, advocacy, and legislation.

The Health Continuum and Dental Hygiene Care

The dental hygienist is an oral health professional who, as a member of the healthcare team, facilitates meeting clients' human needs through oral disease treatment, oral disease prevention, and oral health promotion. In providing care in all three areas, the dental hygienist facilitates client health through a continuum of care (Figure 4-1). If the entry point of care is disease treatment, then the dental hygienist and other healthcare professionals treat the disease and help the client move along the continuum toward prevention of disease recurrence and promotion of health and wellness. Provision of care or professional intervention may take place in many settings, such as primary healthcare clinics, private dental and/or dental hygiene clinics, and residential facilities and hospitals. No matter the setting, the philosophic approach to health and health promotion is one of enabling persons or communities to be healthy, have access to healthcare, and experience quality of life. Effective dental hygiene care requires the dental hygienist to think critically of the client as a holistic being and to listen and respond to clients regarding how they relate their oral health with overall health and wellness. When the dental hygienist does so, the client and the dental hygienist develop an understanding of the factors and determinants of client health. Consider the following scenarios.

In Scenarios 4-1 and 4-2, the dental hygienists are thinking about their clients' oral health in relation to the clients' overall state of being. They are considering how the interrelationship of many variables (e.g., life events, diagnosed disease, healthcare, and personal lifestyle) results in the achievement of the

SCENARIO 4-1

George Fountaine is 30 years old. During the health history interview he informs Phyllis, the dental hygienist, that he is a self-employed graphic designer with regular clients. George leads an active lifestyle. He has just been diagnosed with multiple sclerosis, which he states explains many of his problems. George is beginning to work with an occupational therapist, who is helping him adapt his lifestyle to accommodate the disability that will accompany the disease and its progression. Phyllis acknowledges George's optimistic frame of reference and suggests he consider shortening the time between his periodontal maintenance appointments. This will allow her to assess the state of his periodontal health at intervals that will better able him to maintain his oral health. George has a good perspective on how he plans to manage his condition, and he feels this fits perfectly with his intentions to continue to live his life to the fullest by engaging in behaviors conducive to health.

SCENARIO 4-2

Sherry Gilmore is 28 years old. She and her husband have two sons, both of whom are doing very well in school and in their extracurricular activities. The family moved to the town of Riverview 14 months ago. Because of the move, Sherry had to resign from counseling young mothers at her previous town's community health clinic. Riverview Health Clinic is not able to hire another counselor, so Sherry is unemployed currently. During the dental hygiene assessment she tells Jennifer, the dental hygienist, that although she has been busy with the family, it has been more than a year since she worked as a counselor and she feels distraught about it. Sherry is recognizing she is short-tempered, tired, and disinterested in activities she formerly found fun. Jennifer asks Sherry if she has a good support network, to which Sherry replies, "Not really. I just have been busy getting the family settled and haven't been thinking about making friends." Jennifer knows that having a social support network is important to health, so she suggests that Sherry may want to visit the local community center, because there are a lot of programs being offered at a reasonable price for people to meet and share in similar interests. Jennifer also wonders if Sherry may benefit from speaking to a counselor; she asks Sherry if she wants to connect with one. Sherry is grateful for Jennifer's attentive listening and tells her so as they continue with the dental hygiene assessment.

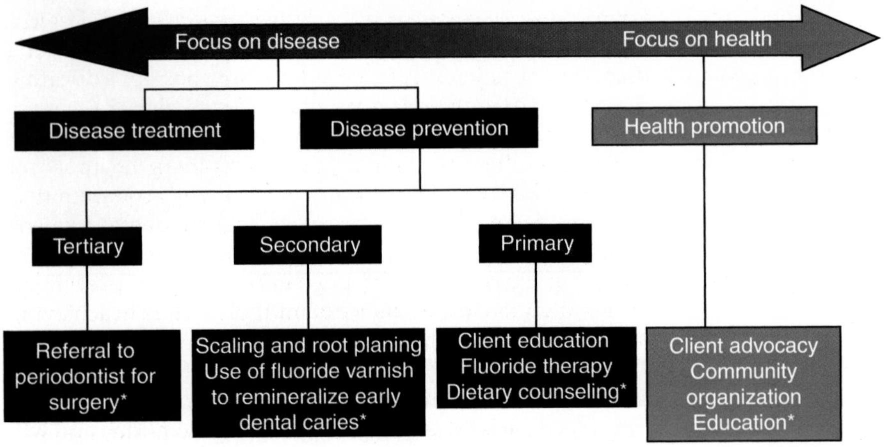

Figure 4-1. Continuum of dental hygiene care: disease treatment, disease prevention, and health promotion.

state of health. The dental hygienists, Phyllis and Jennifer, are thinking of oral health and health in an inclusive manner. What constitutes being healthy? How does a client achieve health and maintain it? Exploring these questions helps dental hygienists to conceptualize their role in healthcare and their view of the health of their clients.

In Scenario 4-1 George shares with the dental hygienist his disease and condition, and yet he expresses his intent to cope with it, knowing it will change his present lifestyle. He has no intention of letting the disease rob him of living his life. Sherry, in Scenario 4-2, also is experiencing a life-altering event. The dental hygienist hears her story and understands that Sherry's oral health may be in jeopardy. Sherry appears to not be coping well with the changes in her life, and this could affect her health. The dental hygiene care plan for Sherry and George will take into consideration the client's respective needs. George's dental hygienist offers to help him maintain his oral health despite a diagnosis of multiple sclerosis, which may hinder him from performing effective self-care; she will likely consider modification in daily oral hygiene practices in addition to suggesting an increase in the frequency of his dental hygiene appointments. Similarly, the dental hygienist will assess Sherry's oral health and work with Sherry to develop a plan according to Sherry's oral health need; but the dental hygienist with a health promotion perspective will respond to Sherry's comments about being short-tempered and tired, and no longer finding fun where she would have before. The dental hygienist embraces a full continuum of care from promoting oral health, preventing oral disease, and, if need be, treating existing disease.

Health

What is **health**? The World Health Organization (WHO) in 1948 defined health as "a state of complete physical, social and mental well-being, and not merely the absence of disease or infirmity" but over the decades, the concept of health has come to be much more. It is about being able to realize aspirations and satisfy needs, as well as being able to change and cope with an ever-changing environment; health is an investment in and resource for living.[1] This broader conceptualization of health evoked a perspective on achieving health that recognizes personal lifestyles as just one determinant of health and that others such as where a person/community lives, education, and social supports are broader determinants with significant impact on a person's health. Health promotion is a positive concept based on the process of enabling people to increase control over, and to improve, their health. All persons have the right to be healthy. Actions and decisions, locally, nationally, and globally are being held accountable to the impact on the health of others. Worldwide the call for action for "health for all" and "global health" is moving not just the health professions but all agencies, such as government and communities, to make a difference with respect to the determinants of health.

Oral systemic health and periodontal medicine is valued increasingly by health professionals and social advocacy groups, not just oral health professionals, as part of the assessment, planning, implementation, and evaluation of disease treatment planning and health promotion strategies. Challenges such as oropharyngeal cancer, poor nutrition, chronic disease and conditions, dental and periodontal infections, lack of access to oral healthcare services, and health literacy affect health. The mouth is part of the body; the body is responsive to the mind; and the mind is intertwined with the spirit. Oral health is viewed as a resource for being able to live a good quality of life. This view is illustrated in the following three examples:

- Having a sound dentition and oral soft-tissue integrity enables a person to enjoy a variety of foods, which support good nutrition, enabling the body to build and repair tissue. A person must have access to foods that enrich and fortify the body. High nutritious food costs, knowing what is a nutritious food, and having readily available foods all play a role in "access to food." Good nutrition is part of being able to be healthy.
- Having freedom from oral pain enables a person to engage fully in the day's activities. The person is productive, and being productive brings a sense of accomplishment and wellness. Consider the child with early childhood caries who is unable to perform in school because of toothache or the worker who misses days of work because of oral pain. Dental care is costly and an out-of-pocket expense for many. In these two cases, early childhood development and income, respectively, affect the person's ability to have freedom from oral pain.
- **Health literacy**, having accurate knowledge and decision-making skills to maintain the oral cavity free of disease or disability, enables individuals to keep their teeth for a

lifetime. Health literacy is a valuable ability. Reading and writing are life skills that all have the right to enjoy, but not all are provided or nurtured with this right. Even with the skills, health behaviors may not be learned or marketing and social forces may be of such strong influence that a person adopts behaviors not conducive to health, such as use of tobacco.

The Continuum of Dental Hygiene Care

Dental hygiene care is a continuum of client-centered care that includes the following:

- Disease treatment
- Disease prevention
- Health promotion

For the purpose of this chapter, the focus of discussion of the continuum is of individual dental hygienists working with their clients in a clinical setting; however, actions along the continuum are far more reaching than the individual client-dental hygienist encounter. Health is determined by more than access to healthcare. Each dental hygienist has a responsibility to the "call for action" to the broader determinants of health, and this can start with the individual client-dental hygienist encounter. This start can be thought of as each person doing his or her part by acting locally but thinking globally.

Figure 4-1 illustrates the continuum of dental hygiene care and provides sample dental hygiene actions in each approach to care. Movement along the continuum may begin with disease prevention or disease treatment, but the broader determinants of health ultimately affect the client's health. Simply offering disease prevention interventions does not promote health. Depending on clients' needs, they may enter dental hygiene care at the health-promotion phase, the oral disease–prevention phase, or the oral disease–treatment phase. The direction or purposeful movement of care on the continuum is toward health promotion, although the encounter initially may require one of the other approaches to the dental hygiene care provided.

Treatment of Disease

Disease treatment in healthcare is about caring for the client's health; when disease, disability, or adversity challenges health, this condition is treated so that the client's health is reestablished or in some way bettered as a result of the treatment or intervention. Access to healthcare is a determinant of health. Disease treatment is critical on the continuum of dental hygiene care and is likely what the client most strongly identifies the clinical dental hygienist with in terms of client–dental hygiene encounters. Dental hygienists recognize, however, that to confine their practice to disease treatment ignores the synergy of care that results when disease is not only treated but prevented and health is promoted. For example, in the case of Sherry Gilmore in Scenario 4-2, emotional stress as a result of unemployment has the potential to affect adversely her periodontal health.

Disease Prevention: Primary, Secondary, Tertiary Prevention

The dental hygienist who practices disease prevention focuses on avoiding or eliminating the disease's causative agent(s) to prevent the disease from recurring or progressing. For example, the dental hygienist considers the effect oral biofilm has on the dentition and periodontium of a person who is taking multiple medications for hypertension. Dental hygienists who are working with a client community, such as at a diabetes education resource center, may consider educating the group about the role good oral self-care plays in managing diabetes as well as maintaining oral health. Another example is when the dental hygienist considers the impact of where clients live on their health. If the client's community is a remote town with little access to regular dental hygiene care, this factor may have a significant influence on oral disease progression or its prevention. Disease prevention brings attention to the balance of multiple factors in achieving health and maintaining it.

The levels of disease prevention are as follows: primary, secondary, and tertiary (Table 4-1).[2] A fourth, termed *primordial prevention,* is synonymous with health promotion and will be addressed as health promotion in this chapter.

- **Primary prevention** consists of interventions to prevent the onset of disease or injury. This level is a major focus of dental hygiene practice. Examples of such dental hygiene actions include tobacco cessation counseling, dietary counseling for the prevention of dental caries, and mouth guard fabrication for preventing sport-related injury.
- **Secondary prevention** consists of early identification of disease and interventions designed to stop or minimize the progression of early disease. Examples of such dental hygiene actions include client education regarding daily mouth care for an individual with gingivitis, recommending daily fluoride gel for persons with incipient dental caries, and applying desensitizing agents for dentinal hypersensitivity.

TABLE 4-1

Modes of Oral Health Intervention for the Three Levels of Prevention

Level	Focus	Activity
Primary	No disease, condition, or injury; prevent it from occurring	Daily mouth care Tobacco-use abstinence Athletic mouth protectors Water fluoridation Fluoridated dentifrice Pit and fissure sealants (no caries activity)
Secondary	Early detection and prompt intervention	Detecting disease as a result of early oral screening programs, self-examination, or professional examinations Tobacco-use cessation Pit and fissure sealants (incipient caries) Oral physiotherapeutic aids for periodontal pockets
Tertiary	Treatment and rehabilitation	Surgical and nonsurgical rehabilitation Periodontal therapy Restorative, prosthodontic, reconstructive therapy

- **Tertiary prevention** consists of interventions to prevent disability and to improve or restore function and prevent further deterioration. A key dental hygiene action in tertiary prevention is nonsurgical periodontal therapy. This level of prevention also is treatment of disease, hence treatment is viewed as part of prevention of disease.

Health Promotion

Health promotion is the process of enabling people to increase control over and improve their current and future health.[3] Everyone and every entity (e.g., individuals, healthcare organizations, and government) is seen as responsible for the creation of environments that predispose and enable people as individuals and communities to achieve health and realize their own and collective aspirations. WHO Health Promotion Logo[3] (Figure 4-2), Population Health[4,5] (Figure 4-3), and Healthy People 2020[6] (Figure 4-4) are examples of models or frameworks guiding health promotion. What determines health is much more than personal lifestyles or individual behaviors. Health also is determined by the impact of social and economic forces, education, where a person lives, and other determinants, known worldwide as the **social determinants of health**.[7] Specifically, health is determined by income and socioeconomic status; social support networks; education and literacy; employment and working conditions; social environment; physical environment; personal health

SCENARIO 4-3

Mary Marks, 50 years old, is a single mother who financially supports her two children attending college. She smokes 20 cigarettes per day and has done so for almost 35 years. Chris Lee, her dental hygienist, recommends she consider joining the tobacco cessation program she is running at the Klein Dental Center. Chris encourages Mary to do so because Mary is at risk for oral cancer. Mary says, "I know I should quit. I realize I should because it is likely killing me. I just can't even consider doing it right now."

Scenario 4-3 provides a good example of the dental hygienist using a disease-prevention approach. Blaming Mary for putting herself at risk for cancer is an oversimplification of why Mary smokes. Being a fair-minded, critical thinker, the dental hygienist can help Mary process her tobacco-use habit considering factors such as the following:

- Mary is physically and psychologically addicted to nicotine.
- When Mary began smoking, it was a socially acceptable thing to do. Although this is no longer the case, she is addicted to nicotine in tobacco.
- Society has taken a strong anti–tobacco-use stance, as is evident by many policies now in effect to reduce tobacco use in public places such as airplanes, restaurants, and workplaces, but tobacco is highly addictive and many find it difficult to quit its use.
- Significant healthcare dollars are spent on the treatment of tobacco-related diseases, but additional research and funding for tobacco cessation programs is required to help many tobacco users overcome their addiction.

The dental hygienist would do well for Mary by recognizing the complexity of Mary's smoking habit (see Chapter 36). It is much more than a simple choice for Mary to quit smoking. Helping her find solutions for her tobacco use involves all three levels of prevention.

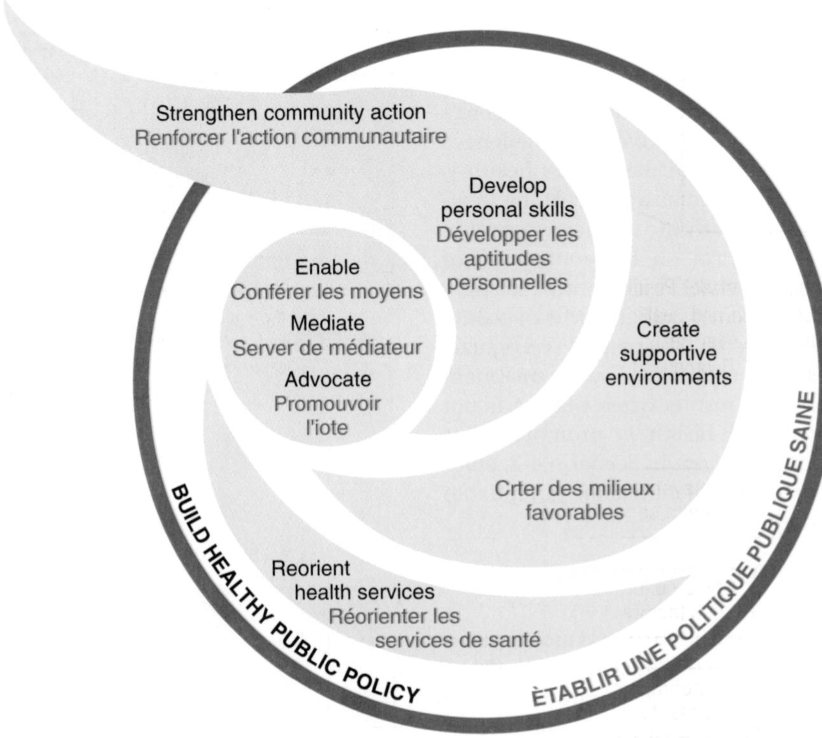

Figure 4-2. World Health Organization health promotion logo. (Reproduced with permission from World Health Organization Press.)

practices and coping skills; healthy child development; biology and genetic endowment; health services; and gender and culture (see Figure 4-3).[5]

Consider asking the client, "What makes you healthy?" This is not the same as asking the client, "What makes you sick?" Population Health explains why a young boy named Jason is in the hospital[5] (Box 4-1). Similarly, the scenario could be layered to understand why Jason has rampant tooth decay. The approach aims at promoting health for all by accepting specific challenges, identifying mechanisms, and implementing health-promotion strategies to meet these challenges. Dental hygienists who base their practice approach on Population Health consider the determinants of health—for example, the client's lifestyle and personal health practices (What does the client believe regarding oral disease and oral hygiene?); where the client lives (Does the community have fluoridated water?); access to healthcare (Is the client able to afford oral healthcare?); and the client's childhood growth and development (Is the client genetically predisposed to periodontal disease?). The goal of health promotion is to lessen inequities by addressing the determinants of health and work to strengthen those so that people are more likely to be healthy than to develop disease. Health promotion builds an environment supportive of health.

To ensure health for all, inequities must be reduced so that each child grows up in healthy environments and receives a quality education; all can engage in meaningful and productive employment; all communities flourish in green and enriching environments; all have access to healthcare; and all have social protection. The World Health Organization principles for taking action with respect to the social determinants of health are outlined in Table 4-2.[7] Significant effort by leading organizations such as the World Health Organization, the United States Department of Health and Human Services, and Health Canada ensured oral health as part of the health promotion initiative of "health for all." For example: the U.S. Surgeon General's Report on Oral Health,[8] the WHO Oral Health Report,[9-11] the United States Healthy People (Oral Health),[12] and Canada's Federal, Provincial, Territorial Dental Working Group Oral Health Strategy[13] are reports based on the interaction between oral health and general health and well-being through the life span, and on evidence that oral health is more than an outcome of individual lifestyle and behaviors—that societal and environmental forces greatly affect oral health. Boxes 4-2 and 4-3 show the evidence related to oral health burdens and disparities and strategies, for oral disease prevention and health promotion, respectively.[8,9] What determines oral health disparities? Why are some populations more at risk for disease than others? Why are some populations healthy and others not?

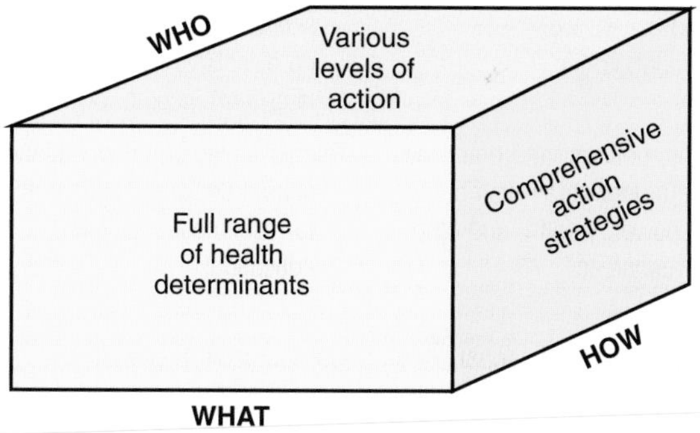

Figure 4-3. Population health promotion model. Population health approach: an integrated model of population health and health promotion. (All rights reserved. An integrated Model of Population Health and Health Promotion Public Health Agency of Canada, 2001. Reproduced with permission from the Minister of Health, 2013.)

BOX 4-1

Determinants of Health

- Why is Jason in the hospital?
  - Because he has a bad infection in his leg
- But why does he have an infection?
  - Because he has a cut on his leg and it got infected
- But why does he have a cut on his leg?
  - Because he was playing in the junkyard next to his apartment building, and there was some sharp, jagged steel there that he fell on
- But why was he playing in a junkyard?
  - Because his neighborhood is kind of run down; a lot of kids play there and there is no one to supervise them
- But why does he live in that neighborhood?
  - Because his parents can't afford a nicer place to live
- But why can't his parents afford a nicer place to live?
  - Because his Dad is unemployed and his Mom is sick
- But why is his Dad unemployed?
  - Because he doesn't have much education and he can't find a job

But why?...

Toward a Healthy Future, page 7 http://www.phac-aspc.gc.ca/ph-sp/report-rapport/toward/pdf/toward_a_healthy_english.PDF Cat H39-468.1999E. ISBN 0-662-27625-6. Public Health Agency of Canada, 1999. Reproduced with the permission of the Minister of Public Works and Government Services Canada, 2012.

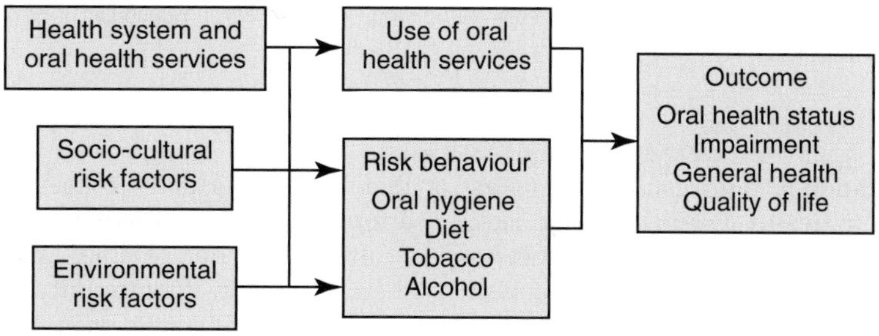

Figure 4-4. WHO risk factor approach in promotion of oral health. (Reproduced with permission from World Health Organization Press.)

SCENARIO 4-4

Meghan Woo, 17 years old, was born a Canadian citizen. She was raised in a middle-class–income household along with two younger siblings. Her parents were able to afford for one of them to stay home during her early childhood development. Meghan sees her family's healthcare team on a regular basis for immunizations and during benchmark periods of growth and development. When the family experienced the tragic loss of a cousin from suicide, they attended grief counseling sessions available through the community health center. Meghan had one hospital stay 3 days in length for recovery from an appendectomy. This hospitalization was completely covered by the national healthcare plan. When Meghan was 13 years old her parents took her to the orthodontist because it looked like her teeth were growing in crooked. The family tree shows many relatives with maligned teeth. Meghan wore orthodontic appliances for 2 years, like more than half of her friends. The cost for care was covered by her parents' health insurance plans, given to them as benefits of their employment. After that experience, Meghan is thinking she might want to become an orthodontist. The family enjoys "quality time" together, and they regularly participate in community activities. Their neighborhood has plenty of green space, walking and cycling paths, dog parks, and an active neighborhood watch program. Meghan plays soccer and belongs to a youth group. She and her family are part of a spiritual community. She has learned to be a good team player, respectful and mindful of her actions on others and the environment. Meghan has never had a toothache, has a strong stance against using tobacco and other substances, eats a good breakfast every day, has chosen to abstain from engaging in sex, wears protective shields when playing sports, and breathes the fresh air enjoyed by her community. She is healthy.

TABLE 4-2

Three Principles of Action with Respect to the Social Determinants of Health

Principle of Action	Meaning	Elaboration	Example
Improve conditions of daily life	People are born, grow, live, work, and age in a variety of circumstances that determine their health	Equity from the start: policy, programming, and education that ensures all children have a healthy start to life Healthy places, healthy people: quality housing, clean water, and sanitation Fair employment and decent work Social protection throughout life Universal healthcare	Born into poverty, live in substandard housing in high-crime neighborhood, work at an early age to bring in household income, "drop out" of school, sustain workplace injury, no disability insurance, no long-term income for elder years
Tackle inequitable distribution of power, money, and resources	Power, money, and resources at all levels (globally, nationally, and locally) determine daily life existence	Address social norms, policies, and practices that enable and promote unfair distribution of and access to power, wealth, and other necessary social resources	Gender equity in the workplace; shared decision making; access to resources (e.g., food, education)
Measure the problem, evaluate action, expand knowledge base, train a workforce to address social determinants of health; and create public awareness of them	Assess, plan, implement, and evaluate actions to reduce the inequities and enable all to enjoy quality of life	Shared and accountable global, national, local, private, interagency efforts to assess determinants of health with effective strategies based on quality decision making	Collaboration; person and community-centered focus; evidence-based best practice; health literacy; healthy public policy

Adapted from Commission on Social Determinants of Health (CSDH): *Closing the gap in a generation: health equity through action on the social determinants of health.* Final Report of the Commission on Social Determinants of Health. Geneva, World Health Organization, 2008. Available at: http://www.who.int/social_determinants/thecommission/finalreport/en/indexhtml, specifically http://whqlibdoc.who.int/publications/2008/9789241563703_eng.pdf. Accessed August 2012. Permission to adapt granted from WHO Press.

The World Health Organization recognizes the risk factors to oral health as being access to health systems and services, sociocultural risk factors, and multiple environmental factors (Figure 4-5).[9] The interplay of these factors leads to risk behavior such as the use of tobacco, which in turn affects oral health. Rather than blaming the client for behaving in a way that is not conducive to health, the oral health–promotion approach looks to discover the factors in place that result in healthy behavior. Dental hygienists, whether providing their services in a community-based clinic, online through an educational Web page, or in a dental hygiene or dental clinic, are integral to the health-promotion movement. Just as

BOX 4-2

United States Oral Surgeon Report, Burden of Oral Disease: Key Issues Cited

Children

- Dental caries (tooth decay) is the single most common chronic childhood disease; it is five times more common than asthma and seven times more common than hay fever.
- Striking disparities in dental disease exist by income.
  - Poor children experience twice as much dental caries as their more affluent peers, and their disease is more likely to be untreated.
- Unintentional injuries, many of which include head, mouth, and neck injuries, are common in children.
- Tobacco-related oral lesions are prevalent in adolescents who currently use smokeless (spit) tobacco.
- Professional care is necessary for maintaining oral health.
  - 25% of poor children have not seen a dentist by the time they enter kindergarten.
- Medical insurance is a strong predictor of access to dental care.
  - Uninsured children are two and a half times less likely than insured children to receive dental care.
  - Children from families without dental insurance are three times more likely to have dental needs than children with either public or private insurance.
  - For each child without medical insurance, there are at least 2.6 children without dental insurance.
- Social impact of oral diseases in children is substantial.
  - More than 51 million school hours are lost each year to dental-related illness.
  - Poor children suffer nearly 12 times more restricted-activity days than children from higher-income families.
  - Pain and suffering resulting from untreated diseases can lead to problems in eating, speaking, and attending to learning.

Adults

- Most adults show signs of periodontal or gingival diseases.
- Pain is a common symptom of craniofacial disorders and is accompanied by interference with vital functions such as eating, swallowing, and speech.
- Population growth and diagnostics enabling earlier detection of cancer mean that more patients than ever before are undergoing cancer treatments. More than 400,000 of these patients will develop oral complications annually.
- Employed adults lose more than 164 million hours of work each year owing to dental disease or dental visits.
- For every adult 19 years of age or older without medical insurance, there are three without dental insurance.
- A little less than two thirds of adults report having visited a dentist in the past 12 months.

Older Adults

- 23% of 65- to 74-year-olds have severe periodontal disease.
- About 30% of adults 65 years of age and older are edentulous, compared with 46% 20 years ago. These figures are higher for those living in poverty.
- Oral and pharyngeal cancers are diagnosed in about 30,000 Americans annually.
  - 8000 die from these diseases each year.
  - They are primarily diagnosed in the elderly.
  - The prognosis is poor.
- Most older Americans take both prescription and over-the-counter drugs.
  - Likely at least one of the medications used will have an oral side effect—usually dry mouth.
- At any given time, 5% of Americans aged 65 and older (currently some 1.65 million people) are living in a long-term care facility where dental care is problematic.
- Many elderly individuals lose their dental insurance when they retire.

From U.S. Department of Health and Human Services: *Oral health in America: a report of the Surgeon General (executive summary),* Rockville, Md, 2000, U.S. Department of Health and Human Services, National Institute of Dental and Craniofacial Research, National Institutes of Health.

BOX 4-3

World Health Organization Strategies for Oral Disease Prevention and Oral Health

The goals of the World Health Organization (WHO) are to build healthy populations and communities and to combat ill health. Four strategic directions provide the broad framework for focusing WHO's technical work; they also have implications for the Oral Health Programme.

1. Reducing oral disease burden and disability, especially in poor and marginalized populations
2. Promoting healthy lifestyles and reducing risk factors to oral health that arise from environmental, economic, social, and behavioral causes
3. Developing oral health systems that equitably improve oral health outcomes, respond to people's legitimate demands, and are financially fair
4. Framing policies in oral health, based on integration of oral health into national and community health programs, and promoting oral health as an effective dimension for development policy of society

From World Health Organization, Programmes and Projects: *Strategies for oral disease prevention and health promotion.* Available at: http://www.who.int/oral_health/strategies/en/.
Reproduced with permission from WHO. Accessed August 2012.

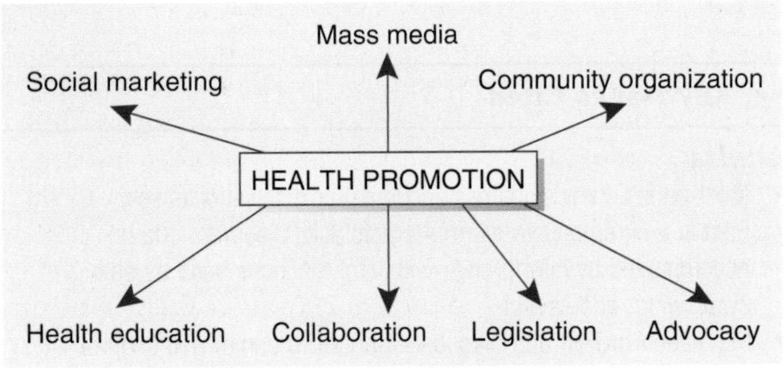

Figure 4-5. Health-promotion strategies.

individuals can do their part in reducing the greenhouse effect, dental hygienists as clinicians can do their part in promoting health, working either one-on-one with an individual client, or with a community of clients. The health-promotion movement challenges health professionals to realize that they are a part of the whole, that what happens to populations happens to people, and that those people (hence populations) are the health professionals' clients. By virtue of a position in health promotion, the health professional is in a leadership role to help clients recognize that oral health is an outcome of who they are, where they live, how they live, why they live the way they do, and who and what affect and influence their lives, from an individual perspective and a much larger global one. Consider why people are healthy. People are healthy because they have the knowledge base to engage in healthy behaviors. They have the knowledge base because they are educated. They are educated because they live in a country in which the law states that all people have the right to receive an education. Dental hygienists must recognize that clients are a product of the environment as much as they are individuals with personal lifestyles and behaviors.

The health-promotion movement calls to more than the health professional. It calls to all levels of influence—individuals, communities, institutions, and governments (see Figure 4-2). The call is to take action by building public policy that honors health; strengthens community action by empowering communities to assume ownership and control of their own destinies; reorients health services to be health promotion–focused; creates supportive environments; and on an individual level facilitates the development of personal skills. The call around the world is for collaboration among individuals, healthcare systems and services, communities, and policymakers to attend to the determinants of health, to enable, mediate, and advocate for people and communities to achieve a high quality of health. Dental hygienists, being health professionals with a body of knowledge and expertise, are ethically obligated to integrate oral health promotion within practice, even if that practice is focused on disease prevention (primary, secondary, and tertiary) and disease treatment. The health-promotion movement shifts the way of thinking from one of treating disease to preventing it and to promoting health.

Some may argue that the health-promotion movement is the responsibility of the public health dental hygienist and that the clinical dental hygienist, responsible for providing care to individual clients, is not integral to the movement. Health promotion, however, is about the individual client who is part of a community of people who are influenced by and who influence their environment and other communities. It is also about policies developed by communities for support of healthy environments and services for the individual client and the community. Therefore health promotion calls all people, not just those health professionals working in community health centers or public health agencies. The call is to think about the determinants of health for the client and not just the risk of disease. Consider how oral and craniofacial cancer reported by *Healthy People* tend to not be diagnosed at an early phase when prognosis is better.[12] The call to action is for the oral health professions to ensure that a head and neck examination is conducted at regular intervals, with frequency dependent on the individual client's risk factors. Although performing a head and neck screening for oral cancer is a secondary prevention measure, if a lesion is discovered early, the prognosis for recovery is improved and the person is able to return to health, thus moving along the health-promotion continuum. Each dental hygienist makes a difference when accepting the health-promotion call.

In Scenario 4-3, Mary Marks informs the dental hygienist that she knows smoking cigarettes is harmful to her, yet she is not able to quit. On an intrapersonal level, she does not believe she could quit. Her dependency on tobacco reflects physical and psychologic addiction. On an interpersonal level, her family may want her to quit, but they also realize how hard it will be for her and enable her to continue because of their sympathy. At the community level, policy is in effect that prevents her from smoking in public places, so she is forced to limit her use to nonpublic places such as her car and home. She has noticed more and more people frown at her smoking in her car, making her increasingly uncomfortable to be seen smoking while driving. Mary also says she has heard that smoking in one's own car is now considered at the public policy level to be illegal. The impetus for Mary to successfully quit cigarette use may very well be the public policy. As with Jason's condition described in Box 4-1, Mary's decision to quit actually originated from social forces at the public policy level—much broader than her own intrapersonal level. The dental hygienist's statement to Mary—"You need to quit"—becomes one of many influences that may help Mary quit tobacco use.

At this point it may seem that there is little difference in dental hygiene actions between disease prevention and oral health promotion, however, there is a difference. Disease prevention is focused on preventing disease. Health promotion aims at establishing a healthy environment so that all people can achieve their aspirations because of engagement in lifestyle behaviors conducive to health and because where they live and how they live are conducive to health. Thinking in terms of health promotion is different from thinking in terms of disease prevention. It is a shift in thinking, much like looking at a glass half-full versus a glass half-empty. Health promotion is a positive, inspirational perspective that enables people to be all they can be because they are healthy.

Health Promotion: a Challenge to the Health Professions

Achieving health for all is a challenge for health professionals, one that can be met by employing strategies of health-promotion: marketing, health education, collaboration, mass media, community organization, advocacy, and legislation.

Dental hygienists, no matter their practice site, can engage in each of these activities and thereby actively participate in the challenge as client advocates, educators, and oral health promoters. Doing so requires dental hygienists to think of their clients as part of the community from which they came, susceptible to and influenced by forces much bigger than themselves. It requires the dental hygienist to think in terms of oral health promotion and not just in terms of disease prevention and disease treatment.

Marketing

SCENARIO 4-5

Karen Fraser recently became a licensed dental hygienist. She was enjoying her practice in a large downtown shopping center. Soon enough, Karen realized she was reaching only those clients who came to her practice. She knew that accessing oral health services was a determinant of health, and she felt ethically responsible to ensure the community knew about the value of professional oral health services for oral and systemic health. Karen developed a website on the oral-systemic-health connection and invited people in the community to contact her with their concerns and questions. In no time, she realized the impact she'd had on raising the awareness of the importance of professional care, because many of the people who visited her site sought out her professional care.

SCENARIO 4-6

Bruce Front has been practicing dental hygiene for 5 years. Within 2 years of his graduation, he established a mobile dental hygiene service and now provides dental hygiene care to residents in more than 15 large facilities. Bruce realized the need and demand for dental hygiene services for the older adults residing in long-term care facilities and marketed his services to them. The result is the provision of regular dental hygiene care that otherwise was not provided by the oral health profession community.

Both Karen (Scenario 4-5) and Bruce (Scenario 4-6) know that access to health services is a determinant to health. They are marketing oral health to their surrounding communities in response to the call for health services to be accountable to the client community. What Bruce and Karen are doing (whether they realize it or not) is part of marketing oral health, by designing, implementing, and controlling programs intended to provide better access to dental hygiene care.

Marketing oral health is marketing an intangible product, unlike marketing a new toothbrush, which is a tangible item. When a concept is marketed, such as health, it is referred to as **social marketing**. Promotion of oral health behaviors and environments requires the dental hygienist to market a concept that, if accepted, results in a product, that being oral health. Examples of social marketing include campaigning against spouse, child, and elder abuse, drinking and driving, tobacco and substance abuse, and promoting breast-feeding.

Social marketing is essential for promoting oral health. It persuades people, through exposure, awareness, reinforcement, and provision of knowledge and skills, to accept responsibility for their health and that of their community. The Surgeon General's report on oral health states that to reduce oral health disparities and promote oral health for all, there is a need to increase understanding of the health–oral health connection by the public, practitioners, and policymakers. Consider a healthy tooth development campaign aimed at parents and caregivers of babies and young children. If the campaign reaches the public through media outlets but the practitioner does not reinforce it at the individual level, the importance or value of the message misses a critical one-on-one interface among the credible health professional, the caregiver, and the message itself. An example of a social marketing strategy applied to dental hygiene practice that considers the relationship of product, promotion, place, and price in promoting oral health is described in Table 4-3.

Health Education

Health education is "any combination of learning experiences designed to help individuals and communities improve their health, by increasing their knowledge or influencing their attitudes."[1] Health education can be provided at the individual level, at community level, and even at the level of legislation and advocacy. All three approaches to health education support the concept of health promotion. Table 4-4 provides examples of health education: The individualistic approach enhances self-help, the community level identifies with people helping people, and the legislative/advocacy

TABLE 4-3
Marketing Applied to Oral Health

Marketing	Oral Health Example
Product	Oral health as part of total health Name of campaign, e.g., "Smile" Make "Smile" a tangible product, e.g., with photographs
Promotion	Radio and television announcements Free preventive oral health services offered during national dental hygiene campaign Bus poster announcements Website development
Place	Workplace and public school locations Information telephone hotlines Booth display at local mall Social media
Price	Psychic costs (client's fear and anxiety) Monetary considerations Resource costs (childcare while parent attends oral healthcare appointment, time for parental supervision of children's oral health behaviors)

TABLE 4-4
Health Education Examples

Approach	Health Promotion Strategy	Health Education Example
Individual	Develop personal skills	One-to-one oral health education on relationship between diabetes and periodontal disease Basic oral hygiene skills education Tobacco-use cessation counseling
Community	Strengthening community action	Holding informational town hall meeting on community water fluoridation Creating "Basic Oral Hygiene" certification program for caregivers of persons requiring assistance with daily living skills
Legislative/ advocacy	Reorient health services Create supportive environments Build healthy public policy	Letters to legislators or members of parliament regarding universal oral healthcare Lobbying for self-regulation of dental hygiene practice

approach considers the creation of healthy public policy and programming.

Collaboration

Interprofessional collaboration is an important element of healthcare. The health professional who collaborates with others—including other health professionals and other individuals and groups who influence health—is the health professional who realizes that oral health is a holistic achievement.

SCENARIO 4-7

Harriet Bezu takes Mr. Smith's blood pressure, as she routinely does, and finds that despite his medication to control his hypertension, his blood pressure is higher than normal. She asks Mr. Smith if he would like her to call his physician. She does so, and the physician schedules Mr. Smith for an appointment in a week's time. The physician asks Harriet about Mr. Smith's salivary flow rate, wanting to know if Harriet detected any salivary changes or noted any oral lesions resulting from the medication. During Harriet's dental hygiene dietary assessment, Mr. Smith told her that he really detests cooking and has come to rely on toast and soup as his mainstay meal. He misses the wonderful foods his wife made for them, but she died a few months ago and he is now on his own. Harriet tells him about an agency that can bring a prepared hot meal to him every day. He thinks that would be a marvelous idea; in fact, the social worker at the community health center had suggested this, and he just hadn't followed through with it.

Harriet is demonstrating collaboration with other health professionals as follows:

- Being aware of a client's holistic health to enhance the person's capacity to adopt preventive and promotional practices
- Interacting with other professionals to avoid territorial boundaries over disease, which limit the opportunity to enhance a client's self-care, mutual aid, and coping ability

In the spirit of collaboration, health professionals provide clients with information on health-promoting resources and programs in the community, such as smoking-cessation programs, cardiovascular fitness programs, fat-free cooking programs, and various support groups.

Collaboration also must occur among decision makers and society outside of the healthcare arena to create healthy environments. An illustration of this collaboration would be mandating elder-abuse as a reportable condition. If dental hygienists' head and neck examinations lead them to suspect that clients are being abused, they are required to report their suspicions to the appropriate authority. Society does not tolerate abuse, and healthcare professions are in the position of possibly detecting abuse. Government bodies (on behalf of the people) require action to be taken to help abuse victims.

Collaboration fuels the health-promotion movement by encouraging discussion among healthcare providers, promoting linkages among them, and creating enabling environments for the achievement of health. Dental hygienists are linking with other healthcare providers to facilitate high-quality care. At the Health Science Center, Winnipeg Regional Health Authority, the Diabetes Education Resource Center for Children and Adolescents (Canada), the healthcare team invited a dental hygienist to join them, because they valued the knowledge base that the dental hygienist brings to the resource center regarding the oral health–diabetes bidirectional relationship. This collaboration enhanced the quality of care for the clients.

Mass Media

Mass media allows for many people to receive a message at one time, thus creating an awareness of a concept or engaging people in thinking and talking about the message. There are many forms of mass media, and each has pros and cons. Not everyone reads the newspaper, so use of newspaper announcements reaches only some people; in addition, the reader's literacy must be considered in the announcement. Many people are using the Internet as a source of health information, so it has become a popular mass media outlet for health promotion. Practicing dental hygienists can use media sources as resources for oral health education; as well, they can participate in media activities to promote oral health as follows:

- Serving as contributing health editors to household magazines
- Creating a webpage on the oral-systemic-health-connection
- Holding press conferences during local, state, or national dental hygiene gatherings
- Performing radio and television spots

Community-Centered Organization: Building Capacity

Community-centered organization aims at developing the skills and abilities of groups of people for the purpose of self-led improvement. It focuses on building capacity from within the community for self-sustaining and longevity of the change. It creates supporting environments and strengthens community action.

SCENARIO 4-8

Mary Donald, a dental hygienist working in a dental clinic in a northern remote community that had primary health-care center, found herself involved in a health promotion initiative. She was approached by the public health nurse about baby first oral health visits and immunization schedule. In the recent past nurses had enjoyed having dental therapists as part of the interprofessional healthcare team that offered babies a series of visits promoting healthy child development. Because of changes in contractual dental services to the community, the dental therapist was no longer part of the team. The nurses looked to Mary as an oral health promotion consultant, and Mary accepted the invitation to join the team. The team met with mothers, public health professionals, community resource workers, health directors, and other key individuals/groups for guidance regarding how the team could help the community ensure healthy early childhood development for all children in the community. All persons in the group were residents of the community, thus promoting strengthened community action and supportive environments. They wanted the dental hygienist to consult about what they should include in an oral health kit to distribute to parents, including some oral health education literature, and how to access dental products. The kits were assembled according to the developmental needs of the child, plus included an oral health tool and message for parental oral health.

Advocacy, Legislation, and Public Policy

Advocacy, legislation, and public policy are essential tools for achieving health for all, the mission of health promotion. The call to action in health promotion is a call to each dental hygienist to take steps in the direction of promoting environments conducive to health so that all people can realize their aspirations because they have their health. Oral health is part of overall health. Oral disease prevention and treatment enable the client to achieve oral health, which promotes general health.

SCENARIO 4-9

The dental practice that employs dental hygienist Roland Pantel is situated in a predominantly Hispanic neighborhood. The practice has surveyed the neighborhood and knows that only about half of the 5-year-olds have had an oral health screening, referral, and follow-up. Roland takes the initiative to find dental hygienists to perform oral screenings in the community school. He confers with his dental hygiene colleagues, the mayor of the community, and the parent council of the school, all of whom sign a petition to be taken to the Health Authority for their approval of funding and other resources. Roland continues to advocate for regulatory changes for his profession. Where Roland lives and practices dental hygiene, the settings in which he can provide dental hygiene care are limited. He is required to practice under direct supervision of a dentist. Knowing that access to care by the 5-year-olds in need of oral healthcare in his community is limited by his scope of practice, Roland becomes an active member of his professional association's legislative committee. Advocacy and legislation are intertwined; advocacy is generally the precursor to legislation. Advocacy, in this context, is the education of decision makers to provide the essential political support for changes, whereas legislation makes these behaviors mandatory. Examples of public policy for health instigated through advocacy and legislation include the requirement that smokers must extinguish their cigarettes before entering public places, that traffic stop signs must be placed at street intersections, and that schoolchildren must be immunized against numerous childhood diseases before attending school. Roland, in taking action to enable access to dental hygiene care for all people, is part of the creation of a healthy public policy.

Dental hygienists are responsible to the call for action in enabling, mediating, and advocating for health promotion so that all can realize health as a resource for quality of life. Through engaging in disease treatment, disease prevention, and health promotion strategies, dental hygienists join the health promotion movement taking place around the world to ensure health for all.

CLIENT EDUCATION TIPS

- Discuss with clients the concept of health as an investment in and resource for living.
- Explore with clients the role oral health plays in their ability to achieve aspirations and realize goals.
- Inform clients about best practices for personal oral hygiene skills.
- Serve as a client advocate, enabling the client to access interventions that promote enablement and decision making by and for the client.
- Share with clients best practice for primary, secondary, and tertiary disease prevention.
- Offer expertise and skill to clients to facilitate strengthening community action, creating supportive environments, and building healthy public policy.

LEGAL, ETHICAL, AND SAFETY ISSUES

- Health is a fundamental right of all people.
- Oral health is part of overall health and wellness.
- Access to dental hygiene care enables disease treatment, disease prevention, and health promotion.
- Health promotion is everyone's responsibility.

KEY CONCEPTS

- Health is the extent to which an individual or group is able to realize and satisfy its needs and to change and cope with the environment.
- Quality of life is affected by oral disease and oral conditions.
- Dental hygienists have an important role to play in promoting oral health as integral to overall health, preventing oral disease, and reducing inequities among population groups.
- Three levels of prevention are primary, secondary, and tertiary.
    - Tertiary prevention treats existing disease, conditions, or injury and rehabilitates a person to recovery of health.
    - Secondary prevention identifies early signs and symptoms of disease, conditions, or injury and aims at prompt intervention and lessening of disability.
    - Primary prevention focuses on preventing the existence of disease, conditions, or injury. The dental hygienist has roles and responsibilities in all areas of prevention.
- Health promotion enhances health by enabling, mediating, and advocating for healthy public policy; creating supportive environments; strengthening community action; developing personal skills; and reorienting health services.
    - Strategies include marketing, health education, collaboration, mass media use, community organization, and advocacy and legislation.
- Dental hygienists collaborate with individuals, groups, and other health professionals to prevent oral disease and promote health.
- Dental hygiene, like all health professions, is called to facilitate the worldwide mission to achieve health (oral health) for all.

CRITICAL THINKING EXERCISES

1. Create a concept map of the determinants of your own health. Why are you healthy? Be sure to focus on health as opposed to disease, injury, or ill condition.
2. Contact a local health-promotion agency, such as a well-baby clinic. Interview the agency employees about their philosophy of care. Consider what the role and responsibility of a dental hygienist could be (or are) with the agency.
3. Using a digital camera, walk around your community and take photographs of elements that create a healthy environment. Make a poster using these photos, and decide on a poster title and text that best addresses oral health promotion.

REFERENCES

1. World Health Organization: *Health promotion glossary*. WHO/HPR/HEP/98.1 Geneva. 1998. Available at: http://whqlibdoc.who.int/hq/1998/WHO_HPR_HEP_98.1.pdf. Accessed August 2012.
2. The Association of Faculties of Medicine of Canada Public Health Educators' Network: *Stages of prevention. AFMC primer on population health*, Available at: http://phprimer.afmc.ca/Part1-TheoryThinkingAboutHealth/Chapter4BasicConceptsInPreventionSurveillanceAndHealthPromotion/Thestagesofprevention. Accessed August 2012.
3. World Health Organization (WHO): *Milestones in health promotion. Statements from Global Conferences*, Switzerland, 2009, WHO Press. Available at: http://www.who.int/healthpromotion/milestones.pdf. Accessed August 2012.
4. Hamilton N, Bhatti T: Public Health Agency of Canada, Canada Health, Population Health: *Population health approach: an integrated model of population health and health promotion, 1996*. Available at: http://www.phac-aspc.gc.ca/ph-sp/index-eng.php. Accessed August 2012.
5. Epp J: *Achieving health for all: a framework for health promotion, 1986*. Ottawa, ON: Health and Welfare Canada. Available at: http://www.hc-sc.gc.ca/hcs-sss/pubs/system-regime/1986-frame-plan-promotion/index-eng.php. Accessed August 2012 from Public Health Agency of Canada.
6. U.S. Department of Health and Human Services: Office of Disease Prevention and Health Promotion: *Healthy People 2020 framework*. Available at: http://healthypeople.gov/2020/Consortium/HP2020Framework.pdf. Accessed August 2012.
7. Commission on Social Determinants of Health (CSDH): *Closing the gap in a generation: health equity through action on the social determinants of health*. Final Report of the Commission on Social Determinants of Health. Geneva, 2008, World Health Organization. Available at: http://whqlibdoc.who.int/publications/2008/9789241563703_eng.pdf. Accessed August 2012.
8. U.S. Department of Health and Human Services: *Oral health in America: a report of the Surgeon General (executive summary)*, Rockville, Md, 2000, U.S. Department of Health and Human Services, National Institute of Dental and Craniofacial Research, National Institutes of Health.
9. World Health Organization (WHO): *The World Oral Health Report 2003. Continuous improvement of oral health in the 21st century: the approach of the WHO Global Oral Health Programme*, Geneva, 2003, WHO Press.
10. World Health Organization (WHO): *Oral health, programmes and projects*. Available at: http://www.who.int/oral_health/en/. Accessed August 2012.
11. Hobdell M, Petersen P, Clarkson P, et al: Global Goals for Oral Health 2020. *Int Dental J* 53:285, 2003.
12. U.S. Department of Health and Human Services, National Institutes of Health: *Healthy people 2020*. Retrieved August 2012 from http://www.healthypeople.gov/2020/default.aspx; specifically Oral Health at http://www.healthypeople.gov/2020/LHI/oralHealth.aspx.
13. Federal, Provincial, Territorial Dental Working Group: *Summary report on the findings of the oral health component of the Canadian Health Measures Survey 2007-2009*, 2010, Health Canada. Available at: http://www.fptdwg.ca/assets/PDF/CHMS/CHMS-E-summ.pdf. Accessed August 2012.

EVOLVE RESOURCES

Please visit http://evolve.elsevier.com/Darby/hygiene for additional practice and study support tools.

CHAPTER 5

Changing Behaviors

Margaret M. Walsh

COMPETENCIES

1. Explain the basic elements of the communication process.
2. Describe factors that influence interpersonal communication.
3. Identify the forms of communication.
4. Describe professional dental hygiene relationships, including the CARE principle.
5. Discuss therapeutic communication techniques.
6. Describe factors that inhibit communication.
7. Identify communication techniques appropriate throughout the life span.
8. Explain motivational interviewing as a client-centered approach to addressing behavior change.

Effective client communication is essential for providing optimal dental hygiene care. For example, during the assessment phase of the dental hygiene process of care, the dental hygienist communicates effectively with the client to obtain and validate information concerning medical, dental, personal and social histories and oral health status and behaviors. Dental hygienists' communication skills also influence client adherence to preventive and therapeutic recommendations. In an environment of rapport, confidence, and trust, a client is more likely to share confidential information and to follow specific oral healthcare recommendations. If dental hygienists possess technical skills and knowledge but are unable to communicate effectively with clients, they may fail to reach important goals related to client oral health, comfort, and long-term behavioral change. This chapter presents foundational concepts about communication and highlights motivational interviewing,[1] a recommended approach to resolve client issues that inhibit positive behavior change. Motivational interviewing actively engages the client in the communication process.

Basic Elements of the Communication Process

Sender, Message, and Receiver

Interpersonal communication is the process by which a person sends a **message** to another person with the intention of evoking a response. Basic communication elements[2] are shown in Figure 5-1. The **sender** is the person who constructs a message to initiate the **interpersonal communication**. The message construction process is known as **encoding**. The message contains information the sender wishes to transmit. It must be in a format of symbols that are understandable to the other person, organized clearly and well expressed, and may be composed of verbal and nonverbal content. The message is sent via a channel that involves visual, auditory, and tactile senses. For example, facial expression uses a visual channel, spoken words use an auditory channel, and touch uses a tactile channel. The **receiver** is the person who accepts the message and deciphers its meaning, a process known as **decoding**. The receiver must share a common language with the sender to decode the message accurately. Communication is most effective when the receiver and the sender accurately perceive the meaning of each other's messages.

Feedback

Communication generally does not stop with one encoded and decoded message. The receiver is prompted to respond and provides a feedback message. The receiver then becomes the sender and the cycle repeats. The feedback communication model illustrates how each person has an encoding and a decoding role in the communication process (Figure 5-2). In a social situation, both persons assume equal responsibilities to seek openness and clarification. In the dental hygienist–client relationship, however, the dental hygienist assumes primary responsibility. Dental hygienists must seek verbal and nonverbal feedback to make sure good communication has occurred. Message transmission is influenced by the sender's and receiver's physical and developmental status, perceptions, values, emotions, knowledge, sociocultural background, roles, and environment.

Factors That Influence Interpersonal Communication

Many **contextual factors** (Box 5-1) can affect interpretation of the messages sent and received by dental hygienists and their clients as discussed in the following sections.[2]

Environmental Factors

The physical surroundings in which communication takes place influence the communication process. For example, people are more likely to communicate effectively in an environment that is comfortable. Factors such as lighting, heating, ventilation, and acoustics may affect the communication process. In the oral healthcare setting, confidentiality may be important if clients are revealing sensitive information about their health. A bustling environment may pose annoying distractions that could block communication.

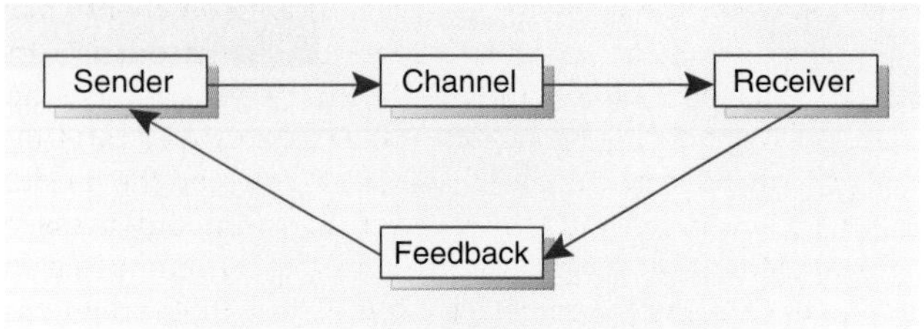

Figure 5-1. Basic communication model.

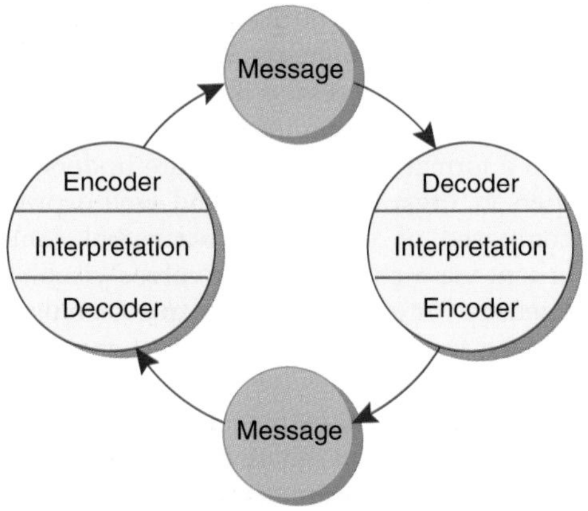

Figure 5-2. Wilbur Schramm feedback model. (Adapted from Schramm W, ed: *The process and effects of mass communication,* Urbana, 1955, University of Illinois Press.)

Internal and Relationship Factors

A person's perceptions, knowledge, values, emotions, and level of need fulfillment influence the way messages are sent and received.[2]

Perceptions

Perceptions can vary greatly from person to person. One individual's analysis of a situation may differ entirely from another's, even though all basic elements are the same. As an example, it is possible for a dental hygienist to take an aggressive approach to oral health education. The hygienist may communicate strong demands for client response and loud, clear warnings about the progression of disease if recommendations are not followed. Some clients may perceive the dental hygienist as an authority figure they can respect and respond to favorably. Others, however, may be offended, perceive the dental hygienist as "pushy" and judgmental, and have a generally adverse reaction to the hygienist's attempts to influence their behavior or health.

Perceptions are formed based on past experience and are difficult to change. If clients had previous contact with a dental hygienist who communicated respect and warmth, they would be more likely to respond well to the hygienist's attempt to resolve a health issue that has become more pressing. When a hygienist takes an aggressive stance with a new client, however, the risk of blocked communication from the client's negative perception of the dental hygienist is great.

Values

Values are personal beliefs that may have moral and ethical implications. Whatever is considered important in life influences the way ideas and feelings are communicated. Each

BOX 5-1

Contextual Factors Influencing Communication

Psychophysiologic Context

The internal factors influencing communication are as follows:

- Physiologic status (e.g., pain, hunger)
- Emotional status (e.g., anxiety, anger)
- Growth and development status (e.g., age)
- Unmet needs (e.g., emotional stress, physical pain)
- Attitudes, values, and beliefs (e.g., meaning of oral health)
- Perceptions and personality (e.g., optimist or pessimist, introvert or extrovert)
- Self-concept and self-esteem (e.g., positive or negative)

Situation Context

Reasons for the communication include the following:

- Information exchange
- Goal achievement
- Problem resolution
- Expression of feelings

Relation Context

The nature of the relationship between the participants involves the following:

- Social, helping, or working relationship
- Level of trust between participants
- Level of self-disclosure between participants
- Shared history of participants
- Balance of power and control

Environmental Context

The physical surroundings in which communication takes place involve the following:

- Privacy level
- Noise level
- Comfort and safety level
- Distraction level

Cultural Context

The sociocultural elements that affect the interaction are as follows:

- Educational level of participants
- Language and self-expression patterns
- Customs and expectations

Adapted from Potter PA, Perry AG: *Fundamentals of nursing,* ed 7, St Louis, 2009, Mosby.

individual has a unique set of values that has been shaped by personal experiences. The hygienist can influence the communication process by exercising tolerance for and understanding of the wide differences of opinion that exist.

Not all clients value oral health. Individuals have reasons, known and unknown, for holding their respective values. A person from an impoverished background may have to prioritize values to survive. Oral health and education may not be highly valued when food, shelter, and clothing are not readily available. On high school campuses, a sugar-free diet may not be valued when candy and soft-drink machines beckon. Water fluoridation may not be valued by people who have been deluged with information from antifluoridationists.

Values can be changed, but experts suggest that they are slow to form and to change. For value change to occur in the oral healthcare environment,[2] oral healthcare professionals must do the following:

- Be aware of their own values and how they affect the choices they make in planning and implementing oral health behavioral change programs.
- Understand the client's values through careful observation and analysis of behavior.
- Avoid imposing their values on a client who has a different set of values.

Sometimes client values related to oral health and disease can be changed by education. The methods used to produce change and the degree of success are dependent on how wide the gap is between the desired value and the client's current value.

Emotions

Emotions are influential in everyday communication. Emotions are strong feelings people have about other people, places, and things in their environment. Fear, wonder, love, sorrow, and shame are examples of strong human emotions that touch all individuals at some time in their lives.

Hygienists who are empathetic may become emotionally involved in their clients' lives. Dental hygiene clients may have serious general health problems that are causing them grief and suffering. The hygienist must be compassionate but must act professionally throughout the process of care.

In contrast, emotions rooted in the hygienist's own personal life should not interfere with client care. For example, Scenario 5-1 is an interesting hypothetic situation.[2]

The hygienist goes to work angered by her husband's lack of understanding. The first client she sees is a 24-year-old mother of three who is divorced and living on welfare. The hygienist cannot allow herself to transfer her anger at her husband to the client's situation. This transfer would prevent her from understanding this client as an individual. If the hygienist is to communicate effectively with the client, she must be aware of her emotions.

SCENARIO 5-1

A young hygienist had an argument with her husband before coming to work. Her husband is just out of law school and is establishing his practice. The hygienist's income is needed for the family's survival. Her husband has proposed that they begin having children. The hygienist knows that she and her husband would have difficulty rearing a family now, particularly because she would soon have to take a leave from work.

Knowledge

Communication can be hindered when knowledge levels differ between the participants. Dental hygiene clients may be highly educated but have an expertise area outside the realm of oral health. A highly technical vocabulary is inappropriate with a client unless terms are explained carefully. Most clients have no need to distinguish between the mesials and distals of their teeth. However, this terminology is essential in professional communication and is commonplace for members of the oral healthcare team. If the dental hygienist uses language the client cannot understand, or "talks down" to the client, the hygienist loses that client's attention and cooperation and lessens the chances that goals will be achieved. The effective dental hygienist monitors client feedback to guide the appropriate level of language usage.

Sociocultural Background

Sociocultural differences are important in social interaction and communication. A dental hygienist who has a broad understanding of cultural diversity is better prepared to communicate with clients from varying backgrounds (see Chapter 6).[3]

Forms of Communication

Interpersonal communication is never static but rather is a dynamic, ongoing process. Messages may be verbal or nonverbal. In nonprofessional communication people rarely analyze the meaning of every gesture or word. In the professional role, however, the dental hygienist must use critical thinking to focus on each aspect of communication to ensure that interactions are purposeful and effective.

Verbal Communication

Using the spoken word to convey a message is **verbal communication**. The most important aspects of verbal communication are vocabulary, **intonation**, clarity, and brevity.[2]

Vocabulary

For communication to be successful, sender and receiver must be able to translate each other's words. Dental jargon sounds like a foreign language to most clients and is to be used only with other oral healthcare professionals. Technical terms must be simplified to an appropriate level to enable clients to know what the dental hygienist is saying. If clients do not understand, they often tune out, and a total breakdown of communication results. By using simple, common language devoid of all superfluous terminology, the hygienist is understood easily and is more likely to give accurate, straightforward, meaningful information. When dental hygienists provide care to clients who speak a different language, an interpreter usually is needed.

Intonation

Intonation is the modulation of the voice. The whisper of confidentiality, the rising crescendo of anger, and the dull tones of despair are examples of how tone of voice dramatically affects a message's meaning.[3] The dental hygienist must be aware of voice tone to avoid sending unintended messages. Moreover, clients' voice tone often provides valuable information about their emotional state.

Clarity

Communication is enhanced when messages sent are simple, brief, and direct. Speaking slowly, enunciating clearly, providing examples to make explanations easier to understand, and repeating the most important part of the message help to achieve clarity. Using short sentences and familiar words to express ideas simply enhances clarity. For example, asking, "Where is your pain?" is better than saying, "Please point out to me the location of your discomfort."[1]

Nonverbal Communication

Nonverbal communication is the use of body language rather than words to transmit a message. Effective nonverbal communication complements and strengthens the message conveyed by verbal communication so that the receiver is less likely to misinterpret the message.

Nonverbal communication includes body movement such as facial expression, eye behavior, gestures, posture and gait, and touch. Because body language is hard to control, it often reveals true feelings. It takes practice, concentration, and sensitivity to others for the dental hygienist to become an astute observer of body language. For example, there probably is something wrong with a client who says she is "fine" but is wringing her hands. Dental hygienists also should be aware of their own body language to avoid sending mixed messages to clients. Saying, "It's good to see you," while frowning does not establish trust and may cause anxiety. To facilitate communication, various aspects of body language are discussed in the following sections.

Facial Expression

The face is the most expressive part of the body. Facial expression often reveals thoughts and feelings and conveys emotions such as anger, fear, sadness, surprise, happiness, and disgust. Clients closely watch the dental hygienist's facial expression. A dental hygienist may frown when concentrating, and a client may interpret the facial expression as anger or disgust. Although it is hard to control facial expressions, the dental hygienist must avoid showing shock or disgust in the client's presence.

Eye Behavior

Eye behavior can be discussed separately from facial features and body movements, but obviously the messages sent depend on all behaviors collectively. Generally, Western culture encourages making eye contact with people while speaking to them. Eye contact often is made before the first spoken word. Thus it is the first message sent when two people meet. The eye can convey trust, interest, or attention. Eye contact is avoided when people feel uncomfortable and is maintained steadily when people are taking an offensive approach as opposed to a defensive approach.

Along with the forehead and eyebrow muscles, the eyes are extremely expressive. Raising an eyebrow can imply a question. Raising both eyebrows may indicate shock or surprise. Narrowed eyes may suggest skepticism, whereas wide-open eyes show amazement.

A dental hygienist works in close proximity to a client's eyes and should always monitor them for nonverbal messages that convey pain or discomfort. In addition, the dental hygienist's eyes are likely to be watched by the client for signs of approval, disapproval, kindness, or displeasure. A face mask hides most of the hygienist's face; therefore eyes become an even more important source of expression and communication.

Gestures

Gesture usually refers to movement of the arms, hands, head, or possibly the whole body. These movements may reveal much about a person's feelings. For example, a client's hands clenching the arm of the dental chair is a cue that the client is experiencing pain, fear, or stress.

Posture and Gait

Posture and body movement may be considered another category of gesture. The way a person moves can tell whether that person is comfortable or uncomfortable, bold or timid. A shift in posture can be an indication of a changing emotional state. Movement toward someone suggests trust and liking. Movement away sends a negative message. The speed at which people move can mean something definite. A slow movement suggests uncertainty; a rapid movement can indicate eagerness, playfulness, or possibly impatience. Posture is affected by a person's size and overall physical appearance. An erect posture and a sharp, snappy step can do much to draw respect to a person of any size.

Touch

Touching is one of the most sensitive means of communication and is related most closely to the human need for freedom from stress. Touch can be reassuring in some contexts. A hand gently placed on a shoulder may mean more to a client than any verbal expression of support. However, people have different attitudes toward being touched. Some are not accustomed to it and may cringe or pull away as the hygienist attempts to comfort them. Touch must be used discriminately to avoid misinterpretation.

The nature of the dental hygiene process of care requires touching clients. The way in which the hygienist touches the client can communicate feelings about the client and the practice of dental hygiene. Rough, jerking movements may send a message of careless indifference, resulting in uncooperative behavior from a client. Accidental touching, such as bumping a person's nose or hitting his or her front teeth with the mouth mirror, also can carry a negative message such as carelessness or haste. A professional, careful approach to touching is appreciated and respected by clients.

Professional Dental Hygiene Relationships

Having a philosophy based on caring and respect for others helps the dental hygienist to establish helping relationships with clients.

The **CARE principle** is used as a simple mnemonic, or memory-assisting technique, to identify aspects of care important to effective dental hygienist–client helping relationships (Box 5-2).

Comfort

Comfort (*C* in the mnemonic) refers to the hygienist's ability to deal with embarrassing or emotionally painful topics related to a client's health; to be aware of the client's physical and emotional response during dental hygiene care; and to

BOX 5-2

CARE Principle

C = Comfort
A = Acceptance
R = Responsiveness
E = Empathy

BOX 5-3

Zones of Personal Space and Touch

Zones of Personal Space

Intimate zone (0 to 18 inches)
- Performing physical assessment
- Placing and removing dental napkin or radiation shield
- Performing intraoral procedures

Personal zone (18 inches to 4 feet)
Sitting next to the client's chair
Taking the client's health, dental, and personal and social histories
Providing oral hygiene education to an individual client

Social zone (4 feet to 12 feet)
- Sitting at a conference table
- Conducting a tobacco-cessation support group

Public zone (12 feet and greater)
- Speaking at a community forum
- Testifying at a legislative hearing
- Lecturing to a class of students

Zones of Touch

Social zone (permission not needed)
- Hands, arms, shoulders, back

Consent and vulnerable zone (permission and special care needed)
- Mouth, neck, head, face

Adapted from Potter PA, Perry AG: *Fundamentals of nursing,* ed 7, St Louis, 2009, Mosby.

provide verbal support to a client who fears oral healthcare procedures. Aspects of dental hygiene practice related to client comfort and communication include effectively addressing a client's loss of teeth and need to wear a prosthetic appliance, a client's inability to seek oral healthcare because of financial difficulties, a client's fear of injections, and clients' discomfort from having their personal space "invaded" during care.

Personal space is invisible and travels with a person. Territoriality refers to the need to maintain and defend one's right to this personal space. During interpersonal communication individuals maintain varying distances between each other depending on their culture, their relationship, and the circumstance. Touching the head and neck area usually is reserved for intimate relationships such as between lovers or a parent and a child. When personal space is violated, people often become defensive and communication becomes ineffective. Because dental hygienists work within the client's intimate zone of personal space, it is important to convey professional confidence, gentleness, and respect when doing so. Zones of personal space and touch are listed in Box 5-3. To meet the client's human need for freedom from stress, the hygienist strives to keep the client's comfort a top priority.

Acceptance

Acceptance refers to the dental hygienist's ability to accept clients as the people they are without allowing any judgment of the clients' attitudes or feelings to interfere with communication. For example, a client may appear unwilling to assume responsibility for his or her health and may be critical or untrusting. The client's poor oral health may seem self-imposed and related to an unhealthy lifestyle. But the client's appearance and attitudes may have deep cultural roots that are unfamiliar to the hygienist. The dental hygienist must develop an attitude of acceptance toward individuals whose values and sociocultural backgrounds seem unusual or foreign (see Chapter 6).

Responsiveness

Responsiveness in a healthcare provider is the ability to reply to messages at the moment they are sent. It requires sensitive alertness to cues that something more must be said. When a client arrives for a dental hygiene appointment and mentions oral discomfort, the comment should be pursued immediately. Scaling and root planing may have been scheduled, but other problems may be an immediate priority and supersede the planned care.

Empathy

Empathy is said to result when "we place ourselves in another's shoes." Empathy means perceiving clients as they see themselves, sensing their hurt or pleasure as they sense it, accepting their feelings, and communicating this understanding of their reality.[2]

In expressing empathy the dental hygienist communicates understanding the importance of the feelings behind a client's statements. Empathy statements are neutral and nonjudgmental. They can be used to establish trust in difficult situations. For example, the dental hygienist may say to an angry client who has lost mobility after a stroke, "It must be very frustrating to know what you want and not be able to do it." This perception of clients' viewpoints helps the dental hygienist to better understand them, their reaction to dental hygiene care, and their capabilities for taking responsibility for their own health.

Therapeutic Communication Techniques

Dental hygiene practice is based on helping relationships. In such relationships the dental hygienist assumes the role of professional helper. The dental hygienist uses therapeutic communication to promote a psychologic climate that facilitates positive change and growth.

Therapeutic communication is a process of sending and receiving messages between a client and a healthcare provider that assists the client to make decisions and reach goals related to comfort and health. No single communication technique works with all clients. One individual may be encouraged to express feelings when the dental hygienist is silent, whereas another may need coaxing with active questioning. Practice and experience, based on a strong theoretic foundation, are required for choosing communication techniques to

BOX 5-4

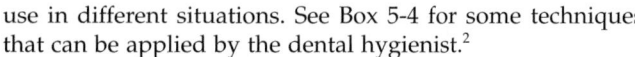

Therapeutic Communication Techniques

- Silence
- Attentive listening
- Humor
- Conveying acceptance
- Related questions
- Paraphrasing
- Clarifying
- Focusing
- Stating observations
- Offering information
- Summarizing

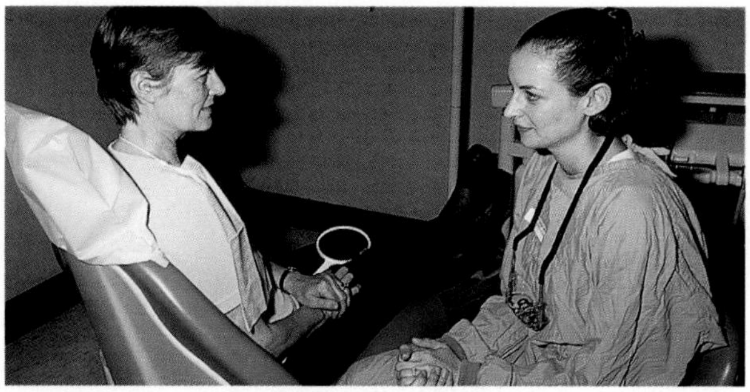

Figure 5-3. Dental hygienist using eye contact to communicate reassurance.

use in different situations. See Box 5-4 for some techniques that can be applied by the dental hygienist.[2]

Silence

Silence can be used effectively in communication because it provides an opportunity for the message senders and receivers to gather and reorganize their thoughts and feelings. During silent moments, nonverbal messages such as loss of eye contact or a wrinkled brow can be sent. Remaining silent may be uncomfortable, but adhering patiently to silence demonstrates the hygienist's willingness to listen and encourages clients to share their thoughts. Skill and timing are required to use silence effectively. The tendency for some is to want to break the silence too soon. Poor timing can interrupt prematurely clients' efforts in choosing words and frustrate their attempts to communicate.

The nature of dental hygiene care often precludes talking by the client. A common complaint, usually shared good naturedly among clients, is that their dental hygienist asks them questions when the hygienist's hands are in their mouths. This typical scenario is unfair to the client. Common courtesy dictates that immediately on asking a question the hygienist removes hands, instruments, and saliva ejectors from the client's mouth to allow the client an opportunity to respond through speaking, not just grunting.

Listening Attentively

Caring involves an interpersonal interaction that is much more than two persons talking back and forth. In a caring relationship, the dental hygienist establishes trust, opens lines of communication, and listens to what the client has to say. Listening attentively is key because it conveys to clients that they have the hygienist's full attention and interest. Listening to the meaning of what a client says helps create a mutual relationship.

The dental hygienist indicates interest by appearing natural and relaxed and facing the client with good eye contact (Figure 5-3). Whatever the services being rendered, the client should remain the center of attention, with the hygienist's ears available to evaluate and respond. Interpersonal attending skills shown in Table 5-1 facilitate active listening and communication.

TABLE 5-1

Checklist of Interpersonal Attending

Skill Area	Criterion
Eye contact	Listener consistently focuses on the face and eyes of the speaker
Body orientation	Listener orients shoulders and legs toward the speaker
Posture	Listener maintains slight forward lean, arms maintained in a relaxed position
Silence	Listener avoids interrupting the speaker and uses periods of silence to facilitate communication
Following cues	Listener uses verbal and nonverbal cues to facilitate communication and indicate interest and attention
Distance	Listener maintains distance of 3-4 feet from speaker
Distractions	Listener avoids distracting behaviors such as pencil tapping, looking at a clock, and extraneous movements

Adapted from Geboy MJ: *Communications and behavior management in dentistry*, Baltimore, 1985, Williams and Wilkins.

Conveying Acceptance

Conveying acceptance requires a tolerant, nonjudgmental attitude toward clients. An open, accepting approach is needed to foster a helping relationship between hygienist and client. Care is taken to avoid nonverbal behavior that may be offensive or that may prevent free-flowing communication. Gestures such as frowning, rolling eyes upward, or shaking the head may communicate disagreement or disapproval to the client. The dental hygienist shows willingness to listen to the client's viewpoint and provide feedback that indicates understanding and acceptance of the person.

Humor

Humor can help decrease client anxiety and embarrassment. Humor is a communication technique that must be used comfortably and naturally with clients of all ages and stages of

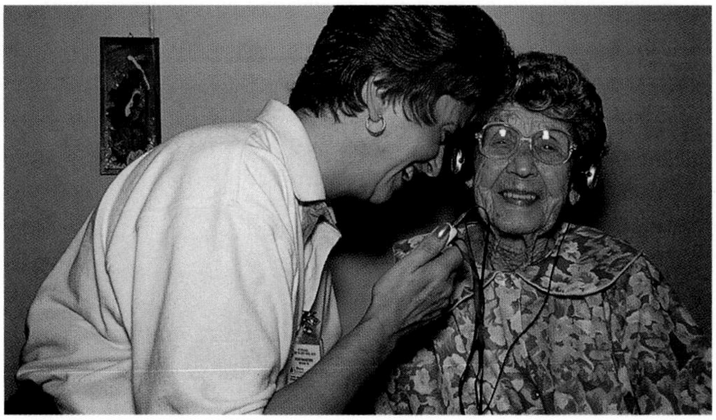

Figure 5-4. Sharing a joke or laughing with clients can assist in reducing stress and support a therapeutic relationship.

development (Figure 5-4). The therapeutic advantages of humor and laughter have been documented. Laughter decreases serum control levels, increases immune activity, and stimulates endorphin release from the hypothalamus. In so doing, it relieves stress-related tension and pain. Cousins described the role of humor in his recovery from two life-threatening illnesses.[4] His experience suggests that laughter and positive emotions are vital to the success of any medical treatment as well as to life in general.

Healthcare personnel and facilities can be perceived as frightening by clients of all ages. Humor as a technique of communication can put people at ease. Even a simple smile can help establish a warm social bond. In her book *Communication in Health Care,* Collins states, "Humor has childlike qualities of playfulness. If one can be playful, one still has vestiges of youth and vigor."[5] The unexpected, the incongruous, the pun, and the exaggeration or understatement are examples of humor that can be effective with younger and older clients.

Asking Questions

One of the most critical and valuable tools in the dental hygienists' arsenal of communication skills is the art of questioning. Among the many types of questions, there are only two basic forms: closed-ended questions, which are directive, and open-ended questions, which are nondirective.

Closed-Ended Questions

Closed-ended questions require narrow answers to specific queries. The answer to these questions is usually "yes" or "no" or some other brief answer. An example is, "Do you want to bleach your teeth?"

Open-Ended Questions

Open-ended questions generally are used to elicit a wide range of responses on a broad topic. Open-ended questions usually have the following characteristics:

- Cannot be answered with a single word or a simple "yes" or "no."
- Begin with *what, how,* or *why.*
- Do not lead the client in a specific direction.
- Encourage dialogue by drawing out the client's feelings or opinions.

BOX 5-5

Examples of Open-Ended Questions

How do you feel about your oral health?
What are you currently doing each day to care for your mouth?
Why do you feel you will never be able to floss regularly?

Open-ended questions are usually more effective than questions that require a simple "yes" or "no" answer. Open-ended questioning allows clients to elaborate and show their genuine feelings by bringing up whatever they think is important (Box 5-5). Skillful questioning by the dental hygienist promotes communication.

Paraphrasing

Paraphrasing means restating or summarizing what the client has just said. Through paraphrasing the client receives a signal that his or her message has been received and understood and is prompted to continue a communication effort by providing further information. The client may say, "I don't understand how I could have periodontal disease. My teeth and gums feel fine. I have absolutely no pain." The hygienist could paraphrase the statement by saying, "You're not convinced that you have periodontal disease or any gum problems because you have no discomfort?" The client may respond, "Right, I just can't believe anything is wrong with my mouth." By actively listening and paraphrasing, the dental hygienist's response allows further analysis of the problem and opens the conversation for communication and problem solving.

The dental hygienist actively listens and analyzes messages received, however, so that the paraphrase is an accurate account not only of what the client actually says but also of what the client feels. For example, if a client sends verbal or nonverbal messages of anger or frustration about being told to floss more, the dental hygienist could say, "It sounds like this situation has really upset you and that you are frustrated with me for not recognizing your efforts." This response encourages clients to communicate further about health problems. Passive listening or silence on the part of the dental hygienist, with no attempt to decode the message, could result in an uncomfortable impasse in the communication process.

Clarifying

At times the message sent by the client may be vague. When clarification is needed, the discussion should be stopped temporarily until confusing or conflicting statements have been understood. For example, consider Scenario 5-2, in which a client has come to the oral care environment for an oral prophylaxis.

SCENARIO 5-2

Client: My mother had pyorrhea and lost all her teeth at a young age. I'm sure it's hereditary. I can only hope to stall it.

Hygienist: Mrs. Thompson, are you having some problem with your teeth or gums now?

In responding this way the hygienist is trying to get clarification. The client's rush of words seems to be related to her own problems, but the hygienist cannot be sure until the client states it clearly (see Table 5-2 for the subcategories of open-ended questions that enhance communication). In addition, the hygienist should be aware that statements made to the client may need clarification. To fulfill their human need for conceptualization and problem solving, clients need to understand why they are asked to comply with a specific home care regimen. In Scenario 5-3, the dental hygienist has completed therapeutic scaling and root planing on the mandibular left quadrant, which has been anesthetized. The more specific the hygienist can be, the clearer the message to the client.

SCENARIO 5-3

Hygienist: Mr. Johnson, after you leave, try not to chew on your left side for awhile.
Client: Do you mean today or for several days?
Hygienist: Oh no, I just mean for a few hours.
Client: What might happen if I do chew on that side? Will it hurt my teeth or gums?
Hygienist: Oh no, I was referring to your anesthesia. I'm afraid you might bite your cheeks or tongue if you chew on that side, because everything is numb. The numbness should be completely gone by about 5:00 PM.

Focusing

Sometimes when clients discuss health-related issues the messages become redundant or rambling. Important information may not surface because the client is off on a tangent. Dental hygienists ask questions to clarify when they are unsure of what the client is talking about. In focusing, however, the hygienist knows what the client is talking about but is having trouble keeping the client on the subject so that data gathering and assessment can be completed. In such cases the dental hygienist encourages verbalization but steers the discussion back on track as a technique to improve communication. Rather than a question, a gentle command may be appropriate, such as, "Please point to the tooth that seems to be causing your discomfort," or "Show me exactly what you do when you floss your back teeth" (Table 5-2).

Stating Observations

Clients may be unaware of the nonverbal messages they are sending. When a client is asked, "How are you, Mrs. Jones?" as a friendly greeting, she may respond, "Oh, just fine." Her appearance, gait, and mannerisms may indicate something different. She may look slightly unkempt, walk with a slow shuffle, and display generally unenthusiastic gestures and facial expressions. When nonverbal cues conflict with the verbal message, stating a simple straightforward observation may open the lines of communication. The hygienist may say, "You appear very tired, Mrs. Jones." This is likely to cause the person to volunteer more information about how she feels without need for further questioning, focusing, or clarifying.

To promote positive communication, however, the dental hygienist uses respectful language. The client may feel sensitive about how observations are worded. Saying a person looks "tired" is different from saying he looks "haggard," which could embarrass or anger him. Other observations that can soften a client's response are stating that teeth are "crowded" rather than "crooked," that a troublesome tongue is "muscular" not "fat," and that gingiva is "pigmented" not "discolored."

Offering Information

Providing clients with detailed information facilitates communication. Although providing information may not be enough to motivate people to change health behaviors, clients have a right to receive information based on the hygienist's

TABLE 5-2

Subcategories of Open-Ended Questions That Enhance Communication

Type	Purpose	Example
Clarifying questions	To seek verification of the content and/or feeling of the client's message	If I am hearing correctly, your major concerns are ____________. Is that so? From what you are telling me, I get the impression you are frustrated, or am I misreading your feelings?
Developmental questions	To draw out a broad response on a narrow topic	Would you please elaborate on that point? Can you give me an example of what you mean by that?
Directive questions	To change the conversation from one topic to another	What was the other issue you wanted to discuss with me?
Third-party questions	To probe indirectly by relating to a client how others feel about a situation and then asking the client to give an opinion or reaction	A lot of people feel our fees are reasonable. What's your opinion?
Testing questions	To assess a client's level of agreement or disagreement about a specific issue	How does that strike you? Do you think you could live with that?

expertise so that they can make health-related decisions based on that information. In any setting, a dental hygienist has a professional obligation to provide health information to all clients, not just to individuals who request information.

Summarizing

Summarizing points discussed at a regularly scheduled appointment focuses attention on the major points of the communicative interaction. For example, the dental hygienist may conclude the appointment with, "Today we discussed the purpose of therapeutic scaling and root planing and the periodontal disease process, and we practiced flossing technique. Remember, you decided to floss daily and to try to slip the floss carefully down below the gum line." If the client is coming in for multiple appointments to receive quadrant or sextant scaling and root planing, the discussion from the previous appointment is summarized before new information is given. Documentation in the client's chart at each appointment reflects topics discussed at the appointment as related to the client's goals.

The summary serves as a review of the key aspects of the information presented so that the client can ask for clarification. Adding new information in the summary may confuse the client; however, a comment about what will be discussed at the next appointment is appropriate. Such a statement may be, "At your next appointment, we will talk about use of the Perio-Aid and continue discussion of the periodontal disease process."

Factors That Inhibit Communication

The dental hygienist unintentionally may impede communication. **Nontherapeutic communication** is a process of sending and receiving messages that does not help clients make decisions or reach goals related to their comfort and health (Box 5-6). These nontherapeutic communication techniques should be avoided by the dental hygienist because they inhibit communication.[2]

Giving an Opinion

A helping relationship fosters the clients' ability to make their own decisions about health. A hygienist may be tempted to offer an opinion, which may weaken the clients' autonomy and jeopardize their need for responsibility for oral health. Clients may volunteer personal information about themselves and may ask for the hygienist's opinion. It is best in such a situation to acknowledge the individual's feelings but to avoid the transfer of decision making from client to hygienist. Scenario 5-4 is a hypothetic situation presenting two possible responses by the dental hygienist in an interaction with a client.

BOX 5-6

Factors That Inhibit Communication

- Giving an opinion
- Offering false reassurance
- Being defensive
- Showing approval or disapproval
- Asking why
- Changing the subject inappropriately

SCENARIO 5-4

Hygienist: Mrs. Smith, you look troubled today.
Client: Well, actually, I'm feeling quite down in the dumps. Yesterday was my birthday and I didn't hear a word from my daughter. I'm sure you wouldn't do such a thing to your mother!
Hygienist: (Response #1) Heavens, no! How terribly inconsiderate of her.
The hygienist may have answered differently:
Hygienist: (Response #2) You seem to feel really disappointed. I'm sorry you're so distressed.

The latter response by the dental hygienist recognizes the client's feelings without expressing an opinion that could make the client feel worse by confirming a doubt she has about her daughter, as in the first response.

Offering False Reassurance

Hygienists may at times offer reassurance when it is not well grounded. It is natural to want to alleviate the client's anxiety and fear, but reassurance may promise something that cannot occur. For example, the dental hygienist should not promise clients that they will experience no discomfort during an anticipated dental treatment. Although the dental hygienist may feel confident that the oral surgeon or periodontist is competent and kind, discomfort may be unavoidable. In addition, when clients are distraught about having periodontal disease it is best not to say, "There's nothing to worry about. You'll be fine." Indeed, depending on the amount of bone loss present and the client's disease susceptibility, the periodontist may not be able to control the disease, even with extensive therapy. Scenario 5-5 illustrates how the dental hygienist can listen to and acknowledge a client's feelings without offering false assurance that the problem is a simple one.

SCENARIO 5-5

Mrs. Frank, a 75-year-old woman, has been told by the dentist that her remaining teeth are hopeless and must be extracted for a full denture placement. The hygienist enters the room as the dentist leaves.
Mrs. Frank: I can't believe this is happening to me. I don't deserve it. I've tried to take good care of my teeth. I'm so distressed. Oh, I'm sorry, I know you don't want to hear about my problems.
Hygienist: Mrs. Frank, I am interested in your feelings about this.

Being Defensive

When clients criticize services or personnel, it is easy for the hygienist to become defensive. A defensive posture may threaten the relationship between dental hygienist and client by communicating to clients that they do not have a right to express their opinions.

In Scenario 5-6 the dental hygienist's response ignores the client's real feelings and hurts future rapport and communication with him.

SCENARIO 5-6

Mr. Tucker has been a regular client in the dental practice for many years. At the last appointment the dental hygienist noted a 2-mm circumscribed white lesion in the retromolar area. Mr. Tucker was a former smoker, and the dentist referred him to an oral surgeon for consultation and possible biopsy of the lesion. The following describes the hygienist-client interaction when Mr. Tucker returns for his periodontal maintenance appointment.

Client: I hope I don't have to see Dr. Herman today.

Hygienist: What's wrong, Mr. Tucker? Dr. Herman usually sees you after your periodontal maintenance care.

Client: He sent me to the oral surgeon and it was a complete waste of my time.

Hygienist: Of course it wasn't. Dr. Herman is an excellent dentist.

Client: You may think so, but he didn't send you for a biopsy for no reason.

Hygienist: Mr. Tucker, that lesion looked very unusual. I'm sure Dr. Herman made a good decision in sending you.

Instead, it would have been better for the hygienist to use the therapeutic communication techniques of active listening to verify what the client has to say and to learn why he is upset or angry. Active listening does not mean that the dental hygienist agrees with what is being said but rather conveys interest in what the client is saying. This latter approach is illustrated in Scenario 5-7.

SCENARIO 5-7

Client: I hope I don't have to see Dr. Herman today.

Hygienist: You sound upset. Can you tell me something about it?

Client: I just don't think he should have sent me to that oral surgeon.

Hygienist: You think the visit there was unnecessary?

Client: Yes. I didn't mind the biopsy, the results were negative, but first I got lost trying to find the place, then I couldn't find a parking place, then they made me wait for 2 hours, and finally they charged me a fortune for the procedure. Actually, I didn't mind the cost as much as the inconvenience.

Some care in listening led to discovery of the source of the client's anger, which was the inconvenience of a particular oral surgeon's location, parking, and office procedures. By avoiding defensiveness and applying active listening and paraphrasing, the hygienist allowed Mr. Tucker to vent his anger. Therefore communication was facilitated, not blocked.

Showing Approval or Disapproval

Showing either approval or disapproval in certain situations can be detrimental to the communication process. Excessive praise may imply to the client that the hygienist thinks the behavior being praised is the only acceptable one. Often clients may reveal information about themselves because they are seeking a way to express their feelings; they are not necessarily looking for approval or disapproval from the dental hygienist. In Scenario 5-8 the hygienist's response cannot be interpreted as neutral.

SCENARIO 5-8

Client: I've been walking to my dental appointments for years. My daughter offered to drive me today and I accepted. She feels the walk has become too much for me.

Hygienist: I'm so glad you didn't walk over. You definitely made the right decision. Your daughter should drive you to your appointments from now on.

The discussion in Scenario 5-8 is likely to stop with the dental hygienist's statements. The client probably sees the hygienist's viewpoint as supportive of her daughter's. Perhaps the woman is better off having her daughter drive her. It is also possible that she is capable of walking, likes the exercise, and enjoys the independence of getting to her own appointments. The dental hygienist's strong statements of approval may inhibit further communication.

In addition, behaviors that communicate disapproval cause clients to feel rejected, and their desire to interact further with the dental hygienist may be weakened. Disapproving statements may be issued by a dental hygienist who is not thinking carefully about how the client may react. Scenario 5-9 exemplifies a dental hygienist's response that communicates hasty disapproval.

SCENARIO 5-9

Client: I've been working so hard at flossing! I only missed 2 or 3 days last week.

Hygienist: Two or 3 days without flossing! You'll have to do better than that. Your inflammation will not improve at that rate.

Instead of this response the dental hygienist may have said, "You're making progress. Tell me more about your activities on those 3 days when you weren't able to floss. Perhaps together we could find a better way of integrating flossing into your lifestyle."

Asking Why

When people are puzzled by another's behavior, the natural reaction is to ask, "Why?" When dental hygienists discover that clients have not been following recommendations, they may feel a natural inclination to ask why this has occurred. Clients may interpret such a question as an accusation. They may feel resentment, leading to withdrawal and a lack of **motivation** to communicate further with the dental hygienist.

Efforts to search for reasons why the client has not practiced the oral healthcare behaviors as recommended can be facilitated by simply rephrasing a probing "why" question. For example, rather than saying, "Why haven't you used the oral irrigator?" the hygienist may say, "You haven't used the oral irrigator. Is something wrong?" For anxious clients, rather than asking, "Why are you upset?" the hygienist may say, "You seem upset. Would you like to talk about it?"

Changing the Subject Inappropriately

Changing the subject abruptly shows a lack of empathy and could be interpreted as rude. In addition, it prevents the client from discussing an issue that may have important implications for care. Scenario 5-10 is a sample client–dental hygienist interaction.

SCENARIO 5-10

Hygienist: Hello, Mrs. Johnson. How are you today?
Client: Not too well. My gums are really sore.
Hygienist: Well, let's get you going. We have a lot to do today.

The dental hygienist's response shows insensitivity and an unwillingness to discuss Mrs. Johnson's complaint. It is possible that the client has a periodontal or periapical abscess or some other serious problem. The dental hygienist is remiss in ignoring the client's attempt to communicate a problem. Communication has been stalled, and the client's oral health jeopardized. The client should be given an opportunity to elaborate on the message she is trying to send.

Communication Across the Life Span

Dental hygienists assume the role of educator when clients have learning needs. The communication and the teaching and learning processes are applied across the life span but must be tailored to each client's age level. **Andragogy** is the art and science of helping the older person learn, whereas pedagogy is the art and science of teaching children. **Pedagogy** assumes that the learners are young, dependent recipients of knowledge and that subject matter has been decided arbitrarily by a teacher who is preparing them for their future. The teacher is the authority in this model, and little regard is given to how learners feel about the material or to their contribution to the process. Andragogy, on the other hand, assumes that the initiative to learn comes from the learner, who is viewed as entering the learning process with a background of prior knowledge and experience. The teacher is a facilitator who learns along with the student, who in turn benefits from the teacher's contribution. The adult learner has a diverse history of experiences and is, in general, independent and self-directed. Pedagogy assumes that the child learner is moving toward becoming a fully matured human being, whereas andragogy assumes that the learner has arrived at this point.[6] The purpose of this section is to address considerations for communication with clients throughout the life span. Table 5-3 summarizes the key developmental

TABLE 5-3

Techniques for Communicating with Clients Through the Life Span

Level	Developmental Characteristics	Communication Techniques
Preschoolers	Beginning use of symbols and language; egocentric, focused on self; concrete in thinking and language	Allow child to use his or her five senses to explore oral healthcare environment (handle a mirror, feel a prophy cup, taste and smell fluoride, etc.) Use simple language and concrete, thorough explanations of exactly what is going to happen Let child see and feel cup "going around" or compressed air before putting in his or her mouth
School-age children	Less egocentric; shift to abstract thought emerges, but much thought still concrete	Demonstrate equipment, allow child to question, give simple explanations of procedures
Adolescents	Concrete thinking evolves to more complex abstraction; can formulate alternative hypotheses in problem solving; may revert to childish manner at times; usually enjoy adult attention	Allow self-expression and avoid being judgmental Give thorough, detailed answers to questions Be attentive
Adults	Broad individual differences in values, experiences, and attitudes; self-directed and independent in comparison with children; have assumed certain family and social roles; periods of stability and change	Appropriately applied therapeutic communication techniques: maintaining silence, listening attentively, conveying acceptance, asking related questions, paraphrasing, clarifying, focusing, stating observations, offering information, summarizing, reflective responding
Older adults	May have sensory loss of hearing, vision; may have high level of anxiety; may be willing to comply with recommendations, but forgetful	Approach with respect, speak clearly and slowly Give time for client to formulate answers to questions and to elaborate Be attentive to nonverbal communication

Adapted from Potter PA, Perry AG: *Fundamentals of nursing: concepts, process, and practice,* ed 3, St Louis, 1993, Mosby.

characteristics at different age levels over the life span and those communication techniques appropriate at each level.[7]

Preschool and Younger School-Age Children

Communicating with children requires an understanding of the influence of growth and development on language, thought processes, and motor skills. Children begin development with simple, concrete language and thinking and move toward the more complex and abstract. Communication techniques and teaching methods also can increase in complexity as the child grows older.

Nonverbal communication is more important with preschoolers than it is with the school-age child whose communication is better developed. The preschooler learns through play and enjoys a gamelike atmosphere. Therefore dentists often call the dental engine their "whistle" or the "buzzy bee," and hygienists often refer to their polishing cup as the "whirly bird" and the saliva ejector as "Mr. Thirsty." Imaginary names help lighten the healthcare experience for small children. Oral health professionals are advised to use simple, short sentences, familiar words, and concrete explanations.

The Guidance-Cooperation Model

Five principles for communicating with young children are suggested in the Guidance-Cooperation Model.[8] Because the model is neither permissive nor coercive, it is ideally suited for the preschool or young school-age child. According to this model, health professionals are placed in a parental role whereby the child is expected to respect and cooperate with them. The principles inherent to the Guidance-Cooperative Model follow.

Tell the Child the Ground Rules Before and During Treatment

Let the child know exactly what is expected of him or her. A comment such as, "You must do exactly as I ask and please keep your hands in your lap like my other helpers," prepares the child to meet expectations. Structuring time so that the child also knows what to expect may be useful. For fluoride treatments, a timer should be set and made visible so that the child knows how long it will be before the trays will come out of his or her mouth.

Praise All Cooperative Behavior

When children respond to a directive such as, "Open wide," praise them with, "That's good! Thank you!" When children sit quietly, remember to praise them for cooperation. It is a mistake to ignore behavior until it is a problem.

Keep Your Cool

Ignore negative behavior such as whining if it is not interfering with the healthcare. Showing anger only makes matters worse. Showing displeasure and using a calm voice for statements such as, "I get upset [or unhappy, etc.] when you …" is likely to communicate the point more successfully.

Use Voice Control

A sudden change in volume can gain attention from a child who is being uncooperative. Modulate voice tone and volume as soon as the child begins to respond.

Allow the Child to Play a Role

Let the child make some structured choices. For example, ask, "Would you like strawberry or grape flavored fluoride today?" Most younger children enjoy the role of "helper" and are happy to hold mirrors, papers, and pencils and to receive praise for their good work.

Avoid Attempting to Talk a Child into Cooperation

Do not give lengthy rationales for the necessity of procedures. Rather, acknowledge the child's feelings by making statements such as, "I understand that you don't like the fluoride treatment; however, we must do it to make your teeth stronger. I understand that you would rather be outside playing, but we need to polish your teeth now." Then firmly request the child's attention and cooperation and proceed with the service.

The preschool and school-age child are eager to learn and explore but may have fears about the oral healthcare environment, personnel, and treatment. Studies have shown that dental fears begin in childhood, and making early oral care a positive experience is necessary if the dental hygienist is interested in the client's long-term attitude toward oral health.[4] Rapport must be established as a foundation for cooperation and trust. The best teaching approaches for younger children follow behavioral rather than cognitive theory. Positive reinforcement used as immediate feedback, short instructional segments with simplified language and content that is concrete rather than abstract, close monitoring of progress, and encouragement for independence in the practice of oral hygiene skills are indicated.

Older School-Age Children and Adolescents

Adolescence is not a single stage of development. The rate at which children progress through adolescence and the psychologic states that accompany the changes can vary considerably from one child to another.[5] In early adolescence (about 13 to 15 years old), children may rather suddenly demonstrate an ambivalence toward parents and other adults, manifested by questioning of adult values and authority. By late adolescence (18 years and older) much of the ambivalence is gone, and values that characterize the adult years have emerged. Friendship patterns in early and middle adolescence are usually intense as the child begins to explore companionship outside the family and become established as an independent person (Figure 5-5).

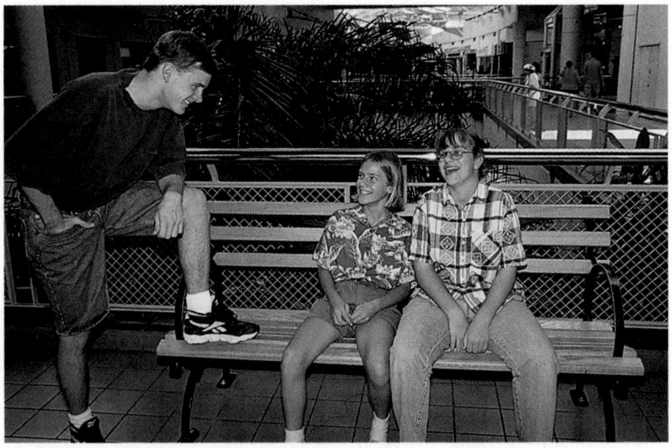

Figure 5-5. Interacting with peers helps to establish independence.

Some common complaints from the adolescent's point of view can sensitize health professionals for positive interactions with this group of young people. First, a frequently voiced complaint of adolescents is that adults do not listen to them. They seem to feel that adults are in too much of a hurry, appear to be looking for certain answers, or listen only to what they want to hear. A second complaint is that too often a conversation turns into unsolicited advice or a mini-lecture. A young person, asked to describe specific experiences in dentistry, related the following[8]:

> My dentist bugged me a lot. He would become angry if I felt pain. He pushed my hair around and lectured constantly about young people and their hair.

Other less-common complaints from adolescents are that they are patronized, that they do not understand questions being asked, and that adults lack humor.

Dental hygienists should consider carefully these complaints and practice behaviors that enhance communication with adolescents. Being attentive and allowing the adolescent time to talk enhance rapport and communication. Some rapport-building questions at the beginning of the appointment may relate to family, school, personal interests, or career intentions. It is useful to have some knowledge of the contemporary interests of adolescents, which may include trends in music, sports, and fashion. They want a sense of being understood and do not want to be judged or lectured.

Adolescents have a strong human need for responsibility. An astute dental hygienist can use these unfulfilled needs to motivate the adolescent client to adopt oral self-care behaviors. This educational approach, based on human needs theory, can enhance adolescents' sense of personal responsibility toward the care of their mouths. So that adolescents do not feel singled out, a dental hygienist may say, "We encourage all of our adult clients to floss daily. This is because we know it works. We've seen the results." Teenagers do not feel patronized or confused if questions and advice are offered in a sincere, straightforward manner.

Adults

Havinghurst delineated three developmental stages for adults and listed common adult concerns at each stage.[7] Although communication techniques may not differ greatly for the adult stages, knowledge of general differences in characteristics among age groups can enlighten the hygienist about typical concerns of clients at different periods of adulthood. An awareness of how priorities in life change for adults as they develop can help the hygienist identify learning needs and "teachable moments" for different clients. The Havinghurst adult stages are summarized in Box 5-7 according to early adulthood, middle age, and late maturity. The dental hygienist should be aware, without asking personal questions, that young adults may be trying to institute oral self-care behaviors while adjusting to major life stresses such as bringing up young children, managing a home, or starting a demanding career. Adults in the middle years may be more settled in careers and have less responsibility for child care but may be involved heavily in social responsibilities, adjusting to their personal physical changes, or the demands of caring for aging parents. Older adults may be adjusting to decreasing physical strength, a chronic health problem, retirement, or death of a spouse. The elderly population is a highly diversified group (Figure 5-6). The wide variations in health and psychologic states dictate the necessity of careful assessment of each individual (see Chapter 55).

Communication approaches appropriate for adults are the therapeutic communication techniques discussed previously

BOX 5-7

Havinghurst's Description of the Adult Developmental Stages

Early Adulthood

Selecting a mate
Learning to live with a marriage partner
Starting a family
Bringing up young children
Managing a home
Getting started in an occupation
Taking on civic responsibilities
Finding a congenial social group

Middle Age

Achieving adulthood and social responsibilities
Establishing and maintaining an economic standard of living
Assisting one's children to become adults
Developing durable leisure-time activities
Relating to one's marriage partner as a person
Accepting and adjusting to physical change
Adjusting to one's aging parent

Late Maturity

Adjusting to decreasing physical strength and to death
Adjusting to retirement and to reduced income
Adjusting to death of one's marriage partner
Establishing an explicit affiliation with one's age group
Meeting social and civic obligations
Establishing satisfactory physical living arrangements in light of physical infirmities

Adapted from Darkenwald GG, Merriam SB: *Adult education: foundations of practice*, New York, 1982, Harper and Row.

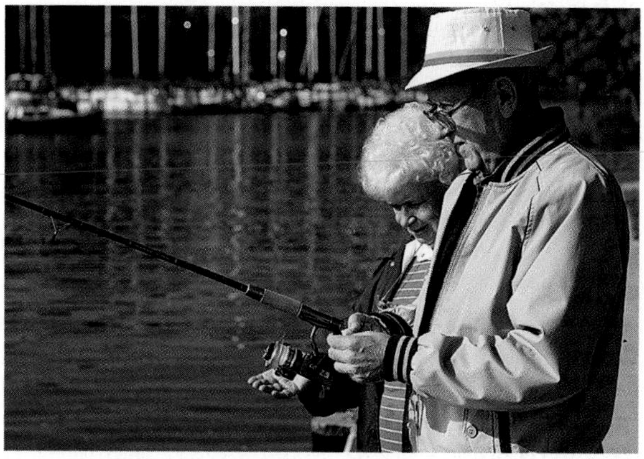

Figure 5-6. A retired couple enjoying fishing together.

in this chapter. In using the techniques, the dental hygienist must be familiar with the adult developmental stages and aware of what demands may be preventing adults of the different stages from easily making oral healthcare behavioral changes. Modern adult learning theory has been supported by some basic assumptions (Box 5-8). Keeping these assumptions in mind facilitates communication with adults who become "learners" as dental hygienists become "teachers" in the healthcare setting. These assumptions can enhance communication and the dental hygiene educator's approach to teaching adults.

For more specific details about individual behavioral theories to promote behavior change, visit the Evolve website Chapter 5 supplemental resources and materials.

BOX 5-8

Assumptions Related to Adult Learners

- Adults are motivated to learn as they experience needs and interests that learning will satisfy; therefore these are the appropriate starting points for organizing adult learning activities.
- Adults are more likely than children or adolescents to acknowledge their needs readily. Mature adults know from past experience how to recognize needs and are motivated to seek information (education) to satisfy these needs.
- Adult's orientation to learning is life-centered; therefore the appropriate units for organizing adult learning are life situations, not subjects.
- Adults are used to learning from everyday events rather than from books and formal lectures. They respond well to anecdotes about other clients' experiences with oral hygiene regimens because they identify with those individuals and their experiences. The dental hygienist may remark, "I have heard such good testimonials from my clients who have begun to floss regularly. They say their mouths feel so much healthier and do not feel really clean unless they floss every day." This statement is likely to have more impact on the client than simply providing information on the subject of flossing.
- Experience is the richest resource for adults' learning; therefore the core methodology of adult education is the analysis of experience.
- When adults return for their maintenance care, the dental hygienist should help them analyze their experiences in trying to institute new self-care procedures. For example, if clients are experiencing difficulty in flossing technique or in incorporating flossing into a busy schedule, they should be encouraged to discuss the problem and receive help from the dental hygienist in developing solutions.
- Adults have a deep need to be self-directing; therefore the role of the teacher is to engage in a process of mutual inquiry with them rather than to transmit his or her knowledge to them and then evaluate their conformity to it.
- The dental hygienist engages adults in discussions that lead to problem solving with participation. The hygienist does not dictate solutions or expect adults to follow rules of oral hygiene that they have had no part in developing.
- Individual differences among people increase with age; therefore adult education must make optimal provision for differences in style, time, and pace of learning.
- The dental hygienist expects people to differ widely in their responses to a particular educational methodology. Although adults are similar in that learning for them is life centered, their individual histories of life experiences differ greatly.

Motivational Interviewing

In the communication process a dental hygienist is striving constantly to influence the client's motivation to perform recommended oral health behaviors. Motivation can be defined as the impulse that leads an individual to action. This section highlights motivational interviewing[1] as a recommended approach to promote client behavior change.

Motivational interviewing[1] is an approach designed to facilitate resolution of client issues that inhibit positive behavior by actively engaging the client in the communication process.

The motivational interview is a form of client-centered communication to help clients get "unstuck from the ambivalence that prevents a specific behavioral change." It is a philosophic approach to client-centered education that emphasizes the following:

- Collaboration, not persuasion
- Eliciting information, not imparting information
- Client's autonomy, not authority of the expert

In this approach to behavioral change, the client does most of the talking with the dental hygienist listening carefully. The goal of motivational interviewing is to have the client voice the arguments for positive change, which is called "**change talk**." Examples of "change talk" would be reasons for concern about their current behavior, or talking about the good things to be gained if they made the recommended behavior change. An example of change talk would be a client saying, "I know I need to floss more because I am really concerned that I have bad breath." Another example of change talk would be a client saying, "I know if I brushed and flossed more, my gums would not bleed so much. My mother had to have a denture because she had gum disease. I do not want that to happen to me." Thus, any time a client voices an advantage of desired change, the dental hygienists affirms the client's comment by saying something such as, "Well, that's a really important point."

Tools for eliciting change talk in motivational interviewing are the following:

- Open-ended questions because they allow clients to express themselves
- **Affirming change talk** is critical to reinforce the client's statement about the advantage of making the recommended change
- **Reflective responding** (repeating back what the client said) to communicate "Here is what I heard you say." Acknowledging the clients by reflecting back what you heard them say, decreases resistance and opens up opportunity for further dialogue
- **Summarizing** results of dialogue
  - The Process of Addressing Ambivalence in Motivational Interviewing

Motivational interviewing "engages" clients to help them resolve ambivalence so that they can make a decision to perform the recommended behavior. In this client interaction the dental hygienist explores both sides of the ambivalence by asking clients, for example, the benefit of flossing and then asking if they have any concerns about not flossing. The dental hygienist should never argue with the client. Raising only one side of the argument causes an ambivalent person to defend the opposite point of view, which may cause what is known as the paradoxical effect. The **paradoxical effect** occurs when the client becomes more committed to refrain from doing the recommended desired behavior. In psychology, there is a saying: "As I hear myself talk, I learn what I believe." Therefore it is important to explore BOTH sides of the ambivalence and to resist the "yes, but ..." syndrome when the client voices what is good about not flossing (or whatever the undesirable behavior may be). When the dental hygienist tries to persuade ambivalent clients to adopt the dental hygienist's point of view, it causes these clients to defend the opposite point of view, which often results in a behavioral outcome that is the opposite behavior the dental hygienist intended to promote.

Therefore, if a client refuses to follow the dental hygienist's oral health recommendation, it is important to support the client's decision by the following:

- Stating that the dental hygienist understands the client is not ready to engage in the recommended behavior now
- Offering some written information on the benefits of engaging in the recommended behavior perhaps for clients to read at their leisure
- Informing clients that the hygienist is ready to help when, and if, they become ready to make the recommended behavioral change
- Asking clients' permission to revisit the issue in the future to assess where they are in their decision-making process
- Noting in the client's electronic record to ask again about the issue at the next visit

In summary, motivational interviewing[1] is an approach designed to facilitate resolution of client issues that inhibit positive behavior change by actively listening to and engaging the client in the communication process. Becoming comfortable with motivational interviewing as a client behavior-change tool enhances client communication and positive outcomes in terms of compliance with recommendations to promote oral health.

CLIENT EDUCATION TIPS

- Establish a partnership to maintain optimal oral hygiene health for the client.
- Provide the most accurate oral health information and feedback on the client's healthcare options, but respect the client's wishes regarding healthcare decisions.
- Consider cultural and age-appropriate needs of the client in all health education efforts.
- Consider theoretic research in all health promotion efforts.

LEGAL, ETHICAL, AND SAFETY ISSUES

- Clients have the right to accept or reject the dental hygiene care plan and still retain the respect of the dental hygienist.
- It is important to meet the client's need for conceptualization and understanding of health information to promote health literacy and informed oral healthcare decisions.
- The client has the right to personalized, up-to-date, evidence-based recommendations and care from the dental hygienist.

KEY CONCEPTS

- Communication during the dental hygiene process of care is a dynamic interaction between the dental hygienist and the client that involves verbal and nonverbal components.
- Factors that may affect the communication process include internal factors of the client and the dental hygienist (e.g., perceptions, values, emotions, and knowledge), the nature of their relationship, the situation prompting communication, and the environment.
- Some communication approaches are therapeutic and helpful in assisting clients to make decisions and attain goals related to their comfort and health. Other approaches are nontherapeutic and unsuccessful in helping clients make decisions and attain goals related to their comfort and health.
- Communication techniques used by the dental hygiene clinician must be flexible to relate to the full range of client ages through the life span.
- Motivational interviewing is an approach designed to facilitate resolution of client issues that inhibit positive behavior by actively engaging the client in the communication process.
- Motivational interviewing emphasizes collaboration, eliciting information from the client, and respecting client autonomy.
- The goal of motivational interviewing is to have the client voice the arguments for positive change which is called "change talk."
- The tools of motivational interviewing are open-ended questions, affirming change talk, reflective responding, and summarizing the results of the dialogue.
- Motivational interviewing can be useful in addressing behavioral problems dental hygienists face every day.

CRITICAL THINKING EXERCISES

1. Identify therapeutic and nontherapeutic communication techniques by name as two people role-play the following client–oral healthcare educator sessions.
   - In the first session, the "client" should improvise a story of frustration with his or her current oral hygiene regimen by explaining that a heavy workload, family responsibilities, or other interference makes it difficult to maintain a good home care regimen. While glancing at a list of the possible responses as a prompt, the "dental hygienist" tries to respond with only therapeutic comments. Classroom listeners should try to determine which specific categories of therapeutic communication fit the educator's comments.
   - In the second session, the "dental hygienist" glances at the list of possible responses, and answers with mostly nontherapeutic responses. Classroom listeners should try to determine which specific categories of nontherapeutic communication fit the dental hygenist's comments.
2. Considering your personality, identify an unhealthy behavioral practice of your own. Engage in motivational interviewing with a student-partner to consider why you continue the unhealthy behavior.

REFERENCES

1. Miller W, Rollnick S: *Motivational interviewing: preparing people for change*, ed 2, New York, 2002, Guilford Press.
2. Potter PA, Perry AG: *Fundamentals of nursing*, ed 7, St Louis, 2009, Mosby.

3. Heineken J, McCoy N: Establishing a bond with clients of different cultures. *Home Healthcare Nurse* 18:45, 2000.
4. Cousins N: *The healing heart*, New York, 1984, Avon Books.
5. Collins M: *Communication in health care: understanding and implementing effective human relationships*, St Louis, 1977, Mosby.
6. Dembo MH: *Teaching for learning: applying educational psychology in the classroom*, ed 4, New York, 1991, Longmans.
7. Havinghurst RJ: *Developmental tasks and education*, New York, 1952, McKay.
8. Weinstein P, Getz T, Milgrom P: *Oral self-care: strategies for preventive dentistry*, Reston, Va, 1991, Reston.
9. National Cancer Institute: *Theory at a glance: a guide for health promotion practice*, ed 2, NIH Publication No. 05-3896, Bethesda, Md, 2005, U.S. Department of Health and Human Services, National Institute of Health.

ACKNOWLEDGMENT

The author acknowledges Sandra K. Rich and Hope Oliver for their past contributions to this chapter.

EVOLVE RESOURCES

Please visit http://evolve.elsevier.com/Darby/hygiene for additional practice and study support tools.

CHAPTER 6

Cultural Competence

Devan Leonardi Darby, Ron J.M. Knevel

COMPETENCIES

1. Reflect on the influence of cultural differences in the interaction between the oral health professional and client.
2. Discuss the concepts of culture, cultural competence, and cultural sensitivity, including subcultures, ethnocentrism, and stereotyping, and do the following:
   - Apply the diversity continuum in communication.
   - Apply creative solutions for culturally sensitive care.
3. Describe and identify cultural barriers to oral healthcare and achievement of optimal health, including shared decision making and inequality and poverty.
4. Explain the importance of culture and health literacy in health communication.
5. Describe how to implement the dental hygiene process in a cross-culture environment, including:
   - Develop cultural competence through self-awareness and exploration of cultural self-identity and the identity of others.
   - Acquire a transcultural perspective.

Globalization has lead to more culturally diverse societies. Regularly the oral health professional encounters clients with different backgrounds, belief systems, cultures, values, attitudes, norms, traditions, and languages. Cultural differences between the clinician and the client can serve as a barrier to effective communication; as a consequence this can lead to client and clinician dissatisfaction, decreased trust, poor adherence, and adverse health outcomes. An important skill that should be acquired by all health professionals is cultural competence. Improved communication among cultural groups improves the quality of the health care. Merely increasing the knowledge of health professionals of cultural differences is not very effective. The development of cultural competence and acquiring a transcultural perspective is essential. **Cultural competence** is "the ability of a care provider to interact with clients who are different from them."[1] Oral health professionals must understand local cultures and culturally influenced healthcare practices to communicate with, educate, and motivate people from diverse racial and ethnic groups so that they can achieve optimal health.

Culture, Cultural Competence, and Cultural Sensitivity

"Understand the differences; act on the commonalities."

Andrew Masondo, African National Congress, 1993

Culture includes the rules of behavior that each person learns to adapt successfully to live within a particular group. **Culture** is a set of guidelines that one can inherit as a member of a particular group or society. It influences the way the members of that society or group view the world. Each cultural group has mechanisms for the transmission of agreed guidelines and views to the next generation. Members slowly acquire a group-specific cultural lens, or way of viewing the world, which influences how members behave in relation to others. Not all individuals who are born and raised within one culture embrace its normative values and attitudes. Culture is a fluid concept, changing and adapting to different developments and environments (Figure 6-1).

A **subculture** is a group of people who have developed interests or goals different from the primary culture, based on occupation, sexual orientation, age, social class, or religion. Although individuals within the same culture may share commonalities in lifestyles and basic beliefs, differences may exist between individuals from different subcultures, especially in attitudes, interests, goals, and dialects. For example, dental hygienists can be viewed as members of a subculture (dental hygiene) with unique philosophic attitudes, practices, beliefs, and values. Many overlapping subcultures may be used to classify a single individual within the predominant culture.

"If you approach each new person you meet in a spirit of adventure, you will find yourself endlessly fascinated by the new channels of thought and experience and personality that you encounter."

Eleanor Roosevelt (1884-1964)

Culture and Health

Often cultural norms contribute to how members of a specific group determine explanations for ill health, health expectations, and to whom they turn for treatment if they become ill. Health and illness not only are physical conditions but also are based on perceptual judgments. The way a person understands illness—oral or systemic—largely is determined culturally. For example, clients in certain cultures may believe that poor oral health is predetermined, that tooth loss is an expected part of aging, or that their oral health status is a result of moral or religious behavior. These beliefs and practices can facilitate or act as barriers to accessing health care services. The oral health professional must realize that clients within any cultural group have wide individual variability: sometimes with sociocultural health beliefs that do not match the clinician's perspective (Figure 6-1).

Cultural differences exist in every clinical encounter and must be assessed conscientiously. Awareness of the biases

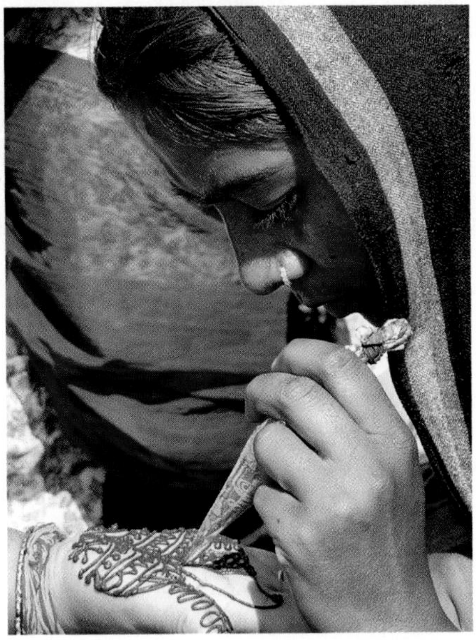

Figure 6-1. Role of symbols in culture: creating henna tattoos during a holy festival in Nepal. (Courtesy Ron J.M. Knevel, RDH, B. Health, Med.)

inherent to one's own culture and subculture is critical to gaining the trust of any client. Becoming self-aware is important when trying to understand the culture of another person. Only a self-aware clinician is able to reflect and understand his or her own reactions to a client and to reflect on the extent to which personal bias may influence the situation. Ethnocentrism refers to the belief that one's culture is superior to that of others. Ethnocentric behavior is characterized as judgmental, condescending, insulting, and narrow-minded, and it makes it difficult for healthcare providers to care for clients who are different from them. It is easy to fall prey to ethnocentrism if blinded to the prejudices, conscious or subconscious, that may influence the clinician's thinking and behavior. The clinician must continually self-assess and reflect on how personal values and beliefs affect daily practice to avoid the pitfalls of ethnocentrism and engage a diverse selection of clients.

Another pitfall in cross-cultural communication is stereotyping. Stereotyping is the often-erroneous assumption that a person possesses certain characteristics or traits simply because he or she is a member of a particular group. Stereotyping fails to recognize the uniqueness of the individual and prevents accurate and unbiased perceptions of those who appear different. Stereotyping clouds perceptions and makes dental hygienists less effective as professionals and human beings. Although stereotyping may provide a comfortable foundation in a strange environment with new people, an accurate assessment always should be made of another human being without the bias inherent in stereotyping. Taking the time to learn about other people rather than relying on popular generalizations is an important step toward eliminating stereotypic thinking.

Developing a genuine interest in learning about traditions, characteristics, and beliefs of other cultures is the best way to ensure that culturally competent care is provided. This means being sensitive to the fact that there are basic differences in the ways people from different cultures communicate, such as through the use of different words, vocal inflection, and body language. For example, different hand gestures may be misinterpreted in some cultures. Calling a client by first name may be considered inappropriate. Differences may be experienced in relation to eye contact or the comfort level with proximity and physical contact. The care provider must take an active role in gaining an understanding of the client's culture and health beliefs. Clients are usually willing to share their ideas and customs with those who express a willingness to understand them. Clinicians do not need extensive knowledge of every cultural practice and belief. By displaying genuine interest and by asking clients to share their beliefs, clinicians increase their cultural knowledge as they practice, without stereotyping. People from most cultural groups react positively to many nonverbal behaviors associated with respect and genuine interest.

Describe at least five stereotypes.

Developing Cultural Competence

"Knowing yourself is not so much about introspection and interaction. To know yourself is to realize that you are more than the little self that has been given to you by your history—the pattern that others made—that your true self is, in truth, much larger and includes other people, other cultures, other species even. That life is less about being and more about interbeing. We come to know ourselves, then, through coming to know each other. And the deeper that knowledge, the richer and more creative the world we build together."

Dr. Daniel Martin,
International Communities for the Renewal of the Earth, 1999

Cultural competence involves awareness of one's own biases or prejudices and is rooted in respect, validation, and openness toward differences. Cultural competence begins with the awareness of one's own cultural beliefs and practices, and the recognition that others have different beliefs than one's own. It also implies that there is more than one way of doing the same thing in the correct manner.[2] The culturally competent clinician views all clients as unique individuals and is aware that experiences, beliefs, values, and language affect the perceptions of clinical service delivery and overall clinical outcome. Lack of familiarity with non-Western medical philosophies and traditions can create a barrier to effective care and communication. For example, a Muslim client's refusal to have his teeth polished and treated with topical fluoride on a day of fasting should not be interpreted erroneously as a lack of interest in professional care but rather as a manifestation of his strong faith. Clients from various cultures may have different definitions of human attractiveness and may have vastly different opinions about what constitutes a wholesome facial image. It is the responsibility of the culturally competent clinician to elicit and understand the client's perspective and social context and to apply a variety of communication strategies to appeal to the client's individual cultural identity. With culturally sensitive care, the oral health professional resolves confusion, reconciles points of disagreement, and strives to achieve a common understanding of the health condition and treatment options.

Cultural sensitivity means being aware that cultural differences and similarities exist that affect values, learning, and behavior.[3] Culturally sensitive care starts with the clinician. The characteristics of culturally sensitive communication are summarized in the diversity continuum in communication model (Figure 6-2). The model emphasizes self-awareness and self-exploration of the clinician as a first requirement to provide culturally competent care. The clinician is encouraged to ask clients about their health beliefs and their cultural backgrounds. This ongoing cycle leads to improved adherence and health outcomes, while at the same time increasing the cultural knowledge of the care provider. Taking these steps in the initial phase of the client encounter results in negotiating a final treatment decision or care plan based on mutual understanding of the client and the provider.[4-6]

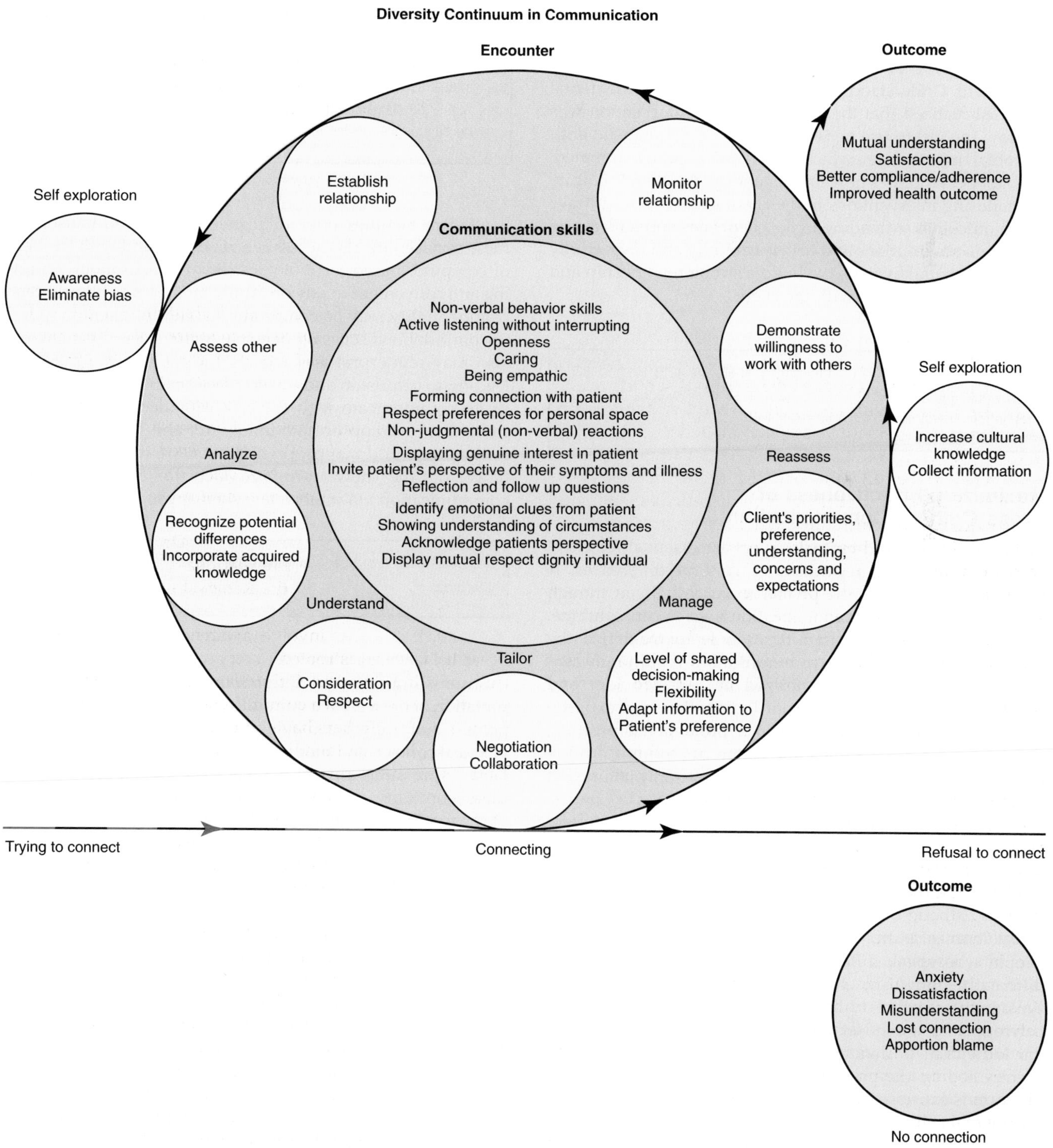

Figure 6-2. Diversity continuum in communication model.

Building Relationships

The oral health professional uses cultural competency and cultural sensitivity to support a positive client-provider relationship. This allows the client to understand best the oral health problem and participate in treatment decisions to a degree that he or she wishes. The dental hygienist may need to remain open minded, make compromises, and implement creative solutions. For example, a dental hygienist practicing in West Africa encountered a young girl with poor oral health whose family refused to accept standard oral hygiene recommendations such as toothbrushing or flossing. On further questioning, the hygienist learned that the girl's family believed that she was cursed and that any items placed in her mouth would become a danger to family members who may touch them. Understanding their cultural context, the dental hygienist realized that the only acceptable intervention was to allow the girl to use her own finger and commercial antimicrobial mouthrinse, which the family readily accepted. This story exemplifies how understanding the client's culture and tailoring interventions to the client's needs can improve health outcomes. Attending to the client cues and addressing inaccurate assumptions and beliefs carefully and respectfully allows the dental hygienist to build a strong relationship and make a real connection with the client.

> Describe a breakdown in communication that you have experienced. How would you describe the communication style? How could the interaction have been more culturally sensitive?

Maximizing Effectiveness of Cross-Cultural Communication

Openness, caring, and mutual respect are essential for effective communication, regardless of cultural differences. A nonjudgmental attitude is pivotal to success. Even though differences may exist, communication always can continue. The goal of effective communication is to maximize the understanding between the communicators. A culturally sensitive environment is characterized by care provider and client informing each other about their beliefs and expectations. The care provider, being in a professional position, should initiate the cultural encounter by **communicating facts and not judgments**. Developing a culturally competent attitude is an ongoing process.

Using communication strategies that are sensitive to language and incorporating cultural or religious values promotes the change of behavior and accommodates various degrees of cultural identification.

Verbal Communication

People who speak different languages perceive the world differently. Linguistic variations in grammatic structure, syntax, and vocabulary have important implications for the native speaker's mindset and values. For example, in English, the individual is denoted as a private, singular entity, as exemplified by the pronoun *I*. In Japanese, the first-person pronoun is expressed differently, depending on the situation and whether the language is written or oral.

When language is a barrier, it is most appropriate to use a medical interpreter with no relationship to the client. Many healthcare facilities offer interpreter services in-house, but these services are also accessible via phone and with the help of computer-based technologies (Box 6-1). Although tempting and convenient to rely on family members as interpreters, confidentiality may be compromised, and the client may feel uncomfortable discussing personal matters. Family members also may reinterpret and modify the client's true message, leading to confusion and misinformation. Because the inability to communicate with the care provider can undermine trust, decrease appropriate follow-up, and may cause diagnostic errors and inappropriate treatment, it is the responsibility of the healthcare provider to ensure effective communication via interpreter when appropriate.

BOX 6-1

Tips for Using an Interpreter

- Interpreter should be professionally certified and unrelated to client.
- Interpreter should be the same sex as client if culturally required.
- Extend appointment time.
- Discuss focus of session with interpreter before client arrives.
- Be clear about aim of session with the client.
- Assess client's health literacy.
- Speak in short sentences or phrases for easier translation.
- Ask client to repeat message in his or her own words to ensure comprehension.
- Focus on and make appropriate eye contact with the client, not the interpreter.
- Ask if the client has any additional questions, because these will be difficult to answer when the interpreter leaves.

> Describe when and how you would use the services of a professional interpreter.

Nonverbal Communication

Culture is important in determining the meaning and interpretation of nonverbal communication. Various ethnic groups possess culturally acceptable gestures, etiquette, eye contact, physical contact, and methods of effective listening. Although facial expressions are universal, a smile can signify different ideas: cordiality, embarrassment, or happiness. In most parts of the world, shaking the head from left to right means "no," but tossing the head to the side means "no" in parts of the Middle East, Bulgaria, Greece, Turkey, and Bosnia-Herzegovina. Some South Asians employ a side-to-side head bobble to signify "yes."

Eye contact is another domain of nonverbal communication with a cultural foundation. Culture dictates the appropriate amount of eye contact. Staring or continuously looking at another person may be considered rude. Lack of eye contact may be interpreted as disinterest in Western cultures but as polite in non-Western cultures. When working with clients of diverse cultural backgrounds, the dental hygienist should be cognizant of eye contact, adjusting when appropriate to maximize the effectiveness of nonverbal communication.

Similarly, physical contact requires a cultural basis for interpretation. A jovial slap on the back may be seen as friendly or insulting. In the clinical setting, touch can be divided into necessary touch, such as the intraoral examination, and nonnecessary touch, such as holding a client's hand while explaining a procedure. Nonnecessary touch can convey feelings of empathy, closeness, and comfort.[7] When done in a culturally appropriate fashion, this type of touch can relieve tension and anxiety while instilling confidence and courage. However, touch can be misinterpreted. For example, in East Asian cultures, touching an older person may be interpreted as a sign of disrespect unless initiated by the elder. Unnecessary body touching also can be viewed as a sexual advance. When in doubt, it is best to restrict physical contact to necessary touch only.

Culture also determines the personal space that must be maintained between individuals during an encounter. This distance may be based on degree of respect, authority, religious beliefs, and friendship. Muslims may refuse healthcare from a provider of the opposite gender for religious reasons. In the role of educator and clinician, dental hygienists invade spatial territories of clients. When prescribed territory is invaded, clients may communicate their discomfort through hesitation or by actively attempting to readjust to a more comfortable distance. Because the acceptable personal space is influenced culturally, the dental hygienist interested in making clients comfortable during healthcare encounters must do so with cultural sensitivity in mind.

> Describe a list of aspects of nonverbal communication skills that you think play a role in the daily practice of the oral health professional.
>
> Explore at least three personal characteristics that would interfere in your culturally sensitive communication attempts.
>
> If you noticed that your client found it difficult to make eye contact during a conversation, what would you do?

Shared Decision Making in Cross-Cultural Settings

In most Western countries, law requires clients to sign informed consent, indicating full understanding of the information provided in relation to their health and disease, their ability to decide freely, and their agreement with a treatment plan. For some ethnic groups, this concept of choice may conflict with cultural values and specific life circumstances. The client or family may believe that discussing possible health events could cause these events to take place, making signing consent forms a frightening experience. Illiteracy, lack of familiarity with the healthcare system, and financial concerns also may impair client autonomy and participation in shared decision making.

In some cultures, decisions are not made independently but as a group. In a **collectivist** environment, the group is viewed as the fundamental unit of society (Figure 6-3). A client with a collectivist attitude expects a high degree of interdependence between the members of the group and would like to make decisions through collaboration between family members and friends, perhaps across several generations. From a collectivist perspective this idea of "free choice" may be completely inadequate, because the client may believe that illness does not happen to a single individual but to the group. A client from a collectivist culture may therefore feel threatened and disoriented by informed consent and autonomous decision making. In contrast, a client from an **individualistic** culture appreciates and feels empowered by this process. Individualists view the single person as central with autonomy and self-determination as essential to medical and dental care. Individualists expect personal responsibility for decision-making, personal well-being, and happiness. Characteristics of individualistic and collectivistic cultures are described in Table 6-1, together with a comparison of Western and Non-Western views of the individual, society, health, and disease.

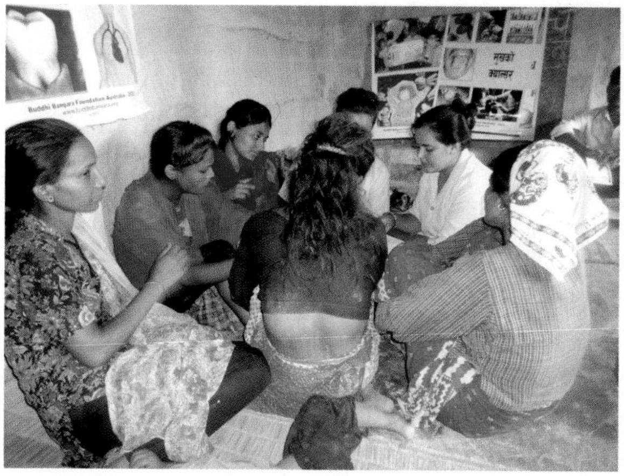

Figure 6-3. Nepalese dental hygienists perform oral health promotion activities in a remote village. The culture is this rural village can be characterized by a collectivist attitude. (Courtesy Ron J.M. Knevel, RDH, B. Health, Med.)

> Do you relate more to an individualist or a collectivist outlook? Reflect on how this influences the decisions you are making.

Inequality and Poverty

A major emphasis of culturally competent care is ensuring equitable, high-quality care among diverse and disadvantaged groups.[4] Knowledge of health inequalities is essential to understanding the different determinants of health (Figure 6-4). The World Health Organization defines health inequalities as differences in health status or the distribution of health determinants between different population groups. **Health inequities** are the result of complex interactions between biologic, lifestyle, environmental, social, and economic factors.[7] Poverty is a major contributor to health disparities and a barrier to individuals meeting their basic human need for systemic and oral health. Other barriers to healthcare associated with poverty are disenfranchisement, lack of transportation, homelessness, seasonal work, prejudice, low literacy, inadequate levels of education, and a lack of culturally competent healthcare personnel. Individuals from low socioeconomic groups are, on average, more intimidated by the healthcare system than individuals of higher socioeconomic

TABLE 6-1

Characteristics of Individualist and Collectivistic Cultures, Compared to Western and Non-Western Views of the Individual, Society, Health, and Disease

Collectivistic	Individualistic	Non-Western Values	Western Values
Stress group goals over individual goals	Emphasize goals of individuals over group goals	Fulfillment of the needs of the group	Fulfillment of individual needs
Tend to belong to in-groups that look after them	Tend to assume responsibility only for themselves and their immediate family	Independence	Compliance
Involves cooperation and solidarity with fellow members of one's group	More self-centered	Group decision making	Freedom of choice
Tend to identify with the group they are in	Clearly see themselves as an individual	Group commonality	Uniqueness of the individual
Work and social life intertwined	Personal privacy is protected	Conformity	Nonconformity
Failure means losing face	Failure means did not live up to one's own expectations		
Harmony and loyalty within company is very important	Emphasize success in job or private wealth	Harmony	Interdependence
Wealth of company more important than one's own	Aiming to reach more or better job position	Cooperation	Competition
Do not disagree with someone in public, avoiding confrontation	Prefer clarity and being direct to the point	Control of one's feelings	Expression of feelings
Family and friends are involved in decision-making patterns, group can determine who will be responsible for healthcare decisions	The individual tends to make the final decision, based on his/her own expectations and values, also in relation to healthcare decisions	Body is viewed as a union of flesh and soul	Body is divided into organ systems with identifiable functions; dichotomous body and mind
		Disease occurs as a result of disharmony or an imbalance of life forces	Body is viewed objectively and is relatively immune to non-somatic influences

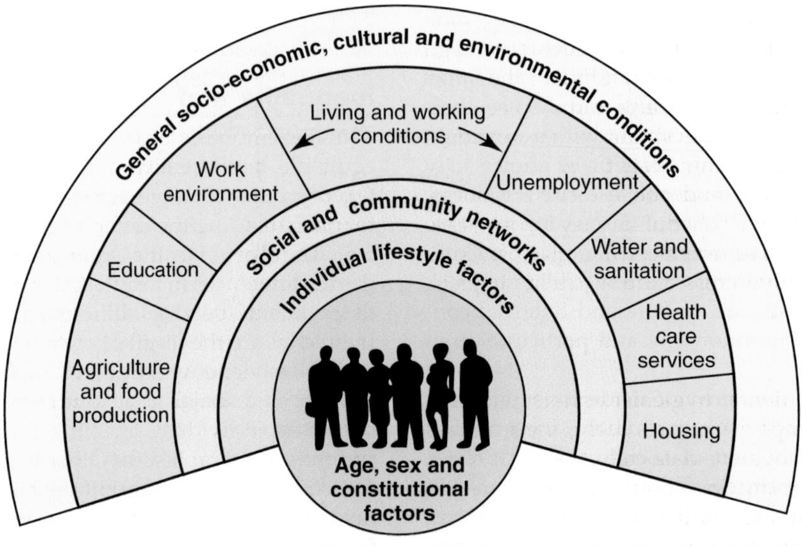

Figure 6-4. Determinants of health. (Adapted from Dahlgren G, Whitehead M: Policies and strategies to promote social equity in health. Stockholm: Institute for Futures Studies, 1991.)

status. They may have more difficulty verbalizing their concerns, asserting their needs, determining their level of participation in care, and seeking second opinions. Greater responsibility and action is required to rectify these health inequalities caused by determinants such as poverty. The oral health professional should take the responsibility to reduce barriers to improve quality of and access to care.

> Identify an underserved population that interests you. Use the Internet and the World Health Organization's website to identify the oral and general health status of this population. Identify the cultural identity, values, and expectations. Describe the delivery of and access to oral health services in this population.

Healthcare Literacy

Healthcare literacy is the ability to understand health, disease, and how the healthcare system works. People with low healthcare literacy also may experience low dental health literacy. Children with the most advanced oral disease are found within minority, poor, homeless, and immigrant populations. These factors are associated with but do not necessarily directly cause poor oral health.[8] Cultural beliefs and practices can influence the oral health status such as appreciation of the importance of healthy primary teeth or expectations about preventive or therapeutic interventions. Underlying cultural beliefs and practices influence the condition of the teeth and mouth, through diet, care-seeking behaviors or use of home remedies.[9] However, being part of an ethnic minority group does not automatically lead a person to have poor oral health. Within all racial or ethnic groups are substantial differences in beliefs and behaviors. This inevitably leads to varying health status.

The Dental Hygiene Process in the Cross-Cultural Environment

Culturally sensitive dental hygiene is the effective integration of clients' diverse cultural backgrounds into the process of care. The oral health professional recognizes that the care of clients from different cultures or ethnic groups takes more time than does caring for clients from similar cultures. Longer time should be scheduled to accommodate the need for translation, repetition, clarification, and socialization to dental hygiene care. Sometimes careful scheduling may be necessary to accommodate clients from different cultural groups. Additional guidelines for effective cross-cultural dental hygiene practice are listed in Box 6-2.

Assessment, Diagnosis, and Care Planning

The culturally competent dental hygienist understands that values and experiences shape everyone's perceptions, beliefs, and attitudes. Most dental hygiene data collection tools direct the hygienist to gather information about the client's health; however, a complete evaluation of the client's condition can only be obtained from assessment of the client's values and beliefs of the culture, ethnic group, or subculture. Therefore, assessing clients to identify culture-specific information is essential.

BOX 6-2

Guidelines for Cross-Cultural Dental Hygiene

- Approach each client as a valued, unique individual.
- Be sensitive about asking intimate health history questions.
- Reflect on your own personal characteristics, values, and life experiences. Understand how cultural factors have influenced your outlook. Identify biases and prejudices in your own life that influence your effectiveness as a healthcare provider, educator, administrator-manager, researcher, and advocate.
- Become a lifelong student of other culture, particularly cultures in the community where you practice.
- Assess clients' culturally influenced practices, attitudes, values, and beliefs as part of the process of care. Do not assume you understand until you ask.
- Display an accepting, nonjudgmental demeanor when presented with diversity.
- Demonstrate knowledge and recognition of the client's cultural practices throughout the interaction.
- Encourage clients to continue cultural health practices that can bring no harm; provide support, show understanding, and allow time when trying to change potentially harmful health practices.
- Consider dietary practices. Provide nutritional counseling within the framework of the client's cultural values and norms.
- Develop collegial relationships with healthcare providers from different ethnic and minority groups.
- Promote cultural exchanges that contribute to the quality of care.

An ethnic and cultural assessment guide is presented in Table 5-6. This guide need not be a separate form but may be incorporated into existing data collection documents, interactions, and procedures. The dental hygiene diagnosis should identify the client's unmet human needs that can be fulfilled through dental hygiene care, the cause of disease, the client's perception of the cause of disease, the evidence for the diagnosis, and related cultural factors. With this detailed focus, an individualized care plan can be developed and appropriate interventions selected. Using a nonjudgmental, nonethnocentric approach, the dental hygienist assesses the client's level of acculturation, English language skills, cultural health practices, and home remedies. Factors such as language comprehension, dietary preferences, and attitudes about the predominant culture can provide important cues for assessing the influence of the client's cultural background. By synthesizing this information, the dental hygienist can conduct more positive, culturally informed interactions with the patient (see Tables 5-2 and 5-4). The dental hygienist who is able to demonstrate acceptance of diversity can establish trust with the client and achieve improved outcomes.

Implementation

Dental hygiene interventions, whether educational, technical, or interpersonal, must be congruent with cultural values. Client values and needs guide the selection of interventions. As demonstrated by the anecdote about the Liberian girl at the beginning of this chapter, oral hygiene interventions must be culturally acceptable if they are to result in successful uptake by the host culture. Successful dental hygiene programs are often given legitimacy by coupling them with culturally accepted values or respected figures. In Sri Lanka, "[o]ral hygiene exercises are performed in Sunday schools run by the monks to propagate the teachings of Buddha. The religious leadership provided in the village gives the needed credibility to the program, and the villagers adhere strictly to the oral hygiene practices taught by the monks because of the respect they command in the villages."[9] In predominantly Muslim countries, people are taught that prayers from a clean mouth are received more favorably by Allah; therefore oral hygiene self-care compliments prayer rituals.[10]

These vignettes underscore the need to understand different cultures if client oral health is to be achieved. As long as cultural beliefs or practices cause no harm, the dental hygienist can determine their importance to the client and recognize that their continued practice might assist in maintaining an effective client-provider relationship (Figure 5-5). Even if the behavior is ineffective, the client's comfort with and belief in its effectiveness can support a situation in which the person might otherwise feel alienated. Go to the website at http://evolve.elsevier.com/Darby/hygiene to view resources for understanding people within various cultures. Obviously, not all people within a culture will subscribe to these beliefs; however, this guide can serve as a starting point for understanding people of diverse cultures.

Evaluation

In cross-cultural interactions, the evaluation phase of care calls for an awareness of the client's cultural perspective of success. Frequent solicitation of the client's perspectives, level of understanding, psychomotor skill development, and self-care practices is particularly important. Evaluation should determine whether dental hygiene services are meeting the client's needs. Urging clients to talk about their oral health practices and status helps with cross-cultural communication. In addition to clinical indicators of health, validation occurs via feedback from the client and client's family that the client's needs are being met.

Implementation Phase

Oral hygiene interventions should be culturally acceptable for optimal adherence. Client values and needs guide the selection of interventions. Oral health therapy and promotion strategies, including the planning of interventions and the implementation of the care plan, also must be delivered in relation to the cultural environment of the client. In fact, successful initiatives often are given legitimacy by coupling them with culturally accepted values or respected figures (Figures 6-5 and 6-6). In Sri Lanka oral hygiene exercises are performed in Sunday schools run by the monks to promote the teachings of Buddha. The religious leadership provided in the village gives credibility to the program, and the villagers adhere strictly to the oral hygiene practices taught by the monks because of the respect they command in the villages.[10] In predominantly Muslim countries, people are taught that Allah receives prayers from a clean mouth more favorably.[11] They learn that the Prophet said:

> *"Your mouth is the pathway of the Qur'an, so make them fragrant. Had it not been difficult for my followers, I would have ordered them to use tooth stick before every prayer."*

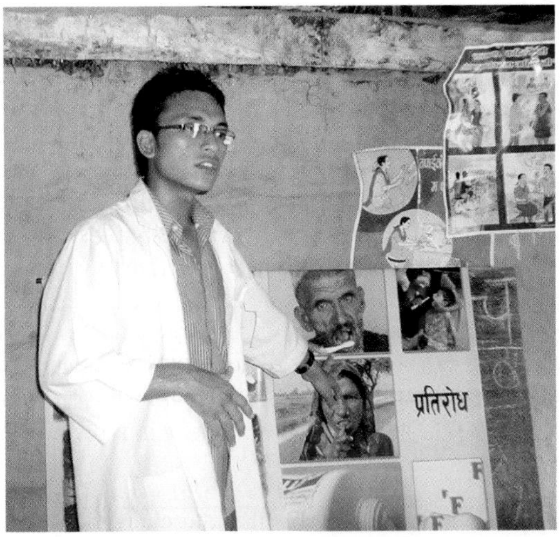

Figure 6-5. Oral health promotion for a rural community in Nepal; the poster allows cultural identification. (Courtesy Ron J.M. Knevel, RDH, B. Health, Med.)

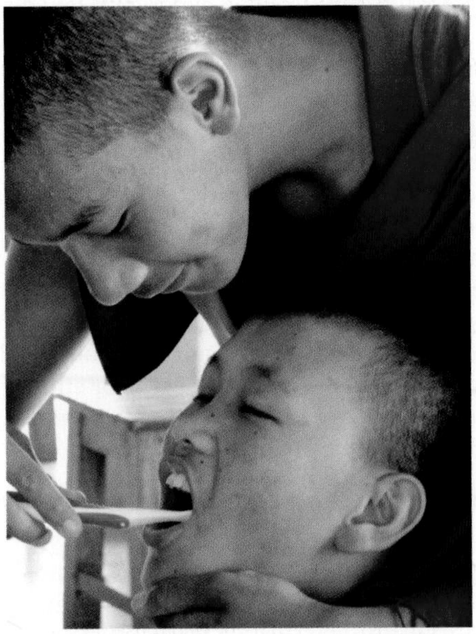

Figure 6-6. Monk performing oral hygiene exercises. (Courtesy Ron J.M. Knevel, RDH, B. Health, Med.)

By connecting an oral health intervention to traditional health practices, the intervention becomes more effective.

Demonstrating willingness to incorporate traditional treatments or to cooperate with alternative healers also can be important. This is especially true if the cultural belief or practice does not cause harm and if continued practice is important to the client and may assist in maintaining an effective client-provider relationship. For example, oral hygiene is important to most Hindus, especially those who practice Ayurvedic principles. Many Hindus prefer to brush their teeth immediately after waking in the morning and before having breakfast. Tongue scraping can be part of the morning ritual to avoid ingestion of impurities that have built up in the mouth during sleep. Building on these Ayurvedic principles could reinforce these rituals while advising the client to brush after meals as well. Likewise, Muslims may have to be advised to alter their oral care habits during Ramadan because nothing with flavorings may be put into the mouth while fasting during the day. Exposure to dentifrices, mouth rinses, prophylaxis paste, dental sealants, or professionally applied fluorides could be moved to evening hours. Oral care appointment scheduling also may have to be modified during Ramadan. In summary, dental hygiene interventions, whether educational, technical, or interpersonal, are most effective when congruent with cultural values.

Table 6-2 provides a guide with characteristics of different cultures which can serve as a starting point for understanding people of diverse cultures. Not all people within a culture subscribe to these beliefs.

Evaluation

It is important to gain insight into the client's perspectives, level of understanding, psychomotor skill development, and self-care practices. Evaluation determines whether the oral health services are meeting the client's needs. Inviting the clients to talk about their oral health practices and status helps with improving culturally sensitive communication. In addition to clinical indicators of health, validation occurs via feedback from the client and client's family. The evaluation phase of care incorporates the awareness of the client's cultural perspective of success. The oral health professional must learn how the client wants to be treated. Although not a comprehensive list, Table 6-2 provides some basic guidelines for working with people from various cultural groups, including many with non-Western medical philosophies.

Documentation

It is critical to record completely and accurately all collected data, treatment planned and provided, recommendations, and all information relevant to client care. Documentation relates to all components of the dental hygiene process of

TABLE 6-2

Guide to Working with People of Various Cultural Groups*

Cultural Group	Basic Beliefs and Concepts	Healthcare Practices, Beliefs, Common Health Problems, and Remedies
African/African American	Life is a process rather than a state No division among physical, emotional, and spiritual needs Present oriented Strong religious and community group support networks	Health occurs when there is harmony with nature; illness is disharmony Belief in both white magic and black magic Living and dead things influence health Employ faith healers, root doctors, and spiritualists to cast out evil spirits and demons Voodoo can cause or prevent malevolent forces Illness can be preventive by avoiding people who carry evil spirits, eating a good diet, and prayer *Remedies:* May use home remedies or folk healing Bangles: thin silver bracelets that let evil out and prevent it from entering the body; sound of bangles frightens evil spirits Talismans: drawn symbols that are worn or carried to ward off sickness Asafetida: known as "incense of the devil"; rubbed on to ward off colds and evil Snake: dehydrated, ground to a powder, and mixed with water; applied to skin lesions
Hispanics or Latin Americans (Spaniards, Cubans, Mexicans, Central and South Americans)	*Curanderos, espiritista, partera, senora:* folk healers, some of whom use the premise of humoral pathology *Humoral pathology:* basic functions of body are regulated by body fluids (humors) defined by temperature and wetness: Blood (hot and wet) Phlegm (cold and wet) Black bile (cold and dry) Yellow bile (hot and dry) "Evil eye" is harmful magic Strong influence of Catholic Church and family Flexible sense of time Respect for tradition Belief in bad magic, spells, and other harmful magic	Good health means balance among four humors Holistic understanding of emotional, physical, spiritual and social factors Health is the result of good luck or rewards from God Can maintain health and avoid disease via a balance among four humors Foods are classified as hot or cold unrelated to their temperature; hot and cold food must be eaten or avoided at certain times Illness is caused by an improper diet of hot and cold foods, dislocation of body parts, the supernatural, or envy *(envidia)* from others Illness can be prevented by proper diet, wearing of amulets, use of candles, prayer, avoiding too much success and harmful people Illness is the result of bad luck, punishment from God, or an imbalance among four humors Important decisions may require consultation among whole family *Remedies:* Burning candles to ward off evil spirits Amulets worn to ward off evil and as a protection against the evil eye *Manzanilla* (chamomile), an herb used to treat stomach disorders, anxiety, and insomnia May adhere to hot/cold theory

Continued

TABLE 6-2
Guide to Working with People of Various Cultural Groups—cont'd

Cultural Group	Basic Beliefs and Concepts	Healthcare Practices, Beliefs, Common Health Problems, and Remedies
Asian or Pacific Islanders (Chinese, Hawaiians, Filipinos, Koreans, Japanese, Southeast Asians, e.g., Laotians, Cambodians, Hmong, Vietnamese)	The body is a gift that must be cared for and maintained Seldom complain about pain Strong family ties Preference for humility, modesty, self-control Respect for authority and tradition	Health is a state of harmony among body, mind, spirit, and nature (Taoism) Illness is caused by an upset in the balance (among body, mind, spirit, and nature) or by the weather, overexertion, or prolonged sitting Illness can be prevented by proper diet, exercise, avoiding temperature changes, and taking certain remedies May be disturbed by loss of blood, because they consider it to be body's life force May refuse surgery because they believe the body should remain intact *Remedies:* May use acu-massage, acupressure, and acupuncture Jen Shen Lu Jung Wan: tonic taken to strengthen the entire system Thousand-year eggs: old uncooked eggs eaten daily for good health Huo Li Jian Mei Su: pills taken to maintain youth, health, and beauty Tiger balm: all-purpose salve to relieve minor aches and pain Ginseng root: most famous all-purpose Chinese and Korean medicine Acupuncture: use of metal needles at certain points in the body to treat and control pain *Nonverbal communication:* Gentle touch may be acceptable in conversation Avoiding eye contact has sign of respect Head nodding does not mean understanding or approval
Native Americans and Alaskan Natives	Both nature and the body must be treated with respect Great respect for elders Value placed on working together Present-oriented Accumulation of wealth and goods is frowned on Living in the presence might conflict with appointment schedules	Health is the result of total harmony with nature Prevention of illness is achieved through harmony of the body, mind, and spirit Illness can be associated with evil spirits, displeasing the holy people, disturbing nature, misusing a sacred ceremony Illness is the result of disharmony among the body, mind, spirit, and nature Autonomy is highly valued; however, large extended families who expect to be included in the healthcare process *Remedies:* Sand painting by medicine man Mask: to hide from evil spirits Sweet grass: burned as a rite of purification Thunderbird: a charm worn for protection and good luck Estafiata: leaves used to treat stomach ailments Use of herbs, ceremonies, fasting, meditation, heat, and massage *Nonverbal communication:* Keep respectful distance Respect can be communicated by avoiding eye contact
Whites	Youth valued over age Punctuality, physical attractiveness, competitiveness, cleanliness, achievement valued Control of emotion Emphasis on the nuclear family versus the extended family	Health is viewed as freedom from illness and disease; illness is the presence of disease symptoms, pain, disability, malformations Illness may be the result of punishment from God, breaking religious rules, drafts, climate *Remedies:* Varied because of the influence of multiple European cultures, e.g., malocchio—horn-shaped amulet used by Italians to ward off the "evil eye"
South Asian	May follow Hinduism, Christianity, Sikhism, Islam, Zoroastrianism Modesty is highly valued Arranged marriages still common Elders and education highly valued Primary body forces (dosha): Vata, Pitta, Kapha	Balance of the dosha yields health May prefer same-gender healthcare provider Indian system of medicine known as Ayurveda emphasizes prevention and herbs The belief that pain and suffering are the result of karma may make symptom control difficult *Remedies:* Herbal remedies of Ayurveda Yoga *Nonverbal communication:* Use of eyes to express care more important than touch Eye contact can be considered rude or disrespectful Acceptance or approval can be expressed by silence

TABLE 6-2

Guide to Working with People of Various Cultural Groups—cont'd

Cultural Group	Basic Beliefs and Concepts	Healthcare Practices, Beliefs, Common Health Problems, and Remedies
Developing countries	Use of "magic" for good and evil throughout culture Believe in the "here" world and "nether" world Avoid certain people, cold air, and evil eyes Distrust in nature Faithful to punitive god Suspicious of other people Distrust friends, relatives, and strangers	Protective and evil magic determine illness, come from supernatural Spells and sacrifices will bring back health Will use healers from more than one healthcare system Good health centers on personal rather than scientific behaviors Explain emotional and physical illness in terms of imbalance between individual and physical, social, and spiritual life *Remedies:* Herbs and home remedies
West Indies	Little value placed on time Present-oriented Belief in voodoo	Obeah (witchcraft, black magic) power is very strong: scientific proof of sticking needles into people with bleeding or pain and frightening victims to death *Remedies:* Folk medicine, traditional healer (root worker)
Arab/American culture	On time is for official business, more spontaneous for social events Health defined as a gift of God Western medicine respected and sought after	Illness can be defined by evil eye or bad luck Regarding to pain, very expressive, especially in presence of family Pain can cause panic Being overweight often associated with health and strength Families make collective decisions *Remedies:* Home and folk remedies may be used *Nonverbal:* Respect professionals Other orientated and expressive

*Not all people from a given culture act in a standard manner. Great variability exists within cultural groups based on socioeconomic status, level of education, and overall life experiences. This chart is not meant to be generalized to all people within a specific culture, but rather to serve as a beginning guide.

care. It is important to recognize the legal and ethical responsibilities of documentation including following guidelines outlined in state regulations and statutes and ensuring compliance with the Federal Health Information Portability and Accountability Act (HIPAA).

KEY CONCEPTS

- Culture is the set of behaviors learned for a person to adapt successfully to life within a particular group; it includes beliefs, traditions, experiences, customs, rituals, and language.
- Culture is integral in oral care because an individual's conception of oral wellness, disease, and illness can be determined culturally.
- Culture influences how people view their health and the healthcare services they receive. Clinicians should be aware of these differences and respect them. The parameters are set by the client's values, and clinicians have to work within them.
- Focusing on characteristics of cultural groups as the basis for culturally appropriate action can lead to stereotypes and risk of cross-cultural misunderstanding. Clinicians should strive to understand cultural practices of diverse groups by asking questions and avoiding assumptions.
- Stereotyping is the erroneous behavior of assuming that a person possesses certain characteristics simply because he or she is a member of a particular group.
- Cultural competence is essential for quality of oral healthcare; it is essential to reach desired health outcomes.
- The clinician must respect differences in other people, including customs, thoughts, behaviors, communication styles, values, traditions, and institutions.
- Cultural competence starts with the clinician exploring his or her own position and attitude before assessing the individual client. Clinicians must recognize their own cultural values and draw parallels where possible. In addition they must be able to identify the prejudice and stereotypes that prevent them from communicating effectively with clients from different cultural backgrounds.
- A culturally competent oral health professional regards all clients as unique and is aware of the fact that the client's experiences, beliefs, values, and language affects the perception of the clinical service delivery, diagnosis, and adherence.
- Many nonverbal behaviors associated with respect, genuine interest, and openness are appropriate for most clients regardless of their cultural background, even when a clinician's cultural knowledge is limited.

- Poverty is a key predictor of poor oral and systemic health; it affects where one lives, how one spends money, where one receives healthcare, and ultimately, one's general and oral health status.
- The oral health professional has a responsibility to reduce barriers to improve access to care.

CLIENT EDUCATION TIPS

- Use models and educational materials that are culturally appropriate.
- Assess and verify client's beliefs and practices.
- Review common healthcare beliefs and practices in the client's culture as a starting point.
- Integrate self-care and professional-care therapies for oral disease management with client's culture; traditional or non-Western approaches may be encouraged if not harmful.
- Provide nutritional counseling within the context of the client's culture.

LEGAL, ETHICAL, AND SAFETY ISSUES

- Investigate the clients' expectations and beliefs; one can minimize risk of clients apportioning blame by establishing a trusting relationship.
- If the client is not satisfied, care cannot be of high quality.
- Barriers to access and participation must be identified and addressed.
- Investigate culturally based therapies to ensure safety and efficacy.
- Document client's use of culturally based therapies and client's response to professional care, instructions, and recommendations, as well as the level that the client (or the environment of the client) wants to be involved in the decision-making process.
- Clients have a right to an interpreter. When language is a barrier, an interpreter enhances and validates communication.

CRITICAL THINKING EXERCISES

1. Explain how culturally sensitive communication complements motivational interviewing strategies.
2. Choose a developing country that interests you. Use the Internet, in particular the World Health Organization's website, to identify the oral and general health status of the people in the selected country. Identify the cultural groups that live there and the behaviors to use and avoid in daily interactions. Describe the delivery of oral health services and the access to these services.
3. Describe a breakdown in communication that you have experienced.
4. Describe at least five stereotypes.
5. If you noticed that someone found it difficult to make eye contact during a conversation, what would you do?
6. Describe a list of aspects of nonverbal communication skills that you think play a role in the daily practice of the oral health professional.
7. Explore at least three personal characteristics that would interfere in your culturally sensitive communication attempts.
8. Describe how you would use the services of a professional interpreter.
9. Determine if you are from an individualist or a collectivist environment and how this influences the decisions you are making.

REFERENCES

1. Dy CJ, Nelson CL: Diversity, cultural competence, and client trust. *Clin Orthop Relat Res* 469:1878, 2011.
2. Kohli HK, Huber R, Faul AC: Historical and theoretical development of culturally competent social work practice. *J Teaching Social Work* 30:252, 2010.
3. Stafford J, Bowman R, Ewing T, et al: *Building culture bridges*, Bloomington, Ind, 1997, National Educational Service.
4. Kutob RM, Senf JH, Harris JM: Teaching culturally effective diabetes care: results of a randomized controlled trial. *Fam Med* 41(3):167, 2009.
5. Kleinman A: *Client and healers in the context of culture*, Berkley, Calif, 1980, University of California Press.
6. Teal CR, Street RL: Critical elements of culturally competent communication in the medical encounter: a review and model. *Soc Sci Med* 68:533, 2009.
7. Routasalo P: Physical touch in nursing studies: a literature review. *J Adv Nurs* 30:843, 1999.
8. Dahlgren G, Whitehead M: *Tackling inequalities in health: what can we learn from what has been tried?* Working paper prepared for the King's Fund International Seminar on Tackling Inequalities in Health, Oxfordshire, England, Ditchley Park, 1993.
9. Butani Y, Weintraub JA, Barker JC: Oral health-related cultural beliefs for four racial/ethnic groups: assessment of the literature. *BMC Oral Health* 8:26, 2009.
10. Saparamadu KDG: The provision of dental services in the Third World. *Int Dent J* 36:194, 1986.
11. Shams M: Concepts of health and hygiene in Islam. Available at: http://www.biharanjuman.org/health_islam.htm. Accessed October 2012.

EVOLVE RESOURCES

Please visit http://evolve.elsevier.com/Darby/hygiene for additional practice and study support tools.

Professional Portfolios

CHAPTER 7

Phyllis Spragge, Catherine Kelly Draper

COMPETENCIES

1. Define the professional portfolio.
2. Describe the various types and formats of portfolios and their uses.
3. Describe the process for creating a student portfolio, including the role of reflection within the portfolio.
4. Discuss portfolio authorship and ethical principles.
5. Discuss transitioning the student portfolio to the professional world.

Portfolios are becoming an integral part of the dental hygiene education and career process. Beginning as a way to showcase student work while in the dental hygiene program, the portfolio demonstrates the growth and achievements throughout the career of the dental hygienist. Portfolios can help students track their progress while in the dental hygiene program by providing a place to archive, reflect upon, and share their best work with faculty members. In addition, portfolios strengthen applications and may be required by scholarship, degree completion, and graduate program review committees. Maintaining a professional portfolio also is a critical component of the employment process for the new graduate, as well as for the seasoned professional. A professional portfolio provides the potential employer with evidence of a candidate's range of skills and experiences extending far beyond the traditional resume. Professional portfolios also are being considered by some states for initial licensure as well as a requirement for the demonstration of professional competency throughout the licentiate's career.

What Is a Professional Portfolio?

A **professional portfolio** is defined as a careful collection of physical evidence, or **artifacts**, which have been selected carefully to document an individual's growth and accomplishments over time. Many portfolios include a reflection component, providing an opportunity for an individual to thoughtfully comment or reflect on their ongoing personal growth and professional goals. Reflection plays an important role in the self-assessment process and evaluation of one's competency. Historically, portfolios have been used by students in fields ranging from art and photography to journalism and education as a means to display visually actual examples of their student work as part of the application process for admission into specialty or graduate programs.

Types of Portfolios

Academic

Today, portfolios are used by more than half of the 4-year universities and one third of the community colleges in the United States alone, as a means to document student learning outcomes, or as a capstone or final project designed to evaluate student skills and content mastery.

Employment

Looking beyond academia, professional portfolios are now being used by individuals seeking employment in a variety of disciplines as a way to expand beyond the 1-page résumé with a more complete visual record of the candidate's abilities and accomplishments. The professional portfolio also can be used as a marketing tool to potential employers, illustrating the applicant's knowledge, skills, and relevant experiences. A portfolio can serve as a visual prompt in the interview process, highlighting an experience or area of expertise that may go unnoticed or forgotten during the verbal interview. A 2008 study of potential job seekers demonstrated that candidates who had created electronic portfolios discovered that they had a better understanding of their skills and attributes in addition to an increased self-confidence when marketing themselves to potential employers.[1]

Demonstration of Ongoing Competency

Healthcare professionals are also turning to the professional portfolio as a way to document and demonstrate competency and professional development throughout their careers. Competency at the time of initial licensure is no longer being accepted as adequate proof for a lifetime of practice. Registered nurses now use professional portfolios for seeking new positions and career ladder promotions as well as for documenting continued competency within their field of expertise. Some nursing boards in the United States also have joined their international counterparts in requiring the submission of a portfolio for licensure renewal.

Pathway to Initial Clinical Licensure

The professional portfolio also is being used to measure clinical competency in dentistry and dental hygiene. In 2011 the California legislature approved the hybrid portfolio as a pathway for initial licensure for general dentists applying for licensure by the Dental Board of California. Although the regulations are still being adopted at this time, in the future, dental students will have the option to take a licensure examination based on a portfolio of completed clinical experiences and competency examinations in seven subject areas evaluated over the entire course of the final year of dental school. Once all of the clinical experiences and assessments have been completed to the satisfaction of calibrated faculty members, students must submit their finished portfolio to the Dental Board of California for final review followed by licensure to practice. Although several other states, including Connecticut, New York, Minnesota, and Washington, have adopted alternative pathways to licensure that have eliminated the use of live patients, California is the first state to adopt the professional portfolio as a means to demonstrate clinical competency for initial licensure in dentistry.[2]

Professional Development Measure

Although initial licensure by portfolio is not an option for dental hygienists in the United States at this time, the state of Minnesota currently requires all dental professionals to maintain a professional development portfolio documenting competency in the subject areas of ethics, patient communication, medical emergencies, diagnosis and treatment planning, record keeping, and infection control. Dentists, dental therapists, hygienists, and assistants must complete a biennial self-assessment test from the Minnesota Board of Dentistry covering these core subject areas and tailor their continuing education professional development courses to address any areas of weakness. Actual portfolio submission is not required as part of the licensure renewal process; however, licentiates may be audited randomly and required to submit their portfolio to the Minnesota Board of Dentistry for review.[3]

In summary, the student portfolio lays the foundation for the future dental hygiene professional. It can serve as an effective tool for the new graduate in seeking entry-level employment, or as part of the application process for a degree completion or post-graduate program. More important, maintaining a professional portfolio is becoming a requirement for licensure and specialty certification boards across all disciplines in healthcare. Developing the necessary skills to demonstrate competency via a professional portfolio begins early in the dental hygiene education process.

Portfolio Formats

The most common types of portfolios used in education and beyond are the traditional paper-based formats and the electronic versions.

Paper Formats

The paper-based portfolio typically is organized in a binder or folders. This method is relatively easy and inexpensive to start; however, the paper portfolio is limited to exclusively print-based artifacts and projects.

Electronic Formats

The electronic versions, e-portfolios, are either Web- or computer-based (Figure 7-1). Electronic formats have the advantage of communicating an individual's work and accomplishments not only through text but also by incorporating graphics, audio, and video formats. The work then can be stored electronically and distributed on a website or on a personal computer. Creating a computer-based e-portfolio may require purchasing additional software and a scanner. The various printed portfolio contents can be scanned or saved as electronic files. Once the computer-based e-portfolio is completed, it can be stored virtually on the cloud or downloaded to a flash drive or CD-ROM. Once a computer-based e-portfolio is stored on the cloud, it becomes Web-based. Although there are no recurring set-up or maintenance fees with this type of portfolio, a computer-based e-portfolio is not as easily accessible as the Web versions. Web-based e-portfolios are created on dedicated websites, often with help of design templates and user-friendly software for uploading files. Annual user fees for accessing the Web domain are common for this type of e-portfolio. Examples of e-portfolio websites can be found in Box 7-1. This chapter focuses on the creation of a dental hygiene student portfolio with specific examples adaptable for electronic formats.[4,5]

Creating the Student Portfolio

Selecting the contents for a dental hygiene portfolio depends on a number of factors, in particular the purpose of the portfolio. Most student portfolio projects are based on the guidelines, learning outcomes, and competencies developed by the specific dental hygiene program, college, or university (Box 7-2). General examples of the elements common to any student portfolio include biographic data, examples of core clinical competencies, student research and projects, summaries of patient/client experiences, professional activities, community service experiences, and related projects outside of the classroom. A strong portfolio should be built with the key projects or assignments that demonstrate achievement of the dental hygiene program competencies as well as examples of the student's critical thinking and problem solving skills. The portfolio is meant to be a dynamic documentation of growth and development. Web-based e-portfolios often have an interactive feedback box where faculty or other site visitors can provide comments to the portfolio owner. Based on the

BOX 7-1

Electronic Portfolio Website Resources

Myefolio: www.myefolio.com
PebblePad: www.pebblepad.co.uk/about.asp
Weebly: www.weebly.com
Wordpress: www.wordpress.org

BOX 7-2

Portfolio Development Guidelines

- Portfolio purpose
  - Best work versus professional development or combination
- Portfolio audience
  - Dental hygiene faculty versus potential employers
- College or university guidelines
  - Institutional required elements
- Dental hygiene program requirements
  - Demonstration of program competencies

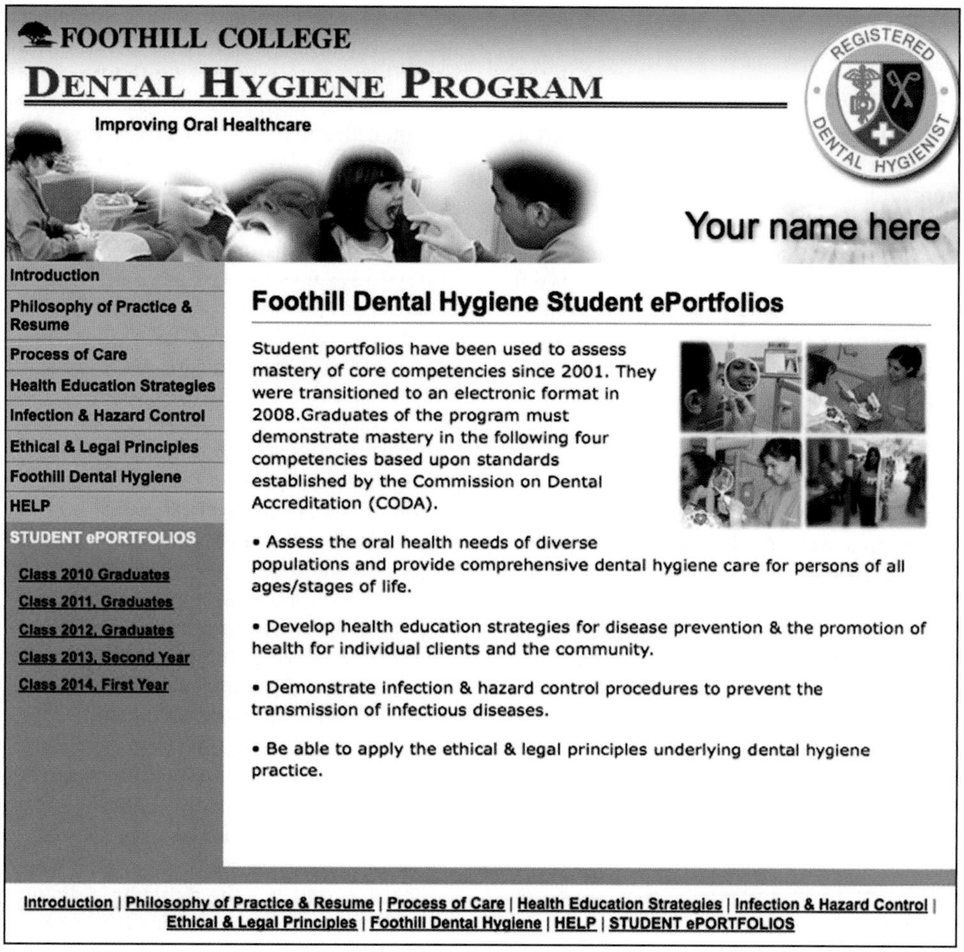

Figure 7-1. Sample template for the organizational structure of a student electronic portfolio. (Provided with permission from Foothill College Dental Hygiene Program, Los Altos Hills, California.)

feedback provided, the student may choose to change or enhance the portfolio content. Examples of best work chosen at the beginning of the dental hygiene program may change over time and should be updated regularly as the student progresses towards graduation.

Portfolios created for the purpose of documenting professional development or ongoing continuing education should include a comprehensive record of all relevant coursework, conferences, workshops, and related activities. **Reflection** is also an important component of any portfolio, adding depth extending beyond the description of the project or activity. Without meaningful reflection, the portfolio is little more than a filing system for projects and activities.

The first step in the portfolio process is to begin to collect the contents or artifacts (Figure 7-2). Regardless of whether the e-portfolio is Web based or computer based, it is important to choose an organizational structure or template to display effectively the artifacts to fit the portfolio's purpose. The design and accompanying photographs and images always should project the image of a healthcare professional. The portfolio is not a digital scrapbook, photo album, or social media page. Although the specific organizational requirements for a student portfolio vary depending on the school and the dental hygiene program, the sample

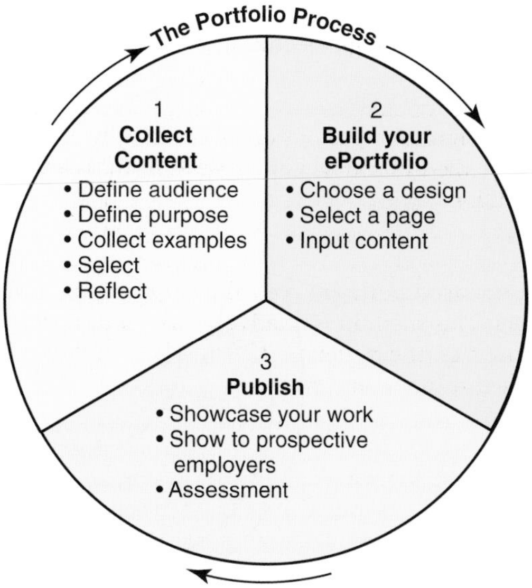

Figure 7-2. The portfolio process: from content collection to publication. (Reprinted with permission from San Francisco State University, http://eportfolio.sfsu.edu.)

template in Box 7-3 can be used to help guide the organizational process.

Reflection and the Professional Portfolio

The ability to think deeply and critically has been defined as a desirable attribute in the competent healthcare professional.[6] Reflection and critical thinking are key components of self-evaluation and guide lifelong learning, growth, and development. Figure 7-3 illustrates how reflective thinking contributes to desirable qualities in a healthcare professional. Students who develop reflective learning skills have demonstrated that they are more proactive in their learning and are better able to identify the areas where they need more self-improvement and skill development. Rather than simply focusing on learning rote clinical skills, the reflective professional is more focused on critical thinking, problem solving, and self-motivated change.

Reflecting on experiences in the clinical setting, as well as outside of the dental hygiene classroom, often is challenging for the beginning student. Expressing thoughts and feelings in written reflection statements can be difficult for seasoned professionals, as well as students, but it is a process that can be developed with practice. The reflection statement is not simply a summary of the activity or assignment; reflection is deeply personal. Meaningful reflection comes by moving past the activity to a deeper level of thinking, and focusing on one's feelings, values, or assumptions surrounding the activity or event. The difference between a nonreflective, factual journal entry as compared with a thoughtful reflection of the same activity is illustrated in Box 7-4. It can be helpful to consider the 4 Rs of reflection: Revisit, React, Relate, and

BOX 7-3

Portfolio Sample Template

I. Portfolio introduction and biographic data
- Philosophy of practice statement
- Career goals
- Résumé
- Curriculum vitae

II. Professional competencies
- Infection control
- Client care
- Client care logs and statistics
- Health education
- Community service
- Legal and ethical principles

III. Professional development and activities
- Continuing education log
- Additional professional activities

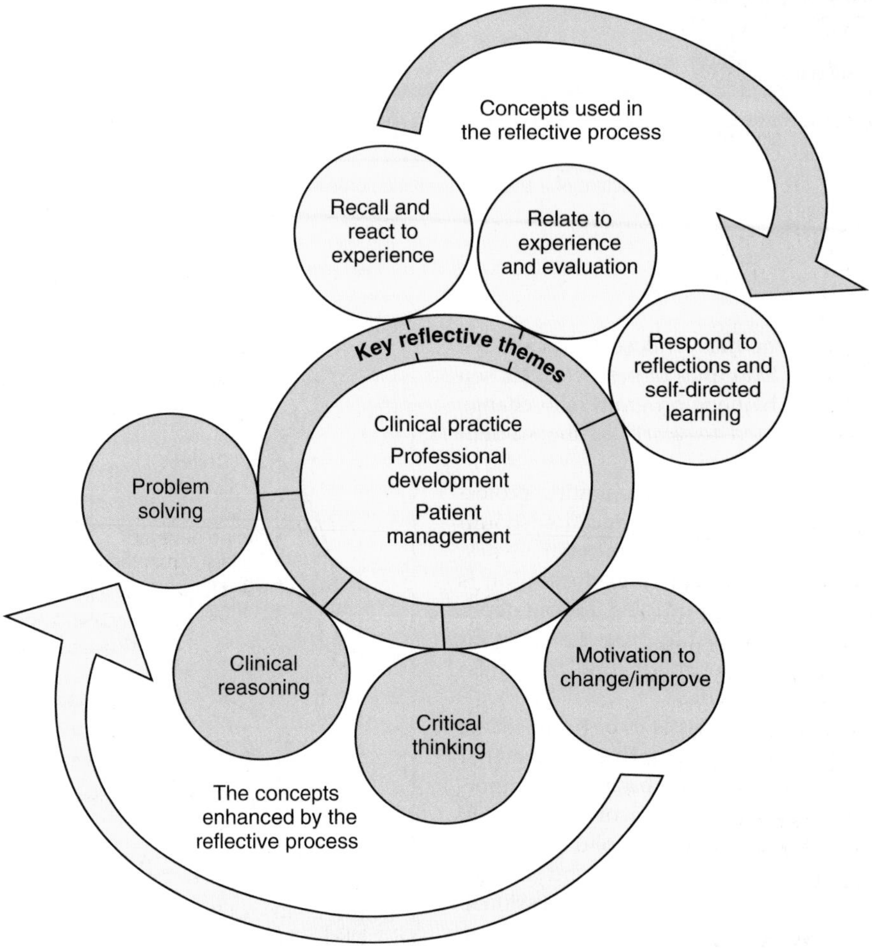

Figure 7-3. **Clinical reflection and the oral healthcare professional. Key reflection themes for healthcare providers and their role in supporting lifelong professional growth and development.** (Data from Tsang AK, Walsh LJ: Oral health students' perceptions of clinical reflective learning-relevance to their development as evolving professionals, *Eur J Dent Educ* 14:99, 2010.)

BOX 7-4

Example of Student Journal Log versus a Reflection

Journal Log Entry

This quarter I had a patient who is legally blind and required special accommodations for her care. I learned a lot about working with a visually impaired patient and I will use this case for my special needs competency.

Reflective Entry

I recently had the experience of working with a patient who is blind. Working with this patient required me to re-think everything I do automatically in clinic. From the simple task of escorting the patient to my chair, to taking x-rays and giving oral hygiene instructions, I had to put myself into her shoes and adapt my approach to meet her unique needs. This was especially challenging since I did not know in advance that I would be caring for a patient who is blind. Working with this amazing patient was rewarding and inspirational. She showed me how far a few minor accommodations can go to help a blind person maintain oral health and independence.

BOX 7-5

Formulating Reflection Statements

- Revisit
  - Briefly describe the activity or situation.
- React
  - How did the activity or situation make you feel?
  - What actions did you take?
  - What choices did you make?
- Relate
  - What was the meaning of your actions or choices?
  - How did your actions or choices challenge your value system?
- Respond
  - What did you learn from this activity or situation?
  - How can you prepare or improve your ability to respond to this situation or activity in the future?

Respond as described in Box 7-5 as helpful guidelines for reflective thinking and constructing a written reflection statement.[7]

Reflection statements can be inserted in a variety of places depending on the specific purpose of the portfolio. Student reflections are often part of each competency section and should be updated at the end of each academic term. Reflections also can be used as part of an introduction to an artifact giving more depth than a simple explanation of a project or activity. If the portfolio is used as evidence of competency for the licensed oral healthcare professional, reflection is an integral part of the clinician's self-assessment of competency and guides the selection of future continuing education and professional development activities.

Introduction and Biographic Data

The portfolio should begin with a brief introduction designed to orient the reader followed by biographic information on the portfolio's owner. Introductions to dental hygiene student portfolios often include a brief description of why the student chose dental hygiene and their personal career goals. This page undoubtedly will change as the student progresses through the program (Figure 7-4).

The biographic data section is the ideal place to keep a current résumé and curriculum vitae. A **résumé** should be a brief document succinctly summarizing an individual's education, employment history, and experiences relevant to a specific employment position. The purpose of a résumé combined with a cover letter is to get an interview. Résumés should be written in a concise style, using bulleted lists rather than sentences or paragraphs and are designed to fit on a single page. It is advisable to maintain a general résumé on file and then tailor it with the most relevant professional experiences that meet the specific requirements of the employment position. Additional information on résumé writing can be found in Chapter 63. The **curriculum vitae** (CV), as the Latin term implies, is an overview of a person's lifetime of professional activities. The CV is an ongoing documentation of one's employment, education, teaching, publications, honors, and volunteer activities. Educators in all disciplines are required to maintain a current CV as part of the institution's accreditation process. In the United States, a CV is usually necessary when applying for academic appointments, grants, fellowships, and scholarships. Outside of the United States, almost all employers expect a CV as part of the application process. The résumé and the CV should be part of the professional portfolio and must be updated regularly to remain current.

Portfolio Artifacts

Artifact is the term commonly used for the evidence used in a portfolio. An artifact for an e-portfolio may be an electronic file of a student-created brochure, research paper, community service project, or any other document that demonstrates a particular competency. Documents and artifacts must be selected carefully and organized to support the portfolio purpose. Remember, the portfolio should not be a display of every assignment or class project, but rather a well-documented, selective collection of evidence designed to illustrate a particular competency (Figure 7-5). Each artifact must be accompanied by a label or caption clearly explaining its significance in relationship to the competency or skill, the title of the artifact, the author(s) and the date it was completed. Reflective statements in the form of sentences or short paragraphs can also be included in the descriptive label (see Figure 7-5). Client care experiences can also be included as an artifact in the student portfolio (Figure 7-6, *A*). A graphic summary of the various types of clients treated as a dental hygiene student can later serve to demonstrate competency as a new graduate (Figure 7-6, *B*).

References and Citations

All documents and artifacts used in the professional portfolio must have appropriate referencing and attribution. If another person's work or research contributed to the project, the work must be appropriately cited. As stated in the *Chicago Manual of Style*, "ethics, copyright laws, and courtesy to readers require authors to identify the sources of direct quotations and of any facts or opinions not generally known or easily checked."[8] Citations not only give credit to others for their work but also allow the reader to further explore the topic by

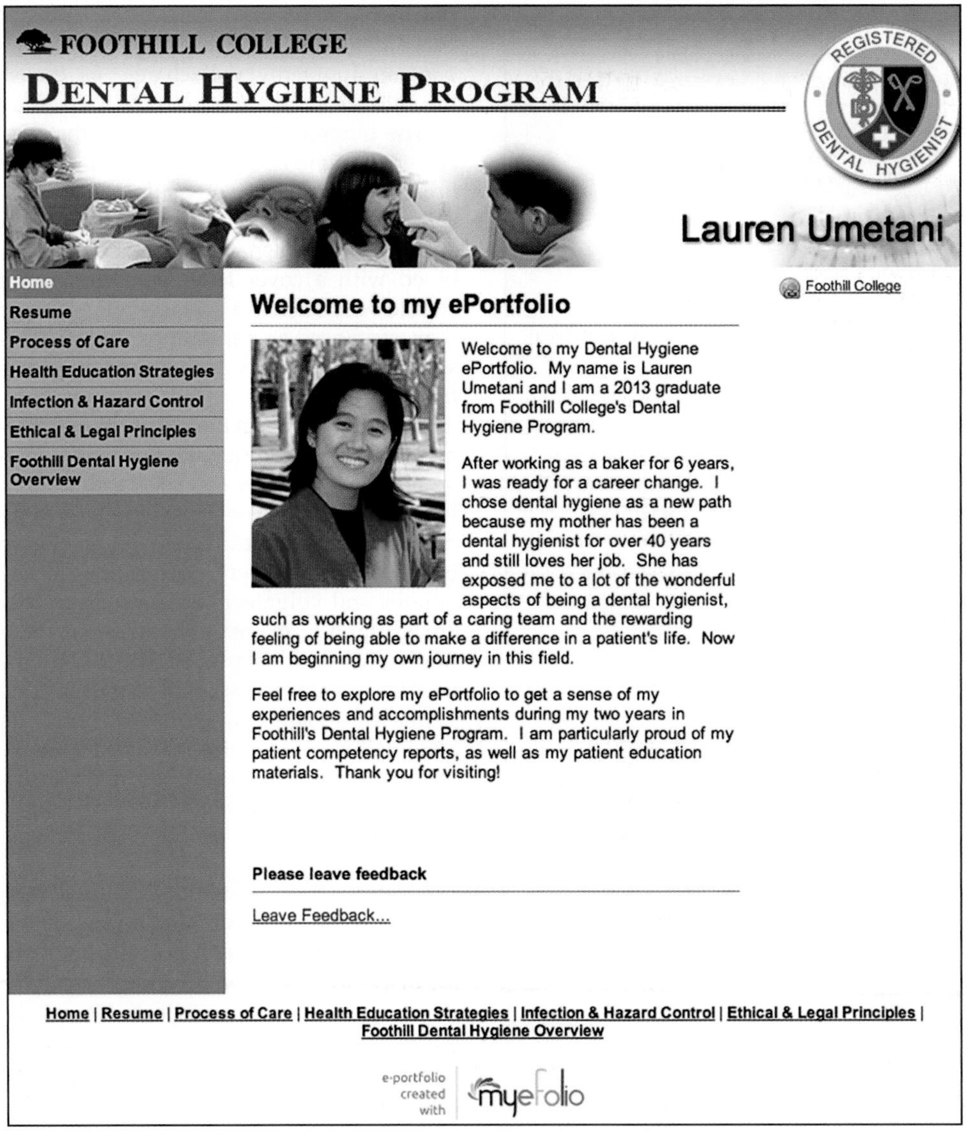

Figure 7-4. Introduction page to a first-year dental hygiene student's electronic portfolio. (Provided with permission from Foothill College Dental Hygiene Program, Los Altos Hills, California.)

providing the information to locate the original resource. Multiple references also add evidence and credibility to support the project or artifact.

There are numerous ways to reference resources. Many medical or biomedical publications require authors to use the National Library of Medicine (NLM) style, whereas nursing publications frequently use the American Psychological (APA) style guidelines. *Citing Medicine,* complete with comprehensive examples of all types of NLM citations, is available free of charge on the National Library of Medicine website, www.nln.nih.gov. Examples of NLM referencing style can be found in Figure 7-7. The particular system for listing references and the specific citation style guidelines for student projects depends on the individual school, department, or dental hygiene program.

Confidentiality and Permissions

Images used in portfolio artifacts can present challenges with patient privacy and copyright laws. Photographs of actual patients must be used with caution. Written permission in the form of a model or photograph release must be obtained to use original photographs, videos, or any other media in which the individuals depicted can be identified. Eliminating names or any identifying information by substitution with initials or pseudonyms can protect the privacy of the individual and institution. Care must be taken in the selection of artifacts particularly in online, Web-based portfolios to preserve confidentiality of the patients, faculty, fellow students, and clinical sites that may be described in the artifacts or reflections.

Copyright and Fair Use

Copyright is a widely enacted legal concept, which in the simplest of terms means "right to copy." Copyright protects the authors and creators of all types of original work including writing, composing, graphic and visual arts, and architectural and industrial designs from others copying their work. It also grants the creator of the work, or copyright holder, the right to be credited for their work, to determine who may

How do I remove plaque from my teeth?

Flossing technique:

Flossing should be done before you brush.

1. Begin with a 12-18 inch piece of floss. Wrap floss around middle fingers two to three times.
2. Grasp floss with index finder and thumb leaving about 1 inch of floss between fingertips.
3. Insert floss between teeth with a gentle seesaw motion until it reaches the gum line.
4. Wrap each tooth in a "C" shape and move the floss up and down and be sure to floss below the gum line.

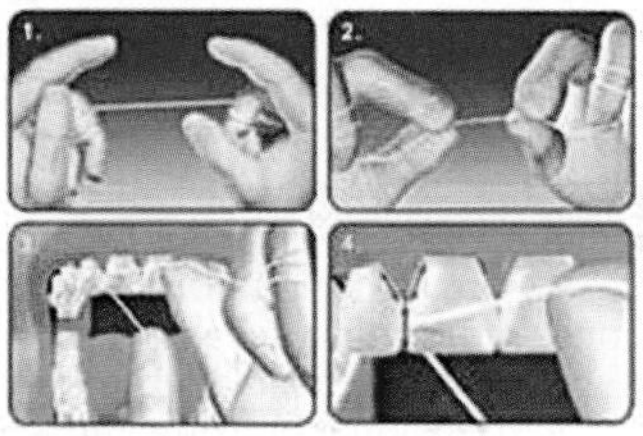

Brushing technique:

Brush for 2 minutes at least twice a day.

1. Use a soft bristle toothbrush and toothpaste.
2. Angle bristles toward the gums at a 45° angle.
3. Use short side to side and rolled strokes on all surfaces of the teeth and apply gentle pressure.
4. Brush outside and inside surfaces and at gum line.
5. Brush chewing surfaces and tongue.

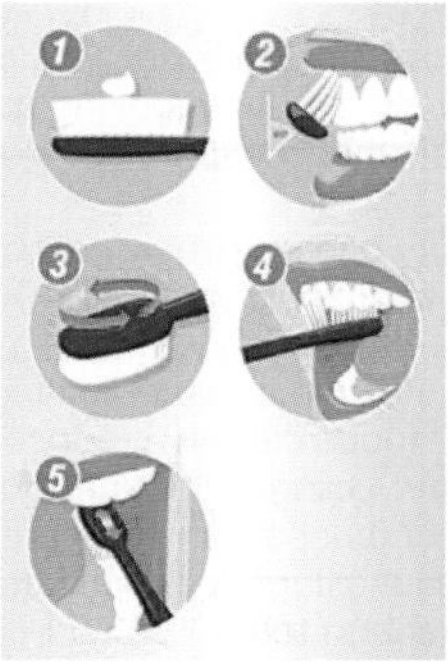

Recommendations

Toothbrush:

Toothpaste:

Floss:

Mouth rinse:

Other instructions:

____

____

____

____

References

Darby ML, Walsh MM. Dental hygiene theory and practice. 3rd ed. St. Louis, MO: Saunders; 2010. 1276 p.

Nield-Gehrig JS. Patient assessment tutorials: a step-by--step guide for the dental hygienist. 2nd ed. Philadelphia, PA: Wolters Kluwer Health; 2010. 695 p.

Aspiras M, Stoodley P, Nistico L, Longwell M, de Jager M. Clinical implications of power toothbrushing on fluoride delivery: effects on biofilm plaque metabolism and physiology. Int J Dent [Internet]. 2010 Apr 15 [cited 2012 Jan 28]; 2010: 651869. Available from: http://www.ncbi.nlm.nih.gov/pmc/articles/PMC2855952/pdf/IJD2010-651869.pdf

Rooban T, Vidya K, Joshua E, Rao A, Ranganathan S, Rao U, Ranganathan K. Tooth decay in alcohol and tobacco abusers. J Oral Maxillofac Pathol. 2011 Jan-Apr; 15(1): 14-21.

Furusawa M, Takahashi J, Isoyama M, Kitamura Y, Kashima T, Ueshima F, Nakahama N, Araki M, Rokukawa Y, Takahashi Y, Makiishi T, Yatabe K. Effectiveness of dental checkups incorporating tooth brushing instruction. Bull Tokyo Dent Coll. 2011 Jun 4; 52(3):129-133.

All images from Google Images and www.dentalcare.com

Your Oral Health

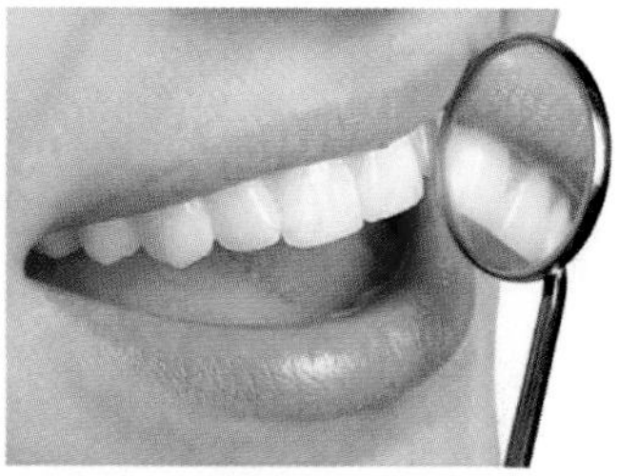

Things to Know to Maintain a Healthy Smile

Karen Wong
Dental Hygiene Student
Foothill College

A

Figure 7-5. A, Student description of health education artifacts created as part of the overall Health Education Competency section of the electronic portfolio. (Provided with permission from Foothill College Dental Hygiene Program, Los Altos Hills, California.)

Continued

adapt or use the work and who may financially benefit from the work. Although copyright does not protect facts, ideas, systems, or methods of operation, it may protect the way these concepts are used or expressed. Copyright protection is available to published and unpublished work and lasts the lifetime of the creator plus a specified number of years.

Copyright does not always prohibit all forms or replication or copying. The fair use doctrine in the United States permits some copying and distribution without asking direct permission of the copyright holder. Under certain conditions, fair use can grant educators and students instructional rights to use copyrighted materials while still preserving the rights of the creator and not financially benefitting the user. Although there are no limits to the number of words, images, text, or sounds that can be used safely without prior permission under fair use it is still best to obtain permission before using copyrighted material when possible. The guidelines defining fair use for educational purposes can be found in Box 7-6. In general, students and professionals creating a portfolio post their own original work in the portfolio. However, there may be occasions in which the portfolio author may want to use an image, link to a website, or quote from a source of literature. It is best to get written permission from the owner of the image and always use the appropriate attribution and reference.[9]

A number of resources for photos and other images do not fall under copyright protection. Creative Commons, a non-profit organization, has developed a standardized licensing approach for individuals wishing to make their creative works available for public use via the Internet. Images licensed through Creative Commons can be found through a number of search engines including Google, Yahoo, and

What is plaque biofilm?

Plaque biofilm is a layer of **bacteria** that sticks to teeth, gums, and other surfaces of the mouth. *Plaque biofilm* forms naturally as soon as **1 hour** after brushing, which is why it is important to brush at least twice a day and floss daily. Plaque buildup can trap stains on teeth and is the main cause of gum disease and tooth decay. Plaque that remains on the teeth can harden and become *calculus*, or *tartar*.

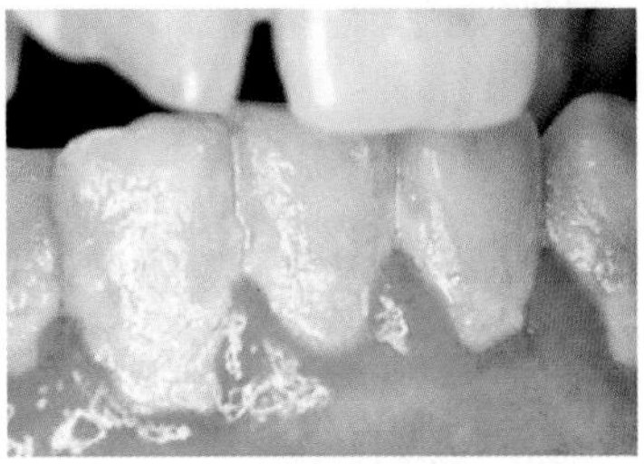

Heavy plaque buildup

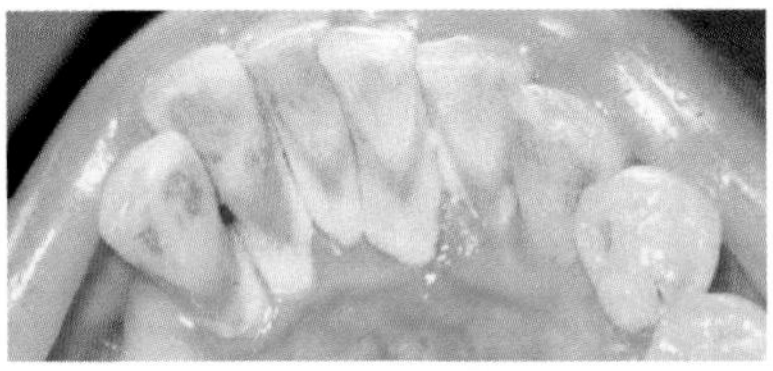

Calculus (tartar)

What is gum disease?

Gum disease is an **infection** of the gums and can be caused by the accumulation of plaque biofilm. It begins with *gingivitis*, which is a mild inflammation of the gums. *Gingivitis* usually presents as red, swollen gums and bleeds when brushing or flossing. *Gingivitis* is reversible with proper brushing and flossing and regular professional cleanings. If left untreated, *gingivitis* maylead to more serious periodontal disease. Periodontal disease, or *periodontitis* , is an irreversible infection that damages the bone and tissue that support the teeth, which can lead to tooth loss. Treatment by a dental professional will keep *periodontitis* from progressing.

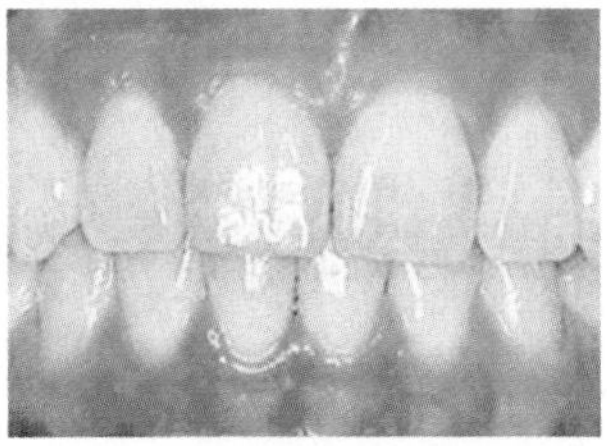

Healthy gingiva (gums)

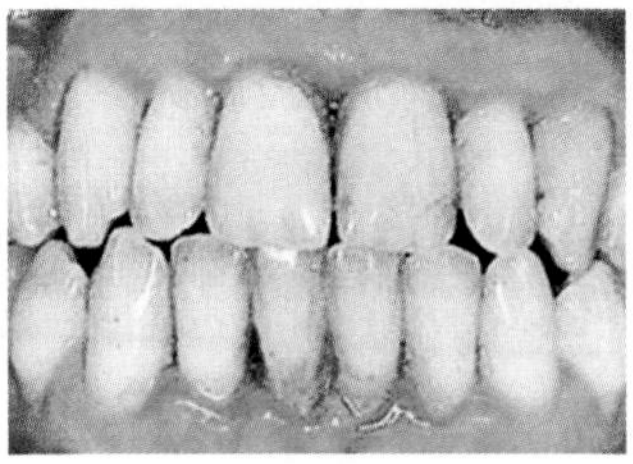

Periodontitis

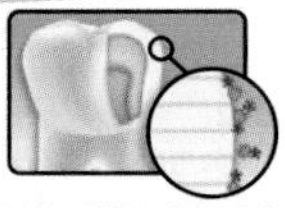

Acid and food particles "attack" the enamel causing it to weaken.

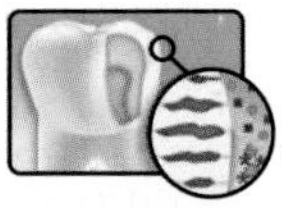

Saliva washes away the acid and food particles while introducing minerals.

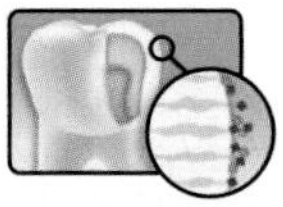

The minerals from the saliva help rebuild tooth enamel

What causes tooth decay?

Tooth decay, commonly known as cavities or dental *caries*, is caused by bacterial plaque. The bacteria feed on the food and beverages you consume and produce acids as waste products. These acids breakdown, or *demineralize*, the tooth structure which is composed of different minerals such as calcium. **Saliva** washes away and neutralizes the acid and rebuilds, or *remineralizes*, the areas attacked by acid by replacing minerals. If the acid level becomes too high, such as when a person is constantly snacking or consuming a high sugar diet, then saliva flow cannot keep up to repair demineralization, thus causing tooth decay.

Risk factors for tooth decay include: high sugar diet, dry mouth, smoking and tobacco use, and alcohol consumption.

Tooth decay can be **prevented** by regularly brushing and flossing to remove plaque. Drinking water frequently, rinsing or brushing after meals, and limiting intake of high sugar foods can also reduce the risk of tooth decay. Using a fluoride toothpaste or fluoride mouthrinse can help prevent tooth decay because fluoride is a mineral that aids in remineralizing teeth

B

Figure 7-5. B, Patient education handout artifact created by a dental hygiene student. (Provided with permission from Foothill College Dental Hygiene Program, Los Altos Hills, California.)

BOX 7-6

General Guidelines for Fair Use in Education[9]

FAIR USE	NOT FAIR USE
Teaching, scholarship, education	Commercial purposes, profit
Non-fiction based, factual information	Creative work (art, music, films, plays, books)
Commentary or criticism	Entertainment
Small sample of work used	Large part of work is used
Limited or restricted access	Open access on Internet or a public forum

Flickr. Appropriate credit must still be given for images and content licensed by Creative Commons.

Portfolio Authorship and Ethical Principles

The ethical principle of **veracity** applies to the creation of a professional portfolio. Veracity is defined as the adherence to the truth or conformity to factual evidence. The student dental hygienist or professional is bound by the American Dental Hygienists' Association Code of Ethics[10] to present artifacts or documents that are the work or accomplishments of the portfolio owner. Work done by others, such as images and outside research, always must be attributed and properly cited. One of the core values in the ADHA Code of Ethics is **confidentiality**, the responsibility to keep patient information private. Applying this concept to a portfolio means that there must not be any identifiable patient information used in the portfolio.

Patient Experiences Log						
Patient initials	**AAP**	**Calculus class**	**Completion date**	**Ethnicity**	**Age and lifestage**	**Summary of treatment and learning experiences**
C.C.	I	II	4/24/07	Hispanic	5. Early childhood	Pediatric competency. Assessments, OHI (Fones), plaque debridement with toothbrush, partial coronal polish. Difficult patient due to age, language barrier and attention span. This experience helped me better understand patient management.
L.T.	II	III	4/26/07	Caucasian	29. Early adulthood	Assessments. OHI (Stillmans), probe evaluation, hand scaling. 2% NaF. There were no surprises with this patient, the appointment went smoothly. I learned that although the focus is on removing subgingival calculus, one should not forget the supragingival plaque.

A

B

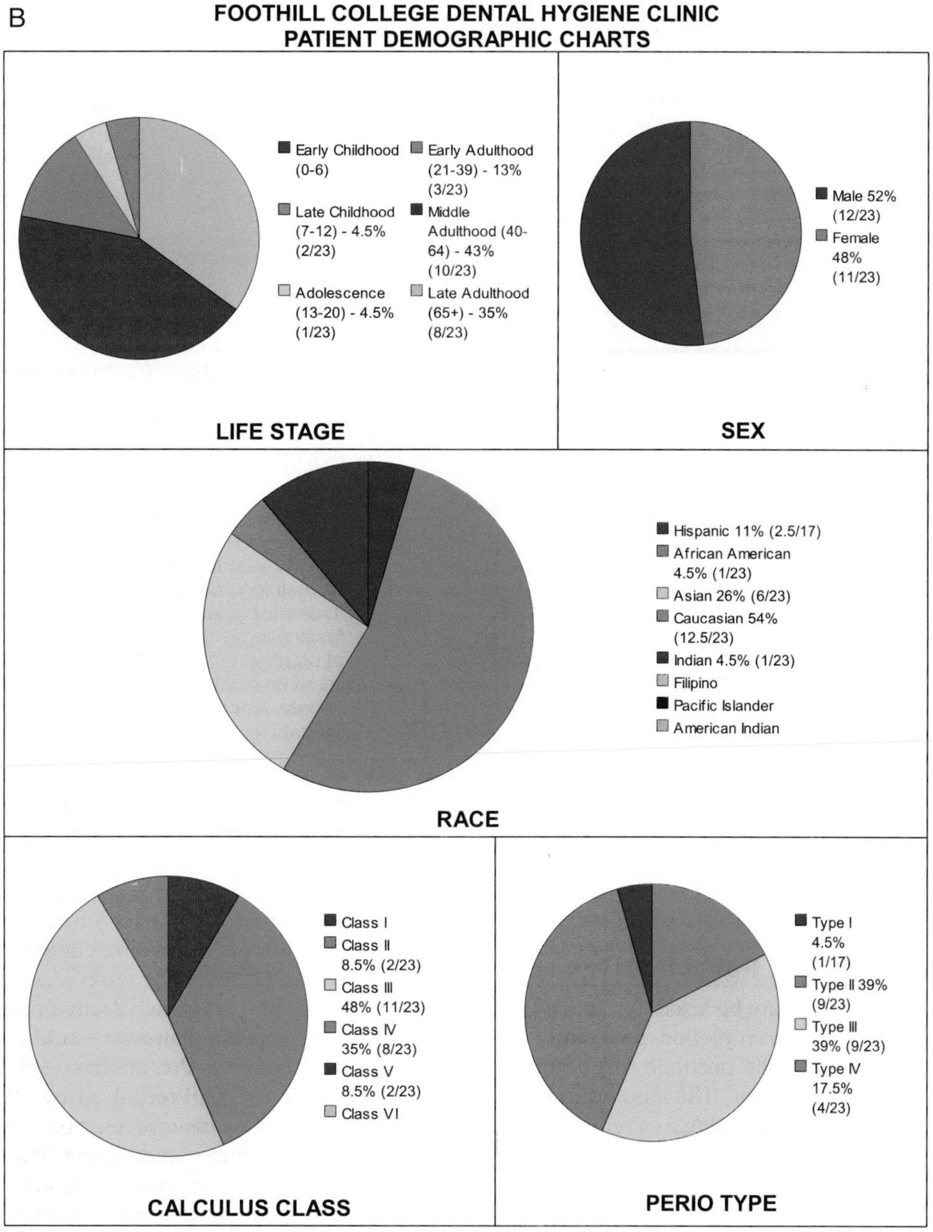

Figure 7-6. A, Sample of a student electronic portfolio patient experiences log. **B,** Sample of client demographic summary from a student electronic portfolio. (Adapted from Patrias K, Wendling D, editor: *Citing medicine: the NLM style guide for authors, editors, and publishers,* ed 2, Bethesda, Md, 2007, National Library of Medicine.)

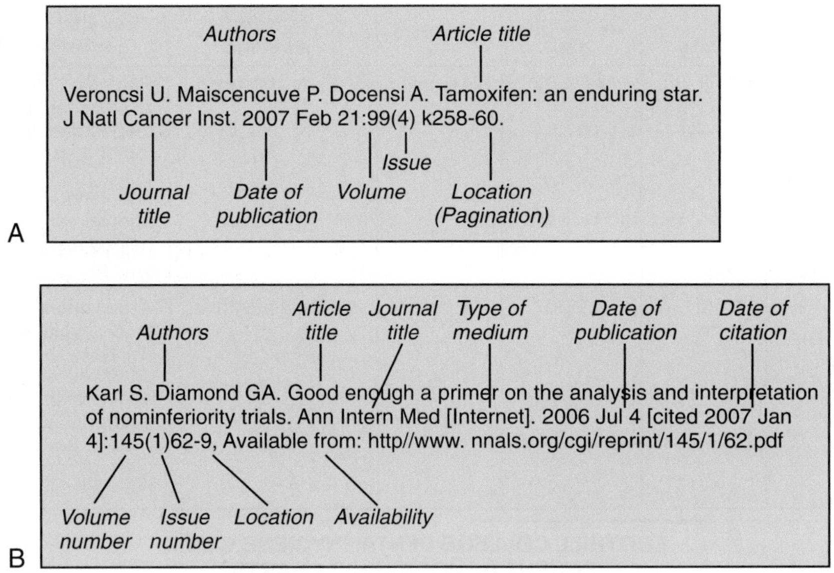

Figure 7-7. Example of National Library of Medicine Citation Style, citing a reference journal, print version (**A**), and an electronic version (**B**). (Adapted from Patrias K, Wendling D, editor: *Citing medicine: the NLM style guide for authors, editors, and publishers,* ed 2, Bethesda, Md, 2007, National Library of Medicine.)

Professional Development Log Template			
Date	Course Title and Presenter	Contact Hours/Units	Course Description/Evaluation
9/20/2011	Dr. Eric Phelps, DDS, MS/What Am I Looking At?	2	Dr. Phelps, an orthodontist, gave a fascinating presentation about some of the interesting cases in his practice. We learned more about orthodontics and some of the changing ideas and new technologies in the field.
10/6/12	Gloria Monzon, RDH – Lasers and Dental Hygiene	2	Ms. Monzon lectured on the developing practice of laser therapy in dental hygiene. This was a fascinating lecture that shows a lot of promise with periodontally involved patients. While the therapy cannot confirm bone regeneration, the radiographs seem to show some regeneration. More research should be done in this area.

Figure 7-8. Sample professional development log template.

Transitioning the Student Portfolio

Initially, the student portfolio can be used for entry-level employment interviews, degree-completion programs, and post-graduate study. Over time, the portfolio can be transitioned to fulfill a variety of purposes. The student portfolio can become a "working portfolio," serving as a repository for organizing and storing artifacts acquired during one's professional life. Looking back to the core competency areas for the student hygienist related to infection control, patient care, health education, and legal and ethical principles, the graduate hygienist could choose to continue to organize artifacts or evidence of ongoing competencies in these areas. The American Dental Hygienists' Association's "Standards for Clinical Dental Hygiene Practice"[11] also can be used as a guideline for demonstration and self-assessment of clinical competencies. Professional development should be ongoing even for the recent graduate. Logs chronicling courses, workshops, in-services, and other activities, including the date, presenter, and a short summary/reflection on the activity, should be created for this section. Once the templates for the professional development log has been created regularly, adding the content becomes an easy task (Figure 7-8).

BOX 7-7

Writing a Healthcare Philosophy of Practice Statement

A healthcare philosophy of practice statement should be a succinct written paragraph or bulleted highlights that serve as the foundation for one's professional beliefs. Reflection on the following topics can guide the philosophy statement:

- Definition of personal objectives and role
- Career goals: short term and long term
- Healthcare values
- Ethical considerations of practice
- Commitment to cultural diversity, special needs, vulnerable populations
- Definition of excellence
- Vision for the future

The portfolio introduction and biographic data section is another area that should be customized to fit the specific purpose of the portfolio. This is the ideal area to state the portfolio owner's philosophy of practice or career goals. Writing a philosophy of practice takes thought and reflection and may change over time and experience. The philosophy of practice also varies, depending on the purpose of the portfolio. A portfolio used to interview for a clinical position in private practice differs from one used for a position in education or the corporate world; the philosophy should be written according to the specific purpose. A well-written introduction and philosophy of practice should pique the interest of the reader to review the portfolio in addition to leaving a professional impression. Guidelines for writing a philosophy statement can be found in Box 7-7.

Transitioning the student portfolio is an excellent way to showcase the professional's strengths and experiences in addition to validating his or her clinical competency, ongoing professional development, and self-reflection.

LEGAL, ETHICAL, AND SAFETY ISSUES

- Always obtain permission to use images or work of other authors in the portfolio and give appropriate credit to the author or source.
- Protect the confidentiality of clients, co-workers, and facilities.
- Apply the core principles of the ADHA Code of Ethics when creating a portfolio.
- Honesty and accuracy are key elements of a student or professional portfolio.

KEY CONCEPTS

- Portfolios are becoming an integral part the dental hygiene education and development of the healthcare professional. The foundation of the portfolio begins with the student dental hygienist and should transition to a professional portfolio, reflecting the growth and achievements throughout the career of the dental hygienist.
- Healthcare professionals must be able to provide ongoing evidence of competency throughout their careers. Maintaining a professional portfolio with artifacts documenting professional development activities is a requirement for licensure renewal for dental professionals in some states. Licensure by portfolio is an alternative for the live patient exam for dental students in California and may be considered in other states as well.
- Reflective thinking supports problem solving, critical thinking, and self-directed learning, key characteristics of a professional. Reflection statements should be integrated into the professional portfolio to support each competency or section of the portfolio and to direct self-assessment and the lifelong learning process of the healthcare professional.
- A professional portfolio can serve as a visual tool to guide or support the interview process. A well-organized portfolio can assist the practitioner in articulating his or her philosophy, experiences, education, and ongoing professional growth.
- The professional portfolio must be an honest representation of the individual. Artifacts must have appropriate attribution and follow all the appropriate ethical and legal guidelines.

CRITICAL THINKING EXERCISES

1. Have a class discussion about appropriate content/artifacts for a dental hygiene portfolio. Discuss the differences between a portfolio and a social media site such as Facebook.
2. Using the following competency subject areas, describe an artifact that could be used to demonstrate mastery of each competency.
   - Infection control
   - Health education
   - Patient care
   - Legal and ethical principles
3. Create an artifact for your portfolio. Write an introduction statement describing the artifact and include an appropriate photograph.
4. Remember caring for your very first patient in clinic. In what ways have you grown as a student dental hygienist? Write a one- to two-paragraph reflection statement on how you have changed and the challenges you still face as a student hygienist.
5. You are a recent graduate getting ready to look for your first position in private practice. Reflect on your professional values and career goals to write a philosophy of practice statement to include as part of your portfolio.
6. Role-play with a student partner an interview for a position as a clinician in a dental practice. Integrate the supporting artifacts of your portfolio into the interview process.

REFERENCES

1. Stevens H: The impact of e-portfolio development on the employability of adults aged 45 and over. *Campus-Wide Information Systems* 25(4):209, 2008. Available at: http://www.emeraldinsight.com/journals.htm?articleid=1742082. Accessed November 2, 2011.
2. Fox K: *California OKs nation's first portfolio exam for licensure*, Chicago, 2010, American Dental Association. Available at: http://www.ada.org/news/4890.aspx. Accessed November 2, 2012.

3. Minnesota Board of Dentistry: *Professional development*, Minneapolis, Minn, 2012, Minnesota Board of Dentistry. Available at: http://www.dentalboard.state.mn.us. Accessed October 30, 2012.
4. Dennision R: What goes into your professional portfolio and what you'll get out of it. *American Nurse Today* 2(1):42, 2007.
5. Cangelosai P: Learning portfolios giving meaning to practice. *Nurse Educator* 33(3):125, 2008.
6. Kardos RL, Cook JM, Butson RJ, et al: The development of an ePortfolio for life-long reflective learning and auditable professional certification. *Eur J Dent Educ* 13:135, 2009.
7. Bourner T: Assessing reflective learning. *Edu Train* 45:267, 2003.
8. University of Chicago Press Staff: *Chicago manual of style*, ed 15, Chicago, 2006, University of Chicago Press, p 594.
9. Library of Congress: *Copyright law of the United States of America* [Internet] Washington (DC), 2012, US Government Bookstore [cited 2012 Nov 7]. Available at: http://www.copyright.gov/title17/.
10. American Dental Hygienists' Association: *Bylaws and code of ethics* [Internet] Chicago (IL), 2011 American Dental Hygienists Association June 20 [cited 2012 Nov 20]. Available at: http://www.adha.org/downloads/adha-bylaws-code-of-ethics.pdf.
11. American Dental Hygienists' Association: *Standards for clinical dental hygiene practice*, Chicago, 2008, American Dental Hygienists Association. Available at: http://www.adha.org/downloads/adha_standards08.pdf. Accessed November 20, 2012.

EVOLVE RESOURCES

Please visit http://evolve.elsevier.com/Darby/hygiene for additional practice and study support tools.

CHAPTER 8

The Dental Hygiene Care Environment

Denise Michelle Claiborne

COMPETENCIES

1. Discuss the dental hygiene care environment in a private office setting, including the components of the dental hygiene treatment area.
2. Discuss the dental hygiene care environment in a dental hygiene care facility (college setting), including the use of electronic health records and simulation technology.
3. Discuss the dental hygiene care environment in a hospital setting, including who the main clients are in this setting.
4. Name an example of a mobile dental facility.

The dental hygiene care environment is the physical setting that contains equipment and instruments where the dental hygienist delivers professional oral care. This chapter identifies the structural components of a conventional treatment area **(operatory),** in addition to community, hospital, and school settings. The equipment and powered instruments the dental hygienist uses and maintains, computer software used (e.g., electronic health records [EHR]), and legal and ethical issues associated with equipment maintenance are discussed.

Settings

Private Practice

Office Design

The ***reception area*** is the first room a client enters and where check-in occurs. Décor, lighting, temperature, sound, and smell influence the environment in an office. These factors also leave a lasting impression to the client and set the tone for the visit. Décor should be calm and relaxing, moreover, with no overwhelming color schemes. The lighting should be adequate enough for reading, and reading material should be available for clients.

Business Area

The business area is located near the entrance of the facility. It contains computer terminals, phones, and intraoffice communication systems; in addition, the client records, appointment schedules, and office supplies are maintained. This area should remain private because of the exchange of client information. The complexity of this area depends on the size and needs of the practice. Adjacent is often the reception area, in which clients can relax before their appointments.

Dental Hygiene Treatment Area

Floor Plan

A private oral healthcare practice or clinic maintains treatment areas for dental units, general structural fixtures, radiographic equipment, a radiographic processing area, an instrument processing area, a laboratory, supply storage, business office, reception area, and a restroom. Some offices also have staff areas and private consultation rooms.

Stools and Chairs

The treatment area, where professional oral care is provided, contains stools, the dental chair, the dental unit, and equipment (Figure 8-1). The operator stool can be adjusted for seat height and back support with controls located under the seat cushion (Figure 8-2). It should provide ergonomic support, especially in the lumbar region of the back, and allow for the operator's feet to be flat on the floor to maintain proper circulation in legs and feet. Stool designs range from saddle stools with no back or arm rests to traditional stools with back and both arm rests. The benefits of saddle stools in dental hygiene are numerous. The stools are lightweight, portable, and easily adjustable to solve a multitude of ergonomic problems. A saddle stool can be adjusted easily with one lever and lends itself to multiple users (Figure 8-3). Raised, tense shoulders are one of the primary problems leading to neck and shoulder pain among dental hygienists. The saddle stool helps to solve this problem by placing hygienists halfway between standing and sitting, increasing the hip angle up to 135 degrees. Lower positioning of the client and a more relaxed shoulder posture results. Regardless of the stool chosen, it is important that the stool is adjusted properly for an operator's body stature to prevent musculoskeletal disorders. The dental assistant stool, taller than an operator stool, differs in function and usually has a bar to support the feet and a torso support bar to allow the dental assistant to lean forward over the client while assisting the operator (Figure 8-4). The dental chair, a reclining elongated lounge, has arm supports and is adjustable by switch, touch pad, or foot control for height, head rest, swivel, and tilt. Coverings on dental stools and chairs are durable and easily cleaned and disinfected.

The Dental Unit

The dental unit contains the delivery system and a dental light (Figure 8-5). The delivery system, attached to a bracket table, moveable arm, or mobile cart, typically contains the air-water syringe, the high-speed and low-speed handpiece tubing, and a radiograph view box. Wireless handpieces

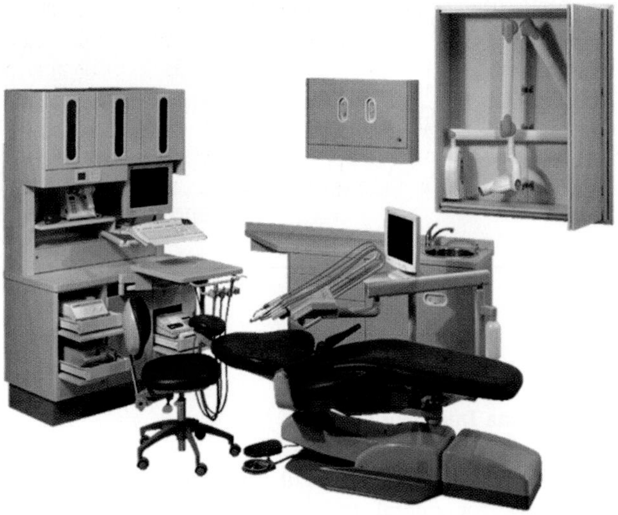

Figure 8-1. The treatment area. (Courtesy A-dec, Inc, Newberg, Oregon.)

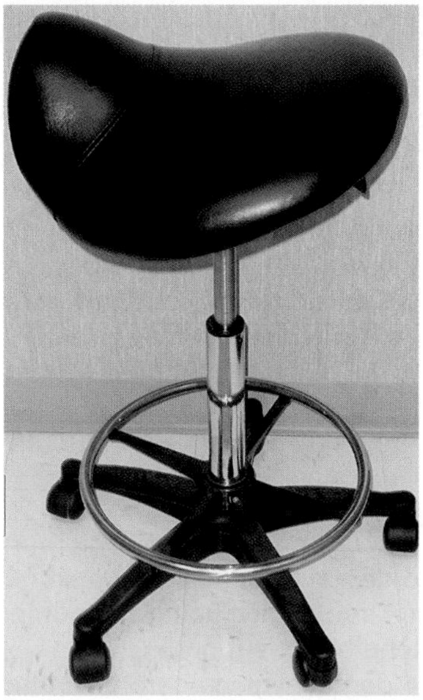

Figure 8-3. The saddle stool. (Courtesy Tracy Martin, LWSS Family Dentistry Norfolk, VA.)

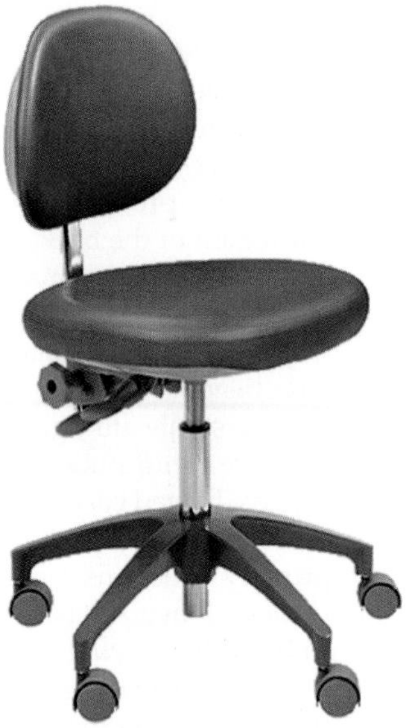

Figure 8-2. The operator stool. (Courtesy A-dec, Inc, Newberg, Oregon.)

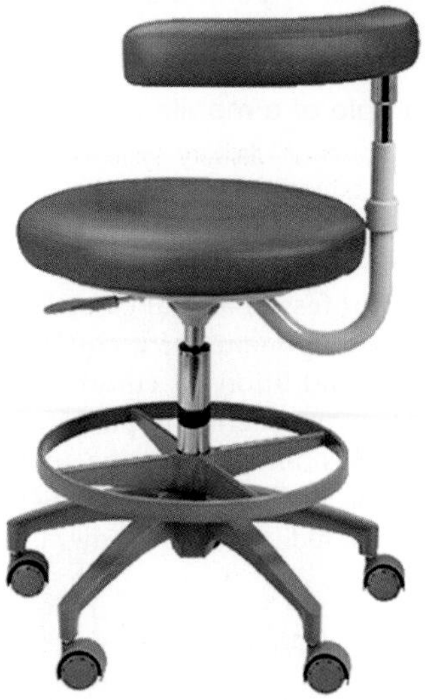

Figure 8-4. The dental assistant stool with torso support bar. (Courtesy A-dec, Inc, Newberg, Oregon.)

allow for use outside of the traditional dental setting (Figure 8-6). The dental light can be mounted on a ceiling track or on a pole attached to the dental unit. Wireless light-emitting diode (LED) headlights also can be worn by an operator. Electrical power, light, and water are controlled by switch or rheostat (foot control); most units have separate power and water switches independent of each other. Some delivery systems have touch pads mounted on the bracket or instrument table that operate components of the system (Figures 8-7 and 8-8). There are a number of variations in design for a bracket or instrument table, which can hold instruments and the components of the delivery system for the clinician and dental assistant. The Dental R.A.T 2.0 is a foot-operated mouse that enables hands-free access to periodontal charting, an intraoral camera, and digital x-rays. The Dental R.A.T requires no additional software and can be wireless or wired. It allows a hygienist to run the operatory's dental software without needing an assistant or increasing the risk of cross-contamination (Figure 8-9).

Additional mounted tubing on the delivery system arm may include an ultrasonic, piezoelectric, or sonic scaler; an air polishing handpiece or unit; a fiberoptic light; a composite curing light; and a laser, all of which may be activated by switch or rheostat. Mounted on the delivery arm could be a monitor for a computer to display electronic client records. These pieces of equipment could be mounted in front of the clinician for a 9 o'clock seating position or behind the client's head for a 12 o'clock delivery system and a seating position for the clinician behind the client's head (Figure 8-10).

High-volume evacuation (HVE) and low-volume evacuation (LVE) tubing or suction lines facilitate client rinsing and maintain visibility and oral fluid control during care.

Adapters and devices are available for suction lines that accommodate narrow and wide suction tip inserts and saliva ejectors. Dental units have a separate water bottle supply (closed water system) for the unit (Figure 8-11) or a facility-wide water treatment system. The Center for Disease Control and Prevention (CDC) recommends all dental devices connected to the water system (handpieces, ultrasonic scalers, and air/water syringe) are flushed at least 30 seconds between clients and several minutes before the start of the clinic day. Water used for dental treatment should meet the nationally recognized standards set by the EPA for drinking water (<500 CFU/mL for heterotrophic plate count) for routine

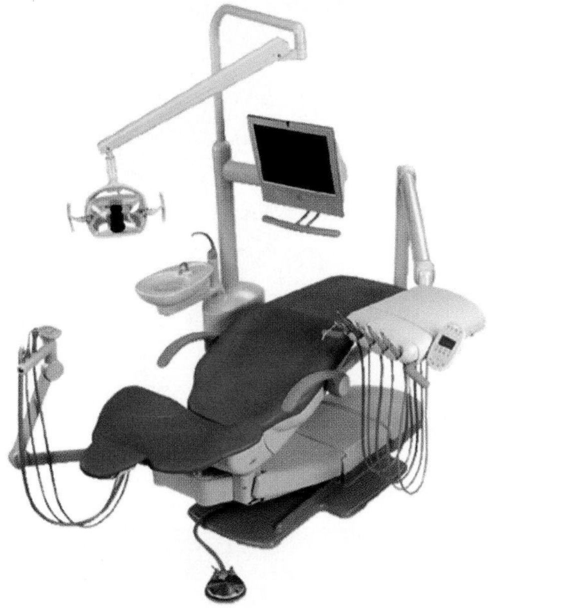

Figure 8-5. The dental chair, delivery systems, monitor, rheostat, light. (Courtesy A-dec, Inc, Newberg, Oregon.)

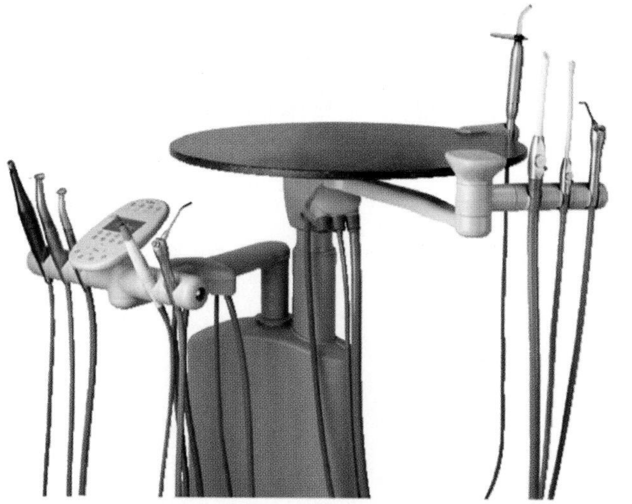

Figure 8-7. Two dental delivery systems. (Courtesy A-dec, Inc, Newberg, Oregon.)

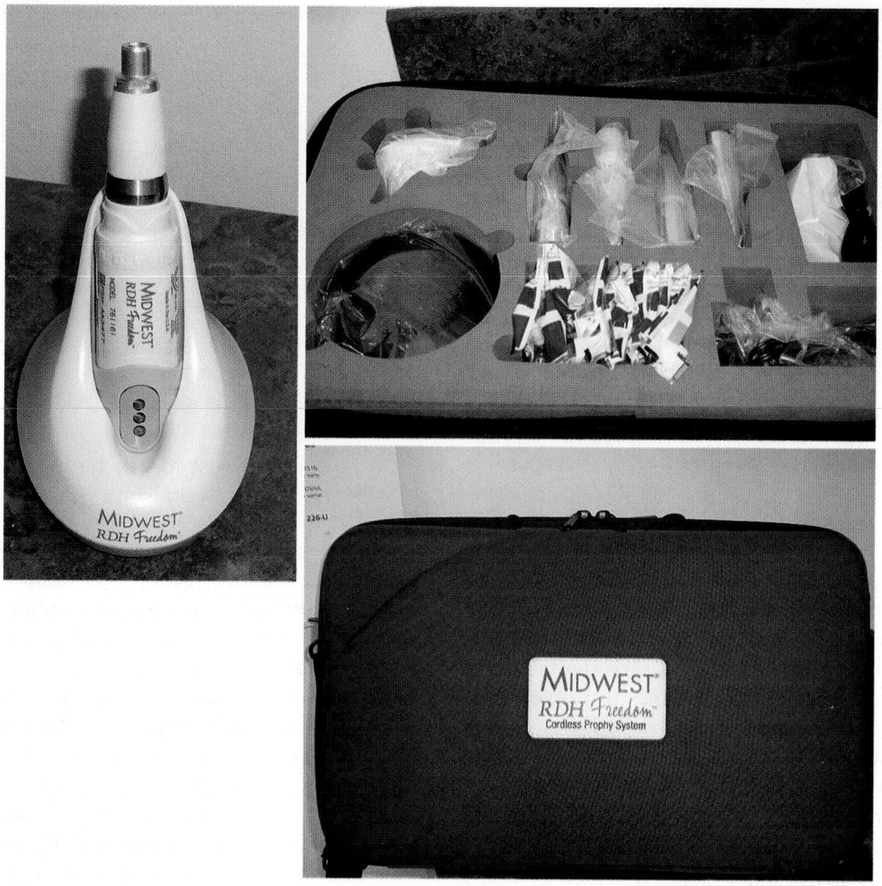

Figure 8-6. Wireless handpiece. (Courtesy Thomas Nelson Community College, Williamsburg, VA.)

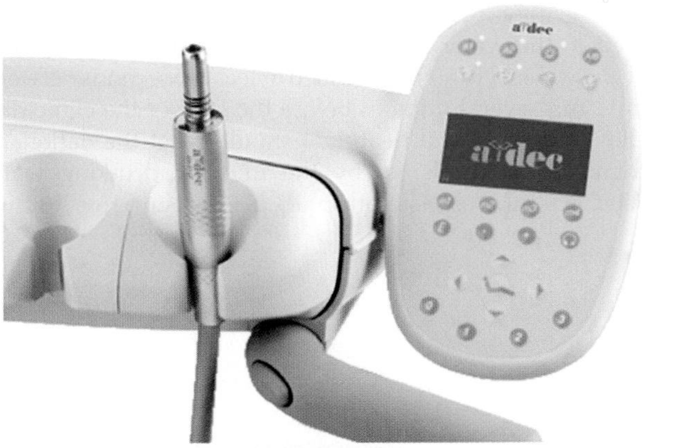

Figure 8-8. A dental unit touch pad. (Courtesy A-dec, Inc, Newberg, Oregon.)

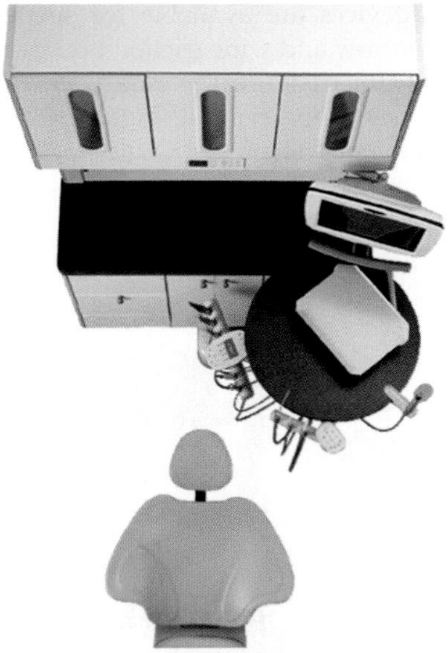

Figure 8-10. A 12:00 dental delivery system. (Courtesy A-dec, Inc, Newberg, Oregon.)

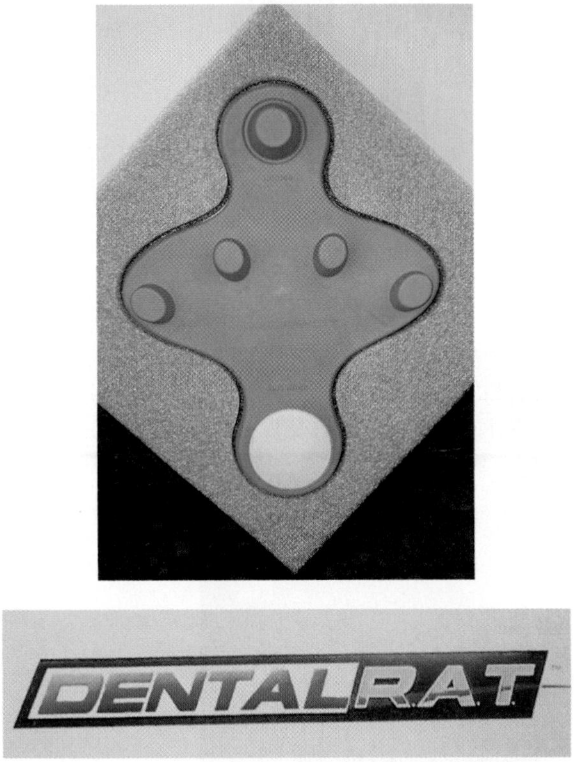

Figure 8-9. The DentalRAT. (Thomas Nelson Community College, Williamsburg, VA.)

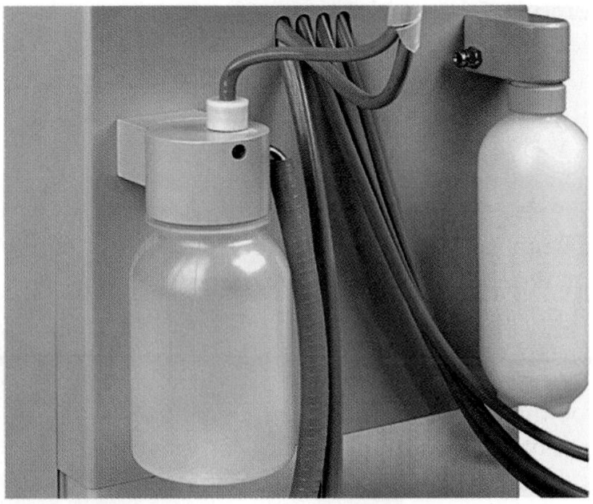

Figure 8-11. Dental unit water bottles. (Courtesy A-dec, Inc, Newberg, Oregon.)

dental treatment output water. In either case, daily treatments such as iodine tablets for water bottles or suction line chemical treatments are necessary to prevent biofilm formation in the water tubing or lines. Most contemporary dental units have anti-retraction valves on the water lines to prevent the backflow of contaminated water into the waterlines of the unit. Water line disinfection products are available that require no daily chemical treatment of the water lines and act as a filter. For example, Sterisil Straw has been approved by the Environmental Protective Agency (EPA) to produce quality water less than or equal to 10 CFU per mL bacteria. Treated water using this product is 50 times lower than the American Dental Association (ADA), CDC, and EPA recommendations (Figure 8-12).

Structural Fixtures

Most treatment areas have storage cabinets, a sink, paper towel dispensers, and alcohol hand rub and antibacterial soap dispensers with manual, foot, or laser controls. Infection-control standards mandate an emergency eye wash station attached to the faucet of a sink in the facility. A biohazard sharps container to collect contaminated needles and sharp objects is in the treatment area to help prevent needle stick exposures during disposal. This counter also can hold the client's dental chart, models, or other reference materials during treatment. The walls and flooring in the treatment area are functional, easily cleaned, and sturdy. Draperies, carpeting, and delicate furnishings are not appropriate in treatment areas because they hold contaminants and are difficult to disinfect.

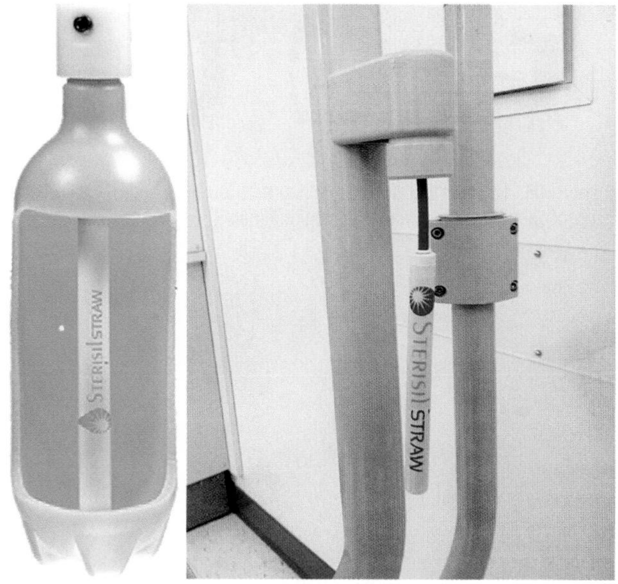

Figure 8-12. The Sterisil Straw. (Courtesy Old Dominion University, Norfolk, VA.)

A compressor provides compressed air to run the dental handpieces and suction. Because of its size and noise production, the compressor may be housed in a mechanical room with other devices such as circuit breakers, fuse box, central suction, water heater, and heating and air conditioning units.

Instrument Recirculation Area (see Chapter 9 on Infection Control)

The instrument recirculation area is where contaminated instruments are processed for reuse. Contaminated instruments must be carried to this area in a covered container or cassette. The area should have a clearly demarcated entrance point to bring in contaminated instruments and an exit point for the sterile instruments. Demarcated areas prevent the accidental exposure of sterile instruments and people to blood and bodily fluids from contaminated instruments. This well-ventilated area contains ultrasonic instrument cleaning device(s); dry heat, steam-pressure or chemical-pressure and/or flash sterilizer(s); products used in preparing instruments for sterilization; and a container with a high-level liquid chemical instrument disinfectant (Figure 8-13). Another biohazard trash and sharps container is located in the contaminated section of the processing area or isolated area.

Sterilized instruments are stored in wrapped preset trays or cassettes away from the contaminated processing area. Following manufacturer's directions for all equipment is necessary so that procedures are implemented consistently to ensure the optimum performance of the equipment. Cleaning and disinfection supplies may be stored in this area.

Equipment Maintenance

Delivery of high-quality dental care requires equipment maintenance; regular cleaning of the dental unit's traps, filters, and lines prevents biofilm contamination and disease transmission. Dental equipment suppliers publish information on the use and maintenance of their products, which should be followed. If these documents are not available, most manufacturers publish maintenance information on their websites.

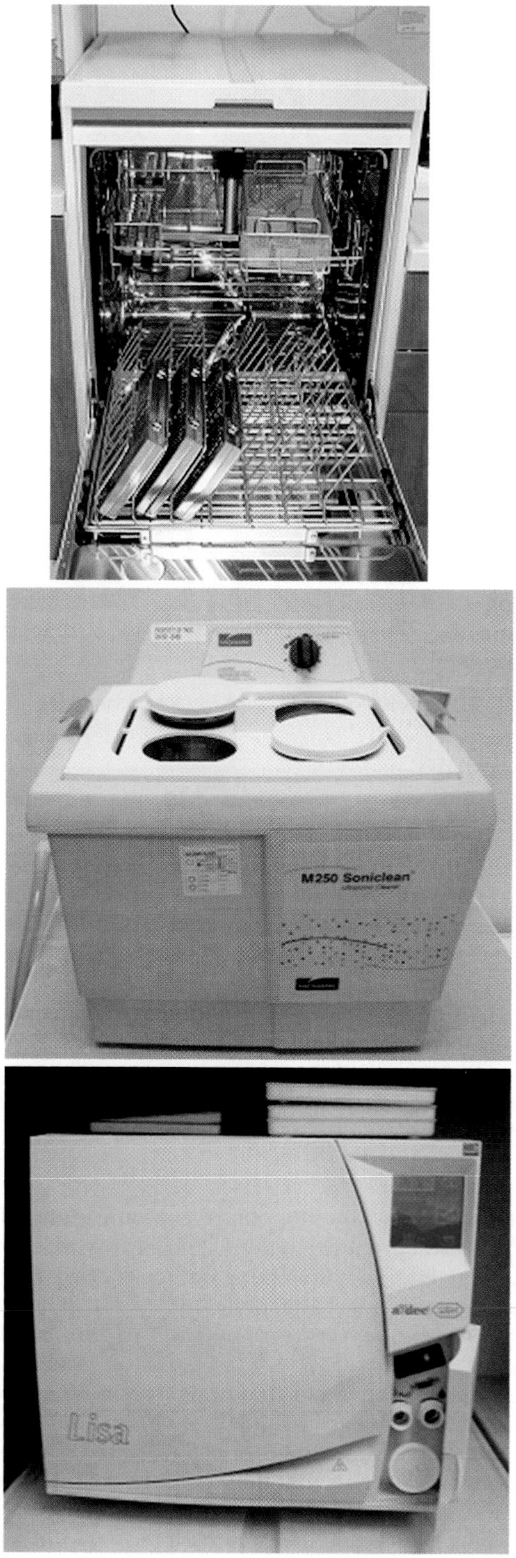

Figure 8-13. Types of ultrasonic cleaners and autoclave machine. (Thomas Nelson Community College, Williamsburg, VA.)

Radiographic Equipment

Radiographic equipment consists of a wall-mounted control panel with an on-off switch, an indicator light, exposure settings, an x-ray tube mounted on a long moveable arm with an open cylinder or rectangular position-indicating device

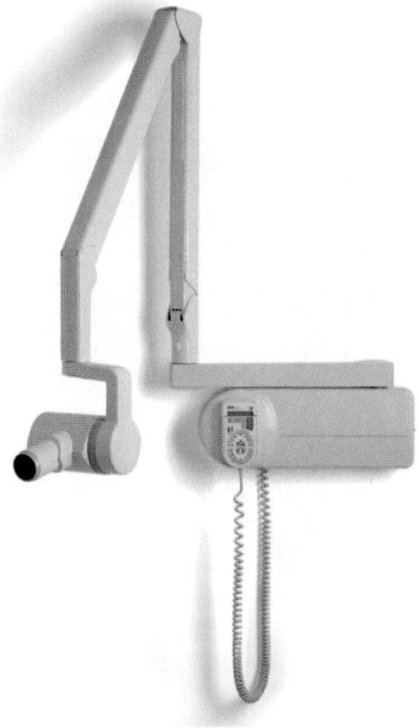

Figure 8-14. A dental unit x-ray tube. (Courtesy Practice Works Systems, LLC, the exclusive maker of Kodak Dental Systems, Atlanta, Georgia.)

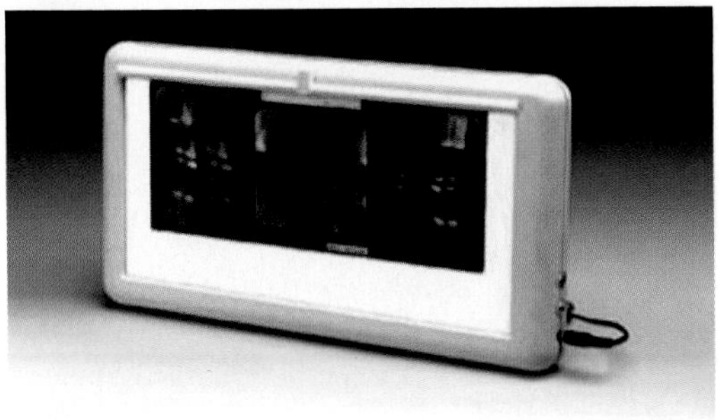

Figure 8-15. Radiograph view box. (Courtesy DENTSPLY Rinn, a division of DENTSPLY International, Elgin, Illinois.)

(PID) at the end and a wall-mounted exposure button (Figure 8-14). The lead apron with a thyroid collar is worn by clients during x-ray exposure; it is hung on hooks or a bar located in the treatment area. The radiograph view box may be mounted on the delivery system, wall, or counter (Figure 8-15).

Digital technology uses the same x-ray tube as conventional methods; however, a charged photoreceptor sensor, the size of 0, 1, or 2 film, is used in lieu of a conventional film packet. Images appear on the computer monitor almost instantaneously after exposure. Digital radiographic images can be viewed on a computer screen, stored, transmitted electronically, or printed (Figure 8-16). Intraoral cameras (IOCs) were first used in dentistry in 1987. Since then IOCs have evolved from oversized mobile units to pocket-sized lightweight wands. The IOC magnifies teeth 40 to 60 times their original size, which allows for the identification of defects within the oral cavity. Dental and dental hygiene schools as well as private offices are using intraoral cameras for chairside client education, oral examinations, comparisons, and specialist referrals (Figure 8-17).

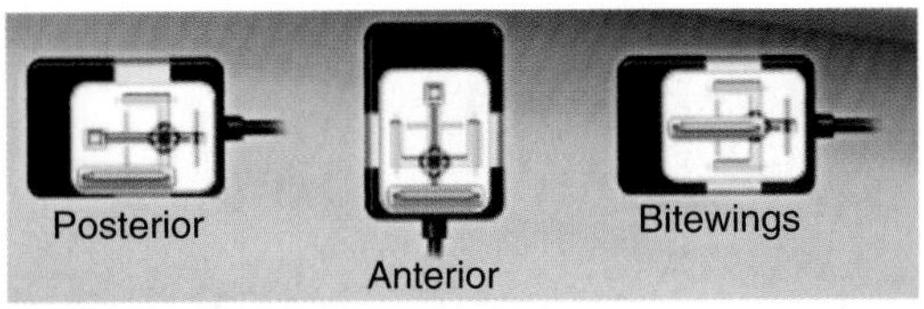

Figure 8-16. Digital radiographic sensors. (Courtesy DENTSPLY Rinn, a division of DENTSPLY International, Elgin, Illinois.)

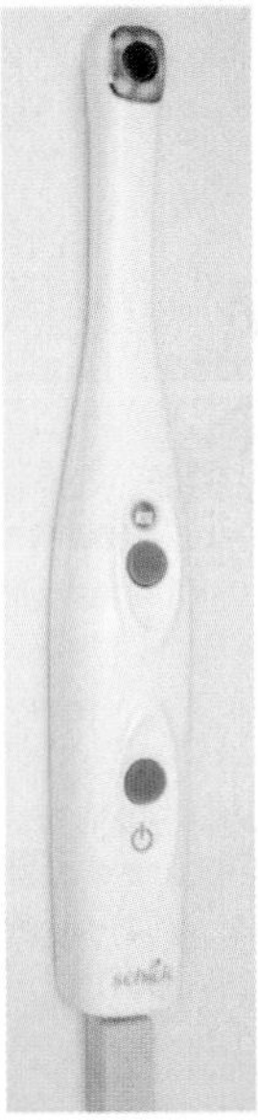

Figure 8-17. The intraoral camera. (Courtesy Old Dominion University, Norfolk, VA.)

Panoramic radiography produces a film or digital image of the maxillary and mandibular jaws. A digital panoramic image appears on the computer monitor while exposure is in progress. The image can be saved to the computer software, transmitted electronically, or printed. Some treatment areas may be large enough to house the panoramic x-ray machine; some facilities have separate rooms for this machine.

Darkroom or Radiograph Processing Area

A film processing area houses automatic dental radiographic film processing units that provide standardized processing of films using premixed solutions, automated time and temperature exposure, and rinsing and drying of films. Safe lights located in the processing room should be 4 feet away from processors. Automatic processors with a daylight loader do not require a dark room. In addition to overhead lighting in the room, an outside warning light prevents accidental entry into the darkroom while films are being processed (Figure 8-18).

Dental Laboratory

The dental laboratory is a well-ventilated area where dental work not directly performed with the client takes place. Personal protective equipment (PPEs) should be worn at all times while working in the laboratory. The dental laboratory is used for pouring impressions and trimming study models. The storing of impression trays, rubber bowls, alginate, spatulas, dental plaster, dental stone, tray formers, and a model vibrator to eliminate air bubbles in the models. A model

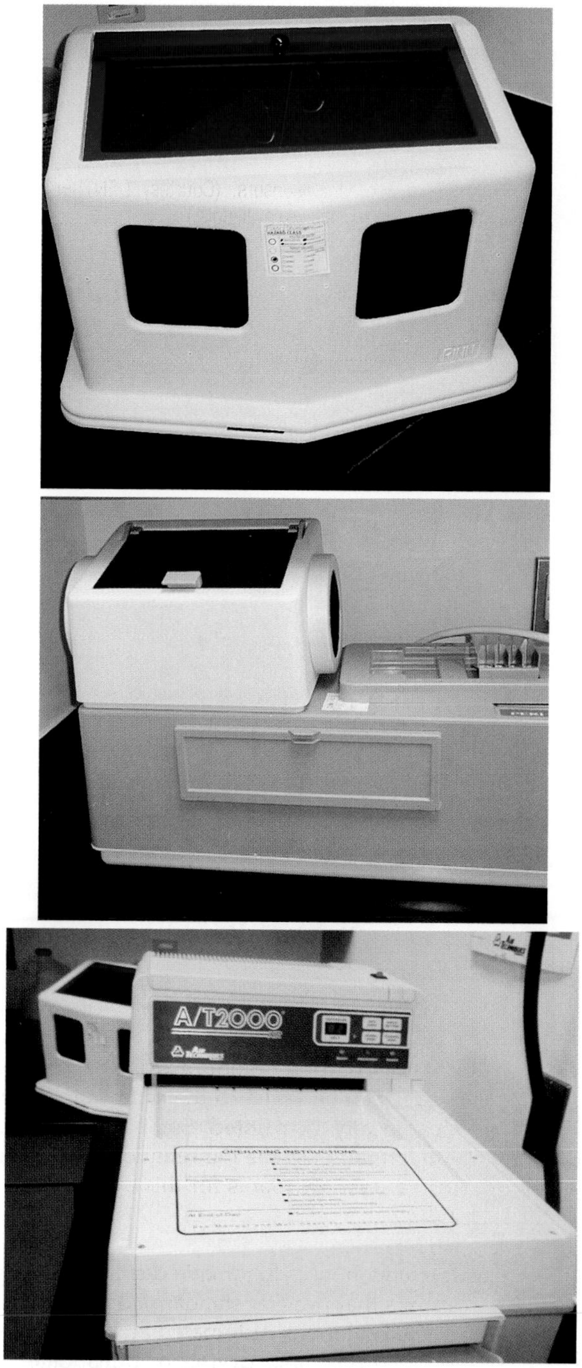

Figure 8-18. Automated film processors. (Thomas Nelson Community College, Williamsburg, VA.)

trimmer, used to trim the excess plaster or stone from the study models, a sink, and a water source with temperature controls are standard dental laboratory features.

Many treatment facilities finish (final stage of polishing or fabrication) crowns or bridges, adjust dental appliances, or fabricate mouth guards, night guards, or custom whitening trays. To accomplish these tasks, a model articulator, dental lathe, a lathe hood, a vacuum machine to shape acrylic, shears and nippers, and a dental engine with a laboratory handpiece are needed, along with air and gas outlets, gas torch, alcohol or Bunsen burners, casting ovens and waxing units to make

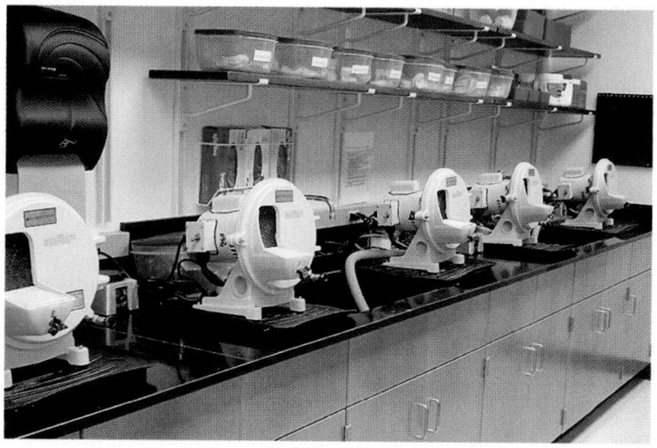

Figure 8-19. A dental laboratory in an educational setting. (Thomas Nelson Community College, Williamsburg, VA.)

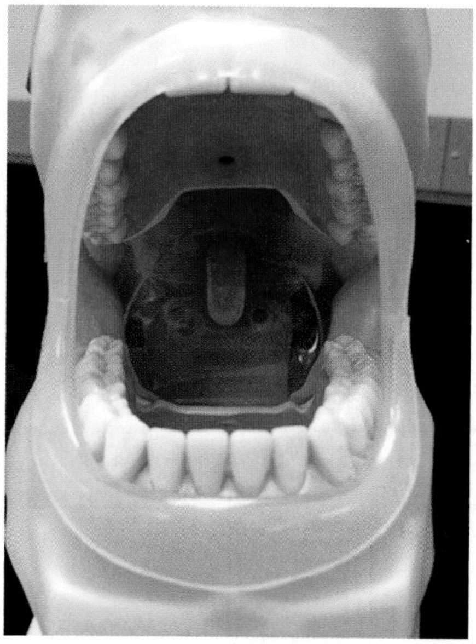

Figure 8-20. A typodont used for local anesthesia training in an educational setting. (Thomas Nelson Community College, Williamsburg, VA.)

templates, base plates, waxing spatulas, copings, and waxed patterns for casting procedures. In some facilities, preparation of impressions or prostheses for transmittal to a commercial laboratory takes place in the laboratory. This area is usually where dust, by-products from procedures, and noises are present. Whenever possible, the dental laboratory is accessible to the treatment areas but out of sight and hearing range of clients (Figure 8-19).

Dental Hygiene Care Facility (College Setting)

In a college setting, dental hygiene students encounter most of the structural fixtures, equipment, and instruments of a private practice. Dental and dental hygiene schools are using mannequin simulation for preclinical teaching. The simulation lab is an asset to academia, especially in the dental setting. For example, some are media equipped and are used to view and record instruction from professors. Subsequently, a dentoform or typodont (replica of the oral cavity) allows students to practice outside of the school setting (Figures 8-20 and 8-21). Electronic Health Records (EHR) are components

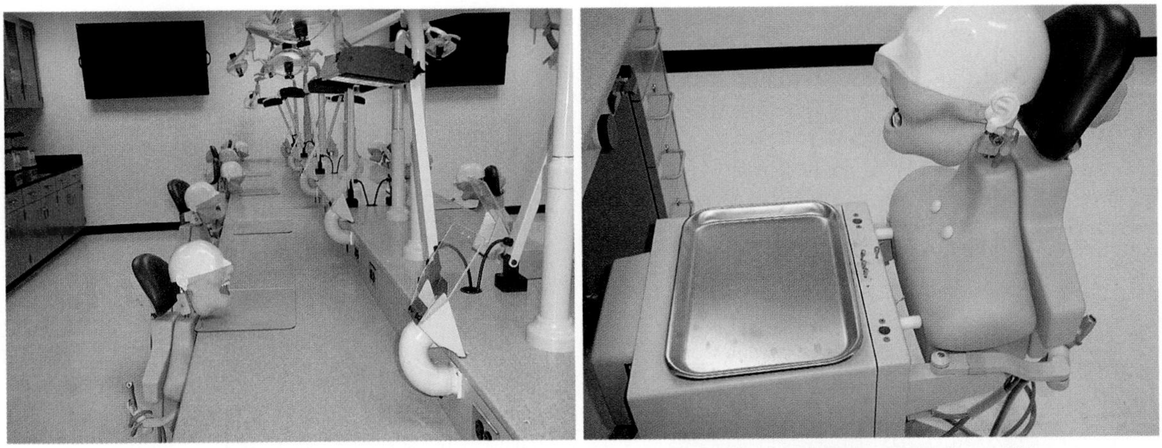

Figure 8-21. Educational setting client simulator. (Thomas Nelson Community College, Williamsburg, VA.)

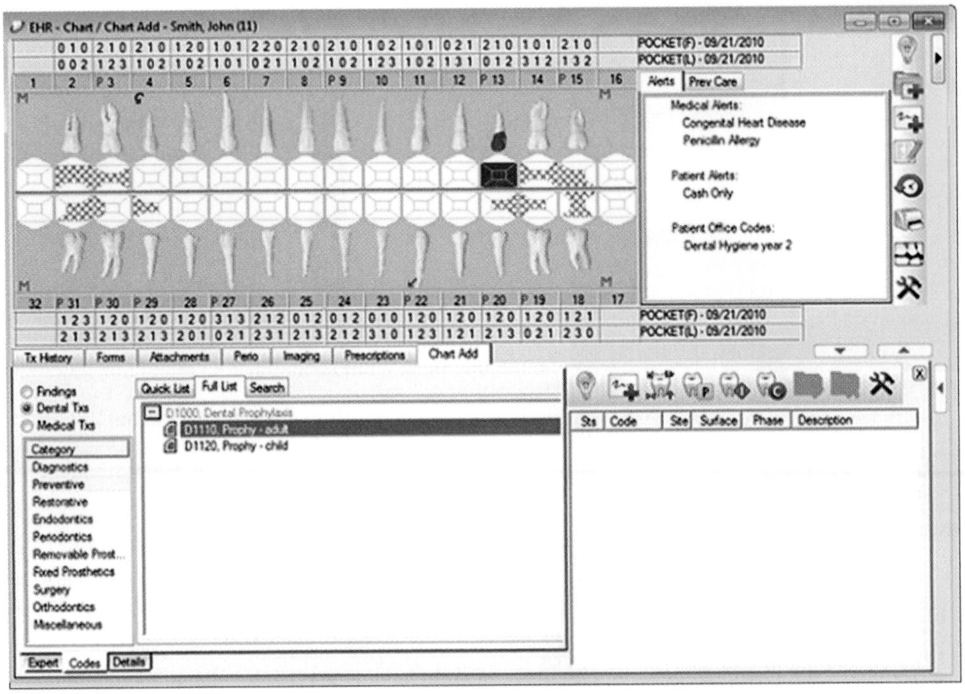

Figure 8-22. A screenshot of Axium 2 Odontogram. (Courtesy Exan, Las Vegas, NV.)

of the technology in academic and oral healthcare practice settings. Axium 2 or (A2) software is a complete dental hygiene clinic management program that allows students to perform clinical services electronically from medical history to treatment planning (Figures 8-22 and 8-23).

Hospital Setting

As part of a specialized oral healthcare team, dental hygienists provide therapeutic services to cognitively challenged and medically complex individuals. In acute and chronic care settings, dental hygienists may provide bedside care to clients too ill to be transported to the dental clinic. Care for persons who are homebound, bedridden, or wheelchair-bound requires the clinician to use hand-activated methods of instrumentation or portable dental equipment (Figures 8-24 and 8-25).

Mobile Dental Facility

Some community health agencies and private foundations own fully equipped mobile dental vans for providing preventive and therapeutic services to underserved populations (Figure 8-26). Fully equipped train cars travel on the existing rail systems, bringing high-quality oral care to underserved areas. An example of this type of mobile dental facility is the Smile Train.

CLIENT EDUCATION TIPS

- Teach the client what to look for in a high-quality dental care facility.
- Teach clients the danger of closing their lips around the saliva ejector to avoid backflow into the mouth from dental line biofilm.

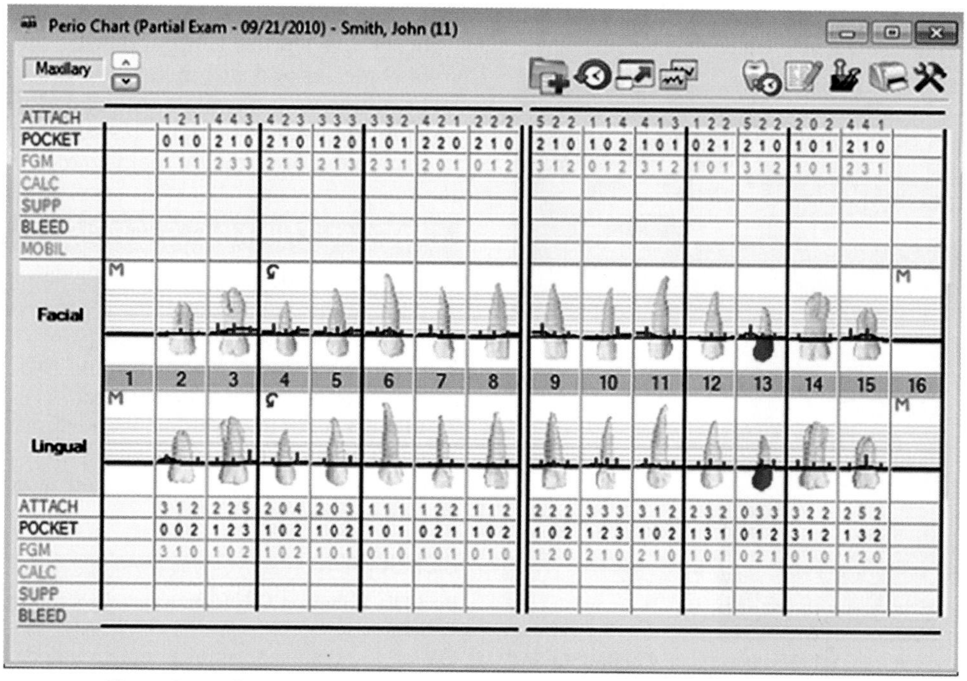

Figure 8-23. A screenshot of Axium 2 Perio Charting. (Courtesy Exan, Las Vegas, NV.)

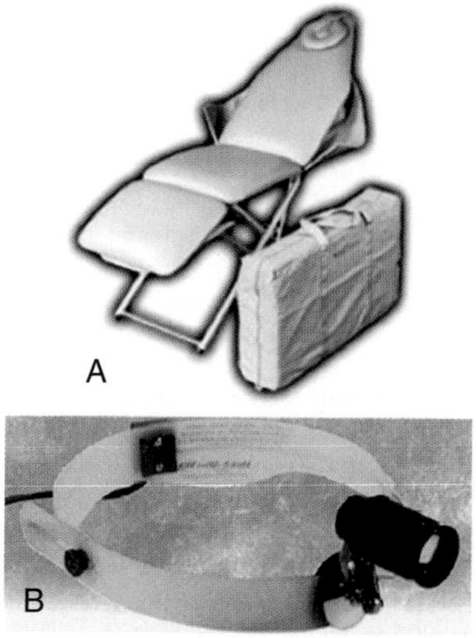

Figure 8-24. **A,** Portable dental chair. **B,** Headband light. (Courtesy DNTLworks Equipment Corporation, Centennial, Colorado.)

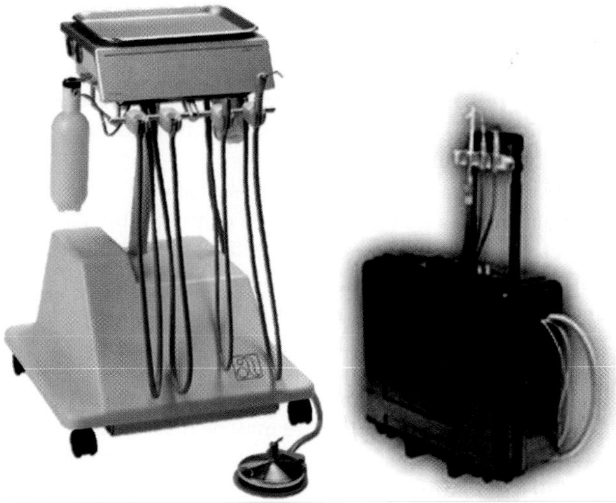

Figure 8-25. Portable dental delivery systems. (Courtesy A-dec, Inc, Newberg, Oregon.)

- Teach clients about instrument processing in the dental care environment.

LEGAL, ETHICAL, AND SAFETY ISSUES

- Assume professional responsibility with the client, co-workers, and the community for maintaining and using effective and safe equipment, supplies, and instruments in the delivery of high-quality care.
- Minimize liability via regular equipment maintenance procedures and documentation.
- Report equipment problems to the facility administrator.
- Stay informed of regulatory issues affecting the dental hygiene care environment.
- Assess the treatment area for potential hazards to protect the client and others.
- Assume responsibility for injuries or damages resulting from faulty equipment or negligent maintenance procedures.
- Practice the six basic ethical principles outlined in the American Dental Hygienists' Association's Code of Ethics, including beneficence, nonmaleficence, autonomy, veracity, societal trust, and justice.
- Always practice according to legal requirements and ethical guidelines.

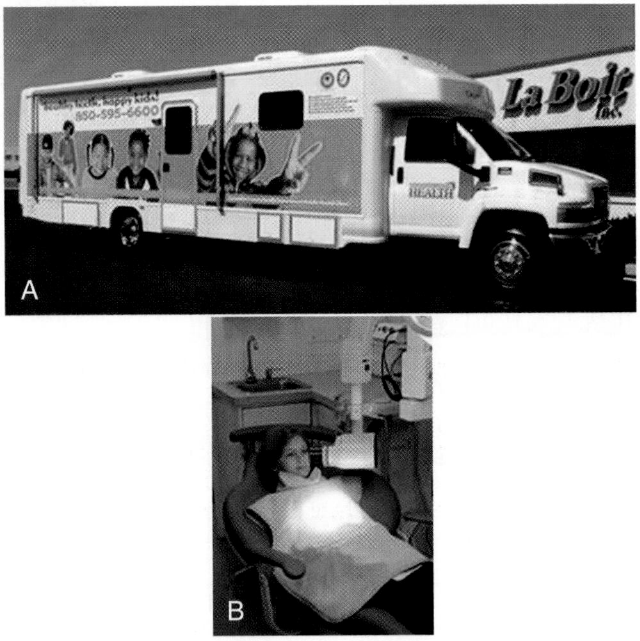

Figure 8-26. A, Mobile dental van. **B,** Treatment area. (Courtesy La Boit, Inc, Gahanna, Ohio, www.laboit.com.)

KEY CONCEPTS

- A dental hygiene care environment is the physical setting in which professional care is delivered; defined areas are designed for the delivery and support of professional care. The environment may be stationary or mobilized to place-bound or underserved populations.
- The treatment area is where professional oral care is delivered; it includes specially designed chairs for the client, the clinician, and the assistant; bracket tables; delivery systems; dental light; sink; an x-ray machine; an ultrasonic, piezoelectric, or sonic scaler; an intraoral camera; and a computer monitor.
- Additional space for instrument and film processing is created in separate rooms or in clearly designated areas.
- High-quality professional care may be delivered in private practices, college campus care facilities, hospitals, research facilities, community clinics, mobile vehicles, elementary schools, long-term care facilities, military bases, penal institutions, and private homes.
- The dental hygienist is responsible for learning effective, safe usage practices for the equipment, supplies, and instruments used in the delivery of care.
- Inadequate equipment and supplies undermine the quality of services rendered and jeopardize the health and welfare of clinicians and clients.
- Practitioners and dental facility administrators are responsible for injuries or damages resulting from inadequate equipment or negligent maintenance procedures.

CRITICAL THINKING EXERCISES

1. Go into the dental treatment area and identify all of the parts of the dental unit. How are the water lines treated to prevent the spread of infection?
2. Go into the dental laboratory and identify the equipment and supplies that are used there.
3. Identify all of the equipment and supplies associated with taking radiographs.
4. How are instruments recirculated in your dental hygiene care environment?

BIBLIOGRAPHY

Bird DL, Robinson DS: *Modern dental assisting*, ed 10, St Louis, 2012, Saunders.

Center for Disease Control and Prevention: Medical and Dental Equipment. Available at: http://www.cdc.gov/healthwater/other/medical/med_dental.html. Updated April 10, 2009. Accessed August 28, 2012.

Finkbeiner B, Finkbeiner C: *Practice management for the dental team*, ed 7, St Louis, 2011, Mosby.

Gottlieb R, Lanning S, Gunsolley J, et al: Faculty impressions of dental students' performance with and without virtual reality simulation. *J Dent Educ* 75(11):1443, 2011.

How the Dental RAT Works. Available at: http://www.dentalrat.com/. Accessed August 20, 2012.

Meet the new standard in dental software. Exan/Axium. Available at: http://www.exangroup.com/axium-dental-software. Accessed September 4, 2012.

Obrochta JC: *Efficient and effective use of the intraoral camera*. Available at: http://www.dentalcare.com. Updated: March 4, 2011. Accessed September 8, 2012.

Pearson Dental: Sterisil Straw. Available at: http://www.pearsondental.com/catalog/product.asp?majcatid=21&catid=3735&subcatid=14642&pid=59386&dpt=0. Accessed August 28, 2012.

Valachi B: Creating the ergonomic operatory: evidence-based strategies for dental hygienists and those who travel. *Access* 26(6):14, 2012.

Williams L, Wilkins E: *Lippincott Williams & Wilkins comprehensive dental assisting*, Maryland, 2012, Lippincott Williams & Wilkins.

EVOLVE RESOURCES

Please visit http://evolve.elsevier.com/Darby/hygiene for additional practice and study support tools.

Infection Control

Eve Cuny, Kathy J. Eklund, Helene S. Bednarsh

CHAPTER

9

COMPETENCIES

1. **Discuss standard precautions and basic infection-control concepts.**
2. **Explain the similarities and differences between the infection-control model and model of dental hygiene care.**
3. **Identify the government agencies that play key roles in regulations of infection control standards.**
4. **Discuss the standard of care, including assessment of risk of disease transmission in oral healthcare, and planning of appropriate control measures.**
5. **Explain the principles of infection control, including:**
   - **Select appropriate protective attire for dental hygiene client care.**
   - **Prepare the dental environment before and after client care.**
6. **Discuss strategies to prevent disease transmission, and how healthcare personnel can take action to stay healthy.**

Standard Precautions and Basic Infection-Control Concepts

Infection control refers to a comprehensive, systematic program that, when applied, prevents the transmission of infectious agents among persons who are in direct or indirect contact with the healthcare environment. The goal of infection control is to create and maintain a safe clinical environment to eliminate the potential for disease transmission from clinician to client, client to clinician, or client to client. Infection control relies on the premise that transmission occurs when an infectious agent has a portal of entry to a susceptible host.

Although the challenge remains to meet the comprehensive needs of diverse clients, the premise of standard precautions goes beyond the individual to eliminate the potential for transfer of disease-causing microorganisms during the delivery of oral health services. **Standard precautions** are a set of infection-control precautions that when used consistently ensure the safe delivery of oral healthcare.

Human needs theory relates directly to standard precautions in the following ways:

- Universality of human needs transcends all ages, cultures, nationalities, genders, sexual orientation, and behaviors. Standard precautions, the practice of infection control, rely on the universal application of precautions in the treatment of all clients regardless of the individual or the client's infectious disease status.
- A link exists between human needs and health as defined by the World Health Organization. The World Health Organization defines health as "the extent to which an individual or group is able, on the one hand, to realize aspirations and satisfy needs and, on the other hand, to change and cope with the environment." Infection control is truly the ability to change and cope with the environment.
- Of all the human needs, infection control is most applicable to protection from health risks. Although infection-control practices cannot reduce unintended harm from the care itself, it can prevent unintended harm to the dental hygienist, client, and other staff. Protection from health risks begins with the client (client assessment), but standard precautions do not depend on the health, dental, and pharmacologic histories, because clients may not always be aware of their health risks, conditions, or emerging concerns. Standard precautions treat all clients as potentially harboring disease-producing organisms and apply evidence-based protocols to reduce the potential harm associated with these organisms. Standard precautions apply to all body fluids, excretions, and secretions with the exception of sweat and tears. The hygienist uses client assessment findings to make decisions about appropriate interventions. With infection control the hygienist considers procedures and behaviors indicated to reduce risk of disease transmission.
- Freedom from fear and stress is another human need related to standard precautions. People need to feel safe in the healthcare environment. Part of this safety comes from the immediate recognition of applied infection-control principles.
- Many human needs are fulfilled by a variety of client services and policies, but the need for conceptualization and problem solving underlies every behavior relative to client care. There must be evidence of the use of sound and appropriate infection-control practices, and there must be an explanation of rationales before care is delivered. Clients need to realize that their safety is paramount; this instills the belief that subsequent care is most appropriate, as well.

Infection control begins with assessment of the healthcare delivery environment, ensuring it is free from infectious hazards. There are steps to take to prevent exposure to potential infectious hazards. Dental hygienists conduct infection-control assessment based on the care plan as follows:

1. How will the client be treated, and what infection-control implications are associated?
2. How will the client understand the infection-control practices and take comfort in their use?

3. What infection-control protocols will protect the client, clinician, staff, and their significant others from inadvertent disease transmission?

Infection-Control Model

A model of infection control parallels the model of dental hygiene care. For example, clients must understand the selection and use of infection-control procedures and the protective outcomes. However, the infection-control model differs from the traditional client care model in that it focuses on tasks and procedures rather than on the client.

Scrutinizing each individual health history does not determine the degree of risk for disease transmission. A person may be infected subclinically with an infectious microorganism and not know it. However, they can be clinically contagious before having the detectable clinical symptoms. Examples include the common cold, influenza, and other highly contagious infectious diseases. Dental procedures generate widely variant amounts of body fluids, and the dental instruments used vary in their tendency to release body fluids. Therefore infection control is procedurally based, not client based. Cognitive goals in the infection-control model relate to the explanation of infection control, the protective intent of infection control, and its benchmark status as a standard of care. Effective goals in the infection-control model are designed to change a client's attitude in a positive manner and reduce fear or anxiety associated with dental hygiene care. The client must see infection control as protective, not punitive.

Government Agencies and Infection Control

Two agencies of the U.S. government play key roles in infection control. Guidelines and regulations developed by both of these agencies have established national standards for infection control.

The Centers for Disease Control and Prevention (CDC) is one of eight federal public health agencies within the U.S. Department of Health and Human Services. Its mission is to promote health and quality of life by preventing and controlling disease, injury, and disability. The CDC develops guidelines and recommendations; among these are infection-control recommendations for healthcare settings. The CDC is not a regulatory agency and does not enforce the guidelines it develops.

The Occupational Safety and Health Administration (OSHA), within the U.S. Department of Labor, protects persons by ensuring a safe and healthy workplace. OSHA enforces workplace safety regulations, including those for infection control in healthcare settings. In approximately half of the states, there are state-administered OSHA agencies. The remainder of the states falls under the rule of federal OSHA. Where there is a state plan, if it is more stringent than the federal, then the state plan must be followed.

The U.S. Food and Drug Administration (FDA) and the U.S. Environmental Protection Agency (EPA) also provide regulatory oversight in the area of products used in the application of infection-control procedures. The FDA regulatory mission is to do the following:

- Promote and protect the public health by helping safe and effective products reach the market in a timely way.
- Monitor products for continued safety after they are in use.
- Help the public obtain accurate, science-based information needed to improve health.

The FDA's regulatory approaches are as varied as the products it regulates. Some products, such as new drugs and complex medical devices, must be proven safe and effective before companies can put them on the market. Other products, such as x-ray machines and medical sterilizers, must measure up to performance standards.

The FDA regulates all medical devices, from simple items such as tongue depressors and thermometers to complex technologies such as heart pacemakers and dialysis machines. Different levels of approval are required based on the complexity and use of products or devices. These differences are dictated by the laws enforced and the relative risks that the products pose to consumers.

The EPA's regulatory mission is to protect human health and the environment. Since 1970 the EPA has been working for a cleaner, healthier environment for the American people. Areas of the EPA's regulatory authority that affect infection control include the following:

- Regulation of medical and chemical waste
- Registration of chemical germicides used for healthcare (e.g., surface disinfectants)

Standard of Care

Standard of care is the level of care that a reasonably prudent practitioner would exercise. It is not a maximum standard; rather it is the minimum level acceptable in all aspects of client care. Infection-control regulations, evidence-based guidelines, government agencies, licensing boards, other dental practitioners, and expert opinion determine the standard of care for appropriate infection-control practices in dentistry. The standard of care provides a basis from which to promote excellence and encourage performance improvement to develop and implement best practices.

The goal of infection control is to prevent healthcare-associated infections among clients and injuries and illnesses in dental healthcare personnel (DHCP). Dental clients and DHCP can be exposed to pathogenic (disease-producing) microorganisms. Human pathogens include cytomegalovirus (CMV), hepatitis B virus (HBV), hepatitis C virus (HCV), herpes simplex virus types 1 and 2, human immunodeficiency virus (HIV), *Mycobacterium tuberculosis* (TB), staphylococci, streptococci, influenza, and other viruses and bacteria that colonize or infect the oral cavity and respiratory tract. These organisms can be transmitted in dental healthcare settings by the following means:

- Direct contact with blood, oral fluids, or other client materials
- Indirect contact with contaminated objects (e.g., instruments, equipment, or environmental surfaces)
- Contact of conjunctiva, nasal membranes, or oral mucosa with droplets (e.g., spatter) that contain microorganisms generated from an infected person and propelled a short distance (e.g., by coughing, sneezing, or talking)
- Inhalation of airborne microorganisms that can remain suspended in the air for long periods

Infection through any of these routes requires that all of the following conditions be present:

- A pathogenic organism of sufficient virulence and in adequate numbers to cause disease
- A reservoir or source that allows the pathogen to survive and multiply (e.g., blood)
- A mode of transmission from the source to the host

- A portal of entry through which the pathogen can enter the host
- A susceptible host (i.e., one who is not immune)

The chain of infection occurs when these events are present. Effective infection-control strategies prevent disease transmission by interrupting one or more links in the chain.

Four Principles of Infection Control

The CDC identifies four principles of infection control that help protect the health of all individuals in the dental environment.

Principle 1: Take Action to Stay Healthy

All persons must take positive steps to maintain their own health. This is especially true for persons working in any healthcare setting, including DHCP. The following are important considerations for DHCP:

- Immunizations for vaccine-preventable diseases
- Hand hygiene
- Postexposure management
- Education and training

Principle 2: Avoid Contact with Blood and Other Infectious Body Substances

Avoid contact with blood and other potentially infectious body fluids by using a combination of safe work practices and behaviors and engineering controls. Infection-prevention and infection-control measures include the following:

- Effective use of personal protective equipment (PPE) (e.g., gloves, face masks, protective eyewear, protective gowns) (Figure 9-1)
- Safe handling of sharp instruments and objects

Principle 3: Make Client Care Items (Dental Instruments, Devices, and Equipment) Safe for Use

Instruments, devices, and equipment used to provide direct client care become contaminated. Appropriate infection-control measures must be taken to prevent transmission of infectious agents from client to client through these contaminated items. Methods of appropriate infection-control measures include the following:

- Cleaning, sterilization, or disinfection of reusable client care items
- Appropriate containment and disposal of all single-use items

Principle 4: Limit the Spread of Blood and Other Infectious Body Substances

Although environmental surfaces and waste products are less likely to provide an efficient mechanism for transmission of infectious agents, they are subject to contamination in oral healthcare settings. Examples of infection-control measures to limit the spread of contamination include the following:

- Environment infection control
  - Protective surface covers or barriers (Figure 9-2)
  - Cleaning and surface disinfection
- Effective management of regulated waste
  - Nonsharp infectious waste
  - Sharps
  - Hazardous waste

Strategies to Prevent Disease Transmission: Take Action to Stay Healthy

A basic strategy for healthcare personnel (HCP) to take action to stay healthy is to develop a personnel health program based on the CDC 2003 dental infection-control guidelines, including medical evaluation, health and safety education and training, management of work-related illness and postexposure management, counseling, work restrictions, and immunization.

Immunizations for Vaccine-Preventable Diseases

Immunization is one of the most effective means of preventing disease transmission. Once a person has acquired immunity through vaccination, the disease no longer poses a threat. In addition to standard childhood immunizations, hygienists should obtain immunizations specifically recommended for HCP. The CDC Advisory Council on Immunization Practices (ACIP) routinely reviews, updates, and revises immunization recommendations. Therefore the most current ACIP recommendations must be used when making immunization decisions (Table 9-1).

HCP in specific geographic locations or with underlying medical conditions may need immunizations in addition to those currently recommended by the CDC. It is important for each individual to consult with his or her physician to determine which immunizations are appropriate based on disease risk in the specific location. All children in the United States and most other countries receive immunization for diphtheria, pertussis, and tetanus (DPT) as a combined vaccine. Adults must receive the tetanus-diphtheria (Td) booster

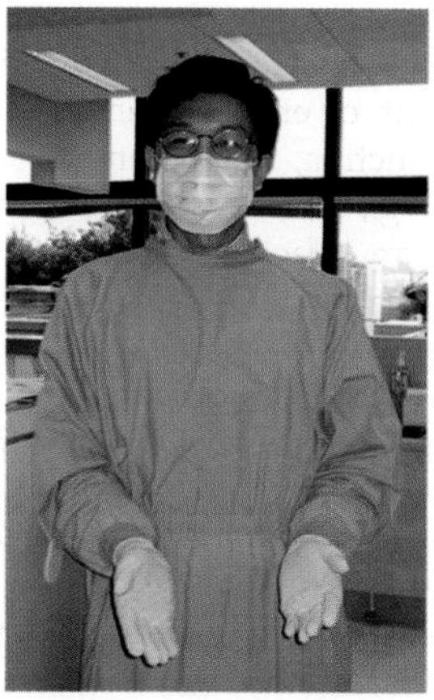

Figure 9-1. Personal protective equipment worn by dental hygienist.

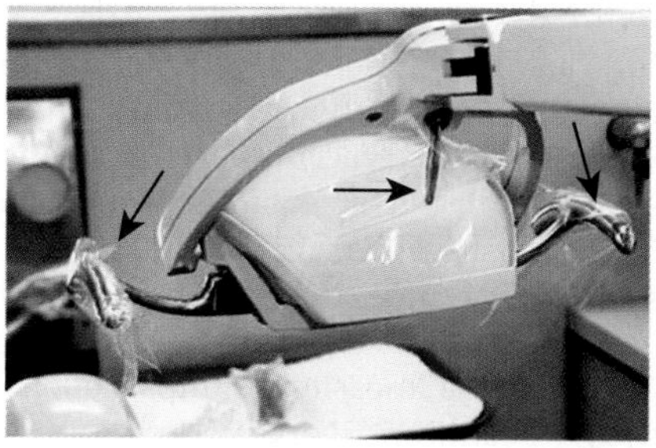

Figure 9-2. Equipment barriers *(arrows)* on dental light.

TABLE 9-1

Immunizations Strongly Recommended for Healthcare Personnel

Hepatitis B	Give 3-dose series (dose #1 now, #2 in 1 month, #3 approximately 5 months after #2). Give IM. Obtain anti-HBs serologic testing 1-2 months after dose #3.
Influenza	Give 1 dose of TIV or LAIV annually. Give TIV intramuscularly or LAIV intranasally. *Follow 2010 recommendations from CDC.*
MMR	HCP born in 1957 or later without evidence of immunity or prior vaccination, give 2 doses MMR, 4 weeks apart. Give SC. If born before 1957, 1 dose. Two doses for all HCP during mumps outbreak.
Varicella	HCP with no serologic proof of immunity, prior vaccination, or history of varicella disease, give 2 doses of varicella vaccine, 4 weeks apart. Give SC.
Tetanus/diphtheria/pertussis	All HCP need Td every 10 years after completing a primary series. Give 1 dose of Tdap IM if not previously received and resume Td thereafter.
Meningococcal	Give 1 dose to microbiologists who are routinely exposed to isolates of *N. meningitis.*

Adapted from CDC: Immunizations of health-care personnel. Recommendations of the Advisory Committee on Immunization Practices (ACIP), *MMWR* 60(7):2011.
LAIV, Live-attenuated influenza vaccine; *TIV*, trivalent inactivated influenza vaccine.

HEPATITIS B VACCINE DECLINATION

I understand that due to my occupational exposure to blood or other potentially infectious materials I may be at risk of acquiring hepatitis B virus (HBV) infection. I have been given the opportunity to be vaccinated with hepatitis B vaccine at no charge to myself. However, I decline hepatitis B vaccination at this time. I understand that by declining this vaccine, I continue to be at risk of acquiring hepatitis B, a serious disease. If in the future I continue to have occupational exposure to blood or other potentially infectious materials and I want to be vaccinated with hepatitis B vaccine, I can receive the vaccination series at no charge to me.

Name:______________________________

Signature:______________________________

Job Title:______________________________

Date:______________________________

Figure 9-3. Required hepatitis B virus vaccine declination form.

every 10 years, and more often if recommended or indicated because of exposure. In addition, a tetanus, diphtheria, and acellular pertussis (Tdap) vaccine is recommended for all adolescents and adults. It is a one-time booster given in place of the Td booster. After receiving the one-time Tdap, individuals should resume the schedule of Td boosters. Additional vaccines recommended for all HCP include hepatitis B, annual influenza, measles, mumps, rubella, and varicella, unless the healthcare worker has naturally acquired immunity stemming from a past infection. In addition, the CDC recommends pneumococcal vaccine for all adults age 65 or older. OSHA requires employers to offer all personnel at risk of exposure to blood and other potentially infectious materials HBV vaccination unless they have verification of previous hepatitis B immunization or are infected with HBV. If the employee declines immunization, he or she must sign a specific OSHA-designated declination waiver (Figure 9-3). An employee must have received information on the safety and efficacy of the vaccine, the benefits to receiving the vaccine, and the risks associated with not receiving vaccination before they may decline. The vaccination is in a three-part series with post-vaccine testing for hepatitis B surface antibodies (anti-HBs) 1 to 2 months after the third dose of vaccine. Persons who fail to respond should be offered a second three-dose series; when completed, the titer is retested for antibody response. Those who fail to develop detectable anti-HBs after six doses should be considered non-responders and tested for hepatitis B surface antigen (HBsAg), which indicates active infection or carrier status. If the result of this test is negative, the individual is considered as susceptible to HBV infection and counseled on precautions to avoid exposure and appropriate postexposure management.

Work Restrictions

DHCP should be aware of their personal health and take action to stay healthy. Within a written infection-control plan it is necessary to discuss those conditions that require a restriction or exclusion from direct patient care. The U.S. Public Health Service recommends work restrictions for HCP with specific infections and following exposure to some diseases (Table 9-2). Many of these infections are preventable with vaccines. The following precautions help protect HCP and clients:

- HCP diagnosed with diphtheria should refrain from working until the illness resolves.
- HCP with mumps or measles should refrain from working during the acute illness phase, as well as after exposure and during the incubation phase if not immunized.
- HCP diagnosed with hepatitis A should refrain from direct client contact and avoid handling food others will eat.
- HCP with an upper respiratory infection should avoid contact with medically compromised persons as defined by the ACIP for complications from influenza.
- HCP with active herpes zoster (shingles) may continue to work unrestricted but should cover lesions to protect against exposure of nonintact skin to blood and body fluids.
  - In 2012 the CDC published *Updated CDC Recommendations for the Management of Hepatitis B Virus–Infected Health-Care Providers and Students*. Before these guidelines were established, it was recommended that healthcare providers who are hepatitis B e-antigen positive (indicating an elevated risk of transmission) consult with an expert review panel before performing exposure-prone invasive procedures. Because of the lack of documented infected healthcare worker-to-patient transmission of hepatitis B in recent years, the CDC now recommends no restrictions and no expert review for practitioners performing dental procedures with the exception of major oral or maxillofacial surgery.

TABLE 9-2

Work Restriction Guidelines for Healthcare Personnel with Infectious Diseases

Disease or Problem	Work Restriction	Duration
Conjunctivitis	Restrict from client contact and contact with client environment.	Until no discharge
Cytomegalovirus infection	No restriction	
Diarrheal disease	Restrict from client contact, contact with client's environment, and food handling.	Until symptoms resolve
Enteroviral infection	Restrict from care of infants, neonates, and immunocompromised people and their environments.	Until symptoms resolve
Hepatitis A	Restrict from client contact, contact with client environment, and food handling.	Until 7 days after onset of jaundice
Hepatitis B		
Personnel with acute or chronic hepatitis B surface antigenemia who do not perform exposure-prone procedures	No restriction*; refer to local regulations. Standard precautions always should be followed.	
Personnel with acute or chronic hepatitis B e-antigenemia who perform major oral or maxillofacial surgery	Do not perform exposure-prone invasive procedures until counsel from a review panel has been sought; panel should review and recommend procedures that personnel can perform, taking into account specific procedures as well as skill and technique. Standard precautions always should be observed. Refer to local regulations or recommendations.	Until hepatitis B e-antigen status is negative
Hepatitis C	No restrictions on professional activity.* HCV-positive healthcare personnel should follow aseptic technique and standard precautions.	
Herpes simplex (hands)	Restrict from client contact and contact with client's environment.	Until lesions heal
Herpes simplex (orofacial)	Evaluate need to restrict from care of clients who are at high risk.	

TABLE 9-2

Work Restriction Guidelines for Healthcare Personnel with Infectious Diseases—cont'd

Disease or Problem	Work Restriction	Duration
Human immunodeficiency virus infection; personnel who perform exposure-prone procedures	Do not perform exposure-prone invasive procedures until counsel from an expert review panel has been sought; panel should review and recommend procedures that personnel can perform, taking into account specific procedures as well as skill and technique. Standard precautions always should be observed. Refer to local regulations or recommendations.	
Measles (active)	Exclude from duty.	Until 7 days after the rash appears
Measles (postexposure of susceptible personnel)	Exclude from duty.	From fifth day after first exposure through twenty-first day after last exposure or 4 days after rash appears
Meningococcal infection	Exclude from duty.	Until 24 hours after start of effective therapy
Mumps (active)	Exclude from duty.	Until 9 days after onset of parotitis
Mumps (postexposure of susceptible personnel)	Exclude from duty.	From twelfth day after first exposure through twenty-sixth day after last exposure, or until 9 days after onset of parotitis
Pediculosis	Restrict from client contact.	Until treated and observed to be free of adult and immature lice
Pertussis (active)	Exclude from duty.	From beginning of catarrhal stage through third week after onset of paroxysms, or until 5 days after start of effective antibiotic therapy
Pertussis (postexposure-asymptomatic personnel)	No restriction; prophylaxis recommended.	
Pertussis (postexposure-symptomatic personnel)	Exclude from duty.	Until 5 days after start of effective antibiotic therapy
Rubella (active)	Exclude from duty.	Until 5 days after rash appears
Rubella (postexposure-susceptible personnel)	Exclude from duty.	From seventh day after first exposure through twenty-first day after last exposure
Staphylococcus aureus infection (active, draining skin lesions)	Restrict from contact with clients and client's environment or food handling.	Until lesions have resolved
Staphylococcus aureus infection (carrier state)	No restriction unless personnel are epidemiologically linked to transmission of the organism.	
Streptococcal group A infection	Restrict from client care, contact with patient's environment, and food handling.	Until 24 hours after adequate treatment started
Tuberculosis (active)	Exclude from duty.	Until proven noninfectious
Tuberculosis (PPD converter)	No restriction.	
Varicella (active)	Exclude from duty.	Until all lesions dry and crust
Varicella (postexposure-susceptible personnel)	Exclude from duty.	From tenth day after first exposure through twenty-first day (twenty-eighth day if varicella-zoster immune globulin [VZIG] administered) after last exposure
Zoster (localized, in healthy person)	Cover lesions, restrict from care of clients[†] at high risk.	Until all lesions dry and crust

TABLE 9-2

Work Restriction Guidelines for Healthcare Personnel with Infectious Diseases—cont'd

Disease or Problem	Work Restriction	Duration
Zoster (generalized or localized in immunosuppressed person)	Restrict from client contact.	Until all lesions dry and crust
Zoster (postexposure-susceptible personnel)	Restrict from client contact.	From tenth day after first exposure through twenty-first day (twenty-eighth day if VZIG administered) after last exposure; or, if varicella occurs, when lesions crust and dry
Viral respiratory illness, acute febrile	Consider excluding from the care of clients at high risk‡ or contact with such clients' environments during community outbreak of respiratory syncytial virus and influenza.	Until symptoms resolve

Adapted from Bolyard EA: Hospital Infection Control Practices Advisory Committee. Guidelines for infection control in health care personnel, 1998, *Am J Infect Control* 26:289, 1998.

Adapted from recommendations of the Advisory Committee on Immunization Practices (ACIP).

*Unless epidemiologically linked to transmission of disease.

†Those susceptible to varicella and who are at increased risk of complications of varicella (e.g., neonates and immunocompromised persons of any age).

‡Patients at high risk as defined by ACIP for complications of influenza.

- HCP with HIV are not specifically restricted, but it is possible that some modifications would be necessary for certain procedures. An expert review panel and physician should be consulted.

It is important to consult current CDC recommendations for HCP and specific state laws or recommendations for additional information about workplace restrictions, if applicable.

Standard Precautions

Standard precautions are the practices by which healthcare personnel follow the same infection-control protocols for all clients regardless of infectious status or health history. Health history alone will not identify reliably all persons with HIV infection, HBV infection, or other blood-borne diseases. Some infected individuals are unaware of their status, and others may choose not to disclose their disease status on the health history. Certain precautions prevent the transmission of these viruses when applied during client care. These precautions protect the HCP and the patient from disease transmission.

Standard precautions are a synthesis of the major features of universal precautions and body substance isolation precautions and apply to the following:

- Blood
- Other bodily fluids, secretions, and excretions except sweat regardless of whether they contain visible blood
- Nonintact skin
- Mucous membranes

Therefore standard precautions apply to blood and all moist body substances.

Transmission-Based Precautions

Certain diseases require measures in addition to universal precautions, based on the route of transmission. Expanded or transmission-based precautions may be necessary to prevent potential spread of certain diseases (e.g., TB, influenza, and varicella) that are airborne or transmitted by droplet or contact (e.g., sneezing, coughing, and contact with skin). Persons acutely ill with these diseases usually do not seek routine dental care. Nonetheless, a general understanding of precautions for diseases transmitted by all routes is critical for the following reasons:

- Some DHCP are hospital based or work part time in hospital settings.
- Persons infected with these diseases may seek urgent treatment at outpatient dental offices.
- DHCP may become infected with these diseases. Necessary transmission-based precautions may include client placement (isolation), adequate room ventilation, respiratory protection (N-95 masks) for DHCP, or postponement of nonemergency dental procedures.

The CDC has identified three categories of transmission-based precautions, as follows:

- Contact precautions
- Droplet precautions
- Airborne precautions

Transmission-based precautions are used when the routes of transmission are not interrupted completely using standard precautions alone. For some diseases that have multiple routes of transmission (e.g., severe acute respiratory syndrome [SARS]), more than one transmission-based precaution category may be used. Whether transmission-based precautions are used singly or in combination, universal precautions always apply as well.

In the case of clinically active TB, the level of protection afforded by standard precautions is not sufficient to prevent transmission. TB transmission is affected by a hierarchy of measures that include administrative controls, environmental controls, and personal respiratory protection. For clients known or suspected to have active TB, the CDC recommends the following:

- Evaluate the client away from other clients and DHCP. When not being evaluated, the client should wear a surgical mask or cover mouth and nose when coughing or sneezing.
- Defer elective dental treatment until the person is noninfectious.
- Refer clients requiring urgent dental treatment to a previously identified facility with TB engineering controls and a respiratory protection program.

Health History

The health history is an important tool for the following:

- Understanding the client's overall health
- Assisting in making appropriate care and referral decisions

DHCP should be aware of signs and symptoms of infectious diseases and cognizant of the steps required to minimize risk of transmission. This is particularly important if a client has active TB, signs and symptoms of which may include coughing, chest pain, sweating, weight loss, and fever. Coughing, especially if persistent and if blood is present, is a key indicator of infection. A client with active TB or suspected of having active TB should be isolated from other clients, asked to wear a face mask, and educated to contact his or her physician of record for definitive medical diagnosis (e.g., presence or absence of TB).

The Tuberculin Skin Test (TST), previously known as the Mantoux test, is the most common and accurate test for TB. The CDC recommends this tuberculin skin test, which involves an intradermal injection of purified protein derivative (PPD) into the skin of the forearm. The area is observed for 48 to 72 hours after the injection for development of a wheal that is red, is raised, and measures at least 10 mm across. If it has been several years since the last time a person had a TB skin test, the physician may recommend repeating the test to rule out the potential for a false-negative result. For HIV-infected individuals, a 5-mm wheal is an indication of infection owing to the tendency of immunocompromised individuals to develop a lesser reaction. A positive skin test result is an indication of infection with the bacterium but is not an indication of active disease. In fact, the majority of individuals with a positive skin test result do not have active TB. About 10% of infected individuals develop active TB in their lifetime. About 5% develop the active disease shortly after exposure, and 5% develop active disease later in life, usually owing to a compromised immune system.

Most people who experience a positive skin test result receive preventive chemotherapy for 6 months. The standard drug for prevention of active infection is isoniazid (INH). To treat an active infection (i.e., in a symptomatic person), physicians use INH in combination with other medications (e.g., rifampin, pyrazinamide). Rare cases of TB do not respond to traditional therapy. These cases, referred to as drug-resistant TB, are more likely to result in death of the infected individual.

Engineering Controls

Engineering controls are devices or equipment that reduce or eliminate a hazard (Figure 9-4). In the context of oral healthcare, these include the following:

- Devices that contain or remove sharp items
- Anesthetic syringes that contain shielding or encapsulation mechanisms

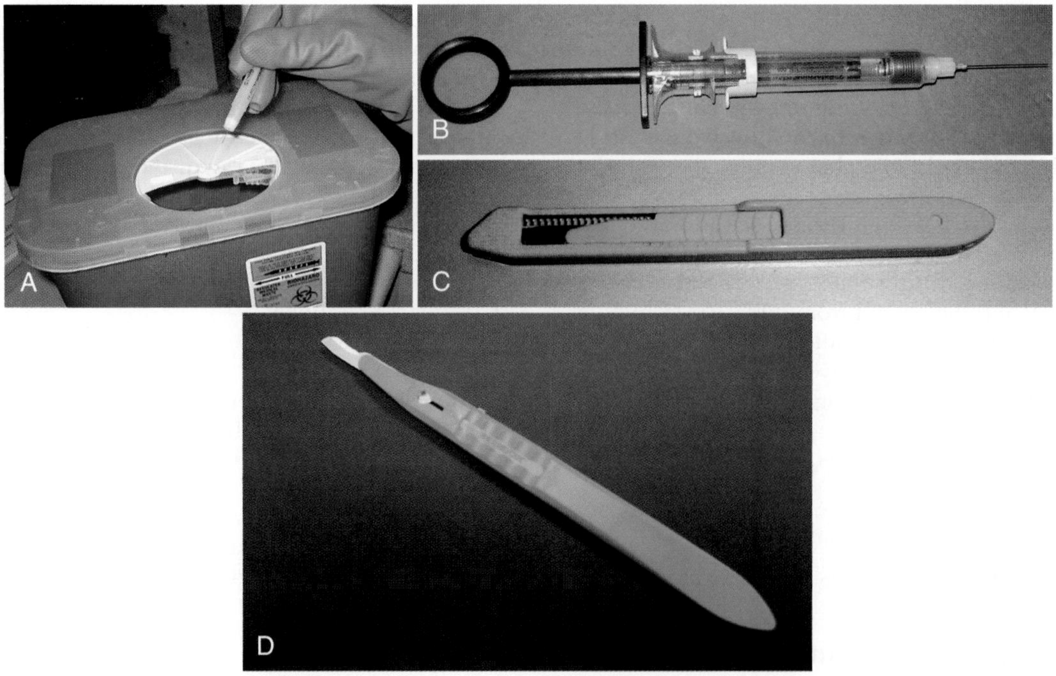

Figure 9-4. Examples of engineering controls. **A,** Sharps container with biohazard warning label. **B,** Dental safety syringe. **C,** Safety scalpel with retractable blade. **D,** Disposable scalpel.

- Anesthetic needles that contain shielding mechanisms
- Disposable scalpels that do not require removal of a used blade
- Scalpel handles with retractable blades
- Safety IV needles and needle-free ports for adding medications to IV lines

Consider the use of engineering controls when it is reasonable to believe that the control measure will reduce the potential for exposure to a client's blood or body fluids. OSHA requires the use of sharps with engineered sharps injury protection when available and when found to provide superior protection compared with the standard devices. Examples include syringes with retractable needles or needle guards, scalpels with retractable blades or blade guards, and other devices that render the sharp safer through blunting, encapsulation, guarding, or destruction.

Work Practice Controls

Work practice controls are precautionary measures that reduce the likelihood of exposure to bloodborne pathogens by altering the way a task or procedure is performed. Figure 9-5 shows improper positioning of fingers, placing the dental hygienist at risk. Proper client positioning that allows a 14- to 18-inch focal distance may reduce the hygienist's exposure to contaminated droplets generated during certain procedures. Proper client positioning also increases visibility and access to the mouth, further decreasing the risk for accidental injury. Use of a high-speed evacuator while spraying a client's mouth with air and water reduces the amount of droplet splash compared with the use of low-speed suction or no suction. Using an ultrasonic cleaner, washer, or washer/disinfector to decontaminate used dental instruments before sterilization is another example of work practice controls. Use of automated instrument cleaning reduces the need for the DHCP to handle contaminated instruments.

Personal Protective Equipment

The term **personal protective equipment (PPE)** refers to garments, eye protection, airway protection, and other attire worn with the intent to protect the worker from blood and body fluid exposure. Work practice controls and engineering controls are the preferred method of protection. PPE is indicated when those controls will not prevent exposure to blood and body fluids. The PPE selected should protect the worker from exposure to the skin, clothing, eyes, mouth, and other mucous membranes during the normal course of his or her duties (see Figure 9-1).

Always base the selection of protective attire on the nature of the procedure and anticipated exposure risks. Procedures that generate spray or droplets of blood or saliva (e.g., scaling and root planing, air polishing) require a higher level of protection than procedures that do not produce body fluids (e.g., x-ray examinations). Do not base the selection of PPE on the infectious disease status of the client. The infection-control precautions for any given procedure should be the same for each client.

Eye and Face Protection

Appropriate eye protection includes goggles, glasses with solid side shields, or a face shield that protect the eyes from exposure to infectious, chemical, and physical hazards (Figure 9-6). The CDC recommends and OSHA regulates that protective eyewear meet the **American National Standards Institute (ANSI)** standards for spatter protection and impact protection. HCP who wear prescription eyeglasses should consult an eyecare professional to ensure that the style and materials of the eyewear meet ANSI standards for protective eyewear or should purchase ANSI-certified goggles or face shields that fit over the prescription eyewear.

When laser technologies are used, additional eye protection may be required. Every pair of safety goggles or safety glasses intended for use with laser beams must bear a label with the following information:

- Laser wavelengths in use
- Optical density of those wavelengths
- Visible light transmission

Masks

A surgical mask protects the mucous membranes of the nose and mouth from exposure to spatter generated under a variety of dental procedures. Wear masks under the same circumstances that warrant the use of eye protection (Figure 9-7). Base the selection of masks on comfort, how well the periphery of the mask conforms to the contours of the face, and the level of filtration the mask provides. In general, a mask rated as surgical has a filtration rating superior to that of masks rated as procedure masks.

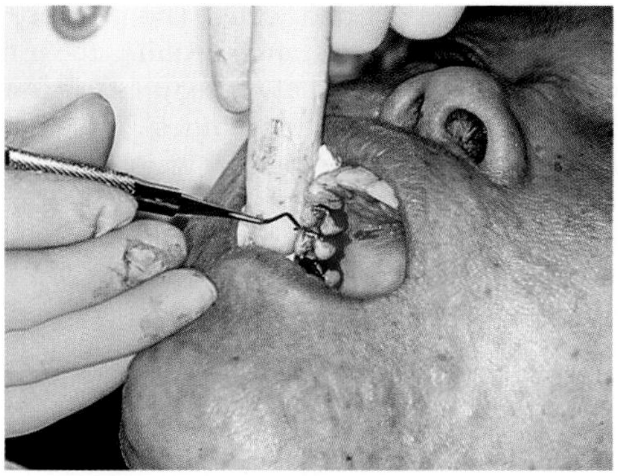

Figure 9-5. Example of improper positioning of operator's fingers, placing the dental hygienist at risk of a puncture wound.

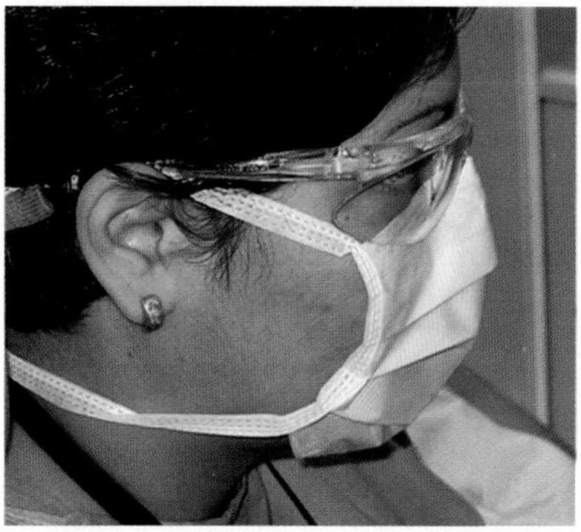

Figure 9-6. Eye protection with side shields and surgical face mask.

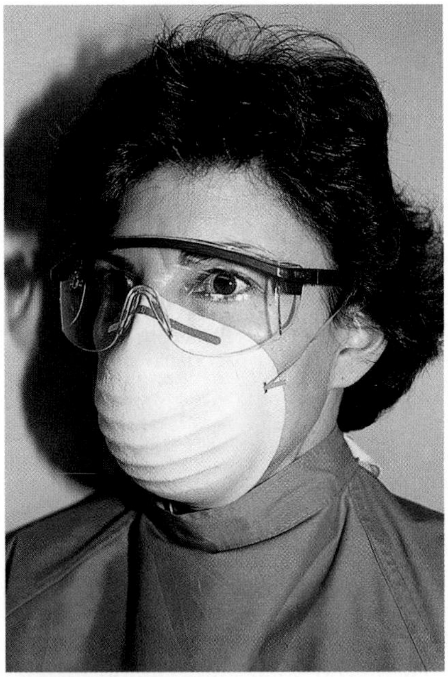

Figure 9-7. Personal protective equipment: barrier gown, eyewear with side shields, and face mask.

Protective Clothing

Protective clothing should shield intact and nonintact skin from spray or splash of body fluids during the course of treatment. In addition, the protective clothing must provide a barrier to protect work clothes or street clothes from exposure. In most dental settings a long-sleeved lab coat that falls below the knees is adequate. However, during exposure-prone procedures, such as surgical procedures, the hygienist may need a more fluid-resistant material. Protective clothing is removed before the hygienist leaves the work area, such as during lunch and other breaks. OSHA restricts HCP from taking protective attire home for laundering. It is the employer's responsibility to arrange for laundering or use of disposable garments, in addition to providing adequate protective attire.

Gloves

Gloves used for dental and dental hygiene procedures fall into three categories, as follows:

- *Medical examination gloves*—nonsterile gloves that are available in a variety of sizes and materials, powdered and unpowdered, and either ambidextrous or right- or left-hand specific (Figure 9-8)
- *Sterile surgeon's gloves* (indicated for oral surgical procedures)—sterile gloves individually packaged in sized pairs. To maintain sterility of gloves, do not open package until ready to use for surgical procedures.
- *Heavy-duty utility gloves*—puncture-resistant gloves (Figure 9-9), used during cleaning and disinfection procedures to reduce risk of accidental puncture injury

Hand Protection and Hand Hygiene

HCP increasingly are reporting allergic and nonallergic dermatitis of the hands. Many of these reactions are the result of contact with chemicals used in the manufacture of latex.

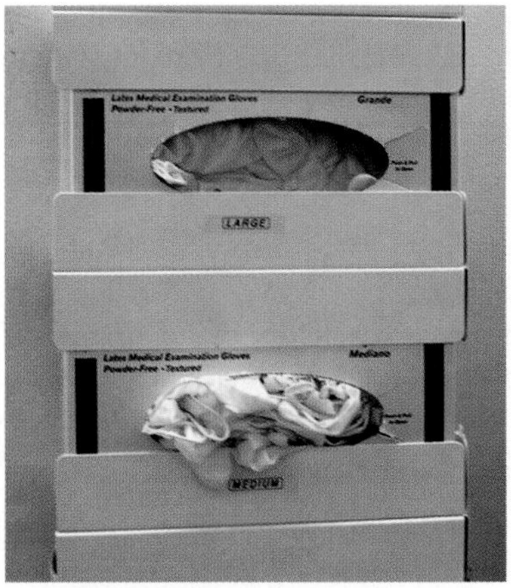

Figure 9-8. Examination gloves.

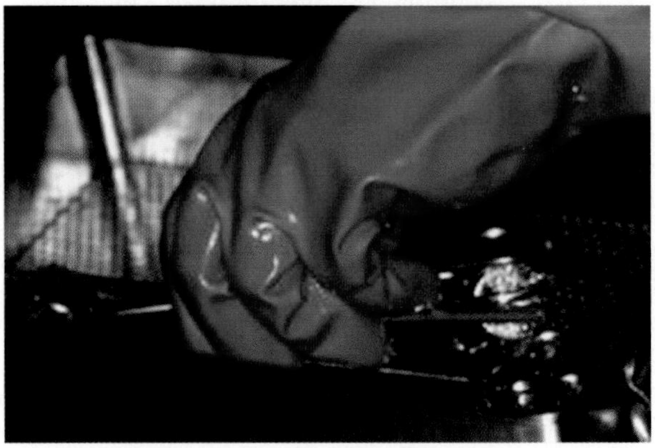

Figure 9-9. Heavy-duty utility gloves.

However, a small percentage involves a potentially serious allergic reaction to the proteins found in natural rubber latex. It is important to seek the advice of a qualified healthcare professional (e.g., physician with specialty in dermatitis and allergies) when experiencing dermal problems related to the use of medical gloves.

Hand hygiene is the most important behavior in the prevention of disease transmission.

The preferred method for hand hygiene depends on the type of procedure, the degree of contamination, and the desired persistence of antimicrobial action on the skin (Table 9-3). Remove transient microbial flora and debris by cleaning the hands with detergent and water. The presence of colonized or resident flora on the hands requires the use of antiseptic agents. For routine dental procedures (e.g., screening, examination, and nonsurgical procedures), wash hands with either plain or antimicrobial soap and water. If the hands are not visibly soiled, an alcohol-based hand rub is adequate. Hand hygiene for surgical procedures (e.g., periodontal surgery, surgical extraction of teeth, biopsy) requires surgical hand antisepsis to eliminate transient flora and reduce resident flora.

Antiseptic agents for surgical procedures should have a lasting antimicrobial effect on the hands for the duration of a procedure, to do the following:

- Prevent introduction of organisms in the operative wound if gloves become punctured or torn.

TABLE 9-3

Types of Hand Hygiene

Methods	Agent	Purpose	Area	Duration (Minimum)
Routine handwash	Water and nonantimicrobial soap (i.e., plain soap[a])	Remove soil[b] and transient microorganisms	All surfaces of hands and fingers	15 seconds[c]
Antiseptic handwash	Water and antimicrobial soap (e.g., chlorhexidine, iodine and iodophors, chloroxylenol [PCMX], triclosan)	Remove or destroy transient microorganisms and reduce resident[d] flora (persistent activity)[e]	All surfaces of hands and fingers	15 seconds[c]
Antiseptic handrub	Alcohol-based handrub[f]	Remove or destroy transient microorganisms and reduce resident[d] flora (persistent activity)[e]	All surfaces of hands and fingers	Until hands are dry
Surgical antisepsis	Water and antimicrobial soap (e.g., chlorhexidine, iodine and iodophors, chloroxylenol [PCMX], triclosan)	Remove or destroy transient microorganisms and reduce resident flora (persistent activity)	Hands and forearms[g]	2-6 minutes
	Water and nonantimicrobial soap (i.e., plain soap[a]) followed by an alcohol-based surgical hand scrub product with persistent activity			Follow manufacturer's instructions for surgical hand scrub product with persistent activity[h]

From Centers for Disease Control and Prevention (CDC): *Frequently asked questions. Hand hygiene.* Available at: www.cdc.gov/oralhealth/infectioncontrol/faq/hand.htm. Accessed February 2008.

[a]Pathogenic organisms have been found on or around bar soap during and after use. Using liquid soap with hands-free controls for dispensing is preferable.

[b]Transient microorganisms often acquired by healthcare personnel during direct contact with patients or contaminated environmental surfaces. Transient microorganisms most frequently associated with healthcare-associated infections and are more amenable to removal by routine hand washing than resident flora.

[c]Time reported as effective in removing most transient flora from the skin. For most procedures a vigorous, brief (at least 15 seconds) rubbing together of all surfaces of premoistened, lathered hands and fingers followed by rinsing under a stream of cool or tepid water is recommended. Hands always should be dried thoroughly before gloves are donned.

[d]Waterless products (e.g., alcohol-based hand rub) are especially useful when water facilities are unavailable (e.g., during dental screenings in schools) or during boil-water advisories. Alcohol-based hand rubs should not be used in the presence of visible soil or organic material.

[e]Persistent activity. Prolonged or extended activity that prevents or inhibits proliferation or survival of microorganisms after application of a product. Previously, this property was sometimes termed *residual activity.*

[f]Resident flora are species of microorganisms that are always present on or in the body; not easily removed by mechanical friction; and less likely to be associated with healthcare-associated infections.

[g]Removal of all jewelry, washing as described above, holding the hands above the elbows during final rinsing, and drying the hands with sterile towels.

[h]Before beginning surgical hand scrub, remove all arm jewelry and any hand jewelry that may make donning gloves more difficult, cause gloves to tear more readily, or interfere with glove usage (e.g., ability to wear the correct-sized glove or altered glove integrity).

- Prevent skin bacteria from multiplying under surgical gloves

However, frequent hand washing and the use of gloves may contribute to the development of nonallergic dermatitis. It is important for DHCP to practice protective hand care as follows:

- Thorough drying of hands after hand washing and before donning gloves
- Use of powder-free gloves (or low amounts of powder)
- Frequent use of appropriate lubricating hand lotions
- Use of cool water when washing hands
- Protecting hands from chapping and drying during cold weather
- Protecting hands from cuts and scratches when performing household chores

Limit the Spread of Blood and Other Infectious Bodies

Environmental Surface Disinfection

Environmental surfaces are less likely to provide an efficient mechanism for transmission of infectious agents than contaminated instruments; however, they can become contaminated in oral healthcare settings. Environmental surfaces are disinfected between clients, as well as at the beginning and end of the day.

Cross-Contamination

Cross-contamination is the transfer of oral fluids and debris from a client to surfaces, equipment, materials, workers' hands, or another person. Because saliva is invisible yet capable of containing high bacterial and viral particle loads, cross-contamination is particularly problematic in oral healthcare. Pathogenic organisms, potentially present in oral fluids, may survive on environmental surfaces for days, weeks, and even months if left untreated with a germicidal product.

Cross-contamination may be by direct or indirect means:

- **Direct cross-contamination** occurs when a worker fails to change gloves between patients or fails to clean and sterilize instruments properly between uses. An example of direct cross-contamination is the use of a disposable dental product such as a saliva ejector on multiple clients.
- **Indirect cross-contamination** occurs when handling a container, armamentaria, or equipment with contaminated gloves and failing to disinfect the items between clients.

Numerous strategies prevent contamination. It is difficult or impossible to sterilize most items and surface areas in the oral care environment. Therefore the best way to manage environmental surfaces in the clinical environment is to clean and disinfect with an EPA-registered disinfectant or protect surfaces with fluid-impervious barriers (e.g., plastic covers). To be effective the disinfectant must come into direct contact with a *precleaned* surface.

The CDC designates environmental surfaces in the oral healthcare setting into two categories:

- **Housekeeping surfaces:** Areas that may be difficult or impossible to clean include switches, knobs, hoses, brackets, and many other items used in the delivery of care. Protect these surfaces by covering them with fluid-impervious barriers (see Figure 9-2). Always change barriers between clients.
- **Clinical contact surfaces:** Surfaces that become contaminated from spray or droplets of oral fluids or by touching with gloved hands during the procedure. These surfaces may be difficult to clean and can subsequently contaminate other instruments, devices, hands, or gloves. Disinfect or barrier-protect clinical contact surfaces including the following:
  - Touch areas on the dental chair
  - Touch areas on the operator chair
  - Dental unit
  - Dental light handle(s)
  - X-ray unit touch areas
  - Countertops that are contacted by contaminated items
  - Air and water syringe handle and tubing
  - Pencils, pens, face
  - Keyboards, pointing devices, monitors
  - Mirror for client education
  - Dental unit suction controls and disposable tip connection tubing
  - Saliva ejector holder and tubing
  - Bracket tables and bracket tray
  - Portable equipment (e.g., ultrasonic cleaner and scaler, airpolisher, curing light, vitalometer, laser)

In the absence of barriers, clean and disinfect surfaces and equipment between clients with an EPA-registered hospital disinfectant (low-level disinfectant) or an EPA-registered hospital disinfectant with a tuberculocidal claim (intermediate-level disinfectant). Use intermediate-level disinfectant for surfaces with visible blood or other potentially infectious materials (OPIM) (Figures 9-10 and 9-11).

General cleaning and disinfection are recommended for clinical contact surfaces, dental unit surfaces, and countertops at the end of daily work activities and are required if surfaces have become contaminated since their last cleaning. Keeping treatment areas free of unnecessary equipment and supplies facilitates daily cleaning.

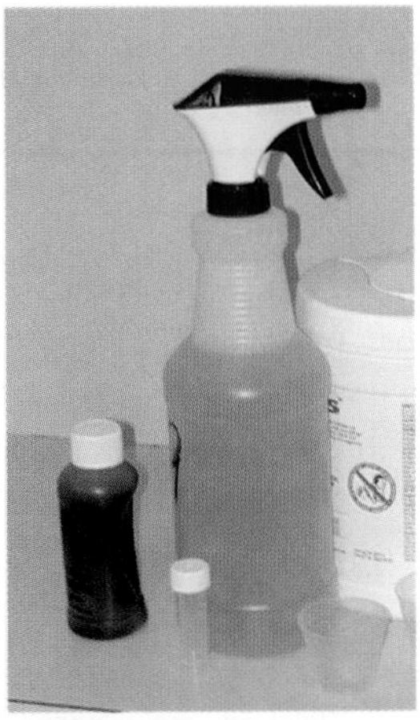

Figure 9-10 Spray disinfectant.

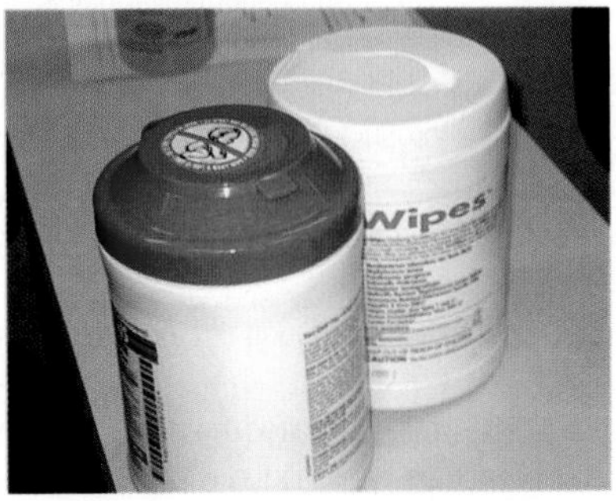

Figure 9-11. Disinfectant wipes.

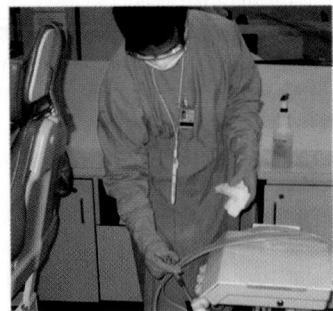

Figure 9-12. Use of PPE during disinfection of treatment area.

Follow manufacturer directions for the handling, use, and storage of all disinfectant and cleaning products. Manufacturers of dental devices and equipment should provide information regarding material compatibility with liquid chemical germicides, precautions regarding immersion of devices for cleaning, and how to decontaminate the item if servicing is required. DHCP who perform environmental cleaning and disinfection should wear gloves and other PPE to prevent occupational exposure to infectious agents and hazardous chemicals. Chemical- and puncture-resistant utility gloves offer more protection than patient examination gloves when hazardous chemicals are used (Figure 9-12).

Sterilization and Sterility Assurance—Make Client Care Items Safe for Use

Client care items are either single-use disposable items or reusable items that require sterilization between uses. Sterilization is the destruction of all living organisms, including highly resistant bacterial spores. Properly performed cleaning and sterilization procedures offer the highest level of assurance that no pathogenic organisms remain on instruments and devices. The intent of instrument and equipment sterilization is not to establish a sterile care environment. Indeed, such an environment would be impossible to establish. Rather, the sterilization process ensures the destruction of all organisms transferred to an item during use on one client before reuse of the item on a subsequent client.

Instrument Classification

Dental instruments fall into three broad categories for determining the minimum level of management between clients (Table 9-4):

- Critical instruments are instruments that penetrate soft tissue or bone. Critical instruments must be heat sterilized between each use or discarded if disposable. Examples of critical instruments and devices include periodontal probes, explorers, scaling and root planing instruments, and tip insert of an ultrasonic scaling unit.
- Semicritical instruments are not intended to penetrate soft tissue or bone but contact oral fluids. Examples include mouth mirrors, ultrasonic scaling handpieces, impression trays, and oral photography retractors. These instruments also should be heat sterilized between each use. The use of high-level disinfectants is indicated for semicritical instruments that cannot be heat sterilized. These germicides are chemical disinfectants that provide sterilization under certain conditions. Chemical germicides are not as reliable as heat sterilization methods and raise worker safety concerns; therefore heat-stable or disposable alternatives are preferred.

TABLE 9-4

Infection-Control Management of Instruments and Devices Based on Classification

Category	Definition	Process	Examples
Critical	Penetrate soft tissue or bone	Sterilization	Surgical instruments, periodontal scalers, surgical dental burs
Semicritical	Contact mucous membranes or nonintact skin	Sterilization or high-level disinfection	Dental mouth mirrors, amalgam condensers, dental handpieces, most hand instruments
Noncritical	Contact intact skin	Low- to intermediate-level disinfection	X-ray head or cone, blood-pressure cuff, facebow

- Noncritical instruments and devices are those items that come into contact only with intact skin. Examples include an x-ray head, light handles, high- and low-volume evacuators, tubing for handpieces, instrument trays, countertops, and chair surfaces. Disinfect these items with an EPA-registered low- to intermediate-level disinfectant.

Heat Methods of Sterilization

Heat-based sterilization methods are more time efficient and reliable than chemical germicides. It is important to determine the method of sterilization that provides a safe and effective outcome for the type of devices.

DHCP must use an FDA-approved sterilization device and follow the manufacturer's instructions for cycle time, temperature, and other parameters involved in achieving sterilization. For satisfactory results, thoroughly clean instruments before placing into appropriate packaging and sterilizing. Three major types of heat sterilization are available:

- Autoclave, the most common method of heat sterilization in the dental office, uses steam in a pressurized chamber to sterilize heat-stable instruments and devices. The user places distilled water into a chamber that dispenses the amount needed to provide steam for the process. Most autoclaves require several minutes to achieve the temperature necessary to begin the sterilization process. Additional time at the end of the sterilization cycle allows depressurization of the chamber. Two methods of air evacuation are available in autoclaves: prevacuum and gravity displacement.
  - A **prevacuum** (also known as *class B sterilizer*) usually consists of a sterilization chamber surrounded by a secondary jacket. When the sterilization cycle is initiated, the air is "pumped" out of the chamber, creating a vacuum into which steam is injected. Once the chamber reaches the desired temperature and pressure, the sterilization process begins. In many prevacuum sterilizers, the actual sterilization time is 4 to 5 minutes, followed by a 20-minute drying cycle. When using a prevacuum sterilizer, conduct an air removal test (one such test is the Bowie-Dick test) at the beginning of each day to ensure the process removes all air from the chamber (Figure 9-13). Pockets of air remaining after the prevacuum may result in incomplete sterilization of the contents.
  - Gravity displacement sterilization relies on gravity to evacuate the air from the sterilizer chamber. Pressurization of the autoclave relies on the effective removal of all air. As steam enters the gravity displacement sterilizer, gravity forces the air out through ventilation ports in the chamber. Gravity displacement is usually a longer process than prevacuum air displacement.
- An unsaturated chemical vapor sterilizer uses a process similar to that of the autoclave; however, in place of steam, a chemical vapor enters the pressurized sterilization chamber. The use of chemical vapor instead of steam reduces the humidity of the sterilization process, reducing the risk of instrument rust and corrosion (primarily carbon steel instruments).
- Dry-heat sterilization uses high heat for a specific amount of time to achieve sterile results. Temperatures often reach 350° F; therefore dry heat is likely to damage heat-sensitive items such as dental handpieces and some plastics.

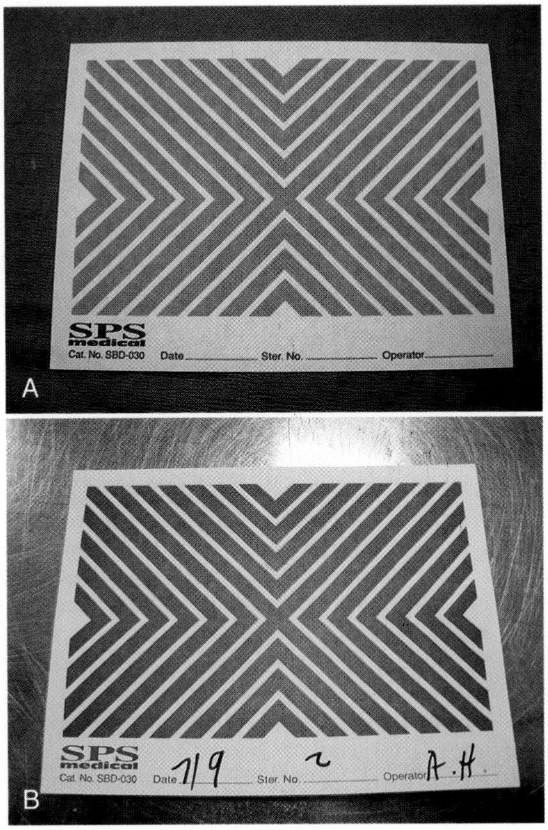

Figure 9-13. Bowie-Dick air removal test. **A,** Test before use. **B,** Test indicating successful air removal.

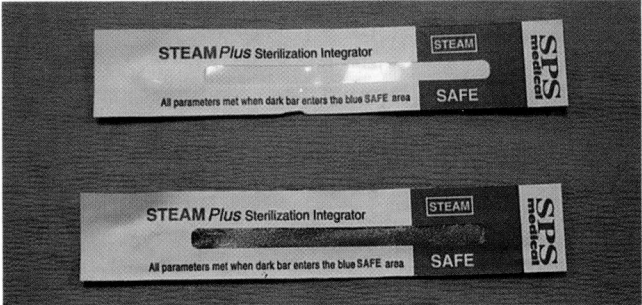

Figure 9-14. Chemical indicator for steam autoclave.

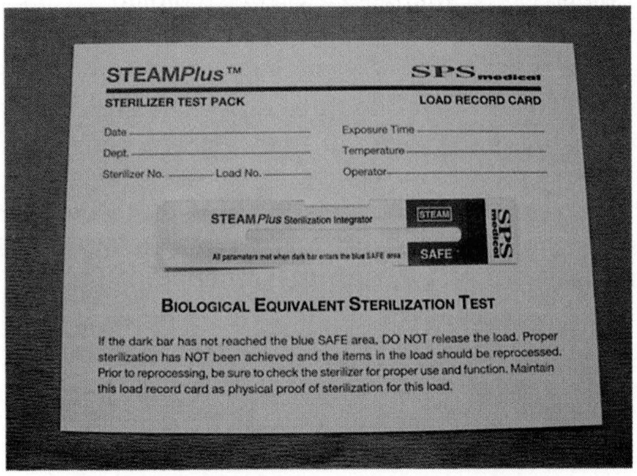

Figure 9-15. Multiparameter integrator.

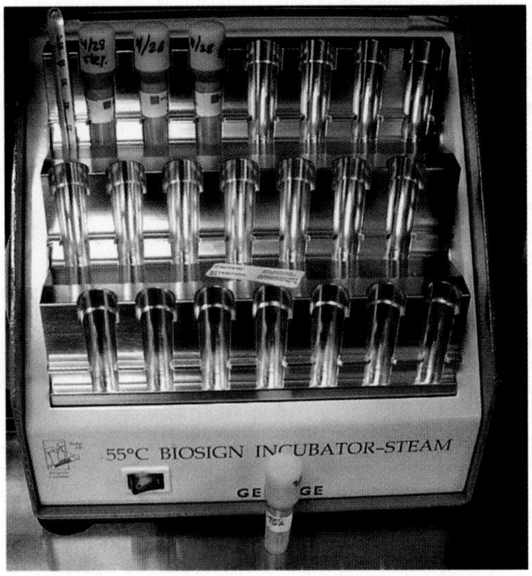

Figure 9-16. Biologic indicator (spore test).

Chemical Disinfectants and Sterilants

Several classes of chemical agents are available that provide high-level disinfection and sterilization under given conditions. Varying degrees of corrosion and damage to certain materials occur if instruments or devices are in prolonged contact with the chemical agent. In addition, the CDC discourages the use of these chemicals because of their toxic properties.

Sterility Assurance

To ensure effectiveness of sterilization, several levels of sterility assurance are available, and a combination approach is best.

- **Chemical indicators** allow the operator to determine the presence of certain necessary parameters such as heat or steam. These indicators often appear as arrows or color-change indicators on pouches used to package instruments during sterilization (Figure 9-14). They are also available as tape imbedded with stripes that change color or indicator strips. One should use chemical indicators with every packet of instruments as a signal to the user that the particular packet completed a heat sterilization process. The indicator is not an indication of effectiveness of the sterilization process itself because many factors may interfere with adequate sterilization.
- **Multiparameter indicators**, also called **integrators**, are a higher level of sterilization assurance and indicate that more than one parameter required for sterilization was present (Figure 9-15). Different levels of integrators provide different levels of sterility assurance. Class V indicators are equivalent to a biologic indicator. The product manufacturer must establish the efficacy of the class V indicator with the Food and Drug Administration (FDA).
- **Biologic indicators (BIs)**, also called **spore tests**, are the highest level of verification (Figure 9-16). BIs use nonpathogenic spores that are especially resistant to the sterilization process embedded on a strip or in a solution that is placed in the sterilizer with a load of instruments. Incubation of the spore test confirms the destruction of the

spores by the sterilization process, which indicates a successful sterilization process.

- *Geobacillus stearothermophilus* is a standard organism for testing steam and chemical vapor sterilization.
- *Bacillus pumilus* spores are the organisms most resistant to dry heat sterilization.
- For monitoring a combination of sterilization methods, dual species biologic indicators (containing both types of spores) would be an appropriate choice.

Destruction of spores resistant to the specific sterilization methods indicates the elimination of all of the organisms of concern. Spore test at least weekly and with each implantable device to verify the proper functioning and operation of the sterilizer. Maintain records of spore testing and their results in the dental office. Many states require biologic monitoring (spore testing) and specify the length of time to maintain the test result records.

Exposure Prevention and Management

The risk of infection with a blood-borne disease after an occupational exposure to blood-borne pathogens in dental settings is low. However, every exposure to blood and body fluids carries some risk for transmission of blood-borne pathogens. Risk reduction strategies include the use of safer work practices, safer devices, PPE, proper policies and procedures, awareness of personal health status, attention to standard precautions, and a program of ongoing education. The majority of exposures are preventable. The CDC defines an **occupational exposure** as a percutaneous injury or contact of mucous membrane or nonintact skin with blood, saliva, tissue, or other body fluids that are potentially infectious. Exposure incidents may pose a risk of HBV, HCV, or HIV infection and are a matter of medical urgency.

Every dental facility must have a postexposure management program for occupational exposures. There should be a written program that identifies the specific steps to follow after an exposure incident and includes training and education regarding the types of exposure that put DHCP at risk and procedures for prompt reporting and evaluation (including counseling, testing, and follow-up) according to the most current U.S. Public Health Service (USPHS) guidelines. These policies should be in compliance with the OSHA blood-borne pathogen standard and with any state or local laws or regulations.

Prevention and management of injury programs follow the **public health doctrine of prevention**:

- **Primary prevention** strives to prevent the injury in the first place.
- **Secondary prevention** strives to contain the injury.
- **Tertiary prevention** strives to return to a functional state of no exposure and prevent similar injuries from occurring again.

Steps for Risk Reduction

Primary prevention involves all efforts to avoid injury during each facet of delivering oral healthcare services, including setting up a treatment room, providing care, and performing post-treatment cleanup. This includes being familiar with the written infection-control plan and all policies, procedures, and best practices to avoid injury. Prevention of injuries may include the use of engineering controls, including safer devices, work practice controls, PPE, and other methods of hazard abatement and risk reduction such as standard precautions. Therefore the first step for risk reduction is to assess risks as environmental, administrative or procedural, and personal. After the risk is assessed, it is important to determine if actions can be taken to remove or at least reduce risk by modifying policies, procedures, or practices or choosing alternative devices.

Risk assessment involves determining what is done, by whom, how it is done, and with what products and devices. Risk reduction then involves the selection of engineering or work practice controls appropriate to the anticipated procedures. The ultimate lesson is that it is far better to prevent the exposure in the first place than to deal with the consequences of an exposure, such as counseling, testing, and medical follow-up. The underlying theme of risk reduction is standard precautions.

Risk Reduction Protocols

Several risk reduction protocols center on the need to prevent percutaneous injuries:

- Use medical devices with engineered safety features designed to prevent injuries and/or use of safer techniques.
  - Never recap needles by hand.
  - Never disengage needles from a reusable syringe.
  - Use disposable needle systems.
  - Dispose of needles and sharps in appropriate sharps disposal containers.
- Avoidance of hand contact with sharps
  - Never wipe instruments on gauze in a hand or wrapped around a finger; use a single-hand technique instead, such as cotton rolls taped to an instrument tray or a commercial safe wipe device.
  - Announce instrument passes to warn others of sharps and exposure potential.
  - Create a neutral zone for sharps to avoid passing directly between healthcare workers.
  - Use appropriate cleanup procedures to minimize hand contact with sharps.

Work practice controls have some of the greatest impact on preventing blood-borne disease transmission. Given the types of exposures found in dental settings, more than 90% are associated with needles or other sharp devices. The CDC determined that most occur outside the mouth and on the hands and fingers of the worker. Many of these are preventable with proper caution and the use of safer devices.

Postexposure Management

When an injury occurs, the goal is to contain the injury as soon as possible to reduce risk of transmission (secondary prevention). If an exposure occurs, offer the exposed worker immediate postexposure management in accordance with the most recent USPHS guidelines. It is critical to select a **qualified healthcare provider (QHCP)** trained to evaluate and treat infectious diseases, including HIV infection. For the QHCP to provide appropriate treatment and assess the need for follow-up, he or she must receive specific information regarding the exposure incident. This information includes the circumstances, devices, degree, and severity of exposure. If the source client consents, the QHCP determines the source client's infectious disease status through testing. Basic steps of postexposure management are as follows:

Step 1

Perform immediate first aid (no extraordinary measures). If an injury occurs, there are basic first aid measures to apply immediately, such as washing an area of percutaneous exposure or flushing nose, mouth, eyes, or skin with clean water, saline, or sterile irrigants. There is no scientific evidence that the use of antiseptics for wound care or bleeding the wound reduces the risk of transmission of a blood-borne pathogen. The exposed worker should not use caustic agents such as bleach.

Step 2

Report the incident to a designated individual. That individual must complete an incident report form (Figure 9-17). This includes the source patient's name and the nature of the exposure. The completion of a report should not cause a delay or defer treatment.

Step 3

A designated individual should discuss the incident with the source patient.

Step 4

Initiate immediate referral to a QHCP capable of treating an exposed individual.

Step 5

Begin medical evaluation and follow-up in accordance with the most recent USPHS guidelines. Medical follow-up should include counseling and testing as indicated and determined

BLOODBORNE EXPOSURE REPORT FORM

Exposed Employee Information:

Name________________ SS#______________Job Title____________

Employer name____________________Address__________________

Time of Occurrence________Time Reported________Date____________

Hepatitis B vaccination Yes_____ No_____

If yes, dates of vaccination: 1.______ 2.______ 3.______

Post-vaccination status, if known: Positive______Titer_______ Negative______

Last tetanus vaccination date:__________

Review of *Exposure Incident Follow-Up Procedures:* Yes_________

Exposure Incident Information:

If sharps-related injury:
Type of sharp:____________________ Brand__________________

Work area where exposure occurred:____________________________

Procedure in progress:____________________________________

How incident occurred:____________________________________

Location of exposure (e.g., right index finger):________________________

Did sharps involved have engineered injury protection? yes:_____ no:_____

If yes:
Was the protective mechanism activated? yes_____ no:_____

If yes, did the injury occur: before activation of protective mechanism__________
during activation of protective mechanism__________
after activation of protective mechanism___________

If no:
Employee's opinion:

Could a mechanism have prevented the injury: yes_____ no_____

How could a mechanism have prevented the injury:___________________________

1 of 2

Figure 9-17. Exposure reporting form.

BLOODBORNE EXPOSURE REPORT FORM

Employee's opinion:

Could any engineering, administrative, or work practice control have prevented the injury?
yes___ no___

Explain:____

____

Source Patient Information:

Name______________ Chart No.______________ Telephone No.______________

	Yes	No
Release of information to evaluating healthcare professional?	___	___
Patient's signature______________		

	Yes	No
Review of source patient medical history:	___	___
Verbally questioned regarding:		
• History of hepatitis B, hepatitis C or HIV infection	___	___
• High risk history associated with these diseases	___	___
• Patient consents to be tested for HIV, HCV and HBV	___	___

If HIV-positive source patient:

List all current medications patient is taking for HIV infection:
1.________ 2.________ 3.________ 4.________

List all medication previously taken by patient to which he or she was resistant or medications that were ineffective:
1.________ 2.________ 3.________ 4.________

Provide most recent viral load: ______________ date:______________

CD4 count if known:______________ date:______________

Healthcare worker referred to:______________

Questionnaire completed by______________

Bill for fees to:______________

Retain one copy in employee's confidential medical record; send one copy to evaluating healthcare professional. Retain copy with employee's and source patient's name removed as sharp's injury log.

2 of 2

Figure 9-17, cont'd

by the infection potential of the exposure. Testing may be for HIV, HBV, or HCV; the QHCP may need to repeat testing at certain intervals. A rapid test for HIV is available in many settings. The QHCP must have access to this test. Results from a rapid test are available in less than a half hour rather than in days. Use of rapid testing results can assist in decision making for medical management.

Exposure Follow-Up Guidelines

- HBV: Follow-up of occupational exposure to HBV depends on the HBsAg status of the source client and the vaccination and anti-HBs response of the exposed worker. If the exposed worker is unvaccinated for HBV, it is likely that the vaccination series will be initiated. A prevaccination titer test is not necessary. If the source individual has a history of HBV infection, administration of hepatitis B immune globulin will likely be part of the management protocol. Treatment should begin as soon as possible, preferably within 24 hours and in less than 1 week. If the exposed DHCP has been vaccinated and is a known responder, no action is necessary because the HBV vaccine has strong immunologic memory. However, if the immune status is unknown or the individual is a known nonresponder to the vaccine, other actions must be taken.
- HCV: There is neither preexposure vaccination nor postexposure prophylaxis (PEP) for occupational exposure to HCV. The most current recommendation for follow-up of occupational exposure to HCV is to test the source client for antibodies to hepatitis C virus (anti-HCV) and to

test the exposed worker for anti-HCV and alanine aminotransferase (ALT) activity. Recommendations include repeated testing at 4 to 6 months. It is important to identify HCV infection early, should transmission occur and to refer the exposed individual to a specialist. Limited data suggest that antiviral treatment initiated early in the course of infection may be beneficial.
- HIV: Recommendations for HIV PEP are based on situations in which there has been an occupational exposure to a source patient who either has or is considered likely to have HIV infection. If indicated, the worker should begin postexposure treatment as soon as possible (within 2 hours). The course of treatment usually involves a 4-week regimen of two or more antiretroviral drugs, depending on the nature of the exposure and the medications being taken by the source patient, if the client is known to be HIV positive.

Postexposure management is an area of rapidly changing recommendations. As new antiretroviral agents become available, some are replacing drugs previously used. Therefore it is important to seek the advice and care of an appropriate provider who is familiar with the most current USPHS recommendations for testing and PEP. Counseling as to the potential side effects and reporting of illness are essential to the appropriate medical management of an occupational exposure to HIV.

The CDC recommends counseling as to the risks and benefits for the pregnant worker and extensive follow-up. Pregnancy may affect the selection of antiretrovirals because some of these drugs are contraindicated in a pregnant woman.

Risk of Exposure

Exposure risk varies with the amount of blood, the titer of virus in the patient, and the depth of the injury with the contaminated device or instrument. Immediate initiation of treatment is important, preferably within 2 hours. The goal is to prevent viral replication in the exposed worker, and there is biologic evidence that this is possible. Postexposure management with antiretroviral drugs may reduce risk of infection by about 80% but will not prevent all cases of infection. Postexposure management may fail owing to a resistant virus, an increased titer of virus, an increased dose of blood, or host factors. Postexposure prophylaxis may not be effective unless promptly initiated.

Follow-up also involves counseling regarding signs and symptoms of infection, the importance of measures to not infect others, and the importance of seeking advice if illness occurs:
- For HCV, it may be necessary to monitor liver function and have tests for HCV antibody. Testing is recommended at baseline and then again at 4 to 6 months. An HCV-RNA test may be conducted at 4 to 6 weeks for more rapid diagnosis.
- For HIV, baseline testing is part of the standard protocol, and repeat testing may be indicated at 6 weeks, 12 weeks, and 6 months. If the worker is taking antiretroviral drugs, the exposed person may need to have drug toxicity tests.

Risk of Infection

Most exposures do not lead to infection, and the risk of seroconversion may vary depending on the agent, the type of exposure, the amount of blood involved, and the amount of circulating virus in the source client. When assessing an occupational exposure and determining the management and follow-up, QHCP review the following:
- Type of exposure (percutaneous, mucous membrane, nonintact skin, or bite) exposure
- Type and amount of fluid (blood versus fluids containing blood)
- Infectious status of the source such as presence of HBsAg, presence of HCV antibody, and/or presence of HIV antibody
- Susceptibility of exposed person with consideration to the HBV vaccine response status and the HBV, HCV, and/or HIV status

For HBV the risk of infection ranges from 6% to 30% in persons not protected by vaccination or previous infection. Source individuals who are hepatitis e-antigen positive are potentially more infectious and more likely to transmit diseases. The best protection is vaccination against HBV.

For HCV the risk is about 1.8% on average for percutaneous exposures. There are no exact estimates of the number of healthcare workers occupationally infected with HCV, but the risk to a healthcare worker is no higher than the average community risk.

For HIV, average risk after a percutaneous exposure is about 0.3%. The risk after exposure to eyes, nose, or mouth is about 0.1%, and the risk to skin is estimated to be less than that unless the skin is damaged or compromised, in which case the risk would be higher.

In tertiary prevention the healthcare professional learns from the exposure incident, restores those exposed to a state of no infection, and takes all steps to reduce future exposure risk by the following:
- Evaluating the circumstances of the exposure
- Reviewing policies, procedures, products, devices, and practices; perhaps modifying policies or procedures and/or selecting safer devices
- Discussing appropriate modifications
- Determining how to communicate these to others

Maximum effort should be aimed at injury prevention because preventing an exposure is far better than dealing with the consequences of an exposure. These include medical management and follow-up as prescribed. Preventive strategies include the routine use of barriers when anticipating contact with blood or OPIM, adherence to hand washing, and the careful handling and disposal of sharps during and after use. Therefore avoiding occupational exposure involves the use of engineering controls, work practice controls, and PPE.

CLIENT EDUCATION TIPS

- Explain infection-control protocols used in the delivery of dental hygiene care and their underlying rationale.
- Explain that infection control is done to protect and not to keep an unnatural distance between client and clinician.
- Discuss postexposure protocols at the initial appointment in case of an exposure.

LEGAL, ETHICAL, AND SAFETY ISSUES

- Using evidence-based infection-control protocols is an ethical and a legal requirement for dental hygienists.

- Beneficent dental hygiene care requires appropriate infection control standards be used for all clients to prevent disease transmission and provide safe, quality care.
- Nonmaleficence requires that dental hygienists prevent harm to their clients by compliance with all infection control standards.
- Societal trust of oral healthcare professionals is related to proper infection control practices and the clients' understanding of them.
- Evidence-based standard precautions are a standard of care. Healthcare personnel who fail to render services using current standards of care place themselves at risk for civil and criminal violations.
- The *reasonably prudent dental hygiene practitioner* must stay current with regard to changing infection-control concepts, protocols, and governmental guidelines; this is a matter of state law or regulation in some jurisdictions.
- It is unethical and illegal to refuse treatment to a client of record because that person has an infectious disease or to refuse to treat a person based on the presence of an infectious disease.
- Adhere to state and federal laws that protect against discrimination based on race, religion, gender, sexual orientation, or disability, including infectious disease.

KEY CONCEPTS

- Sterilization and surface disinfection can be achieved by physical or chemical means based on the equipment, type of procedure, and level of exposure risk.
- Hand washing is the most effective strategy in the prevention of infection and disease transmission.
- The Centers for Disease Control and Prevention recommendations for standard precautions indicate that healthcare personnel use personal protective equipment when exposure to body fluids is likely.
- The basic tenet of standard precautions is that all clients should be viewed as potentially infected.
- Healthcare practitioners who adhere to infection prevention and control strategies reduce the risk of infection for themselves, their families, and their clients.

CRITICAL THINKING EXERCISES

You have been hired by one of the most reputable dental practices in the community. On the second day of employment, while treating your client, you accidentally insert a used hypodermic needle percutaneously into your thumb after administering a local anesthetic agent. Because your client is a high-profile state legislator and you do not want to appear incompetent to your new employer or the client, you say nothing about the exposure incident. After 3 days of thinking about the situation, you report the incident to the office manager. Use the principles of postexposure management to determine the following:

1. What should the office manager do to protect the health and safety of the new dental hygienist?
2. What errors in judgment were made by the dental hygienist?
3. What steps of the postexposure management protocol should have the dental hygienist taken?
4. What tertiary preventive strategies must be initiated by the office manager for the practice to ensure that a similar exposure incident does not occur?

BIBLIOGRAPHY

Barker CS, Soro V, Dymock D, et al: Time-dependent recontamination rates of sterilised dental instruments. *Br Dent J* 211(8):E17, 2011.

Centers for Disease Control and Prevention (CDC): Updated CDC recommendations for the management of hepatitis B virus-infected health-care providers and students. *MMWR Recomm Rep* 6:61(RR-3):1, 2012. Erratum in: *MMWR Recomm Rep* 61(28):542, 2012.

Cleveland JL, Barker L, Gooch BF, et al: Use of HIV postexposure prophylaxis by dental health care personnel: an overview and updated recommendations. *J Am Dent Assoc* 133:1619, 2002.

Cleveland JL, Barker LK, Cuny EJ, et al: National Surveillance System for Health Care Workers Group. Preventing percutaneous injuries among dental health care personnel. *J Am Dent Assoc* 138:169, 2007.

Cleveland JL, Foster M, Barker L, et al: Advancing infection control in dental care settings: factors associated with dentists' implementation of guidelines from the Centers for Disease Control and Prevention. *J Am Dent Assoc* 143(10):1127, 2012.

Cleveland JL, Griffin SO, Romaguera RA: Benefits of using rapid oral HIV-tests in dental offices. *J Dent Res* 84:3196, 2005 (Special Issue A).

Dental Health and Hepatitis C. Available at: http://www.ashm.org.au/publications. Accessed January 2013.

Kohn WG, Harte JA, Malvitz DM, et al: Guidelines for infection control in dental health-care settings, 2003. *J Am Dent Assoc* 135:33, 2004.

November-Rider D, Bray KK, Eklund KJ, et al: Massachusetts dental public health program directors practice behaviors and perceptions of infection control. *J Dent Hyg* 86(3):248, 2012.

Smith GW, McNeil J, Ramage G, et al: In vitro evaluation of cleaning efficacy of detergents recommended for use on dental instruments. *Am J Infect Control* 40(9):e255, 2012.

Trochesset DA, Walker SG: Isolation of Staphylococcus aureus from environmental surfaces in an academic dental clinic. *J Am Dent Assoc* 143(2):164, 2012.

Vassey M, Budge C, Poolman T, et al: Quantitative assessment of residual protein levels on dental instruments reprocessed by manual, ultrasonic and automated cleaning methods. *Br Dent J* 210(9):E14, 2011.

EVOLVE RESOURCES

Please visit http://evolve.elsevier.com/Darby/hygiene for additional practice and study support tools.

CHAPTER 10

Medical Emergencies

Denise M. Bowen, Margaret M. Walsh

COMPETENCIES

1. Discuss prevention of medical emergencies, including how to recognize persons at high risk for a medical emergency.
2. Delineate protocols for performing Basic Life Support in adults, children, and infants.
3. Discuss cardiac arrest and the protocol for management of the situation.
4. Describe protocols for managing victims with mild (partial) airway obstruction and severe (complete) airway obstruction.
5. Discuss the administration of oxygen.
6. Discuss appropriate use of equipment and drugs included in a basic kit for managing medical emergencies in the oral care environment.
7. Identify signs and symptoms of specific medical emergencies and appropriate treatment for each.

Life-threatening emergencies can and do happen in the oral healthcare setting. Although these emergencies are infrequent, many factors increase the likelihood of such incidents during oral healthcare. These factors include the increasing number of older, medically compromised adults seeking care, medical advances in drug therapy, increased number of surgical procedures (e.g., dental implants), longer appointments, and the increasing use of drugs in the oral healthcare setting such as local anesthetics, sedatives, analgesics, and antibiotics.[1] Fortunately, prevention can minimize life-threatening incidents. Prevention is based on a client's **comprehensive health history and risk assessment**, defined as a thorough health history questionnaire with special attention to medication usage and vital signs; an interview dialogue history; anxiety recognition; and use of the American Society of Anesthesiologists (ASA) physical status classification as a medical assessment framework (Box 10-1). Steps for prevention also include dental-related stress reduction protocols and possible modification of care to minimize medical risks[1,2] (see Chapters 12, 13, 14, and 41). All assessment findings are documented in the client's record and updated at each subsequent visit.

The four main risks associated with oral healthcare are related to hemostasis, susceptibility to infection, drug reactions and interactions, and ability to tolerate the stress of the appointment and procedure planned.[2] The dental staff must be prepared to assist in the recognition and management of any potential emergency situation. Should a medical emergency arise, updated and complete client-related information, thorough knowledge of medical emergency protocols, well-trained office personnel, and availability of appropriate, well-maintained emergency equipment are vital to the best possible outcome.

Preventing Medical Emergencies

Office Personnel and Environment Preparation

Preparation of all dental staff members and the office for medical emergencies should include the following:

- Training and current certification in Basic Life Support (BLS), practice in medical emergency drills, and an annual refresher course in emergency medicine that includes all conditions related to increased risk
- Posting of emergency assistance numbers
- Stocking, regularly checking, and updating of emergency drugs and equipment

Client Assessment

Dental hygienists have a duty to use information from the comprehensive health history and risk assessment to create a care plan that will reduce the likelihood of a medical complication. If a client is found to be at high risk, the dentist and/or the client's physician of record are consulted as needed (Box 10-2). Medical consultation is obtained after the client's dental and physical evaluation has been completed. The dental professional should be prepared to provide the physician with detailed information about the proposed oral healthcare plan and any anticipated problems. Based on this consultation, the care plan or medications can be used to reduce the risk of emergencies. Reduction of the stressful environment by careful appointment planning, good communication and client rapport, and administration of conscious sedation or antianxiety premedication also can improve clinical outcomes. The primary goal in the client assessment process is to determine the client's physical and psychologic ability to handle the stress of the planned oral healthcare.[1,2]

Most health history forms include a medical alert box. This blank box usually appears on the top corner of the health history form. If a client has a condition (e.g., allergy, hypertension, requirement for antibiotic prophylaxis) that, if unrecognized, places the client at risk for a medical emergency, this condition is written in red in the medical alert box clearly visible on the top of the health history form. The practitioner and other staff members involved in client care can consider this condition as the care plan is implemented.

Anxiety Recognition and Management

Heightened anxiety and fear of dental care can lead to an acute exacerbation of medical problems such as heart attack, stroke, angina, seizures, and asthma, as well as other

BOX 10-1

The American Society of Anesthesiologists (ASA) Physical Status Classification

- ASA 1: Normal, healthy; no systemic disease
- ASA 2: Mild systemic disease
- ASA 3: Severe systemic disease that limits activity but is not incapacitating
- ASA 4: Incapacitating systemic disease that is a constant threat to life*
- ASA 5: A moribund patient not expected to survive without an operation
- ASA 6: Declared brain dead and having organs removed as donor. Emergency operation of any variety, with E preceding the number to indicate the patient's physical status (e.g., ASA E-III or ASA E-IV)

Data from ASA Relative Value Guide, 2012.

*Normally, oral healthcare is received in a specialty or hospital setting because of the high-risk nature of the health condition.

stress-related problems such as hyperventilation and syncope (fainting). One of the goals of client assessment is to determine whether a client is emotionally and psychologically capable of tolerating the stress associated with the planned care. Recognizing anxiety in a client can be as easy as asking the patient about fear, anxiety, and past traumatic or painful dental experiences during the comprehensive health history and interview. Many patients underestimate or do not want to acknowledge dental anxiety, so direct observation of signs and symptoms is an important component of assessing anxiety (Box 10-3). Some practitioners use anxiety questionnaires to assess each client.

Direct Observation

Careful observation may permit recognition of unusually anxious individuals. Severely anxious individuals may be recognized by the following:

- Increased blood pressure and heart rate
- Trembling
- Excessive sweating
- Dilated pupils
- Overall appearance of extreme uneasiness

Severely anxious persons most commonly appear in the dental office when they have an oral infection or by a severe toothache. Although these individuals wish to have their dental problems alleviated, their underlying dental fear often makes it impossible for them to tolerate the procedure. As a result, severely anxious individuals usually are candidates for the use of either intravenous (IV) sedation or general anesthesia for dental treatment. A moderately anxious client (see Box 10-3), however, is usually managed effectively by stress reduction protocols and conscious sedation (see Chapter 41).

Stress Reduction Protocols

Many medical emergencies are associated with stress. The stress-reduction protocols, or steps taken to reduce dental anxiety and fear, listed in Box 10-4, are based on the belief that the prevention or reduction of stress should start before the dental appointment, continue throughout treatment, and follow through into the postoperative period, if necessary.[1,2] Multiple approaches are most effective.

BOX 10-2

Medical Consultation

- Obtain the client's medical, dental, and pharmacologic histories.
- Complete the physical assessments, including oral examination and vital signs.
- Provide a tentative care plan based on the client's oral needs.
- Make a general ASA physical status assessment.
- Consult the client's physician, when appropriate. This consultation can be completed via telephone or in writing. The verbal form is more expedient, whereas the written form provides direct legal documentation of the physician's recommendations. Confidentiality is to be protected according to requirements of the Health Insurance and Portability and Accountability Act of 1996.

Verbal form:

- Once the physician is available, introduce yourself.
- Give the client's name, date of birth, and the reason for the visit to you.
- Relate briefly your summary of the client's general condition.
- Ask for additional information about the client's diagnosis and current status.
- Present your care plan briefly, including medications to be used and the degree of hemorrhage and/or stress anticipated.
- Obtain information to address any concerns or potential emergencies.
- Ask the physician to follow-up with written recommendations.
- After consultation, write a complete report of the conversation for the client's record, and obtain a written report from the physician if possible.

Written form:

- Provide information about the patient (e.g., name, date of birth, reason for appointment with you).
- Note the client's self-reported information about his or her health condition(s), including their understanding of diagnosis, current status, and any expressed concerns of the client.
- Explain the procedures planned for this series of appointments and include anticipated drugs to be used, anxiety or fear of client, and potential medical emergencies.
- Ask the physician for very specific information such as level of control, most recent test results (e.g., HbA1c, electrocardiogram findings) that you need to decide appropriate protocol to follow in treatment plan, and provide a place for the physician to make notes.
- Use of a facsimile machine facilitates quick and confidential correspondence.

Recognition of Unresponsiveness

Unresponsiveness, also called unconsciousness, whatever its cause, must be recognized quickly and managed effectively. In all cases when a person is found to be unresponsive, Basic Life Support steps must be implemented as soon as possible (Figure 10-1).

BOX 10-3

Clinical Signs of Moderate Anxiety

Reception Area	*In Dental Chair*
Questions receptionist regarding injections or use of sedation	Unnaturally stiff posture
Nervous conversations with others in reception area	Nervous play with tissue or handkerchief
History of emergency dental care only	White-knuckle syndrome
History of canceled appointments for nonemergency treatment	Perspiration on forehead and hands
Cold, sweaty palms	Overly willing to cooperate with clinician
	Quick answers

BOX 10-4

Stress-Reduction Protocols

Normal, Healthy, Anxious Client (ASA I)

- Recognize the client's level of anxiety.
- Premedicate with a sedative or anti-anxiety medication and/or use behavioral relaxation techniques the evening before the dental appointment, as needed.
- Premedicate with a sedative or anti-anxiety medication immediately before the dental appointment, as needed.
- Schedule the appointment in the morning.
- Minimize the client's waiting time.
- Use reassuring, calm communication; explain what the client can expect; encourage relaxation and use of distraction techniques (e.g., earphones, personal music players, breathing); inform clients that they can stop the procedure by raising their hand during treatment.
- Avoid triggers such as sights and sounds associated with previous negative experiences.
- Consider conscious sedation or pharmacologic and/or behavioral interventions during therapy.
- Administer adequate pain control during therapy.
- Length of appointment is variable but allows sufficient time for anxiety management.
- Follow up with postoperative pain and anxiety control.
- Telephone highly anxious or fearful clients later the same day that treatment is delivered.

Medical Risk Client (ASA II, III, IV)

- Recognize the client's degree of medical risk.
- Complete medical consultation before care, as needed.
- Schedule the client's appointment in the morning.
- Monitor and record preoperative and postoperative vital signs.
- Use reassuring, calm communication; avoid aggression; explain what the client can expect; encourage relaxation and use of distraction techniques (e.g., earphones, personal music players, breathing) and inform clients that they can stop the procedure by raising their hand during treatment.
- Avoid triggers such as sights and sounds associated with previous negative experiences.
- Consider conscious sedation, pharmacologic and/or behavioral interventions during therapy.
- Administer adequate pain control during therapy.
- Length of appointment variable; do not exceed the client's limits of tolerance but allow enough time to avoid rushing and manage anxiety.
- Follow up with postoperative pain and anxiety control.
- Telephone the higher medical risk client later on the same day that treatment was delivered.
- Arrange the appointment for the highly anxious or fearful, moderate- to high-risk client during the first few days of the week (Monday through Wednesday in most countries; Saturday or Sunday through Monday in many Middle Eastern countries) when the office is open for emergency care and the treating doctor is available.

Basic Life Support

Basic Life Support (BLS) is the level of care or intervention used for victims of life-threatening illnesses or injuries until they can be given full medical care at a healthcare facility offering such services. Emergency medical personnel are notified before initiation, or someone is asked to do so immediately. Cardiopulmonary resuscitation (CPR) is an emergency procedure, performed to manually preserve brain function until further actions are taken to restore spontaneous blood circulation and breathing in a person who is not breathing, not breathing normally (only gasping), and has no pulse. BLS formerly was known as A-B-C (airway, breathing, circulation); however, this protocol was revised in 2010 by the American Heart Association as C-A-B (chest compressions, airway, breathing).[3] Evidence has shown that the most important aspect of BLS is providing early and effective chest compressions and defibrillation. Compressions (C) must be maintained at a rate of at least 100 per minute (formerly approximately 100 per minute). The first cycle of compressions (30 per 18 seconds) is delivered without the delay that previously resulted from the need to check and open the airway, check breathing, find a barrier device, and deliver rescue breathing. When an automatic external defibrillator (AED) is used by a health professional, one shock (rather than

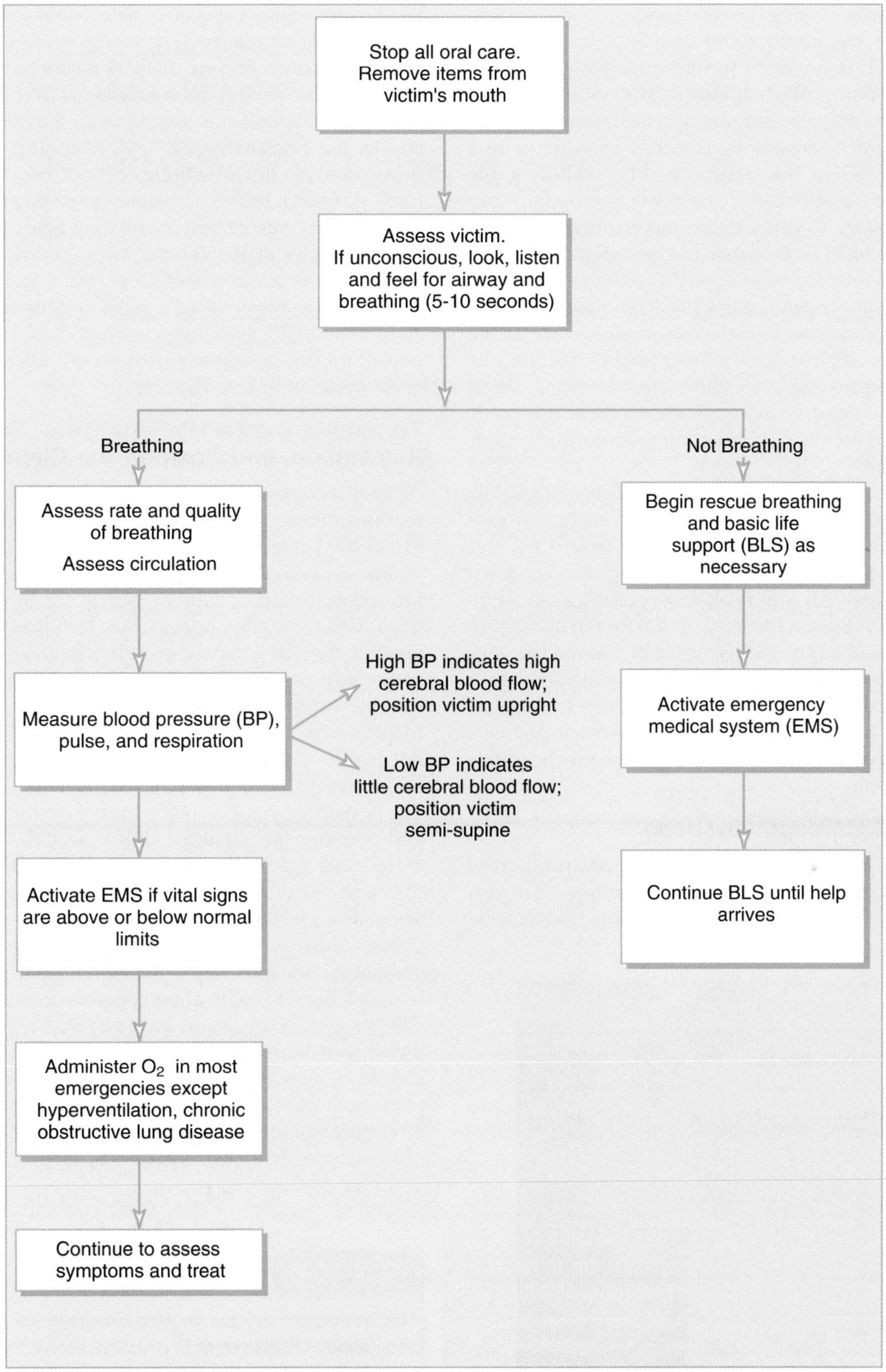

Figure 10-1. Dental hygiene actions taken in an emergency situation.

the former three) is delivered before beginning chest compressions. The depth of chest compressions was revised from 1½ to 2 inches to at least 2 inches in children and adults (1½ inches in infants) with emphasis on allowing full recoil between compressions. Minimizing delays in intervals between compressions improves success and patient survival. These changes affirm the importance of stronger emphasis on compressions of adequate rate and depth, allowing complete chest recoil after each compression, diminishing interruptions in compressions, and avoiding excessive ventilation.[3] After the first round of compressions (C), the airway (A) is opened and two rescue breaths (B) are given.

When more than one trained healthcare provider is present, the person not delivering CPR can perform other procedures, such as activating the emergency response system (EMS), retrieving the resuscitation mask, retrieving and assembling the AED and placing the electrode pads, or relieving the CPR provider as needed. Health professionals assisting in rescue efforts may use judgment in this sequencing, for example, when directly observing someone collapse or in a case of drowning when the traditional BLS including the C-A-B could have some benefit. Untrained lay rescuers can use only compressions to avoid delay and errors in the more complicated form of BLS. Evidence suggests that CPR with chest compression only (hands-only CPR) achieves outcomes similar to those of conventional CPR (compressions with rescue breathing) in adults with cardiac arrest outside of the hospital. However, for children, conventional CPR may be superior.[3] This alternative also eliminates concerns about rescue breathing without a barrier, if one exists, and encourages individuals to deliver CPR via compressions until emergency personnel arrive.

These BLS procedures are applied until recovery, until the victim can be stabilized and transported to an emergency care facility, or until advanced life support is available. CPR and emergency cardiac care including AED are part of BLS for healthcare providers.[3] All oral healthcare personnel must be currently certified at least at the level of BLS for the healthcare provider. In addition, all co-workers must be trained together at least annually so that they may interact effectively as a team when medical emergencies arise. BLS courses are sponsored by many organizations, including the American Heart Association, the American Red Cross, and many hospitals and fire departments.

Recognition of Unresponsiveness

The unresponsive (unconscious) person does not respond to sensory stimulation such as shaking and shouting, "Are you alright?" (Figure 10-2). Pain is another stimulus that may be used to determine the client's level of consciousness. Pinching of the suprascapular region usually evokes a motor response from a conscious person.[1] Lack of response to this stimulation indicates the person is unconscious. When an apparently unconscious person is discovered, the health professional checks for responsiveness and breathing. If the patient is unresponsive, not breathing, or not breathing abnormally (only gasping), BLS is activated immediately.

The healthcare provider also may take up to 10 seconds to detect a pulse at the carotid artery. Evidence shows that a pulse is difficult to detect, even for a trained professional; therefore the detection of a pulse was deemphasized by the AHA when BLS guidelines were revised in 2010.[3] The most important life-saving step is delivery of chest compressions without delay or interruption.

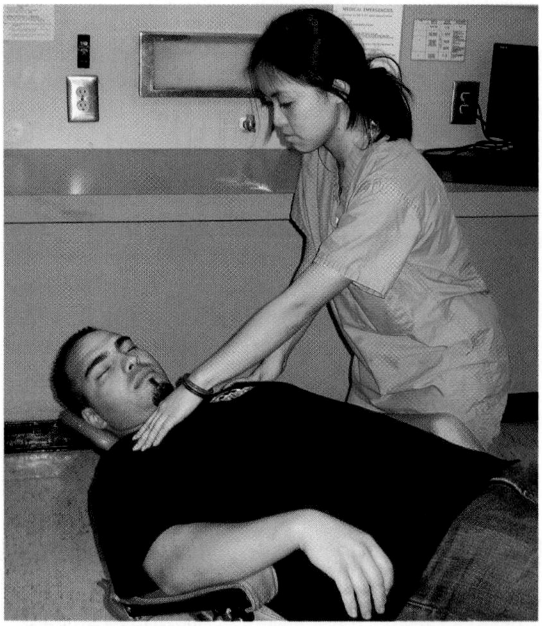

Figure 10-2. Unconsciousness is determined by performing the "shake-and-shout" maneuver, gently shaking the shoulders and calling the client's name. (From Malamed SF: *Medical emergencies in the dental office*, ed 6, St Louis, 2007, Mosby.)

Terminate Dental Hygiene Care, Summon Assistance, and Position the Client

As soon as unresponsiveness is recognized, the hygienist terminates dental hygiene procedures and activates EMS (e.g., 911 in the United States and Canada; 000 in Australia; 119 in Japan; 112 or 999 in the United Kingdom; and 112 in most of Europe; standard on Global System for Mobile Communications [GSM] mobile phones). Box 10-5 lists information to be given to the EMS dispatcher. When available, the office emergency team also is notified. The unconscious person is placed into the supine (horizontal) position. In the supine position, the brain is at the same level with the body positioned on a flat plane. A major objective in the management of unconsciousness is the delivery of oxygenated blood to the brain. The horizontal position helps the heart to accomplish this task and prepares the client for CPR if needed (Figure 10-3). Any extra head supports such as pillows must be removed from the headrest of the dental chair when the client loses consciousness, so the position of the body is supine. After the unconscious person without an easily detectable pulse is positioned, the next step is to begin life support by delivering high-quality CPR with chest compressions at a rate of at least 100 per minute (30 in 18 seconds) and a depth of at least 2 inches in children and adults, $1\frac{1}{2}$ inches in infants. The chest should be allowed to recoil fully after each compression, with interruptions to compressions minimized. CPR is begun with 30 compressions (C). A trained rescuer then opens the airway (A) and provides two breaths (B) (see Procedure 10-1 and

BOX 10-5

Information Given to the Emergency Medical Services Dispatcher

- Your name
- Location of the emergency (with names of cross-streets, if possible)
- Number of telephone from which the call is made
- What happened (e.g., heart attack, seizure)
- Condition of the victim
- Aid being given to the victim
- Any other information requested

Caller should hang up only when told to do so.

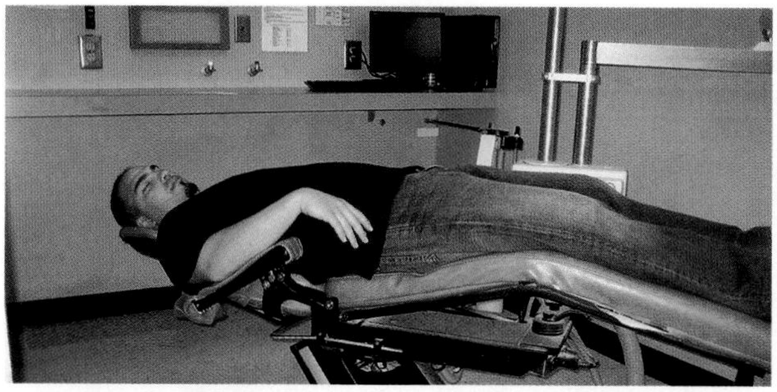

Figure 10-3. Placement of unconscious client in the supine position with feet slightly elevated. (From Malamed SF: *Medical emergencies in the dental office,* ed 6, St Louis, 2007, Mosby.)

corresponding Competency Form). CPR is continued with sequences of 30 compressions and 2 breaths until EMS arrives or the victim recovers.

When office personnel are available to assist, they can be directed to notify EMS while CPR is started and to obtain the AED for the rescuer. If the second rescuer is trained, he or she sets up the AED and prepares it for use, places the electrode pads on the client's chest, and clears the area for shock delivery. One shock of the AED is delivered by the first rescuer, before compressions or as soon as possible, to minimize interruptions in compressions. Other items from the medical emergencies kit also can be obtained by assisting personnel as needed (e.g., oxygen, bag-valve mask, aspirin). When the

Procedure 10-1 Overview of Basic Life Support for an Unresponsive Victim

EQUIPMENT

- Resuscitation or bag mask
- Other protective barriers
- Automatic external defibrillator (AED)

STEP 1

Tap the person on the shoulder and shout, "Are you okay? Are you okay?" (for an infant, gently tap the shoulder or flick the foot) and check to see if the person is breathing normally (see Figure 10-2.). The healthcare provider may take up to 10 seconds to check for a pulse at the carotid artery.

STEP 2

If no response, no breathing, or abnormal breathing (gasping only), activate EMS. If another person is available, summon help to call emergency medical services (EMS) (e.g., 911) and to bring an automated external defibrillator (AED) in case it is needed. If unassisted, perform these steps before continuing.

STEP 3

Place the unconscious client in the supine position (see Figure 10-3).

STEP 4

If the patient is unresponsive, is not breathing, or abnormal breathing (i.e., only gasps):

- Initiate CPR immediately (see Procedure 10-2).
- After one shock with AED, if available, and/or one round of compressions (30 per 18 seconds, at least 100 per minute), the airway may be opened and two breaths are given by a trained rescuer.
- If the AED is not immediately available, begin chest compressions and deliver the AED shock as soon as it can be retrieved and assembled by an assistant.

STEP 5

Open victim's airway:

- Tilt the head back and lift the chin. Place one hand on the victim's forehead and apply firm, backward pressure with the palm to tilt the head back. Place fingers of other hand under the bony part of the jaw near the chin, and lift to bring the chin forward and the teeth almost to occlusion (Figure 10-4). Irregular, gasping, or shallow breathing is not normal breathing.

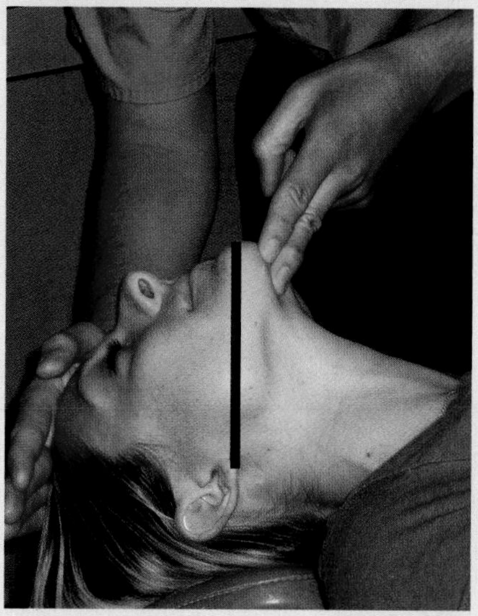

Figure 10-4. For an adult, when the unconscious person's head is extended properly, the tip of the chin points up into the air in line with the earlobes *(black line),* lifting the mandible and tongue off the pharyngeal wall. (From Malamed SF: *Medical emergencies in the dental office,* ed 6, St Louis, 2007, Mosby.)

STEP 6

- Perform rescue breathing: Position the resuscitation mask over the victim's nose and mouth, tilt the head back, and lift the chin to open the airway.
- Form an airtight seal with the mask against the face, and give two rescue breaths by breathing into the mask (Figure 10-5).
- Each rescue breath should last about 1 second and make the chest clearly rise.
- Note: For a child, the head is only slightly tilted past the neutral position. One breath is delivered every 3 to 5 seconds (Figures 10-6 and 10-7).
- Note: For an infant (1 to 12 months), the chin is lifted to open the airway but the head is kept in a neutral position (Figure 10-8). Also, the mask is inverted if there is no infant mask available. One slow gentle breath (a puff) is delivered every 3 seconds.

Continued

Procedure 10-1 Overview of Basic Life Support for an Unresponsive Victim—cont'd

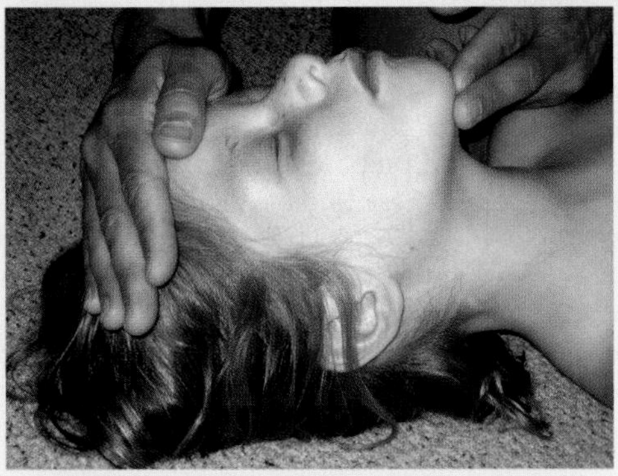

Figure 10-5. Head tilt–chin lift position in a child. (From Malamed SF: *Medical emergencies in the dental office,* ed 6, St Louis, 2007, Mosby.)

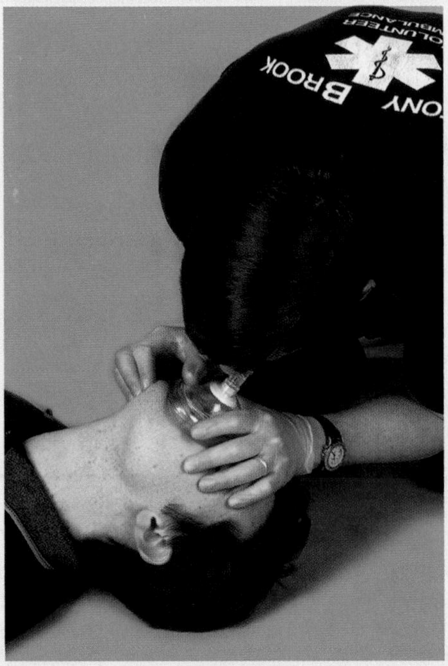

Figure 10-6. Position the resuscitation mask, and breathe into the mask while tilting the head and lifting the chin to open the airway. (From Henry M, Stapleton E: *EMT: prehospital care,* ed 3, St Louis, 2007, Mosby/JEMS.)

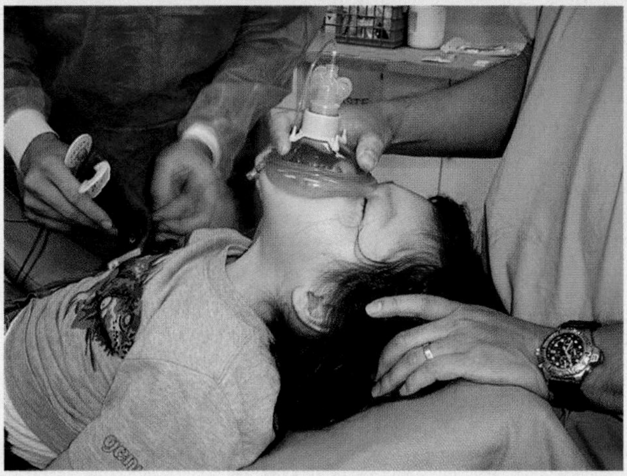

Figure 10-7. Holding pocket mask on face of child. (From Malamed SF: *Medical emergencies in the dental office,* ed 6, St Louis, 2007, Mosby.)

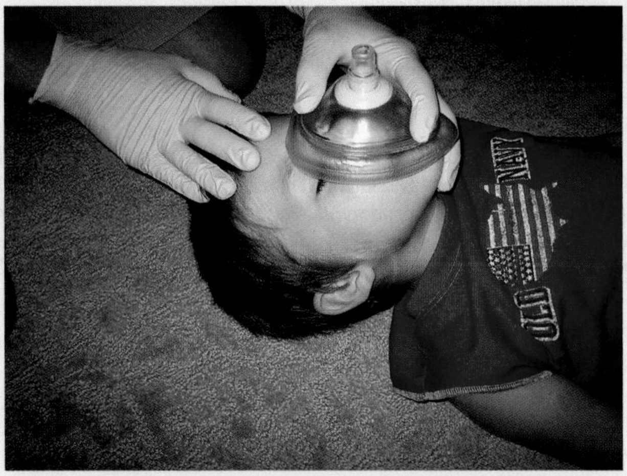

Figure 10-8. Mouth-to-mask rescue breathing in an infant. (Courtesy Sedation Resource, Lone Oak, Texas, http://www.sedationresource.com.)

- If the chest rises and falls with delivery of two rescue breaths, remove the resuscitation mask, recheck breathing, and check for the presence of a pulse for no more than 10 seconds.
- If the chest does not rise and fall with delivery of two rescue breaths, continue with chest compressions (at least 100 per minute, 2 inches in depth for adults and children and 1½ inches for infants) until EMS arrives.

STEP 7: WHAT TO DO

If victim is responsive and there is breathing and a pulse:

- Continue to monitor the vital signs until help arrives.
- Administer emergency oxygen, if available.

If victim is nonresponsive and there is no breathing or abnormal breathing (only gasping):

- Continue with 30 chest compressions followed by two rescue breaths until help arrives or second rescuer assists.

STEP 7

After emergency care, document the situation on an incident report form (see Figure 10-28) and in the client's chart. Provide a copy of incident report to EMS technician if victim is being transferred to a hospital.

second rescuer is ready, he opens the airway and begins rescue breathing or assists with use of the bag-valve mask. After five cycles or about 2 minutes, the second rescuer switches places with the first rescuer and resumes compressions for CPR; the second rescuer also can substitute for the first rescuer if exhausted (see Procedure 10-3).

In an unconscious person, the tongue falls backward against the wall of the pharynx and may produce an airway obstruction. The **head tilt–chin lift technique** is the most important step in maintaining an open airway for rescue breaths. The technique is performed by placing one hand on the unconscious person's forehead and applying a firm, backward pressure with the palm; then the tips of the index and middle fingers of the other hand are placed on the symphysis of the mandible, lifting the mandible as the forehead is tilted backward. For an adult, the victim's head is extended so that the chin points up into the air in line with the earlobes, lifting the mandible and tongue off the pharyngeal wall (see Figure 10-4). This position also allows for use of a rescue breathing device if needed (Figure 10-5). For a child, the head is only slightly tilted past the neutral position (see Figure 10-5). The most important consideration is the delivery of chest compressions with minimal interruption; therefore opening an airway for the delivery of rescue breaths is secondary to that objective. Any extended or unnecessary interruptions in compressions (including longer than needed pauses for rescue breathing) decreases the life-saving effectiveness of CPR.[3] The second trained provider is valuable in achieving this goal and allows for simultaneous delivery of needed procedures.

Rescue Breathing and Bag Mask Ventilation

Rescue breathing is a technique for breathing air into a victim to give him or her oxygen needed to survive. The air the healthcare provider exhales or administers contains enough oxygen to keep a person alive. The entire process of opening the airway and providing two rescue breaths should be less than 18 seconds to avoid interruptions in chest compressions. Although there are several techniques for rescue breathing, this chapter emphasizes the mouth-to-mask ventilation (see Figures 10-6, 10-7, and 10-8). When giving rescue breaths, the rescuer takes a normal breath and then breathes into the victim's mouth and nose using a resuscitation mask (see Figure 10-6). Each breath should last about 1 second and make the chest clearly rise. For an adult, one breath is given every 5 to 6 seconds (10 to 12 breaths per minute) (see Figure 10-6). For a child (see Figure 10-7) or infant (see Figure 10-8), one breath is given every 3 seconds. If the client also needs circulation support (no pulse), chest compressions (30 per 18 seconds) followed by two rescue breaths are continued until one of the following occurs:

- The victim begins to breathe independently.
- Another trained rescuer takes over.
- The rescuer is too exhausted to continue.

Resuscitation Masks

Resuscitation masks are flexible, dome-shaped devices that cover a victim's mouth and nose and allow the healthcare provider to breathe air into a victim without making mouth-to-mouth contact (Figure 10-9). It is recommended that dental hygienists have their own resuscitation mask in their operatory, so one is always available during client care in the event of an emergency requiring CPR. Resuscitation masks have several benefits:

- They supply air to the victim more quickly through both the mouth and nose.
- They create a seal over the victim's mouth and nose.
- They can be connected to emergency oxygen if they have an oxygen inlet.
- They protect against disease transmission when rescue breaths are given.

A resuscitation mask should have the following characteristics (Figure 10-10):

- Be easy to assemble and use.
- Be made of transparent, pliable material that allows the clinician to make a tight seal over the victim's mouth and nose.
- Have a one-way valve for releasing exhaled air away from the rescuer.

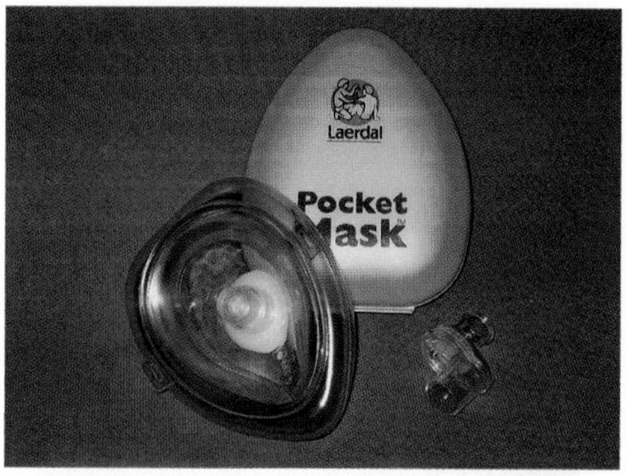

Figure 10-9. Pocket mask. (Courtesy Sedation Resource, Lone Oak, Texas, http://www.sedationresource.com.)

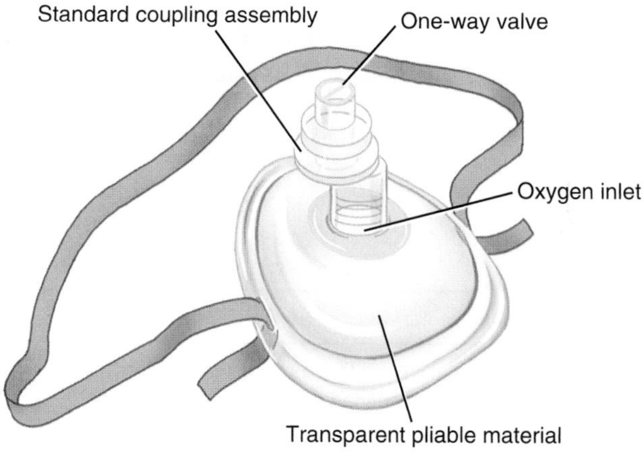

Figure 10-10. A resuscitation mask with required characteristics.

Mouth-to-Mask Ventilation

For **mouth-to-mask ventilation** to be performed, head tilt–chin lift must be maintained. The mask is placed on the victim's face with the narrow portion over the bridge of the nose and the wider part in the cleft of the chin (see Figure 10-6). Using the hand that is closer to the top of the victim's head, the rescuer places an index finger and thumb along the border of the mask while the thumb of the other hand is placed along the lower margin of the mask (Figure 10-11). The remaining fingers of the hand closer to the victim's neck are placed along

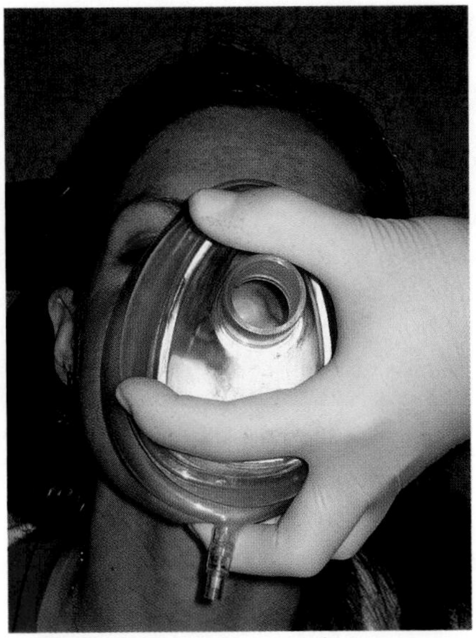

Figure 10-11. Mouth-to-mask ventilation demonstrating finger positioning. (From Malamed SF: *Medical emergencies in the dental office*, ed 6, St Louis, 2007, Mosby.)

BOX 10-6

Pulse Check

- If the rescuer is unsure whether the victim has a pulse, chest compression should be started.
- Unnecessary cardiopulmonary resuscitation is less harmful than not performing chest compression when the victim truly needs it.

Adapted from American Heart Association: Part 1: executive summary: 2010 American Heart Association Guidelines for Cardiopulmonary Resuscitation and Emergency Cardiovascular Care, 2010.

the bony inferior border of the mandible, which is then lifted. Head tilt–chin lift is then performed to establish a patent airway. While head tilt–chin lift is maintained, the rescuer presses firmly and completely around the outside margin of the mask to obtain an airtight seal, with the remaining fingers along the lower margin of the mask to seal the mask against the victim's face. The mask is held in position with one or two hands as needed, maintaining an airtight seal and a patent airway. The rescuer's mouth is placed on the breathing port of the mask, and air is forced into the victim until the chest is seen to rise (see Figure 10-6). The rescuer positions himself or herself at the victim's side, enabling a lone rescuer to perform chest compressions if needed. Air is delivered over 1 second while watching the victim's chest rise (Box 10-6).

- If the victim has a pulse, a breath is delivered every 5 to 10 seconds for an adult and every 3 to 5 seconds for a child using a resuscitation mask.
- If the chest does not rise and air is not entering the victim's lungs, the head is repeated with the head-tilt-chin lift.
- If two rescuers are available and the victim has a pulse, the breath is delivered every 6 to 8 seconds for an adult, and the second rescuer operates the bag mask.
- When the victim has a pulse and needs only rescue breaths, the pulse is checked about every 2 minutes.

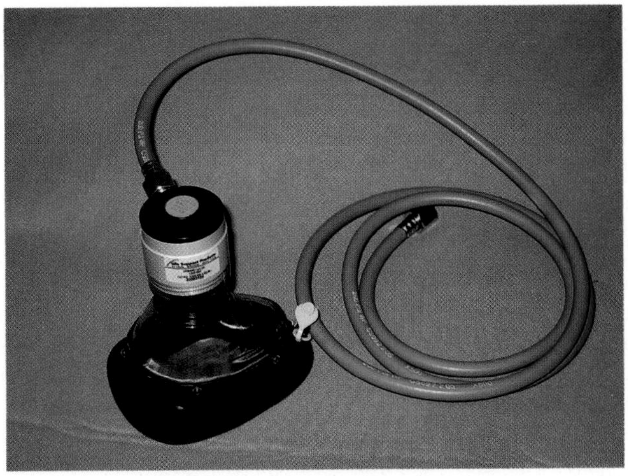

Figure 10-12. Positive-pressure demand valve. (Courtesy Sedation Resource, Lone Oak, Texas, http://www.sedationresource.com.)

- If the victim has no pulse, one-rescuer CPR (see Procedure 10-2) or two-rescuer CPR (see Procedure 10-3) is delivered.

Oxygen-Enriched Ventilation

Whenever possible, the rescuer should ventilate with supplemental oxygen (O_2); however, rescue breathing must never be delayed until supplemental O_2 becomes available. It is recommended that every oral healthcare setting have at least one portable E cylinder of O_2 with adjustable O_2 flow and a positive-pressure demand-valve mask unit (Figure 10-12). The E cylinder of O_2 provides approximately 30 minutes of O_2. Although O_2 is beneficial to the unconscious patient, the healthcare professional should receive adequate training in airway management through mouth-to-mask ventilation; administration of enriched O_2 is effective only as long as O_2 remains in the compressed gas cylinder.

A bag valve mask, sometimes known by the brand name Ambu bag, is a hand-held device used to provide positive pressure ventilation to a client who is not breathing or who is breathing inadequately (only gasping). Use of a bag valve mask requires at least two rescuers; one holds the mask in place while the other operates the bag. The bag-valve mask has flexible air chamber called the bag (about the size of a small American football) attached to a face mask via a one-way valve. When the face mask is sealed properly around the victim's face, nose, and mouth by the first rescuer, the bag is squeezed by the second rescuer, so air is forced into the victim's lungs. Releasing the bag allows it to self-inflate, drawing in either ambient (surrounding) air or a low pressure oxygen flow supplied by a regulated cylinder, while also allowing the lungs to deflate to the surrounding area rather than the bag past the one-way valve. Bag valve masks also can be used for intubation in emergency care centers; however, intubation is not within the scope of practice for dental hygienists.

Cardiac Arrest

Each year, approximately 500,000 people die of cardiac arrest, which stops respiration and blood circulation. Cardiac arrest may result from an acute reaction to medication, myocardial infarction, respiratory arrest, electric shock, drowning, trauma, asphyxiation, shock, or cardiac arrhythmia. The heart's electrical system controls its pumping action.

The Heart's Electrical System

Under normal conditions, (1) specialized cells of the heart initiate and transmit electrical impulses that travel through the upper chambers of the heart (the atria) to the lower chambers of the heart (the ventricles) and (2) electrical impulses reach the muscular walls of the ventricles and cause the ventricles to contract. This contraction forces blood out of the heart to circulate through the body. The contraction of the left ventricle results in a pulse. The pauses between the pulse beats are the periods between contractions. When the heart muscles contract, blood is forced out of the heart. When they relax, blood refills the chambers.

Any damage to the heart from disease or injury can disrupt the heart's electrical system, which can stop circulation. The two most common treatable abnormal rhythms, or cardiac arrhythmias, initially present in sudden cardiac arrest victims are ventricular fibrillation (V-fib) and ventricular tachycardia (V-tach). V-fib is a state of totally disorganized electrical activity in the heart, resulting in quivering of the ventricles. In this state, the ventricles cannot pump blood; there is no movement or breathing and no pulse. V-tach is very rapid ventricular contraction. Although there is electrical activity resulting in a regular rhythm, the rate is often so fast that the heart is unable to pump blood properly. As with V-fib, there is no movement or breathing and no pulse.

Clinical death is cessation of the heart and respiratory effort; it may be reversible with CPR if initiated within 4 minutes. Brain death can begin as soon as 4 minutes after the heart stops beating. A person who is unconscious, is not moving or breathing, and has no pulse is in cardiac arrest and needs CPR. When started promptly, CPR can help by supplying oxygen to the brain and other vital organs. In many cases, such as cardiac arrhythmias causing V-fib or V-tach, CPR by itself cannot correct the underlying heart problem. These irregular rhythms of the heart can be corrected by early defibrillation. Delivering an electrical shock with an AED (Figure 10-13) can disrupt the electrical activity of the V-fib or V-tach

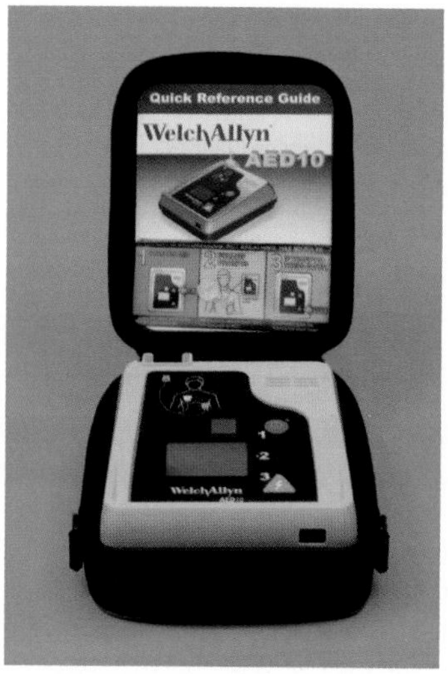

Figure 10-13. Automated external defibrillator. (From Sorrentino SA: *Mosby's textbook for long-term care nursing assistants*, ed 6, St Louis, 2011, Mosby.)

Procedure 10-2 One-Rescuer Cardiopulmonary Resuscitation (CPR) for Adult, Child, and Infant

EQUIPMENT

- Resuscitation mask
- Other protective barriers
- Automated external defibrillator (AED)

STEPS 1 THROUGH 3

Complete Steps 1 through 3 for Basic Life Support (see Procedure 10-1). If the victim is nonresponsive, not breathing or not breathing normally, activate EMS and begin CPR.

STEP 4

Deliver 1 shock with AED if available or send someone to retrieve it (see Box 10-7 and Figures 10-13, 10-19, 10-20).

STEP 5

Deliver chest compressions effectively:

- Find the correct hand position to give compressions.
- Remove clothing covering the victim's chest.
- Place the heel of one hand on the lower half of the breast bone.
- Place the other hand on top. Keep fingers off the chest when giving compressions.
- Position your shoulders over your hands with your elbows locked (Figure 10-14).
- Use your body weight, not your arms, to compress the chest.

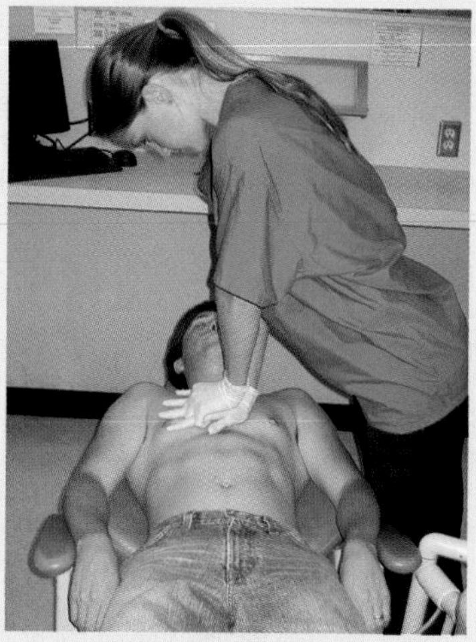

Figure 10-14. Proper rescuer position for adult chest compression. (From Malamed SF: *Medical emergencies in the dental office*, ed 6, St Louis, 2007, Mosby.)

Continued

Procedure 10-2 One-Rescuer Cardiopulmonary Resuscitation (CPR) for Adult, Child, and Infant—cont'd

STEP 6

Give 30 chest compressions.

- For an adult and child, compress the chest about 2 inches.
- For an infant, compress the chest about 1½ inches.
- Let the chest fully recoil to its normal position after each compression.
- Compress at a rate of at least 100 compressions per minute.
- Count out loud to keep an even pace ("1 and 2 and 3 and …").

STEP 7

Replace the resuscitation mask and give two rescue breaths.

- Each rescue breath should last about 1 second.
- Give rescue breaths that make the chest clearly rise (see Figure 10-5).

STEP 8

Continue cycles of 30 compressions and two rescue breaths.

STEP 9: WHAT TO DO

Continue CPR until:

- Another trained rescuer arrives and takes over
- An AED is available and ready to use if one was not available initially, then resume CPR after one shock if the victim remains unconscious
- You are too exhausted to continue
- You notice an obvious sign of life

STEP 12

After emergency care, document the situation on an incident report form (see Figure 10-28) and in the client's chart. Provide a copy of incident report to EMS technician if victim is being transferred to a hospital.

Procedure 10-3 Two-Rescuer Cardiopulmonary Resuscitation (CPR)—Adult and Child

EQUIPMENT

- Resuscitation or bag mask
- Other protective barriers
- Automated external defibrillator (AED)

STEP 1

Assessment for responsiveness is completed by Rescuer 1 (see Procedure 10-1).

STEP 2

Designate a team leader, usually Rescuer 1 if a trained health professional.

STEP 3

If the victim is unresponsive, not breathing, or breathing irregularly, and a pulse is not detected, rescuer 1 immediately begins chest compressions using correct technique.

- Places the heel of one hand on the lower half of the breastbone
- Places the other hand on top
    - Adult: 30 compressions; compress the chest about 2 inches
    - Child: 15 compressions; compress the chest about 2 inches
    - Infant: 15 compressions; compress chest about 1½ inches
- Allows the chest to fully recoil to its normal position after each compression
- Compresses at a rate of at least 100 compressions per minute

Rescuer 2 notifies EMS and retrieves the resuscitation mask and retrieves and assembles the AED, if available, for use by rescuer 1.

STEP 3

After completing one round of chest compressions (30 within 18 seconds maximum), Rescuer 1 places the resuscitation mask and gives two rescue breaths.

Rescuer 2 prepares the AED for use, turning the device on and placing pads on the victim (see Procedure 10-4).

STEP 4

Rescuer 1 provides 1 shock with the AED (see Procedure 10-4).

Rescuer 2 prepares to assist with CPR positioning on the opposite side of the victim.

STEP 5

Rescuer 1 continues with chest compressions without interruption.

Rescuer 2 continues with rescue breaths (2 breaths every 15 compressions).

STEP 6

The two rescuers switch positions; rescuer 2 takes over providing chest compressions (15 compressions and 2 breaths) after about 2 minutes.

- Rescuer 1 calls for a position change by using the word "change" at the end of the last compression cycle.
- Rescuer 2 gives two rescue breaths. If a bag mask is available, it can be used.
- Rescuer 1 moves to the victim's head with his or her own mask.
- Rescuer 2 moves into position at the victim's chest and locates correct hand position on the victim's chest.
- Changing positions should take less than 5 seconds.

STEP 7

Rescuer 2 finds the correct hand position to give compressions.

- Places the heel of one hand on the center of the chest
- Places the other hand on top
- Gives compressions
    - Adult: 30 compressions; compress the chest about 2 inches
    - Child: 15 compressions; compress the chest about 2 inches
    - Infant: 15 compressions; compress the chest about 1½ inches
    - Allows the chest to fully recoil to its normal position after each compression
    - Compresses at a rate of at least 100 compressions per minute

STEP 8

Continue CPR until:

- Help arrives
- An AED is available and ready to use
- You are too exhausted to continue
- You notice signs of life

STEP 9

After emergency care, document the situation on an incident report form (see Figure 10-28) and in the client's chart. Provide a copy of incident report to EMS technician if victim is being transferred to a hospital.

TABLE 10-1

Summary of Techniques for Adult, Child, and Infant Cardiopulmonary Resuscitation

	Adult	Child	Infant
Hand position	Two hands on top of one another (parallel without the fingers touching the chest) with the heel of the bottom hand on the lower half of the breast bone	Two hands on top of one another (parallel without the fingers touching the chest) with the heel of the bottom hand on the lower half of the breast bone	Two-thumb encircling hands technique (with fingers around back of infant and thumbs on chest) in the center of the breast bone
Compress	About 2 inches	At least ⅓ the depth of the chest, about 2 inches	At least ⅓ the depth of the chest, about 1½ inches
Breathe	Until chest clearly rises (about 1 second per breath)	Until chest clearly rises (about 1 second per breath)	Until chest clearly rises (about 1 second per breath)
Cycle (one rescuer)	30 compressions, two breaths	30 compressions, two breaths	30 compressions, two breaths
Cycle (two rescuers)	30 compressions, two breaths	15 compressions, two breaths	15 compressions, two breaths
Rate	At least 100 compressions per minute	At least 100 compressions per minute	At least 100 compressions per minute

long enough to allow the heart to spontaneously develop an effective rhythm on its own. If V-fib or V-tach is not interrupted, all electrical activity eventually will cease (asystole), a condition that cannot be corrected by defibrillation. AEDs provide an electrical shock to the heart, called **defibrillation**. The sooner the shock is administered, the greater the likelihood of the victim's survival.[4] Effective AED intervention is delivered immediately after notifying EMS when an unresponsive victim is found.

Effective Emergency Response

To effectively respond to cardiac emergencies, it helps to understand the importance of the cardiac chain of survival. The four links in the cardiac chain are as follows:

- *Early recognition of the emergency and early access to EMS.* The sooner the local emergency number is called, the sooner advanced EMS personnel arrive and take over.
- *Early CPR.* CPR helps supply oxygen to the brain and other vital organs to keep the victim alive until an AED is used or advanced medical care is given.
- *Early defibrillation.* An electrical shock called *defibrillation* may restore a normal heart rhythm. Each minute defibrillation is delayed reduces the victim's chance of survival by about 10%.
- *Early advanced medical care.* EMS personnel provide more advanced medical care and transport the victim to the hospital.

Early Recognition and Cardiopulmonary Resuscitation

If a person is seated in the dental chair at the time of collapse, the dental hygienist first activates EMS (see Box 8-5), and positions the chair in a supine position for effective CPR delivery. If available, an AED is used to deliver one shock before beginning chest compressions to keep blood flowing from the heart. CPR follows the American Heart Association's recommended sequence of steps C-A-B. Following the first round of chest compressions (30 per 18 seconds) (C), the health professional checks the airway (A) and delivers two rescue breaths (B) (Table 10-1). Effective chest compressions are essential for high-quality CPR capable of circulating blood to the victim's brain and other vital organs. CPR prolongs the period of time that the myocardium remains in ventricular fibrillation, increasing the likelihood that defibrillation will terminate ventricular fibrillation, and allows the heart to resume an effective rhythm.

To ensure high-quality CPR, the following requirements must be met:

- Chest compressions should be performed at a rate of at least 100 compressions per minute.
- Chest compressions should be deep: 1½ to 2 inches for an adult or a child, and 1½ inch for an infant.
- The chest should fully recoil to its normal position after each compression before the next compression is started.
- Minimal interruptions between chest compressions should occur.

The rescuer compresses the lower half of the sternum in the middle of the chest. The heel of one hand is placed on the middle of the sternum between the nipples with the heel of the other hand placed on top so that the fingers of two hands are overlapped and parallel. Only the heel of the lower hand remains in contact with the victim's chest.

To maximize chest compressions, the rescuer's shoulders must be directly over the victim's sternum, and the rescuer's elbows are locked straight. The dental chair is lowered to allow the rescuer to bring shoulders directly over the victim's sternum (see Figure 10-14). Bending of the elbows greatly decreases effectiveness and leads to rapid rescuer fatigue (Figure 10-15).

See Procedure 10-2 and corresponding Competency Form for a summary of one-rescuer CPR. A compression-ventilation ratio of 30 compressions to 2 breaths currently is recommended for one-rescuer resuscitations. A 30:2

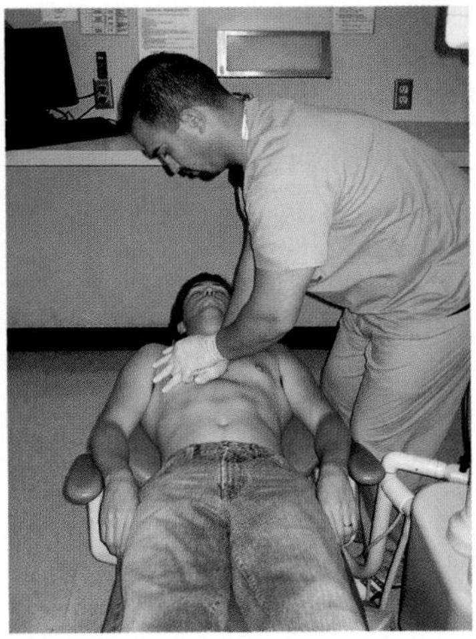

Figure 10-15. Improper positioning (elbows bent, shoulders at angle to chest). (From Malamed SF: *Medical emergencies in the dental office*, ed 6, St Louis, 2007, Mosby.)

compression-ventilation ratio is tiring. Therefore, when an additional rescuer is available, two-rescuer CPR is provided (Procedure 10-3 and corresponding Competency Form). As mentioned previously, in two-rescuer or multiple-rescuer CPR, the goal is completion of multiple tasks simultaneously. A team leader is designated, usually the first rescuer. The first rescuer can begin BLS while the second activates EMS and acquires the AED and barrier or bag mask if available. The first rescuer delivers CPR (30 compressions per 18 seconds followed by opening the airway and 2 rescue breaths) while the second assembles the AED and applies the electrode pads to the victim's sides, and turns the device on to prepare for use. The first rescuer delivers the shock as soon as possible and resumes chest compressions while the second rescuer delivers rescue breaths. If three or more rescuers are available, each person would take one task: activating EMS, chest compressions, AED retrieval and assembly, bag mask retrieval, and airway opening and rescue breaths. It is recommended to switch the compressor after about 2 minutes, so the first rescuer notifies the next of the impending switch of positions and roles, and the change is made after the next 5 cycles of compressions (see Procedure 10-3). Every effort is made to accomplish the switch as quickly as possible, definitely in less than 5 seconds. When providing two-rescuer CPR to an adult, rescuers perform 30 compressions and two rescue breaths (ratio 30:2) during each cycle. When performing two-rescuer CPR on a child or infant, rescuers change the compression to ventilation ratio to 15:2 to provide more frequent respiration for children and infants.

Use of an Automated External Defibrillator

An **automated external defibrillator (AED)** is an automated device that checks the heart rhythm in an unconscious person. If an abnormal heart rhythm is detected, the device delivers a shock to develop a normal heart rhythm by defibrillation (see Figure 10-13). When a cardiac arrest occurs, an AED should be used as soon as it is available and ready to use.

The AED charges itself and prompts the operator if it is necessary to deliver a life-saving shock to the victim by pressing a button. If the AED advises that a shock is needed, the rescuer follows protocols to provide one shock followed by five cycles (about 2 minutes) of CPR.

When a single rescuer encounters a nonresponsive person with no pulse, he or she immediately asks for help to summon EMS (e.g., 911), which is critical for the person's survival, and to bring an AED if available. The single rescuer starts with 2 minutes (four or five cycles) of CPR. The AED is used after four or five cycles of CPR, *only* if the victim is not breathing and has no pulse (see Procedure 10-4 and corresponding Competency Form for one rescuer using AED). Chest compressions increase the likelihood that a successful shock can be delivered to a victim who has experienced a sudden cardiac arrest, especially if more than 4 minutes have elapsed since the victim's collapse. See Box 10-7 for the two-rescuer AED technique for an adult.

The entire dental team should conduct semi-annual cardiac arrest drills. Practicing a variety of scenarios prepares the staff to respond rapidly and effectively in a real emergency.

BOX 10-7

Automated External Defibrillator Two-Rescuer Technique

- First rescuer provides CPR chest compressions.
- Second rescuer retrieves and prepares the automated external defibrillator (AED).
- Second rescuer does the following while minimizing interruptions in chest compressions (no more than 10 seconds):
  - Removes clothing covering the victim's chest to allow rescuers to provide chest compressions and to apply the AED electrode pads.
  - Places the AED at the victim's side near the rescuer who will be operating it (i.e., the side of the victim opposite where the rescuer performing chest compressions).
  - Turns on the AED (POWER ON) and follows voice prompts.
  - Attaches adult or pediatric AED electrode pads as appropriate.
  - Removes the backing from the adhesive electrode pads.
  - Attaches the adhesive electrode pads to the victim's bare skin according to manufacturer's directions.
  - Attaches the electrode cable to the AED.
  - Ensures that no one is touching the victim or resuscitation equipment while the AED is analyzing the heart rhythm (ANALYZE) and when the AED prompts delivery of a shock.
  - Pushes ANALYZE button as needed.
  - Starts CPR immediately (beginning with chest compressions) after delivery of shock.
  - If no shock is indicated, as per AED voice prompts, resumes CPR, beginning with chest compressions.

Use of an AED for Infants

For infants, a manual defibrillator is preferred to an AED for defibrillation. If one is not available, an AED equipped with a pediatric dose attenuator is preferred. If neither is available, AED without a pediatric dose attenuator may be used.

Obstructed Airway

An **obstructed airway** is defined as partial of complete blockage of the breathing passages to the lungs when an object

Procedure 10-4 Single Rescuer Using an Automated External Defibrillator (AED)—Adult and Child*

EQUIPMENT

- Automated external defibrillator (AED) (see Figure 10-14)

STEPS 1 THROUGH 3

Verify unresponsiveness, the absence of breathing, or abnormal breathing (gasping only), and no pulse when checking carotid artery (Figure 10-16); activate EMS and obtain AED (see Procedure 10-1).

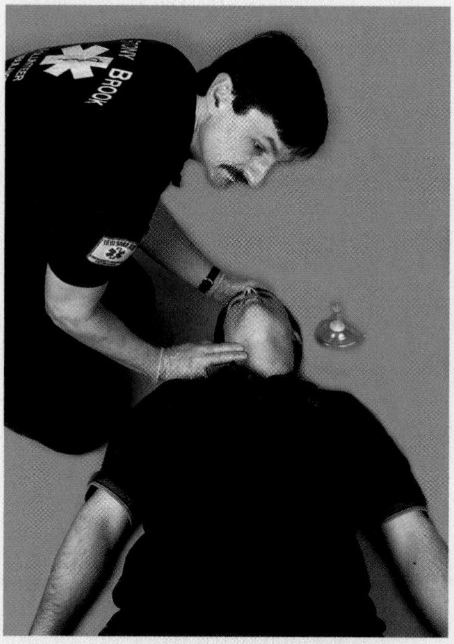

Figure 10-16. Rescuer checking pulse at carotid artery. (From Henry M, Stapleton E: *EMT: prehospital care,* ed 3, St Louis, 2007, Mosby/JEMS.)

STEP 4

- Position the defibrillator machine on the left side of the victim's head.
- Turn on the AED.

STEP 5

- Wipe the chest dry.

STEP 6

- Attach the electrode lines to the pads (Figure 10-17).

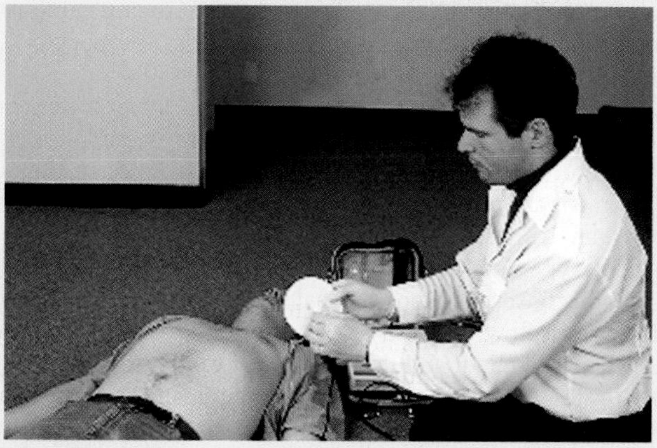

Figure 10-17. Rescuer attaching the electrode lines to the pads. (From Henry M, Stapleton E: *EMT: prehospital care,* ed 3, St Louis, 2007, Mosby/JEMS.)

STEP 7

- Attach the pads to the victim.
- Remove the cover from the adhesive side of the pads.
- Place one pad on the upper right side of the victim's chest above the nipple area.
- Place the other pad on the victim's lower left side at the left sternal border (Figure 10-18). Make sure the pads are not touching.

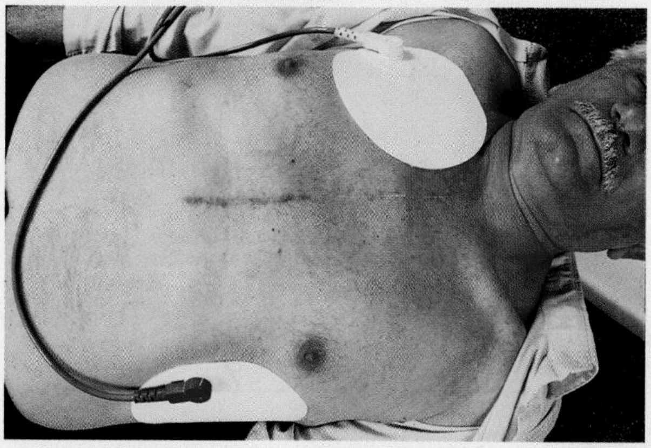

Figure 10-18. Placement of pads on upper right side of the victim's chest and on the lower left side at the left sternal border. (From Henry M, Stapleton E: *EMT: prehospital care,* ed 3, St Louis, 2007, Mosby/JEMS.)

- For a child, use pediatric AED pads if available. Make sure the pads are not touching.
- For infants, a manual defibrillator is preferred to an AED for defibrillation. If one is not available, an AED equipped with a pediatric dose attenuator is preferred. If neither is available, AED without a pediatric dose attenuator may be used. Ensure the pads are not touching.

Note: If the pads risk touching each other on a child, place one pad on the child's chest and the other pad on the child's back (between the shoulder blades).

STEP 8

- Plug the connector into the AED, if necessary.

STEP 9

- Clear the victim.
  - Make sure that nobody, including you, is touching the victim.
  - Tell everyone to "stand clear."

STEP 10

- Push the "analyze" button. Let the AED analyze the heart rhythm (Figure 10-19).

Continued

Procedure 10-4 Single Rescuer Using an Automated External Defibrillator (AED)—Adult and Child—cont'd

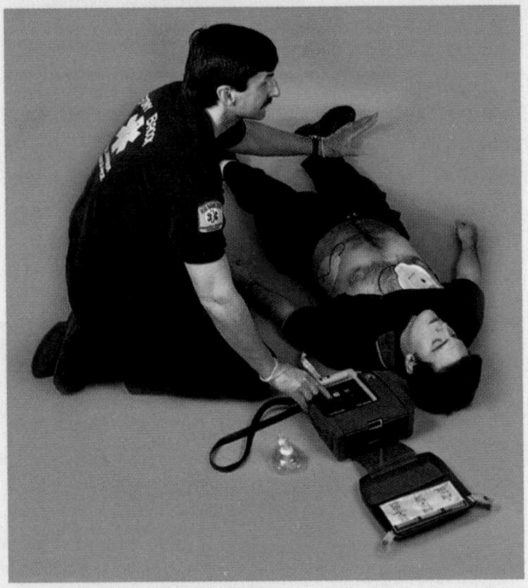

Figure 10-19. Rescuer pushing the analyze button to allow the AED to analyze the heart rhythm. (From Henry M, Stapleton E: *EMT: prehospital care,* ed 3, St Louis, 2007, Mosby/JEMS.)

STEP 11
- If a shock is advised, push the "shock" button.
- Look to see that nobody is touching the victim.
- Tell everyone to "stand clear."

STEP 12
After the shock or if no shock is indicated:
- Give CPR for about 2 minutes. Continue to follow prompts from AED.
- If at any time you notice an obvious sign of life, stop CPR and monitor the responsiveness, breathing and pulse. Administer emergency oxygen, if it is available.

STEP 13
After emergency care, document the situation on an incident report form (see Figure 10-28) and in the client's chart. Provide a copy of incident report to EMS technician if victim is being transferred to a hospital.

Adapted from American Red Cross: *CPR/AED for Professional Rescuers and Health Care Providers Handbook. 2011*, Washington, DC, American Red Cross.
*Note: If two trained responders are present, one should perform CPR while the second responder operates the AED.

prevents the exchange of air in an individual. A foreign-body obstruction may occur in the following situations:
- During eating (food particle blocks airway)
- During a dental procedure (aspiration of a dental instrument or piece of equipment)
- During resuscitation (aspiration of vomitus or blood)
- When unconscious (tongue falls backward, blocking pharynx)

A victim with a mild (partial) airway obstruction:
- Has good air exchange
- Can cough forcefully
- Sometimes wheezes

In this case, the hygienist should not interfere by trying to dislodge the object but should remain with the victim until it is dislodged or help arrives.

Signs of a victim with a severe airway obstruction include the following:
- Poor or no air exchange
- A weak cough or no cough
- Possible cyanosis
- A high-pitched noise or no noise while inhaling
- Increasing respiratory difficulty
- Unable to speak
- Makes the universal choking sign, clutching the neck with the thumb and fingers (see Figure 10-20).[4]

See Procedure 10-5 and corresponding Competency Form for management of partial airway obstruction with poor air exchange and complete airway obstruction in the conscious victim. See Procedure 10-6 and corresponding Competency Form for management of the unconscious victim with complete airway obstruction. See Procedures 10-7, Procedure 10-8, and their corresponding Competency Forms for management of the conscious and unconscious infant with severe (complete) airway obstruction.

Oxygen Administration

During a medical emergency the body tissues may have an increased demand for oxygen or a diminished ability to receive or use oxygen, thus necessitating the administration of higher oxygen concentrations than exist in room air. Indications for oxygen administration include syncope, cardiac problems, and some respiratory difficulties. Oxygen should not be administered to a person experiencing an episode of hyperventilation. High levels of oxygen are contraindicated for individuals with chronic obstructive pulmonary disease (COPD) such as emphysema (see Chapter 50).

As discussed earlier, the E cylinder is the recommended portable oxygen tank for in-office use. A bag-ventilation mask (see Figure 10-13) used to deliver the surrounding air to the victim is particularly valuable to prevent disease transmission between rescuer and victim. Competence in the use of the office oxygen system before an emergency occurs is essential.

For a conscious client, a nasal cannula or face mask (Figure 10-27) at a flow rate of 10 adequately delivers supplemental oxygen. The client should be allowed to breathe at his or her own rate while respiration rate and vital signs are monitored and medical assistance is summoned (see Chapter 13).

The unconscious client with adequate respiratory effort should receive the same type of oxygen administration, with careful observation should the respiratory effort diminish. An

Procedure 10-5 Conscious Choking—Adult and Child

EQUIPMENT

- Resuscitation mask
- Other protective barriers

STEP 1

Ask the person, "Are you choking?"

- If the person is coughing forcefully, encourage continued coughing.
- A conscious victim who is clutching his or her throat with one or both hands is usually choking (Figure 10-20).

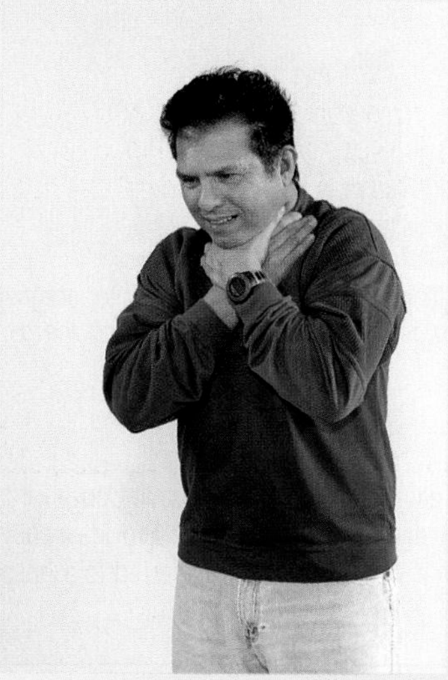

Figure 10-20. Conscious choking victim clutching his throat. (From Chapleau W: *Emergency first responder: making the difference,* St Louis, 2004, Mosby.)

STEP 2

- If the person cannot cough, speak, or breathe, have someone else activate EMS.

STEP 3

- Ask the person if he is choking and obtain nonverbal consent before helping a conscious choking victim (e.g., "Is it OK if I try to help you?").

STEP 4

- Use abdominal thrusts (the Heimlich maneuver) to relieve choking in a responsive victim 1 year of age or older.
  - Adult: Stand behind the victim.
  - Child: Stand or kneel behind the child depending on the child's height. Use less force on a child than you would on an adult.
  - Use one hand to find the navel.
  - Make a fist with your other hand and place the thumb side of your fist against the middle of the victim's abdomen, just above the navel and well below the tip of the xiphoid process (Figure 10-21).

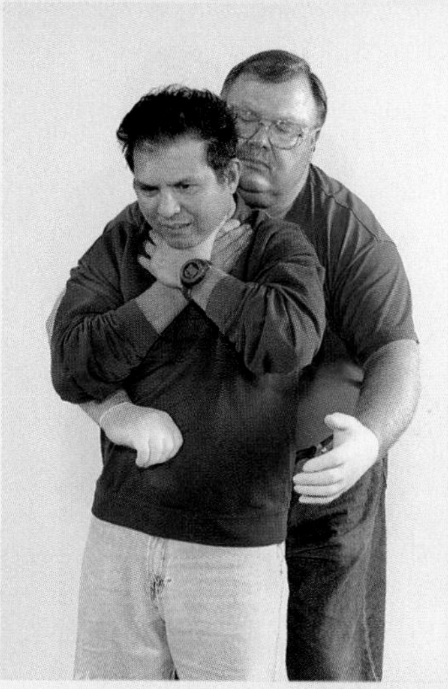

Figure 10-21. Rescuer making a fist against the middle of the victim's abdomen. (From Chapleau W: *Emergency first responder: making the difference,* St Louis, 2004, Mosby.)

- Grab the fist with your other hand (Figure 10-22).
- Press the fist into the victim's abdomen with a brisk inward and upward motion. Give a quick upward thrust.

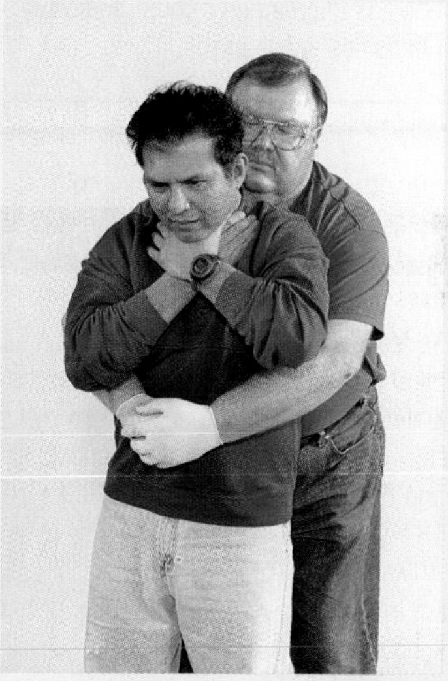

Figure 10-22. Rescuer grabbing the fist with his other hand and giving an abdominal thrust. (From Chapleau W: *Emergency first responder: making the difference,* St Louis, 2004, Mosby.)

It may be necessary to repeat the thrust several times to clear the airway. Each thrust should be a distinct attempt to dislodge the object (Figure 10-23). Note: Use chest thrusts if

- You cannot reach far enough around the victim to give abdominal thrusts
- The victim is pregnant (Figure 10-24)

Continued

Procedure 10-5 Conscious Choking—Adult and Child—cont'd

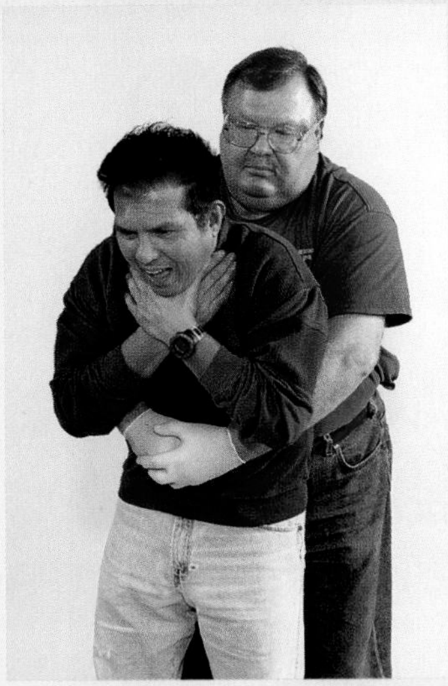

Figure 10-23. Each thrust should be a distinct attempt to dislodge the object. (From Chapleau W: *Emergency first responder: making the difference,* St Louis, 2004, Mosby.)

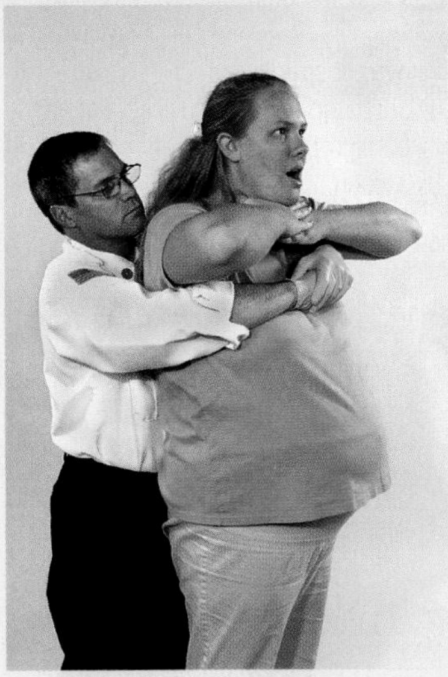

Figure 10-24. Rescuer giving chest thrust to pregnant vicitim. (From Chapleau W: *Emergency first responder: making the difference,* St Louis, 2004, Mosby.)

STEP 6

Continue giving abdominal (or chest) thrusts until

- The foreign body is forced out.
- The victim begins to breathe or cough forcefully.
- The victim becomes unconscious.

STEP 7

After emergency care, document the situation on an incident report form (see Figure 10-28) and in the client's chart. Provide a copy of incident report to EMS technician if victim is being transferred to a hospital.

Procedure 10-6 Unconscious Choking—Adult and Child Over 1 Year of Age

SITUATION

At times, a victim is responsive when choking and then becomes unresponsive. In this case, you know that choking has caused the victim to become unresponsive. If a victim has become unconscious by choking before you arrive, you would have no way of knowing, so you would activate EMS and begin CPR using the C-A-B sequence (see Procedure 10-2).

STEP 1

- Place the victim in the supine position with his or her head in neutral position and send someone to activate EMS.

STEP 2

- Begin CPR, starting with chest compressions using the C-A-B sequence (see Procedure 10-2).

STEP 3

- For an adult or child victim, each time you open the airway to give breaths, open the mouth wide and look for the object.
- If you see an object that can easily be removed, remove it with your fingers. If there is no visible object, continue CPR.

STEP 4

- After about five cycles or 2 minutes of CPR, activate EMS if someone has not done so.

STEP 5: WHAT TO DO

- Continue CPR until the victim recovers or EMS arrives. You know the obstruction has been dislodged and the victim is recovered if you can:
  - Feel air movement and see the chest rise when you give breaths.
  - See and remove a foreign body from the victim's throat.
  - If the victim recovers, continue to monitor vitals and breathing and provide BLS if needed.
- Encourage the victim to seek immediate medical care to ensure no damage occurred during abdominal or chest thrusts.

STEP 6

- After emergency care, document the situation on an incident report form (see Figure 10-28) and in the client's chart.
- Provide a copy of incident report to EMS technician if victim is being transferred to a hospital.

Procedure 10-7 Conscious Choking—Infant

SITUATION

Infants with a mild airway obstruction will be able to make sounds and have a good air exchange, although they may wheeze. If the infant cannot cough, cry, or breathe; makes high pitched sounds; or is cyanotic, the infant has a severe airway obstruction.

STEP 1

- While sitting or standing, carefully position the infant face down on your lap.
- Support the infant's head and neck with your hand.
- Lower the infant onto your thigh, keeping the infant's head lower than his or her chest.

STEP 2

- Give five back blows.
  - Use the heel of your hand.
  - Give five back slaps forcefully with the heel of the hand between the infant's shoulder blades (Figure 10-25).

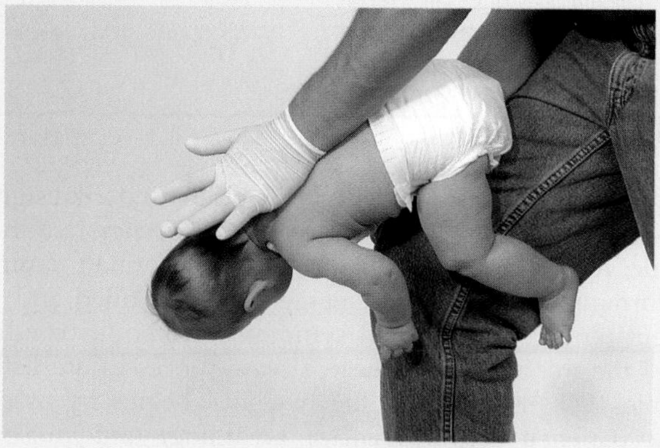

Figure 10-25. Rescuer giving back slaps with the heal of the hand between infants shoulder blades. (From Chapleau W: *Emergency first responder: making the difference,* St Louis, 2004, Mosby.)

STEP 3

- Position the infant face up along your forearm.
  - Before turning the infant, position the infant between both of your forearms, supporting the infant's head and neck.
  - Turn the infant face up.
  - Lower the infant onto your thigh with the infant's head lower than his or her chest.

STEP 4

- Give five downward chest thrusts.
  - Using the two-thumb encircling hands technique, if possible, or placing two fingers on the center of the chest over the middle half of the breast bone just below the nipple line, the same as for chest compression in CPR for an infant (Figure 10-26).
  - Deliver five quick downward chest thrusts at a rate of 1 per second.
  - Each chest thrust should be forceful enough to dislodge a foreign object from the airway.
  - Do not perform finger sweeps or attempt to remove dislodged objects from an infant's throat area because this attempt is likely to push the object back into the airway.

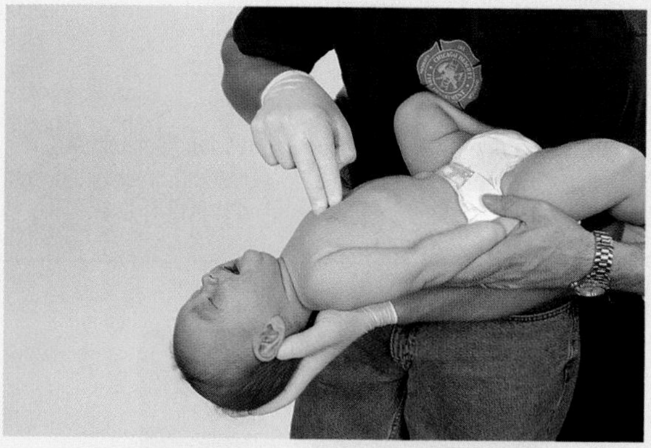

Figure 10-26. Rescuer places two fingers in the center of the chest for chest compressions for an infant. (From Chapleau W: *Emergency first responder: making the difference,* St Louis, 2004, Mosby.)

STEP 5:

- Continue giving five back blows and five chest thrusts until
  - The object is forced out.
  - The infant begins to cough or breathe on his or her own.
  - The infant becomes unconscious (see Procedure 10-8).

STEP 6

- After emergency care, document the situation on an incident report form (see Figure 10-28) and in the client's chart.
- Provide a copy of incident report to EMS technician if victim is being transferred to a hospital.

unconscious client without adequate respiratory effort should be placed in a supine position and the airway opened with the head tilt–chin lift maneuver (see BLS). The clinician then secures the mask over the client's face to cover the nose and mouth, starts the oxygen flow from the cylinder so that the flow inflates the positive-pressure bag, compresses the positive-pressure bag once every 3 to 5 seconds to inflate the victim's lungs, observes for chest movement and exhalation, repositions the victim's head if lungs are not adequately inflating, proceeds with the ABC assessment of BLS, and activates EMS.

Basic Dental Emergency Kit

The dental emergency kit contains all drugs, equipment, and supplies needed to handle a medical emergency in the oral healthcare setting. The emergency kit should contain only drugs that the dental hygienist or dentist is trained to administer. For example, if IV medications that are used for advanced life support are in a dental office emergency drug kit, the dentist or professional staff would need training to ensure they can be administered competently (e.g., in an oral surgery office with an anesthetist). These medications, however, would not normally be used in a dental or dental hygiene

Procedure 10-8 Unconscious Choking—Infant

SITUATION
The infant does not move or breathe and does not respond to sensory stimulation.

STEP 1
- Call for help. If help arrives, ask that person to activate EMS.

STEP 2
- Place the infant on a flat surface and begin CPR chest compressions (C-A-B sequence).
  - Use the two-thumb encircling hands technique when possible, or place two fingers on the center of the breast bone just below the nipple line (see Figure 10-26).
  - Compress the chest approximately 1½ inches.
  - Each chest compression should be a distinct attempt to dislodge the object.

STEP 3:
- Compress at a rate of at least 100 compressions per minute
- Open the airway and look for object in the mouth. If visible in front part of mouth remove it. If not, continue CPR.

STEP 4
- Place the resuscitation mask (if available) and give two rescue breaths.

STEP 5: WHAT TO DO
- If the rescue breaths still do not make the chest clearly rise and there is still a pulse, resume chest compressions and rescue breathing for about five cycles or 2 minutes.
- If the infant remains unresponsive, activate EMS if no one has done so.
- Continue CPR until the infant is responsive or EMS arrives.
- If there is movement, breathing, and a pulse:
  - Continue to monitor response, breathing and pulse, and provide BLS if needed.

STEP 6
- After emergency care, document the situation on an incident report form (see Figure 10-28) and in the client's chart.
- Provide a copy of incident report to EMS technician if victim is being transferred to a hospital.

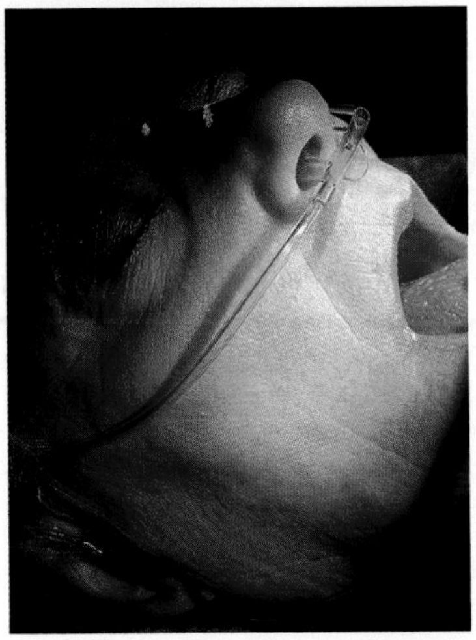

Figure 10-27. The conscious client may receive supplemental oxygen via nasal cannula or the nasal hood (not shown) of an inhalation sedation unit. (From Malamed SF: *Medical emergencies in the dental office*, ed 6, St Louis, 2007, Mosby.)

practice setting without advance training in sedation and anesthesia. Maintaining IV medications in the dental emergency kit without the training to administer them could subject the dental hygienist or dentist to liability claims. The emergency kit should contain the basic drugs and items listed in Table 10-2. In the event of an emergency, the hygienist stops all dental procedures and uses the steps found in Figure 10-1 to take action.

Management of Specific Medical Emergencies

Recognition of certain medical emergencies is essential for early intervention and appropriate treatment. When a medical emergency arises, the client's symptoms and vital signs must be assessed rapidly. Guided by symptoms and vital signs, an assessment of the client's state of consciousness and neurologic, respiratory, or cardiac status is performed. From this information, the type of emergency is identified and treatment rendered. Signs and symptoms of various conditions and the treatments for these disease processes are listed in Table 10-3. In all cases, the hygienist begins by assessing the patient's responsiveness, breathing, and pulse (see Figures 10-1 and 10-2). If the client is unresponsive, the C-A-B sequence BLS should be followed:

- Circulation maintained using CPR chest compressions
- Airway assessed and maintained
- Breathing assessed and maintained with ventilation support provided as needed

Proper documentation of the emergency is required. The medical emergency incident report form in Figure 10-28 can be used for this purpose. A member of the oral care team should be assigned the responsibility to record information on the medical incident report form during the emergency situation. The form is kept in the client's record. In the event that the victim is transferred to a hospital, a copy of the incident report and health history forms should accompany the victim.

CLIENT EDUCATION TIPS

- Explain the importance of having an accurate health, dental, and pharmacologic history in medical emergency prevention.
- Explain the importance of taking prescribed medications for medical emergency prevention.
- Teach stress reduction strategies.
- Explain that complying with medication schedules, seeking regular preventive care, and reporting unusual symptoms immediately to a healthcare professional can prevent emergencies.

Client name ______________________ Date __________ Time __________

Address ______________________ Home phone ______________

______________________ Work phone ______________

Incident described:

Vital signs

Time	BP	Pulse	Resp	Oxygen delivery	Medications administered

Treatment administered	Healthcare provider rendering care

Client response to treatment

____

Figure 10-28. Medical emergency incident report form.

TABLE 10-2
Basic Dental Emergency Kit

Drug/Route Administered*	Action	Indications
Aromatic ammonia/inhaled	Chemical irritant	Syncope (fainting)
Epinephrine pen/subcutaneous	Cardiac stimulant and bronchodilator	Acute allergic reaction (anaphylaxis): acute bronchospasm (asthma)
Nitroglycerin/sublingual	Relaxes smooth muscle and dilates coronary arteries	Angina pectoris
Bronchodilator/inhaled (albuterol, proventil, terbutaline)	Dilates bronchi	Bronchospasm; asthma
Antihistamine/oral (Benadryl)	Decreases the allergic response	Mild or localized allergic reaction
Aspirin 81 mg chewable tablets	Fibrinolysis effect to reduce clotting	Chest pain or discomfort
Equipment and Supplies	**Action**	**Indications**
Automatic external defibrillator (AED)	Provides shock to heart to allow for correction of irregular, ineffective rhythm of heart beat	Unresponsive victim; cardiac arrest
Oxygen tank, mask and cannula	Delivery of free flowing oxygen to a conscious person with inadequate respiration	Syncope, following stabilization in an emergency
Pocket mask (bag mask or positive pressure ventilation device optional)	Provides a barrier for safety during rescue breathing	Basic Life Support
Blood pressure cuff and Stethoscope	Monitoring blood pressure	Before dental hygiene care or administration of drugs, prevention of emergencies, following stabilization in an emergency, following use of conscious sedation or other sedatives
Glucose/oral as sugar cubes, orange juice, or non-diet soft drink	Elevates blood sugar	Hypoglycemia

*Other medications may be included for use in advanced cardiac life support, but advanced training is needed to administer them.

TABLE 10-3
Management of Specific Medical Emergencies

Condition	Signs and Symptoms	Management
Syncope (fainting)	Feeling of warmth, flushed skin, nausea, rapid heart rate, perspiration, pallor Sudden, transient loss of consciousness	Place in *Trendelenburg position* (client's head lower than legs about 15 degrees); for pregnant women, roll on left side: loosen any binding clothes; maintain airway; administer oxygen (10 L/min flow); if unresponsive, pass crushed ammonia capsule under victim's nose; place cold compress on forehead; reassure; monitor and record vital signs.
Shock	Skin pale and clammy, change in mental status and eventual unconsciousness if untreated, drop in blood pressure, increase in pulse and respiratory rate	Position in Trendelenburg, activate EMS, assess breathing responsiveness, breathing, and pulse, administer BLS based on assessment using C-A-B sequence, maintain airway, monitor vital signs, administer oxygen (10 L/min flow).
Hyperventilation	Rapid or excessively deep breathing, light-headedness, dizziness, tingling in extremities, tightness in the chest, rapid heartbeat, lump in throat, panic-stricken appearance	Terminate procedure, use a quiet tone of voice to calm and reassure the client; encourage slow, normal breaths; have client breathe into cupped hands; *do not administer oxygen.*
Asthma	Coughing, shortness of breath, wheezing, pallor, anxiety, use of accessory muscles for breathing, cyanosis, increased pulse rate	Assist client to a position that facilitates breathing (upright is usually best), have client self-medicate with inhaler with instructions to inhale and exhale slowly. If the client recovers, care can be continued. If not, terminate dental hygiene services, have patient self-medicate one more time with inhaler, administer oxygen, monitor vital signs, if necessary activate EMS and initiate BLS.
Angina pectoris	Transient ischemia (lack of oxygenated blood) of the myocardium (heart muscle) manifested by crushing, burning, or squeezing chest pain, radiating to left shoulder, arms, neck, or mandible and lasting 2 to 15 minutes; shortness of breath; diaphoresis (sweating)	Terminate procedure, position client upright, administer oxygen (10 L/min flow), have client self-medicate with personal nitroglycerin supply (0.4 mg tablets or spray) every 5 minutes for maximum of three doses. If client does not have the medication, obtain nitroglycerin from the emergency kit. Monitor and record vital signs, put patient at rest and reassure; if pain is not relieved, activate EMS and treat as a myocardial infarction.
Myocardial infarction (heart attack)	Mild to severe chest pain; pain in the left arm, jaw, and possibly teeth, not relieved by rest and nitroglycerin; cold, clammy skin; nausea; anxiety; shortness of breath; weakness; perspiration; burning feeling of indigestion	Terminate procedure, place client in most comfortable position, usually semi-supine or upright; administer oxygen (10 L/min flow), activate EMS; if possible have patient chew 162 to 325 mg of aspirin, calm and reassure client; initiate BLS as needed; monitor and record vital signs.
Cardiac arrest	Ashen, gray, cold clammy skin; no pulse; no heart sounds; no respirations; unconscious	Activate EMS and initiate BLS using the C-A-B sequence.
Congestive heart failure	Shortness of breath, weakness, cough, swelling of lower extremities, pink frothy sputum, and distention of jugular veins	Terminate procedure, place chair in upright position, administer oxygen (10 L/min flow), monitor vital signs, provide BLS, and activate EMS if necessary.
Stroke or cerebrovascular accident (CVA)	The supply of oxygen to the brain cells is disrupted by ischemia, infarction, or hemorrhage of the cerebral blood vessels; sudden weakness of one side, difficulty of speech, temporary loss of vision, dizziness, change in mental status, nausea, severe headache, and/or convulsions.	Terminate procedure, activate EMS, position patient in semi-supine position or on side with head elevated to maintain open airway, administer oxygen (10 L/min flow), monitor vital signs, monitor and maintain airway and suction if needed, keep client quiet and still, initiate BLS as needed, have client transported to hospital as soon as possible.
Adrenal crisis (cortisol deficiency)	Confusion, weakness, lethargy, respiratory depression, headache, shock-like symptoms—weak, rapid pulse and low blood pressure—abdominal or leg pain, possible loss of consciousness	Terminate procedure. If unresponsive, place in supine position, activate EMS and BLS following C-A-B sequence as needed, administer oxygen (10 L/min flow), transport to nearest hospital emergency room. If responsive, position client semi-supine; monitor and record vital signs; administer oxygen; and activate BLS and EMS if needed.

TABLE 10-3
Management of Specific Medical Emergencies—cont'd

Condition	Signs and Symptoms	Management
Hemorrhage	Arterial blood is red in color and "spurts." Venous blood is darker in color and "oozes."	Compression over hemorrhage, usually with gauze: for bleeding from a dental extraction or surgical site, pack the area with gauze and have the client bite down until bleeding stops or pack site with absorbable material, if trained; if unsuccessful, apply topical thrombin or have client rinse with tranexamic acid; for nosebleeds, apply pressure to bleeding side, or pack the bleeding nostril with gauze; for severe bleeding, watch for signs of shock and activate EMS if bleeding continues.
Foreign body obstruction	If partial, coughing, choking, and grasping throat with hands If complete, no coughing or speaking, possible high pitched noise, grasping throat with hands	Evaluate breathing; if unable to breathe, speak, or cough, position yourself behind patient and use abdominal thrusts (Heimlich maneuver) until dislodged; if pregnant or obese client, use chest compressions until dislodged; administer oxygen (10 L/min flow); maintain supine position and have client transported to hospital to ensure no complications from thrusts or compressions. If client becomes unresponsive, activate BLS and EMS.
Seizure or Convulsions		
Generalized tonic-clonic (grand mal) seizure	Aura (change in taste, smell, or sight preceding seizure), loss of consciousness, sudden cry, involuntary tonic-clonic muscle contractions, altered breathing, and/or involuntary defecation or urination	Terminate procedure, lower dental chair and protect patient from personal damage including clearing area of all sharp and dangerous objects, make no attempts to restrain the person. After convulsion, assess and monitor airway, administer oxygen (10 L/min flow), monitor and record vital signs, support respiration. If unresolved (status epilepticus), initiate BLS and activate EMS. If stable, allow client to rest, arrange for medical follow-up, and arrange for assistance in leaving the dental facility.
Nonconvulsive (petit mal) seizure	Sudden momentary loss of awareness without loss of postural tone, a blank stare, and a duration of several to 90 seconds, muscle twitches	Terminate procedure, observe closely, ensure client safety, clear area of sharp objects, provide supportive care, may need physician evaluation.
Diabetic Emergency		
Hypoglycemia (hyperinsulinism)	Mood changes, hunger, headache, perspiration, nausea, confusion, irritation, dizziness and weakness, increased anxiety, possible unconsciousness	Terminate procedure, place chair in supine position, administer oxygen; if patient is unconscious, administer oral sugar (sugar cube or glucose paste under tongue) and activate BLA and EMS. If client conscious, ask when ate last and whether has taken insulin. Raise chair upright and give concentrated form of oral sugar (e.g., sugar packet, cake icing, concentrated orange juice, apple juice, sugar-containing soda). Monitor and record vital signs and responsiveness; if recovery not rapid, have transported to emergency facility.
Hyperglycemia (ketoacidosis)	Polydipsia (excessive thirst); polyuria (excessive urination); polyphagia (excessive hunger); labored respirations; nausea; dry, flushed skin; low blood pressure; weak, rapid pulse; acetone breath ("fruity" smell), blurred vision, headache, unconsciousness	Terminate procedure, activate EMS and provide BLS if necessary. If client is conscious, ask when ate last, whether has taken insulin, and whether client brought insulin to the appointment. Retrieve client's insulin. If able, client should self-administer the insulin; monitor and record vital signs.
Allergic Reaction		
Localized skin response	Mild pruritus (itching), mild urticaria (skin rash, hives)	Call for assistance; administer diphenhydramine antihistamine (e.g., Benadryl) 25 mL for child or small adult, 50 mg for normal adults; have client consult physician about repeat dose every 6 hours for 2 days following and discontinue drug if related to allergic response, be prepared to administer BLS if needed.

Continued

TABLE 10-3
Management of Specific Medical Emergencies—cont'd

Condition	Signs and Symptoms	Management
Anaphylaxis	Rapid and severe urticaria (hives) and/or pruritus, angioedema (swelling of mucous membranes such as lips, tongue, larynx, pharynx), respiratory distress, wheezing, laryngeal edema, weak pulse, low blood pressure; may progress to unconsciousness and cardiovascular collapse	Terminate procedure; immediately activate EMS; administer epinephrine 0.3-0.5 mg, repeat every 5 minutes up to 10 minutes if qualified; establish and maintain airway; administer oxygen (10 L/min flow); place in supine position; monitor vital signs; initiate BLS as needed.
Reactions to local anesthesia	See Chapter 39 *Toxicity from local anesthesia:* light-headedness, blurred vision and slurred speech, confusion, drowsiness, anxiety, tinnitus, bradycardia, tachypnea *Toxicity from vasopressor or vasoconstrictor:* anxiety, tachycardia, tachypnea, chest pain, dysrhythmias, cardiac arrest	Assess circulation, airway, and breathing; initiate BLS as needed, administer oxygen, activate EMS as needed.

LEGAL, ETHICAL, AND SAFETY ISSUES

- Taking a complete health, dental, and pharmacologic history is one step to reduce the risk of emergencies.
- Ensure that clients seek prompt medical care when signs and symptoms of potential disease are evident.
- If a client is conscious, he or she is asked and permission is obtained before providing any assistance. If a client is unconscious, permission can be assumed.
- A **good samaritan** is a legal term that refers to someone who renders aid in an emergency to an injured person on a voluntary basis. Usually, if a volunteer comes to the aid of an injured or ill person who is a stranger, the person giving the aid owes the stranger a duty of being reasonably careful. If the person providing care is a health professional, he or she is not liable for any civil damages as a result of acts or omissions in rendering first aid or emergency care, nor liable for any civil damages as a result of any act or failure to act to provide or arrange for further medical treatment or care for the injured person. Certain stipulations apply:
  - Emergency care is provided at the scene of the emergency.
  - The health care professional has proper training for care provided.[4,5]
  - The volunteer acts gratuitously and in good faith, and without remuneration or expectation for remuneration. As such, good samaritan statutes generally provide immunity from civil prosecution for those rendering care in emergency situations. These statutes were enacted so that health professionals and volunteers can render care to victims and be protected from lawsuits for negligent harm. They vary from state to state, but gross negligence or willful misconduct is not covered in most jurisdictions. Gross negligence is the intentional failure to perform a task with reckless disregard of the consequences that affects the life of another, or a conscious act or omission that may result in grave injury.
  - Under good samaritan statutes, emergency care also cannot be denied if providing such care is a part of a person's job responsibilities. Dental hygienists have a duty to deliver emergency services within the scope of their training. All dental professionals also have a duty to remain competent through training, re-training, certification, and practice so that they can handle a medical emergency in the practice setting. The dental team should practice its medical emergency plan annually and be familiar with how to use all of the basic equipment, supplies, and drugs contained in the dental emergency kit maintained within the dental practice setting.
- Someone should be designated to monitor contents regularly and resupply and update the dental emergency kit (at least quarterly and following any emergency).
- A medical emergency incident report form must be completed to document the situation, the victim's response and vital signs, treatment and medications administered, and emergency response time. A copy of this form, along with a copy of the client's health history form, should be kept in the client's record and, if applicable, accompany the victim to the emergency room.
- Every dental hygiene work setting should have a medical emergency plan. Each member of the oral care team should have a specific role to play in the event of an emergency. These roles should be reviewed and practiced periodically.

KEY CONCEPTS

- Complete assessment of the client, including health, dental, and pharmacologic history and vital signs, is essential in the prevention of medical emergencies. Conditions that place a client at risk for a medical emergency should be written in red in the medical alert box of the health history form.

- Assess the potential for a medical emergency by considering the risk level of the client, the procedure planned, and the anxiety level of the client.
- Use stress reduction protocols to prevent anxiety-related emergencies.
- If a client is found to be at high risk, consult the client's physician and the care plan and appointment schedule adjusted to avoid possible emergency situations.
- The office staff must be competent in using the emergency equipment and emergency drug kit and should practice medical emergency drills using a variety of scenarios.
- When a medical emergency arises, rapid assessment of signs, symptoms, and vital signs leads to the appropriate diagnosis and treatment. Document any client response that may lead to an emergency situation; document any client emergency.
- Complete a medical emergency report form for documentation in the client's record and to accompany the client to the hospital emergency room if applicable.

CRITICAL THINKING EXERCISES

1. Syncope is one of the most common medical emergencies occurring in the dental setting. Discuss steps to prevent an episode of syncope in a client. Review the signs and symptoms of syncope and the management of this condition.
2. A client complains of squeezing chest pain and shortness of breath and exhibits significant diaphoresis. What condition(s) should you suspect? Discuss appropriate management for this client's condition. What steps could have been taken to reduce the risk of this medical emergency occurring?
3. Visit a local facility where dental hygiene care is delivered. Locate the dental emergency kit in the healthcare facility. Identify all equipment, supplies, and drugs in the kit and describe its intended use. Check the expiration dates on all items. How is the dental emergency kit systematically updated to ensure currency of all items? How is the staff trained to ensure that all contents of the emergency kit can be used when necessary? What is the emergency protocol in the healthcare facility? Does each member of the healthcare team have a clear role to play in the event of an emergency? Define these roles.
4. Role-play these emergency situations: cardiac arrest, insulin shock, diabetic coma, seizure, reaction to the local anesthetic agent, anaphylactic shock, obstructed airway, syncope.
5. Use the Internet to locate a Quick Reference Card for Basic Life Support.
6. A client complains of a severe headache, and you notice his speech seems blurred. What medical emergency should be suspected? What steps should be taken in response to these symptoms? During periodontal debridement the tip of your instrument breaks off and your client aspirates it. What is the appropriate response to this situation? What steps could have been taken to prevent it?

REFERENCES

1. Malamed SF: *Medical emergencies in the dental office*, ed 6, St Louis, 2006, Mosby.
2. Patton LL, editor: *The ADA practical guide to patients with medical conditions*, Oxford, 2012, Wiley-Blackwell.
3. Travers AH, Berg MD, Billi JE, et al: Part 1: executive summary: 2010 American Heart Association Guidelines for Cardiopulmonary Resuscitation and Emergency Cardiovascular Care. *Circulation* 122(suppl 3):S640, 2010.
4. American Red Cross: CPR/AED for the professonal rescuer, 2006.
5. American Heart Association: BLS for Healthcare Providers Online part 1, 2011. www.onlineaha.org.

ACKNOWLEDGMENT

The authors acknowledge Lynn Utecht for her past contributions to this chapter.

ⓔ EVOLVE RESOURCES

Please visit http://evolve.elsevier.com/Darby/hygiene for additional practice and study support tools.

CHAPTER

11

Ergonomics

Lori J. Drummer

COMPETENCIES

1. Apply ergonomic principles in dental hygiene practice, including:
   - Discuss environmental factors leading to repetitive strain injury (RSI).
   - Describe modifications in the work environment that minimize RSI and stress.
   - Relate proper grasp and instrument factors to ergonomic principles.
   - Relate proper hand stabilization to ergonomic principles.
   - Modify client positioning based on ergonomic principles and client needs.
   - Demonstrate neutral shoulder, elbow, forearm, and wrist positions.
2. Demonstrate strengthening and chairside stretching exercises.
3. Describe common RSIs in terms of symptoms, risks, prevention, and treatment.

Principles of Ergonomics

Ergonomics is the study of human performance and workplace design (Figure 11-1). Ergonomists focus on a wide spectrum of workplace situations ranging from physical aspects of the environment to psychologic threats to health (Table 11-1). Dental hygienists are at risk for repetitive strain injuries (RSIs): musculoskeletal disorders involving the tendons, tendons sheaths, muscles, and nerves of hands, wrists, arms, elbows, shoulders, neck, and back. When ergonomic principles are applied, a dental hygienist can practice comfortably and avert disability.[1,2] When ergonomic principles are ignored, RSIs may occur. Minimizing occupational risks increases the likelihood of long-range health and wellness for the practitioner (Figure 11-2).

Environmental Factors

Flexibility of muscles and tendons, important for reducing the occurrence of RSI, is accomplished through physical exercise (discussed later in the chapter) and comfortable room temperatures. Cold room temperature is related to less relaxed, less flexible muscles and tendons. Stress and strain of stiff muscles and tendons lead to RSI. Relaxed atmospheres with minimal background noise contribute to a positive psychologic state for clinician and clients.[3]

Equipment Factors

See Chapter 8.

Dental Unit

The treatment area consists of the dental unit and chair, the dental light, and the clinician's chair. The dental chair, a contoured chair for the client during dental care, supports the client's head, torso, and feet. The dental chair also provides for easy maneuvering of the client via an articulating headrest and foot and side power controls. The dental light transmits illumination to maximize the clinician's view of the client's oral cavity. The dental unit contains essential treatment equipment such as the handpiece lines, water lines, self-contained water source, air and water syringe, evacuation lines, and instrument tray(s). A liquid crystal display (LCD) monitor also may be part of the dental unit.

Clinician's Chair

The chair is one of the most important pieces of equipment for the delivery of care (Figure 11-3). It should have a broad, heavy base and be readily mobile, with a minimum of five free-rolling casters to maneuver around the client's head during care. The chair seat should allow for adequate body support and be adjusted easily for proper height so that the clinician's feet are flat on the floor with thighs parallel with the floor. New ergonomically designed chairs put the clinician in the proper position and lend total body support to reduce strain on the spine, lower back, shoulders, and arms (Figure 11-4). Too high a chair position causes the body weight to be supported by the spine, back, and shoulders. Too low a position causes the clinician to slump and sit with a curved spine (Figure 11-5).

Cords on Powered Instruments

Dental units are equipped with power-driven instruments and air and water syringes. These may be attached to the dental unit via the following:

- Retractable cords: retract into the dental unit to save space and avoid tangling
- Curly cords: coiling characteristics allow cord to hang down a shortened distance and save space
- Straight cords: straight, free-hanging cord

The retractable and curly power cords[2] are encumbering and require constant pulling by the clinician. This repetitive pulling motion increases fatigue and hand, arm, and shoulder muscle strain. A straight cord creates no tension while the clinician is using the motor-driven instrument.

Performance Factors

Five Categories of Motion

Motions and movements can be stressful to the physical well-being of dental clinicians. Stresses caused by movement

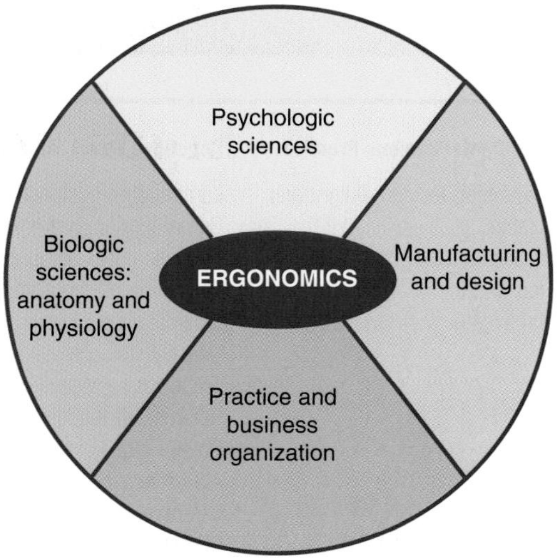

Figure 11-1. Multidimensional nature of ergonomics.

1. Environmental Factors
- ✔ Comfortable temperature
- ✔ Comfortable noise level

2. Equipment Factors
- ✔ Properly designed clinician chair with freedom of movement
- ✔ Properly designed dental chair
- ✔ Bracket tray and dental light within reach

3. Positioning Factors
- ✔ Proper clinician positioning
- ✔ Proper client positioning

4. Performance Factors
- ✔ Proper grasp and fulcrum
- ✔ Maintained neutral wrist, elbow, and shoulder position
- ✔ Maintained neck and back support
- ✔ Proper wrist motion; limited digital motion and wrist extension and flexion
- ✔ Appointment management

5. Instrument Factors
- ✔ Properly maintain cutting edge
- ✔ Use ergonomic handles
- ✔ Variations in handle diameter and shape
- ✔ Use balanced instruments
- ✔ Use ultrasonic and sonic instruments
- ✔ Avoid curly or retracting cords on motor-driven instruments and air/water syringes
- ✔ Limit the use of instruments that cause vibrations

6. Exercises
- ✔ Strengthening exercises
- ✔ Chairside stretching exercises

Figure 11-2. Ergonomic checklist for dental hygienists.

can harm the back, neck, arms, and wrists. There are five categories of motion[3] based on the amount of movement and the bone and muscle support needed to carry out the movement (Table 11-2). Dental clinicians should limit their movements to class I, II, and III.

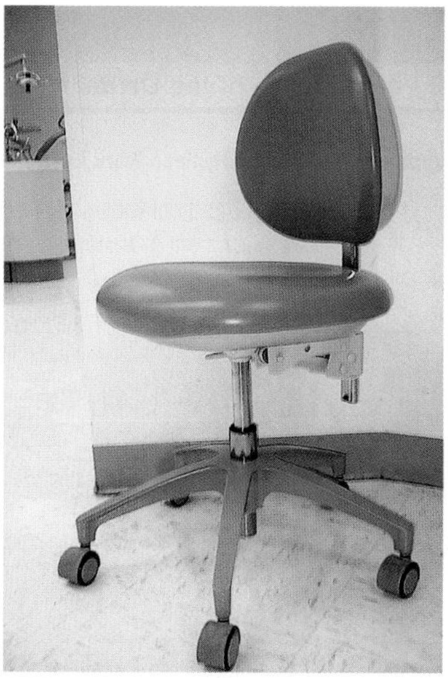

Figure 11-3. Traditional clinician's chair.

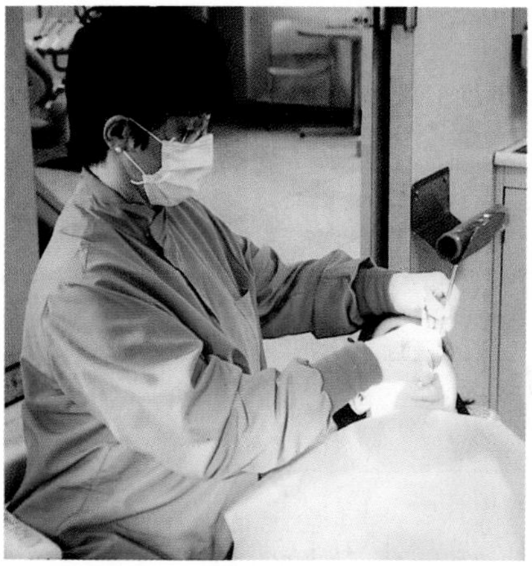

Figure 11-4. Neutral position of clinician. Note shoulders level and held in most relaxed position, elbows close to body, and forearms in same plane as wrists, hands, and client's mouth. (Courtesy Nordent Manufacturing, Inc, Elk Grove Village, Illinois.)

Grasp and Fulcrum

Fundamentals of grasp include holding the instrument firmly, maintaining a secure grip, and maintaining control of the instrument without causing undue strain or fatigue to the clinician's hand, arms, and shoulders. The modified pen grasp is a three-finger grasp using the thumb, index finger, and middle finger. A space must be maintained between the index finger and thumb to facilitate freedom of movement when rolling the instrument into interproximal spaces and around line angles of the teeth during instrumentation. Rolling the instrument between the index finger, middle finger, and thumb eliminates turning and twisting of the wrist, which can lead to an RSI such as carpal tunnel syndrome (CTS).

Holding the instrument with all four fingers wrapped securely around the handle is the palm grasp. The modified pen grasp and palm grasp may be firm or light depending on

TABLE 11-1

Ergonomists' Perspectives of the Dental Hygiene Workplace

Workplace Environment	Dental Hygiene Work Environment	Alterations to Dental Hygiene Practice	Repetitive Strain Injuries
Ergonomic design and layout	Layout and convenience of equipment placement in treatment area	Eliminate stretching for dental light and bracket table Reduce twisting motion of the back, shoulders, and elbow while reaching for dental hygiene instruments	Lumbar joint dysfunction Carpal tunnel syndrome Thoracic outlet compression Tension neck syndrome Cervical spondylolysis Cervical disk disease Trapezius myalgia Rotator cuff tendonitis Rotator cuff tears Adhesive capsulitis Lateral epicondylitis Radial tunnel syndrome Cubital tunnel syndrome
Worker and equipment crossing point	Dull hand instruments Vibrations and stress from rotary instruments Improperly designed hand instruments	Maintain hand instruments Use principles of selective polishing Do not use handpieces with curly or retracting cords Use balanced instruments	Carpal tunnel syndrome Thoracic outlet compression Strained pronator muscle Guyon's canal syndrome Trigger finger nerve syndrome De Quervain's syndrome
Tasks and work to be performed	Repetitive movements and hand fatigue Clinician fatigue and stress on body	Change clinician positions Alternate instrument handle design and diameter Use proper client and clinician positioning	Lumbar joint dysfunction Carpal tunnel syndrome Thoracic outlet compression Tension neck syndrome Cervical spondylolysis Cervical disk disease Trapezius myalgia Strained pronator muscle Guyon's canal syndrome Trigger finger nerve syndrome De Quervain's syndrome
Psychologic aspects and factors	Practice management and appointment scheduling	Alternate involved dental hygiene treatments with less-complicated maintenance appointments Increase continued-care intervals Lengthen appointment times	Lumbar joint dysfunction Carpal tunnel syndrome Thoracic outlet compression Tension neck syndrome Cervical spondylolysis Cervical disk disease Trapezius myalgia Rotator cuff tendonitis Rotator cuff tears Adhesive capsulitis Lateral epicondylitis Radial tunnel syndrome Cubital tunnel syndrome Strained pronator muscle Guyon's canal syndrome Trigger finger nerve syndrome De Quervain's syndrome

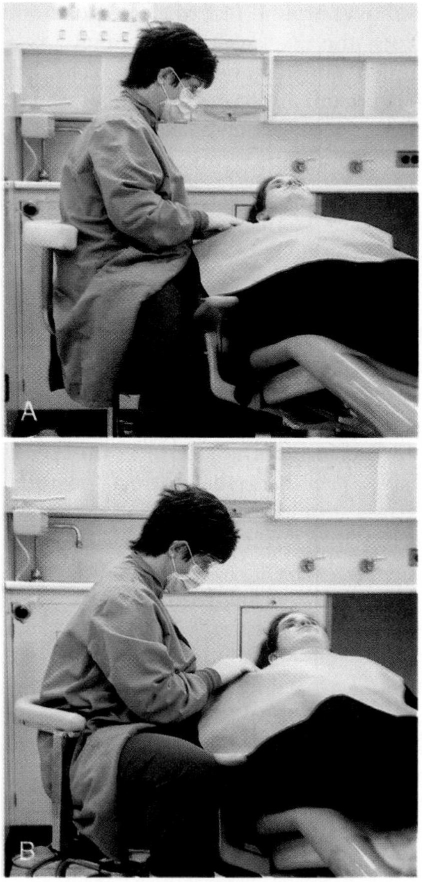

Figure 11-5. **A,** Clinician's stool positioned too high. **B,** Clinician's stool positioned too low. (Courtesy Nordent Manufacturing, Inc, Elk Grove Village, Illinois.)

TABLE 11-2

Five Categories of Motion

Classification	Motion
Class I	Using fingers only
Class II	Using fingers and wrist
Class III	Movement of fingers, wrist, and arm
Class IV	Movement of the entire arm and shoulder
Class V	Movement of arm and twisting of body

the procedure being performed. See website for additional resources and Chapters 26 and 27 for a thorough discussion of instrumentation principles.

Fulcrum and Hand Stabilization

The fulcrum is the area on which the finger rests and against which it pushes while instrumentation is performed. The fulcrum provides a basis for steadiness and control during stroke activation. Proper fulcrum and hand stabilization reduces RSIs.

The intraoral fulcrum is established by resting the pad of the ring finger (fulcrum finger) inside the mouth against a tooth surface. The fulcrum finger must remain locked during instrument activation. A locked fulcrum allows the clinician to pivot on and gain strength from the fulcrum finger. Pivoting on the fulcrum finger helps to maintain a firm grasp, stability, and proper wrist motion. Middle and fulcrum fingers work together to add support during instrument activation. Splitting of the middle and fulcrum fingers decreases instrument control, strength, and stability. With less control, strength, and stability, the clinician automatically tightens the grasp, contributing to RSI. Placing the fulcrum close to the working area is not always possible owing to space limitations in the mouth, teeth alignment, pocket depth, or the angle of access. A variety of intraoral fulcrums may be necessary. See Chapter 26, section on the fulcrum, for a detailed explanation.

The extraoral fulcrum is used when using instruments on deep periodontal pockets. It is accomplished by placing the broad side of the clinician's palm or back of the hand against an outside structure of the client's face such as the chin or cheek (see Chapter 26). Benefits of an extraoral fulcrum are as follows:

- Easier, less strenuous accessibility to deep periodontal pockets and difficult access areas
- Stability and control
- Less twisting of wrist during activation of maxillary posterior areas
- Decreased chance of RSI to the nerves, tendons, and ligaments in the clinician's wrist and elbow (e.g., action of the activation or pulling stroke is transmitted to the arm and shoulder and away from the wrist)

When no fulcrum is used, lateral pressure on the instrument during activation causes the instrument to slip in the hand. To stabilize and control the instrument, the clinician automatically tightens the grasp. Tightening the grasp places stress on hand and arm muscles, tendons, and ligaments, leading to an increased occurrence of RSI.

Wrist Motion During Instrument Activation

Wrist motion[1,2,4] and the fulcrum are related. Safe wrist motion is vital to the health of the clinician's hand, wrist, and forearm muscles, tendons, and ligaments. Pivoting on the fulcrum causes the hand, wrist, and forearm to move in one unified motion. Failing to handle instruments using the unified motion causes the clinician to extend or flex the wrist (Figure 11-6). Continued flexion or extension of the wrist contributes to a variety of RSIs.

Digital motion during instrument activation is also a factor contributing to RSI. Digital motion is the push-and-pull motion of the instrument using fingers only. Muscle fatigue results quickly with digital motion, and a decrease in instrument power and stability occurs.

Appointment Management

Control of appointment procedures and time greatly reduces possible RSI.[2] The dental hygienist should do the following:

- Alternate new clients with continued clients.
- Alternate root debridement and therapeutic scaling with maintenance appointments.
- Alternate difficult appointments with less taxing ones.
- Shorten continued-care intervals.
- Allow for "buffer time" in the daily schedule.

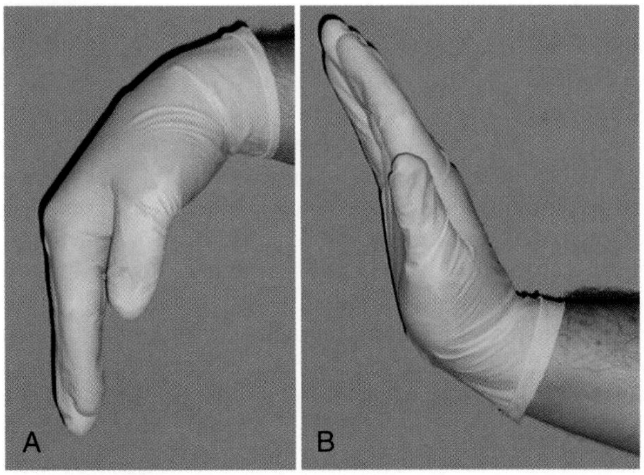

Figure 11-6. **A,** Flexion of the wrist. **B,** Extension of the wrist. Both movements can cause repetitive strain injuries.

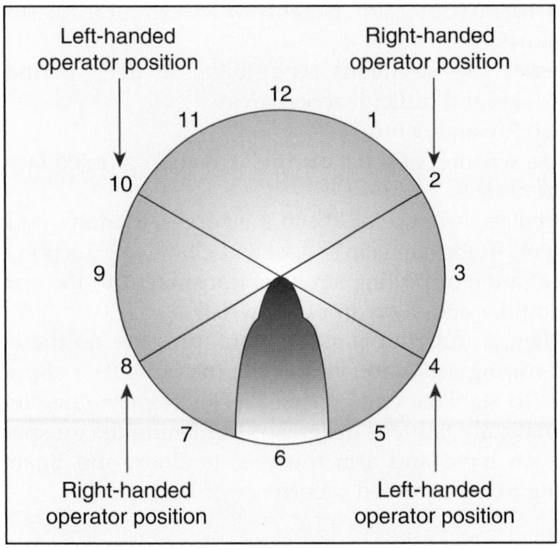

Figure 11-7. Possible clinician positions around the client. Right-handed clinician: 8 to 2 o'clock. Left-handed clinician: 4 to 10 o'clock.

Client-Clinician Positioning Factors

Commonly used client positions are the following[2,4]:

- Upright for interviewing and educating
- Semiupright for treating persons with some cardiovascular and respiratory diseases
- Supine for treating most clients
- Trendelenburg for persons experiencing syncope

In the supine position the client's mouth should be at about the height of the seated clinician's elbow. Distance from the client's mouth to the clinician's eyes should be about 14 to 16 inches. The headrest can be adjusted for maxillary or mandibular arch visibility. During treatment of maxillary teeth, the maxilla should be perpendicular to the floor; during treatment of the mandibular teeth, the mandible should be parallel to the floor.

Clinician-client positioning is best explained using the face of a clock (Figure 11-7):

- Client's head is the center of the clock.
- Clinician moves around face of clock, positioning between the 8 o'clock and the 4 o'clock positions.
- Right-handed clinician uses the 8 o'clock to 2 o'clock range. When teeth are out of alignment, the right-handed clinician may work in the 4 o'clock position.
- Left-handed clinicians work predominantly in the 10 o'clock to 4 o'clock range, with variations necessary at times to the 8 o'clock position.

Figure 11-8 presents a variety of client positions used during dental hygiene care.

Position of the Clinician

Clinician comfort and safety cannot be sacrificed for the client. Repetitive use of incorrect clinician positioning causes stress and fatigue. Therefore client positioning should allow the operator to perform intraoral procedures without increasing RSI. Table 11-3 lists the correct positioning of the clinician's arms, shoulders, legs, feet, back, head, and eyes during care.

Wrist, Arm, Elbow, and Shoulder Position

Maintaining a neutral position of the wrist, arm, elbow, and shoulder reduces clinician fatigue and injury during care.[5] Neutral positions are basic to the prevention of occupational pain and risks related to RSI.

Neutral positions include the following (see Figure 11-4):

- Shoulders: level and held in their lowest, most relaxed position
- Elbow: held close to the clinician's body at a 90-degree angle
- Forearm: held in same plane as wrist and hand
- Wrist: should never be bent; it is held straight

Back and Neck Support

Adequate back and neck support reduces the occurrence of musculoskeletal injuries to the spine. Intervertebral disks in the spine resemble a jelly donut. When uneven pressure is put on an intervertebral disk, the effect is the same as if you pushed down on one side of a jelly donut: the contents of the disk (jelly donut) are pushed out. Poor posture of the clinician results in uneven support of the spine and rupture of an intervertebral disk (see Figure 11-5). Maintaining a straight back, straight neck, and erect head, with feet flat on the floor and thighs parallel to the floor, properly supports the spine.

Eye loupes (telescopes) are magnification devices worn instead of traditional eyeglasses to improve the clinician's operative field of vision, visual accuracy, and posture during client care[6] (Figure 11-9). Use of multilens telescopic loupes in the 2× to 2.5× magnification range offers the necessary depth of field and ensures a specific physical distance between the dental hygienist and client, keeping the dental hygienist's back and spine straight and preventing occupational pain caused by cumulative trauma. If the clinician is too close to or too far away from the client, the visual field seen through the magnification device is blurred. Once back into the proper position, the clinician's field of vision is clear.

Instrument Factors

Hand Instrument Cutting Edge Sharpness

Sharp instruments are essential to the elimination of fatigue and stress on the clinician's hand, wrist, arm, and shoulders that cause RSI.[2] Therefore any instrument with a cutting edge

TABLE 11-3
Correct Clinician Positioning

Feet, Leg, and Thigh Position	Body Weight	Arm and Shoulder Position	Back Position	Head Position	Eyes
Feet flat on the floor	Centered on the seat of the clinician's stool	Shoulders are relaxed and in the neutral position (parallel to the floor)	Back is straight	Aligned with the spine (sit tall in the clinician's stool)	Directed downward
Thighs parallel with the floor	Supported by the legs and thighs	Upper arms are relaxed Elbows are in the neutral position (close to the body)	Lumbar curve is supported	Head is erect	Distance from eyes to client's oral cavity is approximately 14-16 inches

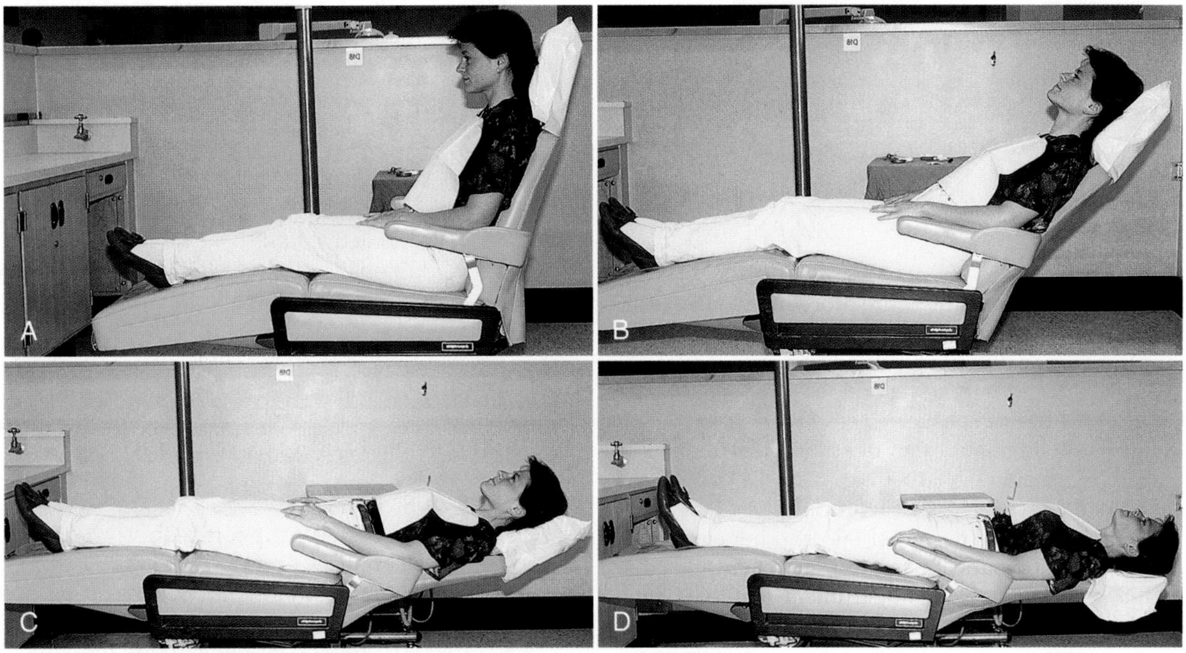

Figure 11-8. **Basic client body positions used during the dental hygiene process of care. A,** Basic upright position; client is seated in an 80- to 90-degree angle. **B,** Semiupright position; client is seated in a 45-degree angle. **C,** Supine position that has been modified for mandibular instrumentation. **D,** Supine position that has been modified for maxillary insertion.

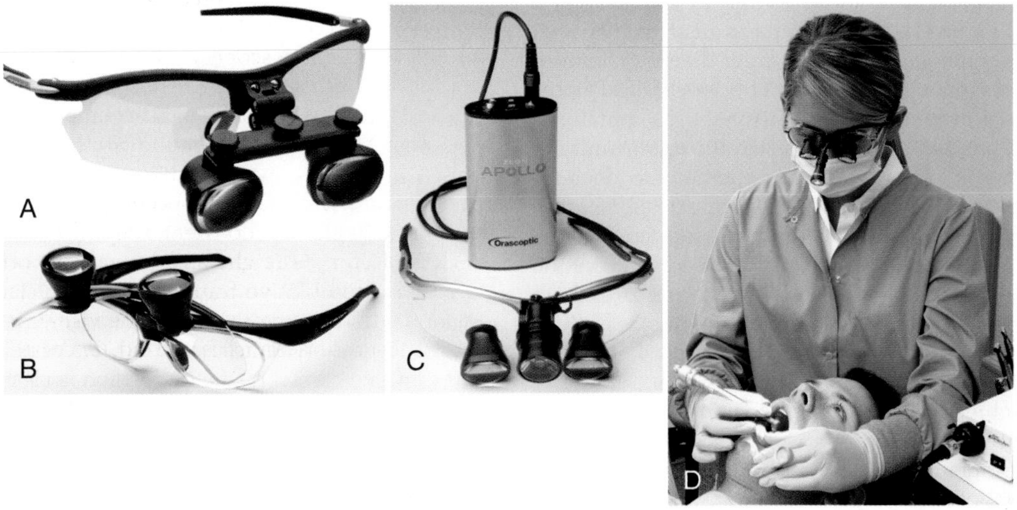

Figure 11-9. **A,** Flip-up loupe on a black Rudy sport frame. **B,** Revolution through-the-flip loupe with insert available for prescription. **C,** Rudy loupe with Apollo LED light. **D,** Correct clinician position when using loupes. (**A** to **C,** Courtesy Orascoptic, Middleton, Wisconsin.)

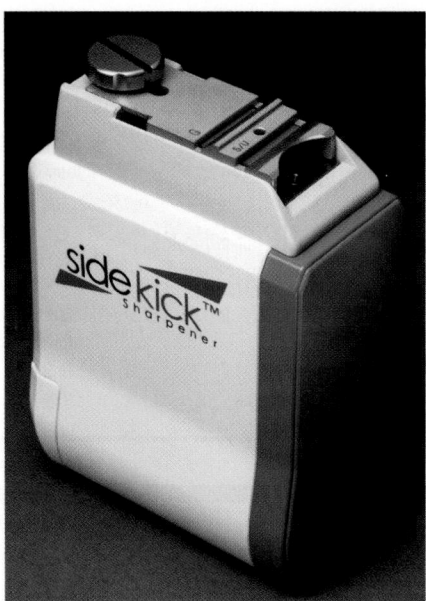

Figure 11-10. Sidekick used to sharpen instruments. (Courtesy Hu-Friedy, Chicago, Illinois.)

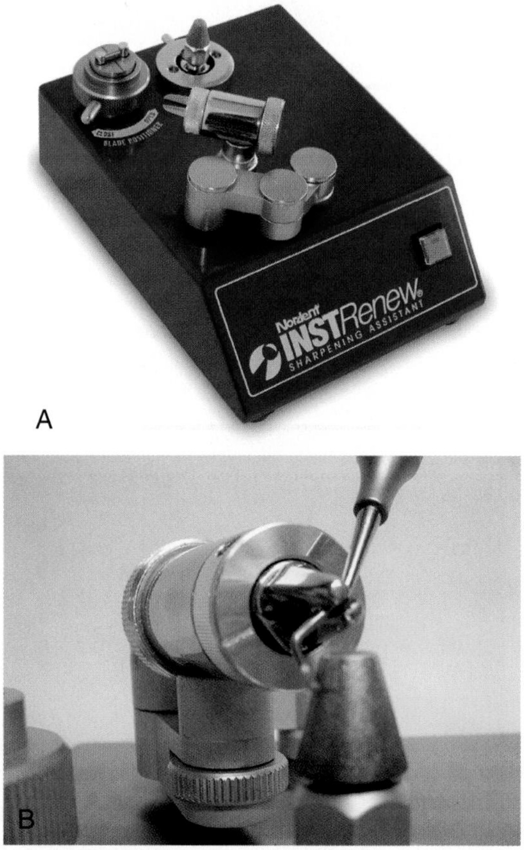

Figure 11-11. **A,** InstRenew Sharpening Assistant used to sharpen instruments. **B,** InstRenew being used to sharpen a curet. Correct cutting-edge angle is maintained. (Courtesy Nordent Manufacturing, Inc, Elk Grove Village, Illinois.)

should be kept sharp during the entire procedure. Dull instruments that deviate from their original design cause the clinician to apply additional force, resulting in increased lateral pressure applied, excess stroke repetitions, and a tightened grasp. Fatigue and RSI can ensue.

Maintaining the original design of scaling instruments is accomplished by manual sharpening using a hand-held sharpening stone or powered sharpening devices that assist in maintaining the original design of the working end of the instrument as well as producing an even, sharp, cutting edge (Figures 11-10 and 11-11). Dental instrument materials have been developed that require no sharpening or reduce the need for sharpening (see Chapter 26, section on instrument sharpening).

Ergonomic Instrument Handles

Ergonomic instrument handles[2] are large in diameter and light in weight. Figure 11-12, *A*, compares instruments with standard versus ergonomic handles. Larger-diameter handles open the grasp just enough to dissipate the mechanical forces over a larger area of muscles. Instrument setups containing several styles of handles give the clinician the opportunity to rest different muscle groups while completing care, decreasing the occurrence of RSI. Another ergonomic design feature to consider is the use of instruments with padded handles (Figure 11-12, *B*). Padded instrument handles cushion the fingertips while the handle is grasped (see Chapter 26, section on parts and characteristics of dental instruments).

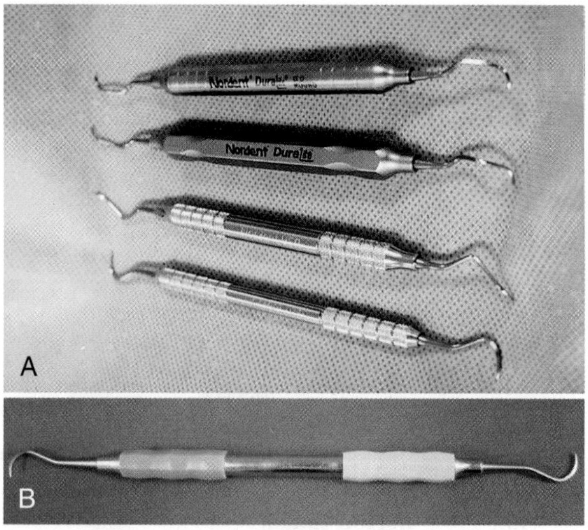

Figure 11-12. **A,** Variety of instrument handles. **B,** Padded handle. (Courtesy Nordent Manufacturing, Inc, Elk Grove Village, Illinois.)

Balanced Instruments

Single- and double-ended instruments should be balanced. This means that the working end is centered over the long axis of the instrument handle. When the instrument is balanced, the lateral pressure placed on the instrument handle and shank during instrument activation will be aimed toward the working end (Figure 11-13). When an instrument is not balanced, the lateral pressure placed on the instrument when activated causes the instrument to turn slightly in the clinician's fingers. To compensate, the clinician grasps the instrument handle more tightly. Use of balanced instruments decreases occurrence of RSI.

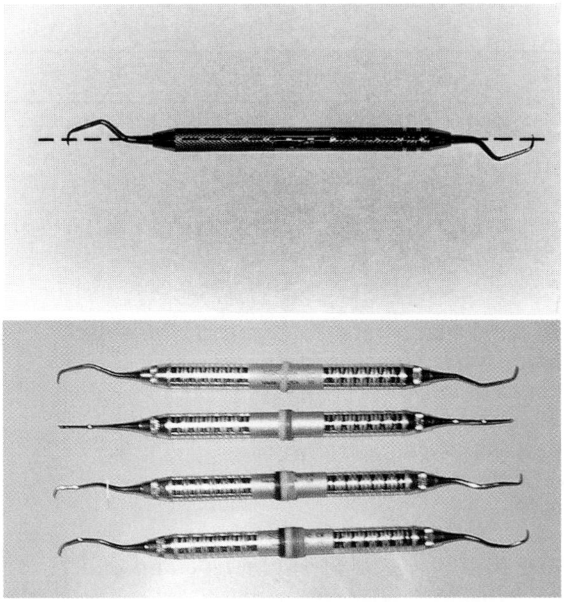

Figure 11-13. Balanced instrument. Note that when the working end is centered over the long axis of the handle, the instrument is balanced.

Mechanized and Vibrating Instruments

Use of ultrasonic and sonic instruments significantly reduces repetitive hand-wrist-forearm motions (see Chapter 27). Oral debridement requires numerous repetitive strokes and significant lateral pressure when using hand-activated instrumentation techniques.

Instruments causing vibrations, such as the motor-driven handpiece, cause fatigue and hand, arm, and shoulder muscle strain. Application of the principles of selective polishing limits the time during which the clinician uses a vibrating instrument. A common RSI caused by vibratory instruments is Raynaud's syndrome, which results in blanching (often painful) fingers.

Dental Mirrors

The mouth mirror is held in the nondominant hand. Practitioners focus on the hand, wrist, and arm position of the dominant hand during instrumentation with limited regard for the nondominant hand. Ergonomic adaptations in mouth mirror handles were associated with increases and decreases in muscle activity. The clinical impact of this increase or decrease in muscle activity amplifies as force is exerted.[7] In comparison of the function of the dominant and nondominant hands during dental hygiene procedures, there is a significant difference between the techniques of the scaling hand and the hand holding the mirror. The nondominant hand holding the mirror functions to increase access and visualization by retracting the tongue and cheeks. Unlike the multitasking dominant hand, the static nondominant hand often requires a forceful grip, retracting the tongue and cheek throughout care.[8] This continuous static position of the nondominant hand decreases blood flow to the hand and fingers, increasing risk of RSI. Ergonomic adaptations to instrument handles (weight, diameter, and padding) vary muscle activity throughout the day to reduce RSIs for dental hygienists.[7]

Physical Exercise

Strengthening Exercises

No one would consider performing strenuous exercise without stretching and doing strengthening maneuvers first. However, oral care providers subject their muscles to strenuous activity daily without properly preparing their bodies for the workplace. Maintaining a healthy musculoskeletal system through daily exercise has the following effects:

- Improves strength and flexibility
- Improves lumbar spine, neck muscle, and lower back health
- Stretches and extends back muscles
- Strengthens abdominal muscles
- Strengthens finger, hand, and arm muscles

Strengthening exercises can be performed regularly to repair and maintain a healthy musculoskeletal system (Box 11-1).

Chairside Stretching Exercises

Stretching and warm-up exercises[6] reduce muscle and joint soreness and injury and prepare the individual psychologically for activities requiring skill and dexterity. Before work and throughout the day, dental hygienists should perform the following tendon gliding exercise (TGE) (Figure 11-14), which diffuses **synovial fluid**, the lubricant around the hand and finger tendons:

1. Hold hand and fingers straight, pointing upward.
2. Bend fingers into a 90-degree angle from hand.
3. Close fingers into hand.
4. Arch hand back toward top of wrist.
5. Further arch fingers in same direction.
6. Hold briefly and release.
7. Repeat four times.

Repetitive Strain Injuries

See Table 11-4.

Hand, Wrist, and Finger Injuries

Carpal Tunnel Syndrome

Carpal tunnel syndrome (CTS),[2,4,9] the most common RSI reported by dental hygienists, has the following causes:

- Congenital: anatomic structure and development
- Self-limiting conditions: pregnancy
- Systemic conditions: edema or arthritis
- Nonmedical reasons: occupational or work related

About one third of dental hygienists report symptoms of CTS, which occurs when the median nerve becomes compressed within the carpal tunnel (Figure 11-15). Function of the median nerve is sensory and motor:

- It supplies sensation to the thumb, index finger, middle finger, and half of the ring finger.
- It supplies a branch to the thumb (thenar) muscles.

The carpal bones of the wrist and the transverse carpal ligament form the carpal tunnel. The carpal bones and transverse carpal tunnel ligament form a furrow, allowing the flexor tendons and the median nerve to pass through to the hand. Repetitive force and motion to the wrist cause tendon inflammation and swelling within the carpal tunnel. The enlarged tendons and lack of space in the carpal tunnel place undue pressure on the median nerve, causing pain. Once the nerve is compressed, CTS begins. Repeated wrist flexion and

BOX 11-1

Strengthening Exercises

Pelvic Tilt: Strengthens Lumbar Spine
1. Lie on your back ideally or, if at work, stand flat against the wall.
2. Keep knees slightly bent.
3. Flatten and press back into floor (or wall).
4. Hold briefly.
5. Repeat.

Hyperextension: Safeguards Lumbar Curve
1. Lie on your stomach.
2. Arch body backward, in an upward direction.
3. Hold briefly.
4. Repeat.

Knee-to-Chest: Stretches Lumbar Spine
1. Lie on your back.
2. Bring both knees to your chest.
3. Hold briefly.
4. Return to original position; avoid straightening legs.
5. Repeat.

Sit-Ups: Strengthen Abdominal Muscles
1. Lie on your back.
2. Bend knees.
3. Support neck.
4. Gently raise shoulders toward knees.
5. Hold briefly and return.
6. Repeat.

Suspend From a Bar: Relieves Lower Back Pain
1. Firmly grasp bar.
2. Suspend your body from bar; lift feet slowly.
3. Hold for a short time.
4. Repeat.

Doorway Stretch: Reverses Poor Posture
1. Stand in front of an open doorway.
2. Place hands on either side of doorframe.
3. Gently allow your body to lean forward through doorway.
4. Hold briefly and return.
5. Repeat.

Neck Isometric: Stretches Cervical Spine and Relieves Neck Muscle Strain
1. Grasp hands behind head.
2. Gently press your head back.
3. Do not allow any backward movement.
4. Hold briefly.
5. Repeat.

Rubber Ball Squeeze: Strengthens Hand and Finger Muscles
1. Grasp a rubber ball firmly in your hand.
2. Gently squeeze.
3. Hold briefly.
4. Repeat.

Rubber Band Stretch: Strengthens Hand and Finger Muscles
1. Extend rubber band between fingers of hand.
2. Gently stretch rubber band until you feel resistance.
3. Hold briefly.
4. Release rubber band.
5. Repeat.

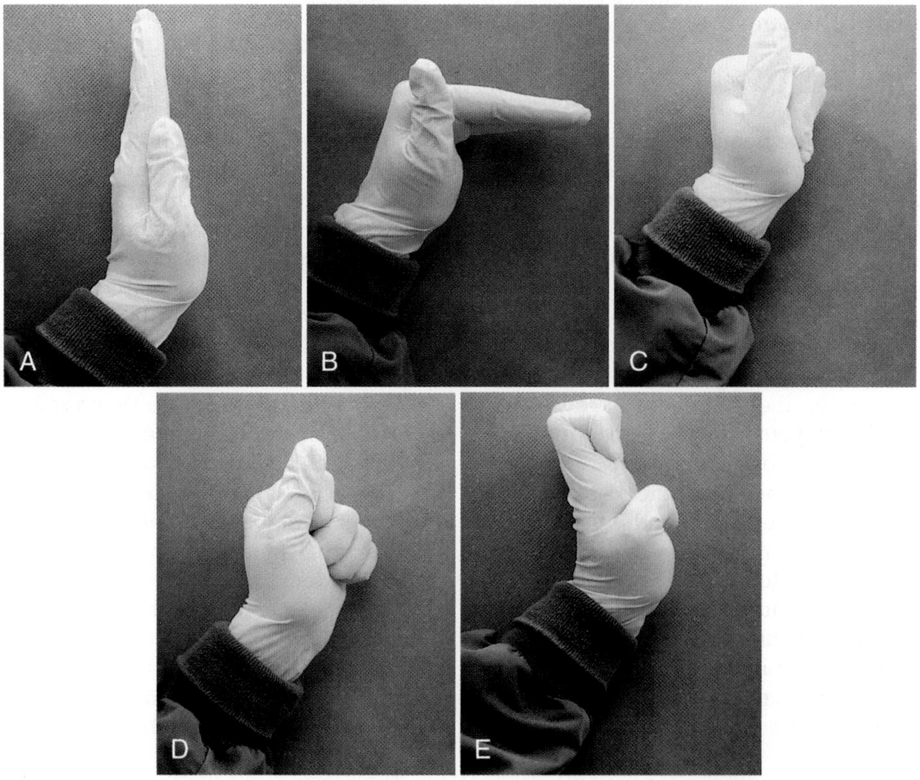

Figure 11-14. Tendon gliding exercises.

TABLE 11-4
Effects of Repetitive Strain Injuries

Common Repetitive Strain Injuries in Dental Hygiene	Area of the Body Affected
Carpal tunnel syndrome	Wrist, forearm, hand, fingers (index finger, middle finger, and half of ring finger and thumb)
Thoracic outlet compression	Shoulder, arm, hand
Surgical glove–induced injury	Hand, fingers, wrist
Guyon's canal syndrome	Lower arm, wrist, fingers (half of ring finger and little finger)
Strained pronator muscle	Elbow
Trigger finger nerve syndrome	Tendons in the fingers
De Quervain's syndrome	Base of the thumb
Tension neck syndrome	Neck, between shoulder blades, arm
Cervical spondylolysis	Neck, scapula, and shoulders
Cervical disk disease	Neck and arm
Trapezius myalgia	Shoulders
Rotator cuff tendonitis	Shoulders
Rotator cuff tears	Shoulders
Adhesive capsulitis	Shoulders
Lumbar joint dysfunction	Spine
Lateral epicondylitis	Elbow and forearm
Radial tunnel syndrome	Elbow and forearm
Cubital tunnel syndrome	Elbow and forearm

hyperextension during instrumentation aggravate tendons and cause further swelling.

Signs and Symptoms

The signs and symptoms of carpal tunnel syndrome are the following:

- Numbness in the areas supplied by the median nerve (earliest sign)
- Pain in the hand, wrist, shoulder, neck, lower back
- Nocturnal pain in hand(s) and forearm(s)
- Pain in hand(s) while working
- Morning and/or daytime stiffness and numbness
- Loss of strength in hand(s); weakened grasp
- Cold fingers
- Increased fatigue in fingers, hand, wrist, forearm, shoulders
- Nerve dysfunction

Risk Factors

Repetition is the foremost risk factor causing CTS. Holding the instruments tightly places too much force on the wrist and hand. Vibrating instruments, including low-speed handpieces and ultrasonic scalers, have been identified as risk factors for CTS.[1] Cold temperatures in the dental treatment area decrease flexibility of the clinician's finger, hand, arm, shoulder, neck, and back muscles. This inflexibility causes stiffness, making workplace performance stressful. Also, wearing gloves that are too tight can pinch the median nerve at the wrist.

Chairside Preventive Measures

The following measures can be taken to prevent carpal tunnel syndrome.

- Maintain good operator posture: the client's mouth should be even with clinician's elbow; the elbow should be held in the neutral position (90-degree angle created by the upper arm and forearm).
- Maintain proper position to support clinician's body, with thighs parallel to floor and feet flat on floor.
- Neutral forearm and wrist position: avoid pinching median nerve in the carpal tunnel.
- Keep shoulders relaxed.
- Use a unified motion (wrist, hand, forearm) during scaling and polishing; avoid flexion and extension of wrist.
- Avoid extremes in temperatures.
- Avoid or limit exposure to vibrating instruments.
- Avoid forceful pinching and gripping of instrument handles.
- Wear properly fitting gloves.
- Alternate clinician positions.
- Perform TGEs.

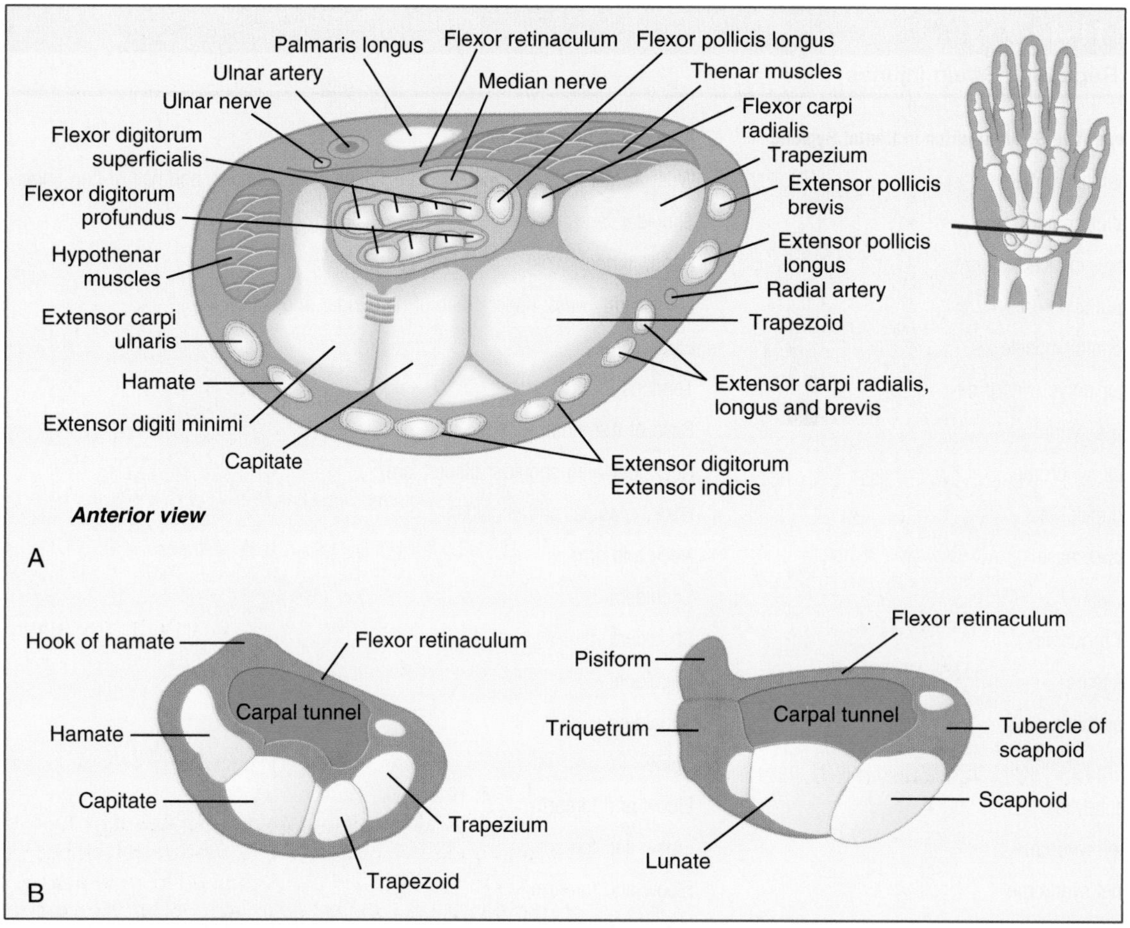

Figure 11-15. Carpal bones. The carpal bones form a trough through which the flexor tendons and median nerve traverse into the hand. **A,** Transverse section of the wrist and carpal tunnel. **B,** Diagram of transverse section through the carpal tunnel. (Redrawn from Agur A: *Grant's atlas of anatomy,* ed 9, Baltimore, 1991, Williams and Wilkins.)

Assessing Symptoms

CTS affects the median nerve, which supplies the thumb, index finger, middle finger, and half of the ring finger. If the symptoms are felt in the little finger and right half of the ring finger, CTS may not be the problem or the operator may have CTS along with another RSI. Two simple tests can be performed to indicate symptoms of CTS:

- Phalen's test: Place the back of hands against each other. Hold flexed wrists together at a 90-degree angle for 1 minute. Subjective sensory changes will be felt within 1 minute. These sensory changes indicate a positive test result (Figure 11-16, *A*).
- Tinel's sign: Tap the median nerve at the ventral side of wrist. If nerve compression is present, sensation is felt in the fingers. The sensation could range from a tingling feeling to an electrical-type shooting pain (Figure 11-16, *B*).

Treatment

Conservative treatment includes corticosteroid injections to reduce tendon inflammation. Iontophoresis, delivery of corticosteroid via an electrical current delivery system, also can be used. The electrical current increases penetration of the corticosteroid through skin and into the carpal tunnel. This method is less painful but is not as effective as the injection of corticosteroid. CTS also can be treated with anti-inflammatory medications and vitamins.

Wearing a wrist brace during the early stages of CTS decreases symptoms by minimizing inflammation. The wrist is kept in the neutral position simply by the brace holding the carpal tunnel in the most open position, allowing nerves and tendons to relax and heal.

Surgical treatment may be performed if conservative therapies fail. In surgery the transverse carpal ligament is cut to relieve pressure on the median nerve. Some surgical procedures for CTS use an endoscope or small fiberoptic camera plus a traditional surgical procedure except that no incision is made in the palm. With only a small incision made in the wrist to access the carpel tunnel, healing time is decreased.

Thoracic Outlet Compression

Thoracic outlet compression (TOC) is an RSI resulting in compression of the brachial artery and plexus nerve trunk at the thoracic outlet. TOC affects the hand, wrist, arm, and shoulder. Compression of the neurovascular bundle (brachial plexus, subclavian artery, and subclavian vein) results in

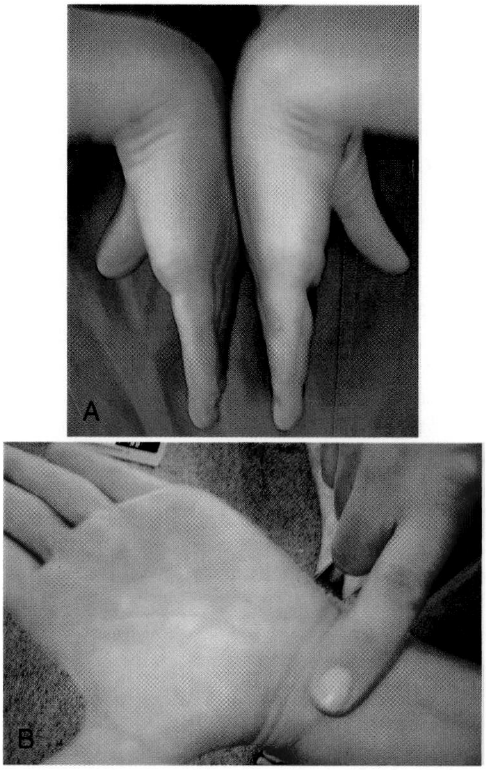

Figure 11-16. **A,** Phalen's test. **B,** Tinel's sign.

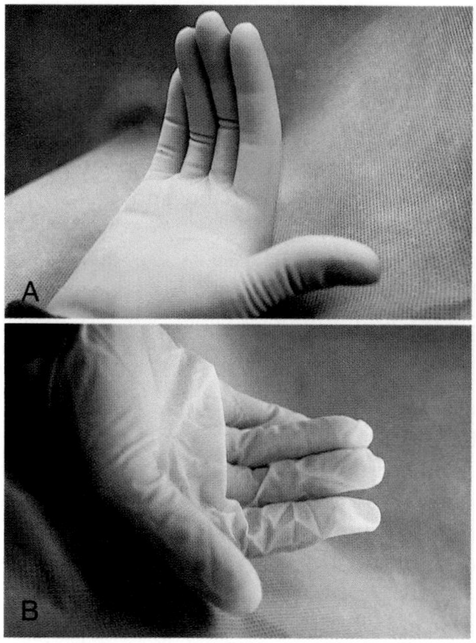

Figure 11-17. **A,** Glove is too tight. **B,** Glove is too loose.

decreased blood flow to the nerve functions of the arm. The compression occurs at the neck, where the scalene muscles create an outlet or tunnel. The nerves and blood vessels run from the neck into the arm and hand.

Symptoms

The symptoms of thoracic outlet compression are the following:

- Numbness and tingling along the side of arms and hands
- Neck and shoulder muscle spasms
- Weakness and clumsiness in hand and fingers
- Cold extremities
- Absence of radial pulse

Risk Factors

Poor posture is the main cause. Tilting the head too much, hunching the shoulders, and positioning the dental chair too high are risk factors for TOC.

Chairside Preventive Measures

The following measures can be taken to prevent thoracic outlet compression.

- Maintain proper clinician positions: head erect, back straight, shoulders in neutral position.
- Maintain proper height of dental chair and client positioning.

Assessing Symptoms

Signs relate to decreased motor function (nerve compression) and arterial symptoms (decreased blood flow).

Treatment

Initially, physical therapy, strengthening of posterior trunk and shoulder muscles, and posture retraining exercises are recommended. If the recommended treatment fails, surgery aimed at reducing the source of compression may be required. Scar tissue or, in some cases, a congenital extra rib may be the cause of compression. An incision is made under the arm where the nerves and brachial plexus are located.

Surgical Glove Injury

Ill-fitting gloves can contribute to surgical glove injury (SGI).[2] The glove should fit the hand and fingers snugly but be neither too tight nor too loose from fingers to forearm (Figure 11-17).

Symptoms

SGI is commonly mistaken for CTS and TOC because so many of the signs and symptoms, as follows, are similar:

- Tingling in fingers
- Cold extremities
- Loss of muscle control and hand strength
- Numbness or pain in fingers

Risk Factors

Wearing properly fitting gloves during dental care reduces RSI. When gloves are too tight, proper circulation to the clinician's hands and fingers is compromised, and pressure is placed on the carpal tunnel across the wrist. Wearing gloves that are too loose causes the clinician to grasp the instrument handle more tightly to compensate for the feeling of lack of control. Excess glove material at the fingertips hinders the clinician's ability to adequately roll the instrument in the fingers to adapt around line angles. The clinician compensates by twisting the wrist or by flexing and hyperextending the wrist.

Chairside Preventive Measures

The following measures can be taken to prevent surgical glove injury:

- Wear properly fitting gloves. Evaluate if gloves fit properly around fingertips, between fingers, between thumb and index finger, across palm of hand, and around wrist.
- Do TGEs and stretch the hand and fingers (see Figure 11-14).

Assessing Symptoms

Gloves that do not fit properly cause SGI. If symptoms arrest when gloves are taken off or when different gloves are worn, SGI may be determined.

Treatment of Surgical Glove Injury

Simply wearing properly fitting gloves may be the only treatment necessary. If pressure to the wrist and compression of the median nerve in the carpal tunnel continue, treatment as in CTS cases may be necessary.

Guyon's Canal Syndrome

Guyon's canal syndrome (GCS),[2] caused by ulnar nerve entrapment at the wrist, differs from CTS in that the ulnar nerve does not pass through the carpal tunnel. Rather the ulnar nerve passes through a tunnel formed by the pisiform and hamate bones and the ligaments that connect them.

Symptoms

The symptoms of Guyon's canal syndrome are the following:

- Numbness and tingling in little finger and right side of ring finger
- Loss of strength in lower forearm
- Loss of movement of small muscles in hand
- Clumsiness of hand

Risk Factors

During instrumentation it is important to hold the little finger close to the fulcrum finger for stability and control. Maintaining this position of the two fingers avoids RSI. Holding the little finger a full span away from the hand and fulcrum finger causes nerve entrapment and symptoms of GCS.

Chairside Preventive Measures

Attention placed on hand and finger position during instrumentation reduces GCS and includes the following:

- Repositioning of little finger during scaling and extrinsic stain removal
- Performing periodic hand stretches

Assessing Symptoms

During instrument adaptation and activation, symptoms will affect the little finger and half of the ring finger. If all digits are affected, GCS may not be a problem or may be one of several problems.

Treatment

Conservative treatment includes performing hand strengthening exercises; wearing a hand and wrist splint at night to decrease pinching of ulnar nerve and allow a decrease in inflammation; and taking prescribed anti-inflammatory medications. If these therapies fail, surgery may be indicated to relieve ulnar nerve entrapment. During the surgical procedure, cutting of the roof of the Guyon's canal is completed.

Trigger Finger Nerve Syndrome

Trigger finger nerve syndrome[2] (TFNS, or triggering) affects movement of the tendons as the fingers and thumb are bent (flexion) and moved. The tendons are held in place on the bones by a series of ligaments called *pulleys*. Friction is reduced by a slippery coating called *tenosynovium*, allowing the tendons to glide easily through the tendon sheaths. When the tendons and tendon sheaths are inflamed and tenosynovium thickens, a nodule forms from the constant irritation of the tendon being pulled through the pulley. As the finger is flexed, the nodule passes under the ligament and becomes stuck. The finger cannot be extended back to its original position.

Symptom

The primary symptom of trigger finger nerve syndrome is the inability to extend the fingers or thumb after flexing.

Risk Factors

Repetitive use of fingers and hands causes overuse of finger and thumb tendons. Overuse often results from fingers and thumb being flexed against resistance. Digital motion during instrumentation results in overuse of finger and thumb tendons. Also, pinching the instrument handle causes fingers and thumb to flex against resistance (Figure 11-18).

Chairside Preventive Measures

Minimizing finger motion and using proper grasp, fulcrum, and unified motion of the hand, wrist, and forearm decrease risk of TFNS.

- Maintain appropriate modified pen grasp for the procedure.
- Grasp instrument handle using finger and thumb pads instead of pinching with tips of fingers.

Assessing Symptoms

When a nodule forms on the fingers or thumb tendons, a palpable click will be felt as the nodule snaps under the finger pulley.

Treatment

Initial treatment with corticosteroids may reduce inflammation and shrink the nodule to relieve the triggering. In most cases a small surgical incision is made in the palm of the hand to locate the pulley in question. Once the pulley is located, it is cut, eliminating the triggering and nodule involvement.

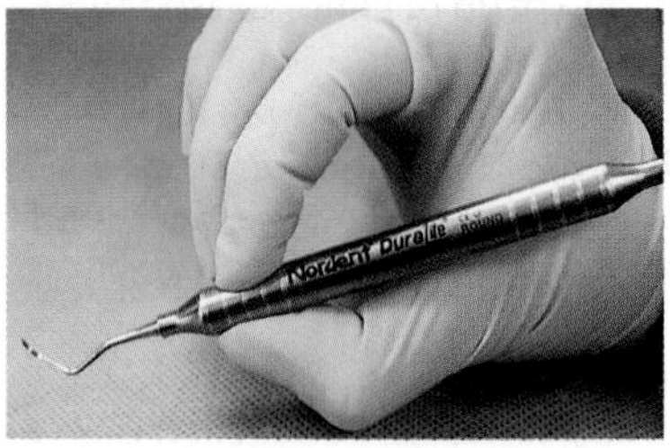

Figure 11-18. Pinched fingers on the instrument handle.

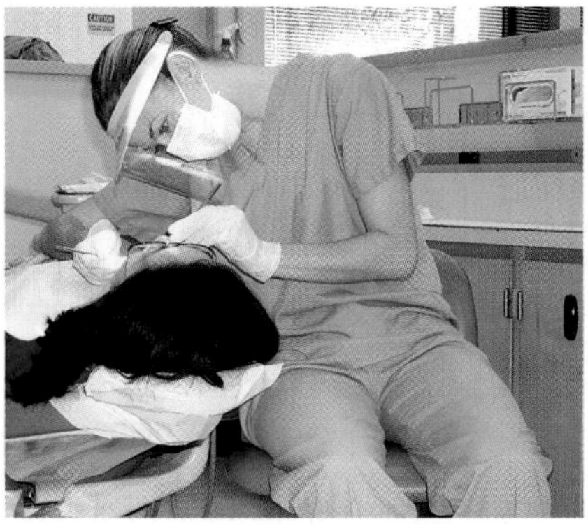

Figure 11-19. Wrist in ulnar deviation. Spine and neck out of alignment. (Courtesy Sarah Talamantes Carter, University of California at San Francisco.)

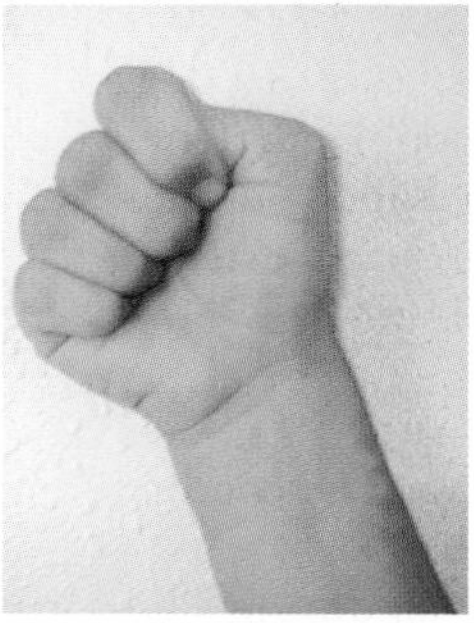

Figure 11-20. Finkelstein's test.

De Quervain's Syndrome

De Quervain's syndrome[2] is an inflammation of the tendons and tendon sheaths at the base of the thumb (the "anatomic snuff box"). This condition occurs from repetitive motion combining hand twisting and forceful gripping along with prolonged work with the wrist held in ulnar deviation (Figure 11-19). Symptoms occur when the pollicis longus and extensor pollicis longus tendons are unable to glide through the tunnel on the side of the wrist.

Symptoms

The symptoms of de Quervain's syndrome are the following:

- Aching and weakness of thumb (along the base)
- Pain migrating into forearm

Risk Factors

Repetitive ulnar deviation of the wrist while reaching for instruments or during instrumentation is the biggest risk factor causing de Quervain's syndrome. Twisting and bending the wrist in an ulnar direction (toward little finger) and using a forceful grip on instrument handles are also risk factors.

Chairside Preventive Measures

The following measures can be taken to prevent de Quervain's syndrome:

- Avoid ulnar wrist deviation during instrumentation.
- Eliminate twisting of wrist when reaching for dental instruments.
- Maintain a neutral wrist position and unified motion during dental care.

Assessing Symptoms

Finkelstein's test is a simple way to assess symptoms (Figure 11-20):

- Bend thumb into palm of hand. Grasp thumb with the four fingers.
- Place wrist in ulnar deviation position by bending wrist toward little finger.

Pain over tendons and tendon sheaths at the base of thumb indicates possible de Quervain's syndrome.

Treatment

Milder cases may simply require rest, prescribed anti-inflammatory medication, immobilization of wrist with a splint, and/or ergonomic adjustments to work environment. If the simple measures fail, corticosteroid injections and progressive physical and occupational therapy may be recommended. In severe or chronic cases, surgery to relieve pressure on the tendon, allowing more space for that tendon, may be in order.

Elbow and Forearm Injuries[10]

Strained Pronator Muscle

The muscle involved in a strained pronator muscle (SPM) injury is an elongated, narrow pronator muscle in the forearm and flexor of the elbow joint. The pronator muscle wraps around the anterior aspect of the elbow. SPM injury is caused by compression of the median nerve as it passes under the pronator muscle.

Symptoms

Compression of the median nerve causes symptoms similar to those experienced by clinicians with CTS.

Risk Factors

Repetitive and constant holding of the arms away from the body with the palm and thumb side of the hand rotated downward during instrumentation is a risk factor. This position commonly occurs during instrumentation of the maxillary right posterior sextant. With the palm in a downward position, the clinician's arm must rotate and twist. Hyperextension of wrist also occurs (see Figure 11-6, *B*).

Chairside Preventive Measures

The following measures can be taken to prevent a strained pronator muscle:

- Maintain neutral arm position: hold arms close to body.
- Maintain neutral wrist position during dental care procedures.
- Avoid rotation and twisting of forearm.

Assessing Symptoms

Symptoms are similar to those of CTS, but performing Phalen and Tinel tests would rule out compression of median nerve at the wrist (true CTS) because with this condition, compression occurs at the elbow. If the clinician is experiencing CTS symptoms but the tests rule out true CTS, SPM may be the cause.

Treatment

Therapy includes rest, anti-inflammatory medication, corticosteroid injections, environmental changes in workplace, and repositioning of clinician's body during instrumentation.

Lateral Epicondylitis

Lateral epicondylitis[11] (LE) is a degenerative elbow disorder. In spite of its common name (tennis elbow), the majority of cases are not from sports injuries. Rather it results from inflammation of the wrist extensor tendons on the lateral epicondyle of the elbow.

Symptoms

The symptoms of lateral epicondylitis are the following:
- Aching or pain in elbow
- Sharp shooting pain during elbow extension

Risk Factors

Repetitive and constant use of a forceful grip or grasp, forceful wrist and elbow movement, and extension of wrist during dental care increase risk.

Chairside Preventive Measures

The following measures can be taken to prevent lateral epicondylitis:
- Avoid wrist extension during dental care.
- Maintain proper neutral wrist position during instrumentation.
- Use proper clinician positions, allowing neutral body positions to be maintained.

Assessing Symptoms

Diagnosis of LE can be made by palpating the wrist extensor muscles at the lateral epicondyle of the elbow during resisted wrist extension. Pain during this exercise may indicate LE.

Treatment

Therapy includes rest, use of anti-inflammatory medications, alterations in work environment, a wrist splint to eliminate wrist extension, physical therapy, and corticosteroid injections.

Radial Tunnel Syndrome

Radial tunnel syndrome[12] (RTS) is a condition affecting the radial nerve entrapped in the radial tunnel. The radial nerve starts at the side of the neck and travels through the armpit and down the arm to the hands and fingers; the nerve passes in front of the elbow through the radial tunnel and allows the hand to turn in a clockwise direction.

Symptoms

Increased tenderness and pain at the lateral side of the elbow when arm and elbow are used may indicate RTS.

Chairside Preventive Measures

As with LE, maintaining proper wrist position and motion during care must be considered.

Assessing Symptoms

Unfortunately, RTS often is mistaken for LE. A history must be taken and assessed by the physician. Electrical tests also should be performed on the radial nerve.

Treatment

Therapy includes rest, anti-inflammatory medications, and possible surgery to relieve tension and pressure on radial nerve. A small incision is made on the outside of the elbow near area where the radial nerve travels into the forearm.

Cubital Tunnel Syndrome

Cubital tunnel syndrome[12] is a condition affecting the ulnar nerve as it crosses behind the elbow. The ulnar nerve controls the muscles in the right half of the ring finger and little finger of the hand. The ulnar nerve starts at the neck and runs through the armpit and down the arm to the hand and fingers. At the elbow the nerve crosses through a tunnel of muscle, ligament, and bone (cubital tunnel). When elbow is bent, the nerve is pulled up between bones, causing compression and entrapment of the ulnar nerve. When nerve compression occurs, impulses are slowed.

Symptoms

The symptoms of cubital tunnel syndrome are the following:
- Pain and numbness on outer side of ring and little fingers
- Pain sometimes relieved when elbow is straightened

Risk Factors

The clinician should avoid all prolonged gripping or grasping of instruments in palm of hand and holding the elbow in a flexed position during procedures.

Chairside Preventive Measures

The following measures can be taken to prevent cubital tunnel syndrome:
- Maintain a neutral elbow position during procedures.
- Alter instrument grasps; avoid prolonged use of palm grasp.
- Avoid repetitive crossing of arms across the chest.
- Avoid leaning on elbow when sitting at table.

Assessing Symptoms

To assess if pain and numbness in fourth and fifth fingers are being caused by ulnar nerve compression in the elbow, simply straighten the elbow. Pain or numbness usually disappears when the elbow is straight.

Treatment

Therapy consists of physical and occupational therapy, anti-inflammatory medications, and use of an elbow extension splint. If prescribed treatment fails, surgery may be required to create a new cubital tunnel for the ulnar nerve.

Shoulder Injuries[1,5]

Trapezius Myalgia

Trapezius myalgia[2,10] (TM) is caused by static loading in the shoulder or stabilizing muscles over a long period of time. This condition commonly is found in workers in repetitive action occupations.

Symptom

Pain and tenderness in descending part of trapezius muscle may indicate TM.

Risk Factors

Long dental procedures cause the clinician to remain in one position, resulting in static loading on muscles supporting the clinician's body weight.

Chairside Preventive Measures

The following measures can be taken to prevent trapezius myalgia:

- Manage appointment times: alternate long and short appointments.
- Take stretching breaks during long procedures.
- Change body positions.
- Maintain proper clinician positions to ensure proper body support.

Assessing Symptoms

Consistent pain and tenderness in area of trapezius muscle may indicate TM.

Treatment

Therapy consists of rest, physical therapy, massage, stretching exercises, and heat and ice regimens.

Rotator Cuff Injuries

Rotator cuff injuries (RCIs) include rotator cuff tendonitis and rotator cuff tears. Both affect the connective tissue in the shoulder and cause common shoulder pain. Most often affected is the supraspinatus tendon. RCIs are associated with repetitive motion and excessive, forceful exertion of shoulder and arm.

Symptoms

The symptoms of rotator cuff injuries are the following:

- Pain when lifting the arm 60 to 90 degrees
- Functional impairment

Risk Factors

Static loading on the shoulder muscles and improper body support leads to RCIs.

Chairside Preventive Measures

The following measures can be taken to prevent rotator cuff injuries:

- Avoid repetitive twisting and reaching.
- Maintain neutral shoulder and arm positions.
- Use proper clinician positions during dental care.

Assessing Symptoms

Constant shoulder pain and increased pain when raising arms may indicate an RCI. Physical therapy assessment, magnetic resonance imaging (MRI), and further medical testing may be needed for diagnosis.

Treatment

Therapy depends on degree of injury. Once tendon tears occur, treatment becomes complex. Physical therapy, corticosteroid injections, and anti-inflammatory medications may be required. If conservative therapy fails, surgery may be performed.

Adhesive Capsulitis

Adhesive capsulitis (AC), also known as *frozen shoulder,* results from immobility of the shoulder because of severe shoulder injury or repeated occurrences of rotator cuff tendonitis.

Symptoms

Symptoms are similar to those of RCIs:

- Pain in shoulder
- Limited range of shoulder motion

Risk Factors

Static loading and improper strain placed on shoulder joint owing to static loading increase risk for AC.

Chairside Preventive Measures

The following measures can be taken to prevent adhesive capsulitis:

- Avoid repetitive twisting and reaching.
- Maintain proper shoulder and arm positions: neutral positions.
- Use proper clinician positions and movement during instrumentation.

Assessing Symptoms

Limited range of motion and constant shoulder pain during lifting of arms along with a history of rotator cuff tendonitis may indicate AC.

Treatment

Therapy includes physical therapy and rehabilitation, anti-inflammatory drug therapy, electrical stimulation, and heat and ice regimens. If therapy fails, a noninvasive treatment of forced shoulder movement may be required with use of a general anesthetic.

Neck and Back Injuries

Lumbar Joint Dysfunction

Lumbar joint dysfunction[2] (LJD) occurs from repetitive and continued twisting and rotating of spine. With improper spine support during dental care delivery, the intervertebral disks experience tremendous pressure, possibly resulting in rupture or injury.

Symptoms

Spinal discomfort and pain in the lumbar region may indicate LJD.

Risk Factors

Right-handed clinicians sitting in the 8 o'clock position (4 o'clock for left-handed clinicians) find accessing specific areas of the client's mouth easier. However, too much rotation of the midsection of the clinician's body while in this position strains the lumbar curve. Care must be taken to avoid RSI while sitting in the 8 o'clock (4 o'clock) position.

Chairside Preventive Measures

The following measures can be taken to prevent lumbar joint dysfunction:

- Avoid twisting back and spine.
- Properly support body weight.
- Modify equipment placement to avoid twisting to reach.

Assessing Symptoms

Indications of LJD include constant lower back pain and limited movement of back and spine.

Treatment

Therapy includes rest, workplace adjustments, physical therapy, occupational therapy, drug therapy, and possibly surgery.

Tension Neck Syndrome

Also called *tension myalgia,* tension neck syndrome (TNS) involves the cervical muscles of the trapezius muscle.

Signs and Symptoms

The signs and symptoms of tension neck syndrome are the following:

- Pain or stiffness around cervical spine (neck)
- Pain between shoulder blades that may radiate down arms
- Muscle tightness and tenderness in neck
- Palpable hardness in neck
- Limited neck movement

Risk Factors

Risks include improper positioning of clinician's head and neck during dental care. The head must be held erect because bending the neck puts tremendous pressure and stress on cervical spine.

Chairside Preventive Measures

The following are measures that can be taken to prevent tension neck syndrome:

- Maintain proper clinician head and neck position to support neck and spine.
- Maintain proper height of dental chair and client position.
- Support weight of head over entire spine, not just cervical portion of spine.
- Keep back straight during dental care.
- Take periodic breaks and perform stretching exercises.

Assessing Symptoms

If limited neck motion partnered with pain and discomfort are experienced, TNS may be indicated.

Treatment

Treatment may include physical therapy, stretching exercises, and massage therapy. To increase blood flow, ultrasonic and electrical muscle stimulation may be required.

Cervical Spondylolysis and Cervical Disk Disease

Cervical spondylolysis (CS) and cervical disk disease (CDD)[1] lead to degeneration of the cervical spine. These RSIs affect the neck, scapula, shoulders, and arms, causing osteoarthritis of the cervical spine, disk degeneration, and herniation.

Signs and Symptoms

The signs and symptoms of cervical spondylolysis and cervical disk disease are the following:

- Stiffness and limited motion of neck
- Crepitus during active or passive neck movements
- Pain in upper and middle cervical region of spine
- Pain in scapula of shoulder regions
- Muscle spasms

Risk Factors

Repeated stress and strain placed on neck and cervical spine are risk factors.

Chairside Preventive Measures

The following measures can be taken to prevent cervical spondylolysis and cervical disk disease:

- Maintain proper clinician head and neck position to support neck and spine.
- Position clients for easy access to the mouth.

Assessing Symptoms

Monitor occurrence of pain and crepitus in cervical spine during neck motion.

Treatment

Therapy includes posture retraining exercises to restore normal curvature of spine, strengthening exercises for neck and back muscles, periods of rest, use of anti-inflammatory drugs, a cervical collar, and physical therapy.

To Change or Not to Change

Recognition of RSIs in dentistry was reported as early as 1946. Sixty-six percent of dentists complained of back pain after as little as 1 to 5 years of practice, and overall 78% felt they would eventually develop posture problems.[13] However, current literature documents that pain and discomfort continue among oral healthcare providers. Recognition of unsound ergonomic practices helps to stop the cycle of occupational pain for dental workers.

About 78% of practicing hygienists in Washington reported pain or discomfort in the neck, shoulders, arm, wrist, or hand.[14] Compliance with ergonomic principles is the foundation for a long, successful career in practice.

CLIENT EDUCATION TIPS

- Use of proper body mechanics during appointments contributes to client comfort and safety, and a successful therapeutic outcome.

LEGAL, ETHICAL, AND SAFETY ISSUES

- Dental hygienists have an ethical obligation to prevent disability and disease in themselves.
- Working while experiencing an untreated physical disability and pain may have ethicolegal implications if poor-quality care is the outcome.

KEY CONCEPTS

- Using ergonomic principles in the workplace reduces risk of repetitive strain injury (RSI).
- Client positioning is dependent on clinician positioning.
- Ergonomically designed equipment and proper positioning of clinician and client decrease risk of RSI to the dental hygienist.
- Grasp and hand stabilization during instrumentation reduce occurrence of RSI.
- Neutral wrist, arm, elbow, and shoulder positions decrease occurrence of RSI.
- Instrument maintenance, handle design, instrument manufacturing, and instrument choice affect clinician comfort and health.
- Regular strengthening and stretching exercises increase the flexibility and strength of muscles and tendons, reducing the risk of RSI in the clinician.
- If signs and symptoms of RSI occur, assessment of the environment and workplace practices should be conducted, and prompt medical attention sought.

CRITICAL THINKING EXERCISES

Practice positioning a client in the dental chair. The clinician must be positioned for access to and visibility of the client's mouth without compromising personal health and comfort.

1. Position the client in a semisupine position. If no adjustments are made to the clinician's position, what aspects of body dynamics are compromised? How can the clinician reposition and still follow ergonomic principles?
2. Position a small child in the dental chair. If no adjustments are made to the position of the clinician, what aspects of body health are compromised? How can the clinician reposition self, client, and chair to follow ergonomic criteria?
3. Position the client in the upright and Trendelenburg positions. When are these positions used?

REFERENCES

1. Michalak-Turcotte C: Controlling dental hygiene work–related musculoskeletal disorders: the ergonomics process. *J Dent Hyg* 74:41, 2000.
2. Michalak-Turcotte C, Atwood-Sanders M: Ergonomic strategies for the dental hygienist. *J Pract Hyg* 9:39, 2000.
3. Bird DL, Robinson DS: *Torres and Ehrlich modern dental assisting*, ed 9, St Louis, 2008, Saunders.
4. Sanders M, Turcotte C: Ergonomic strategies for dental professionals. *Am J Prev Assess Rehabil* 5:55, 1997.
5. Valachi B, Valachi K: Preventing musculoskeletal disorders in clinical dentistry: strategies to address the mechanisms leading to musculoskeletal disorders. *J Am Dent Assoc* 134:1604, 2003.
6. Pencek L: Vision and magnification for clinical dental hygiene practice. *RDH Mag* 27:50, 2007.
7. Slimmer-Beck M, Bray K, Branson B, et al: Comparison of muscle activity associated with structural differences in dental hygiene mirrors. *J Dent Hyg* 80:8, 2006.
8. Horstman S, Horstman B, Horstman F: Ergonomic risk factors associated with the practice of dental hygiene: a preliminary study. *Prof Saf* 42:49, 1997.
9. Mahoney J: Cumulative trauma disorders and carpal tunnel syndrome: sorting out the confusion. *Can J Plast Surg* 3:185, 1995.
10. Novak CB, Mackinnon SE: Repetitive use and static postures: a source of nerve compression and pain. *J Hand Ther* 10:151, 1997.
11. American College of Sports Medicine: *The American College of Sports Medicine fitness book*, ed 3, Champaign, Ill, 2003, Human Kinetics Publishers, Inc.
12. Tishler-Liskiewicz S, Kerschbaum W: Cumulative trauma disorders: an ergonomic approach for prevention. *J Dent Hyg* 7:162, 1997.
13. Dylia J, Forrest J: Fit to sit: strategies to maximize function and minimize occupational pain. *Access* 20:16, 2006.
14. Guignon AN: Comfort zone: turning the prevention spotlight on ourselves. *RDH Mag* 27:72, 2007.

EVOLVE RESOURCES

Please visit http://evolve.elsevier.com/Darby/hygiene for additional practice and study support tools.

CHAPTER 12

The Health History

Frieda Atherton Pickett

COMPETENCIES

1. **Explain the purpose of the health history, including legal and ethical issues regarding health record documentation.**
2. **Gather information pertinent to the health history by utilizing the technique of patient-centered interviewing.**
3. **Discuss decision making after the health history is obtained, including:**
   - **Recognize implications of client health status for dental hygiene care.**
   - **Understand the rationale and indications for preprocedure prophylactic antibiotics.**
   - **Identify the need for consultation and collaboration with other healthcare professionals in order to develop an individualized dental hygiene care plan.**

Purpose of the Health History

Collecting a complete **health history** allows the dental hygiene practitioner to assess a client's level of oral and systemic wellness, both past and present (Figure 12-1). By serving as a record of physical, emotional, and social health, the health history, in conjunction with the physical exam, provides the foundation for clinical decision making. When obtained in a culturally sensitive, patient-centered fashion, the health history allows the dental hygiene practitioner to establish a therapeutic relationship and improve quality of care. Information from the health history is used to determine health status, contraindications to care, and need for medical consultation before dental hygiene procedures are implemented. The health history allows for identification of existing health conditions that may influence clinical outcomes, such as healing, predisposition to infection, or oral disease progression. The health history also constitutes a legal document that provides past and present information about the client's personal, social, dental, and health status.

Health history assessment enables the dental hygiene practitioner to do the following:

- Understand client concerns, attitudes, and goals for the visit.
- Establish rapport with the client.
- Document baseline information about the patient's health status, including overall physical and emotional health, nutritional status, and vital signs.
- Identify key risk factors that affect the provision of dental hygiene care[1] and medical conditions that require special management before, during, or after care.
- Prepare for and prevent possible medical emergencies.
- Facilitate the medical and dental diagnoses of various conditions
- Recognize special physiologic states, such as pregnancy or menopause.
- Maintain legal documentation for managing client and practitioner risks and minimizing potential litigation.

Health History Assessment

Because health status is dynamic, the health history is monitored for changes at the beginning of each appointment to learn about changes in health since the last dental visit. A complete health history includes appropriately documenting a written health history, building rapport through patient-centered interviewing, and verifying key elements of the patient health status.

Documentation of Written Health History

In most practice settings, the client (Figure 12-2) completes a health history questionnaire at each visit before receiving professional services. This client-generated health information can be helpful in facilitating the gathering of the client health history; however, it is important then to clarify and validate the information during the interview. Issues of client illiteracy and poor reading comprehension make verbal confirmation of key health information on client-generated forms especially important. Regardless of the approach used, the dental hygiene practitioner must review the client's responses, assess their significance, and determine their implications for professional care and referral to the dentist or physician of record.

Although many formats for the written health history questionnaire are available, a preferable design includes a clearly demarcated area, usually at the top of the form, to identify critical medical information. This section includes high-risk conditions, such as allergies, hypertension, or antibiotic prophylaxis orders, to be considered before oral care is initiated.

Health History Oral Interview

The health history interview is the first step toward establishing rapport and trust to promote evidence-based interventions that follow. One of the primary objectives of the health history interview is to form a positive **dental hygiene practitioner–client relationship**. The dental hygiene practitioner–client relationship is a partnership with a mutual concern—the patient's well-being. Clients respond more completely to a friendly, caring, nonjudgmental interviewer. Therefore the practitioner must demonstrate verbally and nonverbally acceptance of the client's values. If a positive relationship has been established, the client will feel

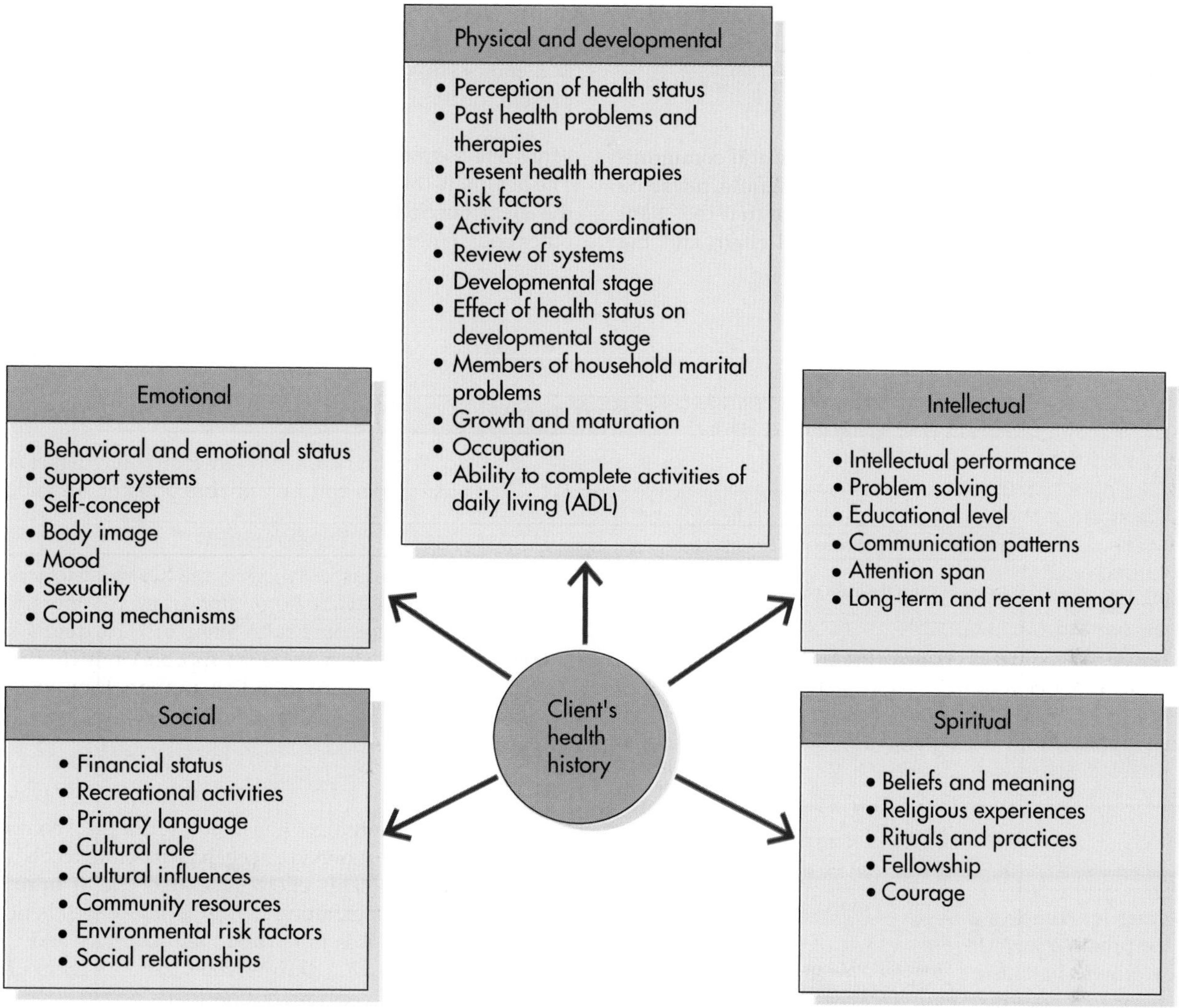

Physical and developmental
• Perception of health status
• Past health problems and therapies
• Present health therapies
• Risk factors
• Activity and coordination
• Review of systems
• Developmental stage
• Effect of health status on developmental stage
• Members of household marital problems
• Growth and maturation
• Occupation
• Ability to complete activities of daily living (ADL)
Emotional
• Behavioral and emotional status
• Support systems
• Self-concept
• Body image
• Mood
• Sexuality
• Coping mechanisms
Intellectual
• Intellectual performance
• Problem solving
• Educational level
• Communication patterns
• Attention span
• Long-term and recent memory
Client's health history
Social
• Financial status
• Recreational activities
• Primary language
• Cultural role
• Cultural influences
• Community resources
• Environmental risk factors
• Social relationships
Spiritual
• Beliefs and meaning
• Religious experiences
• Rituals and practices
• Fellowship
• Courage

Figure 12-1. Dimensions of the health history.

comfortable asking questions about treatments and will trust the practitioner's responses and recommendations.

Patient-Centered Interviewing

Preparing for the practitioner-client interaction begins when the client enters the healthcare setting. The dental hygiene practitioner should be attuned to identifying potential barriers to effective communication. Such barriers may include language or cultural differences, the presence of a physical or mental disability (i.e., hearing loss, dementia), or lack of familiarity with the healthcare system. Early recognition of these barriers is vital, because it enables the dental hygiene practitioner to gather all necessary personnel such as interpreters or social workers, and to plan an appropriate amount of time for the client interaction. There is heightened awareness, as the population becomes increasingly more culturally diverse and medically complex, that understanding and addressing these barriers to quality care should not be overlooked.[2]

Patient-centered interviewing is a technique in which clinicians seek to elicit the patient's emotions and personal health agenda to better understand the psychosocial context for disease. In contrast to solely gathering disease and symptom data in traditional clinician-centered interviewing, the patient-centered approach shifts focus on uncovering client concerns, anxieties, and perceptions of their disease.[3] Components of patient-centered interviewing include allowing the client to establish the agenda of the office visit ("What brought you in today?" and "What particular concerns do you have?") and engaging in emotion-seeking language ("How did that make you feel?" or "Why do you think this is happening to you?"). Patient-centered interviewing also involves using open-ended questions, or questions that require more than a yes/no response. For example, the dental hygiene practitioner may investigate a symptom by saying, "Tell me more about the chest pain you reported on the questionnaire." (See Chapter 5 for more detail.) This technique leads to a discussion in which the client describes the issue, often providing more relevant details, which help determine the risks of providing oral care and whether physician or dentist consultation is indicated.

Patient-centered interviewing is meant not to replace but to complement the clinician-centered technique. Incorporating elements of patient-centered interviewing enables the clinician to better appreciate the client as a person rather than a disease, thus improving the therapeutic relationship while increasing client and provider satisfaction.[4]

Interview Setting

A private setting ensures client confidentiality and communicates respect. The health history interview should never be conducted in hearing range of others. Ensure that the client is comfortably seated upright in the dental chair, and the dental hygiene practitioner is adjacent at eye level with the client. The interview should occur in private unless the client is a minor, in which case the parent or legal guardian is present, or if an interpreter is needed.

Verbal and Nonverbal Communication

The health history interview is also an opportunity to observe the client's use of eye contact, nonverbal communication, and other body language. Close observation of the client's written,

DENTAL HISTORY

Name ______________________________ Date ______________________________

Part I. Dental Experiences and Symptoms

1. What is the main reason for your visit?

____

2. When you look inside your mouth, do you know what to look for?

	Yes	No
Tooth Decay	☐	☐
Oral Cancer	☐	☐
Gum Disease	☐	☐
Cold Sores	☐	☐

3. Have you had dental x rays in the past 2 years?

☐ Yes Type ______________ ☐ No

4. Have you had any complications or negative experiences associated with previous dental treatment?

☐ Yes Explain ______________________________
☐ No

5. Generally, how have you felt about your previous dental appointments?

☐ Very anxious and afraid
☐ Somewhat anxious and afraid
☐ Don't care one way or the other
☐ Look forward to it

6. How much do you agree or disagree with this statement: oral health affects general health.

☐ Strongly agree ☐ Agree ☐ Disagree ☐ Strongly disagree

7. Are you experiencing any of the following symptoms? (please check all that apply)

☐ Sensitive teeth
☐ Bleeding gums
☐ Bad breath
☐ Swelling inside mouth
☐ Sinus problems
☐ Sore jaw
☐ Difficulty chewing
☐ Burning sensation
☐ Tartar buildup
☐ Difficulty swallowing
☐ Toothache
☐ Filling fell out
☐ Abscess
☐ Yellowing teeth
☐ Sore gums
☐ Dry mouth
☐ Recession

8. Do you clench or grind your teeth in the daytime or at night?

☐ Yes ☐ No
If yes, do you wear a bite guard? ________ For how long? ________

9. In the past two years, have you been concerned about your breath or the appearance of your teeth or face?

(If yes, please check all that apply)

☐ Yellowing/graying teeth
☐ Stains
☐ Crowded, crooked teeth
☐ Spacing between teeth
☐ Gums
☐ Facial profile
☐ Bad breath

10. Have you experienced any injuries to your teeth, face and jaw?

☐ Yes Explain ______________________________
☐ No

11. Have you experienced any of the following?

☐ Root planing
☐ Tooth extractions
☐ Dental implants
☐ Root canals
☐ Gum surgery
☐ Orthodontics/braces
☐ Head and neck radiation therapy
☐ Jaw surgery
☐ Severe pains of face/head
☐ Bad reaction to a local anesthetic
☐ Prolonged bleeding after dental treatment
☐ Other

A

Figure 12-2. **Sample dental history questionnaire. A,** Dental experiences and symptoms.

Part II. Oral Self-Care

1. Check the following you regularly use at home:

☐ Soft toothbrush	☐ Dental floss	☐ Floss threader	☐ Fluoride rinse or gel
☐ Hard toothbrush	☐ Special brush	☐ Toothpick	☐ Fluorideted drops/tablets
☐ Medium toothbrush	☐ Floride toothpaste	☐ Mouth rinse	☐ Fluoridated water
☐ Oral irrigator	☐ Rubber tip	☐ Whitening products	☐ Fluoridated water at day care
☐ Denture adhesive	☐ Powered interdental cleaner		☐ Bottled water
☐ Denture cleaner	☐ Power brush		☐ Other ______

2. Check the type of toothpaste you use:

☐ Fluoride	☐ Tartar control	☐ Gum benefit	☐ Multiple benefit
☐ Sensitivity protection	☐ Baking soda	☐ Peroxide	

3. Estimate how long it takes you to clean your teeth and gums each time:
Please indicate your best and most reliable estimate.

Brushing ______ (time) Flossing ______ (time)

4. About how many times each day/week do you brush and floss?

brush about ______ times per day OR ______ times per week
floss about ______ times per day OR ______ times per week

5. Do you find it difficult to maintain an oral hygiene schedule due to your job or other reasons ?

☐ Yes ☐ No

6. Do any conditions make it difficult for you to adequately clean your teeth?
(If yes, please check all that apply)

☐ Hold a toothbrush ☐ Use dental floss ☐ Brush/floss for any length of time ☐ Poor vision

7. Do you perform a monthly self-exam for oral cancer? ☐ Yes ☐ No

Part III. Between-Meal Snacks

Please check which sweets and starches you eat between meals frequently

Food	Frequency	Food	Frequency
☐ Breath mints	______	☐ Canned/bottled beverages	______
☐ Cough drops	______	☐ Sugared liquids	______
☐ Chewing gum	______	☐ Chips	______
☐ Dried fruits	______	☐ Crackers	______
☐ Cookies	______	☐ Others	______

B

Part IV. Beliefs About Oral Health

1. In your opinion, compared with the average person, how likely do you think you are to have cavities or other problems with your teeth and/or gums?

☐ Much more likely ☐ About average ☐ Much less than average
☐ More than average ☐ Less than average

2. How important is it for you to prevent cavities, gum problems, or other diseases of the mouth?

☐ Very important ☐ Somewhat important ☐ Not at all important

3. I believe that I have control over the condition of my mouth. ☐ Yes ☐ No

4. I believe that my oral health is

☐ Excellent ☐ Good ☐ Fair ☐ Poor

C

Comments ______________________________

____

Figure 12-2, cont'd B, Oral self-care and between-meal snacks. **C,** Beliefs about oral health.

verbal, and nonverbal communication can provide important clues that may assist in management. For example, if the client reports no fear of dental care but grasps the arms of the dental chair and appears anxious, the data conflict. This identifies the need to gather more information to resolve the apparent conflict of information with the goal of preventing a medical emergency such as **vasovagal syncope**, a common cause of fainting.

The client interview is also an opportunity for the dental hygiene practitioner to use strong verbal and nonverbal communication skills. The use of eye contact and listening skills enhances communication. A listening technique called **back channeling** includes neutral, encouraging responses such as "I see" or "uh-huh," or nonverbal cues such as nodding and attentive gaze, which indicates the dental hygiene practitioner is actively listening and has understood

BOX 12-1

Strategies to Enhance Communication

Silence provides the patient with time to organize thoughts and shows respect.
Attentive listening demonstrates interest in client's needs, concerns, and problems. Maintain eye contact, remain relaxed, and use appropriate "back channeling" techniques.
Conveying acceptance demonstrates the interviewer's willingness to listen to client's beliefs, values, and practices without being judgmental.
Paraphrasing, or repeating what the patient has said in more specific words, provides an opportunity to validate information without changing the meaning of the client's statement.
Clarifying facilitates accurate communication of information (e.g., asking the client to restate the information or provide an example). When *asking questions,* try to use an open-ended format with words and word patterns the client would understand.
Focusing eliminates vagueness in communication, limits the area of discussion, and helps the interviewer direct attention to the pertinent aspects of a client's message.
Stating observations provides the patient with feedback about observed behavior, action, facial expression, or activities. It also allows the interviewer to gauge the client's reaction.
Offering information allows the interviewer to clarify treatments, initiate health education, and identify and correct misconceptions.
Summarizing condenses and validates data; client has opportunity to confirm data are correct. Summarizing indicates the end to a particular part of the interview.

Adapted from Potter PA, Perry AG: *Fundamentals of nursing,* ed 7, St Louis, 2009, Mosby.

the client. In addition, the dental hygiene practitioner may use other communication strategies to facilitate communication (Box 12-1).

Completing a Comprehensive Health History

Before asking clients to share personal information, dental professionals may want to explain that this additional health information helps plan optimal care. The dental hygiene practitioner also assures the client that all information will be held in confidence. A comprehensive health history should contain the following information:

- **Demographic information.** This includes the client's name, current address, phone numbers (cellular, home, and business), date of birth, gender, referral source, types of insurance coverage, emergency contact information, and names of the dentist and physician of record with addresses and phone numbers. Such information is necessary for conducting the business aspects of the dental practice, establishing a familiarity with new clients, and facilitating follow-up care. Table 12-1 explains items included in client demographics and identifies implications for professional oral care.
- **Chief complaint.** The chief complaint is the client's primary reason for seeking the oral healthcare appointment and is recorded in the client's own words. Inquiring about the reason for the appointment clarifies the patient's needs and identifies potential topics for education or community resources required to meet the client's chief complaint and expectations. The patient's primary concern should be addressed early in the care plan, no matter how minor, to facilitate patient satisfaction, trust, and cooperation.
- **Dental history.** The dental history is important for planning care and oral health education. A separate dental history form may be used to collect this information (see Figure 12-2). Items included in the dental history are explained in Table 12-2. Information collected about the client's experiences with dentistry includes the following:
  - Previous dental treatments, frequency of treatments, related complications, and negative experiences
  - Current symptoms and concerns (e.g., fear of dental care, bleeding gums, loose teeth, oral malodor, toothache, swelling inside the mouth, appearance of teeth)
  - Current oral habits (e.g., bruxism, nail biting, thumb-sucking, cheek biting, tobacco use)
  - Oral self-care practices (e.g., products or home remedies used; methods, frequency, and duration of use)
  - Fluoride history (e.g., use of fluoridated community water; home water filtration; bottled water; fluoride toothpaste, rinses, drops, tablets)
  - Other oral care products used (e.g., antimicrobial mouth rinse, moisturizing mouth rinse, saliva substitute, amorphous calcium phosphate, xylitol gum, or mints)
  - Frequency and type of between-meal snacks
  - Beliefs and values related to oral health, noting if family members wear dentures
- **Medical history.** Medical history documents the client's overall medical health and identifies need for physician consultation. Medical history includes diagnosed medical conditions, current symptoms suggestive for undiagnosed conditions, medications taken on a regular basis (see Chapter 14 for more on the pharmacologic history), alcohol and other drug use, and allergies or unusual drug reactions. For example, a client with history of an aortic valve replacement would require antibiotic prophylaxis against bacterial endocarditis before dental procedures.[5] Systemic conditions such as high blood pressure, hemophilia, or diabetes should be discussed so that safe care can be planned. A comprehensive explanation of medical history items is provided in Table 12-3.
- **Social history.** This includes marital status, occupation, children or dependents, living situation, cultural practices related to health and disease, and any identifiable barriers to seeking or delivering adequate health care.

Legal and Ethical Issues Related to the Health History

The client's health history is confidential and is required by law to be protected from others unless the client's permission is obtained. Office policies to ensure client privacy are required by the **Health Insurance Portability and Accountability Act** (HIPAA). HIPAA protects all "individually identifiable" personal health information, or health-related information that can be reasonably linked to a client using name, birth date, address, or Social Security Number, from being provided to others without the written approval of the client or client's guardian.[6] One exception to this HIPAA "Privacy Rule" is in the case of an emergency situation in

Text continued on p. 179

TABLE 12-1

Demographics Explained

Items	Rationale	Implications for Professional Care
Name, address, email, telephone and fax numbers, gender, marital status, emergency contact, date of form completion	Conduct business aspect of the practice. Establish rapport with patient. Indicate date of most recent update of information. Determine emergency contact information.	Address is used to facilitate communication and send relevant information where patient resides. Health history should be updated at each appointment. Contact information is needed in case of emergency.
Insurance information	Determine who is responsible for payment for dental care. Identify financial barriers related to treatment plan.	Appropriate assessment planning will be needed to manage financial matters.
Date of birth	Indicate the client's age accurately. Assist in identifying age-related conditions. Legal issues for consent of care	The client who is a minor or who lacks decision-making capacity will need parent or guardian to consent for treatment. Older adults (≥age 65) may be prone to orthostatic hypotension. Follow protocol to prevent orthostatic hypotension, raise chair back slowly. Allow upright positioning for several minutes before moving from dental chair.
Height, weight	Consider when calculating drug dosages. Assess risk for medical complications related to obesity or overweight (risk for cardiovascular disease, diabetes, etc.).	For overweight clients, question about risk for diabetes and hypertension. Monitor vital signs to assess cardiovascular status. Maximum dose limitations for local anesthetic agent with vasoconstrictor may be a consideration (less for very old or very young or for a client with severe cardiovascular disorder). Marked weight change may be sign of an underlying disease; physician referral may be indicated.
Previous dentist, address, and phone number	Provide for acquiring prior client dental records and radiographs. Provide for consultation with previous dentist.	Client records can be used for prior dental treatment and current needs. Radiographs must be current to assess current needs adequately, but former radiographs provide basis for comparison and monitoring change.
Physician's name and phone number	Assist in medical consultation. Assist in emergency management should medical emergency occur.	Physician orders or consultation notes are incorporated into treatment plan for dental hygiene care. Physician is contacted rapidly in case of medical emergency.
Referral source	Identify who should receive acknowledgment.	Assist in establishing rapport. Send letter of appreciation to referral source.

TABLE 12-2

Health History Items Explained

Item	Purpose	Relevant Questions	Implications for Professional Care
1. Chief complaint	Identify purpose of dental appointment.	What brings you in today?	Address chief complaint to improve client satisfaction.
2. Prior dental care	Identify types of preventive, restorative, surgical, rehabilitative care. Indicate if client has regular dental care or wears appliances.	When was your last visit to have your teeth cleaned? What treatment was provided? Any problems with prior dental treatment? Have you ever had braces, root canals, teeth removed, dental appliances, dental implants, or any other type of special care? Do you feel anxious about this appointment?	Provide overview of prior dental care and client/family experience with dentistry. Identify specialized maintenance-care needs (orthodontic wires, abutments, prosthesis, implant care, etc.). Fearful, anxious client may be identified; need for stress-reduction protocol is established.

Continued

TABLE 12-2

Health History Items Explained—cont'd

Item	Purpose	Relevant Questions	Implications for Professional Care
3. Radiation history	Identify if recent radiographs have been taken or must be requested from previous dentist. Alert: Limit oral radiographic exposure to necessary films. Alert: If large exposure to radiation is reported (e.g., cancer therapy), limit exposure to minimally necessary films.	When was the last time you had dental x-rays taken? What areas were exposed? How many films taken? Have you had radiation treatment? If so, were the head and neck exposed? What areas of the body received radiation?	Request prior oral radiographs from former dentist. Take only films necessary to diagnose current problem. Consider amount of radiation exposure from past dental and medical sources.
4. Complications during dental treatment	Avoid similar complications. Identify allergy-related complications.	What problem occurred? Do you know why it happened? How was it treated? What was the outcome? Do you have allergies to any medicines or other substances? What reaction do you have?	Complications can be a source of client dissatisfaction; avoid repeating the complication. Avoid using substances that may incite allergy.
5. Dental treatment anxiety	Identify patients prone to anxiety reactions. Identify need for stress-reduction protocol. Alert: Physician consultation if cause of reaction is unknown Alert: Fear is a strong predictor for a medical emergency (syncope, hyperventilation).	Many clients have anxiety about dental care; how do you feel about it? What caused you to fear dental treatment? Have you ever taken a drug to reduce your anxiety? Does it work? How can I help you accept oral care?	Be empathetic and caring regarding client anxiety. Establish confidence and trust. Invite patient to alert you if patient wants treatment to stop. Tell client you will try to prevent pain from occurring; use local anesthesia, and consult with dentist about anxiolytic drug therapy. Fears of parents about dental treatment are often transferred to children.
6. Client's perception of relationship between health and oral health	Assess client's understanding of relationship between oral health and systemic health. Assess expectations surrounding oral health and maintaining teeth.	What do you know about how your oral health affects the rest of your body? How do you feel about keeping your teeth the rest of your life? Do you think you can?	Educate client on role of oral health in total well-being. Consider medical conditions that are affected by poor oral health (diabetes, history of infective endocarditis).
7. Adverse oral symptoms reported by patient	Indicate conditions (sensitivity, pain, abscess, cracked tooth, receding gums, gingival ulceration).	What causes the problem? When did it start? Is there any pain? When does it occur? Ask about situations that may provoke, worsen, or improve the symptom (when biting down, cold foods, hot foods, soft foods, crunchy foods). Assess for traumatic self-care.	Examine oral tissues for evidence of disease. Avoid air from syringe in area. Inform client about cause of problem, if known, and necessary treatment. Recommend oral products to relieve symptoms (desensitizing agent, fluoride). Observe self-care and correct as needed.
7a. Chewing ability	Identify conditions that impair chewing (e.g., ill-fitting denture or appliance, missing teeth, extensive decay).	What causes the difficulty? How do you feel about getting the missing teeth replaced?	Refer to dentist for correction of problem. Consider nutritional counseling until problem is resolved.

TABLE 12-2
Health History Items Explained—cont'd

Item	Purpose	Relevant Questions	Implications for Professional Care
7b. Periodontal health	Indicate medical conditions related to loss of periodontal health (e.g., leukemia, neoplasm, immunosuppression, poor nutrition). Identify cause(s) of periodontal disease.	Do your gums bleed when you brush or floss? How often do you clean your teeth? Do you have loose teeth? Bad taste? Receding gums? How long has this occurred? Do you know why?	Correlate health history information to determine potential causes. Complete periodontal assessment for biofilm control and gingival architecture, and recommend appropriate oral hygiene devices. Recommend appropriate maintenance care interval.
7c. Sores in mouth	Identify cause of lesion (e.g., trauma, herpes virus, aphthae, trauma, leukemia, blood dyscrasia, syphilis). Identify malignancy or medical disorder.	Where are the sores? How long have they been present? Is cause known?	Take appropriate precautions for infectious lesions. Determine differential diagnosis and make appropriate referrals or delay treatment. Poor healing requires referral to medical facility or oral-maxillofacial surgeon.
8. Oral habits	Identify habits that reduce oral health, and make recommendations to stop habit. Alert: Identify potentially dangerous habits (e.g., holding nails or pins between teeth, biting fingernails).	Do you clench or grind your teeth? Do you suck your thumb? Does your child use a pacifier? Do you know what is causing this problem?	Try to determine impact of oral habit and counsel to stop habit behavior.
9. Satisfaction with teeth, face, breath	Identify conditions that relate to dissatisfaction (e.g., periodontal disease, lack of regular dental care, medical problems, developmental issue).	What causes dissatisfaction? What have you considered to improve situation? How do you feel about getting your teeth repaired? Treatment to correct abnormality?	Based on cause of disorder, schedule appointment for orodental evaluation. Provide options for cosmetic procedures or dental care to correct situation (e.g., orthodontic procedure, crown, bridge).
10. Injury to teeth, face, jaw	Identify temporomandibular joint (TMJ) dysfunction, difficulty opening jaw, fracture, malocclusion.	Can you open your mouth wide? Have you had a blow to your face or jaw? Treatment?	Short appointment to reduce time that jaw is opened, reduce fatigue. Use mouth prop as needed for client comfort.
11. Oral biofilm control	Identify efficiency of oral hygiene technique. Determine the need for caregiver intervention.	Tell me what you do currently to care for your teeth. Can you show me how you brush? How often do you floss? What do you use to clean your teeth? What type of brush do you use (manual, powered, soft, hard)? How often? How long usually? When do you replace your toothbrush? Any other devices (oral irrigation)? Use mouth rinse? What dentifrice?	Determine the need for product recommendations. Determine topics for oral health education plan. Determine need to educate caregiver.

Continued

TABLE 12-2

Health History Items Explained—cont'd

Item	Purpose	Relevant Questions	Implications for Professional Care
12. Fluorides, sealants	Determine need for supplemental fluoride or placement of dental sealant.	Do you use fluoride products? How often do you drink bottled beverages? Did you have fluoridated water growing up? Do you want a topical fluoride treatment today? Have you had sealants placed on teeth?	Consider potential for fluorosis and educate appropriately. Provide appropriate caries control recommendations. May need to discuss use of xylitol or amorphous calcium phosphate products.
13. Sugar and beverage consumption	Identify source of related disorder (caries; stain from coffee, tea; erosion). Alert: Note consumption of caries-promoting foods.	How often do you snack between meals? How often do you drink sugar-sweetened beverages or juice? Do you drink sugar-free drinks? Use bottled water often? Drink coffee or tea? Use sugar or honey in it? How often each day?	Counsel about caries risk based on habits and products consumed. Suggest strategies to avoid snacking or healthier between-meal snack options. Seek client agreement on need to reduce snacking to reduce caries risk.
14. Beliefs about oral health	Identify motivational strategies based on human needs theory.	How do you feel about keeping your teeth all your life? Do you think you can? How important is your oral health to you?	Consider client value system for oral health and develop persuasive strategy to promote a desire for maintaining teeth and reducing oral disease. Try to get client to set personal goals to maintain oral health.

TABLE 12-3

Medical History Items Explained

Item	Purpose	Relevant Questions	Implications for Professional Care
I. General Health			
1. Estimation of general health	Determine client's estimate of personal health. Identify incongruent data in client vs. clinician assessment of health status.	How is your health?	Conflicting information compared with health history information requires investigation; client may misunderstand health status. Modifications must be made if a significant disability or medical condition is reported.
2. Change in general health	Investigate response and consider relevance of explanation.	Has there been any recent change in your health? What has happened?	Determine if medical consultation is warranted for more acute changes.
3. Last physical examination	Identify client who does not seek regular medical care and has risk for undiagnosed disease.	When was your last physical exam? What were the results? Who performed the examination?	Many patients have infrequent physical examinations. Determine if client health is monitored for health risks. Monitor vital signs to assess health.
4. Currently under medical care and reason	Identify current health status. Determine if chronic health problems exist. Determine risk for medical emergency.	For what conditions do you see a doctor? How are you being treated? Any complications?	Consider care modifications for medically compromised conditions. Determine physician treating condition and make consultation relevant to oral care.

TABLE 12-3

Medical History Items Explained—cont'd

Item	Purpose	Relevant Questions	Implications for Professional Care
5. Serious illness, hospitalization in past 5 years	Identify recent surgeries or hospitalizations. Identify potential condition needing antibiotic prophylaxis, e.g., cardiac valve replacement. Client may be self-administering drugs.	When were you last hospitalized? Why? Are you recovered? Any complications? Ever had surgery? Do you take any special medication as a result of the illness or hospitalization?	Identify medical condition that may affect oral care plan. Pharmacologic effect and possible interactions of drug is investigated. Identify condition that may require antibiotic prophylaxis before dental hygiene procedures. Determine if stress-reduction protocol is indicated.
6. Medical radiation or x-ray examination in past 5 years and explanation	Identify cancer therapy or other medical problem (e.g., hyperthyroidism). **Alert:** Limit oral radiographic exposure.	What type of x-ray examinations and for what purpose? Was this diagnostic radiation or treatment for a disorder? Do you have any complications from radiation therapy? If so, describe them.	Determine current health status based on reason for radiation therapy. Determine need for oral care product recommendations based on oral needs. Digital oral radiographs have lower ionizing radiation exposure compared to traditional films. Take only films necessary for diagnosis.
7. Medications including nonprescription, herbs	Identify current drug or herbal effects relevant to oral care. Consider effects of drug or herb and potential side effects relevant to oral care.	Ask why each drug or herb is being taken, dose, and frequency. Have you noticed any side effects from drug? (Use drug reference for potential side effects relevant to oral procedures.)	Identify preparations to investigate in drug reference. Drug effects or side effects may influence patient management (xerostomia, bleeding, drug-influenced gingival enlargement, vital sign changes). Consider medical conditions being managed pharmacologically and their effect on oral care (e.g., interaction with local anesthesia).
8. Allergies and reaction	Identify allergy to drugs and substances used in dental and dental hygiene care. Differentiate between true allergic reaction and side effect.	Did you have hives, rash, or itching, or become short of breath? Did you report this to your physician?	True allergic reactions usually involve rash, itching, or anaphylaxis (facial swelling, bronchial constriction, hypotension, shock). Antibiotic: Use appropriate agent from a different class. If client is allergic to penicillin, select clindamycin. Avoid offending drug (and drug class) when allergy exists.
II. Medical Conditions			
9(a). Cardiovascular disease Artificial heart valves or prosthetic material for cardiac valve repair, prior infective endocarditis, unrepaired cyanotic congenital heart disease, repaired CHD with prosthetic material within 6 months of procedure, valvular disease in a cardiac transplant	These are cardiac conditions that may be indicated for antibiotic prophylaxis before dental hygiene procedures. **Alert:** Medical consultation may be necessary.	Do you have any medical problems with your heart? Tell me about the cardiac condition and when it developed. Has your physician told you to take antibiotics before dental treatment? Did you take your antibiotic? What did you take? What dose, and how long ago did you take it?	Investigate cardiac condition and current outcome; may need medical consultation. If applicable, record antibiotic agent, dose, and time administered in record. Current regimen suggests taking appropriate antibiotic ½ to 1 hour before appointment; if inadvertently forgotten, can be administered at dental appointment or within 2 hours of appointment. Advise client to notify dentist if fever develops within 2 weeks of appointment, as this is a sign of possible endocarditis.

Continued

TABLE 12-3
Medical History Items Explained—cont'd

Item	Purpose	Relevant Questions	Implications for Professional Care
9(b). Vascular disease (heart trouble, heart attack and coronary artery disease, chest pain [angina], hypertension, arteriosclerosis, stroke, cardiac bypass, cardiac surgery)	Identify cardiac disease, specific condition. Determine functional capacity and extent of cardiac muscle damage.	Have you experienced any medical problems with your heart or blood vessels? When? What was the outcome? Is the condition controlled? Do you take any medication for it? Did you have complications from the condition or the medical therapy? Has your physician warned you about receiving dental care?	Monitor vital signs and functional capacity to assess cardiovascular recovery.[5] Determine time since cardiovascular event and physician recommendations regarding dental care. Recent event may require physician consultation. Prior MI (myocardial infarction; heart attack) requires 1 month for convalescence; stroke requires 6 months' convalescence before dental hygiene care can be provided.
9(b) 1. Do you have chest pain on exertion?	Identify coronary arteriosclerosis and reduced blood flow to cardiac muscle. **Alert:** There is an increased risk for unstable angina or heart attack. Identify nitroglycerin therapy.	Tell me more about your chest pain. When does it occur? What do you do for it? What makes it better? Worse? Do you have a recent prescription for nitroglycerin? When was your last attack of chest pain? What were you doing? Has it occurred at a dental appointment?	Determine the risk for an anginal attack during the appointment. Ensure nitroglycerin is brought to all appointments by nitrate-dependent client and that date on bottle shows prescription is current. If angina occurs, administer no more than three sublingual tablets over 10 minutes. Ensure client is lying or safely seated, as hypotension and syncope can occur. Monitor blood pressure every 5 minutes during angina management. Record management procedure in record.
9(b) 2. Are you ever short of breath after mild exercise or when lying down? Can you walk up a flight of stairs without stopping to rest?	Determine client's functional capacity.	What does your physician say about your shortness of breath or problem in walking up stairs? Let me know if you begin to feel any problem as I provide treatment.	Cardiologists report that in patients with history of myocardial infarction (MI) or heart failure, the degree of functional capacity relates to ability to receive noncardiac procedures.[5] Adequate functional capacity to receive dental procedures includes ability to walk a block at a moderate speed or ability to climb a flight of stairs without stopping.[5] A contraindication to dental care exists if MI occurred less than 1 month previously.
9(b) 3. How many pillows do you need to sleep?	**Alert:** Identify uncontrolled congestive heart disease. Determine reason for needing upright position to sleep.	Have you always used that number of pillows to sleep? Why do you need to be upright to sleep? Have you been evaluated for heart failure?	Inability to sleep in a supine position may be a sign of congestive heart failure. Investigate if medical evaluation has been completed and, if so, results of that evaluation. Stress can exacerbate heart failure. Consider medical consultation and implementing stress-reduction protocol.
9(b) 4. Do your ankles swell?	Identify initial signs of heart failure. Leg and ankle swelling also may relate to noncardiac reason such as venous varicosities or pregnancy.	Do you know why your ankles swell? Have you seen your physician about it? Any pain associated with swelling?	Determine reason for swelling. Pain is not a feature of swelling in extremities associated with heart failure. Determine if condition has been medically evaluated.

TABLE 12-3
Medical History Items Explained—cont'd

Item	Purpose	Relevant Questions	Implications for Professional Care
9(b) 5. Do you have an implanted cardiac pacemaker or defibrillator?	Indicates cardiac disorder but no need for antibiotic prophylaxis. Ultrasonic scaler is not contraindicated for shielded pacemakers.	When was your last pacemaker implanted? Any complications since the procedure?	Medtronic, St. Jude, or Guidant brands of pacemaker are not disrupted by electromagnetic ultrasonic scaler or unit. Monitor pulse rate for regularity, qualities. No indication for antibiotic prophylaxis.
9(b) 6. Have you recently had severe headaches?	**Alert:** Identify signs of prestroke condition.	Have you seen your physician to learn the cause of headaches? Have you ruled out sinus issues and migraine?	Try to identify the cause of the severe headaches. Medical consultation may be indicated. Monitor blood pressure, as severe hypertension increases risk of stroke.
10(a). Allergy, hives, skin rash	**Alert:** Identify dentally related allergens.	Do you have any allergies? What reaction do you have? How do you treat it?	Avoid using a product to which client is allergic. Monitor vital signs, client appearance, and respiration characteristics.
10(b). Sinus trouble, hay fever, cold	Determine risk for airway constriction.	Do you have any cold symptoms? Any trouble with your sinuses? Any postnasal drainage today?	Consider need for semisupine chair position. Determine risk for spread of infection.
11(a). Respiratory problems (emphysema, bronchitis, chronic obstructive pulmonary disease [COPD]) 11(b). Asthma	**Alert:** Stress may cause an acute attack. **Alert:** Identify risk for constricted airway. **Alert:** Identify client who cannot tolerate supine position for care. **Alert:** Nitrous oxide–oxygen analgesia may be contraindicated (COPD).	How do you control signs and symptoms of your breathing disease? What makes your respiratory disease worse? Better? Do you carry a rescue inhaler? When were you diagnosed? What are your asthma triggers? Can you tolerate being placed in a supine position?	Monitor respiration. Determine need for semisupine positioning. Continuous oxygen ventilation by nasal cannula may be needed. Avoid aerosol production. Avoid nitrous oxide for analgesia. Bronchodilator must be present at every appointment.
12. Fainting spells	Identify risk for emergency involving loss of consciousness.	What causes you to faint? When was the last time it occurred? Have you fainted during a dental appointment?	Determine cause, and prevent reoccurrence. Fainting can be associated with some cardiac and neurologic disorders.
13. Epilepsy or other neurologic disorder	**Alert:** Recent attack is strong risk factor for emergency situation. **Alert:** Failure to take antiseizure medication is a risk factor for recurrent seizures. Investigate side effects of seizure pharmacotherapy (e.g., drug-influenced gingival enlargement, bleeding).	Do you have a history of seizure disorder or any problems with your nervous system? Are you taking antiseizure medication? Did you take it today? What type of seizure disorder do you have? Do you know when a seizure is about to happen? When was your last seizure? Have you ever had to go to the hospital because of a prolonged seizure?	Determine risk for seizure during oral care appointment. Avoid flashing overhead light in client's eyes and use of any device that may precipitate a seizure. Plan for seizure management and watch patient for signs of seizure (loss of consciousness, abnormal movements, stiffness, fluttering eyelids, blank stare). Move dental equipment so that patient is not injured during seizure; immediately notify medical personnel.

Continued

TABLE 12-3

Medical History Items Explained—cont'd

Item	Purpose	Relevant Questions	Implications for Professional Care
14. Low blood pressure	**Alert:** Risk for postural (orthostatic) hypotension and syncope is increased.	Have you ever lost consciousness after lying down or rising from a chair? Have you consulted a physician about it?	Low blood pressure may be normal for individuals with good physical stamina and may represent "normal limits" for that client. Consider collecting supine, sitting, and standing blood pressures. Determine risk for postural hypotension and follow protocol to prevent it at end of appointment.
15. Bowel and bladder problems	Identify need for planning restroom breaks. Symptom associated with a variety of disorders (urinary tract infection, neurologic disease, acquired immunodeficiency syndrome [AIDS], malignancy, bowel disorders, febrile illness).	Do you have any problems with your bowel or bladder function? Which condition? How do you manage the condition? Do you need to go to the restroom before we begin? Let me know if we need to stop during the appointment.	Determine the cause, and manage care appropriately and respectfully. Assess need for bathroom break during appointment.
16. Diabetes mellitus (DM)	**Alert:** Determine risk for hypoglycemia emergency. Patient with controlled diabetes is treated same as normal patient. Uncontrolled DM may cause reduced healing, greater periodontal destruction. Prophylactic antibiotics are not indicated.	Have you been diagnosed with diabetes or prediabetes? When were you diagnosed? When was your last medical evaluation for diabetes? What was your last A_{1c} value? How do you manage your diabetes (i.e., diet, exercise, medication)? Do you have low blood sugar ("hypoglycemic") episodes? Do you use a glucose meter? What was your reading this morning? Did you eat before coming in today?	Controlled DM is characterized by a recent hemoglobin A_{1c} test result of <7%. Blood sugar usually is monitored in evening and morning by pricking the finger and placing blood on a test strip to be inserted in the blood glucose meter. Score of 70-130 (morning) is goal for treatment. Levels >200 should be referred for medical evaluation. Determine risk for hypoglycemia (glucose <70) and keep sugar at chair to reverse hypoglycemia should it develop. Appointment scheduled for morning hours after meal is consumed.
16(a). Do you have to urinate (pass water) more than six times a day? More than three times during night? 16(b). Are you thirsty much of the time? 16(c). Have you had a recent weight change of more than 10 pounds? 16(d). Are you slow to heal, or do you get frequent infections?	**Alert:** These are signs and symptoms of undiagnosed or uncontrolled DM. **Alert:** Risk for hyperglycemic event (diabetic coma or ketoacidosis) is increased. May need to have medical evaluation before treatment. Cardiovascular disease may be present.	Have you ever been checked for diabetes? Does anyone in your family have diabetes? I recommend that you be checked for diabetes. Do you have high blood pressure?	If cause for symptom cannot be determined, refer for medical evaluation. Examine oral tissues for signs of uncontrolled DM (periodontal abscess, extensive attachment loss, fruity breath odor, and candidiasis). Monitor vital signs, as hypertension and atherosclerosis are associated with DM, especially uncontrolled disease. In case of emergency, call 911.

TABLE 12-3

Medical History Items Explained—cont'd

Item	Purpose	Relevant Questions	Implications for Professional Care
17. Thyroid problems	**Alert:** Uncontrolled thyroid disease poses an increased risk for a medical emergency. **Alert:** Thyroid storm is associated with uncontrolled hyperthyroidism; monitor pulse rate and body temperature.	Are you aware of any problems with your thyroid gland? Are you hypothyroid or hyperthyroid? Are you currently being treated for thyroid disorder? Are there any drugs you cannot tolerate?	Uncontrolled hyperthyroidism is characterized by an increased pulse rate and increased body temperature. Monitor vital signs each appointment. Uncontrolled hypothyroidism is characterized by edema, enlarged tongue, bradycardia, and hypotension.
18. Arthritis, rheumatism, or painful swollen joints	Identify client who may have disabilities of hands or fingers and who may not tolerate supine positioning. Identify pharmacologic therapy with side effects that may complicate oral care (immunosuppression, increased bleeding).	Do you have any problems with your joints? How does this affect your ability to perform oral self-care such as brushing and flossing? What medications do you take? What did you take today? Are you able to lie down without discomfort? When is it best for your appointment, mid-morning or afternoon? Is your jaw (temporo-mandibular joint [TMJ]) affected?	Evaluate drug effects for each drug taken before appointment. Monitor for clotting during care, and use digital pressure to achieve hemostasis during oral procedures. Upper extremity impairments may necessitate oral hygiene modifications (e.g., large handle toothbrush, floss aid). Determine best time for appointment around daily pattern of symptoms. Client may have difficulty opening mouth widely if TMJ affected.
19. Problems of immune system, organ transplant	Identify the immuno-compromised patient who is susceptible to infection and may have reduced healing response. Determine need for physician consultation regarding antibiotic prophylaxis.	Do you have any condition that weakens your immune system or increases your risk for infections? What is the cause of the condition? Has your physician told you to take antibiotics before a dental appointment? What medicines are you taking for it?	Determine potential complications associated with oral care (poor healing, infection). Investigate drug therapy; possible drug-influenced gingival enlargement with cyclosporine.
20. Stomach ulcers or hyperacidity or gastroesophageal reflux disorder (GERD)	Identify patient predisposed to erosion. Note contraindication for aspirin and nonsteroidal anti-inflammatory drugs (NSAIDs) with peptic ulcer disease. Identify positioning modifications.	Do you have problems with your stomach or esophagus? How does lying flat affect the reflux problem? Are your teeth sensitive?	Hyperacid conditions are sometimes associated with reflux of stomach acid into mouth, leading to erosion and caries. Examine dentition for erosion, caries, and chipped teeth. Acetaminophen is indicated analgesic for oral pain. Consider semisupine chair position.
21. Kidney disease	Reveal risk for hypertension and inability to excrete drugs normally. May identify patient who is on hemodialysis.	Do you have any problem with your kidneys? How are you being treated?	Some renal disorders (glomerulonephritis) may require medical consultation before oral care. If patient is on hemodialysis, take blood pressure in arm without fistula or graft. Antibiotic prophylaxis is not indicated for shunts and catheters in hemodialysis.

Continued

TABLE 12-3

Medical History Items Explained—cont'd

Item	Purpose	Relevant Questions	Implications for Professional Care
22. Tuberculosis (TB; positive purified protein derivative [PPD] test result, or chest x-ray film)	**Alert:** May identify client with active, infectious TB. **Alert:** Client with active TB should not receive oral treatment.	Have you been tested for TB infection? What was the result? If test was positive, do you have symptoms such as cough, fever, or weight loss? Was a chest x-ray done? Are you or did you ever receive antibiotics? For how long? Have you had sputum tests?	Medical consultation must be completed to ensure absence of active infection. Anti-TB drugs taken for >2 weeks should render patient noninfectious. Be alert to side effects of anti-TB drugs, (e.g., rifampin may cause red/orange discoloration of saliva and tears).
23. Persistent cough or cough that produced blood	**Alert:** Identify client with infectious lung disease (TB).	Have you sought medical evaluation? What was the medical diagnosis? Are you currently in treatment? Do you know if you are infectious to others?	Medical consultation is needed to rule out infectious TB. If non-TB lung infection is suspected, use hand washing, gloves, and surgical mask to prevent cross-contamination.
24. Sexually transmitted diseases (STDs, e.g., syphilis, gonorrhea, chlamydia)	Identify client with untreated STD who may have oral infectious lesions.	Have you ever been diagnosed with a sexually transmitted infection? When were you diagnosed? Are you currently in treatment? When will you finish antibiotic? Are you infectious to others?	Ensure adequate barrier protection is maintained. If oral STD infection is suspected, defer oral care until medical consultation verifies patient is noninfectious. Medical consultation is needed to verify diagnosis and current medical therapy.
25. AIDS or HIV infection	**Alert:** Identify immunocompromised client. Maintain universal standard precautions.	Have you ever been tested for HIV? When? What was the result? Are you currently taking medications? What was your most recent CD4 cell count?	Consultation with the referring physician may be required when considering antibiotic prophylaxis. Opportunistic infections are more likely at CD4 counts <200 cells/μL. Anticipate oral and/or esophageal candidiasis. Investigate all drugs for side effects relevant to oral care.
26. Oral herpes (cold sores, fever blisters)	**Alert:** Oral treatment is contraindicated when labial lesions are present and risk of cross-infection is high.	Do you have an oral lesion today? What usually causes an outbreak? How do you treat the lesion?	Reschedule oral care if labial (lip) lesion is present. Inform patient that lesion is communicable. Recommend using new toothbrush after lesion resolves to reduce reinfection. Acyclovir or over-the-counter products can be advised.
27. Do you have a blood disorder (e.g., anemia, bruising, or leukemia)? 27(a). Do you have abnormal bleeding? 27(b). Have you required a blood transfusion? If yes, when?	Reveal blood disorder that may complicate healing during oral care. Identify risk for increased bleeding or hemorrhage.	Do bruise or bleed easily? When was the condition diagnosed? Are you receiving medical therapy for condition? What do you do to stop bleeding?	Monitor for increased bleeding and reduced healing. Determine cause of condition, and manage as needed.

TABLE 12-3
Medical History Items Explained—cont'd

Item	Purpose	Relevant Questions	Implications for Professional Care
28. Mental health problems	Identify emotional issues that may complicate oral care and patient self-care.	Have you sought help from a mental health professional in the past? Are you currently being treated for any condition? What medication are you taking?	Show concern and try to encourage self-interest in healthy oral cavity. Identify need to initiate stress-reduction protocols. Investigate medication side effects; xerostomia is common.
29. Cancer, tumors, growths, or persistent swollen glands	Identify malignant disease and need for examination for recurrence at maintenance examinations.	Have you ever been diagnosed with cancer? What type of cancer? What treatments have you been receiving? What is your current white blood cell count?	Chemotherapy often reduces white blood cells; medical consultation is needed to establish the time within chemotherapy to receive oral care. For oral malignancy, monitor tissues every maintenance appointment for a new lesion or recurrence. Investigate drug therapy for relevant side effects (e.g., mucocytis, ulceration, xerostomia).
30. Have you had treatment for a tumor or growth (surgery, radiation, chemotherapy)?	Identify client with prior history of malignancy or neoplastic disease.	What type of tumor did you have? What treatment did you receive? What was the outcome? Did you develop oral complications? Describe them.	Determine cause and treatment success, and manage as needed. For radiation-induced xerostomia, consider salivary substitutes or oral lubricating products. Monitor for oral effects, depending on therapy received.
31. Liver disease	Determine etiology. Determine if blood-borne transmission of viral condition exists. Determine if increased bleeding is probable.	Do you know of any problems with your liver? If HBV: Are you being treated with antiviral agents? Are you contagious? Do you bleed for a long time after a cut?	Liver disease may increase bleeding risk. All practitioners should have immunity to HBV from vaccine verified by a blood test to determine adequate antibody formation. Take care to avoid an injury that may compromise standard precaution of gloves. If a puncture occurs, seek medical evaluation immediately for recommended therapy.
32. Are you allergic or have you had a reaction to the following: Local anesthetics Penicillin or antibiotics Sulfa drugs Barbiturates, sedatives, or sleeping pills Aspirin Iodine Codeine or narcotics Latex Metals (silver, mercury) Other	Identify allergies relevant to products used in dentistry. Indicate medication that should not be prescribed or product that should not be used in oral care.	What type of reaction did you have? Describe it. What antibiotic can you take?	Dental hygiene practitioners do not prescribe medications, but over-the-counter products to which an allergy has occurred should not be recommended or provided to the client. Determine if reaction was a hypersensitivity reaction or side effect. Latex: Select nonlatex gloves, prophy cup, or other product; cover arm with barrier before placing blood pressure cuff.
33. Have you had a serious event associated with previous dental treatment?	Identify patient who may be at increased risk for syncope or other emergency.	What happened? How can it be prevented today?	Investigate the event, and institute procedures to prevent it. For anxious patient, talking about patient interests to keep current treatment "off their mind" may reduce anxiety.

Continued

TABLE 12-3
Medical History Items Explained—cont'd

Item	Purpose	Relevant Questions	Implications for Professional Care
34. Do you have a disease, condition, or problem not listed previously that is important? If so, explain.	Identify a condition not included on history form.	What is the condition? Have you received medical treatment? Outcome?	Determine cause of condition, and manage as needed.
35. Are you wearing contact lenses?	Identify special considerations, remove lenses, and provide protective eyewear.	Do you want to take your contact lenses out during treatment?	Consider possibility of introducing aerosol irritant to eyes. Protective eyewear is standard of care, but prophylaxis paste spatter may cause irritation in some cases.
36. Do you use or have you ever used tobacco? If so, what type? How many years? How much tobacco did you use each day? If you stopped, how long ago did you stop?	Identify issues for tobacco cessation program.	Follow up responses as indicated. How do you feel about stopping smoking? If contemplative or ready to quit: would you like information on local tobacco cessation programs?	Offer information on local counseling programs for tobacco cessation. Counsel that nicotine-replacement drugs may be available from physicians (or from dentists, in some practices). Regardless of interest in quitting, encourage tobacco cessation to avoid lung, cardiovascular, and oral cancer conditions.
37. Alcohol and substance use/abuse	Identify alcohol or substance abusing patient. **Alert:** Identify cocaine interaction with vasoconstrictor.	How often do you drink alcohol? How much do you drink? Has your drinking ever been a problem? Any problems with your liver? When was your last drink? Many patients use recreational drugs—do you use cocaine? How do you use it, and when was last use?	Do not recommend mouth rinse with alcohol to recovering alcoholic. Withdrawal of alcohol in an alcohol-dependent patient can precipitate seizure. Vasoconstrictors (epinephrine) are contraindicated when cocaine has been used within past 24 hours. Cocaine use increases the risk for stroke and cardiac arrhythmias.
38. Are you employed in a facility that exposes you regularly to x-rays or ionizing radiation?	Identify need for reducing exposure to ionizing radiation.	Do you have regular assessments to determine your level of ionizing radiation exposure? Can we take dental x-rays if they are necessary?	Consider if there is a need to avoid or limit dental x-ray exposure.
For women only: 39. Are you pregnant? If yes, due date?	Identify time for appointment plan.	Can we schedule you during your second trimester?	Radiographs can be taken during pregnancy using standard precautions. The second trimester is the preferred time for elective oral care. For third trimester, to avoid supine hypotension, place a pillow under right hip and rotate abdomen to left to avoid compression of vena cava.
40. Do you have problems with menstrual periods?	Identify hormone imbalance.	What problems? What do you do about them?	Determine cause, and manage as needed.
41. Are you nursing?	Identify appointment planning schedule.	Can we schedule you for an appointment after your nursing time?	Schedule for appointment as directed by client.

TABLE 12-3

Medical History Items Explained—cont'd

Item	Purpose	Relevant Questions	Implications for Professional Care
42. Are you taking birth control pills?	Identify potential side effects relevant to oral care.	Do your gums bleed more since you started taking birth control pills? Any side effects?	Monitor blood pressure; there is a risk for increased values when hormones are taken. Avoid antibiotics or use additional birth control when taking antibiotic. Strict biofilm control is useful.
43. Are you taking hormone replacement therapy?	Identify issues of hormone replacements.	Do you have hot flashes or signs of menopause? Have you had bone density testing? If so, what was the result?	Monitor vital signs, increased risk for cardiovascular complications.
44. Have you ever taken bisphosphonates or denosumab?	Identify client at risk for osteonecrosis of the jaw.	Have you had a bone density test? Have you been diagnosed with osteopenia or osteoporosis? How long have you taken antiresorptive agents? Which agent did you take? Was it taken orally or intravenously?	Provide client information on the small risk of osteonecrosis of the jaw when oral agents are taken for 3 or more years or with intravenous bisphosphonates taken for 10 months or longer. Examine oral cavity for signs of osteonecrosis affecting the bone of the jaws.

which disclosure of protected health information is acceptable if it is in the best interests of the client. Dental hygiene practitioners are expected to exercise utmost professionalism required to uphold HIPAA, including refraining from discussing client care with third parties and keeping protected health information in secure areas.

Because of its status as a legal document, the health history form should be completed in permanent ink. Pencil or erasable ink is unacceptable. Recording errors should be lined out neatly, initialed, and dated. Accuracy of the health information is ascertained by having the client sign and date the health history form. Written comments concerning the health history interview are initialed by the client to indicate accuracy. If the client is a minor (younger than 18 years of age), a parent or legal guardian must sign and date the health history form to verify accuracy. A separate signed consent form (Figure 12-3) also could be used to verify permission for services to be rendered during the appointment. Suggestions for managing client records are included in Box 12-2.

Decision Making After the Health History Is Obtained

Tools to Interpret Client Data and Degree of Medical Risk

American Society of Anesthesiologists' Physical Status Classification System

A physical status classification system developed by the American Society of Anesthesiologists (ASA) rates the medical risk of a client who is to receive local or general anesthesia. This system, called the ASA classification system, classifies medical risk from 1 to 6 based on the disease or disorder (Box 12-3).[7]

Oral health professionals use the ASA classification system to determine whether treatment is safe for clients with various medical conditions. A client classified as ASA 4 or greater should not receive elective treatment. Treatment can resume when the condition improves and the status is downgraded. For example, a client with uncontrolled diabetes or angina at rest (ASA 4) should be referred for a medical evaluation and treatment before dental hygiene care. If a client with an ASA 4 status is in need of emergency oral care, then a hospital environment should be used in case a life-threatening emergency occurs. Only palliative care is recommended for a client with an ASA 5 status.

Stress, fear, and anxiety can lead to medical emergencies such as vasovagal syncope, cardiac arrhythmia, or hyperventilation. These triggers also can exacerbate certain medical conditions, leading to an emergency situation. Stress reduction protocols should be part of the dental hygiene care plan as a strategy to avoid an emergency. Chapter 41 provides information on stress reduction protocols.

Assessment of Functional Capacity

Increased medical risk may exist for certain conditions that involve altered cardiovascular function (e.g., myocardial infarction, hyperthyroidism, heart failure). A method for determining cardiac risk has been described by the American College of Cardiology and the American Heart Association (ACC/AHA).[8] The official guideline identified the first month after myocardial infarction (MI) as the time period with most risk. After the first month, the method to determine the degree of recovery from the event is determination of functional capacity. Functional capacity is defined as being able to perform a specific level of activity. It is measured on "metabolic equivalents" (MET). A MET is a unit of oxygen

1. I consent to the recommended procedure or treatment ______________________
____
to be completed by Dr./Ms./Mr.__________.
2. The procedure(s) or treatment(s) have been described to me.
3. I have been informed of the purpose of the procedure or treatment.
4. I have been informed of the alternatives to the procedure or treatment.
5. I understand that the following risk(s) may result from the procedure or treatment:
____
____
______________________.
6. I understand that the following risk(s) may occur if the procedure or treatment is not completed:
____
____
______________________.
7. I do—do not—consent to the administration of anesthetic.
   a. I understand that the following risks are involved in administering anesthesia:
   ____
   ____
   ______________________.
   b. The following alternatives to anesthesia were described: ______________________
   ____
   ______________________.

All my questions have been satisfactorily answered.

Signature: ______________________
Date

Representative: ______________________
Date

Signature of Witness: ______________________
Date

Figure 12-3. Sample consent form.

consumption needed for physical activity. Inability to achieve four metabolic equivalents (METs) increases the risk for occurrence of a serious cardiac event during and after non-cardiac surgery,[9] or medical procedures similar in stress to dental treatment. A client who can walk up a flight of stairs or run a short distance without symptomatic limitations likely meets the four MET level of functional capacity, and it is likely that oral procedures can be completed safely.

Use of Drug References

Before professional care is provided, the dental hygiene practitioner investigates and documents medications currently taken by the client (see Chapter 14). Medications taken by the client can alter treatment outcomes and affect clinical treatment. In addition, prior adverse reaction may indicate the need to change the dental care plan or necessitate consultation with a physician before care is initiated. Several drug information sources published annually include the *Physician's Desk Reference (PDR)*,[10] *Facts and Comparisons*, and *GenRx*. Drug information sources specific to oral healthcare are *Mosby's Dental Drug Reference, Drug Information Handbook for Dentistry*, and *LWW's Dental Drug Reference with Clinical Implications*.[11-13] These focus on drug effects relevant to oral

BOX 12-2

Suggestions for Managing Client Records

- Entries should be legible, written in black ink or ballpoint pen. Changes are reviewed with the client, and the client signs the documented information to verify accuracy.
- When there is more than one person making entries, entries should be signed or initialed.
- When errors occur, they should not be blocked out so that they cannot be read. Instead, a single line should be drawn through the entry and a note made above it stating "error in entry, see correction below." The correction should be initialed and dated at the time it is made.
- Financial information should not be kept on the treatment record.
- Entries should be uniformly spaced on the form (i.e., no unusual or irregular blank spaces).
- On health information forms, there should be no blank spaces in the answers to health questions. If the question is inappropriate, a single line is drawn through the question, or "not applicable" (NA) recorded in the box.
- All cancellations, late arrivals, and changes of appointments are recorded.
- Consents are documented, including all risks and alternative treatments presented to the client and remarks made by the client.
- The client is informed of any adverse occurrences or untoward events that take place during the course of care; a note on the record that the client was informed is necessary.
- All requests for consultations and responses are recorded.
- All conversations held with other health practitioners relating to the care of the client are documented.
- All client records should be retained for at least the period of the statute of limitations equal to that of contract actions. In most jurisdictions it is 6 years. In the case of minors, it is until the person reaches the age of 24 years. Check for special laws in your local jurisdiction. A dental office may consider additional record retention options that may include record storage facilities, microfilm, and/or scanning to electronic records. If possible, keep records forever.
- Computerized dental records are common. There should be a standardized protocol that includes daily backup of records and weekly transfer of records to an encrypted electronic database to ensure that records are not altered.
- No subjective evaluations, such as an opinion about the client's mental health, should be recorded on the treatment record unless the writer is qualified and licensed to make such evaluations.
- Confidentiality of information contained on the record should be guarded. Staff should be trained to follow Health Insurance Portability and Accountability Act (HIPAA) guidelines.
- The original record should not be surrendered to anyone, except by order of a court.
- A record should never be altered once there is some indication that legal action is contemplated by the client.
- Heirs are instructed that they must retain the records of clients and comply with any written request for a copy.

Adapted from Pollack BR: *Dentist's risk management guide*, Fort Lauderdale, Fla, 1990, National Society of Dental Practitioners.

BOX 12-3

American Society of Anesthesiologists (ASA) Physical Status Classification System

ASA 1: A normal, healthy patient
ASA 2: A patient with mild systemic disease
ASA 3: A patient with severe systemic disease
ASA 4: A patient with severe systemic disease that is a constant threat to life
ASA 5: A moribund patient who is not expected to survive without an operation
ASA 6: A declared brain-dead patient whose organs are being removed for donor purposes

Data from the American Society of Anesthesiologists (ASA) Physical Status Classification System.[7]

procedures, interactions with various drugs used in dentistry, and the medical conditions frequently managed by the drug. Figure 12-4 illustrates drug information including the generic and brand names of a drug, the drug's action, indication or approved use, interactions with drugs used in dentistry, adverse drug effects, clinical considerations, and oral health information. The *Merck Manual of Diagnosis and Therapy* is a standard reference book on diseases, including their causes, signs and symptoms, diagnostic indicators, and treatment.[14] Dental hygiene practitioners confronted with unfamiliar medical conditions find readily available, concise descriptions of most diseases in this reference book, which is also available online.

Prophylactic Antibiotic Premedication for Prevention of Infective Endocarditis

The epidemiology and pathophysiology of infective endocarditis is presented elsewhere (see Chapter 43). Transient **bacteremia**, or bacteria within the bloodstream, is common after dental procedures and even chewing and routine oral care such as brushing and flossing. Although the host immune response generally resolves the bacteremia within 15 minutes, infectious microorganisms in the bloodstream may cause distant site infections in individuals with selected predisposing conditions. Specifically, microbes may become lodged on damaged or abnormal areas of the heart valves, lining of the heart, and underlying connective tissue.

Manipulation of gingival tissues or the periapical region of teeth or perforation of the oral mucosa during dental or dental hygiene procedures may cause a transient bacteremia.[5] **Prophylactic antibiotic premedication** is the administration of specific antibiotics ½ to 1 hour before the dental procedure that could cause bacteremia. The theoretical rationale behind antibiotic prophylaxis premedication is to prevent transient bacteremia from developing into fulminant infective endocarditis, a life-threatening infection of the tissue lining the heart.

Prescribing antibiotics, especially for prophylactic use, requires careful consideration of the risks and benefits, including healthcare costs and adverse drug reactions. There is increasing awareness of the adverse effects of antibiotic misuse and overuse, the risk of allergic reactions, and an increase in antibiotic-resistant microorganisms worldwide. Although

---

carvedilol (CAR-veh-DILL-ole)

Coreg

Dilatrend

Drug Class: Alpha-adrenergic blocker; Beta-adrenergic blocker

PHARMACOLOGY

Action

Blocks $alpha_1$-receptors and nonselective beta-receptors to decrease BP.

Uses

Management of essential hypertension; treatment of mild to severe heart failure of ischemic or cardiomyopathic origin. Reduce cardiovascular mortality in clinically stable patients who have survived the acute phase of MI and have a left ventricular ejection fraction of 40% or less.

Unlabeled Uses

Angina pectoris.

DRUG INTERACTIONS RELATED TO DENTAL THERAPEUTICS

COX-1 inhibitors: Decreased antihypertensive effect (decreased prostaglandin synthesis)
- Monitor blood pressure.

Sympathomimetic amines: Decreased antihypertensive effect (pharmacological antagonism)
- Use local anesthetic agents containing a vasoconstrictor with caution.
- Monitor blood pressure.

ADVERSE EFFECTS

⚠ **ORAL:** Periodontitis (1% to 3%); dry mouth.

CNS: Dizziness (32%); fatigue (24%); headache (8%); lung edema (for treatment of left ventricular dysfunction following MI [>3%]); somnolence, vertigo, hypesthesia, paresthesia, depression, insomnia (1% to 3%).

CVS: Bradycardia, postural hypotension, edema (2%).

GI: Diarrhea (12%); nausea (9%); vomiting (6%); melena, GI pain (1% to 3%).

RESP: Upper respiratory tract infection (18%); increased cough (8%); sinusitis, bronchitis (5%); rales (4%); dyspnea (for treatment of LVD following MI [>3%]).

MISC: Asthenia (11%); pain (9%); edema generalized, arthralgia (6%); edema dependent (4%); allergy, malaise, hypovolemia, fever, leg edema, infection, viral infection, back pain muscle cramps, arthritis, hypotonia, flu-like syndrome, peripheral vascular disorder (1% to 3%).

CLINICAL IMPLICATIONS

General

- Determine why drug is being taken. Consider implications of condition on dental treatment.
- Monitor vital signs (e.g., BP, pulse pressure, rate, and rhythm) at each appointment to assess disease control. Do not provide elective dental treatment when BP is ≥180/110 or in the presence of other high-risk CV conditions. Refer to the section entitled "The Patient Taking Cardiovascular Drugs" in Chapter 6: *Clinical Medicine*.
- Evaluate respiratory function.
- Use local anesthetic agents with vasoconstrictor with caution based on functional capacity of the patient and use aspirating technique to prevent intravascular injection.
- Beta blockers may mask epinephrine-induced signs and symptoms of hypoglycemia in patients with diabetes.
- Determine ability to adapt to stress of dental treatment. Consider short appointments.
- *Postural hypotension:* Monitor BP at the beginning and end of each appointment; anticipate syncope. Have patient sit upright for several min at the end of the dental appointment before dismissing.
- If GI or respiratory side effects occur, consider semisupine chair position.
- Chronic dry mouth is possible; anticipate increased caries, candidiasis, and lichenoid mucositis.

Oral Health Education

- If chronic dry mouth occurs, recommend home fluoride therapy and use of nonalcoholic oral health care products.
- Encourage daily plaque control procedures for effective self-care in patients at risk for cardiovascular disease.

Figure 12-4. Illustration of information in *Dental Drug Reference with Clinical Implications*. (From Pickett FA, Terezhalmy GT: *Lippincott Williams and Wilkins' dental drug reference with clinical implications*, ed 2, Baltimore, 2009, Lippincott Williams and Wilkins.)

once prescribed liberally, antibiotic prophylaxis before dental procedures has not been shown convincingly to reduce significantly the risk of infective endocarditis.[5] In fact, infective endocarditis is more likely to arise from day-to-day activities than from a dental procedure, and maintenance of good oral hygiene is probably more effective than antibiotic premedication at reducing the risk of infective endocarditis.[5]

Because of the potentially devastating consequences of infective endocarditis, the current American Heart Association guidelines recommend antibiotic prophylaxis before dental procedures only for clients at highest risk for infective endocarditis. These "high-risk" conditions are listed in Box 12-4. Of note, clients with bicuspid aortic valve, acquired mitral or aortic valve disease, and cardiomyopathy no longer require antibiotic prophylaxis according to these guidelines.

BOX 12-4

Cardiac Conditions* Associated with Highest Risk of Adverse Outcome from Endocarditis for Which Prophylaxis with Dental Procedures Is Recommended

- Prosthetic cardiac valve or prosthetic material used for cardiac valve repair
- Previous infective endocarditis
- Unrepaired cyanotic congenital heart disease (CHD), including palliative shunts and conduits
- Completely repaired congenital heart defect with prosthetic material or device, whether placed by surgery or by other catheter intervention, during the first 6 months after the procedure†
- Repaired CHD with residual defects at the site of or adjacent to the site of a prosthetic patch or prosthetic device (which inhibits endothelialization)
- Cardiac transplantation recipients who develop cardiac valvulopathy

From Wilson W, Taubert KA, Gewitz M, et al: Prevention of infective endocarditis: guidelines from the American Heart Association: a guideline from the American Heart Association Rheumatic Fever, Endocarditis, and Kawasaki Disease Committee, Council on Cardiovascular Disease in the Young, and the Council on Clinical Cardiology, Council on Cardiovascular Surgery and Anesthesia, and the Quality of Care and Outcomes Research Interdisciplinary Working Group, *Circulation* 116(15):1736-1754, 2007.

*Except for the conditions listed herein, antibiotic prophylaxis is no longer recommended for any other form of cardiovascular disease, including previous coronary artery bypass graft surgery, coronary artery stenting, mitral valve prolapsed, cardiac pacemakers (intravascular and epicardial), and implanted cardiodefibrillators.

†Prophylaxis during this period is reasonable because endothelialization of prosthetic material requires 6 months.

BOX 12-5

Dental Procedures for Which Antibiotic Premedication May Be Beneficial in High-Risk Patients (Box 12-4)

- Manipulation of the gingival tissues
- Manipulation of the periapical region of teeth
- Perforation of the oral mucosa during dental procedures*

From Wilson W, Taubert KA, Gewitz M, et al: Prevention of infective endocarditis: guidelines from the American Heart Association: a guideline from the American Heart Association Rheumatic Fever, Endocarditis, and Kawasaki Disease Committee, Council on Cardiovascular Disease in the Young, and the Council on Clinical Cardiology, Council on Cardiovascular Surgery and Anesthesia, and the Quality of Care and Outcomes Research Interdisciplinary Working Group, *Circulation* 116(15):1736-1754, 2007.

*Prophylaxis is not recommended in other instances, including restorative dentistry (operative and prosthodontic with or without retraction cord), local anesthetic injections through noninfected tissue, intracanal endodontic treatment; post placement and buildup, placement of rubber dams, postoperative suture removal, placement or removal of prosthodontic or orthodontic appliances, taking of oral impressions, fluoride treatments, taking of oral radiographs, orthodontic appliance adjustment, shedding of primary teeth

Clients for whom antibacterial prophylaxis is appropriate (see Box 12-4) should receive antibiotic prophylaxis before all dental procedures that involve manipulation of gingival tissue or the periapical region of teeth or perforation of the oral mucosa. Antibiotic prophylaxis is not required in the case of routine anesthetic injections through noninfected tissue, taking dental radiographs, placement of removable prosthodontic or orthodontic appliances, adjustment of orthodontic appliances, placement of orthodontic brackets, shedding of primary teeth, or bleeding from trauma to the lips or oral mucosa. These recommendations are summarized in Box 12-5.

Prophylactic Antibiotic Premedication for Prevention of Prosthetic Joint Infections

Prosthetic joint infection (PJI) is another remote site infection that can arise after bacteremia. Prosthetic joint infections have a much lower mortality rate than infective endocarditis; however, when a prosthetic joint infection occurs, surgical removal and prolonged treatment with antibiotics usually is required. Despite the theoretical risk of prosthetic joint bacterial seeding resulting from dental procedures, there is little evidence that dental procedures actually increase the risk of prosthetic joint infection.[15-16] Furthermore, studies have not shown conclusively that prophylactic antibiotics before invasive dental procedures offer significant benefit in preventing PJI.[17]

Although substantial controversy has surrounded its development,[18] the most recent clinical practice guideline from the American Dental Association (ADA) in collaboration with the American Association of Orthopedic Surgeons (AAOS) has suggested that *there is no conclusive evidence that demonstrates a need to routinely administer antibiotics when a prosthetic joint is in place and dental treatment is planned.*[19] The group was also unable to recommend for or against the use of oral topical antimicrobials (i.e., topical antimicrobial mouthrinse) before dental procedures for preventing PJI. The collaborative group agreed that maintenance of good oral hygiene was an important precaution in all clients with prosthetic joints. Because the evidence base considered only hip and knee replacements, there are no official guidelines for other types of joint prostheses.

It is less clear whether antibiotic prophylaxis also may be appropriate in patients with orthopedic prostheses and an **immunocompromised condition**. Examples of immunocompromised conditions include autoimmune disease, solid organ or bone marrow transplant, HIV/AIDS, malignancy, and chronic use of steroids or immunomodulation therapy. There is some evidence that immunocompromised clients and clients with certain other comorbidities such as obesity, hemophilia, malnutrition, tobacco or alcohol use, prior PJI, and current oral infection may be at higher risk for PJI.[20-23] Although antibiotic prophylaxis premedication may be considered based on a given patient's underlying morbidities and planned procedure,[24] the link between prophylactic antibiotics before dental intervention and prevention of PJI in these clients remains unproven. Therefore the possible benefit of antibiotic prophylaxis should be weighed carefully against risks to the client and costs to the healthcare system. When uncertainty exists, consultation between the referring physician and the oral care team is appropriate.

Antibiotic Premedication Dosage Regimen Guidelines

Because of the general recommendation against the administration of prophylactic antibiotics for prevention of prosthetic joint infection, no official dosage regimen exists for this indication. The standard prophylactic regimen for infective endocarditis prevention recommended by the AHA is shown in Table 12-4.[5] One dose of the appropriate antibiotic ½ to 1 hour before the procedure is recommended. This guideline advises taking the antibiotic within 2 hours of the appointment when the dose is inadvertently not taken by the client. For this reason, some facilities keep a supply of antibiotics available to ensure that oral procedures can be provided with no delay when indicated. Table 12-5 summarizes dental management considerations for all indications for antibiotic prophylaxis.

Individuals who currently are taking an antibiotic in the regimen should receive an antibiotic from a different class. For example, in a patient with a history of infective endocarditis who usually would take amoxicillin for antibiotic prophylaxis but who is taking amoxicillin presently for another medical reason, either clindamycin or one of the macrolides (e.g., azithromycin, clarithromycin) can be used. An alternate suggestion is to delay the dental procedure until at least 10 days after completion of the amoxicillin antibiotic therapy and use the one dose amoxicillin. This 10-day time period may allow time for the usual oral flora to reestablish.

Before initiating dental hygiene procedures in clients for whom antibiotic prophylaxis is deemed appropriate, the dental hygiene practitioner should inquire whether the prescribed antibiotic was taken, if the correct dose was taken, and when the antibiotic was taken. This information is recorded in the client record (see Boxes 12-5 and 12-6). The current AHA recommendation advises that when appropriately indicated, the recommended dose of antibiotic prophylaxis can be administered within 2 hours of the dental appointment.[25]

Physician Consultation and Referral

The physician of record is consulted if the patient reveals a condition that may jeopardize safety during care. Medical consultations are initiated for the following:

- A condition that may need prophylactic antibiotic premedication
- Suspicion of an undiagnosed or uncontrolled medical condition
- Abnormal vital signs (see Chapter 13)
- Precautionary treatment modifications (e.g., local anesthetics with reduced levels of vasoconstrictor [see Chapter 40])
- Persons taking anticoagulant or blood thinner medication (e.g., warfarin [Coumadin])

Clients are referred for medical evaluation when a nonurgent but potentially undiagnosed condition is suspected (e.g., the presence of mild hypertension) or when needed laboratory test results are not available (e.g., blood test to determine risk for excessive bleeding when warfarin is taken). Urgent consultation with the referring physician is indicated if the

BOX 12-6

Protocol for Monitoring Compliance with Antibiotic Premedication

- Identify the prescribed antibiotic.
- Ask patient what dose was taken. and the time of administration.
- Record patient response in the treatment record.
- When the antibiotic was not taken, the prescribed antibiotic can be administered within 2 hours of the appointment.

TABLE 12-4

Antibiotic Prophylaxis Regimens for a Dental Procedure (Single Dose 30 to 60 Minutes Before Procedure)

Situation	Agent	Adults	Children
Oral	Amoxicillin	2 g	50 mg/kg
Unable to take oral medication	Ampicillin	2 g IM or IV	50 mg/kg IM or IV
	or		
	Cefazolin or ceftriazone	1 g IM or IV	50 mg/kg IM or IV
Allergic to penicillin or ampicillin (able to take oral medication)	Cephalexin*†	2 g	50 mg/kg
	or		
	Clindamycin	600 mg	20 mg/kg
	or		
	Azithromycin or clarithromycin	500 mg	15 mg/kg
Allergic to penicillin or ampicillin and unable to take oral medication	Cefazolin or ceftriaxone†	1 g IM or IV	50 mg/kg IM or IV
	or		
	Clindamycin	600 mg IM or IV	20 mg/kg IM or IV

From Wilson W, Taubert KA, Gewitz M, et al: Prevention of infective endocarditis: guidelines from the American Heart Association: a guideline from the American Heart Association Rheumatic Fever, Endocarditis, and Kawasaki Disease Committee, Council on Cardiovascular Disease in the Young, and the Council on Clinical Cardiology, Council on Cardiovascular Surgery and Anesthesia, and the Quality of Care and Outcomes Research Interdisciplinary Working Group, *Circulation* 116(15):1736-1754, 2007.

IM, Intramuscular; *IV*, intravenous.

*Or other first- or second-generation oral cephalosporin in equivalent adult or pediatric dosage.

†Cephalosporins should not be used in a person with a history of anaphylaxis, angioedema, or urticaria with penicillins or ampicillin.

From the American Heart Association Prevention of Infective Endocarditis Guidelines.[5]

TABLE 12-5

Dental Management Considerations When Using Prophylactic Antibiotics

Management of At-Risk Individuals	Management Rationale
Use prophylactic antibiotics during the perioperative period (½ -1 hour before treatment) or within 2 hours of appointment.	This may prevent infective endocarditis.
Establish and maintain the best oral health.	This may prevent infective endocarditis. Educate the client.
Schedule appointments for procedures requiring antibiotic prophylaxis 10 days apart.	This reduces emergence of resistant microorganisms and allows repopulation of the usual antibiotic-susceptible flora.
If appointments for procedures requiring antibiotic prophylaxis are scheduled less than 9 days apart or if a patient is currently on a regimen antibiotic for other reasons, use an alternative regimen antibiotic.	This reduces emergence of resistant microorganisms.
A combination of procedures should be planned for a dental appointment in which the patient is prophylaxed.	This reduces the number of times a client is premedicated, which lowers cost and decreases the likelihood of resistant microorganisms emerging.
Encourage full or partial denture wearers to have periodic oral examinations and return to their provider if discomfort develops.	Ill-fitting removable oral prostheses can cause tissue ulceration with concomitant bacteremia of oral origin.
When antibiotic is inadvertently missed, administer antibiotic prophylaxis within 2 hours after the procedure.	This may provide effective prophylaxis. There is no prophylactic benefit if one administers antibiotic 3 or more hours after an indicated procedure.

Adapted from Wilson W, Taubert KA, Gewitz M, et al: Prevention of infective endocarditis: guidelines from the American Heart Association: a guideline from the American Heart Association Rheumatic Fever, Endocarditis and Kawasaki Disease Committee, Council on Cardiovascular Disease in the Young, and the Council on Clinical Cardiology, Council on Cardiovascular Surgery and Anesthesia, and the Quality of Care and Outcomes Research Interdisciplinary Working Group, *J Am Dent Assoc 2007*;138:739.

patient reveals a condition that precludes dental hygiene care or needs prompt dental or medical attention. Consultations should be documented in the client's dental record and followed up with a written consultation form (Figure 12-5). To expedite the receipt of information, a request for the physician to fax information is acceptable.

When requesting additional medical information from a client's referring physician, the dental hygiene practitioner first should obtain consent for information release from the client, per HIPAA regulations. An entry in the treatment record should document to whom the medical request was sent and the reason for the request. Information obtained from the patient's physician should be placed in the patient's dental record. A formal written request for medical consultation is the preferred procedure for medical-legal documentation. Sample medical consultation forms are shown in Figure 12-6.

Referral

Clients are referred for medical evaluation when an undiagnosed condition is suspected (e.g., presence of signs and symptoms of diabetes mellitus) or when needed laboratory test results are not available (e.g., blood test to determine risk for excessive bleeding when warfarin is taken).

CLIENT EDUCATION TIPS

- Counsel clients predisposed to an emergency situation in the dental setting by using the information in the clients' health history. For example, a client with diabetes mellitus should be counseled to eat after taking his or her indicated dose of insulin (or sulfonylurea) the day of an appointment.
- When a medical consultation is indicated, educate the client about the concerns of the condition and the risks of proceeding with oral care without proper medical advice.
- When antibiotic premedication is indicated, educate clients about the rationale for prophylactic antibiotic premedication before dental hygiene procedures involving gingival or apical manipulation.
- Educate clients about the importance of regular oral examinations to reduce the severity of oral disease and decrease costs associated with oral care.
- Educate clients about the legal justification for particular activities; explain issues of standards of care, scope of practice, and duty to the client.
- Data are recorded to keep accurate records to assist in client care and protect individuals from health risks.

LEGAL, ETHICAL, AND SAFETY ISSUES

- Before making a legal or ethical decision, the dental hygiene practitioner seeks resources that guide the process. The American Dental Hygienists Association (ADHA) and Canadian Dental Hygienists Association (CDHA) each publishes a code of ethics. Dental hygiene practitioners also need to be aware of public health statutes, rules, and

FOOTHILL COLLEGE
12345 El Monte Road, Los Altos Hills, CA 94022-4599
Dental Hygiene Care Facility Telephone #: (650) 949-7335 Fax #: (650) 949-7375

To:

From: Foothill College Dental Hygiene Care Facility

Re: Confirmation of Phone Conversation

This is to confirm our phone conversation on ______________ (Date) regarding our patient ______________ (Patient's name) .

According to our conversation, it is my understanding that: ______________

____

____

____

____

____

Please verify the conversation by completing the attached referral letter. Return the referral letter and the white copy of this letter to:

Foothill College Dental Hygiene Care Facility
12345 El Monte Road,
Los Altos Hills, CA 94022-4599

Thank you for your prompt attention to this matter.

______________ (Dental hygiene student signature) ______________ (Date)

______________ (Faculty signature) ______________ (Date)

white - return to Foothill College yellow - physician copy pink - FC patient chart

(3ref/9-95)

Figure 12-5. Sample scripted suggestions for questions regarding medical health consultation. (From Foothill College, Dental Hygiene Program, Los Altos Hills, California.)

FOOTHILL COLLEGE
12345 El Monte Road, Los Altos Hills, CA 94022-4599
Dental Hygiene Care Facility **Telephone #:** (650) 949-7335 **Fax #:** (650) 947-9788

To:

From: Foothill College Dental Hygiene Care Facility

Re: Need for Antibiotic Premedication

______________________________is being seen at the Foothill College Dental Hygiene Clinic. The treatment we are recommending involves scaling and root planing. This procedure involves the smoothing of the unattached surfaces of the teeth by removing calculus and/or cementum. It is performed with the use of a local anesthetic. The anesthetic of choice is ____________________ ______________________________. Since scaling and root planing procedures do contact the blood stream, causing a transient bacteremia, we are requesting this medical consultation prior to proceeding with dental hygiene treatment.

This patient's health history indicates: ____

____

Please evaluate this/these condition(s). Indicate your recommendations and/or contraindications for patient treatment by checking one of the following sections, and signing below. Please return the white copy to our clinic.

- ❑ Antibiotic premedication is necessary. If so, what regimen? (The patient must receive the prescription from you) ____

  ____
- ❑ Dental hygiene care should be postponed at this time because: ______________________

  ____
- ❑ No special considerations are required. Proceed with dental hygiene care.
- ❑ Other ____

______________________________ ______________________
(Dental hygiene student signature) (Date)

______________________________ ______________________
(Faculty signature) (Date)

______________________________ ______________________
(Physician signature) (Date)

______________________________ ______________________
(Physician address, city, zip code) (Physician's phone number)

white - return to Foothill College yellow - physician copy pink - FC patient's chart

(2premed/11-96)

A

Figure 12-6. **A,** Sample medical consultation form.

Continued

FOOTHILL COLLEGE
12345 El Monte Road, Los Altos Hills, CA 94022-4599
Dental Hygiene Care Facility Telephone #:(650) 949-7335 Fax #: (650) 947-9788

To:

From: Foothill College Dental Hygiene Care Facility

Re: Medical Clearance Prior to Dental Hygiene Treatment

________________________ would like to receive dental hygiene treatment at the Foothill College Dental Hygiene Clinic. It is anticipated that the care may extend over a couple of months with a series of appointments of 3 1/2 hours duration. The treatment we are recommending involves scaling and root planing, which is the smoothing of the unattached surfaces of the teeth by removing calculus and/or cementum. This procedure is performed with the use of a local anesthetic, and the anesthetic of choice is ________________.

When there is any question regarding the patient's health status, it is our policy to obtain guidance from his/her physician prior to proceeding with dental hygiene care. This patient's health history indicates:

____

____

Please evaluate this health condition. Indicate your recommendations and/or contraindications for patient treatment by checking one of the following and signing below. Please return the white copy to our clinic.

❑ Postpone dental hygiene treatment at the present time because: ________________

____

❑ This patient's health status is not a contraindication for proceeding with dental hygiene treatment.

❑ Proceed with dental hygiene treatment including the following modifications: ________________

____

____

❑ Other ________________________________

(Dental hygiene student signature)	(Date)
(Faculty signature)	(Date)
(Physician signature)	(Date)
(Physician address, city, zip code)	(Physician phone number)

white - return to Foothill College yellow - physician copy pink - FC patient chart

(7medcle/9-95)

B

Figure 12-6, cont'd **B,** Sample medical clearance before dental hygiene treatment form. (From Foothill College, Dental Hygiene Program, Los Altos Hills, California.)

regulations governing the practice of dental hygiene in their legal jurisdiction. Public health statutes may identify responsibilities such as mandatory reporting of abuse and neglect, domestic violence, and infectious diseases, as well as particular record-keeping instructions.

- Written office protocols that reflect evidence-based practices protect the healthcare team from litigation if the protocols are used.
- The health history should be recorded in permanent ink only.

- The history form is completed by the client. Information can be added by the client and the dental hygiene practitioner while jointly reviewing the health history information. Emergency phone numbers and physician phone numbers always should be present on the form in the event that a medical emergency occurs, so that appropriate personnel can be notified.
- A space at the top of the health history form can be used to alert the practitioner to medical conditions that require dental hygiene care modifications and to prevent health risks. These important conditions should be written in a way that captures the reader's attention.
- Errors are carefully lined out, dated, and initialed. Explanations may be necessary to avoid confusion. For example, if at a later date the client remembers an allergy to penicillin, the correction should be made at the appropriate location on the form and an explanation added, such as, "Client remembers an allergy to penicillin" (date and initial).
- Document relevant information learned during questioning on the health history form; review written comments with the client, which the client should sign or initial.
- The health history form contains confidential information to be shared only with those involved directly with the client's treatment. Follow state and local regulations concerning protection of medical history information.
- Medical consultation or referrals should outline the medical issue requiring consultation or referral. One copy of the form is sent to the physician. Another copy of the form is kept in the client's chart to document the request for consultation or referral. When necessary, telephone consultations should be documented in the client's chart and followed with a faxed verification from the physician, including details of the conversation and the name of the person providing information at the physician's office.
- Signing the health history form indicates accuracy of information provided by the client. Client approval for treatment is indicated by a signed informed consent form, which always should be used.
- Care should be provided to a minor only after an appropriate signature is obtained on the minor's informed consent form from the parent or legal guardian.

KEY CONCEPTS

- The health history is a legal document that contains protected information about the client's state of health.
- The dental hygiene practitioner–client relationship is a partnership based on trust and has the client's well-being as a mutual focus.
- The client completes the written health history questionnaire at the first visit. The dental hygiene practitioner reviews, discusses, and verifies the information on the health history questionnaire during the client interview. At subsequent appointments the health history is updated; changes are investigated and documented in writing.
- The dental hygiene practitioner builds rapport by incorporating patient-centered interviewing techniques, such as open-ended questioning and back-channeling, as well as excellent verbal and nonverbal communication in the health history interview.
- The American Society of Anesthesiologists (ASA) Physical Status Classification System can be used to identify the medical risk of the client and reduce the probability that medical emergencies will occur. Only clients in the ASA 1 through 3 classifications should receive elective oral care.
- Stress reduction protocols minimize risk of a medical emergency and create a satisfactory experience for the anxious client.
- A dental drug reference should be used to determine drug actions, interactions, contraindications, adverse reactions, and oral health education topics. The *Merck Manual* is a useful reference for information concerning diseases or medical conditions.
- Infective endocarditis (IE) can be a life-threatening condition. Dental procedures including gingival manipulation or perforation of oral mucosa may be a risk factor for IE. Only clients at the highest risk for complications from IE should receive prophylactic antibiotic premedication before dental hygiene procedures.
- Clients with prosthetic joints or orthopedic hardware in place are at risk for prosthetic joint infection. These individuals generally do not require prophylactic antibiotics before dental procedures but may require medical evaluation by the referring physician depending on comorbidities.
- Selection of prophylactic antibiotic agent is based on recommended guidelines, concurrently prescribed antibiotic agents, and client tolerance of the medication.
- A client may have an undiagnosed disease that can be recognized by a comprehensive health history review and observation of signs and reported symptoms. The health history review and physical assessment are monitors of a client's health and risk status.

CRITICAL THINKING EXERCISES

Client Profile: Mr. Smith is a 35-year-old male client referred for oral abscess and periodontal care.

Chief Complaint: "To get my teeth taken care of"

Dental History: Mr. Smith has avoided dentists for more than 10 years until he developed severe oral pain. A local endodontist referred him to the general dentist. The referral letter noted that Mr. Smith has an apical abscess associated with decayed tooth No. 30. The endodontist noted that Mr. Smith placed aspirin directly on the gingival tissues near No. 30, resulting in a chemical burn on the adjacent mucosa and gingiva. Mr. Smith needs extensive restorative and nonsurgical periodontal care. Mr. Smith has rescheduled his first appointment with the general dentist three times because of fear of oral care. The periodontal assessment visit with the dental hygiene practitioner also was rescheduled several times by Mr. Smith for similar reasons.

Medical History: Mr. Smith has a history of asthma, hypertension, and diabetes type 1. His asthma is managed with a bronchodilator (albuterol) inhaler taken as needed. His last asthma attack occurred recently at the endodontist office and was managed with his bronchodilator. Mr. Smith has type 1 diabetes that is controlled by daily insulin and diet, with very rare hypoglycemic episodes which he treats with orange juice or hard candy. He reports his fingerstick glucose measurements have been well controlled, although he can't recall his most recent hemoglobin A_{1c}

test value. He sees a physician on a regular basis for the diabetes and asthma. He brought his albuterol inhaler to the appointment in his pocket. He is also taking medication (Procardia) to control high blood pressure, and he took it last evening. He has no history of heart disease as a child, but recalls that his doctor noticed a heart murmur at his last appointment. All vital signs recorded at the first office visit were within normal limits (WNL), and today's readings are also WNL. On his health history questionnaire, he indicates no prior unpleasant experiences in a dental office or nervousness about treatment.

Social History: Mr. Smith never married, is without children, and is self-employed as a contractor and home builder. He lives alone.

Extraoral Examination: All within normal limits

Supplemental Notes: Client arrived late for the 4:30 PM appointment. At 5:15 PM the dental hygiene practitioner escorted him to the treatment room to review the health and dental history. The hygiene practitioner noticed that Mr. Smith was anxious with perspiration beads on his upper lip, trembling hands; he was grasping the arms of the dental chair. The health history was reviewed, vital signs were measured, and no health history changes have occurred other than the recent asthma attack.

1. Before dental hygiene assessment begins, what is the appropriate step in caring for Mr. Smith?
2. What is Mr. Smith's ASA classification?
3. What ASA protocols apply to Mr. Smith?
4. What type of dialogue should occur before care to prevent an emergency situation (e.g., hypoglycemic episode or syncope) during dental hygiene care?
5. Does Mr. Smith require antibiotic prophylaxis?
6. What client behaviors are suggestive of fear and anxiety? How could the dental hygiene practitioner address these emotions?

REFERENCES

1. Pickett F, Gurenlian J: *The medical history: clinical implications and emergency prevention in dental settings*, ed 2, Baltimore, 2009, Lippincott Williams and Wilkins.
2. Fitch P: Cultural competence and dental hygiene care delivery: integrating cultural care into the dental hygiene process of care. *J Dent Hyg* 78(1):11, 2004.
3. Fortin AH, Dwamena FC, Frankel RM, et al: *Smith's patient-centered interviewing: an evidence-based method*, ed 3, New York, 2012, McGraw-Hill.
4. Brody H: The biopsychosocial model, patient-centered care, and culturally sensitive practice. *J Fam Pract* 48(8):585, 1999.
5. Wilson W, Taubert KA, Gewitz M, et al: American Heart Association Rheumatic Fever, Endocarditis, and Kawasaki Disease Committee, American Heart Association Council on Cardiovascular Disease in the Young, American Heart Association Council on Clinical Cardiology, American Heart Association Council on Cardiovascular Surgery and Anesthesia, Quality of Care and Outcomes Research Interdisciplinary Working Group. Prevention of infective endocarditis: guidelines from the American Heart Association: a guideline from the American Heart Association Rheumatic Fever, Endocarditis, and Kawasaki Disease Committee, Council on Cardiovascular Disease in the Young, and the Council on Clinical Cardiology, Council on Cardiovascular Surgery and Anesthesia, and the Quality of Care and Outcomes Research Interdisciplinary Working Group. *Circulation* 116(15):1736, 2007.
6. *Summary of the HIPAA Privacy Rule.* US Dept of Health and Human Services, Office for Civil Rights. Revised May 2003. Available at: http://www.hhs.gov/ocr/privacy/hipaa/understanding/summary/privacysummary.pdf. Accessed February 2013.
7. American Society of Anesthesiologists: *ASA Physical Status Classification System*. Available at http://www.asahq.org/For-Members/Clinical-Information/ASA-Physical-Status-Classification-System.aspx. Accessed February 5, 2013.
8. Fleisher LA, Beckman JA, Brown KA, et al: ACC-AHA 2007 guidelines on perioperative cardiovascular evaluation and care for noncardiac surgery: executive summary: a report of the American College of Cardiology/American Heart Association Task Force on Practice Guidelines. *Circulation* 116(17):1971, 2007.
9. Reilly DF, McNeely MJ, Doerner D, et al: Self-reported exercise tolerance and the risk of serious perioperative complications. *Arch Intern Med* 159(18):2185, 1999.
10. *Physicians' desk reference*, ed 63, Montvale, NJ, 2009, Medical Economics.
11. *Mosby's dental drug reference*, ed 11, St Louis, 2014, Mosby.
12. Wynn RL, Meiller TF, Crossley HL: *Drug information handbook for dentistry*, ed 13, Hudson, Ohio, 2007, LexiComp.
13. Pickett FA, Terezhalmy GT: *Dental drug reference with clinical implications*, ed 2, Baltimore, 2007, Lippincott Williams and Wilkins.
14. Beers MH, Porter RS, Jones TV, editors: *The Merck manual of diagnosis and therapy*, ed 18, Whitehouse Station, NJ, 2006, Merck. http://www.merckmanuals.com/. Accessed September 13, 2013.
15. Wahl MJ: Myths of dental-induced prosthetic joint infections. *Clin Infect Dis* 20(5):1450, 1995.
16. Zimmerly W, Parham S: Antibiotics for prevention of periprosthetic joint infection following dentistry: time to focus on data. *Clin Infect Dis* 50(1):17, 2010.
17. Berbari EF, Osmon DR, Carr A, et al: Dental procedures as risk factors for prosthetic hip or knee infection: a hospital-based prospective case-control study. *Clin Infect Dis* 50(1):8, 2010.
18. Little JW, Jacobson JJ, Lockhart PB: American Academy of Oral Medicine. The dental treatment of patients with joint replacements: a position paper from the American Academy of Oral Medicine. *J Am Dent Assoc* 141(6):667, 2010.
19. American Academy of Orthopaedic Surgeons and the American Dental Association: *Prevention of orthopaedic implant infection in patients undergoing dental procedures guideline*, Rosemont, Ill, 2012, AAOS.
20. Ching DW, Gould IM, Rennie JA, et al: Prevention of late haematogenous infection in major prosthetic joints. *J Antimicrob Chemother* 23:676, 1989.
21. Poss R, Thornhill TS, Ewald FC, et al: Factors influencing the incidence and outcome of infection following total joint arthroplasty. *Clin Orthop* 182:117, 1984.
22. Brause BD: Infections associated with prosthetic joints. *Clin Rheum Dis* 12:523, 1986.
23. Berbari EF, Hanssen AD, Duffy MC, et al: Risk factors for prosthetic joint infection: case-control study. *Clin Infect Dis* 27:1247, 1998.
24. American Dental Association: American Academy of Orthopaedic Surgeons: advisory statement: antibiotic prophylaxis for dental patients with total joint replacements. *J Am Dent Assoc* 134:895, 2003.
25. Wilson W, Taubert KA, Gewitz M, et al: Prevention of infective endocarditis. Guidelines from the American Heart Association. *J Am Dent Assoc* 138:739, 2007.

ACKNOWLEDGMENT

The author acknowledges Cara Miyasaki for her past contributions to this chapter and Dr. Devan Darby for her thorough review.

EVOLVE RESOURCES

Please visit http://evolve.elsevier.com/Darby/hygiene for additional practice and study support tools.

CHAPTER 13

Vital Signs

Cara M. Miyasaki

COMPETENCIES

1. Discuss vital signs and the importance of minimizing risk of a medical emergency via vital signs assessment.
2. Do the following regarding the assessment of body temperature, including:
   - Assess temperature and record these vital signs measurements.
   - Recognize findings that have implications for care planning, and initiate medical referrals for the health and safety of the client.
   - Compare baseline measurements with current findings, and communicate significant changes to the client and dentist.
3. Discuss the significance of the pulse and do the following:
   - Assess the pulse rate and record these vital signs measurements.
   - Recognize findings that have implications for care planning, and initiate medical referrals for the health and safety of the client.
   - Compare baseline measurements with current findings, and communicate significant changes to the client and dentist.
4. Discuss the assessment of respiration, including:
   - Assess the respiration rate and record these vital signs measurements.
   - Recognize findings that have implications for care planning, and initiate medical referrals for the health and safety of the client.
   - Compare baseline measurements with current findings, and communicate significant changes to the client and dentist.
5. Do the following regarding the assessment of blood pressure, including:
   - Assess the blood pressure and record these vital signs measurements.
   - Recognize findings that have implications for care planning, and initiate medical referrals for the health and safety of the client.
   - Compare baseline measurements with current findings, and communicate significant changes to the client and dentist.

Vital Signs

Temperature, pulse rate, respiration rate, and blood pressure, indicators of health status, are referred to as **vital signs**. Inspection, palpation, and **auscultation** (listening either directly or with a stethoscope for sounds produced in the body) are techniques used to determine vital signs. At the initial client appointment, vital signs help to identify undiagnosed medical problems or establish baseline measurements for comparison at future appointments (Box 13-1). Box 13-2 lists appropriate occasions for the dental hygienist to measure and record the client's vital signs.

Vital signs outside an acceptable range may indicate health problems, undiagnosed conditions, the need for referral to a physician, or the need to terminate dental hygiene care. In addition to illness, age, gender, medications, the temperature of the environment, altitude, body position, physical exertion, diet, stress, improperly used equipment, unreliable equipment, and other factors can affect vital signs. Vital signs are analyzed to interpret their significance and make clinical decisions. If abnormal readings are obtained, the dental hygienist questions the client about possible causes and repeats the measurement. When readings that exceed normal limits are validated, the dental hygienist communicates them to the client, dentist, and physician of record. The following practice guidelines assist in obtaining accurate vital signs:

- Use properly working and appropriate equipment designed for the size and age of the client (e.g., an adult-size blood pressure cuff should not be used for a child or obese person).
- Be familiar with the client's baseline measurements, health status, and pharmacologic history; some illnesses, treatment, behaviors, and medications affect vital signs.
- Minimize environmental factors that may affect vital signs (e.g., do not assess temperature in a warm, humid room).
- Use a systematic approach for each procedure.
- Approach the client in a calm, caring manner while demonstrating competence in vital sign measurement.
- Use critical thinking skills to determine when the dentist should be notified and whether a medical consult is needed.

Body Temperature

Body **temperature** is regulated by the brain's hypothalamic area, which acts as the body's thermostat. The hypothalamus senses changes in temperature and sends impulses out to the body to correct them. On a hot day the hypothalamus detects a rise in body temperature and sends signals to the skin to perspire and lower its temperature. In cold weather the hypothalamus detects a lowering of the body's temperature and signals the body to shiver, increasing body temperature.

No single temperature is normal for all people. The normal range for body temperature is 96.8° F to 100.4° F (or 36° C to 38° C).

BOX 13-1

Vital Signs: Acceptable Ranges for Adults

Temperature

Range: 36° C to 38° C (96.8° F to 100.4° F)

Average oral or tympanic: 37° C (98.6° F)

Average axillary: 36.5° C (97.7° F)

Pulse

60 to 100 beats per minute

Average: 80 beats per minute

Respirations

12 to 20 breaths per minute

Blood Pressure

<120/<80 mm Hg

Adapted from Potter PA, Griffin AG, Stockert P, et al: *Fundamentals of nursing*, ed 8, St Louis, 2012, Mosby.

BOX 13-2

When to Take Vital Signs

- At every continued-care appointment (3-month, 4-month, 6-month, 12-month recall appointment) for a client whose vital signs are within normal limits
- Whenever a significant change occurs in the client's health history
- At each appointment for a client with readings that fall outside the normal limits but who is being monitored by a physician; in a client who is on medication that can affect blood pressure; and/or in a client whose condition indicates a need for monitoring blood pressure (e.g., a pregnant woman)
- Before the administration of a local anesthetic agent, nitrous oxide–oxygen analgesia, or any other medication that could affect cardiovascular, respiratory, and temperature regulation and after nitrous oxide administration
- Before, during, and after surgical procedures
- When the client makes statements about feeling physically ill
- If the client reports symptoms that indicate a potential emergency situation or when a medical emergency is in progress

TABLE 13-1

Factors That Affect Body Temperature

Factors	Effects
Exercise	Increases body temperature
Hormonal influences	Decrease or increase body temperature
Before ovulation	Body temperature decreased below baseline
During ovulation	Body temperature increased to baseline or higher
Menopause	Periodic increase (30 seconds to 5 minutes) in body temperature "hot flashes"
Time of Day Variations	
Early morning	Temperature is lowest
Daytime	Body temperature rises
Evening	Body temperature peaks by 0.5° F to 1° F (0.3° C to 0.6° C)
Stress (physical and emotional)	Increases body temperature
Warm environment	Increases body temperature
Cold environment	Decreases body temperature
Infection	Increases body temperature
Tachypnea (rapid breathing)	Decreases oral temperature
Age	For persons >70 years of age, average oral body temperature is 96.8° F (36° C)
Hot liquids	Increase oral temperature for about 15 minutes
Cold liquids	Decrease oral temperature for about 15 minutes
Smoking	Increases oral temperature for about 30 minutes

Maintaining body temperature requires a balance between heat loss and heat production. With aging, the normal temperature range gradually narrows because the mechanisms that control thermoregulation start to deteriorate. Table 13-1 lists factors that affect body temperature.

Body Temperature Measurement Sites

There are five sites to measure temperature: oral, ear, rectal, axilla, and forehead. The superficial temporal electronic device, used to scan across the forehead and slightly behind the ear, is the easiest and most accurate. Electronic oral devices are also accurate; however, caution should be taken to prevent inaccurate readings if hot or cold foods have been ingested (wait 20 to 30 minutes) or if the client has been smoking. Alternative sites such as the ear (tympanic membrane) or axilla (armpit) should be used when the client's safety is a consideration. For example, unconscious clients, infants, small children, or cognitively challenged clients may have difficulty with the oral thermometer under the tongue or may bite the thermometer and break it.

Thermometers

There are many types of thermometers available for measuring body temperature (Table 13-2 and Figures 13-1 to 13-6). The mercury-in-glass thermometer is no longer the standard of care and is no longer recommended because of the environmental hazard of mercury. Electronic (digital) thermometers are used commonly at home and in professional practice.

Electronic (digital) thermometers consist of a probe or infrared scanner attached to a digital readout (see Figures 13-1 and 13-3) to measure oral, axillary, tympanic (ear)

TABLE 13-2

Types of Thermometers for Measuring Body Temperature

Name	Types Available	Disadvantages	Advantages
Electronic thermometer	Oral	Potential for inaccuracies owing to shorter reading time of 15 to 25 seconds (must control environmental factors such as recent intake of hot or cold substances, smoking)	Decreased client discomfort Efficient for healthcare professional Easy to read
	Axillary (underarm)	Specific research on axillary type is limited	Reasonably accurate Short reading time (25-30 seconds)
	Superficial temporal artery	Readings affected by skin moisture (sweating/perspiration)	Ease of use Accurate and reliable Reliable reading in seconds
	Tympanic membrane thermometer	Questions concerning accuracy in young children	Less invasive Short reading time (2-5 seconds)
	Pacifier	Requires longer (2 minute) reading time	Ideal for baby or toddler (Birth-5 years)
Thermometers for screening	Oral (60 seconds) Axillary (3 minutes)	Potential to overestimate or underestimate true temperature readings	Some are disposable Verify with more accurate thermometer if fever detected

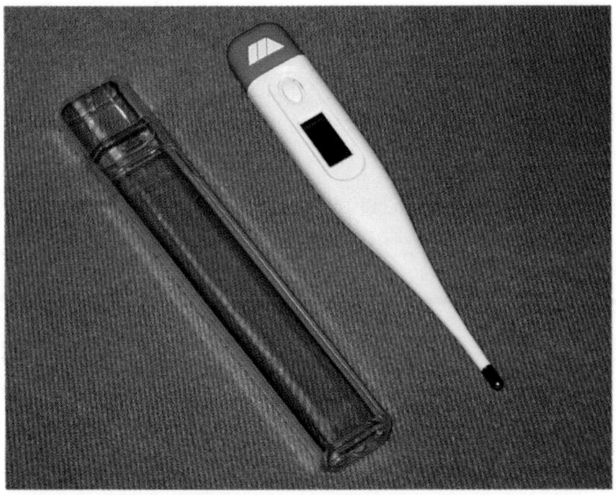

Figure 13-1. Electronic (digital) thermometer. (Courtesy Sedation Resource, Lone Oak, Texas, www.sedationresource.com.)

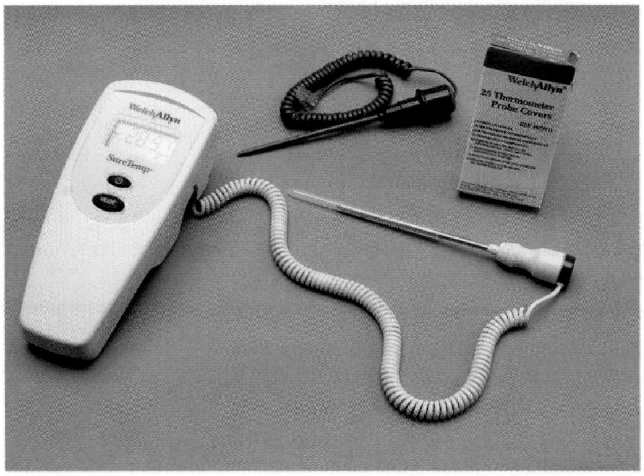

Figure 13-3. Electronic thermometer. Blue probe is for oral or axillary use. Red probe is for rectal use. (From Potter PA, Griffin AG, Stockert P, et al: *Fundamentals of nursing,* ed 8, St Louis, 2012, Mosby.)

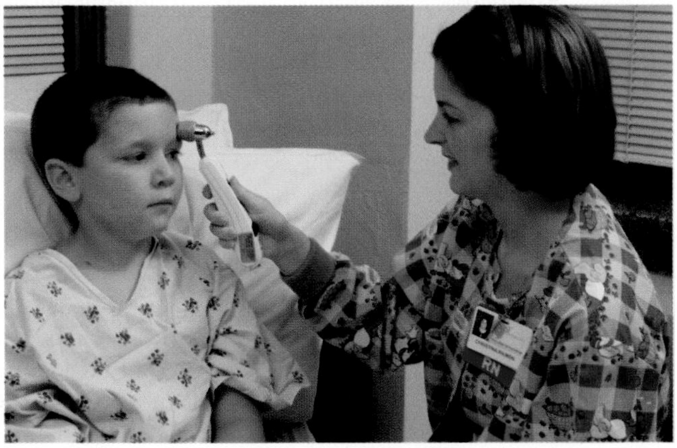

Figure 13-2. Electronic thermometer for superficial temporal artery. (From Potter PA, Griffin, AG, Stockert P, et al: *Fundamentals of nursing,* ed 8, St Louis, 2012, Mosby.)

membrane, and superficial temporal (forehead) artery temperatures. When the thermometer is placed in the mouth, a disposable plastic sheath is used over the oral probe as a protective barrier for infection control. A pacifier thermometer (see Figure 13-4), a type of electronic thermometer, obtains a reasonably accurate reading in younger children within 3 minutes. Underarm (axillary) electronic thermometers (see Figure 13-4), have a short reading time (8 to 30 seconds) and are easy to use in young children. Tympanic membrane (ear) thermometers (see Figure 13-5) are easy to use, less invasive, and achieve a reading within seconds but may not be as reliable as other assessment devices. Oral, axillary, and superficial temporal artery thermometers can indicate a client's temperature within seconds. Disposable single-use thermometers are used mostly for oral temperature screening (see Figure 13-6). See Procedure 13-1 and the corresponding Competency Form for taking basal body temperature. Temperature is recorded in degrees Fahrenheit.

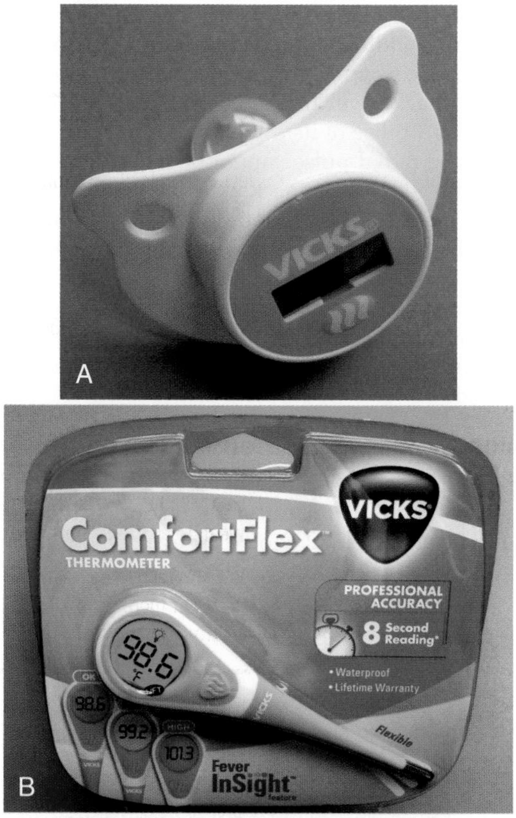

Figure 13-4. **A,** Electronic pacifier thermometer. **B,** Underarm (axillary), oral, and rectal electronic thermometer.

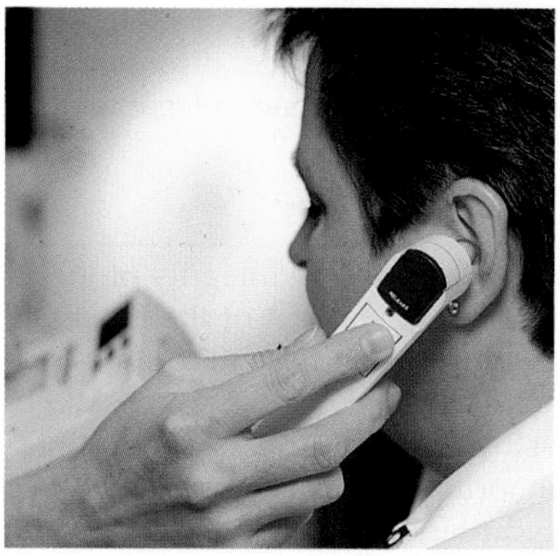

Figure 13-5. Tympanic membrane thermometer. (From Potter PA, Griffin AG, Stockert P, et al: *Fundamentals of nursing,* ed 8, St Louis, 2012, Mosby.)

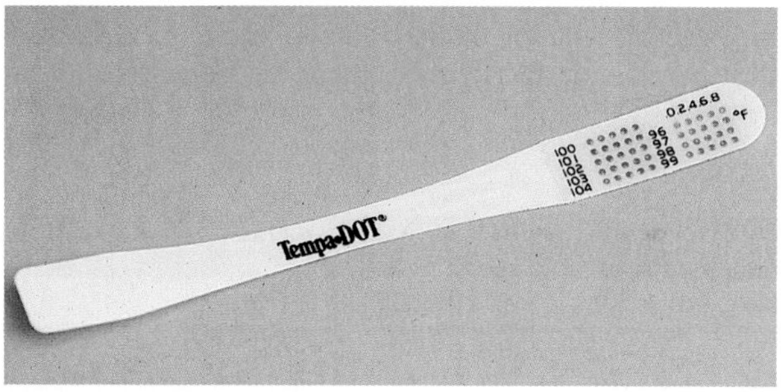

Figure 13-6. Disposable, single-use thermometer strip. (From Potter PA, Griffin AG, Stockert P, et al: *Fundamentals of nursing,* ed 8, St Louis, 2012, Mosby.)

Procedure 13-1 Taking an Oral Temperature Measurement with an Electronic Thermometer

EQUIPMENT

Personal protective equipment for the clinician
Electronic thermometer, disposable sheath

STEPS

1. Wash hands with antimicrobial soap.
2. Explain procedure to client.
3. Ask client if hot or cold substances were ingested or if tobacco was smoked within the previous 30 minutes.
4. Remove thermometer pack from charging unit, check to make sure the oral probe is attached to the unit.
5. Insert the oral probe into the plastic, disposable cover until it locks into place.
6. Ask the client to open his or her mouth, and gently place the probe under the tongue, posterior and lateral to the lower jaw. Avoid placing probe directly under tongue.
7. Ask client to hold the probe with the lips closed.
8. An audible tone will signal that the temperature has been taken; note display.
9. Remove the probe and discard the disposable cover by pushing the ejection button. Place probe back into original storage well in the unit.
10. Return the thermometer to the charger.
11. Record the client's temperature, the date, and the time of day on the chart.
12. Inform client of readings above 37.5° C (99.6° F), and make referral to primary care provider if indicated.
13. Document in the electronic chart the completion of this service in the client's record under "Services Rendered," with the time of day, and date the entry. For example: "8/01/13 client stated that she was not feeling well and felt that she was running a fever. Client's temperature taken at 2:00 PM was 101.5° F. Client referred to primary healthcare provider for evaluation and appointment rescheduled."

Adapted from Potter PA, Griffin AG, Stockert P, et al: *Fundamentals of nursing,* ed 8, St Louis, 2012, Mosby.

Decision Making Based on Observed Temperature

Usually a high body temperature (known as fever or pyrexia) indicates that the body is fighting an infection. Young children (younger than 5 years old) are at risk of febrile seizures if fever exceeds 101.8° F (or 38.8° C). If the client's temperature exceeds 99.6° F (or 37.5° C) or higher, the client should be evaluated for causative factors (see Table 13-1). If the client's temperature is 102.2° F (or 39° C) and the infection is not dentally related, a referral for medical evaluation by the client's primary healthcare provider is indicated. If pyrexia is due to a dental infection, then immediate dental treatment and antibiotic therapy may be indicated. A body temperature of 105.8° F (41° C) indicates a medical emergency, so the EMS system would be activated. Low body temperature can occur with cold exposure, endocrine disorders, sepsis, alcohol intake, eating disorders, and neurologic and neuromuscular disorders.

Pulse

The pulse, an indicator of the integrity of the cardiovascular system, is the intermittent beat of the heart felt through the walls of an artery. Tachycardia (>100 beats per minute [BPM]) is an abnormally elevated heart rate; however, it is a normal response to stress or physical exercise. Bradycardia (<60 BPM) is an abnormally slow heart rate (Table 13-3). Athletes may be bradycardic at rest owing to physical conditioning. Table 13-4 describes factors that influence pulse rate.

Pulse Measurement Sites

Pulse points are body sites where the rhythmic beats of an artery can be felt. The most common site for assessing the radial pulse is on the thumb side of the inner wrist, where the radial artery can be felt (Figure 13-7, See Procedure 13-2 and the corresponding Competency Form). The fingertips of the first two fingers are used to feel for the pulse (a throbbing sensation). (*Note:* Never use the thumb to feel for the pulse, because it has a pulse of its own that can be mistaken for the client's.) If the radial pulse cannot be felt, the carotid pulse, located on the side of the neck over the carotid artery, is an alternative. In emergency situations the carotid pulse should be palpated because the body delivers blood to the brain for as long as possible, whereas peripheral blood supply can decline. The pulse is recorded in beats per minute (BPM). Heart rhythm (regular or irregular) and pulse quality (thready, strong, bounding, or weak) also are assessed when the pulse is measured.

Decision Making Based on Observed Pulse Rate

If the adult client's heart rate falls below 60 BPM or rises above 100 BPM, the client should be evaluated for causative

TABLE 13-3

Acceptable Ranges of Heart (Pulse) Rate

Age	Heart Rate (Beats per Minute)
Infant	120-160
Toddler	90-140
Preschooler	80-110
School-age child	75-100
Adolescent	60-100
Adult	60-100

Adapted from Potter PA, Griffin AG, Stockert P, et al: *Fundamentals of nursing,* ed 8, St Louis, 2012, Mosby.

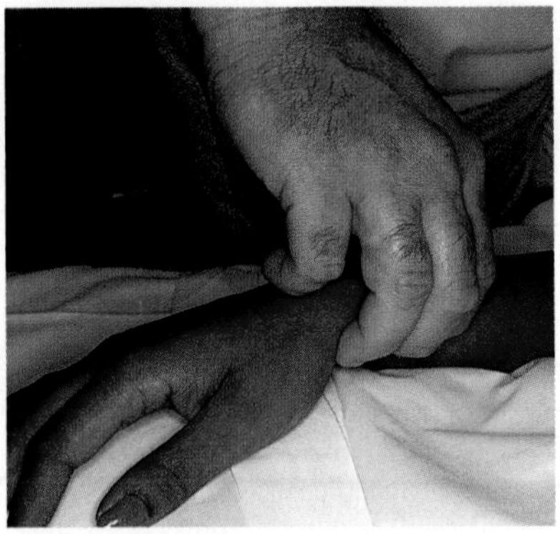

Figure 13-7. Position of the fingers in measuring the radial pulse. (From Potter PA, Griffin AG, Stockert P, et al: *Fundamentals of nursing,* ed 8, St Louis, 2012, Mosby.)

TABLE 13-4

Factors That Influence Heart (Pulse) Rate

Factor	Increased Pulse Rate	Decreased Pulse Rate
Exercise	Short-term exercise	A conditioned athlete who participates in long-term exercise will have a lower heart rate at rest
Temperature	Fever and heat	Hypothermia
Emotions and stress	Acute pain and anxiety increase sympathetic stimulation, affecting heart rate	Unrelieved severe pain increases parasympathetic stimulation, affecting heart rate; relaxation
Medications	Positive chronotropic drugs (e.g., epinephrine)	Negative chronotropic drugs (e.g., digitalis, beta and calcium blockers)
Hemorrhage	Loss of blood increases sympathetic stimulation	
Postural changes	Standing or sitting	Lying down
Pulmonary conditions	Diseases causing poor oxygenation such as asthma, chronic obstructive pulmonary disease (COPD)	

Adapted from Potter PA, Griffin AG, Stockert P, et al: *Fundamentals of nursing,* ed 8, St Louis, 2012, Mosby.

factors or conditions. If no cause can be determined, a medical consultation with the client's physician should be conducted.

A medical consultation is recommended in the following circumstances:

- If a client with risk factors for coronary artery disease is experiencing frequent **premature ventricular contractions** (PVCs) per minute. A PVC is an extra, abnormal heartbeat, which can feel like a skipped beat, fluttering, flip-flops, pounding, or jumpy. An occasional PVC in an otherwise healthy person is usually not of concern; however, if the client experiences frequent symptoms, a medical referral should be initiated.
- If the client is experiencing **pulsus alternans**, alternating strong and weak heartbeats, which may indicate ventricular failure, high blood pressure, or coronary heart disease.

A full, bounding pulse may indicate high blood pressure. A weak, thready pulse may be found in persons with hypotension and also may be a sign of shock.

Procedure 13-2 Measuring the Radial Pulse

EQUIPMENT

Wristwatch with a second hand

STEPS

1. Use a wristwatch with a second hand.
2. Wash hands with antimicrobial soap.
3. Explain purpose and method of procedure to the client. Advise client to relax and not to speak.
4. Have client assume a sitting position, bend the client's elbow 90 degrees, and support the client's lower arm on the armrest of the chair. Extend the wrist with the palm down.
5. Place first two fingers of hand along the client's radial artery (thumb side of wrist) and lightly compress (see Figure 13-7).
6. Obliterate the pulse initially, then relax pressure so that the pulse is easily palpable.
7. Determine rhythm and quality of the pulse (regular, regularly irregular, full and strong, weak and thready).
8. When pulse can be felt regularly, use the watch's second hand and begin to count the rate, starting with 0 and then 1, and so on.
9. If the pulse is regular, count for 30 seconds and multiply the total by 2.
10. If the pulse is irregular, count for a full minute.
11. Record heart rate (beats per minute [BPM]), rhythm of the heart (regular or irregular), the quality of the pulse (thready, strong, weak, bounding), and the date in the chart. Pulse rates outside the normal range should be evaluated by the client's physician.
12. Document in the electronic chart the completion of this service in the client's record under "Services Rendered." Record heart rate (BPM), rhythm of the heart (regular, regularly irregular, or irregularly irregular), the quality of the pulse (thready and weak [not easily felt], strong and full [easily felt]), and the date in the chart. For example: "8/01/13 Client's pulse has a regular rhythm and strong quality with rate of 65 BPM."

Data from Potter PA, Griffin AG, Stockert P, et al: *Fundamentals of nursing*, ed 8, St Louis, 2012, Mosby.

Respiration

Respiration rate is assessed by counting the rise and fall (inspiration and expiration) of the client's chest and is recorded as respirations per minute (RPM). The dental hygienist makes this assessment without the client's awareness to prevent the client from changing breathing patterns.

Respiration Measurement Site

Respiration rate may be measured before or after the client's pulse rate is assessed. The dental hygienist's hand remains on the client's radial pulse while the hygienist inconspicuously counts the rise and fall of the client's chest.

Normal adult range is 12 to 20 respirations per minute (RPM). Children have a more rapid respiratory rate (20 to 30 RPM) than that of adults. Young children also tend to have a less regular breathing cycle. Advancing age produces an increase in the respiration rate. Steps for measuring respirations are shown in Procedure 13-3 and the corresponding Competency Form.

Decision Making Based on Observed Respiration

Alterations in the rate, depth, or rhythm should be noted. If an abnormal respiratory rate is detected, the dental hygienist refers the client to the physician of record for a medical evaluation. Table 13-5 presents acceptable ranges of respiratory rates by age. Tachypnea (rapid breathing) greater than 20

Procedure 13-3 Measuring Respirations

EQUIPMENT

Wristwatch with a second hand

STEPS

1. Use a wristwatch with a second hand.
2. Place hand along the client's radial artery and inconspicuously observe the client's chest.
3. Observe the rise and fall of client's chest. Count complete respiratory cycles (one inspiration and one expiration).
4. For an adult, count the number of respirations in 30 seconds and multiply that number by 2. For a young child, count respirations for a full minute.
5. If an adult has respirations with an irregular rhythm, or if respirations are abnormally slow or fast (<12 or >20 breaths/minute), count for a full minute.
6. While counting, note whether depth is shallow, normal, or deep and whether rhythm is normal or one of the altered patterns.
7. Document in the electronic chart the completion of this service in the client's record under "Services Rendered." Record the date and the client's respirations per minute (RPM) in the chart; a respiration rate with an irregular pattern or that is outside of the normal range should be evaluated by the physician. For example: "8/01/13 Client's respiration has a regular rhythm with rate of 18 RPM."

Data from Potter PA, Griffin AG, Stockert P, et al: *Fundamentals of nursing*, ed 8, St Louis, 2012, Mosby.

TABLE 13-5

Acceptable Ranges of Respiratory Rate According to Age

Age	Rate (Breaths per Minute)
Newborn	35-40
Infant (6 months)	30-50
Toddler (2 years)	25-32
Child	20-30
Adolescent	16-20
Adult	12-20

Adapted from Potter PA, Griffin AG, Stockert P, et al: *Fundamentals of nursing*, ed 8, St Louis, 2012, Mosby.

TABLE 13-6

Average Optimal Blood Pressure According to Age

Age	Blood Pressure (mm Hg)
Newborn (3000 g [6.6 lb])	40 (mean)
1 month	85/54
1 year	95/65
6 years*	105/65
10-13 years*	110/65
14-17 years*	119/75
18 years and older	<120/<80

National Institutes of Health (NIH): *The seventh report of the Joint National Committee on Detection, Evaluation, and Treatment of High Blood Pressure*, Bethesda, Md, 2004, NIH.

*In children and adolescents, hypertension is defined as blood pressure that is, on repeated measurement, at the 95th percentile or higher, adjusted for age, height, and gender (NHBPEP, 2003).

RPM may indicate restrictive lung disease or inflammation of the lungs. An increase in breathing rate and depth could be associated with physical exercise, anxiety, or metabolic acidosis. Bradypnea (slow breathing) may occur with diabetic coma. Obstructed breathing from narrowed airways may occur with asthma, chronic bronchitis, congestive heart disease, and chronic obstructive pulmonary disease.

Blood Pressure

Blood pressure,[1-5] the force exerted by the blood against the arterial walls when the heart contracts, is an important indicator of current cardiovascular function and a risk indicator of future cardiovascular morbidity and mortality. Chronic hypertension causes thickening and loss of elasticity in the arterial walls, which can lead to heart attack, heart failure, stroke, and kidney disease. There are no adverse effects from hypotension (low blood pressure), unless the client is in a state of shock or is affected by a disorder or condition that may lower the blood pressure. In fact, the lower the blood pressure, the better the long-term prognosis for cardiovascular health. An acute change in blood pressure can indicate an emergency situation, such as shock or rapid hemorrhaging.

Blood pressure is measured in millimeters of mercury (mm Hg). The two measurements taken for blood pressure are the systolic blood pressure and the diastolic blood pressure:

- **Systolic blood pressure** measures the maximum pressure occurring in the blood vessels during cardiac ventricular contraction (systole) and is the number on the **sphygmomanometer** (blood pressure cuff) when the first heart sound is heard.
- **Diastolic blood pressure** measures the minimum pressure occurring against the arterial walls as a result of cardiac ventricular relaxation (diastole) and is the number on the sphygmomanometer when the last heart sound is heard.

When documenting blood pressure, the dental hygienist records the date and arm used. Blood pressure is recorded as a fraction. The optimal systolic and diastolic measurements for adults 18 years of age and older is <120/<80 mm Hg. The top number of a given blood pressure is the systolic measurement, and the bottom number is the diastolic measurement ("d for down"). A client has high blood pressure (hypertension) if the systolic blood pressure is 140 mm Hg or greater and the diastolic blood pressure is 90 mm Hg or greater. Table 13-6 presents average optimal blood pressure for different ages. Table 13-7 describes factors that influence blood pressure.

Decision Making Based on Observed Blood Pressure

Hypertension is the major cause of stroke and is a contributing factor for myocardial infarction (heart attack). Although not a disease category, **prehypertension** (systolic 120 to 139 or diastolic 80 to 89) identifies clients who should be counseled to adopt a healthier lifestyle to reduce blood pressure or prevent hypertension entirely. Clients who are prehypertensive are not candidates for drug therapy unless risk factors for hypertension (e.g., diabetes and kidney disease) are present and only after lifestyle modifications fail to reduce the blood pressure to normal levels.

A medical consultation is indicated for persons with abnormal blood pressure (Tables 13-8 and 13-9) before administration of dental or dental hygiene care.

A review of the literature concerning the use of epinephrine on hypertensive clients showed minimal effect; however, caution should be taken for uncontrolled hypertensive surgical clients.

Blood Pressure Equipment and Measurement

Sphygmomanometer (Blood Pressure Cuff)

The aneroid manometer (Figure 13-8) is used to assess blood pressure. The **mercury manometer** (Figure 13-8) is an upright tube containing mercury and was considered the standard for blood pressure measurement. The mercury in the manometer poses a health hazard and is no longer recommended. An **electronic hospital grade blood pressure device** (Figure 13-9) is accurate and can provide pulse rate and oxygen saturation levels but is more costly than a mercury manometer.

TABLE 13-7

Factors Influencing Blood Pressure

Factors	Effects
Age	Blood pressure rises with age. Newborns have the lowest mean systolic blood pressure (115/42 mm Hg). As people age, elasticity in the arteries declines, producing an increase in blood pressure. Hypertension is common in the elderly (≥60 years).
Race	Prevalence of hypertension in African and Hispanic Americans is considerably higher than in the white population, and hypertension tends to appear earlier in life in these groups.
Weight	Blood pressure tends to be elevated in overweight and obese persons. Oversized blood pressure cuffs are necessary for accurate readings.
Gender	Hormonal variation causes females to have lower blood pressure after puberty than males; however, postmenopausal women tend to have higher blood pressure than men of similar age. Preeclampsia is abnormal hypertension experienced by some women during pregnancy. Postmenopausal women experience higher blood pressure.
Emotional stress	Stress stimulates the sympathetic nervous system, which in turn increases cardiac output and vasoconstriction. The outcome is elevated blood pressure.
Severe pain	Pain decreases blood pressure and, if severe, can cause shock.
Oral contraceptives	These can increase blood pressure; however, the change is usually within normal limits.
Exercise	After exercise there is an increase in blood pressure for the first 30 minutes, followed by a decrease in blood pressure.
Eating	Older adults can have a 5- to 10-mm Hg fall in blood pressure 1 hour after eating.
Medications	Medications vary in their ability to increase and decrease blood pressure. Medications must be reviewed at each appointment to determine effects on blood pressure.
Diurnal variation	Blood pressure varies with metabolic rate. Pressure is lowest in the morning, then rises and peaks in the late afternoon or early evening.
Chronic disease	Diseases that affect cardiac output, blood volume, blood viscosity, or arterial elasticity will increase blood pressure.
Tobacco, alcohol, and caffeine use	Elevates blood pressure.
High fat and saturated fat intake	High blood cholesterol, especially high LDL cholesterol, and high triglycerides cause atherosclerosis, which in turn can cause an increase in blood pressure.
Dehydration	Accompanied by sudden changes in posture (lying to standing), can cause orthostatic or postural hypotension.
White-coat hypertension (isolated office hypertension)	Approximately 15% to 20% of clients with stage 1 hypertension may have an elevated blood pressure in the presence of a healthcare worker, especially a physician.[3]
Body position	Blood pressure is lower when a person is lying down.

TABLE 13-8

Classification of Blood Pressure for Adults

Blood Pressure Classification	Systolic Blood Pressure* (mm Hg)	Diastolic Blood Pressure* (mm Hg)
Normal (routine dental treatment recommended)	<120	<80
Prehypertension (routine dental treatment recommended)	120-139	80-89
Stage 1 hypertension (routine dental treatment recommended; assess risk factors, refer for consultation with physician of record)	140-159	90-99
Stage 2† hypertension (refer for consultation with physician of record)	≥160	≥100

National Institutes of Health (NIH): *The seventh report of the Joint National Committee on Detection, Evaluation, and Treatment of High Blood Pressure,* Bethesda, Md, 2004, NIH.

*Based on average of two or more properly measured, seated, blood pressure readings on each of two or more office visits.

†Note that if 160-179/100-109, routine dental care can be provided, but treatment should be delayed if care will be stressful or if client cannot handle stress. If local anesthesia is required, use 1:100,000 vasoconstrictor. If 180/110, delay treatment until blood pressure is controlled. If emergency dental care is needed, care should be provided in a hospital dental clinic where emergency life support personnel and equipment are located.

TABLE 13-9
Adult Blood Pressure Guidelines Used in the Dental Hygiene Process of Care

Blood Pressure (mm Hg)	ASA Physical Status Classification*	Dental and Dental Hygiene Therapy Considerations and Interventions Recommended
<120 systolic and <80 diastolic (normal)	I	No unusual precautions related to client management based on blood pressure readings Recheck at next continuing care appointment.
120-139 systolic and/ or 80-89 diastolic (prehypertension)	I	No unusual precautions related to client management based on blood pressure readings Provide education regarding lifestyle modifications. Recheck at next continuing care appointment.
140-159 systolic and 90-99 diastolic (mild)	II	Recheck blood pressure prior to dental treatment (mild) at next two appointments, if all are in this range or exceed it, refer for medical evaluation. Routine dental hygiene therapy can be continued with stress-reduction protocol. Recommend self-monitoring and lifestyle modifications with continued stress-reduction protocol.
160 to <180 systolic and/or 100 to <110 diastolic	III	Recheck blood pressure in 5 minutes; if still elevated, seek medical consultation before next dental or dental hygiene appointment; continue dental hygiene care if stress or fear is not a factor. No unusual precautions related to client management based on blood pressure readings after medical approval is obtained. Stress reduction protocol, such as administration of nitrous oxide–oxygen analgesia
≥180 systolic and/or ≥110 diastolic	IV	Recheck blood pressure in 5 minutes; discontinue appointment; immediate medical consultation if still elevated. No dental or dental hygiene therapy† until elevated blood pressure is corrected. If blood pressure is not reduced using nitrous oxide–oxygen analgesia, only (noninvasive) emergency therapy with drugs (analgesics, antibiotics) is allowable to treat pain and infection. Refer to hospital if immediate dental therapy is indicated.

Adapted from the National Heart, Lung, and Blood Institute: The seventh report of the Joint National Committee on Prevention, Detection, Evaluation, and Treatment of High Blood Pressure: the JNC 7 report, Bethesda, Maryland, US Department of Health and Human Services, Public Health Service, National Institutes of Health, National Heart, Lung, and Blood Institute, August 2004.

*See Chapter 10 for an explanation of ASA Physical Status Classification.

†When the blood pressure is slightly above the cutoff for category IV and when anxiety is present, the use of inhalation sedation may diminish the blood pressure (via the elimination of stress) below the 180/110 level. The client should be advised that if the nitrous oxide and oxygen succeeds in decreasing the blood pressure below this level, the planned treatment can proceed. However, if the blood pressure remains elevated, the planned procedure must be postponed until the elevated blood pressure has been lowered to a more acceptable range.

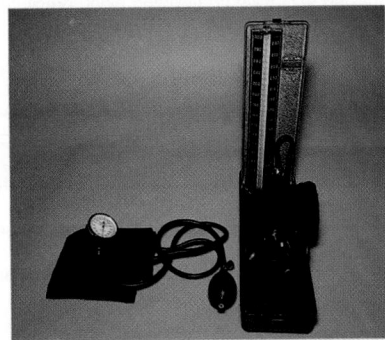

Figure 13-8. Portable sphygmomanometers. Mercury manometer *(right)*. Aneroid manometer *(left)*. (From Potter PA, Griffin AG, Stockert P, et al: *Fundamentals of nursing,* ed 8, St Louis, 2012, Mosby.)

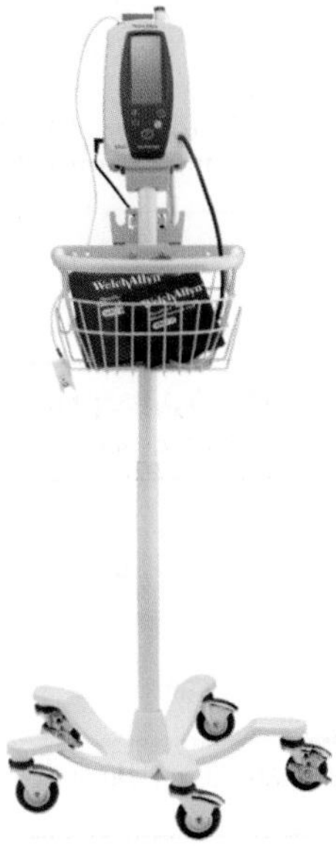

Figure 13-9. Hospital-grade mobile aneroid blood pressure unit. (Courtesy Welch Allyn.)

The sphygmomanometer consists of a pressure-measuring device called a *manometer* and an inflatable cuff that wraps around the arm or leg (see Figure 13-8). Portable and lightweight, the aneroid sphygmomanometer has a glass-enclosed circular gauge containing a needle that registers millimeter calibrations. Aneroid manometers require periodic biomedical calibration to ensure their accuracy. If the patient's blood pressure is unknown, a baseline blood pressure should be obtained by using the auscultatory method for aneroid manometers.

The electronic over-the-counter-type manometer for home use determines blood pressure automatically (Figure 13-10) without the use of a stethoscope. Electronic devices are sensitive to outside interference such as client movement or noise. Such factors interfere with the manometer's sensor signal. An electronic over-the-counter-type manometer easily can become inaccurate and should be recalibrated more than once a year. This manometer is not appropriate for clients with certain conditions (Box 13-3). Regardless of whether the equipment is aneroid or electronic, the equipment should be calibrated at least once a year.

Parts of a manometer are similar regardless of the type and include an occlusive cloth cuff that encloses an inflatable rubber bladder and a pressure bulb with a release valve that inflates the bladder. Large adult cuffs, thigh cuffs, and pediatric sizes are also available.

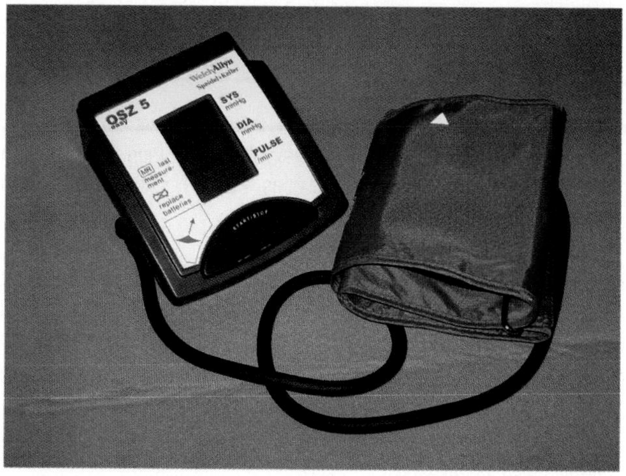

Figure 13-10. Automatic blood pressure cuff for home use. (Courtesy Sedation Resource, Lone Oak, Texas, http://www.sedationresource.com.)

BOX 13-3

Client Conditions Not Appropriate for Electronic Blood Pressure Measurement

- Irregular heart rate
- Peripheral vascular obstruction (e.g., clots, narrowed vessels)
- Shivering
- Seizures
- Excessive tremors
- Inability to cooperate
- Blood pressure less than 90 mm Hg systolic

Adapted from Potter PA, Griffin AG, Stockert P, et al: *Fundamentals of nursing*, ed 8, St Louis, 2012, Mosby.

Proper cuff size is necessary for accurate blood pressure readings. The cuff size selected is proportional to the circumference of the upper arm being assessed. The recommended cuff width should be 20% more than the upper arm (Figure 13-11).

In an adult the bladder within the cuff should encircle at least 80% of the arm, and it should circle the entire arm of a child. Clients with muscular arms that have prominent biceps or obese individuals require use of a large adult cuff. An arm circumference greater than 41 cm requires the use of a thigh cuff (16 × 42 cm).[2] If absolutely necessary, blood pressure for morbidly obese individuals with an arm circumference greater than 52 cm can be measured using the large adult cuff over the forearm with the stethoscope placed over the radial artery.[4] Although cuffs may be labeled newborn, infant, child, small adult, and large adult, the practitioner should not rely on client age as the basis for cuff selection. False readings can occur with faulty equipment and poor techniques (Tables 13-10 and 13-11).

Stethoscope

The stethoscope, an instrument used to amplify sound, consists of two earpieces, plastic or rubber tubing, and a chestpiece. The chestpiece has two sides, the bell and the diaphragm (Figure 13-12).

When the bladder within the occluding cuff is deflated, the blood begins to flow intermittently through the brachial artery (Figure 13-13), producing rhythmic, knocking sounds. These sounds are referred to as Korotkoff (ko-rot-kov) sounds. As the cuff is deflated further, the Korotkoff sounds become less audible, and the pulse eventually disappears. See Figure 13-14 for the five Korotkoff sounds described in phases.

An auscultatory gap, a period of abnormal silence that occurs between the Korotkoff phases, is often present in hypertensive clients. This gap usually appears between the first and second systolic sounds. Failure to recognize the auscultatory gap results in an underestimation of the systolic

TABLE 13-10

Main Types of Manometers Used in Blood Pressure Measurement

Name	Advantages	Disadvantages
Hospital-grade mobile aneroid blood pressure unit (see Figure 13-9)	Most accurate	Cost
Aneroid sphygmomanometer (see Figure 13-8)	Lightweight Portable Compact	Must be recalibrated
Electronic sphygmomanometer (see Figure 13-9)	Easy to use Stethoscope not required	Must be recalibrated Sensitive to outside interference Susceptible to error

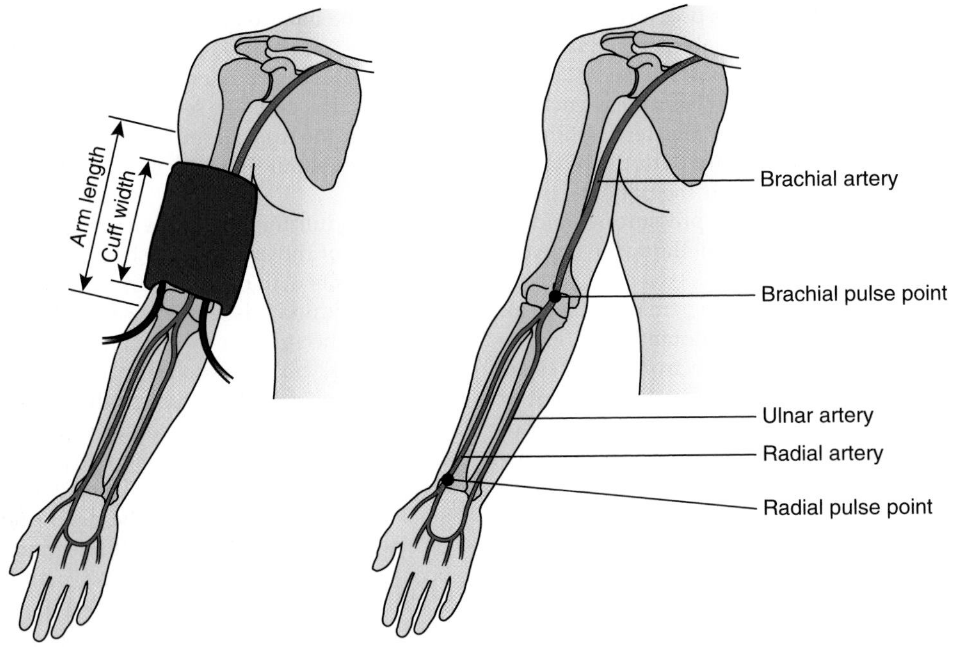

Figure 13-11. Guidelines for proper blood pressure cuff size. Cuff width is 20% more than upper arm diameter or 40% of circumference and two thirds of arm length. (From Potter PA, Griffin AG, Stockert P, et al: *Fundamentals of nursing,* ed 8, St Louis, 2012, Mosby.)

TABLE 13-11

Common Mistakes in Blood Pressure Assessment

Effect	Error
False high reading	Bladder or cuff too narrow Cuff wrapped too loosely or unevenly Deflating cuff too slowly (false high diastolic reading) Arm below heart level Arm not supported Inflating too slowly Repeating assessments too quickly (false high systolic)
False low reading	Failure to identify the auscultatory gap Bladder or cuff too wide Arm above heart level Stethoscope pressed too firmly (false low diastolic) Inadequate inflation level (false low systolic)
False high or false low readings	Multiple examiners using different Korotkoff sounds (false high systolic and false low diastolic) Stethoscope that fits poorly or impairment of examiner's hearing causing sounds to be muffled (false low systolic and false high diastolic) Deflating cuff too quickly (false low systolic and false high diastolic)

pressure. Therefore it is important that the dental hygienist assess the point at which the pulse is obliterated while increasing the pressure in the bladder before taking the blood pressure by auscultation. Moreover, the clinician should increase the bladder pressure 30 mm Hg higher than the point at which the pulse is obliterated when measuring blood pressure (Procedure 13-4 and the corresponding Competency Form). Once taken, blood pressure should be documented in writing and dated in the client's chart under services rendered (e.g., "8/1/13—Blood pressure in right arm, 160/90 mm Hg with auscultatory gap between 160 and 120").

CLIENT EDUCATION TIPS

- Educate client when abnormal vital signs are present; initiate proper physician referral when appropriate.
- Encourage compliance with recommended physician referrals and prescriptive medications to control abnormal vital signs.

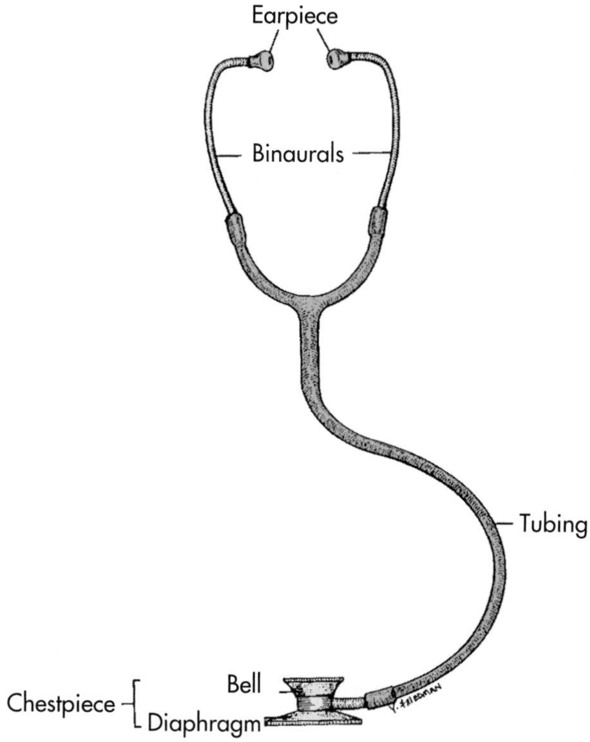

Figure 13-12. Parts of a stethoscope. (From Potter PA, Griffin AG, Stockert P, et al: *Fundamentals of nursing,* ed 8, St Louis, 2012, Mosby.)

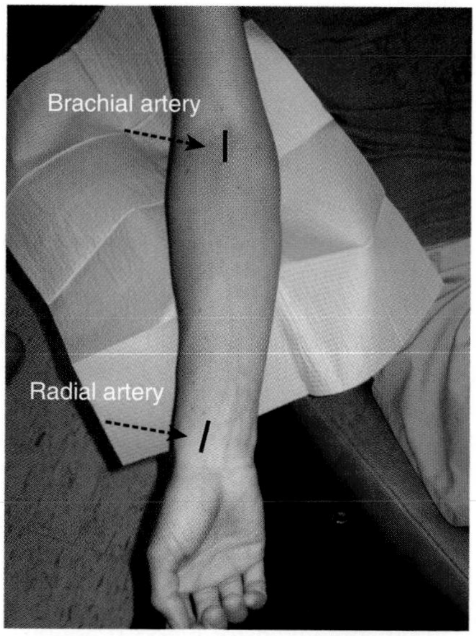

Figure 13-13. Location of the brachial and radial arteries. The brachial artery is located on the medial half of the antecubital fossa, whereas the radial artery is on the lateral volar aspect of the wrist. (From Malamed SF: *Medical emergencies in the dental office,* ed 6, St Louis, 2007, Mosby.)

- Explain risk factors for abnormal vital signs (e.g., clients with high blood pressure may have no overt symptoms yet be at increased risk for cardiac arrest and stroke).

LEGAL, ETHICAL, AND SAFETY ISSUES

- Always record client's vital signs on the treatment record and refer to client's baseline readings for comparison.

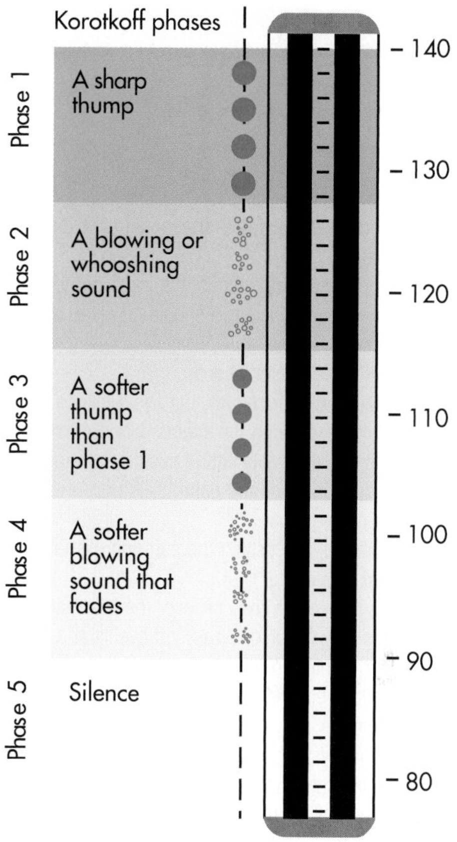

Figure 13-14. The sounds auscultated during blood pressure measurement can be differentiated into five Korotkoff phases. In this example, blood pressure is 140/90. *Phase 1,* The first clear, repetitive tapping sound; recorded as the systolic pressure. *Phase 2,* Brief period of soft, longer swishing, blowing, and whooshing sounds. *Gap,* Sound may disappear altogether in some people (auscultatory gap). *Phase 3,* The return of crisp, sharp, louder thumping sounds. *Phase 4,* The distinct muffling of the sounds, which become soft and blowing. *Phase 5,* The point of silence when all sounds disappear because the blood flow returns to normal; recorded as the diastolic pressure. (From Potter PA, Griffin AG, Stockert P, et al: *Fundamentals of nursing,* ed 8, St Louis, 2012, Mosby.)

These should be performed routinely at continued care appointments and at each appointment when indicated by the client's health and pharmacologic history.
- Refer client to the physician or other primary healthcare provider of record for medical consultation when vital signs exceed normal ranges. Include copies of the referral letter in the client's chart for access and confirmation.
- Disinfect earpiece of stethoscope before and after use to avoid disease transmission.
- Never provide dental hygiene care to a client with medical risk greater than an American Society of Anesthesiologists (ASA) III classification.
- Vital signs must be measured and recorded during a medical emergency.
- Clients in hypertension-prone groups or taking medications that affect blood pressure should have their blood pressure measured at each dental or dental hygiene appointment.
- The dental hygienist is following the ethical principles of integrity and nonmaleficence (do no harm) by ensuring vital signs are taken when necessary. By using the

Procedure 13-4 Assessing Blood Pressure by Auscultation

EQUIPMENT

Blood pressure cuff or sphygmomanometer
Stethoscope

STEPS

1. Ask client about recent activities that could alter the client's normal blood pressure.
2. Determine proper cuff size. Inspect the parts of the release valve and the pressure bulb. The valve should be clean and freely movable in either direction.
3. Wash hands with antimicrobial soap.
4. Explain purpose of the procedure, but avoid talking to client for at least a minute before taking the client's blood pressure.
5. Assist client to a comfortable sitting position, with arm slightly flexed, forearm supported, and palm turned up.
6. Expose the upper arm fully.
7. Palpate brachial artery. Position the cuff approximately 1 inch above the antecubital space.
8. Center arrows marked on the cuff over the brachial artery.
9. Be sure cuff is fully deflated. Wrap cuff evenly and snugly around the upper arm. Center arrow on cuff over artery. If there is no arrow, estimate center of bladder and place over artery.
10. Be sure manometer is positioned for easy reading.
11. If client's normal systolic pressure is unknown, palpate the radial artery and rapidly inflate cuff to a pressure 30 mm Hg above the point at which radial pulsation disappears. Deflate the cuff and wait 30 seconds.
12. Place stethoscope earpieces in ears and be sure sounds are clear, not muffled.
13. Place diaphragm (or the bell) of the stethoscope over the brachial artery in the antecubital fossa. The antecubital fossa is the depression in the underside of the arm at the bend of the elbow. Avoid contact with blood pressure cuff or clothing.
14. Close valve of pressure bulb clockwise until tight.
15. Inflate cuff to 30 mm Hg above client's normal systolic level.
16. Slowly release valve, allowing the needle of the aneroid gauge to fall at a rate of 2 to 3 mm Hg per second.
17. Note point on manometer at which the first clear sound is heard.
18. Continue cuff deflation, noting point on the manometer at which the sound muffles (phase IV) and disappears (phase V). Listen for 10 to 20 mm Hg after last sound.
19. Deflate cuff rapidly. To determine an average blood pressure and ensure a correct reading, wait 2 minutes, then repeat procedure for the same arm.
20. Remove cuff from client's arm. Assist client to a comfortable position and cover upper arm.
21. Disinfect earpieces of stethoscope and fold cuff, and store properly in a cool, dry place.
22. Discuss findings with client.
23. Document in the electronic chart the completion of this service in client's record under "Services Rendered." Record in client's chart the systolic over the diastolic blood pressure reading in mm Hg, the date, cuff size if it was an atypical size, and arm used for measurement (use guidelines in Tables 13-6 to 13-9 to determine need for a referral for medical evaluation by the client's primary healthcare provider). For example: "8/1/13 Client's blood pressure measured with adult size cuff is 110/75 mm Hg right arm sitting."

Data from Potter PA, Griffin AG, Stockert P, et al: *Fundamentals of nursing*, ed 8, St Louis, 2012, Mosby.

equipment properly and following standard procedures, the dental hygienist is following the ethical principle of competence and professionalism.

- The dental hygienist must demonstrate the ethical principle of tolerance by being sensitive to diverse client cultures and beliefs. Inform the client before performing the procedure especially when there will be physical contact. Some cultures may prefer same-sex care providers, and a language barrier may necessitate a family member's presence for moral support and translation assistance.

KEY CONCEPTS

- Abnormal vital signs can be due to client conditions, equipment failure, or operator error. The dental hygienist must take the vital signs accurately and control factors that contribute to errors.
- Blood pressure, pulse, and respiration for baseline measurements should be taken as a comparison for subsequent appointments.
- Temperature is not regularly taken; however, the dental hygienist should take the temperature if the client with signs or symptoms of a fever (pyrexia).
- Pulse rate is recorded in beats per minute (BPM). The pulse in the radial or carotid artery is often measured using the first two fingers of the clinician's hand.
- Normal pulse rate for an adult at rest can range from 60 to 100 BPM. Children usually have a more rapid pulse rate than adults.
- If the client is experiencing frequent premature ventricular contractions (PVCs) per minute, a medical consultation should be considered.
- Respiration rate is determined by observing the rise and fall of the client's chest and is recorded as respirations per minute (RPM).
- Normal adult range for respiration rate is 12 to 20 RPM. Children have a more rapid respiratory rate (20 to 30 RPM for a 6-year-old child) than adults.
- Two measurements taken for blood pressure are the systolic blood pressure and the diastolic blood pressure.
- Optimal systolic and diastolic measurements for adults 18 years of age and older are <120/<80 mm Hg.
- Lifestyle changes are recommended for clients with prehypertension (120 to 139 mm Hg systolic and/or 80 to 89 mm Hg diastolic pressure) with the goal of reducing and/or preventing hypertension.
- Treatment is recommended for stages I and II hypertension with the goal of reducing the blood pressure to <140/<90 mm Hg.
- Rhythmic, knocking sounds heard via the stethoscope when measuring blood pressure are referred to as *Korotkoff sounds*.

Critical Thinking Exercises

1. The client, a 40-year-old medical resident who works at a hospital emergency room, has a history of missing several dental appointments, numerous cancellations, and rescheduled appointments. She is 10 minutes late for her appointment and on arrival is still dressed in scrubs. On inquiry, she wearily states that she has had about 20 hours of sleep in the last week because of her residency assignment. Her health and pharmacologic history reveals migraine headaches, depression, a prosthetic heart valve, and petit mal and grand mal (tonic-clonic) epileptic seizures. She currently is taking a nonsteroidal anti-inflammatory agent for her migraines when needed, a tricyclic antidepressant for depression, and Depakote (an anticonvulsant medication) for her epilepsy. She takes her antidepressant and anticonvulsant on a regular basis and states that she has taken the medications the day of the appointment. She also must take amoxicillin for a prosthetic heart valve and reports an allergy to aspirin products, which has been confirmed by her physician. Her vital signs are pulse 70 BPM, respirations 16 RPM, and blood pressure 120/90 mm Hg.
   A. Before initiating dental hygiene care, what should the dental hygienist do?
   B. The dental hygienist administers 2% lidocaine with 1:100,000 epinephrine for the PSA injection, giving a total of three fourths of the total cartridge with no complications. Proper local anesthetic technique was given to the client, including aspiration that was negative. The client unexpectedly has a petit mal seizure. What is the most likely cause of the seizure?
   C. After the seizure, the client admits that she forgot to take her prophylactic amoxicillin premedication for a prosthetic heart valve. The dental hygienist reschedules the client for treatment, and no treatment other than the local anesthesia administration was given. What recommendation concerning the premedication is indicated before the client is dismissed?
   D. The client calls the next day and reports difficulty with mouth opening and soreness of her jaw. What is the most likely cause of the problem?
2. The dental hygienist takes the client's blood pressure and obtains a reading of 125/90 mm Hg in the right arm. The dental hygienist measures the blood pressure again in 5 minutes, and the blood pressure is 110/70 mm Hg in the right arm. What circumstances could have caused the differences observed in the two readings? Discuss how the problem could be prevented in the future.
3. The dental hygienist takes the client's pulse several times. The client reports an increase in frequency of fluttering or flip-flops in the chest. The finding is discussed with the client, and the client is resistant to seeing his or her physician concerning the problem. Role-play with a partner to demonstrate how to manage the situation effectively.

REFERENCES

1. Chobanian AV, Bakris GL, Black HR, et al: Department of Health and Human Services, National Institutes of Health, National Heart, Lung and Blood Institute, National High Blood Pressure Education Program. The seventh report of the Joint National Committee on Prevention, Detection, Evaluation, and Treatment of High Blood Pressure, 04:4230, August 2004.
2. Malamed SF: *Medical emergencies in the dental office*, ed 6, St Louis, 2007, Mosby.
3. Pickering TG, Hall JE, Appel LJ, et al: Recommendations for blood pressure measurement in humans and experimental animals. *Hypertension* 45:49, 2005.
4. Potter PA, Griffin AG, Stockert P, et al: *Fundamentals of nursing*, ed 8, St Louis, 2012, Mosby.
5. Little JW, Falace DA, Miller CS, et al: *Dental management of the medically compromised patient*, ed 8, St Louis, 2013, Mosby.

EVOLVE RESOURCES

Please visit http://evolve.elsevier.com/Darby/hygiene for additional practice and study support tools.

CHAPTER 14

Pharmacologic History

Ann Eshenaur Spolarich

COMPETENCIES

1. **Discuss the importance of taking a comprehensive pharmacologic history and explain the first step of compiling the medication list.**
2. **Identify fundamental questions to gather a comprehensive pharmacologic history, and do the following:**
   - **Describe adverse drug events, including side effects, drug toxicity, and drug hypersensitivity reactions.**
   - **Describe common side effects caused by medications.**
   - **Discuss strategies to improve client compliance with medication use.**
   - **Discuss dental hygiene interventions to manage the oral side effects of medications.**

Assessment includes taking a comprehensive pharmacologic history, which provides information regarding past and present medications and offers clues about the client's health status and health behaviors. Often a client does not consider a systemic health condition or information about medications to be within the scope of dental hygiene care and simply does not report it on a health history questionnaire. Omission of information about a medical condition or medications may be intentional if the client knows that divulging the information may require that the course of treatment be altered or that additional medical testing or treatment will be required. This situation frequently is encountered with clients who dislike having to take prophylactic antibiotic premedication.[1] Information also may be omitted when the client fears discrimination because of a violation of confidentiality. Sensitive issues such as taking medications for human immunodeficiency virus (HIV) infection, sexually transmitted diseases, or mental illness are managed to ensure client privacy and respect. Conversely, a conscientious client may forget to report certain over-the-counter (OTC) and prescription drugs simply because the client does not view these drugs as "medications." This often is the case with oral contraceptives, antacids, vitamin supplements, herbal supplements, and aspirin. Because many medications interact with drugs used in dentistry or produce side effects, drugs have the potential to compromise client safety and function. The pharmacologic history enables the dental hygienist to assess risks associated with clients taking medications.

Comprehensive Pharmacologic History

Medication List

The first step of the pharmacologic history is compiling a list of all medications that the client is currently taking, including prescription and OTC drugs, as well as herbs, with the name of the medication, the dose schedule (frequency of taking the medication including dosage), and any special instructions for use. A physician consultation may be necessary to verify this information. With the client's informed consent, assistance also may be obtained from the client's pharmacist or caregiver.

The medication list is helpful for assessing the client's attitude toward health and wellness. For example, clients using OTC vitamins and nutritional supplements, or "all-natural" products known as nutraceuticals, may be more interested in nutritional counseling or may seek alternative medicine services. At times, unhealthy behaviors and attitudes may be determined by a client's misuse of drugs, such as abusing OTC stimulants for weight loss or using illegal drugs and alcohol recreationally.

Clients are asked about their own perceptions regarding their medication use to assess their knowledge about their drug therapy. Some people take drugs without understanding why they have been prescribed or knowing the expected outcome of medication therapy. Clients should be encouraged to keep written records of their medications, including dose schedules and the name of the prescribing physician, on their person at all times. This written record is helpful to all health professionals treating the client and may be especially useful during an emergency situation. The dental hygienist helps the client develop this record as a health promotion activity and updates it at each appointment. Box 14-1 lists chairside drug references that contain current drug information.

Eight Fundamental Assessment Questions

See Table 14-1.

Question 1: Why Is the Client Taking Medication?

The dental hygienist assesses why the client is taking medication. Generally, medications are taken for the following reasons:

- To treat an acute systemic condition: Medications taken for acute conditions generally are recommended or prescribed for a defined time frame, usually of short duration, to manage the symptoms of the condition or to eliminate an

BOX 14-1

Chairside Drug References

American Dental Association (ADA): *ADA guide to dental therapeutics,* ed 5, Chicago, 2009, ADA and Thompson PDR.

Physicians' desk reference, ed 66, Montvale, NJ, 2012, Medical Economics.

Physicians' desk reference (PDR) for herbal medicines, ed 4, Montvale, NJ, 2007, Medical Economics.

Pickett FA, Terezhalmy GT: *Dental drug reference with clinical implications,* ed 2, Baltimore, 2008, Lippincott Williams & Wilkins.

Wynn RL, Meiller TF, Crossley HL: *Drug information handbook in dentistry,* ed 18, Hudson, OH, 2012, LexiComp.

TABLE 14-1

Eight Fundamental Questions of the Pharmacologic History

Question	Dental Hygiene Process of Care
1. Why is the client taking the medication(s)? 2. What are the adverse effects of this drug? 3. Are there potential drug interactions? 4. Is there a problem with drug dosage? 5. How is the client managing his/her medications?	Assessment
6. Will any oral side effects of this medication require intervention? 7. Are the client's symptoms caused by a known or unknown condition, or are the symptoms possible side effects of a drug that the client is taking?	Diagnosis
8. Given the pharmacologic history and other assessment data, what are the risks of treating this client?	Planning

From Spolarich AE: Understanding pharmacology: the pharmacologic history, *Access* 9:33, 1995; Spolarich AE, Gurenlian JR: Deductive reasoning with pharmacology: a prescription for quality patient care, *Compend Contin Educ Oral Hyg* 1:3, 1994; College of Registered Dental Hygienists of Alberta: *Elements of prescribing: a pharmacy refresher course for dental hygienists,* 2005.

infection (e.g., cough and cold preparations, antibiotics, antifungals, antidiarrheals, and pain relievers). The assumption is that when the medication is gone, so too will be the cause of the symptoms or the problem in question.

- To treat a chronic systemic condition: Medications may be taken for a longer duration or for extended periods throughout the lifetime (e.g., oral hypoglycemics, allergy drugs, and antihypertensives).
- To prevent a condition from occurring: Medications may be indicated for the prevention of a disease or condition (e.g., oral contraceptives to prevent pregnancy and daily aspirin to prevent stroke).
- To prevent a recurrence of an existing condition: Medications may be used preventively to ward off the recurrence of a chronic problem (e.g., inhaled steroids for asthma and anticonvulsants to prevent seizures).
- To satisfy a habit, with no clinical indication or need: Illegal street drugs have no clinical indication to justify usage. Alcohol, caffeine, and nicotine also may be included in this category. Other drugs, such as daily aspirin and vitamin supplements, may be taken habitually without any documented clinical need or because of a perceived health benefit that may or may not exist. Box 14-2 lists common drug classes with indications for their use.

Question 2: What Are the Adverse Effects of This Drug?

All drugs have the potential to cause harm. When a drug is selected for use, the potential harm must be weighed carefully against its benefits. Drugs are tested extensively and regulated by the U.S. Food and Drug Administration (FDA) to ensure safety and efficacy. The FDA requires the reporting of all known **adverse drug effects**, which can be found in drug reference guides and accessed from the FDA website (see Box 14-1 and information and resources at the Evolve website).

Drugs interact with target tissues to produce a desired effect, also known as the **therapeutic effect**. In addition, drugs also may interact with non-target tissues, resulting in effects that differ from the therapeutic effects. These undesirable effects are also known as drug **side effects**, the severity of which is dose-related. For example, a client takes an angiotensin-converting enzyme (ACE) inhibitor to treat her hypertension, and although it lowers her blood pressure, she experiences a persistent dry cough. All drugs produce side effects, but most are tolerable and disappear when the drug is discontinued (Box 14-3). The FDA requires the reporting of all known side effects, which are organized by body system and the percentage of population affected.

Drug toxicity refers to toxin-induced cell damage and cell death from a medication. Usually a drug does not produce damage directly to the cell. Rather, the damage is caused by an active metabolite formed during metabolic breakdown by the liver or kidneys. Metabolites cause biochemical damage to cellular components, resulting in altered metabolism of the affected cell, cell mutation, or cell death. Unlike side effects, toxicity reactions cannot be tolerated and cause permanent tissue damage on either the microscopic or macroscopic level. These are especially dangerous if major organ systems are involved. Drugs that produce these types of reactions may be labeled as hepatotoxic (causing liver damage), nephrotoxic (causing kidney damage), neurotoxic (causing nerve damage), or cardiotoxic (causing heart damage). Drug toxicity frequently occurs when the drug dosage exceeds the therapeutic level (drug overdose).

Drug hypersensitivity occurs when either the drug or its metabolites act as immunogens, triggering the immune response. Repeated exposure to the same drug produces this allergic response. Signs of a true allergic reaction include skin rash, itching, hives, bronchospasm, and rhinitis. Life-threatening allergic reactions include anaphylaxis, hemolysis, and bone marrow suppression. Allergic reactions are managed

BOX 14-2

Common Drug Classes Associated with Indications for Drug Use

Medications Used to Manage an Acute Condition

Over-the-Counter
- Cold/sinus drugs
- Aspirin
- Acetaminophen
- NSAIDs
- Steroids
- Antiseptics
- Antifungals
- Laxatives
- Allergy drugs
- Cough preparations
- Antidiarrheals
- Antibacterials
- Antacids

Prescription
- Antibiotics
- Antifungals
- Analgesics
- Steroids

Medications Used to Manage a Chronic Condition

Over-the-Counter
- NSAIDs

Prescription
- Antihypertensives
- Antiarrhythmics
- Antidepressants
- Insulin
- Steroids
- NSAIDs
- Antianginals
- Inhalers (asthma)
- Diuretics
- Pain medications
- Oral hypoglycemics

Medications Used to Prevent a Potential Condition

Over-the-Counter
- Aspirin
- Vitamins

Prescription
- Anticoagulants
- Antibiotics
- Anticonvulsants
- Oral contraceptives

Medications Used to Prevent the Recurrence of a Condition

Over-the-Counter
- Allergy drugs

Prescription
- Gastric ulcer medications
- Anticonvulsants
- Antianginals
- Anticoagulants
- Antiplatelet drugs
- Allergy drugs

Medications Taken Habitually (No Clinical Indication)

Over-the-Counter
- NSAIDs
- Alcohol
- Vitamins
- Caffeine

Prescription
- Illegal drugs
- Steroids
- Pain medications
- NSAIDs

From Spolarich AE, Gurenlian JR: Deductive reasoning with pharmacology: a prescription for quality patient care, *Compend Contin Educ Oral Hyg* 1:5, 1994.
NSAIDs, Nonsteroidal anti-inflammatory drugs.

with epinephrine, antihistamines, and corticosteroids, and assistance from emergency support personnel. Allergic reactions are dangerous because they are not predictable and are not dose related. Clients with a history of allergy to a drug in any given class are allergic to all of the drugs in the same class. In addition, some drugs, such as the penicillins and the cephalosporins, show cross-sensitivity to other drug groups with similar chemical structures. The dental hygienist must recognize the warning signs of an allergic reaction so that appropriate treatment interventions can be administered promptly (see Chapter 10).

Other adverse drug effects include negative effects on fetal development, or **teratogenicity**. Many drugs cross the placenta and are secreted in breast milk; therefore drugs are not tested in pregnant and lactating women. The FDA labels each drug with a pregnancy risk factor (A, B, C, D, X) that corresponds to one of five categories indicating the potential of a systemically absorbed drug to cause birth defects (see Chapter 54, Table 54-2). FDA pregnancy category ratings are found in all major drug references and databases.

Occasionally a client experiences a side effect that is completely unexpected or qualitatively different from any known published side effects. This unique response to a drug is called a **drug idiosyncrasy**. Idiosyncratic drug reactions usually are related to a genetic variant. Clients may also report **drug tolerance**, which manifests as the need to take larger doses of the drug to produce the same response, often due to rapid drug metabolism.

BOX 14-3

Common Side Effects of Medications

Central Nervous System Effects
Hyperexcitability
Dizziness
Insomnia
Drowsiness

Cardiac Effects
Hypertension
Hypotension
Orthostatic hypotension or fainting
Edema
Cardiac arrhythmias

Hematologic Effects
Changes in bleeding time
Blood dyscrasias

Gastrointestinal Effects
Weight changes
Appetite changes
Nausea
Vomiting
Diarrhea
Constipation
Xerostomia

Genitourinary Effects
Urinary changes
Sexual dysfunction

Dermatologic Effects
Photosensitivity
Skin disorders

Respiratory Effects
Dyspnea
Coughing

Effects on Special Senses
Blurred vision
Visual disturbances
Taste alteration
Acoustic and balance disorders

Other Effects
Opportunistic infections (yeasts, fungal)

From Spolarich AE: Adverse drug reactions and oral health, *Dimens Dent Hyg* 4(11):22, 2006.

To answer Question 2, the dental hygienist assesses the following:

- What are the known published side effects of the drug(s)?
- Could the symptoms reported by the client be side effects of the drug(s)?
- Are reported symptoms indicative of a drug allergy?

Question 3: Are There Potential Drug Interactions?

Adverse drug effects also can be caused by **drug interactions**, the negative effects that can occur when two or more drugs are taken simultaneously. Drug interactions range in severity from mild alterations in drug action to life-threatening conditions in the client (e.g., alterations in drug efficacy, toxicity reactions, or other dangerous reactions such as hypertensive crisis, extended bleeding time, or respiratory depression). Drugs also may interact with foods and herbal supplements.

Adverse drug interactions are prevented by knowing drug relationships. Dental professionals keep apprised of drug interactions by routinely reviewing lists of known interactions in standard drug reference texts and scientific publications. Drug interactions arise from a variety of mechanisms and result in either a decreased or an increased effect of one or more drugs. The greater the number of medications taken, the greater the likelihood that the client will experience an interaction. Drug interactions also may occur with herbal supplements and foods. To assess whether the client is experiencing a drug interaction, the dental hygienist consults a drug reference text and assesses the following:

- Are there any known drug interactions for this medication?
- Could the client's symptoms be indicative of a drug interaction?

Question 4: Do These Findings Suggest a Problem with Drug Dosage?

Standard drug dosage schedules may be too strong for children and elderly clients and may have to be altered to prevent adverse drug effects. The need to reduce drug dosages in these populations is related directly to drug **pharmacokinetics**, which refers to how the drug is absorbed, distributed, metabolized, and excreted from the body. Children demonstrate an increased skin and mucous membrane permeability; therefore they absorb medications much more readily and more quickly than their adult counterparts. Pediatric dosage is based on the weight of the child. In general, manufacturers' recommended dosages for children are half of the standard adult dose.

In the elderly, normal physiologic changes of aging dictate the need for a reduction in dosage. Increased stomach acidity alters drug absorption into circulation. Normally the liver converts lipid-soluble drugs to water-soluble metabolites, thus inactivating the drug and allowing for filtration and elimination by the kidney. Liver and kidney function declines with age; therefore more drug stays active after passing through the liver, and the portion of the drug that remains lipid soluble is scavenged by the kidneys and either put back in circulation or stored in body fat. Production of plasma proteins, the binding sites for drugs in circulation, also declines with age. The portion of the drug that is unbound in the circulation is the active drug. The amount of active drug in circulation increases when the client takes multiple medications, all of which are competing for fewer binding sites. These physiologic changes manifest as an increased drug effect in the client and contribute to unwanted central nervous systemic side effects, such as sedation, confusion, and extensions of desired therapeutic effects. As with children, doses for the elderly may have to be reduced to half of the standard adult dosage. Liver and kidney function also must be considered when determining proper dosage, especially in clients with hepatic and renal disease. To assess the potential for complications caused by drug dosage, the dental hygienist considers the following:

- Have the client's age and weight been taken into account when determining drug dosage?
- Could the symptoms be attributed to altered drug pharmacokinetics caused by normal physiologic changes of aging?
- Could the symptoms be attributed to altered drug pharmacokinetics caused by hepatic and renal disease?

Question 5: How Is This Client Managing Medications?

Most clients take multiple medications and are treated by many different healthcare providers. The lack of communication among these providers, all of whom may be prescribing medications, results in an increased risk for adverse drug reactions. The dental hygienist, as client advocate, encourages client compliance and assesses risks associated with medication use.

The client's ability to manage medications is confounded by a number of variables. First, the client may be self-medicating with OTC medications, prescription medications, or supplements. Clients are usually unaware of potential adverse drug effects that can occur as a result of mixing medications, altering recommended dosage schedules, or mixing medications with supplements, alcohol, or certain foods. Second, clients may not read the warning labels on the medication packaging or may not understand what they are reading. This is especially true when labels warn against using certain classes of drugs or warn against using the medication because of a preexisting condition. The client may not be aware that he or she has a preexisting condition, such as enlarged prostate, hypertension, or thyroid disease. Other clients simply choose to ignore the warnings and take the medication anyway. The small typeface on many labels poses yet another challenge for the elderly and the visually impaired.

Failure to comply with medication use, intentionally or unintentionally, must be discerned by the dental hygienist. The dental hygienist never assumes that the client intuitively understands the prescribed regimen or reads the instructions from the pharmacy. Whenever a drug is dispensed or prescribed from the dental office, the dental hygienist provides detailed instructions. Even clients who are normally compliant are given instructions and an opportunity to ask questions to reinforce adherence to the prescribed regimen.

Familiarity with a routine can breed laziness in compliance. Just as clients learn proper dosage schedules, they also can learn to give the "right answer" to inquiries about taking their medications. In these instances the dental hygienist must rely on the client's physical presentation as well as personal intuition to discern whether the client truly is following instructions. How well a client complies with medication use can reflect the client's willingness to comply with other professional recommendations, including self-care instructions and referrals.

Dental hygienists also facilitate information transfer between the client and other healthcare professionals. A call to the client's physician can clarify discrepancies in the client's understanding of his or her medications and can confirm that it is safe to provide treatment. Conversations between the dental hygienist and other practitioners should be documented in the services rendered portion of the client record.

When assessing client compliance with medications, the dental hygienist focuses on the following:

- How many medications is the client taking?
- When was the client last seen by a physician? By the physician who prescribed the medication?
- What is the prescribed regimen for the medications?
- How many providers are prescribing medications for the client?
- How long is the client to remain on this medication?
- Does the client understand why the medication was prescribed?
- Have client instructions been provided for taking the medications? If so, by whom?
- Does the client understand the instructions for using the medications?
- Is the client self-medicating? Undermedicating or overmedicating?
- How many refills are there for the medication?
- Has the medication expired?

Question 6: Will Any Oral Side Effects of This Medication Require Intervention?

Management of oral side effects is an ongoing challenge (Box 14-4). Oral side effects cause client discomfort and interfere with the ability to chew, swallow, and digest food. Some oral side effects place the client at risk for oral trauma, and others lead to infection, pain, and possible tooth loss.[2] Dental hygienists must recognize these oral conditions in a timely manner and recommend appropriate treatment interventions. Professional intervention is often necessary to improve client comfort and function.

More than 500 medications cause xerostomia, making it the most commonly reported oral side effect, especially among elderly clients (Box 14-5).[2-4]

BOX 14-4

Common Oral Side Effects of Medications

Xerostomia
Dental caries
Change in taste
Difficulty with mastication
Difficulty wearing appliances
Oral ulcerations
Atrophic mucosa
Hairy tongue
Infection
Mucositis or stomatitis
Burning mouth or tongue
Difficulty with speech
Difficulty with swallowing
Increased periodontal disease progression
Opportunistic infections (candidiasis)
Bleeding
Gingival enlargement

From Spolarich AE: Adverse drug reactions and oral health, *Dimens Dent Hyg* 4(11):22, 2006; Spolarich AE, Gurenlian JR: Drug-induced adverse oral events. In Daniel S, Harfst S, Wilder R, eds: *Mosby's dental hygiene concepts, cases and competencies*, ed 2, St Louis, 2008, Mosby, p 259.

BOX 14-5

Classes of Drugs That Cause Xerostomia

Anorexiants	Anti-inflammatory analgesics
Antiacne agents	Antinauseants
Antianxiety agents	Antiparkinsonian agents
Anticholingerics/antispasmotics	Antipsychotics
Anticonvulsants	Bronchodilators
Antidepressants	Decongestants
Antidiarrheals	Diuretics
Antiemetics	Muscle relaxants
Antihistamines	Opiate analgesics
Antihypertensives	Sedatives

Data from *USP DI drug information for the healthcare professional*, vol 1, ed 26, Englewood, Colo, 2006, Micromedix.

Drug-induced xerostomia is a combination of reduced salivary flow rate and a change in the nature and quality of the residual saliva. Residual saliva is more mucinous and viscous, facilitating food and oral biofilm adherence to tooth surfaces, appliances, dentures, and oral tissues. The client retains more food in the buccal vestibule after eating owing to the loss of natural salivary cleansing. The pH of the mouth becomes more acidic because of the reduction of natural physiologic buffers, which when combined with oral biofilm and food accumulation, places the client at increased risk for dental caries. Xerostomia-induced dental caries are evident along the gingival margin on exposed buccal and lingual root surfaces, at and underneath crown margins, on incisal edges and cusp tips with dentinal exposure from attrition, and in root furcations. Caries can lead to extensive tooth destruction and tooth loss, which is particularly significant for teeth that serve as anchors for dental prostheses. Increased biofilm acidity also contributes to dentinal hypersensitivity. Clients with xerostomia should be placed on supplemental daily fluoride with consideration for use of remineralization therapies to reduce caries and dentinal hypersensitivity risks (see Chapters 33 and 39). Incorporating daily therapeutic doses of xylitol-containing products also may be recommended to reduce *Streptococcus mutans* and stimulate saliva production. Symptomatic relief of dry mouth and dry throat may be obtained through the use of artificial salivary substitutes or by taking pilocarpine (Salagen) or cevimeline (Evoxac), cholinergic drugs that stimulate serous salivary flow (see Chapter 45, Table 45-2 and Box 45-9).

Under normal conditions, saliva maintains the balance of the oral ecosystem with immunologic and antibacterial processes that regulate the population of oral flora. When the ecosystem becomes unbalanced, the proportions of pathogenic and opportunistic organisms increase. Therefore the person is at greater risk for oral infections, including gingivitis, periodontitis, and both viral and fungal infections. People with xerostomia greatly benefit from the use of daily antimicrobial therapy at home. Chlorhexidine and essential oil mouth rinses have demonstrated efficacy against a broad spectrum of oral pathogens and seven species of *Candida* organisms (see Chapter 31).[5] Fungal infections are associated with use of antibiotics, immunosuppressants, and underlying systemic diseases such as diabetes mellitus. Prescription antifungal therapy (e.g., nystatin) is indicated, and often repeated, in xerostomic clients with recurrent fungal infections. Fungal infections may manifest as white plaques overlying red oral mucosa, burning mouth syndrome, symptomatic geographic tongue, and angular cheilitis (see Chapters 55 and 56).

Salivary mucins lubricate the oral mucous membranes, protect against ulceration and penetration of toxins, and assist with wound healing and repair. Xerostomic clients have friable mucous membranes, which are highly susceptible to trauma from toothbrushing, mastication, and rubbing against appliances and dentures. Chlorhexidine and essential oil mouth rinse have been shown to reduce the incidence and severity of aphthous ulcerations when used preventively on a daily basis.[2,5] There are numerous OTC products available for topical pain control associated with aphthous ulcerations and oral mucositis; most contain benzocaine to improve comfort. Prescription lidocaine in the form of a rinse also may be used for pain relief (see Chapter 45, Table 45-1, Box 45-7, and Figure 45-2 for the treatment of oral mucositis).

Salivary mucins also play a role in initiating the breakdown of food in preparation for swallowing and digestion. Often xerostomic clients experience gastrointestinal disorders related to their inability to digest food adequately. These problems are compounded further in clients taking medications that cause taste alteration as a side effect. More than 250 medications alter taste and smell.[6] Saliva is needed to help carry tastants to the taste buds, which is diminished in xerostomic clients. Drugs also may be excreted into saliva and gingival crevicular fluid or may concentrate electrolytes in the saliva. These adverse effects may lead clients to make poor food choices or stop eating because of discomfort, disinterest, or chewing difficulties. Clients may experience weight loss, which alters the fit and comfort of dentures and appliances, leading to a cycle that requires intervention. Weight loss and poor nutritional status are of great concern in those with serious medical conditions or those undergoing cancer therapy (see Chapter 45).

Phenytoin (Dilantin) (seizure medication), cyclosporine (Sandimmune) (organ transplant antirejection drug), and some calcium channel blockers (antihypertensives) cause drug-influenced gingival enlargement as a side effect. Black, hairy tongue typically is associated with antibiotics. Other medication-induced oral side effects include glossitis, erythema multiforme, lichenoid drug reaction, and taste alteration. The dental hygienist should consult a drug reference guide to verify the potential for a drug to produce these adverse effects. For a list of strategies to manage oral side effects associated with medication use, see Box 14-6. To determine the need for intervention, the dental hygienist considers the following:

- Is the client having difficulty speaking, chewing, swallowing, wearing dental appliances?
- Is the client taking medications that could be contributing to these problems?
- Has the client reported changes in weight that could be attributed to a change in nutritional status?
- Are oral assessment findings consistent with known side effects of the drugs that the client is taking?

BOX 14-6

Dental Hygiene Interventions to Manage the Oral Side Effects of Medications

Dental Caries Preventive and Dentinal Hypersensitivity Therapies

Prescription fluorides: dentifrices, gels, and rinses
Professional in-office application of topical fluorides
Amorphous calcium phosphate (ACP, licensed from the ADA Foundation)
Calcium sodium phosphosilicate (NovaMin)
Tricalcium phosphate
Milk casein phosphopeptides (CPP) complexed with ACP (CPP-ACP) (Recaldent)
OTC dentinal hypersensitivity protection dentifrices
Professional in-office treatment for dentinal hypersensitivity
Xylitol

Salivary Replacement Therapy

Artificial saliva
Water

Salivary Stimulation

Pilocarpine (Salagen) (prescribed by dentist)
Cevimeline (Evoxac) (prescribed by dentist)
Sonic toothbrushing

Daily Antimicrobial Therapy

0.12% chlorhexidine mouthrinse
Essential oil mouthrinse
0.07% cetylpyridium chloride mouthrinse

Antifungal Therapy

Prescription drugs: topical ointments, liquids, powders, and troches (e.g., nystatin [Mycostatin]); systemic medications (e.g., fluconazole [Diflucan])
Daily antimicrobial therapy with 0.12% chlorhexidine or essential oil mouth rinse

Antiviral Therapy

Prescription topical ointments, systemic medications (e.g., acyclovir [Zovirax], penciclovir [Denavir])
OTC topical ointments (e.g., docosonol 10% [Abreva], alcohol/benzalkonium chloride [Viroxyn])
OTC topical ointments for pain control

Topical Pain Control for Ulcerations or Mucositis

OTC benzocaine or tetracaine ointments
OTC liquid Benadryl mixed with coating agent
Prescription lidocaine rinse
Prescription amlexanox (Aphthasol) ointment (aphthous ulcerations)

Oral Hygiene Devices

Power toothbrush
Power flosser
Oral irrigator
Interdental cleaning aids

OTC, Over-the-counter.

Question 7: Are Symptoms Reported During the Client's Health History Interview Caused by a Medical Condition, or Are They Drug Side Effects?

Answering this question is a difficult challenge; therefore attention must be paid to findings from the health history interview. The dental hygienist attempts to match the physical findings or symptoms reported by the client with existing medical or dental conditions. Drugs from the medication list should be suitable for the medical and dental conditions for which the client is being treated. Consider that a doctor may prescribe a medication for an off-label use. When symptoms do not correlate with known conditions, the dental hygienist then must discern whether the client's medications may be contributing to the problem or whether there may be an undiagnosed condition, either of which could explain the client's symptoms.

The following questions facilitate problem solving:

- Does the client have a known systemic condition?
- What are the symptoms reported by the client?
- Do these symptoms correlate with the client's known systemic condition?
- Do the symptoms reported indicate the presence of an undiagnosed condition?
- What are the indications for the drugs being taken?
- Could the drug(s) be causing or contributing to the symptoms in question?

Question 8: Given the Pharmacologic History and Other Assessment Data, What Are the Risks of Treating This Client?

Assessing the risk of proceeding with treatment is the final and most important determination made. Treatment risks associated with medication use vary in nature and severity and are not always obvious. To assess risk, the following questions must be considered:

- If treatment is initiated, will the client be placed in a situation that is potentially dangerous or life-threatening?
- Will the planned treatment temporarily or permanently compromise the client's health or ability to function?
- Will the treatment compromise the client's safety or comfort?
- Will the treatment compromise the provider's safety or comfort?

Life-threatening risks are associated with conditions for which the client is taking medication or with side effects. Clients who are immunocompromised from cancer chemotherapy or immunomodulatory drugs, organ transplant antirejection therapy, or acquired immunodeficiency syndrome (AIDS) are at greater risk for developing infections from poor oral hygiene or invasive dental hygiene procedures (see Chapters 45, 46, 48, and 49). Good oral self-care practices, preprocedural antimicrobial rinsing, and prophylactic antibiotic premedication are strategies to minimize the risk for infection. Antibiotic therapy associated with professional care is determined in consultation with the dentist or physician on a case-by-case basis (see Chapter 12).

Risk for hypertensive crisis and stroke is associated with the use of vasoconstrictors, and the dental hygienist must verify the compatibility of administering epinephrine with all medications taken by the client before giving an injection (see Chapter 40). Use of cocaine sensitizes clients to norepinephrine, posing an even greater risk for hypertensive crisis, heart attack, and stroke in the oral care environment. Myocardial infarction, stroke, and anaphylaxis from an unexpected allergic reaction are perhaps the most dangerous risks. Insulin shock, aspiration, and seizures are mostly preventable with proper client assessment and use of safety precautions.

The dental hygienist is exposed to personal health risks when treating clients with medications. Inhalation risks are associated with general anesthetics and nitrous-oxide and oxygen systems with inadequate scavenging systems (see Chapter 41). For example, pregnant practitioners should exercise caution when in the presence of nitrous oxide, a drug that causes spontaneous abortion as a teratogenic effect (capable of producing genetic mutations). However, use of a proper scavenging system significantly minimizes this inhalation risk. Topically applied agents have the potential to come in contact with the skin, mucous membranes, and eyes, requiring the use of personal protective equipment (see Chapter 9). The hygienist also must assess the treatment environment for potential hazards to protect hygienist and client in case a client falls or has a seizure. Risk for falls increases with clients who take medications that cause orthostatic hypotension or central nervous system side effects that alter equilibrium.

All dental hygienists must be currently certified in cardiopulmonary resuscitation (CPR) and managing medical emergencies in the dental office. The dental hygienist can be especially helpful in establishing a safety plan that includes monitoring oxygen tanks to ensure the availability of adequate levels, the expiration dates on emergency medications, and the use of medications dispensed from the office (see Chapter 10).

Dental hygienists should use laboratory test results, medical records, and information obtained from the dentist, physician, and pharmacist to assist with clinical decision making. Maintaining a client's systemic health always takes priority over dental hygiene care needs, and treatment never should be initiated when there is concern about the client's safety (see Chapter 12). The client and the dental hygienist must know about any medication risks associated with treatment, and they should be explained and documented thoroughly in the treatment record.

CLIENT EDUCATION TIPS

- Inform clients about why medications are being prescribed.
- Describe what the client should expect while taking the medications.
- Explain in simple terms what the medication will do, its potential side effects, and proper dosage schedule.
- Explain the difference between side effects and drug allergies.
- Describe the signs of an allergic reaction (itching, hives, shortness of breath, or respiratory distress).
- Explain what to do in case of an allergic reaction.
- Identify known drug interactions ("Do not take drug X when taking drug Y").
- Give any special instructions relevant to the medication (e.g., avoid sun exposure, take the medication until it is gone).
- Suggest ways to minimize side effects (e.g., drink a full glass of water, eat before taking the medication).
- Emphasize that no herbal medication should be taken without a physician's approval.

LEGAL, ETHICAL, AND SAFETY ISSUES

- Ensure that all instructions and answers to client questions are accurate and complete. Ask for assistance if it is necessary to answer questions completely.
- Check each client's health history for known allergies or previous reactions to ensure drug compatibility with existing medications.
- Give written instructions to which the client can refer at home.
- Document in the treatment record what the client was told.
- Caution clients about the dangers of drug interactions and overmedication possible with OTC, prescription, and herbal medications.

KEY CONCEPTS

- The pharmacologic history provides clues regarding a client's general health status and health behaviors and protects the client's health and safety.
- Using a logical, systematic approach to history taking helps the dental hygienist formulate questions and evaluate client responses to safely provide care.
- Interpreting data obtained from the eight fundamental questions of the pharmacologic history enables the dental hygienist to assess the risks of treating clients taking medications.
- All drugs have the potential to cause adverse effects.
- Drug interactions range in severity from mild alterations in drug action to life-threatening conditions in the client.
- Standard drug doses are too strong for children, the elderly and those with hepatic and renal disease, and must be altered to prevent adverse effects.
- The dental hygienist is a client advocate who facilitates client compliance and education on medication use.
- Clients may fail to comply with medication use for several reasons including multiple providers prescribing multiple medications, self-medication, cost, and failure to comply accurately with the prescribed dosage regimens.
- Oral side effects of medications cause client discomfort; interfere with the ability to chew, swallow, and digest food; and increase risk for infection and tooth loss.

CRITICAL THINKING EXERCISES

1. To learn about new medications and known oral side effects, use the computer to access the many drug databases that are available via the Internet. Present to colleagues those sites that appear to be most valuable and explain why.
2. Document recommendations made to clients experiencing oral side effects and monitor clinical outcomes over time.

Interview clients about the efficacy of the products or procedures recommended, personal likes and dislikes about the products or procedures, and factors that influenced the clients' compliance.

3. Read the following two scenarios and try to determine what may be going on with each client's health status and medications being taken. Review the case analyses once you have arrived at your own conclusions.

SCENARIO 14-1

ASSESSMENT OF THE CLIENT'S PHARMACOLOGIC HISTORY

At his appointment, a 46-year-old Caucasian man reports that for the past 2 weeks he has been experiencing headaches on a daily basis and occasional stomach pain that has progressively gotten more frequent and intense. He is scheduled to see his physician at the end of the month for a follow-up on the new hay fever medication that was prescribed 2 weeks ago. The health history review reveals arthritis of the knees, seasonal allergies, and hospitalization 6 months ago for surgery to reset a broken wrist. The client is taking ibuprofen as needed (PRN) for arthritis pain and loratadine daily for allergy symptoms.

On further questioning, the hygienist finds that the client is taking 600 mg of ibuprofen four times per day and has been taking loratadine, 10 mg/day as prescribed, for 2 weeks. The high doses of ibuprofen suggest that his arthritis pain is not well controlled. The client states that he always takes the same amount of ibuprofen, regardless of his pain level, "whether I need it or not, because that seems to keep the pain under control." He saw his physician 2 weeks ago to get a prescription-strength allergy medication because "the over-the-counter stuff just wasn't working anymore."

Case Analysis

The client has two known systemic conditions: arthritis and seasonal allergies. He reports two symptoms that require assessment: daily headaches and stomach pain of increasing frequency and intensity. A possible correlation can be found between the headaches and a sinus-related condition (seasonal allergies). No correlation can be made between stomach pain and arthritis or allergies. Several possible undiagnosed conditions may account for the client's daily headaches, including tooth clenching or grinding, a sinus infection, or hypertension; and a gastrointestinal disorder, stomach virus, or stomach ulcer could explain his stomach pain.

The indications for the drugs taken by the client match his known conditions: ibuprofen for arthritis pain and loratadine for seasonal allergies. Medications may be contributing to the client's symptoms in question. First, chronic use of ibuprofen causes gastrointestinal ulceration and bleeding, known side effects for nonsteroidal antiinflammatory drugs. In this case the client is taking three times the OTC dose for ibuprofen, four times per day, which is most likely contributing to his stomach pain. Second, headaches are a known side effect of loratadine, and the client has experienced headaches only for the past 2 weeks, which correlates with the time he has been taking this medication. The client is referred to his physician for further evaluation of his arthritis pain, a potential stomach ulcer, and his headaches, as these may be medication-related problems.

SCENARIO 14-2

ASSESSMENT OF THE CLIENT'S PHARMACOLOGIC HISTORY

The client is a 36-year-old African American woman with a periodontal abscess associated with a 6-mm pocket on the mesiobuccal surface of tooth No. 30. After thorough periodontal debridement under local anesthesia, the client is given oral hygiene instructions for keeping the site clean. The client also is instructed to take ibuprofen 200 mg for pain as necessary and is given prescriptions for penicillin 500 mg four times daily for 10 days and 0.12% chlorhexidine for rinsing twice daily. The client is scheduled to return in 10 days for evaluation.

When the client returns, the site is still inflamed and exudate is draining from the periodontal pocket. On questioning the client states, "My gum looked so sore that I was afraid to touch it, but the medicine made it feel better after about 3 days, so I didn't think that I needed it anymore. Besides, it was giving me an upset stomach, so I figured that it was all right to stop taking it. The mouthwash left an aftertaste, which didn't help my upset stomach, so I rinsed my mouth out with water, but it made it taste even worse. I used it though, every day." Furthermore, the client took the ibuprofen twice on the day of the procedure only, then stopped, as she reported no additional pain.

Case Analysis

Assessment of the client's compliance suggests that she did not understand the need for the antibiotic or what to expect while taking this medication. The client should have been informed about (1) the gastrointestinal upset that commonly occurs with antibiotic use and how to manage this side effect and (2) the importance of taking the antibiotic until it was gone to ensure that the infection was treated completely and to reduce the risk of bacterial resistance. Also, this client demonstrated willingness to comply with the mouthrinse but should have been informed about taste alteration as a side effect. By rinsing with water after using the 0.12% chlorhexidine mouthwash, the client was rinsing away the flavoring agent and ended up tasting more of the medication that remained. Chlorhexidine will not resolve the remaining infection deep within the pocket. With the incomplete course of antibiotic therapy, the infection persists and now requires re-treatment.

REFERENCES

1. Wilson W, Taubert KA, Gewitz M, et al: Prevention of infective endocarditis: guidelines from the American Heart Association: a guideline from the American Heart Association Rheumatic Fever, Endocarditis, and Kawasaki Disease Committee, Council on Cardiovascular Disease in the Young, and the Council on Clinical Cardiology, Council on Cardiovascular Surgery and Anesthesia, and the Quality of Care and Outcomes Research Interdisciplinary Working Group. *Circulation* 9;116(15):1736, 2007. Erratum in *Circulation* 9;116(15):e376, 2007.
2. Spolarich AE: Xerostomia and oral disease. *Dimens Dent Hyg* 9(11 suppl):43, 2011.
3. Porter SR, Scully C, Hegarty AM: An update of the etiology and management of xerostomia. *Oral Surg Oral Med Oral Pathol Oral Radiol Endod* 97:28, 2004.
4. *USP DI Drug information for the healthcare professional*, vol 1, ed 26, Englewood, Colo, 2006, Micromedix, Inc.
5. DePaola LG, Spolarich AE: Safety and efficacy of antimicrobial mouthrinses in clinical practice. *J Dent Hyg* 81(suppl, pt 2):13, 2007.
6. Pickett FA, Terezhalmy GT: *Dental drug reference with clinical implications*, ed 2, Baltimore, 2008, Lippincott Williams & Wilkins.

EVOLVE RESOURCES

Please visit http://evolve.elsevier.com/Darby/hygiene for additional practice and study support tools.

CHAPTER 15

Extraoral and Intraoral Clinical Assessment

Margaret J. Fehrenbach

COMPETENCIES

1. Discuss the clinical assessment, including recognition of normal head and neck anatomic structures, common signs of oral disease, and deviations from normal.
2. Conduct the extraoral clinical assessment, including proper methods and sequence.
3. Conduct the intraoral clinical assessment, including proper methods and sequence.
4. Describe and document significant findings in the client's record using precise descriptive terms, including appropriate follow-up and referral when atypical or abnormal tissue changes warrant further medical or dental evaluation.
5. Discuss cancers affecting the head and neck, including:
   - Explain oral self-examination techniques to the client.
   - Explain the use of biopsy as well as other methods for early detection of oral cancer.

Careful overall client observation and a thorough assessment of the head and neck as well as the oral cavity are essential to planning and providing optimum client care. The orofacial structures are sensitive general health indicators. Changes in these structures may be the first indication of disease processes in other parts of the body. For example, certain systemic diseases that first may manifest themselves in the oral cavity include diabetes, human immunodeficiency virus (HIV) infection, leukemia, and nutritional deficiencies. The variety of disease-associated skin and oral mucosal lesions observed may or may not be symptomatic.

In addition, orofacial lesions are common in the adult population. An estimated 10% of dental clients have some atypical or abnormal orofacial finding. Although the majority of these findings fall into the category of atypical, some may be abnormal and thus serious and even fatal. It is the dental hygienist's responsibility to recognize oral tissue changes from their normal state and to refer clients with changes to the supervising dentist for further evaluation.

Taking appropriate action after the recognition of an abnormal extraoral or intraoral condition is imperative for promoting optimal client wellness and, in the case of cancer, possibly preventing premature death. In addition, educating clients through instruction in self-examination techniques to identify signs outside of normal in their own mouth engages them in "co-therapy," allowing them to assume some responsibility for the care and control of their own oral and systemic health (see later discussion).

To meet this challenge, the dental hygienist must be thoroughly familiar with normal and abnormal anatomy of the head and neck to recognize abnormal changes. This chapter focuses on the clinical assessment of extraoral and intraoral structures other than those related to tooth structure, oral hygiene status, caries, and the periodontium (see Chapters 16, 17, 18, and 19, respectively).

Clinical Assessment

The skills of **observation**, **palpation**, **auscultation**, and **olfaction** are vital to client assessment. These skills and application examples are described in Table 15-1.[1] Types of palpation techniques (e.g., **digital palpation**, **bidigital palpation**, **manual palpation**, **bimanual palpation**, **bilateral palpation**, **circular compression**) are described in Table 15-2. Anatomic terms that are used regularly in describing head and neck anatomy are defined in Box 15-1 and are discussed later in the chapter (see Describing and Documenting Significant Findings). It is important always to visualize and then palpate to avoid altering the lesion before it is visualized. It is also important always to palpate against a firm structure such as muscles or bones as well as fingers.

Before performing extraoral and intraoral assessments, the dental hygienist reviews clients' histories, radiographs, and any other procedural tests and explains the assessment procedure. Establishing an assessment sequence and following through with it systematically during client assessment reduces the possibility of overlooking any area to be examined. A suggested sequence for a thorough extraoral and intraoral assessment is outlined and illustrated in Procedures 15-1, 15-2, and their corresponding Competency Forms later in the chapter.

Extraoral Clinical Assessment

An extraoral assessment includes an overall evaluation of the client's general characteristics and a thorough evaluation of the head, face, and neck, including the associated skin and regional lymph nodes. Procedure 15-1 with Figures 15-8 to 15-19 lists the steps for examining recommended extraoral structures and examples of normal, atypical, and abnormal findings that may be observed during an extraoral assessment.

Overall Client Evaluation

Initially the client is observed during reception and seating to note any physical characteristics and abnormalities that may require special dental hygiene care modification or medical and/or dental consultation.[2] This overall client

TABLE 15-1

Skills Used in Conducting the Extraoral and Intraoral Assessment

Skill	Definition	Examples of Application
Observation	Act of viewing and watching the client to detect variations from normal and potential disease states	Client movement; body structure and symmetry; skin and mucous membrane color, texture, consistency, contour and form; and client knowledge, attitude, and behavior
Palpation	Act of using the sense of touch to detect variations from normal and potential disease states	Noting tenderness, texture, masses, variations in structure, and temperature
Auscultation	Act of listening to and detecting body sounds to determine variations from normal	Noting sounds made by the temporomandibular joint (e.g., clicking; slurred speech may be due to medications, disabilities such as deafness, or stroke history; hoarseness may be indicative of laryngeal cancer; muffled voice may signal the presence of an oropharyngeal cancer; problems with breathing, may indicate a respiratory or emotional condition; clicking of dentures, indicating a poor fit)
Olfaction	Act of sensing body odors to detect variations from normal and potential disease entities	Noting alcohol breath caused by alcohol abuse; smoker's breath from tobacco use; halitosis associated with dental caries and periodontal disease, especially necrotizing periodontitis; sweet fruity ketosis associated with diabetic acidosis

evaluation includes speech and hearing; the functional level of hands, arms, and legs; and personal hygiene. For example, poor speech quality may indicate problems such as damaged or cancerous vocal cords or history of stroke. Hearing problems may indicate hearing loss resulting from age or injury and compromised hearing resulting from medications, infection, or loss of blood supply to the brain resulting from stroke, high blood pressure, or diabetes. Compromised hand and arm function may indicate the need to modify future oral hygiene instruction. Functional impairment of arms and legs may indicate the need to modify the client seating arrangements or may affect the client's ability to attend easily subsequent appointments. Poor personal hygiene may reflect the client care given to the oral cavity and overall concern about health.

Head, Face, and Neck Evaluation

The client should be seated in an upright position for the head, face, and neck extraoral assessment. Good lighting and exposure of the area being assessed are essential (e.g., remove any neck-related clothing, glasses, dentures, or appliances). Before asking clients to open the mouth, the dental hygienist performs an overall evaluation of the head, neck, eyes, face, lips, and surrounding skin. Normally the head, face, and neck have symmetry, and the skin should be continuous, firm, and pigmented in relation to normal variations.[3]

If lesions are observed initially, clients should be asked how long they have had the lesions, if the lesions have changed, and whether they are painful, with and without palpation. In addition, lymph node location, salivary glands, and the temporomandibular joints (TMJs) should be palpated. Each of these structures is described in depth in the following sections. Suspected atypical or abnormal findings require private consultation with the supervising dentist before the client undergoes further dental examination. The collaborative relationship between dental hygienist and the supervising dentist ensures that the comprehensive treatment needs of the client are identified, addressed, and evaluated.

Lymph Nodes

Lymph nodes are bean-shaped bodies grouped in clusters along the connecting lymphatic vessels, positioned to filter toxic products from the lymph to prevent their entry into the blood (Figure 15-1). In healthy clients, nodes are usually small, soft, and mobile in the surrounding tissue and cannot be visualized or palpated. The nodes can be superficial in position with the superficial veins or deep in the tissue with the associated blood vessels. All the head and neck nodes drain either the right or left tissue in the area, depending on their location (except for the midline submental nodes, which drain the tissue in the region bilaterally).

Palpable lymph nodes are those that have undergone lymphadenopathy (enlargement), resulting from an increase in size and change in consistency of the lymphoid tissue. Changed node consistency can range from firm to hard. Lymph nodes also can become attached or fixed to the surrounding tissue as the disease process progresses. Nodes also can feel tender to the client when palpated because of the pressure on the area nerves from the node enlargement.

Palpable lymph nodes may pinpoint where a disease process (e.g., infection or cancer) is active and may help determine if it has become widespread.[4] Approximately 63% of individuals with oral cancer have palpable enlarged nodes (see Chapter 45). Documentation of palpable nodes assists in the diagnosis, treatment, and prognosis of any disease process that may be present in the client. It is important to understand the relationship between the lymph node location and its drainage patterns. Furthermore, head and neck lymph nodes drain not only intraoral structures such as the teeth but also the eyes, ears, nasal cavity, and deeper areas of the pharynx.

Head and Neck Regions

Client head and neck extraoral clinical assessment begins with visually dividing the head and neck into specific regions and then palpating each region bilaterally in order from the superior to the inferior regions (Figure 15-2).[5]

TABLE 15-2
Palpation Methods for Assessing the Oral Cavity

Type	Definition	Technique	Example
Digital palpation	Using index finger to move or press against tissue	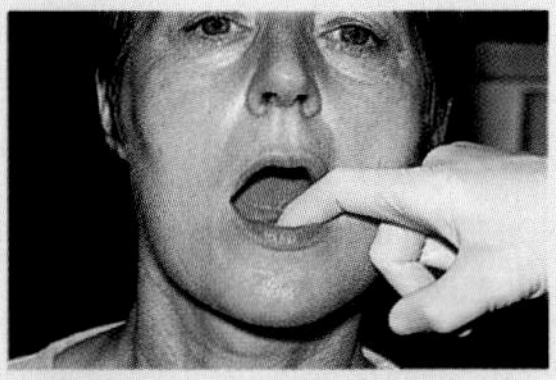	Use to palpate the floor of the mouth and lingual border of the mandible
Bidigital palpation	Using fingers and thumb to move or compress tissue using a rolling motion	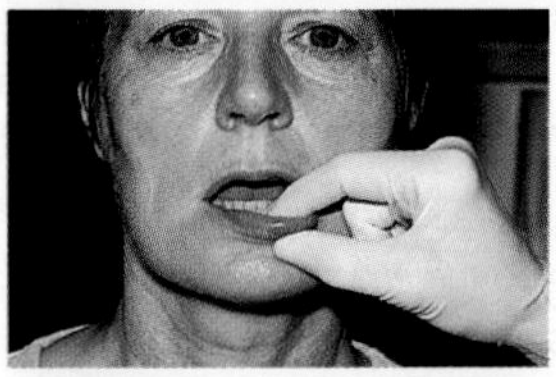	Use to palpate the lips, labial and buccal mucosa, and tongue
Manual palpation	Using all fingers of one hand to simultaneously move or compress tissue	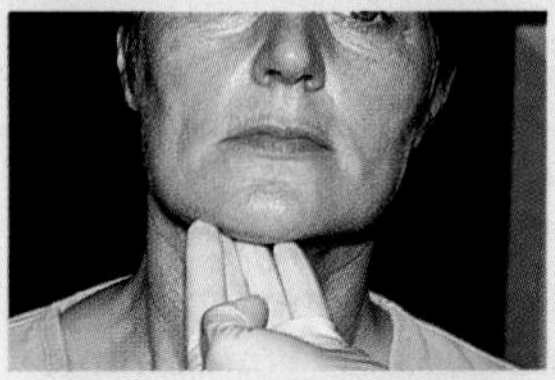	Use to palpate the lymph nodes or thyroid gland
Bimanual palpation	Using index finger of one hand and fingers and thumb of other hand simultaneously to move or compress tissue, holding the fingers closely together to avoid missing areas	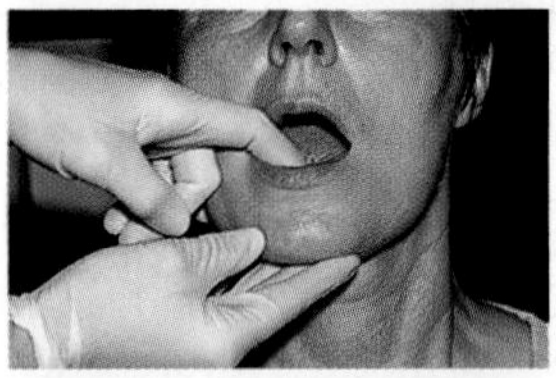	Use to palpate floor of the mouth, submandibular and sublingual glands, and lymph nodes
Bilateral palpation	Using a finger or fingers of both hands simultaneously to move or press tissue on contralateral (opposite) sides of the head and body	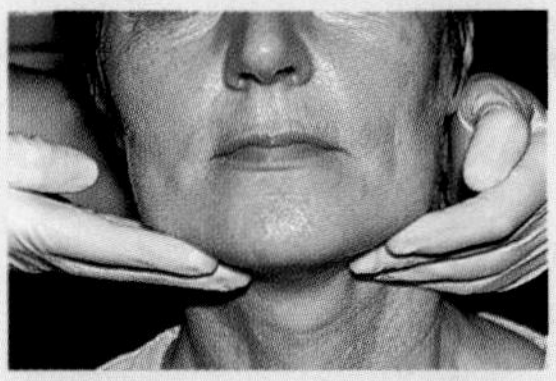	Use to palpate lymph nodes
Circular compression	Moving the fingertips in a deliberate, rotating fashion over tissue to be examined, exerting pressure	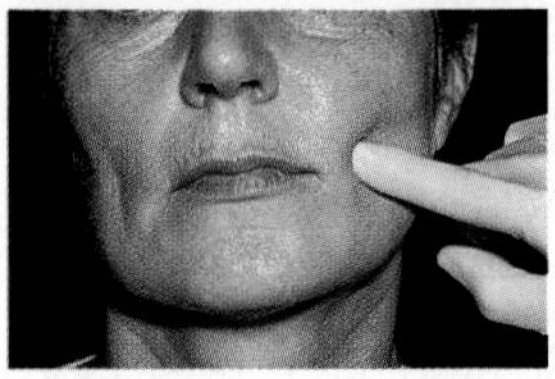	Use to palpate suspected lesion for more information

Parietal and Occipital Regions

The parietal and occipital regions are covered by the scalp overlying the cranium. The occipital nodes are located bilaterally on the posterior base of the head in the occipital region and drain this part of the scalp (see Figure 15-1). The occipital nodes empty into the deep cervical nodes in the neck.

Temporal and Auricular Regions

Within the temporal and auricular regions is the external ear (Figure 15-3), which is composed of an auricle (the larger flap of the ear) and the external acoustic meatus (the tube through which sound waves are transmitted to the middle ear within the skull). The superior and posterior free margin of the auricle is the helix, which ends inferiorly at the lobule (ear lobe). The part of the auricle anterior to the external acoustic meatus is a smaller flap of tissue, the tragus. The other flap of tissue opposite the tragus is the antitragus.

The auricular nodes are located anterior and posterior (retro) to the external acoustic meatus of the ear (see Figure 15-1). These nodes drain the external ear, the lacrimal (tear) gland superior to the eye, and adjacent regions of the scalp and face and then empty into the deep cervical nodes.

Frontal, Orbital, and Nasal Regions

The frontal region includes the forehead and the area superior to the eyes. The paired frontal sinuses are located in the frontal bone just superior to the nasal cavity, and each communicates with and drains into the nasal cavity (Figure 15-4).

In the orbital region the eyeball and all its supporting structures are contained in the bony socket called the *orbit*. On the eyeball is the white area or sclera with its central area of coloration, the circular iris. The opening in the center of the iris is the pupil, which appears black and changes size as the iris responds to changing light conditions. The conjunctiva is the delicate and thin membrane lining the inside of the eyelids and the front of the eyeball.

The outer corner where the upper and lower eyelids meet is called the *outer canthus*. The eye inner angle is called the *inner canthus*. The main nasal region feature is the external nose. Inferior to the apex on each side of the nose is a nostril(s) or naris (plural, nares). The nares are separated by the midline nasal septum. The nares are bounded laterally on each side by a winglike cartilaginous structure(s), the ala (plural, alae) of the nose. The tip is flexible when palpated.

BOX 15-1

Anatomic Terminology

Anterior: the front of an area in relationship to the entire body
Posterior: the back of an area in relationship to the entire body
Superior: an area that faces toward the head and away from the feet
Inferior: an area that faces away from the head and toward the feet
Medial: structures toward the midline of the body
Lateral: structures away from the midline of the body
Unilateral: structures on one side of the body
Bilateral: structures on both sides of the body
Contralateral: structures on the opposite side of the body
Ipsilateral: structures on the same side of the body
Superficial: structures located toward the surface of the body
Deep: structures located inward, away from the body surface

Infraorbital, Zygomatic, and Buccal Regions

The infraorbital and zygomatic regions are located on the face. The infraorbital region is located inferior to the orbital region and lateral to the nasal region. Farther laterally is the zygomatic region, which is composed of the zygomatic arch (cheekbone) (see Figure 15-2). The zygomatic arch extends from just inferior to the eye's lateral margin toward the superior part of the ear.

Facial lymph nodes are positioned along the facial vein and are typically small and variable in number (see Figure 15-1). Each facial node group drains the skin and mucous membranes where they are located and finally drains into the deep cervical nodes by way of the submandibular nodes. The paired maxillary sinuses are each located in the body of the maxillae, superior to the maxillary canine and premolars (see Figure 15-4) and drain into the nasal cavity (mandibular and maxillary anatomy is ilustrated in Chapter 40).

Inferior to the zygomatic arch and just anterior to the ear is the TMJ. The TMJ is where the upper skull forms a joint

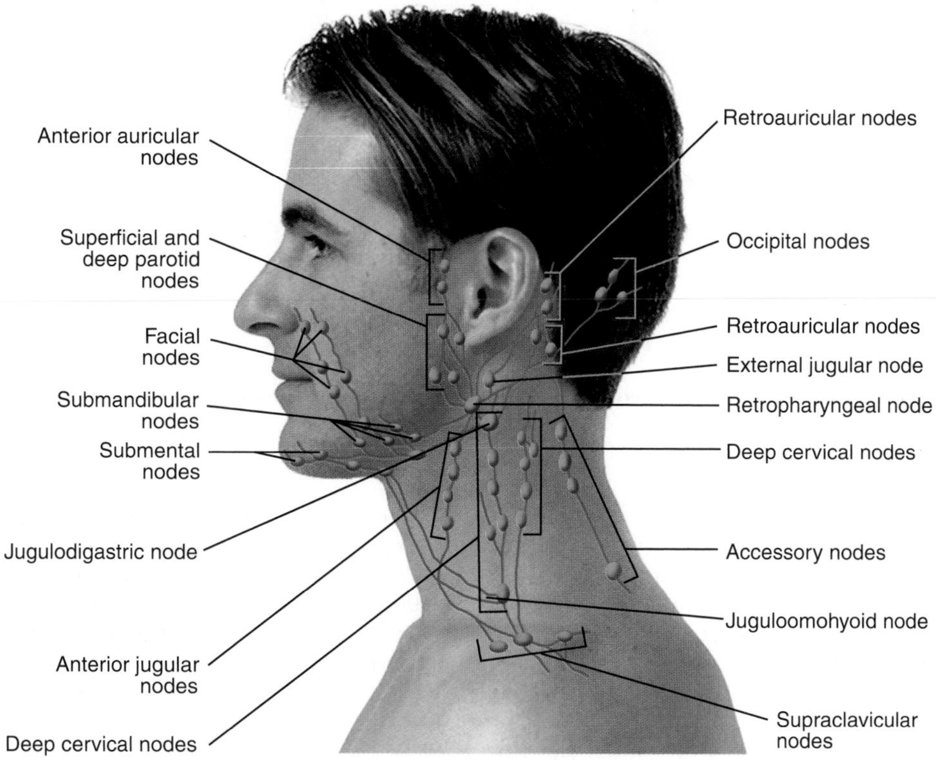

Figure 15-1. Lymphatic drainage system of the head and neck. (Adapted from Seidel HM, Ball JW, Dains JE, et al: *Mosby's guide to physical examination*, ed 7, St Louis, 2011, Mosby.)

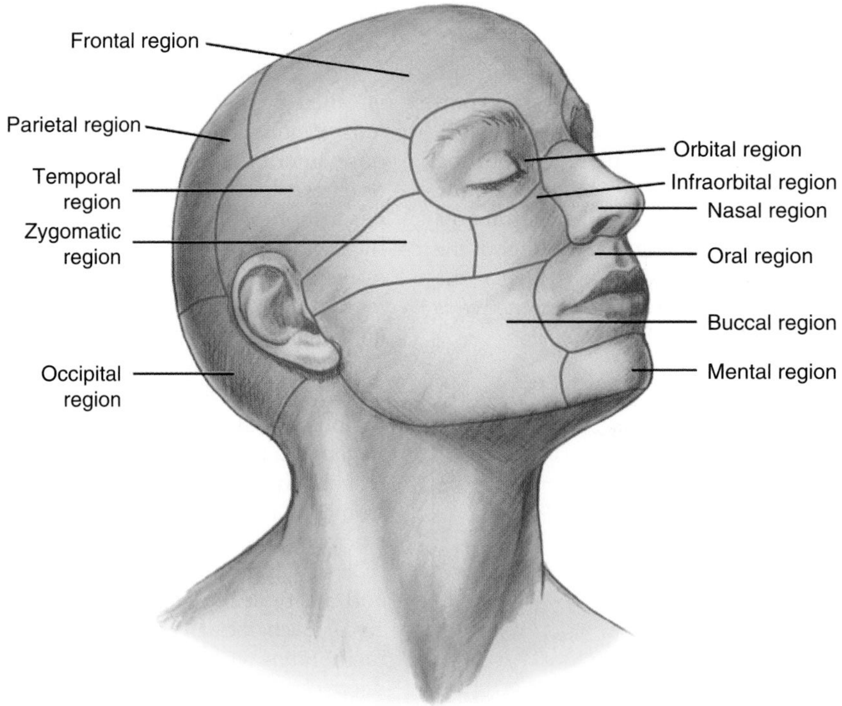

Figure 15-2. Regions of the head for extraoral assessment. (From Fehrenbach MJ, Herring SW: *Illustrated anatomy of the head and neck,* ed 4, St Louis, 2012, Saunders.)

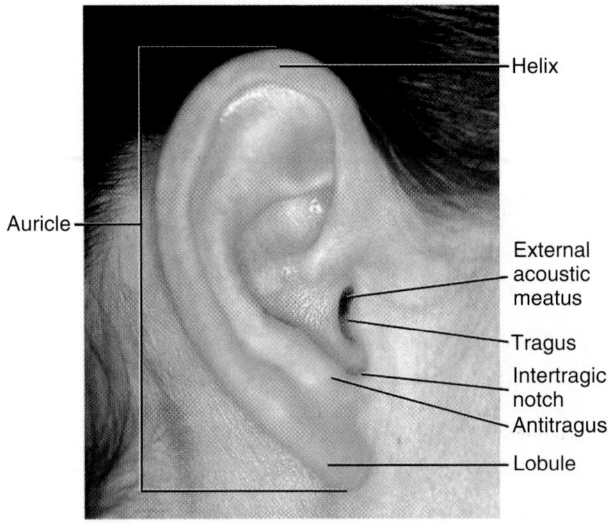

Figure 15-3. Anatomic structures of the external ear. (From Fehrenbach MJ, Herring SW: *Illustrated anatomy of the head and neck,* ed 4, St Louis, 2012, Saunders.)

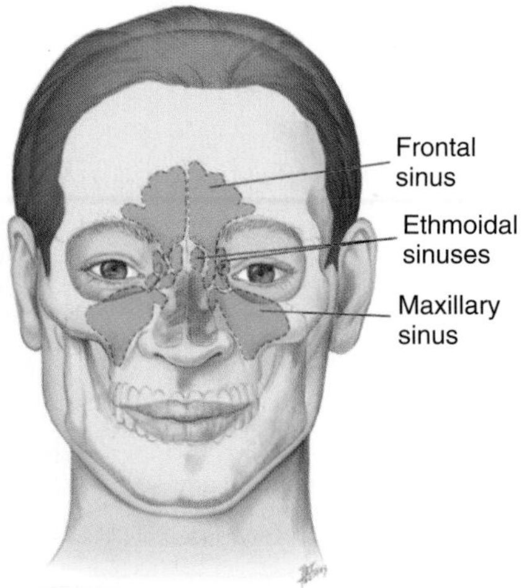

Figure 15-4. Anterior view of the skull and the paranasal sinuses. (From Fehrenbach MJ, Herring SW: *Illustrated anatomy of the head and neck,* ed 4, St Louis, 2012, Saunders.)

with the lower jaw—which involves the two temporal bones of the maxillae and the two condyles of the mandible. Joint movements can be felt when the mouth is opened and closed or the lower jaw is moved to the right, left, and forward. The TMJ should be palpated as well as the movement of the mandible observed as clients open and close the mouth.

The buccal region forms the side of the face and is a broad area between the nose, mouth, and ear (see Figure 15-2). The upper cheek is fleshy, formed primarily by a fat and muscle mass including the strong masseter muscle, which is felt when clients clench the teeth together. The sharp lower jaw angle inferior to the earlobe is the angle of the mandible. Also within this region is the parotid salivary gland, which occupies the area behind the mandibular ramus, anterior and inferior to the ear (Figure 15-5).

Mental Region

The chin is the mental region's major feature. The oral region is discussed later.

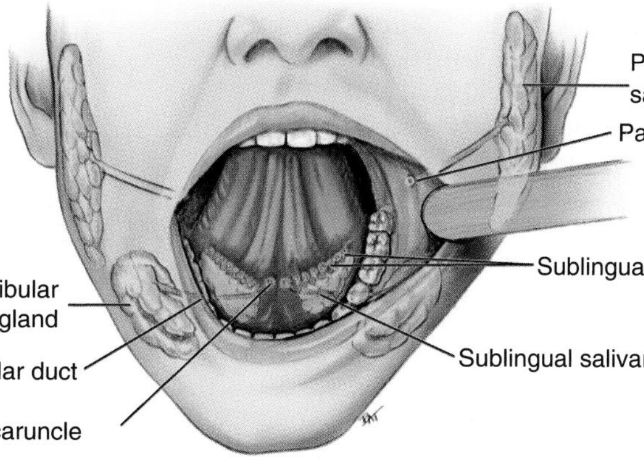

Figure 15-5. Salivary glands and associated structures. (From Fehrenbach MJ, Herring SW: *Illustrated anatomy of the head and neck,* ed 4, St Louis, 2012, Saunders.)

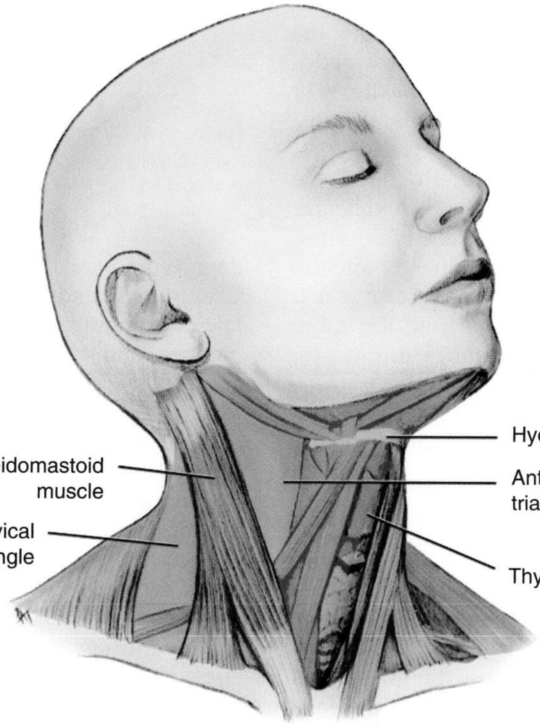

Figure 15-6. Anterior and posterior cervical triangles formed by the sternocleidomastoid muscle. (From Fehrenbach MJ, Herring SW: *Illustrated anatomy of the head and neck,* ed 4, St Louis, 2012, Saunders.)

Submandibular and Submental Triangles

The large strap muscle, the sternocleidomastoid muscle (SCM), divides each side of the neck diagonally into two cervical regions (Figure 15-6). The SCM originates from the clavicle and sternum and passes posteriorly and superiorly to insert on the temporal bone, just posterior and inferior to the ear. When the client's head is tilted to the side, the SCM is more prominent.

The anterior neck region corresponds to the two anterior cervical triangles, which are separated by the midline. The lateral neck region posterior to each SCM forms the posterior cervical triangles. There are many superficial cervical nodes in this region, such as the external jugular nodes, located along the external jugular vein, superficial to the SCM, secondary nodes for the more superior nodal change, and then empty into the deep cervical nodes (see Figure 15-1). Another regional group is the anterior jugular lymph nodes located on each side of the neck along the length of the anterior jugular vein, anterior to the larynx, trachea, and SCM that drain the infrahyoid region of the neck, and then empty into the deep cervical nodes.

The neck's anterior cervical triangle can be further subdivided into smaller triangular regions by parts of neck muscles and the mandible. The submandibular region is the superior part of the anterior cervical triangle on each side of the neck. The paired submandibular salivary glands are located in this region posterior to the paired sublingual glands (see Figure 15-6).

The submandibular nodes are located at the inferior border of the ramus of the mandible, just superficial to the submandibular gland (see Figure 15-1). They drain the cheeks, upper lip, body of the tongue, anterior hard palate, sublingual and submandibular salivary glands, and all the teeth and associated tissue, except the mandibular incisors and maxillary third molars. The submandibular nodes then empty into the deep cervical nodes.

Near the midline of the anterior cervical triangle is the submental region, where both the sublingual salivary glands are located (see Figure 15-6). The sublingual and submental nodes are located inferior to the chin in this region (see Figure 15-1). These nodes drain both sides of the chin, the lower lip, the mouth floor, the apex of the tongue, and the mandibular incisors and associated tissue. They then empty into the submandibular nodes or directly into the deep cervical nodes.

Anterior and Posterior Cervical Triangles

The deep cervical nodes also are located bilaterally along the neck's length, deep to the SCM (see Figure 15-1). These nodes drain the nasal cavity, posterior hard palate, soft palate, base of the tongue, maxillary third molars, esophagus, trachea, and thyroid gland. In addition to the deep cervical nodes, there are also nodes in the neck's most inferior area, the supraclavicular nodes, which are located along the clavicle and drain the anterior cervical triangles (see Figure 15-1), and then empty into one of the jugular trunks or directly into the right lymphatic duct or thoracic duct. These nodes are located in the final endpoint of lymphatic drainage from the entire body; for instance, cancer arising from the lungs, esophagus, and stomach may present in these nodes. Posterior to these are the accessory lymph nodes that drain the posterior scalp and neck regions and then drain into the supraclavicular nodes.

Anterior Midline Cervical Region

Within the anterior midline cervical region is the hyoid bone, which has many muscles attached to it and which controls the position of the base of the tongue (Figure 15-7). The hyoid bone can be palpated effectively inferior and medial to the angles of the mandible because it is suspended in the neck. When palpating the neck, the dental hygienist should not confuse the hyoid bone with the inferiorly placed thyroid cartilage, which also is found in the anterior midline.

The thyroid cartilage is the prominence of the voice box, or larynx. The thyroid cartilage's anterior part is visible as the Adam's apple, especially in adult males. The vocal cords or ligaments of the larynx are attached to the thyroid cartilage posteriorly. The thyroid gland also is located in this region, inferior to the thyroid cartilage, at the junction of the larynx and the trachea. The gland has two lobes on either side of the neck, connected by an isthmus anteriorly. There are no data comparing palpation using the anterior approach for the thyroid gland to the posterior approach, so clinicians should use the approach that they find most comfortable.

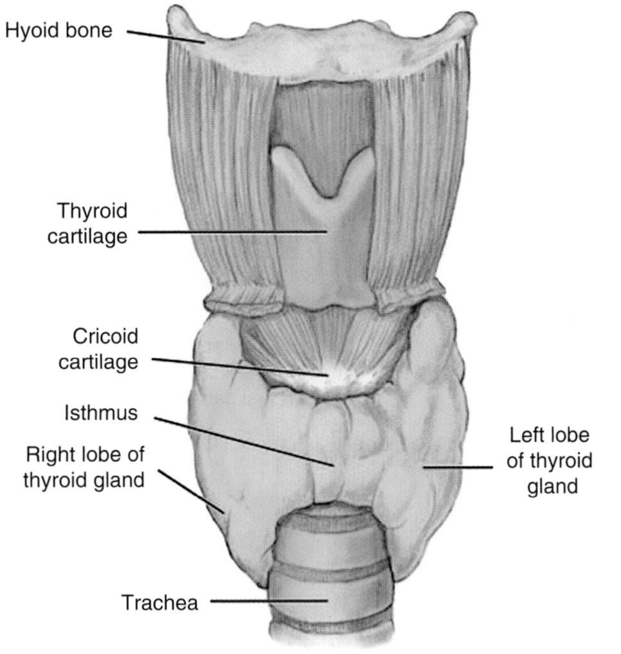

Figure 15-7. Anterior view of the thyroid cartilage, thyroid gland, and associated structures. (From Fehrenbach MJ, Herring SW: *Illustrated anatomy of the head and neck*, ed 4, St Louis, 2012, Saunders.)

Intraoral Clinical Assessment

The intraoral clinical assessment includes evaluation of the oral cavity and associated structures (e.g., the palate, pharynx, tongue, floor of the mouth, dentition, and periodontium). Clients are seated in a supine position. A preprocedural antimicrobial mouth rinse is used, and clients should remove any pigmented lipsticks. Nonpetroleum lubricant is applied to lip areas to make clients more comfortable, and they are asked to remove any removable appliances.

After an initial general inspection is made intraorally with a mouth mirror, client intraoral clinical assessment begins with the systematic assessment of specific regions using visualization and palpation. During assessment of mucosal surfaces, it is important to dry them gently with a gauze or air syringe so that color or texture changes will become more obvious. Ask clients to inform the clinician if they experience any mouth discomfort during any part of the assessment.

Procedure 15-2 details the steps for examining recommended intraoral structures and lists examples of normal, atypical, and abnormal findings that may be observed during an intraoral assessment. After performing this part of the intraoral assessment, the dental hygienist initiates specific dentition assessment, oral hygiene status, caries risk assessment, and periodontal risk assessment, as indicated (see Chapters 16, 17, 18, and 19).

Oral Region

The oral region contains the lips and oral cavity. The lips are outlined from the surrounding skin by a transition, the mucocutaneous junction (Figure 15-20). Each lip's vermilion border has a darker appearance than the surrounding skin. On the upper lip midline, extending downward from the nasal septum, is a vertical groove called the *philtrum*, which terminates in a thicker area or *tubercle*. The upper and lower lips meet at each mouth corner, the labial commissure.

Text continued on p. 225

Procedure 15-1 Conducting Extraoral Assessments

EQUIPMENT

Personal protective equipment
Hand mirror

EXTRAORAL REGIONS	STEPS	NORMAL FINDINGS	ATYPICAL FINDINGS	ABNORMAL FINDINGS
Overall evaluation of the face, head, and neck including the skin 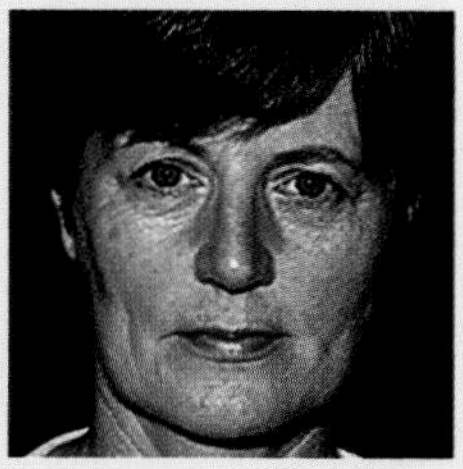 **Figure 15-8.**	Throughout allow the client to look at the hand mirror to understand the steps for self-examination. Visually observe symmetry and coloration of face and neck (Figure 15-8).	Face and head should be symmetric; skin continuous and firm, with normal variations of pigmentation.	Moles, freckles, scars, piercings, or tattoos	Needle marks resulting from drug use, trauma caused by domestic abuse
Frontal region, including forehead and frontal sinuses 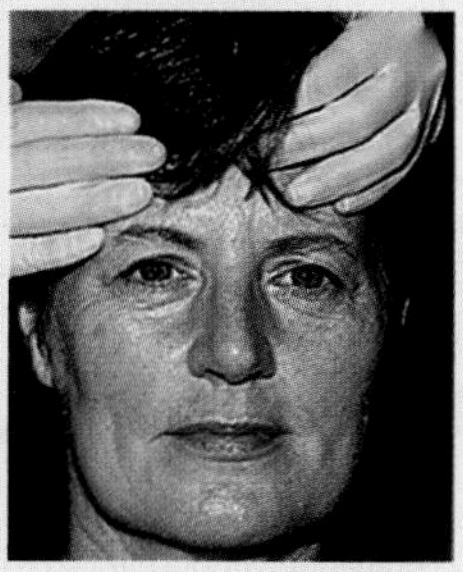 **Figure 15-9.**	Stand near the client to visually inspect and bilaterally palpate the forehead, including the frontal sinuses (Figure 15-9).	Area should be firm and smooth, without tenderness or increased temperature.	Tenderness and increased temperature may indicate frontal sinusitis.	Pigmented, red, or ulcerous lesions may indicate skin cancer.
Parietal and occipital regions, including scalp, hair, and occipital nodes 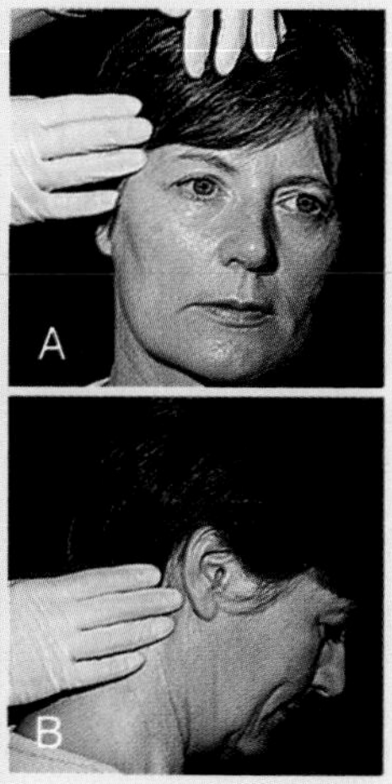 **Figure 15-10.**	Stand near the client to visually inspect the entire scalp by moving the hair, especially around the hairline, starting from one ear and proceeding to the other ear (Figure 15-10, *A*). Stand behind the client, have the client bend the head forward, and bilaterally palpate the occipital nodes on each side of the base of the head (Figure 15-10, *B*).	Scalp should be firm and continuous and without any changes noted, and hair should be free of debris. Nodes should not be clinically palpable or visible.	Debris found on the scalp and in the hair Palpable, nontender node may be the result of scar tissue from a past chronic infection.	Lesions on the scalp that are hidden by the hair, such as pigmented, red, or ulcerous lesions, which may indicate skin cancer; tender, soft, enlarged, and freely movable nodes may indicate an acute infection; hard, nontender, and fixed nodes may indicate a chronic infection or cancer.

Continued

Procedure 15-1 Conducting Extraoral Assessments—cont'd

EXTRAORAL REGIONS	STEPS	NORMAL FINDINGS	ATYPICAL FINDINGS	ABNORMAL FINDINGS
Temporal and auricular regions, including scalp, ears, and auricular nodes 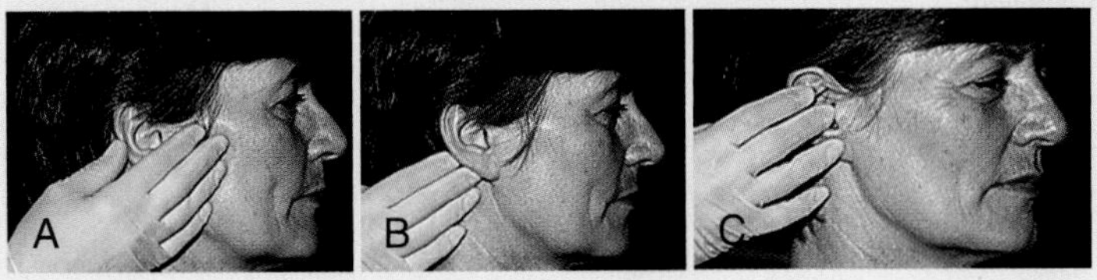 **Figure 15-11.**	Stand near the client, visually inspect and bilaterally palpate the external ear, as well as the scalp, face, and auricular nodes around each ear (Figure 15-11).	Skin should be firm and continuous, without changes noted in the surface. Nodes should not be clinically palpable or visible. Ears should not have discharge or inner canal redness.	Discharge from or redness of the inner canal May have ear piercings	Tender, soft, enlarged, and freely movable nodes may indicate acute infection; hard, nontender, and fixed nodes may indicate a chronic infection, cancer, or trauma resulting from domestic abuse; infections from piercings; pigmented, red, or ulcerous lesions may indicate skin cancer.
Orbital region, including the eyes 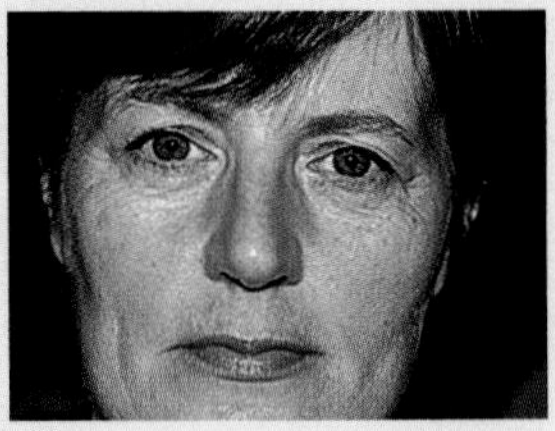 **Figure 15-12.**	Stand near the client to visually inspect the eyes and their movements and responses to light and action (Figure 15-12).	Iris should be clear and exhibit normal responses to light stimulus by the pupil. Sclera should be white. No swelling, bruising, and/or drainage. Client is able to open and close the eyes.	Tearing and eye redness from emotional distress or respiratory condition. Client may wear eyeglasses or contacts or have eyebrow piercings.	Yellowish or bluish coloration of sclera may indicate jaundice or trauma to the eye area; iris may be cloudy because of eye disease or may be pinpoint owing to drug intake; yellowish discharge from eye may indicate infection; excessive tearing and redness may result from drug or alcohol intake or obstructing mass in the maxillary sinus, nose, or facial soft tissue; swelling and bruising from trauma caused by domestic abuse; an inability to close eye on affected side with facial paralysis resulting from Bell palsy or stroke.
Nasal region, including the nose	Stand near the client to visually inspect and bilaterally palpate the external nose, starting at the root of the nose and proceeding to its apex.	Nose should be symmetric and show no signs of discharge or redness or ulceration of the overlying skin.	Nasal discharge may be present, and the surrounding skin may show some redness owing to respiratory conditions such as allergies, colds; loss of symmetry may be due to deviated septum or broken nose.	Inflammation, infection, and necrosis of tissue leading to nasal septum perforation caused by repeated cocaine snorting, possibly forming a saddlenose deformity; pigmented, red, or ulcerous lesions may indicate skin cancer; swelling and bruising from trauma caused by domestic abuse

Procedure 15-1 Conducting Extraoral Assessments—cont'd

EXTRAORAL REGIONS	STEPS	NORMAL FINDINGS	ATYPICAL FINDINGS	ABNORMAL FINDINGS
Infraorbital and zygomatic regions, including the muscles of facial expression, facial nodes, maxillary sinuses, and temporomandibular joints (TMJs)	Stand near the client to inspect visually the inferior to the orbits, noting the use of the muscles of facial expression. Visually inspect and bilaterally palpate each side of the face and the facial nodes, moving from infraorbital region to the labial commissure and then to the surface of the mandible (Figure 15-13, *A* and *B*). Visually inspect and bilateral palpate the maxillary sinuses (Figure 15-13, *C*). To access the TMJ gently place a finger into the outer part of the external acoustic meatus (Figure 15-13, *D*). Ask the client if he or she experienced any pain or tenderness. Note any sounds made by the joint. Then ask the client to open and close the mouth several times (Figure 15-13, *E*). Then ask client to move the opened jaw left, then right, and then forward.	Client should be able to use all of the muscles of facial expression on both sides of the face. Joint movement should be smooth, continuous, and silent; both sides of the joint should function similarly; both joint and associated musculature should be free of pain.	Tenderness and pain associated with maxillary sinusitis; noise or deviation of lower jaw on opening	Facial paralysis resulting from Bell palsy or stroke; temporomandibular disorder (TMD), with limitations of movement and discomfort during appointment; subluxation or pain on TMJ movement
Buccal region, including the masseter muscle and parotid salivary gland	Stand near the client on each side to inspect visually and palpate bilaterally the masseter muscle and parotid gland by starting in front of each ear and moving to the cheek area (Figure 15-14, *A*) and down to the angle of the mandible. Place the fingers of each hand over the masseter muscle surface and ask client to clench the teeth together several times (Figure 15-14, *B*).	Area should be firm and smooth, without tenderness or increased size or firmness.	Overdeveloped masseter muscle in a person with parafunctional habits	Tenderness and pain in the masseter muscle related to TMD; tender, soft, enlarged, and freely movable nodes may indicate an acute infection; hard, nontender, and fixed nodes may indicate a chronic infection or cancer; constant pain in the gland may indicate cancer; pigmented, red, ulcerated lesions may indicate skin cancer; odontogenic infection.

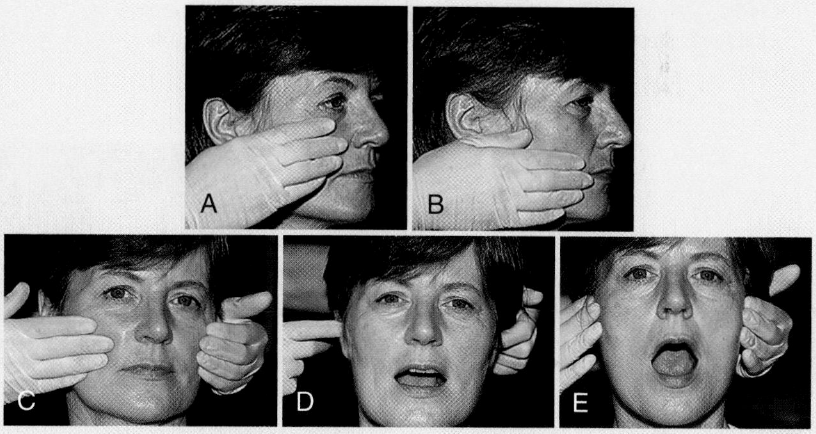

Figure 15-13.

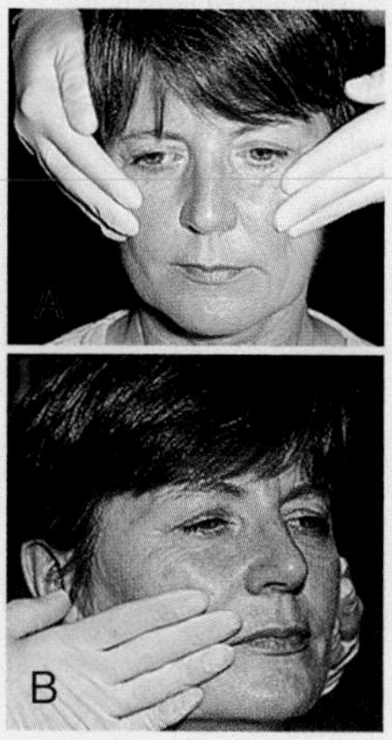

Figure 15-14.

Continued

Procedure 15-1 Conducting Extraoral Assessments—cont'd

EXTRAORAL REGIONS	STEPS	NORMAL FINDINGS	ATYPICAL FINDINGS	ABNORMAL FINDINGS
Mental region, including the chin 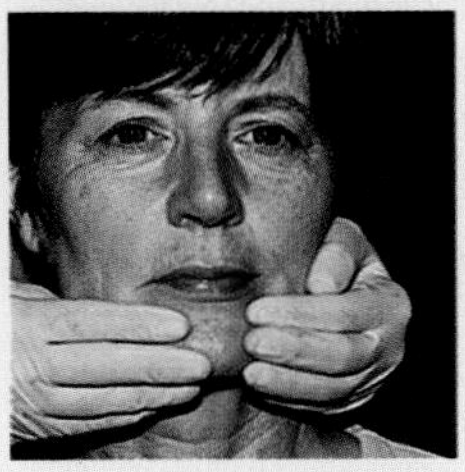 **Figure 15-15.**	Stand near the client on each side to visually inspect and bilaterally palpate the chin (Figure 15-15).	Area should be firm and smooth, without tenderness.	May have dimple or slight cleft associated with mandibular symphysis	Swelling and bruising from trauma caused by domestic abuse or other scars resulting from accidents; odontogenic infection
Submandibular and submental triangles, including submandibular and sublingual salivary glands and associated nodes	Stand slightly behind the client on one side and then the other, and have the client lower chin and manually palpate submandibular and sublingual glands as well as the associated nodes directly underneath the chin and on the inferior border of the mandible (Figure 15-16, *A*). Then push the tissue in the area over the bony inferior border of the mandible on each side, where it is grasped and rolled (Figure 15-16, *B*).	Mandible should be symmetric, with continuous borders. Nodes should not be clinically palpable or visible. 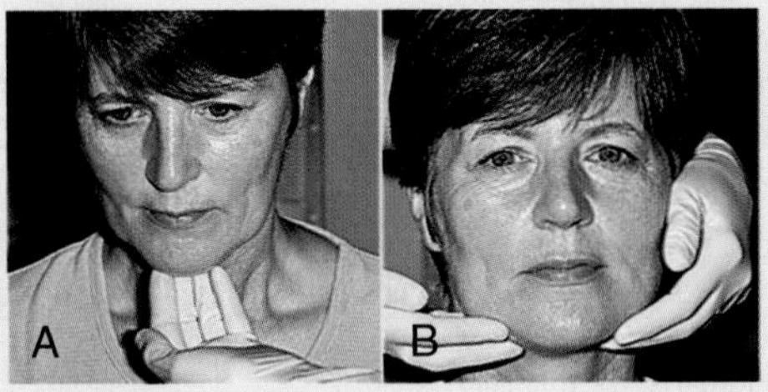 **Figure 15-16.**	Palpable, nontender node may be the result of scar tissue from a past chronic infection.	Sialolithiasis and blocked duct; excessive salivary flow or xerostomia; tender, soft, enlarged, and freely movable nodes may indicate an acute infection; hard, nontender, and fixed nodes may indicate a chronic infection or cancer; odontogenic infection.
Anterior and posterior cervical triangles, including sternocleidomastoid muscle (SCM) and associated nodes 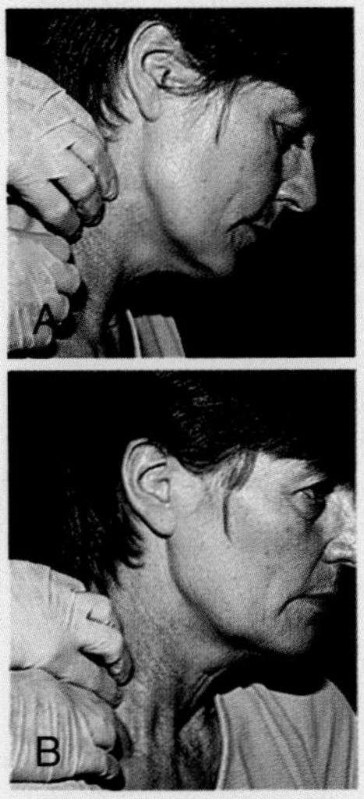 **Figure 15-17.**	With the client looking straight ahead, manually palpate with two hands on each side of the neck the superficial cervical node location. Start inferior to the ear and continue the whole length of the SCM surface to the clavicles (see Figure 15-17, *A*). Then have the client tilt the head to the one side and then to the other to allow palpation of the superior deep cervical nodes on the underside of the anterior and posterior aspects of the SCM. Then have the client raise the shoulders up and forward to palpate over the trapezius muscle surface the inferior deep cervical, accessory, and supraclavicular nodes (Figure 15-17, *B*).	Nodes should not be clinically palpable or visible.	Palpable, nontender node may be the result of scar tissue from a past chronic infection. Jugulodigastric (tonsillar node) becomes palpable when the palatine tonsils and/or pharynx are inflamed.	Tender, soft, enlarged, and freely movable nodes may indicate an acute infection; hard, nontender, and fixed nodes may indicate a chronic infection or cancer, especially if the client has breast cancer (axillary nodes filter breast tissue).

Procedure 15-1 Conducting Extraoral Assessments—cont'd

EXTRAORAL REGIONS	STEPS	NORMAL FINDINGS	ATYPICAL FINDINGS	ABNORMAL FINDINGS
Anterior midline cervical region, including hyoid bone, thyroid cartilage, and gland 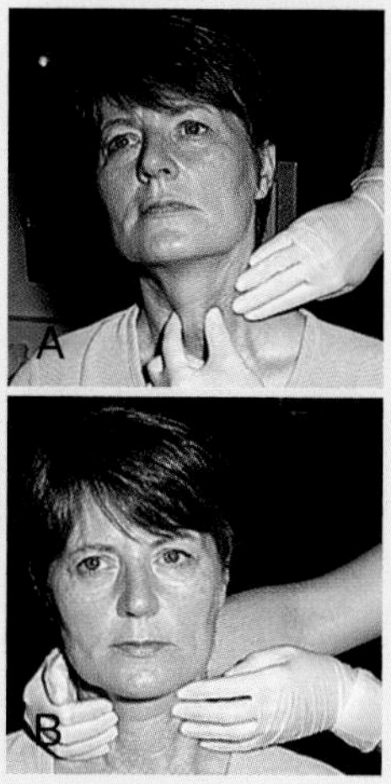 **Figure 15-18.**	Standing near the client, place one hand on each side of the trachea. Then gently displace the thyroid gland tissue to the other side of the neck while the other hand manually palpates the displaced tissue (Figure 15-18, *A*). Then compare the location of two lobes of the thyroid using visual inspection and bimanual or manual palpation (Figure 15-18, *B*). Ask the client to swallow to check for gland mobility by visually inspecting it while it moves superiorly and then back inferiorly. Client may need to use a glass of water to swallow. Then palpate larynx and deliberately move it.	Thyroid gland should not be enlarged, tender, or have unusual texture and should rise up and down during swallowing; larynx should be freely movable when palpated and deliberately moved, also should not have tenderness.	Prominent Adam's apple (thyroid cartilage)	Enlargement of gland with goiter; tender; with unusual texture such as rubbery or hard tissue masses such as with nodules (cyst or cancer); evidence of thyroid surgery with a lack of gland tissue; lack of movement of the gland during swallowing; larynx not freely movable, has stiffness, tenderness, with changes in voice and speech.

Steps from Fehrenbach MJ, Herring SW: *Illustrated anatomy of the head and neck*, ed 4, St Louis, 2012, Saunders. Figures courtesy Margaret M. Walsh, RDH, MS, MA, EdD, UCSF, Master of Science in Dental Hygiene Program Director, UCSF School of Dentistry, San Francisco, CA.

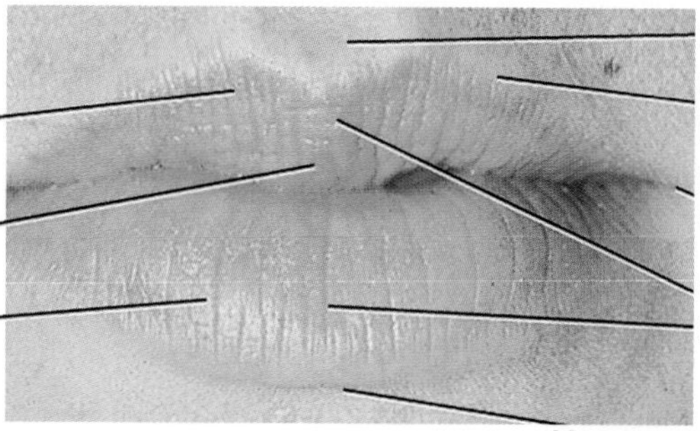

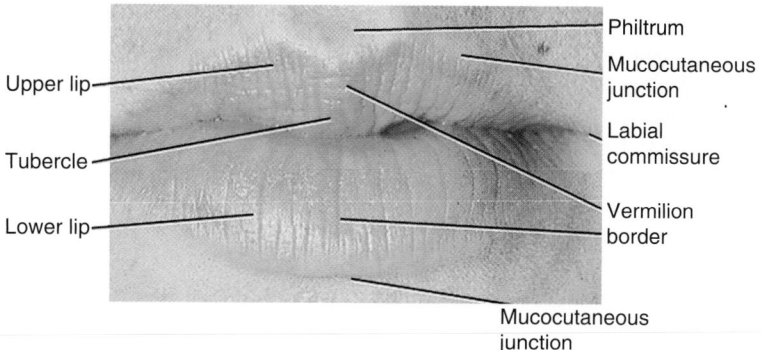

Figure 15-19. Frontal view of the lips and related anatomic landmarks. (From Fehrenbach MJ, Herring SW: *Illustrated anatomy of the head and neck*, ed 4, St Louis, 2012, Saunders.)

The oral cavity is the inside of the mouth. The anatomic landmarks in the oral cavity, as shown in Figure 15-20, can be used as a general point of reference during an intraoral examination.

The oral cavity is lined by nonkeratinized oral mucosa (Figure 15-21). The lip inner area consists of thick labial mucosa that is glistening pink or pigmented with melanin. The labial mucosa is continuous with the equally pink and thick **buccal mucosa** that lines the inner cheek. The buccal mucosa covers a dense inner tissue pad, the buccal fat pad. On the buccal mucosa, just opposite the maxillary second molar, is a small tissue elevation called the **parotid papilla**, which contains the parotid gland opening (see Figures 15-5 and 15-21).

The upper and lower spaces between the cheeks and lips and the gingival tissue are the maxillary and mandibular **vestibules**. Deep within each vestibule the pink and thick labial or buccal mucosa meets the redder and thinner alveolar mucosa at the **mucobuccal fold** (see Figure 15-21). The **labial frenum** is a fold of tissue located at the midline between the labial mucosa and the alveolar mucosa on each jaw. The dentition is located in the upper and lower jaws, the maxillae and mandible. Just posterior to the most distal maxillary tooth position is a rounded elevation, the **maxillary tuberosity**. Just

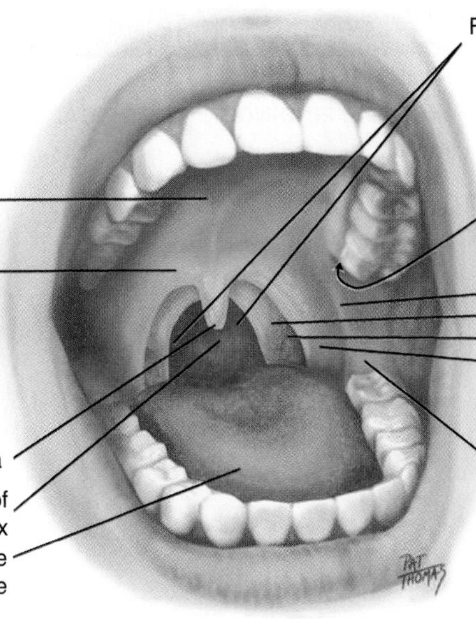

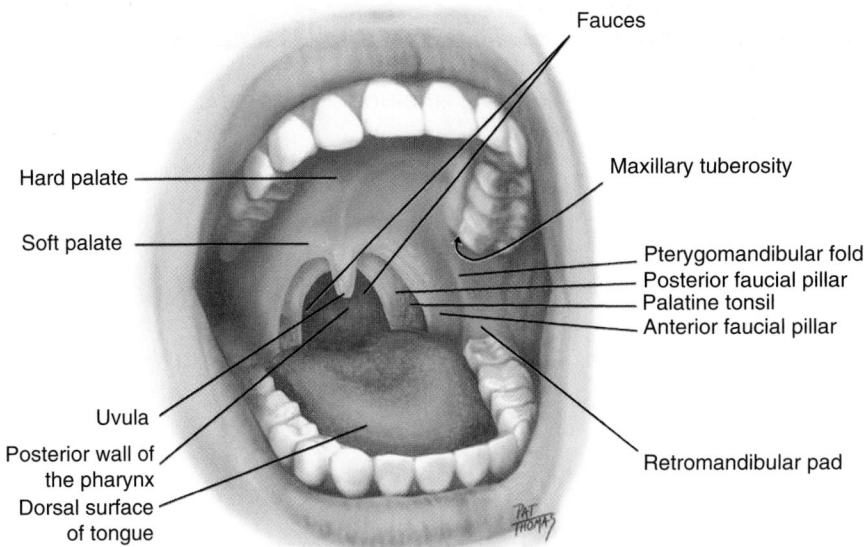

Figure 15-20. Anatomic landmarks in the oral cavity. (From Fehrenbach MJ, Herring SW: *Illustrated anatomy of the head and neck,* ed 4, St Louis, 2012, Saunders.)

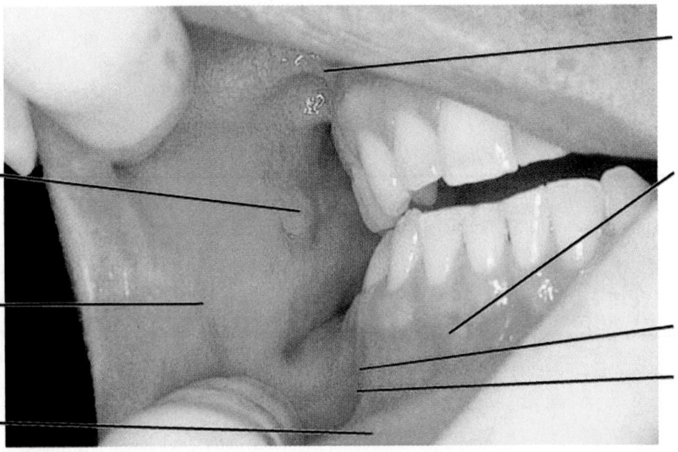

Figure 15-21. View of the buccal and labial mucosa of the oral cavity with anatomic landmarks noted. (From Fehrenbach MJ, Herring SW: *Illustrated anatomy of the head and neck,* ed 4, St Louis, 2012, Saunders.)

posterior to the most distal mandibular tooth is a dense tissue pad, the retromolar pad (see Figure 15-20).

Surrounding the teeth is the attached gingiva, composed of a firm, pink keratinized mucosa that tightly adheres to the bone around the tooth roots, the alveolar ridges. The demarcation line between the firmer and pinker attached gingiva and the movable and redder alveolar mucosa is the scallop-shaped mucogingival junction. The gingiva between the teeth, the interdental papilla, is an extension of attached gingiva (see Chapter 19).

Palate and Pharynx

The mouth roof has two parts: the firmer anterior part is the hard palate, and the looser posterior part is the soft palate (see Figures 15-20 and 15-22). A midline ridge of tissue on the hard palate is the median palatine raphe. A bony projection known as palatal torus is an atypical but normal structure that may be present in this area (Figure 15-23). A small bulge of tissue at the most anterior part, lingual to the anterior teeth, is the incisive papilla, and directly posterior to this papilla are the palatine rugae, which are firm, irregular ridges of tissue.

A midline muscular structure, the uvula, hangs from the posterior margin of the soft palate. The pterygomandibular fold is a fold of tissue that extends from the junction of the hard and soft palates down to the mandible, just behind the retromolar pad. It stretches when clients open the mouth wider, separating the buccal mucosa from the pharynx (see Figure 15-20).

The oral cavity also provides the entrance into the pharynx, which is a muscular tube that serves the respiratory and digestive systems. Parts of the nasopharynx and oropharynx are observable; the laryngopharynx is more inferior and is not observable. The part of the pharynx that is superior to the level of the soft palate is the nasopharynx, which is continuous with the nasal cavity.

The part of the pharynx that is between the soft palate and the opening of the larynx is the oropharynx; the opening from the oral cavity into the oropharynx is the fauces. The fauces of the oral cavity is formed laterally by two folds of tissue, which consists of the anterior and posterior faucial pillars. The palatine tonsils are masses of lymphoid tissue located between these two pillars (see Figure 15-20). Tonsils, like lymph nodes, contain lymphocytes that remove toxic products. Lymphadenopathy also can occur in the tonsils, causing tissue enlargement (see earlier discussion of lymph nodes).

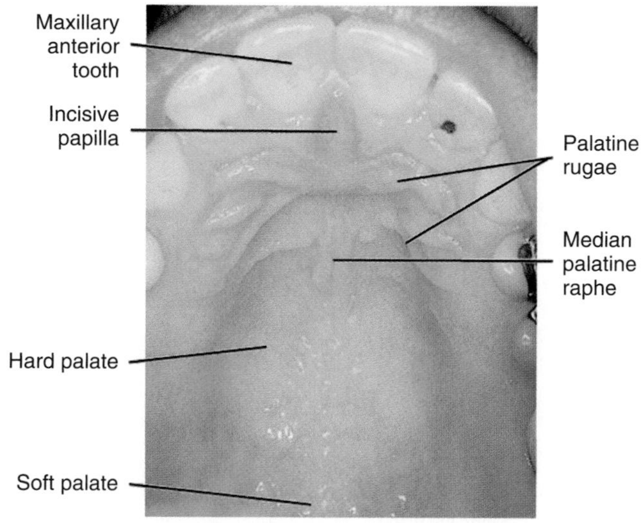

Figure 15-22. View of the palate with its anatomic landmarks noted. (From Fehrenbach MJ, Herring SW: *Illustrated anatomy of the head and neck*, ed 4, St Louis, 2012, Saunders.)

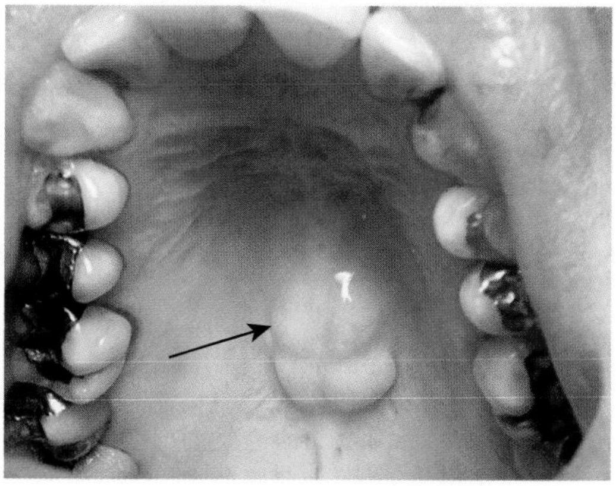

Figure 15-23. Palatal torus.

Tongue

The tongue is an important potential lesion site and must be assessed carefully (Figure 15-24). The posterior third of the tongue is its base, which attaches to the floor of the mouth. The base of the tongue does not lie within the oral cavity, but within the oropharynx. The anterior two thirds of the tongue is its *body*, and it lies within the oral cavity. The dorsal surface (top) of the tongue has a midline depression, the median lingual sulcus. The dorsal surface also has small, elevated structures of specialized mucosa, lingual papillae. The slender, threadlike, whitish filiform lingual papillae give the dorsal surface its velvety texture. The less-numerous red, mushroom-shaped dots are the fungiform lingual papillae. Because of these lingual papillae, the dorsal surface of the tongue should not be exceptionally smooth and allow for taste sensation.

Farther posteriorly on the tongue dorsal surface and more difficult to visualize clinically is a V-shaped groove, the sulcus terminalis (see Figure 15-24). The sulcus terminalis separates the base from the body of the tongue; where it points backward toward the throat is a small pitlike depression, the foramen cecum. The circumvallate lingual papillae (10 to 14 in number) line up along the anterior side of the sulcus terminalis on the body of the tongue. These large, mushroom-shaped lingual papillae also have taste buds. Farther posteriorly on the dorsal surface of the tongue base is an irregular mass of tonsillar tissue, the lingual tonsil, which is more difficult to see clinically. The side or lateral surface of the tongue is noted for its vertical ridges, the foliate lingual papillae (see Figure 15-24), having a large amount of taste buds.

The ventral surface (undersurface) is noted for its visible large blood vessels and the deep lingual veins that run close to the surface on either side (Figure 15-25). Lateral to each deep lingual vein is the plica fimbriata, a feathery fold of tissue.

Floor of the Mouth

The floor of the mouth is inferior to the ventral surface of the tongue (see Figure 15-25). The lingual frenum is a midline

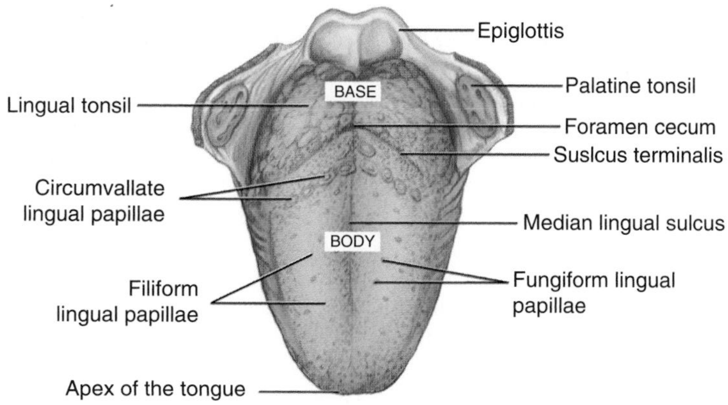

Figure 15-24. Dorsal surface of the tongue and relationship of lingual papillae. (From Fehrenbach MJ, Herring SW: *Illustrated anatomy of the head and neck*, ed 4, St Louis, 2012, Saunders.)

fold of tissue between the tongue's ventral surface and the mouth floor. There is also a tissue ridge on each side of the mouth, the **sublingual folds** that together form a V-shaped configuration from the lingual frenum to the base of the tongue. The sublingual folds contain duct openings from the sublingual salivary gland. The **sublingual caruncle** at the anterior end of each sublingual fold contains the submandibular and sublingual duct openings from the submandibular and the sublingual salivary glands. A bony projection, the **mandibular torus** (plural, tori), is an atypical finding that may be found on the mandibular lingual surface in the premolar area, possibly bilaterally (Figure 15-26).

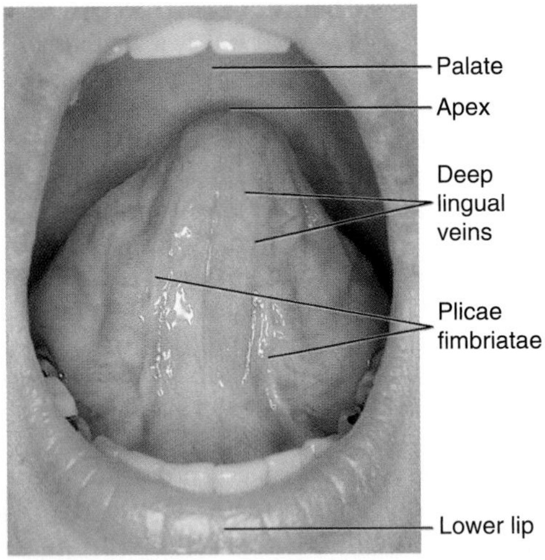

Figure 15-25. Ventral surface of the tongue and associated structures. (From Fehrenbach MJ, Herring SW: *Illustrated anatomy of the head and neck*, ed 4, St Louis, 2012, Saunders.)

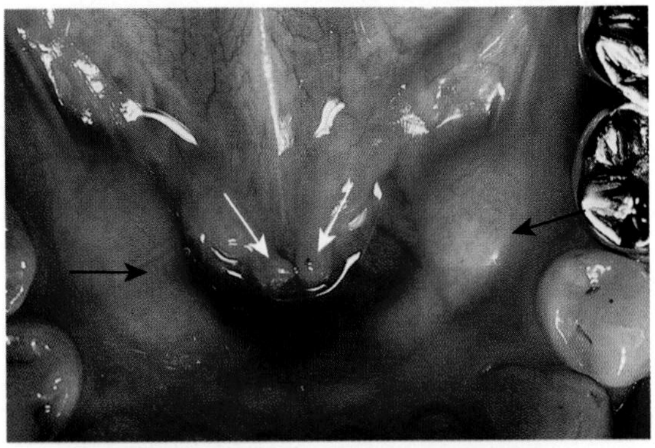

Figure 15-26. Mandibular torus *(black arrows)*. *White arrows* show sublingual caruncles with orifices to submandibular (Wharton) ducts.

Procedure 15-2 Conducting Intraoral Assessments

EQUIPMENT
Mouth mirror
Hand mirror
Gauze
Personal protective equipment

INTRAORAL REGIONS	STEPS	NORMAL FINDINGS	ATYPICAL FINDINGS	ABNORMAL FINDINGS
Lips	Throughout allow the client to look at the hand mirror to understand the steps for self-examination. Look at the lips overall (Figure 15-27, *A*).	Lips should be continuous in color, firm in texture, free of lesions, and semimoist, with an apparent border between the lips and the skin of the face. Commissures should be continuous and intact. Client should be able to make lips meet together.	Lip dryness or cracks that indicate xerostomia; ulcerations, irritation, and scarring that indicate parafunctional habits of biting and chewing lips; inflamed labial commissures that indicate angular cheilitis from parafunctional habits of licking the lips or local and systemic infections; ulcerations or vesicles that indicate herpetic infection	Loss of vermilion border or pigmented, red or white, ulcerated lesions may indicate skin or oral cancer or erosive dermatologic diseases; sagging lips on affected side with facial paralysis resulting from stroke or Bell palsy

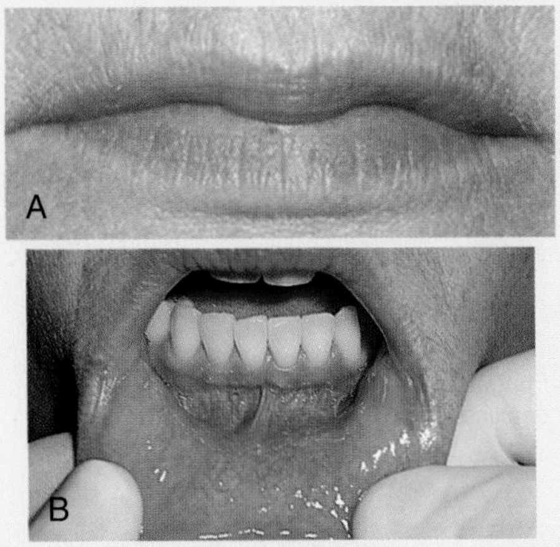

Figure 15-27.

Procedure 15-2 Conducting Intraoral Assessments—cont'd

INTRAORAL REGIONS	STEPS	NORMAL FINDINGS	ATYPICAL FINDINGS	ABNORMAL FINDINGS
	Then have the client smile and then open the mouth slightly and bidigitally palpate, as well as visually inspect the lower lip in a systematic manner from one commissure to the other. Use the same technique for the upper lip. Then gently pull the lower lip away from the teeth to observe the labial mucosa (Figure 15-27, *B*). Use the same technique for the upper lip.			
Oral cavity	Gently pull the buccal mucosa slightly away from the teeth to bidigitally palpate the inner cheek on each side, using circular compression (Figure 15-28). Dry the area with the gauze and then observe the salivary flow from each parotid duct. Retract the mucosal tissue enough to visually inspect the vestibular area and gingival tissue, including the maxillary tuberosity and retromolar pad on each side, and then bidigitally palpate these areas using circular compression.	Oral mucosa should be a continuous pinkish-red color, or pigmented in relation to the normal coloration of the client's skin, firm in texture, free of lesions, and moist. Parotid papilla and duct should be visible and same color and firmness as surrounding mucosa and able to produce saliva. Labial and buccal mucosa should have a pebbly consistency and rough surface texture owing to minor salivary glands. Attached gingiva should have stippling in varying degrees, with a firm consistency and should be anchored tightly to the teeth and underling alveolar bone.	Anterior inflamed tissue that may indicate mouth breathing; ulcerations and scarring from traumatic lesions; whitened areas that may indicate spit tobacco use; tight labial frena attachment, ulceration and scarring that indicate parafunctional habits of biting and chewing oral mucosa; yellow elevated spots from Fordyce spots, white raised line or linea alba at occlusal level from the keratosis; bony projections or exostosis on alveolar ridges; mandibular torus; amalgam tattoo; scarring from oral surgical removal of third molar	Pigmented, red or white, ulcerated lesions may indicate oral cancer or erosive dermatologic disease; whitened areas caused by candidiasis or lichen planus; excessive salivary flow or xerostomia; odontogenic infections; alcohol and smoker's breath; halitosis associated with caries and periodontal disease, especially necrotizing periodontitis; sweet fruity ketosis associated with diabetic acidosis; trauma associated with domestic abuse.

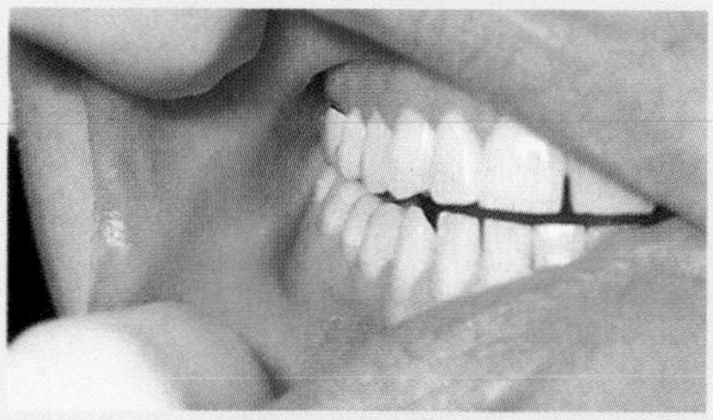

Figure 15-28.

Continued

Procedure 15-2 Conducting Intraoral Assessments—cont'd

INTRAORAL REGIONS	STEPS	NORMAL FINDINGS	ATYPICAL FINDINGS	ABNORMAL FINDINGS
Palate and pharynx, including the hard and soft palates, faucial pillars, palatine tonsils, uvula, oropharynx, and nasopharynx 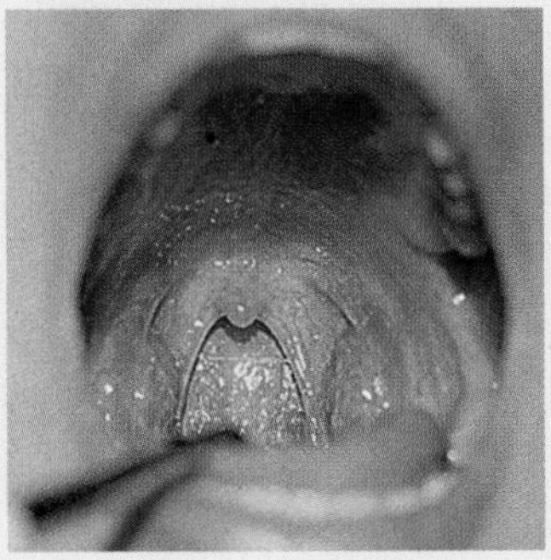 **Figure 15-29.**	Have client tilt the head back slightly. Use mouth mirror to intensify light source and view the palatal and pharyngeal regions. Have client extend the tongue; observe the soft palate. Gently place the mouth mirror (mirror side down) on the middle of the tongue and ask the client to say "ah." As this is done, visually observe the uvula and the visible parts of the pharynx (Figure 15-29). Compress hard and soft palates with first or second finger of one hand. Avoid circular compression on the soft palate to prevent initiating the gag reflex.	Palatal and pharyngeal tissue should be pink or pigmented in relation to the normal coloration of the client's skin (yellowish hue in the soft palate area), well hydrated, and devoid of lesions.	Red dots or petechiae, palatal torus, food burns, red dots on a white background from nicotinic stomatitis; bifid uvula; prominent tonsillar tissue; scarring from surgical removal of third molars; inflammation on soft palate from postnasal drip	Denture stomatitis; pigmented, red or white, ulcerated lesions may indicate oral cancer; trauma caused by child abuse; sagging palatal tissue resulting from facial paralysis from stroke; tonsillitis or tonsillar masses on the tonsils
Tongue 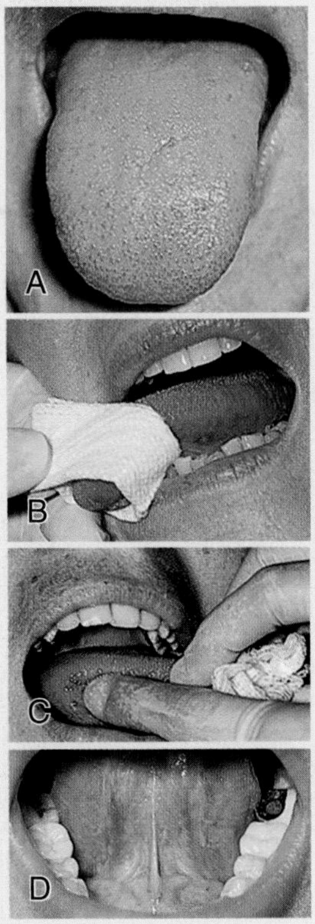 **Figure 15-30.**	To assess the dorsal and lateral surfaces of the tongue, have the client stick his or her tongue out slightly (Figure 15-30, *A*). Then wrap a gauze square around the anterior third of the tongue to obtain a firm grasp (Figure 15-30, *B*). Digitally palpate dorsal surface (Figure 15-30, *C*). If the client is forced to extend the tongue too far, the gag reflex is triggered. Turn the tongue slightly on its side to inspect its base and lateral borders. Bidigitally palpate the lateral surfaces of the tongue. To assess the ventral surface, have the client lift the tongue to permit inspection and digital palpation of the surface (Figure 15-30, *D*).	Bilateral symmetry, extremely vascular, reddish-pink in color all over, and moist; may be pigmented in relation to the normal coloration of the skin. Full range of movement as shown by sticking the tongue out	Clefts on ventral surface resulting from fissured tongue; white and red areas on ventral surface caused by geographic tongue; raised or flat red central area with central papillary atrophy; lingual varicosities; coated or stained tongue, large tongue caused by macroglossia; tongue-thrusting behavior during swallowing; lateral surface may be scalloped or scarred resulting from parafunctional habits of chewing or clenching	Hairy leukoplakia with HIV infection. Tenderness, color changes with tongue; shortened lingual frenum with limited movement resulting from ankyloglossia; any enlargement or induration, or signs of oral cancer; extreme loss of papilla on tongue related to nutritional disorders; trauma caused by child abuse; infection from piercings; difficulty swallowing with dysphagia from certain nerve disorders or oropharyngeal cancers

Procedure 15-2 Conducting Intraoral Assessments—cont'd

INTRAORAL REGIONS	STEPS	NORMAL FINDINGS	ATYPICAL FINDINGS	ABNORMAL FINDINGS
Floor of the mouth, including the submandibular and sublingual salivary glands and ducts 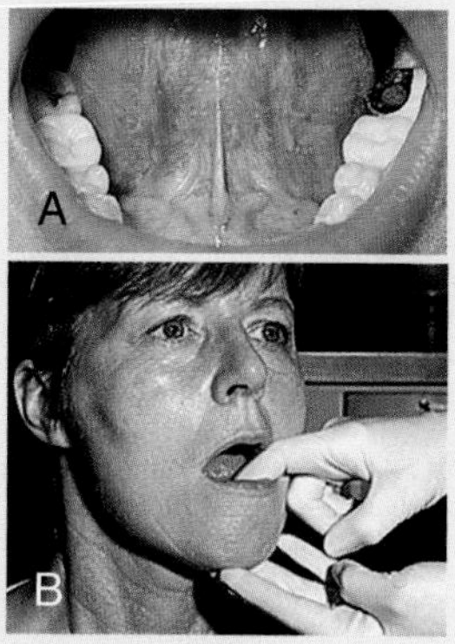 Figure 15-31.	Use the mouth mirror to facilitate lighting and direct observation. While the client lifts the tongue to the roof of the mouth, observe the mucosa of the floor of the mouth for lesions, swelling, or color change (see Figure 15-31, *A*). Check the lingual frenum. Wipe the sublingual caruncle with gauze and observe the saliva flow from the duct. Bimanually palpate the sublingual area by placing the right index finger intraorally and the fingertips of the left hand extraorally under the chin to feel the tissue between the two hands. Use bidigital palpation for the sublingual gland on the floor of the mouth, behind each mandibular canine, by placing the index finger of one hand intraorally and the index finger of the other hand extraorally, with the gland compressed between (Figure 15-31, *B*).	Bilateral symmetry, extremely vascular, reddish-pink, and moist. Sublingual caruncle should be visible and same color and firmness as surrounding mucosa and able to produce saliva.	Tight lingual frenum attachment; mandibular torus Presence of piercings	Blocked duct resulting from sialolithiasis or ranula; excessive salivary flow or xerostomia; tenderness, ankyloglossia; any enlargement or induration or pigmented, red or white, ulcerated lesions may indicate oral cancer; trauma from child abuse

Steps from Fehrenbach MJ, Herring SW: *Illustrated anatomy of the head and neck,* ed 4, St Louis, 2012, Saunders. Figures courtesy Margaret M. Walsh, RDH, MS, MA, EdD, UCSF, Master of Science in Dental Hygiene Program Director, UCSF School of Dentistry, San Francisco, CA.

Describing and Documenting Significant Findings

After the observation of atypical or abnormal findings, the dental hygienist describes and documents them accurately in the client record, forming a dental hygiene diagnosis.

Precise descriptive terms enable the dental hygienist to communicate with the supervising dentist and other healthcare professionals to facilitate an accurate differential diagnosis. A **differential diagnosis** is the identification of a condition by differentiating all pathologic processes that may produce similar lesions. See Table 15-3 for the descriptive categories for oral lesions (e.g., **atrophy**, **bulla**, **macule**, **nodule**, **papule**, **plaque**, **pustule**, **ulcer**, **vesicle**, **wheal**).

A sample form used for collecting data during an extraoral and intraoral assessment is shown in Figure 15-32. In addition, Figure 15-33 has sample lesion descriptions for entry into a client record. Specific descriptive items that must be included in the client record when describing a lesion are discussed in the following sections and are part of the dental hygiene diagnosis of a lesion.

Location and Distribution

When documenting the location of a lesion, the dental hygienist must be as accurate as possible so that follow-up examination by the supervising dentist may be made correctly even if the lesion has healed and no longer remains. The location also is important because some lesions characteristically occur in specific regions or tissue types, and this information can help the supervising dentist formulate a differential diagnosis. For example, hairy leukoplakia (thick white lesions with long fingerlike projections) can occur on the lateral borders of the tongue in clients with an HIV infection. When describing the location of an oral lesion at this level specificity, the clinician identifies the nearest anatomic landmark (e.g., upper lip, labial mucosa, tongue surface, specific teeth) and then notes the lesion's anatomic relationship to the structure (e.g., **anterior** or **posterior**, **medial** or **lateral**, **inferior** or **superior**, **unilateral** or **bilateral**, **contralateral**, or **ipsilateral**).

The description of the lesion's location also must specify whether the lesion is **unilateral** (located on the right side or

TABLE 15-3
Descriptive Categories for Oral Lesions

	Term	Size (cm)	Description	Example
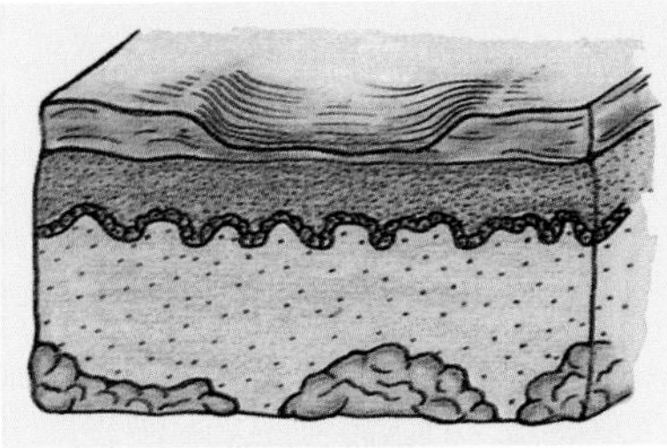	Atrophy	Varies	Thinning of tissue layers, with shiny and translucent appearance	Erosive lichen planus
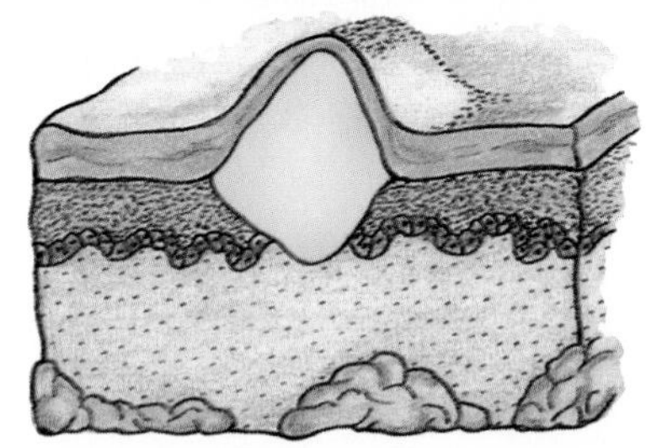	Bulla	>0.5	Larger circumscribed blister containing clear, watery fluid or blood	Pemphigus or pemphigoid
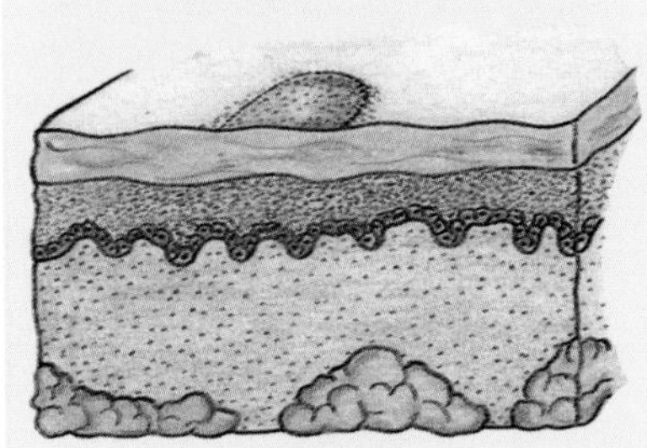	Macule	<1	Flat, nonpalpable	Petechiae
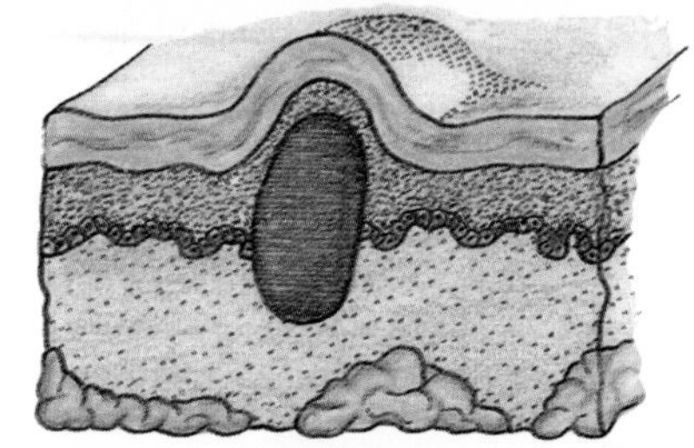	Nodule	0.5-2	Elevated solid mass, deeper and firmer than papule	Torus
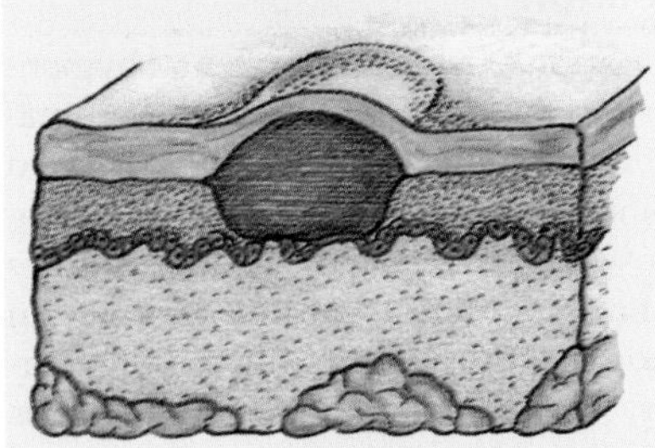	Papule	<0.5	Palpable, circumscribed, solid elevation	Oral fibroma
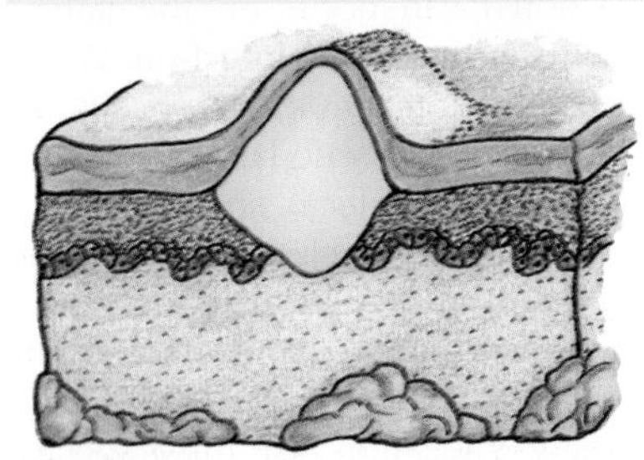	Plaque	>0.5	Discrete, slightly elevated area of altered texture or coloration	Candidiasis

TABLE 15-3
Descriptive Categories for Oral Lesions—cont'd

	Term	Size (cm)	Description	Example
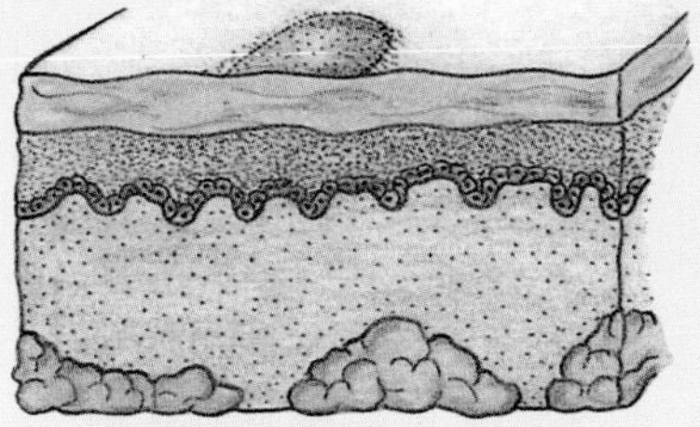	Pustule	Varies	Similar to vesicle but filled with pus	Acne
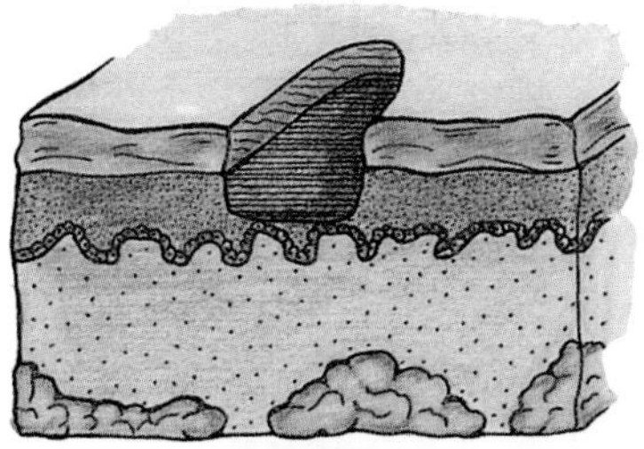	Ulcer	Varies	Deep loss of epithelial layer; may extend to connective tissue layers	Recurrent aphthous ulcer
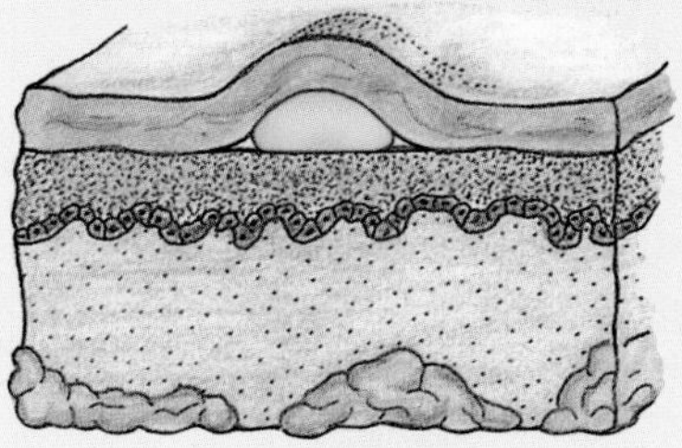	Vesicle	<0.5	Smaller circumscribed blister, filled with clear, watery fluid	Herpes labialis
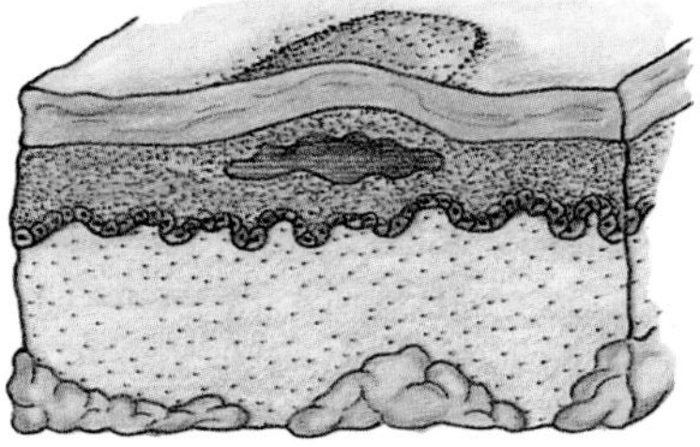	Wheal	Varies	Irregularly-shaped elevated area of superficial localized edema	Type I hypersensitivity

Figures adapted from Potter PA, Perry AG: *Fundamentals of nursing,* ed 8, St Louis, 2015, Mosby.

on the left side) or **bilateral** (located on both sides). Some lesions may be located in the midline. Generally, bilateral structures are normal anatomic structures and thus a unilateral structure may indicate a pathologic lesion. Any additional lesions may be noted as either **contralateral** (located on the opposite side) or **ipsilateral** (located on same side) from the original lesion.

In addition to location, the lesion **distribution** must be described and can be either single or multiple. For example, a mucocele (elevated lesion caused by accumulation of saliva from a blocked duct) is a single lesion, whereas herpes simplex virus infection manifesting on the attached gingival often produces multiple lesions.

Multiple lesions may be described as either separate or coalescing. Multiple lesions that are discrete and do not run together are **separate**, whereas lesions with margins that merge are **coalescing**. In addition, multiple lesions may be localized or generalized. **Localized** refers to lesions that are limited to a single area, whereas **generalized** describes lesions involving more than one area and may indicate a systemic dermatologic disease (e.g., lichen planus).

Size and Shape

Lesion size is determined by using a periodontal probe or small metric ruler to measure the legion's length, width, and height. Oral lesion size varies, but generally a lesion is not apparent to the client when it is smaller than 1 to 2 cm. In addition, lesion height, whether the lesion is a papule (raised) or macule (flat), and the contour of the lesion's borders relate to its shape. Lesion borders must be documented as being either well defined or poorly defined. Generally, noncancerous lesions have well-defined borders and are round or ovoid.

ORAL/FACIAL SOFT TISSUE
EXAMINATION RECORD

PATIENT'S NAME:______________________________
PATIENT'S I.D. No.:______________________________

N 5 Normal   O 5 Other
use "Notes" section

Date:	____		____		____		____	
EXTRAORAL	**N**	**O**	**N**	**O**	**N**	**O**	**N**	**O**
Skin –Face	☐	☐	☐	☐	☐	☐	☐	☐
–Neck	☐	☐	☐	☐	☐	☐	☐	☐
* Vermilion Borders	☐	☐	☐	☐	☐	☐	☐	☐
Parotid Glands	☐	☐	☐	☐	☐	☐	☐	☐
Lymph Nodes	☐	☐	☐	☐	☐	☐	☐	☐
Anterior Cervical	☐	☐	☐	☐	☐	☐	☐	☐
Posterior Cervical	☐	☐	☐	☐	☐	☐	☐	☐
Submental	☐	☐	☐	☐	☐	☐	☐	☐
Submandibular	☐	☐	☐	☐	☐	☐	☐	☐
Supraclavicular	☐	☐	☐	☐	☐	☐	☐	☐
INTRAORAL								
Labial Mucosa	☐	☐	☐	☐	☐	☐	☐	☐
Labial Vestibules	☐	☐	☐	☐	☐	☐	☐	☐
Anterior Gingivae	☐	☐	☐	☐	☐	☐	☐	☐
Buccal Vestibules	☐	☐	☐	☐	☐	☐	☐	☐
Buccal Gingivae	☐	☐	☐	☐	☐	☐	☐	☐
Tongue–Dorsal	☐	☐	☐	☐	☐	☐	☐	☐
* –Ventral	☐	☐	☐	☐	☐	☐	☐	☐
* –Lateral	☐	☐	☐	☐	☐	☐	☐	☐
* Lingual Tonsils	☐	☐	☐	☐	☐	☐	☐	☐
* Floor of Mouth	☐	☐	☐	☐	☐	☐	☐	☐
Lingual Gingivae	☐	☐	☐	☐	☐	☐	☐	☐
* Tonsillar Pillars	☐	☐	☐	☐	☐	☐	☐	☐
* Pharyngeal Wall	☐	☐	☐	☐	☐	☐	☐	☐
* Soft Palate	☐	☐	☐	☐	☐	☐	☐	☐
Uvula	☐	☐	☐	☐	☐	☐	☐	☐
Hard Palate	☐	☐	☐	☐	☐	☐	☐	☐
Palatal Gingivae	☐	☐	☐	☐	☐	☐	☐	☐
Submandibular Glands	☐	☐	☐	☐	☐	☐	☐	☐

* *High risk sites for squamous carcinoma*

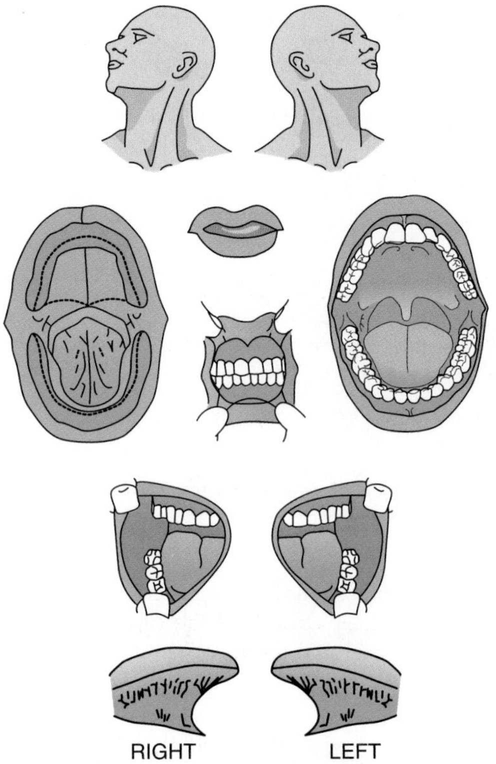

NOTES

RECOMMENDATIONS:

1. Establish an examination sequence and follow it routinely.
2. Tell the patient you are performing a complete Soft Tissue Examination.
3. Examine ALL areas each time.
4. Use visual inspection AND palpation.
5. Record ALL findings—Normal or Abnormal.
6. Remove dental appliances before the examination.
7. Suggested descriptive terms: hard, soft, well-circumscribed, ill-defined, indurated, sessile, pedunculated, hemorrhagic, ulcerated, edematous, normal in color, red, white, speckled, color other than normal.

FOLLOW-UP TAKEN

Biopsy ______________________________

Results ______________________________

Referral to Dr. ______________________________
Other ______________________________

This chart is a general guideline. Neither the American Cancer Society nor the California Dental Association assume liability for individual evaluation or recommendations.

American Cancer Society® California
Developed by the Dental Education Subcommittee American Cancer Society, California Division, Inc.

Figure 15-32. Extraoral and intraoral assessment form. (Courtesy American Cancer Society, Atlanta, GA.)

Example No. 1:

Chart Entry:
Positive finding on intraoral examination: lower right labial mucosa, single white sessile nodule 2 x 3 x 2 mm with a slightly rough surface; nonmobile on palpation. Client is asymptomatic with no associated lymphadenopathy. Client has been informed and will return for follow-up visit in 2 weeks—possible biopsy or referral to oral surgeon if the lesion changes in nature or does not resolve.

Date the entry; have the entry initialed by the dentist and the dental hygienist.

Example No. 2:

Chart entry:
Positive finding on extraoral examination: upper left of the mucocutaneous junction of the upper lip, multiple coalescing vesicles 5 x 3 x 7 mm in total area; slightly red in color with a crust. Lesions have been known to the client for 5 days and began with associated tingling and itching in the area prior to appearance of the lesions. Client reports a history of similar "cold sores" in the area.

Date the entry; have the entry initialed by the dentist and the dental hygienist.

Figure 15-33. Sample descriptions of lesions for entry into the client's dental record.

In contrast, cancers have poorly defined borders and thus an irregular shape as a result of the cancer infiltration process and resulting regional tissue inflammation and fibrosis.

Color

Any unusual color changes in oral tissue may signal an abnormal condition. Lesion colors observed normally are red and white, with white predominating. Other less-common colors include blue, purple, yellow, black, and gray. Lesions even can exhibit the same color as the adjacent tissue. Lesions of a red color (erythema) may be the result of thinning of the superficial epithelium, increased vascularity in the subepithelial tissue, or dissolution of connective tissue. White lesions that cannot be wiped off may be the result of excess keratin in the superficial epithelium making them more opaque, decreased vascularity or an increased amount of fibrous collagen tissue (fibrosis) of the subepithelial tissue.

Brownish, bluish, or black lesions indicate that there is a deposit of melanin, blood, or heavy metal in the tissue, such as amalgam particles (amalgam tattoo). In addition, fluid-filled lesions or lesions with increased or enlarged blood vessels can appear bluish. It is important to remove by biopsy any localized brownish, bluish, or black lesions from the oral cavity because of their risk of being carcinogenic (melanoma). Yellow lesions usually contain sebaceous glands or adipose tissue or presence of purulent suppuration (pus). Sometimes these color modifications can occur simultaneously in the same lesion area, and this must be noted. In addition, it should be noted if the lesion is hemorrhaging (bleeding) spontaneously or easily with palpation.

Texture

Lesion *texture* refers to the surface appearance, which is taken into account when establishing a list of possible differential diagnoses (e.g., **crater**, **crust**, **induration**, **papillary**, **pseudomembrane**, **smooth**, **verrucous**). Terminology used to describe lesion surface texture is listed in Table 15-4. Most of the oral cavity is smooth in texture on the surface, except in the palatal rugae and attached gingival stippling. Superficial epithelial tissue lesions frequently have a rough surface, whereas deep tissue lesions have a smooth surface.

TABLE 15-4

Terminology Used to Describe Surface Texture of a Lesion

Term	Description
Crater	Central depression
Crust	Hard covering, composed of dried serum, pus, blood, or combination
Induration	Hardness of tissue from increased number of surrounding epithelial cells
Papillary	Having rough surface containing small nodulations or elevated projections
Pseudomembrane	Loose membranous surface layer of exudate containing microorganisms formed during inflammatory reaction
Smooth	Deep lesion that pushes up and stretches surface tissue
Verrucous	Having rough, wartlike surface with multiple irregular folds

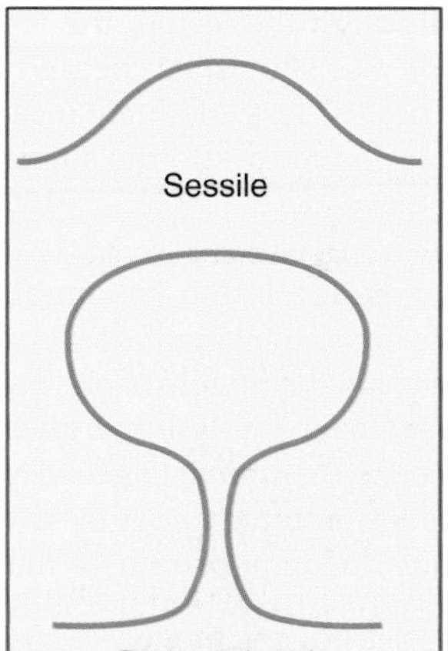

Figure 15-34. Types of base or attachment of a lesion.

Attachment and Depth

If a lesion has a broad base of attachment as wide as the lesion itself, its attachment is described as *sessile*. In contrast, **pedunculated** lesions have a narrow pedicle, or stalklike base of attachment (Figure 15-34). Whether lesions are **superficial** or **deep** is determined by checking with palpation.

Consistency

Consistency refers to the degree of firmness or density of the tissue. This categorization of firmness of the lesion is accomplished by palpating the lesion and then comparing its degree of consistency (e.g., **soft**, **firm**, **hard**) with the consistency of

TABLE 15-5

Terminology to Indicate Consistency of a Lesion

Term	Description	Normal Tissue Comparison
Soft	Composed mainly of cells without much intervening fibrous connective tissue	Adipose tissue, loose connective tissue, or glandular tissue
Firm	Harder than the adjacent softer oral mucosa or skin, indicating presence of increased fibrous connective tissue	Cartilage
Hard	Contains bone or other calcified material	Bone or enamel

normal tissue types of the body. The terminology used to indicate lesion consistency and normal tissue comparisons is described in Table 15-5.

Soft lesions more than 1 cm in diameter also should be tested for **fluctuance** by placing the fingers of one hand on one side of the lesion and gently pressing on the lesion with the fingers of the other hand. If the fingers can detect a wave or force passing through the lesion, the lesion is said to be *fluctuant*. The lesion also should be checked for **emptiability**, which is the temporary loss of fluctuance caused by brief evacuation of the lesion fluid into the surrounding tissue.

Mobility

It is important to note if a lesion has **mobility** (it is free) or **fixation** in relationship to the neighboring tissue. This is done by fixing the lesion with the fingers of one hand while moving the superficial tissue over the lesion with the other hand to see if it is fixed to its overlying tissue. Then an attempt is made to move the lesion independently from its underlying structures or tissue to demonstrate if the lesion is freely movable in all directions. Certain areas of the oral mucosa do not normally allow movement of the oral mucosa separate from the deeper structures such as the attached gingiva, median palatine raphe, or hard palate.

Generally the following aspects of mobility can help the supervising dentist make a differential diagnosis of the unknown lesion:

- If freely movable in all directions, lesion is most likely not a cancer or is encapsulated.
- If fixed to overlying skin or oral mucosa only, lesion originates from the overlying tissue.
- If fixed to underlying structures only, lesion originates from the underlying tissue.
- If fixed to both overlying and underlying tissue or structures, lesion involves either fibrosis or infiltration of a cancer.

Symptomatology

By directing questions to the client, the dental hygienist elicits symptoms related to the finding. A **symptom** is a subjective condition reported by the individual. In contrast, a **sign** is an objective condition that can be observed directly by others. Specifically, the dental hygienist must determine and then document in the client record the following information related to symptoms:

- If the lesion is known to the client, how long it has been present, and if there have been any changes in its size and appearance
- Whether the client has related neurologic symptoms: pain, tingling, burning, or paresthesia (numbness) with and without palpation; generally, painful lesions are due to inflammation
- Procedural test findings such as radiographs, early lesion evaluations for oral cancer or other oral diseases, pathologic report, including any performed by the client's physician

Skin Cancer

The most common types of skin cancer are basal and squamous cell cancers, and about 85% are located on the surface of the head and neck. That is because excessive exposure to sunlight is the single most important factor associated with the development of skin cancer. Fair-skinned people and those who spend more time in the sun are at an increased risk. These skin cancers start as small, pearly, or pale bumps on the skin, and other forms look like a red, scaly, flat patch. Although these types of skin cancer usually do not spread to other parts of the body, if not completely removed, they frequently invade and destroy the skin, muscle, and nerves in their path. Fortunately, these skin cancers usually are recognized in their early stages because of their slow growth, so they generally have a good prognosis.

A less common type of skin cancer and possibly fatal form of skin cancer is melanoma, especially if the initial lesion is detected at an advanced stage.[6] Melanomas frequently develop from or near an existing nevus (mole) but can be found anywhere on the skin including the scalp, oral cavity, and eye. Incidence rates in the United States have risen at a rate of more than 3% in the last decade. Risk factors are the same as for the other more common skin cancers as well as having close relatives with a history of melanoma. In the area, color changes from one area to another, with shades of tan, brown, or black, and sometimes white, red, or blue, presenting a color mixture is one of the more important symptoms, as well as rapid growth and bleeding at the site.

Oral and Oropharyngeal Cancer

More than 75% of head and neck cancers originate in the oral cavity. One of the most serious conditions that can occur in the oral cavity is oral cancer. Oral cancer is a devastating disease when detected in its later stages. Late-stage treatment usually involves major orofacial surgery, radiation, and chemotherapy. More than 54,000 Americans will be diagnosed with oral or pharyngeal cancer this year.[7]

These cancers will cause more than 15,500 deaths per year, mainly because they routinely are discovered late in its development. Even with the death rates for these cancers decreasing since the late 1970s, the rate for oral cancer is still higher than that for cervical or ovarian cancer; Hodgkin lymphoma; leukemia, cancer of the brain, liver, testes, or kidney; or serious skin cancer. Worldwide the problem is now much greater from high global risky behavior, with more than 640,000 new cases being found each year.

These cancers are more than twice as common in men as in women; they are about equally common in blacks and in whites. The average age of most people diagnosed is 62. However, there has been a recent rise in cases of orophayrngeal cancer related to an infection with the human papillomavirus (HPV), especially type 16, in mainly nonsmoking and nondrinking white male dental clients under the age of 55, thus comprising the fastest growing oral cancer segment, around one third of the total cancer cases as diagnosed via DNA tests.

The rising rate of HPV-linked cancers is thought to be due to changes in sexual practices in recent decades, particularly to an increase in oral sex as well as multiple partners. Most people with HPV infections of the oral cavity and phayrnx have no symptoms, but thankfully, only a very small percentage develop oropharyngeal cancer. In fact, oropharyngeal cancers that contain HPV DNA tend to have a better outlook than those without HPV. In recent years, vaccines that reduce the risk of infection with certain types of HPV have become available. These vaccines were meant originally to lower the risk of cervical cancer, but they may appear also to reduce the risk of other cancers linked to HPV. Thus the dental hygienist should encourage vaccination in clients within the high-risk groups for HPV infection according to the latest recommendations by the Centers for Disease Control.[8]

Oral squamous cell carcinoma (OSCC) makes up 94% of all cancers of the oral cavity. The remainder includes salivary gland tumors, lymphoma, and sarcoma. There is a higher risk of cancerous transformation in red and ulcerated areas than in white patches, although the latter often prove to be cancerous. The earliest form of OSCC is termed *carcinoma in situ,* meaning that the cancer cells are present only in the outer layers; this is different from *invasive squamous cell carcinoma,* where the cancer cells have grown into deeper layers of the oral cavity or oropharynx.

In America, OSCC is associated strongly with certain risk factors, such as tobacco use, alcohol abuse, HPV infection, and, for extraoral lesions such as on the lower lip, excessive sun exposure. Tobacco and alcohol related lesions tend to favor the anterior part of the oral cavity (body of the tongue and floor of the mouth) with symptoms possible and HPV-associated lesions tend to favor the posterior part of oral cavity (base of tongue, oropharynx, tonsils) usually without the usual symptoms in the oral mucosa. Thus neck palpation for hard, painless, fixed lymph nodes is an important diagnostic feature for HPV-related cancers. However, 25% of OSCCs occur in people who do not smoke and have no other risk factors.

Although cancer may arise at any site in the oral cavity, the most common sites in the United States for OSCC in order are as follows:

- Lateral border of the tongue (30%)
- Floor of the mouth (14%)
- Oropharyngeal (posterior soft palate, uvula, and faucial arches) (11%)
- Lower lip (38%)

However, the global experience with oral cancers is different: in India, buccal mucosa carcinomas are more common, and in Southeast Asia, nasopharyngeal cancer occurs more frequently.

Cancer does not show healing and resolution within a 2-week window of time, as most traumatic or infective lesions do, and does not respond to treatment. Instead, the cancer shows changes in color, shape, and size over time. See Table 15-6 for the terminology used to describe common signs of OSCC (e.g., **chronicity, erythroplakia, erythroleukoplakia, fissuring, fixation, induration, leukoplakia, lymphadenopathy, ulceration, or erosion**). (For information on dental hygiene care for persons with cancer, see Chapter 45.)

TABLE 15-6

Terminology for Common Signs of Cancer

Term	Definition
Chronicity	Continued presence because of failure to heal
Erythroplakia	Used to identify red patch that is smooth, granular, and velvety and cannot be diagnosed as any other lesion without biopsy
Erythroleukoplakia (mixed)	Having a combination of both red and white color changes; see erythroplakia and leukoplakia
Fissuring	Surface texture may exhibit ridges and irregularities reflecting abnormal cell growth
Fixation	Immobility occurring resulting from abnormally dividing cells invading to deeper areas into muscle and bone
Induration	Hardness primarily resulting from increase in number of surrounding epithelial cells from inflammatory infiltrate
Leukoplakia	Used to identify white, plaquelike lesion that cannot be wiped off and cannot be diagnosed as any other lesion without biopsy
Lymphadenopathy	Involvement of regional lymph nodes (and tonsils) resulting in firm, enlarged, fixed, and painless nodes in cancer cases
Ulceration or erosion	Loss of skin surface layer(s) resulting from destruction of epithelial integrity from cell maturation discrepancy, loss of intercellular attachments, disruption of basement membrane

If a premalignant lesion evolves into a carcinoma, the lesion is entered into various stages based on the TNM system (T = tumor size, N = lymph node spread, M = metastasis), which then allows the best evidence-based treatment for the client:

- Stage I: Lesion is not more than 2 cm but without spread to lymph nodes or metastasis.
- Stage II: Lesion is between 2 and 4 cm but without spread to lymph nodes or metastasis.
- Stage III: Lesion is larger than 4 cm but without spread or metastasis or the lesion is any size and has spread to a single, ipsilateral cervical lymph node that is 3 cm or less but without metastasis.
- Stage IV: One of the following applies:

  A. Lesion of any size has not or has spread locally within the oral cavity or to the lips and has not or has also spread to
  - Single, ipsilateral cervical lymph node that is 3 cm or less
  - Single, ispsilateral cervical lymph node that is between 3 and 6 cm *or* a single, contralateral cervical

lymph node that is not larger than 6 cm *or* spread to one or more cervical lymph nodes, which are no more than 6 cm

B. Lesion has spread locally within the oral cavity or to the lips and has or has not spread to one or more lymph nodes that are larger than 6 cm.

C. Lesion of any size and has or has not spread to lymph nodes but has metastasized from the oral cavity or oropharyngeal region to other body regions, most commonly the lungs (secondly the liver or skeletal system).
  - Recurrent (relapsed)—Cancer returned after treatment, to the same or other body region (see discussion below).

When clients newly diagnosed with oral and oropharyngeal cancers are examined carefully, a smaller group will have another cancer in a nearby area such as the larynx, the esophagus, or the lung. Thus some who successfully treated for oral or oropharyngeal cancer will develop another cancer later in the oral cavity, pharynx, or other nearby regions. This means that clients who survive a first encounter with the disease have up to a 20 times higher risk of developing a second cancer, and this heightened risk factor can last for 5 to 10 years after the first occurrence. For this reason, clients with oral and oropharyngeal cancer always must have annual follow-up examinations. They also need to avoid using tobacco and alcohol, which increase the risk for these recurrent cancers. Again the dental hygienist is in a prime position to help the client with these changes as well as assist them to make a positive decision about their own further cancer treatment options. (For information on tobacco cessation, see Chapter 36.)

Client Self-Examination

The client–dental hygienist interaction is an opportunity to instruct clients in simple self-examination techniques, empowering them with the skills to note any changes in their own extraoral or intraoral conditions.[9] In addition, discussion with clients allows the client to review their risk for OSCC and change their lifestyle, if indicated. Increasingly, dental professionals as well as medical professionals recommend that clients look at their mouth and throat in a mirror every month to check for any abnormal areas, similar to monthly checking other parts of the body at risk for cancer.

Early Detection Discussion

The mortality rate for OSCC is mainly a result of late detection of the disease. More than 52% of these cancers are in advanced stages when diagnosed and show evidence of invasion and metastasis. This late diagnosis of the disease is tragic because the 5-year survival rate is more than 90% when OSCC is detected early (when the lesion is smaller than 2 cm).[10]

Public awareness of OSCC as compared with other cancers continues to be low, and this also contributes to delays in diagnosis and then in obtaining treatment. In addition, many early OSCCs appear clinically normal, and it is not possible to determine with certainty which lesions are cancerous without performing a biopsy. Because biopsy often seems extreme for what appears to be a harmless lesion, many early OSCCs remain undiagnosed and progress to a more advanced stage. Medical professionals now are advised to include the oral cavity and pharynx as part of a routine cancer-related checkup. However, because many clients are seen more regularly for preventive periodontal care than for medical visits, dental hygienists have a unique opportunity during client assessment to detect OSCC while it is still asymptomatic, harmless, and unsuspected. Several techniques have been suggested for early evaluation of lesions to determine whether they show cellular changes that may be cancerous and hence need a biopsy. These early evaluation methods for oral cancer include oral cytology, transepithelial cytology, tissue reflectance and autofluorescence, and toluidine blue dye.[11]

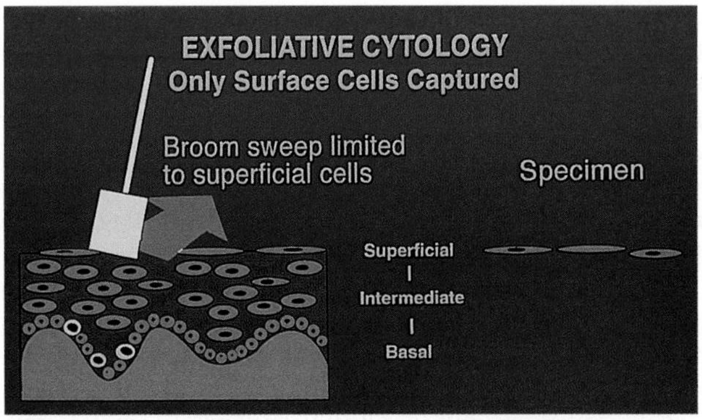

Figure 15-35. Oral cytology. (Courtesy CDx Diagnostics, Suffern, NY.)

Many private practices have instituted one or more of these early detection methods for OSCC as a standard of care as part of the examination procedure resulting from problems with diagnosis. As discussed earlier, it is done yearly for those older than 17 years of age and then twice a year for those with high-risk history. However, these methods are intended as adjuncts to and not a substitute for biopsy. Furthermore, studies now show combining the use of computed tomography and ultrasonography for diagnosis of OSCC is recommended with other methods when indicated because it is a cost-effective, minimally invasive imaging technology to identify premalignancy and malignancy with high sensitivity and specificity. Future methods include saliva screening, blood screening assays, and DNA testing.

To understand and compare the relative value of these adjunctive methods, it is important to comprehend the structure of oral and pharyngeal epithelial tissue.[12] This epithelium consists of three layers: the basal cell layer, the intermediate layers, and the superficial layers. Normally, cell division occurs in the basal cell layer. Cells then move through the intermediate layers to the superficial layers, where they are shed naturally. An important feature of a method for early detection of oral cancer and precancerous lesions is that it evaluates cells from all layers of the epithelium to note any cellular changes.

Oral and Transepithelial Cytology

With oral cytology, the sample cells to be examined are collected by scraping the surface of a lesion with a cotton swab (Figure 15-35). Then they are spread on a slide, fixed and stained, and sent to a pathologist for evaluation. The main disadvantage of this method is that it is likely to evaluate only superficial cells, which may have little diagnostic value as noted earlier. Therefore oral cytology in practice has a minor role in the detection of precancerous and cancerous lesions.

Transepithelial cytology is an evaluation method that uses a specially designed brush to remove sample cells from lesions that may not otherwise be subjected to biopsy because of their more normal-looking appearance (CDx Diagnostics, Suffern, NY). The supplied brush captures cells from all three layers of epithelium (unlike oral cytology) to determine if a lesion is normal or if it should be submitted for further surgical biopsy (Figure 15-36), thus giving validation to the procedure.

However, dental hygienists are permitted to perform transepithelial cytology procedure only in certain states. The technique for transepithelial cytology is described in Procedure 15-3 and the corresponding Competency Form. The brush containing the sample cells then is transferred to a slide that is sent to laboratories for computer-assisted analysis and

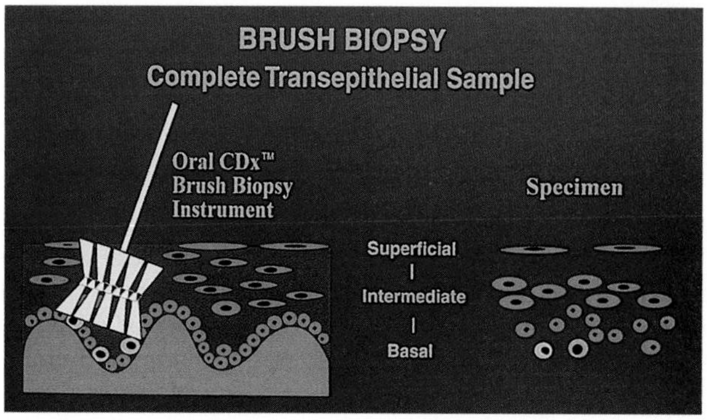

Figure 15-36. Transepithelial cytology. (Courtesy CDx Diagnostics, Suffern, NY.)

Procedure 15-3 Conducting Transepithelial Cytology

EQUIPMENT

Test kit with instructions, return mailing box, barcoded specimen slide and holder, sterile brush instrument, fixative packet (Figure 15-37)
Personal protective equipment

STEPS

1. Put on personal protective equipment before handling brush instrument and slide.
2. Remove brush from kit (Figure 15-38). Slightly moisten the brush with the client's saliva if the lesion is dry. Neither local nor topical anesthetic is required and should not be used because it may distort the sample.
3. Press the brush firmly against the lesion and rotate 5 to 10 times (depending on the thickness of the lesion) until tissue becomes pink or pinpoint microbleeding is observed (Figure 15-39).
4. Transfer the cellular sample from the brush onto the slide by rotating and dragging the brush lengthwise (Figure 15-40).
5. Immediately fix the cells by squeezing the entire contents of one fixative package onto the slide, flooding the slide. Set the slide aside to dry for 15 minutes, and then place in slide holder. Remove personal protective equipment.
6. Complete the test requisition form, and send the specimen to the laboratory in the box provided.
7. Document procedure in the client record, and note on calendar when the pathology report is due back.
8. Read the pathology report from the laboratory, and make sure that findings are shared with the client.
9. Guide the client to receive the appropriate follow-up care as recommended by the supervising dentist.

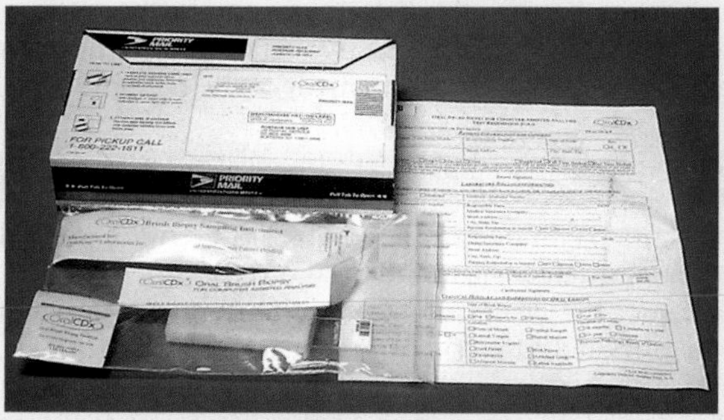

Figure 15-37. Transepithelial cytology test kit. (Courtesy CDx Diagnostics, Suffern, NY.)

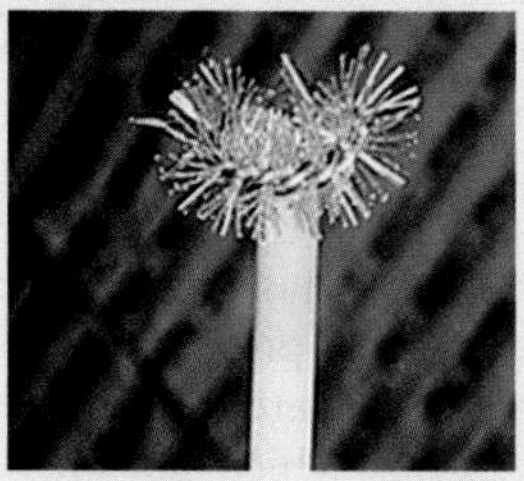

Figure 15-38. Transepithelial brush. (Courtesy CDx Diagnostics, Suffern, NY.)

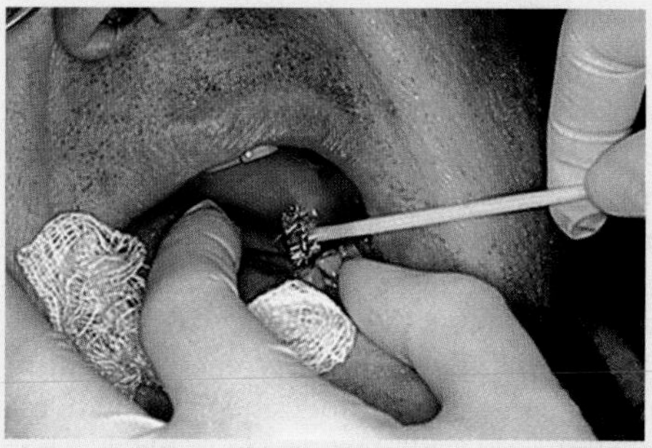

Figure 15-39. Pressing the brush firmly against the lesion. (Courtesy CDx Diagnostics, Suffern, NY.)

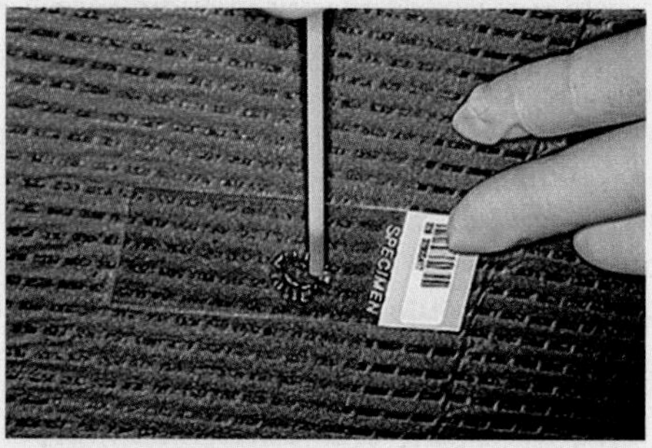

Figure 15-40. Transferring the cellular sample on slide. (Courtesy CDx Diagnostics, Suffern, NY.)

confirmation by a pathologist. Specimens are classified into the following categories:

1. Incomplete specimen: too few cells from all cell layers
2. Negative: no evidence of abnormal cells
3. Atypical: abnormal epithelial cells of uncertain significance
4. Positive: definitive evidence of dysplastic or cancer cells

In the case of atypical or positive results, the company recommends surgical biopsy of the lesion. This is because the test result is limited to reporting the presence or absence of cellular abnormalities and does not provide a definitive diagnosis.

Tissue Reflectance and Autofluorescence for Identification of Abnormal Oral Tissue

A simple test using **tissue reflectance** is now available that improves identification, evaluation, and monitoring of oral mucosal abnormalities in those at increased risk for oral cancer. The test includes either a disposable handheld light (ViziLite, Zila Pharmaceuticals, Phoenix, AZ) or a reusable, battery-powered light-emitting diode (LED) light source that provides a similar blue-white illumination (MicroLux/DL, AdDent, Danbury, CT; Orascoptic DK, Orascoptic, Middleton, WI) as well as a flavored acetic mouth rinse wash before use of its respective light source.

These tests permit detection of abnormalities in the oral cavity that may not be visible to the unaided eye. It is a quick, painless, noninvasive procedure, with the rinse improving visualization of deeper abnormal tissue by removing superficial substances. Normal epithelium absorbs the device's illumination and appears dark, whereas abnormal epithelium reflects it and appears bright white. As a cell becomes more abnormal, the nucleus becomes larger compared with the rest of the cell. The enlarged nucleus reflects light and appears bright white, focusing the attention on lesions that may not be seen otherwise and that may, on biopsy, reveal cancer and precancerous cells.

Also available is a handheld device that provides the direct visualization of **tissue autofluorescence** and the changes in fluorescence that can occur when abnormalities are present (VELscope, LED Dental, Inc, White Rock, BC, Canada). The unit emits a cone of blue light into the oral cavity, creating different fluorescence responses depending on the health of the tissue being screened. Healthy mucosal tissue appears pale green under the light, whereas lesions considered abnormal look dark green to black. The manufacturer cautions, however, that loss of autofluorescence is not limited strictly to epithelial abnormalities and can be seen with prominent surface vascularity, including areas of inflammation, and melanin pigmentation.

A newer product also is available that combines the technologies of tissue reflectance and autofluorescence with a conventional white light source (Identafi 3000, Trimira, Houston, TX). It is claimed to help identify oral mucosal abnormalities that otherwise may not be apparent as well as helping to discern the superficial vascularity of the tissue.

Toluidine Blue Dye

Toluidine blue dye stains cells differentially depending on their nuclear configuration. The dye has selective dye uptake by abnormal cells, which is the premise for its use to confirm clinical impressions of abnormal cellular changes. A drawback to using the dye on the surface of a lesion to detect cellular changes is that inflammatory cells, often present with a lesion, also take up the dye stain and make interpretation of the test difficult. Toluidine blue dye often is used, however, during biopsy to define margins of the lesions and to discover secondary lesions. Also available is a kit that combines tissue reflectance and toluidine blue dye; the light improves lesion visualization and allows identification of abnormal lesions, then the dye allows the documentation of the extent of the lesion for subsequent biopsy (ViziLite Plus, Zila Pharmaceuticals, Phoenix, AZ).

Biopsy

The **definitive diagnosis** is achieved after receiving test results, such as biopsies, that are done to find out if a certain disease or condition is present. **Biopsy** is the surgical removal of a section of tissue or other material from the living body for the purpose of diagnosis, to estimate prognosis, and to monitor the cause of disease when the tissue later undergoes microscopic assessment. **Punch biopsy** is the traditional method of diagnosing a cancer using a tubular surgical instrument that is inserted through to the deeper tissue, to cut the tissue off at the base.

In contrast to the traditional less invasive method of a punch biopsy, **excisional biopsy** indicates that the entire lesion with borders is removed for assessment, whereas **incisional biopsy** indicates that only representative tissue samples are obtained by excising a wedge of tissue. The decision to perform a biopsy after an oral lesion is identified is made by the supervising dentist, or referral is made to an oral surgeon.

After the specimen is obtained and properly packaged for transport, it is sent to a laboratory. A report of the findings then is issued by the pathologist, who assessed the histologic appearance of the suspected lesion in conjunction with the stated differential diagnosis. This report is then sent to the supervising dentist, who determines any further action, such as discussion with the client, which would be noted in the client record along with placement of the report.

CLIENT EDUCATION TIPS

- Discuss the importance of oral assessment for early detection and diagnosis of orofacial diseases.
- Instruct the client in simple self-examination techniques for early detection of orofacial cancer.
- Discuss the elimination of high-risk behaviors and options to change lifestyles that predispose to orofacial cancer, especially in those with a past history of these cancers.

LEGAL, ETHICAL, AND SAFETY ISSUES

- Dental hygienists must perform extraoral and intraoral assessment following the standard precautions of infection control.
- On identification of a lesion, the client must be informed of its existence using appropriate verbal skills, and pertinent information must be provided in writing if the client is referred to a specialist for further treatment.
- Biopsy using surgical instruments with microscopic assessment is the only method for a definitive diagnosis of cancer.

- It is the dental hygienist's legal responsibility to practice within the scope of practice authorized by individual state law concerning performance of any early evaluation methods for oral cancer or other means of an identification of a lesion.
- Dental hygienists have the responsibility to make a dental hygiene diagnosis and then refer all clients with head, neck, or orofacial lesions to the supervising dentist for dental diagnosis.
- All services rendered, including radiographic imaging, as well as interpretation of those services, must be documented in ink and the entry dated in the client's record so as to ensure client record integrity for the client's health and the practitioner's legal protection.
- The collaborative relationship between dental hygienist and the supervising dentist ensures that the comprehensive treatment needs of the client are identified, addressed, and evaluated.

KEY CONCEPTS

- Overall, the orofacial tissue is sensitive and provides general health indicators; these changes may be the first indication of systemic disease.
- Careful overall client observation and a thorough assessment of the head and neck as well as oral cavity are essential to planning and providing optimum client care.
- The dental hygienist must establish an assessment sequence and follow it systematically during client assessment, incorporating the skills of observation, palpation, auscultation, and olfaction.
- During the assessment, the dental hygienist inspects the client carefully for any palpable regional lymph nodes and documents if any are present because they may pinpoint where a disease process is active. Detection assists in the diagnosis and treatment of the disease.
- After the observation of atypical or abnormal findings, the dental hygienist describes and documents them accurately in the client record as a dental hygiene diagnosis.
- Because many clients are seen more regularly for preventive periodontal care than for medical visits, dental hygienists have a unique opportunity during client assessment to detect orofacial cancer while it is still asymptomatic, harmless, and unsuspected.
- The ability to describe an orofacial lesion is critical to the assessment process because precise descriptive terms enable the dental hygienist to communicate with the supervising dentist and other referring healthcare professionals to identify the lesion and facilitate its accurate dental diagnosis.
- It is the responsibility of the dental hygienist to discuss the options of possible lifestyle changes with the client when high-risk behaviors related to either orofacial disease are noted in the client's history or during assessment.
- Methods available for early evaluation of lesions for oral cancer include oral and transepithelial cytology, tissue reflectance and autofluorescence, toluidine blue dye; biopsy is still required if indicated.
- It is the dental hygienist's responsibility after recognizing orofacial tissue changes from normal to collaborate with the supervising dentist regarding these findings.

CRITICAL THINKING EXERCISES

1. *Structure identification exercise: head and neck regions.* When examining a peer, check off the items noted in an extraoral assessment of the head and neck. Note any atypical findings and report any abnormal findings to your supervising instructor.

	IDENTIFIED	ATYPICAL FINDINGS	ABNORMAL FINDINGS
Regions of the Head			
Parietal, Occipital, Temporal, Auricular Regions			
Scalp and hair			
Occipital lymph nodes' location			
Ears			
Auricular lymph nodes' location			
Frontal, Orbital, and Nasal Regions			
Forehead			
Eyes			
Frontal sinuses			
Nose			
Infraorbital, Zygomatic, and Buccal Regions			
Zygomatic arches			
Facial lymph nodes' location			
Maxillary sinuses and maxillary bone			
Facial expression and masseter muscles			
Temporomandibular joints and parotid salivary glands			
Mandible			
Oral and Mental Regions			
Chin			

	IDENTIFIED	ATYPICAL FINDINGS	ABNORMAL FINDINGS
Regions of the Neck			
Anterior and Posterior Cervical Regions			
Sternocleidomastoid muscles			
External and anterior jugular lymph nodes' location			
Superior and inferior deep cervical lymph nodes' location			
Accessory and supraclavicular lymph nodes' location			
Submandibular and Submental Triangle Regions			
Submandibular salivary glands			
Submandibular lymph nodes' location			
Sublingual salivary glands			
Submental lymph nodes' location			
Anterior Midline Cervical Region			
Hyoid bone			
Thyroid cartilage and gland			

2. *Structure identification exercise: oral cavity and associated regions.* When examining a peer, check off the items noted in an intraoral assessment of an oral cavity and associated regions. Note any atypical findings and report any abnormal findings to your supervising instructor.

	IDENTIFIED	ATYPICAL FINDINGS	ABNORMAL FINDINGS
Oral Cavity			
Lips, labial mucosa, and vestibules			
Buccal mucosa and buccal fat pads			
Parotid papillae, parotid salivary glands, and parotid ducts			
Alveolar mucosa and labial frena			
Mucogingival junction			
Maxillary alveolar bone, teeth, gingiva, and tuberosity			
Mandibular alveolar bone, teeth, gingiva, and retromolar pad			
Palate and Pharynx			
Hard palate, median palatine raphe, and incisive papilla			
Soft palate and uvula			
Faucial pillars and palatine tonsils			
Tongue			
Dorsal and lateral surface, lingual papillae, sulcus terminalis, and foramen cecum			
Lingual tonsil			
Ventral surface, lingual veins, and plicae fimbriatae			
Floor of the Mouth			
Lingual frenum			
Sublingual folds and caruncles			
Sublingual salivary glands and ducts			
Submandibular salivary glands and ducts			

Refer to the *Procedures Manual,* where rationales are provided for the steps outlined in the procedures presented in this chapter.

REFERENCES

1. Fehrenbach MJ: Inflammation. Immunity. In Ibsen OC, Phelan JA, editors: *Oral pathology for the dental hygienist*, ed 6, St Louis, 2014, Saunders.
2. *Mosby's dental dictionary*, ed 3, St Louis, 2014, Mosby.
3. Clark N, Sandow P: Comprehensive oral cancer examination of the extra-oral and intra-oral regions of the head and neck, MedEdPORTAL, 2012.
4. Fehrenbach MJ: Dental infections. *J Pract Hyg* 6:2, 1997.
5. Fehrenbach MJ, Herring SW: *Illustrated anatomy of the head and neck*, ed 4, St Louis, 2012, Saunders.
6. National Center for Biotechnology Information: Melanoma. U.S. National Library of Medicine 2012. Available at: http://www.ncbi.nlm.nih.gov/pubmedhealth/PMH0001853/. Accessed January 2013.
7. American Cancer Society: Oral cavity and oropharyngeal cancer, key statistics. Available at http://www.cancer.org/acs/groups/cid/documents/webcontent/003128-pdf.pdf. Accessed January 2013.

8. Centers for Disease Control: Human papillomavirus (HPV). Available at http://www.cdc.gov/hpv/vaccine.html. Accessed January 2013.
9. Elango MJ, Anandkrishnan N, Suresh A, et al: Mouth self-examination to improve oral cancer awareness and early detection in a high-risk population. *Oral Oncol* 47:620, 2011.
10. Rhodus NL: Oral cancer and precancer: improving outcomes. *Compend Contin Educ Dent* 30(8):486, 490, 496, 2009.
11. Rethman MP, Carpenter W, Cohen EE, et al: Evidence-based clinical recommendations regarding screening for oral squamous cell carcinomas. *JADA* 141:5, 509, 2009.
12. Fehrenbach MJ, Popowics T: *Illustrated dental embryology, histology, and anatomy*, ed 4, St Louis, 2014, Saunders.

EVOLVE RESOURCES

Please visit http://evolve.elsevier.com/Darby/hygiene for additional practice and study support tools.

CHAPTER 16

Dentition Assessment

Janice F.L. Pimlott, Joan D. Leakey

COMPETENCIES

1. **Discuss the purpose and methods of documentation including charting and the responsibilities of the dental hygienist.**
2. **Differentiate between the tooth numbering systems.**
3. **Discuss the classification of dental caries and restorations.**
4. **Discuss tooth assessment and detection of signs of dental caries.**
5. **Explain the dentition and periodontal charting, including application of charting symbols to a case study.**
6. **Discuss occlusion and common problems of occlusion.**
7. **Distinguish between the classification of malocclusion and the sub-types.**
8. **Discuss the primary occlusion.**

Tooth assessment is used to determine whether the client's need for a biologically sound and functional dentition is met; assessment also is related to the client's human needs for freedom from pain and for a wholesome facial image. Tooth assessment and its documentation initially occur during the assessment phase of the dental hygiene process and are updated during the implementation and evaluation phases of dental hygiene care. The dental hygienist's tooth assessment goals are to recognize and document signs of dental caries, acquired tooth damage, and developmental anomalies and to call them to the dentist's attention, thus optimizing client care. Documentation of findings must be accurate and complete because it accomplishes the following:

- Visually describes the client's current dental status for use in planning client care
- Enhances communication with the client, other members of the oral healthcare team, and third-party payers, such as insurance companies and health maintenance organizations
- Provides a legal document of the actual care provided that is admissible evidence in a court of law
- Identifies a deceased person during a forensic investigation
- Assists in verifying oral healthcare services provided during financial audits
- Contains a detailed history of the client's clinical examination findings, dental diagnosis, and treatment for quality assurance audits
- Provides a vital record of dental needs that have been or are going to be met

Documentation

Dental charting is the graphic representation of the condition of the client's teeth observed on a specific date. The data recorded are based on clinical and radiographic assessments and the client's reported symptoms. The exact location and condition of all teeth and restorations, including normal and abnormal findings, are documented on an odontogram as part of the client's permanent record.

An ideal dental charting system, electronic or paper based, must be easy to interpret and contain sufficient space for initial recording of data as well as for adding successive findings. To facilitate continuity, sequencing, and ongoing documentation of care, the odontogram should be available for reference during all appointments.

Electronic Health Record

The electronic health record (EHR) is evolving and rapidly becoming the standard for record keeping in healthcare. The EHR is the systematic collection of electronic health information about individual clients; this information, when required, can be shared between health providers. In clinical practice it is used largely as an effective way to manage client records and office systems. It may be possible in the future to develop synchronization of dental electronic systems; if so, this could allow for the secure transfer of client records between treating dental and medical practitioners. Electronic-based charting is one component of the EHR.

Electronic-Based Charting

Paper-based charting was used for more than 100 years. However, over the last decade it is being replaced with electronic-based dental charting systems. As the changeover to electronic formats takes place, some dental offices still employ paper systems. Resources for paper-based charting procedures can be found on the Evolve site.Visit the website at http://evolve.elsevier.com/Darby/hygiene.

To support paperless dental records there are a wide variety of electronic-based charting software. Like many paper-based charts electronic-based charts are generally a two-dimensional anatomic representation. However, with the rapid rate of advancements in electronic technology three-dimensional (3D) chart models have been developed and this technology may be an area of future research and development. The charting information is entered into the computer via a keyboard, mouse, or voice-activated program. The voice-activated approach promotes infection control principles and eliminates the need for an assistant to aid in data entry. Although the data are stored in the computer, a completed charting form can be printed when a hard/paper copy is needed.

The advantages of electronic charting are clear in that not only a paperless office can save space but also electronic charts are readily retrievable chair side. They also allow for the incorporation of digital clinical and radiographic images into the patient record. However, implementing an electronic-based system is not without its challenges. Systems are expensive to implement, and there may be a steep learning curve as practitioners become familiar with the electronic procedures. Also, during this learning time the chance for documentation errors to occur is increased. Input methods or the ease of usability varies and may present challenges such as infection control issues as the dental hygienist moves from client to inputting data, or time issues of inputting data quickly.

Quadrant and Sextant Classification

To facilitate communication about specific dentition areas and individual teeth, the dentition is divided into quadrants and sextants, and each tooth is divided into specific surfaces.

Quadrants

If one were to draw an imaginary line dividing the client's face into two equal halves longitudinally, the maxillary and mandibular arches of the mouth would be divided into two mirror images or halves. This imaginary longitudinal line that bisects the client's face is referred to as the *midline.* If one were to draw horizontally a second imaginary line that divides the upper jaw (the maxillary arch) from the lower jaw (the mandibular arch), the combination of the imaginary horizontal and vertical midlines would divide the client's mouth into four equal sections termed **quadrants** (Q) (Figure 16-1). Each quadrant contains either five or eight teeth, depending on whether the client has a primary or permanent dentition. Permanent dentition quadrants are numbered 1 through 4, and those of the primary dentition 5 through 8. The maxillary right is referred to as *quadrant 1* in the permanent dentition or *quadrant 5* in the primary dentition. Continuing in a clockwise pattern the maxillary left is designated as *quadrant 2* (permanent) or *quadrant 6* (primary). The mandibular left is referred to as *quadrant 3* (permanent) or *quadrant 7* (primary), and the mandibular right is designated as *quadrant 4* (permanent) or *quadrant 8* (primary). In the event that the client has a mixed dentition (primary and permanent teeth), each tooth is identified individually, based on whether it is a primary or a permanent tooth, and is prefaced with quadrant 1 through 4 if it is a permanent tooth or 5 through 8 if it is a primary tooth.

Sextants

Another means to designate sections of the primary and permanent dentition is by drawing additional imaginary lines to create divisions between the front (anterior) and the back (posterior) teeth. Dividing the dentition in this manner creates six areas called **sextants** (S). Each anterior sextant contains incisors and canines, and each posterior sextant contains premolars and molars. Like quadrants, sextants are numbered clockwise beginning at the client's maxillary right (Figure 16-2).

Tooth Surfaces and Zones

The differentiation of tooth surfaces and zones provides a means of pinpointing specific areas of the tooth for accurate assessment, charting, treatment, and evaluation. (See also Chapter 39.) The midline is an imaginary line drawn longitudinally between the central incisors of the maxilla and mandible dividing the arches into two equal halves. Each tooth surface located closest to the midline is called the **mesial** surface and each tooth surface located farthest from the midline is called the **distal** surface. Overall, there are six tooth surfaces (Figure 16-3):

- **Mesial** (M)
- **Distal** (D)
- **Facial** (F) (includes buccal and labial)
- **Lingual** (L) (includes palatal)
- **Occlusal** (O)
- **Incisal** (I)

Tooth Divisions into Thirds

For purposes of describing and communicating the location of landmarks, teeth can be divided into imaginary thirds (Figure 16-4). The root is divided into thirds: the **apical third** (the area involving the root tip or apex), the middle third, and the **cervical third** (the area closest to the "neck" of the tooth crown) (Figure 16-4, *A*). The tooth crown also can be divided into thirds from the facial view, the mesial to distal view, or from the facial to lingual view:

- Occlusocervical division: Dividing the tooth crown horizontally or parallel to the occlusal surface creates the occlusal (for posterior teeth, or incisal for anterior teeth), middle, and gingival thirds (see Figure 16-4, *A*).
- Mesiodistal division: Dividing the crown vertically (or lengthwise) from mesial to distal, creates the mesial, middle, and distal thirds (see Figure 16-4, *B*).
- Faciolingual (or buccolingual) division: Dividing the crown vertically (or lengthwise from front to back) creates the facial (in lieu of labial for anterior teeth or buccal for posterior teeth), middle, and lingual thirds (see Figure 16-4, *C* and *D*).

Types of Teeth

Humans have two sets of natural teeth, commonly referred to as the primary and the permanent dentitions. The primary dentition is made up of 20 teeth, five in each quadrant: two incisors, one canine, and two molars. (See also Chapter 39.)

The permanent, or secondary, dentition has 32 teeth, 8 in each quadrant: 2 incisors, 1 canine, 2 premolars, and 3 molars. The functions of the individual tooth types are similar in the primary and the permanent dentition. The classification of primary and permanent teeth along with age of eruption are provided in Figures 16-5 and 16-6.

Tooth Numbering Systems

Tooth numbering systems were developed to simplify the task of identifying individual teeth without using their full

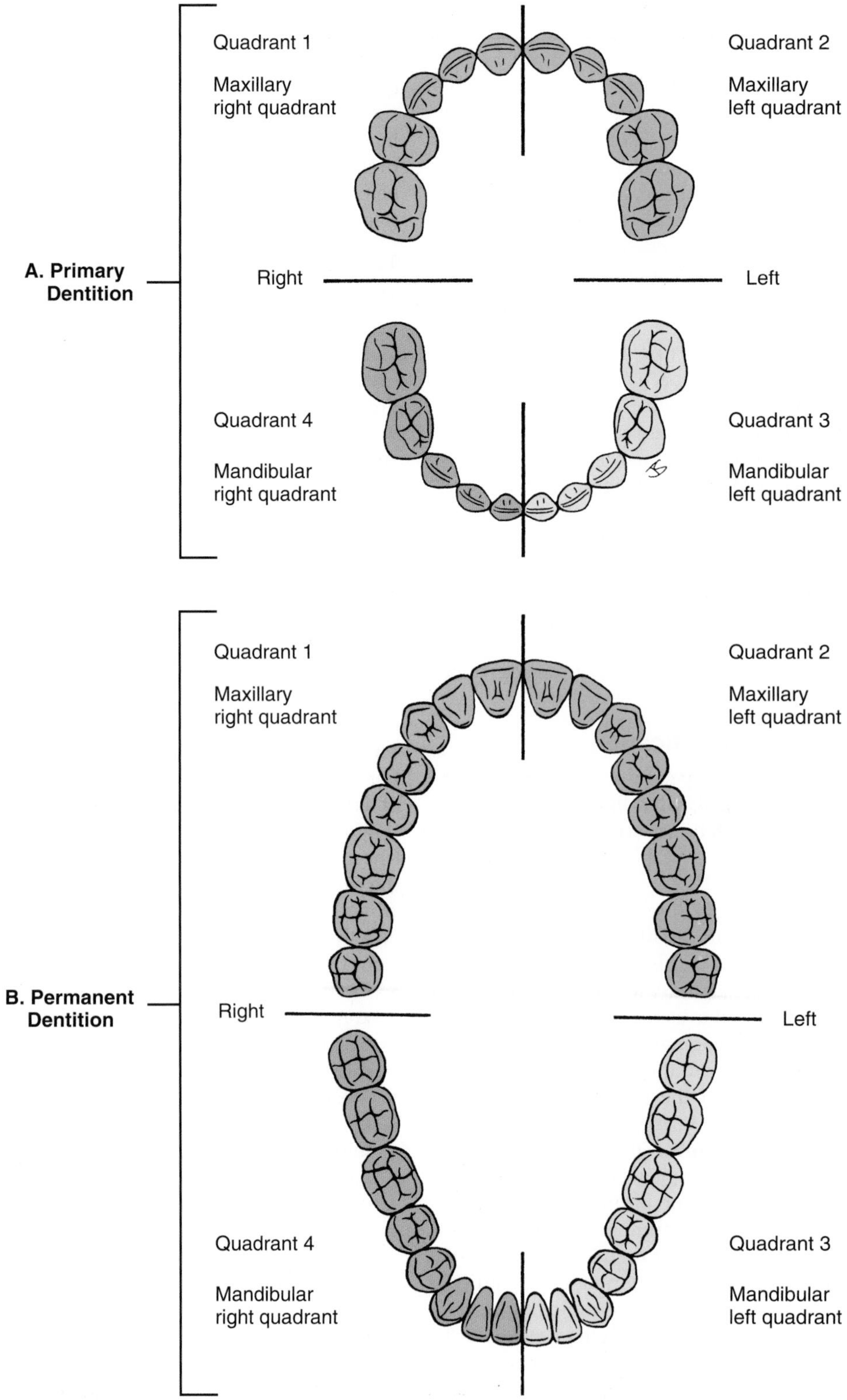

Figure 16-1. Numbering of quadrants in the **(A)** primary and **(B)** permanent dentitions. (From Finkbeiner B, Johnson C: *Comprehensive dental assisting*, St Louis, 1995, Mosby.)

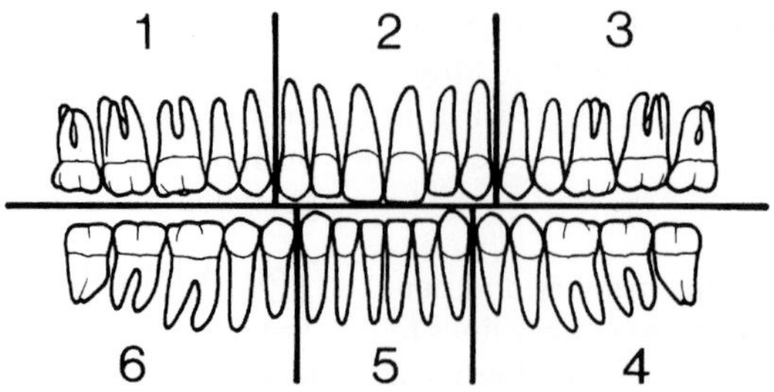

Figure 16-2. Sextant classification in the permanent dentitions.

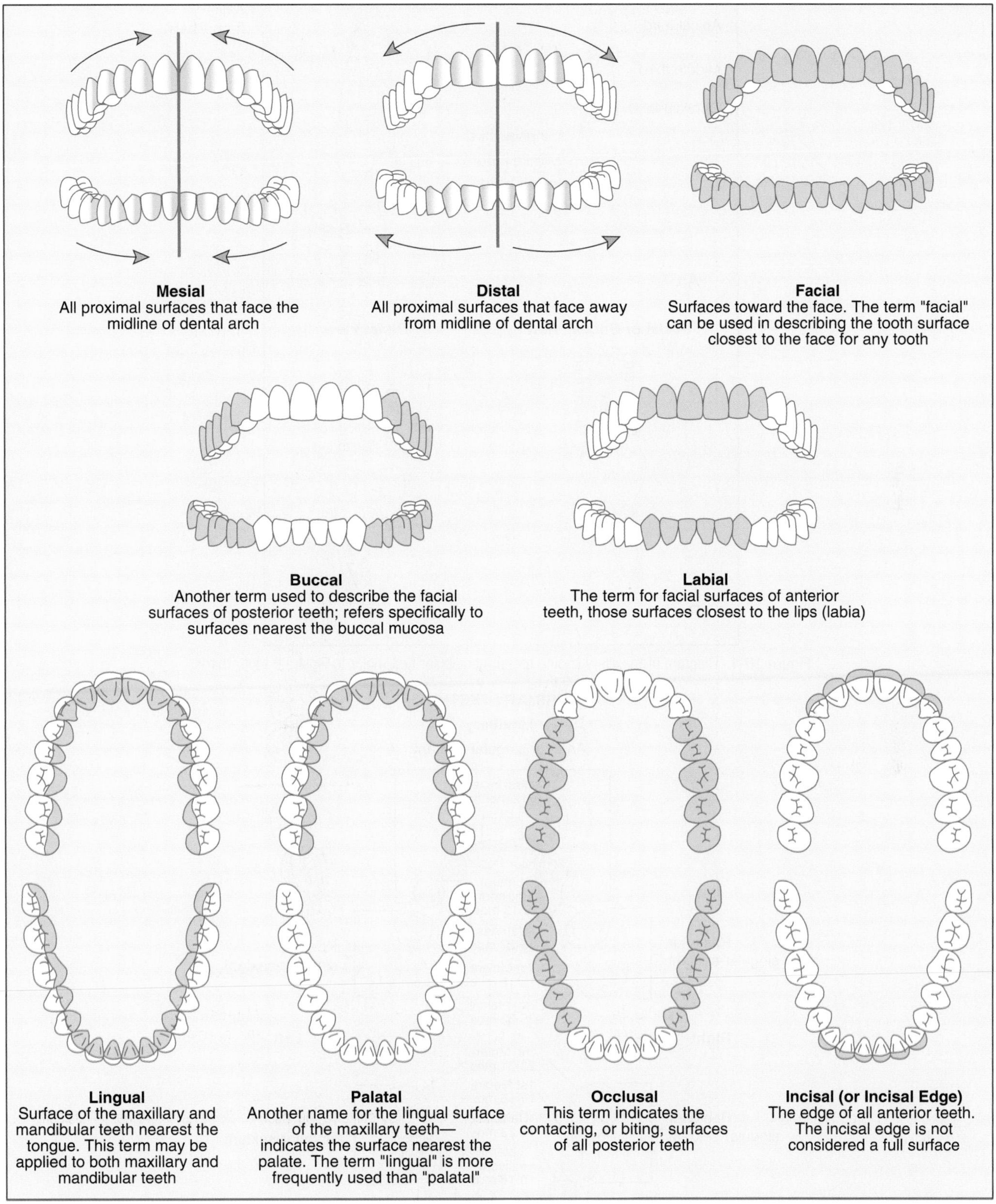
Mesial
All proximal surfaces that face the midline of dental arch
Distal
All proximal surfaces that face away from midline of dental arch
Facial
Surfaces toward the face. The term "facial" can be used in describing the tooth surface closest to the face for any tooth
Buccal
Another term used to describe the facial surfaces of posterior teeth; refers specifically to surfaces nearest the buccal mucosa
Labial
The term for facial surfaces of anterior teeth, those surfaces closest to the lips (labia)
Lingual
Surface of the maxillary and mandibular teeth nearest the tongue. This term may be applied to both maxillary and mandibular teeth
Palatal
Another name for the lingual surface of the maxillary teeth—indicates the surface nearest the palate. The term "lingual" is more frequently used than "palatal"
Occlusal
This term indicates the contacting, or biting, surfaces of all posterior teeth
Incisal (or Incisal Edge)
The edge of all anterior teeth. The incisal edge is not considered a full surface

Figure 16-3. Classification of tooth surfaces. (Adapted from Wootton D: *The art of dental scaling,* Burlington, 1991, University of Vermont.)

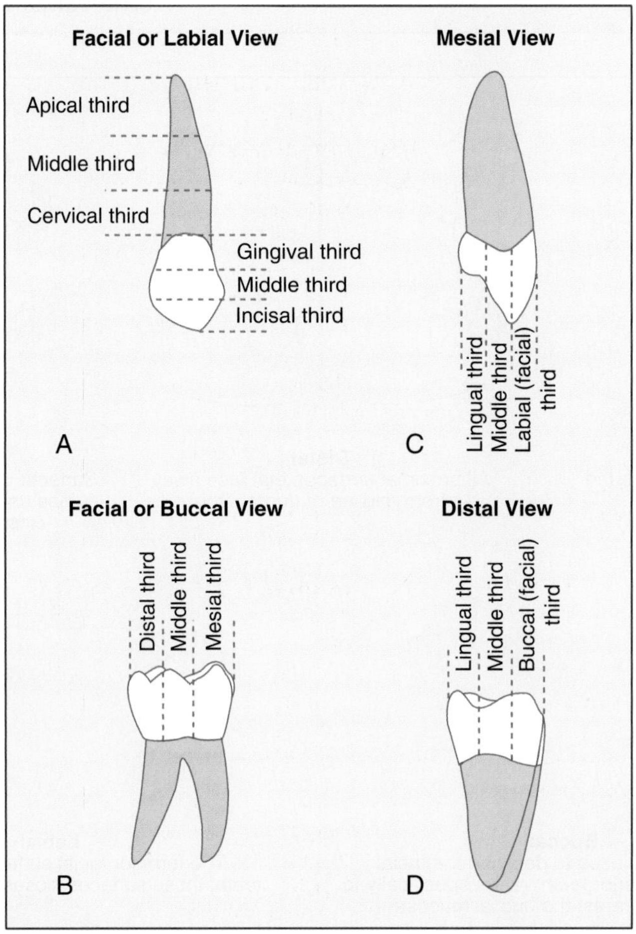

Figure 16-4. Diagram of maxillary canine and a mandibular first molar to illustrate tooth thirds.

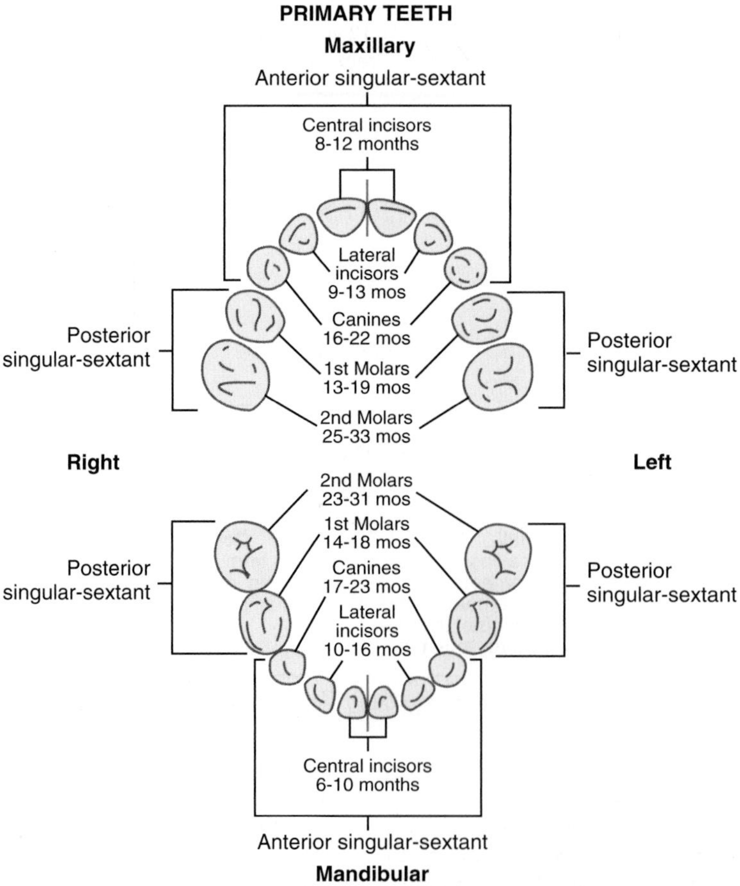

Figure 16-5. Classification of primary teeth and ages of eruption.

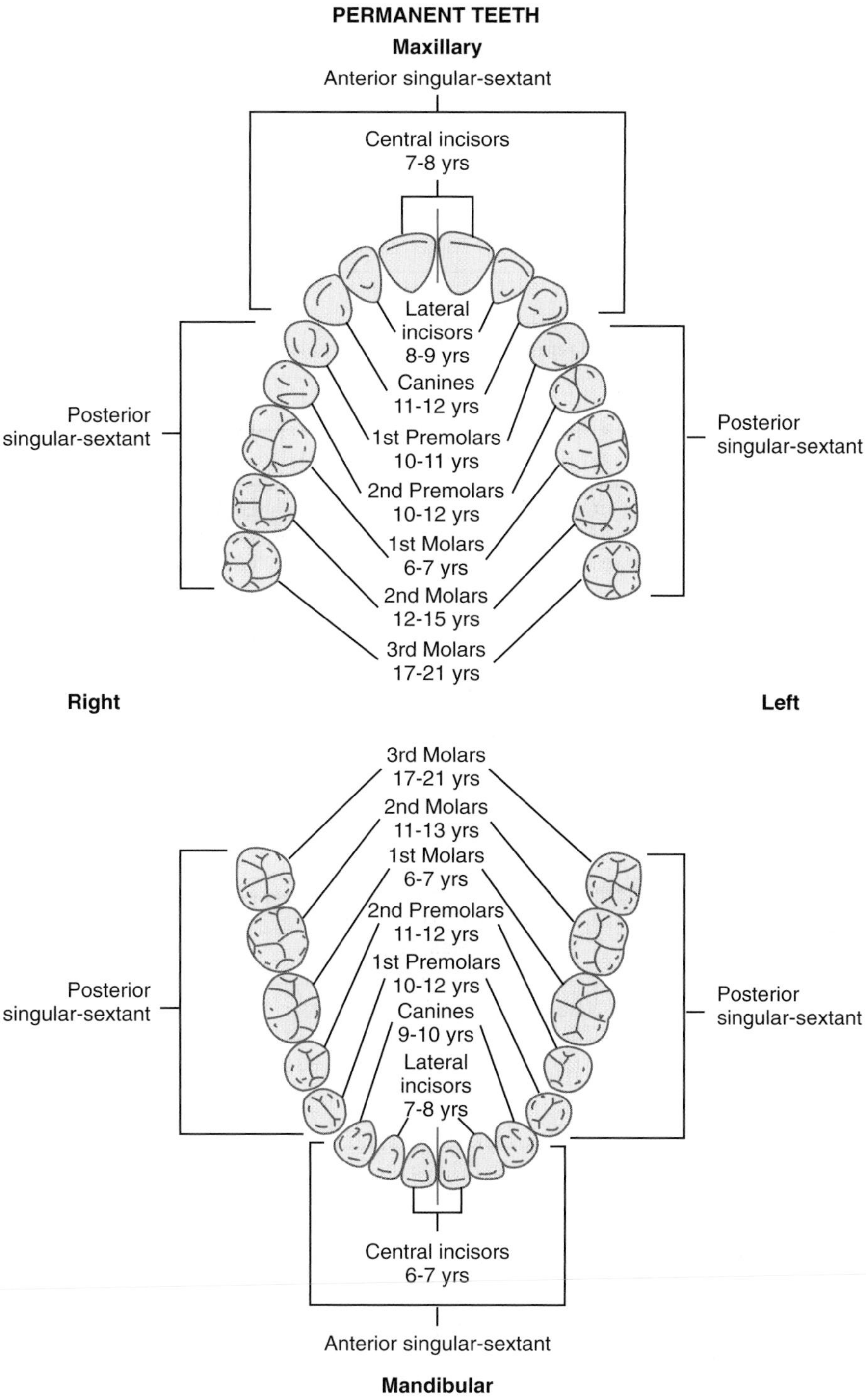

Figure 16-6. Classification of permanent teeth and ages of eruption.

name designations. Such systems are essential for charting and recording procedures. The two most commonly used are the Universal Numbering System and the International Numbering System.

Universal Numbering System

The Universal Numbering System provides a standard sequential numbering system for all permanent teeth numbered 1 through 32. The maxillary numbering follows clockwise from the right maxillary third molar (designated as tooth 1) to the left maxillary third molar (designated tooth 16). The mandibular numbering follows clockwise from the left mandibular third molar (designated as tooth 17), to the right mandibular third molar, designated as tooth 32 (Figure 16-7). The primary teeth are identified by capital letters A to T. In the maxilla, the maxillary right second molar is designated as tooth A across the arch to the left maxillary second molar designated as tooth J. The left mandibular second

Permanent Teeth															
Maxillary Right (Quadrant 1)								Maxillary Left (Quadrant 2)							
1	2	3	4	5	6	7	8	9	10	11	12	13	14	15	16
32	31	30	29	28	27	26	25	24	23	22	21	20	19	18	17
Mandibular Right (Quadrant 4)								Mandibular Left (Quadrant 3)							
Primary Teeth															
Maxillary Right (Quadrant 1)								Maxillary Left (Quadrant 2)							
			A	B	C	D	E	F	G	H	I	J			
			T	S	R	Q	P	O	N	M	L	K			
Mandibular Right (Quadrant 4)								Mandibular Left (Quadrant 3)							

Figure 16-7. Universal numbering system of permanent and primary dentitions.

Permanent Teeth															
Maxillary Right (Quadrant 1)								Maxillary Left (Quadrant 2)							
18	17	16	15	14	13	12	11	21	22	23	24	25	26	27	28
48	47	46	45	44	43	42	41	31	32	33	34	35	36	37	38
Mandibular Right (Quadrant 4)								Mandibular Left (Quadrant 3)							
Primary Teeth															
Maxillary Right (Quadrant 1)								Maxillary Left (Quadrant 2)							
			55	54	53	52	51	61	62	63	64	65			
			85	84	83	82	81	71	72	73	74	75			
Mandibular Right (Quadrant 4)								Mandibular Left (Quadrant 3)							

Figure 16-8. International numbering system of permanent and primary dentitions.

molar is designated by the letter K; following across the mandibular arch, the mandibular right second molar is designated by the letter T.

International Numbering System (Federation Dentaire International)

The International Numbering System uses a two-digit system to identify each tooth. The first digit indicates the quadrant in which the tooth is located, and the second digit identifies the specific tooth. For quadrant designations, numbers 1 to 4 are used to specify permanent quadrants, and numbers 5 to 8 to designate primary quadrants. The second digit identifies the specific tooth in the quadrant: the numbers 1 to 8 are used for permanent teeth, and the numbers 1 to 5 for primary teeth. In each dentition, tooth 1 is the central incisor with the numbers progressing from the midline to the posterior teeth (Figure 16-8). The pronunciation of the International system is pronounced "one six," rather than "sixteen."

Developmental Anomalies

Developmental anomalies arise from a disturbance in the stages of tooth development (odontogenesis), causing one or more of the tooth bud tissues to be disrupted. These disturbances may be the result of local, systemic, or hereditary factors. The extent of the disturbance is dependent on the dental developmental stage at which the disruption occurred and the duration and nature of the assault.

Dental anomalies include anomalies of the number of teeth and anomalies of dental tissues. Tables 16-1 to 16-7 describe the more frequently noted dental anomalies (see also Chapter 30).

Text continued on p. 260

TABLE 16-1
Anomalies of Number of Teeth

Name	Description	Clinical Appearance	Image
Hyperdontia	Extra teeth beyond the normal complement referred to as "supernumerary" or "supplemental" teeth	Supernumerary teeth are extra teeth of abnormal shape Supplemental teeth are extra teeth of normal shape	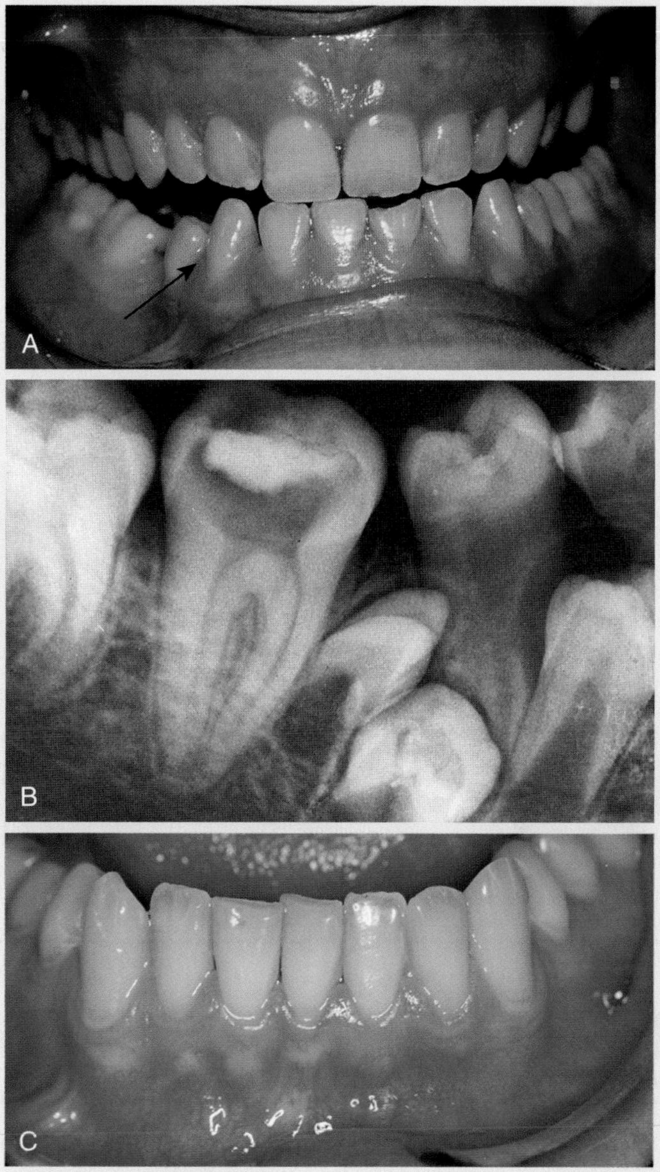
Mesiodens	These supernumerary teeth are usually misshapen, small, and peglike	May be seen as an extra tooth at the midline between the maxillary anterior incisors	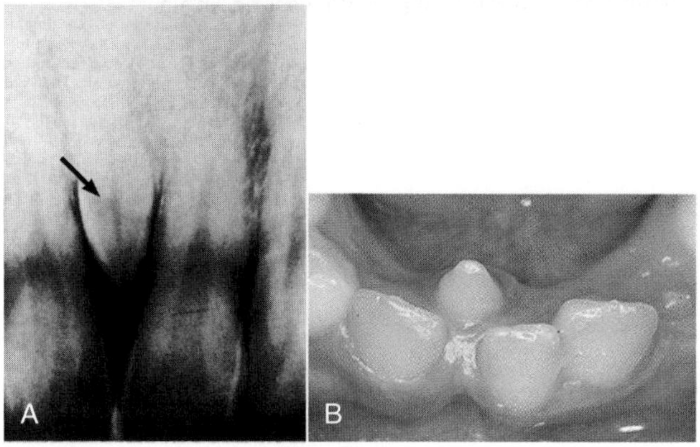

Continued

TABLE 16-1

Anomalies of Number of Teeth—cont'd

Name	Description	Clinical Appearance	Image
Hypodontia (also called *anodontia*)	Absence of one or more teeth Rare condition of complete anodontia is failure of all teeth to develop Partial anodontia is the absence of one or several teeth	Teeth most frequently congenitally missing are the following: Third molars Maxillary lateral incisors Mandibular premolars Teeth least frequently absent are the following: First permanent molars	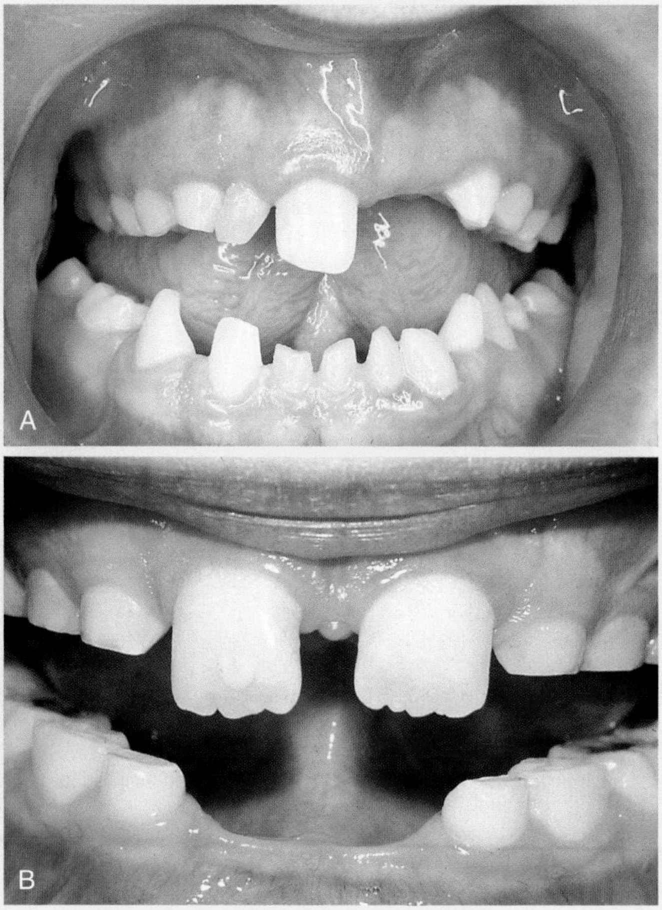

TABLE 16-2

Anomalies of the Whole Tooth

Name	Description	Clinical Appearance	Image
Macrodontia	Larger than normal teeth	May be larger in width, length, or height	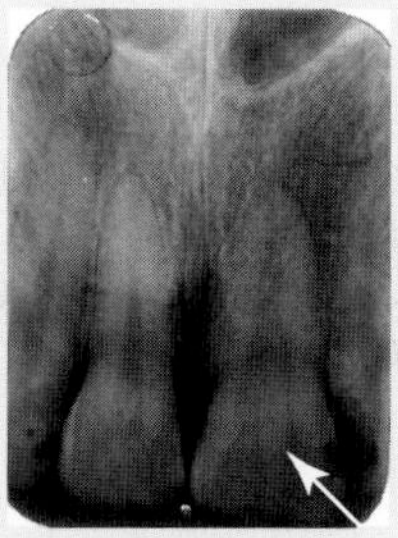 Right central incisor is considerably larger than the left. (Courtesy Steven R. Singer, Rutgers School of Dental Medicine.)

TABLE 16-2
Anomalies of the Whole Tooth—cont'd

Name	Description	Clinical Appearance	Image
Microdontia "Peg-laterals"	Many supernumerary teeth are small and can be classified as microdonts "Peg-lateral" is a term used to describe a type of microdont that can stem from a variety of causes	Smaller teeth than normal; may be one tooth, several teeth, or all teeth within the dentition Seen as conical lateral incisors	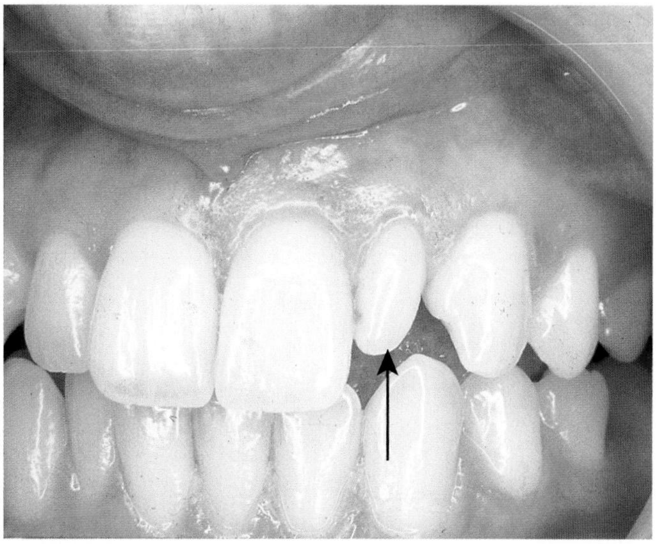 Microdontia *(arrow).* Peg lateral is seen in the previous photograph. (From Ibsen OAC, Phelan JA: *Oral pathology for the dental hygienist,* ed 6, St Louis, 2013, Saunders.)
Gemination	A large tooth resulting from the splitting of a single tooth germ that attempts to form two teeth	Usually results in a partially or completely divided crown attached to a single root with one canal	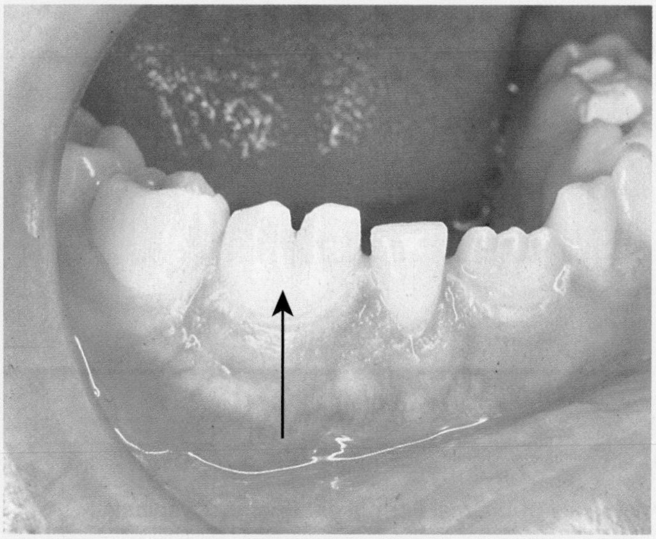 Gemination *(arrow)* in a mandibular cuspid. (From Ibsen OAC, Phelan JA: *Oral pathology for the dental hygienist,* ed 6, St Louis, 2013, Saunders.)

Continued

TABLE 16-2

Anomalies of the Whole Tooth—cont'd

Name	Description	Clinical Appearance	Image
Dens in dente	Defined as a tooth within a tooth Caused by invagination of the enamel organ during development	Most frequently observed on the lingual aspect of the maxillary lateral incisors	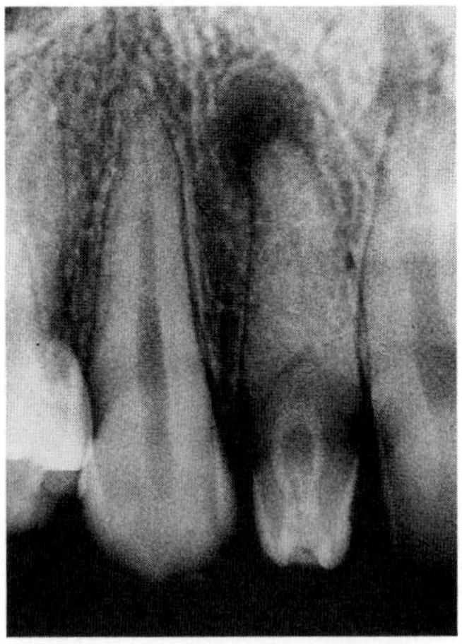 (From Ibsen OAC, Phelan JA: *Oral pathology for the dental hygienist,* ed 6, St Louis, 2013, Saunders.)
Dilaceration	Abnormal distortion of a crown or root caused by trauma during tooth formation. It is usually observed as a severely angulated root.	The root angulation may create extraction challenges for the dentist.[1]	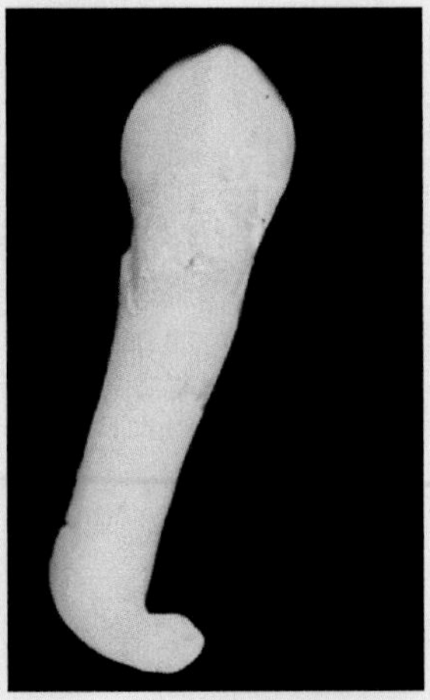 Dilaceration. (Courtesy Oral Pathology University of Alberta, Canada.)

TABLE 16-3

Anomalies of Enamel Formation: Enamel Dysplasia

Name	Description	Clinical Appearance	Image
Enamel hypoplasia	The result of a disturbance of the ameloblasts during matrix formation.	Pitted or rough, striated enamel surface.	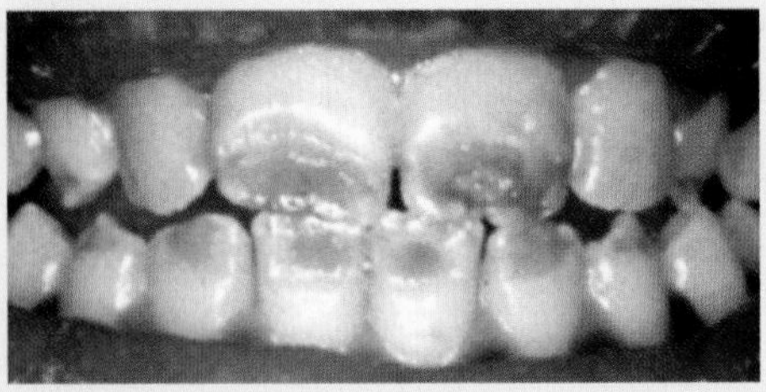 (From Ibsen OAC, Phelan JA: *Oral pathology for the dental hygienist,* ed 6, St Louis, 2013, Saunders.)

TABLE 16-3

Anomalies of Enamel Formation: Enamel Dysplasia—cont'd

Name	Description	Clinical Appearance	Image
Types of Enamel Hypoplasia			
Dental fluorosis	Excessive amounts of systemic fluoride may be responsible for enamel hypoplasia or enamel hypocalcification.	Ranges from mild fluorosis, with white flecking, to severe conditions where the teeth are deeply pitted or brown stained. Notched or screwdriver appearance.	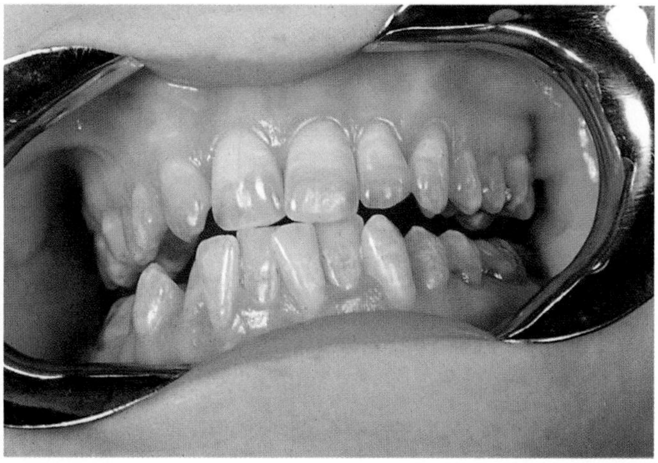 (From Ibsen OAC, Phelan JA: *Oral pathology for the dental hygienist,* ed 6, St Louis, 2013, Saunders.)
Syphilis-related enamel hypoplasia	Congenital syphilis is a rare cause of enamel hypoplasia.	Nodular enamel growths on the cusp surfaces of the permanent molars.	
Hutchinson's incisors	Term used to describe the appearance of syphilitic incisor teeth.		
Mulberry molars	The term **"mulberry molars"** is used to describe the mottled mulberry-shaped molars also associated with congenital syphilis.[2]		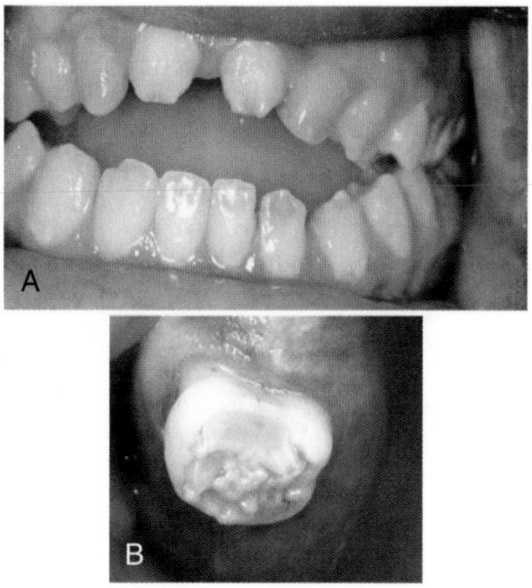 (From Ibsen OAC, Phelan JA: *Oral pathology for the dental hygienist,* ed 6, St Louis, 2013, Saunders.)

Continued

TABLE 16-3
Anomalies of Enamel Formation: Enamel Dysplasia—cont'd

Name	Description	Clinical Appearance	Image
"Peg laterals"	May be associated with syphilitic conditions however as discussed in microdontia can arise from several causes.	Seen as conical lateral incisors.	See microdont photograph in Table 16-2
Enamel hypocalcification	Defect occurring in the enamel as the result of a disturbance during mineralization.	White spotting of the enamel surface; the enamel surface is generally smooth in texture.	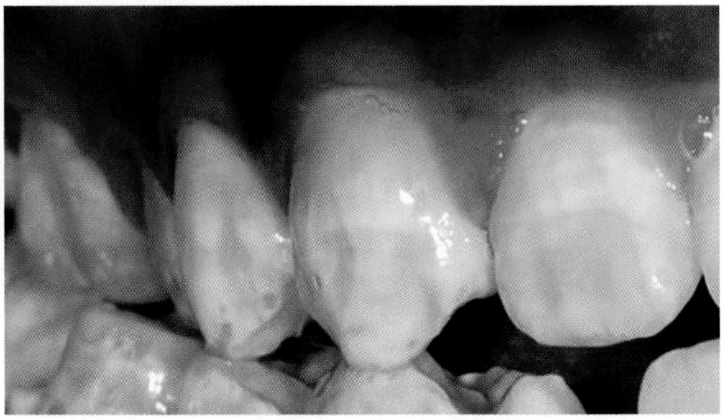 (From Heymann HO, Swift Jr, EJ, Ritter AV: *Sturdevant's art and science of operative dentistry*, ed 6, St Louis, 2013, Mosby.)
Amelogenesis imperfecta	A form of enamel dysplasia resulting from many inheritance patterns such as autosomal dominant, recessive, or X-linked gene.	Partial or total malformation of enamel. The dentin and pulp develop normally, but the enamel is easily chipped or worn away.	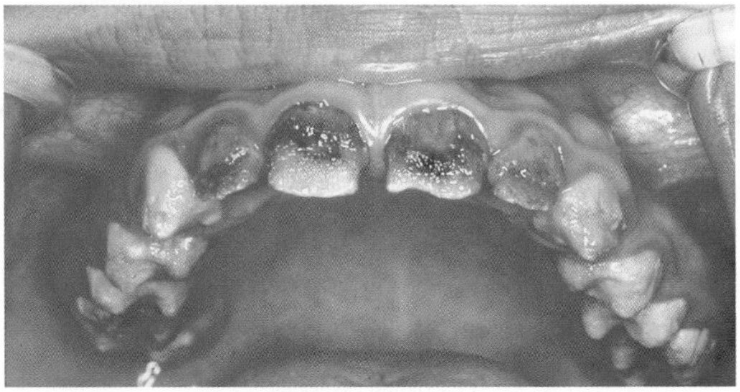 (From Ibsen OAC, Phelan JA: *Oral pathology for the dental hygienist*, ed 6, St Louis, 2013, Saunders.)

TABLE 16-4

Enamel Anomalies Not Classified as Enamel Dysplasia

Name	Description	Clinical Appearance
Dens evaginatus	Also referred to as tuberculated cusp. A rare developmental anomaly caused by proliferation of enamel epithelium that forms an accessory cusp found on the occlusal surface. It is believed to form from an outpouching (evagination) of the enamel epithelium during the early stages of odontogenesis. The tissue mass contains normal pulp and is subject to occlusal wear.	A small mass of enamel or accessory cusp projecting on the occlusal surface of molars and premolars. 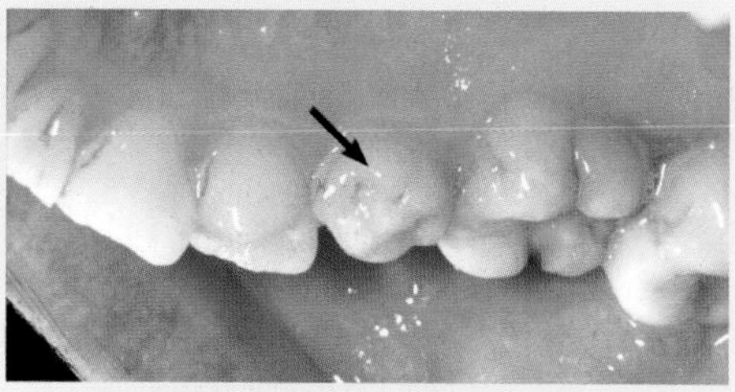 (Courtesy Margot Van Dis.)
Talon cusp	The lingual cusp of anterior teeth was reported to resemble an eagle's talon, and it was named accordingly. The talon cusp has well-developed enamel and dentin and contains a pulp horn.[1]	A well-delineated cusp found on the lingual surfaces of maxillary and mandibular anterior teeth. 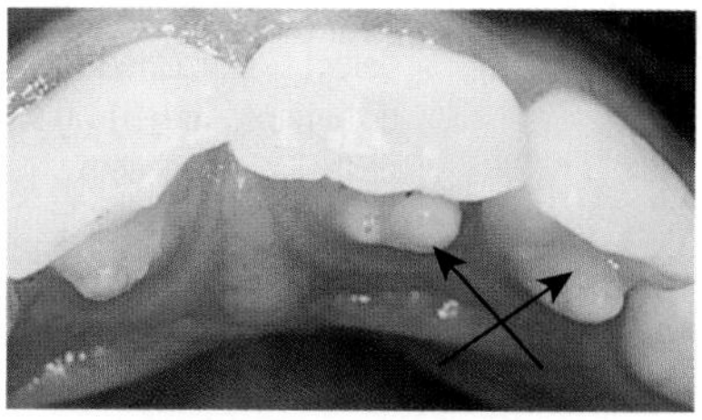 (Courtesy Dr. Geoffrey Sperber, University of Alberta, Canada.)

TABLE 16-5

Anomalies of Dentin Formation

Name	Description	Clinical Appearance
Dentinogenesis imperfecta	Associated with a dominant inherited disorder, characterized by faulty formation of connective tissues. Enamel formation occurs normally, but the enamel easily breaks or chips away, resulting in tooth attrition and dentinal hypersensitivity. Irregular formation or absence of dentinal development.	Displays a softer than normal consistency as a result of increased water and organic content. Larger than normal teeth in width, length, or height. Dental treatment usually includes placement of crowns to preserve existing crown. 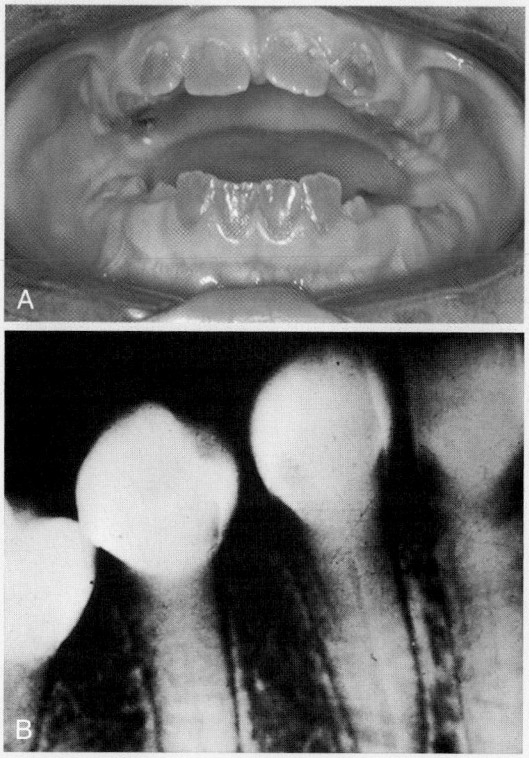 (Courtesy Dr. Edward V Zegarelli.)

Continued

TABLE 16-5

Anomalies of Dentin Formation—cont'd

Name	Description	Clinical Appearance
Dentin dysplasia	Dentin dysplasia has two subdivisions: Type I (radicular dentin dysplasia) and Type II (coronal dentin dysplasia). Type I is an autosomal-dominant inheritance pattern characterized by teeth with normal crowns and abnormal roots. The defect is connected to a disturbance in Hertwig's epithelial root sheath, which guides the formation of the root. Dentin dysplasia Type II has an autosomal-dominant inheritance pattern. There is a mutation in the gene *dentin sialophosphoprotein* (DSPP). Dentinogenesis imperfecta and dentin dysplasia Type II share the DSPP mutation.[2]	Type I: Radicular dentin dysplasia. Total or partial lack of pulp chambers and root canals are seen on radiographs. Primary and secondary dentitions are equally affected. Because the roots are short the teeth are affected easily by any trauma even minor and the teeth are generally lost prematurely. Type II: Coronal dentin dysplasia—obliterated and partial lack of coronal pulp chambers and small root canals.[2] 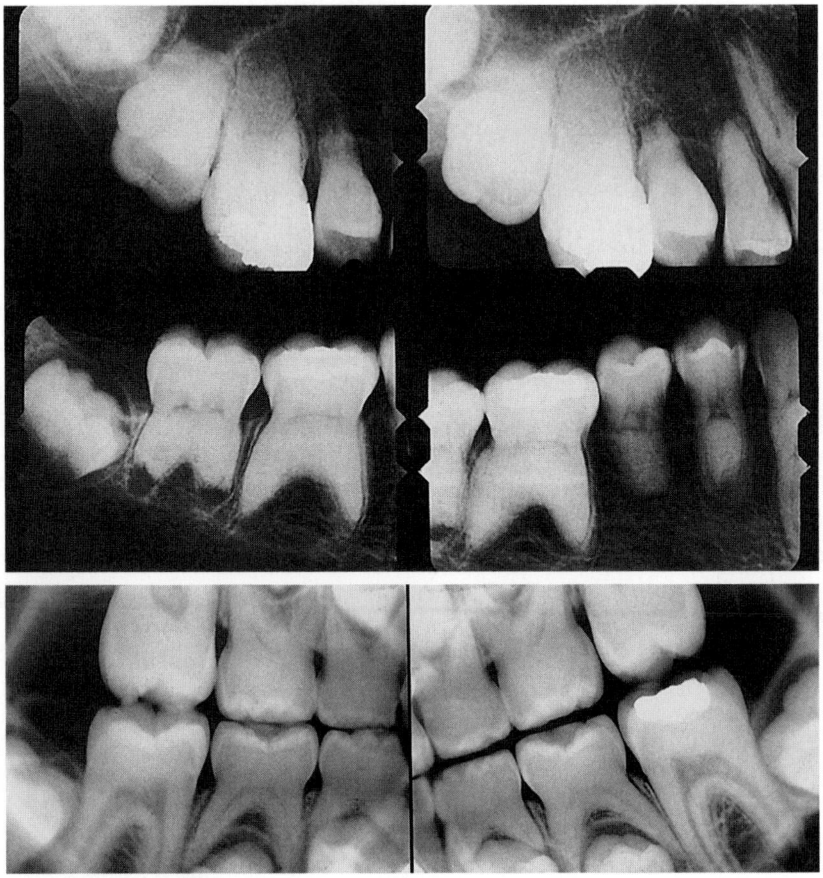 (Courtesy Dr. Carl J. Witkop.)

TABLE 16-6
Anomalies of Pulp Formation

Name	Description	Clinical Appearance	Image
Taurodontism	Meaning bull-like teeth, is an inherited phenomenon and thus is genetically determined.	The crowns of these teeth develop normally; however, the pulp chambers are much enlarged at the expense of the dentinal walls.[1]	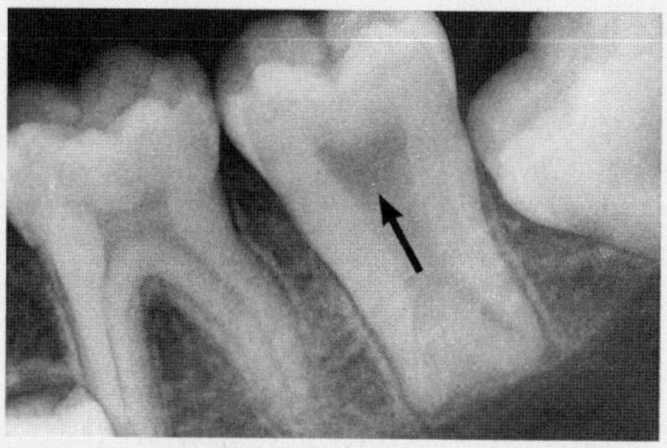 (Courtesy Dr. George Blozis.)

TABLE 16-7
Acquired Tooth Damage

Name	Description	Clinical Appearance	Image
Attrition	Tooth-to-tooth wear of the dentition is pathologic and may be caused by bruxism, grinding, or clenching.	Appears as excessive wear to the occlusal/incisal surfaces. Restoration of teeth with excessive attrition may include complete tooth coverage by a crown.	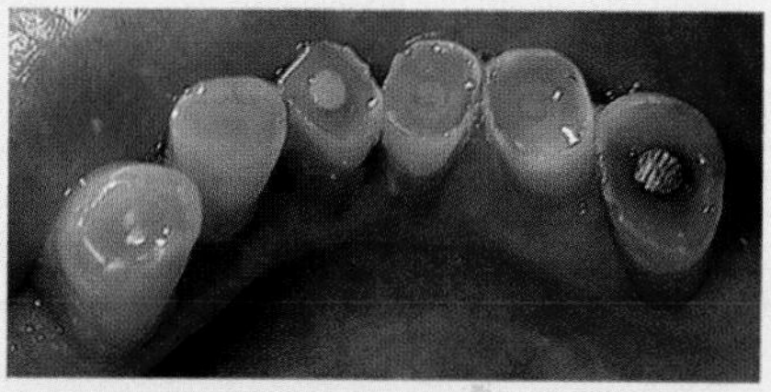 (From Newman MG, Takei HH, Klokkevold PR, et al: *Carranza's clinical periodontology,* ed 11, St Louis, 2012, Saunders.)
Dental abrasion	Pathologic tooth wear caused by a foreign substance, commonly seen as a result of traumatic toothbrushing.	Appears as notches worn into the teeth near the gingival margin.	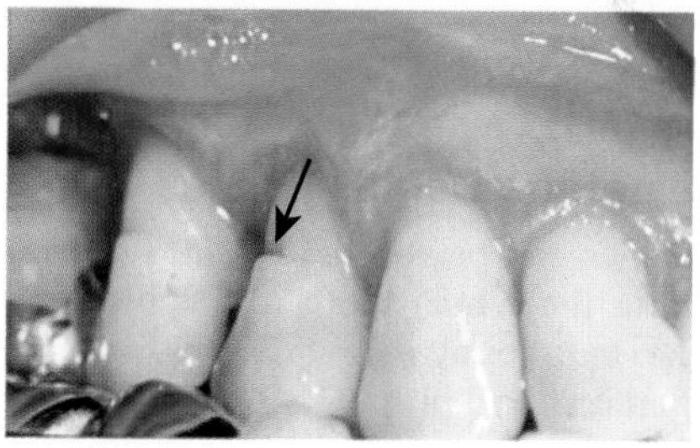 (From Newman MG, Takei HH, Klokkevold PR, et al: *Carranza's clinical periodontology,* ed 11, St Louis, 2012, Saunders.)
Dental erosion	Loss of tooth surface as a result of chemical agents because of the following: acid reflux disease, excessive vomiting with morning sickness, anorexia, and bulimia. Tooth erosion also results from habits such as sucking on lemons, holding mouth fresheners, cough drops, or candies in the mucobuccal fold. The erosive action of these chemicals causes local destruction of tooth enamel.	The repeated regurgitation of stomach acids through the oral cavity results in the dissolution of the dental tissues on the lingual and incisal or occlusal surfaces of the maxillary teeth.	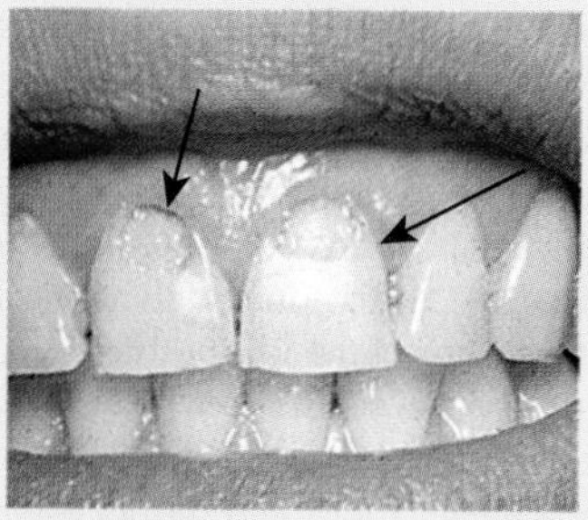 (Courtesy Dr. Margaret Walsh, University of California-San Francisco.)

Continued

TABLE 16-7

Acquired Tooth Damage—cont'd

Name	Description	Clinical Appearance	Image
Abfraction	Abfraction defects are caused by biomechanical forces on teeth, which cause tooth flexure and results in a wedge-shaped or V-shaped loss of tooth structure at the cemento-enamel junction (CEJ); the tooth is more susceptible to toothbrush abrasion.	Cervical stress lesion that is manifested as a V- or wedge-shaped defect at the cementoenamel junction (CEJ).	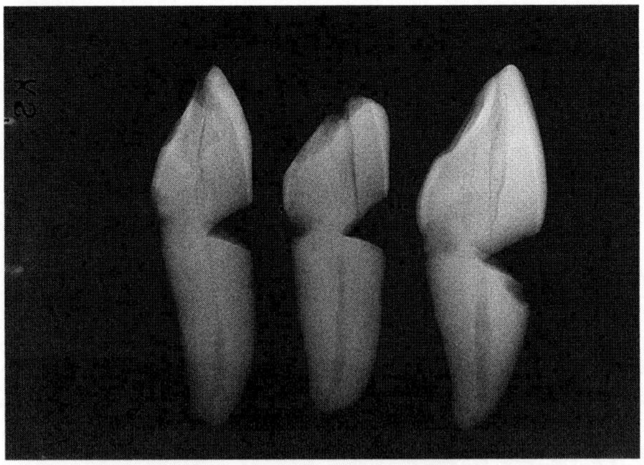 (Courtesy Dr. Geoffrey Sperber, University of Alberta, Canada.)
Tooth fracture	Tooth fractures may range from small chips of the enamel to breaks that penetrate deeply into the tooth.	Minor enamel fractures often require nothing more than the polishing of rough surfaces. More severe fractures require various levels of restoration. Some fractured teeth may not be restorable and, as a result, require removal.	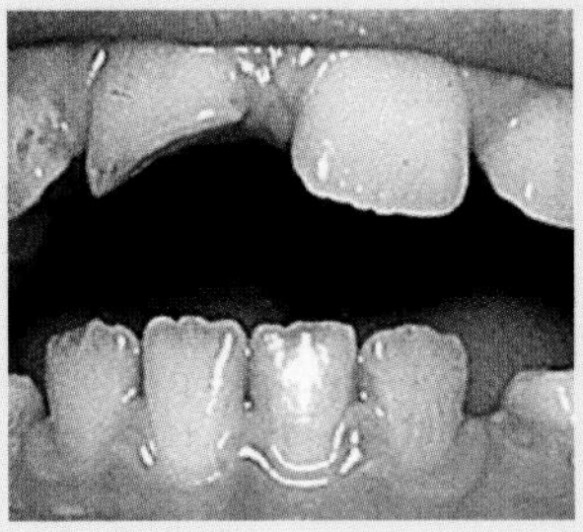 (Courtesy Dr. Margaret Walsh, University of California-San Francisco.)

Anomalies of the Dental Tissues

Tooth anomalies can be subdivided into several categories: those affecting the whole tooth (see Table 16-2) and those affecting the individual dental tissues, including enamel, dentin, cementum, and pulp.

Anomalies of Enamel Formation: Enamel Dysplasia

An insult to ameloblasts during tooth formation may result in abnormal enamel development, referred to generally as enamel dysplasia. Enamel dysplasia encompasses two types of abnormal enamel development: enamel hypoplasia and enamel hypocalcification. Many factors—local (e.g., trauma), systemic (e.g., diseases, nutritional deficiencies, excess systemic fluoride), hereditary, and idiopathic (unknown)—may cause anomalies of enamel formation.

Several anomalies involve enamel but are not classified as enamel dysplasia; these include enamel pearls (see also Chapter 25), dens evaginatus, and talon cusp (see Table 16-4).

Acquired Tooth Damage

Acquired tooth damage can be caused by any process that results in a loss of the integrity of the tooth surface. The most common form of acquired tooth damage is dental caries, an infectious disease caused by bacteria that live in the plaque biofilm and attach to teeth. Other common forms of tooth damage (attrition, abrasion, erosion, and fracture) are the result of mechanical or chemical assault to the tooth structure (see also Chapter 39).

Dental Caries

Dental caries is an infectious and transmissible disease caused by bacterial action on fermentable carbohydrates, which affects the mineralized tissues of the teeth. Dental caries is a multifactorial disease with the primary factors being bacteria (which adhere to all tooth surfaces), the tooth, dietary fermentable carbohydrates, and the host or tooth surface over time (Figure 16-9). *Streptococcus mutans, Streptococcus sobrinus,* and *Lactobacillus* species are the bacteria identified as the primary causative agents in this process, which leads to cavitation and possible tooth loss. *S. mutans* is strongly associated with the initiation of dental caries and is related to the *frequency* of carbohydrate intake. Lactobacilli are considered the secondary invaders responsible for the progression of already established lesions and are related to the *amount* of carbohydrate intake. These bacteria metabolize dietary fermentable carbohydrates (sugars and cooked starch) producing acids, causing the biofilm pH to fall rapidly below

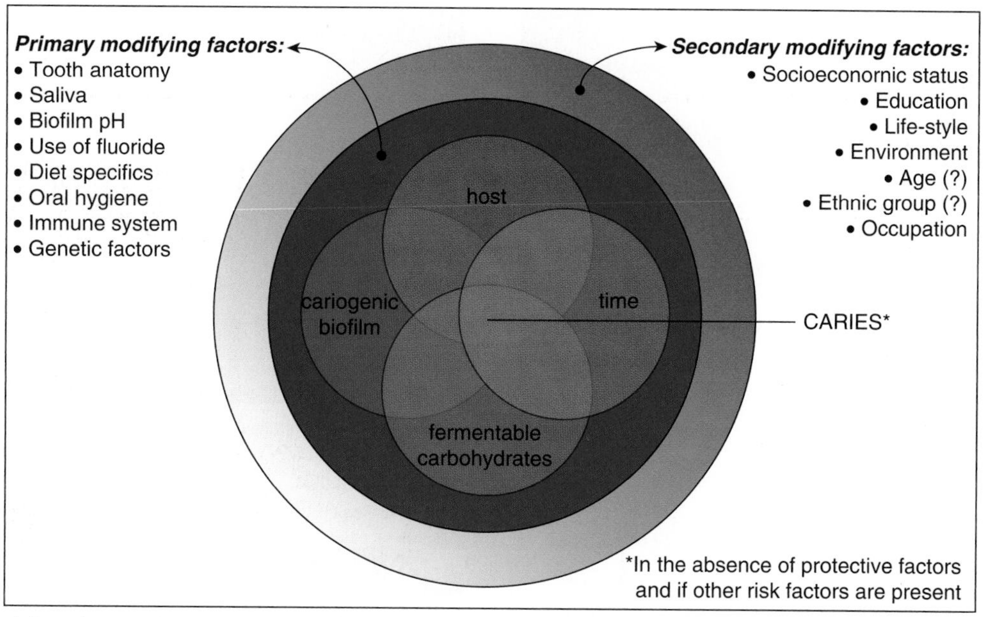

Figure 16-9. Factors influencing initiation and inhibition of dental caries. (Modified from Keyes PH, Jordan HV: Factors influencing initiation, transmission and inhibition of dental caries. In Harris RJ, editor: *Mechanisms of hard tissue destruction*, New York, 1963, Academic Press.)

5 within a matter of minutes. Before eating, pH ranges from 6.2 to 7.0. Critical pH for enamel dissolution ranges from 4.5 to 5.5. Biofilms remains acidic for some time, taking 1 to 2 hours to return to normal pH in the region of 7. These acids diffuse into the tooth to dissolve the calcium and phosphate minerals (carbonated hydroxyapatite), a process called *demineralization*. If the acid attacks are infrequent and of short duration, saliva can assist in repairing the damage by neutralizing the acid and replacing minerals and fluoride lost from the tooth.

However, dental caries is more complex than just the interaction of the key factors with many primary and secondary modifying factors that can influence the caries process in a protective or harmful way (see Figure 16-9). For example, saliva as a primary modifying factor can be protective and initiate remineralization when calcium, phosphate, proteins, and fluoride are in the saliva; there is normal salivary flow; and antibacterial agents if needed are provided (see Chapter 20). Conversely, however, modifying factors can have a harmful component; for example, low saliva flow, frequent and repeated consumption of carbohydrates, and a low biofilm pH may cause demineralization and lead to dental caries. Tooth cavitation, best referred to as a "carious lesion," is more commonly called a "cavity," and the affected tooth is said to be "carious" or "decayed." Thus dental caries involves an interaction among pathologic factors and protective factors.

Tooth susceptible sites that favor biofim retention are particularly prone to decay. These sites are the following:

- Pits and fissures on occlusal, buccal, and lingual surfaces
- Interproximal contacts
- Along the cervical margin but above the free gingival margin
- Areas of recession where root surfaces are exposed
- Deficient or defective margins of restorations
- Surfaces that are adjacent to bridges and dentures

Types of Dental Caries

The classification of dental caries is intended to describe the rate, direction, and/or type of disease progression. The classification terms include *rampant* caries; *chronic* caries; *arrested* caries, and *recurrent* caries. These terms permit the oral healthcare practitioner to communicate the severity or rapidity of the attack and the urgency with which restorative therapy should be delivered. These terms are not specific regarding tooth and surface; therefore they must be combined with other cavity classification terminology to permit location-specific communication.

Rampant Caries

Rampant caries describes sudden, rapid destruction of many teeth that requires urgent intervention. The lesions are usually numerous and may be large. The decayed dentin is very soft and moist and is often light in color (Figure 16-10). Rampant caries often is associated with conditions such as early childhood caries in infants, teens consuming frequent cariogenic snacks and beverages, or with reduced saliva flow in clients, for example, as a result of head and neck cancer radiation therapy.

Early Childhood Caries

Early childhood caries (ECC) is a type of dental caries observed in children under the age of 5 and is characterized by early onset and rapid progression of the disease. As defined by the American Academy of Pediatric Dentistry:

> ECC: The presence of 1 or more; noncavitated or cavitated lesions, missing teeth due to caries, or filled tooth surfaces in the primary dentition in children 71 months of age or younger.[3]

> Severe ECC: (S-ECC): In children younger than 3 years of age any sign of smooth-surface caries is indicative of S-ECC.[3] Between ages 3 to 5 S-ECC is 1 or more:

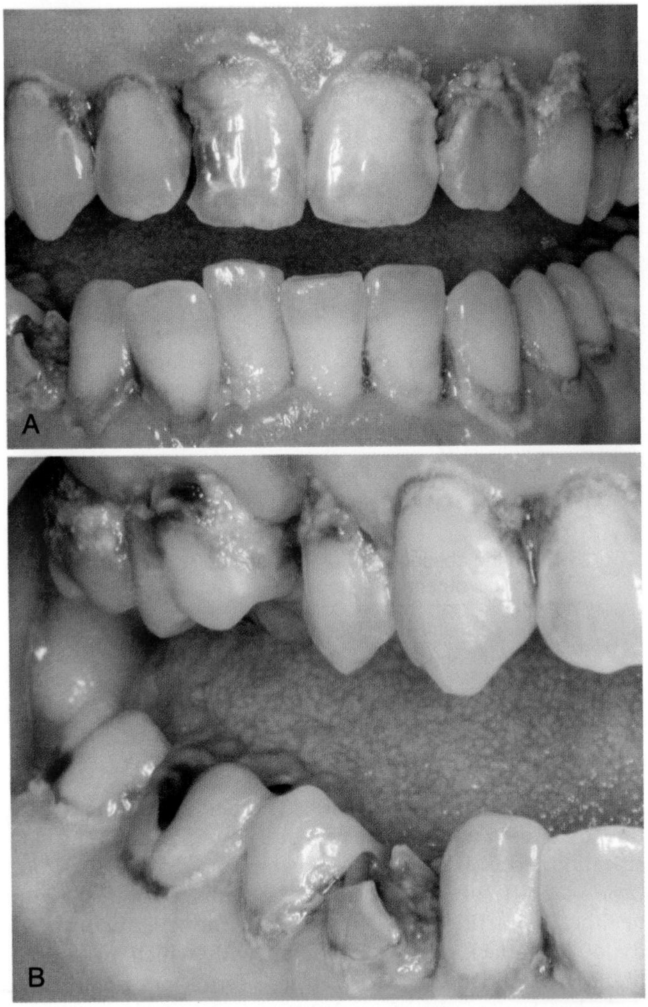

Figure 16-10. Acute, rampant caries in anterior **(A)** and posterior **(B)** teeth. (From Heymann HO, Swift, Jr. EJ, Ritter AV: *Sturdevant's art and science of operative dentistry*, ed 6, St Louis, 2013, Mosby.)

> cavitated teeth, missing teeth as the result of caries, filled smooth surfaces in primary maxillary anterior teeth or a decayed, missing, or filled with a score of ≥4 (age 3), ≥5 (age 4), or ≥6 (age 5) surfaces.[3]

This ECC condition was previously referred to as *nursing caries, nursing bottle syndrome,* or *baby bottle caries*. This type of ECC appears rapidly, commonly affecting maxillary anterior teeth, particularly the facial surfaces not generally considered to be at high risk for decay (Figure 16-11). Lesions may first appear as a cervical band of demineralization, rapidly progressing to overt caries. Mandibular teeth often are not affected, probably because the child's tongue covers these teeth during the caries challenge.[4]

The evidence clearly shows that high levels of *S. mutans* organisms transmitted from the mother are associated with ECC. These elevated bacteria levels combined with frequent carbohydrate intake produce high acid levels over long exposure periods. To provide early intervention strategies the dental hygienist identifies the risk factors for ECC as early as possible (Box 16-1). Several questions to ask parents or caregivers are listed in Box 16-2.

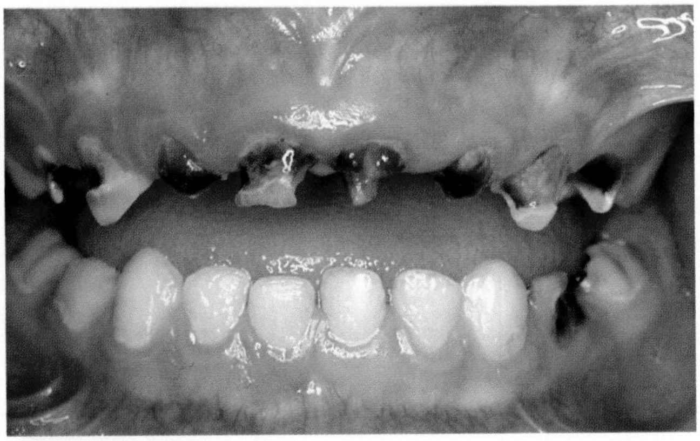

Figure 16-11. Rampant caries in a preschool child. (From Dean JA, Avery DR, McDonald RE: *McDonald and Avery's dentistry for the child and adolescent*, ed 9, St Louis, 2011, Mosby.)

BOX 16-1

Risk Factors for the Development of Early Childhood Caries

- Sleeps with a bottle containing anything other than water
- Snacks three or more times per day
- Visible biofilm on maxillary incisors
- Parents or caregivers do not brush child's teeth
- Siblings or parents have caries
- Drinks low-fluoride water and does not receive fluoride supplements
- Little or no fluoride in diet
- From low-income family

Adapted from Milgrom P, Weinstein P: *Early childhood caries: a team approach to prevention and treatment*, Seattle, 1999, Continuing Education, University of Washington School of Dentistry.

BOX 16-2

Early Childhood Caries: Questions for Parents

- Do the parents clean the child's teeth regularly?
- Do other family members have active dental caries?
- Does the child drink water containing less than the optimal fluoride content or not receive fluoride supplements?
- Does the child sleep with a bottle containing anything other than water?
- Does the child eat more than three cariogenic snacks in a day?
- Does the child drink bottled water or bottled fruit juice?

Adapted from Milgrom P, Weinstein P: *Early childhood caries: a team approach to prevention and treatment*, Seattle, 1999, Continuing Education, University of Washington School of Dentistry.

Chronic Caries

Chronic caries describes a slow progressive decay process that requires regular dental intervention. The carious dentin is firm and often brown to black. In large, open cavities the decayed dentin can be scooped out in large segments and has the consistency of firm leather (Figure 16-12).

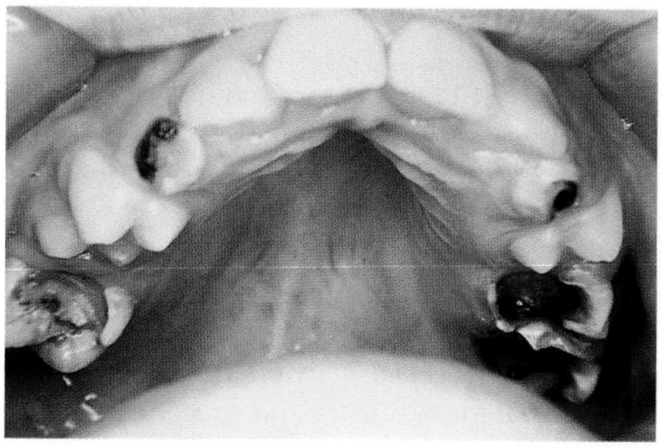

Figure 16-12. Chronic caries.

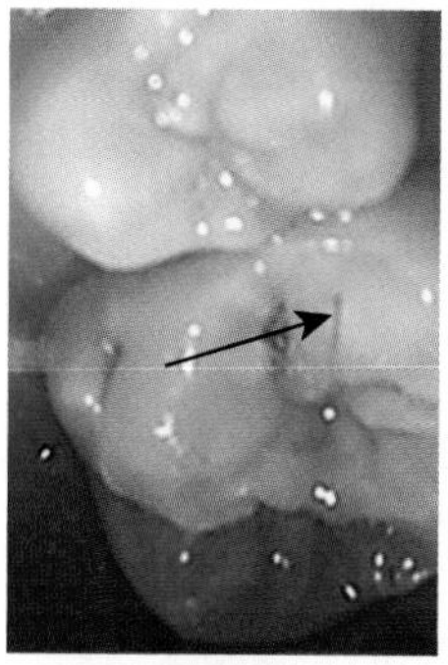

Figure 16-13. Pit and fissure caries.

Arrested Caries

Arrested caries is the halting of the progress of the decay process. It is noted by its dark staining without any breakdown of tooth tissues. Dental decay is not a continuous demineralization process. Evidence supports a continuous demineralization-remineralization process that can be tipped out of balance by changes in diet and oral environment (see Chapter 20). Because saliva provides the constituents that enable enamel to remineralize after an acid attack, a reduction in salivary flow or salivary buffering capacity may cause rapid demineralization. Conversely, demineralized lesions may recalcify as a result of an improved oral environment, especially in the presence of frequent use of 0.05% sodium fluoride mouth rinses. This recalcified lesion resulting from the remineralization process is known as arrested caries. Arrested lesions are characterized by their light or brown color and firm and glasslike surface when evaluated.

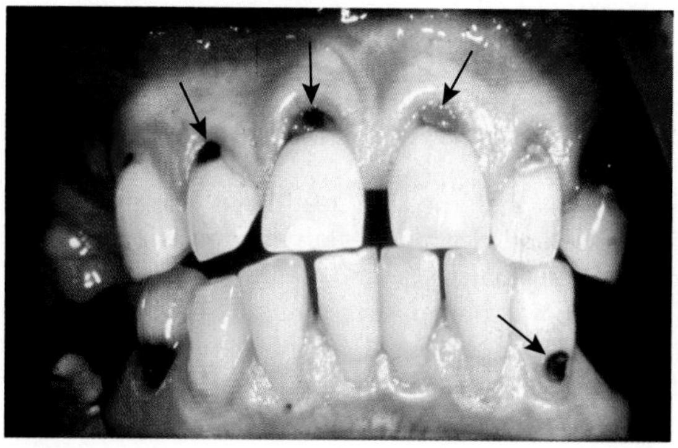

Figure 16-14. Root caries found on the root surfaces of teeth *(arrows)*. (From Bird DL, Robinson DS: *Modern dental assisting*, ed 11, St Louis, 2015, Saunders.)

Recurrent Caries

Recurrent caries describes new decay that occurs under a restoration or around its margins. These lesions pose a special threat because they may go undetected and invade the tissue beneath the restoration.

Types of Carious Lesions by Location

Carious lesions often are referred to by their specific location on a tooth. This descriptive mechanism may be best suited for describing the dental problem to the client. The location description may include anatomic representations such as pit and fissure caries, smooth surface caries, and root caries. Another method of describing the carious lesion location is to identify the specific tooth surface(s) with a lesion. It is not uncommon for noncarious tooth surfaces to become involved in the restoration process because of the need for access or cavity design. For example, a tooth with a carious lesion on the distal surface may require the involvement of the occlusal surface or a disto-occlusal cavity preparation for restoration. Therefore another form of classification is by the number or identification of involved surfaces rather than carious surfaces.

Pit and Fissure Caries

Pit and fissure caries is found most frequently in the grooves and crevices of the occlusal surfaces of premolars and molars (Figure 16-13). It is also found in maxillary incisor lingual pits, mandibular molar facial pits, and maxillary molar lingual grooves. Pits and fissures are particularly susceptible to a carious attack because of the protected bacterial niche provided by the inadequately coalesced developmental lobes of enamel.

Proximal Caries

Dental caries between teeth at the point of their proximal contact (the contact between teeth that stabilizes their position in the dental arch and to prevent food impaction between the teeth) is called **proximal** or approximal **caries.**

Smooth Surface Caries

Smooth surface caries is found on the facial, lingual, mesial, and distal surfaces of the dentition. The proximal smooth surfaces are the most susceptible to dental caries because of the shelter they provide for plaque biofilm development. The gingival third of the facial and lingual surfaces also is more susceptible to caries because of the increased difficulty associated with cleaning this less-bulbous portion of the crown.

Root Caries

Root caries is dental caries involving the tooth root, cementum, or cervical area of the tooth. Root caries is found most frequently in the elderly population, in whom root exposure is common because of gingival recession (Figure 16-14).

Pulpal Damage

The most common causes of pulpal nerve damage are bacterial infection and trauma. Bacterial infection is caused most often by extensive decay. If bacteria reach the nerves and

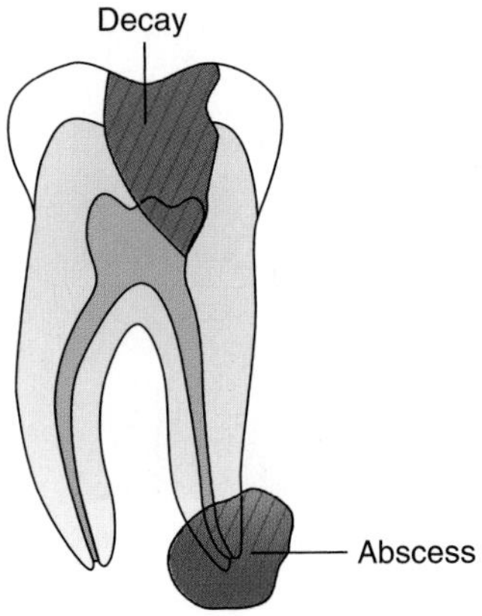

Figure 16-15. Diagram showing extensive decay into the pulp and formation of periapical abscess. (From Bird DL, Robinson DS: *Modern dental assisting*, ed 11, St Louis, 2015, Saunders.)

blood vessels, the infection results in an abscess (Figure 16-15). Endodontics is the specialty of dentistry that manages the prevention, diagnosis, and treatment of the dental pulp and the peri-radicular tissues that surround the root of the tooth. Endodontic treatment, or root canal therapy, provides an effective means of saving a tooth that otherwise may have to be extracted.

Although clients may experience symptoms differently, the most common signs and symptoms of pulpal nerve damage are as follows:

- Pain when biting down
- Pain when chewing
- Sensitivity with hot or cold beverages
- Noticeable facial swelling

Classification of Dental Caries and Restorations

Dental caries and dental restorations are classified commonly either by Black's classification or by the complexity classification system (also see Chapter 39).

Black's Classification System

The most commonly used system to describe the types and locations of dental caries and restorations was established by G.V. Black in the early 1900s. This descriptive system consists of six classifications, shown in Table 16-8.

The Complexity Classification

The complexity classification identifies dental caries and restorations by the number of surfaces they involve. **Simple caries** or restorations are those involving only one tooth surface. Those that involve two surfaces are classified as **compound caries** or restorations, and **complex caries** or restorations involve more than two surfaces. The usual practice is to refer to the caries or restoration using the abbreviation of the surfaces affected, such as *O* for occlusal, *DO* for disto-occlusal, and *MOD* for mesio-occlusodistal. When doing so, the letters are pronounced separately, such as a D-O caries or an M-O-D restoration.

Table 16-9 outlines examples of simple, compound, and complex designations for dental caries or restorations named with nomenclature as described in the following section.

Nomenclature

In describing a cavity or a restoration, specific nomenclature is used that involves the combination of anatomic terms. Basic rules for nomenclature used to describe a cavity or restoration are as follows:

- Rule 1: The terms *mesial* and *distal* precede all other terms, with *mesial* taking precedence (e.g., mesial occlusal distal).
- Rule 2: The terms *labial, buccal, facial,* and *lingual* follow *mesial* and *distal* in that order and precede *incisal* and *occlusal* (e.g., mesial buccal occlusal).
- Rule 3: The terms *incisal* (for anterior teeth) and *occlusal* (for posterior teeth) occur last in any combination, except when they connect two surfaces not connected (e.g., mesial occlusal distal).
- Rule 4: In two-term combinations, the final letters "al" are dropped from the first term and replaced by "o" (e.g., mesiolingual).
- Rule 5: In three-term combinations, the final letters "al" are dropped from each of the first two terms and replaced by "o" (e.g., mesiolabioincisal).
- Rule 6: Whenever dropping of an "al" results in a double "o," a hyphen is added, separating them (e.g., disto-occlusodistal).
- Rule 7: In three-term combinations where two unconnected surfaces are connected by a third surface, the mesial or distal surface is first, followed by facial, lingual, incisal, or occlusal, then the remaining surface (e.g., disto-occlusobuccal).
- Rule 8: In three-term combinations where all surfaces are connected, rules 1 through 3 apply.

Tooth Assessment and Detection of Signs of Dental Caries

Primary approaches to tooth assessment and dental caries detection are direct visual and tactile clinical examination, radiographic evaluation, and evaluation of symptoms described by the client.

Clinical Assessment

Direct clinical examination can be done well only when the teeth are clean and dry and illuminated with good light. Cotton roll isolation can be helpful in maintaining a dry environment, and air-drying of the teeth is essential for the individual examination of each tooth. When plaque biofilm and saliva coat the teeth, defects and signs of disease may go undetected. Tooth assessment proceeds systematically, beginning, for instance, with the most distal tooth in the maxillary right quadrant. The examination continues across the arch, through the last tooth in the maxillary left quadrant. Then the mandible is examined in reverse order, beginning with the most distal tooth in the mandibular left quadrant and ending with the last tooth in the mandibular right quadrant. See Box 16-3 for a description of a systematic approach for dentition charting.

Traditionally in caries detection the clinician examines the tooth surfaces with an explorer to probe questionable tooth surfaces such as pits and fissures, white or brown spot areas, and restoration margins. If the explorer stuck or tugged back on withdrawal, then the area was determined to be positive for caries. The accuracy of this approach is

TABLE 16-8

Black's Classification of Dental Caries and Restorations

Classification	Description
Class I 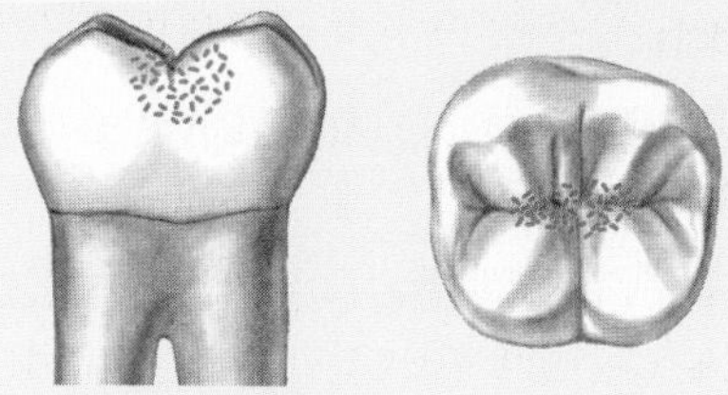	Caries or restoration in the pits and fissures on the occlusal surfaces of molars and premolars, facial (buccal) or lingual pits and molars, and lingual pits of maxillary incisors
Class II 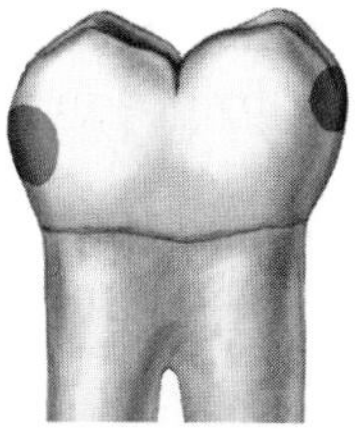	Caries or restoration on the proximal (mesial or distal) surfaces of the premolars and molars involving two or more surfaces
Class III 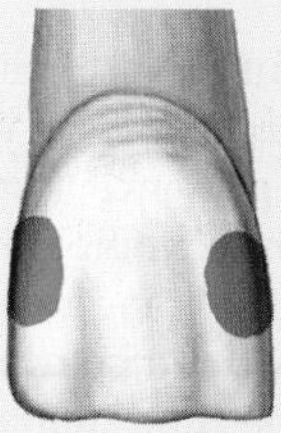	Caries or restoration on the proximal (mesial or distal) surfaces of incisors and canines
Class IV 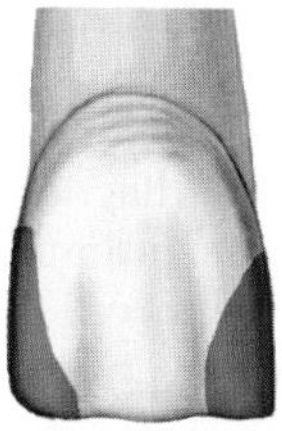	Caries or restoration on the proximal (mesial or distal) surfaces of incisors and canines and also involving the incisal angle
Class V 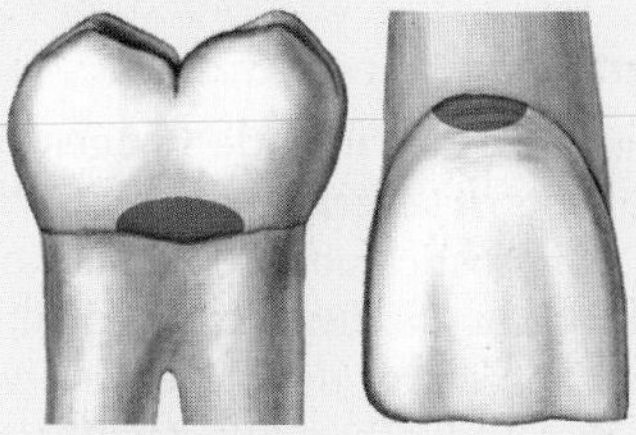	Caries or restoration on the gingival third of the facial or lingual surfaces of any tooth
Class VI 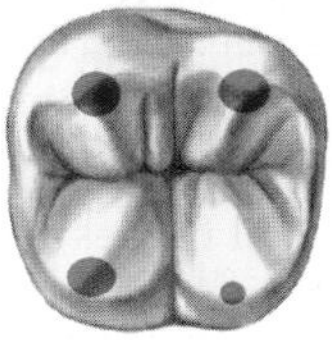	Caries or restoration on the incisal edge of anterior teeth or the cusp tips of posterior teeth

Figures from Bird DL, Robinson DS: *Modern dental assisting,* ed 10, St Louis, 2012, Saunders, an imprint of Elsevier Inc.

TABLE 16-9

Simple, Compound, and Complex Designations for Dental Caries and Restorations

Simple	Abbreviation	Compound	Abbreviation	Complex	Abbreviation
Buccal	B	Mesio-occlusal	MO	Mesioincisodistal	MID
Facial	F	Disto-occlusal	DO	Mesiolinguodistal	MLD
Gingival	G	Occlusobuccal	OB	Mesio-occlusobuccal	MOB
Incisal	I	Distolingual	DL	Mesio-occlusodistal	MOD
Lingual	Li	Disto-occlusal	DO	Mesio-occlusodistobuccolingual	MODBL
Labial	La				
Occlusal	O				

BOX 16-3

Sequential Approach for Dentition Charting

Using the charting symbols outlined in Table 16-10 the following provides a sequential approach to dentition charting.

1. **Tooth identification and position:** Chart all problematic teeth, such as those missing, unerupted, drifted, and rotated, before recording specific tooth-by-tooth information. Use radiographs to chart all unerupted or impacted teeth.
2. **Tooth damage:** Chart signs of tooth damage (dental caries, risk areas, attrition).
3. **Restorative:** Chart existing restorations amalgam, tooth-colored, and temporary restorations; inlays, onlays, and gold foils; crowns, veneers, bridges, and prothestic appliances.
4. **Update the dentition charting** at each re-care visit, and record any areas of change.

now being questioned because the explorer may do the following:

- Rupture remineralizing enamel crystals, causing early carious lesions to become cavitated
- Transfer cariogenic microorganisms from tooth to tooth via the explorer[5]
- Stick or tug back owing to wedging in narrow and deep pits and fissures rather than because of caries
- Fail to reach the base of the pit or fissure owing to narrow, deep pit and fissure morphology, causing the clinician to miss an active carious lesion
- Not improve pit and fissure caries detection compared with visual inspection alone based on evidence-based research findings

Therefore current thinking is that an explorer should not be used when suspected carious lesions are observed visually or on known sensitive areas.[6,7]

Moreover, in terms of caries detection, tooth color is not a foolproof sign of dental caries, because carious dentin can range in color from nearly white to shades of black. If a dark area on a tooth is hard, regardless of the color, it is rarely an active carious lesion. The caries process often undermines otherwise intact enamel, producing a "pearly" appearance. In this case, color may be an indicator of the extent of the carious lesion. Marginal ridges, especially in anterior teeth, should be examined under a well-directed light. The careful use of a nonmagnifying, front-surface mirror for transillumination may show signs of undermining decay, which then can be substantiated by the dentist.

Developing new technologies complement traditional methods of caries diagnosis. The aim of new technologies is to provide objective information about the presence and severity of a lesion. Use of new caries detection technologies complements the clinician's largely subjective diagnosis when conducting a visual examination aided by dental radiographs. It has been well established that by the time dental caries is observed visually or radiographically it is often deeper and larger than it appears and may not be receptive to remineralization strategies.[8] Therefore the aim of using new caries detection devices is as adjunctive techniques used with traditional diagnosis methods to diagnosis caries earlier, implement preventive strategies to promote remineralization and monitor the effectiveness of the interventions by assessing the state of the lesion over time.[8] Table 16-10 presents a few technologies currently available to clinicians.

Radiographic Assessment

Bitewing radiographs (radiographs that include images of the crown and about half of the roots of several posterior teeth in both arches) are standard diagnostic tools for posterior teeth. Bitewing radiographs produce the best image of the tooth crowns, the main area of concern for dental caries and tooth restoration. Dental caries just under the contact between teeth is detected best with bitewing radiographs. Carious lesions appear as radiolucent (black) images on radiographs because dental caries causes localized demineralization and loss of tooth tissue (Figure 16-16). Depending on their density, restorative materials produce relatively radiopaque (white) images. Because of the contrast between the oral tissues and the restorative materials, radiographs readily illustrate the fit and contours of restorations. For example, all suspected overhanging margins of fillings can be verified by radiographs (Figure 16-17).

Periapical radiographs (radiographs that include the tips of roots of teeth in a single arch) may be used for anterior and

TABLE 16-10

Technologies Available for Dental Caries Detection

Technology	Description	Mechanism of Action	Advantages	Disadvantages
Fiber-optic transillumination (FOTI)	A light probe is placed at the gingival edge below the cervical margin of the tooth.[8]	Light passes through the tooth structure and produces a dark shadow. Carious enamel absorbs more light than sound enamel and gives a darker appearance.[8]	The light source used is readily available in dental offices.[8]	Not useful for monitoring caries and it is not sensitive enough to detect early caries.[8]
Digital imaging fiber-optic transillumination (DFOTI)	A computerized version of FOTI; a computer system with monitor, mirror, and light source.[8]	Shines a concentrated beam of visible light on the tooth and, via a mirror, the computer system captures an image on the other side of the tooth that is seen on the computer monitor. Allows for the detection of optical changes at or near the surfaces such as cracks.	A useful adjunct to radiographic assessment and clinical decision making. The computer stores the images and can be compared to future images.	Only measures optical changes near the tooth surface. Does not quantify the images and therefore the examiner makes a subjective analysis based on the appearance of the stored images.[9]
Quantitative light-induced fluorescence (QLF)	A computer system with repositioning software built into the system to enable lesions to be monitored over time.	Blue light shines on the tooth; the enamel is transparent to this light wave length. The dentin fluoresces with the blue light, and the fluorescence passes back through the enamel. A carious lesion is indicated by an area of little or no fluorescence. The system measures the percentage of change in the demineralized defects and produces an image that can be quantified and compared over time.	Can be used for the early detection of carious lesions and for monitoring of demineralization and remineralization of white spots by quantifying the mineral loss and the size of smooth surface lesions. Able to detect surface changes very early, and shows great promise for tracking chemical treatments of early carious lesions over time.[8]	It cannot distinguish between caries, tooth stains, or white spots such as fluorosis and as a result may give false positive results.[8]
DIAGNOdent laser system	Laser fluorescence device with a solid-state diode laser that detects and measures changes in tooth structure.[8]	How it works is not fully understood; two theories exist: **1.** When red incident light connects with the increased porosity of demineralized tooth it stimulates fluorescent light of a different wavelength and this fluorescent light is analyzed. **2.** Metabolites of cariogenic bacteria emit fluorescence. The DIAGNOdent measures the level of cariogenic bacterial activity and works on the assumption that if there is a high level of bacteria there is a high probability of having decalcified enamel.[8]	Useful adjunct to conventional visual and tactile detection methods for lesions on the occlusal surface. The reading gives a guideline when to intervene with preventive measures and the lesions can be monitored at subsequent recall.[8]	There are many substances that can cause fluorescence including stains, plaque and calculus, prophy paste and food, and also some cariogenic bacteria do not produce fluorescence.[8] Therefore in the aforementioned order this can give false positive or false negative results.
Electrical caries monitor (ECM)	Battery powered device with low frequency output of 21 Hz. The ECM probe is directly applied to the tooth typically on an occlusal fissure, and the site is measured.	This technology is based on the differences in electrical conductivity between demineralized and sound enamel. Demineralized enamel has greater porosity and the electrical conductivity increases.	ECM has the potential to monitor lesion progression in depth and mineral content of the enamel. It has good sensitivity in detecting occlusal caries.[9]	It is time consuming and not very feasible to use in a standard dental examination appointment.[8] Also a number of other factors can affect results such as tooth temperature, thickness of enamel and the tissue, the hydration or dryness of the teeth.[9]

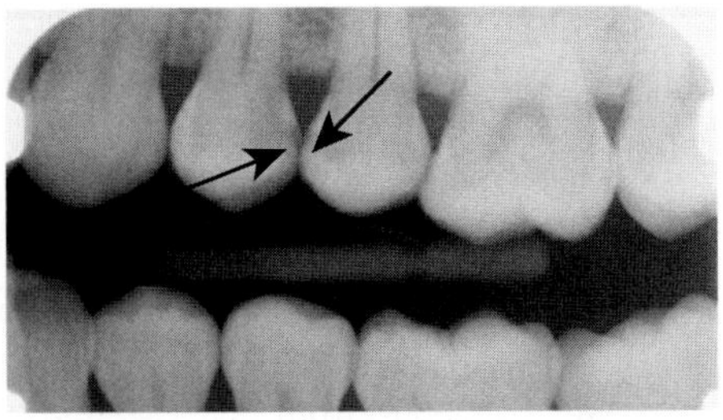

Figure 16-16. Premolar bitewing radiograph. *Arrows* point to sign of proximal dental caries between No. 12 and No. 13. (From Daniel SJ, Harfst SA, Wilder RS: *Mosby's dental hygiene,* ed 2, St Louis, 2008, Mosby.)

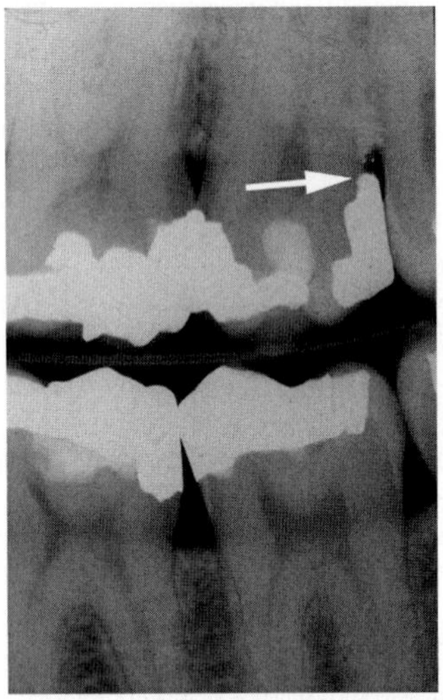

Figure 16-17. Portion of a bitewing radiograph showing restorations and amalgam overhang on the distal surface of maxillary second molar. (From Newman MG, Takei HH, Klokkevold PR, Carranza FA: *Carranza's clinical periodontology,* ed 11, St Louis, 2012, Saunders.)

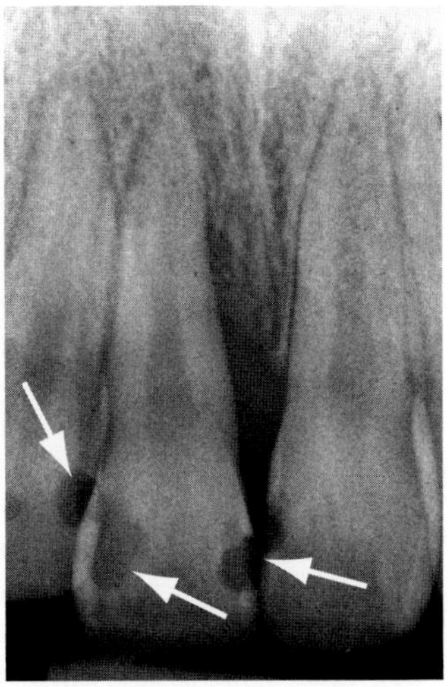

Figure 16-18. Maxillary anterior periapical radiograph. *Arrows* point to signs of dental caries. (From Newman MG, Takei HH, Klokkevold PR, Carranza FA: *Carranza's clinical periodontology,* ed 11, St Louis, 2012, Saunders.)

BOX 16-4

Questions to Determine Quality of Pain

- General: "Tell me about your pain."
- Provoking factors: "Does heat (cold, biting, or chewing) initiate the pain?" (Ask each separately to avoid confusing the client.)
- Attenuating factors: "Does anything relieve the pain?"
- Intensity: "When you have pain, is it mild, moderate, or severe?"
- Location: "Please point to the tooth or area that hurts."
- Duration: "How long does the pain last?"
- Postural: "Do you have any pain when you lie down? Bend over?"
- Quality: "What is the nature of the pain? Sharp? Dull? Stabbing? Throbbing?"

posterior teeth if they are determined to be necessary during the clinical examination (Figure 16-18). In addition, periapical radiographs are required of any tooth in which the health of the pulp and the tip of the root are in question (see Chapter 32).

Client Symptom Assessment

Client report of pain elicited by sugar intake, sensitivity to changes in temperature, and objectionable taste are frequently a result of advanced carious lesions or leaking or defective restorations. Tooth abrasions and erosions may be sensitive to toothbrushing, acidic foods, and cold stimuli. Fractures of teeth may elicit sharp pain during chewing and contact with cold foods. When pain is reported, questioning the client is an important way to gain information about location, duration, postural changes, and qualities of the pain.[10] Questioning should begin with an open-ended question such as, "Tell me about your pain," followed by more specific questions that focus on provoking factors, attenuating factors, frequency, and intensity (Box 16-4). These questions can be followed by further exploration in which the client is asked to expand on previous responses.

Client symptoms are essential to the dental diagnosis and are communicated to the dentist immediately. Factors indicating the need for immediate referral to a dentist for an endodontic diagnosis are listed in Box 16-5.

BOX 16-5

Factors Related to Dental Diagnosis of a Periapical (Endodontic) Abscess

- Sharp, severe, intermittent pain that may be hard to localize
- Clinical and/or radiographic evidence of tooth damage such as caries, tooth fracture, or defective restorations
- Observation of soft tissue redness or swelling and presence of a fistula (sinus tract drainage)
- A rounded radiolucency at the apex of the tooth
- Pulpal vitality test results
- Facial asymmetry caused by swelling
- Skin lesions (occasionally facial lesions may be traced to a tooth source, for example, sinus tract drainage)

Although thermal testing using hot or cold appliances is used to detect vital pulp tissue, electric pulp testers are considered more reliable. Electric pulp testing is based on electric stimulation to create pain to which one can react

(Procedure 16-1). The Competency Form for Evaluation of Electronic Pulp Testing procedures can be found on the Evolve site at http://evolve.elsevier.com/Darby/hygiene. Electric pulp testing may not always be accurate because pulp vitality depends on blood supply, not nerves (Box 16-6).

BOX 16-6

Factors That Affect Client Response to Pulp Testing

- Necrotic pulp: A necrotic pulp gives no response.
- Pulpal inflammation: An inflamed pulp responds in varying degrees from no response to a full normal response depending on degree of inflammation.
- Blockage of nerve transmission: Anesthetics or injury to nerves blocks nerve transmission.
- Metal restorations: Metal restorations or bridgework adjacent to tooth being tested can form a circuit that bypasses the tooth in question.
- Pain perception: Client's reaction to pain depends on such things as pain threshold, premedication, the size of the pulp, and the thickness of dentin, especially secondary dentin.

Dentition and Periodontal Charting

Charting tooth assessment data is conducted at the client's initial assessment appointment and updated at each reappointment. Although no set sequences are required for charting, a systematic approach avoids omitting important information (see Box 16-3 and Box 16-7). Table 16-11 outlines dentition charting symbols, and Table 16-12 outlines periodontal charting symbols from axiUm **dental software** program from Exan Group. (See Evolve site for charting symbols for paper charting.)

Occlusion

Thorough assessment of the dentition includes classifying occlusion and documenting any teeth malrelationships present. (See also Chapter 59.) **Occlusion** is defined as the contact relationship between maxillary and mandibular teeth when the jaws are in a fully closed position, as well as the relationship between the teeth in the same arch. As the primary teeth erupt in the child, occlusion develops and is influenced by the development of facial muscles and

Text continued on p. 274

Procedure 16-1 Use of an Electric Pulp Tester to Determine Pulp Vitality

EQUIPMENT

Personal protective equipment
2 × 2 gauze
Saliva ejector
Cotton rolls
Toothpaste
Electric pulp tester

STEPS

1. Assemble equipment.
2. Review health history.
3. Describe the test's purpose and methods.
4. Explain that the client may feel a tingling or a warm sensation.
5. Identify the suspected tooth and a "control" tooth (preferably an adjacent tooth or the same tooth on the opposite side of the arch) to be tested, then dry these teeth and isolate them with cotton rolls (Figure 16-19).
6. Instruct client to raise a hand or make a sound on feeling a sensation.
7. Set the dial (current level) on the tester to zero.
8. Place a thin layer of toothpaste on the tip of the tester.
9. Test the control tooth first.
10. Apply moistened tip, without pressure but with definite contact, first to the control tooth (Figure 16-20).
11. Place tip on sound tooth structure on the middle third of the crown of a single-rooted tooth and the middle third of each cusp of a multi-rooted tooth.
12. Avoid contact with gingival or other soft tissue.
13. Avoid contact with metallic restorations.
14. Insert a nonconductive plastic matrix strip to separate two metallic restorations.
15. Start with the rheostat at zero and advance slowly but steadily, stopping only momentarily after each number.
16. Test each tooth at least twice. Average the readings.
17. Repeat the procedure on the tooth in question.
18. Record in client's chart the pulp tester used and the lowest number (average) at which a minimal stimulus induced a response for all teeth tested.

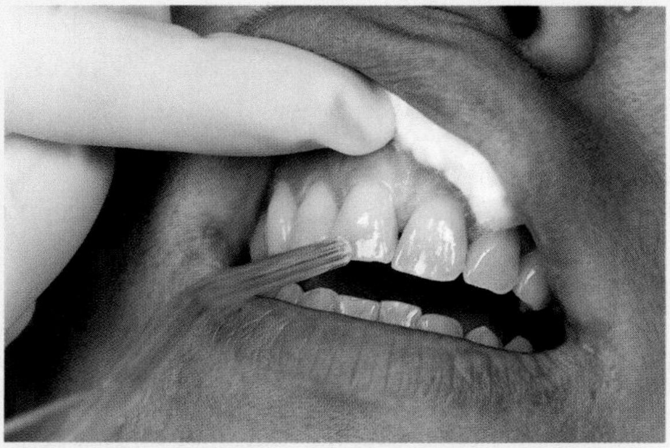

Figure 16-19. (From Bird DL, Robinson DS: *Modern dental assisting,* ed 11, St Louis, 2015, Saunders.)

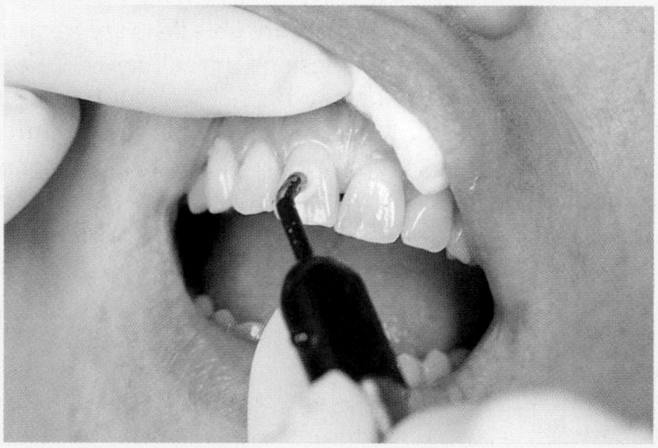

Figure 16-20. (From Bird DL, Robinson DS: Modern dental assisting, ed 11, St Louis, 2015, Saunders.)

BOX 16-7

Sequential Approach for Periodontal Charting

Using the periodontal charting symbols outlined in Table 16-11 the following provides a sequential approach to periodontal charting. For procedural instructions to conduct the following periodontal examination techniques refer to Chapter 19.

1. **Pocket depth:** Measure probing depth on six sites on each tooth.
2. **Bleeding on probing:** Score bleeding points on affected surfaces.
3. **Recession:** Measure free gingival margin to cementoenamel junction: Enter a number for six sites on each tooth.
4. **Clinical attachment loss:** Score a measurement for six sites on each tooth.
5. **Furcations:** Enter the numeric class at the affected site.
6. **Mucogingival involvement:** Enter a Y (Yes) for affected sites.
7. **Mobility:** Enter the numerical class on affected tooth.
8. **Plaque:** Enter a Y (Yes) at affected sites.
9. **Update the periodontal charting at each re-care visit.**

TABLE 16-11

Dentition Charting Symbols

Term	Explanation	Symbol
Tooth Identification and Position		
Missing tooth	Tooth not present because of extraction or congenitally missing	M 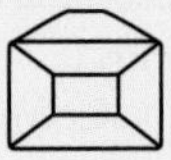
Unerupted or partially erupted tooth	Tooth that has not erupted	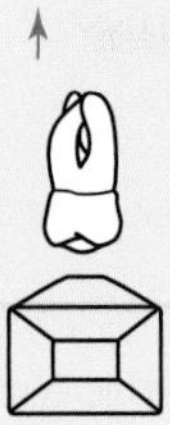
Extruded	Tooth that has erupted past the line of occlusion	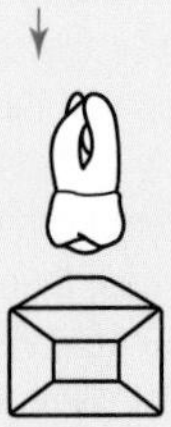
Impacted	Tooth that has not erupted because of impaction	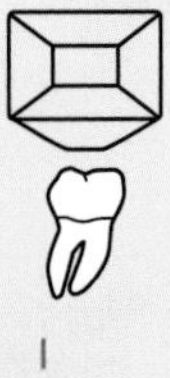
Drifting	Tooth that has shifted from normal position because of missing teeth	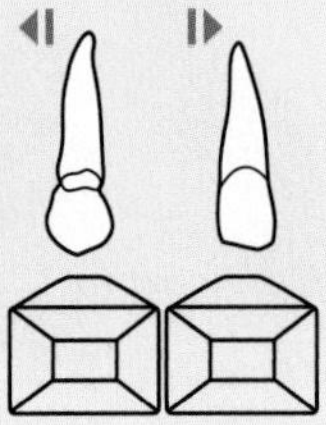

TABLE 16-11
Dentition Charting Symbols—cont'd

Term	Explanation	Symbol
Diastemas	A gap or space between two teeth	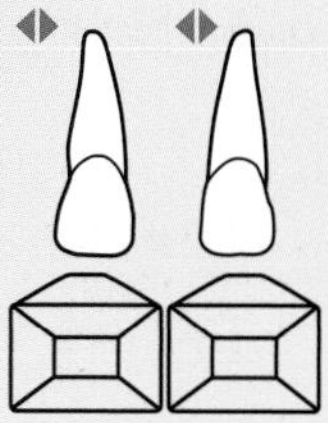
Rotations	The turning of a tooth around its longitudinal axis	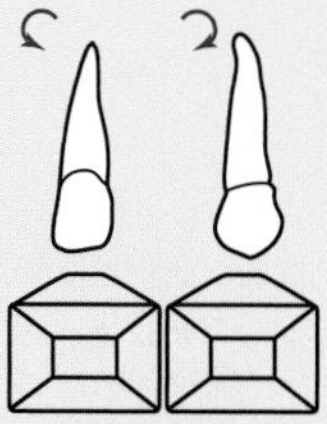
Crowding	Teeth too close together that have abnormal positions such as overlapping or displacement in various directions	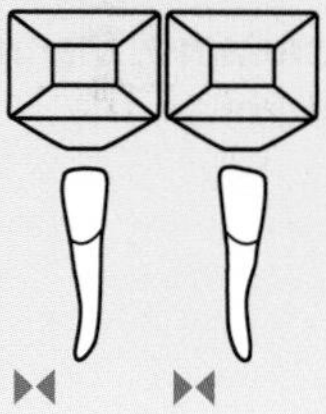
Tooth Damage		
Abrasion	Tooth that exhibits mechanical wear from improper toothbrushing or other abrasive habits	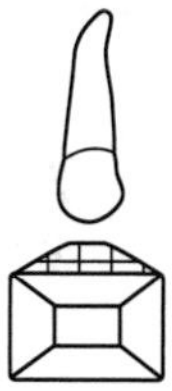
Attrition	Incisal or occlusal surfaces that exhibit wear from occlusal forces	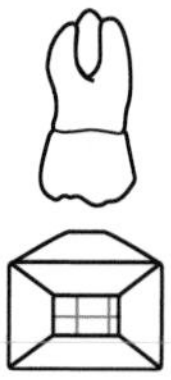
Caries	Surfaces exhibiting caries	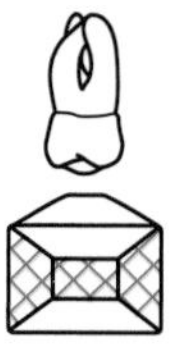
Incipient caries	Areas that have not cavitated and may be remineralized	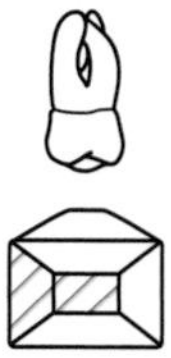

Continued

TABLE 16-11

Dentition Charting Symbols—cont'd

Term	Explanation	Symbol
Observation (watch)	An incipient lesion that has not cavitated and may be remineralized	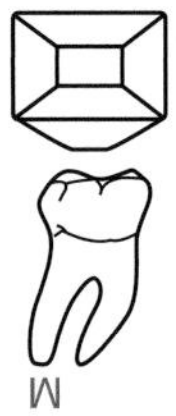
Fracture	Areas of a tooth that have broken because of trauma or extensive caries	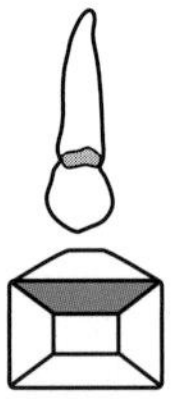
Restorative Therapy		
Amalgam	Alloy of silver and mercury	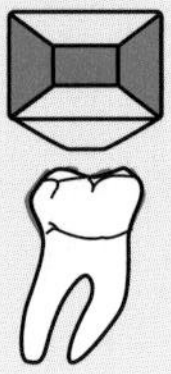
Tooth–Colored Restorations		
Composite resin	Tooth-colored restorative material commonly found on anterior teeth and an acceptable option to amalgam on posterior teeth	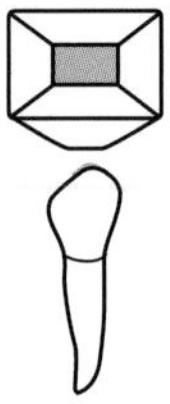
Ceramic/ceramic-metal crowns	Acrylic or porcelain facing bonded over white-gold alloy crown	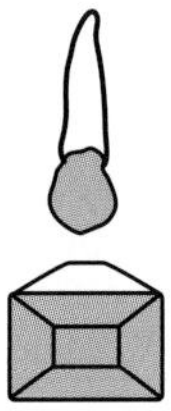
Veneer	Layer of porcelain used on the facial surfaces of teeth	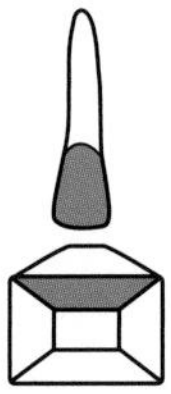
Metal Casting		
A. Full high noble and noble (gold)	Cast yellow-gold crown covering the entire surface or three-quarter crown covering less than three fourths of the surface	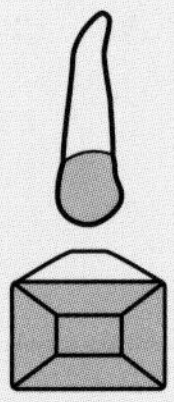

TABLE 16-11

Dentition Charting Symbols—cont'd

Term	Explanation	Symbol
B. Inlay	Cast yellow-gold restoration that does not extend over the cusps	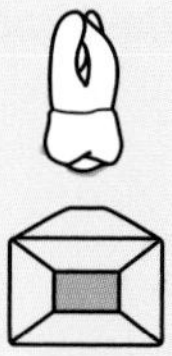
C. Onlay	Cast yellow-gold restoration that extends over the cusp tips	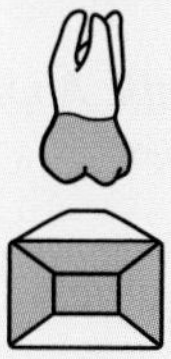
D. Fixed crown and bridge (gold or porcelain)	Functional unit that serves to replace one or missing teeth; consists of an abutment and pontic that are splinted together	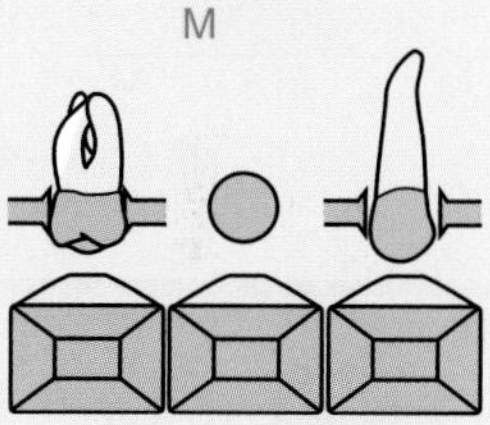
Temporary: restorations crowns	Placed as an intermediary during crown preparation, root canal therapy, or misplaced restoration	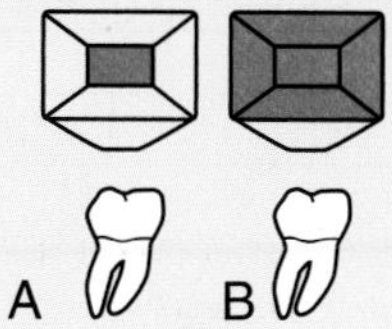
Root canal	A dental procedure to fix a tooth by removing the pulp tissue of the tooth and filling it with a suitable filling material	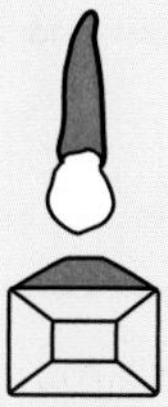
Stainless steel crown	Cast stainless steel crown covering entire tooth surface. Typically prefabricated	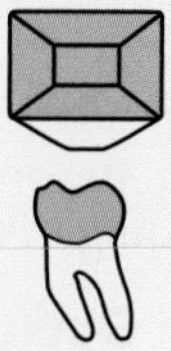
Implants	A surgically placed (osseointegrated) functional replacement for one or more missing teeth; composed of the anchor, abutment, and prosthetic tooth or appliance	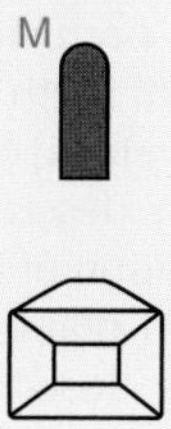
Preventive Therapy		
Sealants	A clear or tinted resin coating that is bonded to the tooth in the pits and fissures	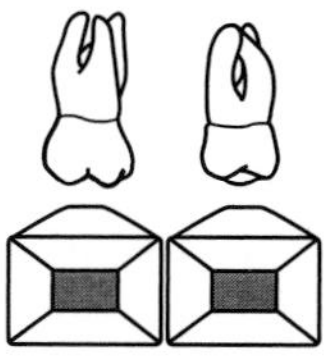

Continued

TABLE 16-11
Dentition Charting Symbols—cont'd

Term	Explanation	Symbol
Faulty Restorations		
Deficient or open margins	Restorations margins that are deficient or open will encourage microbial plaque retention and microleakage and should be replaced.	Make a note in comment section on chart.
Overhangs (Class I, II, or III)	An extension of restorative material beyond the curvature of the tooth; classified by the size of the extension; can be detected both clinically and radiographically.	Make a note in comment section on chart.
Prosthetic Appliances		
Full denture	Removable appliance that replaces missing teeth of an entire arch or both arches.	
Partial denture	Removable appliance that replaces missing teeth.	

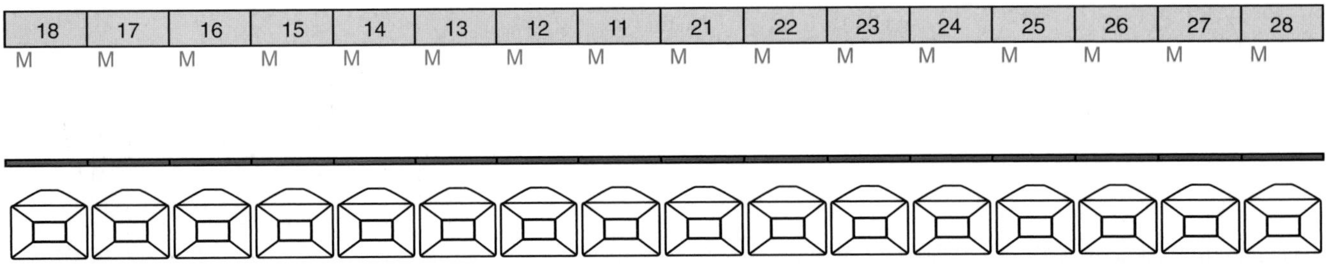

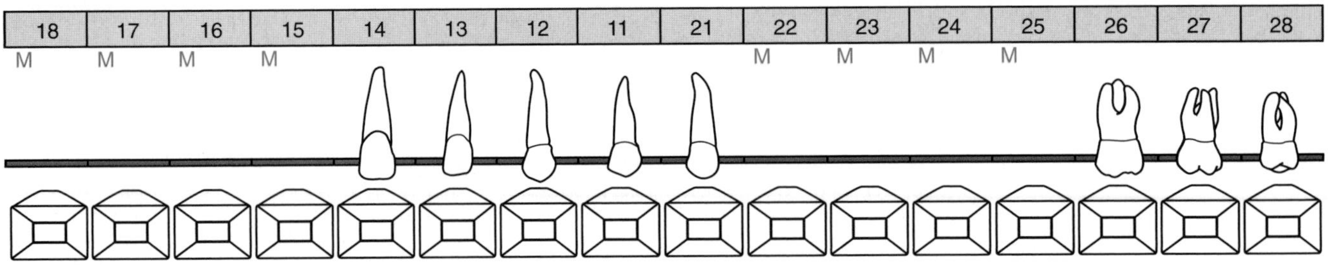

Charting symbols courtesy of axiUm dental software program from Exan Group.

neuromuscular patterns. Among the factors influencing occlusion, the eruption of the permanent teeth is affected by the shedding of the primary teeth.

Centric Occlusion

An ideal occlusion with 138 occlusal contacts when the 32 permanent teeth are in closure, rarely, if ever, exists. Consequently, centric occlusion serves as the standard point of reference for describing a normal occlusion. **Centric occlusion** is the relation of opposing occlusal surfaces that provides the maximum planned contact and/or intercuspation when the teeth are closed. It should exist when the mandible is in centric relation to the maxilla. When the teeth of a normal occlusion are in centric position, each tooth of one arch is in occlusion with two teeth in the opposite arch, except for the mandibular central incisors and the maxillary third molars. This positioning of the teeth equalizes the forces of occlusion. Because of this arrangement, the alignment of the opposing jaw is not disturbed immediately if a tooth is lost. However, if restorative treatment is not performed for a long period, the neighboring teeth begin to drift mesially in an effort to fill the space. The teeth become tilted, and supereruption of the tooth opposite the space in the opposing arch occurs. Thus the loss of one tooth can change the occlusion of the entire dentition.

When teeth do not occlude (come together) properly, unnatural stress is placed on them and the periodontium so that they may be unable to perform their functions. This occlusal disharmony may lead to pain and/or occlusal trauma. Although occlusal trauma does not cause periodontal disease directly, it may be an adverse factor in an already diseased periodontium. An important role of the dental hygienist is to explain to clients the importance of tooth replacement to prevent occlusal disharmonies. To prevent occlusal disharmonies, all clients should have an occlusal evaluation by the dentist before and after completion of their dental treatment.[11]

Overjet

When teeth normally come together in centric occlusion, there is a horizontal projection of the upper teeth beyond the lower teeth, usually measured parallel to the occlusal plane.

TABLE 16-12
Periodontal Charting*

<table>
<tr><th>Term</th><th>Explanation</th><th>Notation/Symbol</th></tr>
<tr><td>Probing depth</td><td>Probing depth is denoted in mm on six sites on each tooth. Program automatically depicts pocket or sulcus status.</td><td>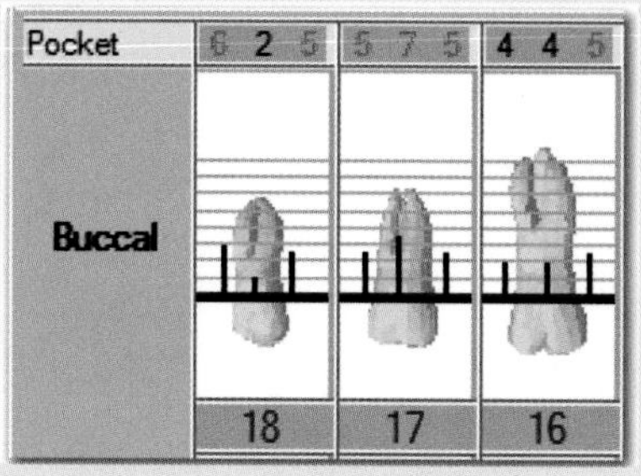
</td></tr>
<tr><td>Bleeding on probing</td><td>Bleeding points are indicated by red asterisks on affected surfaces.</td><td>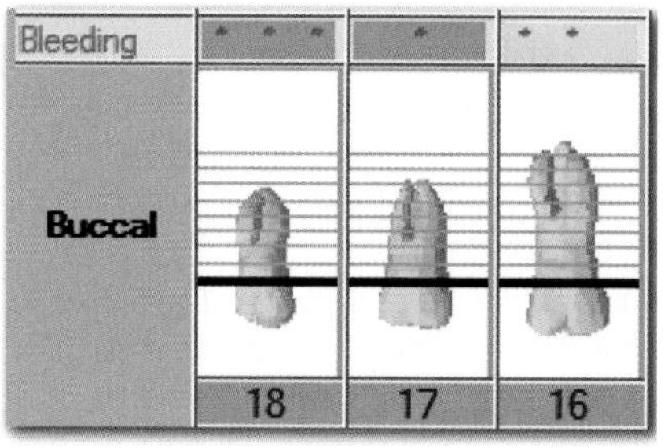
</td></tr>
<tr><td>Recession: Free gingival margin to cementoenamel junction</td><td>(+ #) a. recession
(– #) b. edematous tissue
Enter a number for six sites on each tooth. The program will automatically depict affected sites.</td><td>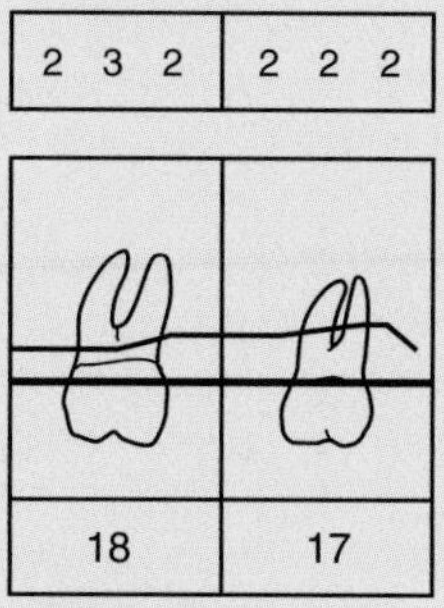

a. Recession
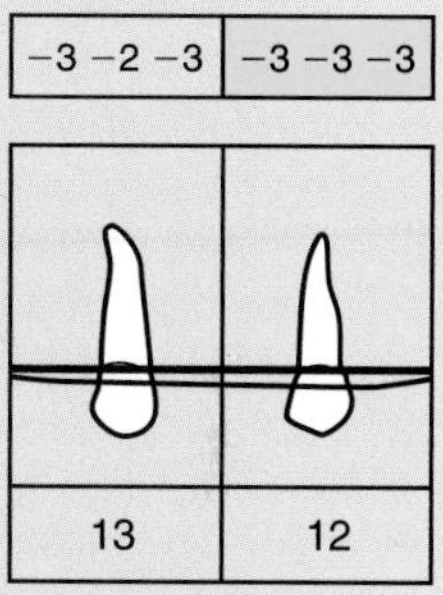

b. Edema</td></tr>
<tr><td>Clinical attachment level:
The position of the attached periodontal tissues at the base of the pocket in relation to the CEJ. This includes location of the gingival margin, probing depth, and recession measurements.</td><td>Enter a number for six sites on each tooth.</td><td>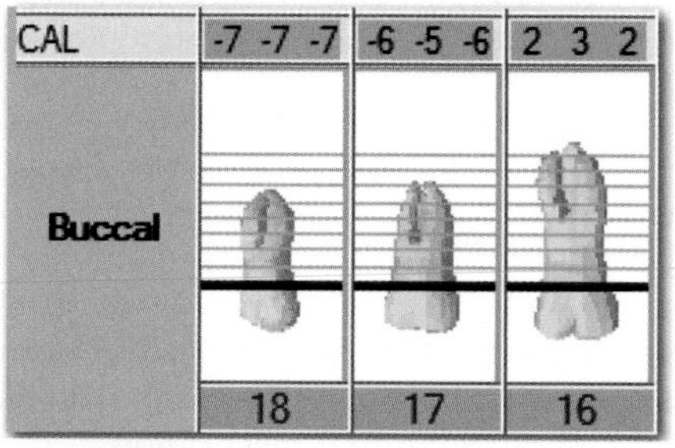
</td></tr>
<tr><td>Classifications of furcation:
<u>Class I</u> Concavity of furcation can be detected with an explorer or probe, but cannot be entered.
<u>Class 2</u> Can enter furcation from one aspect with a probe or explorer but cannot penetrate through to opposite side.
<u>Class 3</u> Can enter furcation all the way through, but is still covered by soft tissue.
<u>Class 4</u> Can enter furcation all the way through, but is not covered by soft tissue.</td><td>Class number is denoted by the numeric class at the affected site. Programs may use Arabic or Roman numerals.</td><td>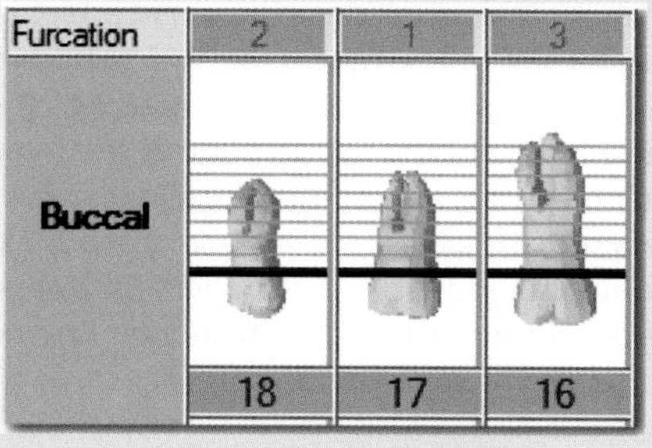
</td></tr>
</table>

Continued

TABLE 16-12
Periodontal Charting—cont'd

Term	Explanation	Notation/Symbol
Mucogingival involvement	Is denoted by a Y (Yes) for affected sites.	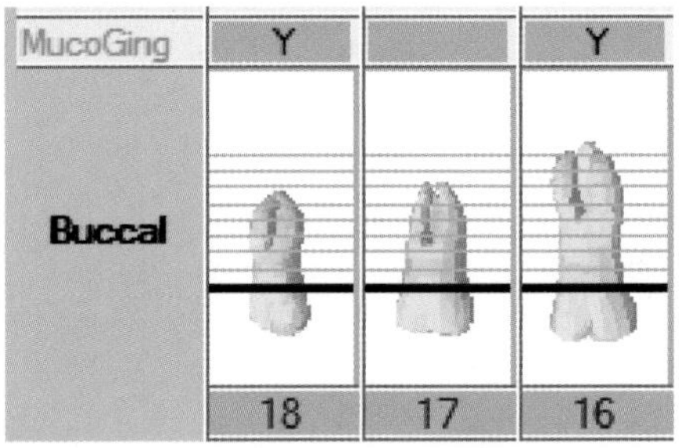
Mobility Classification of Mobility: ***Class I*** Tooth can be moved up to 1 mm in any direction. ***Class 2*** Tooth can be moved more than 1 mm in any direction. ***Class 3*** Tooth can be moved in buccolingual direction and is depressible in the socket.	Is denoted by the numeric class on affected tooth.	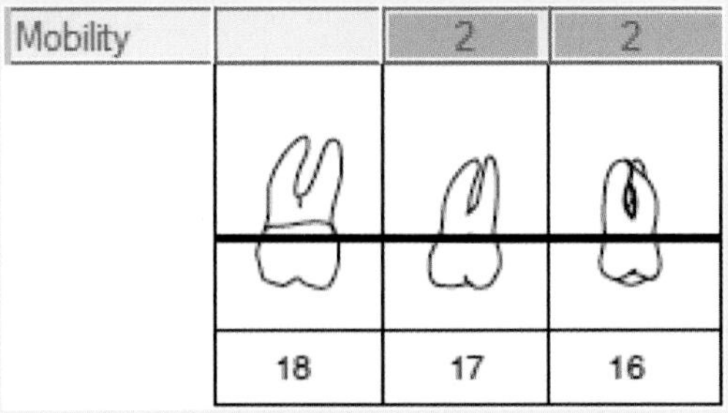
Plaque	Is denoted by a Y (Yes) at affected sites.	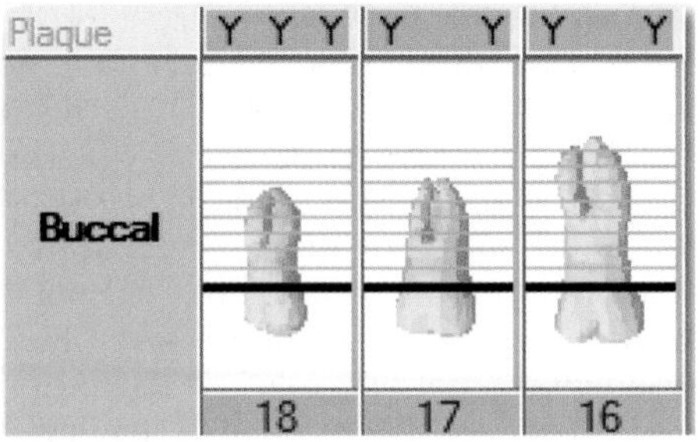

Charting symbols courtesy of axiUm dental software program from Exan Group.

*Periodontal charting is completed on a separate electronic odontogram. Standard periodontal charting notations may include those found in this table.

This is termed overjet (Figure 16-21). This normal horizontal overlap is important because it keeps the soft tissue out of the way of the mandible during mastication.

Overjet is measured when the client's teeth are closed in centric occlusion and the tip of the periodontal probe is placed at a right angle to the labial surface of the mandibular incisor at the base of the incisal edge of the maxillary incisor. The measurement is taken from the labial surface of the mandibular incisor to the lingual surface of the maxillary incisor. The labiolingual width of the maxillary incisor is not included in the recorded measurement. The dental hygienist measures and records the overlap in millimeters.

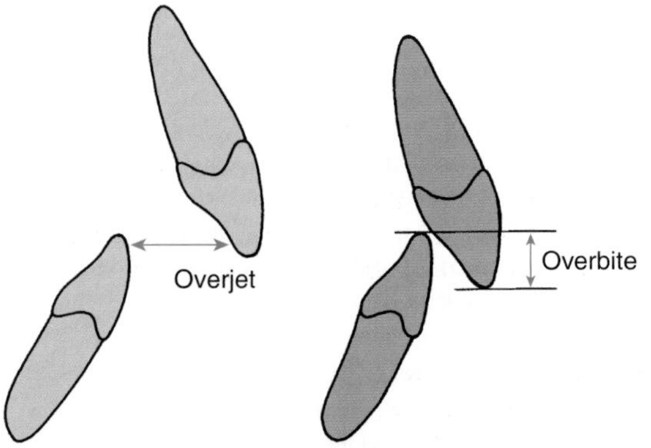

Figure 16-21. Measuring overjet, the horizontal overlap between the two arches, and overbite, the vertical overlap between the two arches. (Adapted from Proffit WR, Fields HW, Sarver DM: *Contemporary orthodontics,* ed 5, St Louis, 2013 by Mosby, an imprint of Elsevier Inc.)

Overbite

In centric occlusion the maxillary incisors vertically overlap the mandibular incisors, a position called overbite. This vertical overlap allows maximum contact between the posterior

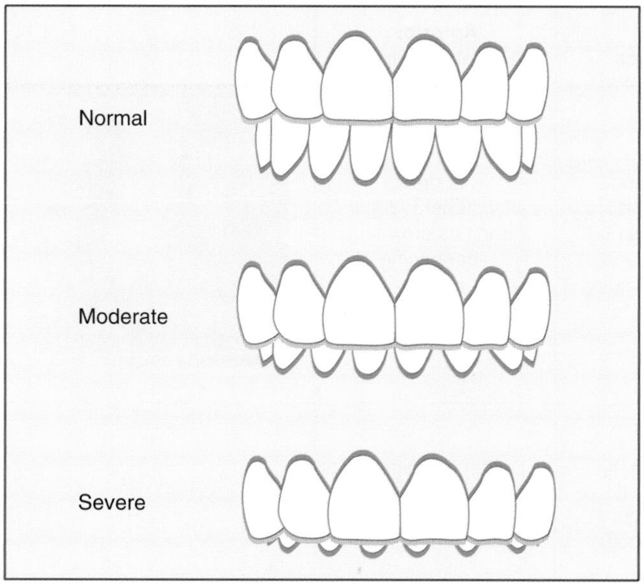

Figure 16-22. Classification of overbite.

teeth during mastication. Overbite is classified as normal, moderate, or severe based on the depth of the overlap. Overbite is considered normal if the maxillary incisors overlap within the incisal third of the mandibular incisors. Moderate overbite occurs when the maxillary incisors overlap to the middle third of the mandibular incisors, and severe overlap when the incisal edges of the maxillary teeth reach the gingival third of the mandibular incisors (Figure 16-22).

Overbite is measured when the client's maxillary and mandibular teeth are closed in centric occlusion. The tip of the periodontal probe is placed at the incisal edge of the maxillary incisor at right angles to the mandibular incisor. As the client slightly opens his or her mouth, the probe then is placed vertically against the mandibular incisor to measure the distance to the incisal edge of the mandibular incisor. It is customary to measure the overbite in millimeters or percentage and to include a classification of normal, moderate, or severe with the recorded measurement. These variations should be documented in writing on the client's chart.[11]

Centric Relation

Centric relation is the relation of the mandible to the maxilla when the condyles are in their most posterosuperior unstrained positions in the fossae. This position allows for lateral movements to be made at the occluding vertical relation normal for the individual. Ideally the mandible is in centric relation when the dentition is in centric occlusion. Usually the teeth slide about 1 mm when clients shift their occlusion from centric relation to centric occlusion.[11]

Contact Areas

In the ideal dental arch are contact areas where the teeth touch their same arch neighbor on their proximal surfaces. These contact areas protect the interdental gingiva and stabilize each tooth in the dental arch. When there is no contact area between teeth, these open contacts can trap food, resulting in gingival inflammation. The use of floss is an effective tool, along with radiographs, in assessing the status of an open contact. The client also may report food impaction issues. Open contacts must be called to the attention of the dentist for evaluation and treatment.[11]

Normal Occlusion

In the late 1800s Dr. Edward H. Angle established a system of classification of occlusion. Angle's method of classification was based on the principle that the maxillary first molars are the keys to occlusion. Because of their stability within the dental arch, the permanent first molars and later the canines were added as the indicator teeth to assess the relationship between the maxilla and the mandible. In a normal molar relationship the mesiobuccal cusp of the maxillary permanent first molar occludes with the buccal groove of the mandibular permanent first molar. In a normal canine relationship the maxillary permanent canine occludes with the distal half of the mandibular permanent canine and the mesial half of the mandibular first premolar.

Malocclusion

Malocclusion is a deviation of the maxillary and mandibular relations of teeth and a lack of overall ideal form in the dentition while in centric occlusion. In addition, excessive overjet or overbite is classified as malocclusion.

Malocclusion may have a negative effect on the client's personal appearance and may make it more difficult for the client to perform effective oral hygiene. Plaque biofilm initiates periodontal disease; therefore individuals with malocclusion are at increased risk for this disease, and malocclusion also may contribute to temporomandibular joint pain. As part of the dental hygiene assessment, occlusion is classified on both the right and left sides of the dentition. Malocclusion and temporomandibular joint dysfunctions, such as pain or popping on opening and closing the mandible, are referred to the dentist for further evaluation (see Chapter 59 for detailed discussion of malocclusion and orthodontic treatment).

In Angle's system there are three types of malocclusion in the permanent dentition: Class I, Class II, and Class III. Class II malocclusion is subclassified into divisions 1 and 2 (Figure 16-23).

Class I Malocclusion

In Class I malocclusion the molar and canine relationships are similar to those in normal occlusion. However, in Class I malocclusion there are malrelationships between individual teeth or groups of teeth. For example, there may be problems with crowding where the teeth are out of line within the dental arch. Some clients with Class I malocclusion have slight, moderate, or severe overbites, or an open bite in which the anterior teeth do not occlude. Some clients have an end-to-end bite in which the teeth occlude without the maxillary teeth overlapping the mandibular teeth, or a crossbite in which the maxillary teeth are positioned lingually to mandibular teeth, an abnormal buccolingual tooth position (Table 16-13). The facial profile associated with Class I malocclusion is classified as straight or orthognathic (see Figure 16-23).

Class II Malocclusion

Class II and III malocclusions are referred to as *skeletal malocclusions* because of the differences in size or the abnormal relationship between the maxilla and the mandible.

Occlusal Relationships in Centric Occlusion	Molar Relationships	Canine Relationships	Anterior Relationships	Face Profile
Normal occlusion 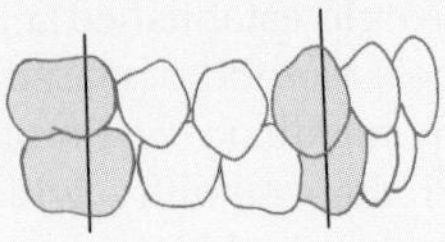	MB cusp of the maxillary first molar occludes with the MB groove of the mandibular first molar	Maxillary canine occludes with the distal half of the mandibular canine and the mesial half of the mandibular first premolar	No dental malalignments present, such as crowding or spacing	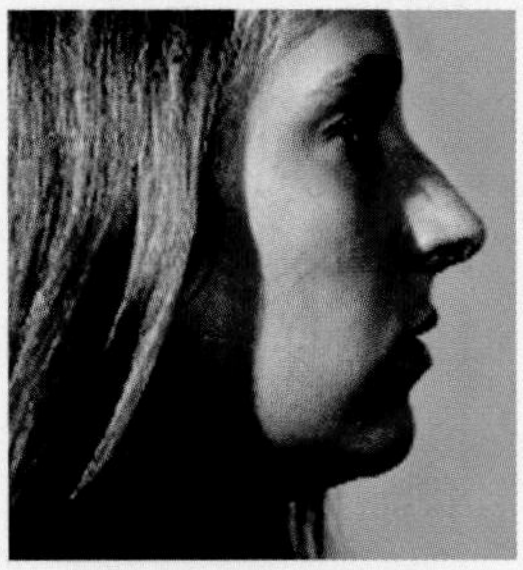 Mesognathic profile
Class I malocclusion 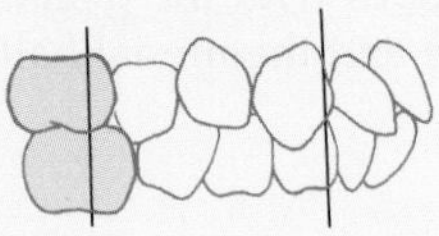	Same as above but malpositions of individual or groups of teeth may occur	Same as above but malpositions of individual or groups of teeth may occur	Dental malalignments present, such as crowding or spacing	Same as above
Class II Distal I malocclusion 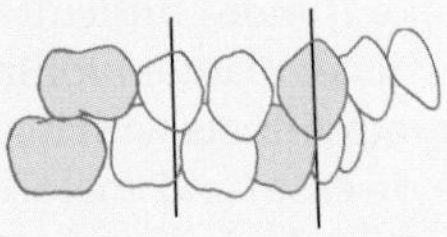	MB cusp of the maxillary first molar occludes (by more than the width of a premolar) mesial to the MB groove of the mandibular first molar	Distal surface of the mandibular canine is distal to the mesial surface of the maxillary canine by at least the width of a premolar	Maxillary anteriors protrude facially from the mandibular anteriors, with deep overbite	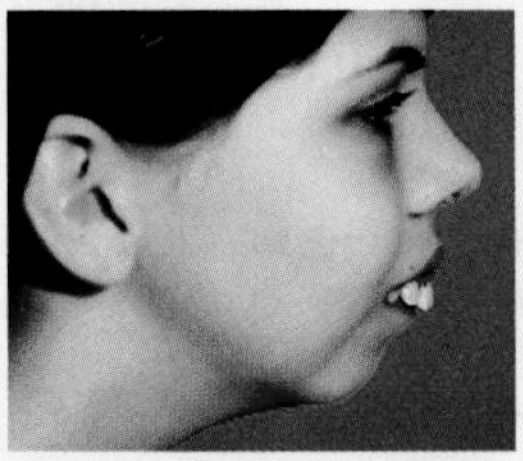 Retrognathic profile with lip incompetence
Class II Division II malocclusion 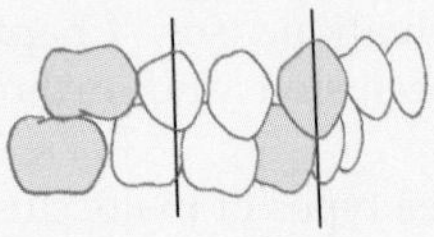	Same as Class II division 1	Same as Class II division 1	Maxillary central incisors are upright or retruded, and lateral incisors are tipped labially or overlap the central incisors with deep overbite	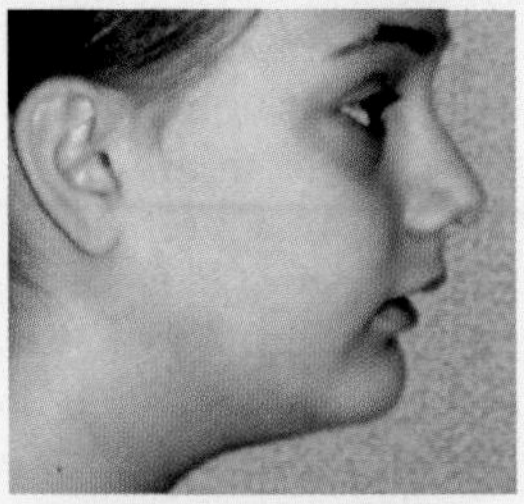 Retrognathic profile
Class III malocclusion 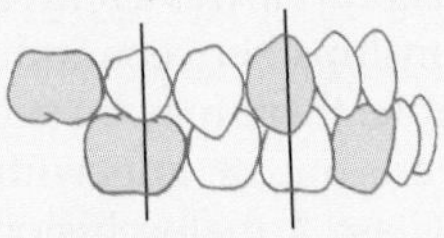	MB cusp of the maxillary first molar occludes (by more than the width of a premolar) distal to the MB groove of the mandibular first molar	Distal surface of the mandibular canine is mesial to the mesial surface of the maxillary canine by at least the width of a premolar	Mandibular incisors in complete crossbite	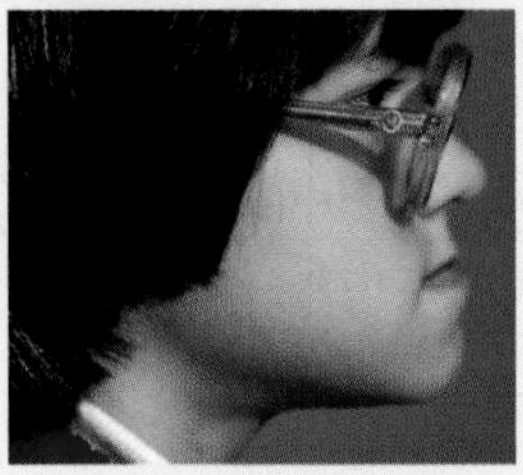 Prognathic profile

Figure 16-23. Classification of malocclusion. *MB*, Mesiobuccal. (Adapted from Bath-Balogh MB, Fehrenbach MJ: *Illustrated dental embryology, histology, and anatomy*, ed 3, St Louis, 2006, Saunders, an imprint of Elsevier Inc. Photographs from Proffit WR, Fields HW, Sarver DM: *Contemporary orthodontics*, ed 5, St Louis, 2013 by Mosby, an imprint of Elsevier Inc.)

Class II malocclusion, also referred to as *distal occlusion,* is characterized by the buccal groove of the mandibular first permanent molar being distal to the mesiobuccal cusp of the maxillary first permanent molar by at least the width of a premolar. The canine relationship is such that the distal surface of the mandibular permanent canine is distal to the mesial surface of the maxillary permanent canine by at least the width of a premolar. If the distance is less than the width of a premolar, it is classified as having a "tendency toward Class II." An individual with a Class II malocclusion usually

TABLE 16-13
Malrelationships of Individual Teeth or Groups of Teeth

Malrelationship	Description
Open bite	Abnormal vertical spaces between mandibular and maxillary teeth most frequently observed in the anterior teeth; however, may occur in posterior areas. 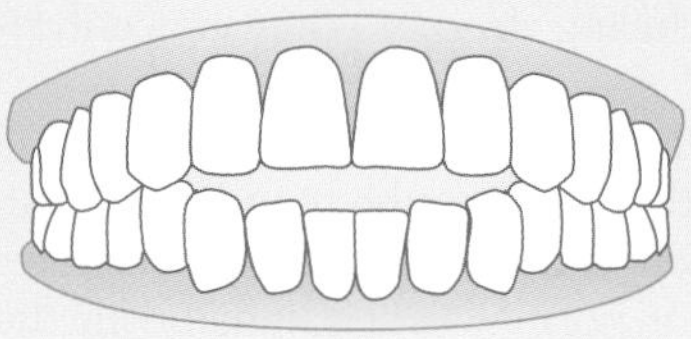
End-to-end (sometimes referred to as *edge-to-edge* in the anterior sextant)	The teeth occlude without the maxillary teeth overlapping the mandibular teeth. An end-to-end bite can occur anteriorly and posteriorly, unilaterally or bilaterally. 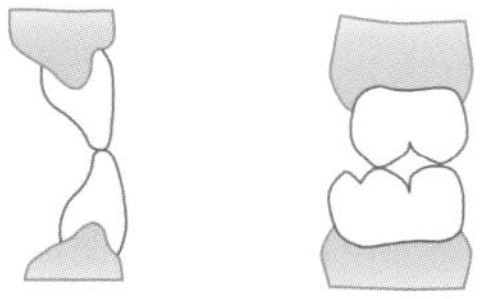
Crossbite	Maxillary teeth are positioned lingually to the mandibular teeth; may occur unilaterally or bilaterally. 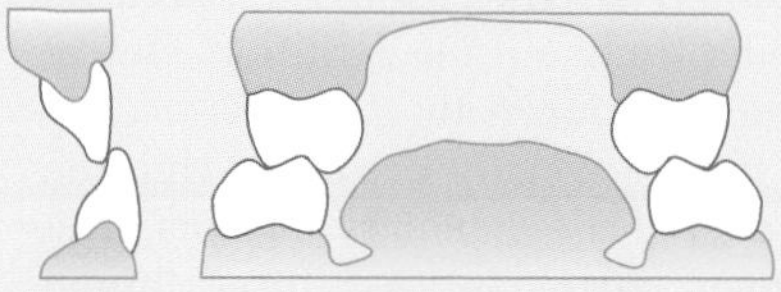
Labioversion	A tooth positioned labial or facial to its normal position. 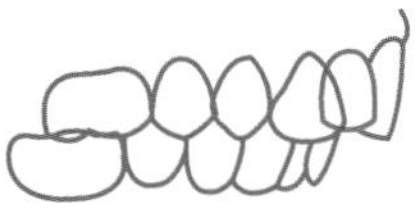
Linguoversion	A tooth positioned lingual to its normal position 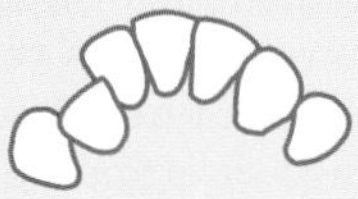

First three figures from Bath-Balogh M, Fehrenbach MJ: *Illustrated dental embryology, histology, and anatomy*, ed 3, St Louis, 2013, Saunders, an imprint of Elsevier Inc.

has a retrognathic facial profile, that is, a small, receded chin because of the apparently small mandible in relationship to the maxilla.

Two subdivisions of the Class II malocclusion are used to indicate the relationship of the anterior teeth. In Class II division 1, the maxillary incisors protrude facially from the mandibular incisors. As a result the mandibular incisors overerupt, causing a severe overbite. Often the palate is deep and narrow and the facial profile includes a protruding upper lip. In Class II division 2, one or more of the maxillary central incisors are lingually inclined or retruded (see Figure 16-23). The maxillary lateral incisors may overlap the central incisors. Overbite is severe, but the palate is wide in comparison with division 1.[11]

Class III Malocclusion

In **Class III malocclusion** the mandible is relatively large compared with the maxilla; thus a prognathic profile results (see Figure 16-23). The molar relationship is such that the buccal groove of the mandibular first permanent molar is situated mesial to the mesiobuccal cusp of the maxillary first permanent molar by at least the width of a premolar, whereas the distal surface of the mandibular permanent canine is mesial to the mesial surface of the maxillary permanent canine by at least the width of a premolar. Similar to the case with the Class II malocclusion, if the distance of movement in the molars or canine is less than the width of a premolar, the classification of occlusion is labeled as "tendency toward Class III."[11]

Primary Occlusion

See Chapter 59, Table 59-1.

Parafunctional Habits

Parafunctional habits are movements of the mandible, such as clenching, bruxism, thumb sucking, and rocking of teeth, which are considered outside or beyond the functions of eating, speech, or respiration. These parafunctional habits often occur subconsciously during sleep or while concentrating deeply on something.

Clenching occurs when the teeth occlude for a long time while in centric position without giving the mandible a rest. Persons who clench their teeth may have enlarged masseter muscles and may consider it normal to feel tension in the facial and masticatory muscles. Directed relaxing of these muscles may help in some cases. Clenching may be due to stress or the way individuals process neurologic impulses.[11]

Bruxism is the forceful grinding of the teeth together, often making an audible noise. Attrition and wear facets of the incisal or occlusal surfaces of the teeth, especially of the canine cusp tips, result from bruxism. Persons who clench or grind their teeth should be referred to a dentist for a "day guard or night guard," which can be worn during waking hours and/or when sleeping. A day guard or night guard is an oral appliance that covers the dentition. It protects the teeth from further attrition and helps to spread the occlusal force generated by the habit throughout the dentition. Newer designs may involve several anterior teeth.

Sucking the thumb or fingers usually occurs in children and can cause extreme overjet of the maxillary incisors, irreversibly stretched lips, a deep palate, and a callused thumb or finger.

Trauma from Occlusion

There are two types of trauma from occlusion: primary and secondary. **Primary trauma from occlusion** results from injury from excessive occlusal forces on a periodontium that has not been altered by disease. There is no attachment loss, apical migration of the junctional epithelium, or loss of connective tissue. Primary trauma from occlusion is caused by "high" restorations, removable partial dentures, insertion of bridges, malaligned teeth, clenching, or grinding and is reversible if the trauma is removed or altered (usually by occlusal adjustment). Signs include the following:

- Widened periodontal ligament space
- Tooth mobility
- Pain

Secondary trauma from occlusion is an injury that occurs from normal occlusal forces placed on a weakened periodontium. It occurs when the surrounding periodontium has been weakened by periodontal disease with evidence of apical migration of the junctional epithelium and loss of connective tissue. With secondary occlusal trauma the clinician may observe rapid bone loss and pocket formation in the client. The client should be referred to the dentist or peridontist for further treatment.

CLIENT EDUCATION TIPS

- Provide oral care strategies to prevent disease onset in areas of developmental anomalies.
- Share information concerning acquired tooth damage, and provide caries preventive strategies based on caries risk (see Chapter 20).
- Interpret and discuss the charted findings for the client.
- Report the factors—local (e.g., trauma), systemic (e.g., diseases, nutritional deficiencies, excess systemic fluoride), hereditary, and idiopathic (unknown)—that may cause enamel formation anomalies.
- Alert the client regarding the need for a dental evaluation and for restorative therapy needed.
- Discuss the importance of tooth replacement to prevent occlusal disharmonies.
- Educate the need for treating open contacts that trap food that may result in gingival inflammation and periodontal breakdown.
- Teach strategies to treat parafunctional habits.

LEGAL, ETHICAL, AND SAFETY ISSUES

- The American Dental Hygienists' Association code of ethics states that clients must be kept informed of their treatment progress and health status.
- It is essential to keep accurate records of care and maintain confidentiality of this information.
- Clients must be informed about their treatment alternatives to meet their oral health needs.
- The client's record is a legal document and is admissible evidence in a court of law.
- Comprehensive charting of tooth assessment findings documents the care provided and is an essential tool for quality assessment.
- During forensic investigations, the record of the client's dentition is often the only means of identifying a deceased person; therefore accuracy and completeness of these records are essential.

KEY CONCEPTS

- Documentation of tooth assessments is important for care planning, communication, legal documentation, and quality assurance.
- Dental charting is the graphic representation of the condition of the client's teeth observed on a specific date. The data recorded are based on clinical and radiographic assessment and the client's report of symptoms.
- The dental chart is a part of the permanent client record and must be accessible for reference during all appointments, thus facilitating continuity, treatment planning, and ongoing documentation of care.
- The goal of tooth assessment for the dental hygienist is to recognize signs of disease, defective restorations, developmental anomalies, and acquired tooth damage and collaborate with other oral health professionals to optimize client care.
- Dental caries and dental restorations commonly are classified either by Black's classification or by the complexity classification system.
- Direct examination can be done well only if the teeth are clean and dry and illuminated with good light. Care should be exercised to avoid exploring early carious lesions and known sensitive areas.

- The dental hygienist may use percussion, a cold stick, or an electric pulp tester to test for pulp vitality. These tests, along with a well-organized and thorough clinical assessment of signs, symptoms, and radiographs, provide additional information to assist in making a diagnosis.
- Thorough dentition assessment includes classifying occlusion and documenting tooth malrelationships and assessing parafunctional habits.
- Malocclusion results when there is lack of overall ideal form in the dentition while in centric occlusion.

CRITICAL THINKING EXERCISES

Marie Smith, a 49-year-old woman, reports that her last dental examination was 18 months ago. Her health history reveals that she currently is being treated for depression and is taking an antidepressant medication. Her chief concerns are the recent sensitivity of several teeth and an uncomfortable dry mouth, which she experiences most of the time. Gingivitis and moderate generalized plaque biofilm are present, with heavy accumulations in posterior lingual areas. On assessment of Marie's teeth, the dental hygienist observes the following:

- Porcelain crowns on teeth No. 7 and No. 10
- Teeth No. 8 and No. 9 have veneers
- Full gold crowns are on teeth No. 18 and No. 31
- Amalgam restorations are found on No. 2 MOD, No. 3 O, No. 4 DO, No. 19 MO, No. 28 MOD, No. 29 DO
- Composite restorations are on No. 6 MO, No. 21 F, No. 22 F, No. 25 F, No. 26 F
- Teeth No. 1, No. 14, No. 16, No. 17, and No. 32 have been extracted
- A porcelain fused to metal bridge is found on teeth No. 13 through No. 15
- Tooth No. 15 has a root canal
- Teeth No. 3 MO, No. 5 D, No. 11 F, and No. 30 MOD have signs of carious lesions
- Attrition is noted on teeth No. 12 through No. 16 and on No. 22 through No. 27

1. Identify the charting symbols or notations that must be entered on the electronic chart.
2. Record your tooth assessment findings on a dental chart for documentation in Marie's permanent record.
3. Propose preventive strategies needed to control the occurrence of future caries.
4. Propose interventions to address the other acquired tooth damage noted.

REFERENCES

1. Sturdevant CM, Roberson TM, Heymann HO, et al, editors: *Sturdevant's The art and science of operative dentistry*, ed 6, St Louis, 2013, Mosby.
2. Ibsen OAC, Phelan JA: *Oral pathology for the dental hygienist*, ed 6, St Louis, 2013, Saunders.
3. American Academy of Pediatric Dentistry: Policy on Early Childhood Caries (ECC)—*Classifications, Consequences, and Preventive Strategies*. 2011. Retrieved November 22, 2012 from www.aapd.org/media/Policies_Guidelines/P_ECCClassifications.pdf.
4. Milgrom P, Weinstein P: *Early childhood caries: a team approach to prevention and treatment*, Seattle, 1999, Continuing Education, University of Washington School of Dentistry.
5. Loesche WJ, Svanberg ML, Pape HL: Intraoral transmission of *Streptococcus mutans* by a dental explorer. *J Dent Res* 58:765, 1979.
6. Featherstone JDB: The science and practice of caries prevention. *J Am Dent Assoc* 131:887, 2000.
7. Featherstone JDB, O'Reilly MM, Shariati M, et al: Enhancement of remineralization in vitro and in vivo. In Leach SA, editor: *Factors relating to demineralization and remineralization of the teeth*, Oxford, England, 1986, IRL Press.
8. Amaechi BT: Emerging technologies for diagnosis of dental caries: the road so far. *J Appl Phys* 105:102047, 2009.
9. Pretty IA: Caries detection and diagnosis: novel technologies. *J Dent* 34:727, 2006.
10. Cohen S: Diagnostic procedures. In Cohen S, Burns RC, editors: *Pathways of the pulp*, ed 10, St Louis, 2011, Mosby.
11. Bath-Balogh M, Fehrenbach M: *Illustrated dental embryology, histology, and anatomy*, ed 3, St Louis, 2011, Saunders an imprint of Elsevier Inc.

ACKNOWLEDGMENT

Portions of this chapter were contributed by Cheryl Cameron, RDH, PhD, and Glen E. Gordon, DDS, University of Washington–Seattle.

EVOLVE RESOURCES

Please visit http://evolve.elsevier.com/Darby/hygiene for additional practice and study support tools.

CHAPTER 17

Oral Hygiene Assessment: Soft and Hard Deposits

Donna Eastabrooks

COMPETENCIES

1. **Discuss the tools and concepts for oral hygiene assessment, including the significance of soft and hard oral deposits.**
2. **Discuss types of oral deposits and explain the oral biofilm formation process.**
3. **Describe the clinical assessment of oral biofilm.**
4. **Explain the skills, motivation, and compliance needed to successfully manage oral self-care.**
5. **Compare the available oral hygiene indices, and list the criteria for an effective oral hygiene index.**
6. **Discuss record keeping and documentation.**

Oral Hygiene Assessment

Oral hygiene is the degree to which the oral cavity is kept clean and free of soft and hard deposits by daily oral self-care or, when necessary, oral care provided by a caregiver. Before the dental hygienist can influence a client's oral health behavior, it is necessary to assess and document the client's current oral hygiene status. Oral hygiene assessment is the process of determining the following about the client:

- Amount of hard tooth deposits (extrinsic dental stain, dental calculus) and soft tooth deposits (food debris, materia alba, oral biofilm)
- Oral hygiene status
- Oral self-care effectiveness
- Motivation related to oral self-care

Assessment Tools

Oral hygiene assessment tools include the following:

- *Light:* Helps to visualize all areas of the mouth
- *Compressed air:* Aids in the detection of supragingival and subgingival soft and hard deposits
- *Mouth mirror:* Permits visualization of entire oral cavity
- *Periodontal explorer:* Allows access subgingivally and, when applicable, to deep pockets (e.g., ODU 11/12 or 3-A explorers) for accurate assessment of subgingival calculus and optimal tactile sensitivity
- *Gauze:* Maintains a clean instrument tip rather than translocating soft deposits around the mouth
- *Disclosing solution* (disclosant): Allows visualization of supragingival plaque throughout the mouth and determines oral self-care effectiveness (see section on disclosing agents)

Concepts for Oral Hygiene Assessment

Soft and hard dental deposits are assessed according to the following:

- Location
  - Supragingival—above the free-gingival margin
  - Subgingival—below the free-gingival margin
- Amount (degree) as indicated by slight, moderate, or heavy accumulations
- Extent and distribution
  - Generalized throughout the dentition (greater than one third of the dentition is involved)
  - Localized to a single tooth or groups of teeth in the anterior or posterior areas but involving less than one third of the dentition

Assessment also involves evaluating the client's knowledge, skill, attitude, and motivation related to oral self-care. Table 17-1 describes the soft and hard deposits that accumulate in the oral cavity. Of these deposits, oral biofilm (bacterial plaque or dental plaque) is a risk factor for dental caries and periodontal diseases. Stain and calculus do not cause oral disease but rather provide irregular surfaces that retain bacterial plaque on teeth, dental appliances, and adjacent periodontal structures and have esthetic implications. The location, amount, and extent of oral biofilm, stain, and calculus, and to a lesser degree food debris and materia alba, are important variables to measure and record during baseline assessment and at continued-care intervals. Clients are informed of oral hygiene assessment findings and encouraged to practice daily of self-care for prevention of oral disease and health promotion.

Bacterial plaque biofilm (see section on oral biofilm) is a major risk factor for dental caries, periodontal disease, and oral malodor; therefore its assessment is key to effective care planning. About 20% of the oral environment is occupied by teeth, the target for toothbrushing and interdental cleaning. The remaining 80% of the mouth includes the oral mucous membrane and specialized mucosa of the tongue. Pathogenic microorganisms can grow on all oral soft tissues and hard surfaces as well as in saliva. By understanding the bacterial load present in the oral cavity, mechanical and antimicrobial interventions can be implemented and recommended to reduce oral biofilm in the entire mouth.

About 50% to 90% of the population exhibit some type of periodontal disease. When disease is present, there is commonly a corresponding need for greater personal

Figures, tables, and boxes marked as "e" are available as supplemental material on the Evolve site. Visit http://evolve.elsevier.com/Darby/hygiene to access these materials.

TABLE 17-1

Soft and Hard Deposits Found in the Oral Cavity

Term	Classification	Definition
Acquired pellicle and exogenous dental cuticle	Acellular, nonmineralized layer	An unstructured, homogenous film adhering to tooth surfaces, firm surfaces in the oral cavity, and old calculus; may be stained by tar products and tannin
Oral biofilm	Cellular, nonmineralized layer	A dense, transparent, nonmineralized, highly organized mass of bacterial colonies in a gel-like intermicrobial, enclosed matrix; a host-associated biofilm
Materia alba	Cellular, nonmineralized layer	Loose deposit of microorganisms, desquamated epithelial cells, and broken down food debris; white to yellowish-white in color; has cottage cheese–like appearance Can be displaced with rinsing and water irrigation
Food debris	Cellular nonmineralized layer	Unstructured particles that remain in the mouth after eating and are removed with irrigation unless impacted between the teeth
Extrinsic stain	Cellular, may be mineralized or nonmineralized	Discolorations that accumulate on the external surface of the tooth via pellicle, plaque biofilm, or calculus; can be removed by power toothbrushing, scaling, and/or polishing
Supragingival calculus	Cellular, mineralized layer	Mineralized bacterial plaque permeated with moderately hard calcium phosphate crystals; superficially covered with bacterial plaque biofilm; usually white or yellowish-white in color but may be stained darker
Subgingival calculus	Cellular, mineralized layer	Mineralized bacterial plaque; adheres to tooth structure in gingival sulcus; organic matrix of bacteria permeated with hard calcium phosphate crystals; may be stained dark green to greenish-black; superficially covered with bacterial plaque biofilm

responsibility for oral health or knowledge about the pathogenicity of oral biofilm and its control. Oral hygiene assessment allows the dental hygienist to determine the client's unmet human needs (e.g., need for responsibility for oral health, conceptualization and problem solving, protection from health risks), communicate these unmet needs to clients, and instruct them in effective self-care behaviors. Individualized oral hygiene instruction is important in motivating a client; no one wants the "one-size-fits-all brush-and-floss lecture."

Oral Deposits

Oral Biofilm

A **biofilm** is a complex, highly organized, three-dimensional communal arrangement of microorganisms adhering to a surface where moisture and nutrients are available. Unlike free-floating (**planktonic**) bacteria, bacteria in a biofilm community are able to maximize nutrients, keep their community clean, communicate with one another when threatened, protect the community when under attack, and even relocate to start new biofilm communities. As a **host-associated biofilm**, **dental plaque** (also known as **microbial plaque**, **dental plaque**, **oral biofilm**, **dental plaque biofilm**, **bacterial plaque biofilm**) is a dense, transparent, nonmineralized mass of bacterial colonies in a gel-like intermicrobial, enclosed **matrix** (**slime layer**) that is attached to a moist environmental surface (Figure 17-1, *A* and *B*). The biofilm lends other protective properties to the associated bacteria, including resistance to antibacterial agents such as chlorhexidine gluconate, fixed combination of essential oils, cetylpyridinium chloride, systemic antibiotics, and host defense mechanisms (immune system and inflammation). A network of slime layers of polysaccharides protects the biofilm bacteria from the host's immune system's defensive cells (neutrophils, leukocytes, macrophages, and lymphocytes) and antimicrobial and antibiotic agents. Bacteria within the biofilm adhere to one another and to tooth surfaces, dental appliances, restorations, the oral mucosa, the specialized mucosa of the tongue, and alveolar bone. Some bacteria are unattached and free floating (Figure 17-1, *C*).

Dental caries and gingival and periodontal infections are caused by microorganisms in oral biofilms. Biofilm-enclosed bacteria benefit from metabolites that are produced by the bacteria and concentrated, retained in the biofilm, the result being enhanced interactions among species of bacteria. The structure of the plaque biofilm includes channels that use the motion of saliva within the oral cavity or gingival crevicular fluid subgingivally for bacterial colonization, nutrition, and transport bacterial wastes. The biofilm creates its own renewing source of lipopolysaccharide (toxins) for long-term

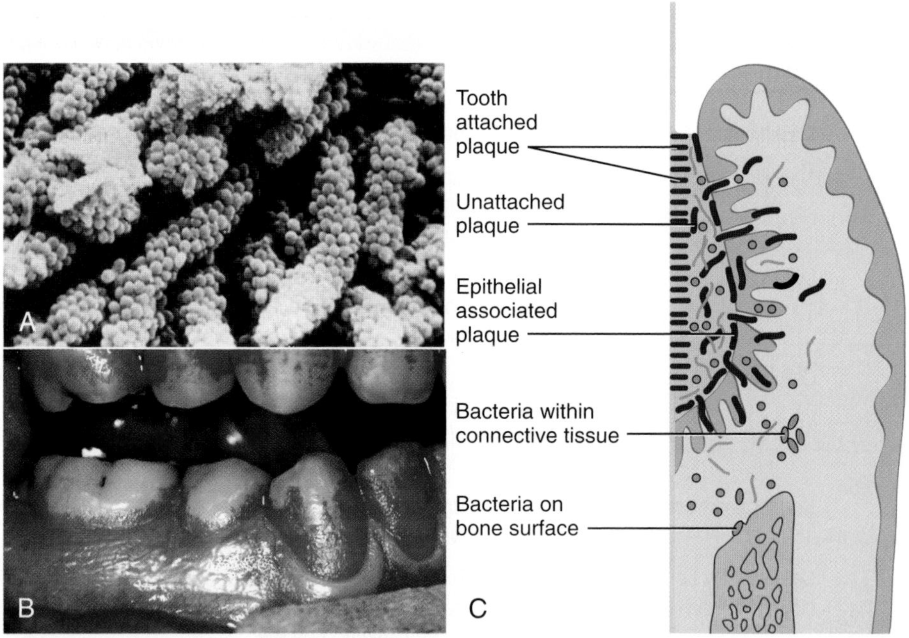

Figure 17-1. Oral biofilm. **A,** Long-standing supragingival plaque near the gingival margin demonstrates "corncob" arrangement. A central gram-negative filamentous core supports the outer coccal cells, which are firmly attached by interbacterial adherence or coaggregation. **B,** Disclosed supragingival plaque covering one third to two thirds of the clinical crown. **C,** Diagram depicting the plaque bacteria associated with tooth surface and periodontal tissues. (From Newman MG, Takei HH, Klokkevold PR, et al: *Carranza's clinical periodontology*, ed 11, St Louis, 2012, Saunders.)

survival of microorganisms. Loosely attached and unattached microbes are found at the surface of the plaque biofilm (see Figure 17-1, *C*). Bacteria within the biofilm store sugars inside their cells and extend the time of their lactic acid production. This prolonged exposure to lactic acid causes the decalcification observed in dental caries. Because of these protective and self-sustaining properties of the biofilm, associated bacteria are likely to survive within the mouth, and oral diseases may become chronic. Recognition of the self-sustaining nature of the biofilm community helps explain why periodontal disease is difficult to control and why periodontal pathogens resist antimicrobial agents, antibiotic therapies, and host-defense mechanisms. Subgingival microorganisms organize themselves into biofilms comprised of complex heterogeneous communities enmeshed in extracellular substances. These microorganisms often coaggregate to colonize and they benefit from metabolic by-products from neighboring species as nutrient sources (eFigure 17-2).

Microorganisms Within Oral Biofilm

See eFigure 17-3.

Supragingival Microorganisms

In healthy mouths, oral biofilm is mainly supragingival and confined to enamel surfaces and oral mucosa. Typically the bacteria associated with healthy plaque biofilm include aerobic gram-positive aerobic rods and cocci, with very few motile species. The bacterial species associated with periodontal health include *Streptococcus mitis, Streptococcus sanguinis, Streptococcus gordonii,* and *Streptococcus oralis,* although these species also may be found in disease. As undisturbed plaque matures, the bacterial population changes to a predominately gram-negative anaerobic flora; this change in bacterial species brings signs of oral infection and inflammation.

Subgingival Microorganisms

In dental plaque–induced gingival disease, there is an increase in the quantity and quality of plaque. As supragingival plaque grows undisturbed, it extends subgingivally. Bacterial species associated with dental plaque–induced gingival disease include gram-negative spirochetes and motile rods such as *Fusobacterium nucleatum,* species of *Prevotella* and *Treponema,* and *Campylobacter rectus.* In advancing periodontal disease, plaque is characterized by a zone of gram-positive organisms attached to the tooth surface, and a loosely adherent zone of gram-negative species adjacent to the pocket wall. Bacteria associated with periodontitis are predominantly anaerobic and include, but are not limited to, *Porphyromonas gingivalis, Prevotella intermedia, Tannerella forsythia, Filifactor* and *Peptostreptococcus*, and *Aggregatibacter actinomycetemcomitans.* Color designations of plaque based on pathogenicity are shown in Figure 17-4. This color coding has been used to differentiate bacterial complexes associated with health and disease severity. Early subgingival colonizers are in the blue, yellow, green, and purple complexes. Late colonizers, the orange and red complexes, are associated with mature subgingival plaque, periodontal pocketing, and clinical attachment loss.

Stages of Oral Biofilm Formation

Plaque formation occurs in four distinct stages: initial adherence, lag phase, rapid growth bacterial colonization, and steady state (see eFigures 17-2 and 17-3). Within these stages, distinct changes take place within the overall biofilm.

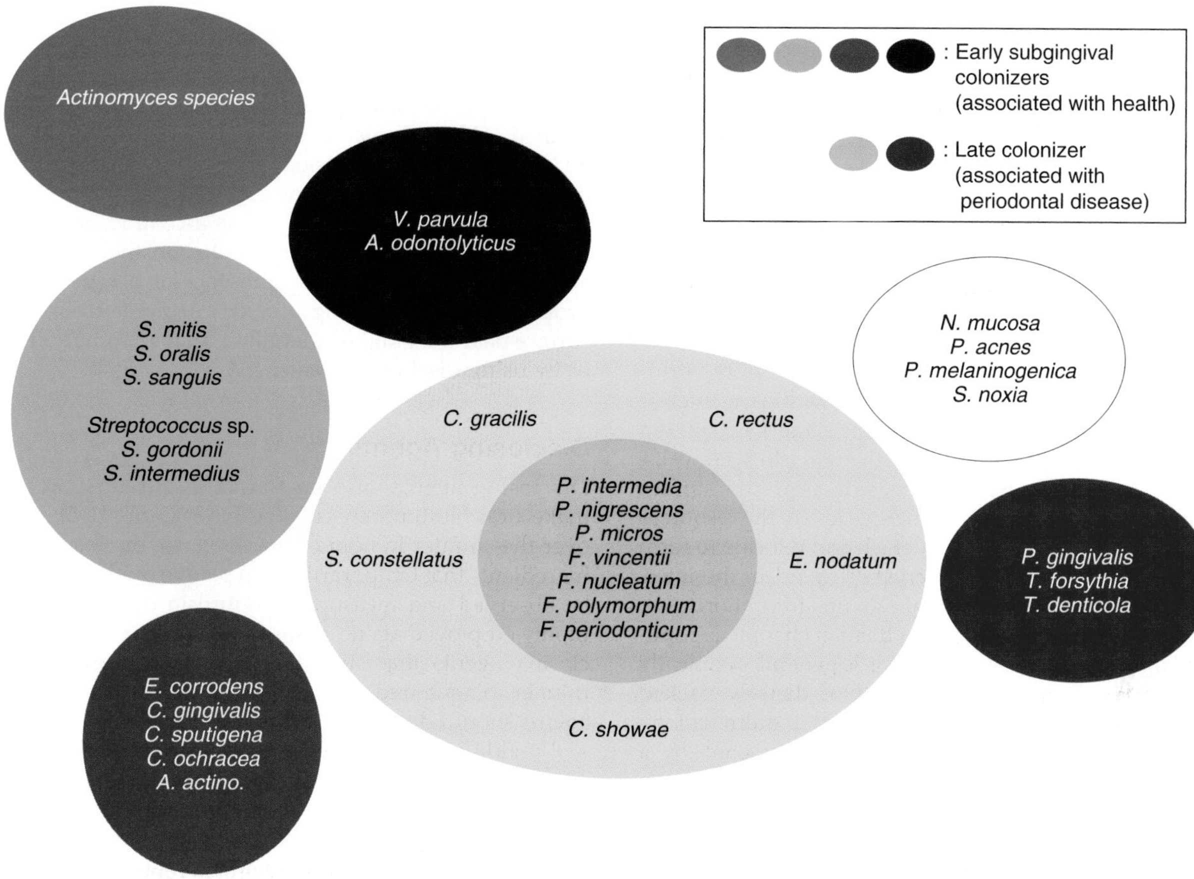

Figure 17-4. Subgingival microbiota in subgingival biofilm. (Adapted from Socransky SS, Haffajee AD, Cugini MA, et al: Microbial complexes in subgingival plaque, *J Clin Periodontol* 25:134, 1998; and Haffajee AD, Bogren A, Hasturk H, et al: Subgingival microbiota of chronic periodontitis subjects from different geographic locations, *J Clin Periodontol* 31:996-1002, 2004. Reprinted with permission from Blackwell Publishing.)

Initial Adherence

The first stage is the deposition of salivary components (the acquired pellicle), a tenacious, insoluble, acellular protein film composed of glycoproteins found within saliva on oral surfaces. Although pellicle performs a protective function, acting as a barrier to acids, it also serves as the initial site of attachment for free-swimming (planktonic) bacteria beginning the first stage of biofilm development. Salivary proteins and peptides promote bacterial adhesion to oral surfaces. Immediately after cleansing the tooth, the pellicle begins to reform on exposed surfaces; within 1 hour, free-floating microorganisms attach to the acquired pellicle and begin sessile colonies. Gram-positive cocci are the first microorganisms to colonize the teeth. Early plaque, 1 to 2 days old, consists primarily of aerobic, gram-positive cocci such as *Streptococcus mutans* and *Streptococcus sanguis.* Primarily because of the methods of bacterial adhesion, plaque is not completely removed by oral irrigation; removal of the entire plaque biofilm requires mechanical action, such as toothbrushing and interdental cleaning with floss, a brush, or a wooden wedge. The significance of this distinction is being studied as it relates to oral health and disease as oral irrigation has been shown to have benefits in reducing plaque biofilm and gingivitis.

Lag Phase

As the planktonic bacteria become sessile (i.e., immobile or fixed in one place), there is a lag in bacterial growth. Bacterial colonization occurs in stratified layers against the tooth surface. On days 2 through 4, filamentous forms of bacteria grow on the surface of the coccal colonies and begin to infiltrate the sessile colonies, replacing the cocci.

Rapid Growth Bacterial Colonization

During rapid growth, adherent bacteria secrete extracellular polysaccharides to form a water-insoluble slime matrix. The matrix is composed of saliva, polymers of host and bacterial origin, and polysaccharides that are adherent. Protected by the matrix and the biofilm, microcolonies begin to form. The matrix is sticky and therefore further facilitates microbial adhesion. A client may experience this phenomenon as the "furry" or "filmy" feeling sometimes detected on the teeth. In addition to providing a method of adherence for the bacterial colonies, the matrix and its polysaccharides trap other nutrients, provide a food source for the bacteria, and contribute to the protective functions of the biofilm. Additional varieties of bacteria coaggregate with the early colonizers, leading to structural stratification within the thickening of the biofilm.

By days 4 through 14, filamentous forms increase and specific types of rods, spirochetes, and fusobacteria increase in number; overall the load of gram-negative anaerobic species and pathogenic spriochetes increases, and white blood cells are found within the plaque. Clinically, signs of inflammation are observed.

Steady State and Detachment

Initial formation is within distinct colonies that form from the indigenous oral microflora, but as the growth process continues, an intermicrobial matrix (protective slime layer) connects the bacterial colonies.

The biofilm is now a fully functioning community of different species living symbiotically. Bacteria within the interior of the biofilm slow their growth or become static. Deep within the biofilm, bacteria show signs of death, disrupted cell walls, and loss of cytoplasm, whereas bacteria near the surface remain intact. The toxic wastes of one species are the resources of another. Some surface bacteria detach and relocate to form new biofilm colonies. Over time crystals found in the interbacterial matrix may become initial calculus formation.

The plaque ages and undergoes a distinct change in population. By days 14 through 24, gingivitis is generally clinically evident, and the biofilm is composed of densely packed gram-negative anaerobic bacteria. As the biofilm colony matures, it blooms into a mushroom shape attached by a narrow base and incorporates channels that capitalize on the fluid movement present in the oral cavity. These fluid channels distribute nutrients, remove wastes, and allow for free-swimming bacteria to leave and begin new biofilm colonies. It is easy to appreciate the importance of thorough, daily mechanical plaque biofilm disruption and removal to inhibit the destructive processes of mature plaque. The longer the oral biofilm remains undisturbed, the greater its pathogenic (disease producing) potential for the host (see Figure 17-4). The host's normal response to injury, inflammation, and foreign bodies, the **immune response**, is activated and eventually overresponds (eTables 17-2 and 17-3). The effects of the proinflammatory mediators and inability of the immune system to reach the site of injury or infection cause the connective tissue and bone destruction in periodontal disease (see Chapter 19).

Clinical Assessment of Oral Biofilm

Clinically, oral biofilm manifests as a transparent film that begins to form within minutes after a surface has been cleaned. Although plaque can be difficult to visualize, it can be detected by direct vision, particularly if there are thick deposits of plaque or if it has acquired yellow, tan, or brown stains. Some people feel plaque as a coating on their teeth; some people do not feel the biofilm on their teeth, dental appliances, and tongue. The presence of plaque is assessed professionally by passing a dental explorer over the tooth surface near the gingival margin to remove some soft deposit or by using disclosing agents.

Disclosing Agents

Disclosing agents, also known as **disclosants**, are used to make oral biofilm clinically visible (Figure 17-5). Available over-the-counter in liquid or tablet form, disclosants contain ingredients that temporarily stain plaque biofilm so that it can be observed and measured. Erythrosin dye, the most commonly employed agent, stains oral biofilm red. Two-tone disclosing agents that stain thicker plaque biofilm blue and thinner plaque red are also available. Ideally, disclosing agents should do the following:

- Provide a distinct staining of deposits that does not rinse off immediately
- Have a pleasant taste
- Be nonirritating to the oral tissues

Because disclosants can camouflage clinical signs of disease, disclosing agents should be applied after the oral and periodontal assessment and after the client sees the oral findings in his or her own mouth. The location of oral biofilm also should be seen by the client before disclosing deposits so that the client understands the correlation among oral hygiene, infection, inflammation, and oral disease risks (see Chapters 18 and 19).

After performing the gingival assessment and instructing the client on the composition and detrimental effects of plaque biofilm, a non–petroleum-based lubricant can be applied to the lips and esthetic dental restorations to prevent them from staining. Petroleum-based products are not

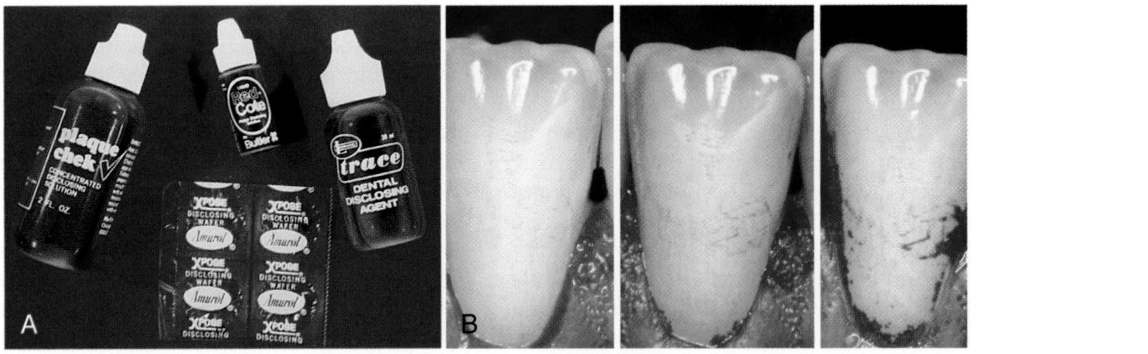

Figure 17-5. Use of disclosing agents to monitor oral biofilm on teeth. **A,** Examples of plaque biofilm disclosants. **B,** Clinical photos of the typical topography of plaque growth. Initial growth starts along the gingival margin and from the interdental space to extend farther in a coronal direction. (**B,** From Newman MG, Takei HH, Klokkevold PR, Carranza FA: *Carranza's clinical periodontology*, ed 11, St Louis, 2012, Saunders.)

recommended because they break down the protective latex barrier of the clinician's gloves.

Disclosing techniques depend on the product used:

- Solutions are applied as a concentrate with a cotton swab or diluted with water in a cup for the client to use as an oral rinse.
- Tablets are chewed and swished around in the mouth by the client.

Clean tooth surfaces do not absorb the dye unless roughness is present (e.g., demineralization, hypocalcification, restorations, cementum). Acquired pellicle, plaque biofilm, debris, and calculus absorb the disclosing agent. This discriminate staining characteristic makes the disclosing agent an excellent oral hygiene aid because the client is able to use it at home for self-evaluation. Seeing, feeling, and smelling the oral biofilm deposits teaches and motivates individuals to improve and monitor their self-care effectiveness.

After application of the disclosant, excess is expectorated or suctioned from the mouth and the client is given a hand mirror to identify the stained deposits. The dental hygienist assists the client in identifying deposits and correlates findings with areas of gingival inflammation, periodontal disease parameters, and dental caries identified before staining. The client then is queried about what he or she wants to do or can do about the oral deposits. Mechanical and chemotherapeutic plaque control techniques are taught to improve oral hygiene and oral health. Instructions from the dental hygienist are followed by direct observation of the client's self-care technique. Each area of concern should be practiced because the client may need guidance adapting the toothbrush or interdental cleaner.

Assessment

The assessment of oral biofilm depends on its location:

- Supragingivally, coronal to the free gingival margin on the clinical crown of the tooth, and subgingivally, apical to the margin of the free gingiva. Supragingival locations include the occlusal surfaces (most common in areas without opposing teeth), buccal or lingual fissures and pits, interproximal tooth surfaces, and free gingival margin.
- Subgingival plaque accumulates in the sulcus or periodontal pocket on all four aspects of the tooth (buccal, lingual, mesial, and distal interproximal spaces).
- On soft tissues such as specialized mucosa (tongue) and oral mucosa.

Next, a determination is made about the amount of plaque present (e.g., is it light, moderate, or heavy?). Extent is an assessment about whether the plaque is generalized throughout the dentition or localized to several teeth. Oral biofilm is influenced by host mediating factors; therefore oral hygiene assessment includes the host's response to the plaque. In health there is a balance point between the plaque and the host where no irreparable damage occurs. If the biofilm bacteria cause tissue destruction that exceeds the reparative ability of the host, disease occurs. Quality of plaque is more important than quantity of plaque. The quality of the plaque (types of microorganisms present) and the client's host response to that bacterial challenge guide clinician and client. For example, a client with a high plaque score in the lingual region of the mouth, plaque-free facial tooth surfaces, and healthy gingival tissue clearly requires instructions targeting the lingual areas, while reinforcing effective techniques in the facial area. A client with a small quantity of plaque accumulation but with severe gingival bleeding requires a different approach to care, perhaps considering systemic factors or regularity of biofilm removal. The client's oral contributing factors influence the growth, retention, and removal of oral biofilm:

- Tight lingual frenum interferes with natural self-cleansing action of the tongue. Papillae on the tongue are conducive to oral biofilm growth (coated tongue).
- Faulty restorations with open or overhanging margins or poorly contoured surfaces readily harbor plaque.
- Missing teeth contribute to plaque retention and inhibit the self-cleaning of occlusal surfaces during mastication.
- Malocclusions result in crowding and tipping of teeth, which can make plaque removal difficult or lead to traumatic occlusion, resulting in widened PDL spaces that lend themselves to greater plaque accumulation.
- Mouth breathing, with its drying effects on oral tissues, favors growth of oral biofilm in the absence of the bactericidal action of saliva. Ropey, viscous saliva is less self-cleansing than watery saliva.
- The rough, porous surface of calculus provides a porous surface where bacteria reside.
- Extrinsic tooth stain provides a rough surface for bacteria to colonize.

All of these factors influence the retention of bacterial plaque and can make oral plaque control challenging.

Tooth Stains

Tooth stain is a discolored accretion or area on a tooth contrasting with the rest of the tooth color (Figures 17-6 and 17-7). Stains are divided into intrinsic stains and extrinsic stains.

- **Intrinsic stains** are incorporated within the tooth structure and cannot be removed by scaling or polishing. Such stains result from alterations during the development of

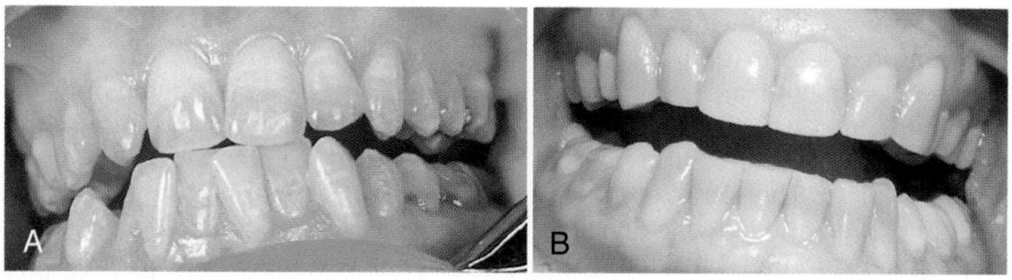

Figure 17-6. Intrinsic tooth stains. **A,** Dental fluorosis. **B,** Tetracycline stain. (From Ibsen OAC, Phelan JA: *Oral pathology for the dental hygienist,* ed 6, St Louis, 2014, Saunders.)

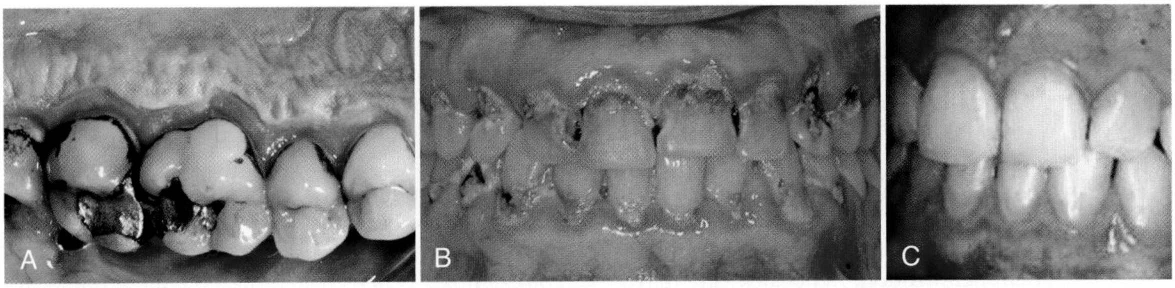

Figure 17-7. Extrinsic tooth stains. **A,** Tobacco stain. **B,** Orange stain in person with poor oral hygiene, severe periodontal disease, and rampant caries. **C,** Green stain. (**A,** From Newman MG, Takei HH, Klokkevold PR, Carranza FA: *Carranza's clinical periodontology,* ed 11, St Louis, 2012, Saunders. **B,** Courtesy Dr. Thomas E. O'Connor, St Louis, Missouri; and Dr. Kevin Thorpe, St Louis, Missouri. **C,** From Scully C, Welbury R, Flaitz C, Paes de Almeida O: *A color atlas of orofacial health and disease in children and adolescents,* ed 2, Oxford, England, 2002, Taylor and Francis.)

the tooth (embryonic to 6 years of age) associated with antibiotic use, fever, trauma, infection, and ingestion of high amounts of systemic fluoride. Examples include dental fluorosis (a mottled, opaque, or brownish discoloration caused by ingesting excessive amounts of fluoride during enamel formation) and tetracycline stain (a yellow, brown, gray, or orange discoloration within the substance of the tooth from ingestion of the antibiotic when the tooth is developing) (see Figure 17-6).

- Extrinsic stains occur on the tooth surface and usually can be removed by coronal polishing or scaling. Method of attachment is the acquired pellicle; without pellicle, stains cannot adhere to the smooth enamel surfaces. Extrinsic stains develop because of the presence of chromogenic bacteria (color-producing bacteria); use of staining substances such as tobacco, red wine, tea, coffee, soda, blueberries, and some drugs; and exposure to metallic compounds (see Figure 17-7).

Of the extrinsic stains, green stain is attributed to chromogenic bacteria, *Penicillium* and *Aspergillus.* Green stain, found in poor oral hygiene, occurs near the cervical third of the teeth. This stain easily can become incorporated within decalcified enamel. Orange stain, less common than other types of stains, also is associated with poor oral hygiene. This stain occurs frequently on anterior teeth and is believed to be due to the presence of chromogenic bacteria *Serratia marcescens* and *Flavobacterium lutescens.*

Chromogenic stain usually can be removed safely with 3% hydrogen peroxide to loosen and bleach the stain, followed by selective polishing and in-office fluoride therapy. If the area under the stain is decalcified, scaling is contraindicated owing to the risk of damaging demineralized tooth surface, and fluoride therapy may be professionally delivered and prescribed for home use to remineralize the tooth surface.

Sources of tooth stain often can be identified by the color of the stain and client self-reported information about lifestyle behavior, diet, work environment, and oral habits. Identification of the stain and its source assists in developing a specific care plan that facilitates stain control and a more esthetic appearance for clients. The client often can reduce stain formation with improved oral hygiene practices and appropriate over-the-counter product selection (e.g., whitening toothpaste, power toothbrushes, frequent tooth cleaning). Table 17-4 describes some common dental stains. See Chapter 29 for professional management of tooth stains.

Brown stains can have multiple causes. Tobacco use causes dark brown, tenacious stains that can become intrinsic; tobacco stains do not necessarily correlate with the amount of tobacco used. Food stains also may be tan to brown and result from the ingestion of foods with tannins, such as red wine, sodas, coffee, tea, and certain fruits. Agents such as 0.12% chlorhexidine gluconate mouth rinse, cetylpyridinium chloride mouth rinse, and stannous fluoride dentifrice or mouth rinse also may impart a brown stain if used twice daily over 2 to 3 months. These stains, related to the substantivity of the product, may be somewhat difficult to remove and often require scaling in addition to polishing. Yellow stain is most commonly associated with heavy plaque accumulation and often can be removed by the client with improved toothbrushing techniques. Black stain (black-line stain) can occur in clients with meticulous oral hygiene. These stains are found on the tooth surface near the gingival margin and are associated with iron in the saliva. Middle-aged females with good oral hygiene are the most likely population to have black-line stain.

Dental Calculus

Dental calculus, commonly referred to as tartar, is oral biofilm that has been mineralized by calcium and phosphate salts from saliva. Although calculus is not the causative factor in periodontal infection, it facilitates the attachment and retention of plaque biofilm; therefore professional calculus removal always is indicated. The dental hygienist removes calculus so that teeth have biologically acceptable smooth surfaces. Like plaque, dental calculus is classified by its location (either supragingival or subgingival), degree (slight, moderate, heavy), and extent (localized or generalized).

Supragingival Calculus

Supragingival calculus, calculus above the free gingival margin, is located most commonly adjacent to the sublingual and parotid salivary gland ducts, resulting in calcified deposits on the mandibular anterior lingual surfaces and maxillary posterior facial surfaces of teeth (Figure 17-8, *A*). However, supragingival calculus can be found in any area of the mouth where there is poor oral hygiene or associated contributory factors such as kidney dialysis, use of 0.12% chlorhexidine mouth rinse, or genetic predisposition.

TABLE 17-4
Types of Tooth Stains

Type	Source	Clinical Approach
Extrinsic Stains		
Green	Chromogenic bacteria and fungi (*Penicillium* and *Aspergillus* species) from poor oral hygiene; most often seen in children with enamel irregularities	Should not be scaled because of underlying demineralized enamel. Have client remove during toothbrush instruction or lightly polish; may use hydrogen peroxide to help with bleaching and removal.
Black stain	Iron in saliva; iron-containing oral solutions; *Actinomyces* species; industrial exposure to iron, manganese, and silver	Firmly scale because of calculus-like nature and selectively polish for complete removal.
Orange	Chromogenic bacteria (*Serratia marcescens* and *Flavobacterium lutescens*) from poor oral hygiene	Lightly scale and then polish selectively.
Brown stains		
Tobacco	Tars from smoking, chewing, and dipping spit tobacco	Lightly scale and then polish selectively.
Food	Food and beverage pigment and tannins	Lightly scale and then polish selectively.
Topical medications	Stannous fluoride, chlorhexidine, or cetylpyridinium chloride mouth rinses	Lightly scale and then polish selectively.
Yellow	Oral biofilm	Have client remove during toothbrush instruction.
Blue-green stain	Mercury and lead dust	Lightly scale and then polish selectively.
Red-black stain	Chewing betel nut, betel leaf, and lime (pan); found in Western pacific and South Asian cultures	Firmly scale and then polish selectively.
Intrinsic Stains		
Dental fluorosis (white-spotted to brown-pitted enamel)	Excessive fluoride ingestion during enamel development	Cannot be removed by scaling or selective polishing.
Hypocalcification (white spots on enamel)	High fever during enamel formation	Cannot be removed by scaling or selective polishing.
Demineralization (white or brown spots on enamel, may be smooth or rough)	Acid erosion of enamel caused by oral biofilm	Cannot be removed by scaling or polishing. Recommend daily 0.05% sodium fluoride rinses for remineralization.
Tetracycline (grayish brown discoloration)	Ingestion of tetracycline during tooth development	Cannot be removed by scaling or selective polishing.

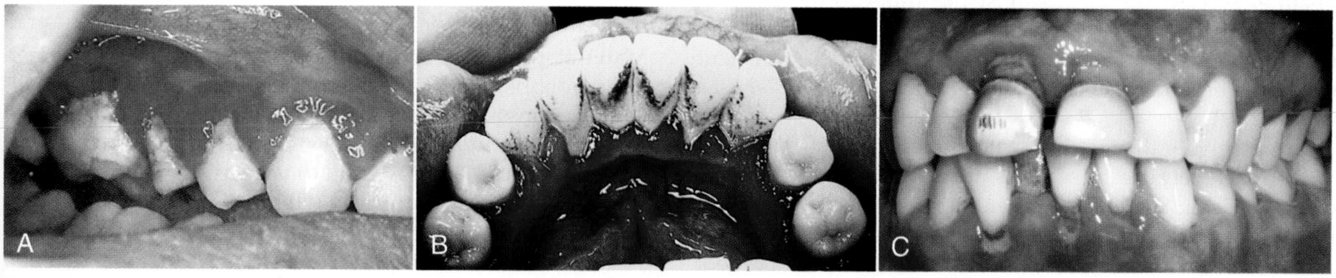

Figure 17-8. Dental calculus. **A,** Heavy calculus on molar and premolars in area opposite Stenson's duct. Note severe gingival inflammation and edema. **B,** Calculus superimposed with tobacco stains in relation to Wharton's ducts. **C,** Generalized supragingival and subgingival calculus and stain in a 31-year-old Caucasian man. (**C,** From Newman MG, Takei HH, Klokkevold PR, Carranza FA: *Carranza's clinical periodontology,* ed 11, St Louis, 2012, Saunders.)

Supragingival calculus is identified using direct visualization and compressed air. Generally the deposits are yellowish-white but may take on surface stains and appear dark yellow or light brown (see Figure 17-8, *B*). Drying the teeth with compressed air allows for a more accurate assessment, because as the calculus is dried it takes on a chalky-white appearance, making it easier to visualize. Supragingival calculus is moderately hard, bridging adjacent teeth or deposited on individual teeth.

Subgingival Calculus

Subgingival calculus is mineralized oral biofilm formed below the free gingival margin, often on the root surface. Unlike supragingival calculus, subgingival calculus is more

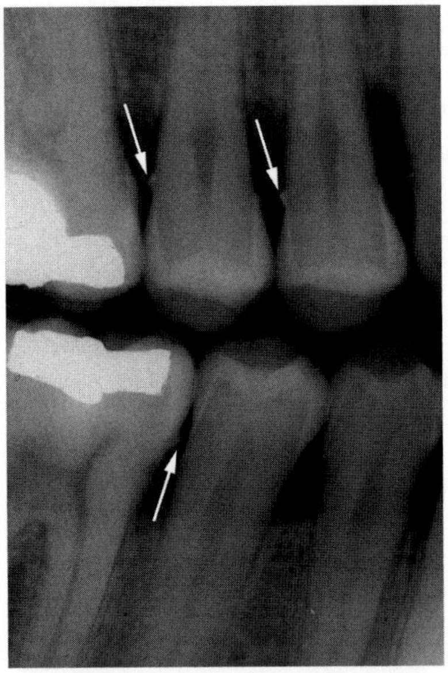

Figure 17-9. Vertical bitewing radiograph illustrating extensive subgingival calculus deposits as interproximal spurs *(arrows)*. (From Newman MG, Takei HH, Klokkevold PR, Carranza FA: *Carranza's clinical periodontology*, ed 11, St Louis, 2012, Saunders.)

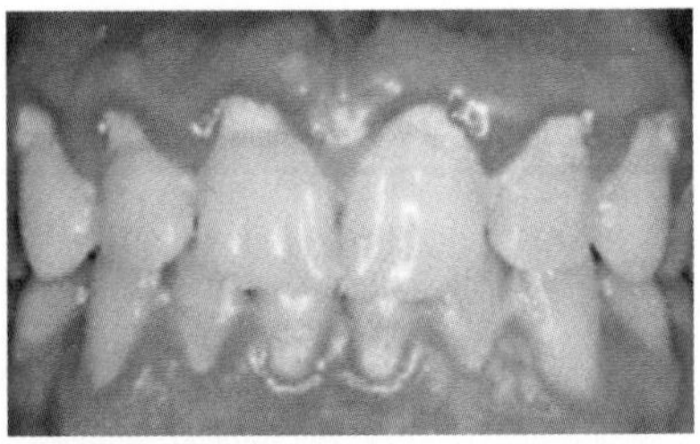

Figure 17-10. Materia alba generalized throughout the mouth, with heaviest accumulation near the gingiva. Note the plaque-induced gingivitis present.

likely to have a dark green–brown-black color owing to the absorption of blood pigments from the gingival sulcus or diseased periodontal pocket (see Figure 17-8, *C*). These deposits may be hard and tenacious and occasionally are visualized within the sulcus or pocket by deflecting the gingival margin with compressed air or seen through thin gingival tissues. The most accurate method of subgingival calculus detection is via subgingival exploration using a periodontal explorer; however, calculus can sometimes be detected during periodontal probing. The quantity of dental calculus is related to personal oral hygiene, diet, and individual biochemistry.

With transillumination, calculus can be observed as a dark, opaque, shadowlike area against the translucent proximal enamel. Heavy calculus deposits are identified easily, as in eFigure 17-8, *D-F*. Some deposits are mineralized to the extent that they become visible on radiographs (Figure 17-9; see Chapter 19).

Subgingival calculus occurs most frequently in interproximal spaces, because these areas are the most difficult for a client to clean. Subgingival calculus may take many forms, including granular deposits, veneers, or thin layers, and spurs or rings that extend around several surfaces of the root and have dimension. The dental hygienist explores this change in tooth surface texture and dimension when assessing for subgingival calculus. Calculus may feel like a ledge or ring around a tooth, nodule, or smooth when it is layered in thin veneers.

Calculus Formation

Because calculus is calcified plaque biofilm, its formation follows the stages of biofilm formation (see section on stages of oral biofilm formation). Calculus forms and grows by the apposition of new layers of biofilm. Mineralization occurs in the intermicrobial matrix of the biofilm. The mineral source for supragingival calculus is saliva, gingival crevicular fluid, and inflammatory exudate. Crystals of hydroxyapatite, octocalcium phosphate, whitlockite, and brushite form in the intercellular matrix, on the surface of bacteria, and within the bacteria. About 10 days (rapid calculus formers) to 20 days (slow calculus formers) are required for undisrupted oral biofilm to change to mineralized calculus, although the mineralization process can begin within 24 to 48 hours. Heavy calculus formers have higher salivary concentrations of calcium and phosphate than light formers. In contrast, light calculus formers have higher levels of pyrophosphate, a known inhibitor of calcification used in an anti-calculus (antitartar) dentifrice.

Calculus Composition

Calculus composition is similar in supragingival and subgingival calculus.

- Inorganic components make up about 75% to 85% of the calculus and include calcium, phosphorus, carbonate, sodium, magnesium, and potassium.
- Organic components make up about 15% to 25% of the calculus and include nonvital microorganisms, desquamated epithelial cells, leukocytes, salivary mucins, cholesterol, cholesterol esters, phospholipids, fatty acids, sugars, carbohydrates, keratins, nucleoproteins, and amino acids.

Materia Alba and Food Debris

Materia alba (white material) is a loosely attached collection of oral debris, desquamated epithelial cells, leukocytes, salivary proteins and lipids, and bacteria that is seen as a whitish to yellowish to grayish mass on the teeth or overlying oral biofilm (Figure 17-10). Typically, materia alba resembles small curds of cottage cheese, is less adherent than oral biofilm, and can be found in areas of poor oral hygiene.

Food debris is composed of remnants of food retained after a meal. Rinsing, use of an oral irrigator, and the self-cleansing action of the tongue and saliva can remove materia alba and food debris. If present in great amounts, materia alba and food debris accumulations impede the dental hygienist's ability to assess accurately the level of oral biofilm and calculus. However, presence of soft deposits may indicate inadequate oral hygiene knowledge and skill, infrequent oral self-care, poor manual dexterity, or low motivation level of the client. The bacteria in the materia alba and the carboxylic acid in the food particles can contribute to oral disease. Materia alba and food debris supply nutrients to the oral biofilm and therefore should be removed regularly.

Skill, Motivation, and Compliance

The client's ability to manage oral self-care must be assessed. A client may be capable of performing the necessary mechanical interventions but have little desire to do so, or the client may be highly motivated but have physical limitations that make self-care difficult. Some clients may be totally dependent on a caregiver for daily oral care. The dental hygienist assesses factors that limit the client's ability to perform daily self-care to make appropriate recommendations that meet individual needs. Assessment occurs through the following:

- Questioning client (or caregiver) about oral care practices
- Direct observation of oral self-care techniques used by client (or caregiver)
- Measurement of client's oral hygiene status and dental history (Procedure 17-1 and corresponding Competency Form)

Once an accurate assessment is made and documented, and the client's readiness to change behavior is determined, the dental hygienist educates and motivates the client (or caregiver) in small steps aimed at changes that will support oral health.

Procedure 17-1 Oral Deposit Assessment

EQUIPMENT

Personal protective equipment
Antimicrobial mouth rinse
Mouth mirror
Periodontal explorer
Gauze
Disclosing solution
Cotton tip applicators
Compressed air
Intraoral light source
Client hand mirror
Oral hygiene assessment form (including a dental index)

STEPS

1. Place the client in supine position; position light source to illuminate client's mouth.
2. Using compressed air, dry the supragingival tooth surfaces a sextant at a time; using a mouth mirror and direct and indirect vision, examine for supragingival calculus deposit.
3. Identify tooth surfaces and soft tissues with supragingival calculus and surfaces with stain; record these areas on the assessment form.
4. Apply disclosing agent, rinse, and dry with compressed air.
5. Examine tooth surfaces and soft tissues with a mouth mirror for areas of stained plaque; have client watch with a hand mirror.
6. Record plaque-covered tooth areas on the assessment form using red ink. Comment about oral biofilm on soft tissues and appliances.
7. Using a periodontal explorer and mouth mirror, explore subgingival tooth surfaces for calculus deposits.
8. Record subgingival calculus deposits on the assessment form.
9. Communicate findings to the client.
10. Record service in "services rendered" section of client record (e.g., "Computed plaque-free score of 75%").

As part of professional care, discussing characteristics of oral soft and hard deposits can serve as a useful motivator for clients having difficulty controlling oral biofilm. Visualization should be combined with the sensory feeling of biofilm on the teeth, the smell of biofilm, and the effects of biofilm (gingival bleeding and demineralization of tooth structure). Client knowledge of the biofilm provides a rationale for frequent professional subgingival root debridement, because biofilm in deep periodontal pockets cannot be reached by toothbrushes, interdental cleaners, and mouth rinses. Teaching the client about the resistant nature of the biofilm and the importance of disrupting and removing oral biofilm daily via mechanical and chemical measures remains the most effective means for its control (see Chapters 25, 26, and 33).

Oral Hygiene Indices

To monitor oral hygiene of an individual or group over time, dental indices are used as quantitative measures of oral status (see Chapter 19, Table 19-9 for periodontal indices and Chapter 58, Table 58-2 for indices used with dental implant clients). A **dental index** is a data collection tool that allows the practitioner (or researcher) to convert specific clinical observations into numeric values that can be quantified, summarized, analyzed, and interpreted. Oral hygiene indices measure levels of oral hygiene to accomplish the following:

- Establish a baseline; monitor, over time, an individual's oral self-care progress; and motivate the client to achieve higher levels of oral wellness
- Survey the oral hygiene status within a population, as is done in epidemiologic research
- Establish a baseline, and monitor, over time, the oral health status of a target population to evaluate the effectiveness of a community-based program or intervention
- Evaluate an intervention, drug, or device, as is found in a clinical trial

The index used must meet criteria for validity, reliability, and usability (Box 17-1).

Indices Used for Assessing Oral Deposits

Use of a standardized method of assessment can be valuable for motivating a client and documenting progress. The ability to show improvement is a powerful positive reinforcement tool that can help a client follow oral care recommendations. An index also can illustrate repeated neglect of a specific area of the mouth and thus guide a client in adhering to a

BOX 17-1

Criteria for an Effective Dental Index

- Simple to use
- Painless to client
- Efficient in terms of time
- Cost effective in terms of time, money, and armamentarium
- Statistically valid (measures what it is intended to measure) and reliable (reproducible)
- Translates clinical descriptions to numeric values on a smooth, graduated scale

self-care regimen. For maximum effectiveness an index performed with an individual should evaluate the entire dentition rather than a specific sample of teeth (e.g., the six Ramford index teeth: maxillary right and mandibular left first molars, maxillary left and mandibular right first premolars, and maxillary left and mandibular right central incisors), as often is used when conducting a randomized clinical trial. Even indices originally designed to measure a sample of teeth in a research subject's mouth can be adapted to measure all teeth present.

A simple plaque index is O'Leary's Plaque Control Record, illustrated in Figure 17-11 and described in eTable 17-5. This index provides a method of recording plaque on the mesial, distal, facial, and lingual tooth surfaces at the gingival margin. Plaque observed is recorded by striking a dash through the appropriate surface or surfaces. After all teeth are examined and scored for plaque, the index is computed by dividing the number of plaque-containing surfaces by the total number of available surfaces. The resulting score is the percentage of tooth surfaces in the mouth with plaque. Use of the index over time allows clients to visualize and monitor their own plaque control progress and therefore facilitates client motivation to improve oral self-care behaviors. This index also can be used to quantify stain in the same manner. eTable 17-5 shows commonly used oral hygiene indices.

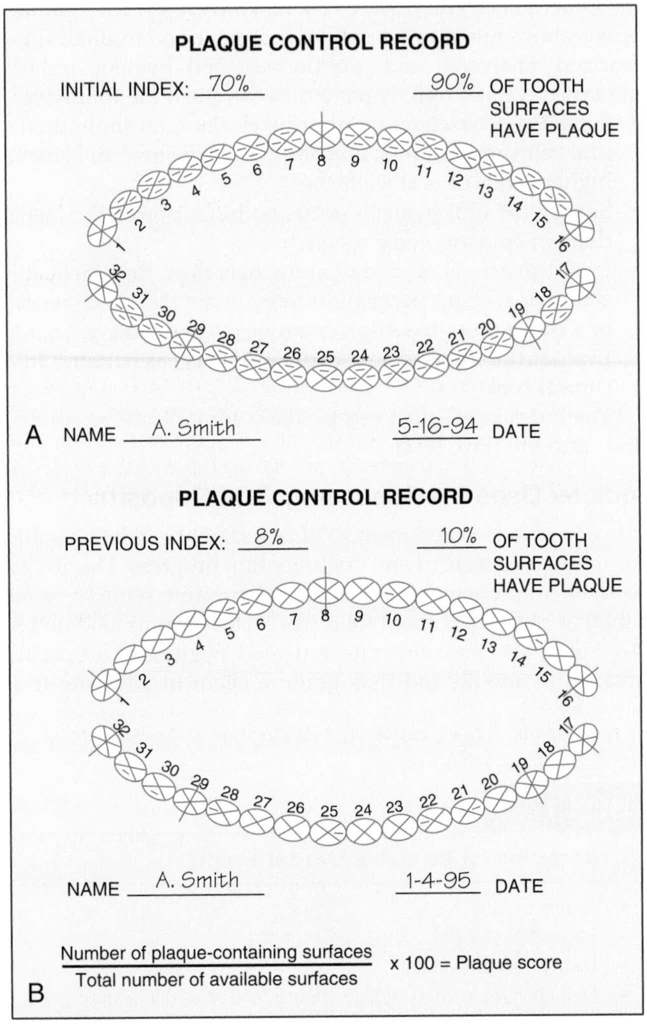

Figure 17-11. Plaque control record form. **A,** Seventy percent of tooth surfaces have plaque at initial appointment. **B,** Eight percent of tooth surfaces have plaque at a follow-up visit. (Redrawn from O'Leary TJ, Drake RB, Naylor JE: The plaque control record, *J Periodontol* 48:38, 1972.)

Record Keeping and Documentation

Maintaining a record of a client's oral hygiene status is part of the assessment phase of care. Such records provide baseline reference for subsequent visits and a basis for making professional care and product recommendations. Documenting oral hygiene products used and previous instruction given to the client provides continuity of care and ensures that educational interventions are appropriate.

Comparing plaque scores at subsequent appointments facilitates client skill development and acceptance of oral hygiene recommendations. Documentation allows the clinician to expand the client's oral health knowledge, reinforce instructions, and encourage effective use of techniques and products. Clients expect a continuing conversation about their success with recommended oral products and devices and an index that documents this information supports such interaction.

CLIENT EDUCATION TIPS

- Explain role of oral biofilm and host response in the development and control of gingival inflammation and periodontal disease progression.
- Explain bacterial plaque as a complex biofilm community that is self-sufficient, secure, and self-sustaining, rather than as a mere accumulation of planktonic bacteria.
- Use disclosing agents, bleeding points, and the senses of smell and feel to identify oral areas that need self-care interventions.
- Discuss how and where calculus is formed and methods of calculus management (e.g., an anticalculus dentifrice or mouth rinse with either a pyrophosphate system or a zinc system).
- Explain contributory factors in oral deposit accumulation.
- Explain relationship between oral hygiene index scores and the client's current oral health status.
- Discuss effective product selection and value of the American Dental Association Seal of Acceptance and the Canadian Dental Association Seal of Recognition.

LEGAL, ETHICAL, AND SAFETY ISSUES

- Prophylactic antibiotic premedication is indicated for clients with highest risk of adverse outcomes resulting from infective endocarditis during invasive dental procedures.
- Dental hygienists have a responsibility to document oral hygiene assessment data over time and clients' compliance with oral hygiene recommendations in the treatment record. Noncompliance may be viewed as contributory negligence in malpractice suits.
- Documenting lack of compliance is a risk management strategy and can be used, if necessary, to establish contributory negligence on the part of the client.

KEY CONCEPTS

- Oral hygiene assessment gives the clinician an accurate understanding of the client's oral hygiene status. Host response (inflammatory and immune responses) to the oral deposits present must be considered in the interpretation of oral hygiene assessment data.
- Oral hygiene assessment yields information that can be used as a teaching tool to motivate the client to achieve or maintain oral health.
- Assessment of soft and hard deposits, their origin, and their location is essential for dental hygiene diagnosis and care planning.
- Many factors contribute to the retention of oral biofilm, including stain, calculus, local predisposing factors, specialized mucosa of the tongue, saliva, and oral contributing factors.
- Oral biofilm creates its own renewing source of lipopolysaccharide for the long-term survival of microorganisms. Biofilm lends protective properties to the associated microorganisms (e.g., resistance to antibacterial and antibiotic agents such as chlorhexidine and systemic amoxicillin, respectively).
- About 20% of the oral cavity is occupied by teeth; about 80% includes the oral mucosa, and specialized mucosa. Oral biofilm grows on all of these surfaces and in saliva.
- Mechanical removal and twice-daily use of an effective antimicrobial mouth rinse is the most effective method to control oral biofilm. Without disruption and removal of the oral biofilm daily and frequent periodontal maintenance therapy (see Chapter 31), antimicrobial and antibiotic therapies may not penetrate the resistant biofilm community.
- Although dental calculus and extrinsic tooth stain are not causative agents in gingival inflammation, they provide an environment for oral biofilm attachment.
- Tracking plaque indices over time gives an objective measure of a client's progress with oral self-care.

CRITICAL THINKING EXERCISES

1. While working with a client, you notice a decrease in the amount of oral biofilm on the posterior lingual surfaces of the mandibular teeth from the last time a plaque index was performed. By reviewing the chart, you note that at the last dental hygiene care visit, particular attention was targeted to these areas during oral hygiene instruction. What is the best means of conveying this information to your client to maximize positive reinforcement?
2. During oral assessment you note a moderate amount of brown stain on a client's teeth, and the client indicates that he is troubled by the appearance of his teeth. What is the most effective way of exploring the nature of the stains and assisting the client in maintaining a more esthetic appearance between professional care visits?
3. Select an appropriate oral hygiene assessment index for a client you are currently treating, and provide the rationale for its selection.
4. For images and information about biofilms, visit the Center for Biofilm Engineering at Montana State University at http://www.erc.montana.edu, the American Society for Microbiology at http://dev.asm.org, and the Microbe Library at http://www.microbelibrary.org. Search for "biofilm."
5. For clinical images and a comprehensive discussion of dental stains, see Kerr AR: *Tooth discoloration*. Available at: http://www.emedicine.com/derm/topic646.htm.

BIBLIOGRAPHY

Greene JC, Vermillion JR: The simplified oral hygiene index. *J Am Dent Assoc* 68:7–13, 1964.

Hunt AA, James GA: *Dimensions Digest of Dental Hygiene, The Periodontal Paradigm: concepts to improve your understanding of biofilm's role in the complex periodontal disease process*. An educational supplement sponsored by Sunstar, 2013.

Löe H: The gingival index, the plaque index and the retention index systems. *J Periodontol* 38(Suppl.):610–616, 1967.

Newman MG, Takei HH, Klokkevold PR, et al: *Carranza's clinical periodontology*, ed 11, St Louis, 2012, Saunders.

Podshadley AG, Haley JV: A method for evaluating oral hygiene performance. *Public Health Rep* 83(3):259–264, 1968.

Rickard AH, Gilbert P, High NJ, et al: Bacterial co-aggregation: an integral process in the development of multi species biofilms. *Trends Microbiol* 11(2):94–100, 2003.

Seneviratne CJ, Zhang CF, Samaranayake LP: Dental plaque biofilm in oral health and disease. *Chin J Dent Res* 14(2):87–94, 2011.

Socransky SS, Haffajee AD, Cugini MA, et al: Microbial complexes in subgingival plaque. *J Clin Periodontol* 25:134, 1998.

Socransky SS, Haffajee AD, Teles R, et al: Effect of periodontal therapy on the subgingival microbiota over a 2-year monitoring period. I. Overall effect and kinetics of change. *J Clin Periodontol* 40(8):771–780, 2013.

ACKNOWLEDGMENT

The authors acknowledge Gwen Essex for her past contributions to this chapter.

EVOLVE RESOURCES

Please visit http://evolve.elsevier.com/Darby/hygiene for additional practice and study support tools.

CHAPTER 18

Dental Caries Management by Risk Assessment

John D.B. Featherstone

COMPETENCIES

1. Explain the team approach in integrating CAMBRA into an oral healthcare practice.
2. Define the disease of dental caries.
3. Explain the dental caries process, including:
   - Explain the process of demineralization and remineralization that occurs in the oral environment.
   - List saliva's beneficial actions.
   - Explain the dental caries balance.
4. Discuss dental caries risk assessment for clients age 6 through adult, including:
   - Explain the caries disease indicators that determine whether the client is at low, moderate, high, or extreme risk.
   - List the caries risk factors.
   - List the caries protective factors.
5. Discuss dental caries risk assessment for children 0 to 5 years of age, including:
   - List the high caries risk factors.
   - List the caries protective factors.
   - Explain the parent/caregiver recommendations for caries prevention.
6. Discuss caries management and identify clinical guidelines for caries management by risk assessment by age.
7. Explain, based on level of dental caries risk, when the following are indicated:
   - Professionally applied and self-applied topical fluorides, which are used to enhance remineralization.
   - Antimicrobial therapy (e.g., chlorhexidine, xylitol, iodine), which is used to reduce levels of pathogenic organisms.
   - Buffering products (e.g., sodium bicarbonate), which are needed to neutralize acid attacks.
   - Calcium and phosphate products, which are needed to replace minerals missing in saliva.

Risk assessment is an estimation of the likelihood that an event will occur in the future.[1] For more than two decades, medical science has recommended that physicians identify and treat patients based on their risk status, rather than treating all patients as if they were the same.[2] Although individual contributing factors to **dental caries** risk have been identified for more than two decades, only recently have combinations been put together in validated procedures for application to everyday clinical practice.[3] Caries risk assessment is the first step in Caries Management by Risk Assessment (**CAMBRA**), an evidence-based disease management protocol. With the CAMBRA methodology the clinician first assesses an individual's caries disease indicators, risk factors, and protective factors and then determines the level of caries risk that the sum of these factors indicates (low, moderate, high, or extreme). Based on the level of caries risk, an evidence-based care plan is developed that includes specific behavioral, chemical, and minimally invasive preventive and therapeutic procedures to manage the individual's dental caries disease.[4,5]

Many of the CAMBRA procedures fall within the purview of the dental hygienist. Dental hygienists must be knowledgeable and prepared to assess caries risk, to implement noninvasive or minimally invasive procedures according to state or province practice acts, and to provide leadership in promoting synergistic relationships with other staff members to create an environment of excellent client care. Every member of the dental team is essential to establishing a CAMBRA prevention-focused practice and to achieving successful client outcomes.[6] This chapter reviews the dental caries disease process and the background, rationale, and step-by-step procedures for the CAMBRA approach to caries management by risk assessment. It also provides an overview of topical fluoride use and other chemical interventions to manage the disease of dental caries based on level of caries risk.

Dental Caries: a Continuing Health Issue

Dental caries is a transmissible bacterial infection that is preventable and in some cases even reversible. Dental decay, however, remains the single most common disease of childhood that is not self-limiting or amenable to a course of antibiotics.[7] Dental caries also is the most common dental disease affecting children and adults in the United States and Canada, and it remains a significant worldwide disease.[8]

Review of Dental Caries Process

Demineralization

Dental caries is caused by mutans streptococci (a group that includes the *Streptococcus mutans* and *Streptococcus sobrinus* species) and lactobacilli that live in the plaque biofilm that attach to teeth. These bacteria metabolize dietary fermentable carbohydrates (sugars and cooked starch) to produce acids. These acids cause a substantial change in the **plaque biofilm** pH. At rest the pH of plaque biofilm is typically neutral. When fermentable carbohydrates are ingested, the plaque biofilm pH drops rapidly to create an acidic environment. The acids diffuse into the tooth to dissolve the calcium and phosphate minerals (carbonated hydroxyapatite). This process is called **demineralization**[9-11] (Figures 18-1 and 18-2).

Cariogenic Bacteria		Fermentable Carbohydrates		Organic Acids
S. mutans	+	Sucrose	→	Which penetrate enamel and dentin
S. sobrinus		Glucose		Dissolve tooth mineral
Lactobacilli		Fructose		
		Cooked starch		

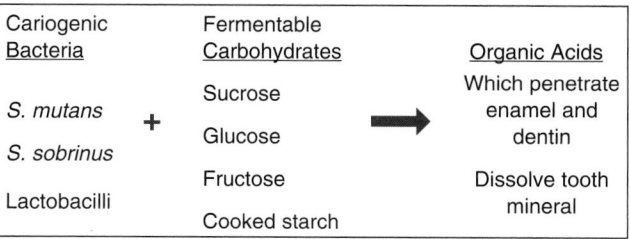

Figure 18-1. Demineralization: step 1.

Dental Mineral	+	Organic Acids	→	Demineralization*
Acid soluble Carbonated hydroxyapatite				Calcium and phosphate dissolve out of the tooth into solution

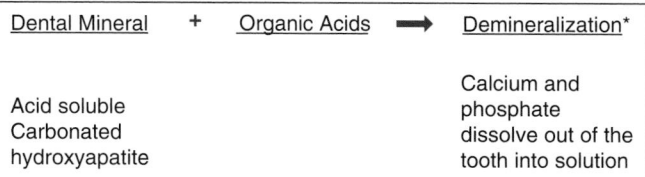

*If fluoride is present in the solution between the crystals, it inhibits mineral loss.

Figure 18-2. Demineralization: step 2.

				Remineralization
Calcium in tooth water (from saliva)	+	Phosphate in tooth water (from saliva)	→	Builds on existing crystal remnants New mineral is less soluble Fluoride speeds up remineralization

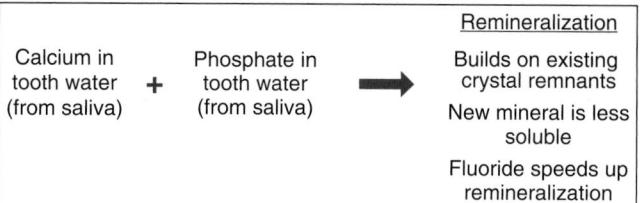

Figure 18-3. Remineralization and tooth repair.

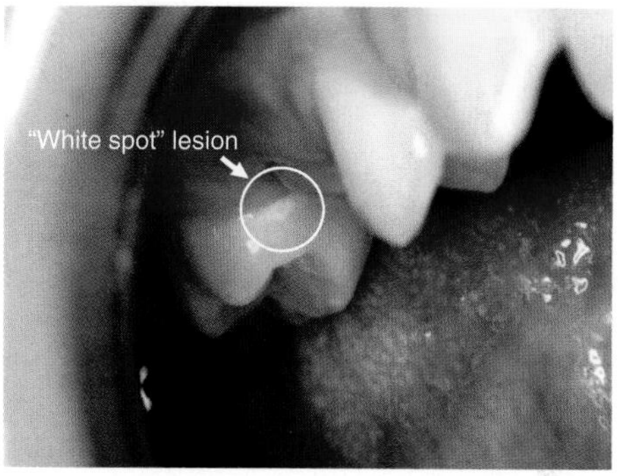

Figure 18-4. A white spot lesion.

BOX 18-1

Saliva's Beneficial Actions

- Provides calcium and phosphate for remineralization
- Carries topical fluoride around the mouth for remineralization
- Neutralizes organic acids produced in plaque biofilm
- Discourages the growth of bacteria, inhibiting infection
- Recycles ingested fluoride into the mouth
- Protects hard and soft tissues from drying
- Facilitates chewing and swallowing
- Speeds oral clearance of food

From Eakle SW, Featherstone JDB: *Caries risk instruction* [course handout], San Francisco, 2002, University of California School of Dentistry.

Remineralization

After the ingestion of fermentable carbohydrates stops, the pH gradually returns to neutral in 30 to 60 minutes provided there is adequate saliva. A variety of factors mediate the return to a neutral pH. Saliva plays a key role in that it neutralizes acids and provides minerals and proteins that protect the teeth (Box 18-1). Once calcium and phosphate are lost from the tooth structure and the pH in the adjacent environment returns to neutral, the area experiences remineralization. Minerals in the saliva and minerals dissolved out of the tooth are available to redeposit onto existing crystal remnants inside the tooth. This deposition of minerals into demineralized areas of tooth structure is called **remineralization**, which repairs the initial carious lesion (Figure 18-3). This ongoing process of destruction and repair occurs with each carbohydrate challenge.

Whether an initial carious lesion progresses and develops into a frank carious lesion (a hole or cavitation) depends on a variety of factors. To prevent the lesion from progressing, there must be enough deposition of salivary minerals to repair and strengthen the area and provide support for the enamel surface and subsurface. Minerals in the saliva initially enable the host to repair demineralized areas. If, however, the flow of saliva is low, the level of acid-producing bacteria is high, and the frequency of eating and/or drinking of fermentable carbohydrates is high, then the tooth mineral lost by acid attacks is too great for repair by natural salivary remineralization. This situation leads to the start of dental caries evidenced clinically as a white spot lesion (Figure 18-4). However, fluoride plays a very important role in the remineralization repair process and the overall prevention of carious lesions. Fluoride works primarily via topical surface mechanisms to inhibit demineralization, enhance remineralization, and inhibit plaque biofilm bacteria.[11]

The White Spot Lesion

Demineralization results in the greatest loss of calcium and phosphate minerals in the subsurface zone of the enamel and the formation of a white spot lesion. The enamel surface of the white spot typically remains intact, but the demineralized area appears white owing to the loss of mineral in the subsurface zone of the enamel (see Figure 18-4). By comparison, the enamel surrounding the white spot appears sound and translucent.[11] Thus a **white spot lesion** is a demineralized area of enamel that usually has an intact surface remaining over the body of the demineralized early carious lesion. It is partially reversible with appropriate topical fluoride intervention. The white spot lesion is a signal to intervene to avoid the development of a frank carious lesion. It is not a signal to do surgery (e.g., place a restoration).[11] The demineralization process for cementum and dentin is similar to that for enamel, except that the process typically does not result in an intact surface remaining over the body of the carious lesion.[8]

The Caries Balance

Dental caries involves an interaction among pathologic factors and protective factors. Pathologic factors include **acidogenic** (acid-producing) **bacteria** (mutans streptococci and lactobacilli), frequent eating and/or drinking of

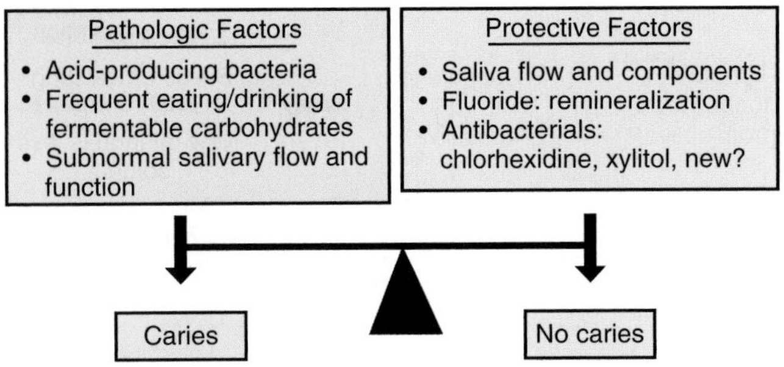

Figure 18-5. The caries balance. (Redrawn from Featherstone JDB: The caries balance: contributing factors and early detection, *J Calif Dent Assoc* 31:129, 2003.)

BOX 18-2

Four Caries Disease Indicators for Caries Risk Assessment

- Teeth with frank cavitations or lesions that radiographically show penetration into dentin
- Approximal radiographic lesions confined to the enamel only
- Visual white spots on smooth surfaces
- Any restorations placed in the last 3 years

fermentable carbohydrates, and subnormal salivary flow and function. Protective factors include calcium, phosphate, proteins, and fluoride in the saliva; normal salivary flow; and antibacterial agents if needed (Figure 18-5).[4] The goal of caries management is to restore and maintain a balance, known as the caries balance, between protective factors and pathologic factors to remineralize early carious lesions and/or prevent future caries.

Dental Caries Risk Assessment for CLIENTS Age 6 through Adult

Caries risk assessment is the first step in CAMBRA. A group of experts from across the United States convened at a consensus conference in 2002 produced a caries risk assessment procedure and form for 6-year-olds through adults that subsequently was validated in a large cohort study.[12,13] Figure 18-6 presents the refined and updated version of that caries risk assessment form for clients 6 years of age or older, which is composed of a hierarchy of disease indicators, risk factors, and protective factors (illustrated in Figure 18-7) that are based on the best scientific evidence available at this time.[4] Use of this caries risk assessment form is discussed later in the chapter.

The goal of caries risk assessment for clients 6 years old or older is to assign a client to a caries risk level for development of future caries as the first step in managing the disease process. This assessment occurs in two phases. First, the clinician assesses an individual's caries disease indicators, risk factors, and protective factors. Second, the clinician then determines the level of caries risk (low, moderate, high, or extreme) based on the presence of caries disease indicators and the balance between pathologic and protective factors.[4,5]

Caries Disease Indicators

Caries disease indicators are four clinical observations from the clinical examination that indicate past caries history and activity.[4] The four caries disease indicators are listed in Box 18-2. Clinicians indicate the presence of each of these caries disease indicators by circling a positive response (i.e., "yes") on the caries risk assessment form (see Figure 18-6).

Presence of any one of these four indicators automatically places the client at high caries risk unless therapeutic interventions are already in place and disease progress has been arrested. The presence of any one of these caries disease indicators in the presence of inadequate salivary flow automatically indicates extreme caries risk.[3]

Caries Risk Factors

Caries risk factors are biologic factors that contribute to the level of risk for developing new carious lesions in the future or having the existing lesions progress. Risk factors are things clinicians can do something about. There are nine risk factors recently identified in studies of caries risk assessment, and these are listed on the caries risk assessment form in Figure 18-6.[4]

These nine pathologic risk factors are as follows:

- Medium or high mutans streptococci and lactobacilli counts
- Visible heavy plaque biofilm on teeth
- Frequent (more than three times daily) snacking between meals
- Deep pits and fissures
- Recreational drug use
- Inadequate salivary flow by observation or measurement
- Saliva-reducing factors (medication, radiation, systemic condition)
- Exposed roots
- Orthodontic appliances

These risk factors also help us to understand the reason behind an ongoing caries problem. If there are no clinical signs of caries disease indicators, the caries risk status (low, moderate, high, or extreme) is determined by the balance between the pathologic factors and protective factors described in the following section (see Figure 18-7).

Caries Protective Factors

Caries protective factors are biologic or therapeutic factors that collectively can offset the challenge presented by the caries risk factors. The more severe the risk factors, the more protective factors are needed to keep the patient in balance or to reverse the caries process.

Currently the following 11 protective factors are included on the caries risk assessment form in Figure 18-6[4]:

- Lives, works, attends school in a fluoridated community
- Uses fluoride toothpaste at least once daily
- Uses fluoride toothpaste at least two times daily (implies an additional benefit over and above once a day or less)
- Uses fluoride mouth rinse (0.05% NaF) daily
- Uses 5000 ppm fluoride toothpaste daily
- Had fluoride varnish applied in the last 6 months
- Had an office fluoride topical application in the last 6 months
- Used prescribed chlorhexidine daily for 1 week in each of the last 6 months

Patient Name: **CHART #:** **DATE:**

Assessment Date: **Is This (please circle) Baseline or Recall**

Disease Indicators (any one YES signifies likely "High Risk" and to do a bacteria test**)	YES = CIRCLE	YES = CIRCLE	YES = CIRCLE
Cavities/radiograph to dentin	YES		
Approximal enamel lesions (by radiograph)	YES		
White spots on smooth surface	YES		
Restorations past 3 years	YES		
Risk Factors (biological predisposing factors)		YES	
MS and LB both medium or high **(by culture**)**		YES	
Visible heavy plaque on teeth		YES	
Frequent snack (>3 times daily between meals)		YES	
Deep pits and fissures		YES	
Recreational drug use		YES	
Inadequate saliva flow by observation or measurement (**if measured, note the flow rate below)		YES	
Saliva-reducing factors (medications/radiation/systemic)		YES	
Exposed roots		YES	
Orthodonic appliances		YES	
Protective Factors			
Lives/work/school fluoridated community			YES
Fluoride toothpaste at least once daily			YES
Fluoride toothpaste at least 2 times daily			YES
Fluoride mouth rinse (0.05% NaF) daily			YES
5000 ppm F fluoride toothpaste daily			YES
Fluoride varnish in past 6 months			YES
Office F topical in past 6 months			YES
Chlorihexidine prescribed/used 1 week each of past 6 months			YES
Xylitol gum/lozenges 4 times daily past 6 months			YES
Ca and PO_4 supplement paste during past 6 months			YES
Adequate saliva flow (>1 mL/min stimulated)			YES
Bacteria/Saliva Test Results: MS: LB: Flow Rate: mL/min. Date:			

VISUALIZE CARIES BALANCE
(Use circled indicators/factors above)

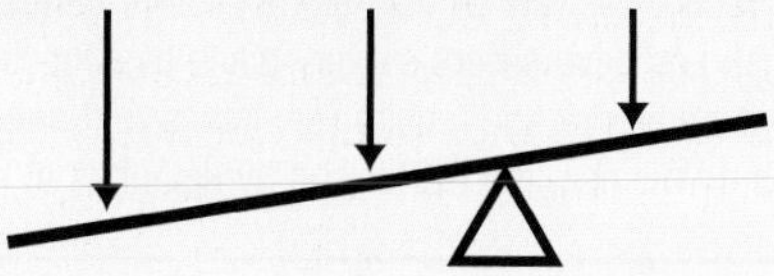

CARIES RISK ASSESSMENT (CIRCLE): **EXTREME HIGH MODERATE LOW**

(EXTREME RISK = HIGH RISK + SEVERE XEROSTOMIA)
Doctor signature/#: **Date:**

Figure 18-6. Caries risk assessment form—children age 6 through adults. (Redrawn from Featherstone JDB, Domejean-Orliaquet S, Jenson L, et al: Caries assessment in practice for age 6 through adult, *J Calif Dent Assoc* 35:704, 2007.)

- Used xylitol gum or lozenges four to five times daily in the last 6 months
- Used calcium and phosphate supplement paste during the last 6 months
- Has adequate salivary flow (>1 mL/min stimulated)

Use of the Caries Risk Assessment Form

Procedure 18-1 and the corresponding Competency Form describes how to use the caries risk assessment form. Box 18-3 summarizes the criteria for high caries risk, and Box 18-4 lists the criteria for extreme caries risk, both for ages

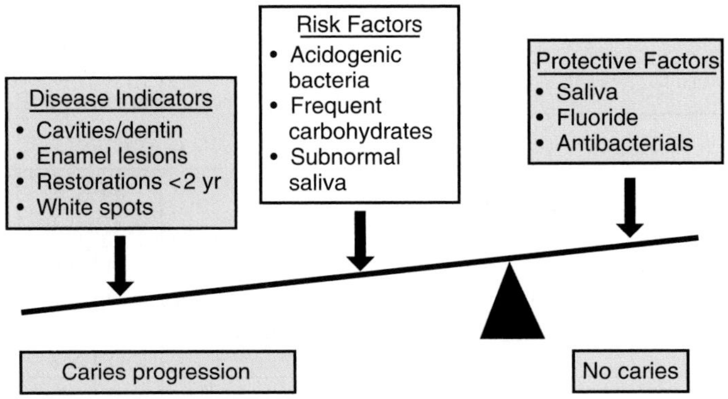

Figure 18-7. Caries imbalance. (Redrawn from Featherstone JDB, Domejean-Orliaquet S, Jenson L, et al: Caries assessment in practice for age 6 through adult, *J Calif Dent Assoc* 35:705, 2007.)

Procedure 18-1 Use of the Caries Risk Assessment Form

STEP 1
Based on data obtained from the health histories and clinical examination, circle the *Yes* categories in the three columns on the form presented in Figure 18-6.

STEP 2
Make notations regarding the number of carious lesions present, the oral hygiene status, the brand of fluorides used, the type of snacks eaten, and the names of medications or drugs causing dry mouth.

STEP 3
If the answer is *Yes* to any one of the four disease indicators in the first column, then take a bacterial culture using the Caries Risk Test (see Procedure 18-2) (Ivoclar Vivadent, Amherst, New York) or an equivalent test.

STEP 4
Make an overall judgment as to whether the client is at low, moderate, high, or extreme risk depending on the balance between the disease indicators or risk factors and the protective factors using the caries balance concept. (Clients who have a current caries lesion or had one in the recent past are at high risk for future caries. Clients who are at high risk and have severe salivary gland hypofunction or special needs are at extreme risk and require very intensive therapy. If the client is not at high or low risk, then he or she by default is at moderate risk.)

BOX 18-3

Criteria for High Caries Risk: Ages 6 Years and Older to Adult

- One or more disease indicators:
  - Cavities
  - Radiographic lesions to dentin
  - Recent restorations
  - White spots

and/or

- Multiple risk factors:
  - Heavy plaque on teeth
  - Frequent (greater than three times per day) between-meal snacks of sugars or cooked starch
  - Appliances present (e.g., orthodontic brackets)

coupled with

- Little or no protective factors

BOX 18-4

Criteria for Extreme Caries Risk: Ages 6 Years and Older to Adult

Same as high caries risk but with saliva-reducing factors, including the following:

- Medications
- Radiation to the head and neck
- Systemic reasons (e.g., Sjögren's syndrome)

BOX 18-5

Moderate Caries Risk: Ages 6 Years and Older to Adult

If you cannot decide whether a client is at high caries risk or low caries risk, then the client should be considered to be at moderate caries risk.

6 years and older. Box 18-5 provides information on clients in this same age group who are considered to be at moderate caries risk.

The California Dental Association caries risk assessment (CDA CRA) form for use with children age 6 and older to adult presented in this chapter is based on a combination of factors related to the caries disease occurrence that are easy to record/assess in everyday practice. The procedure to use the form is straightforward and follows the dental history and clinical examination. A 2011 study was conducted to evaluate the validity of CDA CRA as related to existing caries and to determine its predictive value for future caries. Data were collected retrospectively from electronic and paper charts by a systematic process of chart reviews for 12,954 records over a 6-year period. Findings provided convincing evidence that the CDA caries risk assessment tool is valid in an adult population seeking care and demonstrated that the CDA CRA form can be implemented successfully and used in everyday clinical dental practice. The CDA CRA form accurately identified patients at high caries risk and extreme risk.[14]

Salivary Flow Rate Test

If visually inadequate salivary flow is noticed, or if the client reports having a dry mouth, then a salivary flow rate test should be conducted (Procedure 18-2 and corresponding Competency Form; see Figure 18-9). Saliva neutralizes acids and provides minerals and proteins that protect the teeth from dental caries. Therefore it is essential for controlling dental caries.

The reason for any low salivary flow rate must be determined to plan for caries management. The client should be informed of the results and their implications for dental caries.

Caries Bacteria Testing

If any one of the four disease indicators in the first column of the caries risk assessment form (see Figure 18-6) is present, then a bacterial culture should be taken.[4,5] Currently there are several chairside tests available for caries bacteria testing. Procedure 18-2 describes use of an example bacterial test, the Caries Risk Test (Vivadent, Amherst, New York). This test allows a bacterial culture to be made from collected saliva and is sensitive enough to provide a level of low, medium, or high cariogenic bacterial challenge. The level of bacterial challenge is recorded in the client's record as low, medium, or high. The client is informed of the results and their implications for caries risk and caries management.

Results of this bacterial test also can be used to motivate client compliance with recommended antibacterial regimens.[4,5]

Dental Caries Risk Assessment for Children from 0 to 5 Years of Age[1]

Early childhood caries (ECC) is an infectious disease that affects children from birth to 2 years of age and rapidly destroys newly erupted teeth. Initially ECC appears as bands of demineralized areas usually first seen on the primary maxillary incisors. These areas of demineralization quickly become yellow or brown cavitated areas[7] (Figure 18-8).

The cause of ECC is complex. The primary cause of demineralization in infants and toddlers primarily involves cariogenic bacteria and a diet high in fermentable carbohydrates. Mothers, caregivers, siblings, and other children transmit mutans streptococci to infants and young children. In addition, frequent or prolonged feedings with bottled milk, formula, human breast milk, fruit juice, or sugared drinks are highly cariogenic. Box 18-6 lists high caries risk factors for ages birth to 5 years, and Box 18-7 lists protective factors for the same age group.

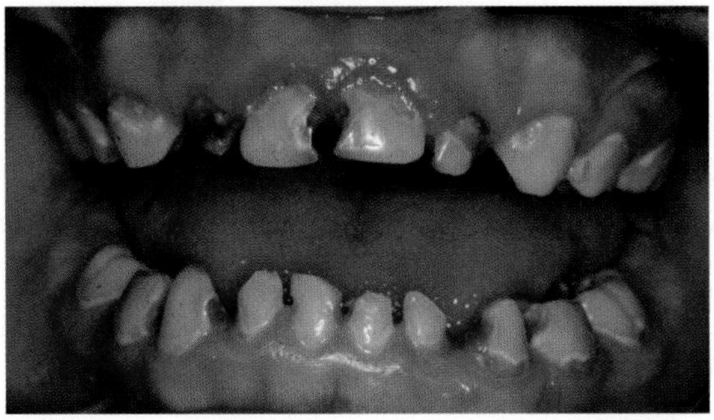

Figure 18-8. Early childhood caries. (Courtesy Dr. Frank Hodges.)

The American Dental Association (ADA), the American Academy of Pediatric Dentistry, and the American Association of Public Health Dentistry recommend all children have their first preventive dental visit by 12 months of age.[15-17] Figure 18-10 presents the CAMBRA assessment form for newborn to 5-year-old infants and toddlers. The protocol for a comprehensive CAMBRA birth-to-5 years oral care visit includes the following components:

- Completion of the caries risk assessment form
- Parent interview
- Examination of the child
- Assignment of caries risk level
- Individualized treatment based on risk level
- If indicated, bacterial culture on parent or caregiver and child
- Sharing of bacterial results with parent or caregiver as the basis for treatment recommendations and to enhance motivation
- Individualized homecare recommendations
- Motivational interview of parent or caregiver for caries control
- Setting of self-management goals with parent and child
- Anticipatory guidance according to a specific age category
- Determination of the interval for periodic oral examination
- Collaboration with other healthcare professionals

BOX 18-6

Factors for High Caries Risk for Ages Birth to 5 Years

- Mother or primary caregiver with active dental decay in the last 12 months
- Sleeps with bottle or nurses on *ad lib* basis
- Bottle contains fluids other than milk or water
- Visible cavities, white spots, or obvious decalcification
- Recent dental restorations (<2 years)
- Bleeding gums or heavy plaque on teeth
- Frequent (more than three times) between-meal snacks of sugars or cooked starch
- Appliances present (e.g., space maintainers, obturators)
- Visually inadequate salivary flow
- Presence of saliva-reducing factors, as follows:
  - Medications, such as for asthma or hyperactivity
  - Medical reasons (cancer treatment) or genetic predisposition

BOX 18-7

Protective Factors for Ages Birth to 5 Years

- Residence in a community with fluoridated water
- Mother or caregiver who cleans child's teeth twice a day with fluoride toothpaste (small amount)
- Dental examination for child combined with oral hygiene instruction for parent or caregiver
- Visibly adequate salivary flow
- Mother or caregiver who uses xylitol gum or mints four to five times daily
- Mother or caregiver who has no caries activity

Procedure 18-2 Testing Salivary Flow Rate and Level of Caries Bacterial Challenge

EQUIPMENT

Paraffin pellets
Measuring cup
Commercially available caries bacterial test kit, such as the Caries Risk Test (Ivolcar Vivadent, Amherst, New York) or an equivalent test
Incubator
Personal protective barriers

STEP 1

Determine salivary flow rate.

- Have the client chew a paraffin pellet for 3 to 5 minutes (timed) and spit all saliva generated into a measuring cup.
- At the end of the 3 to 5 minutes, measure the amount of saliva in milliliters (mL) and divide that amount by time to determine the mL/min of stimulated salivary flow.
- A flow rate of 1 mL/min or higher is considered normal; a level of 0.7 mL/min is low; and anything at 0.5 mL/min or less is dry, indicating severe salivary gland hypofunction.
- Investigate the reason for the flow rate if it is 0.7 mL/min or less (medication, radiation, systemic condition).

STEP 2

Initiate bacterial testing.

- The kit comes with a two-sided selective media stick that assesses mutans streptococci (MS) on the blue side and lactobacilli (LB) on the green side.
- Remove the selective media stick from the culture tube. Peel off the plastic cover sheet from each side of the stick.
- Pour (do not streak) the collected saliva over the media on each side until it is entirely wet.
- Place one of the sodium bicarbonate tablets included in the kit in the bottom of the tube.
- Replace the media stick in the culture tube, screw the lid on, and label the tube with the client's name, registration number, and date.
- Place the tube in the incubator at 37° C for 48 hours (Figure 18-9).* (Incubators suitable for a dental office are also sold by the company.)
- Collect the tube after 48 hours, and compare the densities of bacterial colonies with the pictures provided in the kit indicating relative bacterial levels. The dark blue agar is selective for MS, and the light green agar is selective for LB.
- Record the level of bacterial challenge in the client's chart as low, medium, or high, and inform client of results.

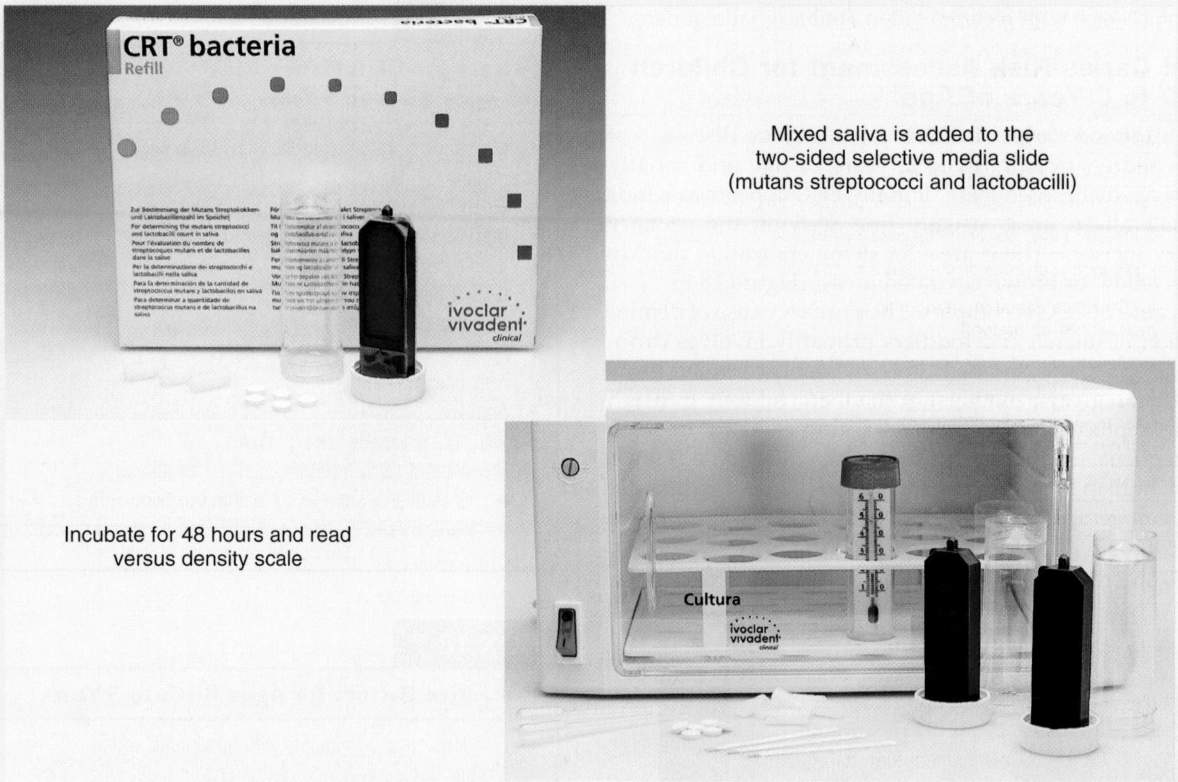
CRT® bacteria
Refill
ivoclar vivadent clinical
Mixed saliva is added to the two-sided selective media slide (mutans streptococci and lactobacilli)
Incubate for 48 hours and read versus density scale
Cultura

Figure 18-9. Bacterial testing equipment. (Courtesy Ivoclar Vivadent, Amherst, New York.)

*Tests have shown that 72 hours' incubation produces more reliable results than the 48 hours recommended by the manufacturer.

CAMBRA for Dental Providers (0-5) Assessment Tool

Caries Risk Assessment Form for Age 0 to 5

Patient Name:____________________ I.D.#________ Age ________ Date________

Initial/base line exam date____________________ Caries recall date____________________

Respond to each question in sections 1, 2, 3, and 4 with a check mark in the "Yes" or "No" column	Yes	No	Notes
1. Caries Risk Indicators — Parent Interview**			
(a) Mother or primary caregiver has had active dental decay in the past 12 months			
(b) Child has recent dental restorations (see 5b below)			
(c) Parent and/or caregiver has low SES (socioeconomic status) and/or low health literacy			
(d) Child has developmental problems			
(e) No dental home/episodic dental care			
2. Caries Risk Factors (Biological) — Parent Interview**			
(a) Child has frequent (greater than 3 times daily) between-meal snacks of sugars/cooked starch/sugared beverages			
(b) Child has saliva-reducing factors present, including: 1. Medications (e.g., some for asthma or hyperactivity) 2. Medical (cancer treatment) or genetic factors			
(c) Child continually uses bottle — contains fluids other than water			
(d) Child sleeps with a bottle or nurses on demand			
3. Protective Factors (Nonbiological) — Parent Interview			
(a) Mother/caregiver decay-free past 3 years			
(b) Child has a dental home and regular dental care			
4. Protective Factors (Biological) — Parent Interview			
(a) Child lives in a fluoridated community or takes fluoride supplements by slowly dissolving or as chewable tablets			
(b) Child's teeth are cleaned with fluoridated toothpaste (pea-size) daily			
(c) Mother/caregiver chews/sucks xylitol chewing gum/lozenges 4-5 times daily			
5. Caries Risk Indicators/Factors — Clinical Examination of Child**			
(a) Obvious white spots, decalcifications, or obvious decay present on the child's teeth			
(b) Restorations placed in the past 2 years in/on child's teeth			
(c) Plaque is obvious on the child's teeth and/or gums bleed easily			
(d) Child has dental or orthodontic appliances present, fixed or removable (e.g., braces, space maintainers, obturators)			
(e) Risk Factor: Visually inadequate saliva flow — dry mouth			

****If yes to any one of 1(a), 1(b), 5(a), or 5(b) or any two in categories 1, 2, 5, consider performing bacterial culture on mother or caregiver and child. Use this as a base line to follow results of antibacterial intervention.**	Parent/Caregiver Date:	Child Date:
(a) Mutans streptococci (indicate bacterial level: high, medium, low)		
(b) *Lactobacillus species* (indicate bacterial level: high, medium, low)		

Child's overall caries risk status: (CIRCLE) Extreme	Low	Moderate	High

Recommendations given: Yes________ No ________ Date given: ________ Date follow up: ________

SELF-MANAGEMENT GOALS 1) ____________________ 2) ____________________

Practitioner signature____________________ Date ____________________

Figure 18-10. Caries risk assessment form for ages 0 to 5. (Redrawn from Ramos-Gomez FJ, Crall J, Gansky SA, et al: Caries risk assessment appropriate for the age 1 visit [infants and toddlers], *J Calif Dent Assoc* 35:687, 2007.)

Parent Interview

A parent interview is conducted before the child is examined to identify caries risk factors, disease indictors, and protective factors already in place. If the mother and/or caregiver has active decay, this automatically places the child at high risk owing to the high likelihood of bacterial transmission from parent or caregiver to child.[1]

Examination of the Child

The examination of the child completes the risk factor–disease indicator list. If the child has obvious decalcification (white spots) or cavities, this places the child at high risk for future caries.[1]

Assignment of Caries Risk Level

Once the risk factor list has been checked, the provider summarizes the risk factors and assigns a caries risk level (low, moderate, or high) based on the balance between pathologic and protective factors. Active decay in the parent or caregiver or in the child automatically places the child at high risk, signaling the need for antibacterial intervention and fluoride treatment for the parent or caregiver and the child.[1]

Individualized Treatment Based on Skill Level

Strategies must be employed to modify the maternal or caregiver transmission of cariogenic bacteria to infants through the potential use of chlorhexidine rinse, fluoride varnish, and xylitol-based products.[1]

Bacterial Culture

If assessments reveal the presence of high caries risk factors and disease indicators, then bacterial cultures of saliva collected from the parent or caregiver and child are indicated.[1] If parents or caregivers have high cariogenic bacterial counts, they should be advised to seek appropriate dental care to reduce their caries risk and control their caries by eliminating the infection source and reducing the early infant inoculation.[1]

Individualized Homecare Recommendations

Once risk level is determined, the provider develops an individualized treatment plan, customizes homecare recommendations, engages the parent or caregiver in the process by conducting a motivational interview,[18] involves the parent or caregiver in setting self-management goals, educates the parent or caregiver about age-specific interventions for prevention (anticipatory guidance), and determines the interval for periodic reevaluation.

Box 18-8 lists parent or caregiver caries prevention recommendations for children birth to 5 years of age. Further information to assist in expansion of related knowledge and skills may be found on the First Smiles website (http://www.first5oralhealth.org) as part of a statewide oral health initiative regarding oral health of children birth to 5 years old, funded by First 5 California and managed by the California Dental Association Foundation and the Dental Health Foundation.

Caries Management

Based on the level of caries risk determined, an evidence-based care plan is developed that includes specific behavioral, chemical, and minimally invasive preventive and therapeutic procedures to manage the individual's dental caries disease. (See Chapters 33, 34, and 35) Caries management is aimed at restoring and maintaining a balance between protective factors and pathologic factors (see Figures 18-5[9] and 18-7).[4] Caries management involves the following:

- Suppressing bacteria that cause the infection
- Remineralizing early noncavitated carious lesions by enhancing salivary flow, using fluorides, and possibly using calcium and phosphate paste products, especially if the client is at extreme caries risk (e.g., low salivary flow)
- Protecting tooth surfaces by using sealants and fluorides
- Decreasing the frequency of sugar intake
- Surgically removing carious lesions that are beyond hope of remineralization and restoring the teeth with minimally invasive techniques and materials[5]

Decreasing pathologic factors involves strategies such as client education, oral hygiene instruction, reduction of the intake of fermentable carbohydrates, and addition of the use of chlorhexidine rinse and/or xylitol gum.[5] Box 18-9 summarizes guiding principles for caries management for high-risk individuals. Box 18-10 summarizes evidence-based therapeutic recommendations for individuals at high caries risk.

After determining the caries risk of an individual, the clinician provides the client with educational material about the caries process (see http://www.cdafoundation.org for a patient information sheet on tooth decay) and makes recommendations based on the caries risk status of the individual as determined by the balance or imbalance between the pathologic factors and the protective factors.[4] Tables 18-1 and 18-2 provide clinical guidelines for caries management by risk assessment for clients age 6 years and older[5] and birth to 5 years,[1] respectively. The client's compliance with recommendations is assessed 3 to 6 months after the initial visit.

BOX 18-8

Parent/Caregiver Recommendations for Caries Prevention: Ages Birth to 5 Years

Daily Oral Hygiene

- Small amount of fluoride-containing toothpaste by cloth or brush twice daily
- Selective daily flossing

Diet

- Elimination of bottles with sugared fluids or juices
- Limited between-meal snacks, limited sodas; substitution of non–caries-causing snacks

Sugar-Free Gum

For parent or caregiver of high-risk infant, use of xylitol-containing gum four to five times daily

Antibacterial Rinse

- For parent or caregiver, use of chlorhexidine gluconate (0.12%) once daily for 1 week every month and use of fluoride rinse (0.05% NaF) daily in intervening weeks

BOX 18-9

Guiding Principles for Caries Management for High-Risk Individuals

- Placing restorations does not reduce the bacterial challenge.
- Fluoride use and concentration should be increased for remineralization.
- Bacterial challenge can be reduced through antibacterial therapy.
- Pathologic factors should be balanced with protective factors.

BOX 18-10

Evidence-Based Therapy for Individuals with High Caries Risk

- Fluoride toothpaste at least two times daily
- Increase of fluoride to 5000 ppm toothpaste for age 6 years through adult
- Fluoride varnish two or three times annually
- Xylitol for mothers and caregivers of newborns to 5-year-olds
- Chlorhexidine (once daily 1 week each month) and xylitol for age 6 years through adult
- Calcium phosphopeptide paste with fluoride (MI Paste Plus)
- Sealants
- Glass ionomer restorations and sealant
- Minimally invasive restorations

If bacterial levels were moderate or high at the initial visit, bacterial assessment is repeated to see if they have been reduced. Recommendations should be modified or reinforced based on bacterial results and patient compliance.[4,5] Chemical therapy is employed to adjust the imbalance between the pathologic factors and the protective factors to reverse or halt the progression of dental caries toward cavitation. Such chemical therapies are discussed later. The evidence base for products used to treat and prevent dental caries should be evaluated and considered before such products are used in practice.

Fluoride Therapies

Fluoride is a naturally occurring element present in many minerals, water supplies, and foods. Fluoride delivered to the tooth surface and the plaque biofilm can have a dramatic caries preventive and reparative effect if delivered at the right concentrations.

Primary Mechanisms of Fluoride Action

Fluoride works primarily and most effectively via topical (surface) mechanisms (whether delivered in the drinking water, foods, beverages, or products) to inhibit demineralization, enhance remineralization, and inhibit plaque bacteria.[8,11]

Inhibition of Demineralization

Fluoride present on the tooth surface and in plaque fluid inhibits acid demineralization by reducing the solubility of the tooth mineral.[8,11]

Enhancement of Remineralization

Fluoride accelerates the remineralization process by adsorbing to mineral crystals within the tooth and attracting calcium ions. In addition, fluoride ions incorporate into the remineralizing tooth structure, resulting in the development of fluorapatite-like crystals. These crystals are less soluble than the original enamel mineral and make remineralized lesions less susceptible to future demineralization. Fluoride levels in the mouth from fluoridated water are sufficient to enhance remineralization. Fluoridated water has primarily a topical effect.

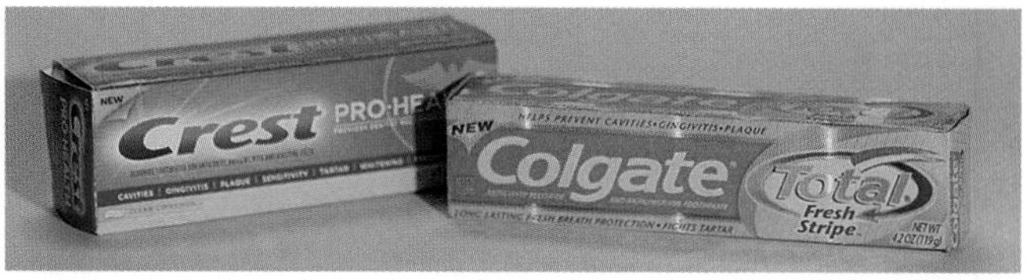

Figure 18-11. Sample sodium fluoride dentifrices that have the American Dental Association Seal of Acceptance for dental caries prevention. (Courtesy Dr. Mark Dillenges.)

Inhibition of Plaque Bacteria

Fluoride present in plaque biofilm is taken up by acid-producing bacteria and interferes with acid production.[8,11]

Topical Fluoride

Beyond the fluoride in drinking water and some beverages, topical fluorides are taken into the oral cavity in the following three primary forms:

- Self-applied by clients in the form of nonprescription products available over the counter
- Self-applied by clients in the form of prescription products
- Professionally applied prescription products

Typically the topical fluoride agents available as self-applied fluoride agents for at-home use are lower in fluoride concentration than those that are applied professionally. In general, the following guidelines apply:

- Low-concentration products are referred to as *low-potency* and usually are applied more frequently.
- High-concentration products are referred to as *high-potency* and typically are applied less frequently.

Self-Applied Dentifrices

Other than the fluoride consumed in drinking water, dentifrices are the most widely used fluoride preparations. ADA-approved fluoride dentifrices for caries prevention provide sufficiently large concentrations of fluoride to facilitate enamel remineralization (Figure 18-11).[8,11] The majority of commercial dentifrices available in the United States contain around 1000 parts per million (ppm) fluoride. Some manufacturers produce higher-strength dentifrices that contain up to 1500 ppm fluoride. Most over-the-counter dentifrices marketed in the United States contain one of the following:

- Sodium fluoride (NaF) formulated with a highly compatible, synthetic-silica base
- Sodium monofluorophosphate (NaMFP)
- Stannous fluoride (SnF_2)

Brushing twice daily with a fluoride-containing dentifrice is one of the most effective ways to control dental decay. Numerous clinical trials report around 30% reduction in caries incidence with fluoride dentifrice containing 1000 to 2800 ppm fluoride.[8] Curnow and colleagues[18] reported 56% reduction with supervised brushing twice daily compared with unsupervised brushing. High–fluoride concentration fluoride products such as 5000 ppm fluoride toothpaste are more effective than 1100 ppm fluoride in high–caries-risk individuals and are proven effective for root caries prevention.[8,19] Such high fluoride concentration dentifrices require a prescription from a dentist and are usually available in

TABLE 18-1

CAMBRA Clinical Guidelines for Patients Age 6 Years and Older

Risk Level*	Frequency of Radiographs	Frequency of Caries Recall Examinations	Saliva Test (Saliva Flow and Bacterial Culture)	Antibacterials, Chlorhexidine, Xylitol†	Fluoride	pH Control	Calcium Phosphate Topical Supplements	Sealants (Resin-Based or Glass Ionomer)
Low risk	Bitewing radiographs every 24-36 months	Every 6-12 months to reevaluate caries risk	May be done as a baseline reference for new patients	Per saliva test if done	OTC fluoride-containing toothpaste twice daily, after breakfast and at bedtime Optional NaF varnish if excessive root exposure or sensitivity	Not required	Not required Optional for excessive root exposure or sensitivity	Optional or as per ICDAS sealant protocol
Moderate risk	Bitewing radiographs every 18-24 months	Every 4-6 months to reevaluate caries risk	May be done as a baseline reference for new patients or if there is suspicion of high bacterial challenge and to assess efficacy and patient cooperation	Per saliva test if done Xylitol (6-10 g/day) gum or candies; two tabs of gum or two candies four to five times daily	OTC fluoride-containing toothpaste twice daily plus 0.05% NaF rinse daily Initially, one or two applications of NaF varnish; one application at 4- to 6-month recall	Not required	Not required Optional for excessive root exposure or sensitivity	As per ICDAS sealant protocol
High risk‡	Bitewing radiographs every 6-18 months or until no cavitated lesions are evident	Every 3-4 months to reevaluate caries risk and apply fluoride varnish	Saliva flow test and bacterial culture initially and at every caries recall appointment to assess efficacy and patient cooperation	Chlorhexidine gluconate 0.12% 10-mL rinse for 1 minute daily for 1 week each month Xylitol (6-10 g/day) gum or candies; two tabs of gum or two candies four to five times daily	1.1% NaF toothpaste twice daily instead of regular fluoride toothpaste Optional 0.2% NaF rinse daily (one bottle) then OTC 0.05% NaF rinse two times daily Initially, one to three applications at 3- to 4-month recall	Not required	Optional: Apply calcium/ phosphate paste several times daily	As per ICDAS sealant protocol
Extreme risk§ (high risk plus dry mouth or special needs)	Bitewing radiographs every 6 months or until no cavitated lesions are evident	Every 3 months to reevaluate caries risk and apply fluoride varnish	Saliva flow test and bacterial culture initially and at every caries recall appointment to assess efficacy and patient cooperation	Chlorhexidine 0.12% (preferably chlorhexidine in water base rinse) 10-mL rinse for 1 minute daily for 1 week each month Xylitol (6-10 g/day) gum or candies; two tabs of gum or two candies four to five times daily	1.1% NaF toothpaste twice daily instead of regular fluoride toothpaste OTC 0.05% NaF rinse when mouth feels dry and after snacking, breakfast, and lunch Initially 1-3 applications of NaF varnish; one application at 3-month recall	Acid-neutralizing rinses as needed if mouth feels dry; after snacking, at bedtime, and after breakfast Baking soda gum as needed	Required: Apply calcium/ phosphate paste twice daily	As per ICDAS sealant protocol

From Jenson L, Brideny AW, Featherstone JDB, et al: Clinical protocols for caries management by risk assessment, *J Calif Dent Assoc* 35:716, 2007.

All restorative work to be done with the minimally invasive philosophy in mind. Existing smooth surface lesions that do not penetrate the dentoenamel junction and are not cavitated should be treated chemically, not surgically. For extreme-risk patients, use holding care with glass ionomer materials until caries progression is controlled. Patients with appliances (removable partial dentures, prosthodontics) require excellent oral hygiene together with intensive fluoride therapy (e.g., high-fluoride toothpaste and fluoride varnish every 3 months). Where indicated, antibacterial therapy should be administered in conjunction with restorative work.

ICDAS, International Caries Detection and Assessment System; *NaF,* sodium fluoride; *OTC,* over-the-counter.

*For all risk levels: Patients must maintain good oral hygiene and a diet low in frequency of fermentable carbohydrates.

†Xylitol is not good for pets (especially dogs).

CAMBRA Clinical Guidelines for Patients Ages Birth to 5 Years

Risk Level*	Saliva Test[†]	Antibacterials	Fluoride	Frequency of Radiographs	Frequency of Periodic Oral Examination (POE)	Xylitol and/or Baking Soda[‡]	Sealant[§]	Existing Lesions
Low risk	Optional (baseline)	Not required or if saliva test was performed; treat main caregiver accordingly	Not required	After age 2: bitewing radiographs every 18-24 months	Every 6-12 months to reevaluate caries risk and give anticipatory guidance		Optional	
Moderate risk	Recommended	Not required or if saliva test was performed; treat main caregiver accordingly	OTC fluoride-containing toothpaste twice daily (a pea-sized amount) Sodium fluoride treatment gels and rinses	After age 2: bitewing radiographs every 12-18 months	Every 6 months to reevaluate caries risk and give anticipatory guidance	Xylitol gum or lozenges Two sticks of gum or two mints four to five times daily for the caregiver Xylitol food, spray, or drinks for the child	Sealants for deep pits and fissures after 2 years of age High-fluoride conventional glass ionomer is recommended	Lesions that do not penetrate the DEJ and are not cavitated should be treated with fluoride toothpaste and fluoride varnish
High risk[‖]	Required	Chlorhexidine 0.12% 10-mL rinse for main caregiver of the infant or child for 1 week each month Bacterial test every caries recall Health provider may brush infant's teeth with chlorhexidine	Fluoride varnish at initial visit and caries recall examinations OTC fluoride-containing toothpaste and calcium phosphate paste combination twice daily Sodium fluoride treatment gels and rinses	After age 2: two size No. 2 occlusal films and two bitewing radiographs every 6-12 months or until no cavitated lesions are evident	Every 3 months to reevaluate caries risk, apply fluoride varnish, and give anticipatory guidance	Xylitol gum or lozenges Two sticks of gum or two mints four to five times daily for the caregiver Xylitol food, spray, or drinks for the child	Sealants for deep pits and fissures after 2 years of age High-fluoride conventional glass ionomer is recommended	Lesions that do not penetrate the DEJ and are not cavitated should be treated with fluoride toothpaste and fluoride varnish ART might be recommended
Extreme risk[¶]	Required	Chlorhexidine 0.12% 10-mL rinse for 1 minute daily at bedtime for 2 weeks each month Bacterial test at every caries recall Health provider might brush infant's teeth with chlorhexidine	Fluoride varnish at initial visit, at each caries recall, and after prophylaxis OTC fluoride-containing toothpaste and phosphate paste combination twice daily Sodium fluoride treatment gels and rinses	After age 2: two size No. 2 occlusal films and two bitewing radiographs every 6 months or until no cavitated lesions are evident	Every 3 months to reevaluate caries risk, apply fluoride varnish, and give anticipatory guidance	Xylitol gum or lozenges Two sticks of gum or two mints four to five times daily for the caregiver Xylitol food, spray, or drinks for the child	Sealants for deep pits and fissures after 2 years of age High fluoride conventional glass ionomer is recommended	Holding care with glass ionomer materials until caries progression is controlled (ART) Fluoride varnish, and anticipatory guidance, self-management goals

From Ramos-Gomez FJ, Crall J, Gansky SA, et al: Caries risk assessments appropriate for the age 1 visit (infants and toddlers), *J Calif Dent Assoc* 35:692, 2007.*ART,* Atraumatic restorative treatment; *DEJ,* dentoenamel junction; *OTC,* over-the-counter.

*For all risk levels: Pediatric patients, through their caregivers, must maintain good oral hygiene and a diet low in frequency of fermentable carbohydrates. Patients with appliances (removable partial dentures, orthodontics) require excellent oral hygiene together with intensive fluoride therapy. Fluoride gel to be placed in removable appliances.

†Pediatric patients with daily medication such as inhalers or behavioral issues will have diminished salivary function.

‡Xylitol is not good for pets (especially dogs).

§ICDAS protocol presented by Jenson et al.[5] This issue may be helpful on sealant decisions.

‖Pediatric patients with one (or more) cavitated lesion(s) are high-risk patients.

¶Pediatric patients with one (or more) cavitated lesion(s) and hyposalivary conditions or special needs are extreme-risk patients.

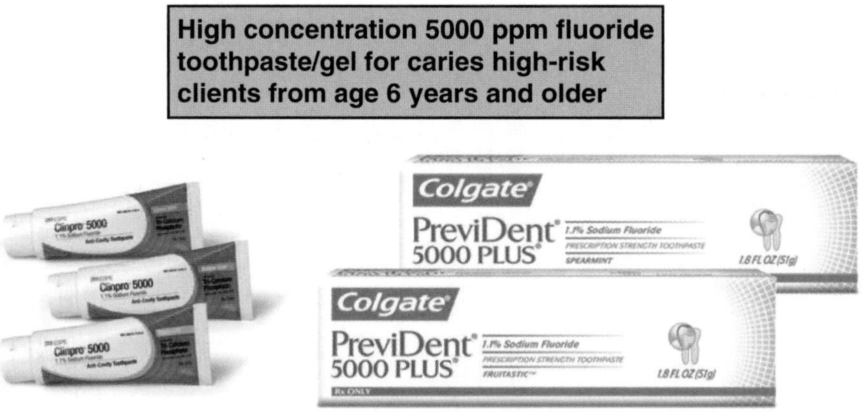

Figure 18-12. Sample prescription fluoride products. (Courtesy Dr. Mark Dillenges.)

the dental office. Figure 18-12 shows examples of high-concentration prescription fluoride products for individuals with high caries risk individuals. Baysan and colleagues[20] reported that 5000 ppm fluoride toothpaste gave statistically significant extra reduction in root caries compared with 1100 ppm fluoride toothpaste. Caries progression, however, still occurred in many subjects even with high concentration fluoride use. Thus a very high bacterial challenge in individuals with high caries risk overcomes the therapeutic effect of fluoride and requires use of additional chemical agents to promote protective factors. (For more information on fluoride dentifrices, see Chapter 25.)

Because carbohydrate and bacterial challenges create daily opportunities for demineralization, the frequent use of additional low-potency fluoride products for the daily management of the caries disease process is recommended.[9] Various other delivery vehicles for fluoride products are available for those individuals whose caries activity or caries risk warrants the use of additional fluoride agents to augment use of an approved fluoride dentifrice.[2,4,5] These systems are discussed later.

Self-Applied Daily Fluoride Mouth Rinses

Low-potency fluoride rinses are available as over-the-counter products. For example, 0.05% NaF rinses have a fluoride concentration of approximately 230 ppm. These products are used as an adjunct to brushing with a fluoride dentifrice. Over-the-counter fluoride rinses (0.05% NaF or 0.4% stannous fluoride; Figure 18-13) are effective when used once or twice daily for 1 minute, along with a fluoride-containing dentifrice.[9,11] Individuals are educated to use the metered dose of the rinse from the bottle, to swish the rinse in the mouth vigorously, and then to expectorate thoroughly. Because there is a risk for young children to swallow fluoride rinses, this product is not recommended for children under 6 years of age. For the same reason, fluoride rinses should be stored out of the reach of young children.[1]

Self-applied fluoride gels also may be used in addition to a fluoride-containing dentifrice to manage dental caries. Like the rinses, the majority of the gels are of low- to mid-range potency and as such are administered with higher frequency. The scientific literature indicates that low-potency fluoride rinses and gels reduce caries by 30% to 35%.[8,9]

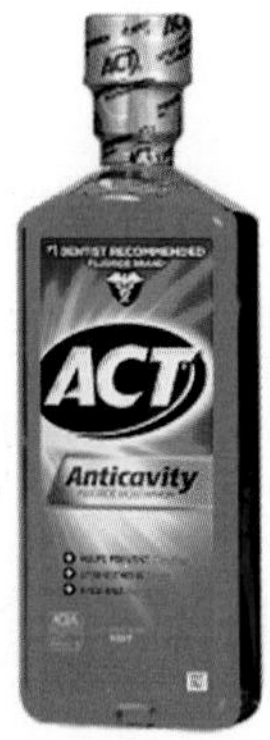

Figure 18-13. Sample of over-the-counter 0.05% NaF rinses with the ADA Seal of Acceptance. (Courtesy ACT.)

Fluoride gels are marketed as stannous fluoride (SnF_2) products at 1000 ppm, neutral (NaF), and acidulated phosphate fluoride (APF) products at 5000 ppm. These products are designed for daily use and typically are brushed on the teeth after toothbrushing with a conventional fluoride dentifrice.[11] In cases in which increased duration of contact with the teeth is desired, the 5000 ppm products can be used in custom trays. Because of the risk for young children to swallow fluoride gels, these products are not recommended for children under 6 years of age. Although few studies document their efficacy, the ADA Council on Scientific Affairs approved SnF_2 gels. In addition, the U.S. Food and Drug Administration (FDA) approved SnF_2 gels for sale over the counter because they contain the same fluoride concentration as conventional dentifrices. Stannous gels do not contain abrasives and should not be substituted for dentifrices that achieve pellicle and stain removal.[11]

Self-applied, prescription strength neutral and APF gels (5000 ppm) are used for individuals with high risk and extreme caries risk such as that resulting from the administration of radiation for head and neck cancers, those with systemic medical conditions, and those who routinely use medications that reduce salivary flow. These products are available as gels without abrasives and as gels with abrasives (marketed as prescription dentifrices). Although the 5000 ppm gels lack ADA Council on Scientific Affairs approval, these products have gained widespread use for individuals with special needs. Careful client education is required when these products are recommended for unsupervised home use. The products should be used as directed in a custom tray or brushed on the teeth, swished in the oral cavity for 1 minute, and then expectorated. Clients should be reminded that these products are available by prescription owing to their moderate levels of fluoride, and therefore they should be stored carefully out of the reach of children.[11]

Professionally Applied Fluoride (In-Office Administration)

Forms of professionally applied topical fluoride supported by evidence of clinical effectiveness for caries prevention include the following[21]:

- Gel
- Varnish (Figure 18-14)

Evidence-based general clinical recommendations are listed in Box 18-10.[21]

Gels

Commonly used professionally applied fluoride gels include APF, which contains 1.23% or 12,300 ppm fluoride ion, and 2% NaF, which contains 0.91% or 9090 ppm fluoride ion. Professionally applied fluoride gels typically are delivered using a tray technique, are one of the last procedures performed in the dental hygiene appointment sequence, and are administered by licensed dental professionals. These high-potency topical fluoride systems have been approved by the FDA for in-office use and have a caries reduction rate of approximately 30%.[21] The 1.23% APF system and the 2.0% neutral NaF are the most widely used. Neutral NaF is recommended when it is inappropriate to use an acidulated product (when a client has tooth-colored restorations and/or dentinal hypersensitivity). Evidence supports the effectiveness of professionally applied fluoride gel in prevention and reduction of dental caries in children and adolescents; however, patient acceptance is not high. Some clinicians have substituted use of fluoride foams which have not been studied extensively. Another alternative commonly employed in practice is fluoride varnish. Evidence supports its use for coronal caries prevention in children and adolescents and for root caries reduction in the elderly. Tray selection[22] and the procedure for administering a professional topical fluoride gel using the tray technique are presented in Chapter 33.

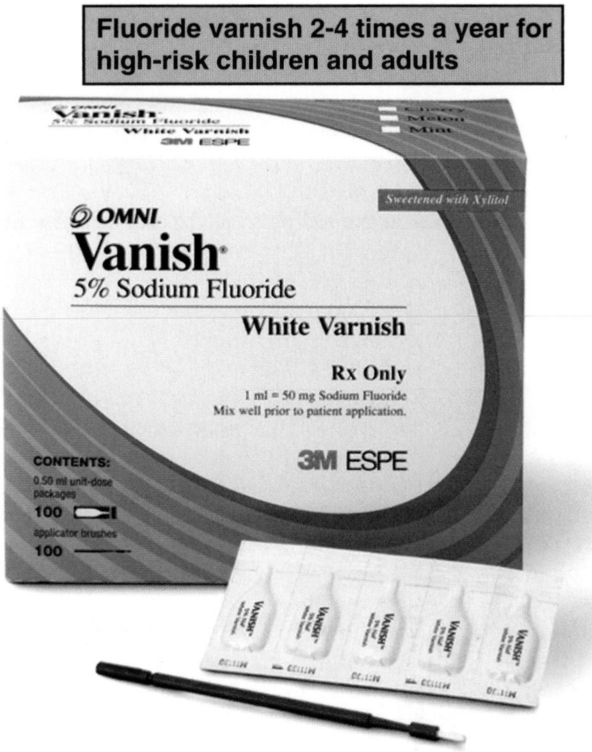

Figure 18-14. Fluoride varnish with tri-calcium phosphate. (Courtesy 3M ESPE.)

Varnishes

Fluoride varnish is a concentrated topical fluoride with a resin or synthetic base that is painted on the teeth to prolong fluoride exposure. It can be used instead of a fluoride gel for risk categories as shown in Table 18-1 (see Figure 18-14). Based on evidence from systematic review of randomized controlled trials, the ADA Council on Scientific Affairs states that two or more applications of fluoride varnish per year are effective in preventing caries in high-risk populations and that fluoride varnish applied every 6 months is effective in preventing caries in the primary and permanent dentition of children and adolescents.[19,23-25]

Fluoride-containing varnishes typically contain 5% NaF, which is equivalent to 2.26% or 22,600 ppm fluoride ion. Some fluoride varnish products also contain remineralization agents (see Chapter 31 for a discussion of remineralization agents). Fluoride varnish applications take less time, create less client discomfort, and achieve greater client acceptability than does fluoride gel, especially in preschool-aged children as well as infants and toddlers.[1,21] In addition, fluoride varnish contains a smaller quantity of fluoride compared with fluoride gels. Therefore its use reduces the risk of inadvertent ingestion in children younger than 6 years.[21] The frequency of application for fluoride varnish should be determined by the client's caries risk. (See Chapter 33 for the procedure for placing fluoride varnish.)

Client Selection

Based on the CAMBRA approach to care, professionally applied fluoride gel application or fluoride varnish application at 3- to 6-month intervals is recommended for individuals with moderate, high, and extreme caries risk (see Table 18-1).

Product Selection

Once it is determined that a client will benefit from a professionally applied topical fluoride treatment, the dental hygienist decides the type of high-potency fluoride that will be used for this procedure. The choice is among neutral NaF gel, APF gel, or fluoride varnish based on clinician and client preference. (There is limited evidence to support effectiveness of the fluoride foam for caries prevention.)

Chlorhexidine as an Antibacterial for Dental Caries

Chlorhexidine gluconate is a broad-spectrum antibacterial agent that works by opening up the cell membranes of the bacteria. It is administered in the United States by prescription. In the United States, only 0.12% chlorhexidine gluconate is available as an antibacterial mouth rinse in the dental treatment setting for the management of dental caries and periodontal diseases (Figure 18-15). For high-risk and extreme-risk individuals, use of 0.12% chlorhexidine gluconate rinse for 1 minute daily for 1 week each month is recommended to reduce mutans streptococci and lactobacilli levels in the plaque biofilm[4,5] (see Table 18-1). This regimen was shown in a recent clinical trial to reduce caries incidence by 24% as compared to a conventional treatment control group.[12] Noting the regimen is very important, because this was developed during the trial and shown to be effective compared to other less-frequent doses that have been proposed by previous authors. Chlorhexidine therapy reduces the bacterial challenge but must be used in conjunction with fluoride remineralization therapy as described in detail previously. Rinsing once daily for 1 week markedly reduces the mutans streptococci levels, but they begin to return quickly. Hence the need to repeat the regimen each month, thereby driving the bacterial levels down to safe regions over a period of 6 months.[12] Minimal staining occurs with this regimen.

In individuals with a high bacterial challenge, this therapy must be continued for approximately 1 year and monitored by bacterial assessment. Problems associated with this compound are that it affects taste, and compliance is often poor.[4,5] Staining also can be a problem with some individuals if used for longer than 1 week at a time.

Remineralization Products

Products are available to deliver additional calcium and phosphate for remineralization (Figure 18-16). Although calcium and phosphate levels present in healthy saliva are sufficient for remineralization, such products could be beneficial to a client with inadequate salivary flow. (See Chapter 31 for a discussion of remineralization agents.)

Other Antibacterial Therapeutics

Xylitol

Xylitol is a sweetener that looks and tastes like sucrose. It inhibits attachment and transmission of bacteria and can be delivered through chewing gum or lozenges as an effective anticaries therapeutic measure (Figure 18-17). Xylitol is not fermented by cariogenic bacteria. In addition, use of xylitol chewing gum (or lozenges) serves the following functions:

- Enhances remineralization
- Inhibits the transfer of bacteria from person to person by altering the way the bacteria stick to surfaces[26]
- Inhibits future recolonization[25,26]

Two tabs of gum or two lozenges four to five times daily are recommended for caries management in individuals with moderate, high, and extreme risk for caries (see Table 18-1).

Sodium Bicarbonate

Sodium bicarbonate (baking soda) neutralizes acids produced by acidogenic bacteria and has antibacterial properties. It can be delivered to extreme-risk clients (those at high risk plus dry mouth or special needs) in gum or toothpaste or in a

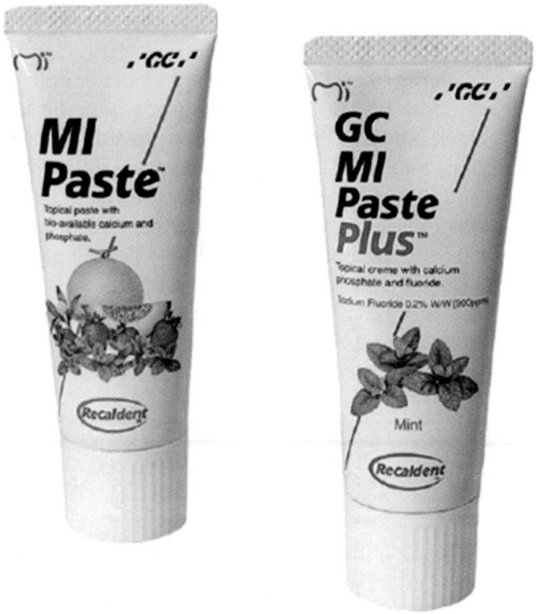

Figure 18-16. A sample calcium and phosphate product. (Courtesy GC America.)

Antibacterial Therapy: Age 6 Years and Older

Chlorhexidine gluconate 0.12%
- Rinse 10 mL daily for 1 week
- Repeat every month for 6 months and reassess
- Continue until cariogenic bacteria are controlled
- Must be used together with fluoride therapy

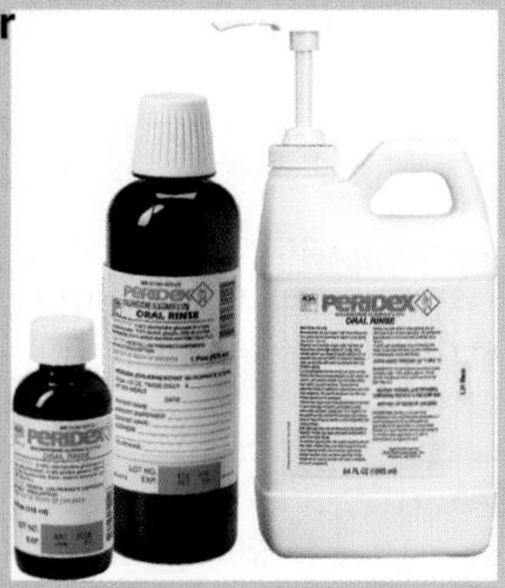

Figure 18-15. Chlorhexidine mouth rinse. (Courtesy 3M ESPE, St Paul, Minnesota.)

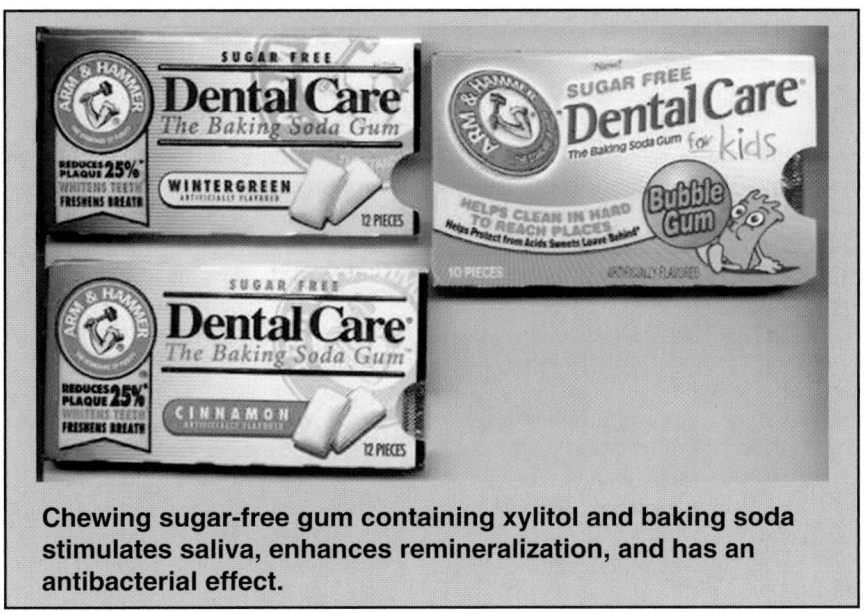

Xylitol Gum, Mints

Xylitol

- Noncariogenic sweetener
- Inhibits transfer of bacteria from mother to child
- Can reduce loading of cariogenic bacteria in the mouth

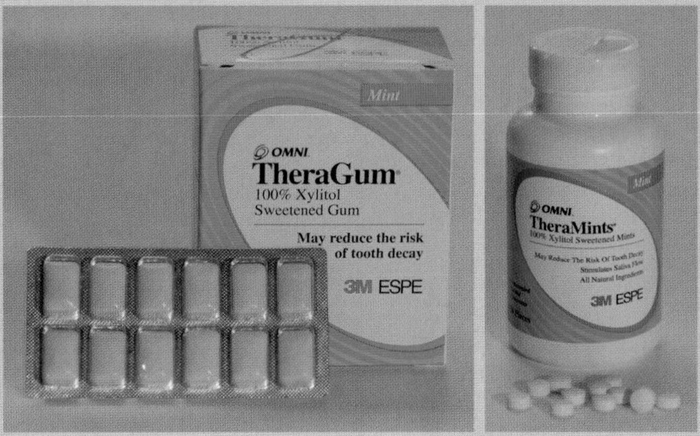

Figure 18-17. Sample xylitol products. (Courtesy Dr. Mark Dillenges.)

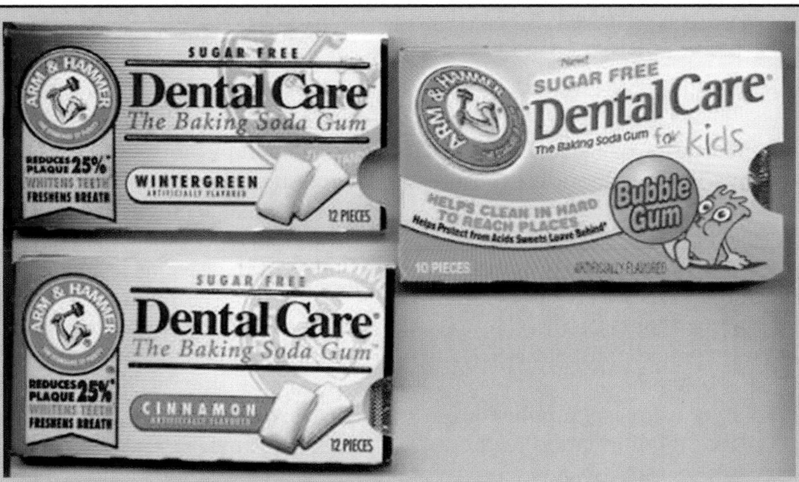

Chewing sugar-free gum containing xylitol and baking soda stimulates saliva, enhances remineralization, and has an antibacterial effect.

Figure 18-18. Sugar-free sodium bicarbonate gum containing xylitol.

solution for individuals with low salivary flow[5] (Figures 18-18 and 18-19; see also Table 18-1).

CLIENT EDUCATION TIPS

- Explain the disease of dental caries.
- Explain that the conventional restorative approach alone does not eliminate the disease of caries.
- Explain the dental caries balance.
- Explain the importance of promoting oral flora to favor health; reducing or eliminating risk factors; enhancing salivary function where needed; enhancing the caries repair process by remineralization; and employing a minimally invasive approach when restorative treatment is needed.

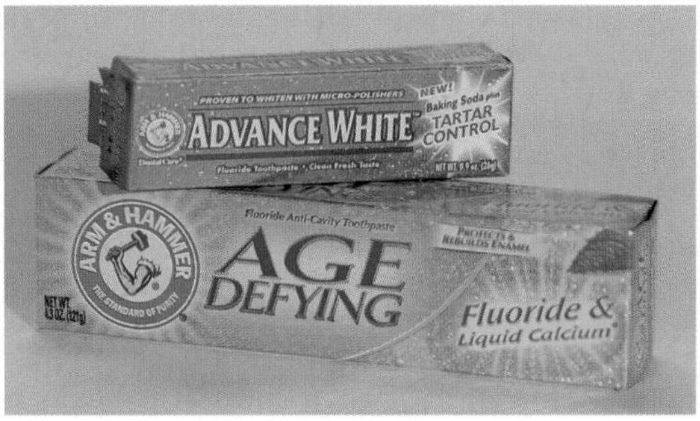

Figure 18-19. Sodium bicarbonate toothpaste. (Courtesy Dr. Mark Dillenges.)

- Explain that dental caries infections can be prevented and controlled with the help of the client and explain preventive and therapeutic choices.
- Inform clients of their current caries risk status and provide an evidence-based care plan based on their level of risk as determined by the balance or imbalance between the pathologic factors and protective factors of each client.
- Explain that caries is an infection that can be transmitted from parent to child or from person to person.
- Emphasize the frequent use of low-dose fluoride-containing products (dentifrices and oral rinses) to repair demineralized areas.
- Explain how certain medications decrease salivary flow and increase dental caries risk.
- Explain that dental caries management is a lifelong issue.
- Teach parents and caregivers that they are critical partners in dental caries management in children under 6 years of age.
- Explain that fluoride is an effective agent in caries management, and it must be used safely and stored.
- Explain that when well water is the primary water source, it should be tested to determine fluoride level.

LEGAL, ETHICAL, AND SAFETY ISSUES

- Carefully assess disease indicators and risk factors to determine dental caries risk level.
- Inform client of current dental caries risk status.
- Carefully analyze the client's overall fluoride exposure; take a fluoride history.
- Make recommendations based on the caries risk status of the individual as determined by the balance or imbalance between the pathologic factors and protective factors of each client; and document in the client's chart.
- Emphasize the safe use of self-applied products, especially with children younger than 6 years of age.
- Document recommendations regarding self-applied products in the client record, including information regarding type of product, frequency of use, safe use, and storage.
- Thoroughly document the administration of in-office products in the client's record.
- Safely store and manage professional-strength fluorides in the dental treatment setting.
- Work in collaboration with other oral care professionals to develop a response plan in the event of an acute fluoride overdose in the dental treatment setting.
- Consult the professional literature regularly for current information and clinical evidence regarding strategies for managing dental caries.

KEY CONCEPTS

- The team approach is essential for the successful caries management program, and the role of the dental hygienist can be critical in the overall management of the program.
- Caries is defined as an infectious, transmissible disease process in which a complex cariogenic biofilm, in the presence of an oral environmental status that is more pathologic than protective, leads to the demineralization and eventual cavitation of dental hard tissues.
- Pathologic factors include cariogenic bacteria (*Streptococcus mutans*, *Streptococcus sobrinus*, and *Lactobacillus* species), frequent ingestion of fermentable carbohydrates (sugars and starches), and salivary dysfunction.
- Protective factors include but are not limited to adequate saliva and its caries-preventive components, fluoride therapy, and antibacterial therapy.
- Saliva plays a key role in that it neutralizes acids and provides minerals and proteins that protect the teeth.
- To determine caries risk, the dental hygienist evaluates disease indicators and risk factors.
- Risk factors are biologic, behavioral, or socioeconomic contributors to the caries disease process that can be modified as part of the care plan.
- Caries management is aimed at restoring and maintaining a balance between protective factors and pathologic factors. The overall aim of the care plan is to reduce the bacterial challenge; reduce or eliminate other risk factors; enhance salivary function where needed; enhance the repair process by remineralization; and employ a minimally invasive approach when restorative treatment is needed.
- High- and extreme-risk individuals require antimicrobial therapy, reduction of identified risk factors, and remineralization therapy. Extreme-risk individuals with severe salivary dysfunction require additional therapy, such as the use of buffering agents and calcium and phosphate supplementation.
- Moderate-risk individuals require improved remineralization therapy and reduction of other risk factors, which may include antimicrobial therapy.
- Caries management includes treatment of the bacterial infection that causes dental caries, rather than just treatment of the carious lesion.
- Caries management involves suppressing bacteria that cause the infection; remineralizing early noncavitated carious lesions by enhancing salivary flow and using fluorides; protecting tooth surfaces by using sealants and fluorides; decreasing the frequency of sugar intake, especially between meals; and referring to the dentist for surgical removal of carious lesions that are beyond hope of remineralization and for restoration of teeth with minimally invasive techniques and materials.
- Levels of cariogenic bacteria in the mouth can be assessed by selective media culturing in the dental office. Saliva that is stimulated by chewing can be used to collect bacteria from the teeth and around the mouth.
- Chlorhexidine is used as a mouth rinse (10 mL once daily for a 1-week period every 2 to 3 months). In individuals with high bacterial challenge, this therapy must be continued for approximately 1 year and monitored by bacterial assessment. Use of the chlorhexidine rinse for a full week, repeated every month is critical for success,[12] as described above. Less frequent use is ineffective, as shown by several studies.
- Demineralization and remineralization occur in the oral cavity on a daily basis.
- Saliva and fluoride are instrumental in the remineralization process.
- Demineralization is an issue from the time the primary dentition erupts into the oral cavity until death or the permanent teeth are prematurely lost.
- Topical fluoride delivery systems play key preventive roles.

- Community water fluoridation is a very important delivery system.
- Fluoridated dentifrices play a key role in fluoride delivery for caries prevention and control.
- Various self-applied dentifrices, rinses, and gels are available, and the market continues to expand in this area.
- Use of professionally applied fluoride gels depends on caries risk.
- Use of fluoride varnish is a key strategy for the management of dental caries.
- It is the dental hygienist's ethical responsibility to document thoroughly the use of and recommendations made regarding chemotherapeutic agents for the management of dental caries.
- It is the dental hygienist's ethical responsibility to read the scientific literature and use it to provide the evidence to substantiate professional decisions.

CRITICAL THINKING EXERCISES

Sue works as a dental hygienist in a large group practice that employs a total of three full-time dental hygienists. This general practice is located in a town that has had community water fluoridation for the past 30 years; nearly all of the clients treated in the office reside in the town. Sue is providing a preventive appointment for a 5-year-old client. The client is new to the practice; her mother is waiting for her in the reception area. The client has the following dental history:

- Mixed dentition
- A healthy diet; infrequently ingests snacks containing fermentable carbohydrates
- Twice-daily brushing with a fluoridated toothpaste (mother monitors toothbrushing at bedtime)
- Fair to good oral hygiene
- Apparently normal salivary flow
- No clinical evidence of demineralization
- No restorations

The office policy is that professionally applied fluorides (tray technique) are administered to all children (3 to 16 years of age) two times annually. As Sue nears the end of her appointment, she explains to the client that she is going to administer a fluoride treatment; the client has never had this procedure before. Sue asks the client what flavor fluoride she would prefer: tooty-fruity, strawberry, or double chocolate. The client says that she loves chocolate, so she selects the double chocolate flavor.

Sue explains the 4-minute tray application to the client, the use of the saliva ejector, and the need to avoid swallowing fluoride during the treatment. Sue selects a small, hinged fluoride tray and fills it two thirds full with 1.23% APF. Sue then dries the teeth, inserts both trays concurrently, inserts the saliva ejector, and begins timing the treatment for 4 minutes. Sue remains chairside during the treatment and distracts the client by talking about her favorite sport.

As Sue removes the fluoride trays, the client immediately begins talking about how much she liked the taste of the double chocolate fluoride. Sue says that she is glad that the client enjoyed her first fluoride treatment and hopes she will look forward to the next appointment in 6 months.

Sue prepares to dismiss the client and return with her to the reception area to talk with the client's mother. As Sue and the client entered the reception area, the client reports to her mother that her stomach "does not feel good" and that she thinks she might "be sick."

1. What aspects of the client assessment did Sue take into consideration when she decided to administer a professional fluoride application to this client?
2. Did Sue's administration technique affect the risk for a fluoride reaction?
3. Is Sue professionally and ethically bound to carry out the office policy regarding professionally applied fluoride applications? Are there any potential legal issues involved?
4. Is the office policy consistent with the evidence in the literature regarding professionally applied fluorides?
5. What should Sue and the mother do to assist the child?
6. How should this appointment be documented in the client record?

REFERENCES

1. Ramos-Gomez FJ, Crall J, Gansky SA, et al: Caries risk assessment appropriate for the age 1 visit (infants and toddlers). *J Calif Dent Assoc* 35:687, 2007.
2. Young DA, Featherstone JDB, Roth JR, et al: Caries management by risk assessment: implementation guidelines. *J Calif Dent Assoc* 35:799, 2007.
3. Featherstone JDB, Adair SM, Anderson MH, et al: Caries management by risk assessment: consensus statement, April 2002. *J Calif Dent Assoc* 31:257, 2003.
4. Featherstone JD, Domejean-Orliaguet S, Jenson L, et al: Caries risk assessment in practice for age 6 through adult. *J Calif Dent Assoc* 35:703, 2007.
5. Jenson L, Brideny AW, Featherstone JDB, et al: Clinical protocols for caries management by risk assessment. *J Calif Dent Assoc* 35:714, 2007.
6. Gutkowski S, Gerger D, Creasey J, et al: The role of dental hygienists, assistants, and office staff in CAMBRA. *J Calif Dent Assoc* 35:786, 2007.
7. Horowitz HS: Decision-making for national programs of community fluoride use. *Community Dent Oral Epidemiol* 28:321, 2000.
8. Stookey GK: Caries prevention. *J Dent Educ* 62:803, 1998.
9. Featherstone JDB: The science and practice of caries prevention. *J Am Dent Assoc* 131:887, 2000.
10. Zero DT: Dental caries process. *Dent Clin North Am* 43:635, 1999.
11. Featherstone JDB: Prevention and reversal of dental caries: role of low level fluoride. *Community Dent Oral Epidemiol* 27:31, 1999.
12. Featherstone JD, White JM, Hoover CI, et al: A randomized clinical trial of anticaries therapies targeted according to risk assessment (caries management by risk assessment). *Caries Res* 46(2): 118, 2012.
13. Domejean S, White JM, Featherstone JD: Validation of the CDA CAMBRA caries risk assessment–a six-year retrospective study. *J Calif Dent Assoc* 39(10):709, 2011.
14. American Dental Association (ADA): *ADA statement on early childhood caries 2004*, Chicago, 2004, ADA. Available at: hwww.ada.org/prof/resources/positions/statements/caries.asp. Accessed August 17, 2008.
15. American Association of Public Health Dentistry: *First oral health assessment policy*, Springfield, Ill, 2004, American Association of Public Health Dentistry. Available at: www.aaphd.org/default.asp?page=policy.htm. Accessed August 17, 2008.
16. American Academy of Pediatric Dentistry (AAPD): *Policy on the dental home*, Chicago, 2004 (rev), AAPD. Available at: www.aapd.org/media/Policies_Guidelines/P_DentalHome.pdf. Accessed August 17, 2008.
17. Weinstein P: Provider versus patient-centered approaches to health promotion with parents of young children: what works/does not work and why. *Pediatr Dent* 28:172, 2006.

18. Curnow MMT, Pine CM, Burnside G, et al: A randomized controlled trial of the efficacy of supervised toothbrushing in high–caries-risk children. *Caries Res* 36:294, 2002.
19. American Dental Association (ADA) Council on Scientific Affairs: Professionally applied topical fluoride: evidence-based clinical recommendations. *J Dent Educ* 71:393, 2007.
20. Baysan A, Lynch E, Ellwood R, et al: Reversal of primary root caries using dentifrices containing 5000 and 1100 ppm fluoride. *Caries Res* 35:41, 2001.
21. Lavigne S: Not all trays are created equal: an analysis of fluoride tray fit. *Probe Sci J* 34:217, 2000.
22. Marinho VC, Higgins JP, Logan S, et al: Topical fluoride (toothpastes, mouthrinses, gels or varnishes) for preventing dental caries in children and adolescents [review]. *Cochrane Database Syst Rev* 4:CD002782, 2003.
23. Moberg Sköld U, Petersson LG, Lith A, et al: Effect of school-based fluoride varnish programmes on approximal caries in adolescents from different caries risk areas. *Caries Res* 39:273, 2005.
24. Weintraub JA, Ramos-Gomez F, Jue B, et al: Fluoride varnish efficacy in preventing early childhood caries. *J Dent Res* 85:172, 2006.
25. Ekstrand J, Fejerskov O, Silverstone LM: *Fluoride in dentistry*, Copenhagen, 1988, Munsgaard.
26. Söderling E, Isokangas P, Pienihäkkinen P, et al: Influence of maternal xylitol consumption on acquisition of mutans streptococci by infants. *J Dent Res* 79:882, 2000.

EVOLVE RESOURCES

Please visit http://evolve.elsevier.com/Darby/hygiene for additional practice and study support tools.

ACKNOWLEDGEMENT

The author wishes to acknowledge Denise Bowen, RDH, MS, for helping to update this chapter for the fourth edition.

CHAPTER 19

Periodontal and Risk Assessment

Susan Lynn Tolle

COMPETENCIES

1. Define risk assessment and its significance.
2. Identify, give examples, and assess modifiable and nonmodifiable risk factors that affect onset, progression, and severity of periodontal disease and health maintenance.
3. Explain the clinical application of risk assessment, including:
   - Identify the six basic tools needed to assess clinical parameters.
   - Describe healthy periodontium by clinical signs and histologic characteristics.
   - Describe diseased periodontium by clinical signs and histologic characteristics.
   - Distinguish among varying types of gingivitis and periodontitis.
4. Discuss radiographic assessment, including evaluation of radiographs for signs of periodontal disease.
5. Discuss assessment of periodontal disease activity, including methods of microbiologic identification of periodontitis.
6. Describe indices for measuring periodontal diseases.
7. Explain proper documentation and record keeping.
8. Define a decision-making matrix and explain its significance.

Risk Assessment Defined

Risk factors influence one's susceptibility to periodontitis.[1,2] Assessment and analysis of risk factors provide information about a client's periodontal disease susceptibility beyond traditional clinical assessment parameters. Although specific pathogenic bacteria are the primary causative agents for periodontal diseases and are necessary for disease initiation, they are not sufficient to cause periodontal destruction. Many host, environmental, and systemic risk factors modify the body's response to bacterial pathogens in oral biofilm, resulting in great variability in individual susceptibility to periodontal disease. The number and type of client risk factors present modulate the onset, degree, and severity of periodontal disease (Box 19-1). Risk factor assessment is important because conditions associated with increased risk may affect treatment, as well as client management. In addition, risk assessment provides the framework to develop treatment plans that target the risk factors, creating opportunities for enhanced treatment outcomes. Risk factor assessment is based on information obtained through client interviews; the comprehensive health, dental, and pharmacologic history; and the clinical and radiographic examination. A wellness model of oral health uses risk in the care paradigm with prevention and treatment focused on targeted patient risk factors as well as reparative treatment interventions.[2]

Figures, tables, and boxes marked as "e" are available as supplemental material on the Evolve site. Visit http://evolve.elsevier.com/Darby/hygiene to access these materials.

Risk Factors

Risk factors are attributes or exposures that significantly increase the risk for onset and/or progression of a specific disease and affect treatment outcomes. Risk factors are categorized as follows:

- Modifiable—those that can be changed
- Nonmodifiable—those that cannot be changed

Modifiable (Mutable) Risk Factors[1-4]

Smoking

Tobacco smoking is one of the most significant risk factors for periodontal disease. Smokers have greater loss of attachment, bone loss, periodontal pocket depths, furcation involvement, dental calculus formation, and tooth loss than nonsmokers. Surgical and nonsurgical interventions are less effective in those who smoke, and disease recurrence is more common than in nonsmokers. The effects of smoking on the periodontium are evident at an early age, usually beginning at age 20 to 30. The onset of disease is earlier in smokers, and the disease progresses more rapidly.

The negative effects of smoking on the periodontium are linked with an altered host response, pathogenic bacterial composition, and direct local (heat and chemical) damage to periodontal tissues. Immunosuppressive effects result from decreased salivary antibodies and impaired neutrophil functioning. Clinically, smokers exhibit gingiva that is thickened and fibrotic with rolled borders and minimal redness. Smoking masks gingival inflammation by reducing gingival blood flow as a result of constriction of blood vessels of the gingiva. Local damage may be related to direct thermal damage. Greater pocket depths and recession are found in the anterior areas and maxillary lingual sites owing to concentrated exposures of heat and toxins from tobacco smoke in these areas.

Length of time used and amount of smoking exposures are important assessment factors. A direct relationship exists between an increased amount of smoking and an increased loss of attachment (called a *dose-response effect*) and vice versa. Heavy smokers are five to seven times more likely to develop severe periodontitis when compared with individuals who have never smoked. Attachment loss is greater in heavy smokers when compared with individuals who are light

BOX 19-1

Risk Factors for Periodontal Disease

Modifiable Risk Factors

- Smoking
- Diabetes
- Specific bacterial pathogens
- Poor self-care
- Osteoporosis
- Human immunodeficiency virus and acquired immunodeficiency syndrome
- Stress
- Bleeding on probing (BOP)
- Medications
- Local factors
- Hormonal variations

Nonmodifiable Risk Factors

- History of periodontitis
- Age
- Gender
- Race
- Genetic disorders
- Genetic marker

BOX 19-2

Bacterial Etiology of Periodontal Disease

Strong Evidence

- *Aggregatibacter actinomycetemcomitans*
- *Porphyromonas gingivalis*
- *Prevotella intermedia*
- *Tannerella forsythia*
- *Campylobacter rectus*
- *Fusobacterium nucleatum*
- *Fusobacterium* spp.
- Treponema denticola–like phylogroup (*Treponema* phylogroup II)
- *Treponema lecithinolyticum, Treponema denticola*

smokers. Smoking cessation seems to elicit a positive response on the periodontium, but previous damage cannot be reversed. Research also links secondhand smoke exposure to increased oral bone loss. Dental hygienists incorporate smoking cessation strategies into care plans as appropriate (see Chapter 36).

Diabetes Mellitus

Diabetes mellitus (DM) is a strong risk factor for periodontal disease. In type 1 and type 2 DM, greater gingivitis and periodontitis prevalence is observed. Prevalence increases significantly when the blood glucose is controlled poorly or uncontrolled. Persons who maintain good control have less attachment and bone loss than those with poor control, and they respond well to therapy. For persons older than age 40 who have diabetes, periodontal disease severity increases with years of disease duration.

With poorly controlled diabetes the increased susceptibility to periodontal infection is linked to immune dysfunction. Neutrophil chemotaxis and phagocytosis, impaired in people with diabetes, inhibits destruction of bacterial pathogens in the pocket, resulting in increased periodontal breakdown. (See the discussion of DM in Chapters 20 and 44.)

Specific Bacterial Pathogens

Specific anaerobic, gram-negative bacteria must be present for inflammatory periodontal disease to occur. (See Chapter 17.) For example, *Aggregatibacter actinomycetemcomitans (AA), Porphyromonas gingivalis (PG), Treponema denticola (TD), Tannerella forsythia (TF),* and *Prevotella intermedia (Pi)* are gram-negative anaerobic bacteria strongly associated with the cause and progression of periodontitis (Box 19-2). These periodontopathic bacteria, also known as *putative bacteria,* can cause direct tissue damage resulting from the production of bacterial enzymes and toxins and play a major role in the immune system's response and ultimate destruction of periodontal tissues. Presence of one or more of the bacteria in oral biofilm does not predict that periodontal disease will occur. Other host and environmental factors must be involved.

Poor Oral Self-Care

Lack of oral self-care has a strong association with periodontitis among all age groups and increases risk for periodontal breakdown. In contrast, good oral hygiene greatly reduces risk for periodontitis. Daily oral biofilm control in conjunction with regular professional care prevents attachment loss in most individuals. Lack of supragingival biofilm control after professional treatment minimizes effective results and interferes with resolution of inflammation and periodontal disease.

Osteoporosis

Evidence indicates an association between alveolar bone loss and osteoporosis. Increased alveolar bone resorption, attachment loss, tooth loss, and edentulousness have been found in women with osteoporosis when compared with women without this condition. The mandible tends to be affected more often than the maxilla. Osteoporosis does not cause periodontitis but may exacerbate existing disease. Estrogen deficiency also has been linked to decreases in alveolar bone density. For women with osteoporosis who smoke, the risk for tooth loss is extremely high. Estrogen replacement therapy (ERT) may be beneficial in preventing tooth loss in women with osteoporosis and may lower gingival inflammation and frequency of attachment loss; however, decisions concerning ERT are based on an individual's history and are decided with each client's medical care provider. Research is ongoing to better understand the effects of osteoporosis on periodontal diseases. (See the discussion of osteoporosis in Chapter 54.)

Human Immunodeficiency Virus and Acquired Immunodeficiency Syndrome

Human immunodeficiency virus (HIV) and acquired immunodeficiency syndrome (AIDS) are suspected risk indicators for periodontal disease. Individuals infected with HIV may exhibit linear gingival erythema, characterized by acute gingival inflammation around the gingival margin that affects all teeth. There is a disproportionate amount of plaque present compared with the degree of inflammation. About 3% to

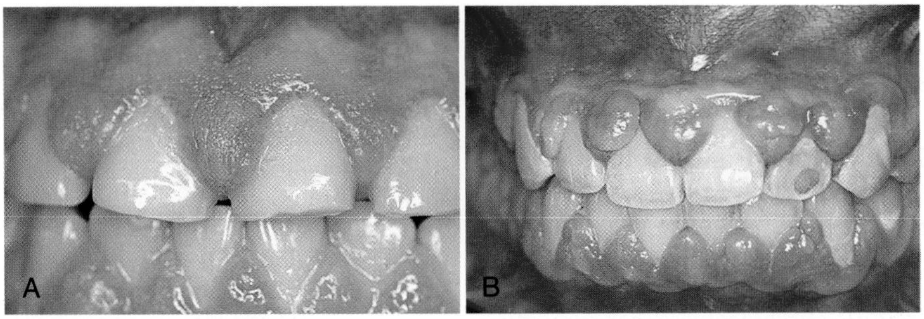

Figure 19-1. Drug-influenced gingival enlargement from cyclosporine use. **A,** Gingival enlargement, particularly on interdental papillae. **B,** Severe cyclosporine-associated gingival enlargement.

17% of persons with HIV disease have necrotizing ulcerative periodontitis, which results in severe, rapidly progressive periodontal destruction (see Chapter 46).

Stress

Epidemiologic evidence suggests that negative life experiences and psychologic factors likely contribute to enhanced susceptibility to periodontitis. Psychologic stress is associated with depression of the immune system; studies suggest a link between stress, poor coping skills, and periodontal attachment loss. Financial stress in adults with poor coping skills is a risk indicator for more severe periodontal disease. Individuals with adequate coping behaviors have less periodontal tissue destruction even with high financial stress than those individuals with inadequate coping skills. Research is ongoing to determine the link between psychologic stress and periodontal disease.

Bleeding on Probing

As a predictor of periodontal breakdown, bleeding on probing (BOP) alone has minimal value. Bleeding is not a predictor of future attachment loss; however, bleeding on probing in combination with increasing pocket depths does increase risk for continued periodontal destruction. Repeated absence of BOP, especially on two or more occasions, generally indicates good periodontal health. Cessation of bleeding correlates with reduced gingival inflammation, repair of gingival connective tissue, and pocket reduction.

Medications

Risk assessment considers client medications (see Chapter 14). Although some medications, such as tetracycline and nonsteroidal anti-inflammatory drugs, have a beneficial effect on the periodontium, others have a negative impact. Xerostomia is associated with more than 500 medications, including diuretics, antihistamines, antipsychotics, antihypertensives, and analgesics. Decreased salivary flow facilitates oral biofilm accumulation, especially at the cervical one third of the tooth, and diminishes resolution of gingival inflammation. Several categories of drugs can cause drug-influenced gingival enlargement. Calcium channel blockers (e.g., nifedipine), immunosuppressive drugs (e.g., cyclosporine), and antiseizure drugs (e.g., phenytoin) have been implicated (Figure 19-1). Sex hormones (e.g., estrogen and progesterone) also have been reported to cause gingival enlargement. Gingival enlargement associated with these types of drugs and hormones is associated with an overproduction of collagen by gingival fibroblasts, is co-dependent on oral biofilm, and generally can be minimized with good biofilm control.

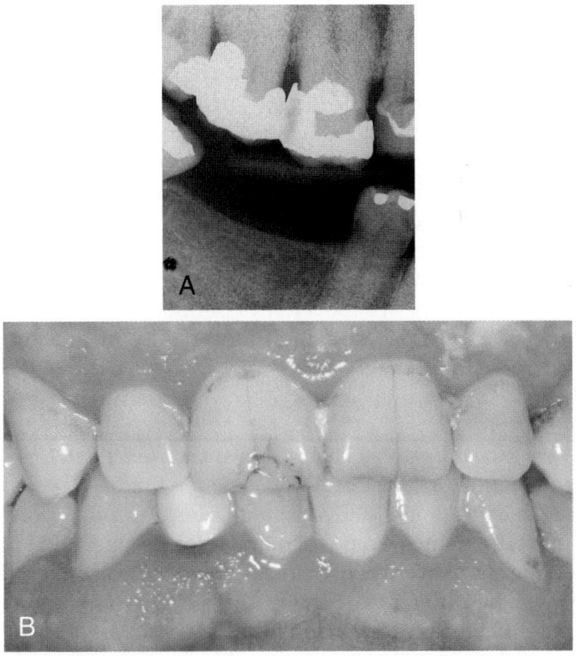

Figure 19-2. Overhanging restoration on the distal aspect of No. 3 contributing to oral bone loss.

Local Contributing Factors

The dental hygienist identifies local contributing factors that may increase the risk for oral disease or augment periodontal disease progression. Because of the biofilm's retentive nature, **iatrogenic factors** (those caused by the practitioner) can contribute to the initiation and progression of periodontal disease. Overhanging restorations (Figure 19-2, *A*), subgingival margin placement of crowns and restorations (Figure 19-2, *B*), orthodontic appliances, and removable partial dentures are examples of iatrogenic factors that may contribute to disease progression because they increase biofilm retention. Other factors include malpositioned teeth, oral jewelry, improper tooth contacts, size and shape of the root, calculus, mouth breathing, minimal amount of attached gingiva, and trauma such as toothbrush abrasion. Local contributing factors serve as biofilm traps, making oral biofilm removal difficult and thus increasing client susceptibility to periodontal disease. The dental hygienist works with the dentist and client to modify these factors.

Nonmodifiable (Nonmutable) Risk Factors

History of Periodontitis

Presence and severity of existing periodontitis are linked strongly with future periodontal breakdown. Persons who have experienced previous episodes of periodontal disease are at a greater risk for future attachment loss than individuals who have not had periodontitis. Because individuals who have existing periodontitis are at great risk for continued periodontal destruction, frequent continued-care appointments are especially important to assist with maintenance of attachment levels.

Age

Aging is associated with enhanced susceptibility to periodontal disease; however, risk factors such as smoking and the presence of specific periodontal pathogens play a much larger role in disease susceptibility. Increased prevalence and severity of periodontal disease in the aging population do not result from changes associated with aging, as once thought. Rather, the cumulative effects of periodontal breakdown over a lifetime cause the increased periodontal disease observed with advancing age. The severity of periodontal disease does not increase with age, although the severity of attachment loss increased with age.

Gender and Race

Background characteristics that may increase the risk for periodontal disease are race and male gender. Studies report significantly more bone loss, attachment loss, and tooth loss in men than in women even when oral hygiene, age, and socioeconomic status were considered. Other studies suggest that oral hygiene differences between men and women account for the differences in periodontal disease risk.

Among racial and ethnic groups Mexican Americans have the highest rate of periodontitis followed by African Americans. This greater disease prevalence and increase in susceptibility to aggressive and chronic periodontitis likely is linked to socioeconomic class, which may be more of a factor than race itself. More research is needed to determine the degree to which periodontal disease susceptibility is a function of race and gender.

Genetic Disorders

Several genetic and inherited disorders are risk factors linked with a depressed immune system and increased periodontal disease susceptibility. Phagocyte dysfunction, cyclic neutropenia, acute monocytic leukemia, Papillon-Lefèvre syndrome, Down syndrome, and Chédiak-Higashi syndrome are highly associated with early-onset types of periodontal disease. (See a current pathology textbook for specific information on these diseases.)

Genetic Marker

An advance in risk factor assessment was the discovery of a genetic marker highly associated with severe periodontal disease. This discovery resulted in the development of a genetic susceptibility test for periodontal disease: the Periodontal Susceptibility Test (PST) analyzes DNA to identify specific variations in interleukin (IL)-1α and IL-1β. A positive result is associated with increased susceptibility to chronic periodontal disease. Studies indicate that approximately 30% of the Caucasian population tests positive for this IL-1 gene type. A key regulator in the inflammatory process, IL-1 in high concentrations causes tissue destruction. Overproduction of IL-1 helps explain the more generalized and severe periodontal disease seen in many genotype-positive clients. The PST can identify potentially high-risk clients and therefore the need for more aggressive treatment and perhaps improved client compliance. The PST is not a diagnostic test but a prognostic test (e.g., some clients test positive for the genotype and never develop severe periodontal disease; some clients who test negative develop severe periodontal disease). Although genetic testing provides important information concerning the risk of periodontal disease in some populations, the best way to use this test clinically has not been determined. The multifactorial nature of periodontal disease must be considered when risk is assessed. The bacterial challenge, smoking, and other risk factors affect the degree to which IL-1 genotype status increases risk for periodontal breakdown. Genotype status is not as important as smoking or DM when risk for periodontitis is evaluated. More research is needed to clarify the role of IL-1 in all population types.

Clinical Application of Risk Assessment

A risk assessment screening form assists in identifying risk factors, determining which are modifiable versus nonmodifiable, and planning evidence-based treatment interventions to optimize care (Figure 19-3). Information to complete the risk assessment screening form is obtained through the comprehensive health and dental history, client interview, and the oral assessment.[3]

A computerized risk assessment tool, available from PreViser Corporation, uses a numeric score from 1 to 5 to predict risk based on nine personal risk factors analyzed via a mathematic algorithm. Evidence suggests the system provides a valid and reliable predictor of periodontitis. This more scientific approach to risk assessment may prove beneficial for developing a plan of care based on risk as well as assessing risk level changes over time.

Risk factors increase client susceptibility for periodontal breakdown; however, even one risk factor may increase substantially the client's degree of risk. The most significant risk factors are as follows:

- Smoking
- Diabetes
- Poor self-care
- Genetics

In fact, heavy smokers (defined as 10 cigarettes or more per day) who also have a genotype-positive status are at the greatest risk for periodontal disease breakdown. Persons with these two risk factors are more than seven times more likely to lose teeth than those without these risk factors. After periodontal and risk assessment, suggestions for eliminating or modifying risk factors are addressed, for example, through consultation with a client's physician to determine if medications not associated with gingival enlargement can be substituted for those that are. Clients who smoke are counseled to quit or enroll in tobacco cessation programs based on their

Periodontal Disease Risk Assessment Form

Patient name: ______________ Chart #: ______________ Date: ______________

Assessment date: (Please circle) is this? Base line or Recall

Disease Indicators	(Please circle)		
Existing or previous periodontitis	NO	YES	% sites:
Gingival bleeding	NO	YES	% sites:
Increasing pocket depths	NO	YES	% sites:
Recession	NO	YES	% sites:
Gingival enlargement	NO	YES	% sites:
Interdental papillary changes (blunting, cratered)	NO	YES	% sites:
Suppuration or purulent exudate	NO	YES	% sites:
Furcation involvement	NO	YES	% sites:
Tooth mobility	NO	YES	% sites:
Radiographic evidence of bone loss	NO	YES	% sites:
	YES circled = increased risk		
Nonmodifiable Risk Factors	(Please circle)		
Past history of periodontal disease	NO	YES	
Race	African American may = increased risk		
Gender	MALE	FEMALE	Male = increased risk
Age	Aging may = increased risk		
Family history of periodontal disease	NO	YES	
Genetic disorders or compromised immune system	NO	YES	
DNA testing for periodontal susceptibility	NEGATIVE	POSITIVE	
	YES circled = increased risk		
Modifiable Risk Factors	(Please circle)		
Adequacy of self-care	GOOD	FAIR	POOR
Xerostomia	NO	YES	
Smoking	NO	YES	Amount per day:
Stress	LOW	MODERATE	HIGH
Medications that affect gingival tissues/cause xerostomia	NO	YES	
Poorly controlled diabetes	NO	YES	
Osteoporosis/osteopenia	NO	YES	
HIV and AIDS	NO	YES	
	YES circled = increased risk		
Local Contributing Factors	(Please circle)		
Overhanging restorations	NO	YES	% sites:
Poorly contoured crown margins	NO	YES	% sites:
Ill-fitting fixed/removable appliances	NO	YES	% sites:
Oral jewelry	NO	YES	% sites:
Malpositioned teeth/contacts	NO	YES	% sites:
Calculus	NO	YES	% sites:
Toothbrush abrasion	NO	YES	% sites:
Inadequate attached gingiva	NO	YES	% sites:
Occlusal trauma/fremitis	NO	YES	% sites:
Mouth breathing	NO	YES	
	YES circled = increased risk		

Figure 19-3. Client risk assessment for periodontal disease. Used with permission from Thomson, Evelyn, *Case Studies in Dental Hygiene,* 3rd edition, Pearson-Prentice Hall, NJ.

state of readiness to change; clients experiencing high levels of psychosocial stress could be provided with stress management strategies and counseled to relieve stress via healthy lifestyle behaviors, for example, exercise, a well-balanced diet, and adequate rest and sleep. Clients with osteoporosis could consult their physicians about use of weight-bearing exercise, bisphosphonate medications, and ERT. Clients who test positive with genetic testing may be scheduled for more request re-care visits. When risk factors are identified in the absence of periodontal disease, the client is educated about his or her increased susceptibility and encouraged to improve self-care, maintain frequent maintenance care, cease tobacco use, and reduce other risk factors as appropriate.

Clients with periodontitis and risk factors are treated aggressively (e.g., scheduled for 2- to 3-month periodontal maintenance care visits; referred for periodontal surgery earlier; and encouraged to follow a rigorous self-care program, including antimicrobial mouth rinse therapy, oral irrigation, systemic antibiotics, local controlled drug delivery, or subantimicrobial doses of doxycycline to control collagenase activity). Eliminating as many risk factors as possible is vital to long-term periodontal health. For more information on the oral-systemic health connection, see Chapter 20.

Periodontal Assessment Instruments

Basic tools to assess clinical parameters include a good source of light, compressed air to dry the tissues, a mouth mirror, an explorer, a periodontal probe, and a current set of radiographs.[5-7]

Many kinds of periodontal probes are available. All are calibrated in millimeters for use in assessing the health of the periodontium and may be made of plastic or metal. Figure 19-4 shows the Marquis probe with colored bands to indicate different measurement levels of 3, 6, 9, and 12 mm, and the Williams probe, which is calibrated with 3-, 5-, 7-, and 10-mm markings. When a probe is inserted into the space between the tooth and the gingiva, the calibrations show the depth of the space in millimeters (Figure 19-5). Probing depths are used to monitor periodontal health and disease. Figure 19-6 displays a plastic periodontal probe with interchangeable plastic tips with varying millimeter markings. (See the discussion of assessment instruments in Chapter 26.)

Computer-assisted, pressure-sensitive, and voice-activated probes are options to manual probing. Probing depths are entered using a computer keyboard and software (Figure 19-7). In addition to probing depths, most computerized systems store and reveal information on attachment levels, recession, mobility, and furcation involvement. The clinician operates the probe by gently probing around the tooth. A foot pedal is used in conjunction with the probe handpiece to select from a list of periodontal data to be entered. The resulting computer-generated chart (Figure 19-8) aids periodontal assessment, may result in time savings over traditional methods, and provides a visual tool for educating clients. Pressure-sensitive probes, mainly used in research, have the

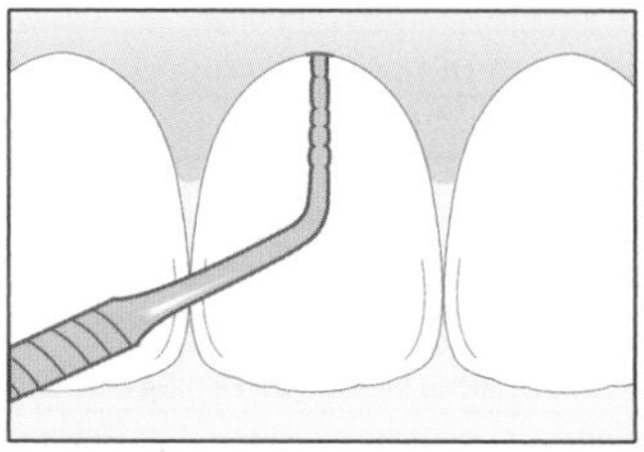

Figure 19-5. Williams probe inserted into a gingival sulcus. Calibrations show a depth of 4 mm. (Probe readings are rounded up to the next highest millimeter. Here, the 3-mm mark is covered up, so the measurement is read "4 mm.")

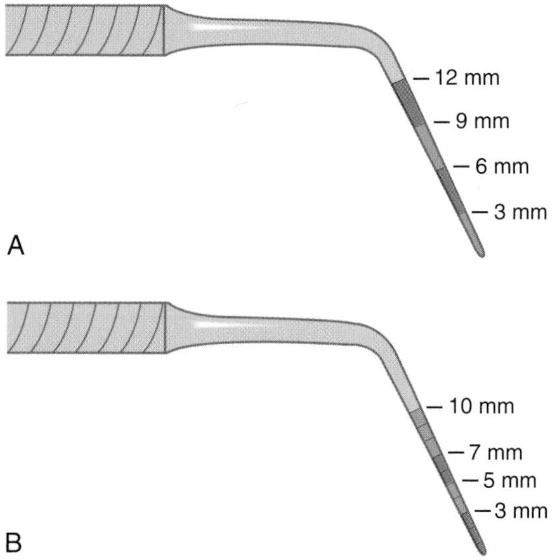

Figure 19-4. **A,** Marquis probe calibrated with color bands to indicate 3-, 6-, 9-, and 12-mm levels of penetration. **B,** Williams probe calibrated in 3-, 5-, 7-, and 10-mm increments.

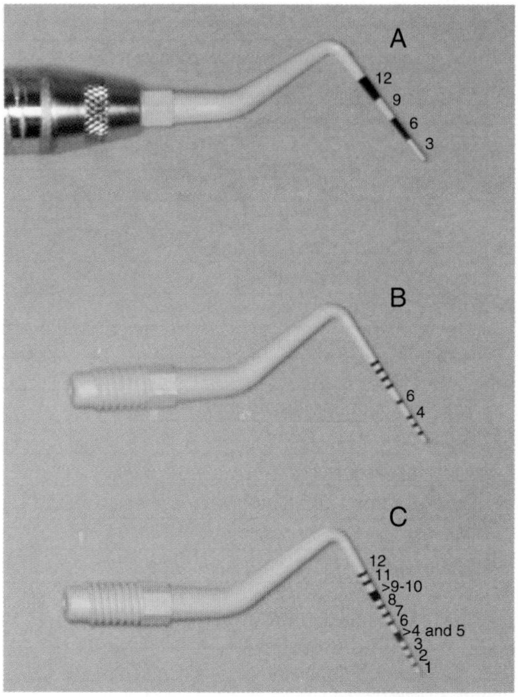

Figure 19-6. Plastic periodontal probe with three different types of interchangeable tips. **A,** Markings at every 3 mm. **B,** Markings at 1 to 10 mm with 4 and 6 absent. **C,** Markings at 1 to 12 mm with 4- to 5-mm band and 9- to 10-mm band.

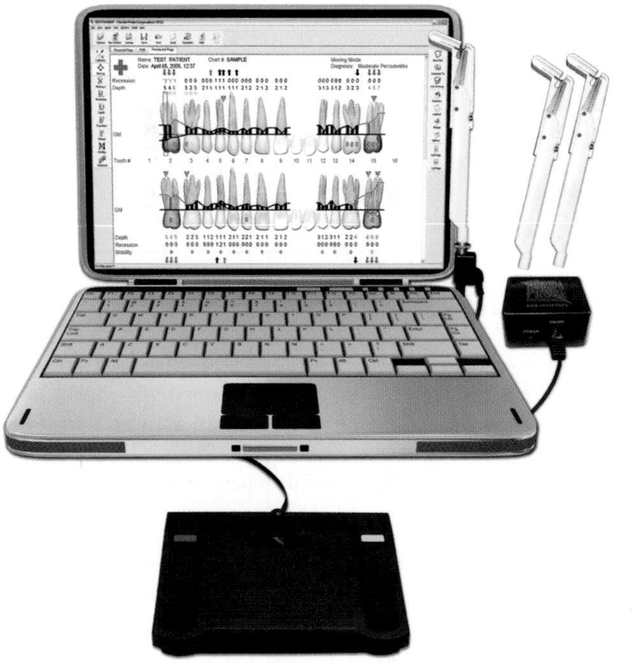

Figure 19-7. Computer-assisted probing device and setup. (Courtesy Florida Probe Corporation, Gainesville, Florida.)

advantage of maintaining a standard probing force, typically 15 g, improving accuracy (Figure 19-9).

A technologic advance in periodontal assessment is the periodontal endoscope, an illuminated fiberoptic instrument that provides high magnification views (24× to 48×) of the gingival sulcus. The instrument consists of a miniature camera attached to a tiny diagnostic explorer or probe. Images of the actual subgingival conditions are exhibited on a monitor. The probe is placed subgingivally, a water irrigation sheath flushes the pocket, and subgingival images (periodontal pocket, root surface, bone, furcation areas, and so on) are displayed immediately on a chairside color screen. Use of this technology assists in visualizing and assessing the extent of the client's periodontal disease (see Chapter 26).

Periodontal Screening and Recording

Periodontal screening and recording (PSR) is a method to screen clients for the presence of periodontal disease. This screening tool requires a specially designed probe that has a 0.5-mm ball tip and is color coded from 3.5 to 5.5 mm. The client's mouth is divided into six sextants, and each tooth is probed by walking the probe around the entire sulcus. At a minimum, five areas of the tooth are examined: mesiofacial, midfacial, distofacial, and the corresponding palatal and lingual areas. Only the highest score is recorded for each sextant according to the codes found in Figure 19-10. Clients found to be at high risk receive comprehensive periodontal examinations. All clients should receive a comprehensive periodontal examination annually.

Healthy Periodontium

Healthy periodontium consists of four physical units: gingiva, periodontal ligament (PDL), alveolar process (supporting bone), and cementum.

Gingiva

Gingiva is masticatory oral mucosa that covers the alveolar process and surrounds the cervical portion of teeth. Histologically, the gingiva has a protective layer of stratified squamous epithelium covering a dense, fibrous connective tissue. Gingiva is divided into four anatomic areas: the free or unattached gingiva; the gingival sulcus; the attached gingiva; and the interdental gingiva or interdental papilla (Figure 19-11).

Gingival tissue closest to the crown is the free or unattached gingiva. Free gingiva is not directly attached to the underlying alveolar bone. In healthy adult dentitions the free gingiva is located on the tooth enamel 0.5 to 2 mm coronal to the cementoenamel junction (CEJ) and fits tightly around each tooth. The edge of the free gingiva nearest the incisal or occlusal area of the tooth is the gingival margin or the gingival crest. The gingival margin marks the opening of the gingival sulcus.

Gingival Sulcus

The space between the free gingiva and the tooth is the gingival sulcus or gingival crevice. A healthy gingival sulcus generally measures 0.5 to 3 mm from the gingival margin to the base of the sulcus. Boundaries of the gingival sulcus are the sulcular epithelium and the tooth. Sulcular epithelium is the nonkeratinized continuation of the keratinized epithelium covering the marginal gingiva. Sulcular epithelium is clinically significant in that it is a semipermeable membrane, which in the presence of oral biofilm may allow bacterial endotoxins to penetrate underlying tissue.

Attached Gingiva

Free gingiva connects with the alveolar gingiva at the gingival groove. The attached or alveolar gingiva, continuous with the free gingiva, is covered with stratified squamous epithelium. Free marginal gingiva joins to the attached gingiva at the gingival groove. This shallow groove is clinically visible in less than half of the population. Attached gingiva covers the crestal portion of the alveolar bone on the facial and lingual surfaces and the roof of the mouth. It is attached firmly to the alveolar bone, unlike the marginal gingiva, which has no attachment fibers. Mandibular facial and lingual attached gingiva and the maxillary facial attached gingiva are demarcated from the alveolar mucosa by the mucogingival junction (MGJ); the width of alveolar gingiva varies throughout the mouth (from 1 to 9 mm). The facial aspect of the maxillary anterior teeth has the widest attached gingiva. In general, at least 1 mm of attached gingiva is sufficient for gingival health. This 1-mm minimum width measurement has significance for planning educational and therapeutic interventions for persons with periodontal disease.

Gingival Papilla

An interdental or gingival papilla is located in the interdental space between two adjacent teeth. The tip and lateral borders of the interdental papilla are continuous with the marginal gingiva, and the center is composed of attached gingiva at the base. The shape of the interdental papilla varies with the space or distance between two adjacent teeth. Given a wide space, the papilla is flat or saddle-shaped. If the interdental space is narrow, the papilla is pointed or pyramidal. When two teeth are in contact, the facial and lingual aspects

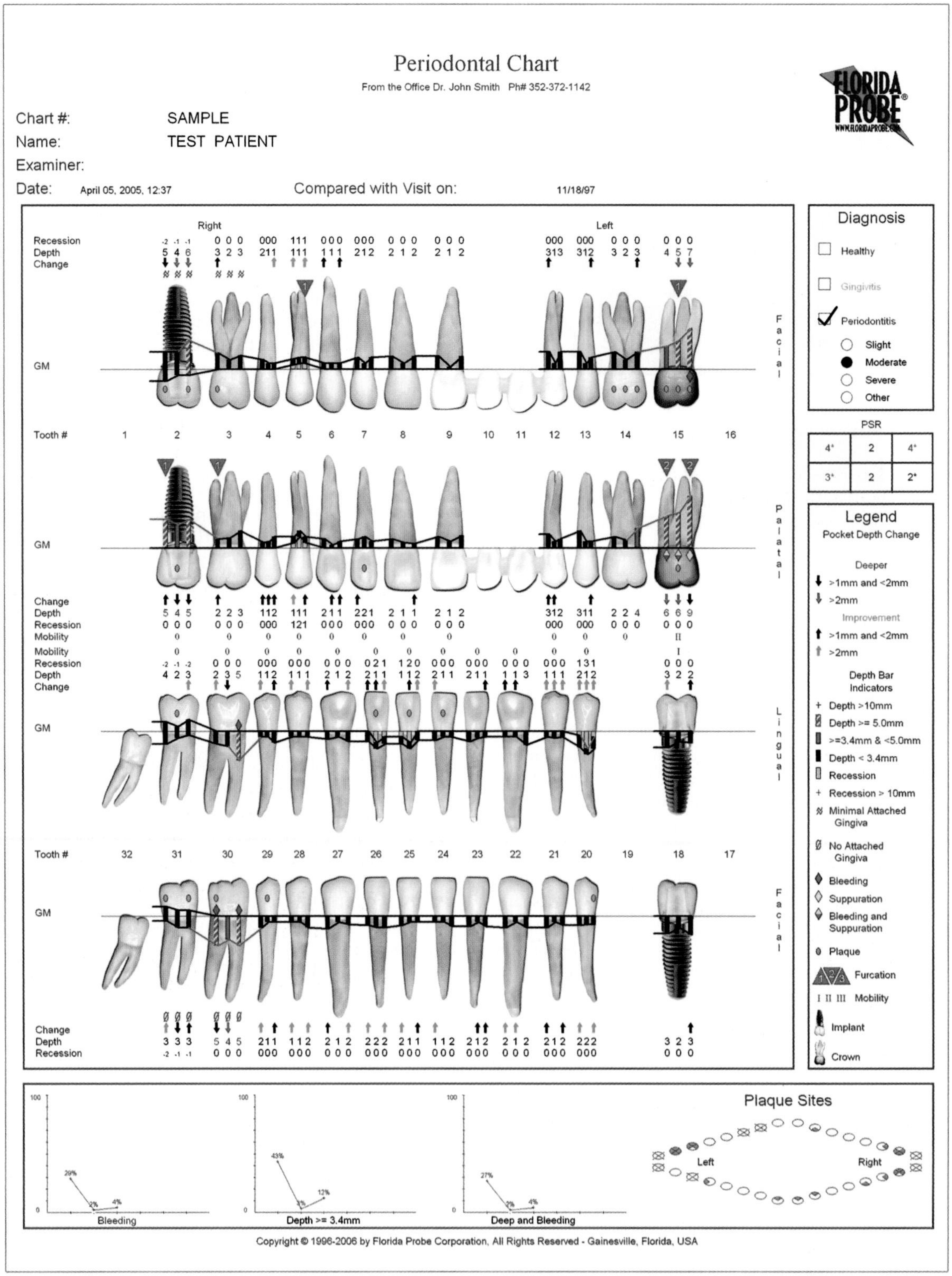

Figure 19-8. Computer-generated periodontal chart. (Courtesy Florida Probe Corporation, Gainesville, Florida.)

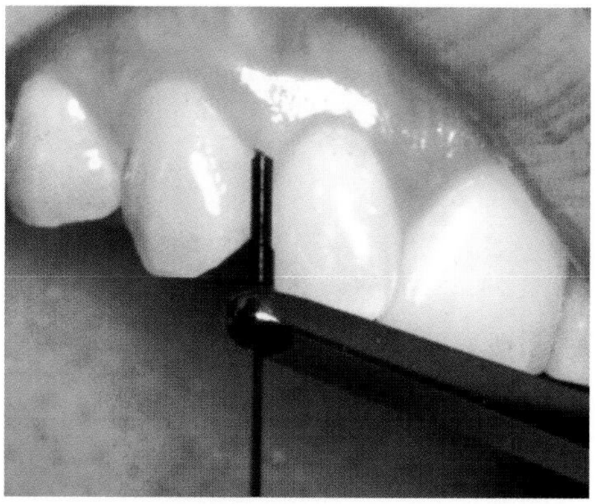

Figure 19-9. Pressure-sensitive periodontal probe. (Courtesy Florida Probe Corporation, Gainesville, Florida.)

of the papilla are connected by the **col,** a nonkeratinized area of interdental gingiva. Because the col is not keratinized, it is highly susceptible to disease (Figure 19-12). Most periodontal infections begin in the col.

Alveolar Mucosa

Alveolar mucosa is movable tissue loosely attached to underlying alveolar bone. Its surface appears smooth and shiny and is composed of thin, nonkeratinized epithelium. The alveolar mucosa is separated from the alveolar gingiva at the MGJ. The alveolar mucosa blends into the palatal gingiva in the maxilla so that no MGJ is distinguishable there. Alveolar mucosa is a darker shade of red than gingiva because of its richer blood supply.

Junctional Epithelium

Inside the gingival sulcus the sulcular epithelium attaches to the tooth at the coronal portion of the junctional epithelium (JE). The JE is a cufflike band of squamous epithelium that completely encircles the tooth and is attached to the tooth. The apex, or base of the sulcus, is formed by the JE (see Figure 19-11). The epithelial attachment is the innermost part of the JE that attaches to the tooth by hemidesmosomes and the basal lamina. A hemidesmosome is half of a dense plate near the cell surface that forms a site of attachment between the JE and the surface of the tooth. The basal lamina is a thin layer of delicate, noncellular material underlying the epithelium, with the principal component being collagen.

Gingival Crevicular Fluid

Gingival crevicular fluid (GCF) is a serum-like fluid secreted from the underlying connective tissue into the sulcular space. Little or no fluid is found in the healthy gingival sulcus, but GCF has been found to flow after 1 day without oral biofilm control and increases with gingival inflammation. The GCF, part of the body's defense mechanism, transports antibodies and certain systemically administered drugs.

Clinical Appearance of Gingiva

In health and disease, gingiva has distinctive color, consistency, surface texture, contour, and size (Table 19-1 and Figure 19-13).

Healthy Gingiva

Gingival color varies according to degree of vascularity, amount of melanin pigmentation, degree of epithelial keratinization, and thickness of the epithelium. Pigment-containing cells in the basal layer of epithelium commonly are present in persons of color (Figure 19-14). Therefore some individuals normally have brown melanin pigmentation throughout the gingiva. Healthy attached gingiva is resilient, firm, and tightly bound to underlying bone by gingival fibers running between connective tissue and the periosteum of the alveolar bone.

Healthy gingiva, when visually examined, air dried, and probed, does not bleed or exude fluids. Healthy attached gingiva usually has an overall stippled texture that varies with individuals and areas of the mouth. The gingival margin in health is located 1 to 2 mm above the CEJ. The gingival contour in health follows the contour of the teeth. In addition, the contour, size, and shape of the gingiva depend on location, tooth size, and tooth alignment (Figure 19-15). Healthy gingiva does not feel hypersensitive to air or touch.

Cementum

Cementum, a mineralized bonelike substance, covers the roots of teeth and provides attachment and anchorage for periodontal fibers. Cementum is usually a very thin cellular layer, not as hard as dentin, and it lacks blood vessels and nerves. In health, cementum is not exposed to the oral environment but is protected by the PDL.

Periodontal Ligament

The PDL is the fibrous connective tissue that surrounds and attaches the tooth roots to the alveolar bone. The width of the PDL, seen in radiographs only as a black (radiolucent) space, depends on age, stage of eruption, function of the tooth, and angle of the film. Collagen fibers of the ligament are inserted into the cementum and prevent tooth mobility by anchoring the tooth into its alveolar socket. The PDL is connected to cementum and bone by collagen fibers called *Sharpey's fibers.* Functions of the PDL also include formation and maintenance of fibrous and calcified tissue, nutritional metabolite transport, and the sensory functions of pain and displacement sensitivity.

Alveolar Bone

Alveolar bone is composed of compact or cortical bone and of spongy bone marked by trabecular spaces seen on radiographs. Compact bone is the outside wall of the alveolar bone, where the PDL fibers are anchored and the rich vascular supply penetrates. Spongy bone is the interior of the alveolar bone. It increases and decreases in response to physical pressure, function, bacterial infection, and inflammation. The alveolar crest—the portion of the alveolar bone located between the teeth—varies in size and shape depending on tooth position.

Diseased Periodontium

Histopathology of periodontal disease is explained in four stages (Table 19-2). Three of the stages describe a sequence of events resulting in gingivitis, and the last stage describes events resulting in periodontitis. Periodontal disease progression involves destruction of connective tissue attachment at the most apical portion of a periodontal pocket. Associated

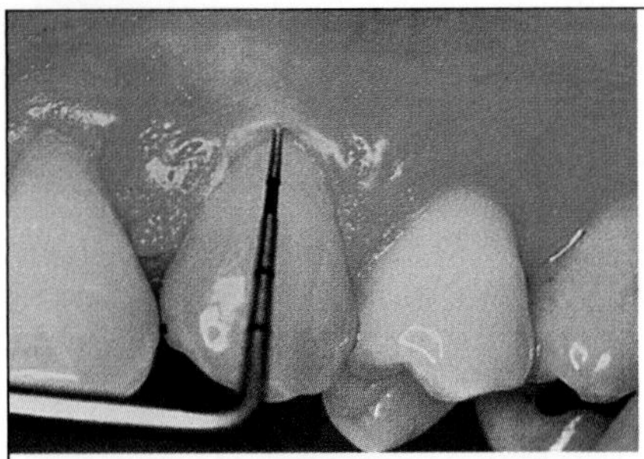

CODE 0

CODE 0

Colored area of probe remains completely visible in the deepest probing depth in the sextant.

- No calculus, bleeding, or defective margins detected
- Gingival tissues are healthy

Treatment recommendations:

Appropriate preventive care

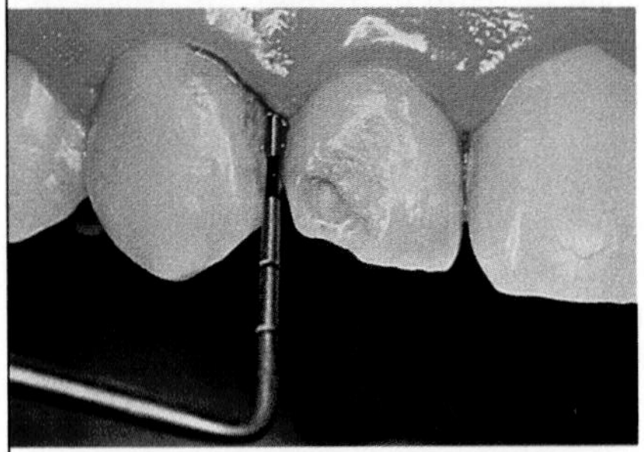

CODE 1

CODE 1

Colored area of probe remains completely visible in the deepest probing depth in the sextant.

- No calculus or defective margins detected
- There is bleeding on probing

Treatment recommendations:

Oral self-care instructions

Appropriate therapy, including:

- Subgingival plaque removal

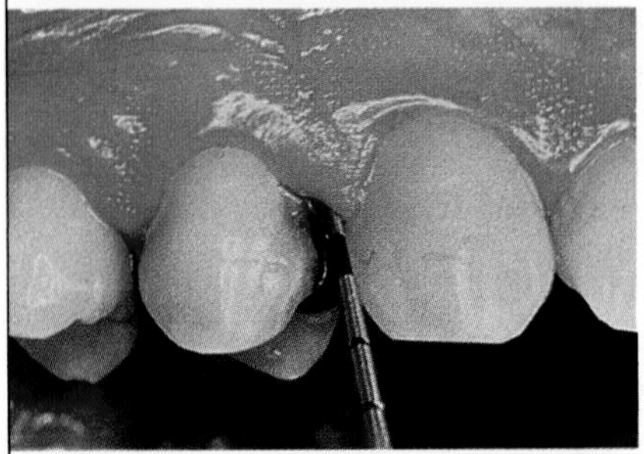

CODE 2

CODE 2

Colored area of probe remains completely visible in the deepest probing depth in the sextant.

- Supra- or subgingival calculus detected, and/or
- Defective margins detected

Treatment recommendations:

Self-care instructions

Appropriate therapy, including:

- Subgingival plaque removal
- Removal of calculus
- Correction of overhanging and defective margins of restorations

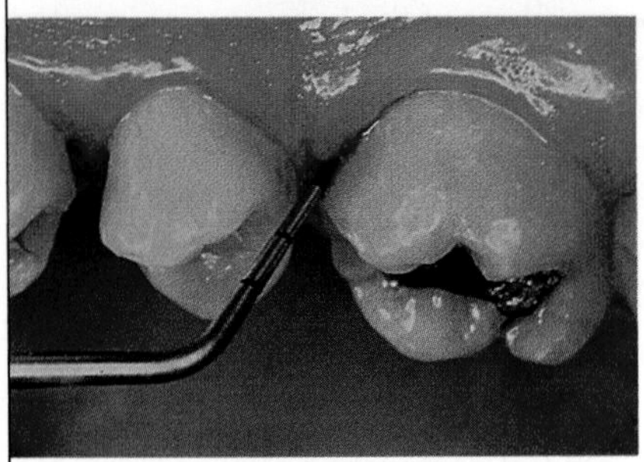

CODE 3

CODE 3

Colored area of probe remains partly visible in the deepest probing depth in the sextant.

Treatment recommendations:

Comprehensive periodontal assessment and charting of the affected sextant are necessary to determine an appropriate treatment plan.

Examination and documentation should include:

- Identification of probing depths
- Mobility
- Gingival recession
- Mucogingival problems
- Furcation invasions
- Radiographs

Note: If two or more sextants score CODE 3, a comprehensive periodontal assessment and evaluation are indicated.

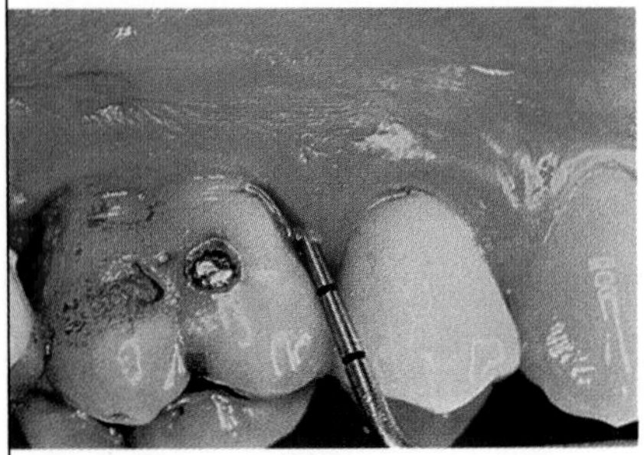

CODE 4

CODE 4

Colored area of probe completely disappears (probing depth greater than 5.5 mm).

Treatment recommendations:

Comprehensive full-mouth periodontal assessment and evaluation are necessary to determine an appropriate treatment plan.

CODE*

The symbol * should be added to sextant score whenever findings indicate clinical abnormalities such as:

- Furcation invasion
- Mobility
- Mucogingival problems
- Recession extending to the colored area of the probe (3.5 mm or greater)

Note: Comprehensive full-mouth examination and charting are necessary to determine an appropriate treatment plan.

Figure 19-10. Periodontal screening and recording (PSR). (From the American Dental Association, Chicago, Illinois.)

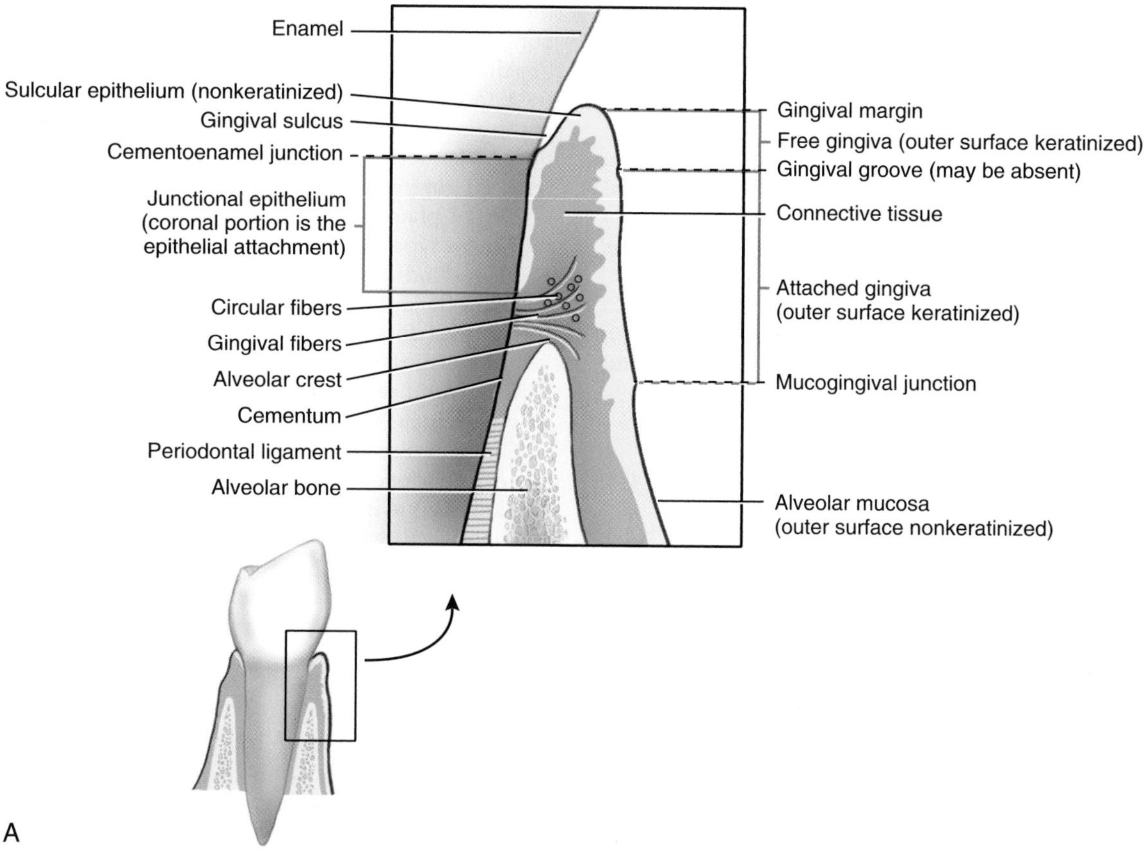

A

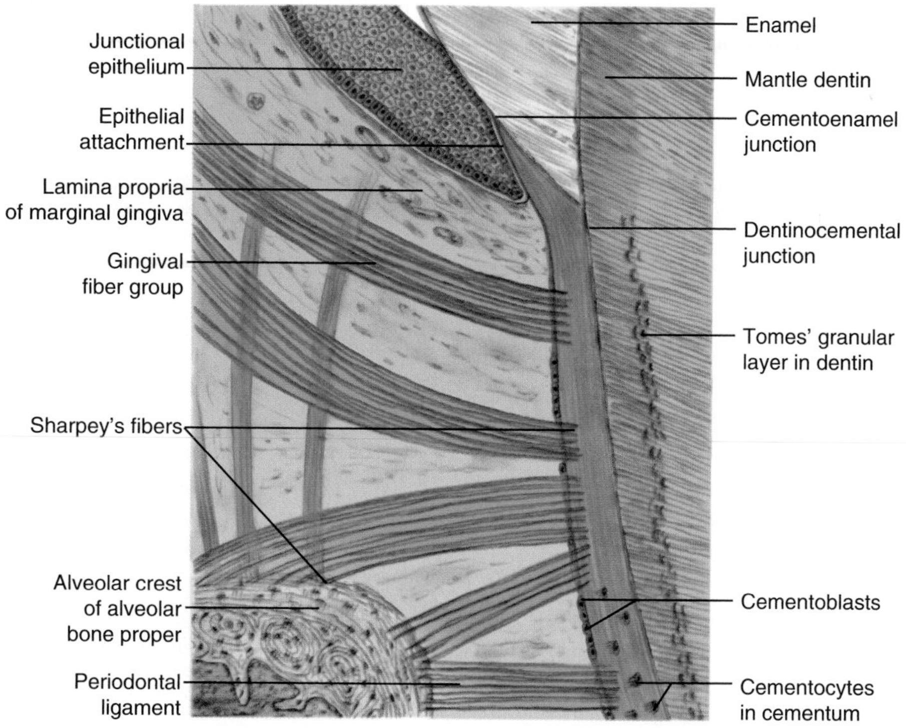

B

Figure 19-11. Gingiva and other periodontal tissues in cross-section.

with this attachment loss is the apical downgrowth of the subgingival flora, apical migration of the JE, and alveolar bone resorption. Table 19-3 compares the clinical characteristics of gingivitis and periodontitis.

Gingivitis

Understanding the characteristics of the healthy periodontium provides a foundation on which to recognize signs of disease and to make evidence-based decisions regarding care. The term *periodontal disease* includes gingivitis and periodontitis. Gingivitis, inflammation of the gingival tissue, is a reversible bacterial infection confined to the gingiva. In gingivitis the free gingiva shows signs of inflammation, but there is no apical migration of the JE beyond the CEJ or bone loss.

Although most forms of gingivitis are plaque induced, host and systemic factors modify the clinical characteristics of the disease. Therefore gingival diseases have two classifications: plaque-induced gingival diseases and non–plaque-induced gingival lesions (Boxes 19-3 and 19-4).

Dental plaque–induced gingivitis includes the following four main types of gingival diseases:

- Plaque-induced gingivitis resulting from dental plaque being the only causative agent (most common type)
- Gingival diseases modified by systemic factors (e.g., endocrine disorders and blood diseases)
- Gingival diseases modified by medications (e.g., anticonvulsive drugs)
- Gingival diseases modified by malnutrition (e.g., ascorbic acid deficiency) (see Box 19-3)

Non–plaque-induced gingivitis includes the following:

- Gingival diseases of viral, bacterial, fungal, and genetic origin
- Gingival manifestations of systemic conditions, such as allergic reactions, traumatic lesions, and mucocutaneous disorders

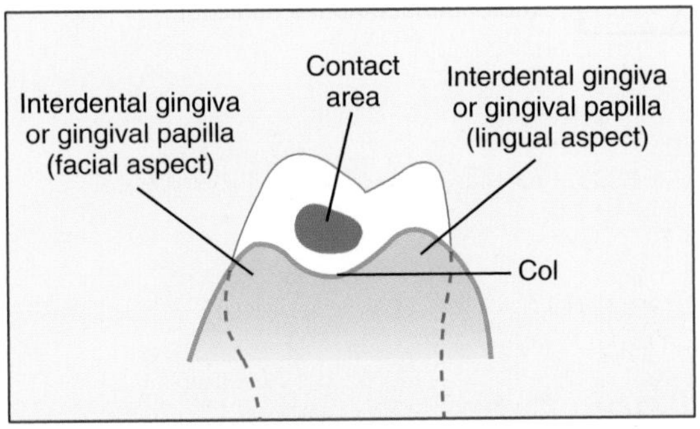

Figure 19-12. The col is significant because it is anatomically predisposed to growth of oral biofilm and hence susceptible to inflammation and disease progression.

Periodontitis

Periodontitis, inflammation of the periodontium, is an irreversible bacterial infection with inflammation extending from the gingiva into the connective tissue and alveolar bone that supports the teeth.[6-8] In periodontitis there is apical migration of the JE with associated loss of attachment and destruction of alveolar bone. To classify periodontal disease, the practitioner decides if gingival disease or periodontitis is present.

TABLE 19-1

Clinical Gingival Characteristics in Health and Disease

Characteristic	Health	Disease
Color	Uniformly pale pink with or without generalized dark brown pigmentation	Bright red Dark red, blue-red Pink if fibrotic
Consistency	Firm, resilient	Soft, spongy, dents easily when pressed with probe Bleed readily on probing
Surface texture	Free gingiva—smooth Attached—stippled	Loss of stippling, shiny Fibrotic with stippling Nodular Hyperkeratotic
Contour	Gingival margin is 1-2 mm above CEJ in fully erupted teeth Marginal gingiva is knife-edge, flat; follows a curved line around the tooth and fits snugly around the tooth Papilla is pointed and pyramidal; fills interproximal spaces	Irregular margins from edema, fibrosis, clefting, and/or festooning May be rounded, rolled, or bulbous; therefore more coronal to CEJ May show recessions so that the anatomic root is exposed Bulbous, flattened, blunted, cratered
Size	Free marginal gingiva is near CEJ and adheres closely to the tooth	Enlarged from excess fluid in tissues or fibrotic from the formation of excess collagen fibers Free marginal gingiva may be highly retractable with air
Probing depth	0-4 mm; no apical migration of JE	More than 4 mm with or without apical migration of JE

CEJ, Cementoenamel junction; *JE,* junctional epithelium.

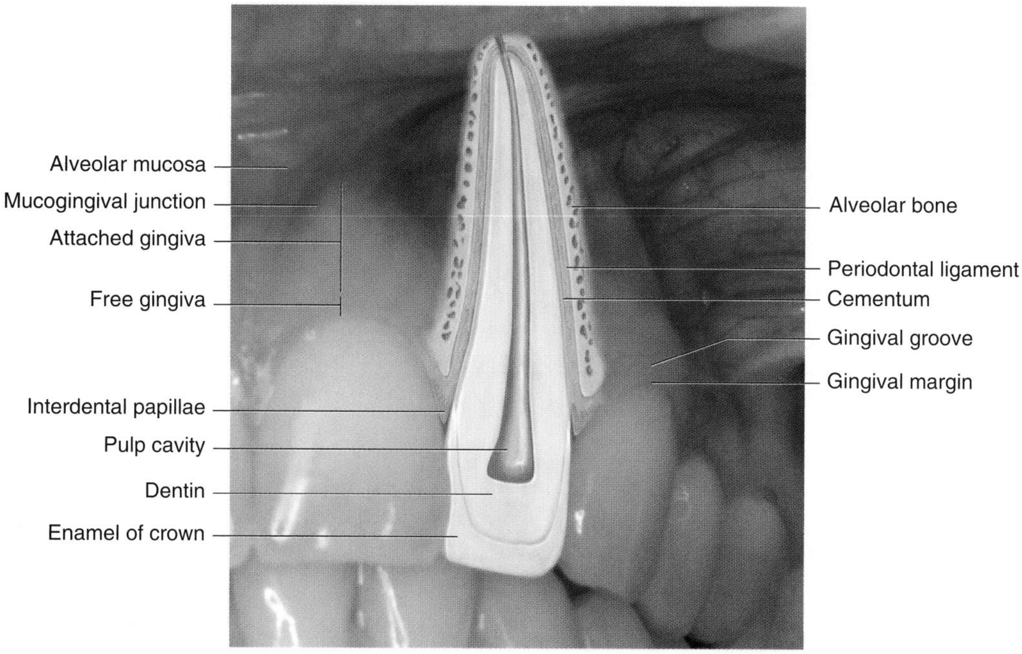

Figure 19-13. Anatomic relationship of normal gingiva. The gingival tissues: alveolar mucosa, mucogingival junction, attached gingiva, free gingiva, interdental papillae.

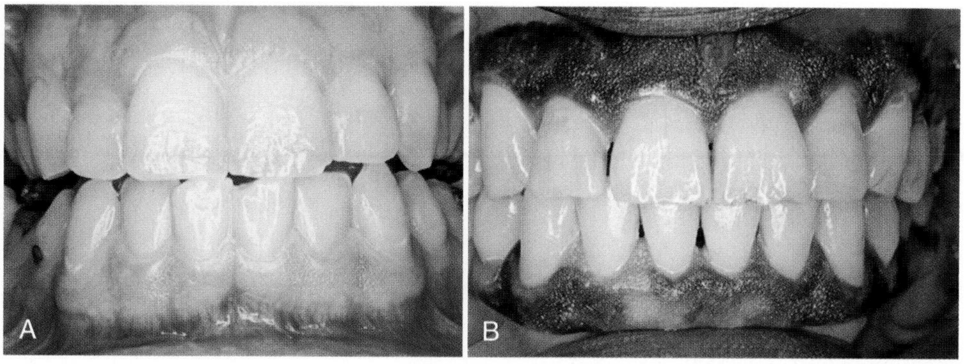

Figure 19-14. A, Clinically normal gingiva in light-skinned individual. **B,** Clinically normal pigmented gingiva in dark-skinned individual. (From Glickman I, Smulow JB: *Periodontal disease: clinical, radiographic, and histopathologic features,* Philadelphia, 1974, Saunders.)

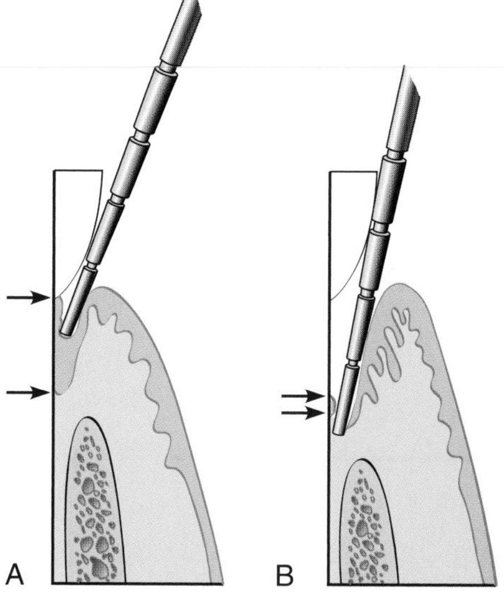

Figure 19-15. Some clinical parameters in health and in periodontitis. **A,** In a normal sulcus with a long junctional epithelium (JE) *(between arrows),* the probe penetrates about one third to half the length of the JE. **B,** In a periodontal pocket with a short JE *(between arrows),* the probe penetrates beyond the apical end of the JE. (From Newman MG, Takei HH, Klokkevold PR, et al, eds: *Carranza's clinical periodontology,* ed 11, St Louis, 2012, Saunders.)

TABLE 19-2

Histopathology of Periodontal Disease: Page and Shroeder Model of Inflammation

Stage	Histopathology	Time	Clinical Signs
Initial lesion	Vasoconstriction followed by migration and infiltration of PMNs into JE and gingival sulcus Alteration of most coronal part of JE Increase in gingival crevicular fluid flow Loss of perivascular collagen	2-4 days of bacterial irritation from oral biofilm accumulation	None Subclinical infection
Early lesion	Accentuation of initial lesion features Chronic inflammatory cells such as lymphocytes accumulate in the connective tissue Junctional and oral epithelium form rete pegs 70% loss of collagen fibers	7-14 days of oral biofilm accumulation with it growing thicker	Acute signs of inflammation Redness Edema Loss of tissue tone Bleeding on provocation
Established lesion	Persistence of acute inflammation manifestations Plasma cells predominate in the connective tissue Increased collagen loss with loss of connective tissue fiber support JE and oral epithelium continue to proliferate with areas of ulceration; epithelium is more permeable JE moves apically with early pocket formation; no bone loss	2 weeks or more	Chronic signs of inflammation Continuation of changes from early lesion; may become more severe Chronic changes such as fibrosis occur over time Condition is reversible
Advanced lesion	Continuation of features in established lesion Pocket epithelium extends deep into connective tissue Extensive destruction of collagen and gingival fibers Extension of irritants into alveolar bone and PDL resulting in bone loss Formation of periodontal pockets Conversion of bone marrow distant from the lesion into fibrous connective tissue Periods of quiescence and exacerbation	Varies, may never progress to this stage; depends on host response	Signs of periodontitis Attachment loss Crestal bone resorption Periodontal pockets Irreversible condition

JE, Junctional epithelium; *PDL,* periodontal ligament; *PMNs,* polymorphonuclear neutrophilic leukocytes.

TABLE 19-3

Clinical Characteristics in Gingivitis and Periodontitis

Characteristic	Gingivitis	Periodontitis
Gingival inflammation	Acute or chronic	Acute or chronic
Position of junctional epithelium	At the CEJ	Below the CEJ (attachment loss)
Position of gingival margin	Greater than 1-2 mm above the CEJ (gingival pocket)	Variable
BOP	Present	May be present
Exudate	May be present	May be present
Furcation involvement	Absent	May be present
Tooth mobility	Absent	May be present
Bone loss	Absent	May be present

BOP, Bleeding on probing; *CEJ,* cementoenamel junction.

BOX 19-3

Classification of Periodontal Diseases and Conditions—Gingival Diseases

*Dental Plaque–Induced Gingival Diseases**

1. Gingivitis associated with dental plaque only
   a. Without other local contributing factors
   b. With local contributing factors
2. Gingival diseases modified by systemic factors
   a. Associated with the endocrine system
      1) Puberty-associated gingivitis
      2) Menstrual cycle–associated gingivitis
      3) Pregnancy-associated
         a) Gingivitis
         b) Pyogenic granuloma
      4) DM–associated gingivitis
   b. Associated with blood dyscrasias
      1) Leukemia-associated gingivitis
      2) Other
3. Gingival diseases modified by medications
   a. Drug-influenced gingival diseases
      1) Drug-influenced gingival enlargements
      2) Drug-influenced gingivitis
         a) Oral contraceptive–associated gingivitis
         b) Other
4. Gingival diseases modified by malnutrition
   a. Ascorbic acid–deficiency gingivitis
   b. Other

Non–Plaque-Induced Gingival Lesions

1. Gingival diseases of specific bacterial origin
   a. *Neisseria gonorrhoeae*–associated lesions
   b. *Treponema pallidum*–associated lesions
   c. Streptococcal species–associated lesions
   d. Other
2. Gingival diseases of viral origin
   a. Herpesvirus infections
      1) Primary herpetic gingivostomatitis
      2) Recurrent oral herpes
      3) Varicella-zoster infection
   b. Other
3. Gingival diseases of fungal origin
   a. *Candida* species infections
      1) Generalized gingival candidosis
   b. Linear gingival erythema
   c. Histoplasmosis
   d. Other
4. Gingival lesions of genetic origin
   a. Hereditary gingival fibromatosis
   b. Other
5. Gingival manifestations of systemic conditions
   a. Mucocutaneous disorders
      1) Lichen planus
      2) Pemphigoid
      3) Pemphigus vulgaris
      4) Erythema multiforme
      5) Lupus erythematosus
      6) Drug-induced
      7) Other
   b. Allergic reactions
      1) Dental restorative materials
         a) Mercury
         b) Nickel
         c) Acrylic
         d) Other
      2) Reactions attributable to
         a) Toothpastes or dentifrices
         b) Mouth rinses or mouthwashes
         c) Chewing gum additives
         d) Foods and additives
      3) Other
6. Traumatic lesions (factitious, iatrogenic, accidental)
   a. Chemical injury
   b. Physical injury
   c. Thermal injury
7. Foreign body reactions
8. Not otherwise specified (NOS)

Adapted from Armitage GC: Development of a classification system for periodontal diseases and conditions, *Ann Periodontol* 4:1, 1999.

*Can occur on a periodontium with no attachment loss or on a periodontium with attachment loss that is not progressing.

The American Academy of Periodontology classifies periodontitis into seven categories (Box 19-5).

Describing the extent (localized or generalized) and severity (slight, moderate, or advanced) of sites affected can identify disease types further as follows:

- If less than 30% of sites in the mouth are affected, the disease is considered localized.
- If more than 30% of sites in the mouth are affected, the disease is considered generalized.
- Disease severity is determined by the amount of clinical attachment loss (Box 19-6) as follows:
  - Slight or early
  - Moderate
  - Severe or advanced

Chronic periodontitis is most prevalent in adults, affecting approximately 47% of the adult population, with those affected averaging about 0.25 mm attachment loss per year.[7] It thus progresses much more slowly than aggressive forms of periodontitis; however, progression rates vary widely. Mild cases of periodontitis affect about 8.7% of the population, moderate cases 30%, and severe cases 8.5%. Periodontitis is cyclic in nature, with extended periods of quiescence or inactivity followed by short periods of exacerbation or activity. Connective tissue attachment loss during the active stage can vary from minor changes to extensive tissue loss. All forms of inflammatory periodontal disease, however, are related to specific gram-negative anaerobic bacteria found in subgingival flora. The mere presence of these bacteria is not sufficient

BOX 19-4

Characteristics of Plaque-Induced Gingival Diseases

Dental Plaque-Induced Gingivitis

Inflammation of the gingiva with plaque present at the gingival margin

Characterized by absence of attachment loss, clinical redness, bleeding on provocation, changes in contour, color, and consistency

No radiographic evidence of crestal bone loss

Local contributing factors may enhance susceptibility

Plaque-Induced Gingival Diseases Modified by Systemic Factors

Endogenous Sex Steroid Hormone Gingival Disease

Includes puberty-associated gingivitis, pregnancy-associated gingivitis, and menstrual cycle gingivitis

Characterized by an exaggerated response to plaque, reflected by intense inflammation, redness, edema, and enlargement with absence of bone and attachment loss; in pregnancy may progress to a pyogenic granuloma (pregnancy tumor)

Diabetes Mellitus–Associated Gingivitis

Found in children with poorly controlled type 1 DM

Characteristics similar to plaque-induced gingivitis, but severity is related to control of blood glucose levels rather than plaque control

Hematologic (Leukemic) Gingival Diseases

Swollen, glazed, and spongy gingival tissues that are red to deep purple in color

Enlargement is first observed in the interdental papilla.

Plaque may exacerbate condition but is not necessary for it to occur.

Drug-Influenced Gingival Enlargement

Occurs as a result of the use of phenytoin, cyclosporine, and calcium channel blockers such as nifedipine and verapamil

Onset is usually within 3 months of drug use and is more common in younger age groups. Characterized by an exaggerated response to plaque resulting in gingival overgrowth (most commonly occurring in the anterior area and beginning in the interdental papilla); found in gingiva with or without bone loss but is not associated with loss of attachment

Gingival Diseases Associated with Nutrition

Associated with severe vitamin C deficiency and scurvy

Gingiva appears red, bulbous, spongy, and hemorrhagic.

Data from Papapanou PN: Periodontal diseases: epidemiology, *Ann Periodontol* 1:1, 1996

BOX 19-5

Classification of Periodontal Diseases and Conditions—Periodontitis

- I. Chronic periodontitis*
  - A. Localized
  - B. Generalized
- II. Aggressive periodontitis*
  - A. Localized
  - B. Generalized
- III. Periodontitis as a manifestation of systemic diseases
  - A. Associated with hematologic disorders
    1. Acquired neutropenia
    2. Leukemias
    3. Other
  - B. Associated with genetic disorders
    1. Familial and cyclic neutropenia
    2. Down syndrome
    3. Leukocyte adhesion deficiency syndromes
    4. Papillon-Lefevre syndrome
    5. Chédiak-Higashi syndrome
    6. Histiocytosis syndromes
    7. Glycogen storage disease
    8. Infantile genetic agranulocytosis
    9. Cohen syndrome
    10. Ehlers-Danlos syndrome
    11. Hypophosphatasia
    12. Other
  - C. Not otherwise specified (NOS)
- IV. Necrotizing periodontal diseases
  - A. Necrotizing ulcerative gingivitis (NUG)
  - B. Necrotizing ulcerative periodontitis (NUP)
- V. Abscesses of the periodontium
  - A. Gingival abscess
  - B. Periodontal abscess
  - C. Periocoronal abscess
- VI. Periodontitis associated with endodontic lesions
  - A. Combined periodontic-endodontic lesions
- VII. Developmental or acquired deformities and conditions
  - A. Localized tooth-related factors that modify or predispose to plaque-induced gingival diseases and periodontitis
    1. Tooth anatomic factors
    2. Dental restorations and appliances
    3. Root fractures
    4. Cervical root resorption and cemental tears
  - B. Mucogingival deformities and conditions around teeth
    1. Gingival soft-tissue recession
       - a. Facial or lingual surfaces
       - b. Interproximal (papillary)
    2. Lack of keratinized gingiva
    3. Decreased vestibular depth
    4. Aberrant frenum or muscle position
    5. Gingival excess
       - a. Pseudopocket
       - b. Inconsistent gingival margin
       - c. Excessive gingival display
       - d. Gingival enlargement
    6. Abnormal color
  - C. Mucogingival deformities and conditions on edentulous ridges
    1. Vertical and/or horizontal ridge deficiency
    2. Lack of gingiva or keratinized tissue
    3. Gingival soft-tissue enlargement
    4. Aberrant frenum or muscle position
    5. Decreased vestibular depth
    6. Abnormal color
  - D. Occlusal trauma
    1. Primary occlusal trauma
    2. Secondary occlusal trauma

Adapted from Armitage GC: Development of a classification system for periodontal diseases and conditions, *Ann Periodontol* 4:1, 1999.

*Can be further classified on the basis of extent and severity.

BOX 19-6

Characteristics of Periodontitis

Chronic Periodontitis

Onset at any age but is most prevalent in adults

Characterized by inflammation of the supporting structures of the teeth, loss of clinical attachment resulting from destruction of the periodontal ligament and loss of adjacent bone

Prevalence and severity increase with age

The following levels of chronic periodontal classifications have been identified.

Slight or Early Periodontitis

Progression of gingival inflammation into the alveolar bone crest and early bone loss resulting in slight attachment loss of 1 to 2 mm with periodontal probing depths of 3 to 4 mm

Moderate Periodontitis

A more advanced state of the previous condition, with increased destruction of periodontal structures, clinical attachment loss up to 4 mm, moderate-to-deep pockets (5 to 7 mm), moderate bone loss, tooth mobility, and furcation involvement not exceeding Class I in molars

Severe or Advanced Periodontitis

Further progression of periodontitis with severe destruction of the periodontal structures, clinical attachment loss over 5 mm, increased bone loss, increased pocket depth (usually 7 mm or greater), increased tooth mobility, and furcation involvement greater than Class I in molars

Aggressive Periodontitis

Occurs before age 35 and is associated with rapid rate of progression of tissue destruction, host defense defects, and composition of subgingival flora

The following subclassifications have been identified.

Prepubertal Periodontitis

Onset occurs between eruption of the primary teeth and puberty; occurs in localized forms usually not associated with a systemic disease and generalized forms usually accompanied by alteration of neutrophil functioning; clinically manifests as attachment loss around primary and/or permanent teeth.

Localized Aggressive (Formerly Juvenile) Periodontitis

Localized and generalized forms:

Generalized form (GJP) occurs late in the teenage years with a variable microbial cause that may include *Actinobacillus actinomycetemcomitans* (Aa) and *Porphyromonas gingivalis* (Pg) and affects most teeth.

Localized form (LJP) is associated with less acute clinical signs of inflammation than would be expected based on the severity of destruction. The localized form is associated with bone and attachment loss confined mostly to permanent first molars and/or incisors. Age of onset is at or around puberty; associated with *A. actinomycetemcomitans* (Aa) and neutrophil dysfunction.

Necrotizing Periodontal Diseases

Necrotizing Ulcerative Gingivitis (NUG)

A gingival infection with complex causes (e.g., plaque, temporary depression of polymorphonuclear leukocyte functioning, stress, poor diet) characterized by sudden onset of pain, necrosis of the tips of the gingival papillae (punched-out appearance), and bleeding

Secondary features include fetid breath and a pseudomembrane covering.

Fusiform bacteria, *Prevotella intermedia,* and spirochetes have been associated with gingival lesions.

Necrotizing Ulcerative Periodontitis (NUP)

Characterized by necrosis of gingival tissues, periodontal ligament, and alveolar bone

Associated with immune disorders such as human immunodeficiency virus (HIV) infection and individuals on immunosuppressive therapies; characteristics include severe and rapid periodontal destruction

Extensive necrosis of the soft tissue occurs simultaneously with alveolar bone loss resulting in a lack of deep pocket formation.

---

for periodontitis to occur because bacterial virulence and host susceptibility are critical contributing factors.

Immunopathology

The following two distinct causative components cause periodontal destruction:

- Gram-negative periodontal pathogens located next to the periodontium
- Host-mediated response to the periodontal pathogens

With adequate removal of oral biofilm and an intact host immune system, pathogen growth is held in check through neutrophil chemotaxis and phagocytosis.[6] When biofilm is not removed adequately, it accumulates at the gingival margin; over several days, biofilm bacteria release byproducts and toxins such as lipopolysaccharides (LPSs) that penetrate the JE, connective tissue, and blood vessels. A host defense system imbalance, a result of bacterial virulence, altered host defense, or other periodontal risk factors, weakens the body's ability to fight the pathogens, and an overproduction of inflammatory mediators occurs. Instead of being protective, the overproduction of inflammatory mediators destroys periodontal tissues. The body responds to the bacteria and their byproducts by triggering the immune system and sending in B and T lymphocytes, macrophages, and plasma cells (Figure 19-16). LPS interacts with monocytes and macrophages to produce cytokines and inflammatory mediators such as IL-1, prostaglandin E_2 (PGE_2), tumor necrosis factor (TNF)–α, and matrix metalloproteinases (MMPs) that lead to periodontal destruction. IL-1 stimulates the synthesis of MMPs and PGE_2. TNF-α, PGE_2, and IL-1 mediate (enhance) bone resorption, thus promoting periodontal destruction. An overproduction of MMPs from the host's inflammatory reaction results in collagen destruction in the connective tissue of gingiva, PDL, and alveolar bone. Degradation of collagenous connective tissue and bone resorption results in the clinical manifestations of periodontal disease. Thus the host's own immunoinflammatory response to the pathogenic microbial challenge, modified by risk factors, is responsible for most of the tissue destruction associated with periodontal disease.

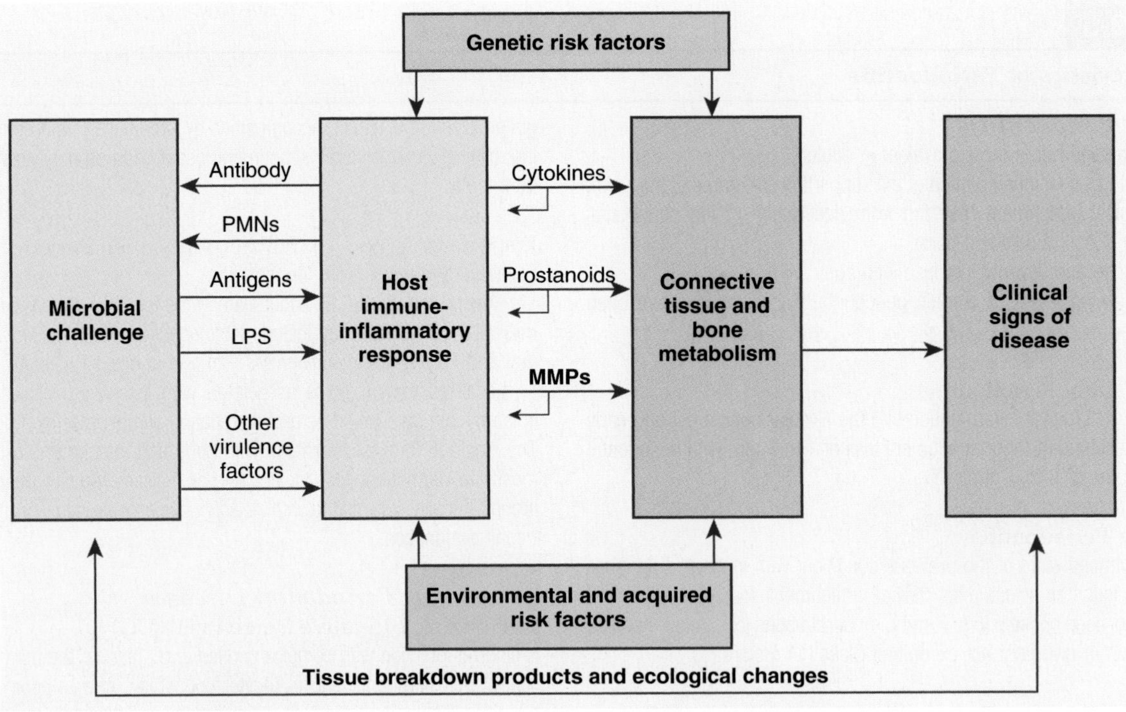

Figure 19-16. Traditional model of host response, risk factors, and microbial challenge in periodontal disease. *LPS,* Lipopolysaccharide; *MMPs,* matrix metalloproteinases; *PMNs,* polymorphonuclear leukocytes. (Adapted from Kornman KS: Host modulation as a therapeutic strategy in the treatment of periodontal disease, *Clin Infect Dis* 28:520, 1999.)

Signs of Gingival Disease

Clinical Signs of Inflammation (Gingivitis)

Inflammation begins in the epithelium of the col and of the marginal gingiva as a result of bacterial invasion or endotoxins (Figure 19-17).[9] Endotoxins and enzymes from gram-negative bacteria break down epithelial intercellular substances, causing sulcular epithelium ulceration. This ulceration permits enzymes and toxins to penetrate further into the underlying connective tissue. Connective tissue inflammation results in dilation and increased permeability of capillaries, resulting in tissue redness, edema, bleeding, and an exudate—that is, the four characteristic signs of gingival or periodontal inflammation:

- Changes in color
- BOP
- Swelling or edema
- Presence of exudate from the gingival sulcus

Oral tissue is assessed for these signs after it has been dried with compressed air.

Color Change. During assessment the first characteristic noted is gingival tissue color. **Erythema** (reddened gingiva), common in inflammation (see Figure 19-17), indicates an increase in the vascular supply as a result of the body's effort to defend itself against bacterial invasion or trauma (e.g., oral biofilm) or foreign objects (e.g., a popcorn shell). Bright red indicates acute gingival inflammation; blue or purple indicates venous congestion (cyanosis) in the connective tissue from chronic inflammation.

Dental hygienists monitor and record the slightest change in gingival color, contour, consistency, and texture, noting the location, distribution, severity, and quality of such changes (Table 19-4). Clients are informed of clinical findings and taught to monitor their gingival health. Using the hand mirror the dental hygienist points out gingival characteristics to the client and compares an inflamed gingival area of the mouth to one that is healthy to teach the client about his or her periodontal status.

Bleeding on Probing. Use of a periodontal probe to measure the depth of a healthy sulcus (one with an intact layer of sulcular epithelium) yields no bleeding. BOP is one of the earliest clinical signs of the presence of inflammation. However, false positive readings may occur if probing is conducted using heavy forces, which result in puncturing of the junctional epithelium. This instrumentation error could result in healthy gingival tissues bleeding. For the most part, the more severe the inflammation is, the more severe the bleeding, except in tobacco users where bleeding may be masked by associated vasoconstriction and altered immune response.

- BOP predicts attachment loss only 30% of the time. Furthermore, fibrotic tissue that results from chronic inflammation may bleed little or not at all.
- Gingival bleeding occurring at several sequential continued-care visits is associated with an increased risk for loss of attachment.
- Absence of bleeding is associated with lack of disease progression; however, the mere presence of bleeding does not predict periodontal breakdown.
- BOP is recorded in the client record and monitored. The dental hygienist explains to the client that BOP is caused by soft-tissue inflammation and gingival infection. Moreover, the hygienist points out that bleeding, or its absence, on brushing or interdental cleaning gives the individual a self-test for monitoring gingival health status at home.

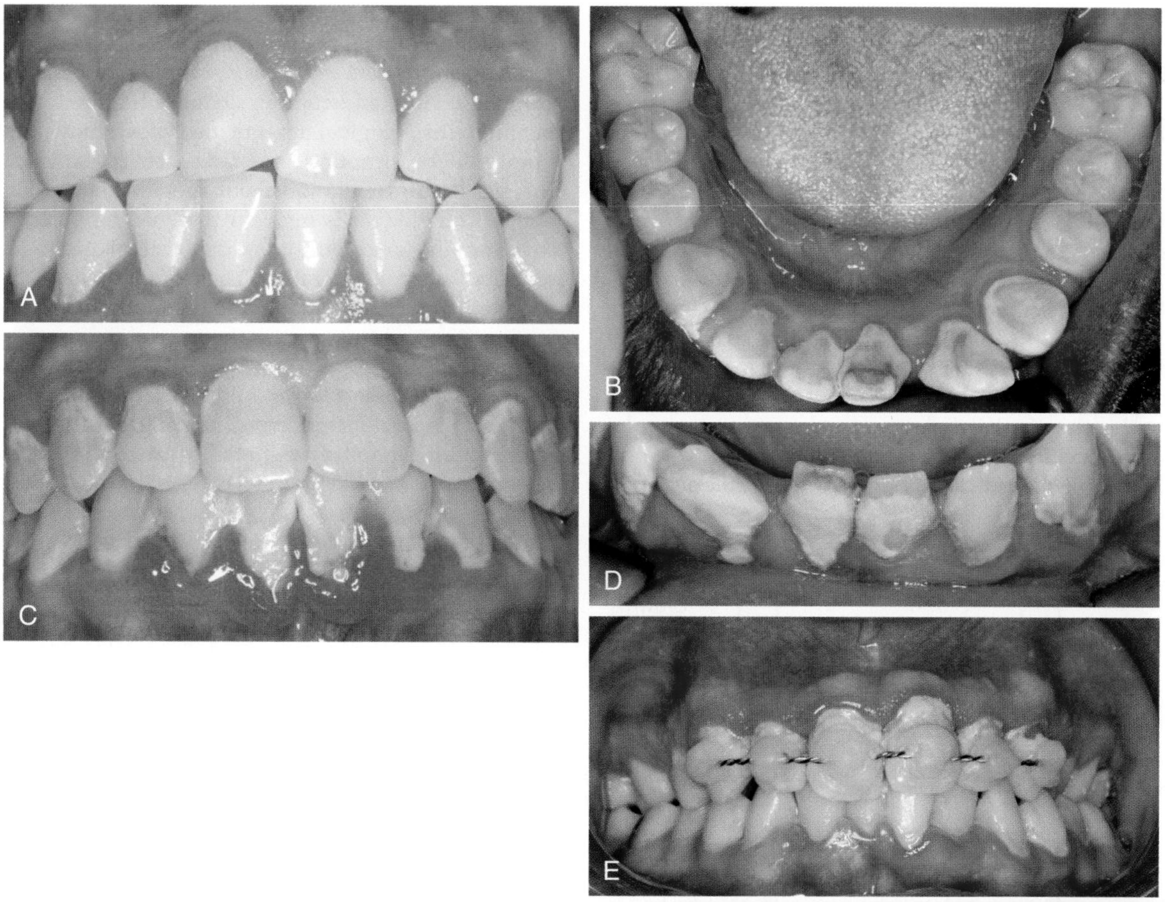

Figure 19-17. **A,** Edema, loss of stippling, and erythema associated with plaque-induced gingivitis. **B,** Life saver–like enlargement of the gingival margin with changes in color, contour, and consistency. Note the large amount of supragingival calculus. **C,** Diffuse enlargement and redness in the mandibular anterior affecting the free and attached gingiva. **D,** Calculus, material alba, and oral biofilm contributing to gingival inflammation; note the lack of stippling, the rolled gingival margins, and the dark red color. **E,** Orthodontics acting as a local risk factor to gingival inflammation. Note the redness, rolled margins, and gingival enlargement with biofilm and material alba localized to maxillary arch.

TABLE 19-4

Terminology Used to Describe Observations Associated with Clinical Assessment of Gingiva

Characteristic	Terminology	Description	Example
Gingival color	Location Distribution Severity Quality	Generalized or localized Diffuse, marginal, or papillary Slight, moderate, severe Red, bright red, pink, cyanotic	Localized slight marginal redness lingual aspects of teeth 18, 19, 30, 31; all other areas coral pink, uniform in color
Gingival contour	Location Distribution Severity Quality	Generalized or localized Diffuse, marginal, or papillary Slight, moderate, severe Bulbous, flattened, punched-out, cratered	Localized moderately cratered papilla teeth 6-11, 22-27; all other areas within normal limits
Consistency of gingiva	Location Distribution Severity Quality	Generalized or localized Diffuse, marginal, or papillary Slight, moderate, severe Firm (fibrotic), spongy (edematous)	Generalized moderate marginal sponginess more severe on facial aspect teeth 8, 9; all other areas coral pink with moderate, generalized melanin pigmentation
Surface texture of gingiva	Location Distribution Quality	Generalized or localized Diffuse, marginal, or papillary Smooth, shiny, eroded, stippling	Localized smooth gingiva on facial aspect teeth 7, 8; all other areas with generalized stippling

Swelling or Edema. Microorganisms in oral biofilm produce harmful toxins, and enzymes increase permeability of blood vessels in the connective tissue underlying the gingival epithelium. Increased blood vessel permeability allows lymphocytes, plasma cells, and extracellular fluid to accumulate in gingival connective tissue. This accumulation results in enlarged, edematous tissue (see Figure 19-17, *C, D, E*). When there is no apical migration of the JE, the sulcus becomes deepened from gingival tissue edema, producing a gingival pocket, also called an *artificially deepened sulcus* or a pseudopocket because the marginal gingiva has moved coronally, not apically (Figure 19-18). Deeper periodontal structures are not involved, and there is no migration of the JE.

A gingival pocket can be reversed to a healthy gingival sulcus by the client's daily plaque control regimen supplemented by professional mechanical therapy. When oral biofilm is controlled and calculus is removed, inflammation subsides; gingival enlargement decreases, with a resultant decrease in gingival pocket depth.

Changes in Texture and Contour. Swelling or edema produces gingival texture and contour changes (Figure 19-19, *A* to *F*). In gingivitis, gingival texture becomes shiny and smooth from loss of stippling and presence of edema. Contour changes occur from gingival enlargement, such that the position of the gingiva is high on the enamel, partly or nearly covering the anatomic crown. Marginal gingiva becomes rounded or rolled (rather than knife-edged or slightly rounded) and closely adapted to the tooth. In chronic inflammation, gingival surfaces may become nodular or fibrotic (see Figure 19-17, *E*).

Interdental Papillae Changes. While examining gingival color, texture, size, and shape, the clinician gives careful attention to the gingival papilla. When the col area is inflamed, epithelial and connective tissue layer degeneration can result in a

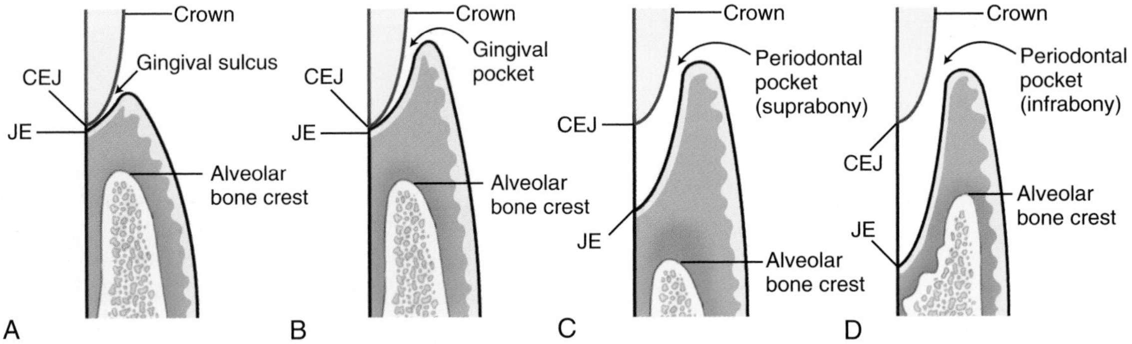

Figure 19-18. **A,** Comparison of the relationship of the junctional epithelium *(JE)* to the cementoenamel junction *(CEJ)* and alveolar bone in health. **B,** Gingival pocket. **C,** Suprabony periodontal pocket (periodontitis), JE above alveolar bone crest. **D,** Intrabony periodontal pocket (periodontitis), JE below alveolar bone crest.

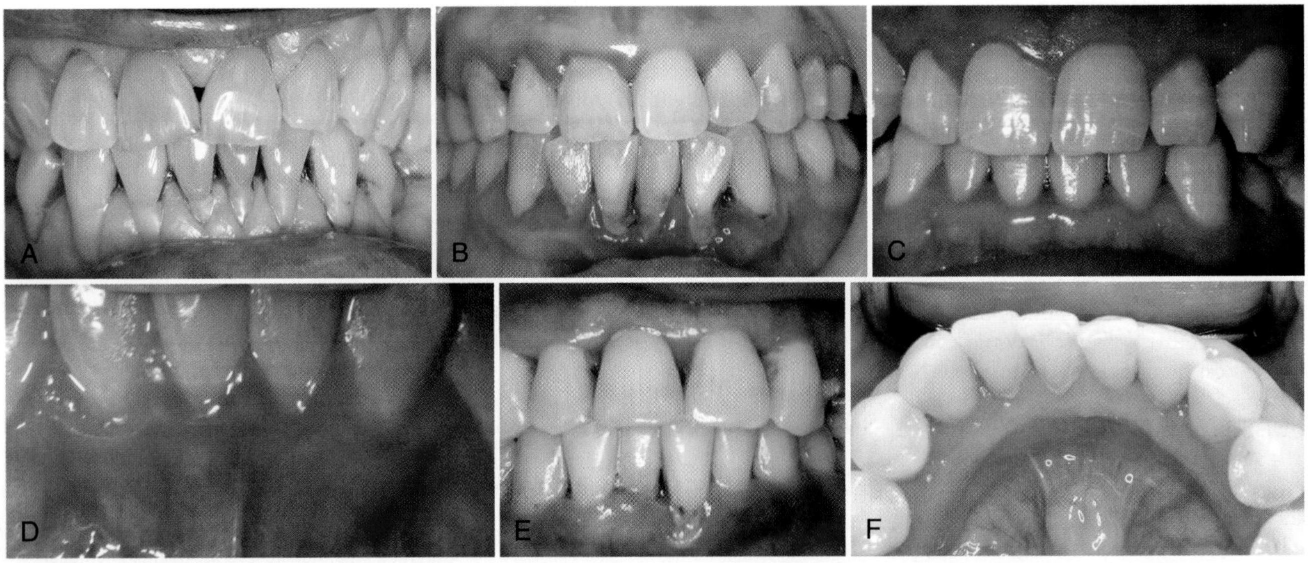

Figure 19-19. **A,** Significant recession of varying degrees throughout the mouth. Note composite restorations at cervical areas on the teeth along with the tobacco stain in mandibular interproximal areas. **B,** Severe inflammation in mandibular anterior tissues. Note blue color. Moderate erythema, edema, and loss of stippling throughout. Note significant recession caused from calculus and oral biofilm in the mandibular anterior. **C,** Generalized marginal erythema with shiny, smooth enlarged gingival tissues. **D,** Plaque-induced gingivitis; interdental papillae has lost its knifelike shape and displays puffy, rolled borders with erythematous tissues. **E,** Loss of interdental papillae in anterior areas with significant recession on tooth 25. Note pigmented gingival tissues. **F,** Slight calculus in the mandibular anterior with slight inflammation of the gingival tissues.

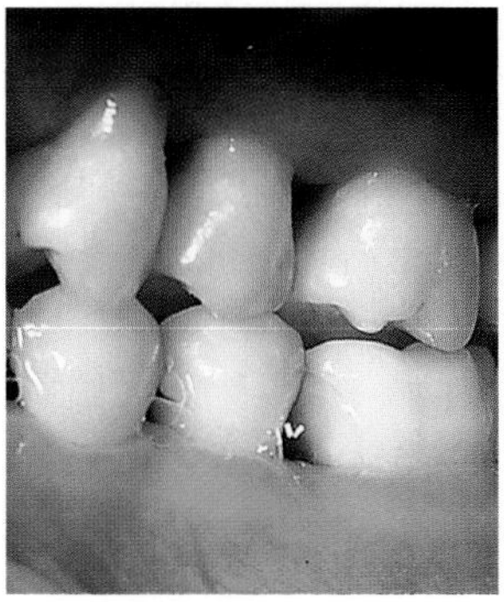

Figure 19-20. Cratered and missing interdental papilla.

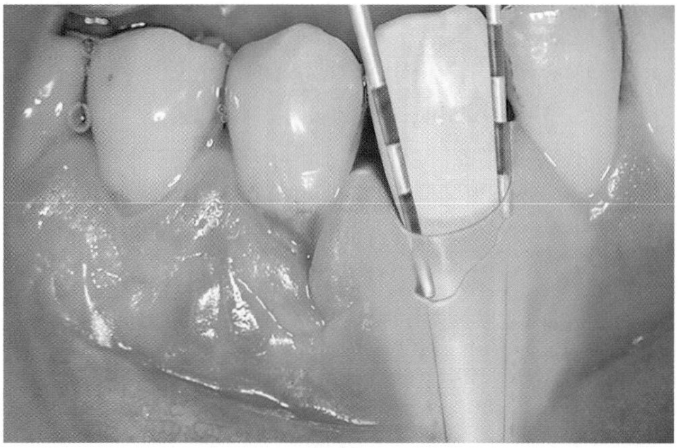

Figure 19-21. Probing depth and attachment loss measurement on same tooth using the Marquis probe. Note that the probe on the left reveals a probe depth of 4 mm and a clinical attachment loss reading of 5 mm. The probe on the right reveals a probe reading within normal limits of 2 mm with no clinical attachment loss. Tooth 28 shows a good example of a gingival cleft. (Adapted from Newman MG, Takei HH, Klokkevold PR, et al, eds: *Carranza's clinical periodontology*, ed 11, St Louis, 2012, Saunders.)

blunted papilla, a split interdental papilla, or a cratered papilla (see Figures 19-17, *B;* 19-19, *E;* and 19-20). Such degradation usually indicates alveolar bone loss. Self-induced trauma from improper use of dental floss may cause laceration of the gingival papillae.

Exudate. GCF rarely is found in healthy gingiva but significantly increases in the presence of inflammation. GCF is measured by isolating a site, drying it with air, and inserting a small paper strip into the pocket or sulcus for 3 to 5 seconds. Electronic devices can measure the GCF volume of the paper strip, although the clinical value of such a test is still under investigation.

GCF is called suppuration when it is a clear, serous liquid and purulent exudate when it contains living and dead polymorphonuclear neutrophilic leukocytes (PMNs), bacteria, necrotic tissue, and enzymes. When purulent exudate is present in the pocket, pus can be noticed during probing and expressed by applying pressure to the base of a pocket with one's finger and moving it coronally. Although purulent exudate is a dramatic sign of inflammation, it does not indicate the severity of inflammation or pocket depth. Some shallow and some deep pockets have pus formation, and some do not. The presence of pus is, however, a good indicator of active periodontal destruction. Suppuration correlates with specific attachment loss 2% to 30% of the time, so it is not a reliable indicator of active periodontal destruction. When suppuration or purulent exudate is observed, it is recorded for each area found.

Documentation of the Clinical Gingival Assessment

When assessing the gingiva, the clinician describes changes in gingival color, consistency, surface texture, contour, and size with regard to the following:

- Location (generalized throughout or localized to a specific area)
- Distribution (diffuse, marginal, or papillary)
- Severity (slight, moderate, severe)
- Quality

(See Table 19-1.)

The term *healthy periodontium* is appropriate for sites that are disease free but have extensive attachment loss and recession resulting from previous episodes of periodontitis. For example, sites that have been treated successfully fall into this category. When successfully treated periodontitis sites become inflamed at the gingival margin, this condition is termed *plaque-induced gingivitis* on a reduced periodontium.

Signs of Disease Progression (Periodontitis)

Periodontal Pocket

Probing depth is the distance from the gingival margin to the base of the sulcus or pocket, as measured by the periodontal probe (Figure 19-21). Unlike a gingival pocket or pseudopocket, a periodontal pocket is a pathologically deepened sulcus caused by bacterial infection. When the coronal end of the JE (the surface that forms the actual sulcus or pocket bottom) comes in contact with oral biofilm, it detaches from the tooth. At the same time the apical end of the JE migrates apically, thus deepening the sulcus into a periodontal pocket. As inflammation causes apical migration of the JE, it also causes gradual alveolar bone resorption, which reduces the level of bone support for the tooth. Periodontal pockets are classified as follows (see Figure 19-18):

- Suprabony periodontal pocket when the JE has migrated below the CEJ but remains above the crest of the alveolar bone. Suprabony pockets are associated most commonly with horizontal bone loss.
- Intrabony periodontal pocket, also known as infrabony pocket, when the JE has migrated below the crest of the alveolar bone. Intrabony pockets are associated with vertical bone loss.

Periodontal pockets may be present in the absence of clinical signs of gingival inflammation. Therefore clinical probing is the only accurate way to assess the gingiva for the presence of periodontal pockets. Because periodontal pockets can develop at any point around a tooth, the probe must be inserted around the entire circumference of the tooth. The deepest reading at each of the six tooth surfaces is the one that should be recorded on the client's periodontal charting form (Figure 19-22). The probe is walked along the pocket bottom and angled to keep the tip in contact with the tooth (Figure 19-23). If calculus is encountered, the probe is teased over the calculus, or the calculus is removed to allow insertion of the probe to the bottom of the pocket (Figure 19-24).

The interproximal area is the most difficult area for the client to clean and therefore is where periodontal pockets

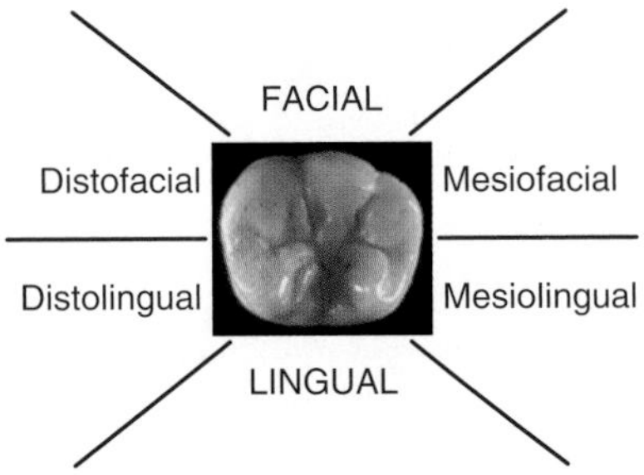

Figure 19-22. Occlusal view of the six surfaces measured in periodontal probing.

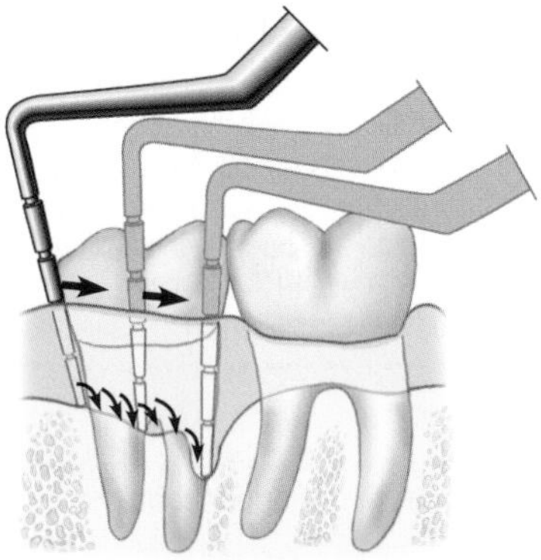

Figure 19-23. Facial view showing how the Williams probe is moved around the tooth in short steps, reestablishing contact with the pocket bottom at each step. (From Newman MG, Takei HH, Klokkevold PR, et al, eds: *Carranza's clinical periodontology,* ed 11, St Louis, 2012, Saunders.)

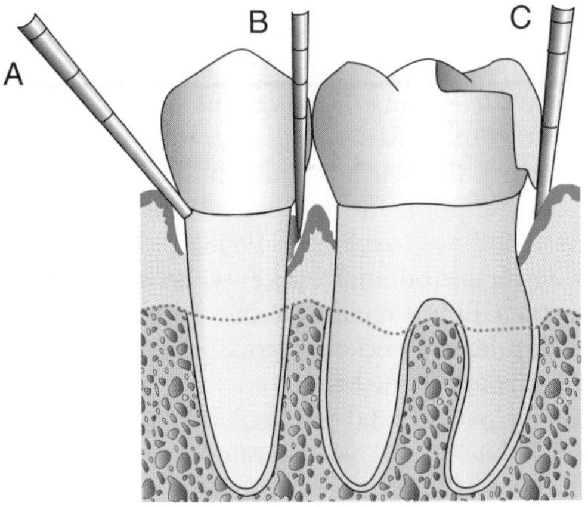

Figure 19-24. Periodontal probing limitations. **A,** Wrong angulation of probe. **B,** Probe blocked by calculus. **C,** Probe blocked by overhanging restoration. (From Newman MG, Takei HH, Klokkevold PR, et al, eds: *Carranza's clinical periodontology,* ed 11, St Louis, 2012, Saunders.)

tend to form. To probe the interproximal area just apical to the contact, place the probe up against the interdental contact and tilt the probe mesially or distally as appropriate to keep the tip touching the tooth (Figure 19-25). Failure to tilt the probe enough to keep its tip in contact with the tooth surface is a common error and causes inaccurate interproximal probing depth readings (Figure 19-26). The interproximal tooth surfaces should be probed from the facial and lingual sides of each tooth as loss of attachment may differ at each site (Figure 19-27).

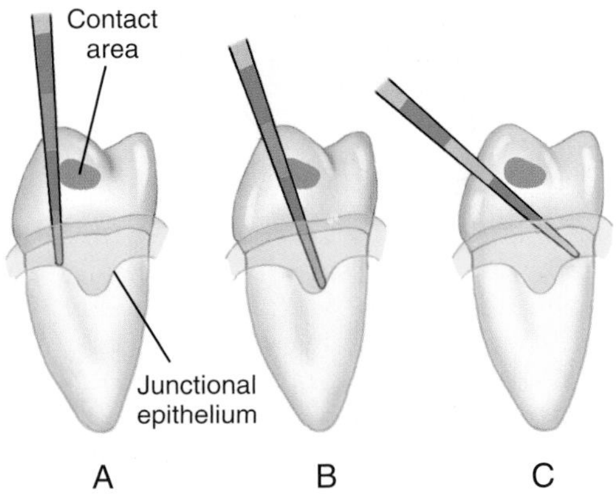

Figure 19-25. **A,** Incorrect technique for probing the interproximal area. **B,** Correct technique. **C,** Incorrect technique. (Adapted from Perry D, Beemsterboer P, Carranza FA: *Techniques and theory of periodontal instrumentation,* Philadelphia, 1990, Saunders.)

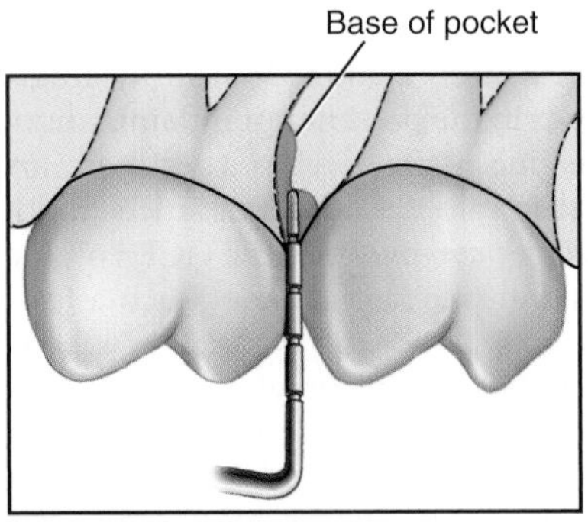

Figure 19-26. Failure to tilt the probe far enough to keep its end in contact with the tooth surface. Probe is resting on the pocket wall, resulting in an inaccurate probing depth measurement. (Adapted from Newman MG, Takei HH, Klokkevold PR, et al, eds: *Carranza's clinical periodontology,* ed 11, St Louis, 2012, Saunders.)

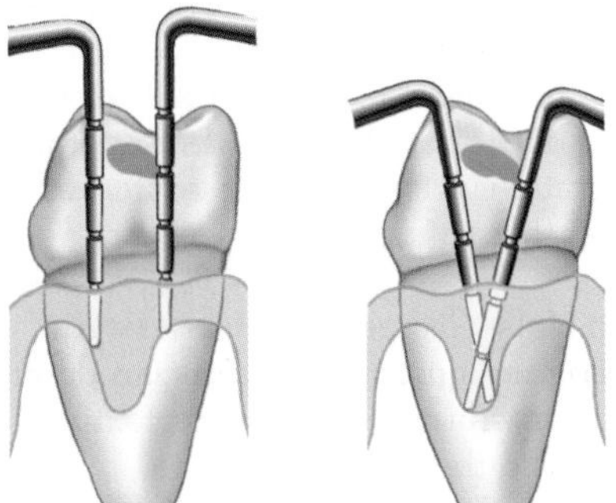

Figure 19-27. Proximal view of tooth being probed. Vertical insertion of the probe *(left)* may not detect interdental craters; oblique positioning of the probe *(right)* reaches the depth of the crater.

Gingival Recession

Gingival recession is a reduction of the height of the marginal gingival to a location apical to the CEJ (see Figure 19-19, *A* and *B*). Recession signifies attachment loss. Causes of gingival recession are numerous. Chronic exposure to bacterial plaque, toothbrush abrasion, abrasives in dentifrices, orthodontic appliances, floss trauma, occlusal trauma, abfraction, and root instrumentation can result in JE migration and recession. Once the root surface is exposed by gingival recession, the connective tissue rarely reattaches because collagen breaks down when exposed to the oral environment, and cementoblasts grow only on root surface adjacent to the PDL. Areas of recession may be sensitive because the exposed cementum may be lost, exposing dentin. Exposed nerve endings in dentin may be stimulated mechanically (e.g., by toothbrushing), chemically (e.g., by acidic foods or bacterial plaque), or thermally (e.g., by cold air or food at extreme temperatures), producing sensitive teeth (see Chapter 39).

Noting areas of dentinal hypersensitivity on the client record provides information for planning care; for example, clients may require more time, a local anesthetic agent, or nitrous oxide–oxygen analgesia for effective tooth instrumentation (see Chapters 40 and 41).

Clinical Attachment Level

Clinical attachment level (CAL), the position of the attached periodontal tissues at the base of the pocket, is determined by comparing the distance from the CEJ to the base of the sulcus or pocket (Figure 19-28). Location of the gingival margin is important in determining the CAL, which includes periodontal pocket depth and recession measurements. When the gingival margin coincides with the CEJ, the CAL and the pocket depth are equal. When the gingival margin is apical to the CEJ, the CAL is greater than the pocket depth and equal to the amount of visual recession plus the pocket depth.

In cases of gingival inflammation or hypertrophy, when the gingival margin is on the enamel, the attachment loss is less than the pocket depth. The gingival margin placement above the CEJ must be measured, and this reading subtracted from the periodontal probe reading to obtain the CAL. For example, if a client has generalized 6-mm probe readings but 2 mm of coronal movement of the gingival margin, the actual CAL is 4 mm. If this 2 mm is not subtracted from the probe reading, a realistic assessment of the CAL cannot be obtained. In this situation a client with only 4 mm of attachment loss may be misclassified as demonstrating a higher periodontal class than what is actually apparent. If a client has generalized 3 mm of recession and 3-mm pocket readings, the recession and the pocket readings are added together to obtain the actual CAL of 6 mm. If they were not added together, the client may be classified as having slight periodontal disease when 6-mm CAL would indicate severe disease.

Attachment loss over time (disease activity), not periodontal pocket readings, indicates actual progression of periodontal disease and is considered its defining feature. Consequently, regular documentation of attachment loss in the client record is important to track periodontal disease activity.

Relative Attachment Level

Relative attachment level (RAL), a record of past disease activity, is the measurement from a fixed reference point on a tooth (CEJ) or a stent to the JE. Such measurements are taken using a periodontal probe.

Furcation Involvement

Furcation involvement (or loss of attachment between the roots of posterior teeth) is identified, classified, and monitored (Figures 19-29 and 19-30, Table 19-5). The client is informed about areas of furcation involvement and taught homecare techniques to manage these areas. The Nabers furcation probe often is used to detect and measure furcation involvement. Radiographs confirm but do not always accurately reveal this condition.

TABLE 19-5

Classifications of Furcations

Class	Description
Class I	Beginning involvement Concavity of furcation can be detected with an explorer or probe, but it cannot be entered Cannot be detected radiographically
Class II	Clinician can enter the furcation from one aspect with a probe or explorer but cannot penetrate through to the opposite side
Class III	Through-and-through involvement, but the furcation is still covered by soft tissue A definite radiolucency in the furcation area on a radiograph visible
Class IV	A through-and-through furcation involvement that is not covered by soft tissue Clinically open and exposed

TABLE 19-6

Classification of Mobility

Class	Description
Class I	Tooth can be moved up to 1 mm in any direction.
Class II	Tooth can be moved >1 mm in any direction but is not depressible in socket.
Class III	Tooth can be moved in a buccolingual direction and is depressible in socket.

Tooth Mobility

Tooth mobility is the degree to which a tooth is able to move in a horizontal or apical direction. Although caused by the loss of PDL and bone support in periodontitis, tooth mobility varies during the day according to diet and stress. Children, young adults, and some women exhibit more movement than other groups. Tooth mobility, which is not a cause of periodontal disease, may contribute to it. Therefore it is assessed along with attachment levels. To test for mobility the practitioner places an instrument handle on the lingual surface of the tooth and gently applies pressure from the fulcrum finger on the facial surface with another instrument and vice versa to rock the tooth in a horizontal motion (e.g., a periodontal probe or mouth mirror). The feeling of movement is most acute at the contact points between two teeth. The classification of mobility should be recorded directly on the dental chart to allow comparative readings at successive appointments (Table 19-6).

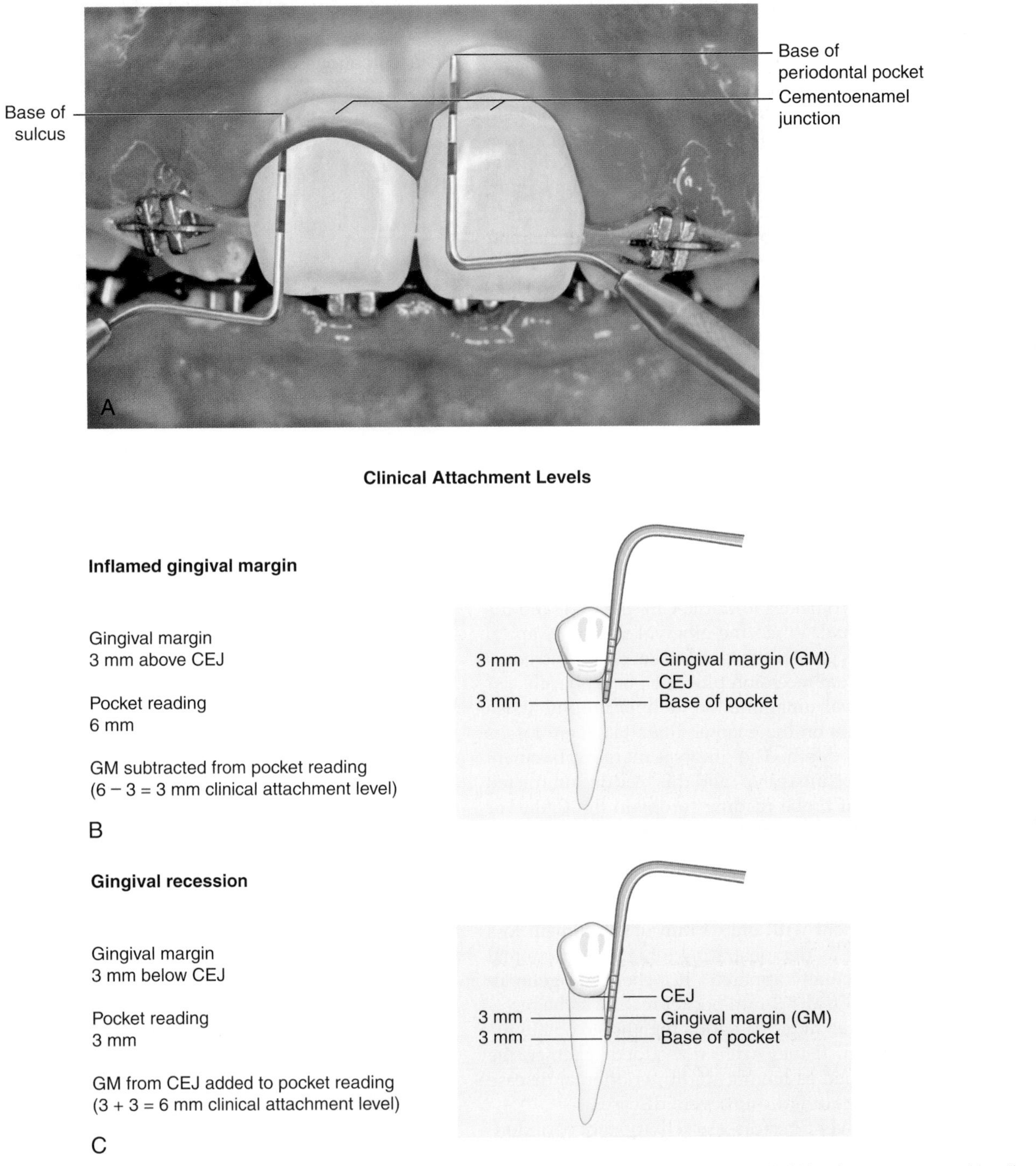

Figure 19-28. Measuring clinical attachment levels. **A,** On the maxillary right central incisor, the inflamed gingival margin hides the cementoenamel junction (CEJ), resulting in a 4-mm pseudopocket (gingival pocket). There is no clinical attachment loss and no bone loss. The base of the sulcus is in a normal relationship to the CEJ and alveolar bone. On the maxillary left central incisor, the gingival margin has receded 2 to 3 mm, exposing the CEJ, and bone loss is evident. There is clinical attachment loss of 6 mm and a 5-mm periodontal pocket. **B,** Gingival margin 3 mm above CEJ. **C,** Gingival margin 3 mm below CEJ (gingival recession). (**A,** Adapted from Newman MG, Takei HH, Klokkevold PR, et al, eds: *Carranza's clinical periodontology,* ed 11, St Louis, 2012, Saunders.)

Fremitus

Fremitus is the vibration or movement of the teeth when in contacting positions from the client's own occlusal forces. To assess fremitus the clinician places his or her index finger along the facial aspects of the cervical one third of each maxillary tooth, and the client is asked to tap the teeth together. Teeth that are displaced are then identified (Table 19-7).

Occlusal Traumatism

Occlusal traumatism is a degenerative, noninflammatory periodontal condition resulting in the destruction of the periodontium because the supporting structures of the teeth cannot withstand the heavy forces. Excessive occlusal force occurs from bruxism, clenching, malocclusion, or iatrogenic factors such as a poorly made dental restoration or appliance.

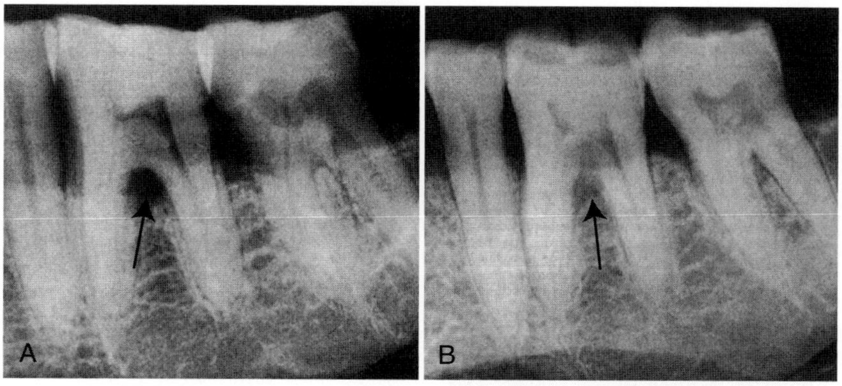

Figure 19-29. Furcation involvement. **A,** Triangular radiolucency in bifurcation area of mandibular first molar indicates furcation involvement. **B,** Same area, different angulation. The triangular radiolucency in the bifurcation of the first molar is obliterated, and involvement of the second bifurcation is apparent. (**A,** From Newman MG, Takei HH, Klokkevold PR, et al, eds: *Carranza's clinical periodontology,* ed 11, St Louis, 2012, Saunders.)

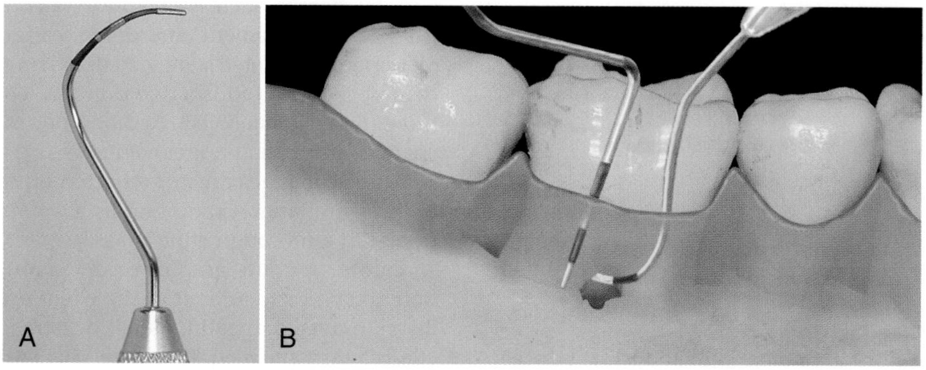

Figure 19-30. **A,** Nabers probe. **B,** Exploring with a periodontal probe *(left)* may not detect furcation involvement. Specially designed instruments (Nabers probe) *(right)* can enter furcation area. (**A,** From Newman MG, Takei HH, Klokkevold PR, et al, eds: *Carranza's clinical periodontology,* ed 11, St Louis, 2012, Saunders.)

TABLE 19-7

Classification of Fremitus

Class	Description
Class I	Mild vibration or movement detected
Class II	Easily palpable vibration but no visible movement
Class III	Movement is clearly visible

BOX 19-7

Signs of Occlusal Trauma

Clinical Signs
- Tooth pain or discomfort on chewing or percussion
- Tooth migration
- Wear facets exceeding expected levels for the client's
- Fremitus
- Chipped enamel
- Tooth mobility
- Root fracture

Radiographic Signs
- Widening of the periodontal ligament space
- Loss of lamina dura
- Radiolucencies at tooth apices in a vital tooth
- Root resorption

Because clinical and radiographic signs and symptoms associated with occlusal traumatism (Box 19-7) often indicate other conditions, pulp vitality testing and evaluation of parafunctional habits is indicated. Figure 19-31 shows widening of the PDL, a primary radiographic sign of occlusal trauma.

Occlusal trauma causing destruction of the supporting structures may be primary or secondary.

- Primary occlusal traumatism is caused by excessive occlusal forces acting on an otherwise normal periodontium.
- Secondary occlusal traumatism is caused by excessive occlusal forces acting on an already diseased periodontium.

Occlusal trauma exacerbates periodontal disease because the supporting structures are weakened already. Elimination of the causative factors of gingivitis and periodontitis comes first, with occlusal therapy a secondary intervention by the dentist.

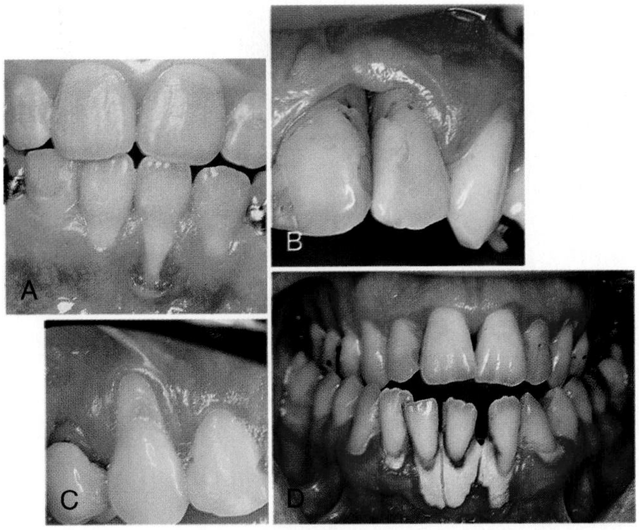

Figure 19-31. Mucogingival defects. **A,** Irregular gingival contours and recession with severe gingival inflammation. **B,** Gingival recession, crater formation, and chronic inflammation with fibrotic tissue. Bottom of the pocket is beyond mucogingival junction. **C,** Recession on maxillary canine with presence of shallow pocket and absence of attached gingiva. **D,** Advanced gingival recession and inflammation caused by heavy plaque and calculus accumulation. (Courtesy Dr. Kenneth Marinak, Adjunct Clinical Instructor, Gene W. Hirschfeld School of Dental Hygiene, Old Dominion University, Norfolk, Virginia.)

Mucogingiva Conditions

Deviations from the normal anatomic relationship between the gingival margin and the MGJ are termed mucogingival conditions (Figure 19-32).[1] Recession, absence or reduction of attached gingiva, and probing depths that reach and extend beyond the MGJ resulting in no attached gingiva are common mucogingival conditions. When pockets extend up to or beyond this point, the area must be monitored closely for tooth loss potential because of reduced periodontium and vascular supply to this defect. Conscientious homecare and precise root debridement are indicated. In the absence of pocket formation, gingival grafts may be performed by the dentist to cover root surfaces with a transplanted piece of gingival tissue from a donor site, such as the palate. In many cases the condition can be maintained nonsurgically.

Frenectomy is a surgical technique to correct a high frenum attachment associated with pocket formation and mucogingival problems. It usually is performed in conjunction with pocket elimination methods.

Inadequate Attached Gingiva

Areas with a limited zone of attached gingiva, termed inadequate attached gingiva (IAG), are noted, shown to the client, and explained during the periodontal assessment. To measure the amount of attached gingiva, a periodontal probe is used to measure the total width of the gingiva from the free gingival margin to the MGJ. Next the periodontal pocket depth is obtained and subtracted from the total width of the gingiva (Figure 19-33). IAG is defined as less than 1 mm of keratinized attached gingiva. Areas with IAG are often sensitive, are difficult to maintain, and can develop into a mucogingival problem because the thin zone of attachment usually reflects a reduced blood supply and a potential for quick loss of supporting bone and connective tissue. Recession and high frenum or muscle attachments may add to the reduction of alveolar mucosa. These chronic conditions must be recorded and monitored. Although good oral hygiene can maintain periodontal health with almost no alveolar gingiva, high frenum attachments or the use of the tooth as a crown and bridge abutment may indicate surgical intervention to widen the zone of attached gingiva (Procedure 19-1 and corresponding Competency Form).

Radiographic Assessment

Clinical Use of Radiographs

Periodontal assessment includes diagnostic radiographs.[10] Good-quality radiographs are indispensable in assessing the amount of alveolar bone present as well as the pattern, location, and extent of alveolar bone loss. Radiographs are also helpful in identifying local causative factors involved in periodontal disease, such as calculus and bone loss (Figure 19-34), furcation involvement, and dental caries (Figure 19-35). Not all periodontal defects are visualized on radiographs because the image produced is a two-dimensional representation of a three-dimensional object. Radiographs indicate alveolar bone changes from past, not current, disease activity. In addition, soft-tissue changes are not reflected on radiographs. Because of these limitations, radiographs always are used in conjunction with a thorough clinical assessment.

Before any radiographic examination, a clinical examination and risk assessment of the client are conducted. Care is taken to consider health, dental, and pharmacologic histories; clinical assessment data; safety concerns; and radiographic history when exposing clients to radiation.

Selection criteria for client radiographic exposures are available from varying professional organizations including the American Dental Association. For most new clients with generalized signs or history of periodontal disease, a complete intraoral radiographic survey is recommended. When disease is localized, selected periapical or bitewing films should be exposed yearly. Dental office radiographic exposure policies that fail to recognize the individual's risk for oral diseases, but rather require annual or biannual radiographs for everyone, border on malpractice.

Selecting Types and Techniques

Periapical and/or vertical bitewing radiographs should be used to evaluate periodontal disease. Vertical bitewing radiographs are recommended over horizontal bitewings because moderate to severe bone loss cannot be adequately imaged on a horizontal bitewing film. When the long dimension of the film packet is positioned vertically instead of horizontally, the area of bone on the radiograph increases by more than 1 cm (Figure 19-36).

Panoramic projections are not recommended for evaluating periodontal disease. Magnification encountered with this type of image minimizes its usefulness in accurately detecting bone changes. The paralleling technique is recommended for periodontal disease assessment over the bisecting angle technique. The paralleling technique produces standardized films that are more anatomically correct, and crestal bone height appears more accurately. The bisecting angle technique can create a foreshortened image, resulting in a film that may show more or less bone than is actually present.

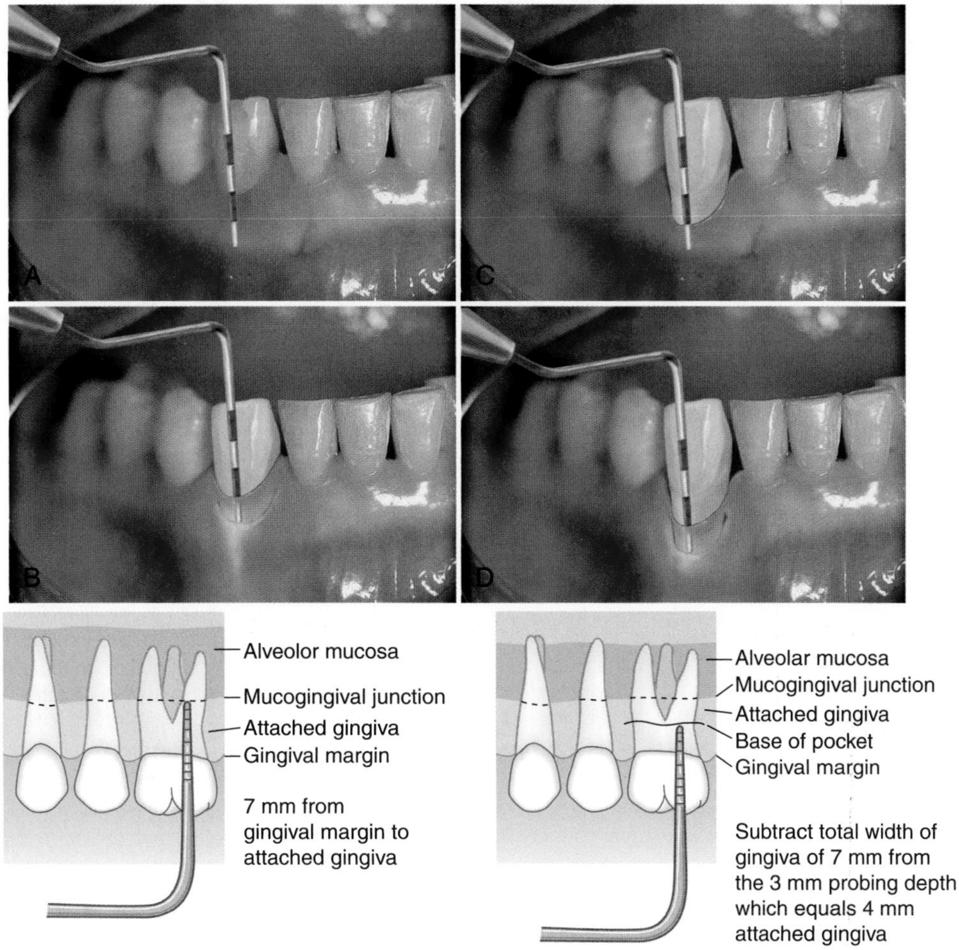

Figure 19-32. Measuring attached gingiva. **A,** Total width of attached gingiva is 6 mm. **B,** Depth of sulcus is 3 mm with no clinical attachment loss. Therefore there is still 3 mm of attached gingiva. **C,** Total width of attached gingiva is 3 mm. **D,** Depth of pocket is 3 mm, and there is 6 mm of clinical attachment loss. Therefore there is no attached gingiva. **E,** Diagram of how attached gingiva is determined.

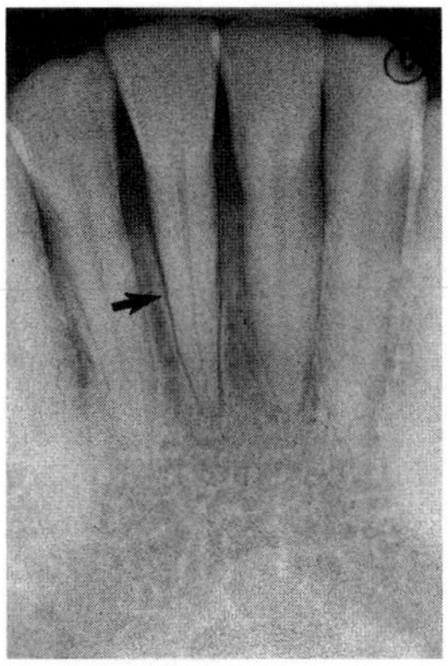

Figure 19-33. Radiograph showing widening of the periodontal ligament associated with occlusal trauma *(arrow).*

Radiographic Interpretation

Radiographically determining changes in the alveolar bone associated with periodontal disease is based on appearance of the crestal lamina dura (Figure 19-37). In health, crestal lamina dura appears radiographically as a continuous, radiopaque line running parallel to an imaginary line drawn between the CEJs of adjacent teeth. In health the difference between the normal alveolar bone crest and the CEJ can range from 0.4 to 2.9 mm. In general, however, a distance greater than 2 mm from CEJ to bone is considered evidence of disease. An early radiographic change associated with periodontal disease is a fuzziness or break in the continuity of the lamina dura at the mesial or distal aspect of the interdental area. This change results from a loss of crestal density. As inflammation spreads, a wedge-shaped widening of the PDL occurs, manifesting as a radiolucent area between the tooth and the crestal bone, known as **triangulation**. The V of the wedge of the triangle points apically. As inflammation spreads deeper into the connective tissue, bone degenerates with a subsequent reduction in bone height.

The pattern of bone loss is described as either horizontal or vertical. The CEJ of adjacent teeth can be used to determine bone loss. If teeth are erupted at varying levels or tilted, the lamina dura crest will be slanted to match the variation in crown level. Normal slanting may be confused with bone loss (Figure 19-38).

- When bone loss is parallel to the CEJ of adjacent teeth, horizontal bone loss is present (Figure 19-39).

Procedure 19-1 Periodontal Charting and Assessment

EQUIPMENT

Personal protective equipment
Periodontal probe
Nabers probe
Mouth mirror
Dental light
Red and blue pencils
Compressed air

STEPS

1. Use direct and indirect lighting, mouth mirror, and compressed air to determine findings.
2. Use proper client and operator body mechanics.
3. Question client about existing conditions.
4. Hold probe with modified pen grasp; establish appropriate fulcrum.
5. Gingival recession: Use periodontal probe to determine location of the gingival margin in relation to the cementoenamel junction (CEJ). Recession of ≥1 mm is recorded; draw gingival margin in blue on chart (see Figure 19-28).
6. Frenal involvement: Determine abnormal muscle pull on gingiva and/or short frenum; draw a right angle in blue pencil with the apex occlusally oriented in area of involvement.
7. Measure periodontal pockets with periodontal probe.
   a. Insert tip to junctional epithelium (JE); maintain tip against tooth structure.
   b. Angle probe slightly on proximal surfaces to reach directly apical to the contact point (see Figures 19-25 and 19-26).
   c. "Walk" tip along JE in 1-mm increments (see Figure 19-22).
   d. Recognize when deposits obstruct probe measurement readings; manipulate probe around calculus deposits (see Figure 19-24).
8. Record proximal, facial, and lingual readings >3 mm (±1 mm) where there is no recession. Where recession is present, record all measurements to reflect clinical attachment level (CAL).
9. Draw clinical attachment level in red throughout dentition.
10. Furcation involvement: Use Nabers probe to determine classification of involvement present (see Table 19-5).
11. Mobility: Use handles of two instruments to rock the tooth; classify amount of movement obtained (see Table 19-6).
12. Evaluate drifting, extrusion, and malalignment.
13. Evaluate areas of food impaction.
14. Evaluate open contacts with dental floss.
15. Assess fremitus, occlusal disharmonies, and wear facets (see Table 19-7 and Figure 19-33).
16. Gingival examination on periodontal chart:
    a. Record gingival disease entity, severity, and location (see Table 19-4).
    b. Use correct dental terminology when describing severity and location (see Table 19-4).
17. Amount of attached gingiva: Subtract the depth of the pocket from the distance from the gingival margin to the mucogingival line (see Figure 19-31); difference is the amount of attached gingiva.
    a. <2 mm should be noted as IAG (inadequately attached gingiva).
    b. <1 mm should be noted as NAG (no attached gingiva) in apical area of the facial aspect of tooth in red pencil.
18. Periodontal examination on periodontal chart:
    a. Record severity of periodontitis.
    b. Record location of periodontitis.
19. Record disease (gingivitis and/or periodontitis).
20. Assign appropriate periodontal classification number according to the American Academy of Periodontology (AAP) Guidelines and record.
21. Use appropriate charting symbols (see Figure 19-43).
22. Correlate radiographic and clinical readings (see Table 19-8).
23. Use appropriate infection control protocols.
24. Record service in client chart under "Services Rendered"—e.g., 9/19/09: periodontal and risk assessment complete. Communicated signs of periodontitis to client. Recommended referral to periodontist.

Adapted from the process evaluation form used at the Gene W. Hirschfeld School of Dental Hygiene, Old Dominion University, Norfolk, Virginia.

- When bone height is oriented diagonally to the CEJ of adjacent teeth, vertical bone loss is present (see Figures 19-34 and 19-35).

Bone loss typically does not occur uniformly throughout the mouth; loss in one area may be more severe than in another. Distribution of bone loss is described as follows:

- Localized destruction—bone loss occurs in a few areas
- Generalized destruction—bone loss is distributed throughout the mouth

Bone loss severity is described as mild, moderate, or severe. Severity is assessed as a percentage loss of the normal amount of bone. To obtain percentage loss, the radiograph and probe are used to measure the total root length (from the CEJ to the root apex). Next, distance from the CEJ to alveolar crest is determined. The percentage of bone loss is a ratio of these two measurements (distance from the CEJ to alveolar crest divided by total root length). For example, a 6-mm distance from the CEJ to the crest of the bone with a 17-mm root length would equal a 25% bone loss (6 mm divided by 17 mm) (Table 19-8).

TABLE 19-8

Relationship Between Periodontal Disease Severity and Radiographic Findings

Disease	Radiographic Evidence
Gingivitis	No bone loss
Slight periodontitis	Slight crestal bone loss
Moderate periodontitis	Approximately 20%-30% bone loss
Severe periodontitis	More than 30% bone loss

Furcation Involvement

Radiographs are used to detect alteration in furcations of multirooted teeth (see Figures 19-34 and 19-35). When bone in a furcation is destroyed, it appears as a radiolucency in the furcal area. Lack of radiolucency in the furcation does not

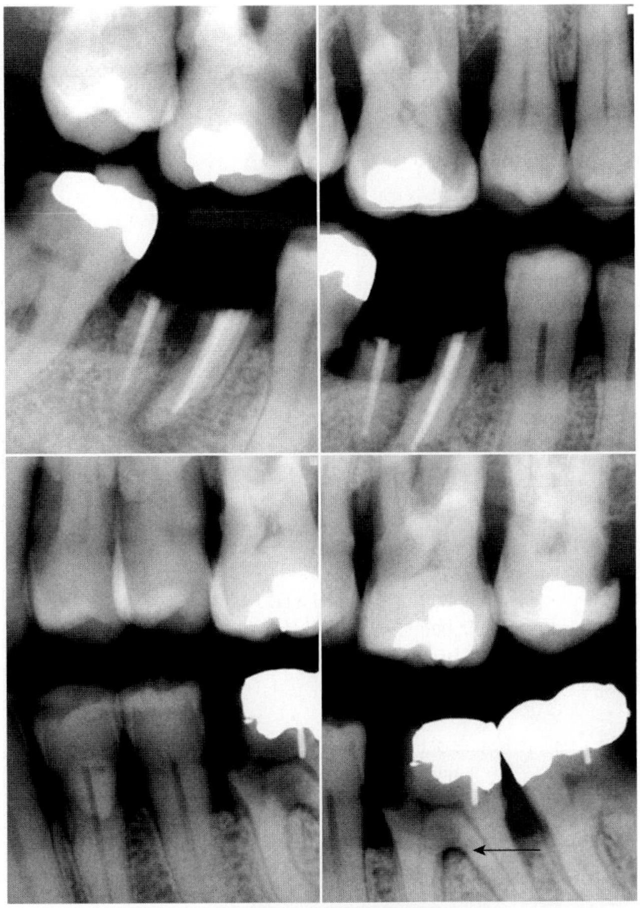

Figure 19-34. Bitewing radiographs showing vertical bone destruction on the mesial of 3 and distal of number 13, generalized calculus on the maxillary teeth, generalized mandibular horizontal bone loss; note the root tips remaining with evidence of endodontics on number 31, through and through furcation involvement of tooth number 19 *(arrow)*.

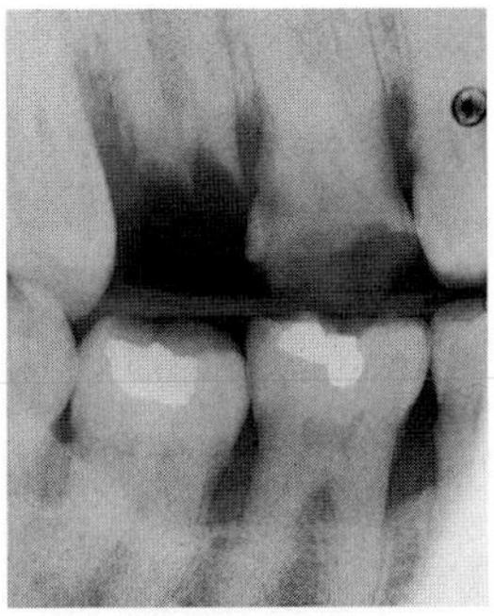

Figure 19-35. Bitewing radiograph showing generalized horizontal bone loss with furcation involvement on tooth 30.

mean that the disease has not spread to the area. Clinical examinations always must be implemented to ensure a true representation of furcation involvement. Exposing radiographs at differing angles also may assist in detecting furcation involvement.

Limitations of Radiographs

Radiographs reveal less severe bone loss than what is actually present, and early bone changes are not visible radiographically. Typically 30% of the bone mineral must be destroyed before it can be seen on a radiograph. Radiographs confirm clinical findings. For example, if the dental hygienist obtains probing depth readings of 2 to 3 mm but observes bone loss on the radiograph, probing depth measurements should be rechecked. In this case, radiographs provide a check of clinical findings for periodontal probing.

Radiographs are a serial record of the client's periodontal status, affording a basis for comparison with new findings, and show the history of disease progression, allowing the dental hygienist to monitor bone levels over time. As part of periodontal risk assessment, absence of bone loss is associated with a lower risk of future periodontal destruction. However, the presence of bone loss on a radiograph does not indicate that the client will experience continued destruction; rather it indicates an increased risk of future bone loss. See Box 19-8 for periodontal conditions observed on radiographs.

> **BOX 19-8**
>
> **Periodontal Conditions Observed on Radiographs**
>
> - Normal anatomy and tooth crown-to-root ratio
> - Confirmation of clinical finding and topography of root surfaces
> - Status of the lamina dura
> - Remaining bone height
> - Changes of periodontal ligament space
> - Local irritants such as calculus and overhanging restorations
> - Pattern or extent of the disease
> - Possible furcation involvement
> - Disease progression or remission by serial radiography

Standardized radiographs of like projections are most helpful in making longitudinal comparisons and providing objective documentation of clinical findings. For example, periapical projections of posterior teeth should not be compared with subsequent bitewing radiographs because an accurate comparison of the bone level cannot be made given two different projection angles. Periodontal probing depths and other clinical findings are subjective assessments, but radiographs present objective data that two or more clinicians can observe at the same time.

Limitations of radiographs in periodontal assessment are as follows:

- Projection factors such as cone-to-film distance, angulation, technique, and film positioning can distort or obscure radiographic images. For example, healthy alveolar bone is located evenly 1 mm apical to the tooth's CEJ, and the alveolar crest should parallel an imaginary line drawn from the CEJ of one tooth to the CEJ of the adjacent tooth. In the radiographic view, this bone position may be distorted by x-ray angulation, erroneously suggesting vertical bone loss.
- Exposure errors such as cone cuts and imbalance of kilovolt peak (kVp) and milliamperage (mA) disguise anatomy and pathosis. Proper exposure uses the widest range of contrast (grays) so that minute changes in bone density and mineralized calculus are shown on the x-ray film. Increased kVp and lower mA produce this broad

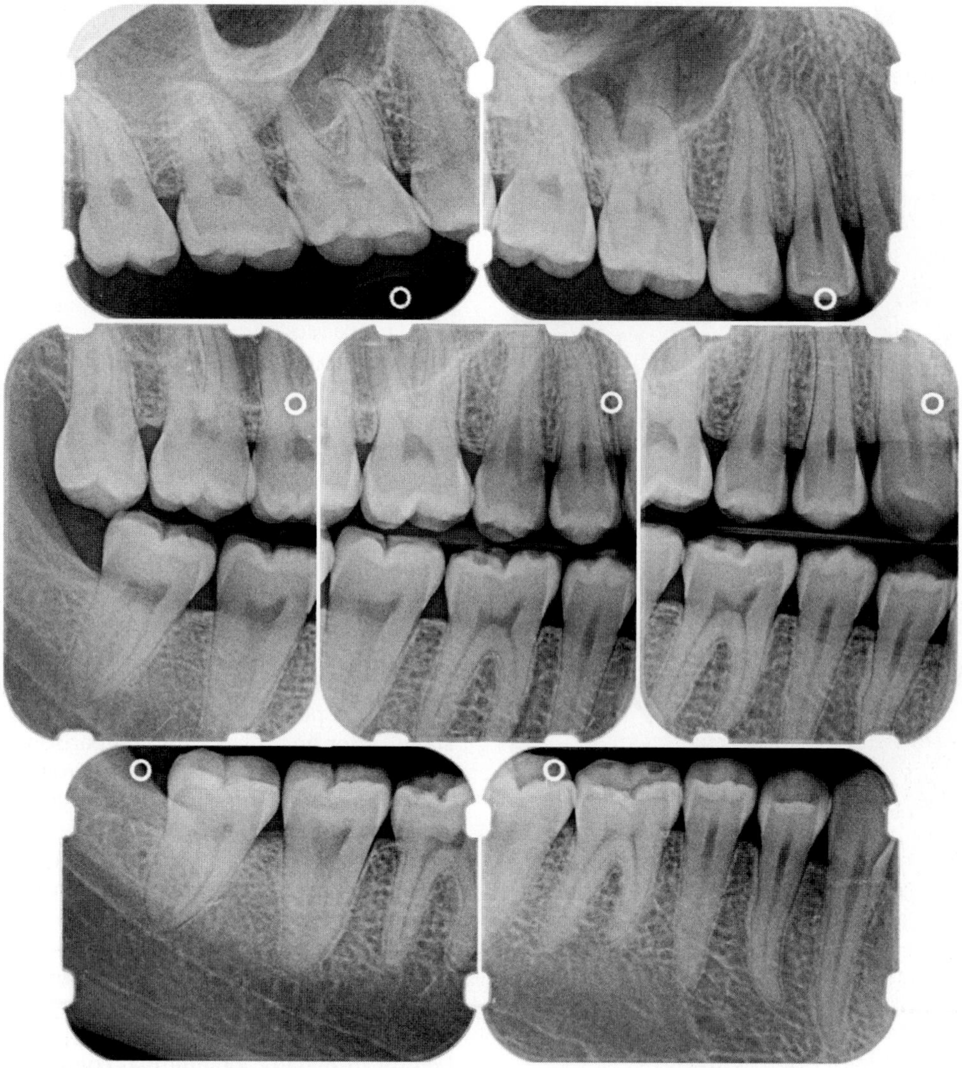

Figure 19-36. Vertical bitewing films can be used to cover a larger area of the alveolar bone. (From Newman MG, Takei HH, Klokkevold PR, et al, eds: *Carranza's clinical periodontology,* ed 11, St Louis, 2012, Saunders.)

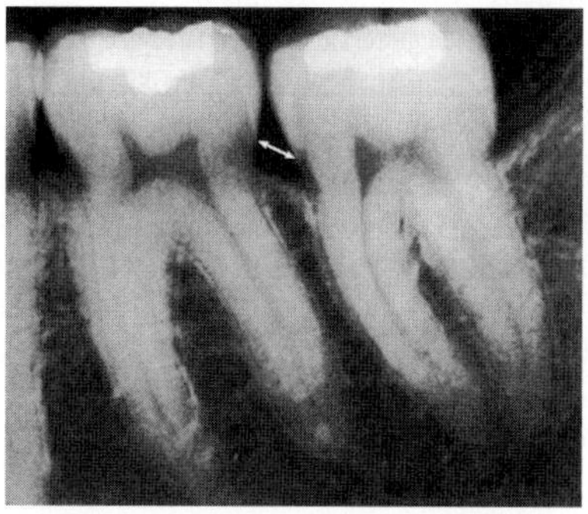

Figure 19-37. Crest of interdental septum normally parallel to a line drawn between the cementoenamel junction of the adjacent teeth *(arrow)*. Note the radiopaque lamina dura around the roots and interdental septa. (From Newman MG, Takei HH, Klokkevold PR, et al, eds: *Carranza's clinical periodontology,* ed 10, St Louis, 2006, Saunders.)

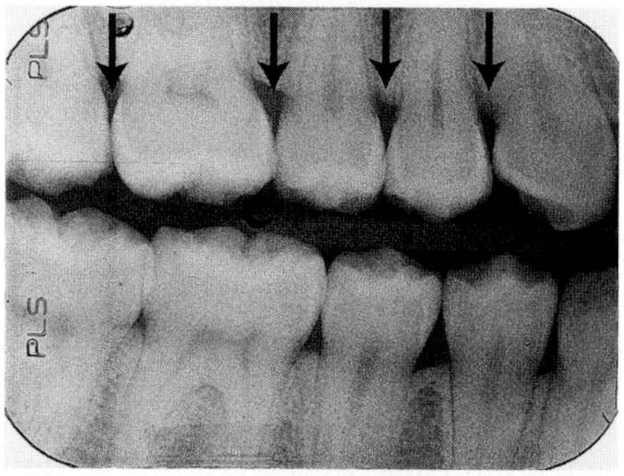

Figure 19-38. Normal bone parallel with bone level and CEJs on teeth 2, 3, 4, and 5; often confused with bone loss.

contrast range and reduce client exposure time, but this combination also lengthens processing time. Shortened processing time decreases contrast and reduces diagnostic information.

- Facial and lingual supporting bone are obscured by the radiodense tooth structure. Therefore facial and lingual bone loss cannot be detected from radiographs.
- Early interdental bone loss is not detectable on radiographs because horizontal alveolar bone loss may not be seen until a significant percentage of the original bone height and density is lost. By the time bone loss is observed radiographically, it is so far advanced that it easily is detected clinically by probing.
- Bony interdental craters, resulting from vertical bone loss, are not well imaged because facial and lingual ridges of the teeth may be superimposed and because the dense facial and lingual walls of bone obscure the crater. Interdental craters therefore are detected only with the periodontal probe.
- Radiographs do not show soft tissues or connective tissue attachment and consequently cannot show soft-tissue changes. Pockets cannot be measured from radiographs except by using radiopaque markers, such as a periodontal probe or silver point placed at the depth of the sulcus before exposure.

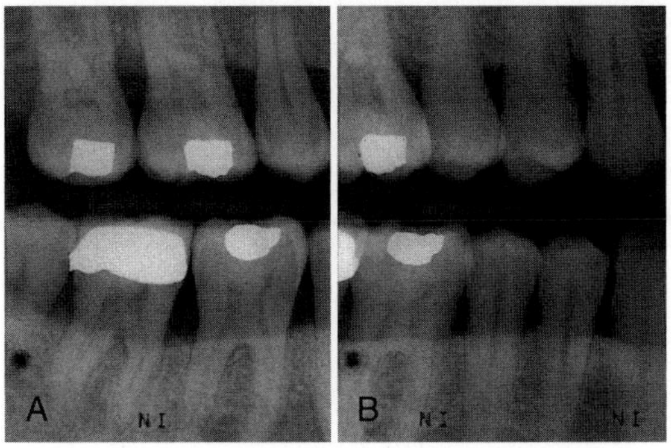

Figure 19-39. Generalized horizontal bone loss.

- Although radiographic images such as a "motheaten" alveolar crest, discontinuous lamina dura, increased trabeculation, and thickened PDL space suggest periodontal abnormality, they are not indicators of periodontitis.
- Normal anatomy can be mistaken for abnormalities on radiographs. Darkened or radiolucent areas, such as the mental and incisive foramina located in apical regions, may masquerade as lesions.
- Although all teeth are radiographically examined for the presence of calculus, radiographs are not the best indicators of calculus because only highly mineralized deposits may be seen as radiopacities.

Digital Radiography

Digital radiography in place of traditional film-based radiography is increasing; many practices are totally digital. The following two types of digital systems are available:

- The first system uses intraoral sensors and a radiation source to display radiographic images on a computer monitor after client exposure (Figure 19-40). A sensor, available in a variety of sizes, is positioned in the client's mouth in place of dental film. Non wireless (Figure 19-41, *A*) and wireless (Figure 19-41, *B*) systems are available. This method requires no chemicals for developing, thus eliminating processing supplies and equipment and trips to the darkroom. Treatment is not interrupted for development of digital radiographic images as with the use of conventional radiographs. Major advantages of digital radiography are reduced client exposure to ionizing radiation by 60% to 80% when compared with E-speed, and film images are displayed on a computer monitor within seconds of a client's exposure. A direct digital imaging system requires a radiation source, typically a conventional dental x-ray unit with the timer modified, an intraoral sensor, and a computer monitor. For infection control the sensor is covered with a protective barrier before

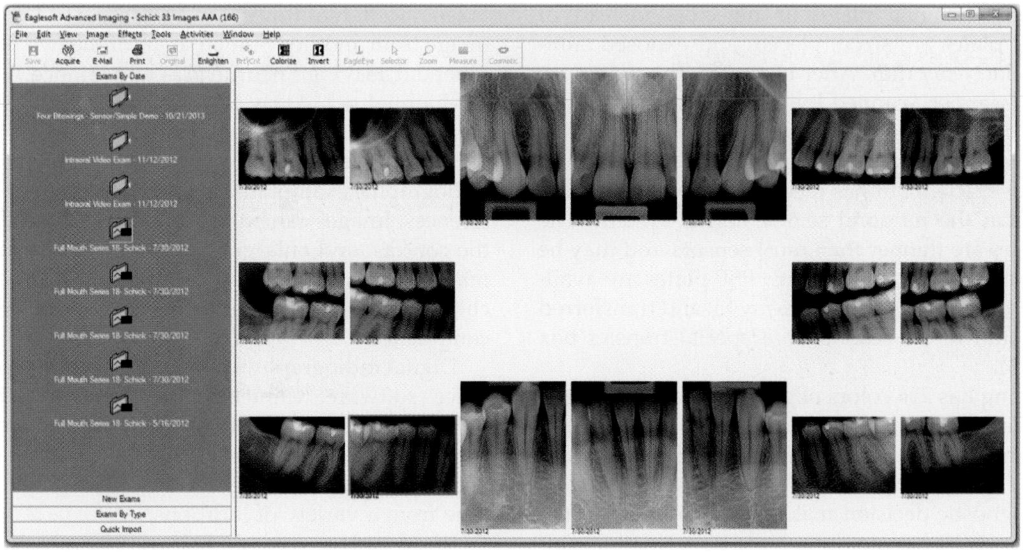

Figure 19-40. Full-mouth series of radiographs displayed on computer monitor using digital technology. (Courtesy Sirona Dental, Inc., Long Island City, New York.)

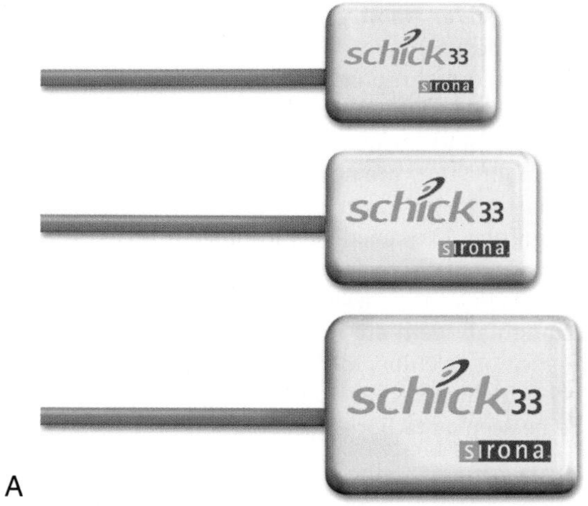

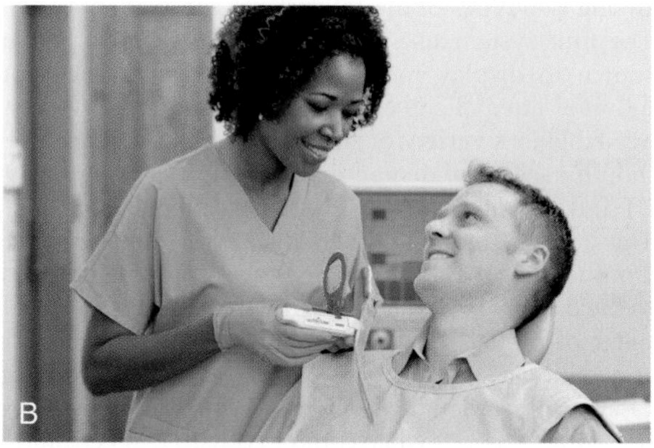

Figure 19-41. A, Digital sensor attachment. **B,** Wireless digital sensor with holder. (Courtesy Sirona Dental, Inc., Long Island City, New York.)

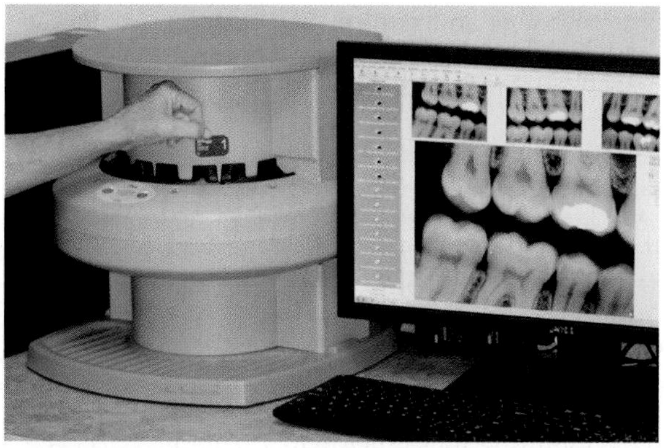

Figure 19-42. Photostimulable phosphor coated (PSP) reusable imaging plates with laser scanner and computer monitor.

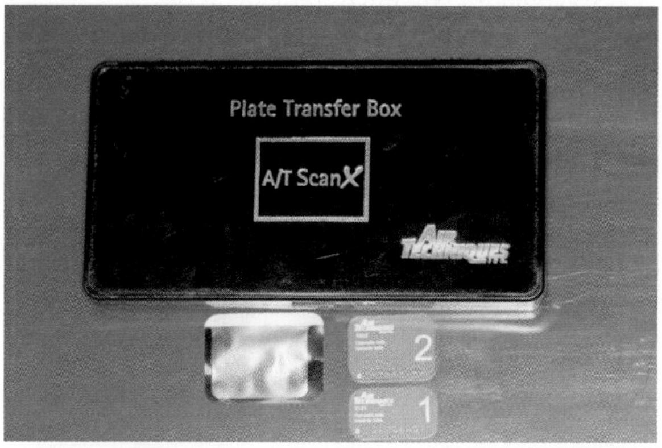

Figure 19-43. PSP size 1 and size 2 plates with transfer box and cover for infection control.

intraoral placement. Sensor-holding devices similar to traditional film-holding devices used for the paralleling technique are recommended (see Figure 19-41, *B*).

- The second system uses photostimulable phosphor coated (PSP) reusable imaging plates as detectors instead of sensors. PSP plates are sized, placed, and exposed similarly to regular x-ray film. After exposure, the plates are placed on a scanner, scanned by a laser beam, and converted into a diagnostic digital radiographic image displayed on the computer screen (Figure 19-42). This method is not as time efficient but has the advantage of being less expensive than the intraoral sensor digital system. The imaging plates are thinner than most sensors and may be more comfortable for some patients. PSP plates are available in a variety of sizes similar to x-ray fill and transferred from the mouth to the scanner in a special transfer box (Figure 19-43).

Digital imaging has 256 colors of gray compared with the 16 to 25 shades of gray found with conventional dental x-ray film. Thus diagnosis is improved with enhanced image contrast. When digital imaging is used as part of periodontal assessment, diagnostic decision making is improved by the excellent images of the lamina dura, bone trabeculation, calculus, furcation involvement, and bone levels produced with minimal distortion (see Box 19-8).

Digital subtraction, another aspect of digital imaging, can improve diagnostic information by comparing a previously stored image with a current image. Subtraction radiography eliminates distracting background information. Radiographs, taken at different times, can be compared by subtracting one image from another. Similar areas of the two films cancel each other out, leaving a neutral gray appearance, whereas changes are highlighted. Areas of bone loss appear darker gray, and areas of bone gain are isolated as lighter gray.

By removing structures that do not exhibit change between radiographic examinations, clinicians easily may identify differences. Images can be manipulated to change and improve the contrast and enlarged for enhanced viewing. This image manipulation affords immediate opportunities to focus on client conditions and improve education, interaction, and compliance.

Digital radiography systems can be integrated with dental office software. Clinicians can archive electronically the dental images and transmit them via modem to insurance companies and specialists. Network-configured workstations allow radiographic images to be accessed by clinicians at any time from a variety of locations.

Disadvantages of digital radiography include startup costs; the bulky sensor, which may result in more client discomfort than with dental x-ray film; and the inability to heat-sterilize the sensor. Controversy surrounds the image quality and image manipulation, which may present legal concerns in lawsuits.

Assessment of Periodontal Disease Activity[10]

Periodontal disease progression is the pathologic process in which connective tissue attachment at the most apical portion of a periodontal pocket is destroyed.[10] Related to attachment loss is the apical migration of the JE and resorption of alveolar bone. Progression of most forms of periodontitis appears to be associated with qualitative changes in the subgingival flora. Currently, no diagnostic tests reliably identify progressing periodontitis lesions other than longitudinal assessments of radiographs and probing attachment levels. Disease activity can be measured by host-modulation tests such as those that test for collagenase associated with connective tissue breakdown. In some circumstances supplemental testing of the GCF and subgingival microflora are performed, although the usefulness of this information in clinical practice has not been validated. More tests designed for this purpose will be marketed in the future; however, only valid data from well-controlled clinical trials justify their use.

Measurement of Attachment Loss

An increase in the distance measured from the CEJ to the base of the sulcus or pocket currently is the best measure for disease progression. Measurement error is related to the fact that the probe's penetration can vary with its thickness, the insertion force, and the degree of tissue inflammation. Also, it is difficult to position the periodontal probe in exactly the same position from one appointment to another. These limitations are minimized by using standardized equipment and techniques.

Clinical Signs of Inflammation

Redness, swelling, BOP, and suppuration have relatively good diagnostic value. Whereas BOP may have some clinical value as an indicator of increased risk of progression when found in conjunction with periodontal pockets, the continuous absence of BOP is a reliable indicator that periodontal health will be maintained.

Supplemental Diagnostic Tests

Salivary Diagnostics

Recent advances in genomic technologies allow for possible saliva based diagnostics.[11] Currently bacterial and genetic tests that use salivary diagnostics are available. More research is needed to determine their practical value in clinical practice. Some salivary diagnostics for periodontal disease are commercially available for the purpose of identifying periodontal disease bacteria. Fragments of bacterial DNA are used in hybridization reactions to "probe" for complementary DNA in subgingival biofilm samples. In-office tests, although available, cannot be used to determine antibiotic sensitivity. Only organisms for which tests are sensitive can be identified.

GCF flow increases with inflammation. The Periotron, a device that measures GCF, has been used in research but has minimal value clinically other than detecting the presence of fluid in the pocket. GCF contains disease markers, such as inflammatory cytokines (PGE_2), enzymes (aspartate aminotransferase and alkaline phosphatase), and tissue breakdown products (proteinases) associated with periodontal disease progression. Tests to identify and quantify these markers in the GCF may prove useful in the future diagnosis of periodontitis owing to their association with active disease. Research is ongoing for valid, cost-effective diagnostic testing devices.

Microbiologic Cultural Analysis

Subgingival plaque is sampled and cultured in the laboratory to determine the presence of specific microorganisms—marker bacteria—associated with the progression of periodontitis (e.g., *Aggregatibacter actinomycetemcomitans* and *P. gingivalis*). The advantage of microbiologic testing is its ability to determine antibiotic susceptibility and resistance; however, this method is time consuming and costly and relies on living anaerobic bacterial samples that must be handled specially to survive transport. Consequently, this test is not used readily in private practice settings.

Immunologic Methods

Antibodies specific for particular bacterial species are applied to plaque samples, and antibody-antigen reactions are detected by a variety of methods (e.g., direct and indirect immunofluorescence, rapid enzyme immunoassay, and latex agglutination tests). Although direct and indirect immunofluorescence is valuable as a research tool, it requires considerable expertise and expense to perform in evaluating plaque.

Periodontal Indices

There are many ways of quantifying periodontal health. If the dental hygienist is to survey the prevalence of periodontal disease in a particular population (epidemiologic research), it is important to use indices used by other researchers so that outcomes can be compared. To assess a single individual's periodontal status for developing a care plan, however, a simple, cost-effective, and easily understood method is warranted.

Indices Used in Client Care

Indices can motivate clients to improve their self-care behaviors and provide an easily understood numeric score for comparison between visits. Once scores are calculated over time, clients can identify changes in their periodontal health. The Gingival Index (GI) and the Plaque Index (PlI) are easy to use in clinical practice (Table 19-9 and see Chapter 17, Table 17-5).

A limitation of indices is that each usually measures only one variable, and thus the GI (Silness and Loe) provides information about the presence and severity of gingival inflammation in a population at a given time, but it provides no information about the cause of the inflammation. In contrast, the PHP (Podshadley) provides information on location and thickness of plaque but does not provide information about inflammation (see Chapter 17, Table 17-5). Moreover, indices that measure the same variable often do not have the same focus. For example, the thickness of plaque is important in the Silness and Loe GI but not in the Turesky modification of the Quigley-Hein Index (see Table 19-9). Also, only a few teeth are evaluated with an index, perhaps missing a problem area in a client's mouth.

TABLE 19-9
Periodontal Indices

Index and Purpose	Procedure for Use	Rating Score and Interpretation
Community Periodontal Index of Treatment Needs (CPITN) (Ainamo, 1982) To assess priorities for periodontal treatment of an individual or a group	For adults (20 years and older), divide the dentition into sextants. Evaluate all teeth except third molars. For children and adolescents (7-19 years of age), divide dentition into sextants but evaluate only first molars in posterior; right central incisor in maxilla; and left central incisor in mandibular anterior. Use WHO periodontal probe (CPITN-E probe) marked at 3.5-, 8.5-, and 11.5-mm intervals and color coding from 3.5-5.5 mm and a ball 0.5 mm in diameter at the working tip. Criteria used: Code 0 = Healthy periodontal tissues Code 1 = Bleeding after gentle probing Code 2 = Supragingival or subgingival calculus or defective margin of filing or crown Code 3 = 4- or 5-mm pocket Code 4 = 6-mm or deeper pathologic pocket Mark one score to represent each sextant. Record only highest code that corresponds with most severe condition. Clients are classified (0, I, II, III) into treatment needs according to the highest coded score recorded during the examination.	Calculations of the number and percentage of individuals with the following can be made: a. No sextant scoring each code b. One or two sextants scoring code 1, 2, 3, or 4 c. Three or four sextants scoring code 1, 2, 3, or 4 d. Five or six sextants scoring code 1, 2, 3, or 4 0 = No need for treatment (code 0) I = Oral hygiene instruction (code 1) II = Oral hygiene instruction plus scaling and root debridement, including elimination of plaque retentive margins of fillings and crowns (codes 2 and 3) III = I + II + complex periodontal therapy that may include surgical intervention and/or deep scaling and root debridement with local anesthesia (code 4)
Gingival Index (GI) (Loe and Silness, 1963) To assess gingival inflammation based on color, consistency, and BOP; based on the assumption that a slight color change is indicative of gingival inflammation	A score of 0-3 is assigned to mesial, distal, buccal, and lingual surfaces of teeth 3, 9, 12, 19, 25, and 28. A blunt instrument, such as a periodontal probe, is used to assess bleeding potential based on the following criteria: 0 = Normal gingival. 1 = Mild inflammation: slight change in color, slight edema. No BOP. 2 = Moderate inflammation: redness, edema, and glazing. BOP. 3 = Severe inflammation: marked redness and edema. Ulceration. Tendency to spontaneous bleeding. Totaling scores around each tooth yields GI score for area; divide by 4, score for tooth is determined. Totaling all scores and dividing by number of teeth examined provides GI score per person. Can be used on selected or all erupted teeth.	0.0 = No gingivitis (excellent) 0.1-1.0 = Mild gingivitis (good) 1.1-2.0 = Moderate gingivitis (fair) 2.1-3.0 = Severe gingivitis (poor)
Periodontal Disease Index (PDI) (Ramfjord, 1967) To measure the extent of periodontal disease (i.e., assesses gingivitis, gingival sulcus depth, calculus, plaque, occlusal and incisal attrition mobility, and lack of contact)	Six teeth are examined: 3, 9, 12, 19, 25, and 28. Criteria used: 0 = Absence of inflammation 1 = Mild to moderate inflammatory gingival changes not extending all around tooth 2 = Mild to moderately severe gingivitis extending all around tooth 3 = Severe gingivitis, characterized by marked redness, tendency to bleed, and ulceration 4 = Gingival crevice in any of four measured areas (mesial, distal, buccal, lingual) extending apically to CEJ but not more than 3 mm 5 = Gingival crevice in any of four measured areas extending apically to CEJ (3-6 mm) 6 = Gingival crevice in any of four measured areas extending apically more than 6 mm from CEJ PDI score is obtained by totaling scores of the teeth and dividing by number of teeth examined.	Group score of 3.5 = Severe gingivitis for epidemiologic purposes. Care must be taken when interpreting the PDI on an individual basis.

TABLE 19-9
Periodontal Indices—cont'd

Index and Purpose	Procedure for Use	Rating Score and Interpretation
Sulcus Bleeding Index (SBI) (Muhlemann and Son, 1971) To assess clinical signs of inflammation; based on the assumption that BOP is the first clinical sign of inflammation	Four gingival units are scored on each tooth: the marginal gingiva, labial and lingual (M units), and the papillary gingiva, mesial and distal (P units). Probe each of the four areas. Hold probe parallel with long axis of the tooth for M units and direct probe toward the col area for P units. Wait 30 seconds after probing and score using the following criteria: 0 = Healthy appearance of P and M, no bleeding on sulcus probing 1 = Apparently healthy P and M showing no change in color and no swelling, but bleeding from sulcus on probing 2 = BOP and change of color caused by inflammation. No swelling or macroscopic edema 3 = BOP and change in color and slight edematous swelling 4 = BOP and change in color and obvious swelling; or BOP and obvious swelling 5 = BOP and spontaneous bleeding and change in color, marked swelling with or without ulceration Scores for the four units are totaled and divided by 4.	Scores may range from 0-5: 0 = Health 5 = Severe gingival inflammation
Eastman Interdental Bleeding Index (Caton and Polson, 1985) To assess interdental gingival bleeding and monitor interproximal gingival health	All interdental gingival areas are examined. 0 = Absence of bleeding when a triangular toothpick is horizontally depressed 2 mm interproximally four times, and checked 15 seconds later 1 = Bleeding after above procedure	Yields a score that reflects the percentage of bleeding sites The higher the percentage of bleeding sites, the more generalized the interdental bleeding

BOP, Bleeding on probing; *CEJ*, cementoenamel junction; *WHO*, World Health Organization.

Indices Used in Research

Periodontal indices are used in epidemiology to quantify the prevalence and incidence of disease and oral debris in specific populations.

- **Prevalence** means the number of cases existing at a specific point in time per specified number of persons. For example, the statement "52% of 1328 college baseball athletes reported using dental floss daily" is a statement of floss use prevalence.
- **Incidence** means the number of new cases or diseases per specified number of persons occurring in a specified period of time, typically 1 year. For example, the statement "50,000 new cases of periodontitis were diagnosed in the United States from 2009 to 2010" is a statement of incidence.
- **Severity** refers to how much destruction is present at one time. For instance, 5 mm CAL is a standard often used to indicate need for periodontal treatment.

Periodontal and oral hygiene indices also are used in research to serve as outcome measures when testing the efficacy of approaches to care, such as when an antimicrobial toothpaste is tested to determine its effectiveness in decreasing gingivitis.

Some periodontal indices used in research are listed in Table 19-9. Usually a subset of teeth described by Ramfjord is used in evaluating groups of people. Based on large-scale studies, Ramfjord determined that measurement of teeth 3, 9, 12, 19, 25, and 28 was representative of the entire dentition. These six teeth, the Ramfjord teeth, are used in many indices. When data are collected on a few representative teeth, the index is called "simplified." Methods of substitution always are calibrated in the simplified index. In some studies, missing teeth are not counted; in others the researcher is required to substitute missing teeth with the next most distal tooth. Other indices require substitution by going mesially or to the contralateral tooth. More than one index often is needed, and examiners must be calibrated before using any oral index in research. With regard to probing depths, examiners are considered calibrated if each one's measurements are within ±1 mm of the others'. Some plaque indices require that disclosing solutions be applied and rinsed away after application, whereas others require no rinsing or no use of a disclosant. Whether in research or practice, the dental hygienist standardizes data-gathering procedures to enable comparable results.

Procedures vary with different indices. The Community Periodontal Index of Treatment Needs (CPITN) is of special interest because it provides information on periodontal status as well as treatment needs. A special periodontal probe with color-coded gradations, designed for this index, has a 0.5-mm ball tip to prevent severing of JE and to allow some tactile sensation as the clinician probes the tooth surface in the pocket. Shallow pockets, represented by reporting a sulcus less than a color-coded gradation from 3.5 to 5.5 mm, indicate that no special treatment is needed. Deeper pockets measuring within the color gradation require therapeutic scaling. The deepest pockets, where the color-coded gradation cannot be seen (more than 5.5 mm), require complex treatment, described as scaling and root debridement under local anesthesia, with or without surgical exposure for access.

Sextants or the full mouth can be assessed by the CPITN, but in epidemiologic studies only 10 teeth are examined and only the worst score per sextant is recorded. This approach may underestimate the number of deep pockets in older adult populations that generally have many areas of attachment loss and may overestimate shallow pockets in younger age groups that have many healthy sulci. Other periodontal indices are shown in Table 19-9; oral hygiene indices can be found in Chapter 17, Table 17-5.

Documentation and Record Keeping

Client information collected throughout care is recorded at each appointment. Documentation allows the hygienist to monitor the client's personal oral hygiene efforts, healing, and ongoing health status. Data collected on periodontal and oral hygiene status facilitate assessment of the client's skin and mucous membrane integrity of the head and neck, a biologically sound and functional dentition, responsibility for oral health, and conceptualization and problem solving.

Legal and insurance regulations require thorough documentation of the client's periodontal and general health status at each visit. Documentation protocols are based on current information related to oral biofilm accumulation and the client's response (e.g., inflammation, attachment levels [probing depth and gingival recession], furcation involvement, tooth mobility, the width of alveolar gingiva, mucogingival problems, and bone loss determined from radiographs). Good records demonstrate the dental hygienist's awareness of the client's periodontal and general health status.

The record must provide a form for baseline documentation of data collected about the client. This form should be organized carefully before the client is seen so that all required data are included and there is one standard location for the information. A well-organized record form eliminates searching for details or critical information, which signals inadequate record keeping to the client or to the healthcare professionals with whom the dental hygienist collaborates. At subsequent client visits, changes in the baseline conditions are further documented; data then are compared with baseline information. Diligent record keeping is key to tracking frequency of care, disease episodes, client response, and outcomes of care. Trend analysis is based on comparing ongoing findings with baseline data. Longitudinal evaluation is critical for providing optimal care, minimizing legal risks, and meeting third-party requirements for periodontal data on client needs and treatment outcomes. Moreover, objective notations of client perceptions, needs, and desires alert other personnel of special considerations and facilitate oral health education and continuity of high-quality, client-focused care.

Documentation

Periodontal status is monitored from appointment to appointment. Findings of inflammation, recession, pocket probe readings, aberrant tissue forms, bleeding, suppuration, minimum attached gingiva, tooth mobility, and furcation involvement are recorded. Initially, complete six-point probing measurements are recorded for each tooth; however, only changes can be recorded at subsequent visits. The practitioner determines improvement or disease progression by comparing assessment parameters and charting data from visit to visit. Comparison of notations facilitates diagnosis, care planning, and long-term monitoring. eFigure 19-44 displays comparisons from two differing dates for the gingival margin *(A)* and attachment levels *(B)*. This visual representation allows the clinician and the client to monitor progress in obtaining periodontal health over time.

The documentation form should list factors that may negatively affect outcomes of care. For example, the dental hygienist notes when gingival inflammation, disease progression, and healing may be affected by modifiable and nonmodifiable risk factors. Client noncompliance, tardiness, cancellations, and missed appointments are recorded to demonstrate that the client may be responsible for a less than satisfactory result (contributory negligence).

Record-Keeping Formats

Recorded findings provide a graphic display of the client's periodontal health status. Other codes, such as for mobility, are added to the form, using the criteria described in Table 19-6, and bleeding often is specified by circling probe readings in red or electronically recorded in red numbers. An electronic periodontal chart recorded using Axium modified for dental hygiene schools is presented in Figure 19-45.

Decision-Making Matrix

Figure 19-46 illustrates a decision-making matrix used in providing dental hygiene care. Decisions are the result of objective clinical and radiographic information collected and recorded during the assessment phase of care, the current research evidence base, and collaboration with the dentist and the client. Objective assessment data can be further evaluated in follow-up assessments.

The health, dental, pharmacologic, and personal history information influences choice of treatment modalities. For example, the host defense mechanisms and presence of systemic disease may compromise care results, as can nutritional status, substance use, medications, oral habits, occlusal trauma, oral appliances, and emotional factors. Orthodontic treatment often entails trauma to gingival tissue and compromises oral hygiene. Client motivation and degree of assumption of responsibility also affect self-care and therapeutic outcomes. Each situation must be assessed to identify the client's perception of his or her needs, the level of dexterity in oral biofilm control, and degree of anatomic access for professional and self-administered maintenance.

The levels of nonsurgical periodontal therapy that the dental hygienist provides are shown in Table 19-10 and explained in detail in Chapter 30. Data collected during periodontal assessment determine the level of care to be recommended to the client. If eliminating inflammation and arresting disease progression can be achieved by therapeutic

PERIODONTAL CHARTING CODE

Tooth Number	Description of Symbols	Tooth Number	Description of Symbols
1	5-mm pocketing with bleeding (fac.)	19	3-mm periodontal pocket on mesial facial (due to gingival enlargement)
2	Class I furcation		
3	2-mm gingival enlargement	20	4-mm pocketing with bleeding (ling.)
4	Gingival margin at CEJ	21	Gingival margin at CEJ
5	Class II mobility	22	2-mm gingival enlargement (fac.)
6	6-mm pocketing with 2-mm of recession equals 8-mm of CAL	23	3-mm probe reading due to gingival enlargement
7	5-mm pocket with 2-mm of gingival hyperplasia equals 3-mm CAL	24	Gingival margin at CEJ
		25	Healthy area on facial
8	2-mm of recession	26	Class III mobility and insufficient attached gingiva
9	Class I mobility		
10	8-mm of recession	27	Healthy area; 2-mm pocketing with no bleeding (ling.)
11	Insufficient attached gingival		
12	4-mm periodontal pocket (fac.)	28	2-mm of recession (fac.)
13	Gingival margin at CEJ	29	5-mm of CAL (mes. fac.)
14	2-mm of recession	30	Class II furcation involvement
15	Class III furcation involvement	31	6-mm periodontal pocket and 6-mm CAL on mes. fac.
16	1-mm of gingival enlargement (fac.)		
17	2-mm of gingival enlargement (ling.)	32	4-mm periodontal pocket (ling.)
18	Class I furcation involvement		

PERIODONTAL CHART

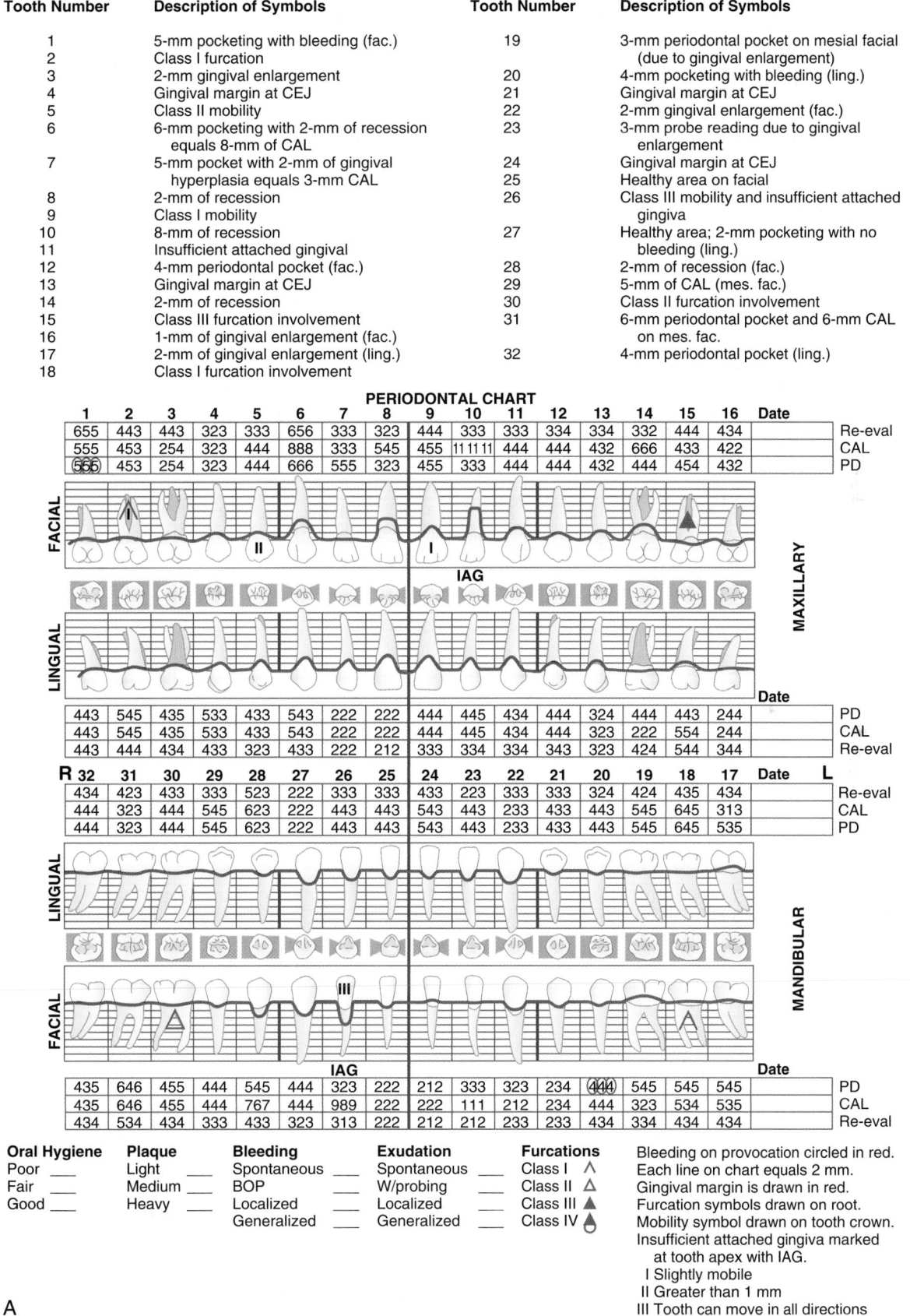

1	2	3	4	5	6	7	8	9	10	11	12	13	14	15	16	Date	
655	443	443	323	333	656	333	323	444	333	333	334	334	332	444	434		Re-eval
555	453	254	323	444	888	333	545	455	11 11 11	444	444	432	666	433	422		CAL
555	453	254	323	444	666	555	323	455	333	444	444	432	444	454	432		PD

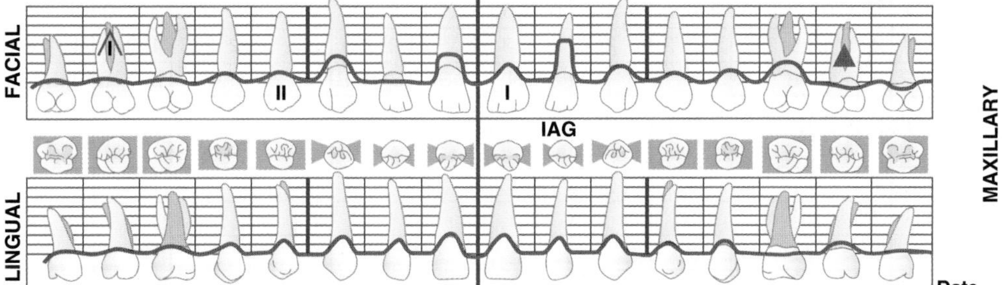

																Date	
443	545	435	533	433	543	222	222	444	445	434	444	324	444	443	244		PD
443	545	435	533	433	543	222	222	444	445	434	444	323	222	554	244		CAL
443	444	434	433	323	433	222	212	333	334	334	343	323	424	544	344		Re-eval

R 32	31	30	29	28	27	26	25	24	23	22	21	20	19	18	17	Date	L
434	423	433	333	523	222	333	333	433	223	333	333	324	424	435	434		Re-eval
444	323	444	545	623	222	443	443	543	443	233	433	443	545	645	313		CAL
444	323	444	545	623	222	443	443	543	443	233	433	443	545	645	535		PD

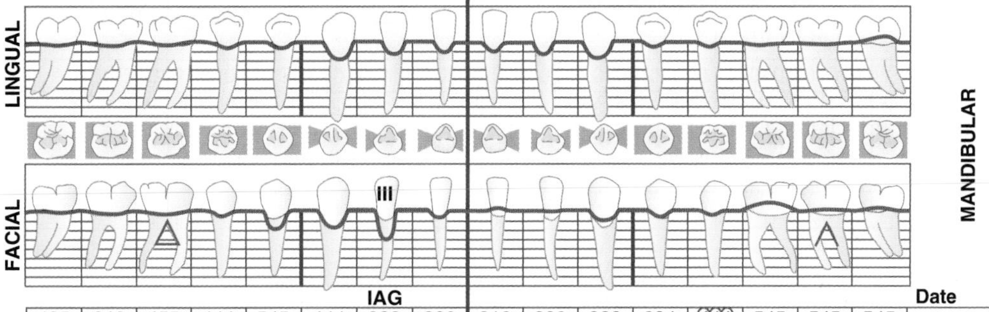

																Date	
435	646	455	444	545	444	323	222	212	333	323	234	444	545	545	545		PD
435	646	455	444	767	444	989	222	222	111	212	234	444	323	534	535		CAL
434	534	434	333	433	323	313	222	212	212	233	233	434	334	434	434		Re-eval

Oral Hygiene
Poor ___
Fair ___
Good ___

Plaque
Light ___
Medium ___
Heavy ___

Bleeding
Spontaneous ___
BOP ___
Localized ___
Generalized ___

Exudation
Spontaneous ___
W/probing ___
Localized ___
Generalized ___

Furcations
Class I Λ
Class II △
Class III ▲
Class IV

Bleeding on provocation circled in red.
Each line on chart equals 2 mm.
Gingival margin is drawn in red.
Furcation symbols drawn on root.
Mobility symbol drawn on tooth crown.
Insufficient attached gingiva marked at tooth apex with IAG.
I Slightly mobile
II Greater than 1 mm
III Tooth can move in all directions

A

Figure 19-45. Periodontal charting. **A,** Printed representation of paper form used for recording.

Continued

	32	31	30	29	28	27	26	25	24	23	22	21	20	19	18	17
Calc																
Attach	4 5 5	7 7 6	3 4 3	3 4 3	2 2 2	3 3 2	2 2 2	2 2 2	2 2 2	3 3 4	6 7 6	3 2 3	3 4 4	4 4 5	4 3 5	5 5 5
Bleed	B B	B B B	B B B				B B	B			B	B	B B	B B B	B	B B B
Pocket	4 5 5	7 7 6	3 4 3	3 4 3	2 2 2	3 3 2	2 2 2	2 2 2	2 2 2	2 2 3	3 2 3	3 2 3	3 4 4	4 4 5	4 3 5	5 5 5
FGM	0 0 0	0 0 0	0 0 0	0 0 0	0 0 0	0 0 0	0 0 0	0 0 0	0 0 0	1 1 1	3 5 3	0 0 0	0 0 0	0 0 0	0 0 0	0 0 0
Lingual	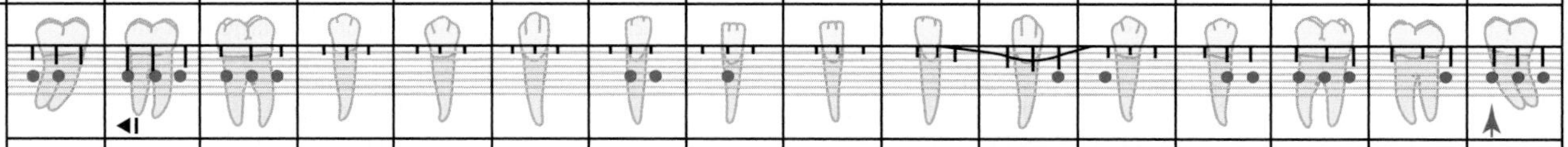															
	32	31	30	29	28	27	26	25	24	23	22	21	20	19	18	17
Facial	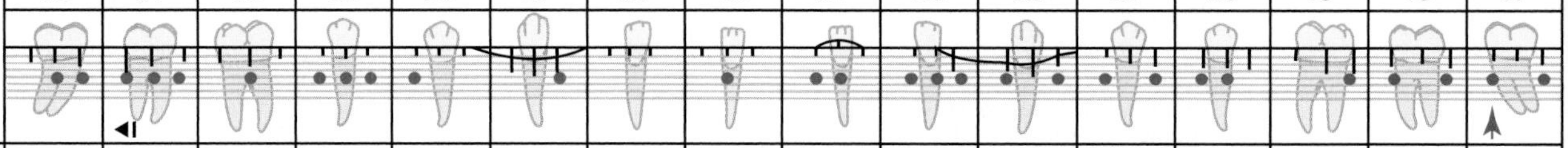															
Calc	1 1 1	1 1							1 1 1	1 1 1	1 1	1 1		1 1	1 1	
IAG						IA					IA					
Furc		2												2		
Mobil																
Attach	4 4 5	7 5 4	4 5 3	2 3 2	2 2 2	7 8 7	2 2 2	2 2 2	2 -1 2	2 2 6	6 8 5	2 4 5	5 5 5	3 7 7	5 4 5	3 3 4
Bleed	B B	B B B	B	B B B	B	B		B	B B	B B B	B B	B B	B B	B	B B	B B
Pocket	4 4 5	6 4 3	3 4 3	2 3 2	2 2 2	4 4 4	2 2 2	2 2 2	2 2 2	2 2 3	2 3 3	2 3 5	5 5 5	3 7 7	5 4 5	3 3 4
FGM	0 0 0	0 0 0	0 0 2	0 1 0	0 0 0	0 0 0	0 1 0	0 0 0	1 2 1	0 0 0	0 0 0	0 0 0	0 0 0	1 -3 2	-2 -2 0	0 0 0

	1	2	3	4	5	6	7	8	9	10	11	12	13	14	15	16
Pocket	4 3 3	5 5 4	5 4 4	4 5 4	5 2 2	2 2 2	2 2 2	2 2 3	2 2 2	2 2 1	2 2 2	2 2 3	4 3 4	4 4 5	5 5 4	6 5 5
Bleed	B	B B B	B	B B B	B			N	B	B B B			B B	B B B	B B	B B
Attach	4 3 3	5 5 4	5 4 6	4 6 4	5 2 2	2 2 2	2 3 2	2 2 3	3 4 3	2 2 1	2 2 2	2 2 3	4 3 4	5 1 7	3 3 4	6 5 5
Mobil																
Furc			1											1		
IAG																
Calc																
Facial	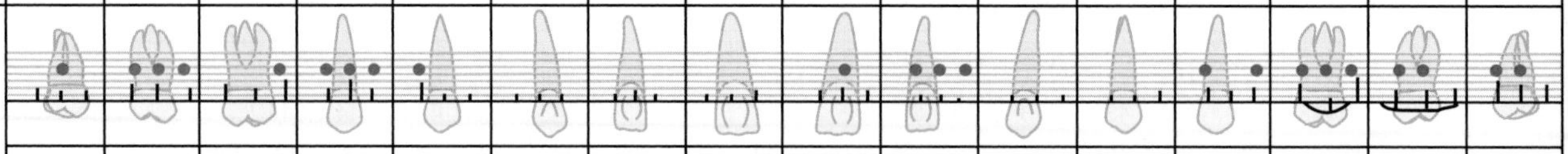															
	1	2	3	4	5	6	7	8	9	10	11	12	13	14	15	16
Lingual	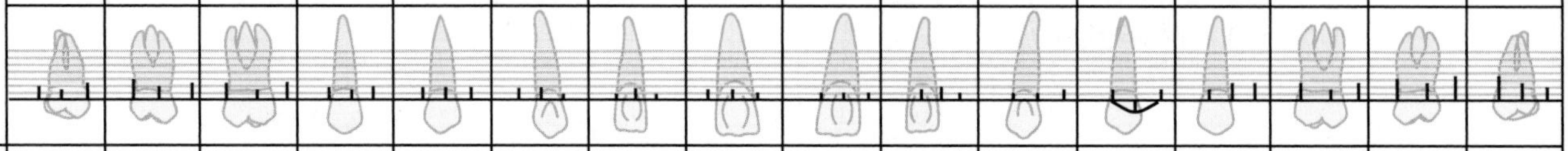															
FGM	0 0 0	0 0 0	1 0 1	0 0 0	0 0 0	0 0 0	0 0 0	0 0 0	0 0 0	1 2 0	0 0 0	0 -3 1	0 1 1	1 1 1	1 1 1	1 1 0
Pocket	4 3 5	6 4 5	4 3 4	4 3 4	4 4 4	3 4 2	2 3 2	3 3 2	2 2 2	2 2 2	2 2 3	3 3 2	3 4 4	4 2 4	5 4 6	6 4 4
Bleed																
Attach	4 3 5	6 4 5	5 3 5	4 3 4	4 4 4	3 4 2	2 3 2	3 3 2	2 2 2	3 4 2	2 2 3	3 0 3	3 5 5	5 3 5	6 5 7	7 5 4
Calc																

B

Figure 19-45, cont'd B, Electronic health record used (Axium).

scaling and root debridement, then no further periodontal treatment is necessary. However, if therapeutic scaling and root debridement fail, then referral for periodontal surgery may be necessary.

CLIENT EDUCATION TIPS

- Explain purpose of the comprehensive periodontal examination and risk factor assessment.
- Show clinical appearance of healthy gingiva, periodontal pocket readings, bleeding on probing, and other signs of disease; use client's radiographs for teaching.
- Enable client to participate in care, self-monitor clinical signs of oral disease, and perform self-examination.
- Explain significance of risk factors so that client understands personal degree of risk for periodontal disease and disease progression and importance of oral self-care and regular professional care.

LEGAL, ETHICAL, AND SAFETY ISSUES

- Comprehensive periodontal assessment including risk assessment is a component of assessment and risk management.

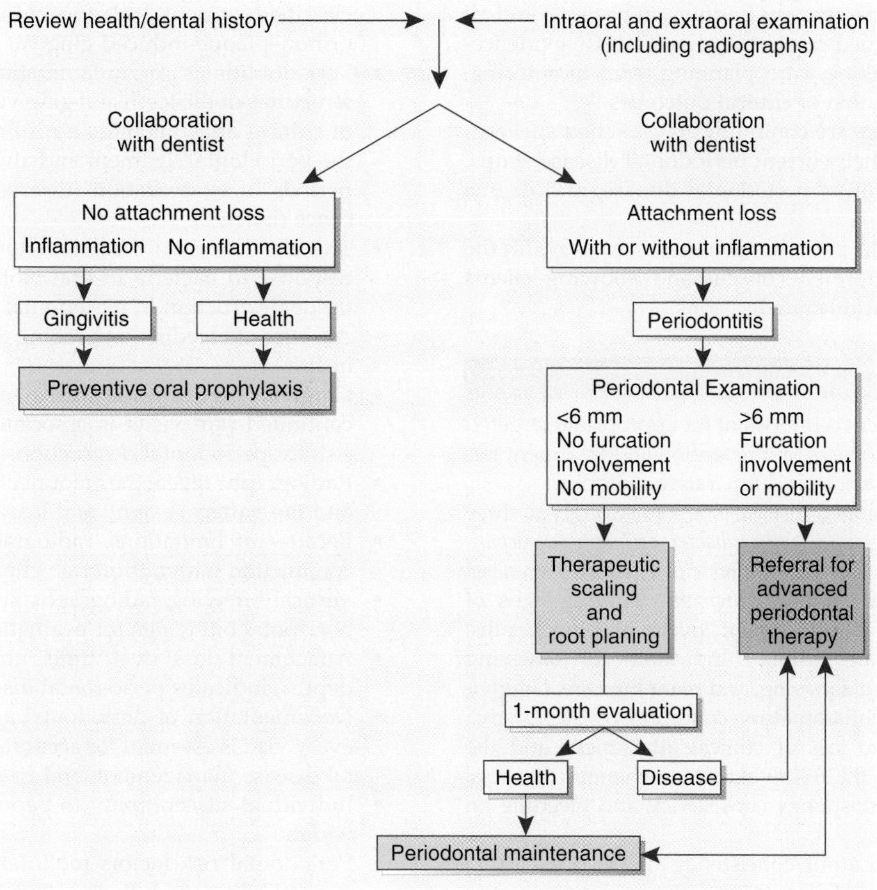

Figure 19-46. Decision tree for periodontal assessment and treatment of the adult.

TABLE 19-10

Professional Mechanical Dental Hygiene Care Modalities

	Preventive	Therapeutic Scaling and Root Debridement	Professional Periodontal Maintenance Care
Objective	To prevent and control gingivitis	To treat periodontitis; to achieve connective tissue reattachment	To maintain attachment level and periodontal health in individuals who have been treated for periodontitis
Continued care interval	3-6 months or as needed	1 month evaluation; repeat as needed	3-4 months or as needed
Dental hygiene action*	Scaling to remove calculus, extrinsic stain, and bacterial plaque to promote a healthy oral environment	Scaling and root debridement to eliminate microorganisms, endotoxins, and calculus to reduce inflammation, promote connective tissue regeneration, and make root surface biologically acceptable to gingival tissues	Closely monitors periodontal status, scaling, and root debridement to prevent return of pathogenic subgingival microflora
Required time	Usually one appointment	Several appointments (up to 8 hours) with use of a local anesthetic	One appointment

*Includes assessment of oral health behaviors and client education.

- Documentation of assessment findings, at baseline and all subsequent continued-care visits, is vital to evidence-based decision making, care planning, care monitoring, referral, and evaluation of clinical outcomes.
- Assessment findings are communicated to clients; clients must understand their current periodontal disease status, potential risk for future periodontal disease, and degree of risk.
- Information from the periodontal assessment provides the basis for client informed consent and allowing clients autonomy is oral healthcare decisions.

KEY CONCEPTS

- Risk factor assessment is important for appropriate targeted care planning that focuses on prevention and treatment targeted specific risk factors and reparative therapies.
- The origin of periodontal disease is linked strongly to three periodontal pathogens: *Aggregatibacter actinomycetemcomitans, Porphyromonas gingivalis, Tannerella forsythia, Treponema denticola,* and *Porphyromonas gingivalis.* Clinical signs of inflammation, clinical attachment levels, probing depths, and radiographs are primary indicators for assessing periodontal health, diagnosing, and planning care. Gingivitis is a reversible inflammatory condition of the gingiva characterized by no loss of clinical attachment and the presence of any of the following tissue changes: redness, edema, enlargement, spongy consistency, and bleeding on probing.
  - Gingival color, contour, consistency, and texture vary in health and disease.
  - Although most forms of gingivitis are plaque induced, host and systemic factors modify the clinical characteristics of the disease. Therefore gingival diseases are classified as dental plaque–induced gingival diseases or non–plaque-induced gingival lesions.
- Periodontitis is an inflammation of the supporting structures of the teeth and gingiva characterized by loss of clinical attachment as a result of the destruction of the periodontal ligament and alveolar bone. It exhibits periods of exacerbation (disease activity) and quiescence (inactivity).
- The host's immunoinflammatory and immunologic response to bacteria in oral biofilm is responsible for tissue destruction in periodontal disease.
- Absence of bleeding on probing is a sign of periodontal health.
- Gingival bleeding occurring at several sequential continued-care visits is associated with an increased risk for periodontal destruction.
- Radiographs reveal the amount of alveolar bone present and the pattern, extent, and loss of bone.
- Because of limitations, radiographs must be used in conjunction with a thorough clinical assessment.
- Vertical bitewing radiographs are recommended over horizontal bitewings for evaluation of periodontitis.
- Attachment loss over time, not periodontal pocket depths, indicates periodontal disease progression.
- Documentation of periodontal assessment findings at every visit is essential for accurate diagnosis, periodontal disease management, and risk management.
- Individual susceptibility to periodontal disease varies widely.
- Periodontal risk factors modulate periodontal disease susceptibility and influence the onset, progression, and severity of the disease.
- The most significant periodontal risk factors are smoking, poor oral hygiene, genetics, and DM.

CRITICAL THINKING EXERCISES

Synopsis of Patient History	**Age:** 64 **Sex:** Male **Height:** 5 feet 6 inches **Weight:** 200	**Vital Signs** **Blood Pressure:** 150/90 mm Hg **Pulse Rate:** 80 bpm **Respiration Rate:** 16 rpm
1. Under care of a physician: Yes ☒ No ■ Condition(s): Hypertension Myocardial infarction 2. Hospitalized within last 5 years: Yes ☒ No ■ Reason(s): Myocardial infarction Colon cancer surgery 3. Has or had the following conditions: Colon cancer Coronary heart disease Asthma 4. Current medications: Plavix Cardizem Albuterol 5. Smokes or uses tobacco products: Yes ☒ No ■		**Health History:** A man reports a heart attack 3 years ago and surgery for a malignant tumor in the colon 2 years ago. He was diagnosed with hypertension 10 years ago and reports his physician has requested he quit smoking but that he just can't stop. **Dental History:** Last visit was 2 years ago when client still had dental insurance. Client reports being told he had periodontitis and needed a "deep scaling." **Social History:** Client reports being highly stressed by mounting medical bills creating financial difficulties for his family. He is a retired school teacher who reports increasing his 30-year smoking habit from about one-half pack of cigarettes a day to a full pack. **Chief Complaint:** "My gums bleed when I brush and I have a bad taste in my mouth."

Supplemental Examination Findings: Client had a full-mouth series of radiographs exposed 2 years ago. Clinical examination reveals pale whitish gingiva in the maxillary anterior and palatal areas and a whitish coat to the gingival margin in the posterior areas, with moderate enlargement. Heavy subgingival calculus is found throughout the mouth with generalized bleeding on probing. Pocket depths have increased from 2 years ago, when the deepest reading was 5 mm.

Periodontal assessment reveals generalized 6-mm pocket depths in all posterior areas, 7-mm pocket depths in the maxillary lingual area, and 4-mm pocket depths in all other areas; and 3-mm recession on teeth 6, 12, and 13 and 6-mm recession on 28.

Use the case information to answer the following questions:

1. List at least five periodontal risk factors for this client. Which risk factors are modifiable, and which are nonmodifiable?
2. Which client medications could cause drug-influenced gingival enlargement? Which could cause xerostomia?
3. What should you teach this client about the effects of smoking on his periodontal health?
4. Based on the periodontal assessment findings, what would be the attachment level on teeth 24 and 26?
5. What is the client's periodontal disease classification?
6. What is the most likely explanation for the increased pocket depths found in the maxillary lingual area?
7. What would be the best type of radiographs to expose for this client?
8. Teach the client about the role of the host response in tissue destruction observed in periodontal disease. Role-play this dialogue with one of your peers.
9. Classify this client's blood pressure reading.
10. The total width of attached gingiva on tooth 6 is 12 mm. Is there mucogingival involvement on this tooth? What is the amount of attached gingiva?
11. Teach the client about the link between periodontitis and coronary heart disease. Role-play this dialogue with one of your peers.
12. What instrument is best for determining if tooth 19 has furcation involvement? Describe a type IV furcation.

REFERENCES

1. American Academy of Periodontology Statement on Risk Assessment. *J Periodontol* 79(2):202, 2008.
2. Kye W, Davison R, Martin J, et al: Current status of periodontal risk assessment. *J Evid Base Dent Prac* 12(Suppl 3):2–11, 2012. DOI: 10.1016/S1532-3382(12)70002-7.
3. Otomo-Corgel J, Pucher J, Rethman M, et al: State of the science: chronic periodontitis and systemic health. *J Evid Base Dent Prac* 12(Suppl 3):20–28, 2012.
4. Buduneli N, Kinane DF: Host derived diagnostic markers related to soft tissue destruction and bone degradation in periodontitis. *J Clin Periodontol* 38(Suppl 11):85–105, 2011.
5. Ad Hoc Committee on Parameters of Care, American Academy of Periodontology: Parameter on comprehensive periodontal examination. *J Periodontol* 71(Suppl 5):847, 2000.
6. American Academy of Periodontology: Comprehensive periodontal therapy: a statement by the American Academy of Periodontology. *J Periodontol* 82(7):943–949, 2011. DOI 10.1902/jop.2011.117001
7. American Academy of Periodontology Research, Science and Therapy Committee: Diagnosis of periodontal diseases. *J Periodontol* 74:1237, 2004.
8. Eke P, Dye B, Wei L, et al: Prevalence of periodontitis in adults in the United States: 2009 and 2010. *J Dent Res* 91(10):914–929, 2012.
9. Armitage G: Development of a classification system for periodontal diseases and conditions. *Ann Periodontol* 4:1, 1999.
10. American Dental Association Council on Scientific Affairs and the U.S. Department of Health and Human Services: Dental radiographic examinations: Recommendations for patient selection and limiting radiation exposure. Available from: www.ada.org/5160.aspx?currentTab=2. Accessed January 2013.
11. Giannobile WV: Salivary diagnostics for periodontal diseases. *JADA* 143(10 Suppl):S6–S11, 2012.

EVOLVE RESOURCES

Please visit http://evolve.elsevier.com/Darby/hygiene for additional practice and study support tools.

CHAPTER 20

Potential Impact of Periodontal Infections on Overall General Health

Gary C. Armitage

COMPETENCIES

1. **Discuss the connection between periodontal infections and overall general health, including why the presence of bleeding upon periodontal probing means that the "door is open" for a wide range of adverse effects on the overall health of the individual.**
2. **Explain the potential connection between periodontal diseases and coronary heart disease (atherosclerosis, myocardial infarction), cerebrovascular disease (stroke), pregnancy complications and adverse outcomes, diabetes mellitus, pulmonary diseases, neurologic diseases, gastrointestinal diseases, and cancer of the stomach and pancreas.**

Background

Emerging evidence implicates periodontal infections as one of several important factors that exert negative effects on overall general health. The potential impact of oral infections on general health has had extensive coverage in the lay press. Accordingly, dental hygienists and other oral healthcare professionals often are asked to explain the potential connection between gum disease and serious medical problems such as atherosclerosis (hardening of the arteries), myocardial infarction (heart attack), cerebrovascular disease (stroke), diabetes mellitus, and adverse pregnancy outcomes. This chapter reviews how periodontal infections may affect overall general or systemic health and provides information needed to answer questions about this important topic.

Box 20-1 lists associations supported by scientific evidence between periodontal infections and adverse systemic outcomes. For most of these associated conditions, the connection begins with the entry of bacteria into the bloodstream from infected periodontal tissues. Bacteria in the bloodstream (bacteremia) is a common occurrence in patients with periodontitis because the epithelial lining of the soft tissue wall of the pocket is ulcerated (i.e., the pocket wall is disrupted and has holes in it) (Figure 20-1). Bacteria infecting periodontal pockets easily enter the bloodstream at these ulcerated sites. "Bleeding gums," a commonly reported symptom of gum disease, often is noticed by the individual after routine daily activities such as eating or toothbrushing. In contrast, healthy gum tissues do not bleed under these normal mechanical stimuli. The presence of bleeding gums strongly suggests sufficient gingival inflammation to cause pocket wall ulcerations that lead to repeated episodes of bacteremia throughout the day. In addition, an important clinical sign of inflammation is the presence of bleeding when the site is examined gently with a periodontal probe (Figure 20-2). Such sites bleed when probed because the epithelial lining of the pocket wall is thin and ulcerated. Therefore the presence of bleeding means that the "door is open" and bacteria from periodontal pockets can enter the bloodstream readily. If bacteremias occur on a chronic basis, the blood-borne bacteria can contribute to a wide range of adverse effects on the overall health of the individual.

Periodontal Diseases and Common Medical Conditions

Coronary Heart Disease (Atherosclerosis)

In coronary heart disease (CHD) the walls of key arteries to the heart (coronary arteries) thicken. Thickening of the arterial walls is not the simple accumulation of fats and lipids. Research clearly indicates that CHD is an inflammatory disease in which the blood vessel walls thicken in response to chronic injury.[1,2] This thickening may become so extensive that the artery becomes completely occluded, thereby blocking the flow of blood to a portion of the heart. When this happens, a myocardial infarction (heart attack) occurs, which may lead to death or disability.

The potential connection of periodontal disease to this process starts with chronic bacteremias. Some blood-borne bacteria attach to, invade, and injure the single layer of endothelial cells that line the circulatory system. Injured endothelial cells trigger inflammation of the blood vessel wall that subsequently leads to the development of an atheroma or intimal thickening of the vessel wall. Well-developed atheromas contain lipids such as cholesterol covered with a fibrous cap surrounding a necrotic core laden with scavenging macrophages. Periodontal bacteria are not the only source of chronic injury to endothelial cells. Other factors can injure endothelial cells and contribute to atheroma formation, including certain viruses, environmental toxins, components of cigarette smoke, hypertension, and diets leading to hyperlipidemia. Therefore CHD is a multifactorial disease in which many risk factors play a role. A common event leading to a heart attack is the disruption of a well-developed atheroma by vascular inflammation induced by one or more of these risk factors. Disruption of the atheroma can lead to the formation of a blood clot that occludes or blocks the vessel (Figure 20-3).

Evidence suggesting that periodontal infections contribute to CHD include the following:

- Epidemiologic studies[3,4]
- Presence of DNA and other components of periodontal pathogens in thrombi[5] and atheromas[6]

BOX 20-1

Potential Associations Between Periodontal Infections and Adverse General Health Outcomes

Heart Diseases
- Infective endocarditis
- Coronary heart disease (atherosclerosis)

Arthritis and Failure of Artificial Joints

Neurologic Diseases
- Nonhemorrhagic (ischemic) stroke
- Brain abscesses
- Alzheimer's disease
- Meningitis

Pregnancy Complications and Outcomes
- Preterm birth
- Low birthweight
- Preeclampsia
- Fetal growth restriction

Diabetes Mellitus

Pulmonary Diseases
- Aspiration and ventilator-associated pneumonias
- Chronic obstructive pulmonary disease

Gastrointestinal Diseases Including Cancer
- Gastric ulcers
- Stomach cancer
- Pancreatic cancer

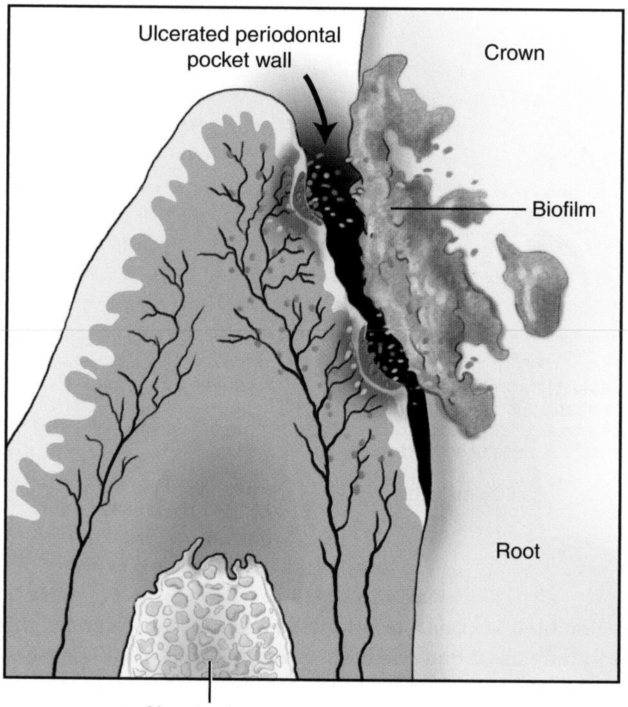

Figure 20-1. Drawing of the interface between the gingival and tooth in a case of periodontal disease. The epithelium of the pocket wall is ulcerated. These ulcerations allow subgingival bacteria in the adjacent periodontal pocket access to the systemic circulation.

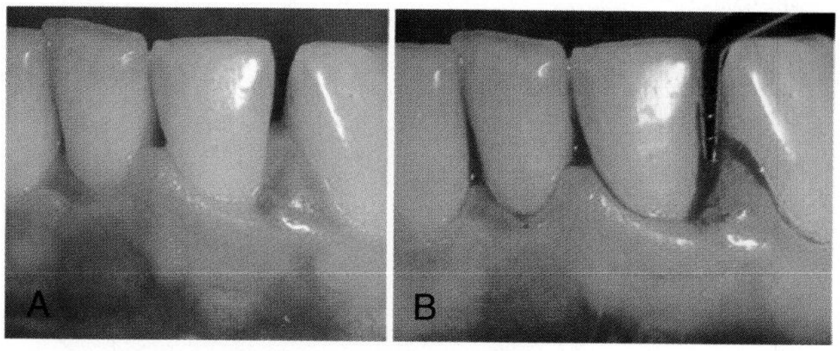

Figure 20-2. **A,** Clinical appearance of a 55-year-old female with chronic periodontitis. Clinical signs of inflammation include redness and swelling (edema) of the gingival papillae. **B,** Bleeding on probing in the same patient shown in **A.**

- Periodontal pathogens, such as *Porphyromonas gingivalis,* are capable of adhering to, invading, and replicating within endothelial cells[7,8]
- Plausible mechanisms by which periodontal pathogens trigger inflammatory reactions that promote the formation and disruption of atheromas[8]
- Preliminary data suggesting that periodontal therapy promotes vascular health[9,10]

Although no conclusive data show an unequivocal cause-and-effect relationship between periodontal infections and cardiovascular disease,[11,12] the association is strong enough that prudent clinicians should include "improvement in overall general health" as one of the possible benefits of treating periodontal disease.

Nonhemorrhagic (Ischemic) Stroke

A stroke is the sudden interruption of the blood supply to part of the brain. There are two general types of strokes: hemorrhagic and nonhemorrhagic. The hemorrhagic type accounts for about 20% of all strokes and occurs when there is bleeding within or around the brain usually resulting from the spontaneous rupture of an artery. The nonhemorrhagic or ischemic type accounts for approximately 80% of all strokes and is caused by a clot or other blockage of one or more of the arteries supplying blood to the brain (e.g., the internal carotid arteries). The process of blocking the artery usually involves the same atherosclerotic changes in blood vessels that lead to coronary heart disease. Indeed, the risk factors for nonhemorrhagic (ischemic) stroke are identical to those for CHD. Atherosclerotic changes in the carotid arteries are associated strongly with the amount of periodontal bone loss.[13] At the present time, however, no intervention data show that treatment of periodontal infections lowers the risk of developing an ischemic stroke. However, a strong circumstantial argument can be made that periodontal therapy may decrease the development of atherosclerotic changes in blood vessels and thereby decrease the risk of having a stroke.

Pregnancy Complications and Outcomes

The presence of infection, particularly in the cervical area of the uterus, increases the risk of delivering a preterm low birth-weight baby (PTLBW). (See Chapter 54.)

Preterm birth is defined as a pregnancy of less than 37 weeks, and low birthweight is less than 5.5 pounds or 2400 grams. One suggested explanation is that endotoxin from

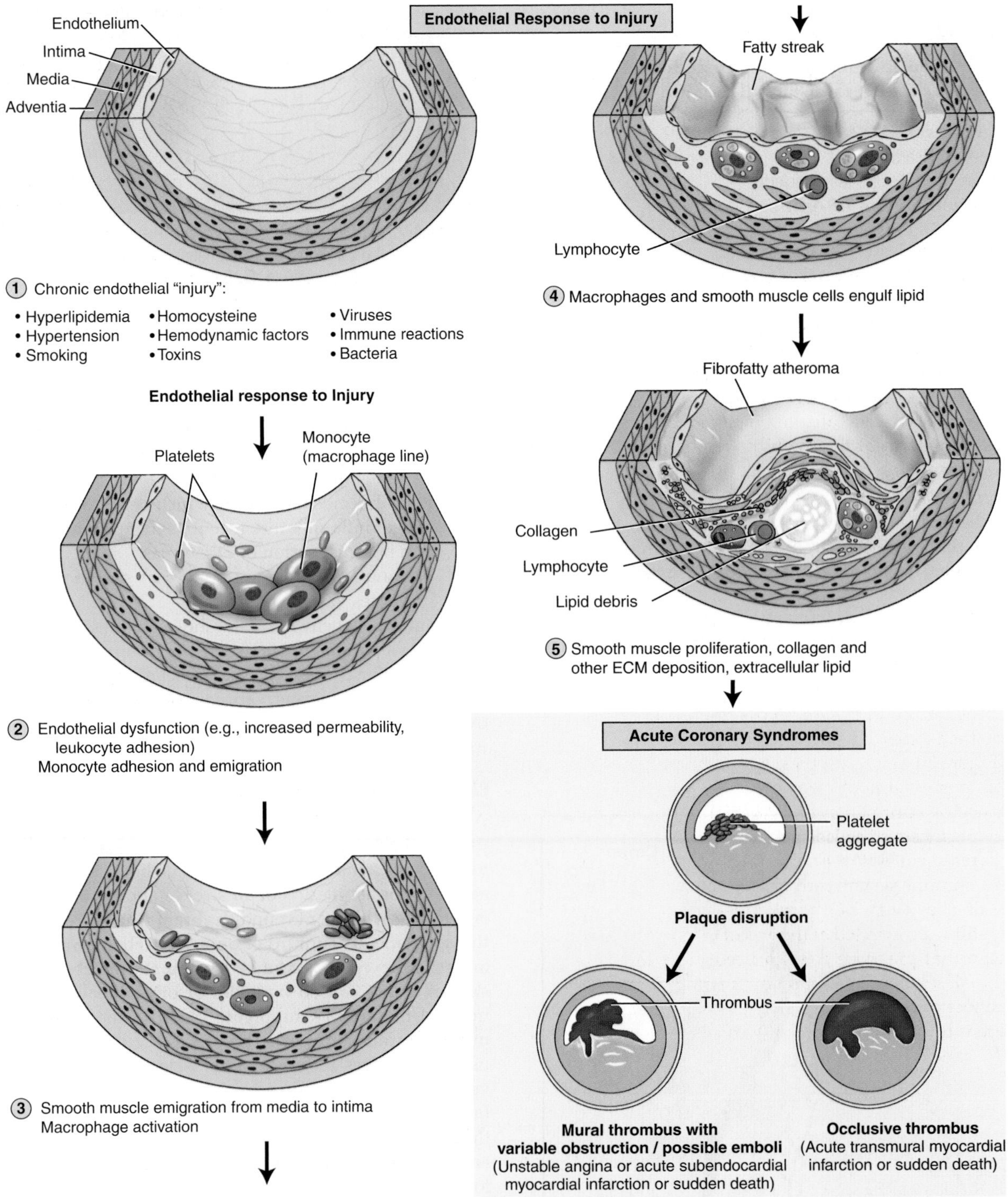

Figure 20-3. Drawing of the development and eventual disruption of an atherosclerotic plaque (atheroma) that can lead to heart attacks and nonhemorrhagic strokes.

gram-negative bacteria enters the circulation at high enough levels to stimulate production of inflammatory mediators, such as prostaglandin E_2 (PGE_2), by the amnion. PGE_2 and other inflammatory mediators are potent inducers of labor.[14] The connection between periodontal infections and adverse pregnancy outcomes is supported by epidemiologic studies.[14,15] The association is even stronger in women whose periodontal disease is progressing or getting worse.[15]

For blood-borne periodontal bacteria to trigger preterm birth they must first reach the amnion and the fetus by crossing the placental barrier. Evidence clearly demonstrates that this does happen because umbilical cord blood from some preterm infants contains antibodies (immunoglobulin M [IgM]) of fetal origin directed against periodontal pathogens such as *Campylobacter rectus* and *Prevotella intermedia*.[16] Intrauterine access of bacteria to the developing baby also appears to retard fetal growth because mothers with moderate to severe periodontitis tend to deliver babies who are small for their gestational age.[17]

A serious complication of pregnancy linked to periodontal infections is preeclampsia.[18] This complication is characterized by hypertension, edema or swelling of the ankles, and proteinuria (protein in the urine). Failure to control these physiologic abnormalities can lead to eclampsia, which may lead to convulsions, coma, and death of the mother.

In spite of a strong relationship between periodontal infections and several adverse pregnancy outcomes, large randomized controlled clinical trials (RCTs) have not shown that routine periodontal therapy decreases the incidence of these outcomes.[19-22] These studies clearly show that the application of standard-of-care periodontal therapy as a public health intervention (i.e., all pregnant individuals with periodontal disease receive oral hygiene instructions + mechanical removal of plaque and calculus) does not alter significantly the rates of preterm birth, low birthweight, or fetal development. However, one positive aspect of these studies was the finding that nonsurgical periodontal therapy during the second trimester is safe.[19-22]

One of the interesting findings from the RCTs dealing with the effects of periodontal therapy on birth outcomes is that standard periodontal therapy is often less effective compared with therapeutic results obtained in nonpregnant individuals.[19,20] For example, data from the Obstetrics and Periodontal Therapy (OPT) study revealed that the treated population experienced a decrease in the percentage of sites with bleeding on probing (BOP) from a pretreatment baseline of 69.6% to a less-than-expected post-treatment value of 45.9% ($P < 0.001$) (Figure 20-4).[19] In a typical nonpregnant population the expected post-treatment percentage of sites with residual BOP should be approximately 10% (Figure 20-5).[23] One of the probable reasons for the less-than-expected response to periodontal treatment is the profound changes that occur in a woman's immune system during pregnancy.[24-26] The high percentage of sites with BOP after treatment means that the patients still were infected at the end of the study. This finding may mean that pregnant women need more intensive periodontal maintenance care than nonpregnant women.

The effect of periodontal therapy on birth outcomes may be different in subpopulations of women who are known to be at high risk of adverse pregnancy outcomes[27] or in those in whom "successful" responses to periodontal therapy are obtained.[28] Periodontal therapy may have positive effects on birth outcomes if the treatment occurs before pregnancy.[29] Future studies are needed to examine these possibilities.

Diabetes Mellitus

Diabetes mellitus (DM) is a group of diseases that results in high levels of glucose in the blood because of either an insufficient supply of insulin or the impaired availability of this pancreatic hormone that regulates carbohydrate metabolism. (See Chapter 44.) In type 1 DM, a severe deficiency of insulin exists usually because of the destruction of the insulin-producing pancreatic beta cells. The disease represents only about 10% to 20% of all cases of DM and occurs with the highest frequency in people of Northern European descent (e.g., those from Sweden and Finland). In type 2 DM, which accounts for 80% to 90% of all cases, there is a chronic hyperglycemia (elevated blood sugar) that causes the exhaustion of pancreatic beta cells. In early stages of the disease there is enough insulin, but it is not able to regulate glucose levels in the peripheral tissues. This condition is known as *insulin resistance*. Obesity is an extremely important environmental risk factor that is linked to the onset of type 2 DM. In many

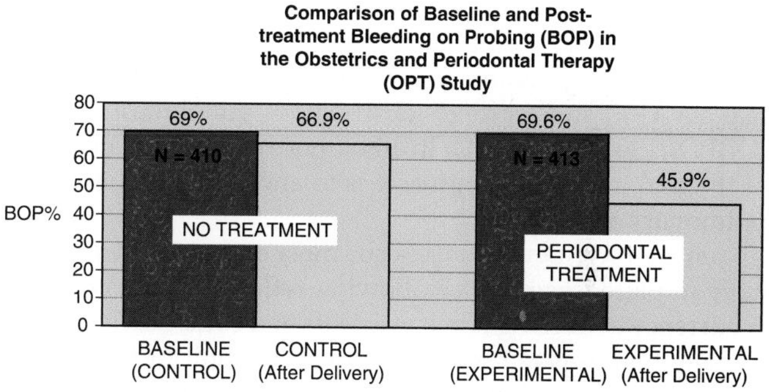

Figure 20-4. Comparison of baseline and post-treatment bleeding on probing (BOP) in the Obstetrics & Periodontal Therapy (OPT) Study.[19] Compared with controls, there is a statistically significant reduction ($P < 0.001$) in the percentage of sites with BOP in the women who received nonsurgical therapy during pregnancy.

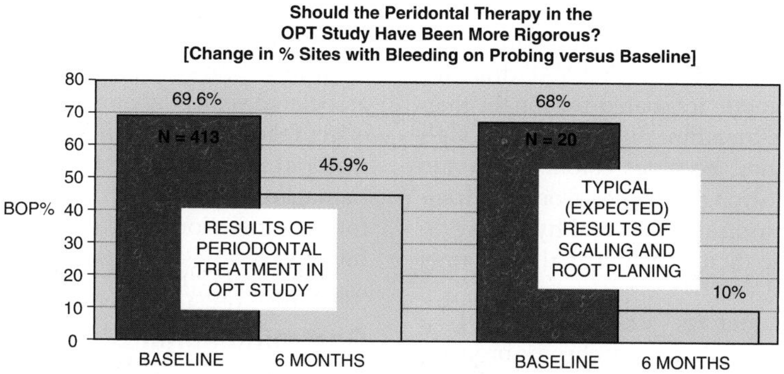

Figure 20-5. Comparison of the percentage reduction in bleeding on probing (BOP) in the treated population in the Obstetrics & Periodontal Therapy (OPT) Study[19] versus what typically would be expected after nonsurgical treatment in a nonpregnant population.[23] The high percentage of sites with residual BOP in the OPT Study (45.9%) versus that expected (10%) in a typical population suggests that pregnant individuals may require more frequent periodontal care than nonpregnant patients.

people with long-standing type 2 DM, supplemental insulin injections are needed because the exhausted pancreatic beta cells eventually die.

People with uncontrolled or poorly controlled DM are more susceptible to infections, including periodontal diseases. This susceptibility to infections is due partly to impaired antibacterial functions of neutrophils and wound healing problems associated with vascular and connective tissue abnormalities. People with diabetes whose disease is under poor metabolic control have more severe periodontitis compared with those who are medically well controlled.[30] Depending on the severity of the DM, the metabolic control of the disease sometimes can be achieved by a carefully planned dietary program. In other people, ingestion of hypoglycemia agents (e.g., tolbutamide [Orinase]) or daily insulin injections are necessary to achieve metabolic control of the disease. Medical regulation of blood sugar levels is hampered by the presence of infections such as untreated periodontitis. Through a number of mechanisms, infections can increase insulin resistance in peripheral tissues and make diabetic control difficult. In some, but not all patients, nonsurgical treatment of periodontitis makes the metabolic control of DM easier.[31] Indeed, physicians sometimes request that oral healthcare professionals treat periodontitis in their DM patients to facilitate metabolic control of the disease.

Pulmonary Diseases

Periodontal infections have been implicated as important in the development of a number of pulmonary diseases, including aspiration pneumonias, ventilator-associated pneumonias (VAP), and chronic obstructive pulmonary disease (COPD). (See Chapter 50.) In all of these conditions, members of the oral microbiota gain access to and infect tissues of the pulmonary tree.

Aspiration pneumonias occur most often in patients who have impaired gag and swallowing reflexes. It is a common occurrence in nursing home residents and sometimes is called nursing home–associated pneumonia.[32] People at the highest risk are those who have dysphagia (difficulty in swallowing) from a stroke, Parkinson's disease, or other neurologic problems (see Chapter 47). The disease develops when oral fluids containing large numbers of microorganisms are aspirated into the bronchial tree and lungs. Some data suggest that periodontal infections alter the local intraoral environment in such a way that the mouth becomes colonized with elevated numbers of respiratory pathogens.[32]

Ventilator-associated pneumonias (VAP) occur most often in patients who need prolonged hospital care in an intensive care unit (ICU). The risk of acquiring VAP dramatically increases in patients who are intubated for longer than 4 or 5 days. In such cases, the breathing tube passes through the mouth and oropharynx and becomes colonized by the microbiota from these sites. Strong evidence from randomized controlled clinical trials indicates that oral hygiene procedures performed on ICU patients by hospital personnel reduce the risk of developing VAP.[32-34]

Chronic obstructive pulmonary disease (COPD), a common respiratory illness characterized by chronic bronchitis and emphysema, is especially prevalent in cigarette smokers. A statistically significant association between COPD and periodontal infections has been demonstrated in a number of epidemiologic studies in which loss of teeth, deep probing depths, and clinical attachment loss were used as surrogate markers for the presence of periodontal disease.[33,35] No studies show that the presence of periodontal infections influences the pathophysiology of COPD. However, a recent pilot study found that periodontal treatment reduced the frequency of occurrence of exacerbations of COPD (i.e., reduced the episodes of difficulty in breathing).[36] Periodontal disease may promote the colonization of the mouth by respiratory pathogens that subsequently lead to chronic bronchitis. It is also possible that there is no causal link between periodontal infections and COPD because smoking is a risk factor shared by the two conditions and the association may be coincidental.

Lung cancer also is linked to periodontal infections. A statistically significant association was demonstrated in a retrospective large national epidemiologic study, even when the data were adjusted for history of smoking. However, problems in accurately measuring smoking history may explain the apparent connection. Perhaps the two conditions have no causal relationship and the association is spurious.[37,38]

Neurologic Diseases

Hematogenous spread of oral infections to the central nervous system (CNS) is a rare occurrence. (See Chapter 47.) CNS infections of oral origin include unusual brain abscesses and extremely rare cases of meningitis. The rarity of these conditions probably is related to the presence of the **blood-brain barrier**, which consists of continuous tight junctions between epithelial cells of the choroid plexus and capillary endothelial cells in the brain. Spread of oral infections to the CNS also can occur locally by a variety of anatomic routes such as the infratemporal fossa through the greater wing of the sphenoid bone near the foramen ovale. Spread of infection by either route is rare and the literature addressing these conditions usually consists of case reports.[39]

Alzheimer's disease (AD) is characterized by a progressive atrophy of the cerebral cortex with a gradual loss of short-term and long-term memory. Characteristic brain lesions contain abnormal proteins that take the form of *senile plaques* with an amyloid core surrounded by dystrophic neurites and *neurofibrillary "tangles"* composed of cytoskeletal intermediate filaments. Components of some microorganisms such as *Chlamydia pneumoniae* and spirochetes (the genus *Treponema*) have been found in brain tissues of persons with AD. In addition, antigens from oral spirochetes have been detected in brain tissues at a higher rate in AD patients (87.5%) compared with non-AD controls (22.2%).[40] Elevated serum antibodies to other oral bacteria also have been demonstrated years before the onset of cognitive impairment associated with Alzheimer's disease.[41] However, a cause-and-effect relationship has not been shown because the microbial material may have been deposited secondarily in previously damaged tissue. Nevertheless, one should not rule out a role for oral infections in AD because a recent long-term epidemiologic study suggests that the development of dementia is associated significantly with tooth loss.[42] (See Chapter 47.)

Gastrointestinal Diseases and Cancer

It is well established that certain gastrointestinal diseases such as chronic gastritis and peptic ulcers can be caused by the overgrowth of *Helicobacter pylori,* a gram-negative microaerophilic, motile, commensal bacterium of the stomach microbiota. (See Chapter 45.) The main suggested connection between these gastrointestinal diseases and oral infections is that the oral cavity can be a reservoir for this opportunistic pathogen.[43,44] In addition, a strong association exists between chronic infection of gastric tissues with *H. pylori* and the development of stomach cancer.[45,46] Data from some epidemiologic studies also suggest an association between periodontal infections, tooth loss, and the development of pancreatic cancer[37,45-48] and even lung cancer.[37] Although a cause-and-effect relationship between periodontal infections and these conditions has not been shown, the epidemiologic associations are a good justification for more research in this area.

CLIENT EDUCATION TIPS

Explain the potential connection between gum disease and
- Atherosclerosis (hardening of the arteries)
- Myocardial infarctions (heart attacks)
- *Cerebrovascular disease (stroke)*
- Diabetes mellitus
- Pulmonary diseases
- Adverse pregnancy outcomes

LEGAL, ETHICAL, AND SAFETY ISSUES

- Periodontal assessment findings must be communicated to clients so that they have an understanding of their current periodontal disease status and potential risk for serious medical problems.
- All assessment findings must be documented, evaluated, and monitored.
- Referrals are made to other health professionals when care required is beyond the scope of dental hygiene practice and skills of the practitioner.

KEY CONCEPTS

- Strong evidence supports that periodontal disease is one of several important risk factors for the development of CHD (atherosclerosis) and nonhemorrhagic (ischemic) stroke. Because these diseases are chronic and multifactorial, it is difficult to prove a cause-and-effect relationship between the development of these diseases and any single risk factor. In addition, it is unlikely that periodontal therapy alone prevents heart attacks and strokes. However, periodontal therapy should be part of a multidisciplinary program of risk reduction that may include smoking cessation, dietary counseling, weight reduction, and treatment of other chronic infections (e.g., chronic bronchitis caused by *C. pneumoniae* and peptic ulcers caused by *H. pylori*). (See Chapters 45 and 50.)
- Convincing data suggest that the presence of moderate to severe periodontitis during pregnancy adversely affects birth outcomes, increases the risk of preeclampsia, and has negative effects on fetal development. Because nonsurgical periodontal therapy during pregnancy has been shown to be safe, it is highly recommended that treatment of periodontal infections should be part of prenatal care programs.
- A two-way relationship exists between periodontitis and diabetes mellitus (DM). Persons with poorly controlled DM are at an elevated risk for developing periodontitis because of a number of DM-associated factors that increase susceptibility to infections. The presence of untreated infections, including periodontitis, makes the metabolic control of DM more difficult. Treatment of periodontitis in persons with DM positively affects oral and systemic health.
- Data from several randomized controlled clinical trials clearly demonstrate that oral hygiene procedures performed by nurses on hospitalized patients in ICUs significantly reduce the risk of developing VAP and certain other nosocomial infections.
- Preliminary data suggest that periodontal diseases have adverse effects on systemic health. The old belief that periodontal infections only have local effects on tissues supporting the teeth is clearly false.

REFERENCES

1. Zakynthinos E, Pappa N: Inflammatory biomarkers in coronary artery disease. *J Cardiol* 53:317, 2009.
2. Choi EY, Yan RT, Fernandes VR, et al: High-sensitivity C-reactive protein as an independent predictor of progressive myocardial functional deterioration: the multiethnic study of atherosclerosis. *Am Heart J* 164:251, 2012.
3. Buhlin K, Mäntylä P, Paju S, et al: Periodontitis is associated with angiographically verified coronary artery disease. *J Clin Periodontol* 38:1007, 2011.
4. Kebschull M, Demmer RT, Papapanou PN: "Gum bug, leave my heart alone"—epidemiologic and mechanistic evidence linking periodontal infections and atherosclerosis. *J Dent Res* 89:879, 2010.
5. Ohki T, Itabashi Y, Kohno T, et al: Detection of periodontal bacteria in thrombi of patients with acute myocardial infarction by polymerase chain reaction. *Am Heart J* 163:164, 2012.
6. Figuero E, Sánchez-Beltrán M, Cuesta-Frechoso S, et al: Detection of periodontal bacteria in atheromatous plaque by nested polymerase chain reaction. *J Periodontol* 82:1469, 2011.
7. Komatsu T, Nagano K, Sugiura S, et al: E-selectin mediates *Porphyromonas gingivalis* adherence to human endothelial cells. *Infect Immun* 80:2570, 2012.
8. Wada K, Kamisaki Y: Molecular dissection of *Porphyromonas gingivalis*-related arteriosclerosis: a novel mechanism of vascular disease. *Periodontol 2000* 54:222, 2010.
9. Tonetti MS, D'Aiuto F, Nibali L, et al: Treatment of periodontitis and endothelial function. *N Engl J Med* 356:911, 2007.
10. Higashi Y, Goto C, Hidaka T, et al: Oral infection-inflammatory pathway, periodontitis, is a risk factor for endothelial dysfunction in patients with coronary artery disease. *Atherosclerosis* 206:604, 2009.
11. Lockart PB, Bolger AF, Papapanou PN, et al: American Heart Association Rheumatic Fever, Endocarditis, and Kawasaki Disease Committee of the Council on Cardiovascular Disease in the Young, Council on Epidemiology and Prevention, Council on Peripheral Vascular Disease, and Council on Clinical Cardiology. *Circulation* 125:2520, 2012.
12. Papapanou PN, Trevisan M: Periodontitis and atherosclerotic vascular disease: what we know and why it is important. *J Am Dent Assoc* 143:826, 2012.
13. Engebretson SP, Lamster IB, Elkind MSV, et al: Radiographic measures of chronic periodontitis and carotid artery plaque. *Stroke* 36:561, 2005.
14. Michalowicz BS, Durand R: Maternal periodontal disease and spontaneous preterm birth. *Periodontol 2000* 44:103, 2007.
15. Offenbacher S, Boggess KA, Murtha AP, et al: Progressive periodontal disease and risk of very preterm delivery. *Obstet Gynecol* 107:29, 2006.

16. Boggess KA, Moss K, Madianos P, et al: Fetal immune response to oral pathogens and risk of preterm birth. *Am J Obstet Gynecol* 193:1121, 2005.
17. Boggess KA, Beck JD, Murtha AP, et al: Maternal periodontal disease in early pregnancy and risk for a small-for-gestational-age infant. *Am J Obstet Gynecol* 194:1316, 2006.
18. Boggess KA, Lieff S, Murtha AP, et al: Maternal periodontal disease is associated with an increased risk of preeclampsia. *Obstet Gynecol* 101:227, 2003.
19. Michalowicz BS, Hodges JS, DiAngelis AJ, et al, for the OPT Study: Treatment of periodontal disease and the risk of preterm birth. *N Engl J Med* 355:1885, 2006.
20. Offenbacher S, Beck JD, Jared HL, et al, for the Maternal Oral Therapy to Reduce Obstetric Risk (MOTOR) investigators: Effects of periodontal therapy on rate of preterm delivery. A randomized controlled trial. *Obstet Gynecol* 114:551, 2009.
21. Newnham JP, Newnham IA, Ball CM, et al: Treatment of periodontal disease during pregnancy. A randomized controlled trial. *Obstet Gynecol* 114:1239, 2009.
22. Macones GA, Parry S, Nelson DB, et al: Treatment of localized periodontal disease in pregnancy does not reduce the occurrence of preterm birth: results from the Periodontal Infections and Prematurity Study (PIPS). *Am J Obstet Gynecol* 202:147, 2010.
23. Apatzidou DA, Kinane DF: Quadrant root planing versus same-day full-mouth root planing. I. Clinical findings. *J Clin Periodontol* 31:132, 2004.
24. Poole JA, Claman HN: Immunology of pregnancy. Implications for the mother. *Clin Rev Allergy Immunol* 26:161, 2004.
25. Tsukimori K, Fukushima K, Komatsu H, et al: Neutrophil function during pregnancy: is nitric oxide production correlated with superoxide production? *Am J Reprod Immunol* 55:99, 2006.
26. Armitage GC: Bidirectional relationship between pregnancy and periodontal disease. *Periodontol 2000* 61:160, 2013.
27. Kim AJ, Lo AJ, Pullin DA, et al: Scaling and root planing treatment for periodontitis to reduce preterm birth and low birth weight: a systematic review and meta-analysis of randomized controlled trials. *J Periodontol* 83:1508, 2012. DOI: 10.1902/jop.2012.110636
28. Jeffcoat M, Parry S, Sammel M, et al: Periodontal infection and preterm birth: successful periodontal therapy reduces the risk of preterm birth. *BJOG* 118:250, 2011.
29. Goldenberg RL, Culhane JF: Preterm birth and periodontal disease. *N Engl J Med* 355:1925, 2006.
30. Mealey BL, Ocampo GL: Diabetes mellitus and periodontal disease. *Periodontol 2000* 44:127, 2007.
31. Faria-Almeida R, Navarro A, Bascones A: Clinical and metabolic changes after conventional treatment of type 2 diabetic patients with chronic periodontitis. *J Periodontol* 77:591, 2006.
32. Raghavendran K, Mylotte JM, Scannapieco FA: Nursing home-associated pneumonia, hospital-acquired pneumonia and ventilator-associated pneumonia: the contribution of dental biofilms and periodontal inflammation. *Periodontol 2000* 44:164, 2007.
33. Scannapieco FA, Bush RB, Paju S: Associations between periodontal disease and risk for nosocomial bacterial pneumonia and chronic obstructive pulmonary disease. A systematic review. *Ann Periodontol* 8:54, 2003.
34. Mori H, Hirasawa H, Oda S, et al: Oral care reduces incidence of ventilator-associated pneumonia in ICU populations. *Intens Care Med* 32:230, 2006.
35. Liu Z, Zhang W, Zhang J, et al: Oral hygiene, periodontal health and chronic obstructive pulmonary disease exacerbations. *J Clin Periodontol* 39:45, 2012.
36. Kucukcoskun M, Baser U, Oztekin G, et al: Initial periodontal treatment for prevention of chronic obstructive pulmonary disease exacerbations. *J Periodontol* 84:863, 2013. DOI: 10.1902/jop.2012.120399.
37. Hujoel PP, Drangsholt M, Spiekerman C, et al: An exploration of the periodontitis-cancer association. *Ann Epidemiol* 13:312, 2003.
38. Fitzpatrick SG, Katz J: The association between periodontal disease and cancer: a review of the literature. *J Dent* 38:83, 2010.
39. Corson MA, Postlethwaite KP, Seymour RA: Are dental infections a cause of brain abscess? Case report and review of the literature. *Oral Diseases* 7:61, 2001.
40. Riviere GR, Riviere KH, Smith KS: Molecular and immunological evidence of oral *Treponema* in the human brain and their association with Alzheimer's disease. *Oral Microbiol Immunol* 17:113, 2002.
41. Sparks Stein P, Steffen MJ, et al: Serum antibodies to periodontal pathogens are a risk factor for Alzheimer's disease. *Alzheimers Dement* 8:196, 2012.
42. Stein PS, Desrosiers M, Donegan SJ, et al: Tooth loss, dementia and neuropathology in the Nun Study. *J Am Dent Assoc* 139:1314, 2007.
43. Dye B, Kruszon-Moran D, McQuillan G: The relationship between periodontal disease attributes and *Helicobacter pylori* infection among adults in the United States. *Am J Public Health* 92:1809, 2002.
44. Umeda M, Kobayashi H, Takeuchi Y, et al: High prevalence of *Helicobacter pylori* detected by PCR in the oral cavities of periodontis patients. *J Periodontol* 74:129, 2003.
45. Stolzenberg-Solomon RZ, Blaser MJ, Limburg PJ, et al: *Helicobacter pylori* seropositivity as a risk factor for pancreatic cancer. *J Natl Cancer Inst* 93:937, 2001.
46. Stolzenberg-Solomon RZ, Dodd KW, Blaser MJ, et al: Tooth loss, pancreatic cancer, and *Helicobacter pylori*. *Am J Clin Nutr* 78:176, 2003.
47. Abnet CC, Kamangar F, Dawsey SM, et al: Tooth loss is associated with increased risk of gastric non-cardia adenocarcinoma in a cohort of Finnish smokers. *Scand J Gastroenterol* 40:681, 2005.
48. Michaud DS, Joshipura K, Giovannucci E, et al: A prospective study of periodontal disease and pancreatic cancer in US male health professionals. *J Natl Cancer Inst* 99:171, 2007.

EVOLVE RESOURCES

Please visit http://evolve.elsevier.com/Darby/hygiene for additional practice and study support tools.

SECTION IV Critical Thinking in Dental Hygiene Practice

CHAPTER 21

Dental Hygiene Diagnosis

Michele Leonardi Darby, Margaret M. Walsh

COMPETENCIES

1. Define diagnosis and differentiate between a dental hygiene diagnosis and a dental diagnosis.
2. Explain the dental hygiene diagnostic process, including:
   - Identify interventions that support various dental hygiene diagnoses.
   - Apply human needs theory to diagnostic decision making.
3. Discuss formulating and validating dental hygiene diagnoses, including:
   - Write dental hygiene diagnostic statements.
   - Explain how to validate a dental hygiene diagnosis.
4. Discuss the outcomes of dental hygiene diagnoses.

Diagnosis Defined

A **diagnosis** is an identification of a condition, problem, or situation based on the analysis of its cause and defining characteristics. The diagnostic process is generic but can be applied to specific disciplines; a diagnosis becomes discipline specific when it is applied to the practice of that discipline. The dental hygienist diagnoses client conditions within the scope of dental hygiene to prevent oral disease, minimize the risk of oral disease, and promote wellness.

Miller introduced the concept of the dental hygiene diagnosis to describe the expression of dental hygiene judgment and decision making.[1] The dental hygiene profession has accepted diagnosis as part of the dental hygienist's role. The American Dental Education Association's Competencies for Entry into Dental Hygiene, the American Dental Hygienists' Association's Code of Ethics and Standards for Clinical Dental Hygiene Practice, and the Commission on Dental Accreditation's Standards for Dental Hygiene Education Programs use the term *dental hygiene diagnosis*.[2-5]

Dental Hygiene Diagnosis

A **dental hygiene diagnosis** is a clinical decision made by a dental hygienist that identifies an actual or potential human need deficit that the dental hygienist is educated and licensed to treat (meet) and/or to refer for care. Using the dental hygiene human needs conceptual model[6] to define the dental hygiene diagnosis as identifying human need deficits defines the scope and domain of dental hygiene practice broadly and clarifies the role of the dental hygienist professionally and legally for other healthcare providers, the public, and legislators. Doing so also clearly distinguishes a dental hygiene diagnosis from a dental diagnosis.

The dental hygiene diagnosis requires analysis of all available assessment data and the use of critical decision-making skills to reach conclusions about the client's dental hygiene care needs.[5]

A dental hygiene diagnosis has the following characteristics:

- Focuses on client conditions, behaviors, or risk factors related to oral health and disease
- Derives from client data collected during assessment
- Requires interventions within the scope of dental hygiene practice
- Is necessary for planning and implementing effective dental hygiene care and evaluating its outcomes

Therefore, after the assessment phase of the dental hygiene process, the diagnostic process begins (Figure 21-1). Making a dental hygiene diagnosis includes identifying the following:

- Unmet human needs that can be met through dental hygiene care
- Factors contributing to or causing the unmet human needs (causes and risk factors)
- Evidence to support the dental hygiene diagnosis (signs and symptoms)

In making a dental hygiene diagnosis the dental hygienist works within the scope of dental hygiene practice. The process requires a concrete understanding of the scope of dental hygiene and collaboration between the dental hygienist and dentist.[7]

Historically, dental hygienists were cautioned to not diagnose but to identify dental problems and then communicate the observations using sentences such as the following:

- "Mr. Jones has suspicious areas on teeth 14, 19, and 32."
- "Ms. Smith has signs of gingival and periodontal disease around teeth 22 to 26."
- "There appears to be a radiolucent area at the apex of tooth 8."

Such observations are neither dental nor dental hygiene diagnoses and create confusion for the client. If state law permits preliminary diagnostic services provided by the dental hygienist, the dental hygienist could say the following:

- "Mr. Jones, my preliminary diagnosis suggests dental caries on several of your teeth; the final dental diagnosis must be made by the dentist."

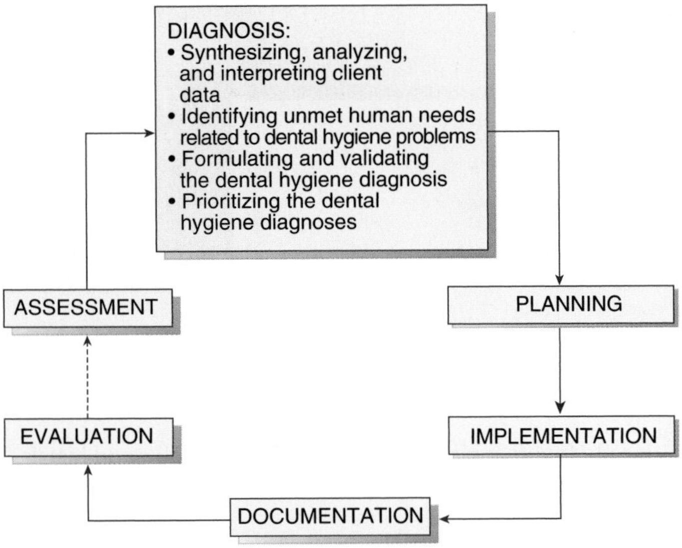

Figure 21-1. The concept of diagnosis within the dental hygiene process. The term *dental hygiene diagnosis* is used to describe actual or potential oral health problems that can be prevented or resolved by dental hygiene interventions. *Broken line* indicates completion of care until next continued care visit.

- "Ms. Smith, the periodontal probing depths of 5 to 7 mm, mobility of 2, and bleeding around the lower front suggest moderate periodontitis; however, the final diagnosis must be confirmed by the dentist."
- "Mrs. Carson, your son has a radiolucent area on the root tip of his top front tooth suggesting a pathologic condition; however, a dental diagnosis must be made by the dentist."

When a dental hygienist identifies oral disease, such as gingivitis or early periodontitis, this is called a *preliminary diagnosis,* which must be referred to a dentist for a definitive diagnosis and treatment or for possible delegation by the dentist back to the dental hygienist for nonsurgical periodontal care. When the client displays signs and symptoms of oral conditions that require diagnosis and treatment by a dentist, a dental consultation and referral are indicated for high-quality client care. When a client displays signs and symptoms of systemic conditions that require medical diagnosis and treatment by a physician, a medical consultation and referral are indicated.

Dental Hygiene Diagnosis versus Dental Diagnosis

Legal, professional, and social responsibilities require clear distinctions between a dental hygiene diagnosis and a dental diagnosis. Diagnostic decision making and therapeutic care fall within precise legal and professional boundaries. Dental diagnoses identify diseases or conditions for which the dentist directs or provides the primary treatment; dental hygiene diagnoses identify unmet human needs (also known as *human need deficits*) that can be met by dental hygienists within the scope of dental hygiene practice. Both types of diagnoses serve different purposes as related to the professional's scope of practice (Table 21-1).

TABLE 21-1

Dental Hygiene Diagnosis versus Dental Diagnosis

Dental Hygiene Diagnosis	Dental Diagnosis
Identifies an unmet human need (human need deficit)	Identifies a specific oral disease
Identifies conditions or problems (unmet human needs) within the scope of dental hygiene practice	Identifies conditions or problems for which the dentist directs the primary treatment
Often deals with the client's perceptions, beliefs, attitudes, and motivations regarding his or her own oral status	Often deals with the actual pathophysiologic changes
May change as the client's responses and behaviors change	Remains the same for as long as the disease is present

Dental Hygiene Diagnostic Classifications

Making a dental hygiene diagnosis that is recognized as separate from a dental diagnosis requires a unique system to classify relevant clinical data about the client.[6] Currently a classification of eight possible diagnoses (i.e., eight human needs) creates a standardized language for identifying client oral health conditions amenable to dental hygiene care. The dental hygiene diagnostic classification uses descriptors that focus on the client's human needs, thus emphasizing the client as an integrated human being rather than as a disease entity. This classification, based on eight human needs, is designed to work synergistically with the diagnosis of the dentist and other healthcare professionals. The diagnostic classification allows dental hygienists to focus on client needs and to communicate this information to the client and other health professionals (Table 21-2).

Dental Hygiene Diagnostic Process

The diagnostic process, a problem-solving approach to clinical decision making, guides the intellectual activity of the dental hygienist (Figure 21-2). The dental hygiene diagnostic process uses eight human needs related to dental hygiene care as its foundation (see Table 21-2). Dental hygiene diagnoses focus on professional care and allow dental hygienists to assess and manage client conditions within their scope of practice. After diagnosis, goals are developed in conjunction with the client interventions then are implemented, evaluated, and documented along with other relevant information. Client goals—the desired outcome of care—clarify what the client needs to do to promote, maintain, or achieve oral health and wellness. Planning care is contingent on the dental hygiene diagnosis (see Chapter 22).

Synthesis, Analysis, and Interpretation of Assessment Data

Dental hygienists begin data synthesis, analysis, and interpretation during assessment. Figure 21-3 provides a tool that can be used to assess the client's unmet human needs. The dental hygienist looks for significant clusters of data that signal the presence of an actual or potential unmet human need, formulates a diagnosis, and develops a care plan (see Chapter 22).

TABLE 21-2

Dental Hygiene Diagnoses: Their Definitions, Causes, Signs and Symptoms, and Interventions

Dental Hygiene Diagnosis	Causes	Signs and Symptoms (Defining Characteristics)	Educational, Preventive, and Therapeutic Interventions
Protection from Health Risks			
The need to avoid medical contraindications to dental hygiene care; includes the need to be protected from health risks related to dental hygiene care	Participation in sports Improper use of oral healthcare product Educational or knowledge deficit Paresthesia, anesthesia Oral habit Potential for infection Potential for oral injury Concern about infection control, radiation safety, fluoride safety, previous negative experience Risky lifestyle behaviors	Evidence on health history for immediate referral to, or consultation with, a physician regarding uncontrolled diseases (e.g., signs of cardiac problem, signs of uncontrolled diabetes, or abnormal vital signs) Evidence of need for antibiotic premedication Evidence that client is at risk for oral injury (e.g., plays a contact sport without an athletic mouth protector or has impaired eyesight, tremor, or limited dexterity) Evidence that client is at risk for oral or systemic disease Evidence that client is in a life-threatening situation	Assess client need for precautions during care. Work to prevent emergencies from occurring. Discuss dental hygiene care plan with client. Address safety factors with client. Use current standards of care.
Freedom from Fear and Stress			
The need to feel safe and to be free from fear and emotional discomfort in the oral healthcare environment	Past negative dental experience Fear of the unknown Lack of financial resources Fear of the cost of care	Client fear Client concerns about confidentiality, cost of care, disease transmission, fluoride toxicity, mercury toxicity, radiation exposure, or dental hygiene care planned	Provide reassurance. Use desensitizing agents. Perform instrumentation techniques with care. Use a topical or local anesthetic agent, and/or nitrous oxide–oxygen (N_2O-O_2) analgesia. Use behavior management strategies.
Wholesome Facial Image			
The need to feel satisfied with one's own oral-facial features and breath	Acquisition of oral prosthesis Visible dental disease or disorder Halitosis Malocclusion Acquisition of orthodontic appliances	Client reports dissatisfaction with the appearance of his or her teeth, gingiva, facial profile, dental prosthesis, or breath	Educate client about dental treatment options such as orthodontics or dental implants to eliminate body image stressors. Refer client to a general dentist, periodontist, prosthodontist, or orthodontist for care beyond the scope of dental hygiene practice. Encourage client to seek other support systems to deal positively with body image stressors, such as individual counseling and group therapy.

Continued

TABLE 21-2

Dental Hygiene Diagnoses: Their Definitions, Causes, Signs and Symptoms, and Interventions—cont'd

Dental Hygiene Diagnosis	Causes	Signs and Symptoms (Defining Characteristics)	Educational, Preventive, and Therapeutic Interventions
Biologically Sound and Functional Dentition			
The need to have intact teeth and restorations that defend against harmful microbes, provide adequate function, and reflect appropriate nutrition and diet	*Streptococcus mutans* infection Nutrition and diet Mutable and nonmutable risk factors Educational deficit Inadequate self-monitoring Lack of regular dental care	Teeth with signs of disease Missing teeth Defective restorations Teeth with abrasion or erosion Teeth with signs of trauma Ill-fitting prosthetic appliances Chewing difficulty	Teach clients strategies for maintaining healthy teeth, including chemotherapeutic (e.g., fluoride, antimicrobial agents, xylitol, amorphous calcium phosphate) and nutritional strategies. Advocate for a healthy dentition. Refer to a general dentist when dental caries or dental dysfunction is evident.
Skin and Mucous Membrane Integrity of Head and Neck			
The need to have an intact and functioning covering of the person's head and neck area, including the oral mucous membranes and periodontium, which defends against harmful microbes, resists injurious substances and trauma, and reflects adequate nutrition	Microbial infection and host response Inadequate oral health behaviors Inadequate nutrition Mutable and nonmutable risk factors Use of tobacco Inadequate control of a systemic disease (e.g., diabetes, human immunodeficiency virus [HIV] infection) Lack of regular dental care	Presence of extraoral or intraoral lesions, tenderness, or swelling; gingival inflammation Bleeding on probing; probing depths or attachment loss 4 mm; mucogingival problems Presence of xerostomia Oral manifestations of nutritional deficiencies	Perform periodontal debridement, chemotherapy to control oral biofilm and gingivitis. Refer client to a specialist (e.g., periodontist, nutritionist). Provide dietary assessment and counseling for oral disease. Discuss link between periodontal and systemic health.
Freedom from Head and Neck Pain			
The need to be exempt from physical discomfort in the head and neck area	Temporomandibular joint (TMJ) discomfort Oral surgery, dental procedure, dental hygiene procedure Untreated dental disease Inadequate access to care or lack of regular dental care	Extraoral or intraoral pain or sensitivity before dental hygiene care Tenderness on palpation during the extraoral or intraoral examination Discomfort during dental hygiene care	Refer client to the dentist for immediate care or pain relief. Initiate pain control strategies that will ensure client's comfort (e.g., reassurance, desensitizing agents, skillful instrumentation techniques). Administer topical and local anesthetic agents, or $N_2O–O_2$ analgesia.

TABLE 21-2

Dental Hygiene Diagnoses: Their Definitions, Causes, Signs and Symptoms, and Interventions—cont'd

Dental Hygiene Diagnosis	Causes	Signs and Symptoms (Defining Characteristics)	Educational, Preventive, and Therapeutic Interventions
Conceptualization and Problem Solving			
The need to grasp ideas and abstractions to make sound decisions about one's oral health	Knowledge deficit Lack of exposure to information	Client has questions, misconceptions, or lack of knowledge about oral diseases. Client does not understand the rationale for daily oral self-care (e.g., oral biofilm and host response or the importance of daily oral biofilm removal). Client does not understand link between some systemic disease and oral disease. Client has misinterpreted information.	Explain rationale for prevention and control of disease. Teach client about disease risk factors and process and how they can be modified if the client is ready to act. Measure client's oral health knowledge and readiness to change, and introduce new concepts accordingly. Promote client self-evaluation of oral cavity and head and neck as a way of maintaining health and client participation in healthcare.
Responsibility for Oral Health			
The need for accountability for one's oral health as a result of interaction between one's motivation, physical capability, and environment	Nonadherence or noncompliance Uses oral care aids or products inappropriately Need for parental supervision of oral hygiene Partial self-care deficit Total self-care deficit Skill deficit Impaired physical, cognitive ability Inadequate oral health behaviors Lack of financial resources	Inadequate plaque control Inadequate parental (guardian) supervision of child's daily oral hygiene regimen Inadequate self-monitoring of health status No dental examination within past 2 years	Teach specific self-care behaviors to maintain oral and systemic health. Evaluate client's oral self-care behaviors and readiness to change behaviors. Appeal to client's sense of self-care. Encourage client's active participation in formulating goals for care. Facilitate choices and decision making by client.

Adapted from Darby ML, Walsh MM: Application of the human needs conceptual model to dental hygiene practice, *J Dent Hyg* 74:230, 2000.

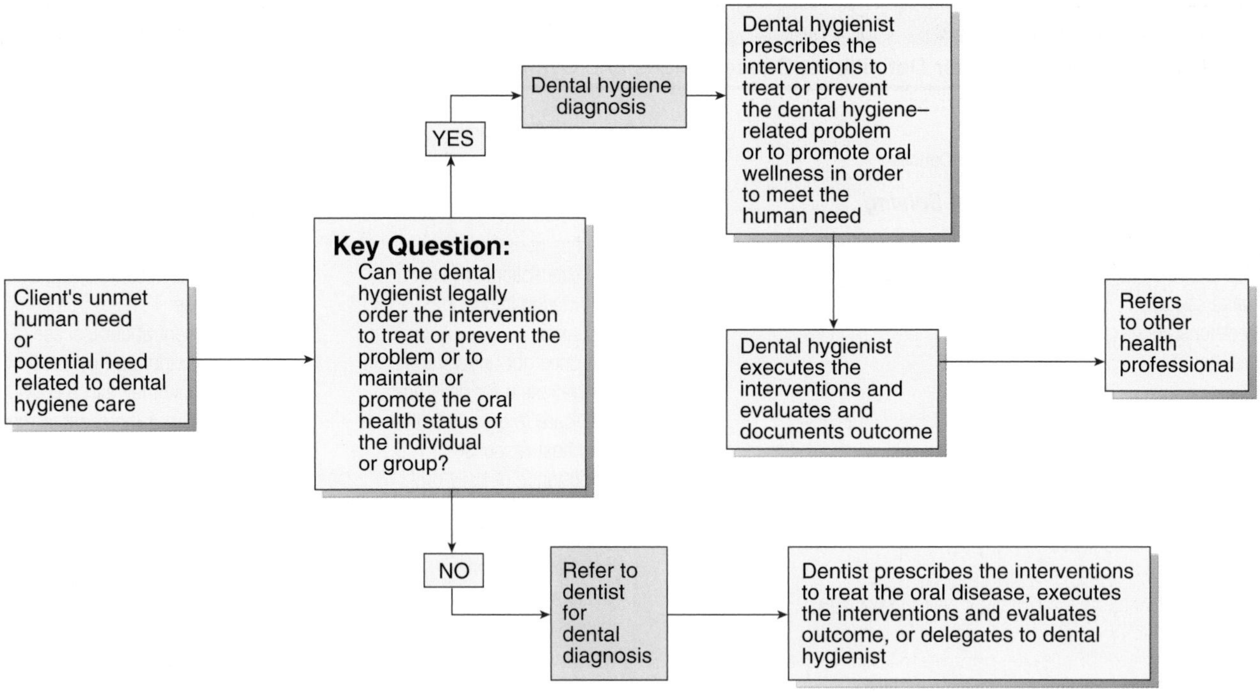

Figure 21-2. Flowchart of the dental hygiene diagnostic process.

Using Standards to Validate Diagnoses

To arrive at a valid dental hygiene diagnosis, the dental hygienist can compare observed data (objective and subjective) with an accepted standard.[8] Appropriate standards include normative values for the client's age and oral status. For example, a child's gingival architecture may be normal given the child's developmental level but may be considered abnormal at another age. Similarly, a blood pressure of 130/90 mm Hg may be within the expected range for an individual with hypertension under the control of a physician, but abnormal for a person not under a physician's care. To recognize significant data, consider the following:

- Changes in a client's usual oral or systemic health patterns that are unexplained by expected norms for growth, development, and maturation
- Oral and systemic health status that deviates from normal limits
- Behavior or condition indicating a developmental lag or risk to health or personal safety

Recognizing Patterns

Dental hygiene diagnoses always should be based on a cluster of significant information rather than on a single sign or symptom. The danger of arriving at a dental hygiene diagnosis from a single factor is evident from this example: The dental hygienist diagnoses an Eastern Indian woman as having an unmet human need for a wholesome facial image. The diagnosis looks to be related to a lack of dental care as evidenced by malpositioned teeth and a prognathic profile, but the observed data may have been misinterpreted. The dental hygienist mistakenly identified the cause as lack of dental care when really it is rooted in the client's culture, which accepts malocclusion as within the range of normal. The woman has had regular dental care throughout her life, but no orthodontic care because of her cultural orientation. Indeed, her human need for a wholesome facial image was met because it was not in deficit from the client's perspective. Gathering complete data to support a recognizable pattern prevents the dental hygienist from formulating an incorrect diagnosis.

Identifying Unmet Human Needs

The next step in the diagnostic process is to determine the client's unmet human needs. The dental hygienist distinguishes between oral health conditions that only a dentist is qualified to treat (dental diagnosis), which requires a dental referral, and oral health conditions that require dental hygiene care (dental hygiene diagnosis). Here, critical thinking determines whether the identified condition requires a dental diagnosis, a dental hygiene diagnosis, or a medical diagnosis.

Clients also may present information during the assessment indicating that they are at risk for developing an unmet human need (i.e., an at-risk problem). For example, the dental hygienist records that a client has signs of possible uncontrolled diabetes mellitus, but a hemoglobin A_{1c} test has not been done for at least 6 months. The dental hygienist then predicts problems this client is likely to experience as a result: a diabetic emergency, longer healing period than normal, continued breakdown of collagen and alveolar bone, and elevated risk for infection. These potential problems are related to the diagnosis of unmet human needs for Protection from Health Risks and for Skin and Mucous Membrane Integrity of the Head and Neck.

Dental hygiene diagnoses have implications for planning interventions. For example, interventions may include

ASSESSMENT (circle signs and symptoms present) 1) PROTECTION FROM HEALTH RISKS *BP outside of normal limits *potential for injury *need for prophylactic antibiotics *risk factors *other ______	5) BIOLOGICALLY SOUND AND FUNCTIONAL DENTITION *reports difficulty in chewing *presents with: –defective restorations –teeth with signs of disease –missing teeth –other ______ –ill-fitting dentures, appliances –abrasion, erosion, abfraction –rampant caries
2) FREEDOM FROM FEAR/STRESS *reports or displays: –anxiety about proximity of clinician, confidentiality, or previous dental experience –oral habits –substance abuse *concern about: –infection control, fluoride therapy, fluoridation, mercury toxicity, other ______	6) CONCEPTUALIZATION AND PROBLEM SOLVING *has questions about DH care and/or oral disease *other ______
3) WHOLESOME FACIAL IMAGE *expresses dissatisfaction with appearance –teeth –gingiva –facial profile –breath –other ______	7) FREEDOM FROM HEAD AND NECK PAIN *extra-/intraoral pain or sensitivity *other ______
4) SKIN AND MUCOUS MEMBRANE INTEGRITY OF HEAD AND NECK –extra-/intraoral lesion –swelling –gingival inflammation –bleeding on probing –pockets >4 mm –attachment loss >1 mm –xerostomia –other ______	8) RESPONSIBILITY FOR ORAL HEALTH *plaque and calculus present *inadequate parental supervision of oral healthcare *no dental exam within the last 2 years *other ______

DENTAL HYGIENE DIAGNOSIS (List the unmet human need, then be specific about the etiology and signs and symptoms evidencing the unmet need)

(Unmet Human Need) due to (Etiology) evidenced by (Signs and Symptoms)

CLIENT GOALS	**INTERVENTIONS** (target etiologies)	**EVALUATION** (goal met, partially met, or unmet)

Appointment Schedule: ______

Continued-care recommendations:

Figure 21-3. Human needs assessment form. (Adapted from Darby ML, Walsh MM: Application of the human needs conceptual model to dental hygiene practice, *J Dent Hyg* 74:230, 2000.)

collaboration with and referral to the dentist and physician of record, analysis of the client's diet and nutrition, review of the client's medication schedule, reduction in length of appointment, prophylactic antibiotic premedication, use of antibacterial dentifrices and mouth rinses to control the bacterial load, and establishment of a personal oral self-care program.

Identifying Strengths (Protective Factors)

At times a client may present no unmet human needs. This situation is an opportunity for the dental hygienist to identify the client's protective factors, build on these strengths for greater levels of oral wellness, and reinforce oral health promotion interventions to maintain and augment wellness. Protective factors may include maintaining good systemic health, living a healthy lifestyle, not smoking, eating a diet rich in fruits and vegetables and low in animal fats, exercising regularly, valuing personal health, seeking regular professional medical and oral care, and meticulously performing daily oral self-care behaviors.

Formulating and Validating Dental Hygiene Diagnoses

Writing Dental Hygiene Diagnostic Statements

After analyzing the client's data, the dental hygienist reaches one of four conclusions, all of which require different actions. These conclusions and actions are shown in Table 21-3.

If the action requires a diagnosis, the dental hygienist formulates, validates, and prioritizes dental hygiene diagnoses before care. Formulation of the dental hygiene diagnosis is based on the identification of the client's human needs as supported by the assessment data. More than one unmet human need may be found, and multiple dental hygiene diagnoses may be identified.

Three components make up a diagnostic statement (Figure 21-4):

- Unmet human need: oral health condition or potential (at-risk) health problem amenable to dental hygiene intervention

TABLE 21-3

Possible Conclusions and Actions Taken by the Dental Hygienist After Analyzing Client Assessment Data

Conclusion	Dental Hygiene Actions
No unmet human needs related to dental hygiene care	Initiate oral health promotion strategies to achieve higher levels of oral and systemic wellness. Reinforce client's oral health beliefs and behaviors.
Possible unmet human needs related to an oral health problem	Collect more assessment data to validate suspected problem, which may require a dental hygiene diagnosis, a dental diagnosis, or a medical diagnosis.
Actual or potential unmet human needs related to dental hygiene care (dental hygiene diagnosis)	Plan, implement, and evaluate dental hygiene care.
Actual or potential unmet human needs requiring a diagnosis by another healthcare professional	Consult with and refer to appropriate healthcare professional; work collaboratively to solve problem.

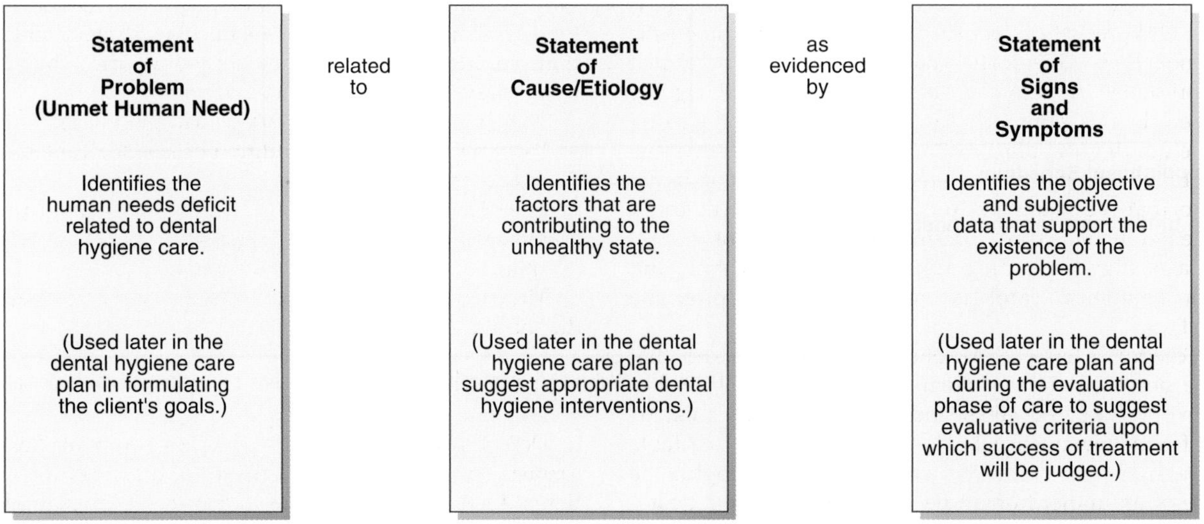

Statement of Problem (Unmet Human Need)
related to
Statement of Cause/Etiology
as evidenced by
Statement of Signs and Symptoms
Identifies the human needs deficit related to dental hygiene care.
(Used later in the dental hygiene care plan in formulating the client's goals.)
Identifies the factors that are contributing to the unhealthy state.
(Used later in the dental hygiene care plan to suggest appropriate dental hygiene interventions.)
Identifies the objective and subjective data that support the existence of the problem.
(Used later in the dental hygiene care plan and during the evaluation phase of care to suggest evaluative criteria upon which success of treatment will be judged.)

Figure 21-4. Three parts of a dental hygiene diagnostic statement. (Adapted from Darby ML, Walsh MM: Application of the human needs conceptual model to dental hygiene practice, *J Dent Hyg* 74:230, 2000.)

TABLE 21-4

Formulation of Dental Hygiene Diagnostic Statements

Dental Hygiene Diagnosis	Cause	Signs and Symptoms/Defining Characteristics
Definitions		
Client's unmet human needs related to dental hygiene care for which the dental hygienist is educated and licensed to treat	Factors causing or maintaining the unhealthy oral state or response, or factors putting the client at risk of a health problem	Subjective and objective data collected during assessment that support existence of a problem or potential problem
Examples		
Skin and mucous membrane integrity of the head and neck	Related to mutable and nonmutable risk factors (e.g., diabetes, smoking, cardiovascular disease, oral biofilm accumulation)	As manifested by moderate gingival bleeding, periodontal probing depths of 5-7 mm
Responsibility for oral health	Related to impaired physical ability	As manifested by heavy oral biofilm accumulation and arthritis in the hands and shoulders
Protection from health risks (potential for oral infection)	Related to the presence of risk factors or risk indicators	*Note:* Potential problems may not have signs or symptoms in the diagnostic statement because the problem has not yet manifested
Protection from health risks (potential for oral injury)	Related to participation in contact sports Client does not wear a mouth protector	*Note:* Potential problems may not have signs or symptoms in the diagnostic statement because the problem has not yet manifested
Responsibility for oral health	Related to inadequate parental supervision of daily oral hygiene	As manifested by heavy oral biofilm accumulation, gingival bleeding, and parent indicating that "John brushes his own teeth"
Wholesome facial image	Related to a Class II, division I malocclusion	As manifested by client's malocclusion and consistent derogatory remarks about her teeth

- Cause: probable cause or risk factors for the actual or potential deficit
- Signs and symptoms (defining characteristics)

A diagnostic statement links the client's problem and its cause, guides the selection of interventions, and facilitates the definition of expected outcomes to evaluate the efficacy of care (see Chapter 22 for a discussion of expected outcomes).

Table 21-4 presents examples of dental hygiene diagnostic statements. Eight diagnostic categories (i.e., eight human needs) presented in Table 21-2 outline possible dental hygiene diagnoses. In this approach to diagnosing, the organizing principle guiding the diagnosis is human needs theory. The diagnostic statement provides a focus on specific client unmet needs so that the routine approach, characteristic of traditional dental hygiene care (a 45-minute appointment for oral prophylaxis, bitewing radiographs, fluoride application, and 6-month continued care) is no longer an appropriate standard.

Each diagnosis has a cluster of defining characteristics that must be observed during client assessment. The **defining characteristics** are the signs and symptoms that must be evident for the diagnostic label to be used correctly (see Table 21-2). The **signs and symptoms** are predictors for judging the presence of an unmet human need related to an oral health condition or a potential problem. The client's signs and symptoms enable the dental hygienist to focus on the true problem and to eliminate others. (The result of this process is referred to as the *differential diagnosis*.)

Sometimes the client may not have a problem yet but has risk factors and risk indicators suggesting that he or she is at risk for a problem. At-risk problems are conditions that also should be diagnosed so that actions can be taken to prevent the potential problem from developing. If the client is at risk for an oral health problem, there may not be signs and symptoms because the problem has not yet occurred; however, it is still preventable if risk factors are modified.

A diagnosis should be accompanied by noting:

- Factors that led to the condition or at-risk problem (cause or causative factors)
- The objective signs observed by the dental hygienist and the subjective symptoms reported by the client (defining characteristics as evidence of the problem)

Thus a dental hygiene diagnosis is written as a three-part diagnostic statement:

- Unmet human need
- Cause (related to or due to)
- As evidenced by signs and symptoms

Dental hygiene diagnoses should be documented as a permanent entry on the client's record. Guidelines for writing dental hygiene diagnoses are in Box 21-1. An example of a diagnostic statement is *an unmet human need for Skin and Mucous Membrane Integrity of the Head and Neck, related to skill deficiency in removing oral biofilm, as evidenced by plaque and gingival bleeding scores of 5 and 3, respectively.*

Potential health problems may not require specification of the cause. In these situations the observed risk factors are the defining characteristics. A dental hygiene diagnosis regarding an at-risk problem is written with its presenting risk factors as the defining characteristics (e.g., a potential unmet need for Freedom from Health Risks, as manifested by the daily use of spit tobacco).

BOX 21-1

Guidelines for Writing Dental Hygiene Diagnoses

- Phrase the dental hygiene diagnosis as a client oral health problem, risk, or alteration in oral health state.
- Indicate what the problem is related to; problem and cause should be linked by the phrase *related to.*
- Indicate evidence for the problem and its cause by stating the defining characteristics as observed in the client; the defining characteristics should be linked to the diagnostic statement by the phrase *as indicated by.*
- Use language that avoids emotionalism or value judgment.
- Be sure that the dental hygiene diagnosis is not a medical or dental diagnosis.

Errors in Writing a Dental Hygiene Diagnostic Statement

The most frequent errors found in dental hygiene diagnostic statements include using emotional terms, including a dental diagnosis, including a medical diagnosis, presenting the cause as the diagnosis, or presenting signs and symptoms as the diagnosis rather than phrasing the diagnosis in terms of the client's unmet needs. These common errors are listed in Table 21-5, with guidelines on how these errors can be corrected. The dental hygienist also must avoid personal beliefs and values in the diagnostic statement by always referring to the documented data as assessed and/or reported by the client and recorded in the dental chart. Nothing should be recorded that insinuates negligence in the treatment rendered by another practitioner. For example, *an unmet need for a Biologically Sound and Functional Dentition, due to poor dentistry, as manifested by overhanging restorations*. Table 21-6 provides examples of conditions that are not dental hygiene diagnoses.

Validation of the Dental Hygiene Diagnosis

Once the diagnosis is formulated, it must be validated. An affirmative response to each of the statements in Figure 21-5 validates the dental hygiene diagnosis.[7] The format in Figure 21-6 can be used to practice the process of diagnostic decision making. The dental hygienist can begin by reviewing Scenarios 21-1 to 21-3, in which the dental hygiene diagnostic process is applied clinically.

TABLE 21-5

Common Errors in Writing Dental Hygiene Diagnoses

Type of Error	Poor Dental Hygiene Diagnosis	Correction Required	Corrected Dental Hygiene Diagnosis
Emotionalism expressed in the diagnosis	Inadequate self-care related to laziness	Eliminate words that express emotionalism.	Unmet need for responsibility for oral health related to lack of adherence to self-care regimen, as evidenced by heavy biofilm accumulation and client's self-report.
Dental diagnosis instead of a dental hygiene diagnosis	Moderate, localized aggressive periodontitis	Avoid using dental diagnostic terms.	Unmet need in skin and mucous membrane integrity because of heavy plaque and cigarette smoking, as indicated by continued loss of clinical attachment since the last 3-month continued-care appointment. Refer to dentist for dental diagnosis.
Citing cause as the diagnosis	Deficit related to nonadherence	Use human need framework.	Unmet need for responsibility for oral health related to a lack of manual dexterity and self-care, as evidenced by a plaque index score of 3 and an inability to grasp a toothbrush.
Identifying signs and symptoms as the client problem	Generalized gingival bleeding and attachment levels of 5-8 mm	Use signs and symptoms to define and validate the actual problem.	Unmet need for skin and mucous membrane integrity related to inadequate oral self-care and smoking, as manifested by generalized, clinical attachment loss of 5-8 mm and signs of nicotine stomatitis.
Writing the diagnosis in terms of what the dental hygienist will do	Needs education on the disease process	Write the diagnosis in terms of the client rather than what the dental hygienist needs to do.	Unmet need in conceptualization and problem solving related to a lack of knowledge about disease process, as evidenced by client's misconceptions about caries cause and prevention.

TABLE 21-6

What a Dental Hygiene Diagnosis Is Not

It Is Not...	Examples	Rationales
A dental diagnosis or pathology	Myofascial pain disorder Class III malocclusion Advanced chronic periodontal disease Oral squamous carcinoma Early childhood caries Necrotizing ulcerative periodontitis Leukoplakia Aphthous ulcer Hyperplastic candidiases	Although dental hygiene care is associated with dental diagnoses, the disease or disorder is not primarily amenable to dental hygiene intervention. Dental hygiene's concern is for the person and the oral health behaviors in which they engage. Dental hygienists must understand pathology underlying disease states to plan appropriate dental hygiene care; however, focus is on the person's response and not the pathology. The person's response to the pathology and its prevention is the domain of dental hygiene.
A diagnostic test, treatment, or appliance	Pulp tester Antibiotic therapy Antimicrobial therapy Oral prosthetic appliances	Dental hygiene's concern is the individual's oral health behavior and response to the diagnostic test, treatment, or equipment. If assessment data or data gathered throughout care reveal an unmet need, this becomes the dental hygiene diagnosis.
A goal of the hygienist or a dental hygiene intervention	To develop the client's responsibility to control oral disease by referring him or her to the dentist and by providing education	The dental hygiene diagnosis should be written from the client's perspective, not the dental hygienist's perspective. Example: unmet need for responsibility for oral health, related to lack of financial resources, as evidenced by no professional care for 5 years and no dental insurance.
A single sign or symptom	Oral biofilm on lingual surfaces of all teeth	A dental hygiene diagnosis is not developed until a pattern or cluster of significant cues is identified. The clustering of signs and symptoms leads to the dental hygiene diagnosis, but it is not the diagnosis. In this situation, no dental hygiene diagnosis is indicated until more data are collected, synthesized, analyzed, and interpreted.
An unvalidated dental hygiene diagnosis	Previous example leads dental hygienist to the dental hygiene diagnosis: unmet need in conceptualization and problem solving.	Unvalidated, a premature dental hygiene diagnosis may not focus on the client's true problem. More defining characteristics (signs and symptoms) must be identified before the dental hygiene diagnosis can be validated.

Dental Hygiene Diagnosis Validation Criteria

1. Database is complete, accurate, and based on scope of dental hygiene. Yes ___ No ___
2. Data reflect the existence of a pattern. Yes ___ No ___
3. Both subjective and objective data support the existence of the unmet human need identified in the dental hygiene diagnosis. Yes ___ No ___
4. Dental hygiene diagnosis is based on scientific knowledge and evidence. Yes ___ No ___
5. Dental hygiene diagnosis can be prevented, controlled, or resolved by dental hygiene interventions. Yes ___ No ___
6. Given the same data, other qualified practitioners would formulate the same dental hygiene diagnosis. Yes ___ No ___

Figure 21-5. "Yes" answers to all of these statements validate the dental hygiene diagnosis.

Outcomes of Dental Hygiene Diagnoses

Dental hygiene diagnoses facilitate the development of professional autonomy and accountability by focusing on phenomena within the scope of dental hygiene practice and by providing a language for communication. By identifying the client's unmet human needs that can be fulfilled through dental hygiene care, the dental hygiene diagnosis clarifies the role of the dental hygienist and allows for a defined scope and domain of dental hygiene practice. "Diagnosis by dental hygienists is not, and should not be, an attempt to move into the domain of the dentist; it is a vehicle for distinguishing roles professionally and legally."[1]

Dental hygiene diagnosis facilitates the delivery of high-quality dental hygiene care and provides a criterion for establishing professional fees. Because dental hygiene diagnoses are based on a diagnostic classification system, communication among oral health professionals is facilitated. Diagnosis facilitates the measurement of clinical outcomes, which has implications for professional accountability, client education, research, regulatory mechanisms, direct access to care, and direct reimbursement. Use of dental hygiene diagnoses

Dental Hygiene Diagnosis	Due to	Evidenced by	Client Goal/Behavior

Figure 21-6. Worksheet for making a dental hygiene diagnosis.

appears promising for the development of a computerized system of dental hygiene diagnosis and care planning, with expansion to a system of cost accounting for dental hygiene. The dental hygienist can review expected outcomes and dental hygiene interventions in Scenarios 21-1 to 21-3 as focused by the dental hygiene diagnoses.

CLIENT EDUCATION TIPS

- Explain the dental hygiene diagnosis so that the client understands the condition or problem and how it can best be resolved.
- Explain how goals established will, if achieved, meet the client's need.

LEGAL, ETHICAL, AND SAFETY ISSUES

- Dental hygiene diagnoses reflect the scope of dental hygiene practice and never the scope of the dentist's practice. Avoid terminology in the diagnostic statement that implies blame or negligence, which could lead to litigation.
- When client manifests signs and symptoms of oral conditions that require dental treatment by a dentist, a dental referral is indicated for high-quality care and legal protection.
- When client manifests signs and symptoms of systemic conditions that require medical evaluation and treatment, a medical consultation and referral are indicated for high-quality care and legal protection.
- Dental hygiene diagnoses must be validated to ensure that the focus of care is accurate.
- Dental hygiene diagnostic statements should be recorded in the client record and used to develop client goals throughout the dental hygiene process of care.

KEY CONCEPTS

- A dental hygiene diagnosis states the client's actual or potential (at-risk) problem related to oral health and disease.
- Diagnosis is a decision-making process that requires critical thinking and professional judgment.
- Current standards (e.g., American Dental Education Association's Competencies for Entry into Dental Hygiene, the American Dental Hygienists' Association's Code of Ethics and Standards for Clinical Dental Hygiene Practice, the American Dental Association Commission on Dental Accreditation's Standards for Dental Hygiene Education Programs) expect dental hygienists to make dental hygiene diagnoses.
- The diagnostic process includes analysis of assessment data; identification of the client's problem, health risks, strengths; and formulation of the diagnostic statements.
- Dental hygiene diagnoses improve communication among the dental hygienist, the client, and other health professionals.
- The *related to* part of the diagnostic statement provides the dental hygienist with direction regarding selecting interventions.
- The *as evidenced by* part of the diagnostic statement provides the dental hygienist with defining characteristics to evaluate the outcome of care.
- *Client goal* reflects the desired outcome of care.
- Dental hygiene diagnostic statements allow the dental hygienist to focus care on the client's unmet needs and individualize care.
- Dental hygiene diagnostic statements should be clear, client centered, and based on reliable assessment data and should reflect only one problem (human need related to oral health and disease).
- Eight dental hygiene diagnoses are based on human needs related to oral health and disease.
- Development of dental hygiene diagnoses is an ongoing project within the profession that requires research.
- Diagnosis by dental hygienists is not, and should not, be an attempt to move into the domain of the dentist.

CRITICAL THINKING EXERCISES

1. Select one new client. Using all of the subjective and objective information from assessment, including data collected

SCENARIO 21-1

YOUNG WOMAN WHO RECENTLY OBTAINED ORTHODONTIC APPLIANCES

Brenda Smith, age 16, Asian American, and a junior in high school, received full orthodontic appliances 1 month ago. Although she wanted the orthodontic appliances to correct the severe crowding of her anterior teeth, she is now experiencing an adjustment problem. Although she was last treated for gingivitis before placement of the orthodontic appliances, she decides to visit her dental office for a 3-month checkup. On assessment, the dental hygienist finds Ms. Smith to have significant loss of weight, slight generalized plaque-induced gingivitis, and fair oral biofilm control. All other findings are within normal limits. Ms. Smith verbalizes that not very many 16-year-olds at her school wear braces, that she can't wait to get them off, and that she can't stand to look at herself in the mirror. One of her high school friends said that she looked weird. She obviously has been experiencing high anxiety since the orthodontic appliances were placed. She said that she has a difficult time eating because food sticks to the appliances, and she feels embarrassed if the appliances are retaining food. She no longer likes to eat with her friends in the school cafeteria or when she is out on weekends.

Dental Hygiene Diagnosis (Unmet Need)	Is Due to or Related to (Causes)	As Evidenced by (Signs and Symptoms)	Client Goal (Expected Outcomes)
Wholesome facial image	Acquisition of orthodontic appliances	Unwillingness to smile Constant negative referral to the appliances and the way she looks	Verbalizes acceptance of appliances after 2 months
Freedom from fear and stress	Inability to eat Acquisition of orthodontic appliances	Loss of weight Anxiety about wearing the orthodontic appliances	Verbalizes acceptance of appliances after 1 month Reports stabilized weight after 2 months

Dental Hygiene Interventions

1. Assess Ms. Smith's perception of her oral condition and appearance before she began to wear the orthodontic appliances.
2. Listen to client's comments. Compliment client on appearance.
3. Assist Ms. Smith in visualizing her altered facial image and the temporary status of the orthodontic appliances. Emphasize that the altered facial image is a normal part of wearing orthodontic appliances.
4. Assist Ms. Smith in concentrating on the positive aspects of her oral health (e.g., no decay, no periodontal disease).
5. Actively reinforce accomplishments such as oral biofilm control, no gingival bleeding.
6. Encourage Ms. Smith to talk with others who wear orthodontic appliances to share concerns and feelings.
7. Conduct nutritional counseling with Ms. Smith to identify healthy foods that can be eaten with orthodontic appliances.
8. Describe the dietary needs of adolescents.
   - Explain using *MyPlate.*
   - Design a basic food plan.
9. Instruct Ms. Smith in how to record a food diary (see Chapter 35). After 1 week, review food diary and lead Ms. Smith to identify areas of concern that may be contributing to undernutrition.
   - Discuss alternative food choices (e.g., foods that are less retentive).
   - Explain how good nutrition will enable her to cope better with the appliances.
   - Consider consultation and/or referral to a nutritionist if necessary.
10. Review oral hygiene care for orthodontic appliances, with specific emphasis on what can be done to keep appliances looking clean while the client is away from home.
11. Continually monitor anxiety level, emotional status, and attitude toward orthodontic appliances.
12. After 1 month, evaluate client's eating habits, body weight, and anxiety level.
13. After 2 months, evaluate client's eating habits, body weight, and anxiety level.

SCENARIO 21-2

CHILD WITH AGGRESSIVE PERIODONTITIS

Devan Prince, age 12, female African American, is a new client in the dental practice and has been scheduled for dental hygiene care. Devan is in the seventh grade and is one of the star players on the girls' soccer team. She is with her mother Margaret (age 32) and her sister Bridget (age 10). After completing health and dental histories, the dental hygienist initiates a baseline assessment of the head and neck, intraoral and extraoral examination, a complete dental and periodontal assessment, assessment of human needs related to dental hygiene care, and client education and skill level assessment. Significant findings include 6-mm probing depths around teeth 19 and 30 and a 4- to 5-mm loss of clinical attachment around teeth 22 to 27. Oral hygiene is generally poor, and tooth mobility of periodontally involved teeth ranges from 2 to 3. Client has a knowledge deficit regarding oral biofilm, periodontal disease process, and status of the oral cavity.

Dental Hygiene Diagnosis (Unmet Need)	Is Due to or Related to (Causes)	As Evidenced by (Signs and Symptoms)	Client Goal (Expected Outcomes)
Freedom from health risks	Participation in contact sport; does not use a mouth protector	Note: Potential problems may not have defining characteristics in the diagnostic statement (no defining characteristics necessary because client is at risk for a problem; problem has not yet occurred)	Verbalizes belief in value of a mouth protector Reports wearing mouth protector at all soccer games and practice sessions by next appointment Verbalizes emergency care protocol for an avulsed tooth
Skin and mucous membrane integrity of the head and neck	Presence of oral biofilm Nonmutable risk factors for juvenile periodontitis	4- to 5-mm clinical attachment loss, poor oral hygiene, tooth mobility of 2 and 3	Decreases bacterial plaque score from 3 to 0 within 1 month Seeks care from periodontist
Conceptualization and problem solving	Knowledge deficit about the periodontal disease process, oral biofilm, genetic risk, and state of oral cavity	Misconceptions about the characteristics of an unhealthy mouth	Identifies unhealthy and healthy signs in her mouth by end of this appointment Explains periodontal disease process by 1 month Seeks care from periodontist

Dental Hygiene Interventions

1. Assess client's present level of knowledge about mouth protectors.
2. Teach client about the value of wearing a mouth protector during contact sports.
3. Teach parent and client emergency care for an avulsed tooth.
4. Construct mouth protector; discuss use and care with the client; fit mouth protector.
5. After 1 week, evaluate fit and client response to mouth protector.
6. Teach child and parent about periodontal disease process.
   - Explain disease process (aggressive periodontitis).
   - Use signs and symptoms of health and disease found in the client's own mouth as teaching aids.
7. Work collaboratively with dentist and periodontist to carry out successful root debridement and antimicrobial therapy. Support therapeutic recommendations of periodontist.
8. Teach child and parent about mutable and nonmutable risk factors.
9. Teach child and parent appropriate self-care (e.g., toothbrushing and interdental cleaning).
10. Evaluate knowledge and skill acquisition after 1 month.
11. Modify plan as needed.
12. Refer client to dentist or periodontist.
13. Establish appropriate continued-care interval that considers periodontal maintenance care from the periodontist.

SCENARIO 21-3

YOUNG CHILD WITH EARLY CHILDHOOD CARIES

Blake Olds, age 4, a Caucasian, is brought to the dental hygiene care facility by his mother Caren, age 28. Caren is unemployed and on public assistance; therefore finances are a major concern. Blake has been in pain associated with his teeth. His mother reported that "he has been crying on and off for about 4 days, saying that his mouth hurt." She indicates that she tries to appease his discomfort with sweets to eat. The dental hygienist conducts a complete health, dental, pharmacologic, and cultural history and initiates the assessment phase of the dental hygiene process. Given the immediate need for relieving the child's pain, she collaborates with the attending dentist, who extracts J, K, and L at that visit and who prescribes an antibiotic to control the infection. Blake's significant findings includes early childhood caries and periapical abscesses on J, K, and L, with caries also on teeth A, B, E, F, I, M, O, P, S, and T. After oral surgery the client is given postoperative instructions and is dismissed, and the dental hygienist analyzes the findings. Because of extraction and interproximal caries, the maintenance of space for the permanent teeth is a major concern. Although no significant periodontal probe depths were found, green and orange extrinsic stain, heavy materia alba, and oral biofilm were present throughout the mouth.

Dental Hygiene Diagnosis (Unmet Need)	Is Due to or Related to (Causes)	As Evidenced by (Signs and Symptoms)	Client Goal (Expected Outcomes)
Freedom from head and neck pain	Untreated caries	Client's expression of pain, mother's report of pain, and signs of severe caries	Parent complies with referral to dentist for emergency care.
Biologically sound and functional dentition	Risk factors for dental disease Lack of dental care and financial resources	Signs of early childhood caries Signs of periapical abscesses on radiographs	Parent complies with referral to dentist for care. Parent lists two dental care resources (e.g., the government-funded Children's Health Insurance Program, local public health dental clinic).
	Cariogenic diet	Space loss that could create a future malocclusion	Parent explains nutritional and chemotherapeutic strategies including xylitol gum and mints to control tooth decay. Parent identifies cariogenic foods to avoid and healthful foods to substitute.
Responsibility for oral health	Lack of parental supervision of daily oral care	Heavy materia alba, oral biofilm, green and orange extrinsic stains present	Decrease plaque index score by 2 within 1 month. Mother reports that client cleans oral cavity once a day by himself by next appointment.
	Skill deficit of parent and client	Lack of a systematic and efficient method of toothbrushing	Mother reports cleaning client's oral cavity once a day by end of next appointment. Mother demonstrates effective mouth cleaning technique on child by end of appointment.
Conceptualization and problem solving	Knowledge deficit of parent about the caries process	Misconceptions about the causes of tooth decay Does not understand oral disease can be prevented cost effectively	Parent explains disease process, cause, and vertical transmission concept; client explains disease process in age-appropriate terms by next appointment. Parent verbalizes value of preventing further tooth loss by next appointment.

Dental Hygiene Interventions

1. Assess oral hygiene knowledge, attitude, and skill level of client and parent.
2. Instruct client and parent on basic daily oral self-care:
   - Knowledge of cause
   - Use of a toothbrush and positioning of client
   - Frequency of toothbrushing
3. Conduct nutritional analysis and counseling for caries control with parent. Discuss concept of vertical transmission of caries.
4. Discuss value of daily fluoride treatment, chlorhexidine mouth rinse, and xylitol until caries are controlled.
5. Discuss reasons for restoring primary teeth:
   - Maintenance of space
   - Prevention of malocclusion and costly orthodontics
6. Compliment client on good job he is doing.
7. Refer parent to community facility where oral healthcare can be obtained on a sliding-scale payment basis.
8. Complete scaling, selective polishing, and fluoride therapy; obtain prescription for daily fluoride therapy and chlorhexidine.
9. In 1 month, evaluate effectiveness of interventions.
10. Modify as necessary; maintain collaboration with treating dentist.

on the form displayed in Figure 19-3, prepare at least one diagnostic statement. What client goals could be established? What dental hygiene interventions will you use to achieve the client goals? Use the information in Table 19-1 to help identify possible causes and defining characteristics. Scenarios 19-1, 19-2, and 19-3 can serve as examples.
2. How would you validate this diagnostic statement?
3. What interventions can be used to elevate a client to higher levels of wellness?

REFERENCES

1. Miller S: Dental hygiene diagnoses. *RDH* 2:46, 1982.
2. American Dental Education Association (ADEA): ADEA competencies for entry into the allied dental professions. *J Dent Educ* 75(7):949, 2011.
3. American Dental Hygienists' Association (ADHA): *Code of ethics*, Chicago, 1997, ADHA.
4. American Dental Association Commission on Dental Accreditation: *Accreditation standards for dental hygiene education programs*, Chicago, 2007 updated effective 2013, Commission on Dental Accreditation.
5. American Dental Hygienists' Association (ADHA): *Dental hygiene diagnosis position paper*, Chicago, 2011, ADHA.
6. Darby ML, Walsh MM: Application of the human needs conceptual model to dental hygiene practice. *J Dent Hyg* 74:230, 2001.
7. Darby ML: Collaborative model of practice: the future of dental hygiene. *J Dent Educ* 47:589, 1983.
8. Price MR: Nursing diagnosis: making a concept come alive. *Am J Nurs* 80:668, 1980.

EVOLVE RESOURCES

Please visit http://evolve.elsevier.com/Darby/hygiene for additional practice and study support tools.

Dental Hygiene Care Plan, Evaluation, and Documentation

CHAPTER 22

Karen M. Palleschi

COMPETENCIES

1. **Discuss the planning phase in the dental hygiene process of care, including:**
   - **Explain the purpose of the planning phase and the client's role in care plan development.**
   - **Identify the sequence for developing a dental hygiene care plan and how each step relates to the dental hygiene diagnosis.**
2. **Do the following regarding the evaluation phase of client care:**
   - **Explain the purpose of the evaluation phase and its significance to the process of care.**
   - **Formulate a client-centered care plan from a dental hygiene diagnosis.**
3. **Discuss documentation, including its significance to the process of care and practitioner liability.**

Care planning, evaluation, and documentation are processes applied daily by the dental hygienist in clinical practice. They are integral to the process of care and dependent on the preceding phases of care, assessing, and diagnosing. Integrating care planning, evaluation, and documentation into dental hygiene care ensures a client-centered approach to care.

Planning

Planning is that phase of the process of care in which diagnosed client needs are prioritized, client goals and evaluative measures are established, and intervention strategies are determined (Figure 22-1). The purpose of the planning phase is to develop a plan of care that results in the resolution of an oral health problem amenable to dental hygiene care, the prevention of a problem, or the promotion of oral and general health. Therefore the term dental hygiene care plan rather than dental hygiene treatment plan is used intentionally to denote the broad range of preventive, educational, therapeutic, and support services within the scope of dental hygiene practice. In keeping with standards of practice and evidence-based interventions, the dental hygienist engages the client in formulating a client-centered plan with clearly defined tangible and measurable outcomes.

To formulate a care plan the dental hygienist must do the following effectively:

- Use parameters or standards of dental hygiene care.
- Collect, analyze, and interpret comprehensive client findings.
- Integrate evidence-based knowledge and theory, professional judgment, and the client's values.
- Develop dental hygiene diagnoses and formulate client-centered goals, which include the action required by the client, a specific date each goal is to be achieved, a criterion-based objective outcome measure, and supportive dental hygiene interventions.
- Synthesize this aforementioned information into a written plan.
- Communicate oral health needs to clients.
- Position the dental hygiene care plan within the context of the total dental treatment plan.

Dental Treatment Plan

The general dentist or dental specialist develops a comprehensive dental treatment plan for the client. This plan includes the dental diagnosis; all essential phases of therapy to be carried out by the dentist, dental hygienist, and client to eliminate and manage disease or promote health; and the prognosis. Components of a dental treatment plan are shown in Table 22-1. The dental hygiene care plan supports the overall dental plan. Ongoing collaboration between the dental hygienist, dentist, physician (when warranted), and client is critical to attaining a successful outcome.

Dental Hygiene Care Plan

The dental hygiene care plan is the written blueprint that directs the dental hygienist and client as they work together to meet the client's oral health goals.[1] The plan encourages the oral healthcare team to work collaboratively to deliver client-centered, goal-oriented care. The plan facilitates the monitoring of client progress, ensures continuity of care, serves as a vehicle for communication among healthcare professionals, and increases the likelihood of high-quality care (Box 22-1).

With the advent of the electronic health record (EHR), the attributes of the dental hygiene care plan can be strengthened. An EHR is a multipurpose health information technology system that compiles comprehensive client information and makes it readily available to the healthcare team. Use of an EHR system has the potential to improve clinical, organizational, and societal outcomes[2,3] (Table 22-2). Therefore it is advantageous to include the dental hygiene care plan within the EHR.

The dental hygiene care plan is written immediately after the assessment and diagnosis phases of the process of care and in conjunction with the overall dental treatment plan

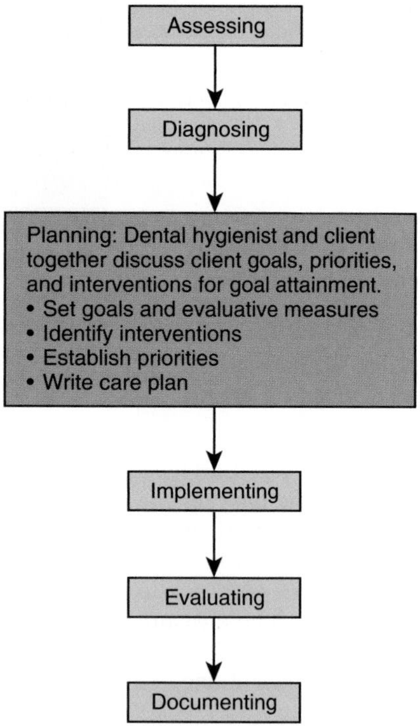

Figure 22-1. Planning phase of the dental hygiene process of care.

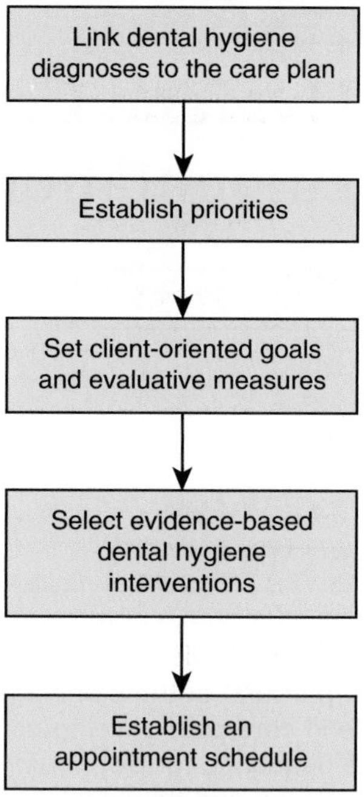

Figure 22-2. Sequence for developing a care plan.

BOX 22-1

Rationale for Developing a Formal Dental Hygiene Care Plan

- Individualize care.
- Focus care on priorities.
- Facilitate communication and collaboration among healthcare professionals.
- Establish client-centered goals.
- Provide foundation on which evaluation of interventions is based.
- Develop roadmap for implementing interventions that will achieve the desired outcome.
- Promote professional practice.

BOX 22-2

Characteristics of a Well-Written Dental Hygiene Care Plan

- Reflects goals of care to (1) develop and maintain the individual's behaviors essential to oral health and the mastery of self-care and the environment; (2) prevent oral disease using primary, secondary, and tertiary preventive interventions; and (3) promote wellness
- Is consistent with client needs and readiness to change
- Identifies a relationship between the dental hygiene diagnoses, client goals, and interventions
- Is compatible with the dental treatment plan prepared by the dentist
- Identifies the dental hygienist's responsibilities, if any, for fulfilling components of the dental treatment plan
- Reflects current standards of evidence-based care
- Meets the client's psychosociocultural and physical needs
- Reflects the dental hygienist's role as clinician, educator, administrator or manager, researcher, and advocate
- Establishes priorities of care

prepared by the dentist. The dental hygiene care plan specifies the following:

- Dental hygiene diagnoses based on assessed deficits in eight human needs related to dental hygiene care
- Client-centered goals
- Dental hygiene interventions
- Appointment schedule

During the planning phase of care, dental hygiene diagnoses are prioritized and each component of the care plan is developed sequentially and linked to the dental hygiene diagnoses. Establishing this link between the dental hygiene diagnosis, client goals, and dental hygiene interventions is critical to the outcome of the care plan (Figure 22-2).

Each dental hygiene care facility may have its own electronic care plan format to document assessment findings, dental hygiene diagnoses, client-centered goals, dental hygiene interventions, appointment schedule, and an evaluative statement of outcome. Although formats may differ, the critical point is that these components are documented in the client's permanent record and are followed to ensure high-quality dental hygiene care. The plan may use standardized abbreviations and key phrases as specified in the policy manual of the healthcare institution with which the dental hygienist is affiliated (Box 22-2). Figure 21-3 in Chapter 21 is a dental hygiene care plan form for documenting unmet human needs.

TABLE 22-1

Components of the Overall Dental Care Plan

Components	Included in the Dental Hygiene Care Plan
Preliminary Phase: Emergency Care	
Relief of pain	
Laboratory tests for suspected pathology	
Emergency needs (e.g., treatment of periodontal or periapical abscess)	
Extraction of hopeless teeth (in some cases may be postponed to later phases of care)	
Provisional replacement to restore function, as needed (in some cases may be postponed to later phases of care)	
Phase I: Nonsurgical Therapy	
Client education and self-care instruction	X
Dietary guidance (e.g., caries risk prevention, tissue healing)	X
Tobacco cessation counseling	X
Fluoride and remineralization therapy	X
Placement of pit and fissure sealants	X
Therapeutic periodontal debridement	X
Hard-tissue desensitization	X
Correction of restorative and prosthetic irritational factors, excavation of caries and restorations (temporary or final as determined by the prognosis of the tooth and location of the caries)	
Antimicrobial (anti-infective) therapy (local or systemic)	X
Occlusal therapy, minor orthodontics	
Coronal polishing	X
Phase I: Evaluation of Response to Nonsurgical Therapy	
Reassessment of gingival and periodontal health, hard and soft deposits, host response, caries risk factors	X
Review and reinforcement of self-care	X
Debridement of residual hard and soft deposits	X
Recommend a schedule for Phase IV: Maintenance Therapy	X
Phase II: Surgical Therapy	
Periodontal surgery	
Implant surgery	
Endodontic therapy	
Phase III: Restorative Therapy	
Restorative care and final management of dental caries	
Fixed and removable prosthodontic appliances	
Evaluation of response to restorative procedures (e.g., periodontal status, host response)	
Phase IV: Maintenance Therapy	
Reassess oral health (e.g., hard and soft deposits, gingival and periodontal inflammation, client adherence to oral self-care, caries risk)	X
Supportive, preventive, and therapeutic periodontal maintenance therapy	X
Self-care education (e.g., review, modify as needed, reinforce)	X
Evaluation and recommendation for schedule of continued-care interval	X

Adapted from Carranza FA, Takei HH: The treatment plan. In Newman MG, Takei HH, Klokkevold PR, et al, eds: *Carranza's clinical periodontology,* ed 11, St Louis, 2012, Elsevier/Saunders; Nield-Gehrig JS, Willmann DE: Decision-making during treatment planning. In Nield-Gehrig JS, Willmann DE: *Foundations in periodontics for the dental hygienist,* ed 3, Philadelphia, 2011, Lippincott Williams and Wilkins.

TABLE 22-2

Potential Benefit of Electronic Health Records to Clinical, Organizational, and Societal Outcome[2,3]

Outcome	Benefits
Clinical	Improves the quality of client care outcomes resulting from improved access to comprehensive health information Able to access and share client information related to direct client care; interdisciplinary approach to eliminate duplication of client services Improves client safety by recognizing drug interactions or client allergies Able to access client education tools from integrated software Able to import, store, and export digital radiographs, oral images, and other electronic assessment documents Able to monitor short-term and long-term client care outcomes by keeping a comparable history of client findings and outcomes
Organizational	Improves efficiency of clinical practice administrative support services (e.g., billing of services, filing insurance claims, continued-care reminders, confirming appointments, scheduling appointments) Improves timeliness of access to client information by real time sharing of client information within clinical practice settings (e.g., health history updates, service provided billing) Improves timeliness of client check in for scheduled appointment by using an electronic check in system Allows for retrieval of a client's record from a central data site for review, entering data and documentation of services rendered (e.g., when away from the practice setting, when a practice setting has multiple practice sites) Allows for sharing of pertinent client information with the client's multidisciplinary healthcare team Supports risk management practice protocols by providing consistency of documents and documentation of client data and services rendered; proving evidence of client-centered care and evidence of standards of care Improves legibility of clinical notes, signatures, documents of consent, prescriptions by eliminating poor penmanship Able to track practice performance and production of client care to improved practice services
Societal	Able to research data that may identify trends in client care and best practices for improved client outcomes

Sequence of Dental Hygiene Care Plan Development

Linking the Diagnosis and the Care Plan

A dental hygiene diagnosis is the foundation for care plan development. Basing dental hygiene care plans on the dental hygiene diagnosis, rather than on oral symptoms alone, ensures that care will be comprehensive, humanistic, and focused on client needs. A care plan may include a single or multiple dental hygiene diagnoses.

A complete dental hygiene diagnosis includes a statement of the problem (unmet human needs related to oral health within the scope of dental hygiene practice), cause of the problem (etiology or contributor), and signs and symptoms of the problem (evidence). By focusing on the causes of the problem and evidence of the unmet human needs, the clinician is able to develop client goals and intervention strategies that best meet the need or eliminate the problem. Therefore client care is individualized rather than generic routine care provided to all. Because signs and symptoms related to dental hygiene problems may have numerous causes, interventions must be selected carefully to ensure that the fundamental cause is addressed in dental hygiene care. For example, a dental hygiene diagnosis of an unmet human need in the area of wholesome facial image may result from the following:

- Client dissatisfaction with the color of his or her teeth
- Client embarrassment because of a disfiguring malocclusion
- Middle-aged client's loss of self-esteem associated with mobile teeth and oral malodor from chronic periodontal disease
- Nursing home resident who no longer wants to interact with friends and family because of lost dentures

These situations require the establishment of unique client goals and dental hygiene interventions to resolve them. Figure 22-3 provides an example of a dental hygiene diagnosis, related client-centered goals, planned dental hygiene interventions, and evaluation statements that focus on the unique needs of a client who is dissatisfied with his tooth color.

Establishing Priorities

In collaboration with the dentist, the dental hygienist considers the dental and dental hygiene diagnoses and determines their urgency.[1] Priorities are based on the degree to which the dental hygiene diagnosis does the following:

- Threatens the client's well-being; it is important to distinguish unmet needs that pose the greatest threat to client safety, health, and comfort from those that are not life threatening and/or related to a current oral disease
- Can be addressed simultaneously with other diagnoses
- Is a client priority (e.g., chief complaint)

Once these criteria are applied to the dental hygiene diagnoses, the dental hygienist ranks the unmet human needs in priority to be addressed. Other than meeting the client's unmet human need for safety (prevention of health risks), which in some instances requires emergency care or referral to a physician, dentists and dental hygienists most likely would identify the client's ability to assume responsibility for oral health as a primary priority. Factors influencing how priorities are established include the following:

- Client values, beliefs, and attitudes
- Healthcare provider philosophy

Client Profile: Personal, dental, medical, and pharmacologic history reveals no significant findings. Assessment reveals slight supragingival calculus, soft deposits, and extrinsic stain. The client verbalized "I wish that my teeth were a whiter color," and "My teeth seem to be darkening with age."		
Dental Hygiene Diagnosis Human need for wholesome facial image *due to* client's dissatisfaction with the color of his teeth *as evidenced by* the client asking if there is anything that can be done to make his teeth whiter.		
Client Goals:	**Intervention:**	**Evaluative Statement:**
♦ Client will seek cosmetic bleaching consultation with dentist by 6/28.	♦ Refer client to dentist for cosmetic bleaching consultation.	♦ Goal unmet. Client did not seek cosmetic bleach consult with dentist.
♦ Client will use tooth whitening dentifrice by 6/14.	♦ Educate client about tooth whitening dentifrice with fluoride and whitening strips available over-the-counter. ♦ Educate client about the normal color of teeth. ♦ Remove all extrinsic stains and deposits from the client's teeth.	♦ Goal met. Client reports using a tooth whitening dentifrice and is satisfied with the results.

Figure 22-3. Example of a dental hygiene diagnosis, goals, interventions, and evaluative statements for a client who wants whiter teeth.

- Collaborating dentist's goals
- Client health status
- Whether the client is experiencing infection, discomfort, anxiety, or pain

Setting Goals

A **client-centered goal** is the client's desired outcome achieved through specific dental hygiene intervention strategies to satisfy an unmet human need related to dental hygiene care.[1] The goal must reflect the signs and reported symptoms of the client's unmet needs. In this way, the clinician establishes a relationship that enables the clinician and client to measure the extent to which a goal has been achieved in terms of changes in the client's initial signs and symptoms. A dental hygiene diagnosis may have one or more defined goals.

A client-centered goal may address cognitive, psychomotor, affective, or oral health status needs:

- **Cognitive goals** target increases in the client's knowledge and understanding.
- **Psychomotor goals** focus on the client's skill development and skill mastery.
- **Affective goals** pinpoint desired changes in client values, beliefs, and attitudes.
- **Oral health status goals** address the signs and symptoms of oral disease (e.g., risk for caries, gingivitis, dentinal hypersensitivity) and reflect a desired health outcome achievable through dental hygiene interventions.

Knowledge and skill development may not result in client adherence to self-care and the resolution of an oral health condition. The client must internalize the desire and make modifications in behavior; therefore a variety of goals are necessary to achieve a positive oral health outcome.

Writing Client-Centered Goals

Adopting a format for writing client-centered goals simplifies the task (Box 22-3). Each client-centered goal should have a subject, a verb, a criterion for measurement, and a time dimension for evaluation:

- The subject is the client or client's caregiver.
- The verb is the client action desired to achieve the desired outcome; it is not the action of the dental hygienist.
- The criterion is the observable behavior or desired tangible outcome.
- Time dimension denotes when the client is to have achieved a goal. This target time may be a specific date or a statement (e.g., by next appointment, by the evaluation appointment, by end of treatment, or by next recare). Assigning a time frame to each client goal gives the client and the clinician a point of reference. Clients need time to do the following:
  - Internalize information
  - Practice new skills
  - Experience physical and attitudinal changes related to oral health and wellness
  - Assess the importance of these changes to their lifestyle
  - Adopt the new behavior

Goals evaluated too early restrict the clinician's and the client's ability to determine the impact of the care provided.

BOX 22-3

Guidelines for Writing Client-Centered Goals

Prepare each goal, or set of goals, from only one dental hygiene diagnosis.
Ensure that goals, if met, will resolve the problem reflected in the dental hygiene diagnosis.
Collaborate with dentist to ensure that the dental hygiene and dental care plans are mutually supportive.
Involve client in goal setting.
Validate that client values and is ready to achieve the delineated goals.
Write observable and measurable goals that include target times when each will be met by the client.
Use active verbs such as the following to denote client behavior expected in the goal:

affirm	detect	plan
attend	discuss	purchase
choose	eliminate	remove
communicate	exhibit	replace
complete	explain	report
decrease	finish	stop
define	guide	use
demonstrate	increase	verbalize
describe	perform	

TABLE 22-3

Sample Dental Hygiene Diagnoses with Related Client-Centered Goals

Dental Hygiene Diagnosis	Goals
Unmet human need for protection from health risk is *due to* blood pressure elevated above normal limits *as evidenced by* a reading of 160/100 mm Hg.	Client will report having blood pressure evaluated by physician before rescheduled visit on 10/5.
Unmet human need in wholesome facial image is *due to* use of chew tobacco *as evidenced by* client dissatisfaction with stained teeth.	Client will complete successfully a formal program for chew tobacco cessation by 12/30.
Unmet human need for skin and mucous membrane integrity of the head and neck is *due to* generalized subgingival biofilm accumulation in 4-mm pockets as *evidenced by* generalized gingival bleeding.	Client will exhibit a gingival bleeding score of no more than 2 by 6/15.

At least one goal should be established for each dental hygiene diagnosis (Table 22-3).

Involving the Client

Client goals are best established by the dental hygienist in collaboration with the client. Too often, individuals receiving care are referred to as "the Class II cavity preparation in treatment room 2" or "the advanced periodontal case at 4 PM." These phrases communicate insensitivity to the individual, who is central in care. The dental hygienist who views the person as the focus of attention is more likely to establish a collaborative, co-therapeutic relationship with the client. This philosophy of care sets the stage for active client participation in identifying needs, readiness to change, priorities, goals, and interventions. Clients encouraged to participate in the process of care are more likely to communicate their wants, needs, and expectations than to relinquish decision making about their care to the dental hygienist. Individuals are more likely to express commitment to a care plan and their willingness to change if they shared in the development of goals, priorities, interventions, and appointment planning (Box 22-4).

At times, specific goals are valued more highly by the dental hygienist than by the client. When this occurs, the dental hygienist explains the professional judgment and decision relative to the goal, with a clear message that the client's readiness to change, wants, and needs are equally important to the overall plan. In addition to improving compliance, respecting the client's autonomy as a co-therapist and partner in decision making is an effective risk management strategy for avoiding legal problems.

BOX 22-4

Common Phrases to Maximize Client Involvement

- "Here is a hand mirror. Let's examine your mouth together."
- "Let's take a look at the images of your mouth on the monitor and review the findings."
- "What was your primary reason for seeking dental hygiene care?"
- "Is this set of treatment priorities acceptable to you?"
- "Is this care plan acceptable to you?"
- "What would you like to achieve as a result of dental hygiene care?"
- "How will you feel if this goal is attained?"
- "Are you satisfied with the plan of care we just discussed?"
- "How important is your oral health?"
- "Where would you like me [the dental hygienist] to start?"
- "When and where is it easiest for you to clean your mouth (or your dependent's mouth)?"
- "Can you think of a better way that we can accomplish this goal?"
- "Let's compare how your gingiva looks today with how it looked 2 weeks ago."
- "What are you willing to do to keep your mouth healthy?"

Selecting Dental Hygiene Interventions

Dental hygiene interventions are the evidence-based strategies, products, and procedures that, if applied, reduce, eliminate, or prevent the oral health problem.[1] Interventions, like client-centered goals, are linked to the dental hygiene diagnosis. However, interventions address the factors contributing to the client's human need deficit. For example, various factors may contribute to a client's unmet need for a biologically sound and functional dentition, including but not limited to the following:

- Lack of knowledge about dental caries process or its infectious, chronic nature
- Lack of knowledge about self-care for dental caries prevention
- Lack of protective factors
- Skill deficit in oral self-care
- Low value on oral health
- Low self-esteem
- Inadequate financial resources
- Culture as a barrier to professional care
- Presence of other risk factors

Therefore not every client with a risk for dental caries is cared for in the same way. For dental hygiene care to achieve the desired outcomes, evidence-based interventions must address specifically the factors contributing to the client's unmet human need. For example, a dental hygiene intervention strategy for a caries risk contributor of "reduced salivary flow from medication" may include an oral self-care recommendation for incorporating a daily salivary substitute product or educating the client on the role of saliva in the caries process. Evidence-based interventions enable the clinician and client to achieve the proposed client-centered goals and resolve the client's unmet human need. Therefore professional dental hygiene care involves the careful tailoring of interventions to meet unique client needs, as directed by the dental hygiene diagnosis.

Appointment Schedule

Once the interventions have been decided, they must be put into action at planned appointments. The appointment schedule becomes a guide for implementing the proposed interventions and specifies the following:

- Number of visits
- Time needed for each visit
- Interventions to be implemented at each visit

Number of visits and sequencing of interventions at appointments vary among clinicians and clients. The following are considered when an appointment schedule is planned:

- Time needed for each intervention (e.g., self-care education, pain management)
- Logic of grouping interrelated procedures
- Status and severity of unmet human needs
- Client's tolerance for long sessions
- Client's scheduling requirements (e.g., early morning only, time limitations)

When unmet client needs and proposed care plan goals are easily attainable, the related interventions may be implemented in one visit. When diagnoses, client goals, and interventions are complex, multiple appointments are necessary.

Scheduling time for educational interventions and the sequencing of self-care strategies must be given consideration during appointment planning. Too often client education is squeezed in at the end of an appointment as time permits. Effectively addressing the client's cognitive, psychomotor, and affective needs influences oral health outcomes and the client's long-term adherence to self-care. Sequencing small increments of instruction into each visit may shape successfully the client's self-care responsibilities. For example, multiple appointment care plans may spread client education over several visits to include time to review and reinforce previously introduced self-care behaviors. Box 22-5 suggests strategies for planning client self-care.

BOX 22-5

Strategies for Care Planning Self-Care Interventions

- Include self-care education in each visit.
- Link self-care education with related dental hygiene interventions.
- Consider variables such as client dexterity, skill, knowledge, disabilities, and personal preferences.
- Involve client during self-care instruction (e.g., have client demonstrate technique intraorally, clarify knowledge with open-ended questions, verbalize opinions).
- Encourage client success (e.g., take small steps, review, monitor, remediate, reinforce).
- Include parent or caregiver when instructing a young child or client with special needs.
- Validate client's ability to obtain recommended oral health aids (e.g., cost, availability).
- Educate client to accept responsibility for health maintenance.

Care Plan Presentation

Before presenting the care plan to the client, the dental hygienist assesses the plan comprehensiveness by answering the following questions:

- Does the care plan address the client's unmet human needs relative to oral health that are amenable to or affect the outcomes of dental hygiene care?
- What are the client's cultural beliefs and behaviors?
- What might the client's response be to the care plan (e.g., interest, commitment, worry, fear, discontent, lack of enthusiasm)?
- How should the care plan be presented to elicit client cooperation?
- How can client involvement be maximized?
- What is the dental hygienist's response if the client refuses care?

When the dental hygienist is satisfied with the completeness of the dental hygiene care plan, the plan is discussed with the client. The dental hygienist must explain all aspects of the care plan and involve the client in the discussion. Presentation and discussion of the dental hygiene care plan will include the following:

- Nature of the condition
- Proposed care plan
- Risks involved (if any)
- Potential for failure
- Expected outcomes if the problem goes untreated
- Alternative procedures

Once agreed on in writing by the client, the care plan becomes a legal contract between the dental hygienist and the client.

By using the EHR and digital images during the care plan presentation, the dental hygienist can strengthen a client's understanding and acceptance of the diagnosed condition and the proposed care plan. Digital images of the client's oral assessment findings (e.g., digital radiographs, dental and periodontal chart, intraoral photographs) can be displayed on a screen and used to provide the client with visual evidence of the condition and factors contributing to the condition. In addition, interactive educational software that is linked to the EHR can be used to familiarize the client with proposed treatment strategies or expected treatment outcomes as well as demonstrate the progression of an untreated condition. The dental hygienist and client can interact with these images to ensure that the client understands the nature of the condition and the proposed care plan. If the care plan is to achieve the desired outcome, the clinician and the client must support it. Therefore enhancing a client's self-awareness of the impact of his or her condition and the proposed treatment outcomes may improve the client's acceptance of the care plan including adherence to self-care recommendations.

Most consumers expect to participate in decision making regarding their healthcare needs and know they have the right to accept or refuse services. Therefore the care plan is presented to the client before preventive and therapeutic dental hygiene services are implemented. Failure to discuss the care plan with the client can result in services being performed without the client's knowledge or informed consent.

Also, the client may not recognize the importance of self-care or may have unrealistic care expectations.

Informed Consent

The process of **informed consent** is the client's acceptance of care after a discussion with the healthcare provider regarding the proposed care plan and risks of not receiving care (Figure 22-4). Informed consent should not be viewed as a one-time activity but as an ongoing process in which the client is informed continuously and reminded of the terms of care. For informed consent to be achieved, the client must be knowledgeable about what the healthcare provider plans to do, have enough information to make a rational choice, and give permission for the plan to be carried out. The client must give consent

- For a specific treatment
- For a procedure that is legal
- Under truthful conditions (e.g., the consent cannot be obtained through fraud, deceit, misrepresentation, or trickery)

In addition to the client being informed, the client must be legally competent to give consent for care. For example, in the case of a minor, consent must be given by the parent or legal guardian (healthcare decision maker). Although **implied consent** is given when a client voluntarily comes to the oral care setting and sits in the dental chair, this consent

EXAN SCHOOL OF DENTISTRY

6170 W Lake Mead Blvd, #1305
Las Vegas, NV 89108
United States

Informed Consent to Treatment

I, Mary Gorski, hereby acknowledge that the procedures(s) or treatment(s) provided by Main Street Dental Institution will be limited to that outlined below, at my request. The recommended procedure(s) or treatment(s) have been described to me. I have been informed of the purpose of the procedure or treatment as well as alternatives to the procedure and treatment. I understand the risks, benefits and reasons for both treatment alternatives. All my questions have been satisfactorily answered. I consent to and accept the following procedure(s) or treatment(s):

1. Oral hygiene counseling
2. Periodontal debridement - UR
3. Periodontal debridement - UL
4. Periodontal debridement - LR
5. Periodontal debridement - LL
6. Local anesthesia - w/o surg
7. Periodontal re-evaluation

Signature: *Mary Gorski*
Name: Mary Gorski
Date: January 27, 2014

Provider signature: *C. Rogers*
Name: C. Rogers, RDH
Date: January 27, 2014

Witness signature: *Helen Smith*
Witness name: Helen Smith
Date: January 27, 2014

Figure 22-4. Example of informed consent in an electronic health record.

applies only to the assessment, diagnosis, and planning components of the dental hygiene process of care. The dental hygienist cannot assume that the client consents to any further care. The client's consent must be obtained for additional services to be implemented and is best documented in writing. Therefore having an automated informed consent document linked to the dental hygiene care plan ensures that this step will not be overlooked. The client's written consent is secured by having the client sign an electronic signature pad that transfers the signature to the informed consent document. This remains a permanent entry into the client's EHR.

Informed Refusal

Given all information necessary for a client to make an informed decision, the possibility exists that a client may decline all or part of the proposed care plan, such as in the following situations:

- Refusal of fluoride therapy, radiographs, or antimicrobial agents
- Noncompliance with referral to a dental specialist or physician
- Nonadherence to a specific oral self-care recommendation
- Decision to terminate care before goal attainment
- Refusal to give up a behavior that increases the risk of periodontal disease progression (e.g., tobacco use)

Although troubling, client refusal must be analyzed to determine how or why the client arrived at that decision. The clinician should engage the client in conversation, listen, and evaluate the client's reasons for declining the services. At this time the clinician may choose to reopen the discussion of treatment needs. If after this discussion the client makes an **informed refusal**, the clinician should have the client sign an electronic declaration of informed refusal that remains part of the client's EHR (Figure 22-5). A copy of the refusal form can be given or e-mailed to the client. Box 22-6 offers suggested client reasons for refusal of care, clinician actions, and documentation of informed refusal as a legal risk management strategy.

BOX 22-6

Client Reasons for Refusal of Care, Dental Hygiene Actions, and Documentation of Informed Refusal

Client Reasons

Cost of service
Fear of pain
Lack of understanding
Low value placed on dental care
Lack of dental insurance coverage

Clinician Actions

Acknowledge client's concerns
Clarify proposed plan of care
Discuss consequences of not receiving recommended care
Recommend alternative treatment options when appropriate

Documentation

Include brief explanation of recommended care
Identify specific treatment procedure being declined
List risks and consequences to client's health without treatment
Indicate date of informed refusal
Include signatures of client, dentist, and a witness

EXAN SCHOOL OF DENTISTRY

6170 W Lake Mead Blvd, #1305
Las Vegas, NV 89108
United States

Informed Refusal of Service

I, Mary Gorski, refuse Periodontal Surgical Consultation as recommended by C. Rogers, RDH. I opt to cooperate in a 3-month maintenance care appointment program for a 9 month period. The risks, benefits and reasons for both treatment alternatives have been adequately explained and my questions answered.

Signature: *Mary Gorski* | Provider signature: *C. Rogers*

Name: Mary Gorski | Name: C. Rogers, RDH

Date: January 27, 2014 | Date: January 27, 2014

Witness signature: *Helen Smith*

Witness name: Helen Smith

Date: January 27, 2014

Figure 22-5. Example of informed refusal in an electronic health record.

Procedure 22-1 Dental Hygiene Care Planning

STEPS
- Link care plan to dental hygiene diagnoses.
- Establish priorities of need.
- Set client-centered goals.
- Select dental hygiene interventions.
- Establish an appointment schedule.
- Present the dental hygiene care plan.
- Have the client sign informed consent statement for the care plan (e.g., signature pad or hard copy that is scanned in).
- Document the completion of this service to the client's EHR by entering a customized electronic note for presentation and client acceptance of the care plan and date and sign the entry; for example, "Care plan was developed to address the client's unmet human need. Clinical and radiographic findings, dental hygiene diagnosis and care plan were presented and discussed with the client. Client asked clarifying questions before acceptance of care plan." A supplemental clinical note may be entered to describe additional relevant events such as client initiated questions or comments.

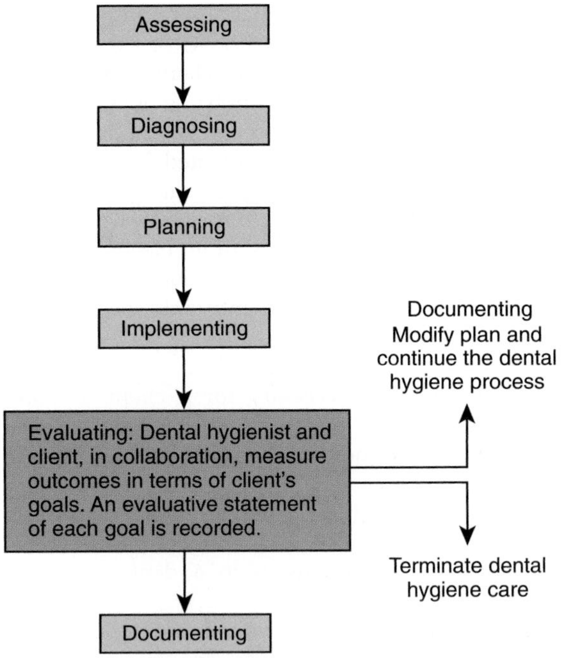

Figure 22-6. Evaluation phase of the dental hygiene process.

In some situations the client may request care that, in the opinion of the dentist or dental hygienist, is unwarranted, inappropriate, or dangerous. If the dental hygienist is faced with this dilemma, he or she should refuse to provide the care and should encourage the client to seek a second professional opinion. As a rule, the client never should be allowed to dictate treatment.

See Procedure 22-1 and corresponding Competency Form for steps for dental hygiene planning.

Evaluation

Goal of Evaluation

The evaluation goal in the process of care is to document success of the care plan intervention strategies at achieving the proposed care plan goals, that is to say, fulfillment of the client's unmet human needs related to oral health and wellness (Figure 22-6). **Evaluation** is a critical component to the successful outcome of dental hygiene care. Specifically, evaluation allows the clinician to measure the short-term achievement of client-centered goals as well as to anticipate the client's long-term prognosis in maintaining the goals achieved.

The evaluation phase of the dental hygiene process is linked inherently to each phase of care. The foundation for formulating an evaluation strategy consists of the baseline signs and symptoms that support the dental hygiene diagnosis. Evaluation strategies are defined by the client-centered goals during the planning phase and applied during the care implementation phase, at the completion of the dental hygiene care planned, and at the subsequent continued-care visit to measure the client's continued success at maintaining the previously achieved outcome. The dental hygienist employs evaluation strategies for the following:

- Ongoing monitoring of client progress during care implementation
- Determining a dental hygiene prognosis and supportive continued cycle of care at termination of the care plan
- Determining continued oral health outcomes and formulating a supportive care plan at the continued-care appointment.

See Procedure 22-2 and corresponding Competency Form for steps for integrating evaluation into client-centered care.

Ongoing Monitoring

As the appointment schedule is put into action and the dental hygiene intervention strategies are implemented, the clinician continually measures client progress toward achieving the goals, or the desired outcomes. During the initial treatment appointment, the clinician implements evaluation strategies to measure the client's newly learned cognitive and psychomotor skills and adapts oral self-care strategies to guide the client's skill development. For example, when multiple treatment appointments are planned to complete phase I nonsurgical therapy, the clinician continues to monitor (reassess) the client's progress towards goal attainment related to oral self-care behaviors, indicators of oral health and disease, and adherence to professional recommendations. At each dental hygiene care appointment, the dental hygienist shares with clients their progress towards achieving the desired care plan goals and reviews and reinforces recommended self-care strategies.

The dental hygienist and the client have an active role in evaluation. For example, a dental hygienist may have performed an intervention competently, but if the intervention or therapy was unsuccessful at helping the client achieve the desired goal, a new strategy must be considered. Therefore evaluation of a client's progress toward achieving a desired outcome is ongoing so that the clinician can do the following:

- Modify the care plan because the client is having difficulty in achieving the goal.

Procedure 22-2 Integrating Evaluation and Documentation into Client-Centered Care

STEPS

Planning

- Define care plan goals, that is, evaluative measures and methodology to address the *evidence* statement of the dental hygiene diagnosis.

Implementing

- Monitor client progress toward achieving care plan goals and modify care plan, as needed, to guide client toward success.

Evaluating

Measure attainment of care plan goals to determine the prognosis of care, to establish continued-care interval and to make referral for additional services, as needed.

CONTINUED CARE: ASSESSING

- Measure and document client's outcome at continued care, that is, the client's long-term success at maintaining the initial care plan goals achieved. When goals have not been maintained, identify contributor to the reoccurrence of the condition and continue with the process of care.

Continued Care: Diagnosing

- Define the dental hygiene diagnosis based upon reassessment findings (e.g., evidence, contributors).

Continued Care: Planning

- Restate or redefine the evaluative measures and methodology as indicated by the evidence statement of the dental hygiene diagnosis.
- Select intervention strategies to support client needs, with consideration to an identified contributor to the reoccurrence of a condition and to previous care plan strategies.

Continued Care: Implementing

Monitor client progress toward achieving care plan goals and modify care plan, as needed to guide client toward success.

Continued Care: Evaluating and documenting

Measure and document attainment of care plan goals to determine the prognosis of care, to establish continued-care interval and to make referral for additional services, as needed.

- Modify the care plan because the client is not ready to achieve the goal.
- Continue the care plan because the client needs more time to achieve the goal.
- Terminate the care plan because the client has achieved the goal.

Evaluation of Client-Centered Goals

Evaluation of client-centered goals determines whether dental hygiene care has achieved the client's unmet human need. Evaluation methods should reflect the intent of the goal

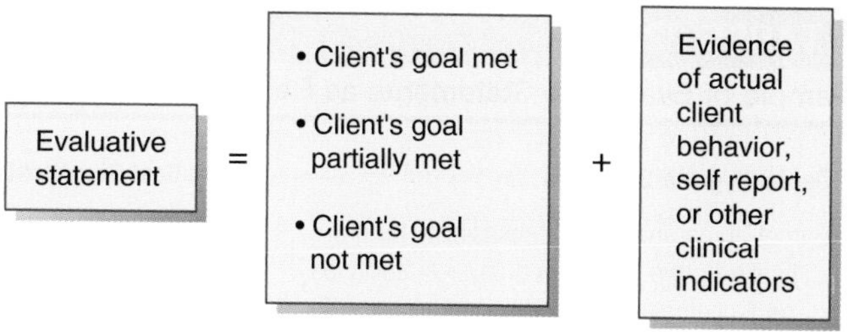

Figure 22-7. Components of an evaluative statement.

statement (e.g., cognitive, psychomotor, affective, or oral health status). An evaluation strategy may be as follows:

- Asking the client open-ended questions to measure acquisition of new knowledge (cognitive)
- Having the client demonstrate a newly learned interdental cleaning technique (psychomotor)
- Having the client report increased motivation to stop smoking by attempting to smoke fewer cigarettes per day (affective)
- Showing the client clinical improvements in oral health, such as decreased probing depth and bleeding points (oral health status)

Each client-centered goal is evaluated to determine the degree to which it has been achieved (Figure 22-7). Based on the new findings the dental hygienist determines one of the following outcomes:

- Goal met
- Goal partially met
- Goal not met

A written evaluative statement includes the dental hygienist's decision on the degree to which the goal was achieved and concrete evidence that supports the decision. This evaluation statement is recorded in the client's permanent record and signed and dated by the dental hygienist. Samples of evaluative statements as they relate to a dental hygiene diagnosis and client goal are displayed in Table 22-4.

Failure to evaluate the client's status after care leaves the clinician unaware of the impact that the care may or may not have had. From a legal perspective, failure to evaluate the outcome of care may be grounds for negligence (malpractice).[8] Unknown to the clinician and the client, the client's oral health knowledge, behaviors, oral health status, or values still may be contributing to an oral health deficit. The dental hygienist demonstrates professional practice by completing the cycle of care by measuring the extent to which client goals have been achieved and recommending continued care based on the evaluation outcomes.

Factors Influencing Client Goal Attainment

Client, dental hygienist, and clinical environment characteristics interact to enhance or hinder client goal attainment. The astute dental hygienist identifies positive and negative factors that may affect goal attainment. To facilitate the desired oral health outcome, positive factors are reinforced and negative factors managed.

Positive factors include the following:

- A client who values oral health, is motivated, and has a sense of inquiry
- A dental hygienist who maintains an evidence-based practice

TABLE 22-4
Sample of Evaluative Statements as Related to the Dental Hygiene Diagnosis and Client-Centered Goal Statements

Dental Hygiene Diagnosis	Goal Statement	Evaluative Statement
Unmet human need for responsibility for oral health is *due to* impaired physical ability *as evidenced by* a plaque-free index score of 30%.	Client will use a manual toothbrush modified with an enlarged, elongated handle at least once daily by 11/1. Client will increase plaque-free index score to 80 by 11/1.	11/1 *Goals met.* Client reported using modified toothbrush twice daily, and plaque-free index has increased to 85%.
Unmet human need for wholesome facial image is *due to* wearing a denture and halitosis *as evidenced by* client's concern with appearance of dentures, and client states that spouse complains she has frequent bad breath.	Client will meet at least two other individuals who successfully wear dentures by 12/1. Client will clean dentures, tongue, and oral cavity with appropriate brushes and dentifrice by 11/25. Client will use an ADA-accepted antimicrobial mouth rinse twice daily for 30 seconds by 11/25.	12/5 *Goal partially met.* Client met one person who successfully wears dentures and verbalized that the dentures looked natural. 11/25 *Goal met.* Client reported cleaning and rinsing mouth twice daily as directed and that spouse no longer complains about her bad breath.
Unmet human need for conceptualization and problem solving is *due to* a knowledge deficit about the periodontal disease process *as evidenced by* bleeding on probing and slight radiographic horizontal bone loss.	Client will verbalize the periodontal disease process and identify oral biofilm as a prime causative agent by 9/20.	9/20 *Goal met.* Client can describe the role of oral biofilm and the periodontal disease process.
Unmet human need for biologically sound dentition is *due to* infrequent dental visits *as evidenced by* signs of four carious lesions.	Client will follow up on a referral made to the dentist of record and have the four carious lesions diagnosed and restored by 8/1.	8/15 *Goal not met.* Client canceled dental appointment.
Unmet human need for skin and mucous membrane integrity of the head and neck is *due to* inadequate self-care *as evidenced by* gingival bleeding.	Client will eliminate bleeding upon probing by 5/8.	5/10 *Goal met.* Client no longer shows clinical signs of gingival bleeding.

- A work environment that values high-quality healthcare and offers incentives for care that meet or exceed recognized standards of practice

Table 22-5 presents common variables that can detract from quality of care. Possible dental hygiene responses are presented to initiate thinking about overcoming factors that impede goal attainment.

Modifying or Terminating the Care Plan

When evaluation reveals that the client has made little progress toward goal attainment (i.e., *goal partially met* or *goal not met*), the dental hygienist reassesses the client's readiness to change, attitudes, beliefs, and practices, and new findings are discussed with the dentist. These evaluation findings may lead to new diagnoses, revised goals, and alternative interventions. Client reassessment identifies barriers that continue to contribute to the client's unmet human needs, such as the following:

- Improperly developed client goals; goals that, if achieved, do not guarantee problem resolution
- Unrealistic goals for the client to achieve; immeasurable goals
- Care plan that does not specifically address the client's goals and unique socioethnocultural characteristics; plan contains only general information
- Care plan that has not been individualized
- Failure to evaluate
- Inadequate documentation

Once it is clear why the client has failed to achieve goals, the evaluative statement can be used to redirect the care plan.

When client goals have been met and no new problems identified, the dental hygienist and client have achieved the outcome of care. The care plan is terminated, and responsibility for continued oral health falls on the individual. Written and verbal instructions are given to the client to take home, and signs and symptoms of any possible future problems should be understood clearly by the client.

Dental Hygiene Prognosis and Continued Care

At the termination of the dental hygiene care plan, a new process-of-care cycle is recommended to the client for continued care. A continued-care interval that will support the client's efforts to maintain the oral health status achieved during active therapy is determined. The dental hygienist determines the cycle of periodic reassessment and continued care from the client's prognosis.

The dental hygiene prognosis is contingent on the following:

- Overall appraisal of the evaluative statements
- Client's continued adherence to recommended self-care
- Level of optimum oral health achieved

TABLE 22-5

Factors That May Detract from the Quality of Dental Hygiene Care

Factors	Possible Dental Hygiene Action
Client Variables	
Client who refuses to cooperate with therapeutic regimen	Determine underlying reason for observed behavior and client readiness to change; consider possible socioethnocultural factors. Counsel and educate appropriately.
Client who rarely communicates needs	Encourage client to ask questions. Be nondirective in the educational approach. Involve primary caregiver, family, or interpreter in communication process.
Dental Hygiene Variables	
Dental hygienist who gives 200% of self when others do not	Learn to leave work on time, avoid assuming work of others, leave work-related concerns at the workplace. Resolve work-related problems positively; seek strategies that improve motivation and morale of colleagues and self. View problems as challenges rather than insurmountable obstacles. Develop a realistic sense of what can be accomplished in amount of time given. When resources do not permit high-quality care and strategies do not result in positive change, explore other employment options.
Dental hygienist is bored	Seek avenues for growth and development; participate in staff development and continuing education; identify a project and become involved; initiate strategies that result in positive change. Evaluate long-term career goals; seek advanced degrees. Participate in professional associations. Search for new position.
Dental hygienist is under stress from outside concerns (e.g., illness or death of significant others; marriage, childbirth, divorce, separation; role conflict as professional, parent, spouse; significant life changes)	Evaluate whether this is the exception or the rule. Assess whether work performance is less than optimal. May need to reduce work hours rather than "cheat" clients. Seek counseling.
Environmental Variables	
Inadequate supplies and equipment	Document problems with supplies and equipment. Identify specific supply and equipment needs and discuss with employer.
Inadequate time allotted to provide high-quality care	Identify and record type of dental hygiene care required. Relate client needs and outcomes to level of care provided. Document how more time can improve client outcomes. Discuss with employer.
Inadequate respect, recognition, and reward from employer	Document incidents when respect, recognition, or reward were withheld. Talk with employer about specific incidents. Give employer suggestions on how situation can be improved. Search for new position. Initiate new policies, procedures, and training in the workplace.

Adapted from Taylor C, Lillis C, LeMone P, Lynn P: *Fundamentals of nursing,* ed 7, Philadelphia, 2011, Lippincott Williams and Wilkins.

A favorable prognosis occurs when risk for a new disease or recurrence of the previous conditions is low. A prognosis is guarded when risk for a new disease or recurrence of the previous condition is moderate to high.

Client-centered goals may be achieved successfully during active therapy; however, the prognosis may be guarded because of risk factors such as smoking or an uncontrolled systemic disease. Therefore the client and dental hygienist would select a frequent continued-care interval to monitor oral health. Periodically the continued-care plan is reviewed and adjusted to meet client needs. Continued-care appointments are scheduled at 2- to 12-month intervals based on client need.

Outcome at Continued-Care Visit

Each continued-care visit begins with reassessment of the client's human needs related to oral health to provide evidence of the long-term outcome of the previous care plan and need for supportive care. Determining *outcomes at the continued-care visit* is critical to ensuring that the client's continued success will be re-enforced and continued need deficits will be recognized and addressed. The goals of evaluation at the continued-care visit are as follows:

- Document client evidence of continued oral health from previous cycle of care.
- Identify a reoccurrence of an unmet need.
- Identify a new condition that may be present.
- Formulate a care plan that supports the client's continued needs.

Therefore the reassessment findings are applied to the previous care plan goals and the outcome at continued care is the foundation for determining a dental hygiene diagnosis and care plan for the continued-care visit (Table 22-6).

Failure to evaluate a client's progress at each subsequent continued-care visit can lead to what has been referred to as **supervised neglect**. Supervised neglect occurs when the client continues to require further dental hygiene care to achieve higher levels of oral wellness or to prevent or control oral disease progression, yet the client has been discharged erroneously from care, thinking that a healthy state was achieved. Supervised neglect can occur in practices that have a **service-oriented approach** to client care rather than a **client-centered approach**. A service-oriented practice applies the same series of services, appointment time, and continued-care recommendations to all clients. The emphasis is on completing the mechanics of a procedure, without considering the needs of the client, risk factors, and the influences of care on the client's health status. In contrast, the dental hygiene process of care supports a client-centered approach, in which the focus is the client and satisfying the client's unmet human needs related to oral disease prevention and health promotion. Integrating evaluation into the process of care demonstrates the dental hygienists' commitment to achievement of the desired client outcomes. Evaluation provides assurance that unmet needs are not overlooked or neglected.

Documentation

Documentation is the complete and accurate recording of all collected data, care planned and provided, recommendations, and other information relevant to client care. The dental hygienist documents all other components of the dental hygiene process of care (i.e., assessment, dental hygiene diagnosis, planning, implementation, and evaluation). This documentation involves objective, accurate, concise, and legible recording of all information and interactions between the client and the dental hygienist (i.e., telephone calls, emergencies, prescriptions, including dates and signatures) to ensure that subsequent providers can understand all clinical information relevant to the client of record.

The processes of **informed consent** and **informed refusal** relate to the client's acceptance or rejection of care after a discussion with the healthcare provider regarding the proposed care plan and risks of not receiving care. The client's consent or refusal must be documented in the client's permanent health record.

A legal risk management strategy is to document evidence of the process of care in each client's permanent record.[4,5] Documentation that demonstrates a relationship among assessment, diagnosis, client-centered care plan, implemented intervention strategies, and evaluative statements of outcomes is evidence that the services rendered reflected client needs. An EHR provides the aforementioned evidence of a

TABLE 22-6

Sample of Evaluative Statements for Continued Health at Continued-Care Visit and Action Plan

Phase I: Dental Hygiene Diagnosis

Unmet human need for skin and mucous membrane integrity of the head and neck is *due to* plaque retention, brushing, and flossing technique *as evidenced by* gingival pockets and moderate spontaneous bleeding.

Goal at Phase I	Evaluation at Phase I	Evaluation at Phase IV Continued-Care Visit	Action Plan
Eliminate bleeding by 6/12. Eliminate gingival pockets by 6/12.	Goal met, no bleeding points Goal met, normal probing depth	Assessment findings show evidence that goals continue to be met, client demonstrates competent brushing and flossing skills.	Share findings with client. Praise and reinforce client's self-care.

Phase I: Dental Hygiene Diagnosis

Unmet human need for protection from health risks is *due to* several predisposing caries risk factors *as evidenced by* generalized supragingival plaque, exposed root surfaces, saliva reducing medication and client reports frequent dry mouth.

Goal at Phase I	Evaluation at Phase I	Evaluation at Phase IV Continued-Care Visit	Action Plan
Client will increase plaque free score to 85% by 7/12. Client will report using OTC salivary substitute by 7/12.	Goal met, plaque-free index score increased to 90% Goal met, client reports daily use of salivary substitute	Assessment findings show evidence that goal for plaque-free index scores has not continued to be met, PFI score is 75%, client reports being inconsistent with recommended plaque removal techniques and goal for OTC salivary substitute continues to be met, client reports using daily.	Share findings with client, identify barrier to client's adherence to recommended self-care and modify diagnosis for *unmet human need for protection from health risks* to address the barrier. Formulate care plan to address the new findings.

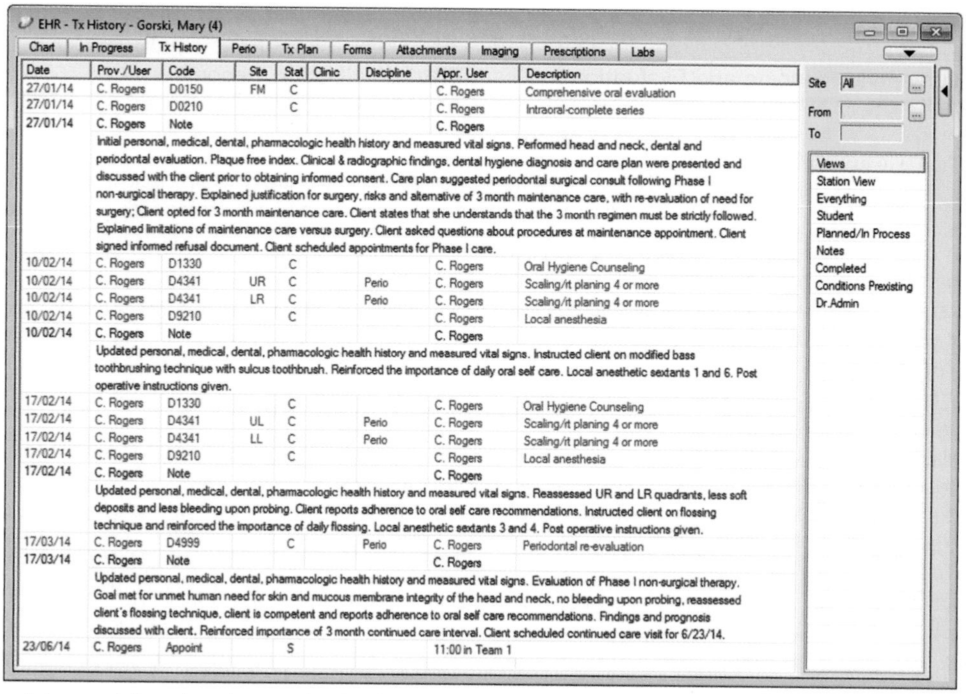

EHR - Tx History - Gorski, Mary (4)

Chart | In Progress | Tx History | Perio | Tx Plan | Forms | Attachments | Imaging | Prescriptions | Labs

Date	Prov./User	Code	Site	Stat	Clinic	Discipline	Appr. User	Description
27/01/14	C. Rogers	D0150	FM	C			C. Rogers	Comprehensive oral evaluation
27/01/14	C. Rogers	D0210		C			C. Rogers	Intraoral-complete series
27/01/14	C. Rogers	Note					C. Rogers	
	Initial personal, medical, dental, pharmacologic health history and measured vital signs. Performed head and neck, dental and periodontal evaluation. Plaque free index. Clinical & radiographic findings, dental hygiene diagnosis and care plan were presented and discussed with the client prior to obtaining informed consent. Care plan suggested periodontal surgical consult following Phase I non-surgical therapy. Explained justification for surgery, risks and alternative of 3 month maintenance care, with re-evaluation of need for surgery; Client opted for 3 month maintenance care. Client states that she understands that the 3 month regimen must be strictly followed. Explained limitations of maintenance care versus surgery. Client asked questions about procedures at maintenance appointment. Client signed informed refusal document. Client scheduled appointments for Phase I care.							
10/02/14	C. Rogers	D1330		C			C. Rogers	Oral Hygiene Counseling
10/02/14	C. Rogers	D4341	UR	C		Perio	C. Rogers	Scaling/rt planing 4 or more
10/02/14	C. Rogers	D4341	LR	C		Perio	C. Rogers	Scaling/rt planing 4 or more
10/02/14	C. Rogers	D9210		C			C. Rogers	Local anesthesia
10/02/14	C. Rogers	Note					C. Rogers	
	Updated personal, medical, dental, pharmacologic health history and measured vital signs. Instructed client on modified bass toothbrushing technique with sulcus toothbrush. Reinforced the importance of daily oral self care. Local anesthetic sextants 1 and 6. Post operative instructions given.							
17/02/14	C. Rogers	D1330		C			C. Rogers	Oral Hygiene Counseling
17/02/14	C. Rogers	D4341	UL	C		Perio	C. Rogers	Scaling/rt planing 4 or more
17/02/14	C. Rogers	D4341	LL	C		Perio	C. Rogers	Scaling/rt planing 4 or more
17/02/14	C. Rogers	D9210		C			C. Rogers	Local anesthesia
17/02/14	C. Rogers	Note					C. Rogers	
	Updated personal, medical, dental, pharmacologic health history and measured vital signs. Reassessed UR and LR quadrants, less soft deposits and less bleeding upon probing. Client reports adherence to oral self care recommendations. Instructed client on flossing technique and reinforced the importance of daily flossing. Local anesthetic sextants 3 and 4. Post operative instructions given.							
17/03/14	C. Rogers	D4999		C		Perio	C. Rogers	Periodontal re-evaluation
17/03/14	C. Rogers	Note					C. Rogers	
	Updated personal, medical, dental, pharmacologic health history and measured vital signs. Evaluation of Phase I non-surgical therapy. Goal met for unmet human need for skin and mucous membrane integrity of the head and neck, no bleeding upon probing, reassessed client's flossing technique, client is competent and reports adherence to oral self care recommendations. Findings and prognosis discussed with client. Reinforced importance of 3 month continued care interval. Client scheduled continued care visit for 6/23/14.							
23/06/14	C. Rogers	Appoint		S			11:00 in Team 1	

Site: All

From

To

Views: Station View, Everything, Student, Planned/In Process, Notes, Completed, Conditions Prexisting, Dr.Admin

Figure 22-8. Example of documentation of services rendered with evidence of the process of care, informed consent to treatment, and informed refusal of service in an electronic health record.

client-centered process of care. Documentation of each component of the process of care in the client's EHR is the best defense against a client's accusation of negligence (Figure 22-8).

Documentation of services rendered represents a legal record of all services performed for the client. Services rendered should be recorded in the client's EHR at the time they are performed. The method of documenting the services rendered may include electronically entering a corresponding **dental procedure code** or a **customized electronic note** and supplementing the entry with a typed narrative describing relevant events of client care. Dental procedure codes denote standardized assessment and treatment codes used by the dental profession to indicate services rendered as defined by the American Dental Association (ADA) Current Dental Terminology (CDT).[6] A customized electronic note is designed specially by an institution to document a frequently used entry to a client's EHR.

All entries must be accurate and factual and provide enough detail to describe how the client progressed through each phase of care to attain the proposed desired outcome. The services rendered and the client's response to those services should be documented by the clinician who performed the services, signed, and dated. The clinician signature may be entered into the EHR by using a signature pad. If an error in documentation is identified after storage, the clinician may correct the error by marking the entry as a *mistaken entry* and entering the correct information.[7] The new entry must be dated and initialed by the clinician.

Table 22-7 suggests guidelines for documentation of care planning and evaluation in the client's EHR under "Services Rendered."

Scenarios 22-1 and 22-2 and care plans are provided as examples.

Additional scenarios can be found on the website for the following examples:

- Preliminary Phase: Emergency Care
- Phase I: Nonsurgical Therapy
- Phase I: Evaluation of Nonsurgical Therapy
- Phase IV: Maintenance Therapy

See Procedure 22-3 and corresponding Competency Form for steps for evaluation of care.

Procedure 22-3 Evaluation of Care

STEPS

1. Identify evaluative criteria and expected outcomes of care.
2. Collect evidence to determine whether goals are being met.
3. Interpret and summarize the findings.
4. Write an evaluative statement.
5. Propose continued care options.
6. Document the completion of this service to the client's EHR by entering a customized electronic note of services rendered for outcome of care and recommendation for continued care, date and sign the entry; for example, "Updated client health history, reassessed client for changes in oral health status and oral health skills. *Goals Met for unmet human need for skin and mucous membrane integrity of the head and neck.*" Add a supplemental clinical note that supports the aforementioned custom note; for example, "follow-up gingival and periodontal assessment indicated that the gingival tissue is pinker and firmer, no bleeding upon probing. Reassessed client's flossing technique and client is competent. Client reports adherence to oral self-care recommendations." Continued-care interval: 6 months.

TABLE 22-7

Guidelines for Documenting Planning and Evaluation in Client Electronic Health Record

Services Rendered	Evidence of Services Rendered
Assessment	Include demographic client data; personal, medical, dental, pharmacologic health history; vital signs; head and neck examination findings; dental and periodontal examination findings; caries risk assessment; oral self-care practices; client chief concern; client readiness to change; oral habits.
Dental hygiene diagnosis	Document a statement of client need supported by related clinical evidence and contributing factors.
Care plan	Document the proposed care plan and a statement of client-centered goals, evidence-based interventions, and supportive appointment schedule. Summarize client involvement in development of care plan.
Presentation of care plan to client	Document client-clinician discussion of proposed care plan, valid informed consent and/or informed refusal.
Implementation of care plan	Document, in detail, implementation of all care provided in chronologic order of appointments (e.g., client self-care education, cognitive and psychomotor skill development, adherence with recommendations; oral self-care aids dispensed for home use; client-clinician interactions; periodontal debridement; anesthesia). Include the client's adherence to the appointment schedule (e.g., late arrival; canceled, failed appointments) and when appointment was rescheduled. Record confirmation of appointments by phone, mail, or electronic communication. Document a narrative of clinician's periodic reassessment to monitor progress toward achieving proposed outcomes. Document recommended continued-care interval and referral; indicate that this was discussed with client.
Evaluative statement of outcome	Document complete evaluative statement of outcome and summary of evaluation methodology. Describe clinician action based on outcome of care. Indicate that outcome and prognosis were discussed with client.
Date and signature of clinician	Conclude each entry with date the service was provided (e.g., month/day/year) and signature of clinician who provided the service and completed the documentation of the services rendered (they should be the same person).

CLIENT EDUCATION TIPS

- Explain the importance of developing a care plan.
- Explain how the dental hygiene care plan is integrated with the overall dental care plan.
- Incorporate client's chief complaint; readiness to change; goals, needs, preferences, and values into the care plan.
- Involve the client in the development of client-centered goals (augments commitment). Use electronic imaging technology and educational materials to enhance clients' awareness of unmet needs and their responsibility in achieving the desired care plan outcomes.
- Explain that clinical outcomes of care will be related to the original goals.
- Reinforce the dental hygienist and client partnership as co-therapists to achieve client-centered goals.
- Explain that the client's readiness to change, wants, and needs are essential to the overall success of the plan.

LEGAL, ETHICAL, AND SAFETY ISSUES

Inherent in the process of care is the legal and ethical responsibility of healthcare providers to do the following:

- Complete a comprehensive assessment of client unmet needs.
- Formulate a diagnosis and care plan based on that assessment.
- Communicate the recommended care plan to the client.
- Secure informed consent before implementing the care plan.
- Implement the care plan.
- Monitor the client's progress toward achieving desired oral health outcomes.
- Evaluate the outcome of care.
- Recommend a continued-care schedule.
- Keep adequate client records that are legible, dated, and signed with the title of the individual making the entry.
- Document clinical and radiographic findings as evidence that the diagnosis and care plan are based on client needs.
- Provide evidence of medical consultation, when needed, and written response with information requested.
- Provide evidence of informed consent before implementation of care, signed and dated.
- Provide evidence of informed refusal when client refuses care or recommendations, signed and dated.
- Document self-care education, status of client compliance, failed or canceled appointments, postoperative instructions provided, modifications made in care plan and supportive facts, referrals, and continued-care schedule.
- Never release client record without written authorization from the client or court subpoena.
- Never share personal password or electronic signature with another member of the staff.[7]

SCENARIO 22-1

CLIENT WITH PLAQUE-INDUCED GINGIVITIS AND DENTAL CARIES AND SAMPLE DENTAL HYGIENE CARE PLAN

Susie S., a healthy 19-year-old single woman without dental insurance, is a second-year student living at the local university. Her last preventive dental appointment was 3 years ago and included a prophylaxis and four bitewing radiographs. She brushes twice daily with fluoride toothpaste and flosses occasionally. Her chief complaint is, "I hate the brown stain on my teeth."

Clinical assessment reveals soft tissues within normal limits, Class I malocclusion with a slight anterior overbite, and crowding in mandibular anteriors. Gingival evaluation indicates localized slight papillary inflammation, sulcus depths within 3 mm, no attachment loss, and slight bleeding on probing in sextant 5. Plaque-free index is 85%. Dental examination indicates that 30 teeth are present, including partially erupted third molars (No. 17/No. 32), extrinsic brown stain from coffee, and slight lingual and proximal calculus in sextant 5. No restorations are present; molars have pit-and-fissure sealants. Bitewing radiographs reveal Class II carious lesions on the mesial surface of teeth 2 and 15 and incipient carious lesions on the mesial surface of teeth 19 and 30. Susie reports that she drinks three to four cups of coffee with 2 teaspoons of sugar daily.

Dental Hygiene Client Goals	Interventions	Evaluation
Dental Hygiene Diagnosis *Unmet human need* for skin and mucous membrane integrity of head and neck is *due to* anterior malocclusion, plaque retention in sextant 5 *as evidenced by* localized papillary inflammation, bleeding on probing, plaque-free score of 85%.		
The Client Will		
Demonstrate proper flossing technique by end of appointment. Eliminate bleeding and inflammation in sextant 5 by next continued-care visit.	Instruct client on relationship between oral biofilm and gingival inflammation. Review client's flossing skills. Perform root debridement.	*Goal met,* client's flossing technique modified. *Goal met,* no evidence of bleeding or inflammation.
Dental Hygiene Diagnosis *Unmet human need* for biologically sound and functional dentition is *due to* frequent coffee and sucrose intake *as evidenced by* smooth surface carious lesions and extrinsic stain.		
The Client Will		
Decrease frequency of sucrose and coffee intake by choosing a noncariogenic coffee sweetener or an alternative beverage with a noncariogenic sweetener by next continued-care visit. Use daily Rx brush-on 1.1% sodium fluoride and therapeutic doses of xylitol to decrease risk for future smooth-surface carious lesions by next continued-care visit. Have current carious lesions restored by next continued-care visit. Use a 0.12% chlorhexidine mouth rinse twice daily for 2 weeks after the restorations are placed to eliminate infection from *Streptococcus mutans* (do not use fluoride at this time).	Instruct client on impact of oral biofilm and frequent sucrose exposure to the caries process. Instruct client on role of fluoride, chlorhexidine, and xylitol in prevention of caries risk. Perform coronal polishing to remove extrinsic stain. Refer to dentist of record for restorative treatment. Recommend use of power toothbrush and an ADA-approved whitening toothpaste to control stain.	*Goal met,* carious lesions restored and no evidence of new lesions. *Goal met,* client reports using daily Rx brush-on 1.1% sodium fluoride, therapeutic levels of xylitol, and noncariogenic sweetener. *Goal met,* client reports completing 2-week regimen of 0.12% chlorhexidine gluconate.

Appointment Schedule

CDT-2013 Dental Procedure Code	Appointment 1 (50 minutes)
D0150	Initial personal, medical, dental, pharmacologic health history, measure vital signs; perform comprehensive oral assessment: head and neck, dental and periodontal; determine plaque-free or gingival index.
D0274	Bitewing radiographs: four films.
	Inform client of clinical findings, diagnosis, and recommended care plan; obtain informed consent (or informed refusal).
D1330	Oral self-care instruction: flossing.
	Client education: oral biofilm and gingival health and caries process, benefits of daily fluoride to prevent smooth surface caries, benefits of a power toothbrush and whitening toothpaste. Use of chlorhexidine mouth rinse to eliminate source of caries infection.
	Discuss need to keep the chlorhexidine rinse and fluoride separate.
D1110	Adult prophylaxis: full-mouth debridement, coronal polishing with mild abrasive.
	Continued-care interval: 6 months.

SCENARIO 22-2

CLIENT WITH PLAQUE-INDUCED GINGIVITIS MODIFIED BY SYSTEMIC FACTORS (PREGNANCY-ASSOCIATED GINGIVITIS) AND SAMPLE DENTAL HYGIENE CARE PLAN

Renee B. is a 29-year-old married woman with a 5-year-old child. Renee, 8 months pregnant and in good health, is taking Pepcid at bedtime for heartburn. She reports that her pregnancy is becoming uncomfortable.

Her last oral prophylaxis was 6 months ago and included oral hygiene instruction. Full-mouth radiographs were taken 1 year ago, and findings were within normal limits. She brushes once daily and flosses sometimes. Her chief complaint is, "My gums are bleeding when I brush and I always have a bad taste in my mouth."

Clinical examination reveals soft tissues within normal limits, Class I malocclusion, generalized moderate marginal gingival erythema and edema, moderately bulbous interdental papilla, spontaneous heavy bleeding on probing, and probing depths of 4 to 5 mm with no attachment loss evident. Plaque-free index is 75.8%. Generalized subgingival calculus can be felt with the explorer and probe; supragingival calculus is visible on the mandibular anterior lingual teeth and facial surface of the maxillary molars. Dental examination reveals 28 teeth present (third molars were previously extracted) and multiple Class I and II amalgam restorations.

Dental Hygiene Client Goal	Interventions	Evaluation
Dental Hygiene Diagnosis *Unmet human need* for conceptualization and problem solving is *due to* client's lack of knowledge about pathogenicity of oral biofilm *as evidenced by* the client's bleeding gums when brushing.		
The Client Will		
Explain composition of oral biofilm and impact on soft tissue and halitosis by 4/16.	Instruct client on composition of oral biofilm and impact on gingival tissues, tongue, and halitosis.	*Goal met,* client verbalized role of oral biofilm and effects on oral health.
Verbalize how pregnancy can enhance gingivitis in the presence of oral biofilm by 4/16.	Instruct client on how pregnancy can enhance the incidence of gingivitis and periodontal disease progression, and how premature birth and low birth weight babies are linked to oral inflammation.	*Goal met,* client explained pregnancy-associated gingivitis and how oral inflammation may be linked to preterm birth.
Dental Hygiene Diagnosis *Unmet human need* for wholesome facial image is *due to* plaque retention plus elevated hormone levels *as evidenced by* plaque-free index of 75.8%, gingivitis, and client's concern about bad taste in her mouth and bad breath.		
The Client Will		
Recognize the importance of daily management of oral biofilm for oral and systemic health by 4/26.	Assist client in identifying plaque-retentive sites with bleeding points and disclosing agent.	*Goal met,* client reports daily flossing, mouth rinsing, and extended brushing time. Client also reports that the bad taste in her mouth is gone.
Use an ADA-accepted antimicrobial mouth rinse twice daily to control oral biofilm and gingivitis by 4/26.	Instruct client on the value of using an ADA-accepted mouth rinse to help control plaque and gingivitis.	*Goal met,* client increased plaque-free index score to 95%.
Increase plaque-free index score to 90% by 4/26.		
Dental Hygiene Diagnosis *Unmet human need* for skin and mucous membrane integrity of the head and neck is *due to* plaque retention, infrequent flossing, and hormones associated with pregnancy *as evidenced by* gingival pockets, spontaneous bleeding.		
The Client Will		
Decrease bleeding by 80% by 5/10.	Instruct client on modified Bass toothbrushing.	*Goal partially met,* bleeding points decreased by 70%.
Decrease probing depths by 1 mm by 5/10.	Use sulcus toothbrush for the disruption of subgingival plaque biofilm.	*Goal met,* decreased gingival pockets by 1 mm.
	Instruct client on flossing to disrupt proximal bacterial plaque biofilm.	
	Instruct client on use of an ADA-accepted antimicrobial dentifrice and mouth rinse to control plaque and gingivitis.	
	Perform therapeutic periodontal debridement: one visit for quadrants 1 and 4; second visit for quadrants 2 and 3.	
	Perform coronal polishing.	

SCENARIO 22-2

CLIENT WITH PLAQUE-INDUCED GINGIVITIS MODIFIED BY SYSTEMIC FACTORS (PREGNANCY-ASSOCIATED GINGIVITIS) AND SAMPLE DENTAL HYGIENE CARE PLAN—cont'd

Dental Hygiene Client Goal	Interventions	Evaluation
Dental Hygiene Diagnosis		
Unmet human need for protection from health risk is *due to* risk of orthostatic hypotension *as evidenced by* client report that her pregnancy is becoming uncomfortable in the eighth month.		
The Client Will		
Identify comfortable chair position at each dental hygiene appointment to prevent orthostatic hypotension.	Position client in semi-upright position (45-degree angle) to alleviate fetal pressure on vena cava. Give client a pillow placed under the right hip while she is in chair.	Goal met, client was asymptomatic of orthostatic hypotension during appointment.

Appointment Schedule

CDT-2013 Dental Procedure Code[8]	Phase I: Nonsurgical Therapy Appointment 1 (1 hour)—4/16
D0150	Update personal, health, dental, pharmacologic health history; measure vital signs; perform comprehensive oral evaluation: head and neck, dental, and periodontal; determine plaque-free index.
	Inform client of diagnosis and recommended care plan, including clinical findings, and obtain informed consent.
D1330	Oral self-care instruction: modified Bass toothbrushing technique.
	Client education: oral biofilm, gingivitis, halitosis, hormone-influenced gingivitis. Instruct client on use of an ADA-accepted antimicrobial dentifrice and mouth rinse to control plaque and gingivitis.
D4341	Therapeutic periodontal debridement of quadrants 1 and 4.
Appointment 2 (1 hour)—4/26	
	Update health history and measure vital signs. Assess tissue response to self-care and periodontal debridement of quadrants 1 and 4, determine plaque-free index.
D1330	Self-care instruction: review toothbrushing if needed and instruct on flossing.
D4341	Therapeutic periodontal debridement of quadrants 2 and 3.
	Phase I: Evaluation of Response to Nonsurgical Therapy Appointment 3 (1 hour)—5/10
D4999*	Update health history and measure vital signs. Assess all quadrants for tissue response to self-care and periodontal debridement, determine plaque-free index.
D1330	Review and reinforce oral self-care.
	In preparation for new baby, dispense literature on preventive oral health for infants, vertical transmission of caries from mother to infant, early childhood caries.
D1110	Adult prophylaxis to remove residual calculus (if any) and extrinsic stain with mild abrasive.
	Continued-care interval: 3 months.

*Indicates unspecified periodontal procedure, may be used to report a periodontal re-evaluation.[7]

- Recognize ethical and legal responsibilities of record keeping including guidelines outlined in state regulations and statutes.
- Ensure compliance with the federal Health Information Portability and Accountability Act (HIPAA).
- Respect and protect the confidentiality of client information displayed on an unattended monitor in your operatory.[7]

KEY CONCEPTS

- A dental hygiene care plan is an evidence-based, client-centered written proposal to meet the unmet human needs of a client that are related to oral health and within the scope of dental hygiene practice.
- The dental hygiene diagnosis provides the foundation for care plan development.
- The care plan reflects the dental hygiene diagnosis, client-centered goals, dental hygiene interventions, detailed appointment schedule, and expected outcomes.
- A well-formulated and executed care plan increases the likelihood of a positive outcome in the dental hygiene care process.
- Evaluation is a critical component of the dental hygiene process and a necessary step to document evidence of care plan success in achieving a desired outcome in the client's oral health status.

- Documentation of the dental hygiene process of care in the client's record is a management strategy to minimize the risk of litigation.
- Without evaluation, a dental hygienist's contribution to the oral health of the client is invisible and undervalued.

CRITICAL THINKING EXERCISES

Client Profile 1

James W., a 50-year-old man, is a long-haul truck driver who is taking hydrochlorothiazide for hypertension, drinks two to three cups of coffee per day, and smokes one pack of cigarettes per day.

Dental History: James' last dental appointment was 1 month ago for extraction of tooth 2, which was periodontally involved; before this time, 10 years had passed since his last dental appointment. He brushes once daily with fluoride toothpaste, and his chief complaint is, "I have pain in the upper left molar region, and I do not want to lose any more teeth."

Assessment: Clinical examination reveals nicotine stomatitis, Class II malocclusion with a moderate overbite, and a coated tongue. Dental examination reveals missing third molars and maxillary right second molar; generalized moderate brown stain; slight subgingival calculus; localized moderate supragingival calculus in sextant 5; and Class I and II amalgam restorations.

Gingival and periodontal assessment findings reveal generalized moderate marginal inflammation, generalized slight recession; localized moderate recession on facial surfaces of sextants 3 and 4; bleeding on probing; pocket depths of 3 to 5 mm with clinical attachment loss at 4 to 5 mm; Class II and III furcations and Class I mobility on teeth No. 14 and No. 15. Full-mouth periapical and vertical bitewing radiographs show evidence of a recurrent carious lesion on tooth 30 and root caries on the distal surface of tooth 14, generalized moderate horizontal bone loss in molar regions, and localized vertical bone loss on the distal surface of tooth 14.

1. Formulate a comprehensive dental hygiene care plan for this client.
2. Refer to Table 22-1 and identify the phase of care that is being planned and implemented for this client.
3. Discuss the client's likely prognosis after implementation of the dental hygiene care plan and propose a continued-care interval to support the client's needs.

Client Profile 2

Mrs. Wilton is a 57-year-old woman who has been married for 35 years. She cares for her two grandchildren, Dayne, age 2, and Katie, age 4, 3 days per week while the children's mother works.

Health History: Mrs. Wilton has type 2 diabetes, controlled by oral hypoglycemic medication and diet, and hypertension, controlled by Avapro. She sees her physician on a regular basis for her diabetes and hypertension.

Dental History: Mrs. Wilton has not seen a dentist in 7 years. She is a client of record at the local university dental hygiene clinic where she has been treated every 4 to 6 months for the past 4 years because she does not have dental insurance. At each past continued-care appointment, she has had generalized slight chronic periodontitis. Each past care plan has indicated the dental hygiene diagnosis: "Human need for skin and mucous membrane integrity of the head and neck *due to* inadequate oral biofilm management by the client and generalized moderate calculus *as evidenced by* generalized bleeding on probing." The care plans have emphasized the same intervention strategies (i.e., modified Bass toothbrushing and flossing followed by a series of quadrant root debridement appointments). Appointment notes indicate that the client keeps her scheduled appointments and properly demonstrates recommended toothbrushing and flossing skills; however, she states she does not like to floss.

Supplemental Notes: Mrs. Wilton arrives today at the dental hygiene clinic for a scheduled continued-care visit. No changes have occurred in her health history; all medications are taken as prescribed; blood pressure is within normal limits. Assessment findings reveal no change in oral health status since the last continued-care appointment. Reason for her visit: "to have my teeth cleaned."

1. Considering the dental hygiene process of care, what legal and ethical issues are present?
2. Discuss possible factors influencing why the client's oral health has *not* improved at each continued-care visit.
3. Suggest alternative dental hygiene diagnoses and formulate a dental hygiene care plan.
4. Role-play a clinician's presentation of the care plan to the client for informed consent.
5. Complete services rendered notes for this scenario that document evidence of the dental hygiene process of care including assessment, diagnosis, and care plan presentation for informed consent.

REFERENCES

1. Darby M, Walsh M: *Application of the human needs conceptual model to dental hygiene practice.* Presented at the 14th International Symposium on Dental Hygiene, Florence, Italy, July 1998.
2. Menachemi N, Collum T: Benefits and drawbacks of electronic health record systems. *Risk Management and Healthcare Policy* 4:47, 2011.
3. Hill HK, Stewart DCL, Ash JS: Health information technology systems profoundly impact users: a case study in dental schools. *J Dent Educ* 74(4):434, 2010.
4. American Dental Hygienists' Association (ADHA): *Standards of practice position paper*, Chicago, 2008, ADHA.
5. Marsh L: Legal issues in dental hygiene. *Access* 24(3):19, 2010.
6. American Dental Association: *CDT 2013 Procedure Codes*, 2012, American Dental Association.
7. Taylor C, Lillis C, LeMone P, et al: Documentation, reporting, conferring, and using informatics. In *Fundamentals of nursing: the art and science of nursing care*, ed 7, Philadelphia, 2011, Lippincott, Williams & Wilkins.
8. American Dental Association: *The ADA practical guide to dental procedure codes, 2011-2012 CDT Current Dental Terminology*, 2010, American Dental Association.

EVOLVE RESOURCES

Please visit http://evolve.elsevier.com/Darby/hygiene for additional practice and study support tools.

CHAPTER 23

Toothbrushing

Denise M. Bowen

COMPETENCIES

1. **Describe characteristics of acceptable manual toothbrush designs.**
2. **Describe characteristics and modes of action of power toothbrush designs.**
3. **Discuss toothbrushing instruction, including differentiation among toothbrushing methods including indications, limitations, and impact on oral tissues.**
4. **Discuss soft- and hard-tissue lesions, including factors that cause tissue lesions, and the significance of a clean tongue and toothbrush.**
5. **Discuss the dental hygiene process of care and toothbrushing, including the sharing of evidence-based decision making with clients regarding selection and use of a toothbrush based on specific client needs.**

Self-care or homecare refers to behaviors that clients perform to achieve, maintain, or promote health or oral health. Oral biofilm or plaque control is the daily removal of bacteria, biofilm, and debris from the teeth, tongue, and adjacent oral tissues as part of an overall preventive program to prevent or control oral diseases. Although 100% removal is not possible, the normal host can tolerate some oral biofilm.

Mechanical removal of oral biofilm via toothbrushing is the most common means for plaque control. Mechanical cleansing devices such as toothbrushes are indispensable because, to date, no chemotherapeutic agents totally prevent the formation of oral biofilm in the mouth.

Toothbrushing also provides for twice daily fluoride application in toothpaste as another important part of a disease prevention program.

Manual Toothbrushes

The most commonly used device for removing oral biofilm, the manual toothbrush, is well designed to remove plaque from the facial, lingual, and occlusal tooth surfaces (Box 23-1). Although many features of toothbrushes and toothbrushing methods have been studied, evidence has not demonstrated that any individual manual toothbrush design is consistently superior in removing plaque or preventing and controlling periodontal diseases.[1,2]

Parts of the Toothbrush

Manual toothbrushes have several parts, as follows (Figure 23-1):

- Head—Contains the filaments (bristles) and is approximately 1 to $\frac{1}{4}$ inches (25.4 to 31.8 mm) long and $\frac{5}{16}$ to $\frac{3}{8}$ inch (7.9 to 9.5 mm) wide. Head size is selected based on the size of the client's mouth rather than age. The head should be large enough to remove plaque efficiently and small enough to reach to all areas of the mouth. Contemporary toothbrush head designs are less rectangular and more tapered and oval in shape.
- Handle—Used for grasping the toothbrush by the hand during use; may be aligned in a straight plane with the toothbrush head, angled like a dental mirror, curved, or offset. Consumers may select their preferred handle shape for comfortable use.
- Shank—Connects the head of the toothbrush to the handle.

Toothbrush Filament Design

The toothbrush head contains tufts typically composed of nylon filaments. Tufts are individual bundles of filaments secured in a hole in the toothbrush head. Number and length of filaments in a tuft, number of tufts, and arrangement of tufts vary with toothbrush designs. Less commonly, in-mold tufting has filaments inserted individually into the head. The brushing plane (surface of the toothbrush head used for cleaning the teeth and tissues) may be flat with all of filaments the same length, bilevel, multilevel, rippled, or crisscrossed with tufts angled in different directions (Figure 23-2).

Filament design affects toothbrushing efficacy, particularly in difficult-to-access approximal areas. Angled, rather than vertical, bristle tuft arrangements have been shown to contribute significantly to more effective plaque removal because they reach farther interproximally.[3] Toothbrushing alone does not clean the entire interproximal tooth surface, so interdental cleaning augments toothbrushing for thorough biofilm removal.

It is unclear whether end-rounding of bristles has a significant benefit for clients' safety. Some toothbrushes that claim to have end-rounding do not have uniformly rounded bristles. Dental professionals often recommend that clients use toothbrushes with soft nylon filaments, believing that they are less traumatic to the oral tissues and remove as much or more plaque than hard toothbrushes; however, the influence of bristle stiffness on plaque removal and trauma remains unclear.[1] Nylon toothbrush filaments have a range of diameters from 0.15 mm to 0.4 mm. Stiffness is related primarily to the filament's diameter and length; shorter and wider diameters result in a harder toothbrush. Traditionally, most filaments have been 10 to 12 mm long. Many manufacturers vary the type, length, and diameter of the filaments within a single toothbrush head. Improvement in efficacy can be achieved with a multilevel bristle tuft configuration.[3]

BOX 23-1

Characteristics of an Effective Toothbrush

Size, shape, weight, and texture meet individual user's needs
Easily held, used, and disinfected
Inexpensive and durable
Functional (flexible, comfortable, effective)
Appropriate strength, rigidity, and weight

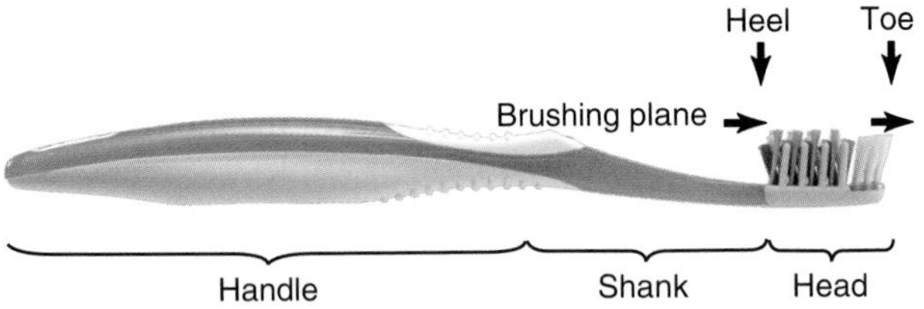

Figure 23-1. Parts of a manual toothbrush. (Courtesy Procter & Gamble, Professional and Scientific Relations, Cincinnati, Ohio.)

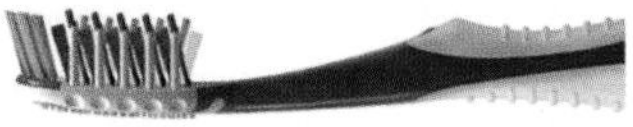

Figure 23-2. Crisscross bristle design of the Oral-B CrossAction Pro-Health toothbrush. (Courtesy Procter & Gamble, Professional and Scientific Relations, Cincinnati, Ohio.)

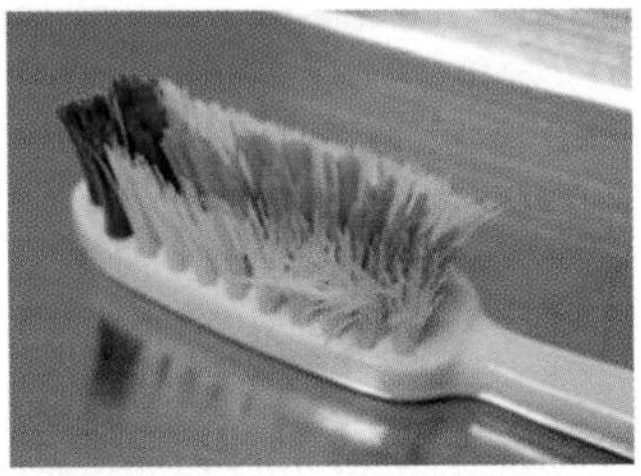

Figure 23-3. Worn out toothbrush.

Toothbrush Bristle Wear

Worn toothbrushes have bristles that are splaying, bending, curling, spreading, or matting (Figure 23-3). Although it makes sense that a worn toothbrush would reduce toothbrush efficacy, evidence supporting this claim is inconclusive. Filament wear varies considerably with different individuals over time; therefore, rather than using the usual 2 to 3 months as an indicator for toothbrush replacement, clients must learn to identify visible signs of worn filaments.

Power Toothbrushes

Rechargeable power toothbrushes, defined by their modes of action, typically are activated by electricity or battery (Table 23-1). When used properly, power and manual toothbrushes are effective in removing plaque and preventing and controlling gingival disease. In a Cochrane systematic review and meta-analysis (Box 23-2), power toothbrushes using several different modes of action were compared with a traditional manual toothbrush (rectangular head with a flat brushing plane). Only the oscillating-rotating design power brush significantly outperformed the manual toothbrush in plaque reduction (7%) and gingivitis reduction (17%) in both short- and long-term studies.[4] Battery-powered toothbrushes and less-expensive rechargeable models increase accessibility of power toothbrushing.

Power toothbrushes have been shown to be safe and effective; therefore a power toothbrush is suitable for almost any client (Box 23-3). Power toothbrushes have a high level of client acceptance, and clients can be assured that power brushes are at least as effective as manual and safe to use.[1,4-5]

BOX 23-2

The Cochrane Collaboration

THE COCHRANE COLLABORATION
Preparing, maintaining and disseminating systematic reviews of the effects of health care

- An international, nonprofit organization dedicated to improving healthcare decision making through the publication of independently conducted health-related systematic reviews
- Makes these reviews widely available through the *Cochrane Database of Systematic Reviews*
- Qualified healthcare professionals conduct the reviews with editorial teams who help ensure high, rigorous research standards

BOX 23-3

Power Toothbrushes: Indications for Use

Any individual, but particularly those with the following:
- Fixed orthodontic appliances
- Decalcification
- Uncontrolled oral biofilm and periodontal diseases
- Extensive prosthodontics or dental implants
- Dexterity and motivational challenges
- Gingival recession or noncarious cervical hard-tissue lesions
- Caregiver responsibilities

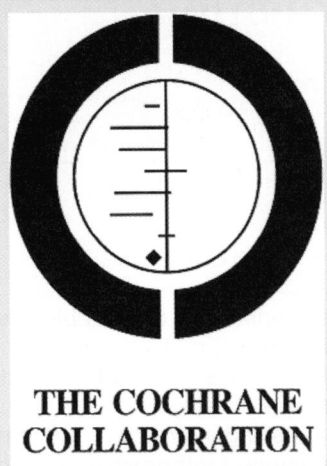

TABLE 23-1

Power Toothbrushes: General Modes of Action

Action	Description	Examples	Diagram
Side-to-side	Brush head that moves laterally	Early power models and sonic	
Oscillating-rotating	Entire brush head rotates in one direction and then the other; some models also pulsate in and out	Oral-B Professional Care and Vitality Conair Opticlean	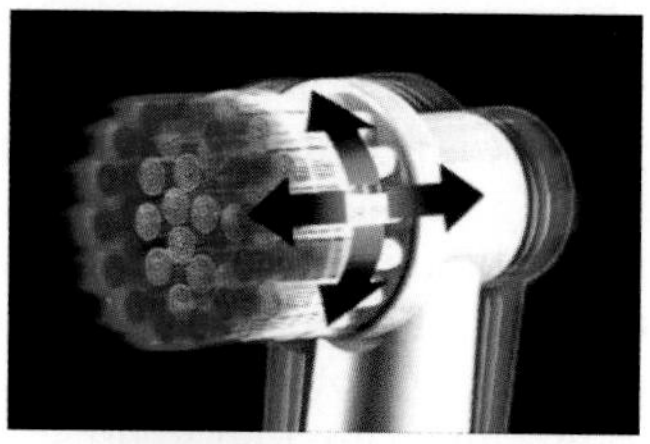
Circular	Entire brush head rotates in one direction	Zila Rotadent Plus*	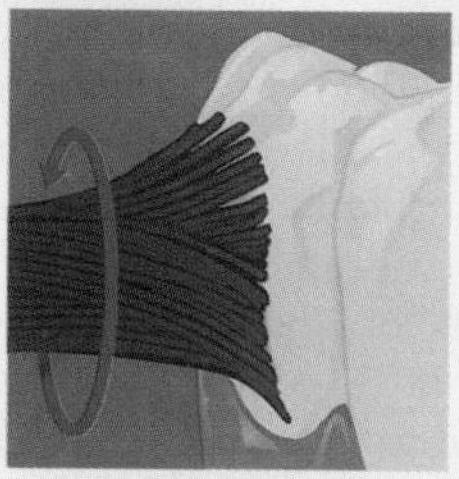
Sonic	Bristles vibrate side to side or up and down with high amplitude and high frequency; sound waves cause fluid motion	Philips Sonicare[†] Oral-B Sonic Waterpik Sensonic Colgate 360° SonicPower	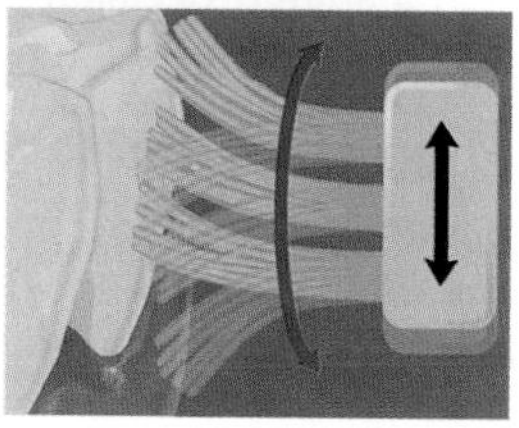
Ultrasonic	Bristles vibrate at ultrasonic frequencies (>20 kHz)	Emmi-dent Smilex	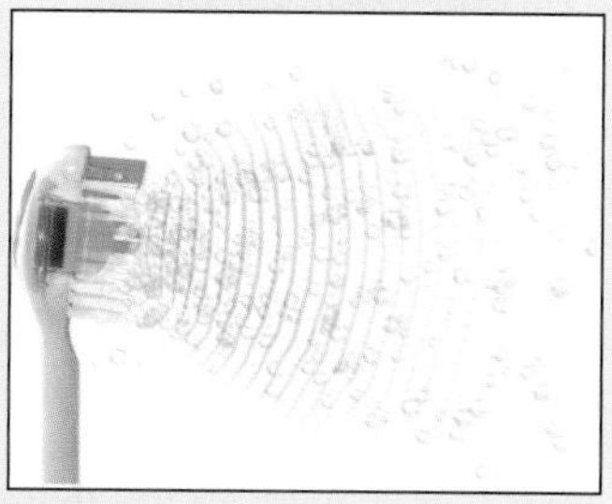

*Rota-dent toothbrush head action. (From Barnes CM: Powered toothbrushes: a focus on the evidence, *Oral Hyg* 7:3, 2000.)
[†]Sonicare toothbrush head action. (From Barnes CM: Powered toothbrushes: a focus on the evidence, *Oral Hyg* 7:3, 2000.)

Toothbrushing Instruction

Toothbrushes require client-specific instructions on thoroughness, duration, frequency, method, and force to achieve an effective technique and adherence. Also, when giving instruction the dental hygienist considers client characteristics such as risk and susceptibility to disease, dexterity, personal values, and preferences. In addition, communication should be appropriate to the client's (caregiver's) age, language, educational level, culture, learning style, and readiness to adopt new behaviors.

Regardless of the toothbrushing method, dental hygienists advise the client to clean the mouth and tongue thoroughly using a systematic approach. Clients also need to understand the link among oral biofilm, oral and systemic diseases, and the importance of controlling plaque and inflammation. Findings from gingival, periodontal, and dental assessments are reviewed with the client and correlated with the presence of oral biofilm. Suggestions for improved technique in these areas help clients enhance effectiveness of biofilm removal. Quantitative plaque, gingivitis, and bleeding indices are used to improve client understanding, monitor self-care, motivate positive behaviors, and measure outcomes of care.

Toothbrushing Duration and Frequency

Dental hygienists teach clients to brush thoroughly for an adequate period of time for efficient and effective biofilm removal. There are many possibilities for sequencing, but the individual should be encouraged to select a logical sequence and to use it consistently to avoid omission of any area. This concept is particularly important to instill early in children.

Research findings suggest the importance of brushing time. The recommended duration often is 2 minutes, and some models of power toothbrushes have 2-minute timers to encourage adherence. The average brushing time is 1 minute or less, but evidence indicates that, as brushing times increase, efficacy also increases.[3] Different teaching strategies can be used to encourage longer toothbrushing such as counting strokes before proceeding to the next area of the mouth or using a timer or a small hourglass.

There is no standard recommendation for how many times per day persons should brush. How often and how much plaque biofilm must be removed to prevent development of dental disease is not known; however, most people do not remove 100% of the plaque biofilm. From a practical viewpoint, clients are told to brush their teeth at least twice daily to remove plaque and to apply fluoride dentifrice to prevent caries. Following this advice also promotes a feeling of oral freshness.[3] Twice-daily brushing commonly is recommended to control plaque biofilm that contributes to oral diseases and **oral malodor (halitosis)**, the condition of having unpleasant breath. Brushing before bedtime and after a period of sleep is encouraged (i.e., in the morning and at night). However, decisions about when and how often to brush must be made through a shared decision-making process based on clinical findings and client preferences.

Toothbrushing Force (Pressure)

Most literature on force applied during toothbrushing has focused on its association with damaging soft tissue (gingival abrasion and recession) and hard tissue (dental abrasion), and fewer researchers have examined the effect of force on plaque reduction. Earlier concerns about excessive force leading to tissue damage with power toothbrushes have not been substantiated. Some power toothbrush designs are equipped with indicators or automatic shut-offs when excessive force is applied to the tooth surface, and some manual toothbrush designs incorporate a flexible shaft to contribute to improved safety. This technologic improvement is important because clients are unable to perceive accurately the pressure used. Some clinicians suggest that clients use a fingertip grasp instead of a palm grasp to reduce force during brushing. Evaluating if a client is exerting excessive toothbrushing force is challenging because of the multifactorial etiology of soft- and hard-tissue lesions.[6] The dental hygienist makes client recommendations based on specific client assessment findings.

Toothbrushing Methods

Table 23-2 summarizes key toothbrushing techniques and indications for use. In general, the Bass and Stillman methods of toothbrushing concentrate on the cervical portion of the teeth and the adjacent gingival tissues. Both methods can be modified to add a roll stroke (i.e., modified Bass and modified Stillman) by rolling the toothbrush bristles occlusally to clean the entire facial and lingual surfaces after cleaning the cervical area. The Bass method emphasizes sulcular cleaning, so it is the most commonly recommended toothbrushing method (Figure 23-4). More than 90% of people use their own "personal toothbrushing method," typically a scrub technique. Although this method removes oral biofilm from smooth tooth surfaces, it is considered to be less effective in other areas and may cause more injury to the soft and hard tissues.

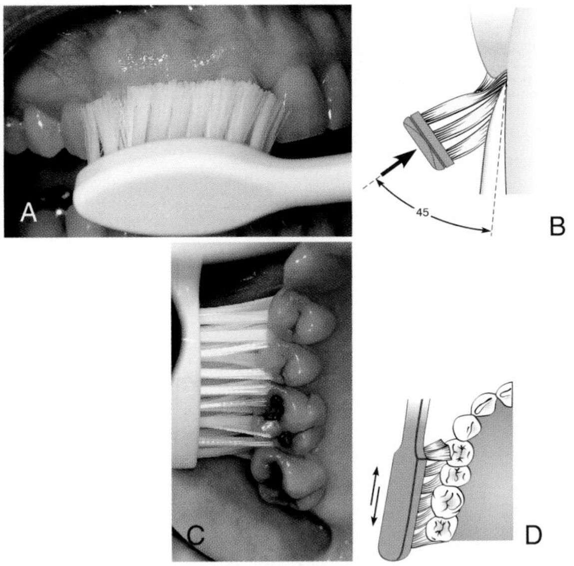

Figure 23-4. The Bass toothbrushing method. **A,** Proper intrasulcular position of brush in the mouth aims the filaments toward and into the gingival sulcus. **B,** Diagram shows the ideal placement with slight subgingival penetration of the filament tips. **C,** Place toothbrush so that filaments are angled approximately 45 degrees from the long axis of the tooth. **D,** Start at the most distal tooth in the arch and use a vibrating, back-and-forth motion to brush. (**B** and **D,** From Newman MG, Takei HH, Klokkevold PR, Carranza FA: *Carranza's clinical periodontology,* ed 11, St Louis, 2012, Saunders.)

Research has not shown convincingly one method to be consistently superior.[6] Specific claims about particular methods producing better outcomes surrounding gingival stimulation, preventing recession, or sulcular cleansing have not been substantiated in the literature.

Selection of the toothbrushing method should depend on client needs, dexterity, and preferences. Dental hygienists have to assess the client's oral hygiene, level of health or disease, and current toothbrushing practices to make meaningful recommendations. No toothbrushing method can clean adequately interproximal surfaces, and the client should be made aware that some means of interdental cleansing, and use of an antimicrobial mouth rinse, as needed, significantly improves oral biofilm and disease control.

For most manual toothbrushing techniques, the toothbrush can be grasped with a fingertip or palm grasp and placed as follows:

- The brush head is moved from one group of teeth (two to three teeth) to the next by overlapping with the previously completed group.
- On facial and lingual surfaces of posterior teeth the toothbrush head is positioned parallel to the arch.
- On anterior teeth the toothbrush head is placed parallel to the arch when the labial surfaces are brushed; on lingual surfaces the brush will likely have to be placed parallel with the long axis of the teeth (or vertically).
- On occlusal surfaces the toothbrush head is pressed firmly into the surfaces so that the filament ends can reach into the pits and fissures as much as possible, and a back-and-forth brushing stroke is used. The brush is advanced section by section until all occlusal surfaces have been cleaned.

TABLE 23-2
Toothbrushing Methods and Indications for Use

Method	Technique	Indications	
Bass (sulcular)	Filaments are directed apically at a 45-degree angle to the long axis of the tooth; gentle force is applied to insert bristles into sulcus; use gentle but firm vibratory strokes without removing filament ends from sulcus.	Sulcular cleansing Periodontal health Periodontal disease Periodontal maintenance	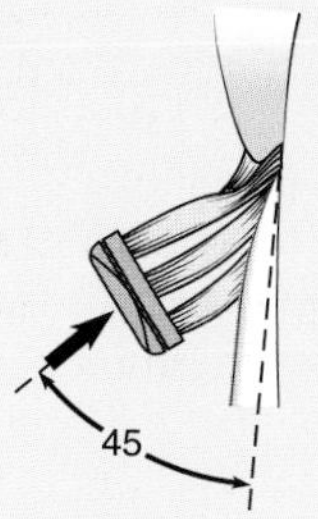
Stillman	Filaments are directed apically and angled similar to Bass method; filaments are placed partly on cervical portion of teeth and partly on adjacent gingiva; short back-and-forth vibratory strokes are employed, and the brush head is moved occlusally with light pressure.	Progressive gingival recession; gingival stimulation	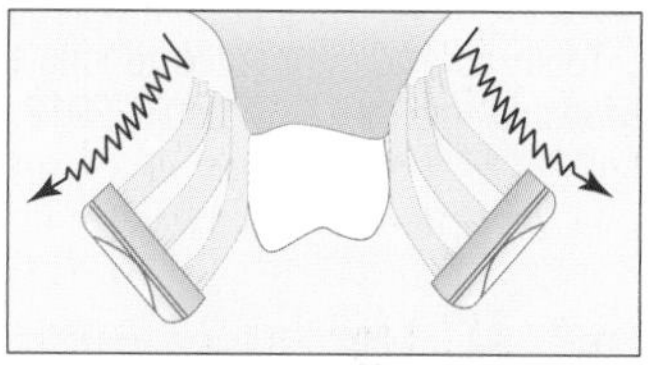
Charter	Filaments are directed toward the crown of the tooth; filaments are placed at the gingival margin and angled 45 degrees to the long axis of the tooth; short back-and-forth vibratory strokes are used for activation. (Distinguished from the Bass and Stillman methods in that the bristles are directed away from the gingiva towards the occlusal or incisal edge.)	Orthodontics Temporary cleaning of surgical sites Fixed prosthetic appliances	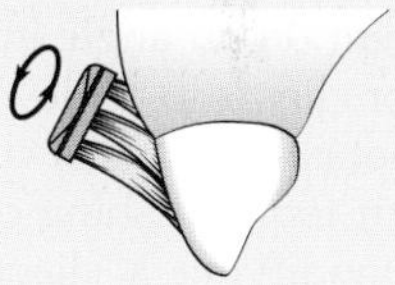
Roll stroke	Filaments are directed apically and rolled occlusally in a vertical motion.	Used in conjunction with Bass, Stillman, and Charter methods	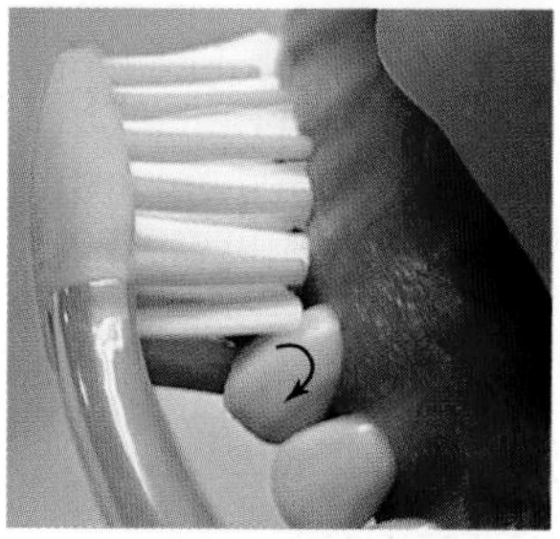
Modified Bass, Stillman, and Charter methods	Add a roll stroke; roll tufts occlusally in a vertical motion after cervical area is cleaned by prescribed method.	Cleaning of entire facial and lingual surfaces	
Fones	Filaments are activated in a circular motion.	Young children with primary teeth; otherwise not recommended	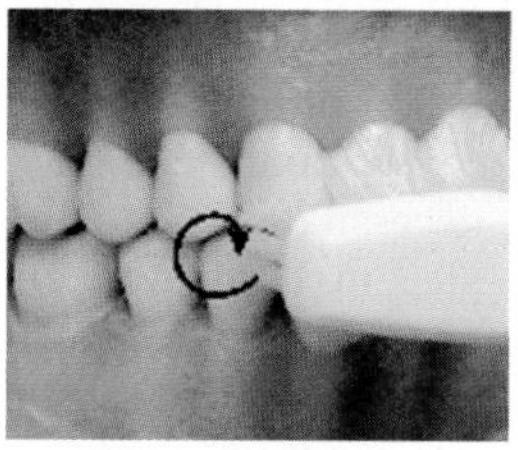

Illustrations from Newman MG, Takei HH, Klokkevold PR, et al: *Carranza's clinical periodontology,* ed 11, St Louis, 2012, Saunders. Photographs from Daniel SJ, Harfst SA, Wilder RS: *Mosby's dental hygiene,* ed 2, St Louis, 2008, Mosby.

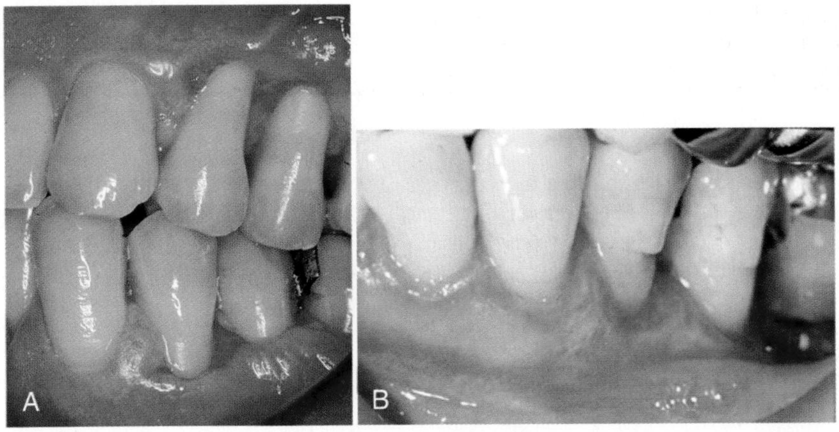

Figure 23-5. **A,** Trauma from vigorous toothbrushing with an abrasive dentifrice. Note trauma to gingival and root surface abrasion and gingival recession. **B,** Tooth abrasion attributed to long-term aggressive toothbrushing. (From Newman MG, Takei HH, Klokkevold PR, Carranza FA, eds: *Carranza's clinical periodontology*, ed 11, St Louis, 2012, Saunders.)

Toothbrushing techniques that require brush filament placement on an angle in relation to the teeth are more difficult for clients to achieve consistently. Effective toothbrushing is not easy for most clients, and this additional challenge can limit toothbrushing effectiveness and client motivation. When modifying a client's toothbrushing technique, clinicians must demonstrate the new technique on a mouth model and then in the client's mouth. This initial demonstration does not replace the need to monitor the client actually performing the new technique and to provide feedback to ensure that the skill is acquired, problems are identified, and errors are corrected over time.

Clients also require instruction with power toothbrushes. Although these instructions vary with manufacturer and design, in general, power toothbrushing is relatively straightforward because the mechanism of action removes the need for the client to manipulate the toothbrush. Most designs recommend that the client hold the brush head with a fingertip grasp in place for a few seconds on each tooth or small group of teeth before guiding the brush head slowly to the next tooth or group of teeth and allowing the brush to do the work. The filaments flare slightly while the brush is activated for cleansing the sulcus (Figure 23-5). The client must apply sufficient but not excessive pressure, focus on the gingival margin, and keep the toothbrush engaged for a sufficiently long period of time before moving to the next area.

An individual's dexterity and vision may deteriorate with time, necessitating ongoing assessment and modifications to suggested methods and toothbrush selection. Over time at maintenance appointments, the reinforcement of instruction, observation of client's technique, and ongoing encouragement are effective means of achieving oral biofilm removal and adherence to professional recommendations.

Soft- and Hard-Tissue Lesions

As part of making toothbrushing recommendations, the dental hygienist assesses soft and hard tissues for damage from toothbrushing. Although clients may be removing oral biofilm adequately, they also may be causing trauma from the toothbrushing technique or toothbrush selection. Negative changes in tissues can be detected anywhere in the mouth, although they often are seen on the facial tooth surfaces at the gingival margin.

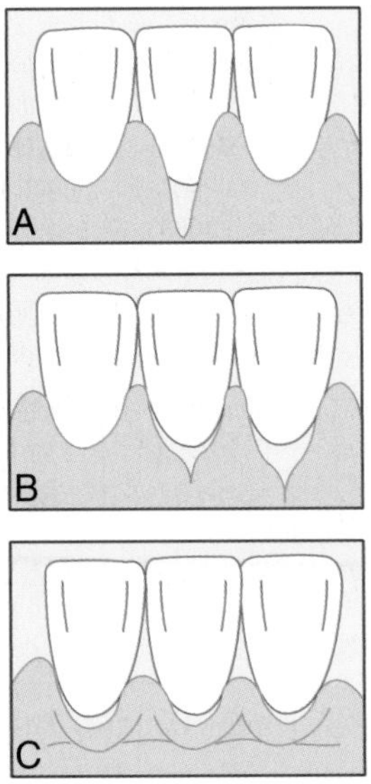

Figure 23-6. **A,** Gingival recession. **B,** Gingival clefting. **C,** Gingival festooning.

Soft-Tissue Lesions

Vigorous toothbrushing in combination with a hard or stiff toothbrush traditionally has been associated with gingival abrasions and recession. However, the cause of gingival trauma is multifactorial, with toothbrushing technique having a less-certain influence. Other factors that may influence abrasion include toothbrush filament stiffness, irregularities, or flexibility; toothbrushing force or duration; and abrasiveness of the toothpaste used. If observed, toothbrush trauma in the form of gingival abrasions can appear as redness, scuffing, or punctate lesions. Over time, if multifactorial influences continue, these early abrasions can lead to more permanent soft-tissue lesions including gingival recession, clefts, or festooning (Figure 23-6).

Although visible gingival abrasions are not a common clinical finding, gingival recession affects 80% to 100% of middle-age and elderly Americans to some degree. Prevalence and severity of recession are associated with increasing age, but younger individuals also can have aggressive levels of recession. Recession is a concern for several reasons, including its association with increased risk of dentinal hypersensitivity, loss of tooth support, root caries, and aesthetic dissatisfaction. The combined benefit of softer toothbrushes, less-abrasive toothpastes, and good toothbrushing technique has the potential to impact positively the prevention of gingival lesions (see Chapter 25 on dentifrices).

The cause of recession is multifactorial. Factors include the following:

- Toothbrushing factors similar to those potentially causing abrasion
- Anatomic factors (e.g., tooth malposition)
- Pathologic factors (e.g., clinical attachment loss from periodontal disease)

Hard-Tissue Lesions

Hard-tissue lesions have been attributed to toothbrushing. Tooth **abrasion** is the wearing away of the tooth surface typically located around the cementoenamel junction (CEJ) (see Figure 23-5). Clinically, tooth abrasions appear as cervical notches surrounding the CEJ, increasing dentinal hypersensitivity and unpleasant aesthetics and possibly requiring restorations. Cervical defect shapes associated with toothbrushing include V-wedged (most common), U-rounded, and combinations; these defects change shape over time.

Tooth abrasions have been considered distinct from dental **abfractions**, similarly shaped noncarious cervical lesions caused by excessive occlusal loading as teeth flex under pressure resulting in subsequent loss of hard tooth structure at the CEJ. Difficulty in determining actual causes of tooth abrasions and abfractions has led to use of the term **noncarious cervical lesion**, reflecting the multifactorial etiology of the condition. Despite studies showing an association between hard-tissue wear and greater brushing frequency and duration, and the use of scrubbing techniques, toothbrushing has only minor influence on cervical wear. In fact, toothpaste is needed to create significant abrasion. Brushing force and bristle flexibility are other possible contributing factors.

Some clients have noncarious cervical lesions from demineralization as a result of chemical erosion. There may be a synergistic effect between toothbrushing and previously eroded hard tissue, resulting in more clinically significant lesions than seen in the absence of dental erosion.

Tongue Cleansing

The dorsum of the tongue is a bacterial habitat. Tongue cleaning reduces the number of organisms, thereby controlling oral malodor, decreasing the opportunity for microorganisms to translocate, improving the client's taste perception, and contributing to overall oral cleanliness.

Although tongue scrapers and cleansers are marketed, tongue cleansing can be achieved with a manual toothbrush or a power toothbrush with a special head. A tongue cleaning device may be preferred to reduce the risk of stimulating the gag reflex (see Figure 23-7).

If a toothbrush is to be used for tongue cleansing, the client does the following:

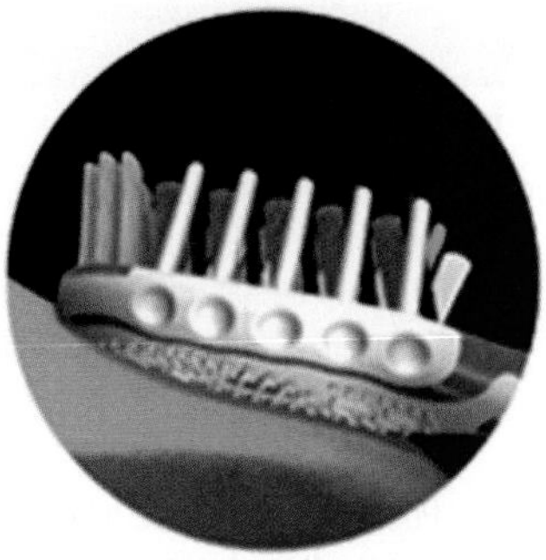

Figure 23-7. Oral-B CrossAction Pro-Health with tongue cleaner on head of brush. (Courtesy Procter & Gamble, Professional and Scientific Relations, Cincinnati, Ohio.)

- Extends the tongue and, with the toothbrush head placed on the tongue and the bristles angled slightly posteriorly, draws the bristles forward with light pressure
- Repeats brushing motion until the tongue is coating free

Clients should be advised not to scrub the tongue with the toothbrush or a tongue cleaner because tissue trauma could result. Use of an antibacterial mouth rinse after mechanical tongue cleaning further improves tongue hygiene.

Toothbrush Contamination

Toothbrushes can be a mode of indirect transmission for pathogenic organisms. The toothbrush can act as a **fomite**, an inanimate object that houses and transmits potentially infectious agents. A systematic review of studies related to toothbrush contamination found that toothbrushes of healthy and oral diseased adults become contaminated with potentially pathogenic bacteria from dental plaque, design, environment, or a combination of factors.[7] The important point to consider in relation to client care is how to reduce toothbrush contamination.

Solid toothbrush designs have been shown to be less conducive to sustaining colonization of microorganisms than hollow designs. Toothbrush caps and holders or plastic coverings further encourage microbial growth, so air drying is preferred.

Some interventions, such as chlorhexidine gluconate 0.12% or antiseptic mouth rinses, toothpaste, and ultrasonic sanitizers, have been shown to reduce toothbrush contamination. Studies are needed to examine specifically contamination in relation to disease transmission in vulnerable populations (e.g., critically ill adults, immunocompromised individuals).

The Dental Hygiene Process of Care and Toothbrushing

Because oral hygiene instruction is part of the implementation phase of care, the dental hygienist completes the client's assessment including current self-care behaviors, type of toothbrush used, frequency and duration of toothbrushing, toothbrush replacement practices, level of satisfaction with tools and technique, and personal values and preferences. As part of oral hygiene instruction, the client should be asked to demonstrate the toothbrushing method used so that the dental hygienist can observe the client's technique, skill, and dexterity.

TABLE 23-3

Shared Decision-Making Model

Knowledge transfer	Direction: Two-way Dental hygienist to client: Technical knowledge Client to dental hygienist: Client preferences, beliefs, values, and current practices
Deliberation and decision making	*Direction:* Bilateral Between dental hygienist and client Possibly may include other healthcare providers, caregivers, and family members

The dental hygienist links information about the client's self-care with clinical and radiographic observations and identifies the client's unmet human need deficits related to oral health (dental hygiene diagnoses), along with the corresponding causes, signs, and symptoms. Through this process the dental hygienist and client, in shared decision making, formulate a plan of care that includes self-care recommendations (Table 23-3; see Chapter 22). Oral biofilm may be present because the client has not been able to brush for several hours; conversely, absence of biofilm may be the result of thorough brushing immediately before the appointment rather than an indication of adequate daily plaque removal. Assessment of the soft and hard tissues for signs of oral disease provides more valid information about the adequacy of self-care.

At times, clients avoid toothbrushing because of discomfort, but avoidance results in oral biofilm maturation. Examples of these clients include those with necrotizing ulcerative gingivitis, acute soft-tissue injuries, healing surgical sites, or new dental appliances. In these situations, special toothbrushing instructions and mouth rinsing with alcohol-free 0.12% chlorhexidine gluconate is indicated.

Clients need positive reinforcement of their attempts to incorporate positive oral health behaviors throughout the process of care. Regardless of the client's situation, instruction, practice, and reinforcement are indicated at all appointments subsequent to the planning phase. Dental hygienists spend the least amount of educational time with clients for whom they hold the lowest expectations—that is, clients with the highest plaque levels. Dental hygienists should be aware of their personal biases and be accepting of all clients' personal abilities and values.[1]

CLIENT EDUCATION TIPS

- Communicate in a manner appropriate to the client's (caregiver's) age, language, culture, readiness, and learning style.
- Discuss toothbrush selection and toothbrushing methods in relation to the client's specific needs and oral assessment findings.
- Incorporate interdental cleansing and, if needed, use of an antimicrobial toothpaste or mouth rinse along with toothbrushing.
- Explain the benefits of tongue brushing.
- Correlate toothbrushing effectiveness with presence of oral biofilm, calcified deposits, and gingival disease.
- Discuss gingival recession and noncarious cervical lesions and explain possible causes with clients who exhibit these conditions.
- Use shared decision making when educating clients about toothbrushing; incorporate client abilities, values, and preferences.

LEGAL, ETHICAL, AND SAFETY ISSUES

- It is the dental hygienist's ethical responsibility to use the highest level of professional knowledge, judgment, and ability to increase public awareness and understanding of high-quality oral health practices, an ethical principle known as beneficence.
- The dental hygienist has an ethical obligation to review scientific literature related to preventive interventions and to apply the knowledge to client care.
- Beneficent dental hygiene care requires allocation of time for self-care instruction, repetition, reinforcement, and continual assessment of each client's oral health practices.
- The ethical principle of autonomy requires dental hygienists to listen to and allow for the client's participation in decision making and to respect the client's right to make a decision.
- The legal standard of care requires that dental hygienists educate clients about oral self-care considering the client's age, language, culture, and learning style.
- Care plans should include evaluation of the presence and distribution of oral biofilm and its retentive factors and client self-care.
- On completion of care, the dental hygienist documents in the client's legal record that clients have been counseled on why and how to perform an effective daily personal oral hygiene program and their level of progress. Confirmation of the client's understanding also is documented.
- Dental hygiene clients must be legally and ethically informed about the relationship between their oral health status and disease risk.

KEY CONCEPTS

- The manual toothbrush is the most commonly used device for removing oral biofilm from the facial, lingual, and occlusal surfaces.
- A toothbrush that has a small enough head to adapt to all areas of the mouth with a comfortable handle designed to secure a good grasp is desirable.
- Damage to soft and hard oral tissues has a multifactorial etiology; although toothbrush selection and toothbrushing variables contribute to negative effects, dentifrice use and other factors are likely to be more influential.
- Manual toothbrushes and power toothbrushes have greater benefit when dental professionals provide advice and instruction for using these devices.
- Toothbrush replacement should be based on individual wear rather than on time of ownership.
- Power toothbrushes are as effective as manual toothbrushes; oscillating-rotating power toothbrush designs have been shown to be more effective than traditional manual toothbrushes in reducing plaque and gingivitis.

- Comprehensive toothbrush instruction includes toothbrush selection and replacement, toothbrushing method, evaluation of toothbrushing effectiveness, and tongue brushing.
- Evaluation of toothbrushing effectiveness includes observation of the client's toothbrushing, disclosing agent use to visualize and quantify plaque, and gingival evaluation for signs of inflammation; corrective measures are undertaken as needed.
- Interdental cleaning, tongue brushing, and, if needed, use of an antimicrobial agent should be planned along with toothbrushing instructions.
- Dental hygienists must be aware of emerging research on toothbrushing and to be able to interpret study results critically.

CRITICAL THINKING EXERCISES

Case Study: Mrs. Truman, a 65-year-old retired schoolteacher, is being treated by the dental hygienist. Assessment findings reveal that the client has generalized heavy oral biofilm, gingival inflammation, and bleeding on probing. Early in the appointment Mrs. Truman says, "Lately my arthritis has been particularly bothersome in my hands, and I find it difficult to brush my teeth." Proceed with your counseling of Mrs. Truman regarding her home care. Consider her age, language, educational level, culture, learning style, and readiness to adopt new behaviors. What type of toothbrush and toothbrushing method should be recommend for Mrs. Truman and why?

Role-Play Exercise: Working in pairs, one student assumes the role of the dental hygienist and the other student acts as the client. The dental hygienist interviews the client about current homecare devices, behaviors, and techniques and provides client-specific education and feedback based on the evidence. Student pairs can use their dental models for demonstration purposes; or if in the clinical setting, demonstrate techniques intraorally. Students can then reverse roles so that both experience the roles.

Case Study: Tommy Dee, a 35-year-old professional golfer, is a new client in your office. His health history findings present no significant findings. Oral examination findings reveal extensive gingival recession, especially on the facial surfaces, minimal gingival inflammation on the lingual of the mandibular anteriors and buccal of the maxillary molars adjacent to calculus deposits, and minimal oral biofilm. No carious lesions are present on his canines, premolars, and molars. His occlusion is normal, but he reports bruxism while sleeping. Tommy's daily oral hygiene regimen includes toothbrushing with a manual brush and fluoride three times, flossing one to two times, and use of a fluoride mouth rinse. You observe Tommy's toothbrushing technique and notice he uses a palm grasp with enough pressure that his biceps are flexing, and his personal method approximates scrubbing.

- What should you discuss with Tommy, and how would you correlate his oral assessment findings with his toothbrushing?
- What would you demonstrate and recommend to Tommy to increase his safety during daily oral hygiene?
- What would you recommend Tommy discuss with the dentist?

REFERENCES

1. Asadoorian J: CDHA position paper on toothbrushing. *Can J Dent Hygiene* 40:232, 2006.
2. Van der Weijden F, Slot D: Oral hygiene in the prevention of periodontal diseases: the evidence. *Periodontology 2000* 55:104, 2011.
3. Slot DE, Wiggelinkhuizen L, Rosema NAM, et al: The efficacy of manual toothbrushes following a brushing exercise: a systematic review. *Int J Dent Hygiene* 10:187, 2012.
4. Robinson PG, Deacon SA, Deery C, et al: Manual versus powered toothbrushing for oral health. *Cochrane Database Syst Rev* (2):CD002281, 2005.
5. Deacon SA, Glenny AM, Deery C, et al: Different powered toothbrushes for plaque control and gingival health. *Cochrane Database Syst Rev* (2):CD004971, 2010.
6. Asadoorian J: CDHA position paper on tooth brushing, *CJDH* 40:(5):232–248, 2006.
7. Frazell MR, Munroe CL: Toothbrush contamination: a review of the literature. *Nurs Res Prac* Article ID 420630, 2012.

ACKNOWLEDGMENT

The authors acknowledge Joanna Asadoorian for her past contributions to this chapter.

EVOLVE RESOURCES

Please visit http://evolve.elsevier.com/Darby/hygiene for additional practice and study support tools.

CHAPTER 24

Mechanical Oral Biofilm Control: Interdental and Supplemental Self-Care Devices

Denise M. Bowen

COMPETENCIES

1. Discuss the selection of self-care devices, including the significance of removing or reducing interdental and subgingival plaque biofilm.
2. Discuss types of nonpowered interdental and supplemental self-care devices, including:
   - Appropriate use of nonpowered self-care devices designed for interdental and subgingival biofilm removal.
   - Recommendations for the appropriate device(s) for clients based on efficacy, client needs, and preferences.
3. Discuss types of powered interdental and supplemental self-care devices, including:
   - Appropriate use of powered self-care devices designed for interdental and subgingival biofilm removal.
   - Recommendations for the appropriate device(s) for clients based on efficacy, client needs, and preferences.

Making individualized recommendations to clients about appropriate selection and use of self-care devices can be challenging. Numerous devices on the market help meet clients' self-care needs; the plethora of products also makes it difficult for clients to decide which is the appropriate device for them. Clients depend on the dental hygienist to help them navigate the "oral healthcare aisle." In many cases several devices potentially can provide the desired outcome for a client. Client preference and likelihood to use the device then becomes a focal point of discussion. Therefore dental hygienists must be familiar with the different devices, the evidence specific to each device, and the expected results from using the device. This knowledge fosters a conversation between the dental hygienist and client that leads to a recommendation that produces the outcomes valued by the client.

Selecting Self-Care Devices

Traditionally, self-care recommendations most commonly have consisted of brushing and flossing. Toothbrushes, either manual or power, continue to be the product of choice for cleaning the facial, lingual, and occlusal surfaces of the teeth. Toothbrushing does not reach the proximal surfaces of teeth or the area immediately under the contact point of adjacent teeth (**gingival embrasure space**). These areas are known as the **interproximal** or **interdental** areas. Dental floss is designed to clean the interdental surfaces of the teeth. In a healthy mouth, brushing and flossing performed effectively on a daily basis can be effective in preventing periodontal diseases in low-risk clients. However, clients who have an increased risk, special needs, or periodontal disease may need other devices.

With the introduction of new technology, several studies have demonstrated that, in some individuals, alternatives to manual floss such as floss holders, interdental brushes, and power flossers are as effective or more effective as dental floss at reducing plaque biofilm, bleeding, gingivitis, and/or pocket depths.[1-3] Evidence also indicates that a dental water jet can be as effective or more effective when compared with manual floss for the reduction of interdental plaque biofilm, bleeding, and gingivitis.[4,5]

Removal of plaque biofilm from the interdental areas where toothbrushing does not reach is important for the following reasons:

1. To prevent periodontal diseases: Most periodontal diseases commonly begin in the interdental col area, a depressed concave area of nonkeratinized gingival tissue under the contact area of two teeth. The col area connects the lingual and buccal papillae, and because of its saddle-like shape it harbors plaque biofilm (Figure 24-1). The epithelial tissue covering the col area is thin and less resistant to infection. When inflammation is present in this area, the papilla may become red, swollen, or enlarged and the col may become deeper (see Chapter 19) as evidenced by increased probe readings.
2. To prevent malodor (bad breath): This problem may be caused by interdental and subgingival plaque biofilm.

Types of Interdental and Supplemental Self-Care Devices: Nonpowered

A wide variety of interdental and supplemental plaque control aids are available. In general, when the interdental gingiva fills the embrasure spaces, plaque biofilm removal from proximal tooth surfaces and shallow pockets can be accomplished with dental floss or tape, provided the client has the dexterity and the inclination to use them. When the interdental gingiva is reduced or missing, however, the embrasures are open (type II and type III) and other methods of interdental cleaning are needed. The dental hygienist evaluates the information gained during the assessment phase of

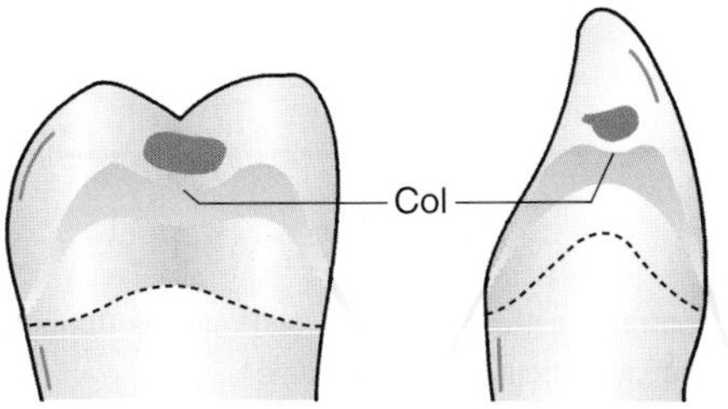

Figure 24-1. Location of the col, the nonkeratinized epithelial depression connecting the buccal and lingual papillae of teeth, apical to the contact area *(in gray).* (From Perry DA, Beemsterboer PL: *Periodontology for the dental hygienist,* ed 4, St Louis, 2014, Saunders.)

care to select the most appropriate interdental and supplemental aids for the client. To accomplish this, it is important to keep in mind the following client conditions and risk factors:

- Contour and consistency of the gingival tissues
- Probing depths
- Gingival attachment levels
- Size of the interproximal embrasures
- Tooth position and alignment
- Condition and types of restorative work present
- Susceptibility of the client to disease (risk assessment)
- Level of dexterity and ability to use a device
- Client motivation
- Cost, safety, and effectiveness of the recommended device
- Client preference

Once an assessment is made, the dental hygienist reviews the care plan and goals with the client to determine which self-care device is most effective. The simplest, least time-consuming procedures that effectively control bacterial plaque biofilm and maintain oral health are recommended. Also, if one device works, the dental hygienist chooses it over two devices that would accomplish the same goal. Studies demonstrate that client acceptance and effectiveness of self-care recommendations improve when the number of devices is limited.

If the client's current self-care regimen is effective in maintaining optimal oral health, the dental hygienist reinforces current practices, documents the products used and frequency of use in the permanent record, and does not introduce anything new to the daily routine. If a client's regimen is not effective, then the dental hygienist asks the client why he or she thinks the recommendations are not working for them. If the problem is difficulty using the device, the dental hygienist can observe the client's use and modify it or select another device that may be easier for that client to use. If remembering to build the new self-care device into the daily schedule is the problem, the hygienist can recommend strategies for developing a new habit such as linking it with something the client already does every day. If the client simply does not want to use the device, other options for interdental cleansing are explored. The dental hygienist reviews assessment data, including risk factors, and presents new recommendations to the client. Tables 24-1 and 24-2 summarize a variety of nonpowered interdental and supplemental self-care devices. These devices can enhance the benefits of a toothbrush, reach areas that the toothbrush is not designed to access, or meet special client needs based on assessment. They include the following:

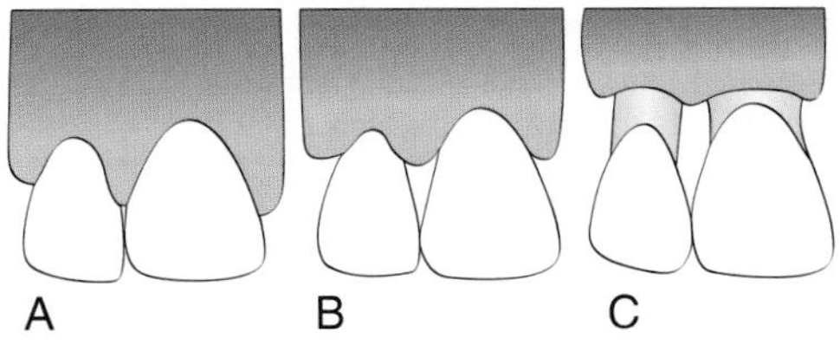

Figure 24-2. **A** to **C,** Interproximal embrasure types.

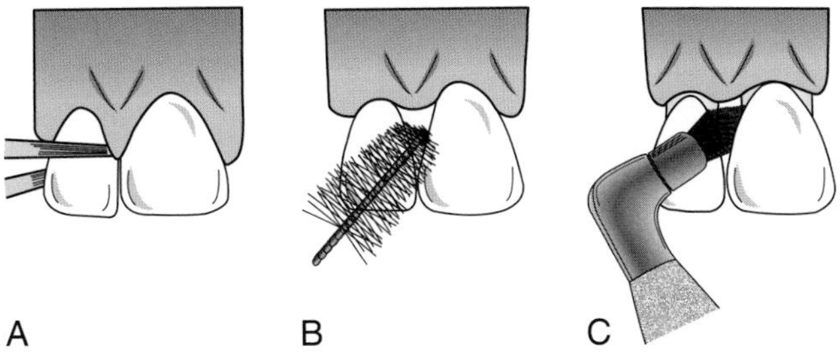

Figure 24-3. Use of interdental plaque control devices in various sizes of embrasures. **A,** Dental floss. **B,** Interdental brush. **C,** End-tuft brush.

- Dental floss and tape
- Floss holders and threaders
- Toothpicks and wooden wedges
- Rubber tip stimulators
- Interdental brushes and tips
- End-tuft, single-tuft brushes
- Tongue cleaners

Dental Floss and Tape

Dental floss is the most frequently recommended product for cleaning proximal tooth surfaces with normal gingival contour and embrasure spaces. Figures 24-2 and 24-3 illustrate the various embrasure types and devices. Dental floss is recommended only for individuals with type I embrasures with normal gingival contour. If blunted papilla or recession is present resulting in a larger embrasure space, floss is less effective.

Most types of dental floss are made of synthetic material (e.g., nylon, polytetrafluoroethylene [PTFE]) and some are impregnated with flavoring, fluoride, or antimicrobial or whitening agents. The following general types of dental floss are available:

- Unwaxed, waxed, and dental tape
- Braided and tufted

Unwaxed and Waxed Floss and Dental Tape

Today **dental floss** is made of waxed or unwaxed monofilaments (e.g., PTFE) or multifilaments (e.g., nylon). The coated monofilament type of floss slides easily between the teeth and does not fray, although cost is generally higher. The multifilament type allows for separation of the fibers. It is available in varying widths and waxed or unwaxed formulations. Studies have shown no difference in the effectiveness of unwaxed versus waxed dental floss. Recommendations are based on client's ease of use or preference. Waxed floss or monofilament floss may be easier to use for those clients who have tight contacts.

Dental tape or ribbon is a waxed floss product that is wider and flatter than conventional dental floss. The flat-sided surface of dental tape is preferred by some, particularly when the surface area to be flossed is large. The choice of

TABLE 24-1
Nonpowered Interdental Self-Care Devices

Interdental Nonpowered Self-Care Products	Description and Types	Indications	Contraindications and Limitations	Common Problems During Use or Misuse
Floss	Unwaxed vs. waxed Dental tape polytetrafluoroethylene (PTFE) Braided Plain vs. flavored Therapeutic agents added (fluoride)	Type I embrasures Floss cleans between papilla and tooth Braided floss is for implants	Type II and III embrasures	Floss cuts Floss clefts Circulation to fingers cut off from wrapping too tight Inability to reach posterior teeth
Tufted dental floss	Regular diameter floss, wider tufted portion looks like yarn, and threader combination	Type II and III embrasures Interproximal surfaces of abutment teeth Under pontics of fixed partial dentures	Type I embrasures	Trauma from forcing threader into tissues Yarnlike portion may catch on dental work
Floss holder	Flossing aid Handle with two prongs in Y or C shape	Type I embrasures Clients lacking manual dexterity, who are physically challenged, or who have a strong gag reflex Caregivers	Type II and III embrasures	Unable to maintain tension of floss against tooth and fully wrap around proximal area Translocation of bacteria from one site to another Need fulcrum to avoid floss cuts
Floss threader	Designs resemble a needle with a large opening to thread floss Floss is pulled through the interproximal space to allow cleaning of the proximal surface	Type I embrasures Floss between and under abutment teeth and pontics, orthodontic appliances, implants, and lingual bars	Type II and III embrasures	Trauma from forcing threader into tissues
Toothpick (wooden or plastic)	Round Triangular	Type II and III embrasures from facial aspect only Accessible furcations Small root concavities	Type I embrasures Healthy tissue	Blunting of papilla from incorrect usage Splaying of wood ends may cause tissue trauma, cuts, or abrasions
Toothpick holder	Plastic handle with opening at the tip to place a toothpick	Type II and III embrasures from facial or lingual aspect Accessible furcations Concave interproximal surfaces Fixed prosthetic and orthodontic appliances Sulcular cleansing in shallow pockets	Type I embrasures Healthy tissue	Blunting of papilla and tissues from incorrect use Splaying of wood ends may cause trauma Possible damage of epithelial attachment if used incorrectly subgingivally
Wooden wedge	Triangular wooden wedge	Type II and III embrasures from facial aspect Accessible furcations	Type I embrasures Healthy tissue	Wearing down of papilla and marginal tissues from incorrect use Splaying of wood ends may cause tissue trauma
Interproximal brush	Bristle inserts: tapered (conical) or straight Variety of sizes Attached to reusable handle or single disposable units	Type II and III embrasures Exposed root furcations Orthodontic and fixed appliances	Type I embrasures Healthy tissue	Trauma to tooth surface or gingiva from sharp wire center of some designs
Interdental tip	Handle with soft absorbent tip or plastic filament	Type II and III embrasures Fixed dental appliances Application of fluoride, antimicrobial agent, or desensitizing agent	Type I embrasures Healthy tissue	Trauma caused by forcing into too small a space

TABLE 24-2

Nonpowered Supplemental Self-Care Devices

Supplemental Nonpowered Self-Care Devices	Description and Types	Indications	Contraindications and Limitations	Common Problems During Use or Misuse
Interdental tip with soft rubber bristles	Small interdental, soft pick with narrow conical shape	Food and bioflim removal interdentally, around crowns, bridges, implants and orthodontic applicances	Tight contacts and embrasure spaces	Ineffective if space is too large (e.g., Type II and III embrasures)
Rubber tip stimulator	Conical rubber tip on the end of a metal or plastic handle	Type II and III embrasures Margins of tissue after periodontal surgery Exposed furcations	Type I embrasures and healthy tissues	Tissue trauma (to papilla and tissues, if used aggressively)
End-tuft brush Single-tuft brush	Flat or tapered end Straight or angled handle	Type III embrasures Fixed dental prosthesis (e.g., orthodontic appliances, implants, pontics, maxillofacial surgery client wired shut) Difficult-to-reach areas (e.g., lingual surface of mandible, molars, abutment teeth, distal surface of terminal teeth, crowded teeth, third molars)	Type I embrasures	Tissue trauma Similar to problems associated with improper toothbrushing methods
Tongue cleaner (also known as *tongue scraper*)	Flat vs. ridged Plastic strip or handle with scraper on the end	Dorsal surface of tongue to remove coating and reduce malodor		If clients press too hard they may traumatize papilla
Tooth towelettes	Gauze treated with mouthwash	Remove plaque from teeth and freshen breath in absence of a toothbrush	Should not replace toothbrushing	Difficult to remove all plaque from teeth; educate clients about limited use
Denture clasp brush	Cylindric brush	Metal clasp of removable partial dentures	Not for intraoral use	Use with nonabrasive denture paste to avoid scratching
Denture brush	Flat, trim, firm nylon design, stiffer than manual toothbrushes Some have double-end, flat side for tooth side of denture, pointed bristle end for tissue side	Tooth and tissue sides of dentures	Not for intraoral use	Use with nonabrasive denture paste to avoid scratching

which floss to recommend or even if dental floss is the best choice is influenced by the following:

- The tightness of the contact area
- The contour of the gingival tissue
- The roughness of the interproximal surface (e.g., margins of restorations)
- The client's manual dexterity and preference

Figure 24-4. Tufted dental floss.

Braided and Tufted Floss

Tufted dental floss, or variable-diameter dental floss, has been found to be equally as effective as waxed or unwaxed dental floss for removing plaque biofilm. Tufted dental floss is designed to have three continuous segments: a length of waxed or unwaxed dental floss; a shorter segment of cylindric, nylon meshwork; and a relatively rigid nylon needle capable of being threaded beneath the contact or under fixed bridges (Figure 24-4). The dental floss segment is used in areas of normal gingival contour, and the other segments are used as indicated in Table 24-2 (e.g., crown and bridge abutments and pontics).

Braided floss, intended for cleaning dental implants, is sold on a spool or as a precut piece with a stiff nylon end for threading. The braided nylon resembles a cord, can be washed after use, and is reused after drying. Some floss has a mesh or gauze appearance and is meant for one-time use. More information on self-care for dental implants can be found in Chapter 58.

String Flossing Methods

The two primary methods of dental flossing are the spool method and the loop method. Procedure 24-1 and the corresponding Competency Form reviews the spool method of flossing, a method used by many teens and adults. The spool method of flossing requires manual dexterity. Children may prefer to use the loop method of flossing as described in Procedure 24-2 and the corresponding Competency Form.

Proper flossing technique is not easy to master, and detailed instructions must be given and demonstrated. If the client does not have the ability to master the technique or does not like or want to floss, other devices should be recommended. Disclosing solution and the presence of plaque biofilm, gingival bleeding, and periodontal indices are parameters used to assess the effectiveness of plaque biofilm removal

Procedure 24-1 Spool Flossing Method: Adults

STEPS

1. Break off a piece of floss 12 to 18 inches long from the spool.
2. Wrap floss around middle fingers; wrap floss around right middle finger two to three times; wrap remaining floss around left middle finger (or vice versa) (Figure 24-5, *A*).
3. For maxillary insertion, grasp floss firmly with thumb and index finger of each hand, using ½ inch of floss between fingertips (Figure 24-5, *B*). For mandibular insertion, direct the floss down with the index fingers (Figure 24-5, *C*).
4. Select area to begin flossing, and establish a pattern to progress throughout the mouth.
5. Set a fulcrum on the cheek or in the mouth.
6. Use gentle seesaw motion to pass through contact area.
7. Wrap tightly in C shape around tooth (Figure 24-6).
8. Move floss up and down on mesial of tooth three to four strokes, then move above papilla (just below contact); wrap in C shape on distal surface of adjacent tooth, moving floss up and down three to four strokes (Figure 24-7).
9. Use a seesaw motion to remove floss through contact.
10. Advance floss to a new area by unwrapping floss from left-hand middle finger and wrapping onto right-hand middle finger (or vice versa; see step 2).
11. Repeat steps 5 to 11 until all teeth have been completed, continuing to grasp the floss with the thumb and index fingers.
12. Dispose of floss in waste receptacle and cleanse hands.

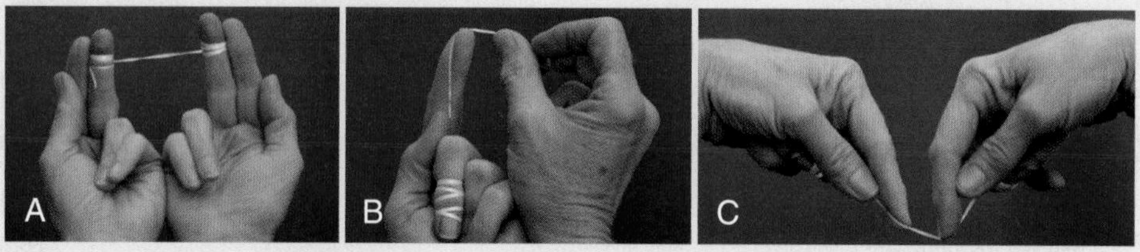

Figure 24-5

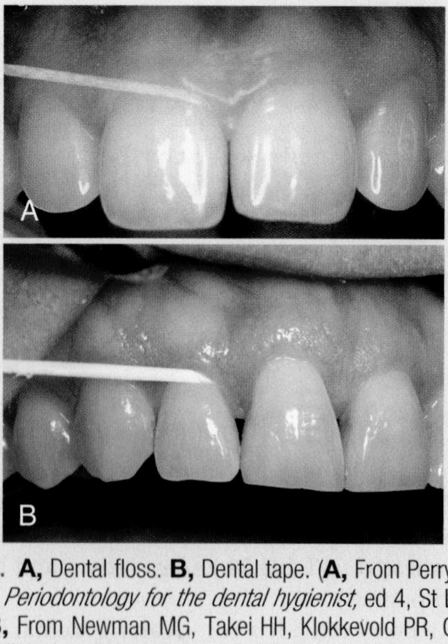

Figure 24-6. A, Dental floss. **B,** Dental tape. (**A,** From Perry DA, Beemsterboer PL: *Periodontology for the dental hygienist,* ed 4, St Louis, 2014, Saunders. **B,** From Newman MG, Takei HH, Klokkevold PR, Carranza FA: *Carranza's clinical periodontology,* ed 11, St Louis, 2012, Saunders.)

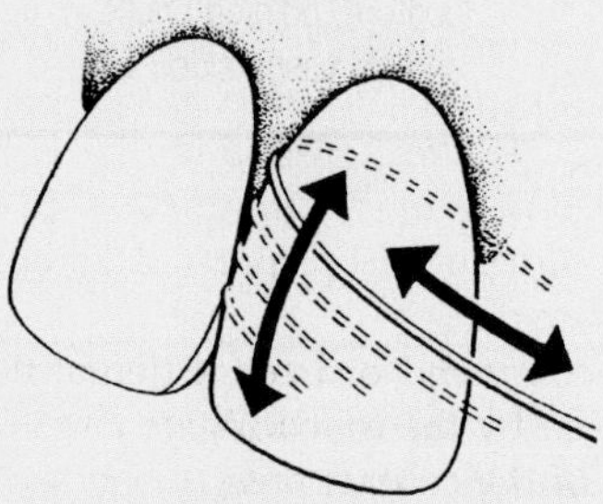

Figure 24-7. Floss wrapped around dental surface. (From Hoag PM, Pawlak EA: *Essentials of periodontics,* ed 4, St Louis, 1990, Mosby.)

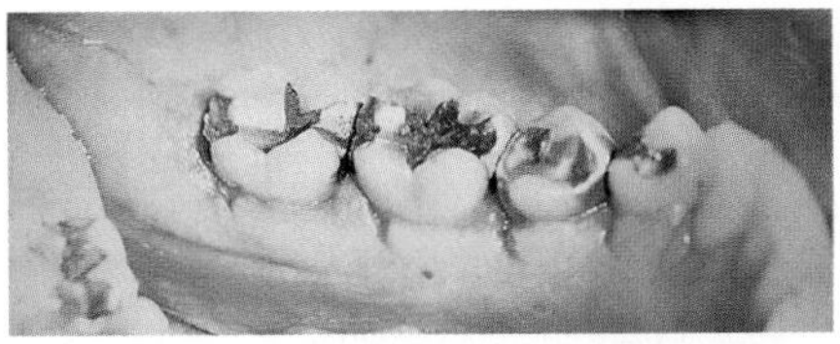

Figure 24-8. Floss cuts. (Courtesy Dr. Margaret Walsh, University of California–San Francisco.)

Procedure 24-2 Loop Flossing Method: Children

STEPS

1. Break off a piece of floss 8 to 10 inches long from the spool.
2. Tie the two ends together in a knot (Figure 24-9).
3. Follow steps listed for spool flossing method (see Procedure 24-1).
4. Advance floss to new area by sliding floss away from the knot.
5. Repeat steps 5 to 11 until all teeth have been completed, continuing to grasp the floss with the thumb and index fingers.
6. Dispose of floss in waste receptacle.

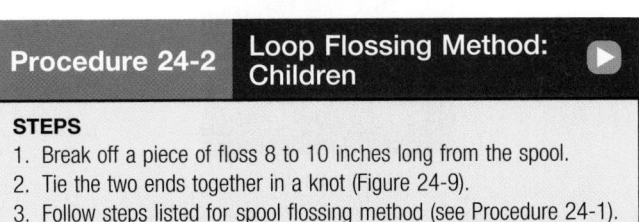

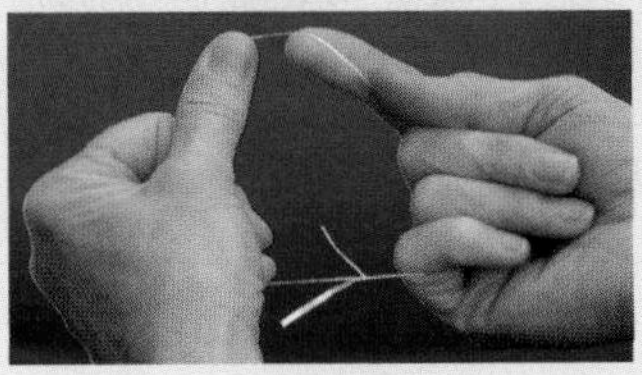

Figure 24-9.

in terms of clinical outcomes. Oral signs of gingival trauma (e.g., floss cuts, gingival clefts, gingival abrasion) are used for the safety evaluation (Figure 24-8). Causes of gingival trauma include the following:

- Using too long a piece of floss between fingers when inserting between teeth
- Snapping the floss in the contact area
- Failing to wrap the floss around the tooth before moving it subgingivally between the tooth and the papilla
- Failing to use a finger rest to prevent undue pressure and to provide control

Gingival bleeding during flossing can be a result of trauma or an indication of inflammation. When clients with gingival inflammation initiate flossing, the gingiva bleeds as a result of the microulcerations in the sulcular lining that occur during the active disease process. Clients must be aware that bleeding in the absence of trauma is not a sign to avoid flossing, but rather an indicator of infection that must be controlled by improved self-care techniques. In most cases bleeding from gingival inflammation subsides with the regular removal of the plaque biofilm and supportive periodontal therapy.

Floss Holders and Threaders

Clients who have difficulty mastering string floss techniques for interdental cleaning may find it easier to use a floss holder (Figures 24-10 and 24-11). **Floss holders** are plastic handles that aid in the placement and movement of floss between the

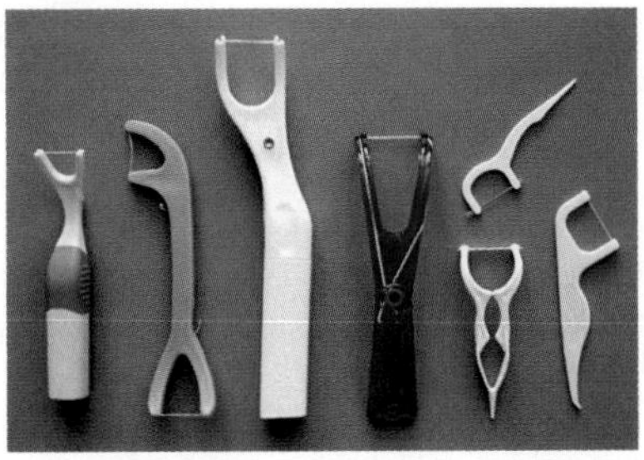

Figure 24-10. Disposable floss devices are convenient for some clients and may enhance plaque biofilm control.

Procedure 24-3 Use of a Floss Holder

STEPS

1. Tightly string floss on holder following the manufacturer's recommendations (see Figure 24-10).
2. Follow steps 4 to 10 for spool method of flossing (see Procedure 24-1).
3. To direct floss in a C shape toward mesial and distal in step 8, use push or pull motion with floss holder (Figure 24-11).
4. To move to a new area of floss (step 11 of the spool method), the holder must be unwrapped, the floss advanced, and the holder rewrapped.
5. Continue until all teeth are completed.
6. Dispose of the floss in waste receptacle.
7. Wash off floss holder with warm water and soap, dry, and store in clean, dry area until next use.

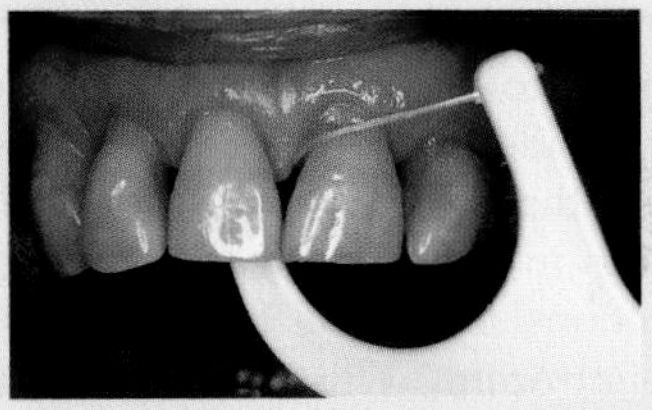

Figure 24-11. Placement of floss holder in mouth. (From Perry DA, Beemsterboer PL: *Periodontology for the dental hygienist*, ed 4, St Louis, 2014, Saunders.)

teeth. Floss holders are described in Table 24-2, and their method of use in Procedure 24-3 and the corresponding Competency Form. Studies have found that use of floss with proper use of a floss holder reduced gingivitis as effectively as use of string floss. In addition, those who used the floss holder preferred using it to traditional flossing techniques.

Another device that assists clients in cleaning under bridges and around abutments or orthodontic appliances is the floss threader (see Figure 24-12). As described in Table 24-2, a **floss threader** assists in introducing floss between an abutment tooth used for support of a fixed bridge and a pontic, the artificial tooth that replaces a missing natural tooth. Procedure 24-4 and the corresponding Competency Form reviews the use of a floss threader.

Benefits of Flossing

The benefit of daily interdental cleaning such as flossing is the reduction or prevention of inflammation caused by the

Procedure 24-4 Use of a Floss Threader

STEPS

1. Determine the need to use a floss threader and appropriate areas for use.
2. Break off a piece of floss 4 to 6 inches long from the spool.
3. Thread floss through eye of floss threader, overlapping floss 1 to 2 inches.
4. Grasp threader with thumb and index finger of one hand.
5. Insert tip of threader from the facial surface through an open interproximal area or area between a pontic and an abutment tooth (Figure 24-12, *A*).
6. Pull floss threader toward the lingual side until threader has passed completely through the interproximal space or under a pontic (only floss is now in the space) (Figure 24-12, *B*).
7. Slide the floss threader off the floss and remove from mouth.
8. Move floss back and forth several times under the pontic. Then follow steps 8 and 9 of the spool method of flossing (Figure 24-13).
9. Remove floss by letting go with the hand that is on the lingual side and pulling floss toward the buccal side.
10. Dispose of floss and threader in waste receptacle.

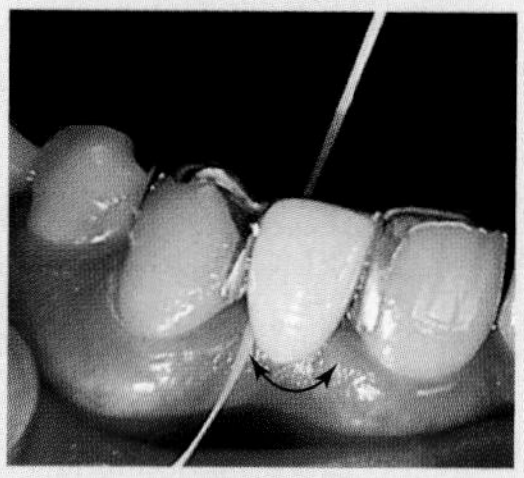

Figure 24-13.

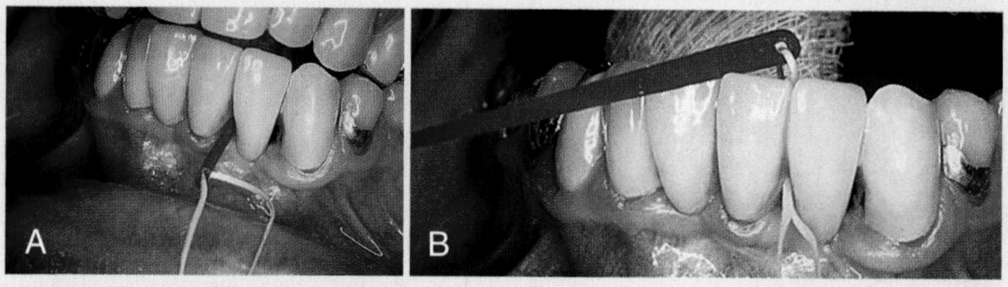

Figure 24-12. A, Facial insertion of the threader tip. **B,** Threader pulled lingually through the interproximal space.

immune response to the toxins produced by interdental plaque biofilm. Evidence from a comprehensive systematic review indicated that flossing in addition to toothbrushing reduces gingivitis in comparison with toothbrushing alone; however, reductions in plaque biofilm over toothbrushing alone are not significant.[6] This finding is difficult to understand based on the strong evidence documenting the relationship between plaque biofilm and gingivitis. Perhaps the additional effect of flossing beyond toothbrushing is related to subgingival plaque in the col area, which is not visible for scoring by dental indices used to measure plaque biofilm.[2] Flossing is a difficult skill for most clients to master, and many clients do not want to floss. As a result, benefits of floss over toothbrushing alone are not always supported by the evidence.[3] There also is no evidence that flossing reduces the incidence of interproximal caries.[6,7] Fluoride therapy has more impact on interproximal caries and studies combining the two interventions show no additional benefit from flossing.[6] For more details on caries risk and prevention see Chapter 18 and 33.

Toothpicks, Toothpick Holders, and Triangular Toothpicks

Some individuals prefer to use toothpicks for control of interdental plaque biofilm, particularly on concave proximal surfaces and exposed furcation areas. **Toothpicks** can be either wooden or plastic. Studies have shown that a household toothpick has no oral health benefit beyond removal of food impacted between the teeth.[3] Safe use of the toothpicks, however, requires sufficient interdental space available (see Table 24-2 for indications) because otherwise they may cause trauma to or blunting of the papilla. Toothpicks are often too long and wide to reach interproximally from the buccal to lingual surface and have the potential to damage tissue. Clients who use toothpicks for food impaction must be taught proper toothpick use to prevent damage to the gingiva, especially the epithelial attachment (Procedure 24-5 and the corresponding Competency Form). An interdental device should not be directed toward the epithelial attachment, or bacteria will be introduced into the nonkeratinized tissue rather than removed. For safe and effective plaque biofilm removal, a toothpick holder or triangular toothpick (wooden wedge) is recommended; however, the same precaution applies. **Toothpick holders** (Figure 24-14) are designed to allow use from the facial or lingual aspect and adapt better interproximally and posteriorly when compared with toothpicks alone.

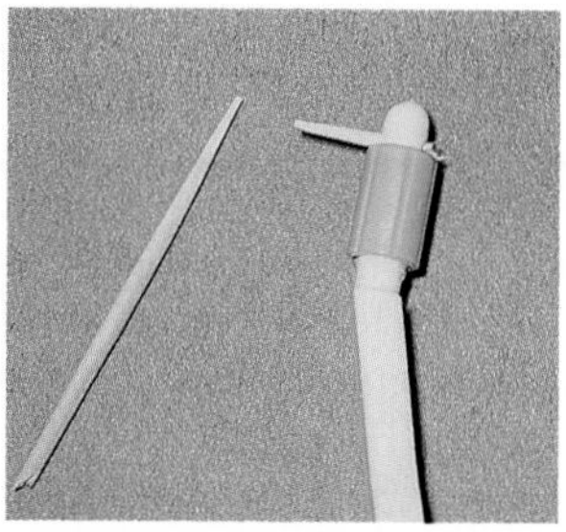

Figure 24-14. Example of toothpick holder.

Triangular toothpicks, also called **wooden wedges**, are designed to remove interproximal plaque biofilm from type

Procedure 24-5 Use of a Toothpick in a Toothpick Holder

STEPS

1. Insert a round tapered toothpick into the end of an angled plastic holder. Twist toothpick securely into holder, and break off longer end of toothpick (see Figure 24-14).
2. Some suggest moistening the end of the toothpick with saliva; others believe it may splinter.
3. Place the toothpick tip at the gingival margin with the tip pointing at a 45-degree angle to the long axis of the tooth. Trace the gingival margin around the tooth (Figure 24-15, *A*).
4. Some clients may be dexterous enough to point the tip at less than a 45-degree angle into the sulcus or pocket and trace around the tooth surfaces and root concavities. The tip should maintain contact with the tooth at all times. Insertion should stop once the toothpick meets a slight resistance in the space without the teeth being forced apart interproximally or the tissue being impinged. Keeping the tip at the tooth, use a gentle up-and-down motion to clean concave proximal surfaces (Figure 24-15, *B*).
5. For exposed furcation areas, trace the furcation and use an in-and-out motion to clean the furcation. The tip should maintain contact with the tooth at all times.
6. If debris accumulates on toothpick, rinse under running water.
7. Once all areas of the mouth are completed, dispose of toothpick in waste receptacle.
8. Holder may be washed with soap and warm water and stored in a clean, dry place for reuse.

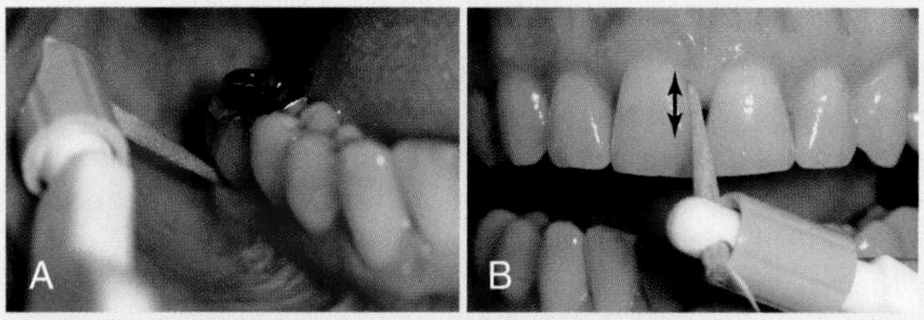

Figure 24-15. A, Toothpick tip placed at gingival margin. **B,** Gentle up-and-down motion keeping tip on tooth. (From Newman MG, Takei HH, Klokkevold PR, et al: *Carranza's clinical periodontology,* ed 11, St Louis, 2012, Saunders.)

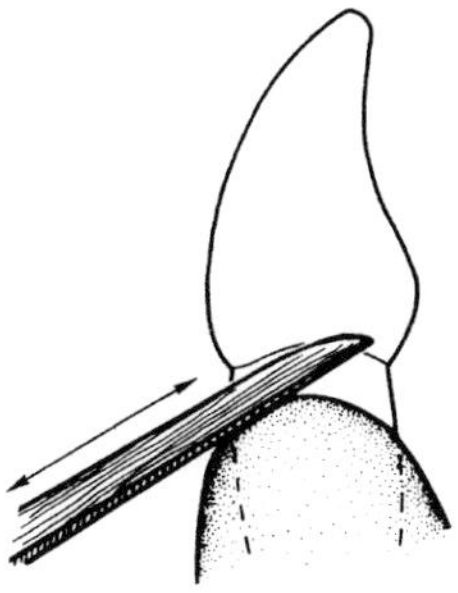

Figure 24-16. Proper placement of the Balsa triangular toothpick (wooden wedge) against the proximal surface of a tooth. (From Hoag PM, Pawlak EA: *Essentials of periodontics,* ed 4, St Louis, 1990, Mosby.)

II and III embrasures. They are recommended for use only from the facial aspect, where the proximal surfaces are exposed to avoid traumatizing gingival tissue. The use of wooden wedges is reviewed in Procedure 24-6 and the corresponding Competency Form. The key difference between the use of toothpicks and wooden wedges relates to the triangular design of the wedge. The advantage over floss is that there is no need for a mirror and use requires only one hand. Space must be available for safe use. Triangular toothpicks are inserted interdentally, with the base of the triangle resting on the gingival side, the tip pointing occlusally or incisally, and the sides of the triangle against the adjacent tooth surfaces (Figure 24-16). Placing the triangle base against the tissue prevents damage, such as gingival cuts and clefts, to the interdental papilla and gingival margins (see Figure 24-17). The triangular wedge fits the interdental area more snugly, covering a larger surface area, thereby allowing for the removal of plaque biofilm. Systematic reviews have shown that triangular toothpicks are as effective in reducing gingivitis as floss or interdental brushes.[2] They are

Procedure 24-6 Use of a Triangular Toothpick

STEPS

1. Determine the need to use a triangular toothpick (wooden wedge) and appropriate areas for use.
2. Establish a rest by placing the hand on the cheek or chin or by placing a finger on the gingiva convenient to the place where the tip will be applied.
3. Place wedge against the proximal surface of a tooth with the base of the wedge triangle toward gingival border and the tip pointing occlusally or incisally at approximately a 45-degree angle (see Figure 24-16).
4. Use an in-and-out motion interproximally from the facial area only. Apply a burnishing stroke with moderate pressure first to the proximal surface of one tooth and then to the other, about four strokes each. Stop once wedge meets a slight resistance in the space (Figure 24-17).
5. Trace margin of tissue to remove marginal debris, again with tip pointing occlusally (away from tissue).
6. If debris accumulates on wedge, rinse under running water.
7. Once all areas of mouth are completed, dispose of wedge in waste receptacle.

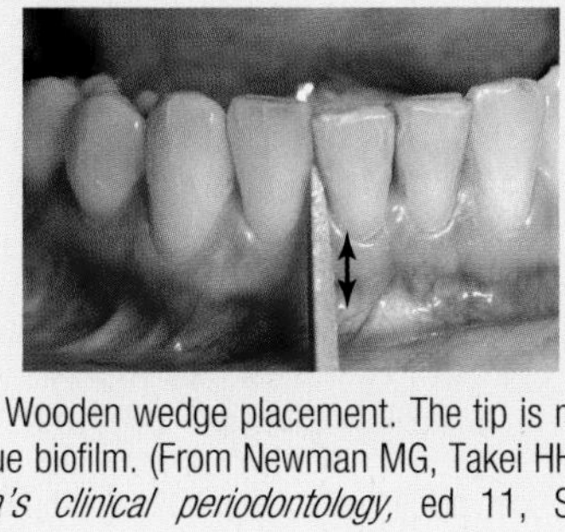

Figure 24-17. Wooden wedge placement. The tip is moved in and out to remove plaque biofilm. (From Newman MG, Takei HH, Klokkevold PR, et al: *Carranza's clinical periodontology,* ed 11, St Louis, 2012, Saunders.)

particularly effective in reducing interproximal inflammation and probing depth in clients with periodontitis because they depress the papilla by 2 to 3 mm and allow for subgingival biofilm removal from the interproximal tooth surface without directing the device toward the epithelial attachment.

Rubber Tip Stimulators

Interdental stimulators are devices designed primarily for gingival stimulation. The rubber tip stimulator, attached to the end of a metal or plastic handle (see Figure 24-18), is used to remove plaque biofilm by rubbing it against the exposed tooth surfaces, to stimulate the gingiva, and to recontour gingival papillae after periodontal therapy (see Table 24-3, Procedure 24-7 and the corresponding Competency Form). Research on rubber tip stimulators is limited and inconclusive regarding the efficacy of plaque biofilm removal and reduction of infection.

Massaging the gingiva with a rubber tip or other device can lead to improved circulation, increased keratinization, and epithelial thickening. Whether these gingival changes provide any clinical benefits has not been studied. Improved gingival health resulting from oral hygiene practices has been shown to be related directly to plaque biofilm removal and reduction of risk factors.

Interdental Brushes and Tips

Interdental brushes are available in various sizes and shapes. The most common brushes are conical or tapered (like an evergreen tree) and designed to be inserted into a plastic, reusable handle that is angled to facilitate interproximal adaptation (see Figure 24-19). Studies have shown that interproximal brushes are equal to or more effective than floss for plaque biofilm removal and for reducing gingival inflammation in type II embrasures, type III embrasures, and exposed furcations.[1] Further indications for use are discussed in Table 24-2. The brush design selected is related to the size of the gingival embrasure or furcation to be cleaned. The interdental brush must be slightly larger than the embrasure space so that it can clean effectively the designated area. Interdental brush use is reviewed in Procedure 24-8, the

Procedure 24-7 Use of a Rubber Tip Stimulator

STEPS

1. Determine the need to use a rubber tip stimulator and appropriate areas for use.
2. Place side of rubber tip interdentally and slightly pointing coronally (45-degree angle) (Figure 24-18).
3. Move in and out with a slow stroke, rubbing the tip against the teeth and under the contact area.
4. Remove from the interproximal space and trace the gingival margin, with the tip positioned just below the margin, following the contour of the gingiva.
5. Once all appropriate areas are completed, rinse stimulator with soap and warm water, then store in a clean, dry place.
6. Replace rubber tip as it becomes worn, cracked, or splayed.

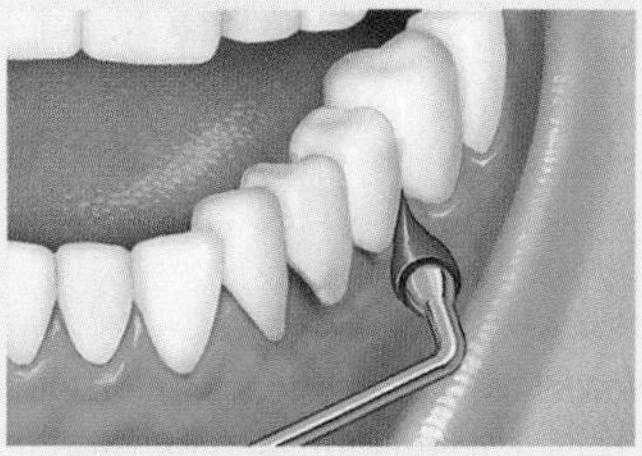

Figure 24-18. Proper placement of a rubber tip stimulator. (Courtesy Sunstar Americas, Inc, Chicago, Illinois.)

Procedure 24-8 Use of an Interdental Brush

STEPS

1. Determine the need to use an interdental brush and appropriate areas for use.
2. Insert bristles into embrasure at a 90-degree angle to tooth surface (long axis of the tooth) (Figure 24-19, *A*).
3. Move brush using in-and-out motion from facial and/or lingual surfaces of appropriate areas (Figure 24-19, *B*).
4. Rinse bristles under running water as necessary to remove debris.
5. On completion of use, rinse entire handle and bristles with warm water.
6. Store in a clean, dry place.
7. Replace bristles as they become worn or splayed.

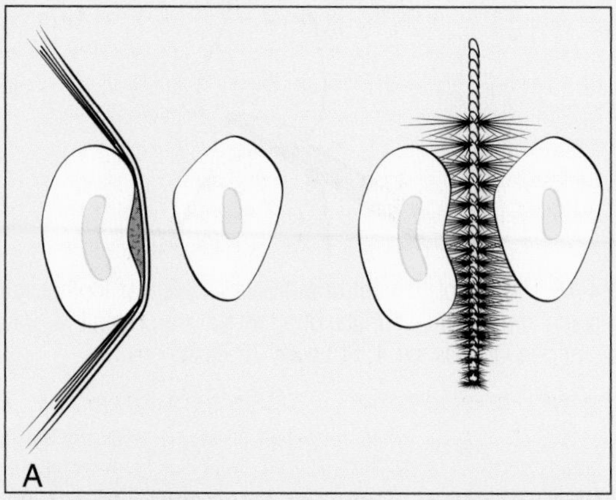

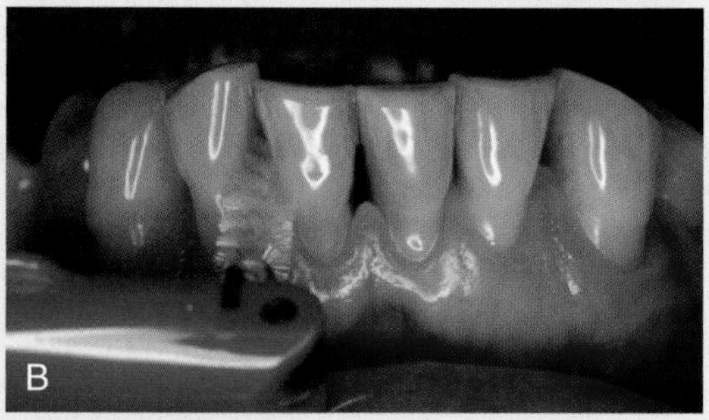

Figure 24-19. **A,** Cleaning of concave or irregular proximal tooth surfaces. Dental floss may be less effective than an interdental brush on long root surfaces with concavities. **B,** Proper placement of inderdental brush. (**A,** From Newman MG, Takei HH, Klokkevold PR, Carranza FA: *Carranza's clinical periodontology,* ed 11, St Louis, 2012, Saunders. **B,** From Perry DA, Beemsterboer PL: *Periodontology for the dental hygienist,* ed 4, St Louis, 2014, Saunders.)

TABLE 24-3
Powered Interdental and Supplemental Self-Care Devices

Powered Interdental and Supplemental Self-Care Devices	Description and Types	Indications	Contraindications and Limitations	Common Problems That May Be Experienced During Use or Misuse
Flossing devices	Single nylon filament or a bow-shaped tip attached to a power handle Special attachment for a power toothbrush that resembles a floss holder Power floss holder with replaceable floss heads	Class I embrasures Clients with physical challenges Clients who cannot master string flossing Client preference	Class II and III embrasures Tight contacts or crowed dentition May not be able to access all proximal spaces	Floss cuts or clefts with floss holder designs Unable to maintain tension or wrap floss completely around proximal area
End- or single-tufted brush	Special attachment for power toothbrush	Type III embrasure depending on design (tapered or flat) Fixed dental prosthesis (e.g., orthodontic appliances, implants, maxillofacial surgery client with jaw wired shut) Difficult-to-reach areas (e.g., lingual surface of mandibular molars, distal surface of terminal teeth, crowded teeth, third molars)	Type I embrasure	Tissue trauma Similar to problems associated with improper brushing technique
Interdental brushes and tips	Attached to a power handle Design similar to nonpower brushes	Type II and III embrasures Exposed root furcations Orthodontic and fixed appliances Maxillofacial surgery client with jaw wired shut Difficult-to-access areas	Class I embrasures	Clients may have difficulty controlling the tip once device is turned on
Dental water jet	Motor-driven pulsating device with a reservoir and specially designed tips to deliver irrigant Nonpulsating devices attach to a faucet or showerhead	Indicated for all patient types	Children need to have the ability and dexterity to use the product	Directing the stream of water under the tongue may damage the soft tissue

corresponding Competency Form, and illustrated in Figure 24-19, *B*.

Other interdental tips (see Table 24-2) are also available in various sizes and material including plastic and foam for plaque biofilm removal in areas similar to interdental brushes. Some interdental tips are designed to fit into smaller areas than a Class II embrasure (e.g., Soft Picks). The tips made of foam or other absorbent material can facilitate delivery of liquid chemotherapeutic agents, such as antimicrobials or desensitizing agents, to the proximal surface. Research in this area is limited. Interdental brushes and tips are available in disposable units designed for travel or use when away from home.

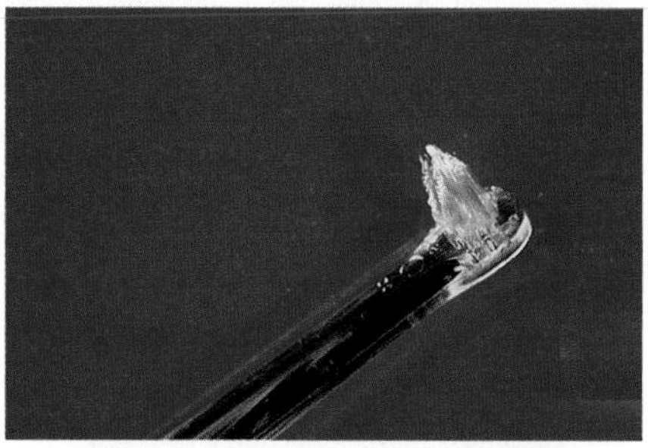

Figure 24-20. End-tufted brush.

End-Tufted or Single-Tufted Brushes

End-tufted or single-tufted toothbrushes, indicated for type II and III embrasures, for difficult-to-reach areas, or around fixed dental appliances (see Table 24-3), are designed with a smaller brush head that has a small group of tufts (end-tufted) or a single tuft (single-tufted) (Figure 24-20). The bristles are directed into the area to be cleaned and activated with a rotating motion, similar to the vibratory motion of Bass toothbrushing. Evidence supporting conical and tapered interdental brushes for effective biofilm removal and reduction in gingivitis; however, data are lacking specific to end-tufted brushes.

Tongue Cleaners

Bad breath, also known as *malodor,* is a common client complaint. Tongue cleaning often is overlooked because clients are not aware that the papillae of the tongue harbor bacteria. Bacteria on the tongue are the primary cause of bad breath. **Tongue cleaners** or scrapers are designed and intended for removal of debris and bacteria from the tongue's dorsal surface (see Figure 24-21). Brushing the tongue with a toothbrush also can remove bacteria and debris. Some clients may find it difficult to reach the tongue's posterior third with a toothbrush, and the bristles may be too soft to remove moderate to heavy debris adequately. Clients may find that a tongue cleaner is easier to use because it does not stimulate the gag reflex as readily as a toothbrush. Tongue cleaners come in many shapes, styles, and colors, from a simple plastic strip to a variety of handled devices. Procedure 24-9 and the corresponding Competency Form outlines use of a tongue cleaner.

Additional Devices

Tooth Towelettes or Finger-Mounted Wipes

Tooth towelettes and finger-mounted wipes are being marketed as a method of plaque biofilm removal when toothbrushing is not possible. The **tooth towelettes** are gauze squares usually treated with some form of mouthwash to freshen breath. The gauze square is held between the thumb and index finger and wiped on the tooth surface, moving from the cervical margin to the incisal or occlusal edge. Facial and lingual surfaces are cleaned at the same time. The finger-mounted wipe is placed over the index finger for the same type of use. These devices are not meant to replace a daily toothbrushing.

Clasp and Denture Brush

Specialty brushes such as the **clasp brush** and **denture brush** have been designed with firm nylon filaments to clean dentures and the clasps of partial dentures (see Table 24-3 and Figures 24-22 and 24-23). Because these prostheses are removable and cleaned outside of the mouth, the firmer filaments cannot cause gingival tissue destruction (see Chapter 56).

Types of Interdental and Supplemental Self-Care Devices: Powered

In the past several years, many new powered oral self-care devices have become available to consumers. The most recognizable is the powered toothbrush (see Chapter 23). Other powered devices include flossers, interdental brushes, dental water jets, and tongue cleaners. Not all products have undergone clinical testing. Table 24-3 describes a variety of powered interdental and supplemental devices.

Flossing Devices

Power flossing devices are available to make interdental cleaning easier. Research has shown that these devices can remove plaque biofilm and reduce bleeding and gingivitis similarly to string floss.[7,8] Some designs are similar to a floss holder, with floss pulled taught between a bow-shaped handle (Figure 24-24). Another design uses a single flexible nylon tip placed interproximally between the tooth and the papilla and is long enough to reach to the lingual aspect of the tooth (Figure 24-25). These products may increase compliance with some clients.

Procedure 24-9 Use of a Tongue Cleaner

STEPS

1. Determine the need to use a tongue cleaner.
2. Hold the handle of the tongue cleaner, or if it is a strip tongue cleaner, wrap in a U shape by holding both ends of the cleaner.
3. Start at the posterior part of the tongue, and drag the tongue cleaner to the tip of the tongue. If gag reflex is triggered, drag from the lateral border of the tongue to the opposite lateral border (Figure 24-21).
4. Rinse tongue scraper with water.
5. Repeat step 3 until tongue cleaner is clean on removal, being sure to cover all aspects of the tongue with overlapping strokes.
6. Rinse tongue cleaner with soap and warm water to clean. Store in a clean, dry place.

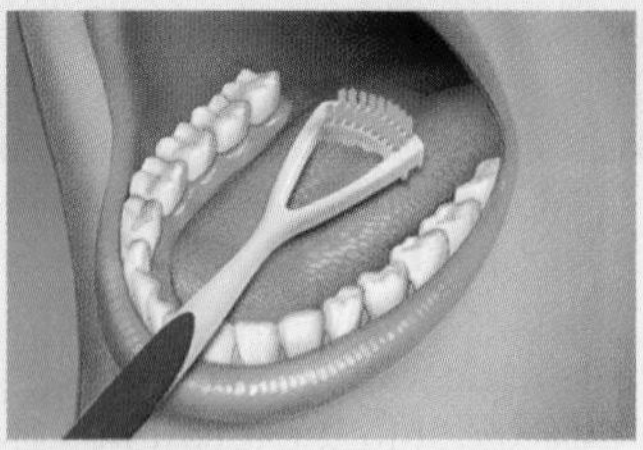

Figure 24-21. Tongue cleaner. (Courtesy Sunstar Americas, Inc, Chicago, Illinois.)

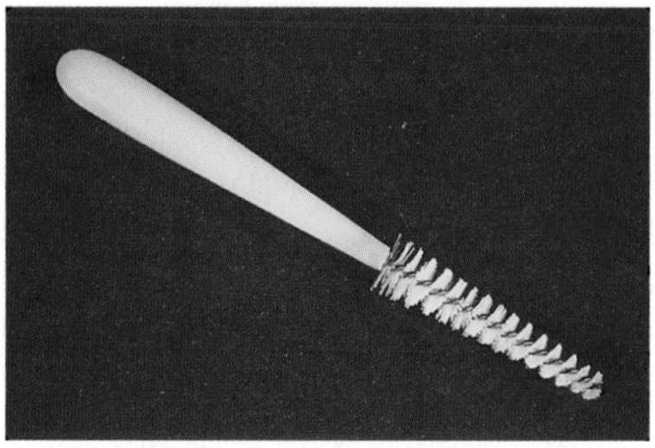

Figure 24-22. Example of denture brushes.

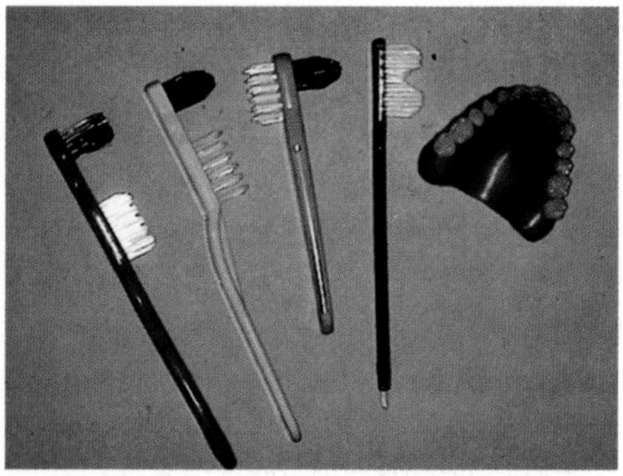

Figure 24-23. Examples of a denture clasp brush.

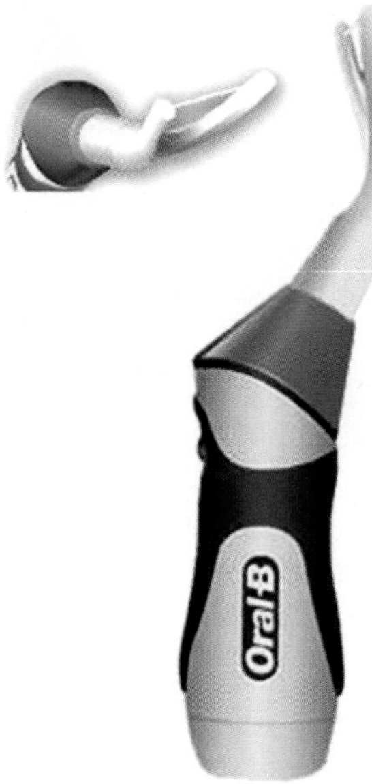

Figure 24-24. Power flosser with bow type tip, similar to nonpower devices. (Courtesy Procter & Gamble, Cincinnati, Ohio.)

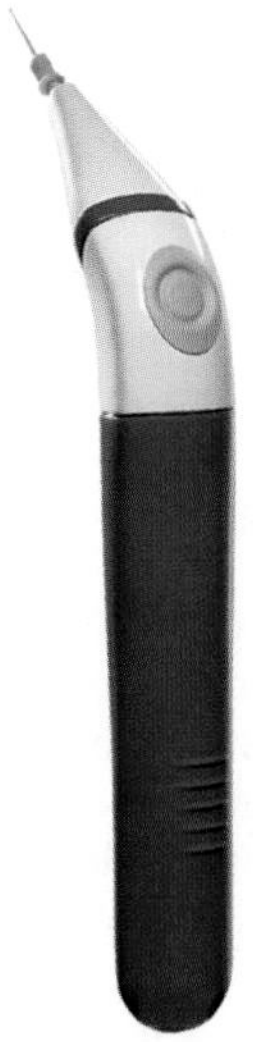

Figure 24-25. Power flosser with a single filament nylon tip. (Courtesy Water Pik, Inc, Fort Collins, Colorado.)

Interproximal Brushes and Tips

Some power toothbrushes come with attachments designed to clean the approximal or interproximal area. Attached to the brush handle, they are activated by turning on the brush and using it according to the manufacturer's directions. These attachments may be similar to a floss holder, an interdental brush, or a single- or end-tufted brush.

Dental Water Jets

In studies of clients with fixed orthodontics, implants, crowns and bridges, and gingivitis and those in a periodontal maintenance program, irrigating the gingival area with a dental water jet, or water flosser, that produces pulsating streams of fluid has been reported to reduce plaque biofilm, bleeding, gingivitis, pocket depth, pathogenic microorganisms, and calculus.[4,5,9,10] In addition, studies have shown that daily water irrigation can reduce inflammatory mediators that promote or enhance the periodontal disease process.[11] These improvements to the inflammatory response potentially may extend to systemic health, as documented by a study on persons with diabetes in which systemic measures of inflammatory mediators were reduced by the addition of oral irrigation to the self-care routine.[12]

On the other hand, dental water jets that produce a steady stream of fluid as seen with such devices that are attached to a shower or faucet have not been tested clinically for efficacy in reducing clinical parameters of periodontal disease.

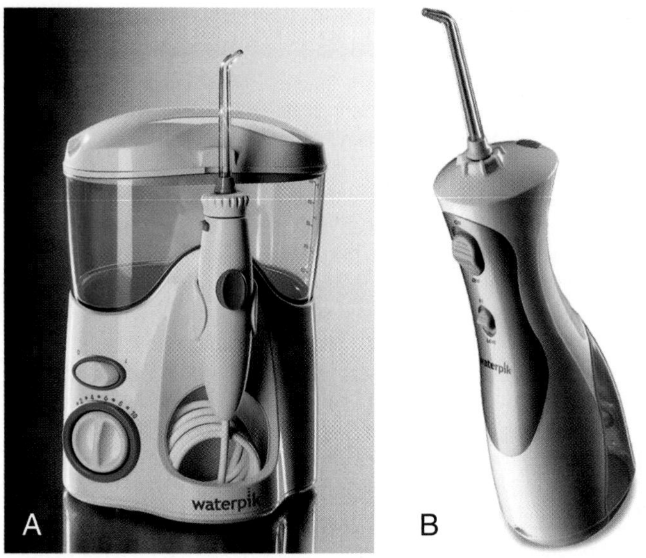

Figure 24-26. **A,** Countertop dental water jet. **B,** Cordless dental water jet. (Courtesy Water Pik, Inc, Fort Collins, Colorado.)

Mechanism of Action

A dental water jet that produces a pulsating stream of fluid (Figure 24-26) works by impacting the gingival margin with the pulsed irrigant (impact zone) and the subsequent flushing of the gingival crevice or pocket (flushing zone). This **hydrokinetic activity** produces a compression and decompression action that allows the irrigant to reach subgingivally. The majority of studies demonstrating safety and efficacy have been done with devices that deliver 1200 pulsations per minute and pressure settings between medium and high (50 to 90 pounds per square inch). Irrigation pressure can be controlled on most devices. Procedure 24-10 and the corresponding Competency Form outlines basic use of a pulsating dental water jet. For additional information on oral irrigation, see Chapter 31.

Depth of Delivery of a Solution

The dental water jet has the ability to reach deeper into the periodontal pocket than a toothbrush, interdental aid, or rinsing. This penetration allows for better subgingival cleaning and deeper delivery of antimicrobial agents. The depth to which the solution can reach depends on the tip used. A standard jet tip has been shown to reach 71% in pockets 0 to

Procedure 24-10 Use of a Dental Water Jet: Jet Tip

STEPS

1. Fill the reservoir with lukewarm water or an antimicrobial agent.
2. Select the appropriate tip and insert into the handle, pressing firmly until it is fully engaged.
3. Adjust the pressure gauge to the lowest setting when using for the first time. Increase as needed or dictated by client comfort.
4. Place the tip in the mouth, then turn the unit on. Lean over the sink and close the lips enough to prevent splashing while still allowing the water to flow from mouth into the sink.
5. Aim the standard tip at a 90-degree angle to the long axis of the tooth (Figure 24-27); follow manufacturer's instructions for other tip designs (e.g., subgingival or sulcular tips, Figure 24-28). Starting in the posterior, follow the gingival margin, pausing between the teeth for a few seconds before continuing to the next tooth. Be sure to irrigate from the buccal and lingual aspects of all teeth.
6. Read manufacturer's instructions for each model of dental water jet before demonstration.

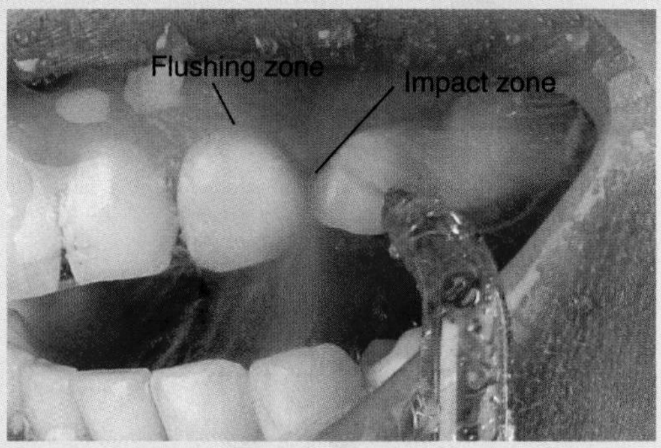

Figure 24-27. Proper placement of a standard jet tip. (From Daniel SJ, Harfst SA, Wilder RS: *Mosby's dental hygiene,* ed 2, St Louis, 2008, Mosby.)

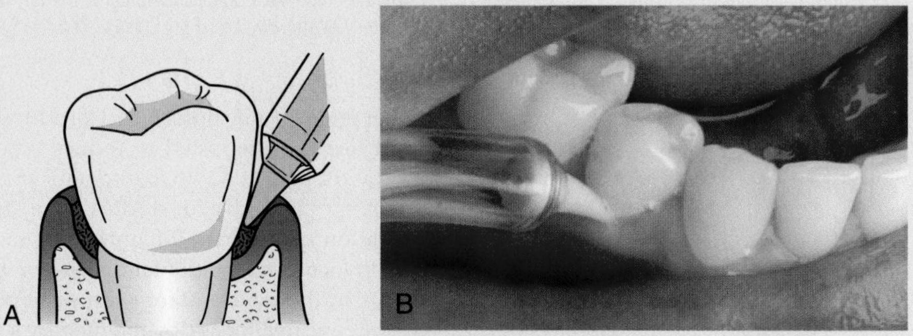

Figure 24-28. A, Irrigation with a specialized subgingival tip. **B,** Proper placement of a specialized subgingival tip. (**B,** From Daniel SJ, Harfst SA, Wilder RS: *Mosby's dental hygiene,* ed 2, St Louis, 2008, Mosby.)

3 mm, 44% in pockets 4 to 7 mm, and 68% in pockets greater than 7 mm. Specialty tips designed to be placed slightly below the gingival margin deliver a solution up to 90% in pockets 6 mm deep and 64% in pockets 7 mm or greater[8] (see Figure 24-28).

Tongue Cleaner Attachments

Powered tongue cleaners have been developed to remove plaque and debris from the dorsum of the tongue and to help control or eliminate malodor. Automation provides a means for additional action that may help clients who have difficulty with dexterity. A tongue-cleaning attachment is available for dental water jets and provides a water flushing action or the delivery of an antimicrobial. Tongue cleaning attachments are also available for some power toothbrushes. No data demonstrate that these devices are better than a manual tongue cleaner.

CLIENT EDUCATION TIPS

- Explain the importance of interdental and subgingival cleaning to the prevention and control of periodontal disease.
- Demonstrate proper use of power and nonpower mechanical self-care devices other than a toothbrush.
- Explain that breath malodor may be improved by cleaning the tongue and periodontal pocket.
- Explain that minor dexterity and visual acuity problems may be compensated through use of power devices.
- Explain how certain devices are better for specific embrasure spaces based on product design and function.
- Explain the limitations of floss, especially with clients who have deeper pockets, loss of attachment, and type II or III embrasures.
- Explain that client-specific self-care is an integral part of achieving and maintaining therapy outcomes.
- Question clients to determine which devices they currently use, the reasons they chose the devices, and whether they feel the devices are effective.
- Instruct clients based on their unique human needs to promote client acceptance.
- Evaluate the client's use of devices recommended at subsequent appointments based on signs of gingival health or disease and assist them with modifications as needed.

LEGAL, ETHICAL, AND SAFETY ISSUES

- The legal standard of care requires that dental hygienists educate clients about oral self-care.
- The legal records of the client should reveal that the client has been counseled on why and how to perform an effective daily personal self-care program. Specific recommendations of products are noted in the legal records.

- The clients' progress and adherence with recommendations are recorded. Alternative methods are recommended and demonstrated if prior instructions are not producing the expected outcomes or if the client is not able or willing to use a recommended device.
- Malpractice cases for failure to recognize and treat periodontal disease can be related to failure to inform clients of oral and periodontal conditions, teach adequate plaque biofilm techniques to clients, and provide adequate care and follow-up. Improper use of devices can cause damage to the hard and soft tissue in the oral cavity. Properly educating and demonstrating the recommended devices to the client are required and noted in the legal records.
- Autonomy is an ethical principle that applies to self-care instruction; patients always should be given choices regarding self-care devices and given evidence-based information to make an informed decision.

KEY CONCEPTS

- Interdental and subgingival plaque biofilm control is essential for the prevention of oral disease.
- Self-care recommendations are based on client's preferences, values, and needs.
- If a client refuses to floss or if floss is not appropriate, the dental hygienist recommends alternatives that will provide similar benefits.
- Flossing is not the device of choice for many clients based on preference and assessment. It is effective when used properly and daily by the clients who have type I embrasures and normal sulcus. It is a good choice for prevention of periodontal disease in clients with a healthy periodontium.
- Risk assessment is an important part of determining which self-care device to recommend.
- Clients must be involved in the selection of self-care devices. Recommendations should be based on the fewest devices that provide the optimal plaque biofilm control for the client.

CRITICAL THINKING EXERCISES

Scenario: A middle-age male client presents with normal gingival contour and localized pockets of 4 to 5 mm in the molar areas. His toothbrushing appears to be effective with healthy gingival tissues buccally and lingually, but bleeding on probing occurs in various areas of the mouth where interdental papillae are inflamed. Localized inflammation also is apparent around the existing crown and bridge No. 2-4.

1. Discuss devices that could be used, and make recommendations for home care.
2. With a classmate practice the following techniques:
   a. Identify and discuss the benefits of the different types of floss provided by your instructor in class or clinic.
   b. Demonstrate proper flossing techniques for spool and loop methods on a typodont. Once mastered on a typodont, demonstrate flossing in your own mouth and then on a partner while using proper infection-control methods.
   c. Identify devices that would benefit clients with orthodontics, and demonstrate proper use of the devices on a typodont with fixed orthodontic brackets and wires.
   d. Role-play providing instructions on the use of floss, floss threader and holder, dental water jet, interdental tips, brush and stimulator, wood or plastic sticks, toothpick and holder, and tongue cleaner.
   e. On a periodontal typodont, demonstrate use of the various devices designed specifically for periodontal maintenance clients.
   f. Divide into groups of two or three, with each group assigned one device or category. Students should deliver oral reports to the class that include features, benefits, expected outcomes based on clinical research, and what types of clients would benefit from using the device. Compare and contrast the assigned device to another category of device that can deliver the same benefits.

REFERENCES

1. Slot DE, Dorfer CE, Van derWeijden GA: The efficacy of interdental brushes on plaque and parameters of periodontal inflammation: a systematic review. *Int J Dent Hygiene* 6:253, 2008.
2. Hoenderdos NL, Slot DE, Paraskevas S, et al: The efficacy of woodsticks on plaque and gingival inflammation: a systematic review. *Int J Dent Hyg* 6:280, 2008.
3. Van derWeijden GA, Slot DE: Oral hygiene in the prevention of periodontal diseases: the evidence. *Periodontology 2000* 55:105, 2011.
4. Husseini A, Slot DE, Van derWeijden GA: The efficacy of oral irrigation in addition to a toothbrush on plaque and the clinical parameters of periodontal inflammation: a systematic review. *Int J Dent Hyg* 6:304, 2008.
5. Rosema NA, Hennequin-Hoenderdos NL, Berchier CE, et al: The effect of different interdental cleaning devices on gingival bleeding. *J Int Acad Periodontol* 13:2, 2011.
6. Sambunjak D, Nickerson JW, Poklepovic T, et al: Flossing for the management of periodontal diseases and dental caries in adults. *Cochrane Datab System Rev* 2011, Issue 12. Art. No.: CD008829. DOI:10.1002/14651858.CD008829.pub2.
7. Hujoel PP, Cunha-Cruz J, Banting DW, et al: Dental flossing and interproximal caries: a systematic review. *J Dent Res* 85:298, 2006.
8. Eakle WS, Ford C, Boyd RL: Depth of penetration in periodontal pockets with oral irrigation. *J Clin Periodontol* 13:39, 1986. doi: 10.1111/j.1600-051X.1986.tb01412.x.
9. Cronin M, Dembling WZ, Cugini M, et al: A 30-day clinical comparison of a novel interdental cleaning device and dental floss in the reduction of plaque and gingivitis. *J Clin Dent* 16:33, 2005.
10. Cutler CW, Stanford TW, Abraham C, et al: Clinical benefits of oral irrigation for periodontitis are related to reduction of pro-inflammatory cytokine levels and plaque. *J Clin Periodontol* 27:134, 2000.
11. Sharma NC, Lyle DM, Qaqish JG, et al: The effect of a dental water jet with orthodontic tip on plaque and bleeding in adolescent patients with fixed appliances. *Am J Orthod Dentofacial Orthop* 133:565, 2008.
12. Al-Mubarak S, Ciancio S, Aljada A, et al: Comparative evaluation of adjunctive oral irrigation in diabetics. *J Clin Periodontol* 29:295, 2002.

ACKNOWLEDGMENT

The authors acknowledge the contributions of Brenda Parton Maddox and Deborah M. Lyle for their past contributions to this chapter.

EVOLVE RESOURCES

Please visit http://evolve.elsevier.com/Darby/hygiene for additional practice and study support tools.

CHAPTER 25

Dentifrices

France Lavoie, Nadia Dubreuil, Louise Bourassa

COMPETENCIES

1. Explain the purpose of a dentifrice and types of effects that it can produce.
2. Discuss choosing the right dentifrice, including role of dentifrices in the demineralization and remineralization process.
3. Explain why each member of a family should have his or her own tube of toothpaste.
4. Describe the different forms of dentifrices and the role of medicinal and nonmedicinal components in dentifrices.
5. Explain the concept of bioavailability.
6. Debate the possible adverse health effects of dentifrices.
7. Explain the impact of the pH level of dentifrices.
8. Recommend dentifrices appropriate for unique client needs and risk factors.
9. Discuss the loss of tooth structures.
10. Compare methods to evaluate dentifrice abrasiveness.
11. Delineate the legal and ethical responsibilities of the dental hygienist with regard to dentifrices.

Purpose of a Dentifrice

Clients look to the dental hygienist to recommend a daily use dentifrice that will meet the clients' unique oral health needs. A **dentifrice** or **toothpaste** is a substance used with a toothbrush or other oral hygiene device to clean the teeth, tongue, and gingiva and to deliver cosmetic and therapeutic agents to the teeth and oral environment. A dentifrice can yield the following types of effects:

- Cosmetic effect: Prevents or removes stains, inhibits supragingival calculus formation, whitens teeth, freshens breath, controls oral malodor
- Hygienic effect: Removes food particles and oral biofilm
- Therapeutic effect: Prevents or reverses dental caries; reduces gingivitis, oral biofilm, or dentinal hypersensitivity[1]

Toothpastes that carry the American Dental Association (ADA) Seal of Acceptance or the Canadian Dental Association Seal of Recognition have been shown through rigorous research to be safe and therapeutically effective (antiplaque, antigingivitis, anticaries, and anti–dentinal hypersensitivity). The ADA Seal also has been awarded to dentifrices that safely and effectively remove tooth stain. (See the discussion of product selection and evaluation in Chapter 29.) The absence of a seal does not mean that the dentifrice is not safe and effective; it implies the dentifrice company did not obtain, or possibly apply for, approval. The dental hygienist should compare the dentifrice without a seal to similar products and/or search for evidence regarding these products before recommending them to clients.

Choosing a Dentifrice

A dentifrice is selected to meet particular client needs, but the array of dentifrices on the market can be confusing to the consumer as well as the professional (Figure 25-1). Manufacturers develop dentifrices for topical intraoral use and for cleaning dentures; nonfoaming to low-foaming dentifrices for use with power toothbrushes and children; ingestible dentifrices for persons with special needs; and dentifrices free of preservatives, sodium lauryl sulfate (SLS), fluoride, dyes, peroxide, and artificial flavors for persons who may be allergic or who desire a "natural" product.

Dentifrices containing calcium and phosphate technologies claim to enhance the bioavailability of calcium and phosphate ions for incorporation into the tooth surface. In theory, this aids in the enhancement of remineralization and reduces dentinal sensitivity, but more clinical trials are needed to substantiate effectiveness in caries management.[2] Fluoride is the ingredient with the strongest evidence supporting its effectiveness in remineralization and caries prevention. Combinations of agents may influence their effectiveness. Some ingredients increase the bioavailability of fluoride (F) in their formulation. For example, toothpaste containing the cocaprophyl betaine as a detergent has better bioavailability of F compared with a product containing SLS. The abrasive particle calcium carbonate binds sodium fluoride to render it less effective as an anticaries agent; in contrast, sodium monofluorophosphate is effective with calcium carbonate.[3]

Other dentifrices have antibacterial ingredients such as chlorhexidine gluconate (CHG or CHX), stannous fluoride (SnF_2), or triclosan with copolymer to control gingivitis and oral biofilm.[3] The addition of the copolymer is intended to increase the substantivity of triclosan, thus prolonging the antibacterial effect for 12 hours.

Some dentifrices containing amorphous calcium phosphate (ACP), calcium sodium phosphosilicate (CSP), or NovaMin, potassium nitrate, or potassium citrate, or a combination of ingredients offer a desensitizing effect. Other dentifrices contain arginine, sodium monofluorophosphate (MFP), and calcium carbonate chloride to reduce dentinal hypersensitivity.[3]

Figures, tables, and boxes marked as "e" are available as supplemental material on the Evolve site. Visit http://evolve.elsevier.com/Darby/hygiene to access these materials.

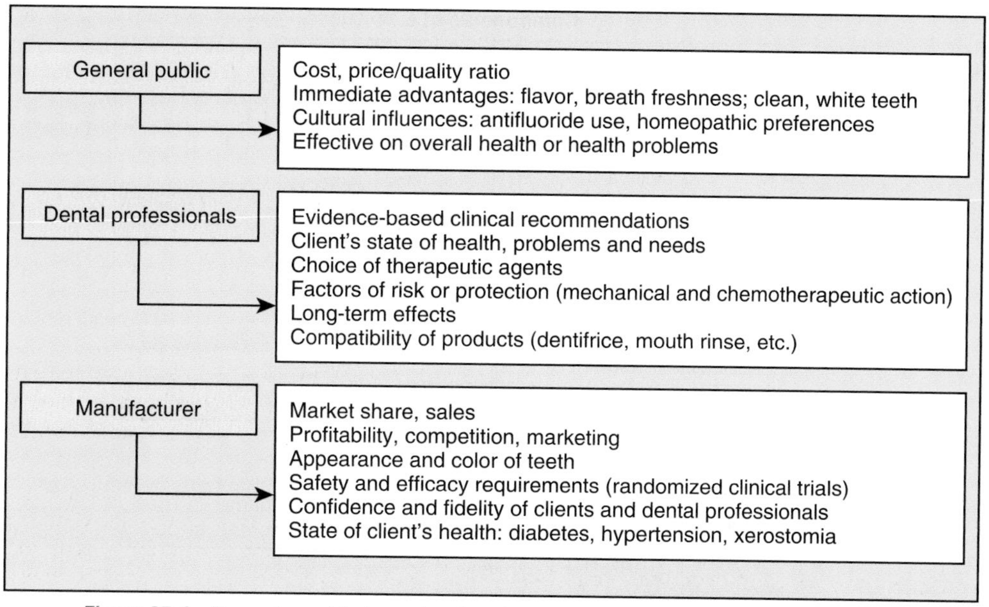

Figure 25-1. Comparison of factors related to choice of a dentifrice. (Courtesy France Lavoie.)

Dentifrices have been formulated for persons with health problems such as diabetes (with sweeteners that have no effect on blood sugar), xerostomia (with salivary enzymes, lubricants, and salivary enhancers), recurrent aphthous ulcers (SLS-free), and hypertension (sodium bicarbonate free or sodium chloride free).

Toothpaste Tube Contamination

The orifice of the tube can be a source of cross-contamination. Transmission of bacteria responsible for oral and systemic disease is possible when family members' toothbrushes come into contact with the neck of the same tube of dentifrice. Each family member should have his or her own tube of toothpaste to prevent cross-contamination, to control infection among people living in the same household or in a daycare center, and to meet his or her unique oral care needs. In Canada in the field of public dental health, it is recommended to file individual portions of the recommended dose of dentifrice on a waxed paper or a cardboard box so that each child takes his or her amount of toothpaste without the risk of contaminating the tube or the other children's toothbrushes. These measures are established to prevent the transmission of infectious diseases such as hepatitis B, gastroenteritis, and the cold or even the flu.

Forms of Dentifrices

Dentifrices come in powders, liquid gels, gels, pastes, foam, and gel-paste combinations (Figure 25-2). Fluoride gel containing potassium nitrate, in contact with saliva and the temperature of the mouth, is transformed into foam and easily infiltrates between the interdental surfaces to better protect them. A fluoridated liquid gel dentifrice is effective in caries prevention, because it reaches the interproximal surfaces and deep grooves of the teeth.[1]

Components of Dentifrices

Toothpastes contain ingredients from natural or synthetic origin (Figure 25-3, Table 25-1, and eTab.e 25-2).[2,3] In general, manufacturers choose these ingredients according to their

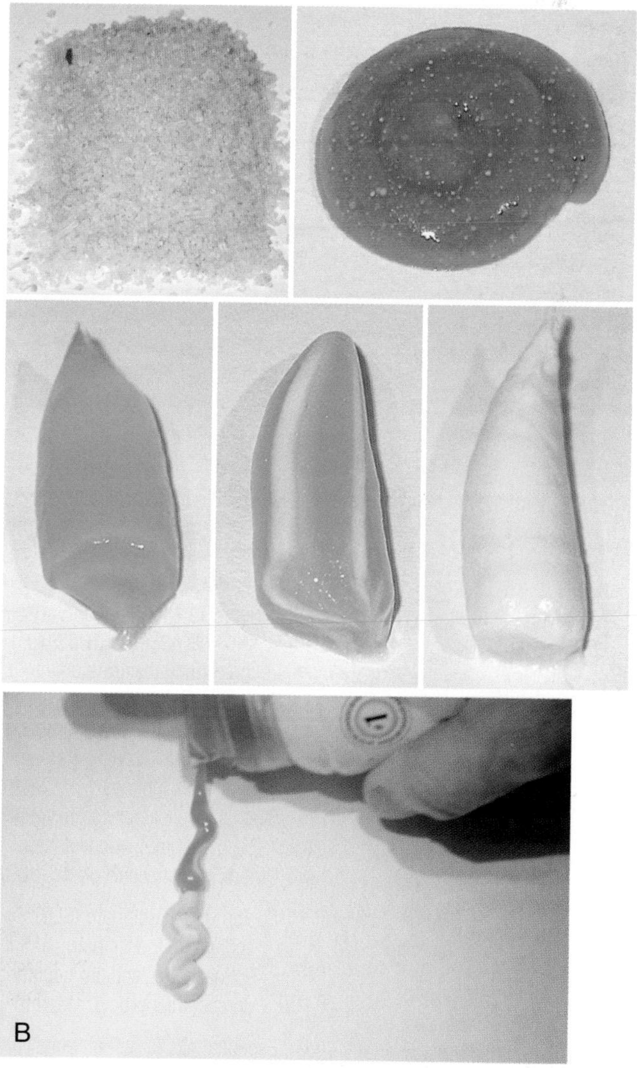

Figure 25-2. Forms of dentifrices. **A,** Powder, liquid gel, gel, gel/paste, and paste. **B,** Foaming gel. (Courtesy Nadia Dubreuil, member of the GREHD (Dental Hygiene Research Group) Cégep Garneau, Québec, Canada.)

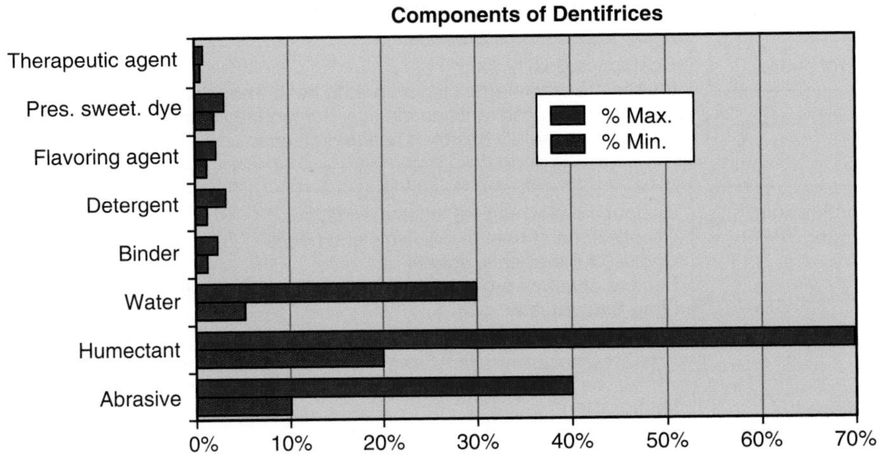

	Abrasive	Humectant	Water	Binder	Detergent	Flavoring agent	Pres. sweet. dye	Therapeutic agent
% Max.	40%	70%	30%	2%	3%	2%	3%	0.50%
% Min.	10%	20%	5%	1%	1%	1%	2%	0.10%

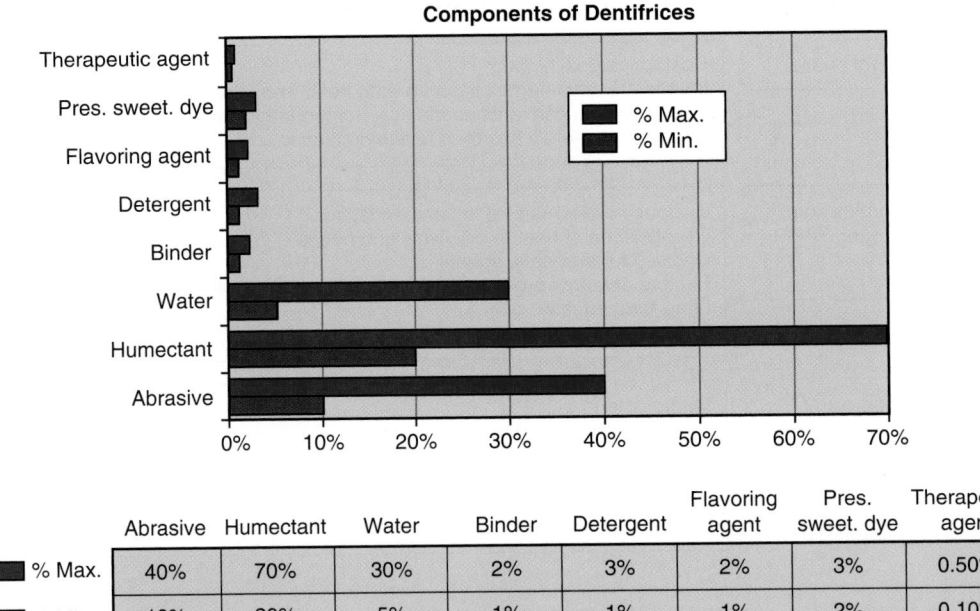

Figure 25-3. Components of dentifrices and percentage by weight. *Pres.*, Preservative; *sweet.*, sweetener.

TABLE 25-1
Components of Dentifrices

Components	Examples	Quantity
Cleansing and polishing agents (10%-40%)	Phosphate: calcium pyrophosphate, dicalcium phosphate dihydrate, anhydrous dicalcium phosphate, insoluble calcium metaphosphate (IMP) Carbonates: calcium carbonate (chalk), sodium bicarbonate Silices: silica, silicates, dehydrated silica gels, synthetic amorphous silicates in gel form, perlite Aluminium compounds: hydrated aluminium oxides, aluminium trihydrates, alumines, amorphous aluminium silicate Others: complex salt of synthetic, methacrylate, argile (pumice, kaolin, bentonite), magnesium carbonate, insoluble materials (herbs)	NA
Humectants (20%-70%)	Glycerin, sorbitol, mannitol, propylene glycol, vegetable oils, synthetic cellulose	NA
Water (5%-30%)	Distilled water, deionized water, spring water	NA
Binders (1%-2%) or gelling agent or thickeners	Mineral colloids: Varieties of clay: bentonite (derived from volcanic ash), china clay, Laponite (inorganic silica clay), kaolin Veegum (magnesium aluminium silicate) Sodium aluminium silicate, viscarine Natural gums: arabic or arabic gum, karaya, tragacanth, guar gum, xanthan Seaweed colloids: alginates (and derivatives), Irish moss extract, gum carrageenan, agar-agar, chitosan Synthetic cellulose: carboxymethyl cellulose, hydroxyethyl cellulose, hydroxypropyl cellulose, methyl cellulose Others: polyethylene glycol (PEG), glycerol carbomer	NA
Detergents (1%-3%) or surfactants or foaming agents	Sodium lauryl sulphate (SLS), sodium *N*-lauryl sarcosinate, *N*-lauryl sarcosinate, dioctyl sodium sulfosuccinate, sodium, streryl fumarate, sodium stearyl lactate, sodium lauryl sulfoacetate, sodium cocomonoglyceride sulfonate, cocamidopropyl betaine or betaine de cocamidopropyl, steareth-30, sodium monoglyceride sulfate, ethionates of fatty acid	NA
Flavoring agents or aromatizers (1%-2%)	Essential oils (menthol, eucalyptus, peppermint, spearmint), clove oil, aniseed, vanilla, wintergreen, caraway, pimento, citrus, nutmeg, thyme, cinnamon	NA
Preservatives (2%-3%)*	Alcohols, sodium benzoates, formaldehydes, phenolics (methyl, ethy, propyl), methylparaben, ethylparaben, polyaminopropyl biguanide	NA

TABLE 25-1

Components of Dentifrices—cont'd

Components	Examples	Quantity
Sweeteners (2%-3%)*	Noncariogenic artificial sweetener, sorbitol, glycerin, sodium saccharin, sodium cyclamate, xylitol, aspartame, acesulfame	NA
Coloring or dye agents (2%-3%)*	Vegetable coloring, titanium dioxide, sodium perborate, chlorophyll, magnesium peroxide, tartrazine, hydrogen peroxide-urea compounds	NA
Therapeutic or medicinal agents	Anticaries agents, désensibilisant, antigingivitis, anticalculus, antistains, antihalitosis	Minimal
Anticaries agents	Fluoride	
	Sodium fluoride (NaF)[†]	*0.24%*
	Sodium monofluorophosphate (MFP)	*0.76%*
	Stannous fluoride (SnF_2)	*0.4%*
	Amine fluoride (AmF)	0.125%
	Nicomethanol hydrofluoride	NA
	Silver diamine fluoride	NA
	Nonfluoride anticaries components	
	Calcium and phosphate derivatives or components:	
	Recaldent	NA
	NovaMin	5%
	Calcium lactate	NA
	Phosphate derivatives (trimetaphosphates, pyrophosphates, glycerophosphates)	NA
	Various antimicrobials	
	Antibacterial enzymes (glucose oxydase)	NA
	Metals (zinc, tin, aluminium, iron, manganese, molybdenum)	NA
		NA
	Xylitol	5%
Desensitizing agents	Chemical or mechanical action	
	Potassium salts (2% minimum to be effective):	
	Potassium nitrate	*5%*
	Potassium chloride	*3.75%*
	Potassium citrate	*5.75*
	Strontium chloride	*10%*
	Strontium acetate hemihydrate	*8 %*
	Stannous fluoride (SnF_2)	*0.4%*
	Sodium fluoride (NaF) (5000 ppm)	*1.1%*
	Sodium citrate	*NA*
	Calcium sodium phosphosilicates (NovaMin)	*5%*
	Amorphous calcium phosphate (Recaldent)	*NA*
	Component of:	
	Arginine	(8%)
	Calcium carbonate	35%
	MFP (1450 ppm)	1.1%
Antigingivitis and oral biofilm reduction agents	*Triclosan with 2% copolymer PVM/MA*	*0.3%*
	Stannous fluoride (SnF_2)	*0.4%*
	Chlorhexidine	*0.12%*
	Essential oils (combination):	
	Eucalyptol	*0.738%*
	Menthol	*0.340%*
	Methyl salicylate	*0.480%*
	Thymol	*0.511%*
	Cetylpyridinium chloride (CPC)	*0.05%*
	Antibacterial enzymes:	
	Lactoperoxidase	*15,000 units*
	Oxydase glucose	*10,000 units*
	Lysozyme	*16 mg*
	Lactoferrin	*NA*
	Potassium thiocyanate	NA
	Triclosan and zinc citrate	NA
	Xylitol	5%

Continued

TABLE 25-1

Components of Dentifrices—cont'd

Components	Examples	Quantity
Anticalculus agents Active ingredients but not considered therapeutic	*Pyrophosphates and derivated:* *Tetrasodium pyrophosphate* Disodium pyrophosphate *Sodium hexamethaphosphate (SHMP)* Sodium tripolyphosphate Tetrapotassium pyrophosphate *Zinc and derivated:* *Zinc citrate* *Zinc chloride* Zinc salts and copolymer of methyl vinyl ether and maleic anhydride	 *1% (ADA) to 5% (CDA)* *2%* *NA* *NA*
Antistain agents: Active ingredients but not considered therapeutic	*Abrasives in dentifrices (remove or prevent stains)* Peroxides (remove or prevent stains, can alter enamel) Hydrogen Carbamide Phosphates and derivatives (remove or prevent stains): sodium tripolyphosphate, sodium bicarbonate, sodium hexametaphosphate Papain (enzyme whitening agent) and sodium citrate Dimethicone (prevents stain formation)	*NA* NA NA NA NA
Antihalitosis or malodor (reduction of oral bacteria and the volatile sulphur compounds [VSC]) Active ingredients but not considered therapeutic	*Antibacterian agents* Triclosan/co-copolymer/sodium fluoride Stannous fluoride and hexametaphosphate (SHMP) *Zinc and derived* *Chlorine dioxide* *Essentials oils* Enzymes	*NA* *NA* *NA* *NA* NA

ADA, American Dental Association; *CDA*, Canadian Dental Association; *NA*, not applicable; *PVM/MA*, polyvinylmethoxyethylene and maleic acid.

*Total for preservatives, sweeteners, and dyes.

†Italic typeface denotes acceptance by the ADA or CDA.

cost of production. On the other hand, official bodies (ADA, CDA) have no requirement in regard to the natural or artificial origin of the product and even less in terms of its labeling. As a result, people with allergy problems are not sufficiently informed and become exposed to these ingredients. The population should be aware of the risks associated with long-term exposure to these ingredients, because these can cause an allergic reaction.

Toothpastes are complex formulas of medicinal (therapeutic or active) and nonmedicinal (inactive ingredients) that must be compatible to be effective. A **medicinal ingredient** is an additive that produces a therapeutic or beneficial effect on either the hard or soft tissues. Some authors use the terms *medicinal ingredient*, *active ingredient*, and *therapeutic ingredient* interchangeably; however, for a medicinal ingredient to be therapeutic, it must improve oral health status in a safe and effective way—for example, fluoride for caries control; triclosan-copolymer for control of gingivitis and oral biofilm; agents such as NovaMin and SnF_2 to achieve desensitization and caries control; and potassium nitrate or potassium citrate to control dentinal hypersensitivity.[3] A medicinal ingredient may be beneficial but still not be therapeutic (e.g., pyrophosphate zinc systems to inhibit calculus formation). A **nonmedicinal** is an additive that is necessary to make the formulation thick, hold together, clean efficiently, or have a particular color or flavor for consumer appeal. Listing specific ingredients on the packaging of oral care products would make it possible to meet client needs and avoid risks of allergies and intolerances. Medicinal and nonmedicinal ingredients found in dentifrices are discussed in the following sections.

Abrasives

Abrasive agents are used to clean and polish teeth to a smooth, lustrous surface; they establish the abrasive capacity of the dentifrice (see Table 25-1, eTable 25-2, Table 25-3 and Figure 25-4). Their origins are natural or synthetic. If abrasive capacity is too low, the abrasive agent is less effective in removing the soft deposits and stains. If it is too high, it may increase abrasion of tooth structure and restored tooth surfaces, especially with excessive toothbrushing force. A client who brushes teeth without dentifrice must brush longer, because there is no abrasive agent on the toothbrush to help remove soft deposits and stains adequately.[1] Dentifrices

TABLE 25-3

Variables Influencing Dentifrice Abrasiveness

Particle size (grit)	The larger the particles, the more they wear on dental surfaces (see Figure 25-5).
Particle shape	The more irregular the shape, the more dental surfaces are worn and abraded. A round particle is less detrimental to the tooth (see Figure 25-5).
Particle hardness	The harder the particles, the more the dental surfaces are abraded.
pH level	The more acidic and abrasive, the more the dentifrice increases tooth surface mineral loss, particularly if dentin or cementum is exposed (see Figure 25-6 and Table 25-6).
Quantity of glycerin and water in dentifrice	The higher the level of glycerin in a dentifrice, the higher its level of abrasiveness, as the dissolution of insoluble materials is reduced. The greater the amount of water in a dentifrice, the more soluble particles can dissolve, making them less abrasive to dental surfaces (see Table 25-2).

Data from Lavoie F, Feeney N, McCallum L, et al: Evaluation of toothpastes and of variables associated with the choice of a product, *CDHA* 41:42, 2007.

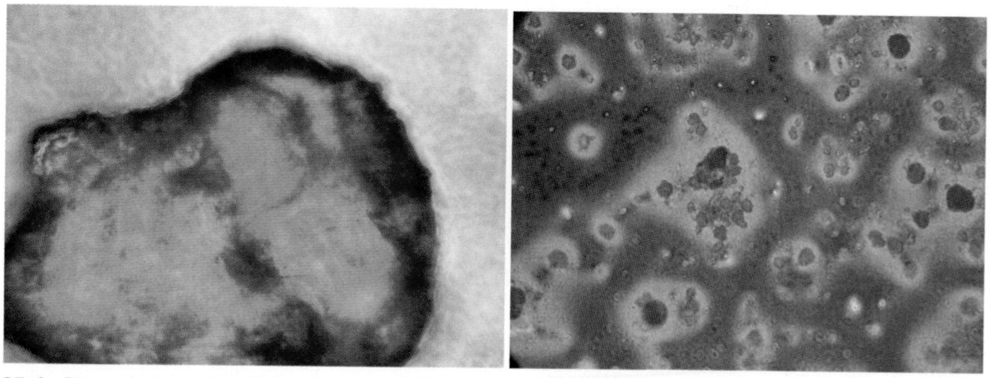

Figure 25-4. Size and shape of particles. (Courtesy GREHD (Dental Hygiene Research Group), Cégep Garneau, Québec, Canada.)

powders, gels, foaming gel, and pastes contain abrasive agents.[1-3]

The five common dentifrice abrasives are phosphates, carbonates, silicas, aluminium compounds, and other substances.

- Phosphates help the dentifrice make the teeth look white and feel clean and include the following:
  - Dicalcium phosphate dihydrate (DCPD)
  - Calcium pyrophosphate (CalPyro)
- Carbonates help to clean and deodorize the mouth and make it smell fresh.
  - Sodium bicarbonate (baking soda)—used in toothpastes with NaF; bactericidal
  - Calcium carbonate (chalk)—used in toothpastes with MFP
- Silicas mechanically clean the teeth, and some thicken the dentifrice. Silicas are chemically compatible with NaF and MFP. Silicas are nonreactive and therefore are used frequently as abrasives in toothpaste.
- Alumina and aluminium compounds. Alumina is an insoluble material with a very high abrasive potential, whose hardness is greater than the tooth.
  - Aluminium trihydrate
  - Alumine
- Other substances. Many substances are used as abrasives. Many are composed of minerals, clay, and synthetics such as vinyl and resins.
  - Clay: Bentonite, China clay, kaolin, volcanic ash
  - Methacrylate

Mohs Hardness Scale described and rated the hardness of materials, with 1 being the softest and 10 being the hardest.[1] The hardness of abrasive agents found in dentifrices and the hardness of a tooth are compared in Figure 25-5. Mohs Hardness Scale is useful for understanding abrasiveness of cleaning and polishing agents. For example, the threshold of 2 to 4 is equal to the hardness of cementum or dentin, often exposed because of gingival recession. Dentifrices whose level of abrasiveness is 2 or less are recommended to avoid tooth structure loss on exposed roots. Children can use a more abrasive dentifrice when their tooth enamel is mature (hardness level of 4 to 5). A dentifrice containing alumina is efficient for stain removal but has a higher risk for damaging tooth surfaces because its hardness level is higher than that of the tooth's enamel. Even hard agents can be made safe by varying their particle size and shape in the manufacturing process.

Humectants

A **humectant** is a substance used to retain moisture, prevent air-drying, and ensure a chemically and physically stable product. Low concentrations of synthetic cellulose are used as a humectant; high concentrations are used as binders to stabilize the gel or liquid gel dentifrice formula and up to 40%, it also acts as a preservative.[5] Other humectants include polyoxyethylene glycol esters (PEG 8), polypropylene glycol ethers (PPG), pentatol, glycerin, and xylitol.

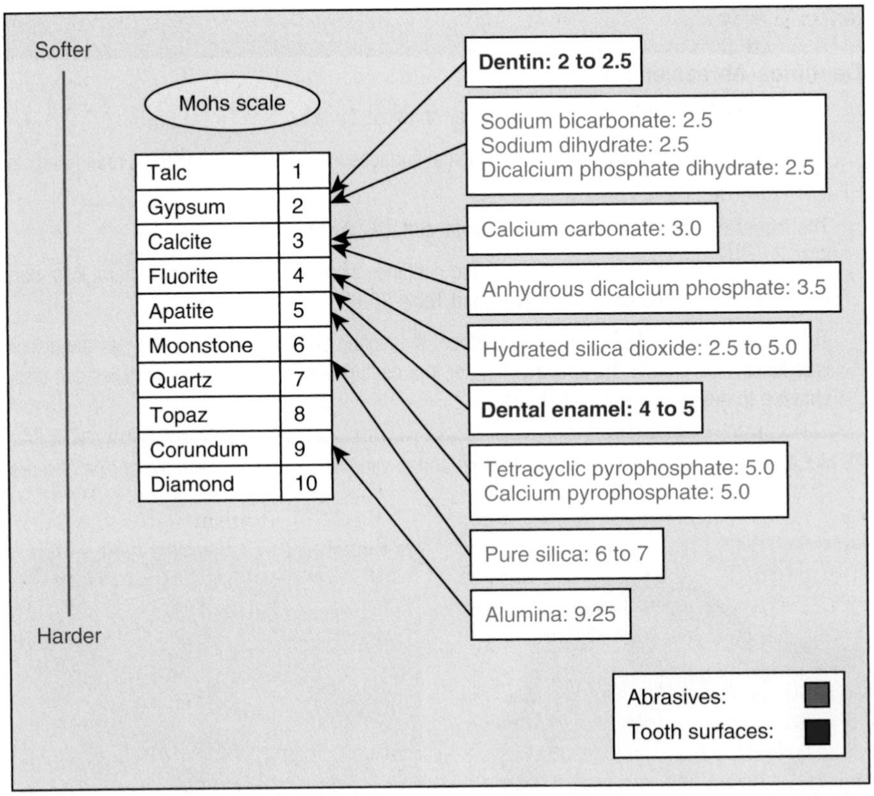

Figure 25-5. Comparison of hardness scales, abrasives, tooth surfaces, dental restaurations, and others. (Courtesy Nadia Dubreuil. Adaptation of Mohs Scale [1812].)

Water

The list of dentifrice ingredients seldom specifies the type of water used (deionized or distilled water) despite the fact that it represents 20% to 30% of the composition of the dentifrice (see Figure 25-3).

Preservatives

Because the risk of microorganism contamination is omnipresent, preservatives such as dichlorinated phenol, sodium benzoate, methylparaben, trisodium phosphate, and alcohols are added to inhibit mold and bacterial growth and prolong shelf life.

Binders

Substances such as sodium carrageenan, xanthan gum, alginates, and synthetic cellulose derivatives (carboxymethylcellulose) are used as thickeners and prevent liquid and solid ingredients from separating in pastes and gels. Gel formulas contain more binders than pastes. "Natural" dentifrice manufacturers tend to replace the oil-based products such as PEG with plant-based products such as algae and agar-agar. A new binder used in Europe, chitosan, also has antibacterial properties.[6] However, associated with stannous chloride (Sn^{2+}) it would provide better protection against erosion.[7]

Detergents

Foaming agents or detergents such as sodium lauryl sarcosinate, SLS, or cocamidopropyl betaine, called *surfactants,* are popular in toothpastes to lower surface tension to loosen debris and stain. SLS[5] can contribute to recurrent aphthous ulcers or irritation of oral mucosa in some people. If such intolerance occurs, it is preferable to use a dentifrice containing cocamidopropyl betaine (e.g., Sensodyne Pronamel or Colgate Luminous). SLS neutralizes the effects of CHG; therefore clients using a dentifrice containing SLS should wait half an hour before using a CHG-containing oral rinse.[5]

Flavoring and Sweetening Agents

Ingredients are added to provide a refreshing flavor and aftertaste and to mask the taste of unpleasant chemical compounds. Typical flavoring agents include oils of spearmint, peppermint, wintergreen, or cinnamon; bubble gum and fruit flavors; and menthol. Certain flavors, such as cinnamon, can cause a burning sensation, tissue sloughing, contact stomatitis, intolerances, or allergic reactions.

Sorbitol and xylitol are sweeteners that contribute to a pleasant taste. In doses greater than 10%, xylitol is an effective antimicrobial agent to combat tooth decay.[8]

Coloring Agents

Dyes, such as vegetable coloring, make the product attractive; tartrazine (yellow #5) in some dentifrices may produce an allergic reaction, especially in persons hypersensitive to aspirin.

Therapeutic Agents or Medicinal Ingredients

Ingredients added for specific preventive, treatment, or beneficial purposes are referred to as *therapeutic agents* or *medicinal ingredients.* For example, CHG is available in different concentrations and is used to control dental plaque formation and gingivitis.[9] GUM Gingidex dentifrice contains 0.06% CHG and GUM Paroex dentifrice contains 0.12% CHG to control gingivitis and plaque. These products vary by country. For a dentifrice to be considered therapeutic the manufacturer must follow strict pharmaceutic standards with regard to the quantity and bioavailability of therapeutic agents used, their safety, and their efficacy. The main therapeutic and medicinal agents found in dentifrices are found in Table 25-1. These agents are divided according to the needs of the population: anticaries, desensitizing, antigingivitis, anticalculus, antistains, and antihalitosis. In addition, each category is subdivided according to these medicinal agents.

Anticaries Agents

Fluoride

Fluoride plays a key role in keeping the remineralization-demineralization process in favor of remineralization. Common fluorides found in daily-use dentifrice formulas include SnF_2, NaF, MFP, and SnF_2-sodium hexametaphosphate. A dentifrice with 0.24% NaF has an efficacy equivalent to a dentifrice containing 0.76% MFP. These two concentrations differ because the agents do not have the same molecular weight. Fluoride levels in dentifrices vary among countries. In Europe dentifrices may contain from 250 ppm to 10,000 ppm of fluoride. In North America the levels are between 400 ppm (for children) and 5000 ppm of fluoride. Most products contain about 1000 ppm. Fluoride neutralizes the antibacterial effect of CHG; therefore a client brushing with a fluoride-containing oral care product should wait for 30 minutes before using a CHG-containing product.[5] Other authors suggest a longer period is 1 to 2 hours.[10]

Nonfluoride Anticaries Components

Some products combine ACP with fluoride and others also add sodium bicarbonate, also known as baking soda (e.g., Arm & Hammer Age-Defying and Whitening Booster Plus Enamel Strengthening formulations). Another calcium phosphate technology incorporated into dentifrices is casein (milk protein) phosphopeptide and amorphous calcium phosphate (CPP-ACP) intended to remineralize teeth and add luster (e.g., Recaldent). Clients who are allergic to milk products would not be candidates for use of this form because the presence of the casein. Calcium sodium phosphosilicate (CSP or NovaMin) releases ions of calcium, phosphate, and sodium when exposed to saliva. The sodium is intended to buffer acid in the oral cavity and, over time, the calcium and phosphate ions are available to assist in remineralization. Examples of NovaMin products include Burt's Bees Natural Toothpaste and Dr. Collins Restore Toothpaste or X-Pur, Revitalizing Paste, and Sensodyne, Repair and Protect. These various calcium phosphate compounds also are used for desensitization. They can be found in sealant materials, desensitizing products, prophy pastes, fluoride varnishes, cements, and chewing gum. Calcium phosphate products may offer clients added protection against carious lesions, but more clinical trials are needed to determine their short-term and long-term effects and to establish their clinical relevance.

Antimicrobial Components Targeting Caries Pathogens

Bacterial flora initiate caries, so some toothpaste contains antimicrobial agents such as xylitol, enzymes, and minerals to act as anticaries.[2] The most popular, xylitol, a sugar alcohol and sugar substitute derived from fruits, mushrooms, and birch bark, has anticaries and antiplaque properties. *Streptococcus mutans* cannot metabolize xylitol; therefore their acids that demineralize tooth structure are decreased. Xylitol in a therapeutic dose of 1.55 g (minimum of 5 g used daily in the oral cavity) decreases *S. mutans* levels and plaque biofilm and its adhesion to the tooth.

Desensitizing Agents

To prevent or reduce hypersensitivity, using Ph neutral and mildly abrasive products is recommended. (See Chapter 39.) Chemotherapeutic agents may be added to do the following:

- Mechanically block dentinal tubules—for example, NovaMin 5%, a calcium sodium phosphosilicate (in Oravive, SoothRx, and DenShield); SnF_2 0.4%; strontium acetate hemihydrate 8% (Sensodyne Rapid Relief); a compound of 8% arginine, calcium carbonate, and 1450 PPM of MFP or a high level of fluoride (10,000 ppm), such as Elmex 1.25% (12,500 ppm), an amine fluoride (AmF) that remineralizes enamel
- Chemically prevent the depolarization of nerve fibers in the tooth (transmission of nervous influx), as potassium nitrate or potassium citrate does
- Acting mechanically and chemically: 5000-ppm fluoride product is efficient in reducing dentinal hypersensitivity (Colgate PreviDent 5000 ppm Sensitive 1.1% NaF and 5% potassium nitrate)

Antigingivitis Agents

Triclosan

Triclosan, a bisphenol, is a broad-spectrum antimicrobial agent that has antiplaque and antigingivitis properties. Polyvinylmethoxyethylene and maleic acid (PVM/MA) copolymer (Gantrez) is added to the triclosan to increase its duration in the mouth (substantively) and hence its antibacterial effect. A dentifrice formulation (Colgate Total) with triclosan, PVM/MA copolymer, and NaF has the ADA Seal of Acceptance for its safety and efficacy as an anticaries, antiplaque, antigingivitis, and anticalculus dentifrice. In North America, triclosan with copolymer PVM/MA (Gantrez), used in Colgate Total, is available as an antigingivitis, antiplaque ingredient.[3-9] Triclosan has been shown to slow periodontal disease progression in periodontal pocket depths greater than or equal to 3.5 mm. (In some countries, triclosan is regarded as an active ingredient with restricted use because of detection of trace amounts in water systems; however, it has not been shown to cause a significant concern for human health.[11] The long-term safety of this ingredient for the microbial ecosystem and general health is unknown.)

Chlorhexidine Gluconate

CHG is an efficacious ingredient for the treatment of gingivitis. Although it cannot be found in over-the-counter dentifrices in North America, a CHG mouthwash is available by prescription. CHG-containing dentifrice is available in Europe.

Anticalculus Agents

Sodium Hexametaphosphate, Tetrapotassium Pyrophosphate, Gantrez, Zinc Compounds

Chlorites, derivatives of sodium, phosphate, and stabilized SnF_2, are accepted by the ADA[9] as supragingival calculus-inhibiting agents (see Table 25-1). Disodium pyrophosphate, tetrasodium pyrophosphate, and tetrapotassium pyrophosphate inhibit the mineralization of biofilm before it is transformed into supragingival calculus. Zinc chloride and zinc citrate prevent or break down calculus formation.

Pyrophosphate and zinc chloride also have minor abrasive properties.

Dentifrice formulations with zinc citrate or pyrophosphates are effective as antitartar toothpastes. Extrinsic stain removal ingredients or whitening agents work mechanically with the help of abrasives such as silicate or alumina. However, the dental hygienist must be cautious in recommending toothpastes containing alumina because this abrasive is harder than enamel and cementum, and if the particle size is large and irregular, the toothpaste may increase tooth surface lost, especially with rigorous toothbrushing or excessive pressure. A dentifrice formulation with SnF_2–sodium hexametaphosphate (Crest Pro-Health) has the ADA *Seal of Acceptance* for its safety and efficacy as an anticaries, antiplaque, antigingivitis, antistain, and anti–dentinal hypersensitivity dentifrice. It also has anticalculus benefits. The ADA Seal is not given for anticalculus properties because calculus does not cause disease.

Antistain Agents

Hydrogen Peroxide

Hydrogen peroxide or carbamide peroxide can remove stains from 0.5% to 1%, chemically whiten teeth, assist in the control of oral malodor, and have antigingivitis properties. Toothpaste whitening used every day should have a neutral Ph. Acid toothpaste used on a daily basis can damage the teeth and dental restorations.[12] If the percentage of hydrogen peroxide in the dentifrice is less than 1%, the product is considered safe. If the percentage of hydrogen peroxide is higher in toothpaste, it can cause dental sensitivity.[12]

Sodium Bicarbonate

Baking soda, a mild abrasive, has been shown to neutralize acids produced by acidogenic bacteria that cause demineralization, effectively control extrinsic staining, reduce oral malodor, and have a mild antibacterial effect. It can be combined with hydrogen peroxide for tooth whitening and fluoride for an anticaries effect. It can be delivered for persons at extreme risk for caries (high risk plus dry mouth or special needs) in gum or toothpaste or in a solution for individuals with low saliva flow.

Antihalitosis Agents

Halitosis is caused by multiple factors such as systemic or topical foods and certain diseases. In the case of systemic diseases, hygienist's intervention is limited, and the professional refers to a specialist. When the cause is topical the hygienist may advise the client more efficiently by recommending appropriate products. Some medicinal agents act directly on oral bacteria and volatile sulfur compounds (VSC) such as complex formulas triclosan-copolymer-sodium and stannous fluoride in combination with hexametaphosphate. In addition, other agents are used, such as zinc and its derivatives or chlorine and its derivatives. Chlorine dioxide has been shown to reduce VSC; however, it has been studied in mouthrinses. The combination of these ingredients in dentifrices requires further study.

Concept of Bioavailability

Bioavailability occurs when the medicinal agent is stable during storage and biologically active when used in the mouth to achieve the desired therapeutic effect. It corresponds to the proportion of the therapeutic agent available in a pharmaceutic substance that produces the desired effect when used as recommended. Some manufacturers use cocamidopropyl betaine as a detergent instead of SLS to increase the bioavailability of fluoride ions. For example, Colgate-Palmolive Canada (Colgate Luminous) and GlaxoSmithKline (Sensodyne Pronamel) use this detergent. The percentage of available fluoride ions can be lower in the case of a dentifrice containing 1000 ppm of fluoride, such as NaF (eTable 25-4). This difference could be attributed mainly to the following three elements:

- Type of fluoride: Some types have less bioavailability, such as SnF_2, than others, such as NaF or AmF.
- A pH lower than 6 in dentifrice or in saliva supports the incorporation of fluoride ions.
- SLS may interfere with fluoride effectiveness.

Some manufacturers, such as Meridol, Homéodent, and Colgate, purport to have more fluoride in their toothpaste by mixing fluorides such as MFP, NaF, and AmF with SnF_2 to make the dentifrice more effective against caries. However, bioavailability is not proportional to the quantity of fluoride contained in the toothpaste. As an example, Colgate Cavity Protection contains 1450 ppm MFP/NaF and has only 839 ppm fluoride (57.8%) available. The bioavailability of fluoride can be different in toothpastes with sources or similar fluoride levels, providing different levels of remineralization of eroded enamel.[13]

Dentifrice: Adverse Health Effects?

Some ingredients in toothpaste can affect the overall health of people who suffer from allergies or intolerances: for example, dyes, natural flavors (e.g., strawberries or cinnamon), milk derivatives, eggs, and even derivatives of aspirin (acetylsalicylic acid as methyl hydroxybenzoate). In addition, there may be negative effects of certain ingredients.[1,3,14] Toothpaste ingredients that are not safe for ingestion may be ingested, especially by children or people with learning disabilities. Some ingredients may contribute to damage to hard tissues (abrasion, staining) and occasionally soft tissues.

Medicinal and nonmedicinal ingredients can cause adverse reactions, such as the following:

- Fluoride-causing fluorosis when used in higher concentrations or from multiple sources
- Soft-tissue reactions
  - Tartar-control (anticalculus) pyrophosphate dentifrices occasionally can cause erythema, scaling, and fissuring of the perioral area, cheilitis, gingivitis, and circumoral dermatitis.
  - Herbal toothpastes may lead to similar reactions as anticalculus ingredients.
  - Sodium lauryl sulfate (SLS) causes mucosal desquamation or ulceration in sensitive individuals.
  - Essential oils (peppermint, anethole, cinnamon, cloves, and spearmint) have been shown to cause cheilitis or circumoral dermatitis in sensitive individuals.
  - Antimicrobial agents may cause staining or soft-tissue irritation.
  - Flavoring, benzoates, carvone, and cinnamon aldehyde manifest as direct irritants or allergic reactions in the mouth or lips, as contact cheilitis. Rarely allergic rhinitis or asthma may occur.[3]

Consequently, the choice of toothpaste is an important element to be considered by the healthcare professional because this product has a direct impact on dental health, overall health, and quality of life of the patient.

A dentifrice can prevent or control an oral disease or condition when it provides a therapeutic function.[1] It also can be a risk factor if it causes dentin hypersensitivity, erosion, or abrasion (Figures 25-6, 25-7, and 25-8). Therefore dentifrices must be selected to meet the needs of each client. For example, a client with root exposures must be given advice regarding abrasiveness, role of pH,[15] and insoluble materials contained in dentifrices.

Insoluble and Soluble Materials

Dentifrices contain insoluble and water-soluble ingredients.[1] Ingredients in toothpaste that cannot dissolve in water are **insoluble materials**. Ingredients that dissolve in water are **soluble materials**, such as sodium bicarbonate. The insoluble abrasives such as silica or alumina remain intact in water. Some plant extracts such as golden seal, lithothamnion (seaweed), horsetail, sage, often found in natural dentifrices, are also insoluble in water. Insoluble ingredients can increase a dentifrice's abrasiveness.

For some dentifrices the level of insoluble materials is less than 20% and/or lower abrasiveness, making them gentle on tooth surfaces (e.g., MI Paste (Recaldent), Aquafresh Whitening).[1-16] For others the insoluble material level is 30% to 55% (e.g., Pearl Drops Whitening toothpaste). Colgate Gel-Kam Fruit and Berry flavor dentifrice contains no insoluble materials, has no abrasiveness, and has a pH of 3.6. Baking soda mixed 1:1 with water has no insoluble materials and low abrasiveness. Refer to the Evolve website for additional resources regarding insoluble materials in dentifrices.

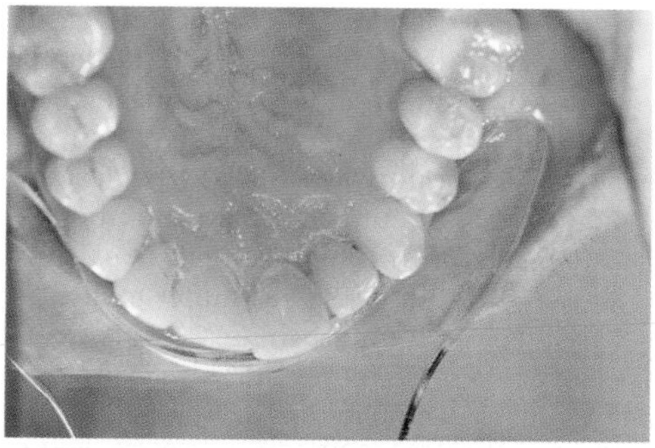

Figure 25-6. Erosion. (Courtesy Nadia Dubreuil.)

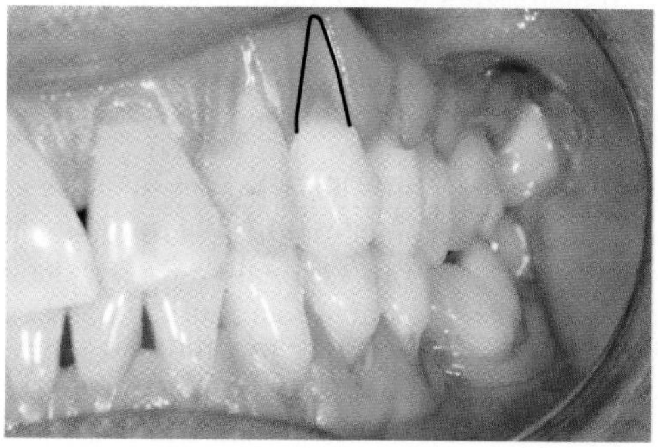

Figure 25-7. Abrasion. (Courtesy Nadia Dubreuil.)

Advantages of Higher Abrasive Levels (More Than 2%)

In a client without root exposure but with heavy quantities of oral biofilm, a more-abrasive dentifrice removes biofilm and acquires pellicle faster than a less-abrasive agent. Fortunately, the acquired pellicle forms quickly and can protect enamel against erosion.[15-17] Many common brands have slightly higher abrasive levels without being excessive for clients needing more abrasiveness (e.g., Crest Multicare Whitening, Colgate Total Advanced Health). Some dentifrices with natural ingredients, such as Jasön Health Mouth Tea Tree Oil Toothpaste, have an abrasiveness of 5.17%.

Disadvantages of High Abrasive Levels

A dentifrice with a high abrasive level can increase abrasion in a client with exposed root surfaces and can cause dentinal hypersensitivity.[16] A dentifrice with low abrasiveness is recommended for persons with esthetic restorations and/or titanium implants to avoid damaging the surface. Smooth intact restorative materials do not retain bacteria easily.

Abrasive Scales Used to Evaluate Dentifrices

Abrasiveness Scale

According to the abrasiveness scale developed by Désautels and used by the team of researchers at the Cégep Garneau (Québec, Canada),[1,18] approximately 72% of dentifrices fall

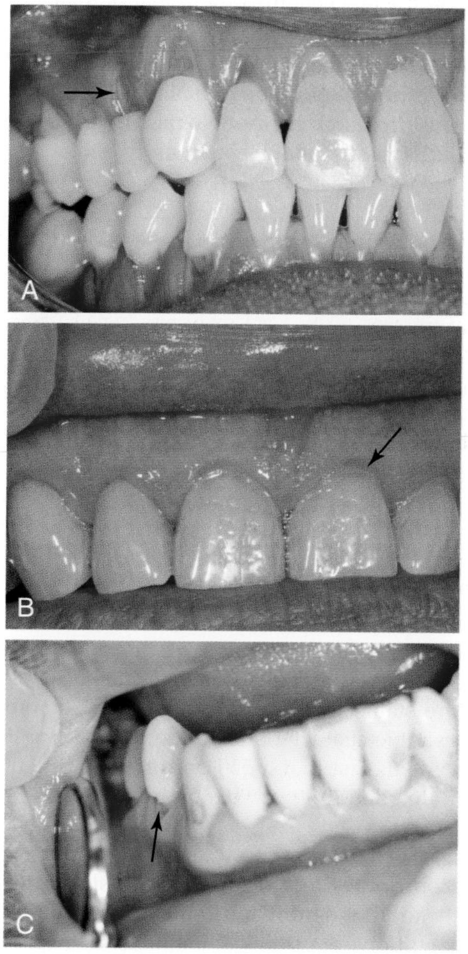

Figure 25-8. Abfraction. (Courtesy Nadia Dubreuil.)

TABLE 25-5
Relative Dentin Abrasivity (RDA) Scale

RDA Score	Level
0-70	Low abrasive: safe for cementum, dentin, and enamel
70-100	Medium abrasive: safe for enamel, dangerous for cementum and dentin
100-150	High abrasive: dangerous for cementum, dentin, and enamel
150-250	Very high abrasive: harmful limit, damaging for teeth
250 and over	Not recommended

below 2% on the Abrasiveness Scale,[1,14] meaning they do not risk damaging dentin or exposing cementum. About 29% of commercially available dentifrices are "not very abrasive" (<0.87%). About 27% of dentifrices are very abrasive (>2%). Dentifrices such as Aquafresh KidzMint triple protection (4.29%), Colgate Total Whitening (4.75%), and Nature's Gate-Creme de Anise (6.18%) are more abrasive than enamel (Mohs Hardness Score of 4 to 5) and can damage tooth structures.

Relative Dentin Abrasivity Scale

Abrasiveness of most dentifrices is determined by the universally used Relative Dentin Abrasivity (RDA) Scale (Table 25-5). The higher the score is, the more abrasive the dentifrice. Unfortunately, there is no link among abrasiveness scales because research methodologies differ. Consequently, research findings cannot always be compared.

Dentifrice pH

The potential of the hydrogen molecule (pH) of a substance is measured on a scale from 1 to 14. Level 1 is very acidic, 7 is neutral, and 14 is basic (alkaline). The pH of a dentifrice can be beneficial or detrimental to dental structures while interfering in the demineralization-remineralization process. Decay caused by acids from the fermentation of sugars by *S. mutans* occurs at a pH of 6.5 on cementum and dentin, at a pH of 5.5 on enamel (hydroxyapatite),[17] and at a pH of 4.5 on fluorapatite enamel.[4] The majority of dentifrices have a neutral pH, but few products have a pH between 3 to 10.

Low or Acidic pH

Advantages for Tooth Enamel

Acidity of a dentifrice promotes the formation of fluorapatite by facilitating the incorporation of fluoride ions into the enamel crystals. Fluorapatite crystals are characteristically larger, more stable, and less acid soluble.[19] Therefore a low pH is a desirable characteristic in fluoride toothpastes. Some studies even suggest that a 550 ppm F pH 4.5 dentifrices is equivalent to a dentifrice at 1100 ppm F pH 7.0.[20]

Disadvantages in the Case of Root Exposure or Titanium Implants

Low pH contributes to erosion of tooth structure. Because demineralization of dentin and cementum occurs at a pH of 6.5[21] the practitioner must pay attention to the client with root exposures to avoid tooth mineral loss and dentinal hypersensitivity. Low pH can tarnish titanium implants.[22] Toothpastes containing a high concentration of peroxide generally have an acidic pH.[12] Peroxide-containing toothpastes pose a risk to increase the roughness of the implants.[22] Other studies show the negative effect of low pH on the pit and fissure dental sealants and on composite restorations.[12]

Neutral and Basic pH

Advantages for Teeth and Mucous Membrane

Because of similarities to healthy saliva, a neutral or basic pH is less irritating for soft tissues and does not demineralize teeth. The saliva and its components are used as a reservoir and ensure the fluoride biodisponibility.[23]

Disadvantages for Teeth and Gums

Neutral or basic pH levels promote the mineralization of biofilm (calculus formation), which in turn supports the retention of biofilm and extrinsic stains.

More than 87% of dentifrices have a neutral or basic pH. The pH of acidic or highly acidic dentifrices (13% of dentifrices) is below the critical threshold of demineralization. A dentifrice with a pH under 6.5 demineralizes and weakens exposed root surfaces. A combination of dentifrice acidity and abrasiveness further increases the loss of dental substance.[12-15] According to the ADA,[9] dentifrices bearing the Seal of Acceptance contain a safe level of abrasives, but the organization makes no mention of pH levels. For example, Crest Pro-Health,[14] which carries the ADA Seal of Acceptance,[9] has a pH of 5.5; some believe that this pH may risk root surface demineralization in persons with gingival recession, yet it is important for fluoride uptake.[1-4] More research is needed on dentifrice pH and its role in tooth remineralization and demineralization.

Thus pH levels are relevant in the analysis of dentifrices. Loss of dental substance of chemical origin (erosion) can be increased further by mechanical actions such as toothbrush abrasion. Table 25-6 provides a comparison of various dentifrices. Persons who experience dietary acid or gastroesophageal reflux should wait 60 minutes[24-25] before toothbrushing to minimize loss of tooth structure. If waiting is not an option, the client should first rinse with water, neutral sodium fluoride-containing mouthwash (0.05%), water and baking soda solution or magnesium hydroxide solution (Maalox).[4] Other products containing a high content of calcium such as milk and cheese also can be used as buffer to create remineralization effects before toothbrushing.[15-26] Persons who have cancer or chronic vomiting from bulimia or pregnancy need the same approach. Persons who take antidepressants, anti-Parkinsonian medications, antihistamines, or antihypertensives that cause chronic xerostomia[9] should use oral hygiene products (moisturizers for dry mouth or substitutes salivary or any products to help them to alleviate dry mouth). These products, which are often acidic, should contain minerals and fluoride to help to strengthen tooth enamel.[27]

Recommending Dentifrices to Clients

A comparison of commercial dentifrices, professionally dispensed dentifrices, and professionally applied dental products is important to recommend and use available products with confidence.[1,2] For example, no commercially available dentifrice is as abrasive as Nupro Fine prophylaxis paste, which is 7.9 on the abrasiveness scale and is alkaline. Products such as water, hydrogen peroxide, and sodium bicarbonate have no abrasiveness and contain no insoluble materials;

TABLE 25-6

Comparison of Dental Products in Terms of Abrasiveness and pH

Dentifrices	Abrasiveness (%)*	pH
Crest Pro-Health, clean mint	2.51	5.5
Mentadent Advanced Whitening, refreshing mint	2.00	8.1
Arm and Hammer, Cow Brand, baking soda, dry	0.98	NA
Gel-Kam, mint flavour	0.24	3.2
Baking soda with water 1:1	0.06	8.4
Water	0.00	6.9
Hydrogen peroxide USP 3%/10 vol	0.00	4.9
Baking soda with peroxide 1 : 1	0.00	8.3

Courtesy GREHD, Dental Hygiene Research Group, Cégep Garneau, Québec, Canada.
**Dry,* Without water or any other liquid; assessed using Desautels Scale.[18]

however, they differ in pH. Water is neutral, peroxide is acidic with a pH of 4.9, and sodium bicarbonate is basic. Thus a client who uses peroxide-containing toothpaste daily increases risk of tooth surface erosion over time. As for sodium bicarbonate, its relatively high solubility contributes to its low level of abrasiveness.[1] It can abrade dentin if used dry because its particles are irregular. Some dentifrices contain micronized abrasive particles to reduce abrasiveness. (The finer the particle size or grit, the less abrasive the material, even if the material scores very high on the Mohs Hardness Scale.)

Loss of Tooth Structures

Saliva plays several roles: lubrication, predigestion (contains ptyalin), immunity, and buffering capacity to neutralize mouth acids. Therefore quality and quantity of saliva affect the demineralization and remineralization process. Medications that cause xerostomia, an individual's condition (stress, fatigue, and dehydration), time of the day (saliva is more abundant in the morning and at mealtimes), and certain health problems (Sjögren's syndrome, radiotherapy in the salivary gland region) influence the quantity and quality of saliva as well.

Loss of dental substance may occur by erosion, abrasion, abfraction, and attrition and has diverse causes such as dentifrice used, frequency of brushing, toothbrush filament hardness, pressure during brushing, the direction of the brush strokes, choice of manual or power toothbrush, the surface substrate being brushed (dentin, cementum, or enamel), and a reduced or an absence of salivary flow or absence of its constituents.[5]

- **Erosion:** Dissolution of organic and inorganic tooth structure as a result of chemical agents (see Figure 25-6)
- **Abrasion**: Pathologic tooth wear caused by a foreign substance that is harder than the tooth structure (see Figure 25-7)
- **Abfraction**: Cervical tooth structure loss of noncariogenic origin caused when the tooth is subjected to a high occlusal load—that is, the occlusal stress is high enough to cause cervical cracking and mineral loss of tooth structure (see Figure 25-8)
- **Attrition**: Loss of tooth structure on surfaces resulting from tooth-to-tooth contact (proximal or biting surfaces) from normal (chewing) or pathologic (bruxing or clenching) friction with adjacent or opposite teeth (see Figure 25-9)

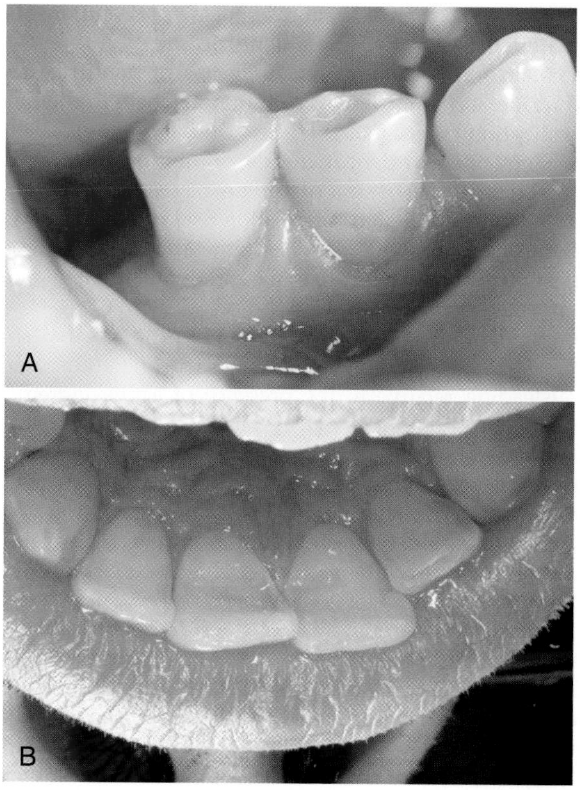

Figure 25-9. A, Lingual attrition. **B,** Attrition and erosion. (Courtesy Nadia Dubreuil.)

Comparison of Methods to Evaluate Dentifrice Abrasiveness

Dentifrice abrasiveness is not easily compared because of the various methods used to evaluate abrasiveness.[26-28] Manufacturers use different protocols and laboratory products, making direct comparisons among dentifrices difficult.[18] Therefore dentifrices may be compared only from the same manufacturer[1-16] or resort to an independent laboratory that conducts testing using the same protocol.

An interdisciplinary team representing dental hygiene, chemistry, physics, and biology independently studied the abrasiveness, the pH, and the insoluble materials found in dentifrices using the Cégep Garneau protocols.[14-16]

CLIENT EDUCATION TIPS

- Link relevant medicinal agents in dentifrices to unique client oral problems.
- Check the risk of allergy or intolerance to certain ingredients in dentifrice such as milk derivatives, certain dyes, natural flavors (e.g., strawberries), cinnamon, seafood derivatives (chitosan), and derivatives of eggs, and the reactions of derivatives of aspirin (acetylsalicylic acid [ASA] as methyl hydroxybenzoate).

- Explain importance of abrasiveness, pH, and insoluble materials when choosing a dentifrice.
- Explain importance of the daily use of dentifrices with fluoride and amorphous calcium phosphate in the remineralization process.
- Understand that dentifrices, depending on the one used, can be a risk factor or a therapeutic agent for clients.
- The American Dental Association Seal of Acceptance and the Canadian Dental Association Seal of Recognition are designed to help the consumer and dental hygienist make informed oral care product choices.
- Be vigilant against the advertising of products that sometimes are identified on the container labeling; they could be misleading relative to the presence of active ingredients, their concentration, its pH, and its rate of abrasiveness.
- Balance risk of dental caries with risk of future dental fluorosis on permanent teeth in young or disabled children who cannot expectorate.
- Analyze the effects of combining over-the-counter fluoride and ingested fluoride to avoid dental fluorosis and acute fluoride toxicity.
- Demonstrate the quantities of fluoride dentifrices recommended for different age groups. Avoid fluoridated dentifrice until children are 2 years of age, then use minimal quantity (pea size or smear on the toothbrush head) for young children with primary teeth. There are established tables that make it possible to determine the maximum tolerated dose (MTD) and the lethal dose (LD), according to the weight and age of the individual[4] (see Chapter 33). Keep oral healthcare products out of young children's reach.
- Keep in mind the child's age and weight in relation to the quantity of fluoride ingested during the period of permanent tooth formation (7 months to 4 years), brushing frequency, and ability to expectorate.
- Distinguish a bleaching agent (abrasive) that acts on the enamel surface versus a whitening agent (peroxide) whose action takes place in the deeper layers as dentin.
- Choose ingredients that act on volatile sulphur compounds (CVS) such as zinc instead of products that have a role that is only cosmetic (cetylpyridinium chloride) because they do not affect the main cause of bad breath and therefore do not solve the problem.
- Choose a low-abrasive toothpaste on dentin hypersensitivity, do not brush more than two times a day, and avoid any beverage or food acid immediately after brushing.[29]
- Give priority, in the presence of an eroded enamel, a toothpaste containing NaF/triclosan/copolymer to a nonfluoride toothpaste and a monofluorophosphate (MFP).[30]

LEGAL, ETHICAL, AND SAFETY ISSUES

- Recognize that persons may be using dentifrices that place them at risk.
- Assess client's health, dental, and pharmacologic histories to make sure there are no conditions, allergies, or medications that would contraindicate a particular dentifrice recommendation.
- Make recommendations based on a client's assessed needs and expectations and product evidence. Use the American Dental Association (ADA) Seal of Acceptance or the Canadian Dental Association (CDA) Seal of Recognition as a guide to help make product recommendations.
- Document recommendations in client's record, including the product, frequency, dosage, and reasons for use. Confirm, with client's signature, that the client understands these recommendations and agrees to the regimen.
- Review client's self-care regimen regularly; offer advice based on evolving research evidence to reach optimal oral health.
- Make sure that products recommended to clients have been accepted by the ADA[9] or CDA[31] and contain ingredients that have been approved by the U.S. Food and Drug Administration,[32] Health Canada,[11] or other regulatory organization. It is therefore of utmost importance to consult these organizations regularly via their websites.

KEY CONCEPTS

- The majority of manufacturers produces dentifrices effective against calculus, gingivitis and oral biofilm, dentinal hypersensitivity, or a combination of the above. Studies to date indicate that these products make toothpastes more therapeutically efficacious but more abrasive than first-generation products.
- When developing a care plan, the clinician must verify the dentifrice and the quantity and frequency with which it is to be used. Evaluate whether the product meets client needs, taking into consideration root exposure, erosion, abrasion, dental caries, stains, calculus, and brushing habits (e.g., pressure applied, soft- or stiff-bristled toothbrush, brushing method).
- Variables about level of abrasion, the pH of dentifrices, and the insoluble materials must be considered when recommending dentifrices to clients. Various sources of references exist, such as the American Dental Association,[9] Radioactive Dentin Abrasivity, and Radioactive Enamel Abrasivity, but the *Descriptive Guide to Mouthwashes and Dentifrices* considers all of these variables, making it useful for comparison of dentifrices.
- Flavoring agents, dyes, and detergents in dentifrices may cause side effects (burning sensation, oral tissue desquamation, aphthous ulcers, intolerance, allergies).
- Health conditions of the client (hypertension, allergies, or intolerance) are considered when recommending a dentifrice.

CRITICAL THINKING EXERCISES

Role-play each of the following case scenarios. One person should be the clinician and one the client. Analyze each scenario by noting the following:

- Client's significant clinical findings
- Medicinal agents used in each case
- Abrasiveness and the pH level of dentifrices used
- State of health

What information should be given to clients (caregivers) regarding safe, effective dentifrice use?

Example: A 3-year-old child with healthy teeth, no composite restorations, a thin biofilm at the lingual surface of the mandibular molars, healthy eating habits, and good oral hygiene comes to the dental hygiene clinic. His mother indicates an allergy to dairy products. The child brushes twice daily with a dentifrice for children with 0.24% NaF, which completely covers bristles of a small-headed toothbrush. Parental supervision of brushing occurs once daily.

Clinical Findings: None except for biofilm on molars.

Medicinal Agent: Fluoride is used as primary prevention against caries. The quantity of dentifrice is equal to the size of a grain of rice to reduce the risk of fluorosis.

Abrasiveness: Low-abrasiveness dentifrice is used for primary teeth, because in this case the child has only a thin biofilm.

Allergy to Dairy Products: Products without milk derivatives are essential to avoid all reactions in this child.

pH: Slightly acidic or neutral to promote fluoroapatite formation (the more acidic a dentifrice, the more it demineralizes, allowing for a greater remineralization and incorporation of fluoride onto dental structures).

Scenario 1: An 8-year-old boy with one area of decalcification (white spot lesion), two untreated carious areas, no sealants, generalized gingival redness, materia alba, and oral biofilm is your client. Daily he chews one package of sugarless chewing gum (nine pieces), and he has variable eating habits, including two glasses of regular cola (pH 3).

Daily Oral Care Regimen: Rapid brushing once daily with whichever dentifrice is available at home

Scenario 2: A 22-year-old woman with four dental sealants, two composite restorations, two areas of gingival recession on maxillary first premolars causing no sensitivity, a slight supragingival calculus, moderate gingivitis, and generally good eating habits

Daily Oral Care Regimen: Uses dental floss once weekly, brushes twice daily using a power toothbrush and a small amount of dentifrice because of too much foam. Choice of dentifrice depends on price.

Scenario 3: A 58-year-old smoker (one pack of cigarettes per day) with generalized moderate tobacco stains, periodontitis (four sites at 4 PSR), heavy subgingival calculus, and occasional bleeding on probing

Daily Oral Care Regimen: Brushes once or twice daily with a dentifrice chosen by his spouse; never uses an interdental cleaning aid

REFERENCES

1. Comité Dentifrice Collège François-Xavier-Garneau, Lavoie F, Feeney N, et al: Evaluation of toothpastes and of variables associated with the choice of a product. *CDHA* 41:42, 2007.
2. Hurlbutt M: Caries management with calcium phosphate. *Dimens Dent Hygiene* 8(10):40,42,44, 2010.
3. Davies R, Scully C, Preston AJ: Dentifrices—an update. *Med Oral Pathol Oral Cir Bucal* (6):e976, 2010.
4. Wilkins E: *Clinical practice of the dental hygienist*, ed 11, Philadelphia, 2013, Lippincott Williams and Wilkins.
5. Harris NM, Garcia-Godoy F, Nathe C: *Primary preventive dentistry*, ed 8, Upper Saddle River, NJ, 2014, Pearson Prentice Hall.
6. Mohire NC, Yadav AV: Chitosan-based polyherbal toothpaste: as novel oral hygiene product. *Indian J Dent Res* 21(3):380, 2010.
7. Ganss C, von Hinckeldey J, Tolle A, et al: Efficacy of the stannous ion and the biopolymer in toothpastes on enamel erosion/abrasion. *J Dent* 40(12):1036, 2012.
8. Council of Clinical Affairs: *Guideline of xylitol use in caries prevention*, American Academy of Pediatric Dentistry (AAPD) Clinical Guidelines; V34/N0 6, Adopted 2011.
9. American Dental Association (ADA): *ADA/PDR guide to dental therapeutics*, ed 4, Chicago, 2006, ADA.
10. Johnson VB, Chalmers J: Guideline summary: oral hygiene care for functionally dependent and cognitively impaired older adults. *Agency for Healthcare Research and Quality*, revised 2011.
11. Health Canada/Santé Canada website. Available at: http://www.hc-sc.gc.ca/ahc-asc/media/nr-cp/_2012/2012-48-fra.php. Accessed September 2013.
12. Price RBT, Sedarous M, Hiltz G: Le pH des produits de blanchiment des dents. *J Can Dent Assoc* 66:421, 2000. Available at: http://www.cda-adc.ca/jadc. Accessed January 2013.
13. Hara AT, Kelly SA, Gonzalez-Cabezas C, et al: Influence of fluoride availability of dentifrices on eroded enamel remineralization in situ. *Caries Res* 43:57, 2009.
14. Lavoie F, Dubreuil N, Turcotte G, et al: *Guide descriptif des rinces bouches et des dentifrices*, Québec, 2011, Cégep Garneau.
15. Zero DT, Lussi A: Érosion—facteurs chimiques et biologiques importants pour le praticien dentaire, *Int Dent J* 55:285, 2005.
16. GREHD (dental hygiene research group): www.grehd.org website descriptive guide coming spring 2014.
17. Lussi A, Schlueter N, Rakhmatullina E, et al: Dental erosion—an overview with emphasis on chemical and histopathological aspects. *Caries Res* 45(suppl 1):2, 2011.
18. Désautels P, Labrèche H: Abrasion relative des dentifrices. Un dentifrice pour chacun. *J Dentaire du Québec* 31:461, 1994.
19. Daniel SJ, Harfst SA, Wilder RS: *Mosby's dental hygiene: concepts, cases, and competencies*, ed 2, St Louis, 2008, Mosby.
20. Buzalaf MAR, Hannas AR, Magalhães AC, et al: pH-cycling models for *in vitro* evaluation of the efficacy of fluoridated dentifrices for caries control: strengths and limitations. *J Appl Oral Sci* 18(4), 2010.
21. Faria ACL, Bordin ARV, Pedrazzi V, et al: Effect of whitening toothpaste on titanium and titanium alloy surfaces. *Braz Oral Res May* 2012.
22. Hossain A, Okawa S, Miyakawa O: Effect of toothbrushing on titanium surface: an approach to understanding surface properties of brushed titanium. *Dent Mater* 22:346, 2006.
23. Naumova EA, Kuehnl P, Hertenstein P, et al: Fluoride bioavailability in saliva and plaque. *BMC Oral Health.* 12:3, 2012. Available at: http://www.biomedcentral.com/1472-6831/12/3. Accessed September 2013.
24. Ontario Dental Hygienists' Association (ODHA): Acid reflux and oral health: dental hygiene facts. Available at: http://www.odha.on.ca. Accessed September 2013.
25. Addy M: Brossage des dents, usure dentaire et hyperesthésie dentaire—existe-t-il un lien? *Int Dent J* 4:261, 2005.
26. Johannsen G, Tellefsen G, Johannsen A, et al: The importance of measuring toothpaste abrasivity in both a quantitative and qualitative way. *Acta Ondontologica Scandinavia*, 2012. Available at: http://informahealthcare.com. Accessed September 2013.
27. Goronvenko MR: *Over the counter xerostomia remedies currently available in Canada*, 2009, The Canadian Dental Hygienists Association.
28. Lutz F, Imfeld T: Relative dentin (RDA) and relative enamel abrasion (REA) of toothpastes and prophylaxis pastes. *Compend Contin Educ Dent* 23:61, 2002.
29. West NX, Hooper SM, O'Sullivan D, et al: In situ randomized trial investigating abrasive effects of two desensitizing toothpastes on dentine with acidic challenge prior to brushing. *J Dent* 40(1), 2012.
30. Passos VF, Santiago SL, Tenuta LM, et al: Protective effect of NaF/triclosan/copolymer and MFP dentifrice on enamel erosion. *Am J Dent* 23(4):193, 2010.
31. Canadian Dental Association (CDA): *CDA reconnaissance de l'ADC*. Available at: http://www.cda-adc.ca. Accessed September 2013.
32. U.S. Food and Drug Administration (FDA): U.S. FDA website. Available at: http://www.fda.gov. Accessed September 2013.

EVOLVE RESOURCES

Please visit http://evolve.elsevier.com/Darby/hygiene for additional practice and study support tools.

CHAPTER 26

Hand-Activated Instrumentation

Joyce Y. Sumi, Michaela Nguyen

COMPETENCIES

1. Discuss basic dental hygiene instrument design and classify an instrument and its use based upon variations in instrument shank length, curvature, flexibility, blade type, and blade-to-shank angulation.
2. Discuss the classifications of instruments, including:
   - Describe assessment instruments, their design, and uses.
   - Customize fulcrum placement for a tooth surface.
   - Describe treatment instruments, their design, and uses.
   - Explain proper instrument blade adaptation and angulation.
   - Define the stroke principles of blade angulation, adaptation, and activation.
   - Describe protective scaling strategies and reinforcement scaling.
   - Identify intraoral and extraoral fulcrums for periodontal instrumentation.
3. Describe the value of dental perioscopy.
4. Describe the methods, techniques, and importance of instrument sharpening.
5. Discuss how to prevent and manage instrument tip breakage.

Hand-activated instruments used in caring for clients with healthy or diseased periodontium are classified as assessment instruments or treatment instruments. **Assessment instruments** provide the dental hygienist with clinical periodontal and tooth assessment information. **Treatment instruments** are used for calculus removal by performing periodontal scaling and root planing. Therefore use of these hand instruments is the focus of this chapter. (See Chapter 27 for ultrasonic instrumentation, Chapter 29 for coronal polishing instrumentation, and Chapter 38 for hand instruments used in restorative therapy.)

Specific examples and use of assessment and treatment instruments are discussed in detail later in this chapter. Because all assessment and treatment instruments consist of similar functional parts, however, this chapter begins by highlighting the common functional parts of all dental hygiene hand-activated instruments. Understanding the variations in these functional parts can aid the clinician in determining the purpose, effectiveness, efficiency, and comfort of use.

Basic Dental Hygiene Instrument Design: Parts and Characteristics

Dental hygiene hand-activated instruments consist of three functional parts:

- Handle
- Shank
- Working end

A good instrument supports all of these functions.

Handle

The handle is typically the longest part of an instrument where clinicians hold or place their grasp. Handles can be designed for single- or double-ended use; some working ends are replaceable.

When an instrument is selected, handle specifications primarily benefit clinician comfort. Nevertheless, handles should not be considered less important than any other instrument part. Handles also function as an information source to the clinician because they transmit vibrations to the clinician's hand when the instrument is in use. In response to a heightened concern for clinician comfort and to lessen the effect of repetitive strain injuries (RSIs), instrument manufacturers offer a variety of handle options relating to the following:

- Material
- Diameter size
- Texture (knurling) and shape
- Weight

Handle Material

Handles of hand-activated instruments used by dental hygienists can be made of metal, resin, or silicone. In general, the resin and silicone materials are more comfortable and have wider diameter grips than the smaller metal handles.

Handle Diameter Size

The handle diameter can range from small to large grips (Figure 26-1, *A*). Larger-diameter handles tend to be more comfortable than the smaller, slender handles. Handles that are too slender can lead to cramping of the hands after prolonged use.[1] However, handles with the extra circumference of larger diameter grips may have difficulty with access to posterior teeth, especially if the client has limited mouth-opening ability. Handles with larger-diameter grips also can limit proper angulation in deeper periodontal pocket depths.

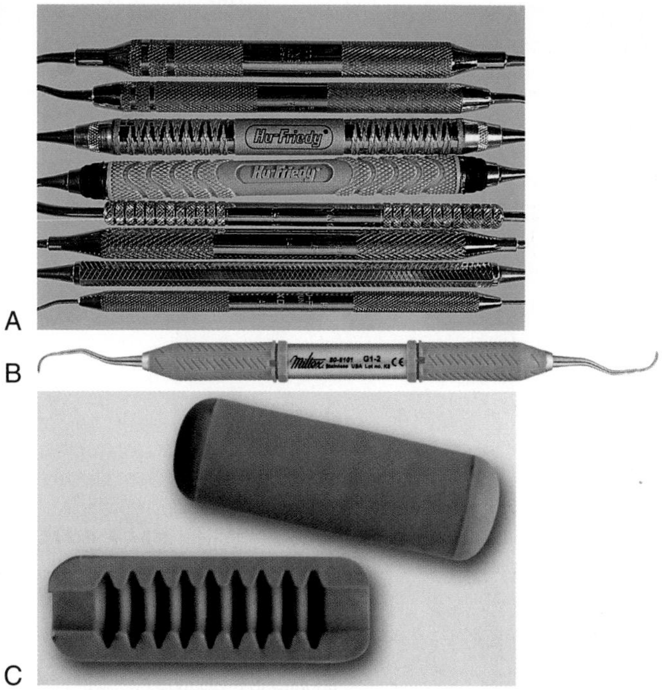

Figure 26-1. **A,** Instrumentation handle variations in size, shape, and pattern. **B,** GripLite handle. **C,** Air Cell grip that goes over a handle. (**B,** Courtesy Miltex, York, Pennsylvania. **C,** Courtesy Tony Riso Company, North Miami Beach, Florida.)

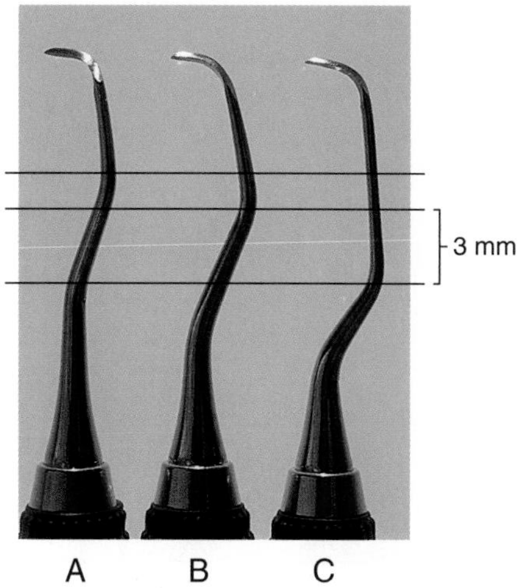

Figure 26-2. Comparison of instrument shank lengths. **A,** Gracey 1/2. **B,** Gracey 5/6. **C,** Gracey After-Five series 5/6.

Handle Texture and Shape

Texture, or knurling, refers to the pattern cut into the handle or the relief. Texture assists in a uniform sure grasp and control of the instrument on an otherwise smooth surface. The depth of the pattern on some handles, however, may affect the practitioner's comfort level. Some patterns are cut so deeply that they feel as if they are biting into the skin when pressure is placed on the instrument. Grips also can be added to instruments to improve comfort (Figure 26-1, *B* and *C*).

Handle shape or circumference may be round or hexagonal. Both are comfortable when a suitable surface pattern and material are used.

Handle Weight

Handle weight is the final consideration in handle selection. For handle selection, there are two basic types:
- Solid handles
- Hollow handles

Most clinicians find that hollow-handled instruments are lighter and less strenuous to use and allow greater tactile sensitivity than solid-handled instruments.

Shank

The shank of an instrument connects the working end to the handle and is the major factor determining the use of each particular instrument.

There are two main parts of the shank:
- The functional shank
- The terminal shank

The **functional shank** is the overall shank that starts from the bend nearest the handle to the tip of the working end.

The **terminal shank** is the portion of the functional shank that is from the last bend or curve closest to the working end.

The position of the terminal shank to the working end is important in determining the correct positioning of the angulation of the curet blade. Most instruments are designed for the terminal shank to be parallel to the long axis of the tooth during usage.

Important differences in shank design among instruments relate to the following:
- Shank length
- Shank angle
- Shank flexibility or strength

Shank Length

Instrument shank length ranges from short to long (Figure 26-2, *A, B,* and *C*). An instrument with a long shank is preferred for use on teeth with deep periodontal pocket depths or recession. It is also an important consideration when the operator needs to fulcrum a great distance from the area being instrumented. An instrument with a short shank is best suited for anterior teeth with shallow pocket depths, supragingival procedures, and a fulcrum close to the area being instrumented.

Shank Angle

The shank of an instrument can be configured with angles as follows:
- Straight
- Curved
- Angled or bent

Most periodontal instruments have shanks that are curved or bent in at least one and usually two places (Figure 26-3). The degree and angle of this curvature also can determine the area(s) in which the instrument is effective.
- The smaller the angle and the fewer the number of shank bends, the more suitable for use on anterior teeth.
- The more acute the angle and the greater the number of shank bends, the more suitable for use on posterior teeth.

However, the implementation of intraoral and extraoral fulcrums enables the clinician the flexibility to use straighter shanked instruments in the posterior areas and curved-shanked instruments in the anterior areas.

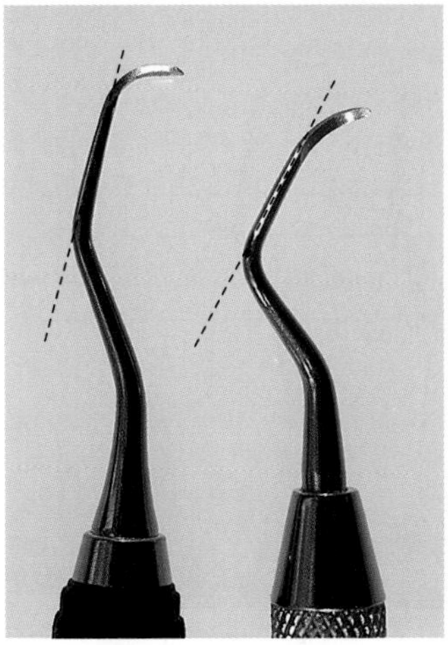

A B

Figure 26-3. Comparison of shank angles or curvatures. **A,** Gracey curet 5/6. **B,** Universal curet.

TABLE 26-1

Assessment Instruments

Assessment Instruments	Basic Use
Mouth mirror 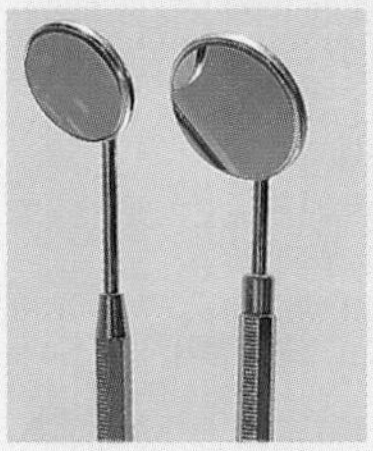	Indirect vision, indirect illumination, transillumination, and retraction of buccal mucosa and tongue; for use throughout appointment
Periodontal probe 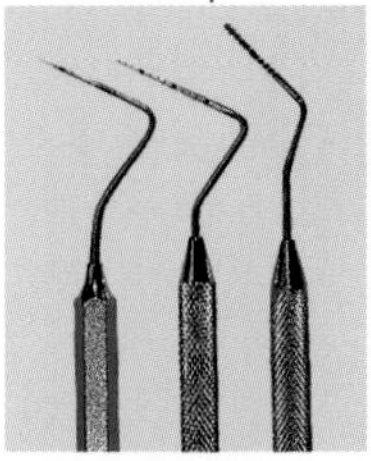	Measurement of probing depth, clinical attachment level, relative attachment level, amount of attached gingiva, gingival recession, and furcation invasion; assessment of oral biofilm, gingival inflammation, bleeding points, and pathologic lesions Used during assessment and again during the evaluation phase of care
Nabers probe 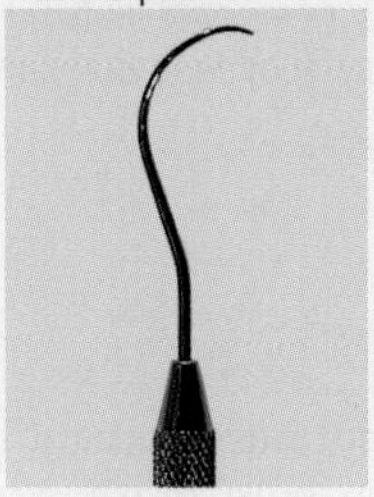	A furcation classification instrument to be used during assessment and again during the evaluation phase of care
Explorer 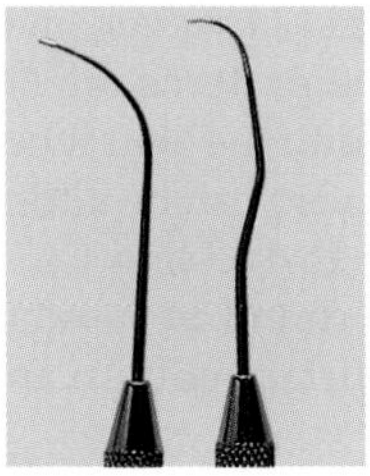	Detection of calculus, irregular cementum, junctional epithelium, dental caries, irregular root anatomy, margins or restorations, external resorption, and osseous exposures. For use during assessment, implementation, and evaluation phases of care

Shank Flexibility (Strength)

All shanks taper in diameter from the handle to the working end. The type of metal used and the shank thickness determine the shank strength. Some manufacturers categorize the degree of their instruments' shank flexibility as follows:

- Flexible
- Moderately flexible
- Rigid
- Extra rigid

The flexibility of the shank of an assessment instrument, such as a wirelike explorer, can be important in transmitting vibrations from the working end to the clinician for increased detection accuracy. In addition, the shank flexibility is an important characteristic that determines the strength of the treatment instrument as it also transfers the clinician's pressure on the handle and shank to the working end against the tooth surface for calculus removal. Shank flexibility is particularly important in dental hygiene procedures.

- *Flexible shanks* are used to detect and remove light subgingival calculus deposits or oral biofilm.
- *Moderately flexible shanks* are ideal for removal of moderate to light calculus, providing adequate resistance against this type of tooth deposit.
- *Extra rigid and rigid shanks* are for removing tenacious and heavy calculus.

Working End

The working end *(terminal end)* of the instrument is the part of the instrument from the terminal shank to the end of the instrument that comes in contact to the tooth or tissue and determines the general purpose of the instrument (Figure 26-4).

Important considerations to understand differences in working ends are the following:

- Design
- Material
- Style

There are slight differences among manufacturers regarding shape, length, cutting edges, width, strength, bend or curvature, and metallurgy or material of the working ends of identically named and numbered instruments. These details are important considerations when instruments are being selected for purchase. Design name and numbers are identifying marks on the handles. The design name usually indicates the manufacturer, person, or institutional origin of the instrument. The numbers usually indicate the type of working end(s) of the instrument. On double-ended instruments, two numbers follow the name, each designating a working end (e.g., Columbia 13/14).

The working end is designed for a specific task. For example, if an instrument is needed for assessing distance between the marginal gingiva and the base of the periodontal pocket, the dental hygienist selects an instrument that has a working end calibrated to measure distance (e.g., the periodontal probe or Nabers probe; Table 26-1).

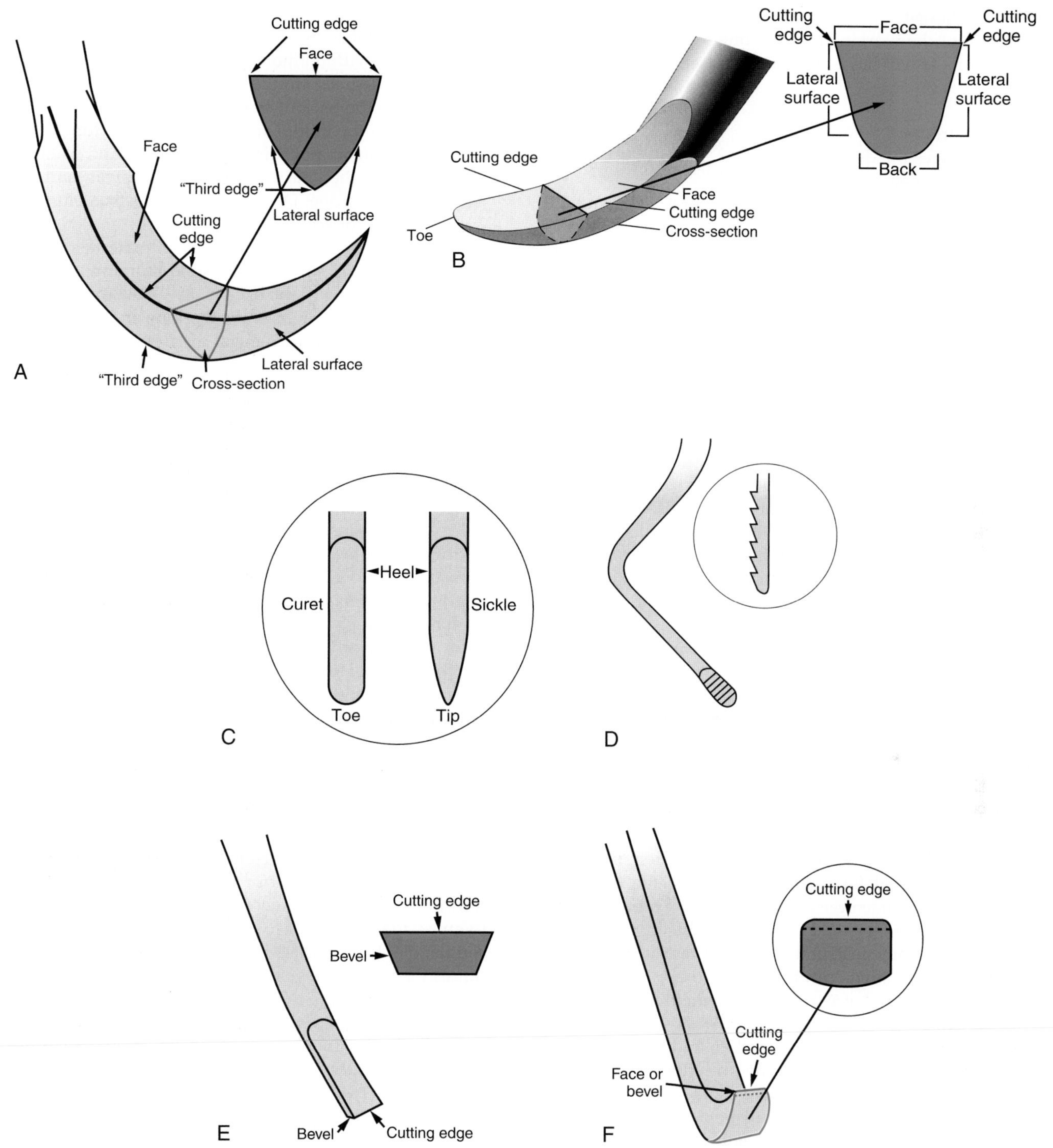

Figure 26-4. Comparison of the working ends of scaling instruments. **A,** Sickle scaler. **B,** Curet. **C,** Comparison of curet and sickle working ends. **D,** File. **E,** Chisel. **F,** Hoe. (**A, C** through **F,** Adapted from Daniel SJ, Harfst SA, Wilder RS: *Mosby's dental hygiene*, ed 2, St Louis, 2008, Mosby. **B,** From Newman MG, Takei HH, Klokkevold PR, et al: *Carranza's clinical periodontology*, ed 11, St Louis, 2012, Saunders.)

The general shape and length of the probe's working end are fairly consistent among all manufacturers. However, there are differences in the working ends of periodontal probes with respect to their thickness, intervals of millimeter markings, materials, and presence or absence of color-coded probe markings for easier reading. The expanding availability of plastic probes for use with implants and client comfort has increased the clinician's choices.

The explorers with curvature bends such as the Gracey 11/12 can improve access and therefore calculus detection. For deeper periodontal pockets, extended shank explorers are a reasonable option.

Working End Design

The design of the working ends among scaling instruments varies, but most will have the following (see Figure 26-4):

- Face
- Back
- Lateral surfaces
- Cutting edges (blades)
- Tip or toe (pointed or rounded)

The **face** is the innermost surface of a curet blade and the ***back*** is the opposite surface to the face.

The **lateral surfaces** are the surfaces on either side of the face. The **cutting edges** are the sharp edges formed where the face and lateral surfaces meet. The **tip** or **toe** is the area where the face, back, and lateral surfaces terminally converge. A pointed end is a tip, whereas a rounded end is a toe.

Working End Material

The material of the instrument's working end is also an important consideration. New materials are emerging continually because of increasing technology and needs for dental implant maintenance.

Instruments can be subdivided further based on metallurgy and materials of the blade. Some are as follows:

- Stainless steel instruments maintain adequate sharpness for scaling and root planing and do not rust or discolor when sterilized with saturated steam or with formalin-alcohol vapor.
- Carbon steel blades tend to feel sharper clinically and hold their sharpened edges longer after prolonged use than do stainless steel blades. However, carbon steel is more brittle and breaks more easily than stainless steel. Carbon steel instruments also may corrode or rust when sterilized. Carbon steel has a tendency to oxidize (rust) after saturated steam sterilization or when moisture content of a formalin-alcohol vapor sterilizer reaches 15% or greater. Because of this tendency for oxidation of the carbon steel metal, commercially available corrosion inhibitors are recommended for use with the autoclave to reduce oxidation. Manufacturer instructions concerning dilution of ultrasonic cleaners and chemical disinfection solutions and length of time instruments should remain in solution must be monitored carefully. Dry heat sterilization, however, does not present a problem for carbon steel instruments.
- Stainless steel alloy that is harder than traditional stainless steel is used in some instruments to reduce the need for sharpening (but do not eliminate sharpening) (EverEdge Technology, Hu-Friedy Manufacturing). Instruments made from this material are available as regular and rigid instruments and can be used for fine scaling as well as for removing heavy tenacious calculus, depending on the instrument design.
- Instruments made of stainless steel impregnated with nitrate (XP Technology, American Eagle Instruments) do not need sharpening and are discarded when the coating is lost and they become dull in about 3 to 4 months. Instruments made with this material are used for debridement, fine scaling, and root planing of areas associated with non-tenacious calculus deposits; however, they are contraindicated for removal of overhangs and tenacious deposits, and for trimming the margins of restorations. The American Eagle sickle is an example of a thin sickle that maintains its shape and sharpness because of its XP Technology (see Table 26-12).
- Instruments with diamond-coated working ends (coating placed 360 degrees around the tip or 180 degrees around the tip with the back of the instrument smooth for placement against the tissue) are designed for performing final root debridement, polishing root surfaces, and scaling furcations and other narrow inaccessible areas and when using an endoscope. Diamond-coated instrument tips are not designed for scaling heavy calculus.
- Implants demand another category of materials for maintenance. Plastic, graphite, gold, solid titanium, and coated titanium are some of the options available to the clinician (Table 26-2). The designs of the working end follow similar characteristics of various metal instruments.

Working End Style

Hand-activated instrument styles are categorized into three basic categories based upon working ends:

- Single-ended
- Double-ended, paired
- Double-ended, unpaired

Single-ended instruments are instruments with only one working end. Some instruments are single-ended that have the practicality to allow the end of the handles as an additional usage. For example, the handle end of a single-ended mouth mirror can be placed facial and lingual to the tooth to test for mobility or tapped on a tooth for clinical indications from percussion. However, single-ended scaling instruments have only one blade and require the practitioner to have twice as many instruments. Single-ended instruments are inefficient because of the necessity of picking up and replacing instruments to and from the work area every time the dental hygienist chooses to work from the opposite aspect of the same tooth. Instrument cleaning, packaging, sterilization, and storage efforts also are doubled.

Instruments with double-ended, paired working ends are instruments with exact mirror images on the opposite ends. These mirror images are necessary because the same blade curvature does not adapt to each side of the same tooth. For example, the distal surface from the facial aspect of the tooth requires the mirror image of the same instrument to scale the distal surface from the lingual aspect.

Instruments with dissimilar working ends that allow two different, distinct functions are instruments with **double-ended, unpaired** *working ends*. These instruments are double ended but have two different instruments on the same handle (Figure 26-5).

Balanced Instruments

A **balanced instrument** is one in which the working ends are in alignment with the long axis of the handle. (See Chapter 11, Figure 11-13 and section on balanced instruments.)

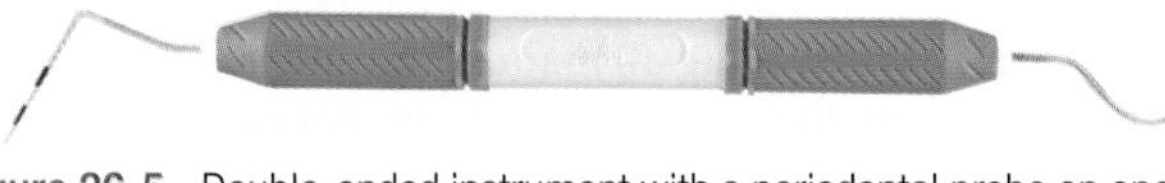

Figure 26-5. Double-ended instrument with a periodontal probe on one end and an explorer on the opposite end. (Courtesy Milltex, York, Pennsylvania.)

TABLE 26-2
Treatment Instruments

Treatment Instruments	Basic Use
Universal curet 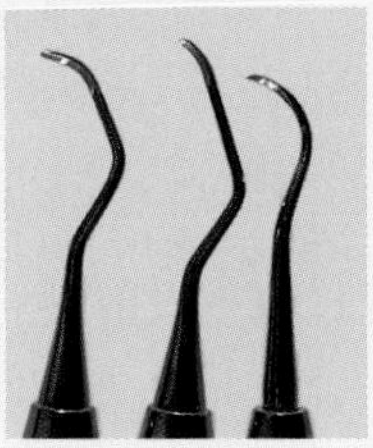	Depending on design, may be used in all areas of mouth for supragingival and subgingival scaling and root planing Used for periodontal scaling and root planing
Gracey curets 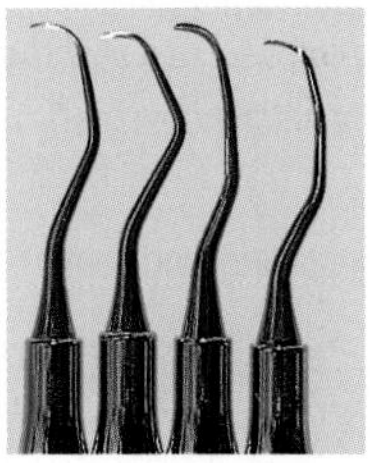	Area-specific curets that, depending on design, may be used in various areas of the mouth for supragingival and subgingival scaling, root planing, and oral biofilm removal Used for periodontal scaling and root planing
Sickle 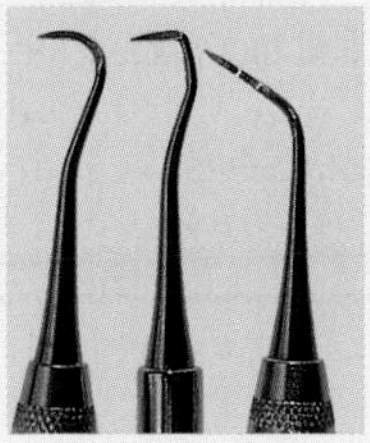	Principally a supragingival calculus removal instrument Used for gross calculus removal This instrument is not used for root planing
File 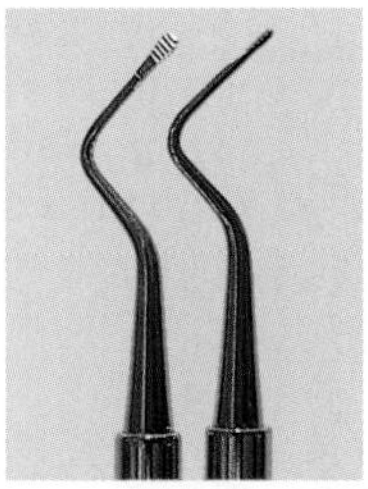	Used for supragingival and subgingival calculus removal where tissue is retractable For use during initial scaling; should not be used for root planing
Hoe 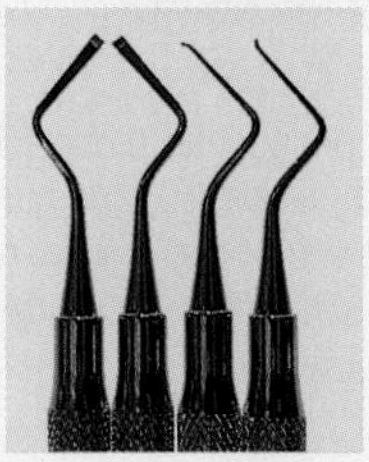	Used for supragingival and subgingival calculus removal where tissue is retractable and during initial scaling; should not be used for root planing

Continued

TABLE 26-2
Treatment Instruments—cont'd

Treatment Instruments	Basic Use
Plastic, graphite, gold, and titanium instruments 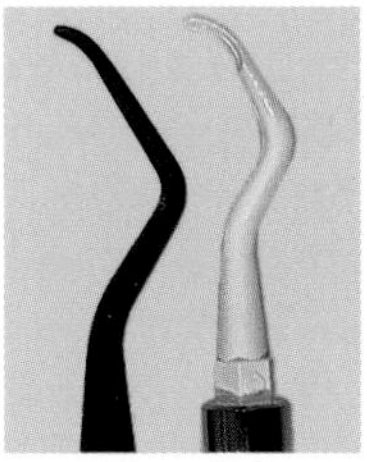 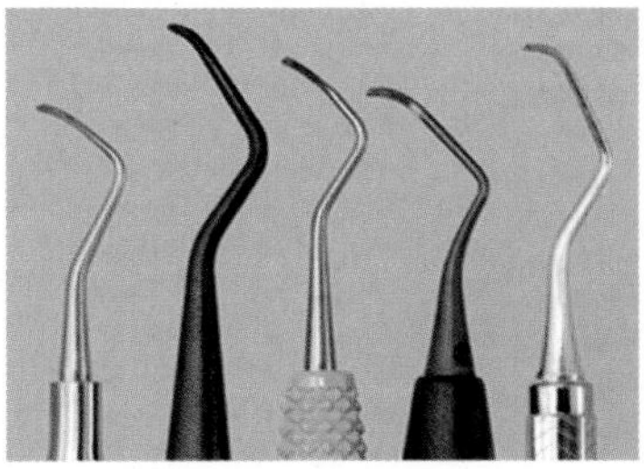	Used for assessment as well as calculus and biofilm removal around titanium dental implant abutment cylinders (see Chapter 58)
Ultrasonic and sonic scaling devices (see Chapters 27 and 58)	Used for supragingival and subgingival calculus removal, oral biofilm Recommendation regarding titanium dental implant abutment cylinders is to use these devices only when working end is a specially designed rubber-coated tip (see Chapter 58)
Low-speed dental handpiece (see Chapter 29)	Used for oral biofilm and extrinsic stain removal after scaling and root planing are completed Recommended for use with a fine abrasive agent for polishing titanium dental implant abutment cylinders Prophylaxis angle, rubber cup, point or brush, and polishing agent are part of the armamentarium
Air polishing or airbrasion system (see Chapter 29)	Used for oral biofilm and stain removal after scaling and root planing are complete Contraindicated for use around titanium dental implant abutment cylinders and in clients with pulmonary disease

Instrument Classification

Dental hygiene care instruments are classified as either assessment instruments or treatment instruments. Examples of assessment and treatment instruments are shown in Figure 26-6.

Assessment instruments provide clinical periodontal and tooth evaluation information. Basic assessment instrument categories are explorers and periodontal probes. Mouth mirrors can be categorized as diagnostic instruments; however, they also are used with treatment instruments (see Table 26-1).

Treatment instruments are used for calculus removal by performing periodontal scaling, debridement, and root planing (see Table 26-2). A more detailed discussion of each instrument category is below.

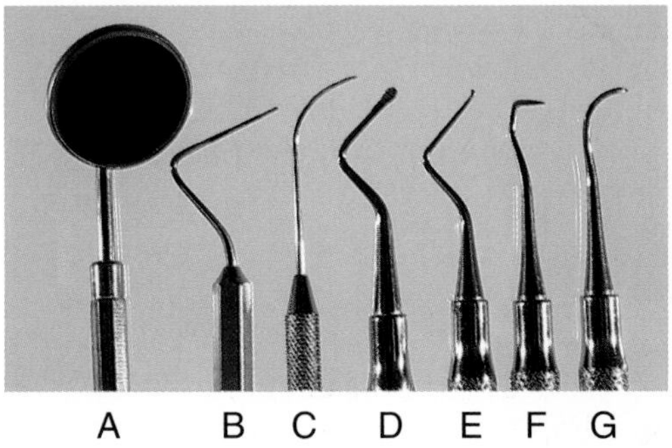

Figure 26-6. Assessment instruments: mirror (**A**), periodontal probe (**B**), explorer (**C**). Treatment instruments: file (**D**), hoe (**E**), sickle (**F**), and curet (**G**).

Assessment Instruments

Mouth Mirror Design and Use

The traditional **mouth mirror** has a handle and mirror, each with a threaded design or cone-socket attachment (see Table 26-1). Mirror heads come in a variety of sizes from ⅝- to 2-inch diameters. Mirror size selection is made according to the size of the client's mouth, the clinician's ability to place the mirror and another instrument within a confined space, and the clinician's comfort in holding and using a certain size mirror head. The most commonly used mouth mirror in dental hygiene procedures is the manufacturer sizing of No. 4 and No. 5, which is approximately ⅞ to 1 inch in mirror diameter.

Three types of mirror reflective faces include the following (Table 26-3):

TABLE 26-3
Types of Mouth Mirror Surfaces

Type	Advantages and Disadvantages
Front surface	Mirror surface is on the front of the glass; therefore the image produced is the mirror image of the area reflected Most commonly used because there is no distortion or magnification of the image
Concave surface	Causes magnification of the image; because each movement visualized with this mirror is magnified, the operator must relate the scale of movement and the image differently from the way it actually appears More difficult to use than the front-surface mirror Does not allow the operator to see as wide a range as the front surface mirror and causes distortion, even dizziness, for some clinicians Not recommended unless eyestrain or vision is a significant problem
Flat surface	The image appears doubled or shadowed Not recommended for periodontal procedures

TABLE 26-4
Functions of the Dental Mouth Mirror

Function	Reason for Use
Indirect vision	Most difficult function to master. Reflection in mirror provides indirect vision of area. Use when it is difficult to view the tooth or area directly (e.g., distal surfaces of last molars or when a direct vision requires a strenuous operator position).
Indirect illumination	Use to catch light and direct increased illumination to intraoral areas. When mirror is being used in this capacity, it cannot be used for indirect vision at the same time. Therefore operator and client position must be adjusted for direct-vision scaling.
Transillumination	Use to reflect light back onto anterior tooth surfaces, which are thin enough to allow light to pass through. Essentially this is a shadowing technique for visualization of teeth. Areas of various density or darkness such as dental caries and calculus will contrast and be visible.
Retraction	A pulling away of soft tissue for illumination, visualization, and protection of client's tissue. Use with the face of the mirror toward the buccal mucosa, lips, or tongue to retract tissues for light to illuminate the working area and/or protect the soft tissues during instrumentation. Face of mirror should be turned toward the working area to provide indirect vision while at the same time retracting the soft tissue.

- Front surface
- Concave surface
- Flat surface

The handle and mirror components should be separated, ultrasonically cleaned, and autoclaved after each appointment. Wrapping the mirror heads with 2-inch × 2-inch gauze squares when packaged with other instruments during sterilization minimizes scratching of the reflective surface. Mirror heads are replaced when they eventually become clouded or scratched, unlike the handles that rarely need replacing.

The dental mouth mirror is used for the following purposes (Table 26-4):

- Retraction of tissues and tongue
- Indirect vision
- Indirect illumination
- Transillumination

Retraction is using the mouth mirror to hold soft tissues such as the client's cheek, lip, or tongue to allow visualization or clearance.

A modified pen grasp should be used for stability when there is resistance to the mirror head, such as during the retraction of buccal mucosa or the tongue (Figure 26-7). The mouth mirror generally is held with a modified pen grasp; however, other grasps also may be used. The pads of the thumb and the index and middle fingers all rest on the shank and handle of the instrument with the modified pen grasp.

When the mouth mirror is used for retraction, care is taken to avoid tissue trauma with the handle or shank of the instrument, particularly at the commissures. This injury may be as slight as soreness, or as serious as initiation of herpetic lesions on the client's lips. Trauma can be avoided by maintaining less pressure on stretched lips. In addition, the mouth mirror never should be allowed to rest on sublingual tissue because doing so causes client discomfort.

Indirect vision is using the mouth mirror to view areas or surfaces that cannot be seen directly.

For indirect vision or illumination and reinforcement of a curet with the nondominant hand, the mirror is held between the middle and ring fingers. This position allows little manipulation of the mirror; however, in areas where indirect vision is needed, positioning changes of the mouth mirror are minimal (Figure 26-8, *A*)

Indirect illumination is using the reflective properties of the mouth mirror to direct additional light into an area (Figure 26-8, *B*).

Transillumination is using the reflective properties of the mouth mirror to pass light through a thin structure such as an anterior tooth (see Figure 26-8, *B*).

When there is no resistance and when indirect vision, indirect illumination, and/or transillumination are the goals, the standard pen grasp is adequate and perhaps desirable. The

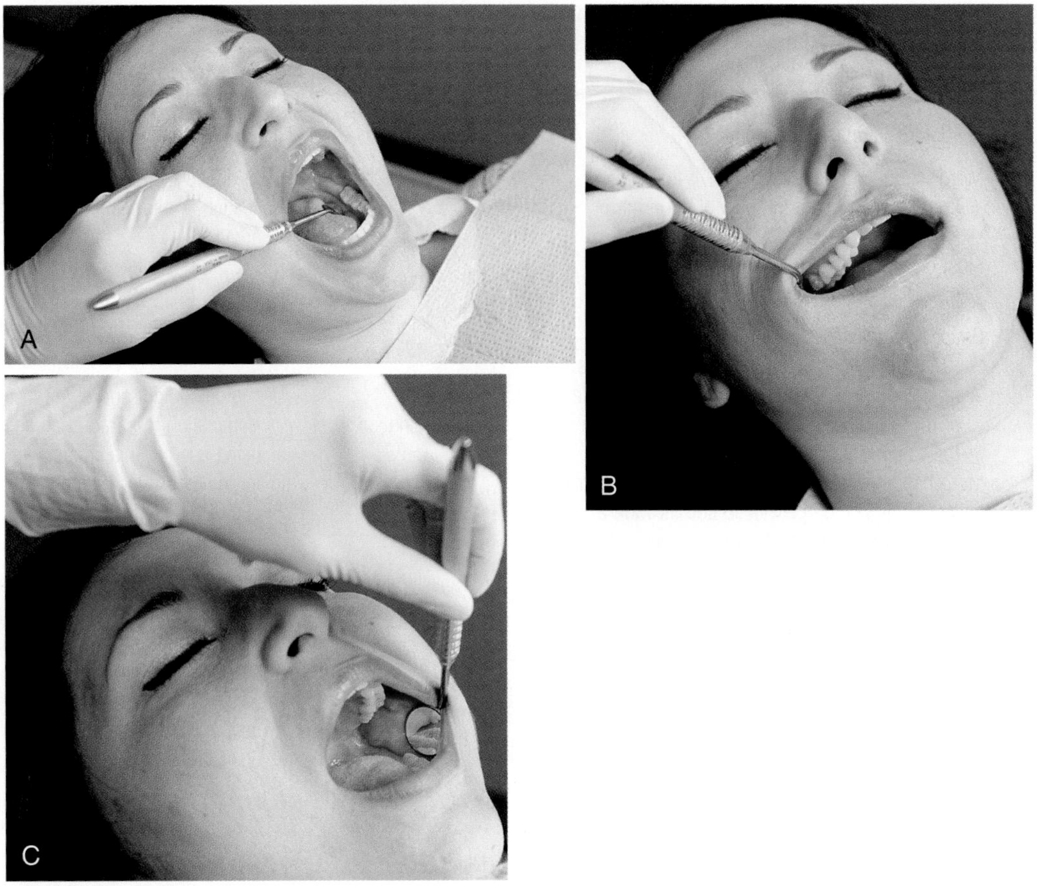

Figure 26-7. **A,** The mouth mirror is used for retraction of tongue. **B** and **C,**The mouth mirror is used for retraction of buccal mucosa.

standard pen grasp yields a very loose grasp that generally allows easy, fluid movement of the mirror head around the mouth. This range of movement is beneficial when large oral areas are examined or compared. Moistening the face of the mouth mirror by gently rubbing it against the buccal mucosa or dipping it in a commercial mouthwash prevents mirror fogging.

Explorer

Design and Use

The **explorer** consists of a very fine, wirelike tip with a sharp point that comes in a variety of lengths, diameters, and bends (Table 26-5). Tactile sensitivity (as described in a later section), the ability to sense the vibrations from the instrument, is a critical element of an explorer. Explorers usually are designed with narrow shank diameters for increased tactile sensitivity to identify physical properties in the mouth. The differences in curvature of the shank, length, and diameter make different explorers useful for specific purposes dependent on tissue, calculus, probing depth, tooth alignment, and other details specific to individual clients.

The explorer, designed for adaptation around the tooth, is used to detect and assess the following:

- Dental caries
- Decalcification
- Irregularities in margins of restorations
- Secondary caries around restorations
- Morphologic crown and root anomalies
- External root resorption
- Supragingival calculus
- Subgingival calculus
- Cemental irregularities

An explorer is selected for the task it is to perform, as follows:

- Heavier-, wider-, or even medium-diameter explorers are best suited for caries detection or exploration around restorations. Such explorers are sturdy and do not deform or bend as they are manipulated under and around caries and metallic margins. Fine, elongated explorers are more difficult to use for caries detection because of the deflection of the instrument during use. The side of the tip of an explorer may be used for caries detection; however, the tip or point should not be used and open cavities can and should be detected without exploration. Current evidence suggests limiting the usage of the explorer to decrease the chance of breaking the enamel's integrity during tactile verification of caries. For caries detection and diagnosis, greater emphasis is now on visual examination, use of compressed air, optional caries detection devices (e.g., Diagnodent Laser Cavity Detection), transillumination, and x-ray examination. If the integrity of the enamel is not compromised in this early stage, interventions can facilitate remineralization (see Chapter 18).
- Fine-diameter explorers are best suited for subgingival exploration of root structure and identification of calculus and allow for increased tactile sensitivity. Explorers that

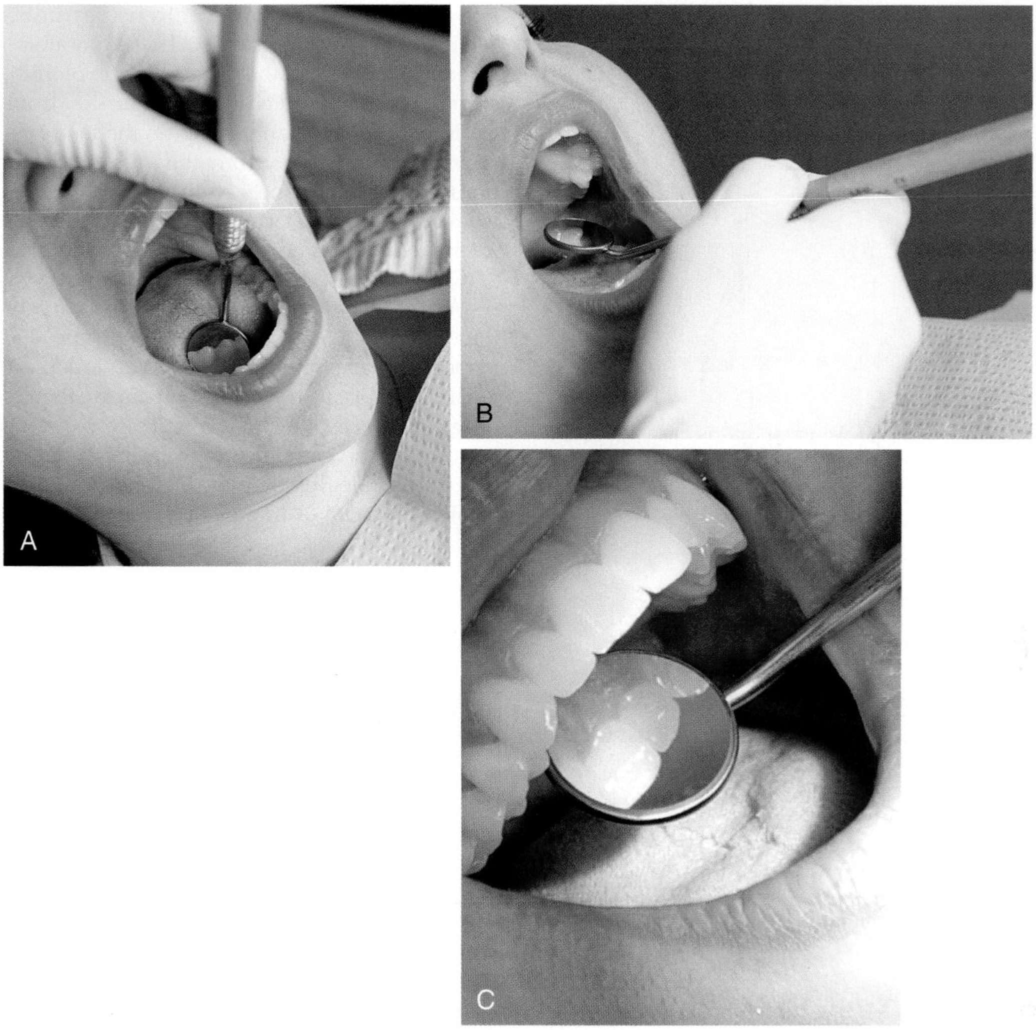

Figure 26-8. **A,** The mouth mirror is used for indirect vision. **B,** The mouth mirror is used for illumination. **C,** The mouth mirror is used for transillumination.

TABLE 26-5

Clinical Outcomes Using Sharp versus Dull Instruments

Outcome	Sharp Instrument	Dull Instrument
Tactile sensitivity	Increased	Decreased
Client safety and comfort	Increased	Decreased
Working efficiency	Increased	Decreased
Control	Increased	Decreased
Lateral pressure	Decreased	Increased
Probability of burnished calculus	Decreased	Increased

are too thin, however, may flex and catch in tissue or on root structure in fibrotic or tight areas, relaying incorrect messages about subgingival deposits.

- For deep periodontal pockets, the explorer should be slightly bent and long enough (such as the Hu-Friedy No. 3-A EXD or the No. EXD 11/12AF) to reach to the apical regions (i.e., 12 mm or deeper).
- For shallow sulcus areas, CEJs, and under contact areas, a short explorer (such as a pigtail explorer) is adapted easily because it is short and acutely bent. These short, curved explorers are usually double ended and area specific—that is, each end works best on specific surfaces of the tooth.

Comparisons of these and other explorers are shown in Figure 26-9. Criteria for design, selection, and procedure for use of the explorer are found in Table 26-3, Procedure 26-1 and the corresponding Competency Form, and Procedure 26-2 and corresponding Competency Form.

Grasp and Fulcrum

The modified pen grasp is used with the dental explorer. When exploring shallow, light, or obvious calculus, the dental hygienist uses a grasp with light to moderate strength. The grasp should become firmer when more pressure must be exerted against the tooth, or when the dental hygienist must distinguish between tooth structure and burnished calculus.

The most important rule governing fulcrum placement when exploring is that the fulcrum be flexible enough to allow the explorer to move from the CEJ to the apex of the pocket with correct insertion and adaptation. Almost any scaling fulcrum could be used as an exploring fulcrum;

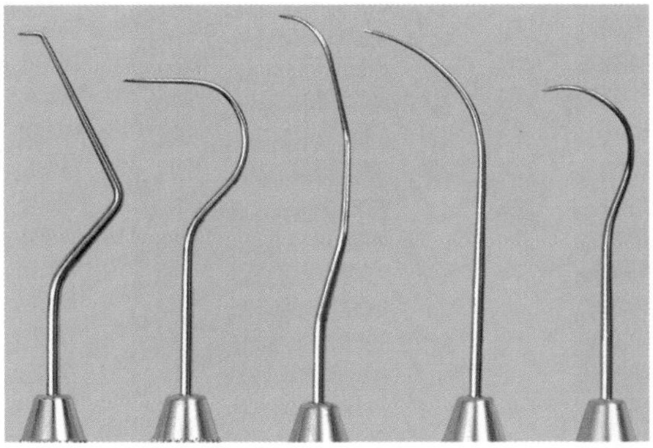

Figure 26-9. Five typical explorers. **A,** No. 17. **B,** No. 23 Shepherd's hook explorer. **C,** EXD 11/12. **D,** No. 3. **E,** No. 3H pigtail. (From Newman MG, Takei HH, Klokkevold PR, Carranza FA: *Carranza's clinical periodontology*, ed 11, St Louis, 2012, Saunders.)

however, the reverse may not always be true because a scaling fulcrum needs more stability. The exploratory fulcrum could be located close to the area being explored, cross-arch, or extraorally. As the fulcrum moves further from the area being explored, the clinician's grasp on the instrument handle also moves further away from the working end. This distance does not diminish one's ability to explore the area, nor does it lessen instrument control. Rather, it enhances access into interproximal regions and deep periodontal pockets.

Clinicians use many diagnostic indicators, such as tissue response, bleeding, and radiographic surveys to determine the presence of subgingival deposits. However, tissue response to calculus varies by individual, and radiographs are limiting because they are two dimensional. Adept explorer usage enhances the quality of care by a dental hygienist because of the difficulty with radiographs to visualize flat, burnished calculus or deposits obscured by restorations or located on facial or lingual surfaces of teeth.

Procedure 26-1 Fundamental Components of Hand-Activated Instrumentation

Equipment	Ergonomic dental chair Ergonomic operator chair Personal protective equipment (PPE) Loupes and coaxial lights, optional Protective eyewear for client	Assessment and treatment instruments Air-water syringe Gauze Evacuation equipment
Client positioning	Mandibular occlusal plane positioned parallel to floor Maxillary occlusal plane positioned perpendicular to floor Client's head turned for maximum direct view of instrumentation when possible without compromising lateral pressure Client (mouth) positioned at the height of clinician's waist	
Operator positioning	For healthy client: Right-handed operator: 8 to 1 o'clock Left-handed operator: 4 to 11 o'clock For clients with moderate/severe mandibular posterior periodontal pockets and for surfaces facing away on anterior teeth: Right-handed: 8 to 5 o'clock Left-handed: 4 to 7 o'clock Occasionally requires extraoral fulcrums. Very challenging deep pockets may necessitate a standing position.	
Grasp	Pen: occasionally assessment instruments, mirror retraction Modified pen: assessment instruments, treatment instruments Extended modified pen: extraoral, cross-arch, opposite arch Palm-thumb: treatment instruments	
Fulcrum	Intraoral (digital): same arch, cross-arch, opposite arch Extraoral (palm): palm-up, palm-down, knuckle-rest, chin-cup, finger-on-finger	
Stroke principles	Insertion and re-insertion during scaling (0-10 degrees) Adaptation: assessment (2-3 mm tip), treatment (lower ⅓ of blade) Angulation: scaling (>45-<90 degrees), root planing (45-60 degrees) Activation: exploratory and scaling/root planing, vertical, horizontal, oblique, basketweave, channel, push, pull	
Lateral pressure	Assessment: light to moderate pressure with thumb Treatment: light, moderate, heavy (firm) pressure with thumb Coordination of grasp, fulcrum, positioning for use of thumb or middle finger	
Reinforcement (protective) scaling	Nondominant hand: stability, enhanced pressure, guides instrument Dominant hand: controls adaptation, angulation, working stroke	

Procedure 26-2 Use of Assessment Instruments

INSTRUMENT	PERIODONTAL PROBE	PERIODONTAL EXPLORER
Equipment	Periodontal probe, mouth mirror	Periodontal explorer (3-A or ODU 11/12), mouth mirror
Steps	Fundamentals (Procedure 26-1)	Same fundamentals as for periodontal probe.
Grasp	Pen or modified pen, light grasp Increase grasp pressure when discerning tooth structure, restorative materials, calculus.	Pen or modified pen, light to moderate grasp Increase grasp pressure when discerning tooth structure, restorative materials, calculus.
Fulcrum and pressure	Light and adjustable fulcrum placement opposite arch, extraoral (see Figures 26-33 to 26-37) Intraoral, adjacent to tooth being instrumented, cross-arch	Light and adjustable fulcrum placement opposite arch, extraoral (see Figures 26-33 to 26-37). Intraoral, adjacent to tooth being instrumented, cross-arch. Same technique as for periodontal probe.
Working end selection	Periodontal probe: Typically one working end but can be on one end of a double-ended unpaired instrument	3-A extended explorer: typically one working end 11/12 extended explorer: paired with two working ends. On posteriors, the first bend angles distally. On anteriors, the first bend angles toward midsection of the tooth.
Insertion, adaptation, angulation	All periodontal probes: Insert parallel to long axis of tooth with lower 1 to 3 mm of probe adapted against tooth until the junctional epithelium is contacted. When probe reaches contact area, angle tip area directly under contact (col), shank touching the contact. Furcation probe: Guided by radiographs, previously recorded probing depths, and root anatomy knowledge. Negotiate furcation probe into the furcation; note extent of penetration and classification. Plastic probe: With very light pressure, insert and adapt plastic probe to implant surface until resistance is met.	Adapting explorer tip to root surface, insert with lower 1 to 3 mm of explorer curved toward tooth until the junctional epithelium is contacted. In anesthetized clients or known pocket topography, reinsert tip parallel to long axis of tooth (downward like a probe) with 1 to 2 mm adapted by curving toward tooth surface. Exploring in the upward and downward direction can help detect burnished or sheetlike calculus.
Activation, stroke	With gentle pressure, walk probe in small, vertical increments along base of sulcus or pocket where the junctional epithelium feels soft and resilient. Insert toward distal of tooth. With one side of probe maintaining contact with tooth surface, walk distally in small 1 mm increments until distal col area (under contact) of tooth is reached with upper portion of probe straightened and touching contact area. Lift probe and reinsert at distal line angle; repeat technique by walking forward to mesial col area. Continue throughout mouth buccally and lingually.	Begin activation with insertion stroke (vertical with both a push and pull stroke). Assess root surfaces with multidirectional strokes to detect calculus, burnished deposits, root caries, or restorative margins. Strokes are long and sweeping to evaluate root smoothness and shortened when encountering pieces of calculus or surface irregularities. Generally longer and fewer strokes during final evaluation phase of care when root surfaces are smooth.
Additional notes	Record deepest readings of distal, buccal or lingual, and mesial surfaces from buccal and lingual approach. Six readings recorded per tooth.	Light pressure: friable tissue, light calculus, final assessment Increased pressure: root irregularities, moderate to heavy calculus, burnished calculus

Periodontal Probe

See the discussion of periodontal probes in Chapter 19.

Design and Use

The **periodontal probe** is a slender, tapered, blunt instrument with millimeter markings (Table 26-6). It is used to determine the following:

- Probing depth
- Clinical attachment level (CAL)
- Relative attachment level (RAL)
- Bleeding on probing (BOP)
- Demarcation of the mucogingival junction
- Amount of keratinized gingiva
- Amount of attached gingiva
- Gingival recession
- Furcation invasion or involvement
- Size of atypical or pathologic lesions
- Distance between teeth

Millimeter markings and other design differences vary among manufacturers. For example, the Marquis probe is marked at the 3-, 6-, 9-, and 12-mm intervals; the Williams probe is marked at the 1-, 2-, 3-, 5-, 7-, 8-, 9-, and 10-mm intervals. Differences in markings, color coding, shapes, materials used, and an automated probe are shown in Figures 26-10 and 26-11.

Personal operator preference determines selection of interval and color-coded markings of the periodontal probe. In the case of failing dental implants, which require the use of plastic probes (see Figure 26-11, *A* and *B*), safety against further injury and scratching of the titanium implants determines instrument selection (see Chapter 58 regarding osseointegrated dental implants).

TABLE 26-6

Periodontal Probe: Use, Technique, and Significance of Results (see Chapter 19)

Measurement	Technique and Significance of Results
Probing depth	Measures probing depth from marginal gingiva to junctional epithelium. Six measurements are taken around each tooth (distofacial, facial, mesiofacial, distolingual, lingual, and mesiolingual). The deepest measurements are recorded for each surface. Within any sextant, it is easier to record all facial surface measurements, then all lingual surface measurements. Probing depth is an important indicator of past disease activity (see Procedure 26-2).
Clinical attachment level	Measurement from the cementoenamel junction to the junctional epithelium. The technique is similar to measurement of probing depth, except that the depth is measured from the junctional epithelium to a fixed reference point. When measuring from a fixed reference point, the clinician can determine a clearer picture of bone loss, especially when recession and minimal probing depths are present.
Relative attachment level	Measurement from a fixed reference point on the tooth or a stent to the junctional epithelium. The technique is similar to assessing probing depth and offers a record of past disease activity.
Amount of attached gingiva	Attached gingiva is the keratinized stratified squamous epithelium firmly attached to the cementum and alveolar bone. Adequate attached gingiva is an important safeguard against future mucogingival defects and recession when there is bone loss.
Gingival recession	Measurement from the gingival margin to the cementoenamel junction. This measurement is another indicator of apical migration of the attachment apparatus.
Furcation invasion	See Chapter 19 for classifications. The No. 2 Nabers probe is a specialized probe used for furcation detection and classification. Detection of furcation invasion is critical to the therapy and long-term prognosis of the tooth and adjacent bone.
Bleeding on probing	Observation of bleeding on light probing is a primary clinical indicator of gingival inflammation.
Pathologic lesions	An important aspect of assessment is an accurate description of the size and shape of the lesion. The periodontal probe is used for measurement of pathologic lesions.
Distance between teeth	The periodontal probe is used to measure the distance between teeth (diastema), overjet, and migration of teeth with severe periodontal disease.

When the periodontal probe design is flat and too thick or wide, it is difficult to manipulate the instrument into and around narrow, tight areas for accurate measurement. Conversely, if the probe is too fine and sharp, there is danger of trauma and perforation through the nonkeratinized junctional epithelium, resulting in inaccurate readings. If too fine a probe is selected, client comfort and safety become important factors to consider. Thin design instruments also are subject to damage during sterilization procedures.

Variations of the periodontal probe and criteria for selection, design, and procedures are found in Table 26-7 and Procedures 26-1 and 26-2. A variation in shank design of the periodontal probe is shown in Figure 26-12. This periodontal probe design (Hu-Friedy Novatech) features a right-angle tip that is color coded. It offers ease of access in posterior distal surfaces.

Computerized periodontal probes are also available, for example, the Florida Probe (see Figure 26-10, *G* and *H*). The tip of the probe is inserted into the sulcus or pocket and, with the use of a foot pedal, the system automatically records pocket depth, attachment loss, bleeding, mobility, and other clinical parameters. Once data are collected, a graphic chart can be printed and used as part of the dental record, for client education and research. The computerized probe applies 15 g of pressure each time it is used. This design feature increases consistency in the probing technique over time and among practitioners. Some computerized probes are accurate to 0.2 mm, exceeding the accuracy of a traditional marked probe.

For information on the measurement of probing depth, clinical attachment, relative attachment, adequacy of attached gingiva, and gingival recession, see Chapter 19 and Table 26-6.

The blunted tip of the periodontal probe makes it ideal to determine (but not measure) bleeding tendencies on probing. If gentle probing elicits bleeding, this observation should be noted on the client's record as a clinical indication of inflammation. Gingival bleeding is associated with inflammation, significant increases in periodontal pathogens, and increased flow of gingival crevicular fluid. Evidence of bleeding has only a 30% predictive value in determining future clinical attachment loss. Cessation of bleeding is related to a significant reduction in gingival inflammation and is used to monitor periodontal treatment outcomes.

By compressing the side of the probe tip against the attached gingiva, the dental hygienist evaluates tissue tone without producing trauma. More information may be

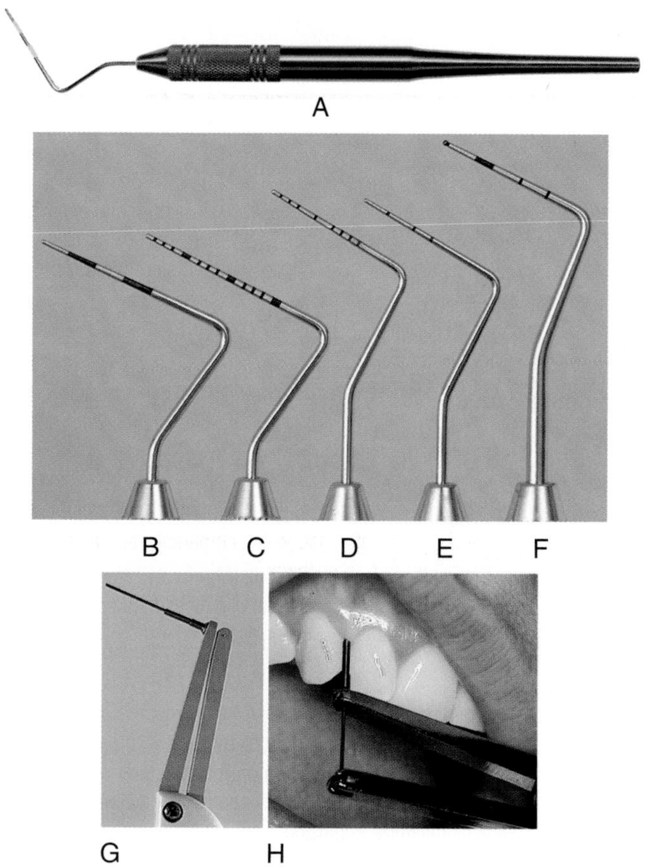

Figure 26-10. Examples of periodontal probes. Note the differences in marking. **A,** AEP12Y/GX Probe with green band at 3 to 6 mm and yellow band at 9 to 12 mm. **B,** Marquis colored probe with markings at intervals of 3, 6, 9, and 12 mm. **C,** UNC-15 probe, a 15-mm–long probe with millimeter markings at each millimeter and color coding at the fifth, tenth, and fifteenth mm. **D,** University of Michigan O probe with Williams markings at 1, 2, 3, 5, 7, 8, 9, and 10 mm. **E,** Michigan O probe with markings at 3, 6, and 8 mm. **F,** World Health Organization probe, which has a 0.5-mm ball at the tip and millimeter markings at 3.5, 8.8, and 11.5 mm and color coding from 3.5 to 5.5 mm. **G,** Florida probe computerized periodontal probing and patient-education system. **H,** Florida probe positioned in periodontal pocket. (**A,** Courtesy American Eagle Instruments, Missoula, Montana. **B** to **F,** From Newman MG, Takei HH, Klokkevold PR, et al: *Carranza's clinical periodontology*, ed 11, St Louis, 2012, Saunders. **H,** Courtesy Florida Probe Corporation, Gainesville, Florida.)

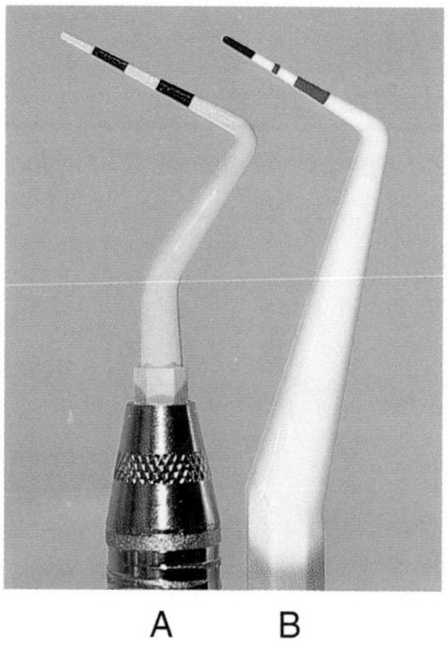

Figure 26-11. Examples of plastic periodontal probes. **A,** Hu-Friedy black and yellow color-coded replaceable plastic periodontal probe tip. **B,** Premier Dental Products reusable plastic periodontal probe.

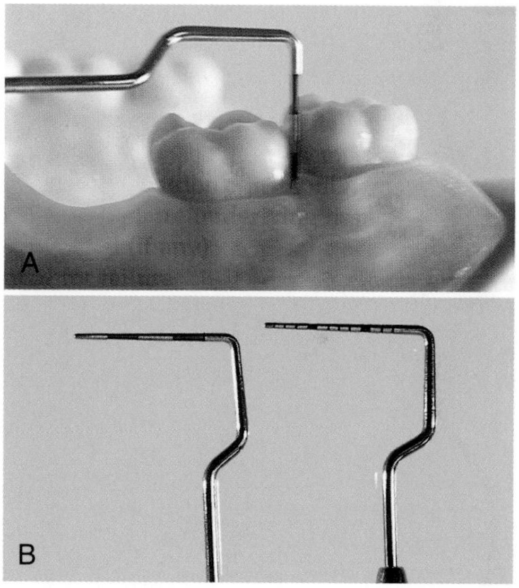

Figure 26-12. **A,** Hu-Freidy Novatech periodontal probe with its upward bend is designed for access in posterior areas. **B,** Type of probe tip may differ, as illustrated in photograph.

obtained from a standard dental index such as the Silness and Löe Plaque Index, which uses the periodontal probe in the assessment (see Chapter 17, Table 17-5). Some practitioners use the periodontal probe to identify subgingival calculus; however, most find a dental explorer such as the ODU 11/12 more reliable for deposit assessment because of its curvature and fine tip.

The probe can be used to establish the location of the mucogingival junction. This landmark allows the measurement of the width of the keratinized gingiva, calculation of the resultant attached gingiva, and determination of mucogingival involvement. When the mucogingival junction is not obvious, the blunt probe also can be used to identify the demarcation of this line. This identification is done by placing the side of a straight-designed probe laterally on the alveolar mucosa and pushing the moveable tissue coronally toward any firm, resilient attached gingiva.

A diagram of the shape and verbal description, including measurements, of intraoral and extraoral suspected pathologic lesions is important for accurate documentation. The periodontal probe is used to measure the dimensions of small lesions, and the side and tip of the instrument are used to palpate, lift, or rub over the lesion to examine other characteristics that may be helpful to the dentist making a differential diagnosis. If not excisionally biopsied, the lesion should be monitored by evaluating the size (with a periodontal probe), shape, and visual description on subsequent appointments (see Chapter 15 regarding extraoral and intraoral clinical assessment).

The periodontal probe also is used to measure the distance between teeth (diastema) and the amount of overjet a person

TABLE 26-7
Periodontal Probe Design

Common Design Specifications of All Periodontal Probes

This slender, often tapered assessment instrument is used to measure sulcus and periodontal pocket depth, clinical attachment levels, and amount of attached gingiva.
Calibrated markings are engraved or color-coded onto the angulated tip design.
Tips are blunted or rounded.
Cross-sectional view is rounded, oval, or rectangular.

Probe Examples	Design and Use Characteristics	
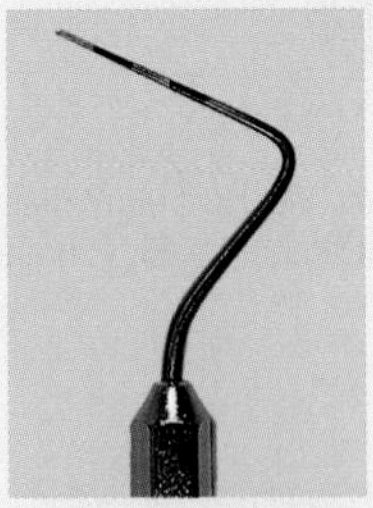	***Marquis Color-Coded Probe***	
	Shank	Thin, round, and tapered
	Measurement	Alternately color-coded at 3, 6, 9, and 12 mm
	Tip design	Thin tip
	Advantages	Color-coding every 3 mm makes it easy to read. Thin shank allows access into tight fibrotic sulci.
	Disadvantages	Markings must be estimated between color bands. Thin tip may penetrate junctional epithelium if too much pressure is applied.
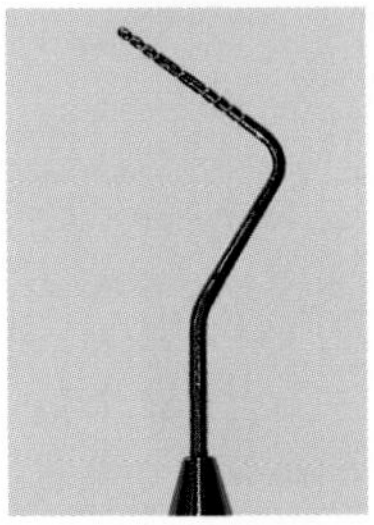	***Williams Probe***	
	Shank	Round and tapered
	Measurement	1, 2, 3, 5, 7, 8, 9, and 10 mm
	Tip design	Thin to thick, depending on manufacturer
	Advantages	Spaces between 3 and 5 and between 5 and 7 minimize confusion.
	Disadvantages	Markings are difficult to read.
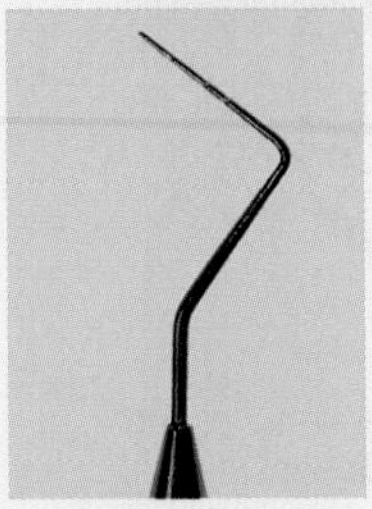	***Michigan O Probe***	
	Shank	Thin, round, and tapered
	Measurement	3, 6, and 8 mm
	Tip design	Thin tip
	Advantages	Thin shank allows access into tight fibrotic sulci.
	Disadvantages	Markings end at 8 mm.
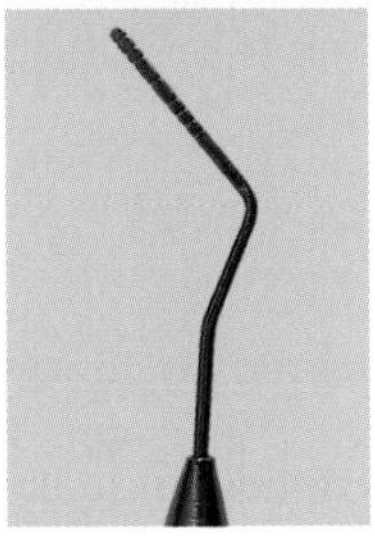	***Goldman Fox Probe***	
	Shank	Flat
	Measurement	1, 2, 3, 5, 7, 8, 9, and 10 mm
	Tip design	Blunt or wide
	Advantages	No mark at 4 and 6 mm
	Disadvantages	Flat shank does not allow easy access into tight fibrotic pockets.

TABLE 26-7
Periodontal Probe Design—cont'd

Probe Examples	Design and Use Characteristics	
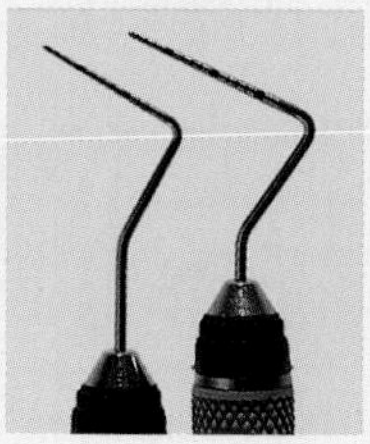	***UNC-12 Probe and UNC-15 Probe (University of North Carolina)***	
	Shank	Thin, round, and tapered
	Measurement	UNC-12: 1, 2, 3, 4, 5, 6, 7, 8, 9, 10, 11, and 12 mm UNC-15: 1, 2, 3, 4, 5, 6, 7, 8, 9, 10, 11, 12, 13, 14, and 15 mm
	Tip design	Thin tip
	Advantages	UNC-12 color-coded at 4 and 9 mm UNC-15 color-coded at 4, 9, and 14 mm Thin shank allows access into tight fibrotic sulci. UNC-12 is used for maintenance and UNC-15 for clients with significant attachment loss.
	Disadvantages	Not applicable
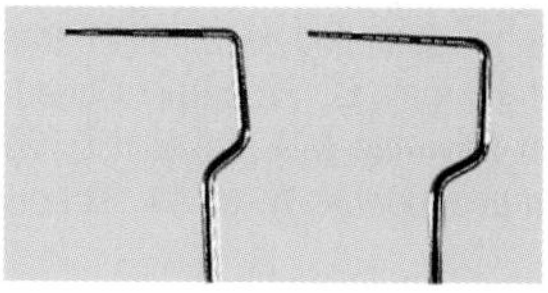	***Novatech Probe***	
	Shank	Upward and right-angled bend
	Measurement	Available in a variety of designs
	Tip design	Available in a variety of designs
	Advantages	Easier access in posterior distal areas
	Disadvantages	May feel bulky because of angulation
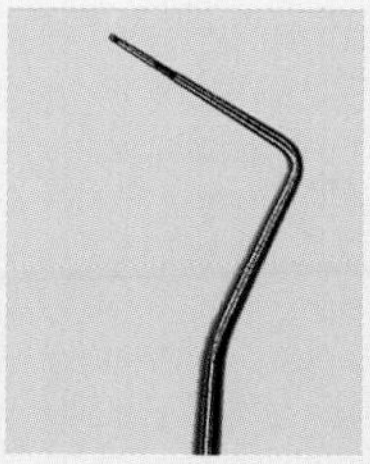	***PSR Screening Probe (World Health Organization Probe)***	
	Shank	Thin, round, and tapered
	Measurement	0.5, 3.5, 5.5, 8.5, and 11.5 mm
	Tip design	Thin tip with ball tip
	Advantages	Ball tip (0.5 mm) for client comfort Color-coded from 3.5-5.5 mm Easy-to-read markings Thin shank allows access into tight fibrotic sulci
	Disadvantages	Markings at 0.5 mm
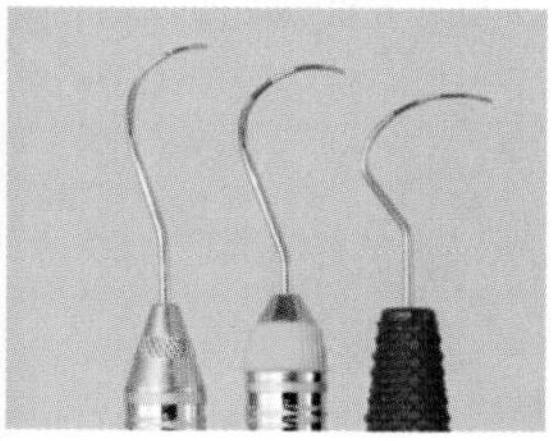	***Nabers Furcation Probe***	
	Shank	Round, tapered, and curved
	Measurement	Available with or without measurement markings
	Tip design	Blunted tip
	Advantages	Ideal for detection of mesial and distal furcations in maxillary molars. Measurement markings are helpful.
	Disadvantages	May feel bulky when clinician is accustomed to using a periodontal explorer for furcation detection
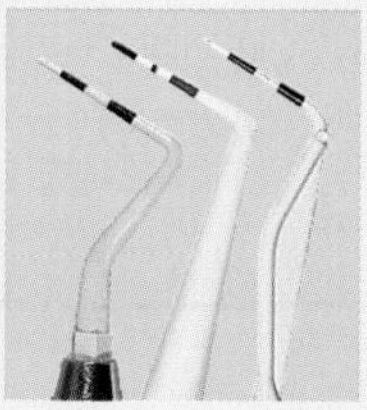	***Plastic Probe (Particularly for Dental Implants)***	
	Shank	Thin, round, and tapered
	Measurement	Color-coded and variable measurements depending on manufacturer
	Tip design	Thin tip or ball tip
	Advantages	Ball tip for client comfort and less chance of penetration Color-coded, easy-to-read markings Thin shank allows access into tight fibrotic sulci. Sterilizable for reuse Will not scratch implants
	Disadvantages	Markings wear away. When this occurs, the entire probe or unscrewed probe tip must be thrown out.

may exhibit. In individuals with severe periodontal disease, tooth migration is an indicator of further loss of support structures, and the stability or degree of movement over time may be monitored with the periodontal probe.

Furcation Probe

(See discussions of furcation involvement in Chapter 19 and furcation anatomy in Chapter 28.)

The **furcation probe** is a specialized probe instrument designed to adapt to the architecture of multirooted teeth to measure the vertical and horizontal depths of a furcation. Typical furcation probe characteristics are a curved shank with a blunted working end. The most widely used furcation detection instrument is the Nabors probe: the 1N and 2N. The 1N is a specialized probe used for the detection and classification of mesial and distal furcations of maxillary molars, whereas the 2N Nabers probe is used for assessing these as well as buccal and lingual furcations. Because classification of furcation involvement is based on the degree of penetration of a probe between the roots of multirooted teeth, the Nabers probe is well suited for subgingival insertion and furcation classification. Its color-coded markings at 3, 6, 9, and 12 mm allow the clinician to classify furcations more accurately (Figure 26-13).

The ACE (Advanced Comprehensive Evaluation) probe is the furcation instrument from Paradise Dental Technology (PDT), whose flexible design allows adaptability to all furcations. It is a nonpaired instrument that has a standard probe on one end with Marquis or UNC markings and a straighter furcation probe on the other, making it an efficient assessment tool because of the universal adaptation to any area (Figure 26-14).

Tactile Sensitivity and Explorer Use

Tactile sensitivity is the ability to distinguish relative degrees of roughness and smoothness on the tooth surface. Experience in detecting light calculus when it is almost completely scaled and in feeling heavy calculus when it has been burnished is a prerequisite for developing tactile sensitivity. The skill may be improved by attention to stroke direction, pressure, type of calculus, and type of root surface being explored.

For calculus detection with an explorer, the practitioner uses a variety of stroke directions (vertical, horizontal, and oblique) to form a "basketweave" of strokes, as described in a later section (Figure 26-15). This use of a variety of strokes is particularly helpful when problems of differentiation between calculus and root structure occur. The dental hygienist should practice different strokes when instrumentation has been particularly difficult in a certain area or when it is

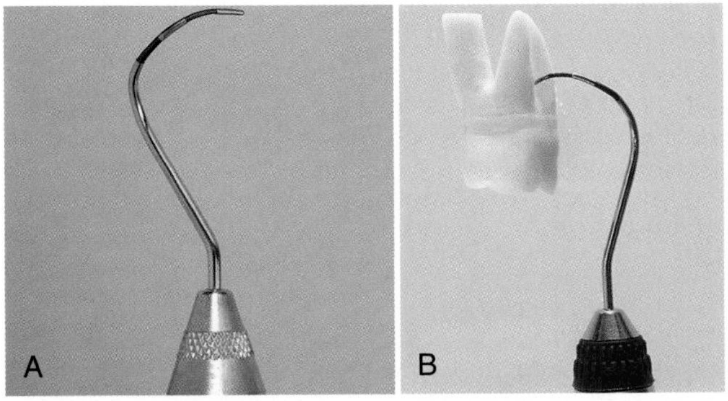

Figure 26-13. A, The No. 2 Nabers probe for detection of furcation areas, with color-coded markings at 3, 6, 9, and 12 mm. **B,** Probe positioned in furca for furcation classification. (**A,** From Newman MG, Takei HH, Klokkevold PR, Carranza FA: *Carranza's clinical periodontology*, ed 11, St Louis, 2012, Saunders.)

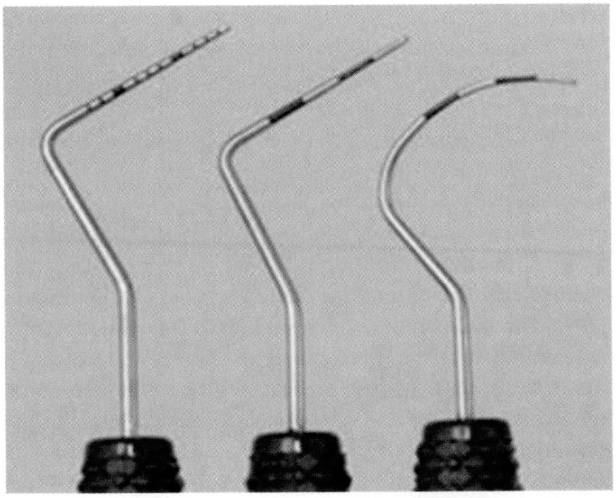

Figure 26-14. ACE Probe is a nonpaired furcation instrument with the option of the opposite working end of UNC 12 or Marquis probe.

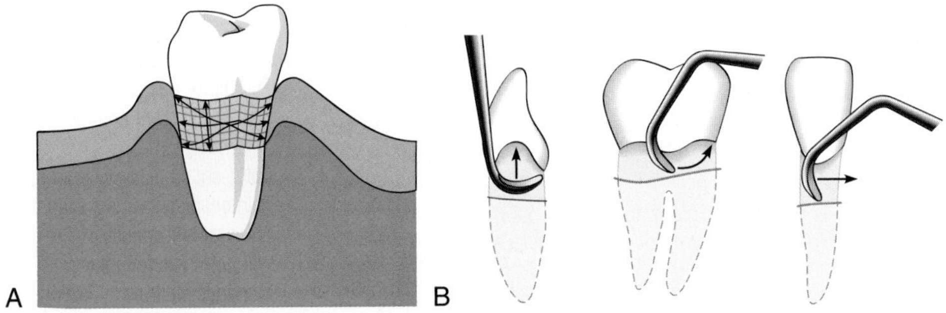

Figure 26-15. A, This diagram illustrates vertical, horizontal, and oblique stroke directions. **B,** Three basic stroke directions: vertical *(left)*, oblique *(middle)*, and horizontal *(right)*. (**A,** Redrawn from Pattison A, Pattison G: *Periodontal instrumentation*, ed 2, Norwalk, Conn, 1992, Appleton and Lange. **B,** From Newman MG, Takei HH, Klokkevold PR, et al: *Carranza's clinical periodontology*, ed 11, St Louis, 2012, Saunders.)

necessary to be particularly thorough in calculus detection (such as in a deep pocket or in an area where there is a periodontal abscess).

Tactile sensitivity also is important in distinguishing between the sulcular soft-tissue wall, the junctional epithelium, and possible osseous exposures. The explorer tip should not stop on the sulcular wall if the instrument is inserted properly and the tip remains well adapted to the tooth surface to the base of the pocket. If the explorer contacts soft tissue, it bounces and snags along the wall until the instrument is adapted properly. As the clinician follows the root of the tooth down to the base of the pocket, the nonkeratinized junctional epithelium is the base of the pocket. The junctional epithelium feels different at different states of periodontal health, as follows:

- In healthy sulci, the junctional epithelium is firm and elastic in nature.
- In the inflamed state, the junctional epithelium is soft and easily penetrable with a sharp-pointed instrument.
- If osseous exposure occurs because of heavy instrumentation and exceptionally friable soft tissue, the sensation at the base of the pocket is much like that of heavy, porous calculus. To differentiate calculus from an osseous exposure, the dental hygienist attempts to move around and under the area. If it is calculus, the junctional epithelium is felt under the deposit. If the roughness is an osseous exposure, it is impossible to move the explorer down and under the area.

The practitioner uses light pressure with the explorer when faced with light calculus, little pocket depth, and friable tissue. Increased pressure is required when trying to distinguish burnished calculus or when overinstrumentation may have caused irregular changes in root structure. Explorer pressure should be decreased, however, after thorough root planing to get an overview of the end product.

Treatment Instruments

Curets

Curets have typically one face, two lateral surfaces (one or two cutting edges), a rounded back, and a face that join to form a rounded toe (see Figure 26-4, *B*). The two main categories of curets are as follows:

- Universal curets
- Area-specific curets

Universal Curet

Design and Use. The universal curet is a double-ended instrument designed with paired mirror-image working ends (Table 26-8). It has two lateral surfaces that form two parallel cutting edges on both sides of the flat face (inner surface) that form a rounded tip (or toe) at the terminal end of the blade. The lateral surfaces converge to form the rounded back of the blade. This design reduces the chances of subgingival trauma to sulcular tissues and tooth structure. Both cutting edges of a universal curet blade are parallel and curved upward toward the toe of the blade (Figure 26-16). The curvature of the blades defines the areas in which the instrument is most useful. (See Table 26-8.)

The face of the universal curet blade is positioned at a 90-degree angle to the lower shank. There is a bend above the lower shank so that the handle is not parallel with the lower shank (Figures 26-17 and 26-18). Therefore, to close

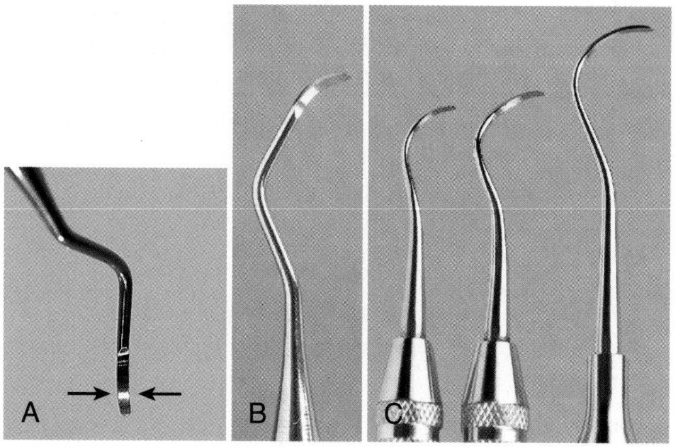

Figure 26-16. A, Both cutting edges of a universal curet blade are parallel and curved upward toward the toe of the blade. **B,** Columbia No. 4R-4L universal curet. **C,** Younger-Good No. 7-8, McCalls No. 17-18, and Indiana University No. 17-18 universal curets. (**B** and **C,** From Newman MG, Takei HH, Klokkevold PR, et al: *Carranza's clinical periodontology*, ed 11, St Louis, 2012, Saunders.)

angulation, the handle and lower shank of the universal curet must be tilted slightly toward the tooth (see Figure 26-18).

The universal curet is a double-ended curet used for supragingival and subgingival scaling and root planing in all areas of the mouth. A universal curet particularly is used for scaling periodontally healthy dentition. Scaling with a universal curet can be more difficult with increased pocket depth. In deeper pockets, combinations of universal curets may be necessary to extend their reach. The Columbia 13/14, for instance, is a short, acutely curved universal curet. This instrument works well in anterior areas or in areas with slight to moderate probing depths and often is paired with the Columbia 4R/4L for use in deeper, more posterior areas. The Columbia 2R/2L is even longer than the Columbia 4R/4L and is ideal for areas of deep facial or lingual pocket depth (Figure 26-19). The Loma Linda 10/11 and the Queen of Hearts by Paradise Dental Technologies also has a longer working end that works well to root plane palatal periodontal pockets and line angles (see Table 26-8).

Blade Selection for Anterior Teeth. In anterior areas the correct side of the instrument is not so critical. Both cutting edges of the universal curet blade may be used for scaling and root planing in anterior areas. Only the angulation or the degree to which the blade is open is different from one end to the other when the ends of the instrument are exchanged. The cutting edge that offers a more open angulation is better for traction and reduces calculus burnishing. However, the type of tissue is a major consideration in selecting the cutting edge for anterior scaling. If the tissue is tight and fibrotic and the pocket depth very shallow, the cutting edge that offers a more closed blade angulation (closer to the tooth surface) is preferable. If the tissue is loose, however, the cutting edge that offers a more open angulation, better traction, and less burnishing action is a better choice because there is less chance of inadvertent soft-tissue trauma against the wall of the pocket.

Blade Selection for Posterior Teeth. Because the ends of a double-ended universal curet are mirror images, they are

TABLE 26-8
Universal Curet Design and Selection

Common Design Specifications of All Universal Curets

Double-ended, mirror image working ends
Two curved cutting edges that end in a rounded toe
Face is at 90 degrees or perpendicular to lower shank
Cross-sectional view is semicircular
Back is round
Differences in shank length, design, and blade size affect use
One curet can be used throughout the healthy mouth of a child, adolescent, or adult

Instrument — **Design, Function, and Recommendation**

Posterior and Anterior Application

(A) Columbia 13/14
(B) Barnhardt 5/6
(C) Younger Good 7/8

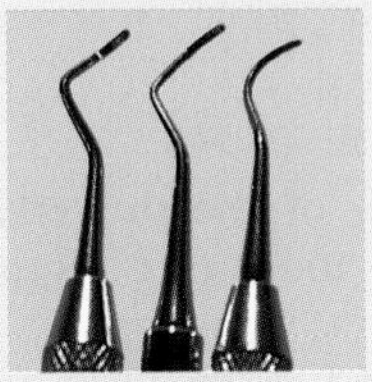

A B C

Design	Short lower shank
Function	Rigid or regular flexibility in shank
Recommendation	Scaling and root planing of supragingival and subgingival biofilm and calculus
	Use on all anterior tooth surfaces
	May be useful in posterior areas of the healthy mouth

Posterior and Anterior Application

(A) Columbia 4R/4L
(B) Columbia 2R/2L
(C) Barnhardt 1/2

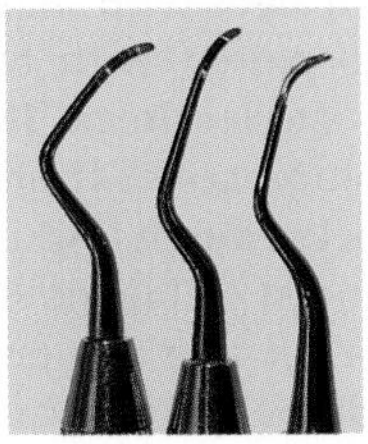

A B C

Design	Long lower shank
Function	Rigid or regular flexibility in shank
Recommendation	Scaling and root planing of supragingival and subgingival biofilm and calculus
	Use on all posterior tooth surfaces in clients with moderate to deep pocket depth.
	The more bent the shank, the easier it is to reach interproximally (*A* and *C*). The straighter the shank, the easier it is to reach buccally and lingually *(B)*.
	May be useful on anterior teeth where there are deep pockets and or recession

Posterior Application

(A) 10/11 Loma Linda
(B) R 144 Queen of Hearts

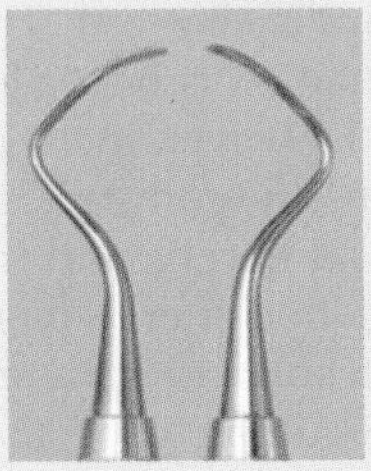

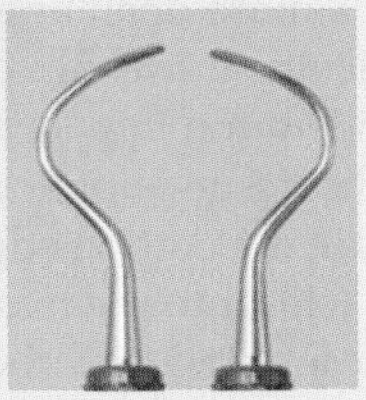

Design	Longer lower shank
Function	Regular flexibility in shank
	Scaling and root planing of supragingival and subgingival biofilm and calculus
Recommendation	Use on posterior areas with moderate to deep pocket depth.
	Blade design is advantageous for line angles.

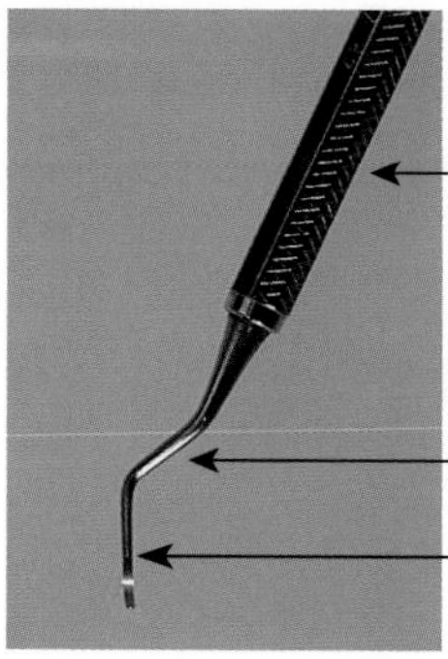

Figure 26-17. The handle of the universal curet is not parallel with the lower shank.

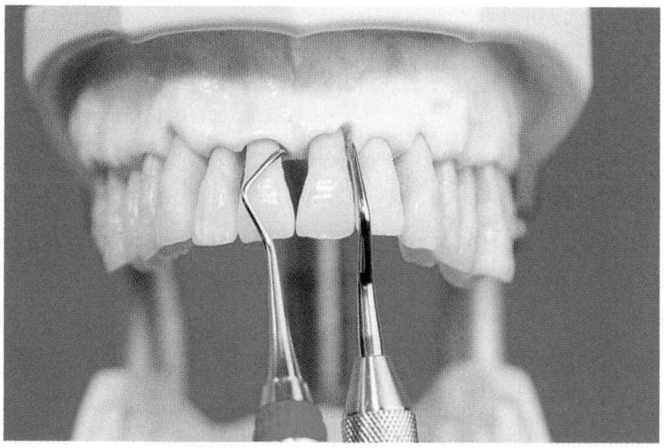

Figure 26-18. Universal Barnhart 5/6 and Gracey 5/6—The angulation of the two instruments are shown as a result of the differences in the relationships of the face of the blade and the lower shanks.

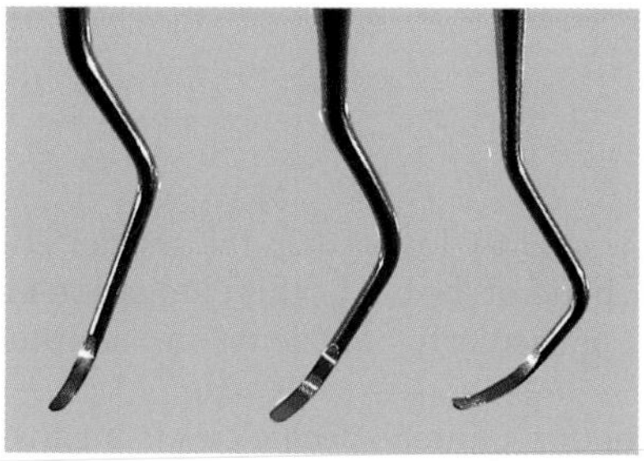

A B C

Figure 26-19. Universal curets. **A,** Columbia 2R/2L. **B,** Columbia 4R/4L. **C,** Columbia 13/14.

used in the same manner but for mirror-image surfaces. This application is especially true in posterior regions. If, for example, one end is used for the distal interproximal surface from the facial aspect, then the opposite end is used for the mesial interproximal surface from the lingual aspect. The end that works best for the straight facial aspect is the same end used for the mesial surface. The end that works best for the straight lingual aspect is the same end used again for the mesial aspect from the lingual surface. Therefore the working ends of the universal curet are not the same for the facial and lingual surfaces in posterior areas.

The basic modified pen grasp and fulcrum placement techniques are used with the universal curet (see Procedure 26-1 and Procedure 26-2).

Area-Specific Curets

Design and Use

Area-specific curets are designed with shanks in a variety of strengths and lengths as well as blades of various sizes (Table 26-9). These variations are to accommodate primarily the subgingival scaling needs of periodontally involved dentitions. Some of the modifications to area-specific Gracey curets are listed below:

- Area-specific Gracey
- Extended shank Gracey
- Minibladed Gracey
- Micro-mini Five Gracey
- O'Hehir New Millennium Series curettes

Like the universal curet, the area-specific curet has two-bladed sides that come together to form a rounded toe. But unlike the universal curet, which has two useful cutting edges because both blades run parallel to each other, the area-specific curet has only one designated cutting edge. The correct cutting edge is determined by examining the curvatures of the blade. The longer curved side is the cutting edge.

The basic modified pen grasp and fulcrum placement techniques used with the universal curet also are used with Gracey curets.

Shank Design

The shank rigidity of curet instruments is an important characteristic to be considered in evaluating the needs of the scaling procedure as mentioned earlier in the description of parts and characteristics of hand-activated instruments.

Certain manufacturers make the Gracey curet with a rigid and even an extra-rigid shank that does not dissipate the power used in a working stroke. This design differentiates the rigid Gracey from the finishing Gracey curet, which has a more flexible shank.

Most clinicians find selection of a rigid-shanked or flexible-shanked instrument is based primarily upon the level and degree of calculus present. The benefits in using instruments with less-flexible shanks when performing heavy scaling and root planing are as follows:

- Improved effectiveness as less lateral pressure is required against the tooth because a rigid shank bends or flexes away from the tooth when pressure is exerted to a lesser degree.
- Savings in operator effort and possible avoidance of injury such as wrist tendonitis are benefits when scaling and root planing teeth with rigid-shanked instruments (see the discussion of hand, wrist, and finger injuries in Chapter 11).
- A stronger shank results in decreased dissipation of pressure exerted by the operator when it is required to fulcrum distant from the working area. The use of extended fulcrums is required when instrumenting deep periodontal defects or when using elongated, specialized Gracey curets.
- When tenacious calculus is present, rigid-shanked instruments prevent the flexing that can contribute to incomplete calculus removal resulting in burnished calculus.

TABLE 26-9

Area-Specific Curet Design Variations

Common Design Specifications of All Area-Specific Curets (see Figure 24-22)

Double-ended, mirror-image working ends
Each blade has two curved cutting edges that end in a rounded toe; however, only one cutting edge per working end is used.
When the lower shank is held vertically, only lower edge of blade is identified as the cutting edge.
Face is offset or tilted at approximately 60 to 70 degrees to the lower shank for perfect working angulation.
Cross-sectional view is semicircular.
Back is round.
Shank design varies with each instrument, making them specific to areas and tooth surfaces where they are used.
All Gracey curets may be used for supragingival and subgingival biofilm and calculus removal and root planing.

Variations	Options	Comparisons	Application
Shank strength	Standard	Slight flexion with moderate to heavy instrumentation pressure	Healthy or maintenance clients
	Rigid and extra rigid	Larger, stronger, less-flexible shank	Moderate to heavy tenacious calculus removal
Shank length	Standard	Area specificity allows for deep scaling, root planing, and periodontal debridement	Healthy or maintenance clients
	Examples by manufacturer: After-Five (Hu-Friedy); Extended Gracey (G. Hartzell & Son)	Terminal shank elongated by 3 mm Deep periodontal pockets	
Blade size	Standard	Offset blade relative to the lower shank, curved upward with a curved blade producing an elongated cutting edge	Healthy to periodontally involved clients
	Examples by manufacturer: Mini-Five (Hu-Friedy); Mini-Extended Gracey (G. Hartzell & Son); Micro-Mini Five (Hu-Friedy)	Terminal shank elongated by 3 mm and blade length reduced by half standard blade 20% thinner blade than the Mini-Five Gracey curets, shank rigidity greater than the Mini-Five Gracey curets	Deep, narrow periodontal pockets and furcations Precise debridement of root and tooth surfaces in challenging periodontal pockets

- The rigid shank enhances control and reduces energy needed to make any stroke direction under any degree of pressure and does not diminish tactile sensitivity.

Arguments against rigid-shanked instruments claim decreased tactile sensitivity compared with flexible shanked instruments. Some clinicians prefer flexible shank instruments for light scaling and root planing, whereas others find the rigid shanks comfortable for all scaling procedures.

The finishing Gracey curet has a more flexible shank and bends under pressure. Because a significant amount of lateral pressure is lost in the flexion that occurs under firm working strokes, this instrument is indicated for light scaling and root planing.

Gracey Curet

Design and Use

One widely used area-specific curet is the **Gracey curet** (Table 26-10). The Gracey curet blade is bent in a curve and is bent so that one cutting edge is elongated. This longer curved side of the Gracey curet, as shown in Figure 26-20, is the correct cutting edge. When the lower shank is held perpendicular to the floor with the face of the blade up, this cutting edge is slightly lower than the shorter edge. Together with the basic bend of the blade, this elongation makes Gracey instruments particularly efficient in adapting to root morphology.

The designation of area-specific curets means that each of the instruments in the collection is designed to scale specific areas of the mouth (e.g., anterior versus posterior) and specific tooth surfaces (e.g., mesial versus distal). Gracey curets are particularly effective for instrumenting teeth with slight to severe periodontitis in individuals who require therapeutic scaling and root planing by quadrant or sextant.

Gracey curets consist of nine mirror-image pairs of instruments: the Gracey 1/2, 3/4, 5/6, 7/8, 9/10, 11/12, 13/14, 15/16, and 17/18. Although Gracey curets are designed for use in designated areas of the mouth (area specific), it is possible to use Gracey curets in a variety of places. Because of this, dental hygiene educators often provide instruction for full-mouth periodontal instrumentation using a select few instruments of the entire collection. The instruments selected usually represent basic anterior-, posterior-, mesial-, and distal-specific instruments. An example of such a selection is the Gracey 5/6, 7/8, 11/12, and 13/14 (Figure 26-21,

A and *B*). Table 26-9 outlines the variations of design in area-specific curets. Table 26-10 summarizes the design of and selection criteria for the use of each of the Gracey area-specific curets. Procedures 26-1 and 26-3 and the corresponding Competency Form outline the steps for their use.

The basic reason Gracey instruments are ideal for instrumenting periodontitis-affected teeth lies with the relationship of the face of the blade to the lower shank. The Gracey curet is honed so that the face is "offset" or at an angle to the lower shank. (The lower or terminal shank is the last bend of the shank closest to the working end.) Whereas the universal curet's face is at 90 degrees, the Gracey curet is at a 60- to 70-degree angle to the lower shank (Figure 26-21, *C*). With this angle of the face to the lower shank, the lower shank is

TABLE 26-10
Area-Specific Curet Design and Selection

Instrument	Design and Selection	
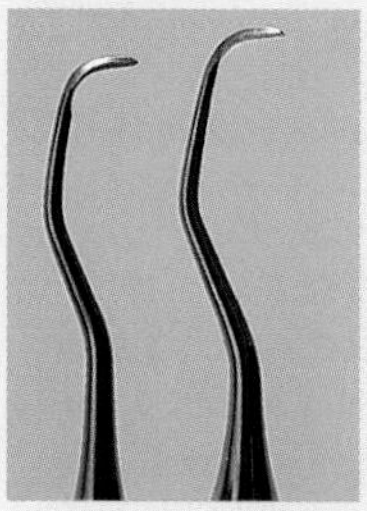 A B	Gracey 1/2 Design Function	Straight shank in the Gracey 1/2 *(A)* similar to that of a Gracey 5/6 *(B)*, but shorter Maxillary and mandibular anterior incisors and canines Shorter shank length limits this instrument to shallower depth than the Gracey 5/6
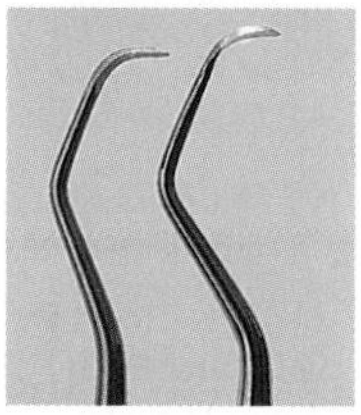 A B	Gracey 3/4 Design Function	Bent shank in the Gracey 3/4 *(A)* similar to that of a Gracey 7/8 *(B)*, but shorter Maxillary and mandibular anterior incisors and canines Shorter shank length limits this instrument to shallower depth than the Gracey 7/8
(See comparison above with Gracey 1/2)	Gracey 5/6 Design Function	Similar straight shank to that of a Gracey 1/2 but longer Maxillary and mandibular anterior incisors, canines, and premolars
(See comparison above with Gracey 3/4)	Gracey 7/8 Design Function	Similar shank bend to that of a Gracey 3/4 but longer Maxillary and mandibular anterior incisors, canines, premolars, and molars Limitations on distal surfaces of molars
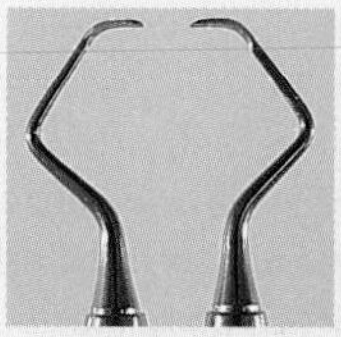 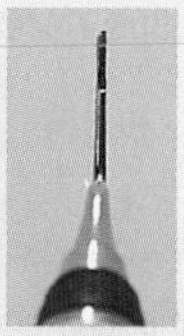 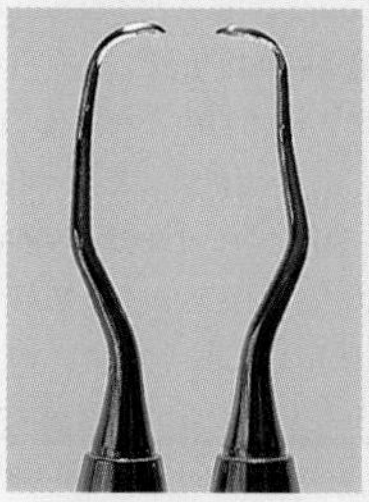 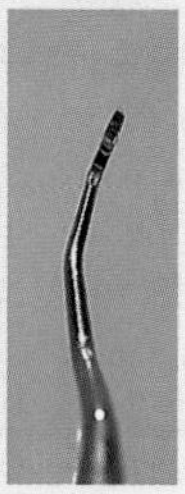	Gracey 9/10 Design Function	Shank bend is more pronounced than on a Gracey 7/8 Maxillary and mandibular molar buccal and lingual surfaces

Continued

TABLE 26-10
Area-Specific Curet Design and Selection—cont'd

Instrument	Design and Selection	
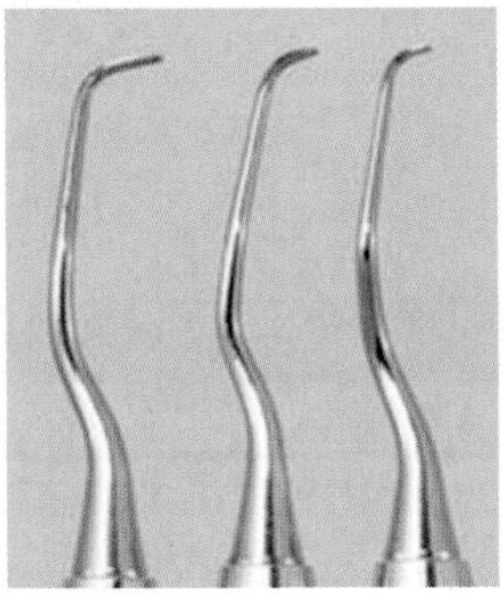 Notes: Gracey 11/12 Category: Replace single instrument with Figure U34	Gracey 11/12 Design Function	Shank is slightly angulated at two points for adaptation to mesial surfaces Maxillary and mandibular molar and premolar mesial surfaces
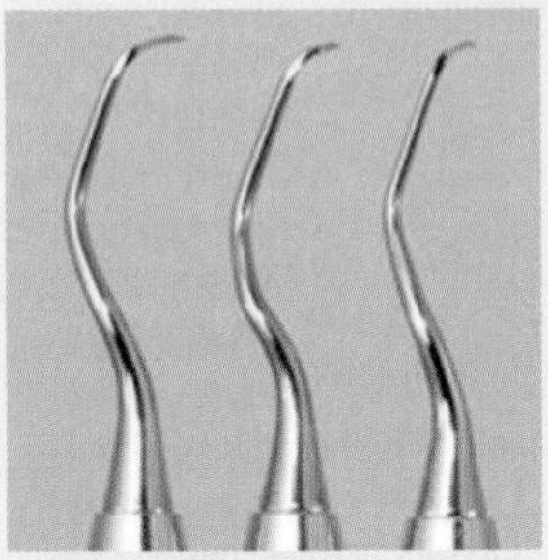 Notes: Gracey 13/14 Category: Replace single instrument with Figure U35	Gracey 13/14 Design Function	Shank is angulated for adaptation to distal surfaces Maxillary and mandibular molar and premolar distal surfaces Using extraoral fulcrums and a variety of operator positions around the client, the clinician also may be able to use the 13/14 in nontraditional areas such as lingual surfaces
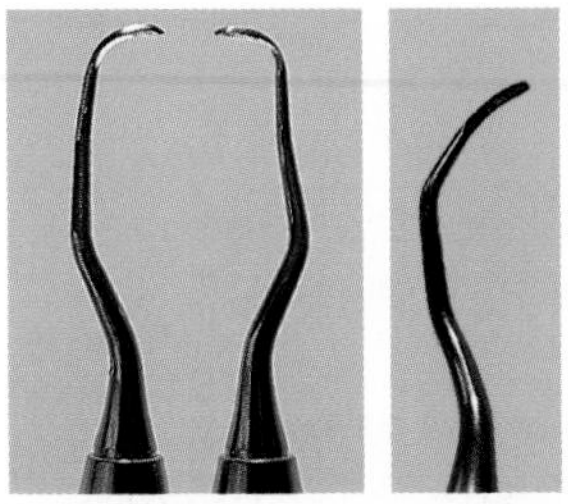	Gracey 15/16 Design Function	Same shank angulation as the Gracey 13/14, but nonworking blade is now the cutting edge, thereby positioned to reach mesial posterior surfaces Maxillary and mandibular molar and premolar mesial surfaces
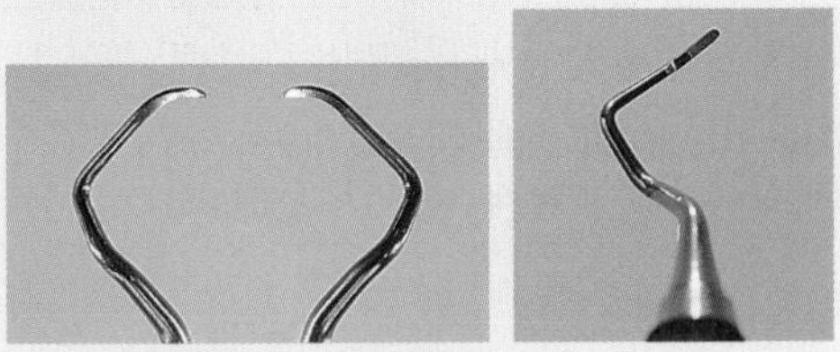	Gracey 17/18 Design Function	Accentuated shank angles for access to distal posterior surfaces Smaller blade and slightly longer terminal shank Maxillary and mandibular molar distal surfaces
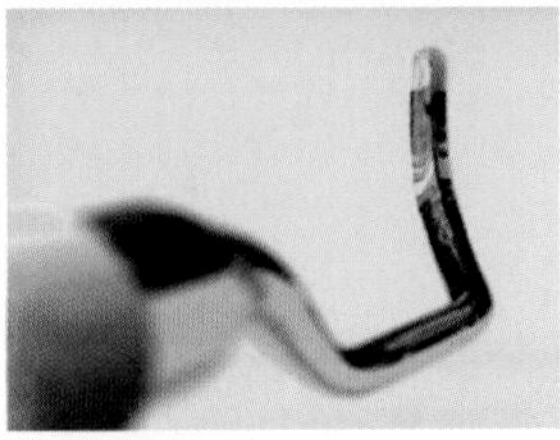 (Courtesy American Eagle Instruments, Inc.)	All-purpose Double Gracey Design Function	All purpose Gracey with two cutting edges on each working end that can adapt to the mesials and distals or buccals and linguals. Regular flexibility in shank. Root planing of supragingival and subgingival biofilm and calculus.

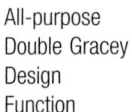

parallel to the tooth surface being scaled when proper angulation of the cutting edge to the tooth surface is achieved. Therefore, when using Gracey curets, the dental hygienist must observe the relationship of the lower shank to the surface being scaled to help determine if correct angulation is achieved.

Another example of area-specific curets are the XP Scandette instruments from American Eagle, an all-purpose, double-ended Gracey designed curet (see Table 26-10). It uniquely has each working end with two faces, a rounded back, and two lateral surfaces with two cutting edges that adapt to mesial and distal surfaces and converge to form a rounded toe.

Extended-Shank Curets

Design and Use

The extended-shank curets are a modified set of Gracey curets that are exactly like the traditional Gracey curets, except that the lower shank of each instrument is 3 mm longer (Figure 26-22). Extended Gracey curets are particularly useful in areas with significant pocket depth or recession. Hu-Friedy calls its extended Gracey curet the *Hu-Friedy After-Five,* and G. Hartzell & Son uses the name *extended Gracey curet.* Some manufacturers offer a blade thinned by 10% for ease in gingival insertion and to reduce tissue distention. Because the shanks are longer than those of the traditional Gracey curets, they often require an extended fulcrum such as an opposite arch, cross-arch, or extraoral fulcrum. Reinforcement with the nondominant hand often may be helpful for additional control.

Minibladed Curets

Design and Use

Another variation of the basic curet is the Gracey minibladed curet, which has a terminal shank that is 3 mm longer than and a working blade that is half the length of the traditional Gracey curet (Figure 26-23, *A* and *B*). Like the extended-shank curets, each manufacturer labels the mini series differently: Hu-Friedy calls their mini–Gracey curet the *Hu-Friedy Mini-Five,* G. Hartzell & Son uses the name *Mini-Extended Gracey* curet, and American Eagle uses *XP Gracey* (double Gracey) +3 Access. The minibladed Gracey curet is particularly useful in areas of narrow, deep pocketing in which it is impossible to insert vertically a long, regular blade straight down into the pocket or vertically instrument interradicular root furcation surfaces. The options in these situations are to use a horizontal stroke with the toe directed to the junctional epithelium or to use a shortened instrument such as a mini-curet with a vertical stroke. This instrument also is used in rounded convexities or concavities found going into and out of root depressions and around line angles.

Micro Mini-Five Gracey Curets

Design and Use

Micro Mini-Five Gracey curets (area-specific) are designed to debride precisely root and tooth surfaces even in the most

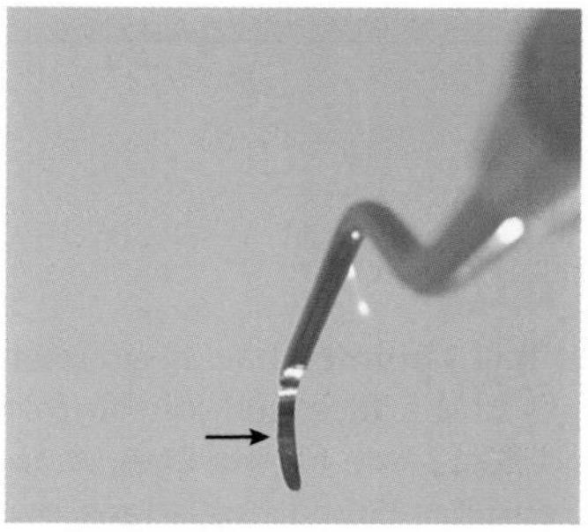

Figure 26-20. The longer curved side of the Gracey curet blade is the cutting edge *(arrow).*

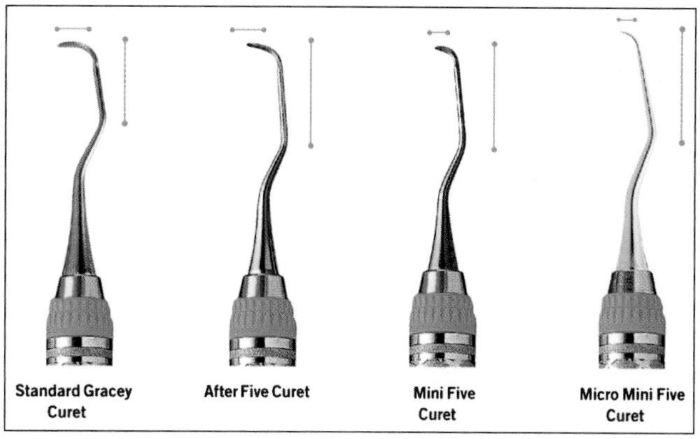

Figure 26-22. Gracey curet tip comparisons. (Courtesy Hu-Friedy Manufacturing, Chicago, Illinois.)

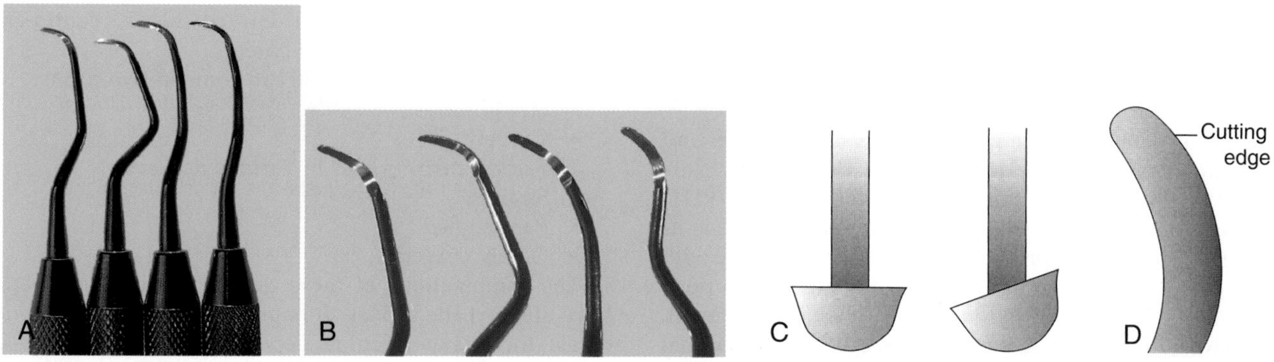

Figure 26-21. **A,** Gracey curets 5/6, 7/8, 11/12, and 13/14. **B,** Close-up of Gracey curets 5/6, 7/8, 11/12, and 13/14. **C,** Face of a universal curet is at 90 degrees to its shank *(left),* whereas the face of a Gracey curet is offset, forming a 70-degree angle with its shank *(right).* **D,** Determining the correct cutting edge of a Gracey curet. When viewed from directly above the face of the blade, the correct cutting edge is the one forming the larger outer curve on the right. (**C** and **D,** From Newman MG, Takei HH, Klokkevold PR, et al: *Carranza's clinical periodontology,* ed 11, St Louis, 2012, Saunders.)

Procedure 26-3 Use of Sickle Scalers

INSTRUMENT	STRAIGHT-SHANKED SICKLE (ANTERIOR)	CONTRA-ANGLED SICKLE (POSTERIOR)
Equipment	Straight-shanked sickle, subgingival explorer, mouth mirror	Contra-angled sickle, subgingival explorer, mouth mirror
Steps	Fundamentals (Procedure 26-1)	
Grasp	Modified pen, moderate pressure grasp	Same as for straight-shanked sickle.
Fulcrum and pressure	Stable, moderate fulcrum pressure Intraoral, adjacent to tooth being scaled Opposite arch	Same as for straight-shanked sickle.
Selection of working ends based on design	Determine working end based on amount of calculus, tissue tone, pocket depth, and correct adaptation. Use straight end of SH 5/33 on anterior interproximal surfaces. Use slight contra-angle design of SH 6/7 in anterior and premolar areas. Thinner tip designed sickles can be used for calculus located just below tight, anterior contacts areas.	Determine working end based on amount of calculus, tissue tone, pocket depth and correct adaptation. Use SCNEVI-4 rather than S204-SD for more periodontally involved clients. While keeping side of tip well adapted to root surface, insert to greatest depth tissue allows. Engage lower edge of supragingival calculus. Engage ledge of subgingival calculus. Use opposite end for alternate sides of tooth.
Insertion	Engage lower edge of interproximal supragingival calculus; may extend 1 to 2 mm subgingivally when soft tissue permits.	Same as for straight-shanked sickle.
Adaptation	Lower third cutting edge and tip of sickle closely adapted to tooth surface.	Same as for straight-shanked sickle.
Angulation	Adjust blade to 80 to <90 degrees against tooth surface.	Same as for straight-shanked sickle.
Activation, stroke direction and efficiency	<u>Supragingival:</u> Engage large calculus deposits with vertical to oblique pull stroke with moderate pressure. Move across tooth surface until all gross calculus is removed. <u>Subgingival:</u> Activate vertical pull stroke using moderate pressure. Move across subgingival area until all gross calculus is removed.	Same as for straight-shanked sickle. Same as for straight-shanked sickle.

challenging periodontal pockets. This curet is another variation of the mini-curet series with ultra slender blades and shank rigidity, manufactured with a special metal (EverEdge technology) that decreases the amount of sharpening required. The blades are 20% thinner than Mini-Five Gracey curets to further reduce tissue distention and ease subgingival insertion. Terminal shanks are elongated for deep access into pockets; they have slightly increased shank rigidity compared with the Mini-Five Gracey curet. Because of the Ever Edge technology, the instruments keep their sharp edge longer, and sharpening time is reduced (Figure 26-23, *B*).

Debridement Curettes

Design and Usage

Debridment curets provide precise access to furcations and concavities for root surface detoxification. The **O'Hehir New Millennium curettes** by Paradise Dental Technologies (PDT) are area-specific instruments with similar shank designs as Graceys that are used supragingivally and subgingivally with a push or pull stroke in multiple directions, although a push stroke should not be directed into the epithelial attachment. They have unique tiny, scooped blades at 280 degrees that allow easier subgingival adaptation to root surfaces, including furcations. Another debridement curet by Hu-Friedy has unique 365-degree cutting edges on a discoid base. Its use is similar to a file (Figure 26-24).

Sickle Scaler

Design and Use

The **sickle scaler** has a pointed back, two lateral surfaces, and two cutting edges and a face that join to form a pointed tip (Tables 26-11 and 26-12, see Figure 26-4, *A* and *C*).

The working end has flat cutting edges, usually 90 degrees to the shank, on both sides of the face. The two lateral sides join together to form the back of the instrument in a V shape. The sickle scaler tip always ends in a sharp point. This tip is the major difference between a sickle scaler and a curet, especially when comparing the curved blade, contra-angle designed sickle scalers with a curet.

The face of the sickle blade can come in two forms:

- Straight
- Curved

The sickle shank comes in various designs:

- Straight
- Bent-angled
- Gently curved

The combinations of these design modification features have allowed the sickles to be an important supplement to curets for heavy calculus deposits and accessibility. The newer curved bladed sickles are used with growing popularity, because many are thinner with slight shank bends that allow anterior and posterior versatility especially when combined with extraoral fulcrums.

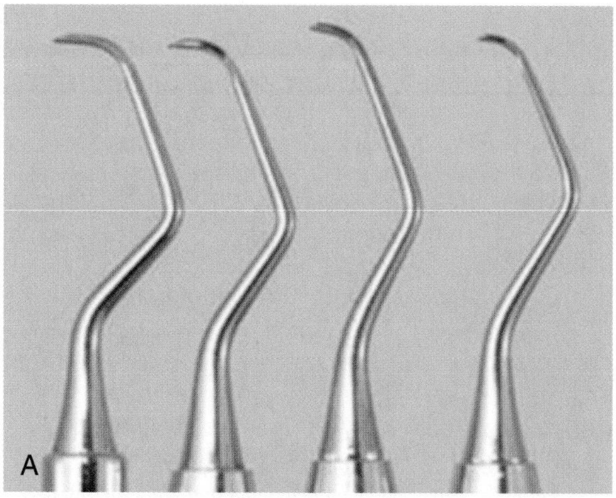

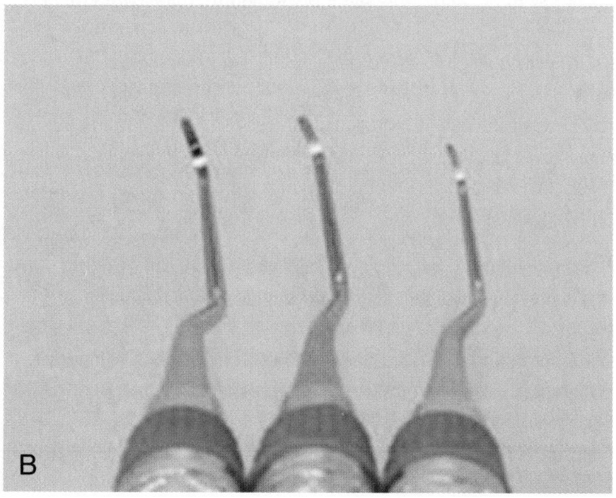

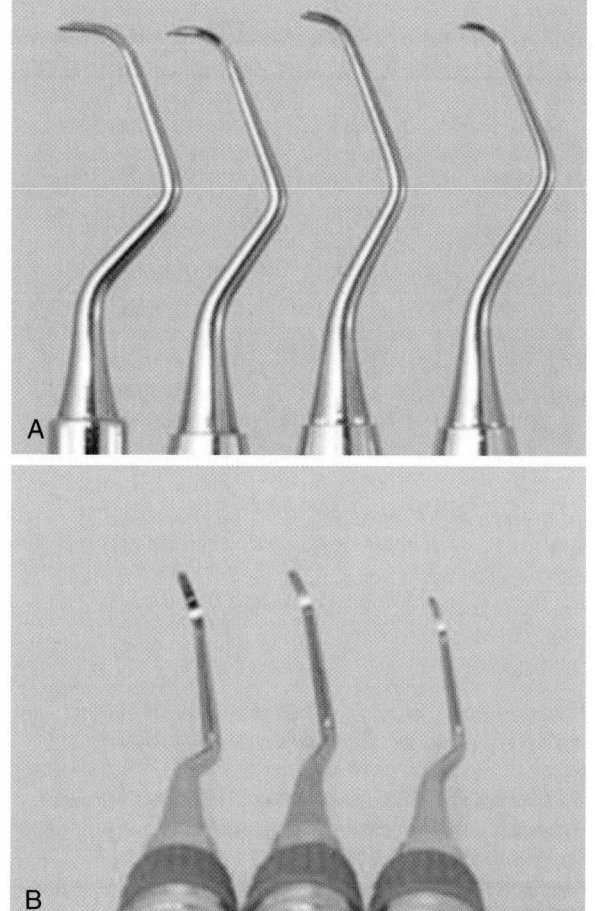

Figure 26-23. **A,** Comparison of regular Graceys, after-five Graceys and mini-five Graceys, and micro mini-five Graceys 7/8 curets. **B,** A close-up working end comparison of regular Gracey, mini-five Gracey, and micro mini-five Gracey 7/8 curets.

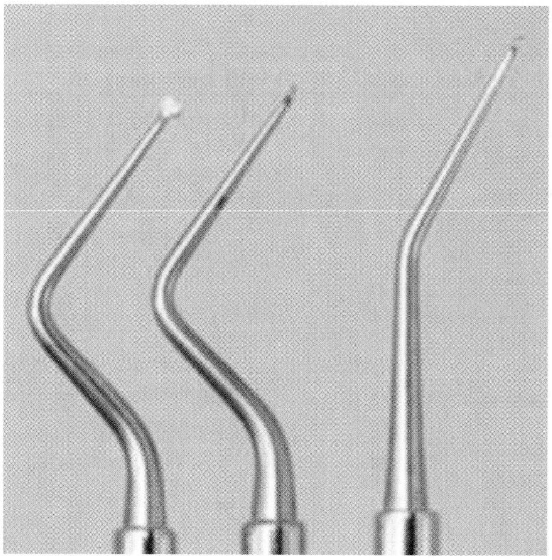

Figure 26-24. Debridement curettes. (Courtesy Hu-Friedy Manufacturing, Chicago, Illinois.)

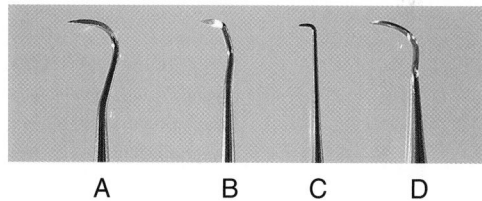

Figure 26-25. Comparison of various sickle scalers. **A,** Curved anterior sickle. **B,** Jacquette (double-ended) sickle. **C,** Morse anterior sickle. **D,** Posterior sickle.

The sickle scaler is designed with either a straight, bent-angled (contra-angle) or curved shank design (Figure 26-25). The straight-shanked sickle scalers are traditionally anterior scaling instruments and are often single ended because the same end may be used mesially and distally (see Procedures 26-1 and 26-4 and the corresponding Competency Form and Table 26-10). The bent or curved shanked sickle scalers may be used for anterior as well as posterior areas of the mouth and are usually double ended, with one end designed for scaling mesial tooth surfaces and the other end for scaling distal tooth surfaces (see Procedures 26-1 and 26-4 and Table 26-11).

The advantage of the sickle scaler is its ability to reach between very tight contacts. The disadvantage is that the sharp tip and straight cutting edge do not adapt well to rounded tooth surfaces; some part of the instrument is always off the tooth. This problem of adaptation and a V-shaped back imposing on the sulcular wall makes the sickle scaler largely a supragingival scaling instrument. Because of the need to control adaptation of the toe and cutting edge of this instrument, instrumentation techniques for sickle scalers require a stable modified pen grasp and fulcrum relatively close to the area being scaled. A pull stroke action in a vertical or oblique direction is made against the tooth surface.

The sickle scaler is valuable for removal of heavy calculus. Because the sides form a V shape, this instrument is sturdy in terms of strength even after it has been sharpened many times.

Only in situations of moderate to heavy subgingival calculus and very loose tissue may the sickle scaler be used subgingivally. Many experienced practitioners who are adept optionally use sickles supragingivally and subgingivally for heavy calculus because of the sturdiness of the instrument. The sickle blade angulation is usually set at 90 degrees and their shank strengths facilitate fracturing and cleaving off deposits. A Gracey curet has a blade angulation of 70 degrees, which, if used improperly, can be overclosed and shave off subgingival calculus resulting in residual burnished deposits. The curved shanked sickle scalers with a curved blade design are effective for moderate to heavy subgingival calculus removal in anterior and posterior areas (see Table 26-12).

Small straight-shanked sickle scalers such as the Morse scaler (see Figure 26-25, *C*) cause even less trauma and may be easier to use for subgingival scaling in tight anterior areas. The extra width from the face to the back of the working end, however, can make it difficult to close the angulation of most sickles without traumatizing the sulcular epithelium with the

TABLE 26-11
Anterior Sickle Scaler Design and Selection

Common Design Specifications of All Anterior Sickle Scalers

Single-ended straight shank
Double-ended, paired design when the shank is slightly bent
Blade, shank, and handle are in the same plane.
Two cutting edges on a straight blade that end in a point or two cutting edges on a curved blade that end in a sharp point
Cross-sectional view is triangular.
Back is a sharp edge of the meeting of the two sides or flattened depending on manufacturer.

Instrument Examples	Design, Function, and Recommendation	
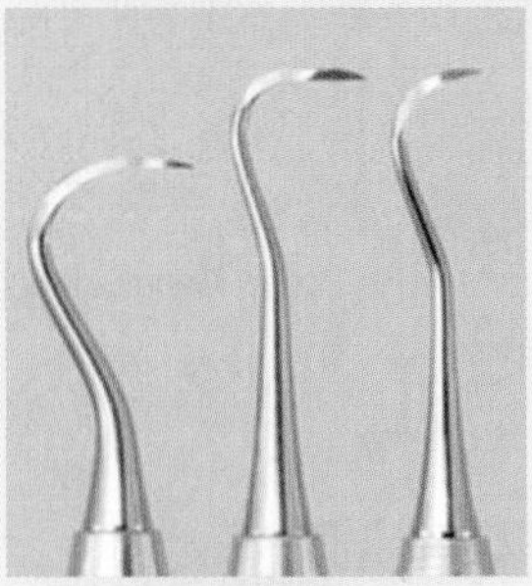	SH 6/7 Design Function Recommendation	Paired, contra-angle, curved sickle design Short lower shank with slight angulation for accessibility; however, blades, shank, and handle should be considered to be within the same plane and therefore are anterior sickles. Blade is long, relatively thin, with a large rounded back. Use for anterior and premolar supragingival and subgingival (1-2 mm) calculus removal. Contra-angle design allows easier access interproximally than with a straight shank. With good adaptation, this instrument could be used to remove heavy ledges of calculus on lingual surfaces of posterior teeth in a horizontal direction. Not recommended for subgingival calculus removal ≥3 mm or root planing
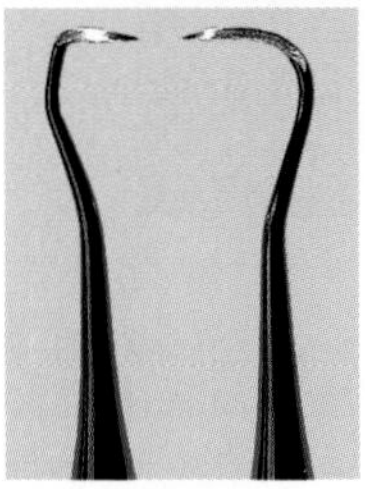	SH 5/33 Design Function Recommendation	Double-ended with a straight sickle on one end and a curved sickle on other end Both blades are within the same plane as the shank and handle. Both blades are relatively thin. Use both ends for anterior supragingival and subgingival (1-2 mm) calculus removal. Not recommended for subgingival calculus removal ≥3 mm or root planing
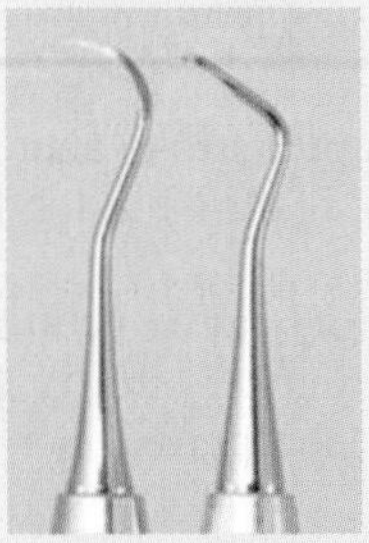 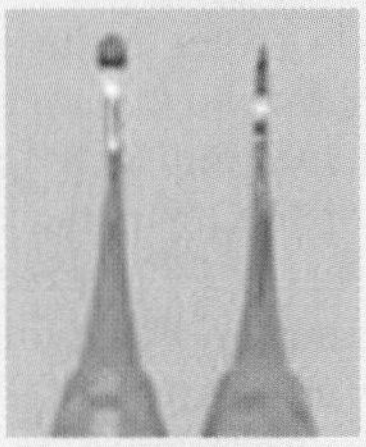	SCNevi 1 Design Function	An elongated disk end and paired with an anterior curved sickle Rigid in shank Anterior lingual stain and calculus removal and a thin curved blade for interproximal scaling of biofilm and calculus

V-shaped back during subgingival instrumentation. This problem is accentuated with large bladed sickle scalers.

The modified pen grasp should be used with the sickle scaler. The cutting edge is positioned under the deposit, and a pull stroke in a vertical or oblique direction is applied to remove the calculus.

Hoe Scaler
Design and Use

The **hoe scaler** has a straight, beveled cutting edge at a right angle (90 degrees) to the shank (see Figure 26-4, *F*). The terminal end of the blade is bent to a 99- to 100-degree angle, and the tip is beveled at a 45-degree angle to form a single

TABLE 26-12
Posterior Sickle Scaler Design and Selection

Common Design Specifications of All Posterior Sickle Scalers

Double-ended, paired design with a bent shank for posterior interproximal access
Two straight or curved cutting edges that end in a sharp point
Cross-sectional view is triangular.
Back is a sharp edge of the meeting of the two sides or flattened depending on manufacturer.

Instrument Examples	Design, Function, and Recommendation	
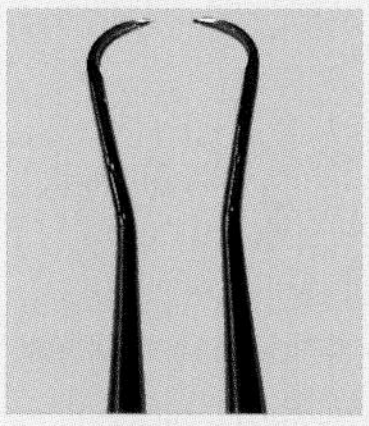	S204SD Design Function Recommendation	Paired, contra-angle, curved sickle design Shank is bent in two places Blade is small, about half the width and length of the anterior SH 6/7 sickle scaler Bent lower shank allows access interproximally in anterior and posterior areas Short narrow blade allows access subgingivally Use for supragingival and subgingival calculus removal (where tissue permits)
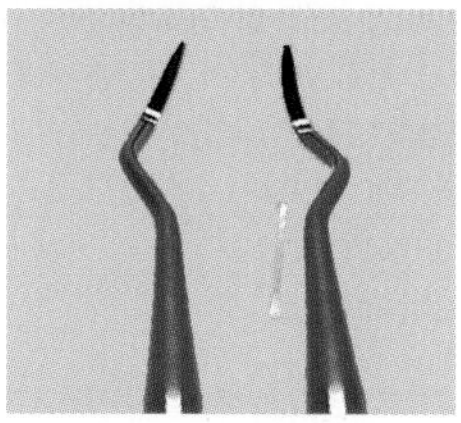	SJ 34/35 Design Function Recommendation	Paired, contra-angle, straight sickle design (Jacquette scaler) Shank is bent in two places The 34/35 is a miniature sickle scaler Bent lower shank allows access interproximally and subgingivally in anterior and posterior areas Access may be limited owing to size of blade
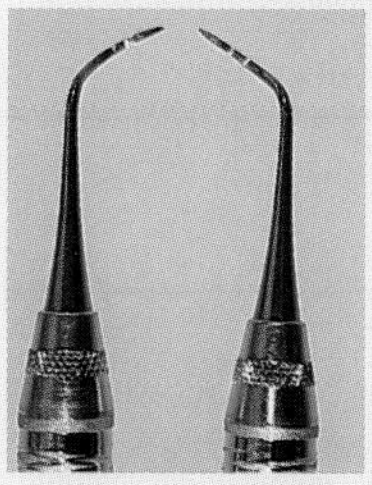	SCNEVI2 Design Function Recommendation	Paired, contra-angle, curved sickle design Shank is acutely bent The blade is long and thin Bent lower shank allows ideal access interproximally in anterior and particularly in posterior areas Use for supragingival and subgingival calculus removal (where tissue permits)
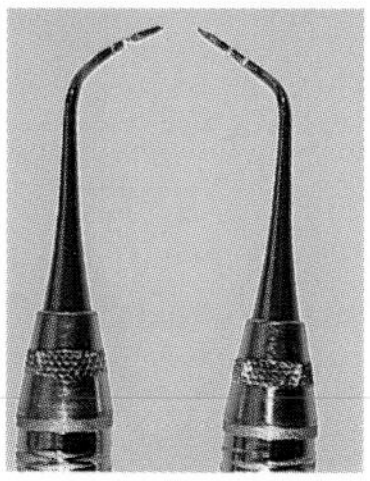	Montana Jack/Nevi 4 Design Function Recommendation	Paired, curved shank, curved bladed sickle design. The blade is long and thin Curved lower shank allows ideal access interproximally in anterior and particularly in posterior areas Use for supragingival and subgingival calculus removal (where tissue permits)

cutting edge. The upper edge forms the actual cutting edge because the hoe scaler is a pull instrument. The cutting edge is a straight, thick, short blade with two sharp corners on each end.

The hoe has paired working ends, and a set of four working ends is needed to instrument each tooth surface. Shank length on a hoe may vary from long to short, and the shank also may be bowed in a slight or more acute angle (Figure 26-26). These variations in shank length and angle help determine the best areas in which to use the hoe scaler. The longer and more angled the shank is, the better suited the instrument is for posterior areas. The shorter, less acutely angled shank is better suited for anterior areas.

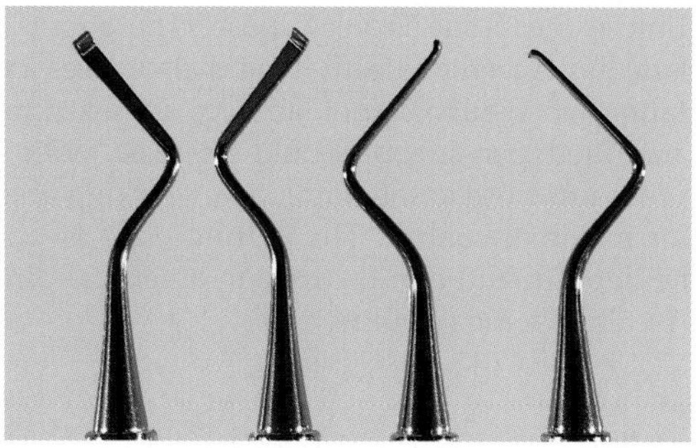

Figure 26-26. Hoe scaler.

Procedure 26-4 Use of Curets

INSTRUMENT	UNIVERSAL CURET	AREA-SPECIFIC CURET
Equipment	Universal curet, subgingival explorer, mouth mirror	Area-specific curets, subgingival explorer, mouth mirror
Steps	Fundamentals Procedure 26-1	Fundamentals Procedure 26-1
Grasp	Modified pen, secure but responsive to changes during calculus removal and root topography such as line angles and concavities Grasp allows handle (hence blade) to fluidly roll around convexities and into concavities.	Same as for Universal Curet
Fulcrum and pressure	Stable, moderate fulcrum pressure with working stroke Intraoral, adjacent to tooth being scaled Cross-arch, opposite arch, extraoral Fulcrum pressure increases with tenacity of calculus	Same as for Universal Curet
Working end selection	See Table 26-11 and Table 26-12 to determine anterior vs. posterior usage. Posterior instrument end selection is made by positioning blade against buccal surface of tooth and choosing end that offers a more closed adaptation. Use this approach for mesial and distal surfaces from the buccal aspect. Repeat above for determining end for the lingual aspect. Anterior instrument end selection can be either end of the universal curet depending on tissue retractability.	See Tables 26-9 and 26-10 for design and selection criteria of area-specific curets. Select correct end of curet by positioning longer, lower cutting edge of blade against tooth. The correct end positions face of blade toward root surface with vertical stroke, the lower shank is parallel to the long axis of the tooth or root surface being scaled.
Insertion	Insert blade in relatively closed position to base of pocket.	Same as for Universal Curet
Adaptation	Adjust first 2 to 3 mm of blade against tooth surface using tactile sensations.	Same as for Universal Curet
Angulation	Open blade to between 60 and 80 degrees.	Same as for the Universal Curet
Activation, stroke direction, and efficiency	Resecure grasp and fulcrum to achieve an effective vertical or oblique, pull, working stroke. Modify pressure against tooth by type, amount and position of calculus, and/or tooth irregularity. Following series of vertical strokes, use a variety of stroke directions to complete calculus removal and root planing.	

The hoe scaler is used for heavy supragingival calculus removal. Because of design limitations, it is best used in subgingival areas where access is easy, such as facial and lingual surfaces (as opposed to interproximal surfaces), and when tissue tone is retractable, loose, and edematous. It is not well suited for fine subgingival scaling and root planing.

When the instrument is inserted subgingivally and the blade is well adapted to the tooth surface, the side of the shank should form a two-point contact with the tooth surface. This improves stability and leverage during instrumentation.

The limitations of the hoe scaler begin with the bow or angle in the shank. This characteristic angle of hoe scalers seriously limits the ability to instrument to the base of the pocket unless the tissue is very loose. The short, straight, bulky blade limits tactile sensitivity and also poses a problem of adaptation when curved root surfaces are instrumented.

The modified pen grasp should be used with the hoe scaler. A fulcrum close to the immediate working area is suggested for maximal control. The cutting edge is positioned under the deposit, and a pull stroke in a vertical direction is applied to remove the calculus.

File Scaler

Design and Use

The file scaler, which is similar in design to the hoe scaler, is a pull stroke instrument. It consists of a series of miniature hoe blades on a pad attached to the shank. Each blade is bent at an angle of 90 to 105 degrees from the shank. Each blade possesses sharp corners that together pose a hazard to tooth structure if adaptation is not maintained during stroke activation. These corners may be rounded slightly with a sharpening stone before the file is used (see Figure 26-4, *D*, and Figure 26-27).

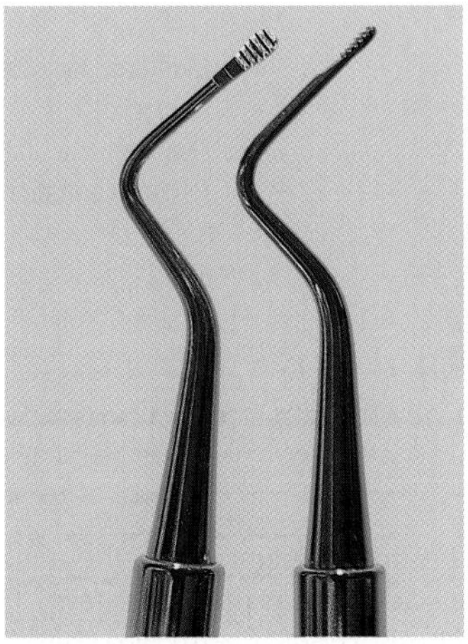

Figure 26-27. File scaler.

The instrument may be double ended or single ended. The file has paired ends, and, as with the hoe, four working ends are needed to instrument each of the four surfaces of a tooth (mesial, distal, facial, and lingual). As with the hoe, the longer, more angled shanks are better suited for posterior areas. The shorter, less-angled shanks are better suited for anterior areas. The shank of the file is fairly rigid, which is advantageous when pressure is applied against the tooth.

The pad or base of the working end of the file may come in a variety of shapes (round, oval, or rectangular) and in numerous sizes, depending on the manufacturer. The larger the base is, the more difficult it becomes to adapt to rounded root surfaces. The size, adaptation, and bend of the shank create problems for working in interproximal areas. As with the hoe, the easiest areas are the facial and lingual surfaces and mesial and distal surfaces, where there are no contacts. Loose, edematous tissue is necessary for reaching areas close to the base of the pocket.

The file scaler is used supragingivally or subgingivally for crushing or breaking up heavy subgingival calculus (Orban or Sugarman). Roughening up tenacious, burnished calculus helps to prepare the surface, making it easier for the curet to latch onto to break the piece away from the tooth. Because this instrument has many of the limitations of the hoe scaler, it should not be used for definitive subgingival scaling and root planing, unless finer, finishing files such as Hirschfeld are used. Finishing files typically have either a smaller pad or slender shape for access to planing root surfaces. Although files traditionally have the rows of parallel blades on a flat working head, a file also can be diamond coated with the surface like an emery board as a finishing instrument.

The modified pen grasp should be used with the file scaler with a fulcrum close to the immediate working area and the entire series of blades positioned against tooth surface.

Chisel Scalers

Design and Use

The chisel scaler is a double-ended instrument that has a straight, (45-degree) beveled single cutting edge on a straight or curved shank designed for push stroke on supragingival calculus. The shank is continuous with the narrow cutting edge blade (see Figure 26-4, *E*, and Figure 26-28). This instrument should be used only on heavy interproximal calculus ledges, especially on lower anterior teeth. It should not be used for scaling and root planing procedures. The chisel is very limited and is not often used by dental hygienists because of the better versatility and advantages of other scaling instruments.

To avoid unnecessary trauma to soft tissues, it should be used only in a horizontal direction. The instrument should be stabilized against a tooth structure and used with a pushing motion to dislodge heavy interproximal, facial, and lingual calculus from mandibular anterior teeth. Because the corners of the chisel are sharp, care should be taken to keep the blade evenly positioned on tooth structures during stroke activation.

A modified pen grasp with an intraoral fulcrum close to the working area aids the practitioner in stabilizing this instrument. Sharpening objectives and procedures for the chisel scaler are similar to those for the hoe scaler.

Furcation Instruments

See the discussion of furcation involvement in Chapter 19, and see Chapter 28 for a review of furcation anatomy.

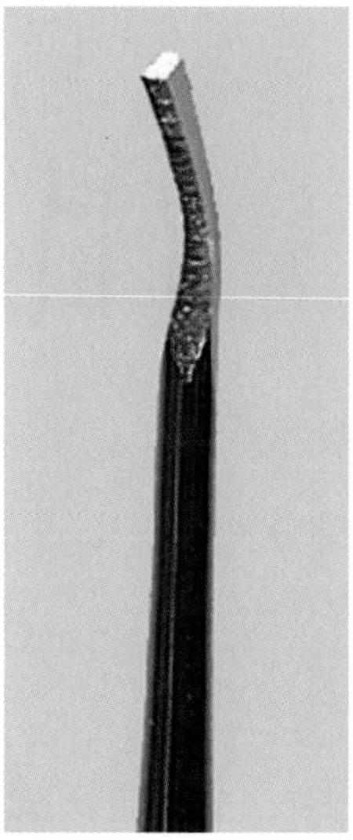

Figure 26-28. Chisel scaler.

Design and Use

Instruments specially designed to access small areas such as furcations and other concave root surfaces are available from a number of manufacturers. Generally, the purpose of these instruments is to remove light deposits and finish surfaces in narrow, inaccessible areas. They are not for heavy calculus removal. Although these instruments are not truly scalers, curets, or files, some are named as such. The following are some examples:

- Diamond Tec File Scalers, Hu-Friedy Manufacturing
- Diamond-Tip Curettes, Brasseler USA
- Diamond Files (not necessarily for only furcations), G. Hartzell & Son
- Furcation Files, LM-Instruments
- Quetin (pronounced *kee-tin*) furcation curets (Hu-Friedy)
- O'Hehir Debridement (Hu-Friedy) and New Millennium Curettes (PDT)

Instruments with diamond-coated working ends are used with push and pull strokes with light pressure in a multidirectional manner. Used in a sanding motion, such instruments remove flat, smooth calculus and significantly reduce root overinstrumentation that may have resulted with curet use.

Buccal and lingual designs (e.g., SDCN7, Hu-Friedy; 209.F1 and 209.F2, Brasseler USA) have paired ends and as such are universal instruments. Mesial and distal diamond-coated working ends have a concave mesial end and a convex distal end on one instrument (Hu-Friedy, Figures 26-29 and 26-30), or concave mesial and distal ends on one instrument (Brasseler USA). These designs are for adaptation to line angles and deep developmental grooves and for final debridement and polishing of root surfaces and furcations.

The LM Furcator (LM-Instruments) has designs to reach concave root surfaces (see Figure 26-29).

Quetins are small hoes with semicircular blades designed to scale a furcation ceiling or floor and are available as a buccal lingual or a mesial distal instrument.

The Hu-Friedy Debridement Curettes are instruments with a small disc blade and a long terminal shank than can be used with a push/pull stroke on any tooth surface. The small size allows adaptation in grooves, depressions, and furcations. This instrument design by Paradise Dental

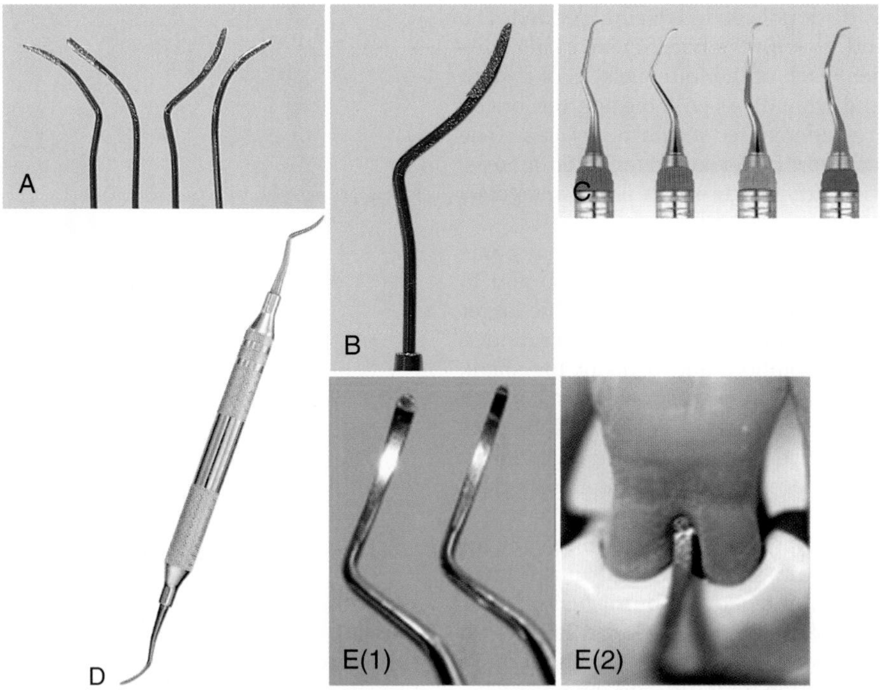

Figure 26-29. Furcation instruments. **A** and **B,** Brasseler diamond-coated instruments. **C,** Diamond Tec file scalers. **D,** Diamond furcation file No. DF1/2. **E,** Quentin furcation curet by Hu-Friedy. (**C,** Courtesy Hu-Friedy, Chicago, Illinois. **D,** Courtesy G. Hartzell & Son, Concord, California. **E,** From Pattison A, Matsuda S, Pattison G: *Periodontal instrumentation*, ed 3, Upper Saddle River, NJ, Prentice Hall [in press].)

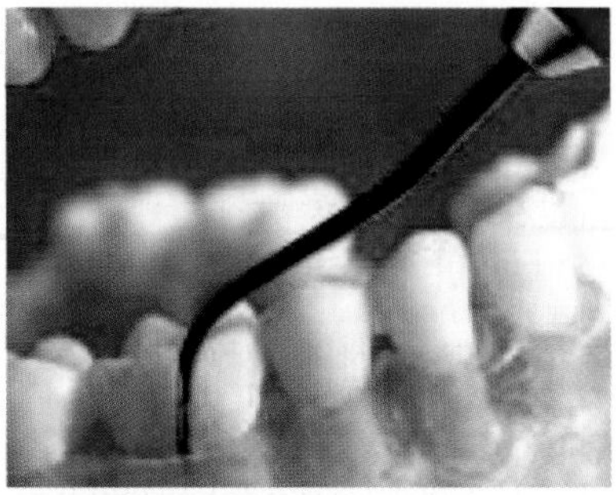

Figure 26-30. Placement of SDCN7 Diamond Tec file scaler into a mandibular furcation. (Courtesy Hu-Friedy Manufacturing, Chicago, Illinois.)

Technologies (PDT), the O'Hehir New Millennium Series Curettes, is discussed previously in the area-specific instrument section (see Figure 26-24).

Implant Scaler

Design and Use

Implant instruments are specially made by various manufacturers with material designed to remove deposits without damaging the titanium implant surfaces. Some of the materials used are plastic composites, graphite, resins, gold, and titanium. Their designs are similar to standard metal curets and the materials determine their effectiveness and rigidity in removing calculus (see Table 26-2).

Fundamental Components

A clinician must know the fundamental components to achieve protective and productive hand-activated instrumentation. Correct application of these foundational principles facilitates desired outcomes and minimizes occupational injury:

- Operator/client positioning
- Body mechanics
- Grasp
- Fulcrum
- Lateral pressure
- Reinforcement scaling
- Stroke principles
- Field of vision

Improper attention to these fundamental components increases the possibility of developing repetitive strain injuries (see Chapter 11). Self-evaluation, done at any time during the instrumentation process, requires that the practitioner monitor the stress effects on the working hand, wrist, elbow, shoulder, neck, back, or spine (Procedure 26-5 and the corresponding Competency Form, and see Chapter 11, Figure 11-2).

Operator/Client Positioning

Correct operator and client positioning facilitate proper instrumentation technique. In operator positioning the dental hygienist attempts to achieve a state of musculoskeletal balance that protects the body from strain and cumulative injury (see the section on positioning factors in Chapter 11).

Operator position relative to the client usually is described as clock positions with the head of the patient at 12 o'clock. Operators should place themselves in the proper clock position around the client that enables them to have either a direct view or an indirect view with a mouth mirror of the site being treated while maintaining correct body mechanics (Figure 26-31).

Procedure 26-5 Self-Evaluation of Operator Basic Body Mechanics Technique

PROBLEM	SOLUTION
Fatigue or stiffness in joints Reduced range of motion in back, neck, or shoulders Pain in the back, neck, shoulders, forearms, wrist, hand Numbness in legs, arms, hands Muscle cramping Loss of strength	Procedure 26-1 Body mechanics 6 components of posture (see below) Self-evaluation questions/criteria Seek medical consultation (See Chapter 11)

SELF-EVALUATION QUESTIONS	EVALUATION CRITERIA
Am I in a balanced and comfortable working position?	6 components of posture: base of support, the pelvis, the lumbar spine, the trunk, the shoulders, the head and neck Feet flat on floor; hips level on stool; tailbone up; trunk, head, and neck within a protective range of 20 degrees of freedom; relaxed shoulders are down and back and stomach pulled in to support the lumbar spine
Am I sitting with a wide base of support?	Placement of the feet: flat on the floor, shoulder-width apart, in front of the hips, knees slightly lower than the hips
Am I maintaining a neutral sitting?	Wide base of support, level pelvis, tailbone up without hinging forward or backward at the hip
Are my back and spine in a neutral position?	Neutral spine position: slight forward curve in the neck, a slight backward curve in the upper back, and a slight forward curve in the lower back
Are my shoulders relaxed?	Shoulders are down and back, not slumped forward, arms not too far in front, or raised greater than 20 degrees from a level plane.
Is my head fairly straight?	Protective range of cervical flexion is 20 degrees with ears generally over shoulder joints.
Am I in a neutral standing position?	Wide stance, trunk vertically aligned without rotation or flexing laterally. Neck not flexed more than 20 degrees. Arms at side and not abducted away from body or extended too far forward
Can I reduce the amount of stress on any musculoskeletal areas?	Prolonged static sitting positioning contributes to fatigue and increased intradiscal pressure in the spine. However, movement should stay within the protective, three-dimensional range of 20 degrees of freedom.

Body Mechanics

Protective Scaling

The term *protective scaling* (established by M. Tsutsui) denotes operator and client positioning, fulcrums, and reinforcements that seek to minimize practitioner injury (see the discussion of Repetitive Strain Injuries in Chapter 11).

According to current literature by J. Dylla and J. Forrest, it is important to understand the basics of body mechanics because dental hygiene procedures require movement and positioning that can challenge physical health. Overloads on muscles, ligaments, and joints by excessive flexation such as twisting, bending, or tilting eventually can cause pain. Protective strategies of adopting a stable and neutral posture and adapting the client and equipment to the procedure enables biomechanical sound practicalities to minimize the risk of injury[2] (Procedure 26-6 and the corresponding Competency Form).

Basic body mechanics concepts to be discussed are the following:

- Neutral positions
- Base of support
- Structural stability
- Degree of freedom

Neutral positions[3] are those in which the body is relaxed and comfortable with normal musculoskeletal alignments. Sound positioning begins with a neutral spine position, which is described as a slight forward curve of the neck, a slight backward curve of the upper back, and a slight forward curve of the lower back. The term *neutral positions* can be vague and should be based upon known biomechanical information. It generally is recognized, however, by the lack of abnormal bending, twisting or tilting of muscles, ligaments, joints, disks, nerves, and bone. Operators should not bend their head from the neck area (cervical flexion) and preferably use capital flexion by unitizing the forward movement of head and neck.

The **base of support**[3] is to create the fundamental structure to support the spine by providing a wide base of support. This support is achieved by the positioning of the feet to be flat on the floor, shoulder width apart, in front of the hips with the knees pointing out and slightly lower than the hips.

Structural stability[3] is the concept of stable positions and movements of the complete body that provide the foundation for maximum function and minimal injury through correct posture. The six components of posture to promote structural stability are the following:

- Base of support
- Pelvis
- Lumbar spine
- Trunk
- Shoulders
- Head and neck

Procedure 26-6 Strategies for Protective Scaling

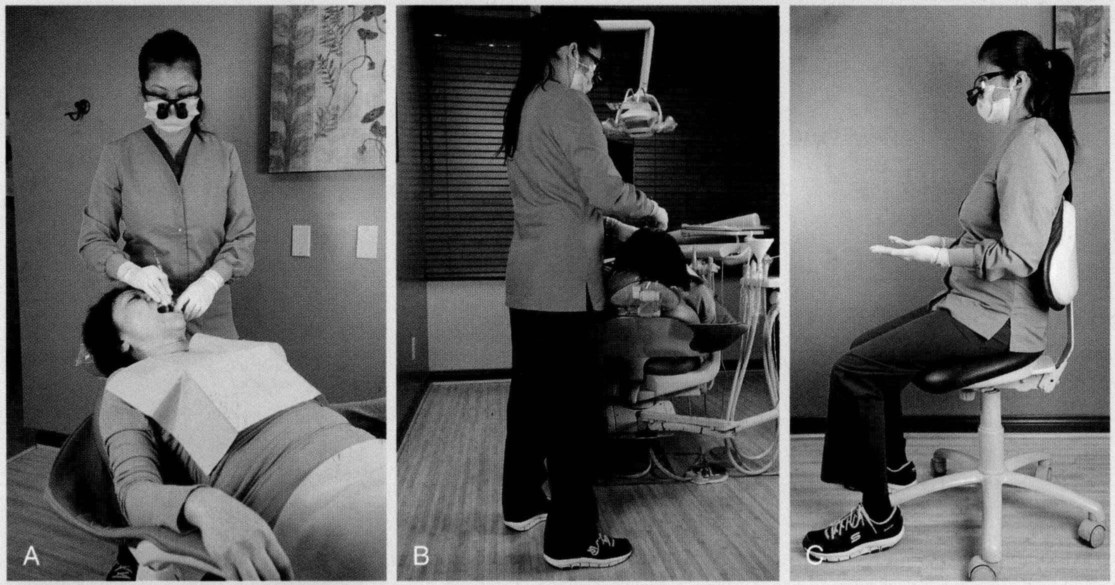

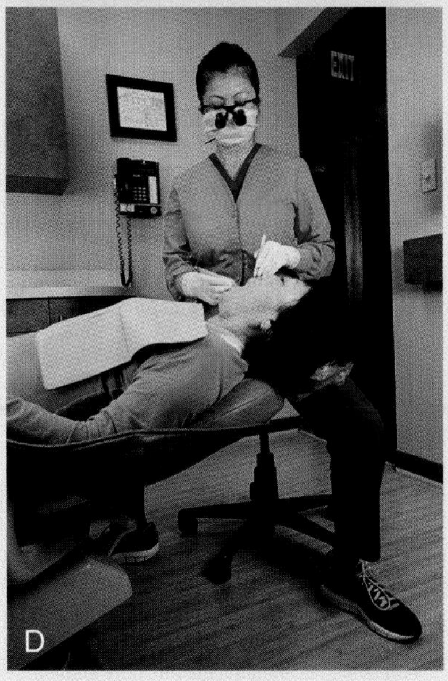

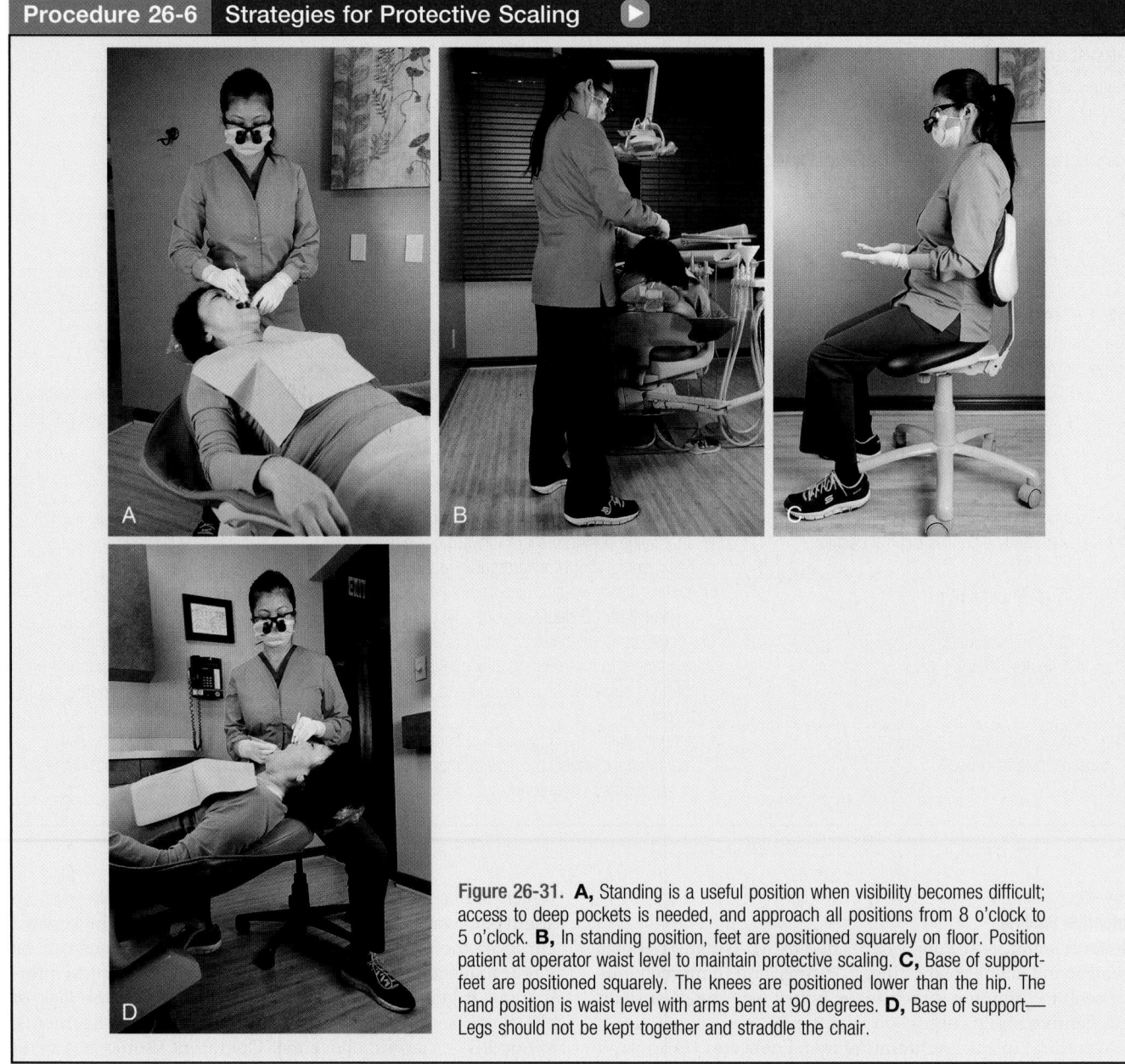

Figure 26-31. **A,** Standing is a useful position when visibility becomes difficult; access to deep pockets is needed, and approach all positions from 8 o'clock to 5 o'clock. **B,** In standing position, feet are positioned squarely on floor. Position patient at operator waist level to maintain protective scaling. **C,** Base of support-feet are positioned squarely. The knees are positioned lower than the hip. The hand position is waist level with arms bent at 90 degrees. **D,** Base of support—Legs should not be kept together and straddle the chair.

Proper posture for structural stability are establishing feet flat on floor, hips level on stool, tailbone up with the trunk, head and neck within a 20-degree range, relaxed shoulders that are down and back, and stomach pulled in to support the lumbar spine. The knees should be slightly less than hips in height and elbows within 20 degrees of the body. Prolonged static sitting can be associated with fatigue as well as injury resulting from increased intradiscal pressure in the spine[1] (Figure 26-31, *C* and *D*).

Degree of freedom[3] means the three-dimensional range of movement by an operator to remain in a protective position. The body has 20 degrees of freedom to help safeguard against injuries.

Gloves and Hand Mechanics

Procedural gloves significantly influence hand mechanics. The glove material and the fit can elevate risk for strain and cumulative injury by compressing joints out of neutral positions.[4] Natural latex had been the glove of choice because of the elastic and adaptive nature of the material. Elastic nitrile, however, has been gaining acceptance as the preferred option. Nitrile has benefits over latex when discussing the increasing attention to repetitive strain injuries and operator protection (see Box 26-1).

Ambidextrous gloves, flat with thumbs in an unnatural position, were designed originally for exams or short procedures. Right/left gloves are designed for more intricate procedures and decrease strain on the thumb and palm,[5] but they are more costly. The common practice of dental hygienists using ambidextrous gloves necessitates that clinicians pay particular attention to the looser fit across the palm to decrease the pull on the thumb. Although manufacturers offer a wide variety of sizes, there is no standardization of the physical dimensions that constitute size labeling. If a glove is too tight in fingers, across the palms or around the wrists, flexibility and movements are restricted. This constraint results in limiting scaling techniques, fatigue, and cumulative injury. A glove that is too large can feel awkward, unwieldy, and uncomfortable and interfere with the safety and efficiency of the procedure.[5] Important value must be placed on the material, style, and size of an operator's procedural gloves because it can affect an operator's safety, clinical efficiency, and effective hand instrumentation.[6]

BOX 26-1

Comparison of Latex to Nitrile Gloves

LATEX	NITRILE
Natural rubber material	Synthetic rubber material
Highly elastic	Less elastic
High compression forces	Lower compression forces
Adapts well to hand	More relaxed fit
High friction rate, but elasticity eases placement and removal	Less elastic, but low friction rate aids placement and removal
Higher hand fatigue	Decreased hand fatigue
Higher restrictions on hand and finger movements	Decreased pressure on blood vessels and nerves in hand and wrist
Commonly powdered	Commonly powder free
More tear-resistant, but more compromised protection with pinhole punctures going undetected	More puncture resistant and splits when punctured giving more awareness of any compromise of protection
Protein in latex can cause allergies	Higher chemical protection
Economical	

Grasp

Table 11-5 in Chapter 11 categorizes grasp by instrument selection.

The basic grasps used in hand-activated instrumentation are listed below:

- Pen grasp
- Modified pen grasp
- Extended modified pen grasp
- Palm-thumb grasp

Pen Grasp

The **pen grasp** (Figure 26-32, *A*) is used when the exacting or directive type of pressure in scaling and root planing is not required. The thumb and index finger pads are well situated on the instrument handle, but the middle finger slips down, and the instrument rests on the side of the finger near the first knuckle. The pen grasp may be used when light, easy probing or exploring into nonperiodontally involved areas is performed. Much heavier pressure also may be used with this grasp on the mouth mirror for retraction of the buccal mucosa, tongue, or other soft tissues.

Modified Pen Grasp

The **modified pen grasp** (Figure 26-32, *B*) is the standard grasp used for dental hygiene instrumentation. When

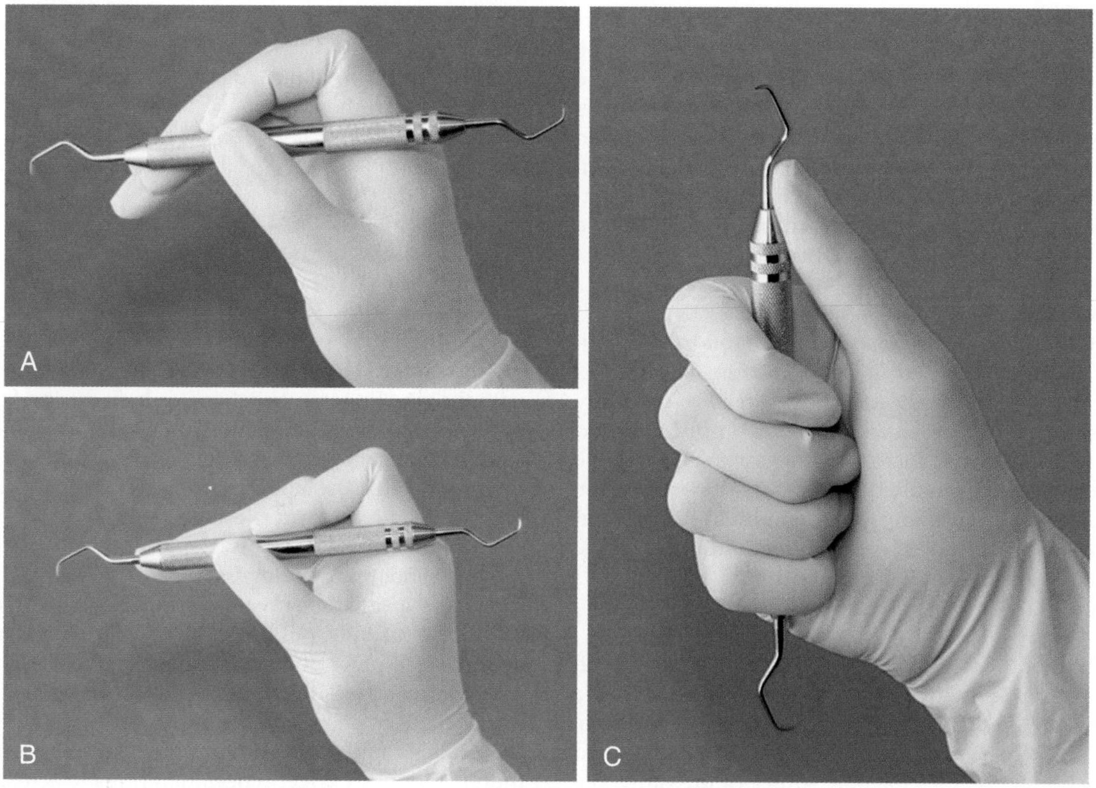

Figure 26-32. A, Pen grasp. **B,** Modified pen grasp. **C,** Palm-thumb grasp.

correctly applied, it is a sensitive, stable, and strong grasp because of the tripod effect produced by the position of the thumb, index finger, and middle finger. The thumb pad must be placed on the instrument handle and the joint bent slightly, depending on the area being scaled. The index finger pad should be on the instrument at a point slightly higher on the handle than the thumb, and the first joint should be slightly bent downward with the second joint cocked upward. The side of the middle finger near the nailbed should be placed opposing the thumb and further down the instrument on the shank toward the working end. The instrument handle should be positioned between the first and second knuckle of the index finger and not in the web of the hand. Rolling of the instrument with proper fingers for adaptation enables grasp consistency.

Once instrumentation is initiated, the modified pen grasp must be reestablished continually on the instrument handle to accommodate the minute rolling of the instrument into and around depressions of tooth structure. Otherwise the instrument can roll and slip out of the grasp, or the thumb and fingers can end up in an undesirable position on the instrument handle, which may not allow for optimal pressure to be placed against the instrument for adequate assessment or instrumentation.

The thumb, index, and middle fingers also are flexed to allow the instrument to be manipulated in various directions around the tooth surface and to allow equal pressure to be applied against root structure during the course of the stroke. Historically, dental hygienists were taught to avoid digital movement during instrumentation, but it now appears that such digital movement, when combined with the movement of the wrist, facilitates accurate, even scaling and root planing strokes in deep periodontal pockets during nonsurgical periodontal therapy. Moreover, the most protective situation for the dental hygienist when scaling in deep pockets occurs when finger movement and wrist (or arm) movement can be used, minimizing stress to one particular area such as the hand or wrist. The degree to which digital movement is required for successful instrumentation varies according to the fulcrum used, the area being scaled, the instrument used, and the periodontal pocket depth. In certain areas, a combination of digital movement and hand/arm movement with a neutral wrist position is used.

Extended Modified Pen Grasp

The **extended modified pen grasp** is considered to be a subcategory of the modified pen grasp. Although the grasp is essentially the same, the middle finger may be slightly straighter and not on the shank. Extraoral, opposite, and cross-arch fulcrums have increased the awareness of the value of an extended modified pen grasp. Extending the grasp further away from the working end on an instrument handle allows improved angulation, adaptation, and leverage in the approach for scaling deeper periodontal pockets.

Palm-Thumb Grasp

The **palm-thumb grasp** (Figure 26-32, *C*) is achieved with all four fingers wrapped tightly around the handle and the thumb placed on the shank in a direction pointing toward the instrument tip. This grasp is awkward and uncontrolled because the thumb provides the only source of pressure. The opposing fingers clumsily wrap around the handle and do not provide a means of turning the instrument or modifying the thumb effect. The palm-thumb grasp provides little in the way of tactile sensitivity during scaling procedures and is not recommended for supragingival or subgingival periodontal instrumentation. Because the palm-thumb grasp is a very stable grasp that does not allow the instrument to move on its own, it is ideal for use during instrument sharpening.

Fulcrum

Applying lateral pressure against the tooth surface with the tip and the anterior third of a sharp blade or pointed instrument necessitates a stable fulcrum. The **fulcrum** is the source of stability or leverage on which the finger rests and against which it pushes to hold the instrument with control during stroke activation. All fulcrums should be on firm tooth or osseous structures for stability and application of force transfer to working strokes. When there is no fulcrum, the instrument uncontrollably slips off the tooth surface when even a slight amount of lateral pressure is exerted. Fulcrums traditionally have been finger rests as intraoral fulcrums rely on digital focal points for stability and leverage. With the choice of alternate application of extraoral fulcrums, the rest is usually a hand or palm rest against a firm facial surface.

The fulcrum plays a major role in directing instrument use, despite the shank angle. Although straighter-shanked instruments are used in anterior areas and the more curved-shanked instruments are used in posterior areas, this does not always have to be the case. For example, clinicians who use a variety of intraoral and extraoral fulcrums to gain working-end access to deep periodontal areas find that shank angle does not limit instrument usefulness. Fulcrum versatility allows greater flexibility in instrument use in nontraditional areas. Therefore, in some cases, straighter-shanked instruments may be used for posterior teeth scaling and considerably more curved instruments may be used in anterior areas.

There are two main fulcrum categories used in hand-activated instrumentation:

- Intraoral
- Extraoral

Intraoral Fulcrum

Established inside the mouth against a tooth surface, the **intraoral fulcrum** is used for scaling in shallow pockets. The ring finger pad usually is positioned on the occlusal, incisal, lingual, or facial surface of a tooth close to the one being instrumented. The middle finger should remain in contact with the ring finger even when it is bent during finger flexing or when making digital movements. If the middle finger splits away from the ring finger, stroke control and strength diminish. With the added support of the middle finger, a built-up stable fulcrum is established (Figure 26-33, *A*).

Intraoral rests are most stable and powerful when the fulcrum and middle fingers stay close together and wrist motion is used to activate the stroke. The middle finger fulcrum is usually not as effective as a ring finger fulcrum because as a pivot point, it shortens the arc of movement on activation and results in a shallow stroke that cannot be extended very deep subgingivally. This pivotal stroke closes the blade angulation and promotes finger flexing by the thumb and index finger when attempting to activate a vertical stroke. The diminished ability to maintain proper angulation,

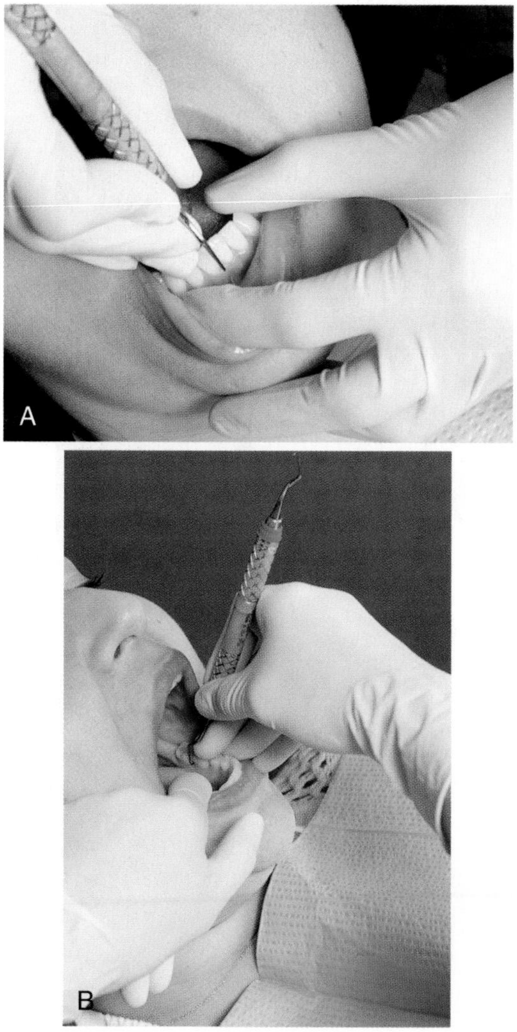

Figure 26-33. A, Same arch fulcrum positioned near area being scaled. **B,** Middle finger fulcrum rest on the lower left occlusals and the ring finger rest on the buccal surface. Operator position is at 9 o'clock. The Gracey curet 13/14 is being used. The upper shank is positioned against the side of the finger nail bed. The thumb is used for distal lateral pressure. Pivot using the middle finger for leverage and power.

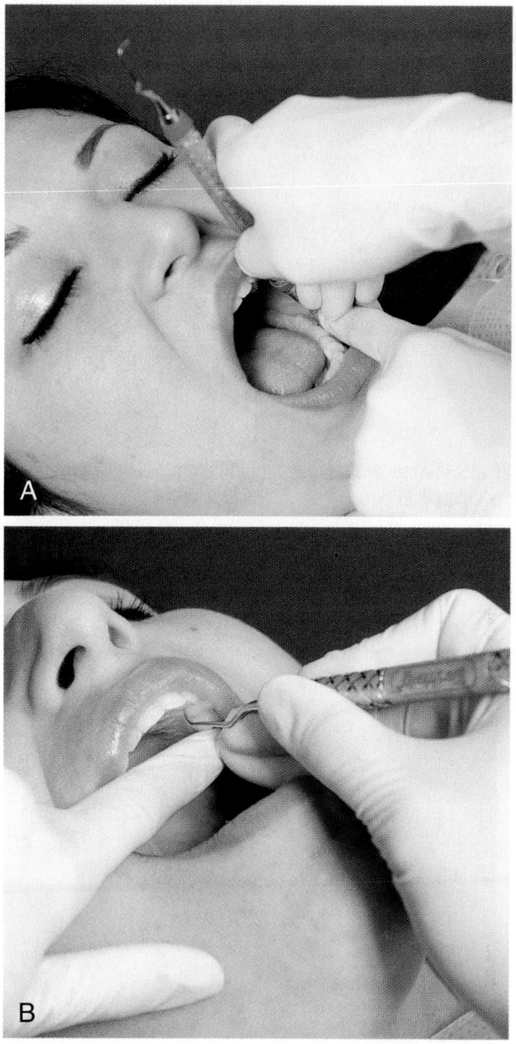

Figure 26-34. A, At 8 o'clock clinician position, nondominant index finger is placed in the vestibule to aid in accessing the distals and buccals with dominant hand using intraoral, same arch fulcrum. **B,** Left index finger is placed across the maxillary arch and the dominant hand fulcrums on the index to aid in accessing lingual approach.

control, and power can result in burnishing calculus and operator fatigue.[10] One exception to this general principle, however, can still produce an effective fulcrum. When working on the distal/linguals of lower left posteriors with a Gracey 13/14, if the ring finger is placed on the buccal of the posterior teeth and the middle finger is placed as an occlusal pivoting point, this allows the principle of keeping the fulcrum and middle fingers together and a wrist motion can be used to create a stable and powerful stroke (Figure 26-33, *B*).

Depending on the area to be scaled, the angle of access, and the pocket depth, intraoral fulcrums may be positioned on the following:

- The operator's own finger (finger-on-finger) (e.g., fulcrum on index or thumb), located within the oral cavity (Figure 26-34, *A* and *B*)
- A tooth surface on the same arch near the area being scaled (same arch fulcrum) (see Figure 26-34, *A*)
- A tooth surface on the same arch but across from the area being scaled (i.e., on the opposite quadrant or cross-arch), creating a cross-arch fulcrum (Figure 26-35)
- A tooth surface on the opposing arch from the arch being scaled (opposite arch fulcrum) (Figure 26-36)

Extraoral Fulcrum

Established outside of the mouth, the **extraoral fulcrum** is used predominantly when instrumenting teeth with deep periodontal pockets. The extraoral fulcrum is placed against the client's jaw, or on a broad surface such as the side of the face (Figure 26-37, *A* and *B*). The extraoral fulcrum does not use a small finger point source, as does the intraoral fulcrum. Rather, the extraoral fulcrum is established by placing the broad side of the palm or back of the hand against the chin or outer cheek. The extraoral fulcrum does not use light pressure against the skin of the client's face. Rather, the palm or

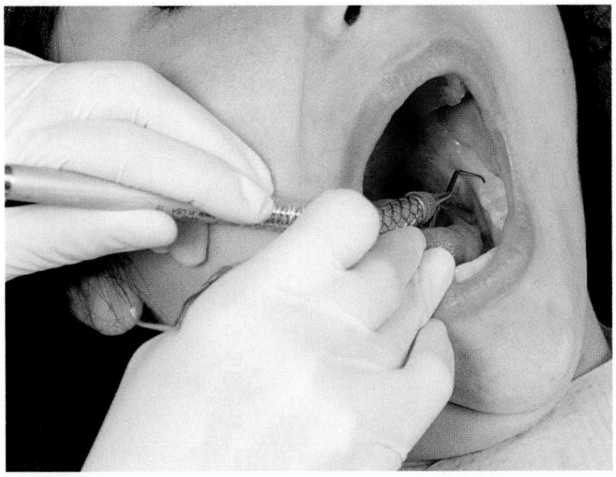

Figure 26-35. Same arch cross-arch fulcrum. Distal of the last molar. Operator position is at 8 to 9 o'clock. Position of the working hand is intraoral fulcrum, palm down, on the occlusal/incisal of the opposite side of the arch being scaled. The Gracey curet 7/8 is being used.

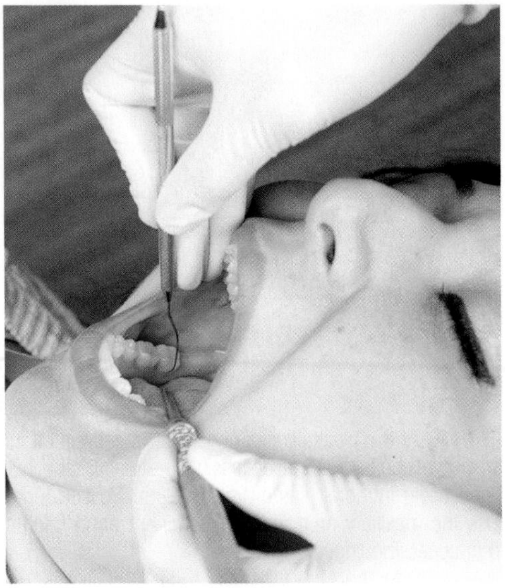

Figure 26-36. Intraoral—opposite arch fulcrum. Operator position is at 1 o'clock. Position of the working hand is intraoral fulcrum, palm down, on the incisal of the opposite arch of area being scaled and reaching down. The Explorer 11/12 is being used.

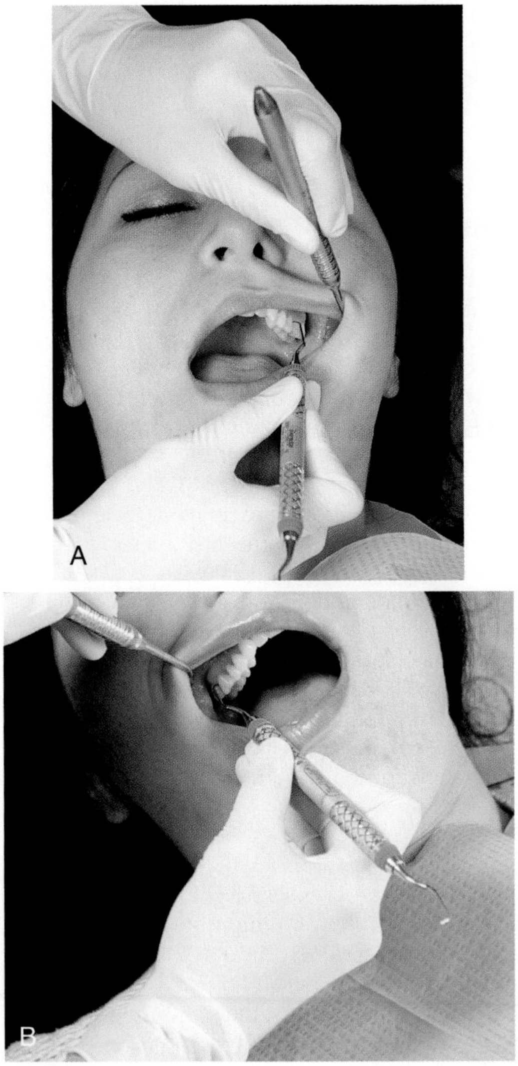

Figure 26-37. A, Extraoral, opposite arch, palm down/cupping the chin fulcrum. The front surfaces of the fingers rest on the left lateral aspect of the mandible while the maxillary left posterior teeth are instrumented. Operator position is at 9 o'clock. The Gracey curet 11/12 is being used. **B,** Extraoral, palm up, opposite arch fulcrum. The backs of the fingers rest on the right lateral aspect of the mandible while the maxillary right posterior teeth are instrumented. Operator position is at 9 o'clock. Position of the working hand is extraoral fulcrum, palm up, extending the instrument to the opposite arch. The Gracey curet 7/8 is being used.

backside of the hand rests with moderate pressure against the bony structures of the face and/or mandible. This extraoral fulcrum may be a palm-up, palm-down, or chin-cup position. The extraoral fulcrum provides an excellent means of control and stability for access into periodontally involved areas that may be cumbersome or physiologically strenuous for the dental hygienist to instrument using intraoral fulcrums. The extraoral fulcrum allows a direct "line of draw" in which the instrument may be pulled straight down, as opposed to rocking with the wrist in areas such as the maxillary posterior regions.

Criticism of extraoral techniques stems from fear of loss of fulcrum stability when fulcruming farther from the working area, when grasping the instrument farther from the working end, and/or when stabilizing the instrument against a slightly mobile surface such as the skin rather than on a solid tooth. In reality, fulcruming away from the immediate working area does not necessarily diminish the stability of the fulcrum.[4] Rather, when instrumenting a tooth surface in a deep periodontal pocket, the clinician may increase and extend the leverage and lateral pressure throughout the length of a long working stroke (scaling or root planing stroke). The control loss from extending the grasp away from the instrument's working end can be overcome easily by using reinforcement from the nonworking index finger or thumb to the shank or handle close to the instrument's working end. Finally, the extraoral fulcrum allows the operator to change the action of pulling the stroke from the wrist to the lower arm, upper arm, and shoulder. It also helps keep a consistent blade adaptation to the tooth surface from the base of the pocket up to the contact when scaling using the pull stroke. Using instrumentation techniques such as these may protect the operator from future injury and stress to the nerves, tendons, and ligaments of the wrist and elbow. (See the section on reinforcement scaling later in this chapter.)

Lateral Pressure

Lateral pressure is the pressure of the anterior third of the working end of the instrument against the tooth. This pressure may range from very light to firm, depending on the nature of the tooth surface roughness. Therefore it is necessary to use gradations of pressure during exploratory, scaling, and root planing strokes. The grasp, fulcrum, and basic control of the instrument is important for lateral pressure as well as the proper clinician and client positioning and practiced coordination of these elements. This is why the beginning student may experience difficulty in physically applying firm lateral pressure. Basic principles with applying lateral pressure include the use of the thumb and middle finger during instrumentation (Figure 26-38, *A* and *B*).

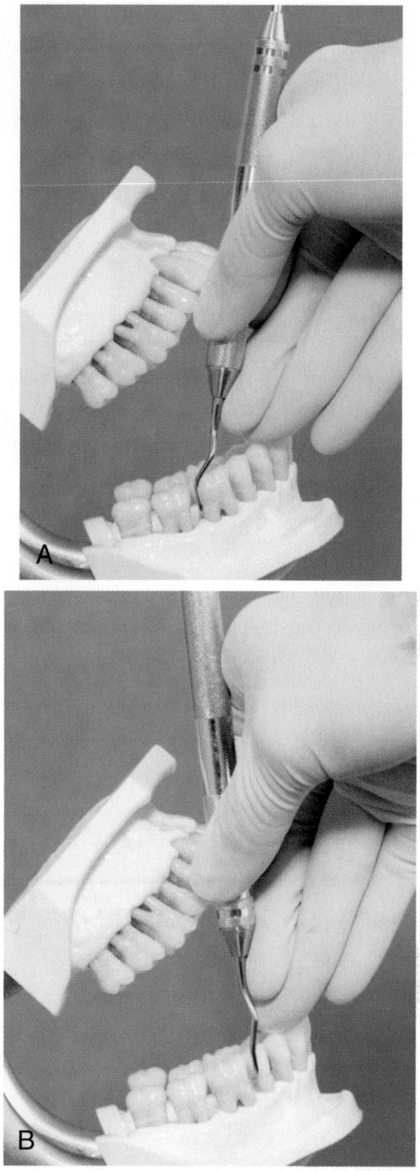

Figure 26-38. **A,** Lateral pressure for No. 30 distal—The thumb is placed against the distal for increase pressure. **B,** Lateral pressure for No. 30 mesial—The middle finger is placed against the mesial for increase pressure.

The degree of lateral pressure affects the tactile sensitivity. Exploratory strokes for detection with assessment instruments benefit with light to moderate pressure. Treatment instruments vary depending on the procedure. Biofilm debridement may require only light pressure, whereas root planing may warrant light to moderate pressure. The removal of calculus deposits can demand light, moderate, and heavy lateral pressure.

Reinforcement Scaling

Reinforcement scaling is used to gain additional instrument stability and control when scaling with the intraoral and extraoral fulcrums. In most cases, reinforcement scaling means that the nondominant hand is used for additional support of the instrument instead of holding the mouth mirror.

The nondominant hand supports the instrument of the working hand, providing additional lateral pressure during instrumentation procedures. The added support from reinforcement may come from the nondominant hand's index finger, thumb, or thenar region (radial palm or fleshy mass on lateral side of palm, thenar muscle; see Chapter 11). The dominant hand must continue to play the major role in adapting and angulating the blade against the tooth surface. It also must exert control over the direction in which the instrument is pulled over the tooth.

Reinforcements are used only with treatment instruments such as curets. They are not necessary with assessment instruments because control and lateral pressure are not difficult with these instruments. Reinforcements provide additional support and lateral pressure in deep periodontal pockets, particularly with extended fulcrums (cross-arch, opposite arch, and extraoral) placed away from the immediate area being scaled. Several reinforcements increase stabilization, which adds control accuracy and pressure enhancing scaling technique discussed later in this chapter. In addition, the reinforcement techniques are protective to the practitioner because it redistributes forces among other components of the musculoskeletal system reducing RSIs.

The benefits of reinforcement are as follows:

- Provides additional lateral pressure in the same direction in which the dominant hand's fingers are directing pressure
- Guides the instrument in a longer pull stroke when an extended extraoral fulcrum is used
- Supports the thenar region of the dominant hand, which provides protective qualities during often strenuous and intensive instrumentation processes

The beneficial aspects of reinforcement scaling are found only when the operator uses intraoral and extraoral fulcrum techniques. The names of the reinforcements tell the operator where the reinforcements originate. The placement of the index finger and thumb may be on or around the instrument between the working end and the dominant hand. The reinforcing thumb also may be positioned against the dominant thumb or thenar region for support and operator comfort. Examples of reinforcement scaling in selected mouth areas are shown in Figures 26-39 and 26-40.

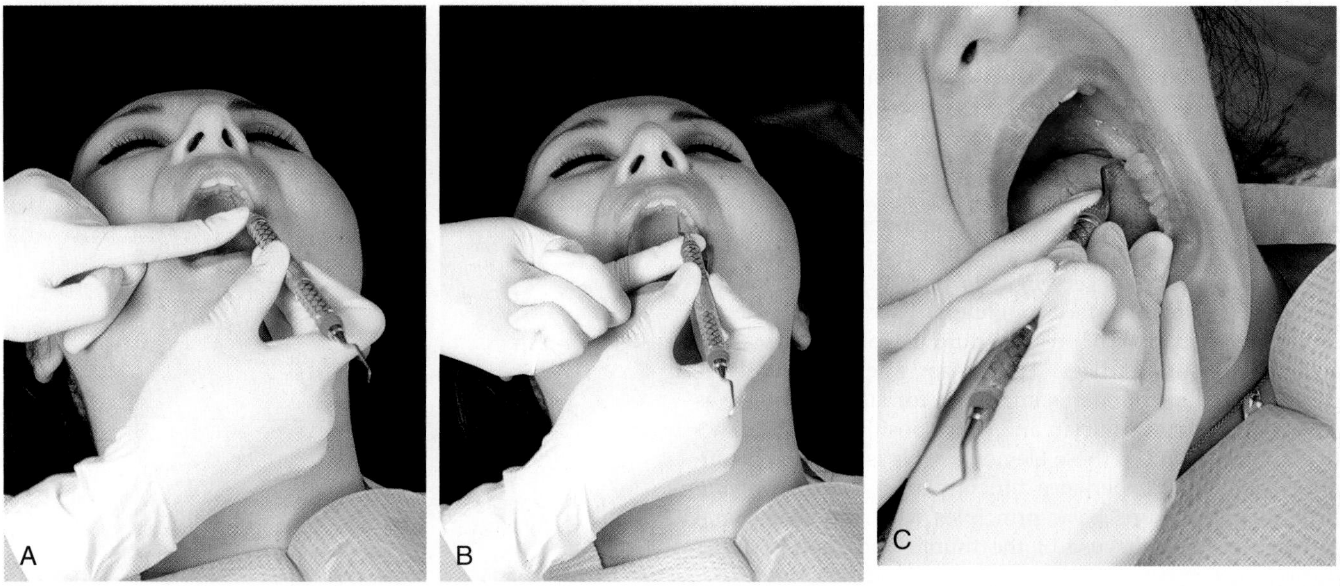

Figure 26-39. **A,** Index finger reinforcement. Left maxillary mesial surface from the lingual approach. Operator is at 9 o'clock. The Gracey curet 7/8 is being used. Position of the working hand is extraoral fulcrum, palm down. The position of the reinforcement hand shows the index finger on the instrument applying pressure in the same direction of lateral pressure in which the dominant hand is working. **B,** Index finger reinforcement. Left maxillary distal surface from the lingual approach. Operator is at 9 o'clock. The Gracey curet 7/8 is being used. The position of the working hand is extraoral fulcrum, palm down. The position of the reinforcement hand shows the index finger on the instrument applying pressure in the same direction of lateral pressure in which the dominant hand is working. **C,** Index finger reinforcement. Mandibular left posterior distal line angle from lingual approach. Operator is at 8 o'clock to 9 o'clock position. The Gracey curet 7/8 is being used. The working hand is positioned cross arch of the area being scaled. The index finger of the reinforcement hand is positioned on the instrument.

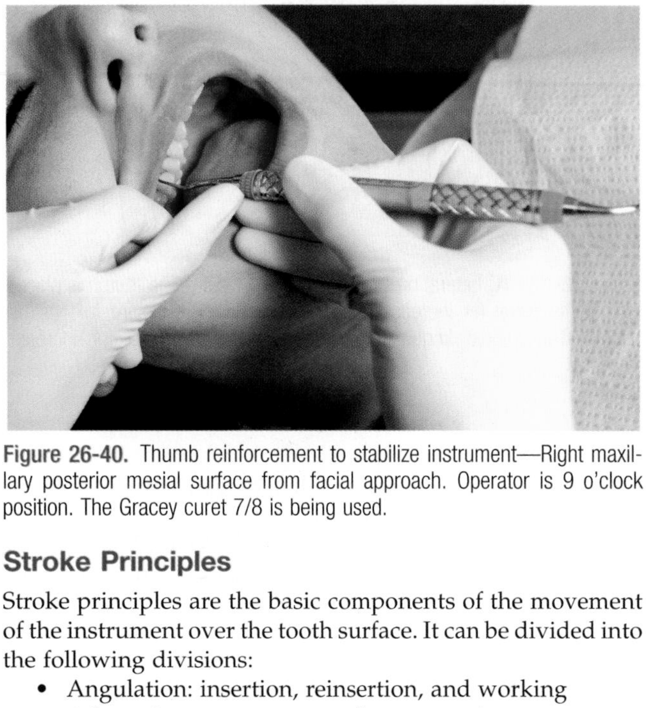

Figure 26-40. Thumb reinforcement to stabilize instrument—Right maxillary posterior mesial surface from facial approach. Operator is 9 o'clock position. The Gracey curet 7/8 is being used.

Stroke Principles

Stroke principles are the basic components of the movement of the instrument over the tooth surface. It can be divided into the following divisions:

- Angulation: insertion, reinsertion, and working
- Adaptation: assessment and treatment instruments
- Activation: exploratory and scaling/root planing

Angulation

Insertion

Insertion is the act of placing an assessment or treatment instrument into subgingival areas. The purpose of insertion may be to measure the sulcus or pocket depth, classify furcation involvement, explore the subgingival areas, or scale and/or root plane subgingival areas. Whatever the purpose is, the procedure must be nontraumatic and accurate. As with all sharp-pointed instruments, extreme care must be taken when the point is inserted directly toward the junctional epithelium. Too much pressure and lack of proper grasp, fulcrum, and contact points with the instrument as it glides subgingivally may cause perforation through the attachment apparatus.

Straight instruments such as the periodontal probe are manipulated easily as long as the side of the tip and the rest of the working end stay in contact with the root when the tip is inserted. A delicate touch using fairly light pressure is required when probing or initially exploring subgingivally. With such exploratory strokes, the junctional epithelium offers a moderate amount of resistance, feels slightly elastic to the touch, and gives with a slight amount of pressure from the instrument. Pressure on the instrument may be increased after the pocket topography is understood, to interpret cemental irregularities, calculus, and restorative margins. When a curved explorer is inserted, the tip should be pointed apically and the side of the tip should be in contact with the tooth surface being explored. Care must be taken to avoid tissue distention with the rounded bend and to avoid directing the point right at the root surface. Inaccurate deposit assessment and possible root surface scratching result if the pointed tip is directed into the root surface. The only time this is done intentionally is when the dental hygienist suspects root caries or furcation involvement and at times to detect burnished subgingival calculus.

Careful insertion of a bladed treatment instrument into subgingival areas involves closing the angle of the cutting edge of the blade relative to the tooth surface to avoid tissue trauma with the opposite side of the blade and to reach the base of the pocket on the downstroke of insertion. With the curet the closed blade angulation is from 0 to 10 degrees. With sickle scalers (sharp-pointed back and triangular design) the angulation of insertion is slightly more than 10 degrees but much less than the more open "working" angulation (defined as the angle of the cutting edge of the blade against the tooth that produces a grip or bite to the tooth surface).

Reinsertion is the act of returning the instrument down into the subgingival areas after an assessment or working stroke has been accomplished. The reinsertion stroke angulation is slightly closed compared with that of a working stroke. The instrument working end should remain in contact with the tooth until instrumentation is complete.

A common error with the reinsertion stroke is lifting the instrument from the tooth surface during the act of reinsertion. The dental hygienist should use the same guidelines of following tooth structure down on reinsertion as in the initial insertion to avoid tissue trauma and to reposition accurately the blade for continuous, overlapping strokes. To ensure reinsertion to base of pocket, the clinician should release the pressure of the working stroke.

Working

Angulation of a bladed instrument refers to the relationship of the cutting edge to the tooth surface (Figure 26-41). Specifically, this is the measurement from the face of the blade to the tooth surface being scaled.

- Angulation between 60 and 80 degrees is ideal for removing calculus and planing roots. This standard allows a range in which to modify the angulation.
- The closer the angulation is to 45 degrees, the more the instrument slides over the tooth surface.
- The closer the angulation is to 90 degrees, the more the instrument bites the tooth surface.
- A more closed angulation (45 to 60 degrees) is recommended when a smoothing, shaving, multidirectional root planing stroke is desired.
- A more open angulation (near 70 to 80 degrees) is recommended when there is heavy deposit to remove and it is necessary to grab the root surface effectively.

It often is necessary to modulate blade angulation. An example of such a situation is when there is heavy calculus only at the base of a 6-mm pocket with smooth cementum directly above. Angulation of the blade is more closed and the pressure applied is heavier at the base of the pocket to remove the calculus. The angulation is more open and the pressure applied is lighter toward the mouth of the pocket for root planing. The procedure is followed by several more strokes at less than 90 degrees for root planing from the junctional epithelium to the cementoenamel junction (CEJ). The likely result of improper instrument angulation is residual calculus.

Adaptation

Assessment Instruments

With regard to pointed assessment instruments, **instrument adaptation** refers to the alignment or placement of the side of the first few millimeters of the periodontal probe or straight explorer against the tooth. Adaptation is important with

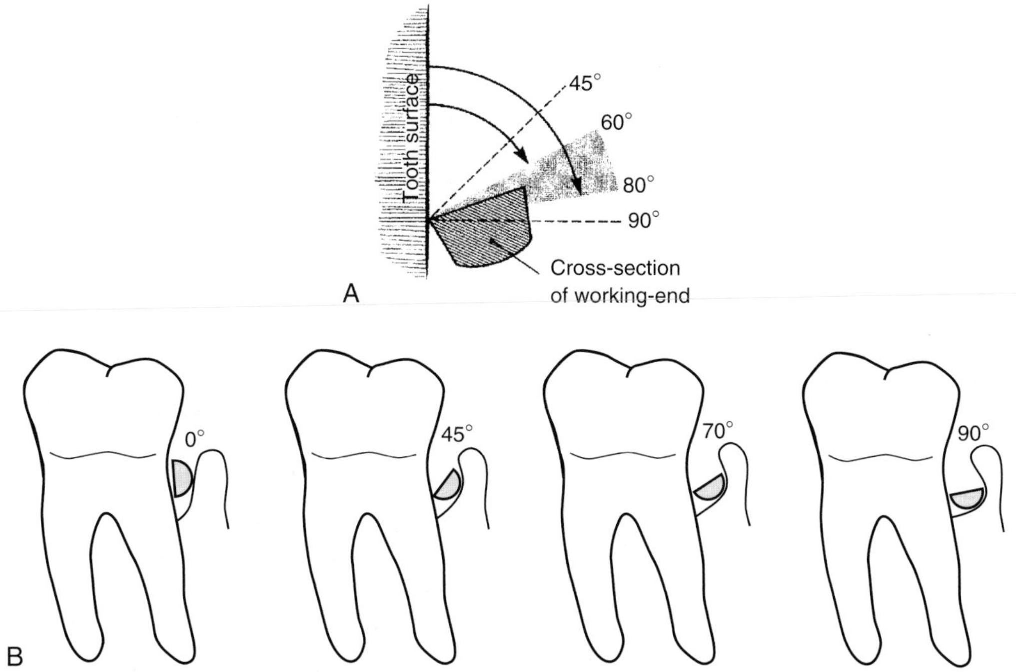

Figure 26-41. A, The correct working angulation of the blade to the tooth should be between 45 and 90 degrees; 60 to 80 degrees is ideal for debridement. **B,** Insertion angle of close to 0 degrees is ideal for insertion of working end into the pocket; a 45-degree cutting edge to tooth angulation is too closed to remove calculus, and burnishing is likely to occur; a 70-degree cutting edge to tooth angulation is ideal for debridement; a 90-degree cutting edge to tooth angulation is too open, with potential for damaging adjacent tissues. (Adapted from Daniel SJ, Harfst SA, Wilder RS: *Mosby's dental hygiene*, ed 2, St Louis, 2008, Mosby.)

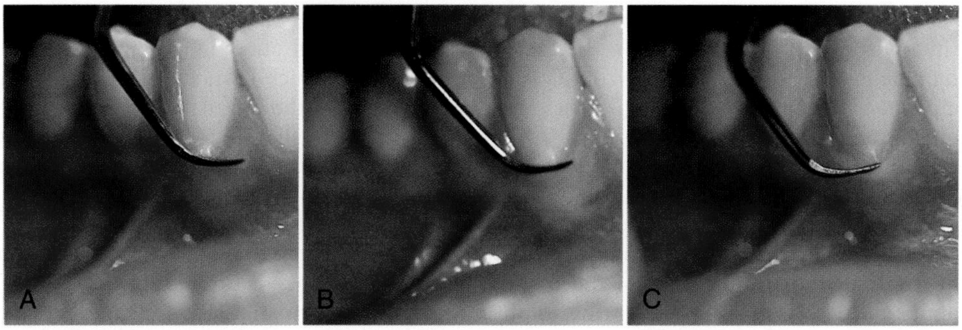

Figure 26-42. Comparison of various adaptations of bladed instrument. **A,** Upper third of blade. **B,** Middle third of blade. **C,** Lower third of blade.

assessment instruments because it provides the clinician with an accurate measurement or with information about the smoothness of the tooth surface. If the instrument is not well aligned against the tooth surface, it will be off the tooth and into soft tissue. This lack of alignment leads to client discomfort as well as to misinterpretations regarding probing depths and the presence of calculus deposits or cemental irregularities.

The periodontal probe and the explorer are always thin, pointed instruments by design to reach deep, sometimes tight subgingival pockets and to facilitate tactile sensitivity. Because they have to reach under tight tooth contacts to detect calculus and root irregularities, explorers have fine, delicate working ends. However, the side of the tip always should be in contact with the tooth structure to avoid tissue trauma when the clinician assesses the presence of cemental irregularities and acquired deposits. The remainder of the explorer's working end should be as closely adapted to the subgingival tooth surface as possible to avoid excessive distention of tissues, excessive pressure against the instrument from the pocket wall, and the possible use of the point instead of the side of the instrument tip. There is only one working end on the straight periodontal probe and explorer. Although the correct working end is automatically determined, proper adaptation to the tooth surface must be maintained.

With a bent explorer such as the double-ended pigtail explorer, there is a correct and incorrect working end for different tooth surfaces. The first 2 to 3 mm of the side of the toe (or side of the tip of the instrument) must adapt to an area between the base of the pocket and the contact of the next tooth. The rest of the working end should not distend excessively the sulcular tissues.

Treatment Instruments

With regard to treatment instruments used for scaling and root planing, **instrument adaptation** is the close relationship of the working blade to the tooth surface. When the working blade is well adapted to the tooth surface, it instruments more root surface than does a poorly adapted blade and causes less damage to root surfaces and/or soft tissues. If only the toe or tip is in contact with the tooth, the tooth surface may become gouged or overinstrumented. If the middle or upper third of the blade is in contact with tooth surface and the lower third is off the tooth, the toe is in an open position and may cause tissue trauma to sulcular epithelium (Figure 26-42, *A* and *B*). The adaptation position most effective and causing the least amount of hard- or soft-tissue damage occurs when the lower third of the working blade remains in contact with the tooth surface during scaling and root planing procedures (Figure 26-42, *C*).

For treatment instruments that have sharp, pointed tips, such as sickle scalers, the dental hygienist uses adaptation guidelines similar to those presented for assessment instruments. Proper adaptation with the side of the tip to avoid tissue trauma is as important with the sickle scaler as it is with the periodontal probe and the explorer.

If the sickle scaler has a bent shank and is double ended, one bladed side is preferable for each tooth surface. The correct end produces the closest blade adaptation to the tooth surface and maintains a shank position parallel to the plane of the tooth surface being scaled. The angulation (relationship of the cutting edge to the tooth surface) should be greater than 45 and less than 90 degrees to the tooth surface (see Figure 26-41).

Adaptation of the curet follows many of the same principles previously discussed. In general, the lower third of the blade is the most desirable portion of the curet blade to contact the tooth surface. However, when broad, flat areas of tooth surface are scaled, the middle third of the blade can be used in addition to the lower third. The principle to adapt the lower third of the blade is critical because most instrumentation difficulties lie in conforming instruments to the varying convexities and concavities found on root surfaces (see Chapter 28). Especially when instrumenting periodontitis-affected teeth, proper adaptation of the curet blade is a continuing process because of root morphology. Instrumentation is further complicated when there is close root proximity on multiple-rooted teeth or from adjacent teeth and furcation involvement. Tooth alignment also complicates procedures. In situations such as these, the most successful adaptation is use of the lower third of the blade. Alternative methods are by scaling with smaller working ends such as a diamond-coated file, or a Micro Mini blade curet (Hu-Friedy Manufacturing).

Activation

Exploratory Stroke

The **exploratory stroke** is used for detection and usually is performed with an explorer or periodontal probe. The curet also may perform an exploratory function to assess the tooth surface during actual scaling or root planing. An exploratory stroke may use light to firm lateral pressure, as follows:

- Light lateral pressure is recommended for detecting light spicules of subgingival calculus (heavier lateral pressure is insensitive for fine-deposit exploration).
- Moderate to firm lateral pressure is recommended for the detection of flat, burnished calculus or distinguishing restorative margins from tooth anatomy.

Scaling Stroke

The **scaling stroke** is used for removing calculus from supragingival and subgingival areas. The curet is the instrument of choice for definitive scaling and root planing. As in the exploratory stroke, the lateral pressure used with the scaling stroke ranges from light to firm. The difference, however, is that the magnitude of what is considered firm is far greater during scaling than during exploring. During scaling, the instrument action may change quickly from a scaling stroke to an exploratory stroke. This change in lateral pressure is done specifically to break off calculus but not to overinstrument a clean area above or below that calculus. It is performed also to assess areas previously scaled without having to stop and pick up an explorer. It is efficient to be able to work in this manner and to reserve the use of an explorer for after major areas have been scaled.

The practitioner uses assessment data on pocket depth, clinical attachment, tissue color, tissue consistency, tissue surface texture, tissue size, bleeding, and bone loss to determine the degree of periodontal involvement and the probable amount of lateral pressure needed for calculus detection and scaling. Generally, the more periodontally involved the client's teeth, the more suspicious the dental hygienist should be of local contributing factors such as subgingival calculus harboring oral biofilm. If the calculus occurs in the form of ledges, any amount of pressure is likely to detect it. If, however, the calculus formation is flat and smooth, medium or even firm exploratory strokes may be necessary to detect the deposit.

Calculus density may be determined by radiographs and most accurately by "hardness" felt with the explorer. Dense calculus appears more radiopaque than lighter, easier-to-remove calculus. Dense calculus feels hard, like tooth structure, as opposed to the porous feel of lighter calculus. In situations in which there is dense calculus and naturally grainy or rough root surfaces, the calculus is likely to be embedded in the root surface. Calculus deposits that are dense and tenacious make scaling more difficult than with light calculus deposits.

The older and more dense the calculus, usually the more tenacious it is. The practitioner increases the lateral pressure of the scaling stroke as the tenacity and density of the calculus increase. Too little lateral pressure on instrumentation may cause burnishing of tenacious calculus on cementum. To avoid indiscriminately applying too much lateral pressure on instrumentation, causing unnecessary gouging and overinstrumentation of root surfaces, the dental hygienist should evaluate the changes occurring on the root surface during instrumentation with the curet using exploratory strokes or by using a dental explorer. Lighter lateral pressure during scaling strokes is indicated for light and easy-to-remove calculus.

Root Planing Stroke

The **root planing stroke** is used for shaving embedded calculus from cemental surfaces and smoothing roots. The rationale for root planing lies in the fact that clean, smooth roots are more biologically acceptable for connective tissue reattachment than are rough roots, accounting for a reduction of periodontopathic bacteria. In addition, the client's ability to maintain soft-tissue health is improved because oral biofilm control is easier when the roots are smooth.

Successful root planing requires extremely good control; dedication to smoothing subgingival surfaces evenly from the junctional epithelium to the CEJ; knowledge of root morphology; and a sense of the dimensions of this subgingival space and the area the curet has covered. The root planing stroke is a longer stroke than the scaling stroke and may begin with firm lateral pressure if there is significant root roughness to smooth. The change to lighter lateral pressure should occur rather quickly as the curet moves to even out the cementum surface.

The cementum thickness varies, but it is thinnest at the cervical third of the tooth (0.02 to 0.05 mm). In scaling and root planing tooth structure with such a thin covering of cementum, it is easy to visualize how cementum removal often occurs during indiscriminate root planing, leading to dentin exposure and dentinal hypersensitivity (see Chapter 39). To avoid client hypersensitivity, the dental hygienist explores the area carefully and uses lateral pressure discriminately during scaling and root planing with the purpose of removing only subgingival calculus and altered cementum, smoothing the root surface, and removing as little healthy cementum as possible to achieve good results. (See the discussion of clinical and therapeutic endpoints in Chapter 30.)

Stroke Direction

Subgingival assessments are aided by direction and pressure of the strokes. For accurate identification and removal of deposits, a combination of three basic stroke directions is used with assessment and treatment instruments, as follows:

- Vertical stroke direction is parallel to the long axis of the tooth.
- Horizontal stroke direction is perpendicular to the long axis of the tooth.
- Oblique stroke direction is diagonal across the long axis of the tooth.

Using combinations of stroke directions is referred to as a **"basketweave"** of strokes (see Figure 26-15, *A*). Varying stroke direction allows a greater possibility that an area of burnished or smooth calculus may be detected because the instrument may catch one side of the calculus when all other sides may be smooth. The explorer and the probe are activated beginning with a gentle insertion or downward stroke into the pocket.

This exploratory stroke is used as part of the detection process as long as the side of the tip is well adapted to the tooth surface.

Besides the direction of the strokes in relation to the tooth axis, the forces also can be defined by the direction of working pressure in relation to drawing toward or away from the operator. These strokes are as follows:

- Pull
- Push

The typical working stroke of the curet, sickle, file, and hoe is performed with a pull stroke. The pull stroke direction may be vertical, horizontal, or oblique, and it is not directed toward the junctional epithelium. Usually the push or insertion stroke with working pressure is not recommended with treatment instruments. This stroke causes unnecessary client discomfort and could violate the integrity of the client's intact junctional epithelium by forcing dental calculus and oral biofilm through the membrane, potentially causing a periodontal abscess. A push stroke with most treatment instruments can promote burnishing calculus because of the blade adaptation. Some treatment instruments, however, are designed effectively for the push stroke.

Once an efficient stroke direction has been established, it is best to keep moving forward in the direction of the toe of the instrument. Short, overlapping strokes for calculus removal and longer, overlapping strokes for root planing maximize root coverage. Channel scaling is the continuous, systematic, overlapping strokes for complete calculus removal.

Stroke Length

Stroke length is limited by tissue tone, tooth morphology, and periodontal probing depth measurements. Loose and inflamed tissue accommodates the movement of long, sweeping, overlapping strokes. However, if the tissue is healthy or fibrotic in tone and positioned tightly against the tooth, short, overlapping, well-adapted strokes are indicated to prevent tissue trauma.

Short, overlapping strokes and a firmly planted fulcrum provide for good operator-controlled strokes. When managing the curvatures common to most root surfaces, shorter strokes do not pass over deposits in root depressions as easily as longer strokes and therefore are more reliable. On relatively flat areas, however, clinicians may use long stroke lengths and still maintain a controlled, effective movement.

Deep periodontal pockets allow for greater flexibility in stroke length than shallow pockets because of greater root surface area from clinical attachment. Recession may be accompanied by significant root surface. Therefore, with greater pocket depth or more exposed root surface area, it is easier to vary stroke length than where pocket depth is very shallow with little recession.

To remove calculus, the scaling stroke is a short pull stroke. The short stroke is best for calculus removal because the increased pressure needed reduces stroke control. A short stroke facilitates a controlled stroke. For root planing, the stroke length should be increased and the pressure lightened once the calculus has been removed.

Field of Vision

A clear **field of vision**, keeping the treatment area visible and accessible, is an important basic concept for the clinician. The benefits of good visibility and accessibility are increased safety of the procedure, increased effectiveness, and decreased eye and body strain.

Achieving a clear vision field requires having a visible treatment area clear from oral tissues, fluids, and debris. Examples of oral tissues that can compromise visibility include the tongue, cheek, and lips. Compromising fluids can be water, saliva, blood, or solutions; compromising debris can be calculus, food, granulation tissues, or even biofilm.[11] The treatment area should remain accessible and unencumbered during the procedure. Having a clear field of vision enhances therapy comfort by decreasing possible tissue trauma and improving the client and operator's experience.

Maintaining a clear field of vision can be achieved through various methods as follows:

- Mirror retraction of oral tissues
- Evacuation of fluids by saliva ejector, surgical evacuator tips, or isolation evacuator devices
- Water syringe use to rinse treatment area
- Air syringe use to dry and eliminate moisture from treatment site
- Mouth props to maintain an open field
- Gauze used adjacent to working site to dry and wick away fluids
- Gauze "packed" into retractable pocket areas for hemostasis and direct root surface vision

Loupes and lights have become common with clinicians for enhanced views of the treatment areas. With use of loupe magnification, the visualized area is called the field of view. Higher magnifications decrease the field of view. Magnification and coaxial illumination (headlights) that focus on the targeted treatment sites have helped decrease eyestrain and improper body mechanics. Reduced overhead light adjustments also have reduced arm/shoulder strains. Other forms of lights such as the fiberoptic handpieces in ultrasonics and even mouth mirrors have augmented improved fields of view.

Treatment Instrument Selection

Curet Selection

Because the curets are critically important instruments in scaling and root planing, the dental hygienist must select the best instruments made from many different manufacturers. As discussed earlier, curets are made in several varieties of metals, each with specific strengths and weaknesses. In addition, the shank strength and blade thickness when new are also instrument selection factors to consider. The most important factor, however, in determining successful subgingival instrumentation is the blade size.[7] Instrument selection decisions are based on experience using different scaling and root planing instruments, the quantity and quality of calculus, the severity of periodontal involvement, gingival retractability, root morphology complexities, and overall accessibility. These factors are important when choosing the width and thickness of a blade (Procedure 26-7 and the corresponding Competency Form). Variations require customization of basic instrumentation technique to treat a particular individual successfully. Customizing instrumentation in periodontitis-affected areas allows the clinician to reach almost any area of the mouth, to reach both sulcus areas and deep periodontal pockets, and to manage difficult root anatomy with the control and strength needed for effective care (Procedure 26-8 and the corresponding Competency Form).

Instrument Blade Selection

After the appropriate instrument has been selected, the hygienist determines the correct instrument working end to use for the tooth surface to be scaled. For some instruments, such as the periodontal probe and the No. 3-A EXD explorer, the working end is universal (i.e., used on all tooth surfaces). For other instruments, such as the straight-shanked sickle scaler, the working end works well on all mesial and distal surfaces, but mainly on the anterior teeth. The majority of

Procedure 26-7 Hand-Activated Scaling Instrument Sequence Guide

SEQUENCE STEPS	PROCESS	REFERENCE
1. Initial grasp	Hold instrument with a modified pen grasp.	Procedure 26-1 Figure 26-32, *B*
2. Operator position	Apply proper body mechanics. Establish effective position around patient for area to be scaled.	Procedure 26-6 Chapter 11, Table 11-7, Figure 11-8
3. Client position	Adjust client height and reclining angle for area to be scaled. Head of client should be at waist-height of operator.	Figure 26-31, *A* and *D*
4. Field of vision	Assess the visibility and accessibility of the treatment site. Establish the lighting and limit obstructions for area.	
5. Initial fulcrum	Find general fulcrum site for intraoral (same quadrant, cross-arch, opposite arch) or extraoral.	Figures 26-33 to 26-37
6. Adaptation*	Insert and adapt tip and lower ⅓ of blade (2-3 mm) to base of pocket.	Figures 26-42, and 26-38
7. Angulation*	Feeling for a bite of the blade against the tooth surface, angulate blade between 60 and 80 degrees for scaling and root planing.	Figure 26-41
8. Adjusted fulcrum*	Assess if the fine-tuning of instrument placement requires minor fulcrum placement adjustment or a need to reestablish the fulcrum to cross-arch, extraoral, etc.	Figures 26-33 to 26-37
9. Adjusted grasp*	Adjust the grasp on handle as incremental changes while adapting, angulating the blade and fulcrum adjustments may require modifications. Increase the grasp pressure and confirm finger positioning for maximum lateral pressure.	Figure 26-32, *B*, and 26-38
10. Adjusted operator/ client positions*	Assess if the small modifications of instrument placement requires operator and/or client positioning adjustments that allow hand, arm, and shoulder to move as one unit upon stroke movements. Body positions (generally 8 to 4 o'clock) are based upon area being scaled and fulcrum being used.	Chapter 11
11. Reinforcement scaling	Apply reinforcements by the nondominant hand as needed.	Figures 26-39 and 26-40
12. Activation*	Initiate working stroke as the final step of the sequence.	Figure 26-15

*Adapted with reference to analytic approaches to root debridement.

treatment instruments, however, are site specific, with a definite side of the blade that should be used against a particular tooth surface.

Criteria Considerations

The criteria in determining the appropriate instrument's design and blade size are as follows (see Procedure 26-6):

- Treatment objective
- Type of calculus
- Tissue assessment
- Tooth surface
- Technique preference
- Task challenges

Treatment Objective

The treatment objective begins to narrow the instrument selection. Primary decision making for the desired outcome includes identifying if a natural tooth, a restored tooth, or an osseointegrated implant is to be scaled. Time constraints and appointment therapy endpoints of removing gross deposits or root planing assist in this decision making.

Type of Calculus

Assess the type of calculus with quantity and quality of the deposits. Quantity includes descriptions such as light, moderate, heavy, grainy, rough, spicules, sheets, ledges, and rings. Quality includes descriptions such as porous, dense, tenacious, and burnished.

In the presence of heavy, tenacious subgingival calculus, one type of treatment instrument option is the rigid curet. Within this category of treatment instrument there is a range in variation among manufacturers of the same instrument (e.g., differences in blade size, length, shape, and metallurgy).

Tissues Assessment

Evaluating the gingival tissues include assessing the consistency, size, and texture for level of retractability for instrument insertion. In addition, periodontal health assessment is important for instrument selection to evaluate considerations such as the pocket depths, amount of attached gingiva and mucogingival involvement.

Tooth Surface

Tooth surface is an important consideration in instrument selection. Instrument selection can vary from those designed for use on multiple tooth surfaces, such as universals, to those that are area-specific curets. This category includes location within the oral cavity (anterior, posterior, maxillary or mandibular), the specific site on the tooth (mesial, distal, buccal, facial, lingual, palatal, and all line angle areas), tooth

Procedure 26-8 Treatment Instrument Selection

FACTOR	ASSESSMENT CONSIDERATIONS
Treatment objective	Natural tooth, restored tooth, osseointegrated implant Time constraints Target therapy endpoint Client profile: child, adult, special needs, geriatric
Type of calculus	Quantity: light, moderate, heavy, grainy, rough, spicules, sheets, ledges, rings Quality: porous, dense, tenacious, burnished
Tissue assessment	Consistency, size, texture, retractability Pocket depth, inflammation, attached gingiva, mucogingival involvement
Tooth surface	Area: supragingival, subgingival Arch: maxillary, mandible Location: anterior, posterior Site: single, multiple, mesial, distal, buccal, facial, lingual, palatal, line angle Morphology: furcations, depressions, prominent CEJs
Technique preference	Fulcrum: intraoral, extraoral, opposite arch, same arch, cross arch Operator trait: finger hyperflexibility Familiarity: positions, instruments, experience
Task challenges	Severity of periodontal disease Tooth alignments Missing teeth Root proximity Client limited jaw opening Overactive lip/tongue

CEJ, Cementoenamel junction.

morphology (furcations, depressions, and prominent cement-enamel junctions), and location of deposits to be removed (supra- or subgingival accumulations).

Technique Preferences

Operator comfort and personal preference relative to which instrument and fulcrum works best with a given instrumentation technique, instrument familiarity, and operator traits also are factors influencing instrument selection. For example, a clinician who prefers to use extraoral fulcrums to scale heavy calculus in deep periodontal pockets will do so and choose familiar instruments to accomplish the treatment objective. If the client has no significant periodontal disease, then the operator may choose to use universal curets to accomplish the scaling with more efficiency in terms of time management rather than select area-specific curets, which require different instruments for different tooth areas. Other factors that may define instrument selection may be if the operator has finger hypermobility or hyperflexibility conditions, or if the operator prefers instruments made with materials that reduce or eliminate the need for sharpening.

Task Challenges

Task challenges that influence instrument selection include the following:

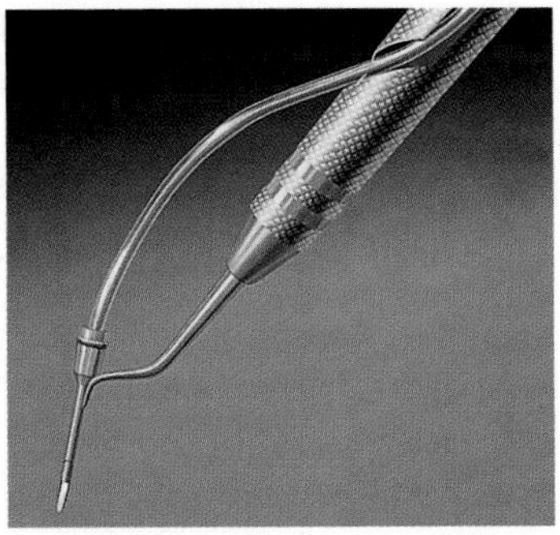

Figure 26-43. The endoscope explorer with sheath and fiberoptic bundle in the "thistle" adapter. (Courtesy DentalView, Irvine, California.)

- Periodontal disease severity
- Tooth alignments
- Root proximity
- Client's limited ability to open the mouth
- Overactive lip and tongue

Customizing Instrumentation for Periodontitis-Affected Teeth

Customizing instrumentation successfully depends on finding the correct fulcrum. The dental hygienist should use an analytic approach in accomplishing this (see Procedure 26-7).

If the tooth surface shape changes to the degree that one fulcrum position no longer works, the fulcrum must be altered to accommodate the change. With experience, adjustments are made within seconds.

It is important to allow for variations in probing depths or alterations in root anatomy, which affect the amount and direction of lateral pressure that can be applied to the root surface. For instance, as probing depth increases on the distal aspect of a mandibular molar from 3 mm to 10 mm, the dental hygienist may find a change in the root surface plane from a vertical to a slightly more oblique or horizontal inclination. Such slight changes in the tooth surface plane alter stroke effectiveness. By readjusting the fulcrum as the instrument maneuvers into deeper pocket depths, the practitioner is able to produce effective lateral pressure.

The more periodontally involved the tooth, the more the dental hygienist needs to fulcrum away from the working site.

Dental Perioscopy

Although costly, **dental perioscopy**, fiberoptic imaging of the periodontal pocket, allows subgingival visualization for diagnosis as well as treatment. Using dental perioscopy, the clinician magnifies, visualizes, and accesses deep subgingival calculus, root fractures, and the periodontal pocket's internal wall. Magnification is from 24× to as high as 46×, depending on the distance between the object and the lens.

The system is composed of a disposable sterile sheath that houses a fiberoptic endoscope, provides continuous irrigation, and has a metal soft-tissue shield that keeps the soft tissue away from the tube (Figure 26-43). The actual size of the handheld sheath and instrument with proper hand grasp is shown in Figure 26-44. The system includes a flat-panel liquid crystal display (LCD) color monitor and a small footprint transport system (Figure 26-45). A composite video-out

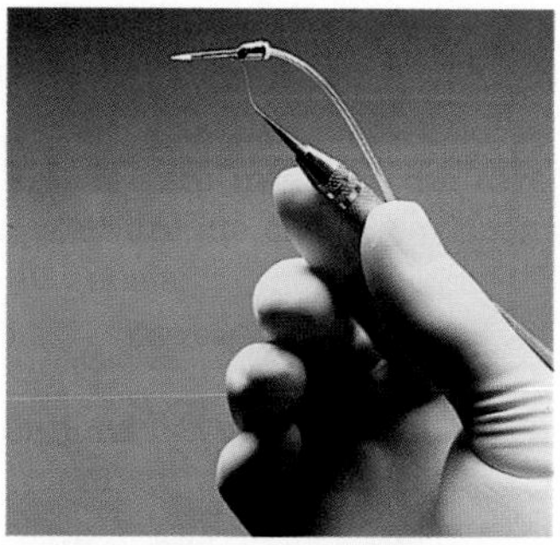

Figure 26-44. Proper grasp for the endoscope explorer. (Courtesy DentalView, Irvine, California.)

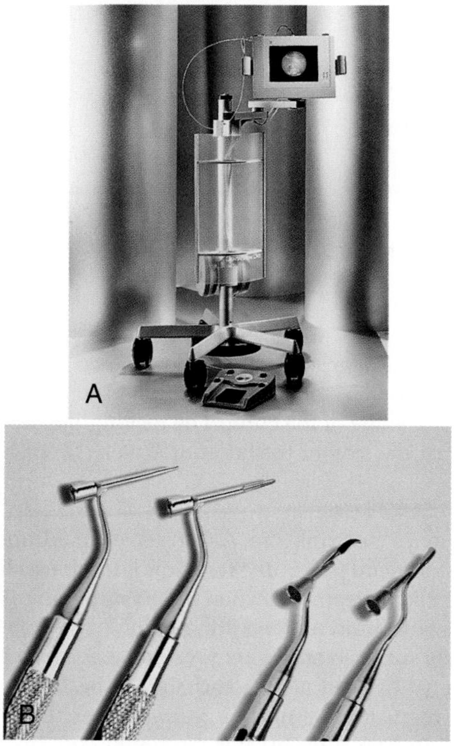

Figure 26-45. **A,** The DentalView 2 endoscope with an image of the subgingival sulcus on the monitor screen. **B,** Viewing periodontal explorers for the perioscopy system. (**A,** Courtesy DentalView, Irvine, California. **B,** From Newman MG, Takei HH, Klokkevold PR, et al: *Carranza's clinical periodontology,* ed 11, St Louis, 2012, Saunders.)

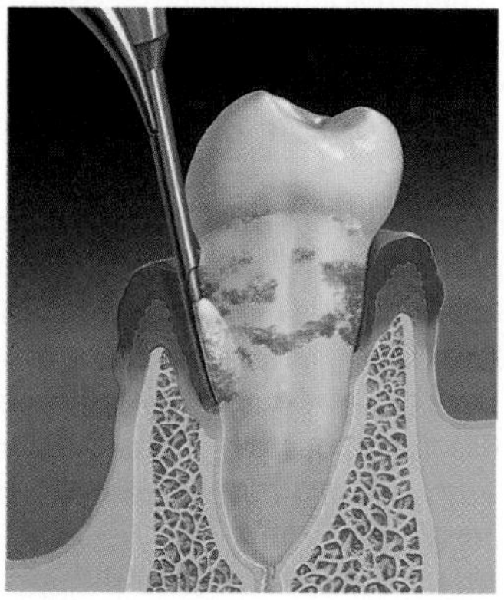

Figure 26-46. Diagrammatic illustration of the endoscope's explorer examining the subgingival root surface and calculus deposits. (Courtesy DentalView, Irvine, California.)

source connection allows users to employ a digital system to record and later view endoscopic images if desired.

Under endoscopic magnification, black calculus ledges are actually white, porous, and crystalline in appearance, and subgingival calculus sheets may occur in colors from golden brown to black. Dental perioscopy has shown the direct relationship of tissue inflammation and the presence of subgingival calculus deposits. Direct visualization has shown the degree of inflammation of tissues is greater in areas of calculus deposits covered with biofilm than areas of biofilm alone.[9]

This system of visualization during root surface instrumentation improves clinical assessment of results over traditional tactile assessment methods. Clinicians experienced with the system indicate an extraordinary ability to visualize and instrument deep, narrow pockets, depressions, line angles, and furcations. The process also is educational, because clients see the intricacies of their disease and treatment on the monitor and judge the effectiveness of oral self-care procedures. Figure 26-46 illustrates a cross-sectional view of the endoscope in place subgingivally.

Periodontal instrumentation with visualization is significantly more accurate and specific than instrumentation without visualization. In addition to traditional treatment instruments, nontraditional periodontal instruments such as diamond-coated instruments (see Figure 26-29) are being used with success when the clinician is able to view areas of burnished calculus. Even with visualization, successful instrumentation is still dependent on the clinician's ability to use a variety of fulcrums, stroke directions, and periodontal instruments.

Instrument Sharpening

(See the discussion of instrument factors in Chapter 11.)

The objective of instrument sharpening is to restore blade sharpness while preserving the original contours and angles of the instrument. The basic clinical outcome of using sharp versus dull instruments is delineated in Table 26-13. Sharp instruments improve client comfort and decrease operator fatigue by working to remove dental deposits effectively and are easier to control than dull instruments because they do not slip as readily over tooth surfaces.

To maintain effectiveness and client care quality, at the first sign of instrument dullness, the dental hygienist should sharpen the instrument. If the instrument is made with a material that requires no sharpening and it becomes dull, the instrument is discarded. The clinician should consider instruments made with materials that require less sharpening

TABLE 26-13

Quality of Clinical Outcomes with Instrument Sharpening

Increases	Decreases
Calculus removal	Burnishing calculus
Tactile sensitivity	Instrument slippage
Client comfort	Operator fatigue
Client safety	Possible tissue trauma
Instrument control	Lateral pressure
Appointment efficiency	Working time

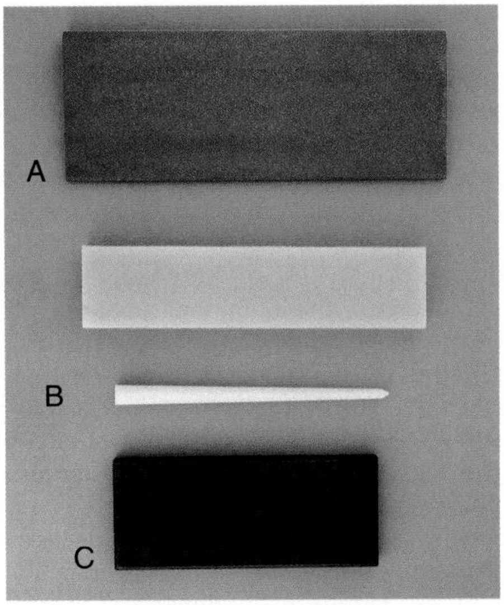

Figure 26-47. Sharpening stones. **A,** India stone. **B,** Arkansas stone (flat and cone shaped). **C,** Ceramic stone. (From Boyd LRB: *Dental instruments: a pocket guide*, ed 4, St Louis, 2012, Saunders.)

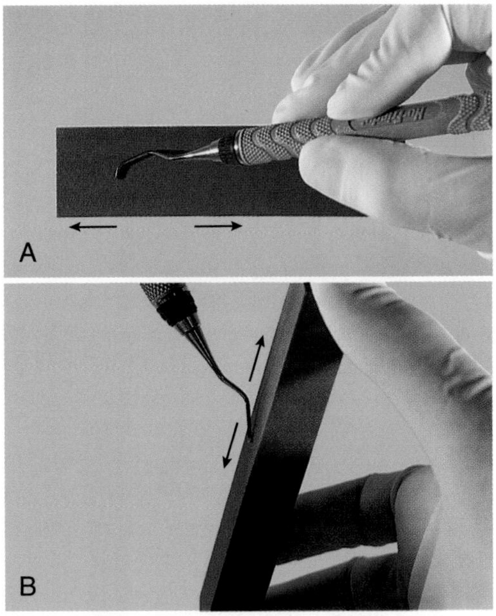

Figure 26-48. **A,** Sharpening by moving the instrument over the sharpening stone. **B,** Sharpening by moving sharpening stone over instrument.

(EverEdge technology) to no sharpening (XP Technology). Traditional sharpening methods for individual instruments are discussed under each instrument subheading. Instruments also can be sharpened with mechanical honing devices such as the Sidekick (Hu-Friedy Manufacturing) or the InstRenew Sharpening Assistant (Nordent Manufacturing). See Chapter 11, Figures 11-10 and 11-11.

Sharpening Stones

Natural and synthetic sharpening stones for sharpening dental instruments are composed of abrasive crystals that are harder than the metal of the instrument (Figure 26-47).

Natural Stones

The **Arkansas stone**, a natural stone with a fine texture, is manufactured in a variety of shapes for sharpening instruments. Conical and cylindric Arkansas stones are used for sharpening the face of curets, a practice that tends to weaken the blade. The **India stone**, also a natural stone, comes in a medium texture that removes metal easily, and therefore sharpening with an India stone should be followed by use of an Arkansas stone to provide a polished edge. Natural stones such as the Arkansas and India usually are lubricated with clear, fine oil to facilitate the movement across the stone, reduce friction, and reduce the problem of metallic particles embedding into the stone surface. Stones should be washed and/or ultrasonically cleaned to remove sludge or the excess oil and mix of metal shavings. The stone is then placed in the instrument cassette for sterilization. Steam, chemical vapor, or dry heat may be used to sterilize these stones.

Synthetic Stones (Composition and Ceramic Stones)

The **composition stone** is a mounted rotary stone, and the **ceramic stone** is manufactured as a handheld rectangular stone. Both stones are of fine to medium coarseness and are lubricated with water rather than oil and thus metal filings rather than a sludge layer must be cleaned from the stone surface. The rotary stone may be adapted to the face as well as the cutting edge of the curet. The rectangular stone is used only against the side of the curet or scaler.

Sharpening Stone Selection

- Fine stones such as the Arkansas or medium-textured India stones are preferable for the novice or for sharpening during client treatment when little sharpening is required for reestablishment of a cutting edge.
- Coarsely surfaced stones remove metal at a faster rate than do finely surfaced stones and should be used on instruments requiring significant recontouring. Less pressure, fewer strokes, and greater accuracy are needed with coarsely textured stones.
- Rotary-mounted stones (e.g., composition stone) are considerably more abrasive than coarse handheld stones because the stone is mounted on a metal mandrel and used in a motor-driven handpiece. The mounted rotary stone should be used only when major instrument recontouring is required. Lack of good control, friction, and rapid wearing of the instrument are disadvantages of the rotary-mounted stone.

Manual Sharpening Technique

To begin instrument sharpening, select the proper sterilized, lubricated stone for the amount of sharpening to be done. Techniques for using handheld sharpening stones consist of either of the following (Figure 26-48, *A* and *B*):

- Moving the instrument over the stone (recommended for sharpening flat surfaces such as the hoe or sickle scaler)
- Moving the stone over the instrument (recommended for sharpening curets)

With either method, movement is initiated by the operator's dominant hand.

To guard against accidental clinician injury when moving the stone against the sharpening instrument, care must be

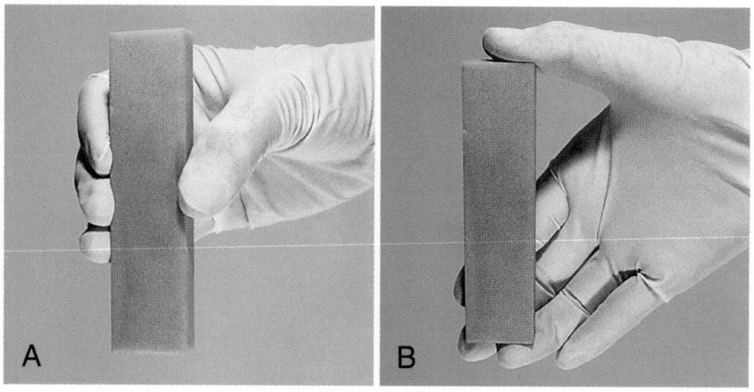

Figure 26-49. **A,** Incorrect finger position on stone; fingertips are exposed to possible injury if stone slips. **B,** Correct finger position on stone.

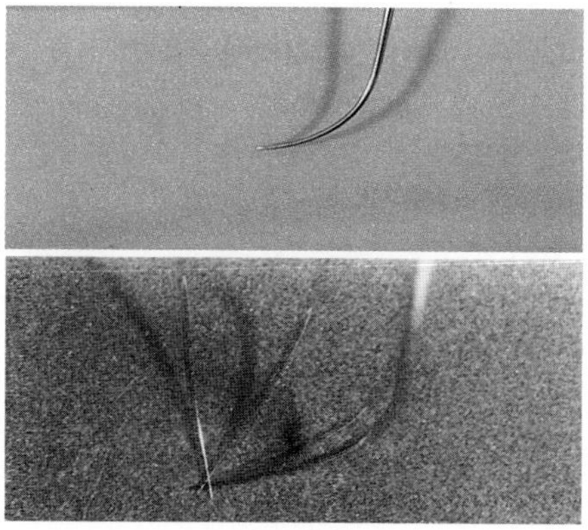

Figure 26-50. The dental explorer is sharpened by lightly dragging and rotating the first 2 to 3 mm along the sharpening stone.

observed in stroke length, stone grasp, and instrument grasp. Short, even, continuous strokes tend to keep the instrument on the stone. The hand holding the instrument should assume a palm-thumb grasp and be supported against a firm surface such as a cabinet top, or the operator's own elbow may be pulled close to the body to support the wrist and hand holding the instrument. The fingers holding the stone should not be wrapped around the stone on the long side exposed to the cutting surface but should be positioned behind the cutting surface or at the short end of the stone (Figure 26-49).

Before the sharpening stroke is initiated, proper angulation of the stone to the surface of the instrument is assumed, and continuous sharpening motions at this constant angle are made across the length of the cutting edge. Stones can be designed to facilitate proper sharpening such as the Gold Edge Sharpener by New Edge Technologies, which is a synthetic stone, shaped to assist with correct angulation and channels to maintain a rounded toe on curets. (Correct angulation of stone to cutting surface is discussed under each individual instrument.) The amount of pressure applied should be determined by the amount of recontouring necessary to produce a sharp blade. Greater pressure exerted against the blade with the stone removes more metal. Prudent advice for instrument conservation is to limit sharpening procedures to what is necessary. The last sharpening stroke(s) should be away from the face of the instrument in a downward motion to remove small metal particles called *flash* that adhere to the instrument edges. The practitioner should wipe the blade with a 2-inch × 2-inch gauze square to aid in removing oil and metal shavings floating on the instrument surface.

Mechanical Sharpening Technique

A number of manufacturers offer mechanical devices, also known as *honing devices,* for sharpening instruments. The Sidekick (Hu-Friedy Manufacturing) is one example of a battery-operated sharpening device that has a ceramic stone and built-in channel guides and vertical stops for maintaining a perfect angulation of the instrument blade against the stone. Once the desired angulation of the working end against the stone is achieved, the stone is automatically activated and moves gently across the working end to create a sharp blade. The device can be used for sharpening sickle scalers, universal curets, and Gracey curets. The device removes metal from the lateral sides of the working end and has a toe guide to maintain the round toe of curets. After instrument sharpening, the ceramic stone, guide plates, and screw can be cleaned in an ultrasonic cleaning unit and then autoclaved.

Testing for Instrument Sharpness

Testing for sharpness is done by visual inspection or by comparing the sharpness before and after the procedure using a plastic testing stick.

- With visual inspection, it is important to have a strong light such as the dental light for viewing. With this test, the sharp instrument does not reflect light at the junction between the face and the lateral side of the instrument. In contrast, the dull instrument is beveled on the cutting edge and reflects light back to the observer.
- With the tactile test, the sharpened instrument blade at the proper working angulation engages a hard plastic stick. When using this method, clinicians must test the instrument fully across the length of the blade and resharpen any area that allows the instrument to slip over the stick.

When testing for sharpness, the dental hygienist examines the sharpened blade's shape. To protect the client against unnecessary instrument breakage, all instruments that have lost their original strength or are too fine to remove heavy deposits or reach deep pockets should no longer be used in such areas. Instruments that have been sharpened down and are of moderate or fine dimensions may be used for the healthier individual with little calculus formation and shallow probing depths. The instrument is retipped or discarded when it is no longer functional or is a danger to the client from possible breakage.

Explorer Sharpening Techniques

Fine explorers become dull through general use and from caries detection in pits and fissures and around restorations. Decreased tactile sensitivity is evident when fine changes in root texture cannot be distinguished, or when the explorer glides over the plastic testing stick instead of catching on irregularities. To sharpen the explorer tip, the instrument is held with a modified pen grasp, dragged, and rotated along the stone at an angle that keeps the tip and 2 to 3 mm of the terminal end in contact with the stone. Two to three rotations around the tip on the stone sufficiently sharpen the dental explorer (Figure 26-50). Because the periodontal explorer's length is important, an explorer shortened through wear should be replaced.

Universal Curet Sharpening Techniques

A curet has lost sharpness if the following occur:

- Tactile sensitivity decreases during light root planing strokes.
- The curet does not grasp tooth structure unless the practitioner uses inordinate lateral pressure.
- The curets angulation must be further closed for the instrument to maintain a working relationship with the tooth surface.

The more accurately the curet has been sharpened (i.e., the angulation of the lateral surface to the face of the blade is correct and a definite cutting edge has been established), the longer the curet remains sharp. Accurate sharpening lengthens the time interval between sharpening and thus preserves the metal. Because the universal curet cutting edge is two sided and includes the rounded toe, sharpening includes all of these areas. It is recommended, however, that the toe of the universal curet be preserved as long as possible because the toe itself is not usually used in instrumentation except occasionally under the floor of furcations or under tooth contacts. When the toe is sharpened each time the lateral surfaces are sharpened, there is unnecessary reduction of the blade length, eventually making the instrument inaccessible to interproximal areas. Both sides of the blade should be sharpened if dull.

Sharpening the Lateral Sides

The universal curet may be sharpened in two ways, as follows:

- Moving the instrument over the stone requires the stone to be placed on a stable surface such as a tabletop, the curet held in a modified pen grasp, angulation of the face to the surface of the stone positioned between 100 and 110 degrees, and the curet blade moved at this angulation from the lower third of the blade to the midline of the toe. Each side of the universal curet blade is sharpened as needed.
- Moving the stone over the blade requires the stone to be held in the dominant hand and the instrument held with a palm-thumb grasp secured against a firm surface (tabletop), or the elbow drawn close to the body for support. The instrument is held with the face of the blade parallel to the floor and the stone positioned on the lateral surface at a 100- to 110-degree angle. The stone is moved with short, light to firm vertical strokes, depending on the amount of sharpening needed, and slowly is passed across the entire cutting edge at consistent angulation. It is important to maintain consistent angulation for an evenly sharpened blade. For this to be accomplished, the stone should not be lifted from the blade; both the upward and downward strokes are used for sharpening. Even pressure should be used along the cutting edge to prevent changing the normal shape of a curet blade.

Figure 26-51 illustrates the cross-sectional views of curet blades resulting from common sharpening errors.

The most common error is to increase the pressure as the stroke nears the toe, producing a blade with converging lateral sides connected by a point instead of parallel lateral sides connected by a rounded toe (Figure 26-52). The method of moving the stone over the instrument is slightly easier than moving the instrument, because as the stone is moved a light film of lubricant and/or sharpening byproducts (sludge) accumulates on the surface of the face, and angulation of lateral surface to stone is easier to visualize. The last stroke(s) should be in a downward motion toward the back of the instrument to reduce the possibility of a wire edge on the face of the blade. Figure 26-48 compares both methods of sharpening the universal curet.

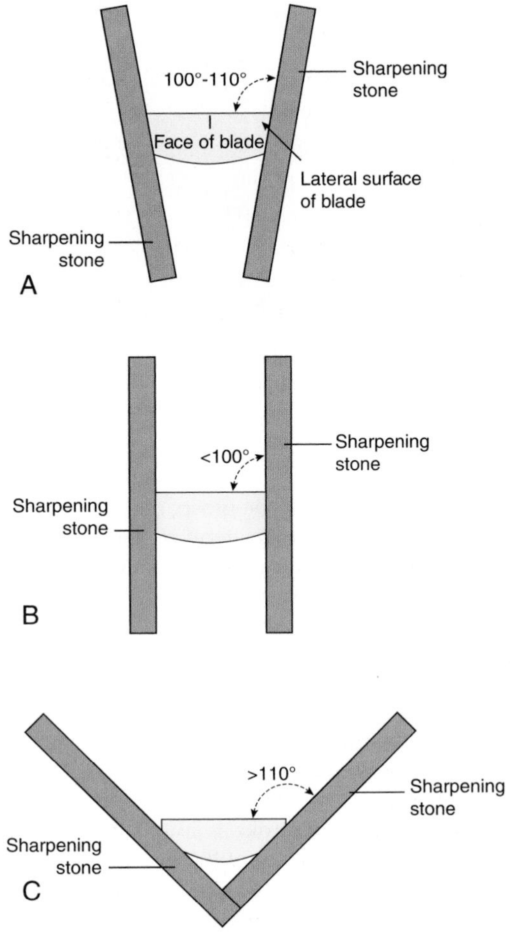

Figure 26-51. A, Correct instrument sharpening. **B** and **C,** Common sharpening errors.

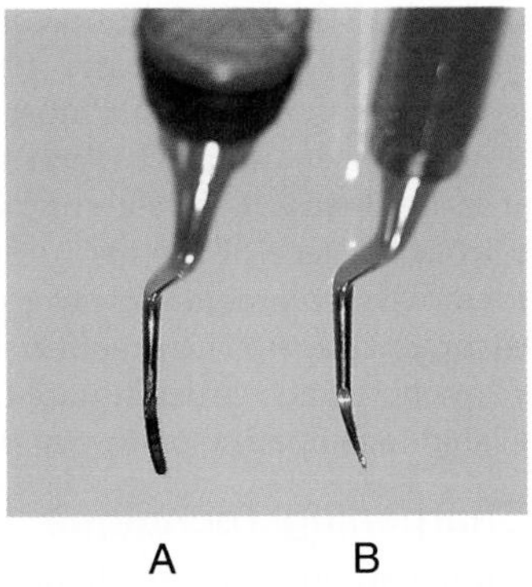

Figure 26-52. A, Parallel lateral cutting edge of a Gracey curet 7/8. **B,** Converging lateral cutting edge resulting from too heavy pressure of the sharpening stone near the toe of the blade of a Gracey curet 7/8.

Sharpening the Face

The face of the curet blade may be sharpened with a cone-shaped sharpening stone, the rounded side of a sharpening stone, or a mounted rotary stone. Often these methods produce unreliable results because it is difficult to maintain even pressure across the face. If too much metal is removed (as with the rotary stone), the blade strength from face to back is weakened. This dimension from face to back is significant because it is an important factor in providing strength to an instrument that uses a pulling action, as does the curet. When all sharpening has been completed, the instrument is wiped with a 2-inch × 2-inch gauze square and tested for sharpness.

Area-Specific Curet Sharpening Technique

The major difference between sharpening the Gracey and the universal curet is that the Gracey curet blade is offset. Both instruments may be sharpened with movement of the instrument or the stone. Grasp positions, angulation of 100 to 110 degrees, and movement across the blade are the same for the Gracey and universal curets. The Gracey curet blade face is offset at 60 to 70 degrees to the shank (as opposed to 90 degrees for the universal curet), which opens the stone angle on the Gracey when the lower shank of each is held perpendicular to the floor. When the Gracey curet blade face is held parallel with the floor (like the universal curet), the stone is positioned like the universal curet, but the handle and shank of the Gracey curet are tilted away from the stone and not perpendicular to the floor. Figure 26-53 shows a comparison of stone and handle when the faces of a Gracey and a universal curet are held parallel to the floor. On the Gracey curet, only the lower, longer cutting edge from the area where blade sharpness begins and occasionally around the toe is sharpened. After sharpening procedures, the blade should be tested for sharpness and wiped clean before instrumentation. These principles of sharpening also apply to the variations of the Gracey curet that follow.

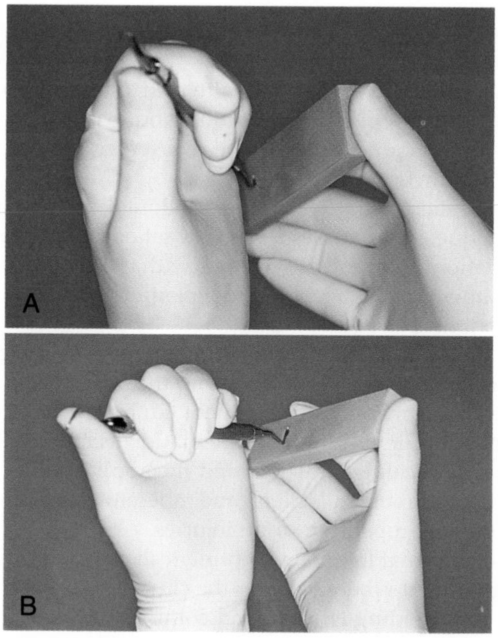

Figure 26-53. Comparison of handle position of a universal curet (**A**) and a Gracey curet (**B**) when the face of the blade is held parallel to the floor for sharpening (from the point of view of the clinician looking down).

Curets are now available in new materials that eliminate the need for sharpening (XP Technology, American Eagle Instruments) or reduce the need for sharpening (EverEdge technology, Hu-Friedy Manufacturing). Currently there is limited research evidence on the advantages of instruments made with these materials and ones currently under development. Dental hygienists must use evidence-based decision making to ensure the best outcome for their clients.

Extended Shank Area–Specific Curets Sharpening Technique

See the discussion of sharpening technique in the section on area-specific curets.

Mini-Bladed Area–Specific Curets Sharpening Technique

See the discussion of sharpening technique in the section on area-specific curets.

Micro Mini-Bladed Area–Specific Curets Sharpening Technique

See the discussion of sharpening technique in the section on area-specific curets.

Sickle-Sharpening Technique

Sharpening the sickle scaler requires the stone to remain stationary and the instrument to move over the stone. The stone is secured with the nondominant hand, the instrument held with a modified pen grasp, and the lateral surface positioned at an angle of 100 to 110 degrees to the stone. The entire lateral surface on a flat-surfaced sickle scaler lies against the stone. For curved sickle scalers, small portions of the lateral surfaces are sharpened at a time, beginning from the portion nearest the shank. The working hand is stabilized with a fulcrum on the stone, and short, firm strokes are applied for sharpening. Because the sickle scaler has two cutting edges, the instrument is turned over and the procedure is repeated for the other lateral surface of the blade. Occasionally the face of the sickle scaler is sharpened. For this surface, the stone must be either positioned near the edge of the table or held up so that the entire face may be sharpened against the stone surface. Tests for sharpness include the visual or tactile methods described earlier.

Hoe-Sharpening Techniques

The hoe is sharpened by placing a stationary stone on a tabletop and positioning the entire blade surface on the stone. It is important to maintain the 45-degree bevel. The instrument is held with a modified pen grasp and stabilized with a fulcrum on the stone. Movement of the instrument across the stone is made in short, moderate pull strokes. A push-pull or grinding stroke is not recommended. The corners at each cutting edge occasionally are rounded with light rolling strokes to prevent grooving or gouging of the tooth structure and soft-tissue injury. The hoe is tested for sharpness on a testing stick and wiped of debris before instrumentation.

File-Sharpening Techniques

The file is a difficult instrument to sharpen because of the miniature size of each blade. Sharpening may be accomplished with a tanged file sharpener positioned against each small, flat-bladed surface (Figure 26-54). For the sharpening

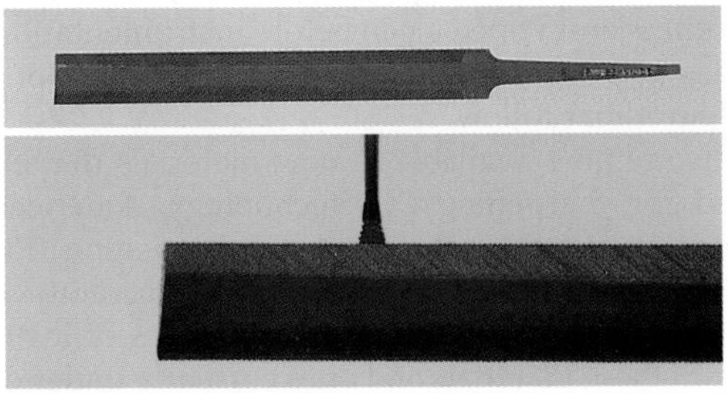

Figure 26-54. A tanged file for sharpening the file.

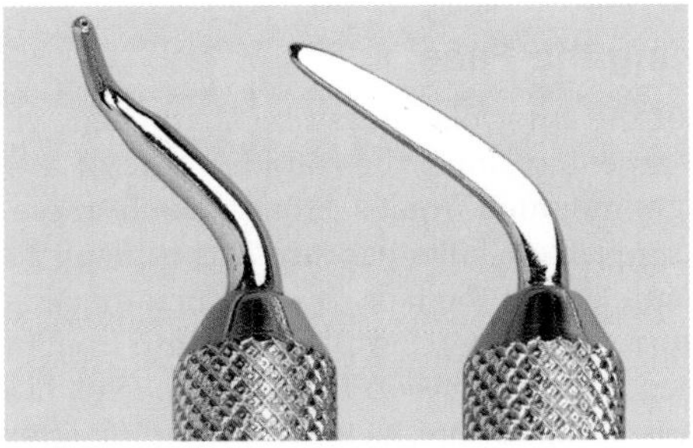

Figure 26-55. Magnetic broken tip retrievers (Schwartz Periotrievers). Contra-angle tip is for use in furcations; the long tip is for use in pockets. (From Newman MG, Takei HH, Klokkevold PR, et al: *Carranza's clinical periodontology*, ed 11, St Louis, 2012, Saunders.)

procedure, the instrument is stabilized on a firm surface (tabletop) and the practitioner stabilizes the working hand near the instrument on the tabletop to perform light, short, push-pull strokes across each blade. Consistently good results are difficult to achieve when sharpening this instrument.

Chisel-Sharpening Techniques

See the discussion of sharpening technique in the section on hoes.

Furcation Instrument–Sharpening Techniques

Refer to various manufacturers for sharpening methods of specific instruments.

Instrument Tip Breakage

Prevention

As sharpening narrows the working end, it is best to discard worn scalers that have become too thin. Instruments that have developed points of weakness possibly because of uneven sharpening, corrosion, or metal fatigue should be discarded because they are subject to easier breakage. Even new instruments, especially curets, break if they are lodged in a tight area such as under a contact and are twisted or pulled in a direction in which the toe may not be released.

Complications

Instrument tip breakage can cause client trauma and distress and liability and stress to the clinician. Managing the incident is important to ensure the tip has not been swallowed or aspirated because this requires medical intervention. Serious medical problems can result if a foreign object is lodged internally.

Managing Instrument Tip Breakage

When an instrument breaks subgingivally, only the tip breaks off, leaving it for the dental hygienist to locate. To retrieve the small metal fragment the dental hygienist stops instrumentation as soon as the instrument tip has broken and informs the client. Until the tip is found, low-speed or high-speed aspiration (suction) should be discontinued and the client should use a cup to expectorate into in the event the tip is floating in saliva. Techniques for locating the broken piece include the following:

- Reinstrumentation with another instrument to tease out from subgingival areas and catch with gauze
- Use of magnetic-tip Periotrievers, shaped like thick explorers or probes, to draw and grab tip fragment (Figure 26-55)
- Open-flap periodontal surgery if attempts are unsuccessful for an identified tip fragment

Radiographic examination is helpful during these exploration techniques to locate the metal tip. If the broken tip cannot be clinically located, or if it is not visible on a radiograph of the area, the tip may be outside of the sulcus. A complete visual inspection of the oral cavity is initiated. Gauze squares are used to wipe out the vestibular areas and areas under the client's tongue. They then are inspected carefully for the broken tip. When the tip is recovered, the client should be informed to confirm the metal tip fragment retrieval.

If the tip cannot be located, the client must be apprised and a chest radiograph is indicated to rule out the possibility of the client aspirating the fragment.

Clinicians should document routinely any instrument tip breakage by noting the specific tooth or site, incident disclosure to client with signature verification, client response, follow-ups or referrals, and procedure results.

CLIENT EDUCATION TIPS

- Teach clients to visualize health and disease by using a mouth mirror, periodontal probe, and explorer in the client's own mouth while the client observes by looking into a hand mirror.
- Inform clients that effective periodontal instrumentation technique encompasses a complex set of skills, assessment of relationships, and movements with the goal of performing subgingival scaling and root planing to treat and arrest periodontal disease.
- Use dental perioscopy, which magnifies the subgingival periodontal pocket for visualizing the area during assessment, instrumentation, and client education.
- Share with clients how instrumentation techniques include protective scaling strategies and the application of proper body positioning of client and operator as a means of minimizing repetitive strain injuries.
- Tell clients that frequent instrument sharpening during the appointment is beneficial for the client as well as the operator in providing efficient and comfortable care.
- Inform clients how high-quality preventive care includes usage of various dental hygiene assessment and treatment instruments.

LEGAL, ETHICAL, AND SAFETY ISSUES

- The clinician has instruments to assess the severity of the client's periodontal condition and is educated to make decisions to recommend referrals to other professionals. Not evaluating the periodontal status by lack of full mouth probing, or the need for referral, can put the client at risk.
- The clinician retrieves broken instrument tips and documents such occurrences in the client record. When broken instrument tips cannot be found, a chest radiograph for the client is indicated.
- Clinicians use appropriate instrumentation techniques to safely, efficiently, and effectively treat clients.

KEY CONCEPTS

- Basic dental hygiene assessment instruments include the mouth mirror, periodontal probe, and explorer.
- Shape, length, and markings of periodontal probes and explorers vary; selection is dependent on the client's oral disease status and clinician preference.
- Periodontal hand instruments are available, and selection is dependent on function, the client's periodontal health status, and clinician preference and experience.
- Periodontal treatment instruments vary in handle size, shape, and pattern.
- Major classifications in blade design, shape, and size dictate use and effectiveness of periodontal instruments; small variations in periodontal treatment instruments in shank length, curvature, and flexibility profoundly affect use and effectiveness.
- Proper grasp and fulcrum placement are essential for safe and effective periodontal instrumentation technique.
- Body mechanics and protective scaling techniques are important to incorporate into hand-activated instrumentation to prevent repetitive strain injuries.

CRITICAL THINKING EXERCISES

1. To simulate the sensation of a probe contacting tissue, practice using the periodontal probe across the resistance of a thick rubber band stretched over a ceramic coffee cup so that it crosses the opening. Do this first with your eyes open, then with your eyes closed.
2. To facilitate the development of tactile sensitivity, take a few coins and practice exploring the relief on the coin with a periodontal explorer designed for calculus detection. Do this first with your eyes open, then with your eyes closed.
3. To simulate hand-instrumentation scaling techniques, apply artificial calculus on models and practice using a variety of assessment and treatment instruments for calculus assessment and removal.
4. To enhance indirect vision skills, stand an open textbook upright with pages facing away from you; peer over and use a mouth mirror to read letters and trace lines with the tip of an explorer. Alternately, you can turn your laptop screen away from you to use a regular mirror to view the screen to read or trace lines of a PowerPoint on the screen with your finger.

REFERENCES

1. Dong H, Barr A, Loomer P, et al: The effects of periodontal instrument handle design on hand muscle load and pinch force. *J Amer Dent Hyg* 80:8, 2006.
2. Dylla J, Forrest JL: Fit to sit—strategies to maximize function and minimize occupational pain. *J Mich Dent Assoc* 90(5):38, 2008.
3. Dylla J, Forrest JL: Practice in motion. Available at: http://www.Dentalcare.com. Accessed October 10, 2012.
4. Drabek T, Boucek CD, Buffington CW: Wearing the wrong size latex surgical gloves impairs manual dexterity. *J Occup Environ Hyg* 7(3):152, 2010.
5. Powell BJ, Winkley GP, Brown JO, et al: Evaluating the fit of ambidextrous and fitted gloves: implications for hand discomfort. *J Am Dent Assoc* 125(9):1235, 1994.
6. Sawyer J, Bennett A: Comparing the level of dexterity offered by latex and nitrile SafeSkin gloves. *Ann Occup Hyg* 50(3):289, 2006.
7. Pattison A, Matsuda S, Pattison G: Extraoral fulcrums: the essentials of using extraoral fulcrums for periodontal instrumentation. *Dimens Dent Hyg* 2(10):20, 2004.
8. Pattison A: The use of hand instruments in supportive periodontal treatment. *Periodontology 2000* 12:72, 1996.
9. Wilson TG, Harrel SK, Nunn ME, et al: The relationship between the presence of tooth-borne subgingival deposits and inflammation found with a dental endoscope. *J Periodontol* 79:11, 2008.
10. Pattison A: Establishing effective extraoral fulcrums. *Dimens Dent Hyg* 6(4):46, 2008.
11. Dofka CM: *Dental terminology*, ed 3, Clifton Park, NY, 2012, Delmar Cengage Learning.

ACKNOWLEDGMENTS

The authors acknowledge Peggy T. Tsutsui for her past contributions to this chapter, Anna Pattison for providing advice on new assessment and treatment instruments currently available, and Jane Forrest for consulting on operator body mechanics to prevent repetitive strain injuries.

Photos generously provided by Kevin Thanh Vu.

Instruments provided by Brasseler USA, G. Hartzell & Son, Hu-Friedy Manufactering, Florida Probe Corporation, American Eagle Instruments, Miltex, Paradise Dental Technologies, L-M Instruments and Premier Dental Products.

EVOLVE RESOURCES

Please visit http://evolve.elsevier.com/Darby/hygiene for additional practice and study support tools.

CHAPTER 27

Ultrasonic Instrumentation

Kathleen O. Hodges

COMPETENCIES

1. Discuss power-driven instrumentation used in oral prophylaxis, nonsurgical periodontal therapy, and periodontal maintenance therapy, including:
   - Discuss strategies for appropriate insert or tip selection based on client needs.
   - Apply correct procedures for ultrasonic instrumentation using standard and thin designs.
   - Compare and contrast magnetostrictive and piezoelectric instrumentation.
2. Explain health-related outcomes of using ultrasonic instrumentation.
3. Discuss ultrasonic instrumentation in practice, including indications, precautions, and contraindications for ultrasonic instrumentation.
4. Demonstrate proper instrumentation technique.

Periodontal Debridement

Ultrasonic instrumentation is referred to as power-driven, *mechanical* or *mechanized* instrumentation. It is used to remove mechanically calculus, biofilm, and root surface constituents in periodontal debridement. There are two types of devices: magnetostrictive and piezoelectric (Figures 27-1, *A* and *B*). Handpieces of magnetostrictive units accept inserts, and handpieces of piezoelectric units accept tips, both with varying working end designs. The large working end of the power-driven insert or tip is described as a *conventional, traditional,* or *standard design.* Narrower working ends for subgingival access are called *microultrasonic, periodontal, slim, precision thin,* or *thin* designs.

Ultrasonic instruments have the following three modes of action:

- Mechanical action, or vibration of the working end, results in deposit removal. Ultrasonic instruments have clinical power, referring to the ability to remove calculus deposits under load. Working-end action that provides clinical power depends on the stroke, frequency, type of motion, and angulation against the tooth surface. Load is the resistance on a working end when placed against the calculus deposit or tooth surface.
- Cavitation is the action created by the formation and collapse of bubbles in the water by high-frequency sound waves surrounding the working end (Figure 27-2). Cavitation results in lavage, which is the therapeutic washing of the sulcus or pocket and root surface to remove endotoxins and loose debris. It may enhance biofilm removal depending on the working end design and load[1]; in vivo research is needed to study the effects of cavitation. Irrigation occurs via the water or the antimicrobial used to replace the water that circulates through the tip or insert from a reservoir or water system.
- Acoustic microstreaming is generated by ultrasound in the presence of a fluid environment and has the potential to destroy or disrupt bacteria.

Ultrasonic Instruments

Ultrasonic instruments convert electrical energy into mechanical energy in the range of 18,000 to 50,000 vibrations per second. The term ultrasonic describes a nonaudible range of acoustic vibrations that are a unit of frequency referred to in cycles per second (CPS) or hertz (Hz). Magnetostrictive and piezoelectric ultrasonic units have four similar components: the electric generator, the handpiece, the insert/tip, and the foot pedal control (Figure 27-3). When the ultrasonic unit receives electrical energy and the foot pedal is activated, an electrical current is sent through the generator, or base of the unit, to the handpiece. The handpiece holds the transducer or insert. The transducer converts the electrical energy to mechanical energy, causing the tip to vibrate. The mechanical action of the working end removes calculus, oral biofilm, and root surface constituents that are contacted directly by the tip.

Manual and Autotuned Units

Ultrasonic units are either manual-tuned or autotuned. These terms refer to how the frequency, or the number of times per second that the tip moves back and forth in one complete cycle (speed of movement of the tip), is adjusted during use. The clinician's ability to control the frequency may assist in deposit removal or debridement. For example, a lower setting may be used for light deposits and a higher setting may be helpful for larger or more tenacious deposits. The most commonly used unit is the autotuned unit, which has a preset frequency within the instrument that automatically tunes the cycles per second to maximum efficiency for each insert used. Therefore no tuning is needed to adjust the speed (frequency) of the working end because the frequency is automatically adjusted to correlate with the power setting determined by the clinician. Many contemporary models have adjustable power settings at the low end of the power spectrum to provide for low-power subgingival debridement or have a power boost feature available on the foot pedal for intermittent use as needed. The majority of magnetostrictive units (e.g., Parkell, Dentsply/Cavitron, Coltene/Whaledent) and all piezoelectric units (e.g., Prodentec, EMS Electro Medical Systems, Amdent Biotrol, Amadent/Satelec) are autotuned. Manual-tuned units are magnetostrictive ultrasonic devices

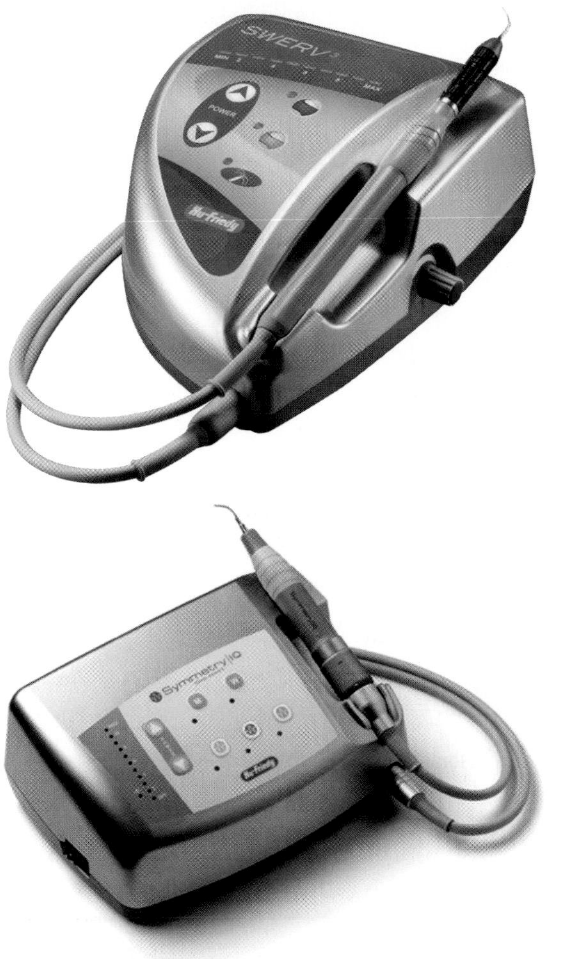

A

B

Figure 27-1. Ultrasonic Units: magnetostrictive and piezoelectric. **A,** Magnetostrictive: Swerv. **B,** Piezoelectric: Symmetry IQ 3000. (Courtesy Hu-Friedy Manufacturing, Chicago, Illinois.)

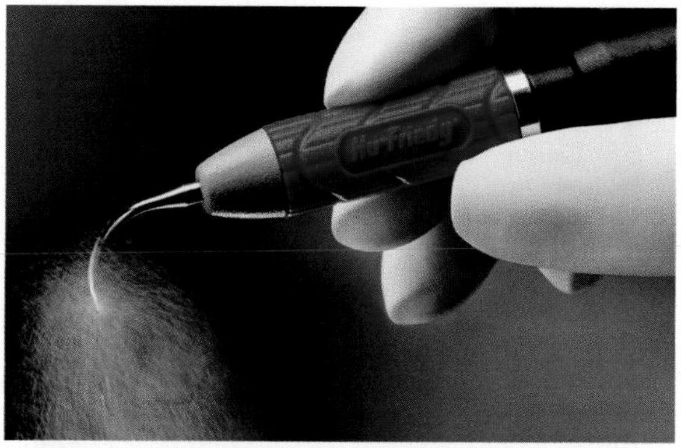

Figure 27-2. Cavitation. (Courtesy Hu-Friedy Manufacturing, Chicago. Illinois.)

only (e.g., Parkell, Ultrasonic Services, Ltd, Tony Riso Co.). The **manual-tuned unit** permits the clinician to adjust the frequency via the tuning knob (see Figure 27-3). However, frequent readjustments of the tuning knob to ensure optimal unit efficiency unit could increase treatment time.

Manual-tuned and autotuned units have power and water control knobs. **Power** (also known as **amplitude**) is the energy in the handpiece that creates movement of the working end. Increasing the power setting increases the distance the working end moves. This is the length of the stroke (Figure 27-4). The distance the working end travels in the single vibration is called **tip displacement**. As amplitude increases, the output of power increases, enhancing the efficiency of the action of the working end.

The water control knob adjusts the volume and temperature of the flow from the handpiece. Water flow does the following:

- Cools the transducer and working end (*Note:* Although a piezoelectric transducer can run without water, the working end generates frictional heat that requires water to keep it cool and flush debris. Also, piezoelectric transducers create heat and lose efficiency without water flow. In clinical practice, magnetostrictive and piezoelectric units always are operated with water.)
- Stems bleeding
- Increases visibility
- Provides lavage
- Removes root surface constituents
- Irrigates sulci and periodontal pockets

Proper water spray is critical to prevent root surface damage. The greater the water flow is, the lower the water temperature. A decreased water flow creates a higher water temperature; therefore water temperature should be adjusted if clients experience heat or sensitivity. Water flow is independent of the energy generated from the tip (i.e., increased water flow does not affect the mechanized energy produced).

Magnetostrictive Units

The insert in a magnetostrictive unit is a core attached to the working end (see Figure 27-1, *B*). (See Procedure 27-1 and the corresponding Competency Form.) The core is either a stack of metal (Permanickel) strips or a ferrite rod, depending on the type of unit. The Cavitron Jet Plus and Cavitron Select SPS with 30-kHz (DENTSPLY Professional) are examples of magnetostrictive technology with a handpiece that houses an insert with metal strips for the core.

Inside the handpiece is a copper wire coil that exposes the core to a varying magnetic field when it receives an electrical current. When magnetized, the core contracts; when demagnetized, the core returns to its original size. The alternating electromagnetic field causes the working end of the insert to vibrate. The **active tip area** is the portion of the working end that performs the instrumentation, as it is affected by the frequency. In the 25,000- to 30,000-Hz unit the active tip area is approximately the last 4.3 mm of the working end (see Procedure 27-1).

Heat is a by-product of the action of the instrument in magnetostrictive units; therefore water is needed to control the heat to prevent pulp tissue damage. When water flows to the end of the insert and contacts the moving working end, tiny droplets and a fine spray result. This phenomenon is called **atomization** (see Figure 27-2).

Insert Selection

When selecting inserts for mechanized instrumentation, the dental hygienist considers the following:

- Working end and handle designs for periodontal debridement
- Compatibility with the frequency (kHz) of the unit
- Compatibility with other units in the practice setting
- Method of fluid (water) delivery

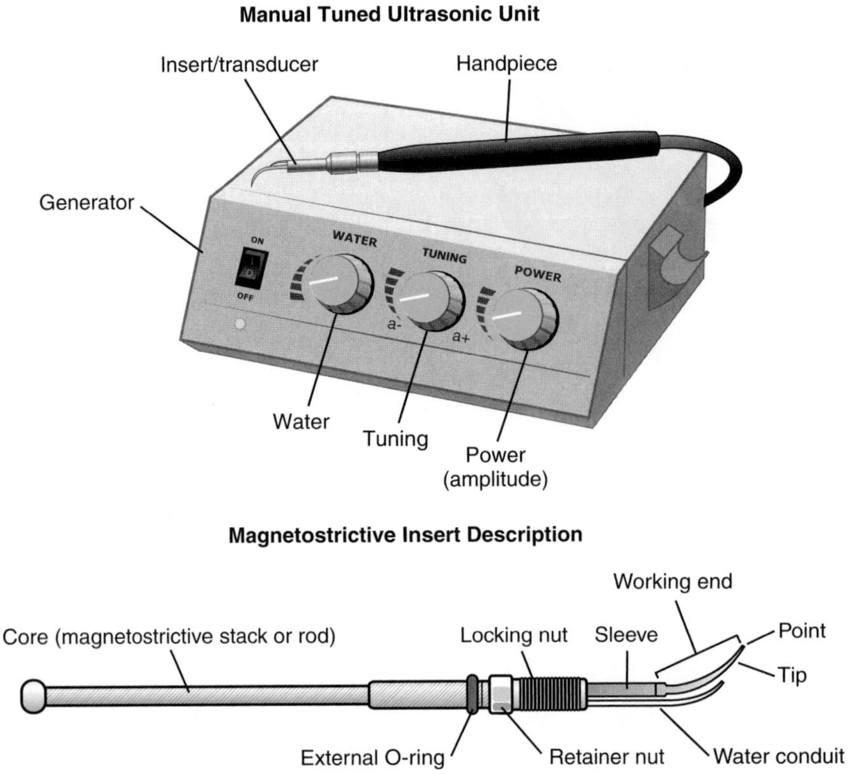

Figure 27-3. Components of an ultrasonic dental unit and insert.

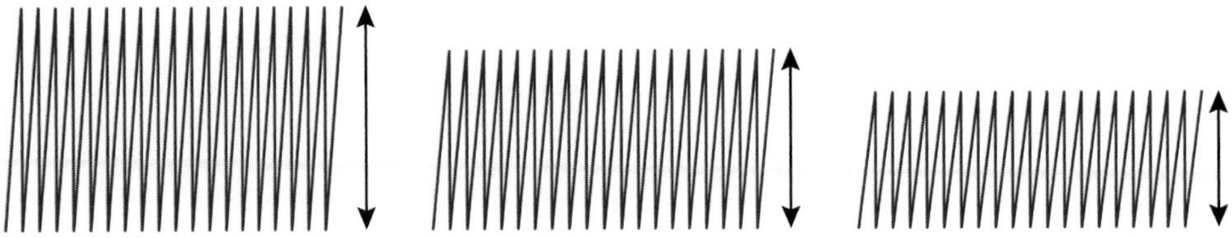

Figure 27-4. Displacement or amplitude. (From Hodges KO: *Concepts in nonsurgical periodontal therapy,* Albany, NY, 1998, Delmar.)

There are two types of magnetostrictive inserts based on the frequency requirements of the unit: either 25 kHz or 30 kHz. The stack of the 30-kHz insert is shorter than that of the 25-kHz insert (Figure 27-5, *A*), and it produces a quicker stroke than the 25 kHz. Insert designs are selected in either type based on the frequency of the equipment being used. Most magnetostrictive units accept their own as well as other manufacturers' 25-kHz or 30-kHz inserts. Some units accept 25-kHz and 30-kHz inserts. Inserts or handpiece cables also may swivel to increase maneuverability (Figure 27-5, *B*). An internal or external fluid hose (conduit) is available in most designs (Figure 27-6). The internal hose does not bend as the external tube can. The external hose is available in two types: a tube that is long and not fixed, and a shorter external tube that is fixed. There are many choices in internal design water flow from various manufacturers. One contemporary choice in internal hose design is the PowerLINE series that is designed to provide an improved view of the area because of the focus of the spray (DENTSPLY Professional) (Figure 27-7). Evidence does not support use of a particular type of water delivery; therefore operator preference influences choice.

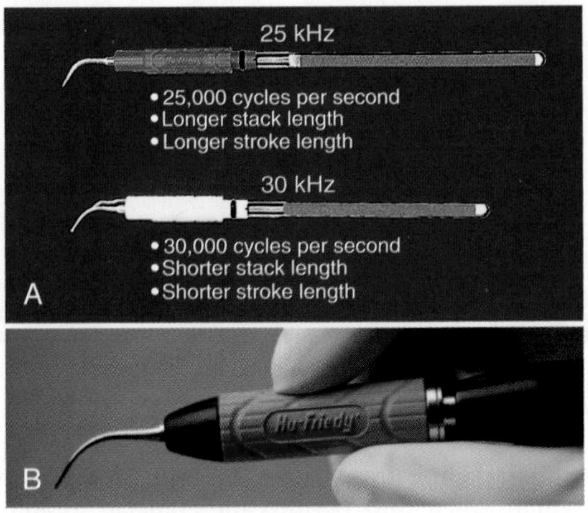

Figure 27-5. **A,** Magnetostrictive inserts: 27-kHz and 30-kHz. **B,** Satin Swivel Ultrasonic inserts with soft silicone grip. Slight swivel increases maneuverability and adaptability. (Courtesy Hu-Friedy Manufacturing, Chicago, Illinois.)

Procedure 27-1 Instrumentation with the Magnetostrictive Ultrasonic Unit

EQUIPMENT

Personal protective equipment, including face shield
Ultrasonic unit (manual or autotuned) tuned appropriately
Inserts (standard and/or precision thin)
Subgingival explorer
Mouth mirror
Files
Curets
High-speed evacuation
Preprocedural mouth rinse of 0.12% chlorhexidine gluconate
Protective eyewear and drape for client

STEPS

Preparation

1. Connect ultrasonic unit to water source on dental unit and electrical power source.
2. Turn ultrasonic unit on, and allow water to flow through handpiece for 2 to 5 minutes (30 seconds between clients).
3. Select a straight-angled working end, and slide insert into water-filled handpiece of ultrasonic unit.
4. Holding handpiece over a water receptacle, adjust water and power to desired setting. Working end emits mist of water without excessive dripping.

Positioning

5. Place client in appropriate supine position: Have client tilt head toward right or left depending on area being treated and place suction appropriately. Provide protective eyewear and plastic drape.

Grasp

6. Use light pen or modified pen grasp.

Fulcrum

7. Employ conventional, opposite arch, cross-arch, or other fulcrum.
8. Use intraoral fulcrum for standard designs and extraoral fulcrum for thin designs.

Mirror Use

9. Prepare mirror to allow water to pool on its surface.

Adaptation

10. Explore or visually locate deposit. Position side of working end on deposit (standard) or at epithelial attachment (thin).
11. Apply working end at no more than a 15-degree angle to tooth surface.
12. Adapt back or lateral surfaces of working end parallel to long axis of tooth.
13. Adapt working end diagonally (bisecting the long axis of the tooth) on proximal surface. Back of thin working end can be adapted in pocket on proximal surfaces or in furcation invasions.
14. Roll insert within handpiece to adapt to various tooth surfaces, unless using a swivel design.
15. Extend working end to midline of proximal surfaces.

Activation

16. Keep insert in motion at all times.
17. Use quick, controlled, eraser-like motions with standard working end. Speed of movement is slower with thin inserts.
18. Use overlapping, multidirectional strokes.
19. Do not apply excessive lateral pressure.
20. Stop periodically to allow complete evacuation.
21. Evaluate progress and product with light, magnification, air, and explorer. Reinstrument areas as necessary.

Documentation

22. Record services rendered in client record (e.g., debridement of mandibular left quadrant using magnetostrictive universal standard and thin designs).
23. Follow current infection control protocol.

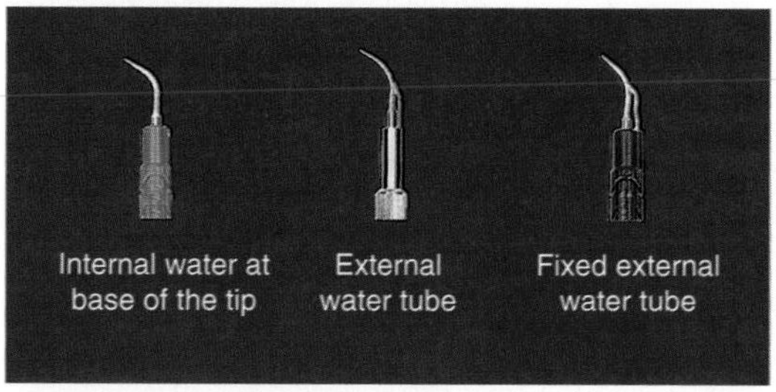

Figure 27-6. Methods of water delivery. (Courtesy Hu-Friedy Manufacturing, Chicago, Illinois.)

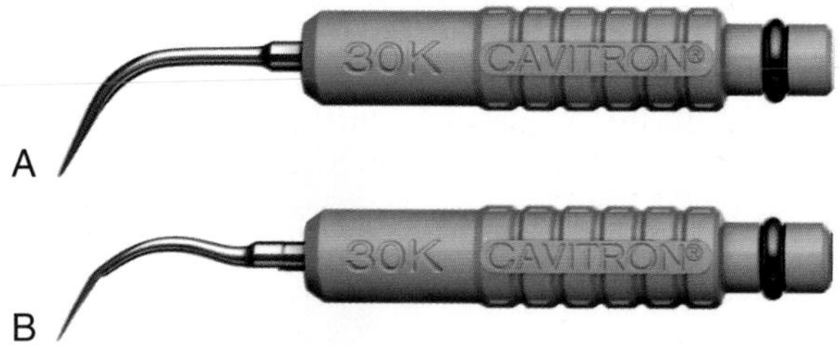

Figure 27-7. PowerLINE series. Formerly known as the Focused Spray Insert (FSI) series. **A,** 10. **B,** 100. (Courtesy Dentsply Professional.)

Insert Design

Design affects the efficiency and quality of the periodontal instrumentation. Refer to Table 27-1 for a review of magnetostrictive inserts manufactured by DENTSPLY Professional, Hu-Friedy, and Tony Riso. Other companies make similar inserts. Some inserts have a grip with a built-in light-emitting diode (LED) to illuminate the working surface (Philips, Insight) and options for the insert to "swivel" or turn in the handpiece with a slight roll of the fingers to aid in effective ergonomics.

Standard inserts are used for supragingival or, depending on access, subgingival debridement of the following:

- Calculus (larger-diameter insert is indicated primarily for removal of moderate to heavy deposits)

TABLE 27-1
Summary of Ultrasonic Insert Designs

Type of Insert	Design	Power Setting	Indications	Adaptation and Activation
Standard	Beavertail 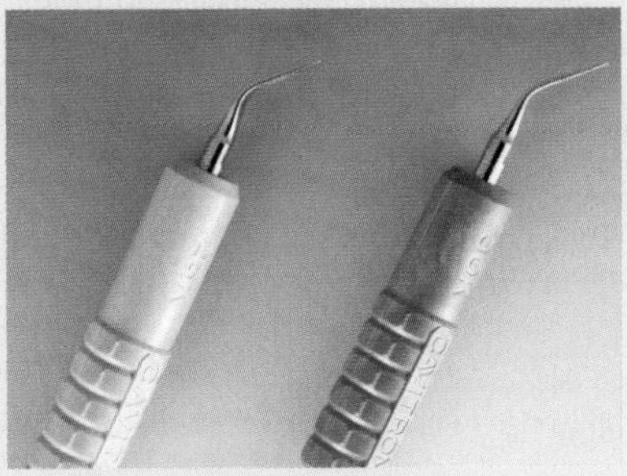 (Courtesy DENTSPLY International, Professional Division, York, Pennsylvania.)	Low to high	Supragingival moderate to heavy calculus, labial and lingual surfaces of teeth (usually anteriors) Removing stain from all accessible tooth surfaces	Work with flat end of insert; avoid using sides or face of this insert. *Stain:* "erasing" motion using very light pressure. *Scaling lingually or buccally:* vertical overlapping strokes using light pressure.
Standard	Universal 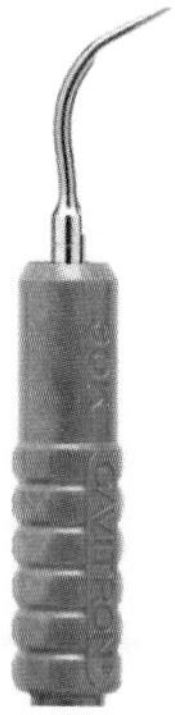 (Courtesy DENTSPLY International, Professional Division, York, Pennsylvania.)	Low to high	Light, moderate, and heavy calculus removal in all areas (universal)	Work with side of working end.
Standard	Universal 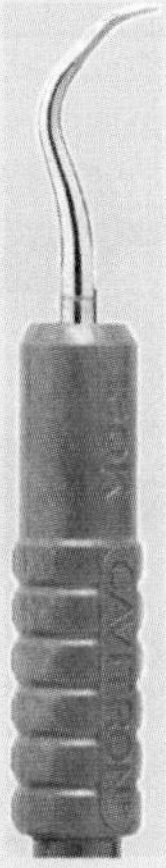 (Courtesy DENTSPLY International, Professional Division, York, Pennsylvania.)	Low to high	Anterior and posterior subgingival moderate and heavy calculus removal	Use sides of working end for complete deposit removal (cross-hatch); horizontal or vertical strokes.

TABLE 27-1
Summary of Ultrasonic Insert Designs—cont'd

Type of Insert	Design	Power Setting	Indications	Adaptation and Activation
Precision thin (straight, left, right designs)	Probelike 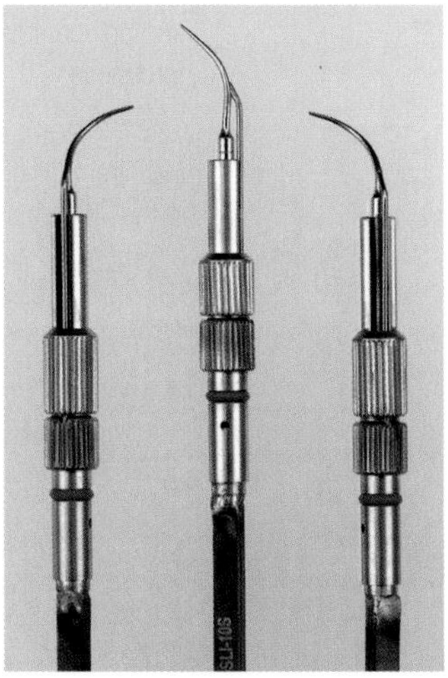 (Courtesy Tony Riso Company, North Miami Beach, Florida.) 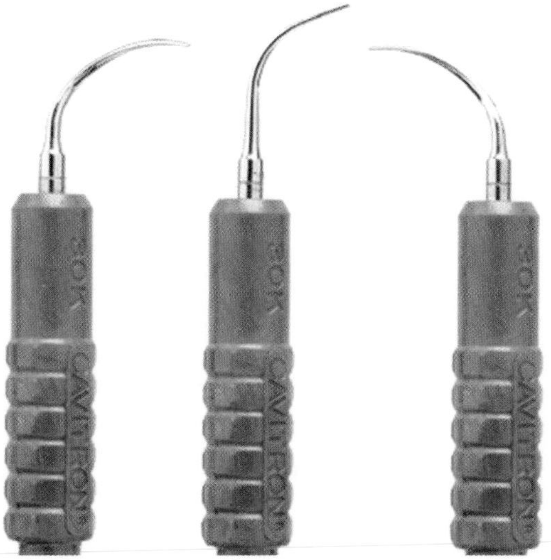 (Courtesy DENTSPLY International, Professional Division, York, Pennsylvania.)	Low to medium	Light subgingival periodontal debridement (calculus and biofilm) Shallow and deep pocket depth Concavities and furcations	Adapt sides and back; horizontal, vertical, and oblique strokes.
Micro-precision thin	Probelike	Low	For light deposit and oral biofilm Subgingival periodontal debridement Furcations Concavities	Adapt sides and back.

Continued

TABLE 27-1

Summary of Ultrasonic Insert Designs—cont'd

Type of Insert	Design	Power Setting	Indications	Adaptation and Activation
Precision thin	Furcation	Low to medium	Periodontal debridement in and adjacent to furcations Concavities	Furcation insert terminates with a small ball at the end.
Implants	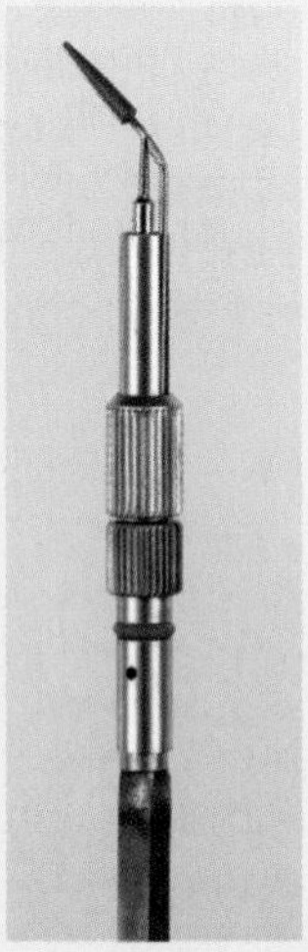 (Courtesy Tony Riso Company, North Miami Beach, Florida.) 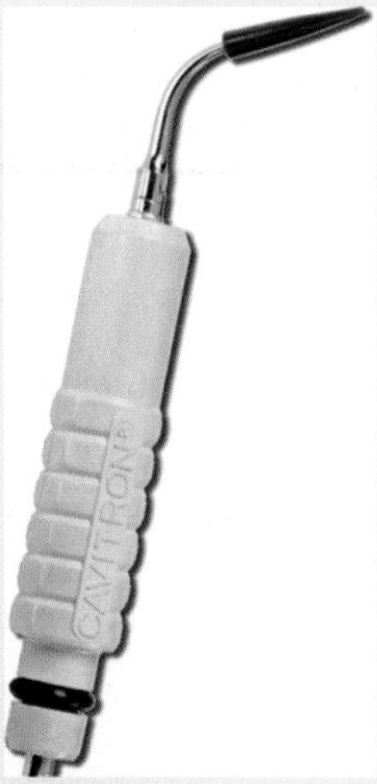 (Courtesy DENTSPLY International, Professional Division, York, Pennsylvania.)	Low	Debridement of dental implants	Adapt sides, using horizontal, oblique, or vertical strokes.

Note: Not all manufacturers make all designs. Designs for piezoelectric tips are similar.

- Oral biofilm (easily removed with ultrasonic instrumentation, so standard insert is not required for removal)
- Extrinsic tooth stain
- Orthodontic cement

Universal inserts (#1000, #100 or #10, DENTSPLY Professional) can be used supragingivally, primarily for initial debridement of moderate to heavy, nontenacious deposits. Depending on access and gingival contour and consistency, these inserts also can be used subgingivally.

Thin inserts have probelike, slim working-end designs (from 0.3 to 0.6 mm wide) indicated for periodontal debridement and removal of light deposits subgingivally, in shallow and deep pockets (e.g., Slimline by DENTSPLY Professional or After Five Ultrasonic Designs by Hu-Friedy). Supragingival applications include light deposits and debridement at the gingival margin, or root surfaces exposed after gingival recession. Thin inserts are at least 40% narrower in diameter than standard inserts, facilitating subgingival access, client comfort, and tactile sense. Micro slim inserts, the thinnest of tips, are also on the market. The slender width of the thin inserts should be considered when treating pockets in nonsurgical periodontal therapy (NSPT). The thinner the instrument, the greater chance of negotiating the pocket topography. Slim and microslim inserts are available in three designs as follows:

- Straight design—indicated for periodontal pockets that are 4 mm or less, although access into deeper areas may be possible depending on gingival contour and tone. It is adapted best to straighter surfaces and is especially useful on anterior teeth and in narrow periodontal pockets.
- Right and left designs—indicated to reach depths greater than 4 mm, concavities, and furcations. Their curved design facilitates adaptation to the curved tooth and root surfaces, including proximal surfaces.

Trends indicate that these thinner inserts debride the apical oral biofilm border in deep pockets. A comparison of pocket penetration with mini-inserts as compared to hand-activated, area-specific curets (i.e., Gracey) revealed that the mini-inserts allowed greater apical access with untreated periodontitis.[2] Even though precision thin inserts create more clinical attachment loss immediately after therapy as compared with the use of standard inserts, this difference does not affect the long-term clinical response to nonsurgical periodontal therapy.[3]

Furcation inserts (also considered thin inserts) have a 0.8-mm ball-end feature, providing more working-end surface area for periodontal debridement of furcations and root concavities where access permits. Furcation inserts also are available in three configurations—straight, right, and left—to enhance subgingival access and adaptation to root anatomy and furcations (e.g., Furcation Designs, Hu-Friedy) (Figure 27-8). Mean buccal furcation entrance dimension of maxillary first and second molars varies from 0.63 to 1.04 mm; openings in mandibular molars vary from 0.71 to 0.88 mm.[4] Standard inserts with an average of 0.56 mm in diameter, or hand-activated Gracey curets measuring 0.76 to 1.00 mm would not be able to access readily a furcation. The use of thin ultrasonic inserts or tips is indicated because a significant percentage of furcation entrances are not treatable by hand curets.[5] These thin tips also are beneficial in deep or narrow periodontal pockets. Diamond-coated inserts (DENTSPLY Professional) are available for furcations and root planing; however, they are recommended for surgical procedures with direct vision because of the rapid removal of deposits and potential for unintentional root surface removal. If used in dental hygiene therapy, the use of an endoscope is indicated.

Specially designed implant inserts are recommended to remove safely oral biofilm and loosely adherent calculus around titanium implants and abutments. Plastic or rubber-coated working ends have a polishing effect, although some can leave plastic residue on the implant surface. Metallic working ends, however, are avoided because they can cause damage to the implant surface.[6]

Function of Inserts

Inserts for magnetostrictive units deliver energy from all four working end surfaces: point, concave surface, convex surface, and sides or lateral surfaces. The point generates the greatest amount of energy and is not used to prevent unwanted surface alterations to the root and sensitivity. The lateral surfaces generate the least amount of energy. (Refer to Figure 27-9 to evaluate the order of energy generated.) The lateral surfaces (sides) and convex back of the working end are the surfaces that are adapted to the tooth.

In addition to the energy generated from the power and the frequency settings of a unit, the following other factors influence the energy emitted from the working end:

- Time of exposure: The longer the time spent on the tooth structure, the greater the amount of energy is expended.
- Pressure: Pressure increases the effects of the working end. When too much pressure is applied, it stops or dampens, and the clinician must reevaluate the pressure used. Calculus removal is less effective when strong lateral pressure is used.
- Shape: The more square the working end, the greater the amount of energy is expended. Blunt or rounded ends are preferred for light periodontal debridement because less energy output enhances comfort and reduces hard- and soft-tissue trauma.
- Angle of application: The greater the angle between the working end and the tooth, the greater the energy output. Typically the tooth-to-end angle should be 15 degrees or less.

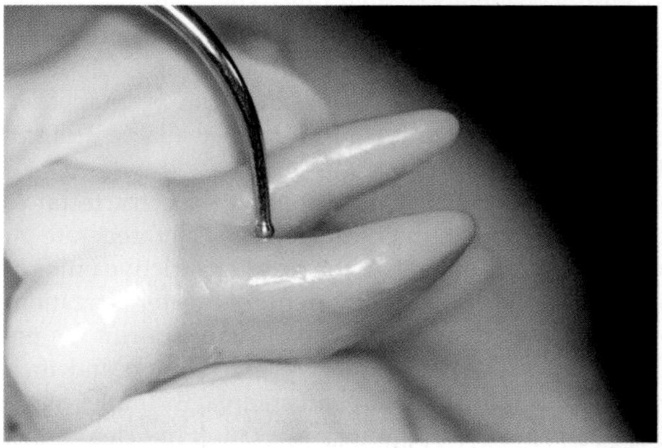

Figure 27-8. Furcation design. Ball-ended insert adapted to a maxillary first molar.

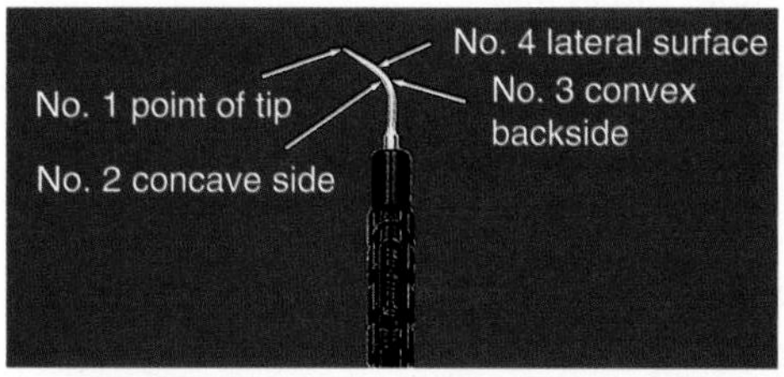

Figure 27-9. Power dispersion of a magnetostrictive insert working end. *(1)* Point generates the greatest amount of energy. *(2)* Concave side generates the second greatest amount of energy. *(3)* Convex backside generates less energy than the point or concave surface. *(4)* Lateral surface generates the least amount of energy. (Courtesy Hu-Friedy Manufacturing, Chicago, Illinois.)

Working end design is related to power setting. In general, the lowest effective power setting is used to accomplish the clinician's goal of biofilm removal or calculus removal. Low power is recommended for biofilm removal and light calculus removal using thin working ends for subgingival access. Medium- or higher-power settings are used for moderate to heavy calculus deposit that is tenacious; standard inserts also may be used, provided they can gain access to the area being treated. The higher the power setting, the more calculus removal; however, at lower-power settings a more favorable relationship occurs between deposit removal, minimal loss of tooth surface (dentin), and surface roughness.[7]

Insert Care and Maintenance

Inserts must be sterilized according to the manufacturer's instructions, which vary. Before autoclaving, most manufacturers recommend that used inserts be rinsed with water and dried. For sterilization, inserts should be placed in an all-paper or combination paper and plastic autoclave bag or preferably a cassette to decrease risk of damage and enhance insert longevity. All-plastic autoclave bags are not recommended, because the bag can build up too much heat during autoclaving and shorten the lifespan of the insert. For sterilization, bagged inserts should be placed on top of other instruments in the autoclave or processed separately to prevent damage. Inserts should not be placed in disinfectants because the chemicals may disintegrate the plastic grips and alter the metal components, resulting in a shorter insert lifespan.

Magnetostrictive inserts require maintenance of the O-ring (see Figure 27-3). To aid in slipping the tip into the handpiece, the ring is lubricated with water and gently twisted into place. O-rings are replaced when worn or cracked to prevent leakage of water at the junction of the handpiece and insert.

Inserts for magnetostrictive units wear out with regular use and should be examined often to ensure that the metal working ends are not bent and that the stacks are not damaged. The length of the working end also should be evaluated because wear over time shortens the end. Worn working ends reduce efficiency, resulting in extended instrumentation time, need for increased power settings, and risk of fracture. Working end wear in the following amounts has the following effects:

- A 1-mm loss results in 25% less efficiency.
- A 2-mm loss results in 50% less efficiency (replacement is recommended).

Efficiency guides provided by or purchased from a manufacturer are used to assess working end loss. Some manufacturers "retip" or refurbish inserts, but if the stack is original, it is still subject to aging.

Piezoelectric Units

A piezoelectric unit (see Figure 27-1) differs from a magnetostrictive unit in the following characteristics:

- Transducer material
- Working-end pattern (Figure 27-10)
- Activated surfaces of the working end
- Working-end and transducer-handpiece design
- Functions of the water source

A piezoelectric unit uses a transducer that consists of ceramic crystals. Vibration occurs when alternating electrical currents are applied to the transducer, creating a dimensional change that is transmitted to the working end as follows:

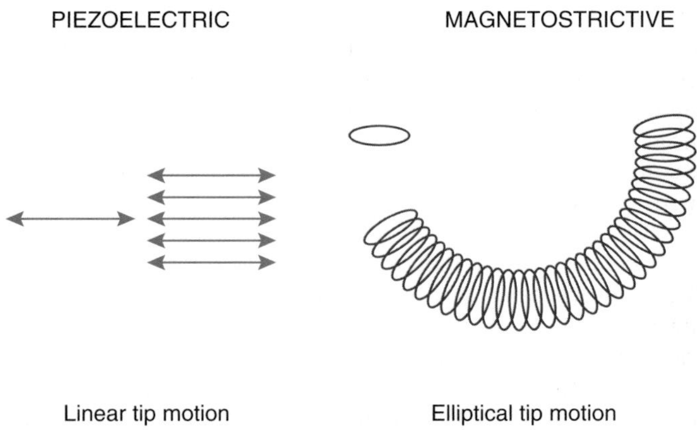

Figure 27-10. Working end motion of the piezoelectric and magnetostrictive units.

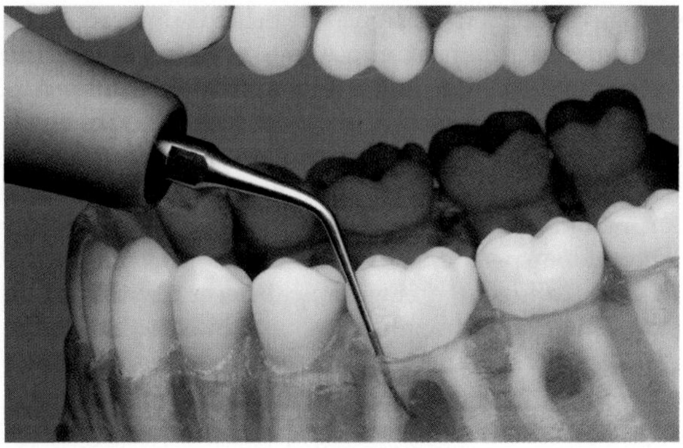

Figure 27-11. Piezoelectric tip adaptation. (Courtesy Hu-Friedy Manufacturing, Chicago, Illinois.)

- The working end moves in a linear pattern.
- All surfaces of the working end are activated; however, only the lateral surfaces are adapted to the tooth surface (Figure 27-11); lateral surfaces emit the least amount of energy. Research, however, demonstrates that once loaded against the tooth, the working end moves in an elliptical pattern similar to the magnetostrictive insert.[8]

The transducer is contained within the permanently sealed handpiece of the piezoelectric unit. The working end is threaded or screwed into the handpiece with a specialized wrench and is not connected to the transducer as is the insert used with a magnetostrictive unit. Therefore working ends for piezoelectric units are not transferable to magnetostrictive units. Piezoelectric units come with working ends designed for the unit; additional working ends can be purchased. If selecting this type of unit, consider the available designs for NSPT.

Cavitation is also a by-product of piezoelectric technology. The quartz crystals in the piezoelectric scaler generate virtually no heat in comparison to the magnetostrictive unit's heat-generating metal stack, which requires water irrigation for cooling. Less heat generation means you can run the piezoelectric device with very little water irrigation and thereby have better visibility of the treatment area. Examples of piezoelectric units are the Symmetry IQ 3000 (Hu-Friedy), Piezon Master 700 (Electro Medical Systems), and Amdent LM Pro-Power (LM Instruments). The active tip area for the 25- to

30-kHz piezoelectric units is from 2.2 to 3.5 mm, depending on tip design. Frequencies of the units vary from 25,000 to 50,000 kHz. Piezoelectric and magnetostrictive technologies appear to be similarly efficacious for ultrasonic instrumentation. Calculus removal immediately after debridement was equal between the piezoelectric and magnetostrictive units with similar tip designs.[9]

Tip Function, Care, and Maintenance

Tips are attached and unattached to the handpiece of the piezoelectric unit with a wrench mechanism. This device also can serve as a protective guard, depending on the manufacturer, and can be used in sterilization and storage of the tip (Figure 27-12). Color-coding is also available; the color of the guard for the tip matches the recommended primary power setting identified by color-coded power buttons on the control panel (Symmetry IQ, Hu-Friedy). Standard, universal, thin, and periodontal designs, as well as diamond-coated and implant tips are manufactured (Figure 27-13). Tips may be interchangeable between units and different manufacturers. Some tips are bladed, similar to a curet. Caution should be exercised when using bladed and diamond coated tips to avoid overinstrumentation. A newly developed piezoelectric tip made from copper and silver is suitable for the peri-implant surface because it has limited effects (roughness) on the titanium surface.[10] Plastic tips and copper alloy are acceptable for implant maintenance.[11] Handpieces are available with a fiberoptic illumination option.

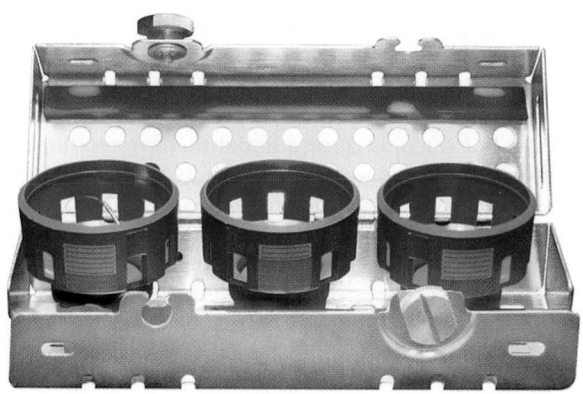

Figure 27-12. Piezoelectric wrench and tip storage.

Care should be taken to avoid using worn or damaged instrument tips. Tip wear guides are available to detect when tips need replacing because of wear. Piezoelectric tip wear has been shown to increase root roughness.[12] Cassettes are recommended to hold the tips, wrenches, and handpieces for sterilization to avoid damage or loss.

Table 27-2 provides a summary of the two types of ultrasonic instruments.

Health-Related Outcomes

Little difference exists between the long-term clinical response achieved with ultrasonic and hand instrumentation.[13] A combination of ultrasonic and hand instrumentation provides choices for clients needing oral prophylaxis, NSPT, and periodontal maintenance therapy. Interproximal areas, furcations, the cementoenamel junction, and multirooted teeth are most likely to exhibit residual calculus regardless of instrument method.

Microbial Findings and Endotoxin Removal

Equal reductions in microbial flora are found with the ultrasonic instrumentation and hand instrumentation.[13] Studies have evaluated periodontal pathogens such as *Porphyromonas gingivalis, Aggregatibacter actinomycetemcomitans, Tannerella forsythia, Prevotella intermedia,* and *Treponema denticola.*

Ultrasonic instrumentation is effective in removing weakly adherent endotoxin. Endotoxin removal is achieved with less time, effort, and root surface removal because of the powered action versus the hand instrumentation that ultimately could result in overinstrumentation.

Oral Biofilm and Calculus Removal

Hand and powered instrumentation seem to be equally effective in removing subgingival oral biofilm and calculus in

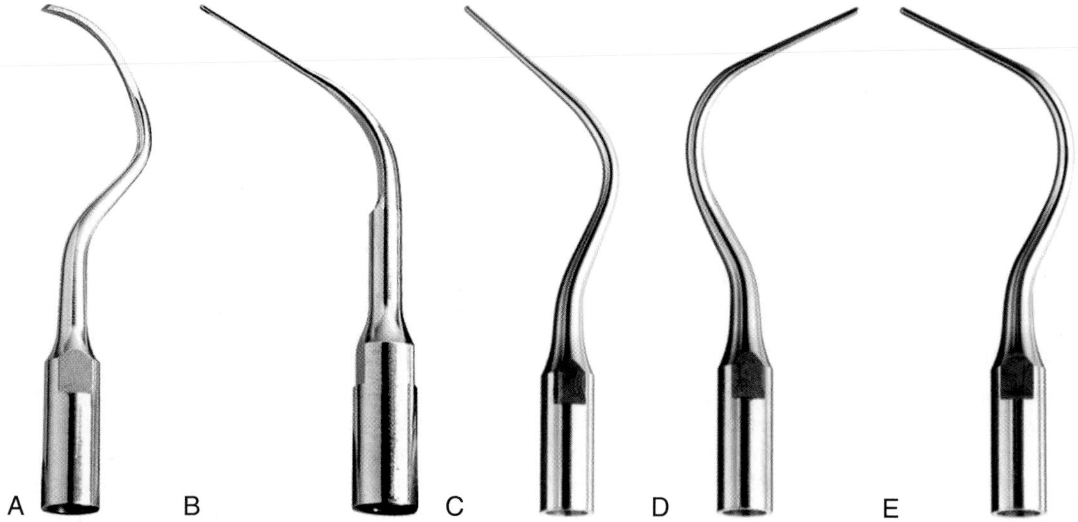

Figure 27-13. Examples of piezoelectric tip designs. **A,** Standard (#3). **B,** Standard (#10). **C, D, E,** Thin (straight, right, and left). (Courtesy Hu-Friedy Manufacturing, Chicago, Illinois.)

TABLE 27-2
Summary of Ultrasonic Instrumentation

Type of Unit	Frequency (cycles per second)	Type of Transducer	Motion of Insert	Activated Surfaces of Working End	Active Tip Area	Water Used as Coolant
Magnetostrictive ultrasonic	25,000-42,000	Stack of metal strips (Permanickel) or ferrite solid rod	Elliptical or orbital	All; back and sides are used most often	4.3 mm (ultimately depends on frequency)	Yes
Piezoelectric ultrasonic	25,000-50,000	Ceramic	Linear to tight elliptical when loaded	The two lateral sides of the tip are more active	2.3-3.5 mm	Yes, but less may be needed

NSPT. Furthermore, both types of ultrasonic instrumentation seem to be equally effective at the clinical endpoint in moderate calculus removal.[9] To date, new designs in powered instruments have not shown an advantage over those of the past; however, it is known that different tips and devices produce different results in vitro.[14]

Aerosols and Spatter

During mechanized periodontal debridement a large amount of contaminated aerosols and spatter are produced.[15] Dental **aerosols** are fine, airborne particles that are liquid, solid, or a combination of both and are 50 μm or less in size. **Spatter** includes particles greater than 50 μm that travel a considerable distance from the source and splash on environmental surfaces, masks, and the operator's skin and clothes. Source of the contamination is the client's blood, saliva, and bacteria, and the water spray coolant provides the means for the aerosols. Airborne particles can be pulled into the nasal passages and respiratory system. The dried residue formed by evaporation of liquid-containing particles, called **droplet nuclei**, can carry potentially infectious microorganisms such as the respiratory bacteria, *Mycobacterium tuberculosis.* Large and small particles contain blood elements with attached viral particles, such as human immunodeficiency virus (HIV) or hepatitis B virus (HBV).

The number of potentially pathogenic organisms in aerosol and spatter produced by ultrasonic instrumentation remains unknown. No epidemiologic studies link dental aerosols to disease transmission; however, the dental hygienist should be concerned about this potential.

A recent study showed that blood-contaminated aerosols are suspended in the air in general dental settings after ultrasonic instrumentation and that extraoral evacuation systems are an advantage in reducing aerosols.[15] Currently, high-speed suction and specially designed evacuation systems are recommended to reduce aerosols for the benefit of the client and clinician.

Root Surface Roughness

Considerable attention has been focused on roughness of the root or implant created by various instrumentation methods.[1] A smoother root or titanium implant surface is assumed to have less chance of biofilm reattachment and recurrent periodontal disease (peri-mucositis or peri- implantitis). Laboratory studies showed similar root roughness between hand and ultrasonic methods.[16] Various methods—copper silver alloy, plastic tips, and piezoelectric metal tips—produce some degree of roughness and the copper silver alloy and plastic tips were favorable over the piezoelectric method.[17] Tip angulation, exposure time, lateral pressure, tip wear,[11] and power settings are critical factors to consider to avoid overinstrumentation. Future research that evaluates the long-term effects of this roughness on clinical outcomes is indicated.

Root Substance Removal

To prevent root surface damage, the piezoelectric tip must be angulated as close to 0 degrees to the root as possible. Lateral force and tip angulation seem to have the greatest influence on the amount of surface removed.

Removal of calculus during initial therapy requires multiple instrument designs and increased instrumentation time compared with periodontal maintenance (PM); however, PM requires frequent visits over the life of the tooth. Preventing root structure damage and loss of substance is a consideration; therefore power-driven instruments are potentially advantageous in PM.

Client Preference

Limited evidence addresses client preference for either magnetostrictive or piezoelectric devices. Participants in a study generally preferred the piezoelectric unit in relation to less discomfort and vibration[18] and indicated they would prefer it for treatment at the next re-care interval.[19] Results of studies such as these may assist clinicians in providing additional client comfort and increased adherence with re-care intervals.

Ultrasonic Instruments in Practice

Advantages

There is increased efficiency of removal for large calculus deposits when compared with hand instrumentation. (See Box 27-1.) Burnished calculus, however, could result if ultrasonic instruments alone are used for tenacious deposit removal. For large and tenacious deposits, the clinical power of the unit is increased and hand instruments, such as the periodontal working file, are incorporated into debridement therapy. Also, it takes less time to debride with ultrasonic instrumentation when compared with hand instrumentation.[14] Overall, the increased efficiency is a benefit for hygienist and client.

Multiple surfaces of the working end can be used to remove deposits rather than the single-surface cutting edge

BOX 27-1

Advantages and Disadvantages of Power-Driven Instruments as Compared with Hand Instruments

ADVANTAGES	DISADVANTAGES
Increased efficiency	More precautions and limitations
Multiple surfaces of tip are capable of removing deposits	Client comfort (water spraying)
	Aerosol production
No need to sharpen	Temporary hearing shifts
Less chance for repetitive stress injuries	Noise
	Less tactile sensation
Handpiece size large	Reduced visibility
Reduced lateral pressure	
Less tissue distention	
Water	
Lavage	
Irrigation	
Acoustic mainstreaming	

of a curet. A single precise curet blade must be adapted at a precise tooth-to-blade angle to remove calculus and extrinsic stain in a channeling fashion—one reason why hand instrument debridement is technically demanding.

Ultrasonic working ends never need sharpening as hand instruments do, saving time and effort for the operator and client. Also, inserts or tips are replaced less often than curets.

A large-diameter handpiece is an advantage for the clinician because it does not require much pinching motion to hold it as compared with a smaller-diameter manual instrument handle. In addition, lateral pressure is not needed to enhance activation of the working end; therefore the chance of developing repetitive strain injuries could be reduced (see Chapter 11).

Water lavage and irrigation may enhance healing and client comfort when compared with hand instrumentation. Enhanced comfort could be a result of the warm lavage and/or the fact that less lateral pressure is needed to remove the deposit. Acoustic mainstreaming associated with water coolant also removes bacteria.

Disadvantages

Water flow can interfere with client comfort because of unavoidable spray on the cheeks and chin. Aerosol production is a concern, although further evidence is needed to study its effects on the clinician and client. (See Box 27-1.)

Temporary hearing shifts from airborne subharmonics have been observed with the ultrasonic instrument. Tinnitus, an early sign of hearing loss, may occur. For the client, ultrasound travels through the tooth to the inner ear via bones in the skull. This is possible via instrumentation on molar teeth. At times the noise produced also may be uncomfortable for the client. Further research on hearing loss in the clinician and client is needed.

Water spray interferes with the operator's visibility and potential contamination is produced. Continued oral evacuation is a must, and commercially prepared solutions to prevent mirror fog may be useful (see section on instrumentation technique for mechanized instruments).

Indications

With precision thin designs, the clinician can remove lighter deposits supragingivally and subgingivally. Subgingival instrumentation for calculus, oral biofilm, root surface constituents, and periodontal pathogens is accomplished primarily with thin designs. Standard inserts, however, probably extend subgingivally about 1 to 3 mm depending on the tissue, access to the area, insert selection, and client sensitivity.

Mechanized instruments also can assist in the removal of excess cement and bonding agents around orthodontic appliances and after appliance removal. In these cases, manual instrumentation is usually not as effective. Other indications include dental hygiene care for necrotizing periodontal diseases, pericoronitis, or treatment during surgical interventions (removal of residual deposits and granulation tissue).

Precautions

Caution should be exercised when a client reports having a cardiovascular implantable device such as a pacemaker or cardioverter-defibrillator.[20] Unshielded pacemakers may be disrupted by external electric fields. Older models were unipolar and less insulated, causing interference from dental equipment. Newer shielded models are bipolar and well insulated, so the small amount of electromagnetic radiation generated by dental equipment is less of a concern. Select electronic devices such as ultrasonic units, ultrasonic cleaning systems, and battery-operated composite curing lights can affect the sensing and pacing activities of pacemakers and ICD in vitro.[21] Evidence is inconsistent and a conservative and practical approach is recommended.[20]

- Encourage clients to carry the implant devices' identification card including the manufacturer, model number, serial number, date of implantation, and mode of operation.
- Consultation with the cardiologist of record provides more information.

In summary, magnetostrictive units are not be recommended depending on model of implant device and shielding; piezoelectric units do not seem to affect these devices, and further in vivo trials are needed. Another consideration is use of ultrasonic instrumentation around individuals with implantable cardiac devices, such as co-workers or other healthcare providers.

Communicable diseases such as hepatitis, tuberculosis, strep throat, and respiratory infections could be transmitted via aerosols. Clients with communicable disease should not receive elective dental hygiene care until the disease has been treated for an appropriate period of time. When it is appropriate based on health status, standard precautions are employed to protect the client and clinician. All clients should be provided with a 30-second rinse of 0.12% chlorhexidine gluconate to reduce the number of organisms in aerosols before care.

- Presence of demineralized tooth structure, dentinal hypersensitivity, restorative materials, and restorations such as veneers, cast crowns, and titanium implants do not prevent the clinician from using powered instruments; however, these localized areas should be avoided or treated properly. Working end placement should occur adjacent to these conditions and not on or within these entities. In the case of implants, the appropriate working end for the needed therapy should be selected (see Table 27-1). The periodontal and dental chart guides decisions about surfaces to treat or avoid. If restorative material is on the clinical crown, and the working end can be placed apical to the restoration, it can be used. Restorative materials can be affected adversely by creating roughness or striations (e.g., on composite restorations, black-colored striations result because the composite material will abrade the metal tip). Also, undue wear to the working end can occur when it is placed against metal restorations.

- Use with children is a concern because vibrations may negatively affect young growing tissue. Primary and newly erupted teeth have large pulp chambers that are more susceptible to heat generated by dental instruments. Water "ow and temperature of the instrument must be appropriate at all times, especially with children. The lowest possible power setting is recommended
- Special precautions are indicated when a client is immunosuppressed from a disease or from chemotherapy; for example, HIV infection, organ transplantation, cancer, systemic lupus erythematous, Crohn's disease, or corticosteroid therapy may increase risk of opportunistic infection from breathing contaminated aerosols and from ingesting contaminated dental unit water.

Contraindications

Mechanized instrumentation should *not* be used with clients who report any of the following conditions:

- Lung/pulmonary disease—Acute pulmonary infections such as bronchitis or pneumonia contraindicate elective dental hygiene care. Unstable conditions such as shortness of breath when resting, a productive cough, or an oxygen saturation less than 91% also are reasons to reschedule elective dental hygiene or dental care and make a medical referral. Chronic pulmonary disease includes asthma, emphysema, cystic fibrosis, and pneumonia. Unstable conditions such as shortness of breath at rest, a productive cough, upper respiratory infection, or an oxygen saturation less than 91% are reasons to reschedule the appointment and make a medical referral. Although no studies have shown direct negative consequences of ultrasonic scaling in clients with chronic pulmonary diseases, caution is exercised during production of aerosols in any client experiencing difficulty breathing. In a small-scale study, clients with COPD (chronic bronchitis and emphysema) and chronic periodontitis were treated with magnetostrictive instrumentation, hand instrumentation, and no instrumentation, and no significant differences were found after care as measured by respiratory and illness questionnaires.[22] Risk versus benefit must be considered in care planning for each client with pulmonary disease.
- Dysphagia or swallowing difficulty caused by water flow (e.g., muscular dystrophy, multiple sclerosis, paralysis, or a psychologic disorder) may affect the client's swallowing.

A summary of the indications, precautions, and contraindications is found in Box 27-2. Box 27-3 provides recommendations for discussion and demonstration of power-driven instruments with a client.

Unit Tuning

Autotuned Units (Magnetostrictive and Piezoelectric)

Frequency is already preset; the clinician controls only energy output by adjusting the power knob. The lowest power

BOX 27-2

Indications, Precautions, and Contraindications

Indications

- Supragingival debridement of calculus and extrinsic stain
- Subgingival debridement of calculus, oral biofilm, root surface constituents, and periodontal pathogens
- Removal of orthodontic cement
- Gingival and periodontal conditions and diseases
- Surgical interventions

Precautions

- Implanted pacemakers and defibrillators
- Infectious diseases: human immunodeficiency virus, hepatitis, tuberculosis (active stages)
- Demineralized tooth surface
- Exposed dentin (associated with sensitivity)
- Restorative materials (porcelain, amalgam, gold, composite)
- Children (primary teeth)
- Immunosuppression from disease or chemotherapy
- Uncontrolled diabetes mellitus
- Pulmonary disease

Contraindications

- Unstable pulmonary disease
- Swallowing difficulty (dysphagia)

BOX 27-3

Recommendations for Discussion of Ultrasonic Instruments with a Client

Operation. Discuss how instrument operates by electrical energy that is converted to mechanical energy (sound waves) to create mechanical tip movement to remove deposits.

Water use. Discuss why water is needed.

Water evacuation. Demonstrate how water will be evacuated using either high-volume or low-volume suction.

Feel of instrumentation. Describe what the instrument will feel like. Clients need to know they should not experience discomfort.

Discomfort. Discuss what to do if it the instrumentation is uncomfortable. Explain that the water, the tip, and heat are factors that can create a problem with client comfort. If any of these factors is present, advise client to raise a hand so that proper adjustments can be made. Assure client that in most cases adjustment can result in comfort.

Sound. Demonstrate what instrument will sound like (high-pitched noise). Any extended noise exposure can produce temporary hearing shifts. If sound is too bothersome, direct the client to let you know. If a hearing aid is worn, it should be turned off.

Adjunct instrumentation. Discuss use of hand instruments because ultrasonic instruments alone will not accomplish clinical and therapeutic goals.

Informed consent. Questions should be answered to the client's satisfaction. A two-way discussion occurs to gain informed consent.

setting that is effective should be selected. For most procedures, a low to medium power setting is usually adequate. Water flow must be adjusted with the water knob to achieve a fine mist or spray.

Manual-Tuned Units

Frequency, power, and water are controlled by the clinician. The option to tune frequency is available only in manual-tuned units; this increases the clinician's control over insert performance. The tuning procedure is repeated for each new insert as follows:

- Power is adjusted to the lowest setting and the frequency knob is adjusted so that no vibration is emitted from the tip.
- External water conduit (if using one) is positioned 1 mm from the back of the tip and not contacting the insert.
- With desired insert in place, the handpiece is held in a horizontal position in relation to the floor.
- Insert tip is pointed upward toward the ceiling; the water is adjusted until an arch from 1 to 1½ inches occurs over the tip. This arch of water ensures adequate water flow.
- Insert tip is pointed downward toward the floor; the frequency knob is adjusted so that a light aerosol of water is emitted from the tip, accompanied by a fluent stream of water.
- Adjustments in power are available at the lower end for light deposits or root surface debridement, and power boosts may be available in the foot pedal for heavier or more tenacious deposits encountered intermittently.

In phase and *out of phase* are terms used to describe the frequency adjustment of an insert:

- **In phase** means that the insert is adjusted to resonance frequency for maximum energy output. This level of tuning puts the insert at peak efficiency suitable for light to heavy deposit removal. Usually the in-phase adjustment is used with standard inserts and a fine mist of water; in phase also is used for thin inserts for removal of light to moderate deposits or periodontal maintenance care.
- **Out of phase** means that the insert is detuned from resonance frequency. The out-of-phase adjustment usually is used with the thin inserts and a fine mist with a water drip for light deposit and biofilm removal (Figure 27-14). Out-of-phase adjustment is thought to enhance client comfort and results in less vibration for debridement procedures.

Instrumentation Technique

Positioning

The client is placed in a normal supine position appropriate for the maxillary or mandibular arch (e.g., if applying an instrument to the mandibular right lingual surface, have client turn to the right). Water pools in the right posterior of the oral cavity, where suction can remove it efficiently, reducing the potential for gagging. The client turns to the right for the right side of the mouth to be treated and to the left for treatment on the left side.

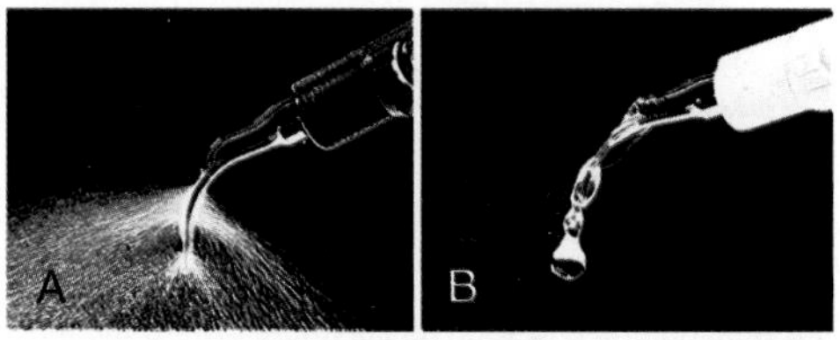

Figure 27-14. Tuning options. **A,** In phase. **B,** Out of phase. (Courtesy Hu-Friedy Manufacturing, Chicago, Illinois.)

Suction and Retraction

High-volume suction that requires assistance from another individual is recommended for the following reasons:

- To reduce aerosols created
- To prevent pathogens and dislodged deposits from being aspirated by client
- If assistance is not available, a low-speed saliva ejector with either a straight saliva ejector or a curved circular ejector is used (Hygoformic, Pulpdent, Orsing, Crosstex) as follows:
  - For a straight device: The client participates by holding and placing the ejector intraorally as needed. Another option is the use of a straight suction tip (Otis Formeject) with a tubing device (Blue Boa) that allows the clinician to use both hands for instrumentation. The client does not participate as much because the suction tip is bent and placed in the oral cavity while instrumentation occurs.
  - For a curved circular ejector: The suction hose is extended behind the dental chair to place the ejector in the mouth. The weight of the hose stabilizes the ejector. This ejector can retract the buccal mucosa when placed between the buccal plane of the teeth and the cheek mucosa. The circular end is twisted to adapt to the contour of the cheek and to expose the holes where the water exits to the suction hose. A long suction hose can be used to connect the high-speed evacuation and the hygoformic ejector (Blue Boa) to enhance instrumentation. Another option to increase visibility is a suction mirror device (EMS Hammer Head).

Retracting the client's lips helps control the water. In the anterior the lips can form a cuplike space between the facial tooth surfaces and mucosa. In the posterior the lips can be retracted away from the teeth to form a space for the water to pool.

Grasp

A light grasp, similar to that used with exploration, is needed because it increases tactile sensitivity and reduces the likelihood of excessive lateral pressure. The light grasp is all that is necessary because tip activation removes the biofilm or calculus deposit, not pressure. The grasp occurs next to the junction of the handpiece and insert, or the grasp may be placed further up the handpiece to enhance access.

The handpiece cord should be straight and not twisted to prevent undue stress on the operator's shoulder, arm, and hand. The cord can be draped over the clinician's shoulder, draped over the light handle, or held between the ring and little fingers. When the clinician is adapting the tip to the tooth and rolling the handpiece within the grasp, strain also is placed on the clinician's arm. The insert therefore should be rotated (using the nondominant hand) within the handpiece of the magnetostrictive unit to minimize this strain. Rotation of the insert within the handpiece occurs when adaptating the tip between the distal and buccal or lingual surfaces, as well as the buccal or lingual surfaces and the mesial surfaces. If the handpiece alone is rotated, the cord could get twisted, causing ergonomic problems.

Using a handpiece that rotates to eliminate twisting of the cord, reduce cable drag, and minimize stress on internal tubings enhances ergonomics. The Swivel Direct Flow Inserts by Hu-Friedy and the Cavitron Steri-Mate handpiece cable with swivel by DENTSPLY Professional have been designed to address this ergonomic issue.

Fulcrum

An intraoral or extraoral fulcrum may be used with standard designs, whereas an extraoral fulcrum is recommended with thin designs because only an extremely light stroke is needed to debride. The extraoral fulcrum enhances the tactile sensitivity. The dental hygienist does not need a firm fulcrum on tooth surface as with hand instrumentation because strength to exert lateral pressure is not indicated. Fulcrum placement is either conventional, opposite arch, or cross-arch, depending on the surface being treated. Grasp relates to the fulcrum placement just as with hand instrumentation. In other words, a cross-arch fulcrum requires the clinician to place the grasp further back on the handpiece.

Dental Mirror Use

The mirror is still used, but visibility is impaired. Operators tend to use direct vision as much as possible while striving to attain ergonomically correct client and operator positioning. Use of magnification lens and headlights also enhances vision.

Adaptation

For adapting the working end, use the correct part of the active tip: 2 to 4 mm. For supragingival debridement the clinician focuses on visible deposit (Figure 27-15). For subgingival debridement all root surfaces usually are covered.

The easiest way to adapt any universal working end to the tooth surface is to think of the application in relation to a universal curet, that is, the tip is directed toward the distal surface when the clinician is inserting the tip at the distal line angle (Figure 27-16). The clinician then activates the tip toward the distal surface while adapting the lateral surface of the tip. To keep the tip adapted, the clinician rolls and pivots it while advancing the tip to extend to the midline of the distal surface.

Next the clinician reinserts the tip, adapting the tip parallel to the long axis at the distal line angle, advances across the buccal or lingual surface, and rolls and pivots (or turns the insert in the handpiece) at the mesial line angle to keep the side of the tip adapted to the tooth surface (Figure 27-17, *A* and *B*). The clinician ensures that the tip reaches the midline of the mesial surface. The tip is applied somewhat diagonally to the long axis of proximal surfaces (Figure 27-17, *C*). Another approach to the buccal or lingual area is to complete the distal surface of each tooth first, then to approach the buccal and lingual surfaces, then the mesial surfaces one by one. This method involves less rolling and pivoting and allows the clinician to move the insert in the handpiece less often.

With magnetostrictive units the convex or back surface of the working end can be used. Adapting the convex surface to

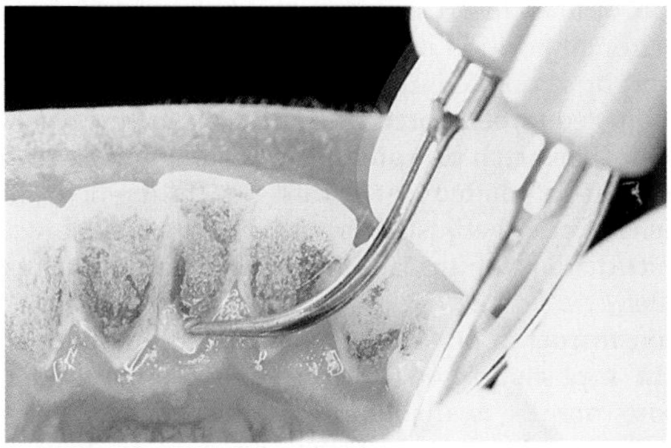

Figure 27-15. Working end adapted for supragingival debridement. (Courtesy Hu-Friedy, Chicago, Illinois.)

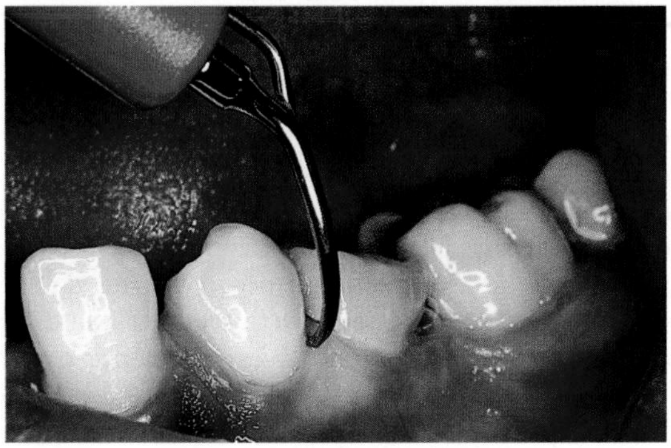

Figure 27-16. Thin working end adapted to distal surface covered with dental calculus. (Courtesy Hu-Friedy, Chicago, Illinois.)

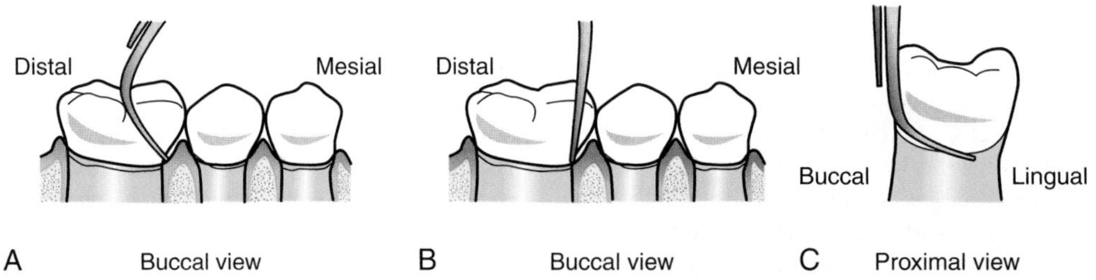

Figure 27-17. Right precision thin working end used to debride the buccal surfaces. **A,** Select working end based on its curvature toward the mesial surface. Adapt working end below contact area. **B,** Roll working end onto the proximal surface. Keep working end against tooth. **C,** Extend working end toward the lingual surface to negotiate the cementoenamel junction and proximal surfaces.

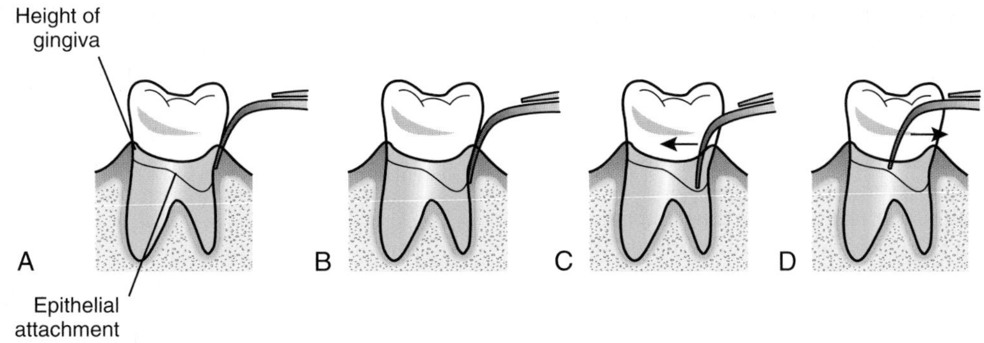

Figure 27-18. Pocket negotiation. **A,** Enter pocket using the back surface. Keep working end in contact with root and parallel to the long axis of the root. **B,** Negotiate working end to the apical extent of the pocket using minute overlapping strokes. *Note:* Weight of the instrument and the oscillations generated guides the working end subgingivally. **C,** To move the working end along the epithelial attachment, use the back and a pushlike stroke to avoid trauma and client discomfort. **D,** Avoid using a pull stroke with front or concave surface when working end is against the epithelial attachment. Place current periodontal charting and radiographs within view for reference during instrumentation.

the enamel and cementum is indicated for loss of clinical attachment, periodontal pockets, root concavities, and furca (Figure 27-18). At all times the tip to tooth angle is 15 degrees or less. The point of the insert or tip is ***never*** placed on the tooth surface because it could cause iatrogenic damage (clinician-caused damage). With standard-size inserts, extension to the epithelial attachment is not an objective.

With piezoelectric units the active sides of the tip are adapted carefully and maintained during the procedure. Again, the terminal portion of the tip is adapted unless manufacturer's directions recommend other aspects of the tip be adapted.

Activation

Tip activation is initiated by wrist movement or rocking from the fulcrum as with hand instrumentation. The tip must be moving at all times to prevent iatrogenic damage to the root or crown of the tooth, excessive heat, or a "shock" effect felt by the client. Strokes are overlapping and multidirectional: oblique and vertical strokes are used primarily; however, horizontal and combination strokes also are employed. Movement in different directions helps break up calculus deposits and aids in treating all root surfaces in periodontal pockets. Removal of large to moderate subgingival deposits occurs from the gingival margin to the epithelial attachment. Removal of lighter deposits and biofilm occurs from the epithelial attachment to the gingival margin. It is important to use the working end like a periodontal probe when removing heavier tenacious deposits and to tap on the top and sides of the deposit to fracture it. If the clinician activates the working end on the outside of the deposit and shaves layers of deposit, instead of fracturing, it causes deposit smoothing (burnishing).

Different designs of inserts/tips require different techniques for instrumentation. (See Table 27-1 and Procedure 27-1 to review the designs, indications, and applications.) Instrumentation with precision thin designs parallels instrumentation with standard designs, keeping in mind differences in purpose of therapy. Right and left inserts are used successfully in the posterior regions and adapted like a universal curet, as previously described. A straight design is used in deep periodontal pockets and furcations and adapts well in anterior regions of the mouth. Instrumentation of furcations is achieved with multiple thin designs. They are adapted using the sides (lateral) or back (convex) into the concavities adjacent to the furcation and on the mesial and distal surfaces of the furcation itself. The tooth is mentally divided into two teeth—one tooth being the distal root and the other tooth being the mesial root. Both distal surfaces are treated first, then the buccal and lingual surfaces of the roots are treated, and finally the mesial surfaces of each root are debrided.

Hand instruments are considered as adjuncts to ultrasonic instruments, and an explorer is used to evaluate the clinical endpoint.

CLIENT EDUCATION TIPS

- A combination of hand and power-driven instrumentation is recommended to obtain optimal results from periodontal debridement in a variety of cases and settings.
- Advantages of power-driven over hand instrumentation include increased efficiency, enhanced comfort, adaptation of multiple surface areas of the tip, less tissue distention, less pressure, and water for lavage.
- Disadvantages of power driven over hand instrumentation include aerosols, possible temporary hearing problems, noise, and the water spray.

LEGAL, ETHICAL, AND SAFETY ISSUES

- The client must be informed of the nonsurgical periodontal therapy and periodontal maintenance care plan, including method of periodontal debridement, and must participate in decision making.
- There is no significant difference in long-term healing between hand and power-driven instrumentation.
- Informed consent should be obtained for this method of instrumentation.
- Consultation with the physician of record may be necessary to evaluate the client's health status before ultrasonic instrumentation.
- The hygienist uses evidence-based decision making to select interventions for care and remains current with information about mechanized instrumentation by reading systematic reviews and attending continuing education courses.

KEY CONCEPTS

- Mechanical pocket therapy is periodontal debridement using hand and/or ultrasonic instrumentation; both methods are efficacious.
- Two modes of ultrasonic instrumentation are magnetostrictive and piezoelectric.
- Manual-tuned ultrasonic units allow the clinician unlimited adjustments to the frequency, but autotuned units do not. Some autotuned units offer an option for adjusting the power at the lower end of the power range and the frequency is automatically adjusted to correlate with the power setting. Both types require the clinician to control power and water.
- Two basic types of working-end are the standard design and thin design.

CRITICAL THINKING EXERCISES

1. Role-playing: Discuss the use of ultrasonic instrumentation for a client who has not experienced this method of periodontal debridement. Include an overview of factors identified in Box 27-3.
2. A client reports tooth sensitivity after ultrasonic instrumentation. Develop a care plan to eliminate dentinal hypersensitivity.

REFERENCES

1. Walmsley AD, Lea SC, Felver B, et al: Mapping cavitational activity around dental ultrasonic tips. *Clin Oral Investig* 17:1227, 2013.
2. Barendregt DS, van der Velden U, Timmerman MF, et al: Penetration depths with an ultrasonic mini insert compared with a conventional curette in patients with periodontitis and in periodontal maintenance. *J Clin Perio* 35:31, 2008.
3. Casarin RC, Bittencourt S, Ribeiro Edel P, et al: Influence of immediate attachment loss during instrumentation employing thin ultrasonic tips on clinical response to nonsurgical periodontal therapy. *Quintessence Int* 41:249, 2010.
4. Hou GL, Chen SF, Wu YM, et al: The topography of the furcation entrance in Chinese molars: furcations entrance dimensions. *J Clin Perio* 21:451, 1994.
5. Al Habashneh RA, Khader YS, Al Masri S, et al: Furcation entrance dimensions of first and second mandibular molars among Jordanians. *Oral Health Prev Dent* 8:401, 2010.
6. Mann M, Parmar D, Walmsley AD, et al: Effect of plastic covered ultrasonic scalers on titanium implant surfaces. *Clin Oral Implants Res* 23:76, 2012.
7. Bless K, Sener B, Dual J, et al: Cleaning ability and induced dentin loss of a magnetostrictive ultrasonic. *Clin Oral Invest* 15:241, 2012.
8. Lea SC, Walmsley AD: Mechano-physical and biophysical properties of power-driven scalers: driving the future of powered instrument design and evaluation. *Periodontology 2000* 51:63, 2009.
9. Brion SL, Hodges KO, Calley KH, et al: A comparison of dental ultrasonic technologies on subgingival calculus removal; a pilot study. *JDH* 86:150, 2012.
10. Seol HW, Heo SJ, Koak JK, et al: Surface alterations of several dental materials by novel ultrasonic scaler tip. *Int J Oral Maxillofac Implants* 27:801, 2012.
11. Baek SH, Shon WJ, Bae KS, et al: Evaluation of the safety and efficiency of novel ultrasonic scaler tip on titanium surfaces. *Clin Oral Implants Research* 23:1269, 2012.
12. Arabaci T, Cicek Y, Dilsiz A, et al: Influence of tip wear of piezoelectric ultrasonic scalers on root surface roughness at different working parameters: a profilometric and atomic force microscopy study. *Int J Dent Hyg* 11:69, 2013.
13. Ioannou I, Dimitriadis N, Papadimitriou K, et al: Hand instrumentation versus ultrasonic debridement in the treatment of chronic periodontitis: a randomized clinical and microbial trial. *J Clin Perio* 36:132, 2009.
14. Walmsley AD, Lea SC, Landini G, et al: Advances in power driven pocket/root instrumentation. *J Clin Periodontol* 35(8 Suppl):22, 2008.
15. Yamada H, Ishihama K, Yasuda K, et al: Aerial dispersal of blood-contaminated aerosols during dental procedures. *Quintessence Inter* 42:399, 2011.
16. Singh S, Uppoor A, Nayak D: A comparative evaluation of the efficacy of manual, magnetostrictive and piezoelectric ultrasonic instruments—an in vitro profilometric and SEM study. *J Appl Oral Sci* 20:21, 2012.
17. Unursaikhan O, Lee JS, Cha JK, et al: Comparative evaluation of roughness of titanium surfaces treated by different hygiene instruments. *J Periodontal Implant Sci* 42(3):88, 2012.
18. Muhney KA, Dechow PC: Patients' perception of pain during ultrasonic debridement: a comparison between piezoelectric and magnetostrictive scalers, *JDH* 84:185, 2010.
19. Brion-Silva L: *Master's thesis. Comparison of dental ultrasonic technologies on subgingival calculus removal and patient preference: a pilot study*, 2008, Idaho State University, p. 254.
20. Stoopler ET, Sia YW, Arthur S, et al: Does ultrasonic dental equipment affect cardiovascular implantable electronic devices? *J Can Dent Assoc* 77:b113, 2011.
21. Roedig JJ, Shah J, Elayi CS, et al: Interference of cardiac pacemaker and implantable cardioverter-defibrillator activity during electronic dental device use. *J Am Dent Assoc* 141(5):521, 2010.
22. Agado BE, Crawford B, Delarosa J, et al: Effects of periodontal instrumentation on quality of life and illness in patients with chronic obstructive pulmonary disease: a pilot study. *J Dent Hyg* 86:204, 2012.

ⓔ EVOLVE RESOURCES

Please visit http://evolve.elsevier.com/Darby/hygiene for additional practice and study support tools.

Root Morphology and Instrumentation Implications

CHAPTER 28

Lynn Bergstrom Bryan

COMPETENCIES

1. Discuss general morphologic considerations, including:
   - Describe the roots of each of the permanent teeth in terms of numbers, shapes, and characteristic landmarks.
   - Discuss significance of root morphology and positioning in the alveolar bone to root instrumentation.
   - Describe variations in root structure that may affect the dental hygiene process of care.
   - Explain how the contour of the cementoenamel junction, root morphology in both horizontal and vertical directions, furcation location, and root concavities influence instrument adaptation on root surfaces.
   - State the importance of tooth alignment to instrument adaptation on root surfaces.
2. Identify variations of root form and explain the significance for root instrumentation.

Various assessment instruments (e.g., the periodontal probe, Nabers probe, dental explorer) are used for assessing root surface characteristics. Current periapical and vertical bitewing radiographs on screen or view box provide information on root number, shape, and alterations; furcation location; bone height and contour; calculus, caries, and defective restorations and other contributing factors that may influence root instrumentation.

An anatomically correct model of the dentition with transparent gingiva is helpful for visualizing anatomy of individual roots and their positioning within the alveolar processes. Models and Table 28-1 can be used for review. See Chapters 19 and 26 for a review of periodontal assessment and assessment instruments.

General Morphologic Considerations

See Table 28-1 (Figures 28-1 through 28-14) for specific information for each tooth.

Root Terminology

The anatomic root of a tooth is that part of the dentin covered by cementum and embedded in the alveolar bone; it begins at the cementoenamel junction. The end of the root is called the root apex, and the area surrounding the apex is the periapex. At the apex is an opening, the periapical foramen, where the blood vessels and nerves enter the pulp (root) canal.

Teeth have one, two, or three roots. Teeth with two or three roots have an unbranched portion called the root trunk. The area where the root trunk branches into two roots is the furcation or furca. The opening into the furcation is the furcation entrance (Figure 28-15). The most coronal portion of the furcation is the furcation roof, which is often more coronal than the furcation entrance. The area between the roots of a two- or three-rooted tooth is the interfurcal or interradicular area.

When the junctional epithelium has migrated apically and there is clinical attachment loss, portions of the anatomic root are included in the definition of a clinical crown, the unattached portion of a tooth. The concept of cervical, middle, and apical thirds is used when discussing root anatomy.

Cementoenamel Junction

The cementoenamel junction (CEJ) or cervical line is a structure that the dental hygienist must be able to identify subgingivally with an instrument. In health the CEJ is located within 1 mm of the free gingival margin and is covered slightly by free gingiva. The CEJ is the fixed landmark in the identification of the amount of attached gingiva. Subgingival identification of the CEJ is a competency that requires knowledge of root anatomy, development of tactile skill, and experience. Tactile, nonvisual indicators of the CEJ may include the following:

- Rougher root texture, because cementum is not as smooth as enamel.
- Location between the convex cervical third of a crown and the flatter root surface.
- Facial and lingual contours of the CEJ on anterior and premolar teeth are convex (Figure 28-16); on molars, the CEJ is much straighter.
- An apical dip of the CEJ, called the *cervical enamel projection* (CEP), may be present toward the furcation on molars.
- Proximal curvature of the CEJ is more pronounced on anterior than on posterior teeth.
  - On anterior teeth the curvature is V-shaped toward the incisal surface and more prominent on the mesial surface of incisors, especially the maxillary central incisor. (These areas are particularly difficult to instrument because of limited proximal access, which may contribute to incomplete deposit removal.)

Root Surface Texture

Surface textures of crowns and roots differ owing to different degrees of enamel and cementum mineralization and how it is altered by oral biofilm, as follows:

- Enamel (anatomic crown) is analogous to glazed pottery—smooth, hard, and glassy when unaltered.

TABLE 28-1

Characteristics of Roots

Maxillary Arch

Central Incisor

One cone-shaped root
Does not have prominent root concavities
Most prominent cementoenamel junction (CEJ) curvature toward incisal on mesial surface
Lingual surface is smaller than facial because proximal surface tapers toward the lingual surface
Cervical cross-section is a "rounded" triangle in shape
Flat mesial surface
Root is approximately one and one third times the length of the crown*

See Figure 28-17, *A*

Tooth No. 8

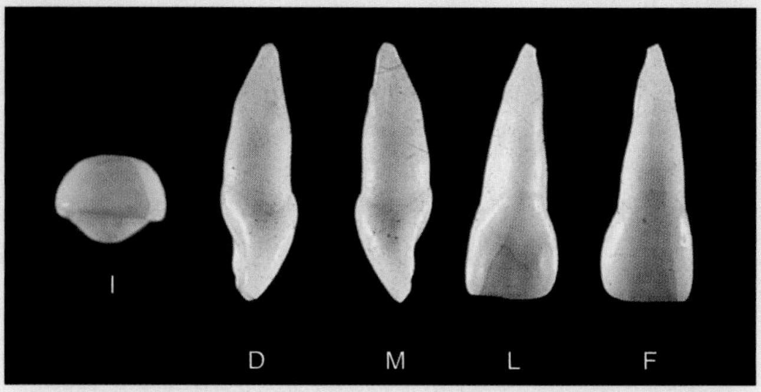

Figure 28-1. (Courtesy former Department of Dental Hygiene, Marquette University.)

Lateral Incisor

One cone-shaped root
May have a palatogingival groove
Lateral root rounder
Lateral root longer than central root*

Tooth No. 7

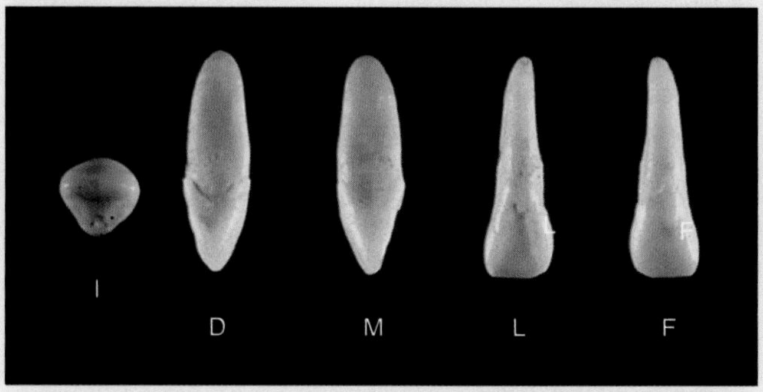

Figure 28-2. (Courtesy former Department of Dental Hygiene, Marquette University.)

Canine

One long cone-shaped root
Generally has proximal root concavities
Distal crest of curvature in the crown may hinder access to the mesial surface of the first premolar
Root length is one and a half times the length of the very long crown*

Tooth No. 6

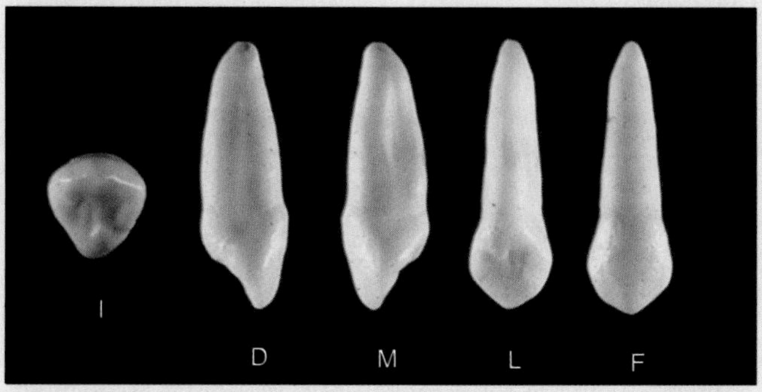

Figure 28-3. (Courtesy former Department of Dental Hygiene, Marquette University.)

TABLE 28-1

Characteristics of Roots—cont'd

Maxillary Arch—cont'd

See Figure 28-17, *A*

First Premolar

Two roots, F and L (may have only one)

Prominent mesial root concavity that extends apically from the mesial contact on the crown

Bifurcated in cervical third to half

Elliptic in shape in cervical cross-section; narrow facial and lingual root surfaces, broad proximal surfaces

Root approximately one and three fourths times the length of the crown*

Tooth No. 5

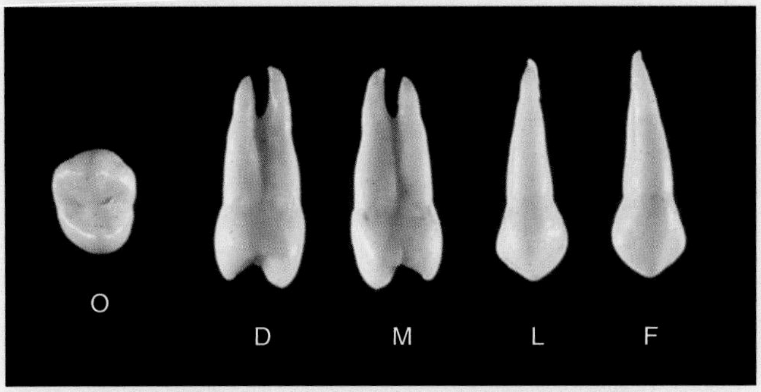

Figure 28-4. (Courtesy former Department of Dental Hygiene, Marquette University.)

Second Premolar

One root

Mesial concavity not as pronounced as in first premolar (may be prominent)

Elliptic in cross-section; broad proximal surfaces

Root is approximately one and one third times the length of the crown*

Tooth No. 4

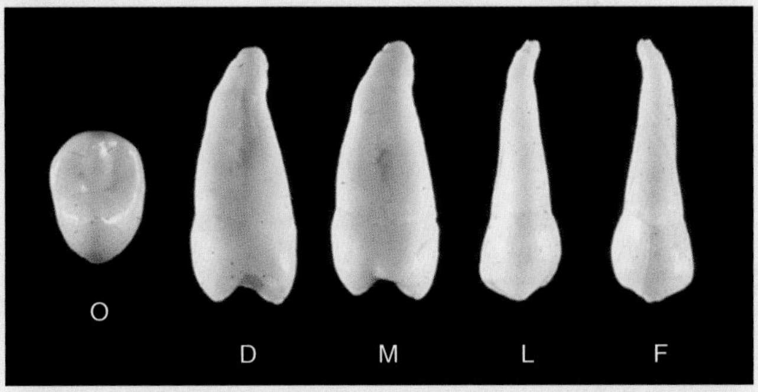

Figure 28-5. (Courtesy former Department of Dental Hygiene, Marquette University.)

First Molar

Three roots: mesiobuccal, distobuccal, and palatal

Palatal root is longest and extends out beyond the lingual surface of the crown (lingual root concavity on its palatal surface)

Root concavities may be present on the mesiobuccal and palatal roots and also on furcal surfaces

Mesiobuccal and distobuccal roots may appear as a "pair" with their apices curved toward each other; look like pliers

Mesiobuccal root has a mesial concavity

Furcations are on the facial, mesial, and distal aspects and begin gradually before the entrance, which is located near the junction of the cervical and middle third of the root

The root trunk on the mesial surface is the shortest and on the distal surface is the longest

Mesial furcation is located more toward the lingual aspect

Roots are one and three fourths the length of the crown*

Tooth No. 3

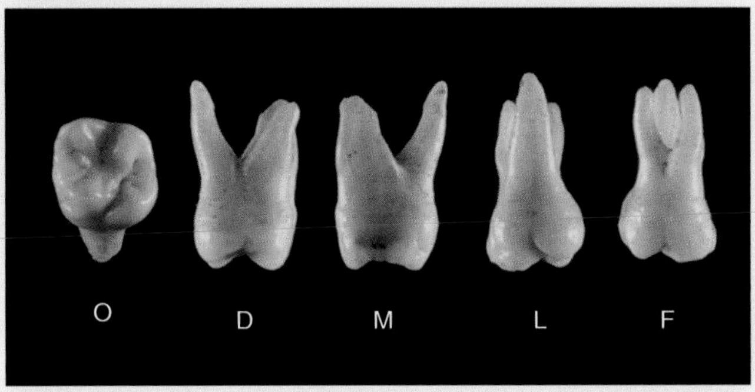

Figure 28-6. (Courtesy former Department of Dental Hygiene, Marquette University.)

Continued

TABLE 28-1

Characteristics of Roots—cont'd

Maxillary Arch—cont'd

See Figure 28-17, *A*

Second Molar

Three roots: mesiobuccal, distobuccal, and palatal
Longer root trunk than first molar
Roots are closer together with more distal orientation
Less interradicular bone than on first molar

Tooth No. 2

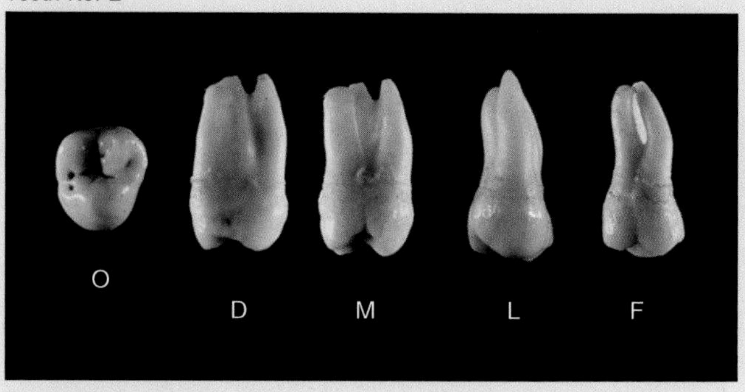

Figure 28-7. (Courtesy former Department of Dental Hygiene, Marquette University.)

Third Molar

Root morphology varies greatly; may be three rooted, roots may be fused and may have accessory roots

Mandibular Arch

See Figure 28-17, *B*

Central and Lateral Incisor

Very similar
One cone-shaped root
Cervical cross-section is elliptic in shape with very narrow facial and lingual surfaces and broader proximal surfaces
Frequently have very shallow root concavities on proximal surfaces
Root one and a half times the length of the crown*

Tooth No. 25

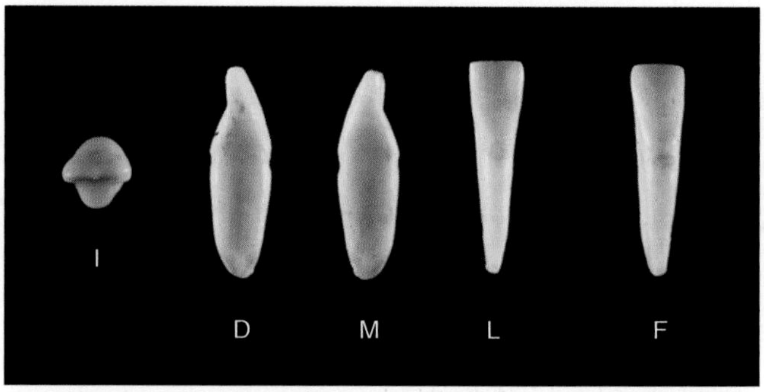

Figure 28-8. (Courtesy former Department of Dental Hygiene, Marquette University.)

Tooth No. 26

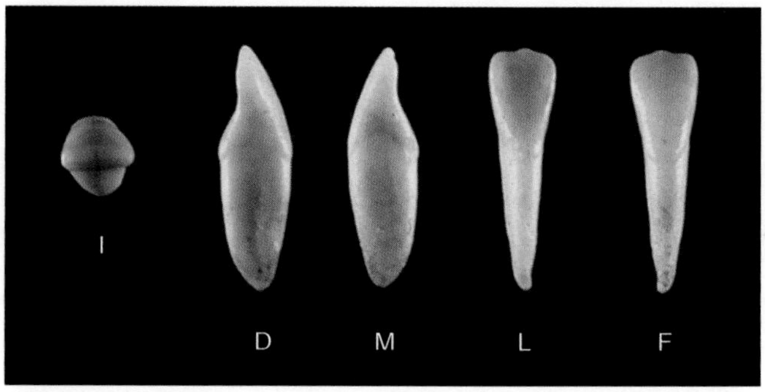

Figure 28-9. (Courtesy former Department of Dental Hygiene, Marquette University.)

TABLE 28-1

Characteristics of Roots—cont'd

Mandibular Arch—cont'd

See Figure 28-17, *B*

Canine

One cone-shaped root
Cervical cross-section is ovoid in shape with small lingual surface
Proximal root concavities are present
Root length about one and a half times the length of the crown*
Occasionally the root apex is bifurcated into a facial and a lingual root

Tooth No. 27

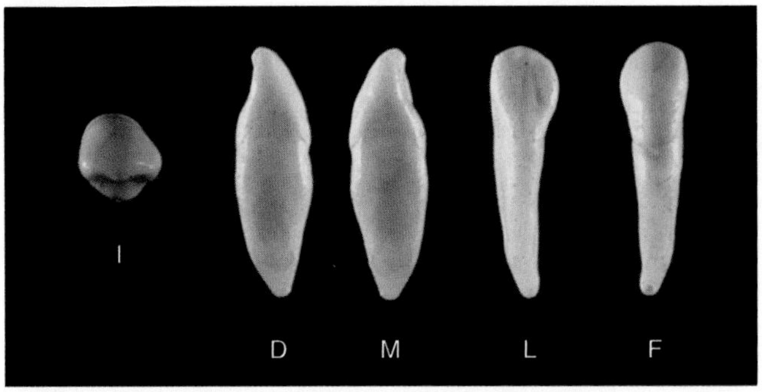

Figure 28-10. (Courtesy former Department of Dental Hygiene, Marquette University.)

First Premolar†

One cone-shaped root
Cervical cross-section may be elliptic or ovoid in shape
Facial and lingual root surfaces converge markedly toward the apex
May have root concavities deep on distal surface
Root length one and two thirds times the length of the crown*

Tooth No. 28

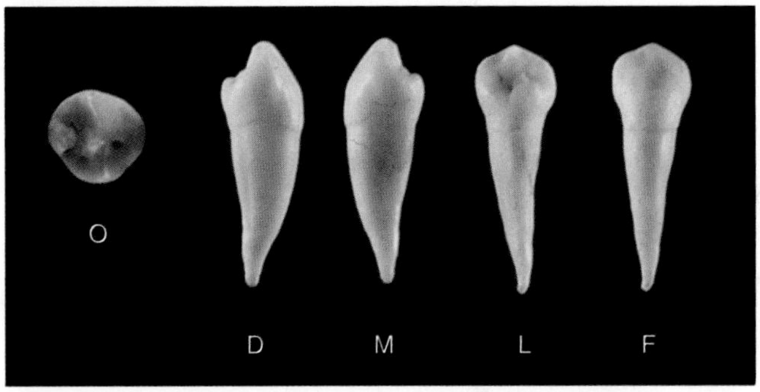

Figure 28-11. (Courtesy former Department of Dental Hygiene, Marquette University.)

Second Premolar†

One cone-shaped root
Cervical cross-section may be elliptic or ovoid in shape
Mandibular premolars may have proximal root concavities
Root length is one and two thirds the length of the crown*

Tooth No. 29

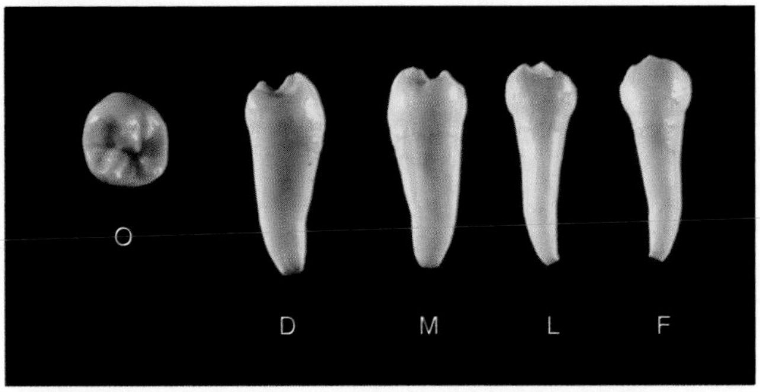

Figure 28-12. (Courtesy former Department of Dental Hygiene, Marquette University.)

Continued

TABLE 28-1

Characteristics of Roots—cont'd

Mandibular Arch—cont'd

See Figure 28-17, *B*

First Molar[†]

Two roots: mesial and distal, which is narrower
Furcations on facial and lingual surface, facial concavity before the furcation begins just apical to the CEJ
Short root trunk, about 3 mm on the facial surface, one fourth the length of root trunk; longer on lingual surface
Large interradicular area
Proximal and furcal concavities on mesial root, furcal concavity on distal root
Roots are one and three fourths times the length of the crown
Cervical enamel projections may be present

Tooth No. 30

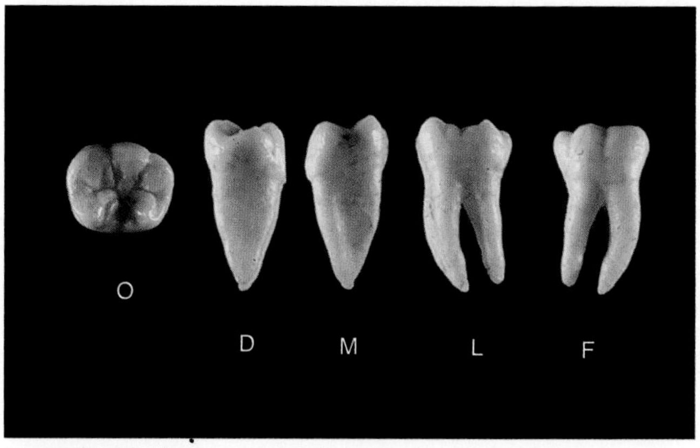

Figure 28-13. (Courtesy former Department of Dental Hygiene, Marquette University.)

Second Molar[†]

Two roots: mesial and distal
Roots are likely to be closer together with a longer root trunk than first molar
Mesial root concavities are not as prominent as in first molar
Roots are one and three fourths times the length of the crown
Cervical enamel projections may be present

Tooth No. 31

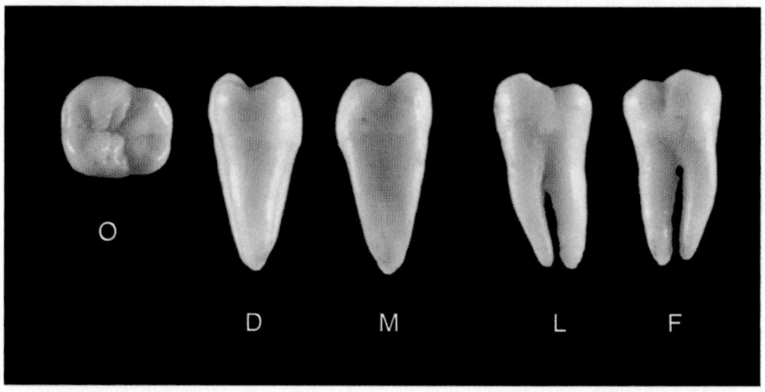

Figure 28-14. (Courtesy former Department of Dental Hygiene, Marquette University.)

Third Molar[†]

Root structure varies greatly
Typically has two roots
Roots are frequently shorter, fused, and dilacerated

D, Distal; *I,* incisal; *F,* facial; *L,* lingual; *M,* mesial; *O,* occlusal.

*Knowing the length of the crown of a tooth is helpful in assessing the length of its root and the amount of attachment:

Maxillary central and lateral incisor crowns are the longest in the dentition, approximately ½ inch in length.

Anterior crowns are approximately 2 to 3 mm longer than posterior crowns. Roots range from approximately 12 to 17 mm in length; incisor roots are the shortest, and canines are the longest.

Proportionally, when the length of roots is compared with the length of crowns, molars have the longest roots (because of their short crowns), and maxillary incisors have the shortest.

[†]Crowns of all mandibular posterior teeth are inclined lingually and make instrument placement more difficult.

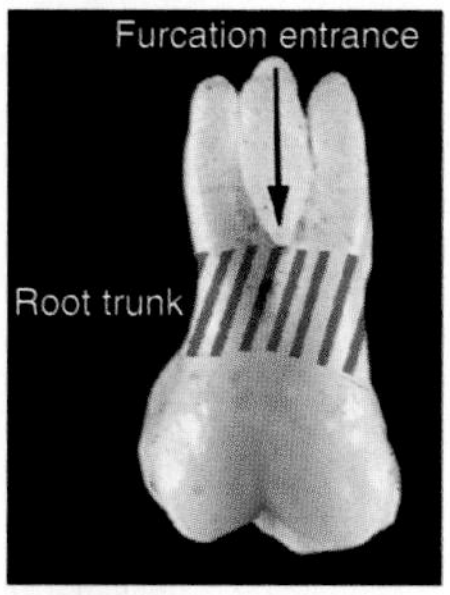

Figure 28-15. Root terminology: root trunk and furcation entrance. (Courtesy former Department of Dental Hygiene, Marquette University.)

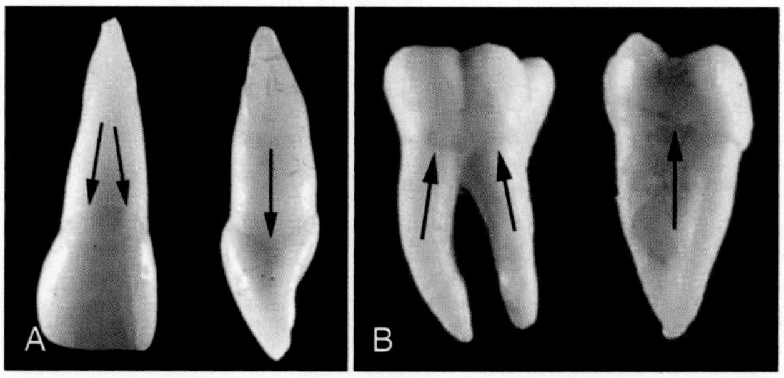

Figure 28-16. Cementoenamel junction contours. **A,** Anterior teeth. **B,** Posterior teeth. (Courtesy former Department of Dental Hygiene, Marquette University.)

- Cementum (anatomic root) is not as smooth, hard, or glassy but is more porous. Cementum can be altered by the following:
  - Loss of periodontal attachment, plaque by-products, and unintentional injury by client or clinician
  - Root planing using ultrasonic instruments and curets
    - Scaling instruments with pointed tips should not be used on root surfaces.
    - During root planing, varying amounts of cementum are removed and dentin may be exposed, resulting in dentinal hypersensitivity (see Chapter 39).

Root Shapes

Permanent teeth roots vary from one individual to another. For instrument placement on root surfaces, the following are considered:

- Individual root morphology
- Position of the teeth in the alveolar bone
- Interference from crown contours
- Client's periodontal status
- Instrument design

Teeth with One Root

All anterior teeth and maxillary second and mandibular premolars have one root. (See Table 28-1 and Figure 28-17.) Characteristics of teeth with one root include the following:

- Cone shape with facial, lingual, and proximal surfaces converging (tapering) apically with different degrees of convergence widest in the cervical third and tapering to a small apex (see Figure 28-16, *A*)
- Distal inclination from a facial (lingual) view
- Cervical cross-sections (i.e., crown cut off the root horizontally at CEJ) are triangular, ovid, or elliptic (see Figure 28-17, *A* and *B*):
  - Triangular: Appears to be three-sided with broad (equal) facial, mesial, and distal surfaces and a narrow lingual surface. Proximal surfaces converge markedly to the lingual surface (e.g., maxillary central incisors). Proximal surfaces of roots that are narrower on the lingual than the facial surface (both triangular and ovoid root shapes in cervical section) are instrumented more readily from the lingual surface because of greater access.
  - Ovoid: Oval, "egg-shaped," with facial surface broader than lingual surface; proximal surfaces are equal and broader than either facial or lingual surface (e.g., canines).
  - Elliptic: Proximal surfaces are relatively equal; facial and lingual surfaces are approximately the same size but smaller than the proximal surfaces. Root dimensions are broad from the facial and lingual view, and narrower from the mesial and distal view. Roots of mandibular incisors and maxillary premolars are elliptic in cervical cross-section.

In midroot sections, root shapes are generally the same as in cervical sections, although smaller.

Roots that are triangular or ovoid in cross-section have smaller lingual than facial surfaces because of proximal surface convergence (taper) toward the lingual surface. Cervical cross-section shapes may be altered by the presence of root concavities. The cervical half of a conical-shaped root has more than 50% of the root surface area because of the convergence of surfaces apically.

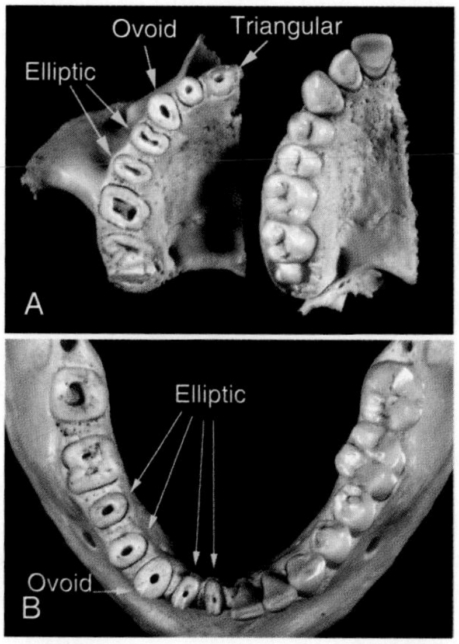

Figure 28-17. Root shapes in cervical cross-section. **A,** Maxillary teeth: triangular, elliptic, and ovoid. **B,** Mandibular teeth: elliptic and ovoid. (Courtesy former Department of Dental Hygiene, Marquette University.)

Teeth with Two or Three Roots

For periodontal assessment and instrumentation, each root of a multirooted tooth must be treated individually—that is, a two-rooted tooth is like having two single-rooted teeth (see Table 28-1). In addition, the complexity of unbranched root trunks and furcas must be considered. Posterior teeth are more difficult to reach, and the clinician's competence influences the therapeutic outcome. Characteristics of the teeth with more than one root are as follows:

- Maxillary first premolars
  - Generally have two roots (facial and lingual)
  - Furcations on the mesial and distal sides (Figure 28-18)
- Maxillary molars
  - Have three roots: mesiobuccal, distobuccal, and palatal (lingual)
  - Furcations on the buccal side between the mesiobuccal and distobuccal roots, on the mesial side between the mesiobuccal and palatal roots, and on the distal side between the distobuccal and palatal roots (Figure 28-19)
  - Radiographic assessment of the roots can be compromised owing to the complex root anatomy of the mesiobuccal, distobuccal, and palatal roots (radiographs show the image only from a facial or lingual view)

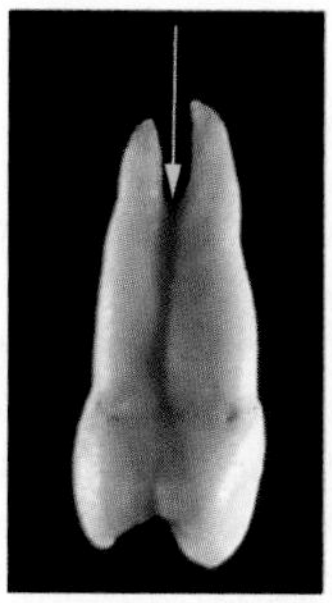

Figure 28-18. Mesial furcation on a maxillary first premolar. (Courtesy former Department of Dental Hygiene, Marquette University.)

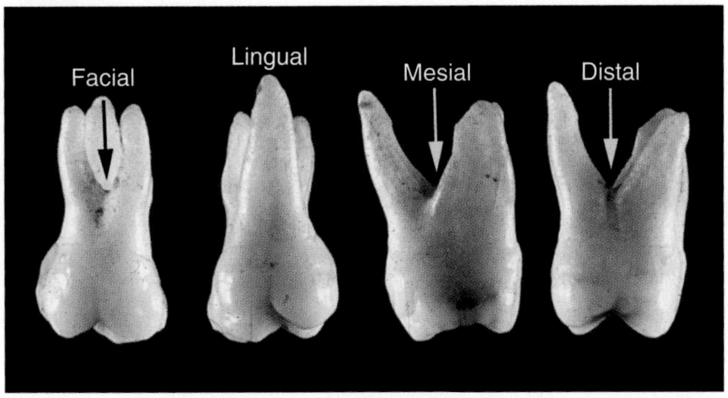

Figure 28-19. Furcations on a maxillary (first) molar. (Courtesy former Department of Dental Hygiene, Marquette University.)

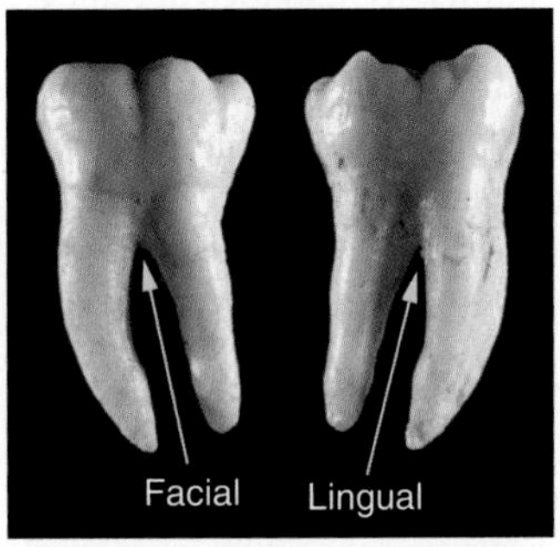

Figure 28-20. Furcations on a mandibular (first) molar. (Courtesy former Department of Dental Hygiene, Marquette University.)

- Mandibular molars
  - Have two roots: mesial and distal
  - Furcations on the buccal and lingual surfaces between the mesial and distal roots (Figure 28-20)
  - Roots on second molars more likely to have longer root trunks, be closer together, and have more distal orientation
- Cervical cross-sections of maxillary and mandibular molar roots are larger and more difficult to describe (see Figure 28-17).
  - Both may show slight depressions where furcations or proximal root concavities begin.
  - The root trunk of maxillary molars has more equal sides; appears somewhat rhomboidal in shape, with the more prominent "corner" being the mesiobuccal.
  - The root trunk of the mandibular molar is more rectangular in shape, with the mesial distal width being greater than the facial lingual width.
  - Generally, roots are elliptic in cervical cross-section after the furcation.

Furcations

Furcations generally begin as a shallow depression on the root trunk that gradually opens into a space between the roots; this opening may be too narrow for instruments. Initially, anatomic changes in root trunk anatomy or beginning furcations can be felt by the working end of a dental explorer and then, as the periodontal status changes and as the space widens, furcations are readily appreciated by a Nabors probe. Furcations are difficult to access with traditional scaling and root planing instruments, because their working ends are too large. Rather, precision thin and furcation inserts for ultrasonic instruments, microbladed and minibladed curets with smaller and narrower working ends, curets with extended shanks, and furcation curets are used to debride furcation areas (see Chapters 26, 27, and 30). A very narrow furcation entrance can be enlarged surgically with burs by a periodontist. Furcation characteristics are as follows:

- The more cervical the furcation is, the more stable the tooth because of root divergence (separation).
- Furcations are generally more cervical on first molars; first molar root trunks are shorter than second or third molar root trunks.
- Furcations close to the CEJ are more likely to become involved with periodontal disease, although access for instrumentation is easier (shallower) and therefore such disease has a more favorable post-therapy prognosis.
- Furcations close to the apex are less likely to result in furcation involvement; however, instrument access is more difficult (deeper) and post-therapy prognosis is less favorable.
- Furcation involvement occurs when there is a loss of attachment apical to the furcation and is classified according to extent (see Chapter 19 and Table 19-5 for classification of furcations).

It is important to know the expected furcation location in horizontal and vertical directions. Horizontally, most furcations are located midway on the root trunk. The mesial furcation of a maxillary first molar generally is located more toward the lingual surface in a horizontal direction, and therefore instrumentation of the mesial furcation of this tooth is easier from the lingual approach (see Figure 28-19). Vertically, furcations on a maxillary premolar are in the apical third to half (see Figure 28-18). Furcations on a maxillary molar are near the junction of the cervical and middle thirds of the root (see Figure 28-19) and on average are the following distance from the CEJ: mesial—3.6 mm, buccal—4.2 mm, and distal—4.8 mm. Furcations on maxillary second and third molars are slightly more apical. Furcations on a mandibular first molar are apical to the cervical one fourth of the root, averaging 3 mm (buccal) and 4 mm (lingual), making this the shortest root trunk in the permanent dentition and the most likely to experience furcation involvement (see Figure 28-20). Furcations on the mandibular second and third molars are slightly more apical than on the first mandibular molar.

Root Concavities

Root concavities are shallow vertical depressions on root surfaces. They protect the tooth from forces that could rotate it in its alveolus and provide more root surface area and direction for periodontal fiber attachment. Root concavities complicate root instrumentation and access and make it more difficult to place the cutting edge of the instrument on the root surface. Root concavities most frequently occur on proximal root surfaces (proximal root concavities) (see Figure 28-15). Maxillary first molars have a concavity on the lingual surface of the palatal root (lingual concavity) (see Figure 28-19). Molars may have root concavities on the surface of their root toward the furcation (furcal concavities).

Tooth Alignment

Assessment of the alignment of the teeth within an arch is essential to adapting instruments subgingivally. Tooth size, prominence of its crown, contact areas, and the convergence of root surfaces determine the amount of space and interproximal bone in health and disease. In health the mandibular anterior teeth have the narrowest amount of space and bone because they are very narrow. In disease, if loss of bone is accompanied by gingival recession, there is more access for instrumentation. When teeth have insufficient space, crowding occurs, making instrument positioning difficult. Teeth with close or altered root proximity may have minimal or no proximal space and long proximal root contact, which may influence significantly oral hygiene, periodontal health, and subgingival instrumentation.

The position of teeth within the alveoli also is a factor in root instrumentation. **Axial positioning** is the relationship of an imaginary vertical line representing the long axis of a tooth in relationship to a horizontal plane. This concept is diagrammed in Figure 28-21. The functions of this positioning are to bring the maxillary and mandibular teeth into an interarch relationship that facilitates incision and mastication and distributes forces throughout the bones of the skull.

Following the vertical lines in Figure 28-21, it is clear that in a faciolingual dimension the roots of all the teeth except the mandibular posteriors have a more lingual inclination than the crowns. Mandibular posterior crowns are more lingually inclined than roots that are more facial in orientation, making plaque biofilm removal in this area especially difficult for clients.

Again following the vertical lines in Figure 28-21, in a mesiodistal dimension the roots of the canines, premolars, and molars have a distal inclination, which is more pronounced posteriorly. Incisor roots do not incline distally.

Variations in Root Form

Root alterations, anomalies, or abnormalities should be recognized and documented in the client record for instrumentation adaptations and subsequent client education.

Fused Roots, Fusion, and Concrescence

Molar roots may be **fused** together, especially second and third molar roots, and are a result of limited space during tooth development (Figure 28-22). Fused roots frequently can be observed on radiographs.

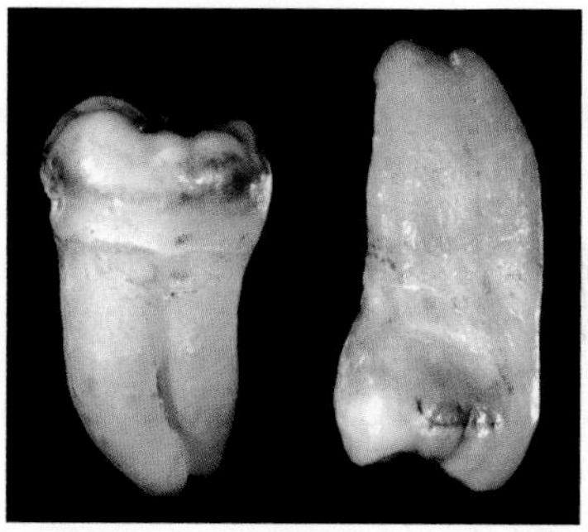

Figure 28-22. Fused roots on a mandibular and maxillary molar. (Courtesy former Department of Dental Hygiene, Marquette University.)

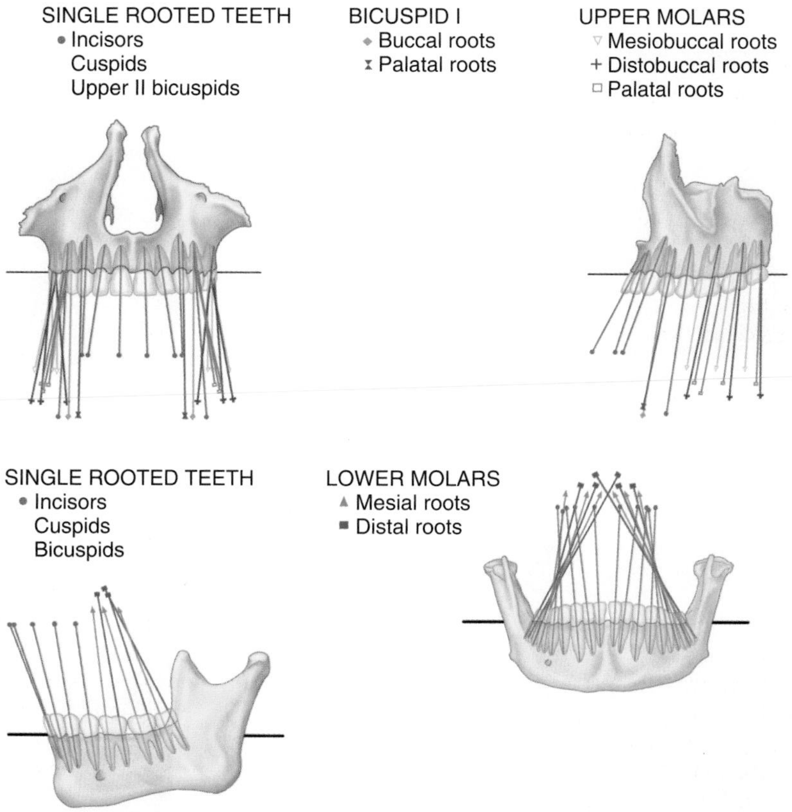

Figure 28-21. Axial positioning of the maxillary and mandibular teeth in an anterior and lateral view. The slant of the roots along their long axis is shown by vertical lines that have been extended to represent the direction of the slant in faciolingual and mesiodistal directions. (From Dempster WT, Adams WJ, Duddles RA: Arrangement in the jaws of the roots of the teeth, *J Am Dent Assoc* 67:779, 1963.)

Teeth may be joined together in an anomaly called *fusion,* in which two tooth buds fuse together during development and form one large tooth with a large crown and a single root that has two pulp canals. This fusion must be confirmed by radiographs. *Concrescence* occurs when two adjacent teeth become joined by cementum after they have been formed.

Accessory Roots

Accessory roots are extra roots. Sometimes the mandibular permanent canines are bifurcated into facial and lingual roots in the apical third (Figure 28-23). Maxillary first premolars can have three roots—two buccal and one lingual. Buccal roots are very thin, which makes treatment difficult if periodontal disease is present. Third molars sometimes have extra roots. Accessory roots may be assessed via radiographs and are instrumented only if the attachment level is apical to their occurrence.

Palatogingival Grooves (Palatoradicular Grooves)

A palatogingival groove (Figure 28-24) extends apically from the lingual concavity of the crown of a permanent maxillary incisor, usually the lateral incisor, onto the root, often resulting in an isolated, narrow pocket. This groove provides challenges in instrumentation, is highly plaque retentive, and is susceptible to periodontal disease.

Hypercementosis

Hypercementosis, the excessive formation of cementum in the apical third to half of the tooth after the tooth has erupted (Figure 28-25), may be caused by trauma, chronic inflammation of the pulp, or metabolic disturbances. It is assessed radiographically. If areas of hypercementosis are exposed with apical migration of the junctional epithelium, decisions about the extent of root instrumentation will be more difficult.

Cervical Enamel Projections

Cervical enamel projections (CEPs) are apical extensions of the CEJ toward the furcation of a molar (Figure 28-26). CEPs are classified by degree of extension, as follows:

- Grade I CEPs slightly extend toward the furcation and occur frequently.
- Grade II CEPs approach the area of root separation.
- Grade III CEPs extend into the furcation.
- Grade IV CEPs are the same as Grade III CEPs, plus the furcation is visible because of recession.

Periodontal attachment loss is more likely in CEP areas because periodontal fibers do not form the same type of attachment to enamel as to cementum. Most isolated furcation involvements in otherwise healthy dentitions are found to be related to CEPs. A CEP can be removed surgically to expose dentin and facilitate reattachment of periodontal fibers.

Enamel Pearls

Enamel pearls, most frequently seen on maxillary molars, are "droplets" of enamel in the furcation area (Figure 28-27). They are thought to be due to a genetic error in the developing root sheath as it reaches the furcation area. Because periodontal fibers will not attach to enamel, enamel pearls may encourage periodontal disease. Exploration of an enamel pearl sometimes can be puzzling if it is not visible on radiographs, because it may feel like subgingival calculus.

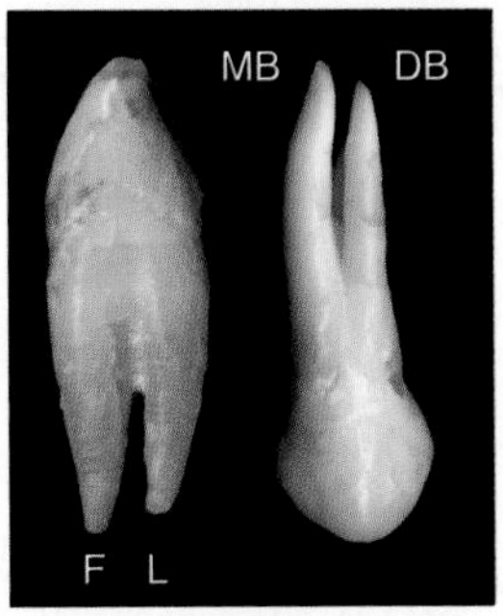

Figure 28-23. Accessory roots on a mandibular canine and maxillary first premolar. *DB,* Distobuccal; *F,* facial; *L,* lingual; *MB,* mesiobuccal. (Courtesy former Department of Dental Hygiene, Marquette University.)

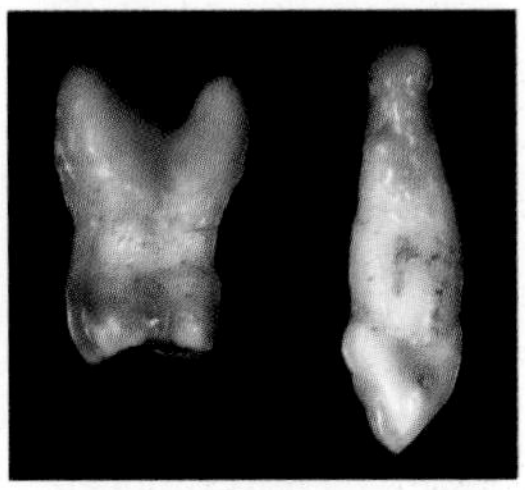

Figure 28-25. Hypercementosis. (Courtesy former Department of Dental Hygiene, Marquette University.)

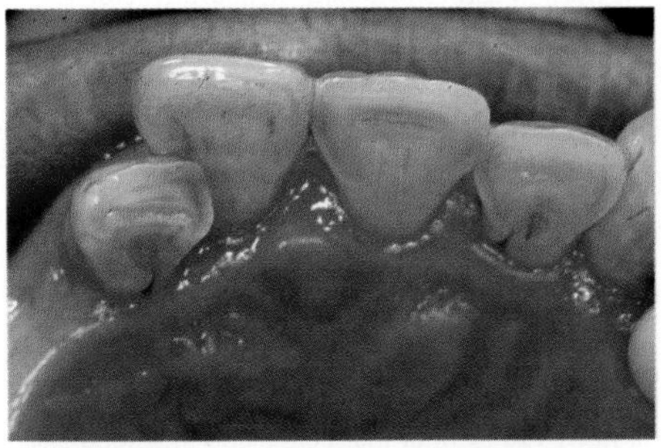

Figure 28-24. Palatogingival groove on a maxillary lateral incisor. (Courtesy Gay Derderian, BA, DDS, MSD, Marquette University School of Dentistry.)

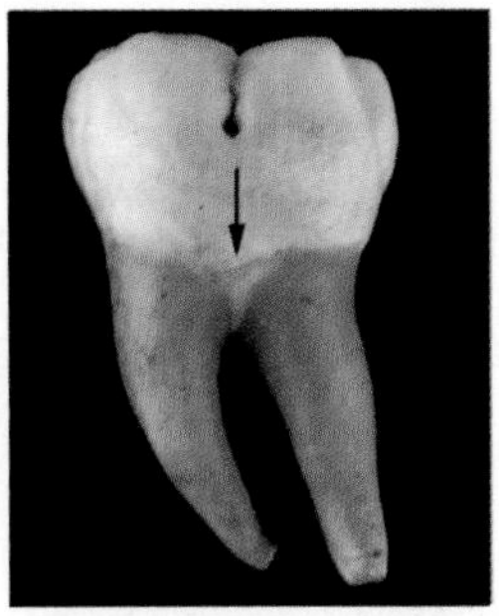

Figure 28-26. Cervical enamel projection on a mandibular first molar. (Courtesy former Department of Dental Hygiene, Marquette University.)

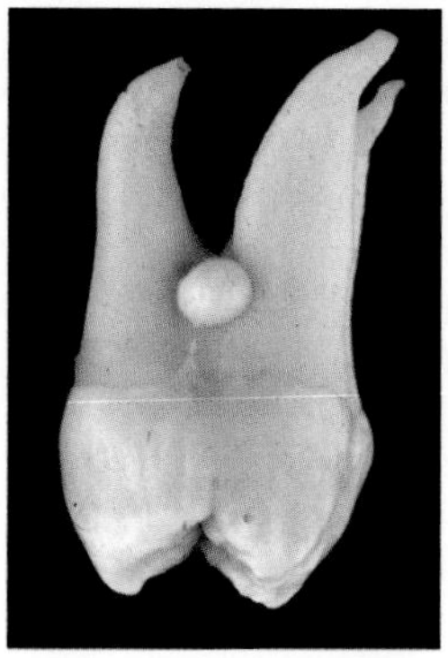

Figure 28-27. Enamel pearls near the furcation of a maxillary molar. (Courtesy former Department of Dental Hygiene, Marquette University.)

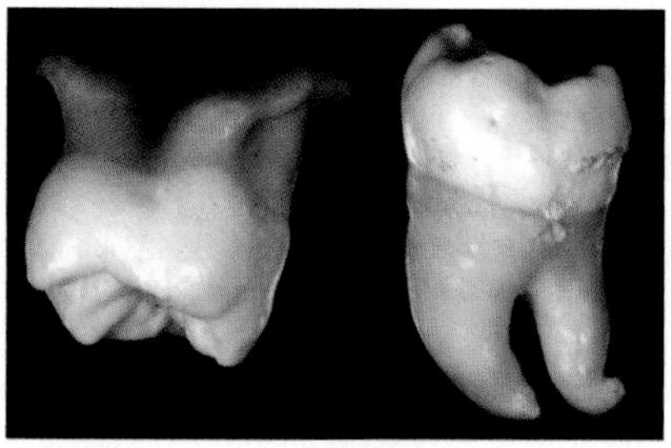

Figure 28-28. Dilaceration. (Courtesy former Department of Dental Hygiene, Marquette University.)

Dilaceration

Dilaceration is a sharp bend in the root surface caused by the displacement of the root during tooth development (Figure 28-28).

See Procedure 28-1 and the corresponding Competency Form on root morphology and implications for root instrumentation.

CLIENT EDUCATION TIPS

- Educate clients about root morphology and related periodontal structures as a rationale for recommended self-care behaviors, products, and devices.
- Individualize oral self-care methods and appropriate adjunctive aids to client's root morphology, oral health status, level of understanding, and capability.

LEGAL, ETHICAL, AND SAFETY ISSUES

- Root variations must be recorded in the client's chart, discussed with the client, and accounted for in the plan of care as they influence treatment, referral, and self-care recommendations.
- Dental hygienists regularly renew and update their knowledge of root anatomy and instrumentation.

KEY CONCEPTS

- Root assessment, instrumentation, and management require thorough knowledge of root morphology.
- Periodontal assessment includes the identification of root anatomy and root surface characteristics before the development of the plan for care.
- Incisors, canines, and all of the premolars except the maxillary first premolars have one root.
- Approximately 60% of maxillary first premolars have two roots (one facial and one lingual), with furcations on the mesial and distal surfaces.
- Mandibular molars have two roots, one mesial and one distal, with furcations on the facial and lingual surfaces.
- Maxillary molars have three roots (mesiobuccal, distobuccal, and lingual), with mesial, facial, and distal furcations.
- Teeth with more than one root have a root trunk before root division.
- The division area is called the *furca;* a furcation entrance may be very narrow.
- The cementoenamel junction on posterior teeth has much less-pronounced curvatures on all surfaces.
- Cementum is not as hard as enamel; only instruments with a rounded toe should be used on it.
- Number and shape of the roots determine the selection and adaptation of assessment, scaling, and root planing instruments.
- Root surfaces converge (taper) apically; there is more root surface area in the cervical third than in the apical or middle thirds.
- More of the proximal surface of a single-rooted tooth with broader facial than lingual surfaces can be reached from the lingual approach because of the proximal convergence toward the lingual side.
- Horizontal and vertical location of the furcation determines selection and placement of instruments.
- Root surfaces may have shallow, longitudinal vertical depressions, which add curvature and dimension to instrumentation.
- Axial positioning of each individual tooth in its alveolus is considered when instruments are adapted on root surface.

CRITICAL THINKING EXERCISES

Root Identification Exercise

Materials: Autoclaved extracted permanent teeth with crowns sectioned off or, if available, anatomically accurate plastic specimens of permanent teeth with crowns cut off. *(When natural specimens are used in this and all other exercises, personal protective equipment and infection control procedures are required.)* Photographs also may be used for this exercise, but specimens have the advantage of being three dimensional and easily manipulated. Refer to Table 28-1 for guidance.

1. Identify roots of the teeth and match them with their description.

   Note: It is not possible to distinguish mandibular central from lateral incisor roots, or mandibular first from second premolar roots. For these, the identification of the root only as a mandibular incisor or mandibular premolar is the expectation. Sometimes it is also difficult to distinguish maxillary and mandibular canine roots.

Procedure 28-1 Root Morphology and Implications for Root Instrumentation

ASSUMPTION

The clinician has mastered instrumentation procedures from Chapter 19, Periodontal and Risk Assessment; Chapter 26, Hand-Activated Instruments; and Chapter 27, Ultrasonic Instrumentation.

Select ultrasonic insert and universal and area-specific curets for use on cementum and root surfaces.

STEPS

1. Make a mental image of the unseen portion of the tooth to be instrumented and the width and height of the adjacent alveolar bone.
2. Review periodontal parameters recorded on the periodontal assessment form.
3. Observe clinical and radiographic alignment of the tooth and adjacent teeth.

General Characteristics of Roots and Their Implications for Instrumentation

1. Adapt instrument so that it follows the long axis of the root and the taper or convergence of root surfaces apically. For curets, use the terminal shank of the instrument as the guide to maintain parallelism. For periodontal probe and universal ultrasonic inserts, use working end to maintain parallelism.
2. Adapt instrument to the taper or convergence of the proximal surfaces toward the lingual surface. If the convergence of the proximal surfaces is pronounced as in maxillary anterior teeth and maxillary molars, approach more of the proximal surfaces from the lingual surface.
3. Adapt instrument so that it also accounts for the position of the tooth in the alveolar bone and the client's position in the chair.
4. Use multidirectional strokes, alternating horizontal, vertical, and oblique stroke directions.
5. Adapt instrument to the lingual inclination of mandibular posterior teeth by slightly angling instrument shank toward the lingual surface.
6. Use alternative instrument placement or an alternative instrument for very narrow spaces (e.g., posterior curet on an anterior tooth or rarely a scaler).

Root Morphology Instrumentation

Specific Characteristics of Roots and Their Implications for Instrumentation (see Table 28-1)

1. Adapt instrument to curvature of the cementoenamel junction (CEJ) on the proximal surface of anterior teeth by turning toe end of a curet or ultrasonic insert into the most incisal portion of it, which may be very narrow. The end of a scaler may be needed to access this area.
2. Adapt toe end of instrument's cutting edge to proximal root concavities with small overlapping strokes that are channeled gradually into the concave area from facial and lingual approaches. If tooth has more than one root, adapt instrument similarly to the slight concave area approaching the furcation.
3. Adapt instrument into furcations.
   a. If there are (anatomic) concavities cervical to or with Class I furcation involvement, scale area with very small strokes and turn toe into concave area that marks the initial stages of division.
   b. With Class II, III, or IV furcation involvement, instrument furcation area as if there were two or three distinct roots. If access is limited, furcation or ultrasonic instruments can be used. Refer to the dentist of record when Class II or higher furcation involvement is found.

Variations

1. For concrescence, use toe end of curet to instrument area of junction of the roots.
2. For palatogingival groove, use toe end of a micro-, mini-, or extended-shank curet to access the groove.
3. Complete progress note. In addition to the date and traditional progress notes inclusions of BP, RR, HR, etc., document completion of the root morphology specific services in the client's record. For example: "08-24-14: No. 30 facial, Class II furcation with 6-mm pocket depth present; used slim ultrasonic insert and 11-14 Gracey used for full furcation instrumentation; spoke with client at length regarding home care requirements, prognosis and need for follow-up treatment; no anesthesia; client tolerated well; reinforced OHI in area; referred to dentist of record." *Or* "06-14-14: No. 3 Class II mesial furcation with 6-mm pocket depth present, used ultrasonics and curets for full furcation instrumentation; access easiest from lingual aspect; reinforced OHI in area; advised on need for periodontal referral/evaluation; referred to dentist of record."

Root Surface and Stroke Coverage Exercise

Materials: One permanent incisor and one permanent maxillary molar typodont or natural tooth; mechanical pencil; tray cover; and gauze square

1. Identify tooth; with nondominant hand, hold it in correct orientation throughout this exercise.
2. In dominant hand, grasp mechanical pencil with traditional pen grasp. Fulcrum as necessary; accounting for height/crest of curvature, orient pencil lead to cervical third of the root. Assume a 6-mm pocket from the cementoenamel junction to the junctional epithelium.
3. Using the side of the pencil lead as a curet toe, "root plane" the facial surface of the root; use vertical, horizontal, oblique, overlapping, and cross-hatching strokes.
4. Identify how each stroke covers (darkens) the surface. Which stroke direction is most successful? How does each stroke direction have to be approached? Are there adaptations that must be made for tooth anatomy? For pocket depth?
5. Observe stroke direction coverage, number of strokes, and length of time it takes to instrument completely the facial root surface.
6. Document and discuss your results and observations.
7. Repeat for the mesial, distal, and lingual aspects of the tooth; pay special attention to the number of strokes, stroke direction, and adaptations necessary for line angles, root trunk, furcations, and concavities.
8. Repeat for one maxillary molar and one incisor tooth.

Root Surface Characteristic Exercise

Materials: Autoclaved extracted tooth with subgingival deposit, curets, dissecting microscope, tray cover, gauze square

1. Observe the root of the tooth under the microscope.
2. Select one area of the root surface; remove the deposit with a curet.
3. Observe the root again, noting the residual deposit microscopically.
4. Root plane the area until it is smooth and hard.
5. Observe the root again; document observations.

Root Anatomy Exercise

Materials: Autoclaved extracted permanent maxillary and mandibular first molars or plastic typodont molars; black nail polish (or liquid paper); glitter (or fine sand); black crayon; 11/12 and 13/14 area-specific curets; tray cover; gauze square

Preparation: Apply nail polish to the root cervical third of the distal half of the tooth; while it is wet, sprinkle glitter on the painted area (simulates deposit, altered cementum); color the mesial half of the root with crayon (simulates subgingival plaque/slime layer).

1. Identify natural or plastic first molar, and hold it in the correct orientation. (May also reinsert the plastic molars into the typodont as an additional exercise.)
2. Select the appropriate curet for an area, and remove deposit from root trunk and roots.
3. Observe how each root is approached as if it were a single tooth, and how each of the surfaces must be approached.
4. Count number of strokes needed to remove the deposit.

BIBLIOGRAPHY

Ash M, Nelson SJ: *Wheeler's dental anatomy, physiology and occlusion*, ed 9, Philadelphia, 2009, Saunders/Elsevier.

Bath-Balogh M, Fehrenbach M: *Illustrated dental embryology, histology and anatomy*, ed 3, Philadelphia, 2010, Saunders/Elsevier.

Brown P, Herbranson E: *3D interactive tooth atlas*, version 6.6, Portola Valley, Calif, 2010, Brown and Herbranson Imaging and Quintessence Publishing.

Darby MD, editor: *Mosby's comprehensive review of dental hygiene*, ed 7, Philadelphia, 2012, Mosby/Elsevier.

Lindhe J, Karing T, Lang N: *Clinical periodontology and implant dentistry*, ed 5, Oxford, UK, 2008, Blackwell Munksgaard.

Newman MG, Takei H, Carranza FA, et al: *Carranza's clinical periodontology*, ed 11, Philadelphia, 2012, Saunders/Elsevier.

Nield-Gehrig JS: *Fundamentals of periodontal instrumentation and advanced root instrumentation*, ed 7, Philadelphia, 2013, Lippincott Williams & Wilkins.

Rose LF, Mealy BL, Genco RJ, et al: *Periodontics: medicine, surgery, and implants*, St Louis, 2004, Elsevier/Mosby.

Scheid R: *Woelfel's dental anatomy: its relevance to dentistry*, ed 8, Philadelphia, 2011, Lippincott Williams & Wilkins.

ACKNOWLEDGMENT

The author acknowledges Merry Greig and Marilyn Beck for their previous contributions to this chapter and the Department of Dental Informatics at the Marquette University School of Dentistry for technical assistance in the preparation of the photographs for this edition.

ⓔ EVOLVE RESOURCES

Please visit http://evolve.elsevier.com/Darby/hygiene for additional practice and study support tools.

CHAPTER 29

Stain Management and Tooth Whitening

Michele Leonardi Darby, Margaret M. Walsh

COMPETENCIES

1. Define extrinsic and intrinsic tooth stains.
2. Discuss extrinsic stain management.
3. Discuss extrinsic stain removal, including:
   - Describe effects of rubber-cup and air polishing on teeth, gingiva, restorative materials, and the dental care setting.
   - Describe indications, contraindications, precautions, and techniques for rubber-cup polishing.
   - Describe selection, maintenance, and infection control for instruments, devices, and armamentaria used for rubber-cup polishing.
   - Explain goal and rationale for selective polishing.
   - Describe effects of air polishing on teeth, gingiva, restorative materials, and implants.
   - Describe indications, contraindications, precautions, and techniques for air polishing.
   - Describe selection, maintenance, and infection control for instruments, devices, and armamentaria used for air polishing.
4. Discuss intrinsic stain management.
5. Discuss whitening agents, including:
   - Identify the advantages and disadvantages of each method of whitening.
   - Describe side effects of tooth whitening.
   - Explain restorative procedures to manage stained teeth.
6. Discuss ethical and legal aspects of extrinsic stain removal and tooth whitening.

Clients dissatisfied with the appearance of their teeth have a human need for a wholesome facial image. Identification of the cause of the client's concern is the first step. If tooth stain is the cause of the concern, determining its cause is the next step because some stains cannot be modified, and others can be altered to varying degrees. During assessment, the dental hygienist identifies types of stain and client factors that contribute to tooth stain (see Chapter 17). With this information the client and dental hygienist formulate the stain management plan. The dental hygienist selects the least damaging method to remove and control stain; more than one method may be indicated for the same client. If the cause of concern is color of the teeth that is unrelated to staining, a management plan for safe and efficacious tooth whitening can be made, or a restorative option can be discussed.

Types of Tooth Stains

Extrinsic Tooth Stains

Extrinsic stains are discolorations of the tooth that can be caused by smoking cigarettes, marijuana, cigars, or pipes; using spit (smokeless) tobacco; and rinsing with antimicrobial agents with substantivity such as chlorhexidine, stannous fluoride, or cetylpyridinium chloride. Other common sources of stains include artificial and natural dyes in foods and beverages (e.g., tea, coffee, cola beverages, red wine, berries, chocolate), iron tablets, chromogenic bacteria in oral biofilm, and poor oral hygiene. Teeth also may become stained from environmental factors such as metallic dust in industrial employment settings (see Chapter 17). Extrinsic stains usually can be removed by scaling with hand-activated, sonic, and ultrasonic instruments and by rubber-cup or air polishing.

Intrinsic Tooth Stains

Intrinsic stains may be hereditary, developmental in nature, or associated with aging. Defects in enamel or dentin during tooth development resulting from high fevers, trauma, excessive intake of fluoride, or tetracycline medication may result in permanently mottled or stained tooth structure (Figure 29-1, *A*). Tooth enamel effects may range from barely noticeable pitting to gross enamel discoloration and defects that fracture easily. Color changes may be slight or severe, including yellow, light to dark brown, blue-gray, and black. Given the translucence of enamel, intrinsic stains may occur adjacent to large restorations, pulpal necrosis, and dental caries. The combined effect of multiple sources of fluoride (e.g., water, toothpaste, mouth rinses, foods, and beverages), fluorosis has been increasing in prevalence in the United States. Advising the parent of a child client about fluoride exposure and providing anticipatory guidance is an important preventive mechanism for intrinsic tooth staining and caries prevention (see Chapter 18).

Extrinsic Stain Management

Extrinsic stain management focuses primarily on oral self-care that may prevent the recurrence of stain. Often, modifying the daily oral care practices is the most long-lasting solution for extrinsic stain management and always should be based on the client's health history, oral assessment, and self-care assessment. Once removed, extrinsic stain may be prevented by a client's change in self-care practices (e.g., using a power toothbrush and whitening dentifrice), smoking

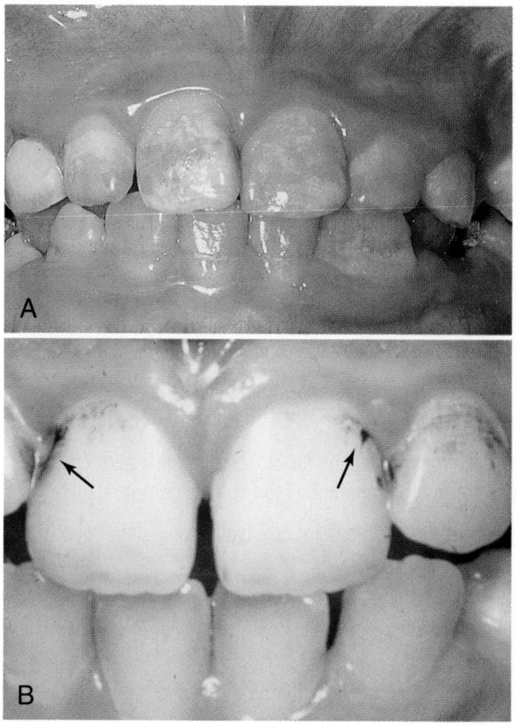

Figure 29-1. A, Intrinsic staining from dental fluorosis. **B,** Brown and yellow extrinsic stain. (Courtesy Dr. Frank Hodges.)

cessation, and avoidance of stain-producing foods and beverages (Figure 29-1, *B*).

Cleansing and Polishing Agents for Managing Extrinsic Stains

Agents used to clean and polish teeth, restored tooth surfaces, and dental appliances contain abrasive agents (see Chapter 25, Figure 25-5). **Abrasive agents** are composed of natural or synthetic materials that vary in hardness, particle shape, and particle size (grit). These agents are used commonly in clinical and laboratory procedures and added to dentifrices, prophylaxis pastes, abrasive strips, and polishing discs. Fine grit abrasive agents are used for cleaning and polishing tooth enamel, whereas fine, medium, and coarse grit abrasives are used to polish dental appliances in the laboratory. A hard abrasive can produce minimal abrasion if its particle size is very fine to superfine.

Abrasives found in dentifrices (e.g., calcium pyrophosphate, dibasic calcium phosphate dehydrate, tricalcium phosphate, hydrated alumina, hydrated silica, sodium metaphosphate) should have extremely low abrasiveness because toothpastes are used for daily cleaning. Abrasives found in prophylaxis pastes (superfine pumice, silicon dioxide, zirconium silicate, calcium carbonate) have a low to moderate abrasiveness to facilitate extrinsic stain removal and polish teeth. Abrasives used in the laboratory and to contour some restorations (rouge, tripoli, cuttle, garnet, emery, coarse pumice) may have low, moderate, or high abrasiveness. Abrasive agents used in the mouth must produce a smooth, clean, lustrous surface with minimal scratches because polished tooth surfaces are more resistant to the accumulation of extrinsic stain and calculus.

Natural abrasives include Arkansas stone, chalk, cuttle, kieselguhr, corundum, pumice, emery, garnet, quartz, sand, tripoli, zirconium silicate, and diamond. Synthetic abrasives include aluminum oxide, tin oxide, silicon carbide, synthetic diamond, and rouge. Common abrasives are listed in Table 29-1. For extrinsic tooth stain removal or the polishing of a restorative material to be achieved, an abrasive agent is applied against the surface to abrade the stain away and/or create a surface with a high luster. The following key characteristics of the abrasive agent affect the size of the surface scratches and the polishing outcome:

- **Hardness** determines whether one abrasive material can scratch the surface of another material. Hardness is assessed using the Mohs Hardness Scale, which ranges from 1 (lowest hardness material) to 10 (highest hardness material). To polish, particles must be 1 to 2 units on the scale harder than the surface being polished. Cleansing a surface requires a material less than or equal to that of the surface being cleaned to prevent scratching.
- **Particle shape** of an abrasive may be angular, blocky, semiround, or round. Sharp angular edges deepen the scratches on the surface being polished.
- **Particle size** (also known as **grit**) affects cleaning rate and scratch pattern produced on a surface. Fine grit yields the least amount of surface abrasion even if the abrasive material is high on the Mohs Hardness Scale, whereas coarse grit, the most abrasive, can scratch and roughen surfaces, making them more likely to accumulate oral biofilm and stain. There is no industry standard for defining superfine, fine, medium, or coarse grit. The meaning of these labels varies from manufacturer to manufacturer.

Bleaching or Whitening Agents and Restorative Options for Intrinsic Stain

Although intrinsic stains cannot be removed by traditional professional methods (scaling and selective polishing), they may be managed by tooth bleaching with a chemical oxidizing agent to lighten tooth discolorations or by restorative procedures such as veneers and crowns. Several commonly used oxidizing agents found in professionally applied, professionally dispensed and over-the-counter (OTC) products include hydrogen peroxide, carbamide peroxide, or papain (an enzyme from papaya fruit) as the active ingredient. A whitening product containing 10% carbamide peroxide is equivalent to another product that contains 3.3% hydrogen peroxide. Recognition of intrinsic staining, the client's perception of tooth color, and referral for appropriate treatment address the client's human need for a wholesome facial image. Intrinsic tooth stain severity and tooth color usually determine which stain management method (i.e., rubber cup or air polishing, tooth whitening, or a restorative option) is recommended, and these methods are discussed later in this chapter.

Extrinsic Stain Removal

Rubber-Cup Polishing

Rubber-cup polishing is the removal of extrinsic tooth stains after scaling using a low-speed dental handpiece, a prophylaxis angle with rubber cup and bristle brush, and prophylaxis paste or other cleaning or polishing agent. Rubber-cup polishing also is known as **coronal polishing** because the

TABLE 29-1

Abrasives Used in Dental Hygiene Practice

Abrasive Agent	Mohs Hardness Value*	Application
Potassium	0.4	Used as a cleaning agent in dentifrices and in desensitizing agents (potassium nitrate); promotes occlusion of dentinal tubules
Sodium	0.5	Used as a cleaning agent in dentifrices; used in some fluoride compounds
Aluminum silicates	2	Used as a cleaning and polishing agent; no excessive abrasion; compatible with dental fluoride compounds; noncorrosive to aluminum containers
Sodium bicarbonate, kaolinite	2.5	Used as a cleaning agent in dentifrices for oral biofilm and stain removal and as an acid-neutralizing agent
Calcium carbonate (whiting, calcite chalk)	3	Used as a cleaning agent in dentifrices for oral biofilm and stain removal; mild abrasive used to polish tooth enamel, gold foil, amalgam, and plastic materials
Phosphate salts (pyrophosphate, dibasic calcium phosphate dehydrate, tricalcium phosphate, sodium metaphosphate)	5	Used as cleaning agents in dentifrices for oral biofilm and stain removal
Rouge (jewelers rouge, iron oxide)	5-6	Used for polishing gold and precious metal alloys in the dental laboratory; blended with soft binders into a cake form; not used in the mouth.
Pumice	6-7	
Superfine pumice (pumice flour)		Used as a cleaning agent in prophylaxis paste for oral biofilm and stain removal; used for polishing tooth enamel, gold foil, dental amalgam, and acrylic resin
Fine pumice		Not for use on natural teeth
Medium pumice		Not for use on natural teeth
Coarse pumice		Not for use on natural teeth
Tin oxide (putty powder, stannic oxide)	6-7	Used extensively for polishing teeth and metallic restorations; mixed with water or glycerin to form a mildly abrasive paste
Silica or sand (silex [silicon dioxide], hydrated silica, sodium potassium aluminum silicate)	6-7	May be applied under air pressure (sandblasting) to remove investment material from base metal alloy castings; coated onto paper discs for grinding metal alloys and plastic materials Used for heavy stain removal; effectively cleans tooth surfaces with low abrasion and high cleaning capability
Zirconium silicate (zircon)	6.5-7.5	Used in dental prophylaxis pastes and to coat abrasive discs and strips
Garnet	6.5-7.5	Used for polishing acrylic dental appliances and composites
Cuttle	7	Originally a powdered calcareous shell of the cuttlefish but now derived from quartz; used to coat paper discs to finish gold alloys, acrylics, and composites
Corundum (aluminum oxide [alumina])	9	Aluminum oxide—used for polishing composite, highly filled hybrid composites, acrylic resin, and porcelain restorations and custom trays; bonded to discs or paper strips; impregnated into rubber wheels and points; air-propelled grit Levigated alumina—used on metals and for grinding metal alloys; used to make white stones
Silicon carbide	9.5	Used as an abrasive in coated disc; can cut metal alloys, ceramics, and plastic materials
Diamond	10	Used in polishing paste; used on ceramic, porcelain, and resin-based composite materials and metal-backed abrasive strips and furcation files

*Mohs Hardness Value: standard for the hardness of abrasives and substrates; the higher the value, the harder or more abrasive the material. For comparison, cementum is 2 to 3, dentin is 3 to 4, and enamel or apatite is 5 to 6. Even a very hard material is minimally abrasive if used with a very fine particle size.

technique is focused on the crowns of the teeth. Tooth polishing is another term used interchangeably with rubber-cup polishing. This traditional method is effective for removal of extrinsic tooth stains, has good client acceptance, and is easy to learn and perform. Five variables influence efficiency, effectiveness, and tooth structure loss during extrinsic tooth stain removal with a rubber cup:

- Abrasiveness of the prophylaxis paste (or other abrasive agent) used during the procedure: The harder the abrasive, the greater the rate of abrasion. Always use the least abrasive agent to accomplish stain removal.
- Quantity of abrasive agent: The greater the amount of abrasive particles applied, the greater the rate of abrasion. Abrasive agent particles should be suspended in a lubricating vehicle such as water or humectants to decrease both quantity of abrasive particles and frictional heat generated by the procedure. Never use a dry abrasive agent on tooth enamel. Always use wet abrasive agents.
- Contact time of the rubber cup or bristle brush on the tooth surface: The longer the contact time, the greater the rate of abrasion and frictional heat. Always use short, intermittent contact between rubber cup and the tooth or restorative materials.
- Speed or revolutions per minute (rpm) of the rubber cup or bristle brush: The greater the speed of the rotating rubber cup, the greater the rate of abrasion and frictional heat generated. Always use low speeds no greater than 3000 rpm.
- Applied pressure or force of the rubber cup or bristle brush on the tooth surface: The greater the force applied to the rubber cup against the tooth, the greater the rate of abrasion and frictional heat generated. Always use a light intermittent (staccato) touch.

To preserve tooth structure and prevent damage to teeth and restorative materials, the practitioner starts with the least abrasive agent and amount of agent, with the least amount of contact time, at the lowest speed, and with the least amount of pressure to remove the extrinsic stain and to avoid tooth surface damage. The clinician always can increase any of these variables if necessary to achieve the desired clinical outcome.

Adverse Effects on Teeth

Rubber-cup polishing removes the outer layer of tooth enamel. Because the highest fluoride concentration is in the outermost layer, performing repeated, routine rubber-cup polishing could remove the fluoride-rich outer enamel layer; however, minerals in saliva continuously remineralize enamel. Use of fluoride-containing toothpaste, gel, or mouth rinse, as indicated, on a daily basis also is important for remineralization. Prophylaxis paste containing fluoride or calcium phosphate also may contribute to remineralization; however, more research is indicated on the efficacy of these products. Research shows that the amount of fluoride lost during rubber-cup polishing is minimal, even when repeated over time; however, root surfaces may be at risk of tooth wear over time because cementum and dentin are softer than enamel. Demineralized tooth areas lose three times more surface structure during polishing than intact enamel. Newly erupted teeth are not fully mineralized, so polishing should be avoided on these teeth. Exposed root surfaces, demineralized white spot lesions, and newly erupted teeth should not be polished with an abrasive agent and require home and professional fluoride therapy because they are at risk for caries regardless of rubber-cup polishing. For clients with moderate, high, or extreme caries risk, professionally applied topical fluoride or fluoride varnish should be applied after tooth polishing, and coupled with recommendations for home fluoride use (see Chapter 18).

Dentin and cementum are less resistant to abrasion than tooth enamel. Because dentin and cementum can be abraded 25 times faster and 35 times faster, respectively, than enamel, polishing roots should be avoided. Moreover, tooth sensitivity to rubber-cup polishing may occur in cervical areas owing to the thinness of enamel in these areas and exposed dentin or cementum. Finally, coarse abrasives never are used on root surfaces. Stain on root surfaces often is removed with ultrasonic, sonic, or piezoelectric scaling devices set on a low power.

Adverse Effects on Restorations

Rubber-cup polishing may damage restorations by making surfaces rough. Gold, amalgam, conventional composites, and microfilled composites exhibit surface roughness after being polished with a prophylaxis paste. Therefore prophylaxis pastes designed for cosmetic restorations are recommended (e.g., Soft Shine Cosmetic Polishing Paste, Waterpik, Fort Collins, Colorado). Polishing of a titanium implant with an abrasive agent is not recommended because it would be damaged, and stain does not readily form on these implants. Plaque can be removed from titanium implants with oral hygiene aids. (Note that neither rubber-cup nor air polishing can be used safely on dental implants.) Restorative materials should be polished with the appropriate agent to maintain restorations.

Adverse Effects on Soft Tissues

Irritation of soft tissues can result from rubber-cup polishing if the tissues are inflamed; particles of the abrasive agent can become embedded in the gingiva and delay healing. Trauma to gingiva also can occur with improper technique, especially if the rubber cup is used at a high speed or with excessive pressure and/or is kept in one place too long. Pressure should be enough to flatten one edge of the cup so that it slips into the sulcus but not enough so that the entire lip of the cup is flattened. Generation of heat with the handpiece and rubber cup may initiate pulpal necrosis, especially in primary teeth with large pulps. Pulpal discomfort also may occur if pressure, speed, and abrasiveness of the polishing paste are sufficient to generate heat.

Adverse Effects on Environment

Aerosol production during rubber-cup polishing may transmit infectious disease to people in the dental care setting. Microorganisms remain suspended in the air for hours and settle on environmental surfaces. Inhalation of contaminated aerosols could be problematic for those with respiratory problems or who are immunocompromised. The clinician also may experience occupational injury from the weight of the handpiece. Most of these problems can be minimized by adhering to appropriate protocols for technique, ergonomic principles and equipment, and infection control and by using rubber-cup polishing selectively.

BOX 29-1

Contraindications and Precautions to Rubber-Cup Polishing

Absence of extrinsic stain
Newly erupted teeth, especially primary teeth
Tooth decalcification, hypocalcification, hypoplasia, demineralization, rampant caries
Areas of recession where cementum or dentin is exposed
Areas of dentinal hypersensitivity
Acute gingival or periodontal inflammation
Immediately after deep scaling, root planing, or curettage
Restored tooth surfaces: composite, bonding, glass ionomer, porcelain, gold, titanium (unless special polishing agent for these materials is used)
Allergy to ingredients in paste
Clients who:

- are highly susceptible to infection (e.g., who have pulmonary disease, are immunosuppressed, are medically complex, or are debilitated)*
- have communicable diseases that could be spread via contaminated aerosols*
- have the highest risk of adverse effects if not premedicated (if so, then antibiotic premedication may be required for polishing)*

*Precautions needed, but these are not strict contraindications.

Risk Management Strategies for Rubber-Cup Polishing

Because of the adverse effects discussed in the preceding section, contraindications to rubber-cup polishing exist (Box 29-1). During or after scaling and root planing, stains and biofilm on teeth can be removed during hand-activated and mechanized scaling; biofilm also can be removed mechanically using a toothbrush and interdental aids. When stains remain after scaling, selective polishing may be indicated.

Selective Rubber-Cup Polishing

Selective rubber-cup polishing, also known as extrinsic stain removal, is the practice of omitting tooth polishing where there is no extrinsic tooth stain and when the procedure could cause loss of tooth structure, damage to restorative materials, or gingival abrasion or undermine the systemic health of the client. The procedure is applied "selectively" by polishing only those tooth surfaces that are stained, avoiding newly erupted teeth, cementum, dentin, demineralized areas, and restored tooth surfaces that could be damaged by the process. Not all teeth must be polished on a routine basis. Enamel is approximately 2.5 mm thick on cuspal surfaces, with considerable thinning at the cervix of the tooth. Polishing with pumice for 30 seconds removes about 4 μm of the fluoride-rich outer layer of enamel. These effects are cumulative over years of polishing during maintenance visits; however, when appropriate technique and low abrasive agents are used, this risk is not clinically relevant.

Tooth polishing (extrinsic stain removal) has no therapeutic value in terms of periodontal health. Although it is a cosmetic concern, tooth stain is not pathologic. Because extrinsic stain and oral biofilm do not block fluoride uptake in enamel, and biofilm has the potential to serve as a reservoir for the fluoride, topical fluoride applications can be provided without first polishing the teeth.

The value of stain removal lies in the client's desire for whiter teeth and a pleasing facial appearance. Therefore selective polishing of only tooth surfaces with stain (instead of the routine polishing of all tooth surfaces) is recommended when localized areas of extrinsic stain are present. For clients to make an informed decision, they must be educated about the choice of selective polishing and its rationale, alternative methods of stain removal and management, the lack of therapeutic value in rubber-cup polishing for stain removal, and the purely cosmetic nature of the procedure. When the dental hygienist prefers to use full-mouth rubber-cup polishing for application of potentially therapeutic agents such as hydroxycarbonate apatite (HCA), calcium phosphate, fluoride, or a desensitizing agent, that option also should be discussed with the client. In those cases, the lowest abrasive agent that can be employed effectively should be chosen.

Preprocedural Rinse

Before selective polishing, like all oral health care procedures that produce aerosols, all clients should rinse with a preprocedural antimicrobial rinse for 30 seconds to decrease infectious organisms present in aerosol production. Protective safety glasses for the client are recommended for all intraoral procedures, especially for those that generate spatter. The dental hygienist follows the Centers for Disease Control and Prevention (CDC) guidelines for infection control to ensure that clients and clinicians are protected from health risks (see Chapter 9).

Postprofessionally Applied Topical Fluoride Therapy

When the client is indicated for selective polishing or a polishing procedure on all teeth and informed consent is provided by the client, the rubber-cup polishing procedure should be followed by professionally applied topical fluoride therapy.

Client Education and Motivation

Often clients with poor oral hygiene are unaware of the look and feel of clean, polished teeth. Teeth with oral deposits may feel and look normal to the individual after a period of time. Scaling and polishing teeth in half of the mouth is an effective strategy because it allows the client to experience the look and feel of clean tooth surfaces and a positive gingival response as compared to what the client is accustomed. When selective polishing is used as a teaching strategy, most clients take notice and cannot wait until the other half of the mouth is treated. Through professional dental hygiene care, a new baseline for the client is established to maintain at home.

Armamentarium for Rubber-Cup Polishing

Prophylaxis Paste

Abrasives used in polishing agents (e.g., prophylaxis pastes) are applied selectively based on amount and type of extrinsic stain, and whether the surface to be polished is a natural or restored surface (Figure 29-2, *A*). Prophylaxis pastes are pleasantly flavored and may contain active ingredients to prevent dental caries (fluoride); enhance enamel

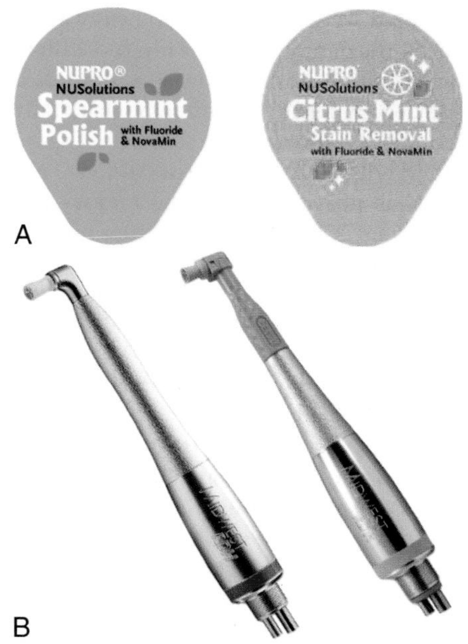

Figure 29-2. **A,** Examples of commercial prophylaxis pastes in unit doses. **B,** Low-speed handpieces. (Courtesy DENTSPLY Preventive Care Division, York, Pennsylvania.)

mineralization, tooth smoothness, and enamel luster (e.g., amorphous calcium phosphate [ACP], casein phosphopeptides [CPP-ACP]); improve tooth whiteness (e.g., hydrogen peroxide), or decrease tooth sensitivity (e.g., fluoride, arginine bicarbonate, CPP-ACP, ACP, bicarbonate or carbonate). Types of prophylaxis pastes are the following:

- Fluoride-containing prophylaxis paste (Nupro, Oral-B)
  - May contain 4000 to 20,000 ppm fluoride ion, so the client must not swallow it
  - May replace some of the fluoride lost by the abrasive action of the polishing procedure
  - Not a substitute for professionally applied fluoride therapy when indicated
- ACP-containing prophylaxis paste (Enamel Pro with ACP)
  - Combines with fluoride and tooth structure to form apatite
  - May seal exposed dentinal tubules; may reduce dentinal hypersensitivity
  - May enhance tooth smoothness and luster of the enamel
  - More research needed
- CPP-ACP–containing paste (MI Paste)
  - Combines with fluoride and tooth structure to form apatite
  - May enhance tooth smoothness and luster of the enamel
  - Promotes remineralization
  - May seal exposed dentinal tubules; may reduce dentinal hypersensitivity
  - Also can be applied with a finger or custom mouth tray
  - Not to be used if client has a casein allergy; can be used in clients who are lactose intolerant
  - More research needed
- Hydrogen peroxide–containing prophylaxis paste (Natural Elegance)
  - May contain up to 35% hydrogen peroxide to provide a whitening benefit
  - Hydrogen peroxide gel can be polished into the tooth surface with a rubber cup and prophylaxis paste
  - Best for maintaining tooth whitening, rather than as a tooth-whitening protocol
  - More research needed
- Arginine bicarbonate, calcium bicarbonate, or carbonate-containing prophylaxis paste (ProClude)
  - May seal exposed dentinal tubules; may reduce dentinal hypersensitivity
  - More research needed
- NovaMin-containing prophylaxis paste (with hydroxycarbonate apatite [HCA], calcium, phosphorus, sodium, and silica) (NuSolutions Prophy Paste)
  - May seal exposed dentinal tubules; may reduce dentinal hypersensitivity
  - More research needed
- Xylitol-containing pastes may be combined with other agents listed
  - Although it is known that xylitol provides a taste advantage because it is sweet, it is dose dependent for caries prevention and effectiveness against plaque biofilm; therefore its therapeutic benefit is less likely than its taste benefit.

Prophylaxis pastes containing microfine white sapphire particles also are marketed to restore the original luster to veneer, composite, gold, and porcelain restorations and also can be used safely on natural teeth (e.g., Soft Shine cosmetic polishing paste). Toothpastes also contain mild abrasives for cleaning with a toothbrush or with a rubber cup and low-speed handpiece. The least abrasive type of paste necessary for stain removal should be used at a low speed with light intermittent pressure.

Prophylaxis Angle and Dental Handpiece

A disposable or stainless steel prophylaxis angle attached to a low-speed, ergonomically designed handpiece is used for coronal polishing (Figure 29-2, *B*).

The head of the prophylaxis angle has one of the following:

- Rubber cup (screw-type, latch-type, or snap-on or on a disposable prophylaxis angle)—used on all tooth surfaces
- Flat or pointed bristle brush (screw-type, latch-type, or snap-on or on a disposable prophylaxis angle)—for stain removal on occlusal surfaces and in fossa (Figure 29-3)

Handpieces and stainless steel prophylaxis angles are cleaned, lubricated, and sterilized according to manufacturers' directions. Disposable prophylaxis angles are discarded after each use. Materials and procedures for rubber-cup polishing are outlined in Procedure 29-1 and the corresponding Competency Form.

Hand Scaling

Hand-activated instruments such as curets and sickle scalers are designed primarily for calculus removal but also can be used for extrinsic stain removal (see Chapter 26). When stain adheres to calculus, it may be removed efficiently along with the calculus. Because hand-activated instruments are small, they can remove stain in areas inaccessible to a rubber cup (e.g., in an embrasure). Hand-activated instruments are not significantly abrasive to enamel surfaces; however, they can remove cementum on root surfaces, so overinstrumentation

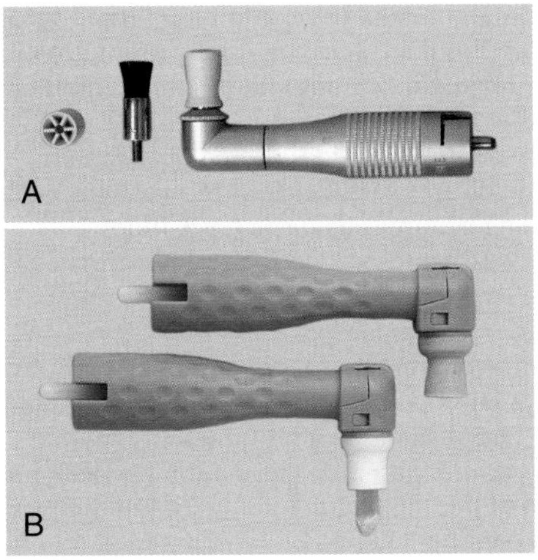

Figure 29-3. **A,** Metal prophylaxis angle with rubber cup and brush. **B,** Disposable plastic prophylaxis angles with rubber cup and with brush. (From Newman MG, Takei HH, Klokkevold PR, Carranza FA: *Carranza's clinical periodontology,* ed 11, St Louis, 2012, Saunders.)

should be avoided. When moderate to heavy stain is present on root surfaces, the dental hygienist is faced with the problem of removing the stain with the least alteration of exposed cementum or dentin. Because stain removal is only cosmetic, the client should be informed that stain is not associated with oral disease and will not harm teeth or gingiva if not removed. As much stain as possible should be removed during root planing with curets. The less root structure removed, the less chance of root surface sensitivity after the procedure. At present, any method capable of removing stain from root surfaces also may remove cementum.

Sonic, Piezoelectric, and Ultrasonic Scaling Instruments

Ultrasonic and sonic, and scaling (see Chapter 27) to remove extrinsic stain has the same advantages and disadvantages as when these processes are used for calculus removal. Efficiency and efficacy are the primary benefits for selecting mechanized instruments for stain removal. In addition, a slender tip is able to remove stain on occlusal surfaces and in

Procedure 29-1 Rubber-Cup Polishing

EQUIPMENT

Polishing paste, aesthetic restoration polishing paste, and low-abrasive toothpaste
Prophylaxis angle and toothbrush
Dental floss or tape
Floss threader (if needed)
Rubber cups and pointed bristle brushes
Low-speed handpiece
Gauze squares
Mouth mirror, air-water syringe
Disclosing solution
Preprocedural antimicrobial mouth rinse
Saliva ejector or high-volume evacuation (HVE) tip
Safety glasses for client
Personal protective equipment (PPE)

STEPS

Preparation and Positioning

1. Evaluate client's health and pharmacologic history to determine need for precautions or treatment alterations.
2. Identify tooth surfaces indicated and contraindicated for polishing. Always polish aesthetic restorations first, then polish teeth.
3. Educate client about selective polishing procedure.
4. Select polishing abrasive based on type of stain and oral restorations and assemble basic setup (see Figure 29-2, *A*).
5. Wear appropriate PPE and provide protective eyewear for client.
6. Provide client with a preprocedural antimicrobial rinse polishing.
7. Have client tilt head up and turn slightly away when polishing maxillary and mandibular right buccal surfaces of posterior teeth (left buccal if left-handed practitioner) and maxillary and mandibular left lingual surfaces of posterior teeth (right lingual if left-handed practitioner).

Grasp

8. Use modified pen grasp (Figure 29-4).
9. Rest handpiece in V of hand.
10. Have all fingers in contact as a unit.

Fulcrum

11. Establish intraoral fulcrum close to working area.
12. Fulcrum on ring finger.
13. Use moderate fulcrum pressure.

Adaptation

14. Angle rubber cup to flare at gingival margin.
15. Adapt rubber cup to reach distal, facial and lingual, or mesial surfaces.
16. Adapt cup to tooth by rotating handpiece or pivoting on fulcrum as necessary.
17. Adapt brush to occlusal surface.

Stroke

18. Fill cup with paste and evenly apply to surfaces to be polished.
19. Place cup on tooth; activate handpiece by gently stepping on rheostat. Stroke from the gingival third to the incisal third with just enough pressure to make the cup flare while using wrist-forearm motion to polish the teeth.

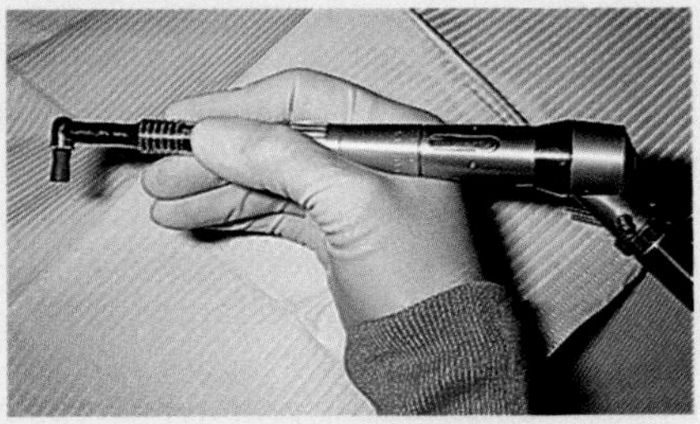

Figure 29-4. Handpiece grasp.

Procedure 29-1 Rubber-Cup Polishing—cont'd

20. **Use low speed and intermittent, dabbing, overlapping** strokes with light to moderate pressure in a cervical to occlusal or incisal direction (Figure 29-5).
21. Remove rubber cup from tooth at completion of stroke; readapt cup for next stroke.
22. Hold mirror in nondominant hand to retract buccal mucosa. Instruct client to close mouth halfway and to tilt head slightly toward the ceiling. Polish buccal surfaces of maxillary right posterior quadrant (Figure 29-6).
23. Polish facial surfaces of maxillary anterior teeth. Palm mirror and retract lip with fingers of nondominant hand (Figure 29-7).
24. Hold mirror in nondominant hand to retract buccal mucosa. Instruct client to close mouth halfway and to tilt head slightly toward the ceiling. Polish buccal surfaces of maxillary left posterior quadrant (Figure 29-8).
25. Polish lingual surfaces of maxillary right posterior quadrant. Use mirror for indirect view and indirect lighting (Figure 29-9).
26. Polish lingual surfaces of maxillary anterior teeth. Use mirror for indirect vision (Figure 29-10).
27. Polish lingual surfaces of maxillary left posterior quadrant. Use mirror for indirect vision (Figure 29-11).
28. Rinse client's teeth.
29. Hold mirror in nondominant hand to retract right buccal mucosa. Polish buccal surfaces of mandibular right posterior quadrant (Figure 29-12).
30. Palm mirror and retract lip with fingers of nondominant hand. Polish facial surfaces of mandibular anterior teeth (Figure 29-13).
31. Retract buccal mucosa with mirror and polish buccal surfaces of mandibular left posterior quadrant (Figure 29-14).
32. Polish lingual surfaces of mandibular right posterior quadrant. Use mirror to retract tongue and for indirect vision and lighting (Figure 29-15).

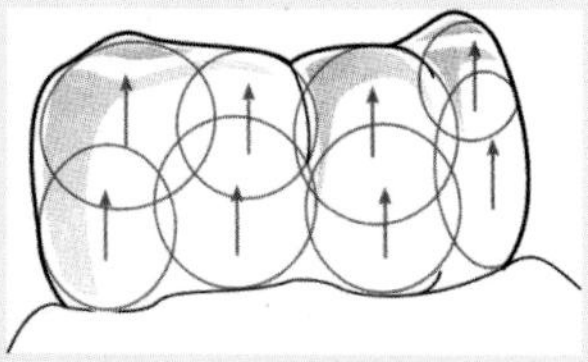

Figure 29-5. Overlapping strokes to ensure complete coverage of the tooth as needed. (From Bird DL, Robinson DS: *Torres and Ehrlich modern dental assisting,* ed 11, St Louis, 2015, Saunders.)

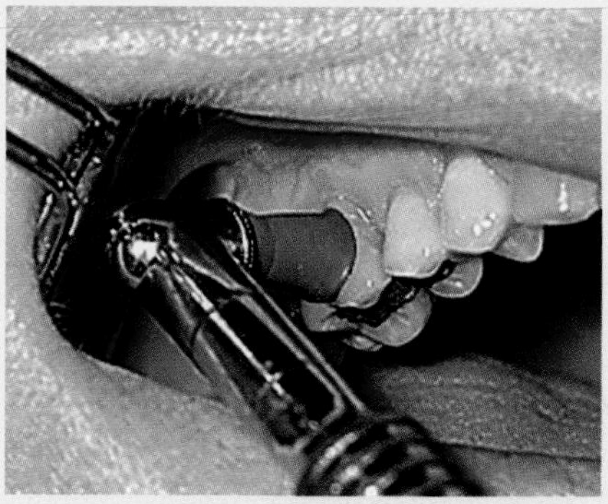

Figure 29-6. Polishing the buccal surfaces of the maxillary right posterior quadrant.

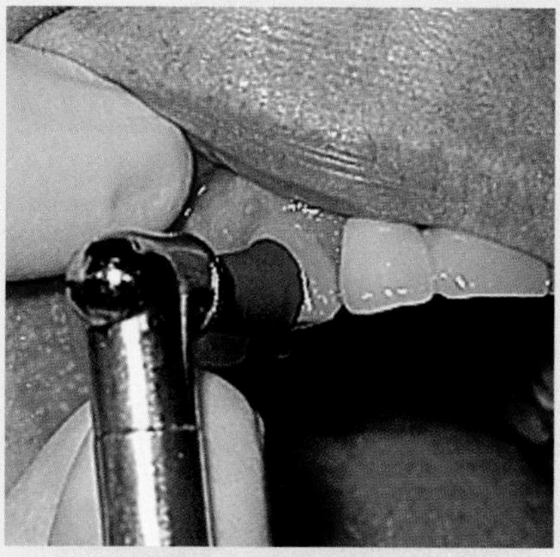

Figure 29-7. Polishing the facial surfaces of the maxillary anterior teeth.

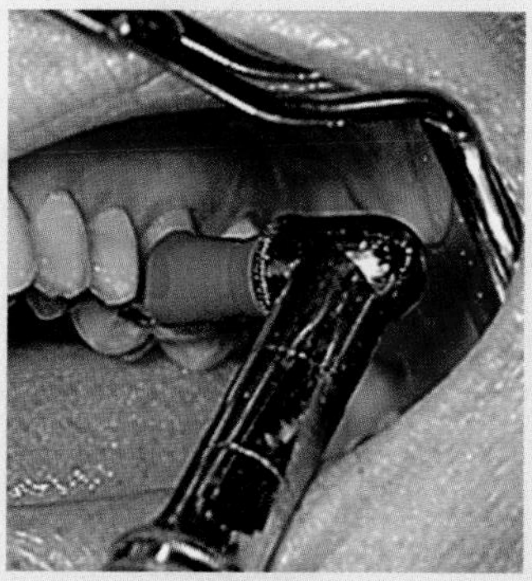

Figure 29-8. Polishing the buccal surfaces of the maxillary left posterior quadrant.

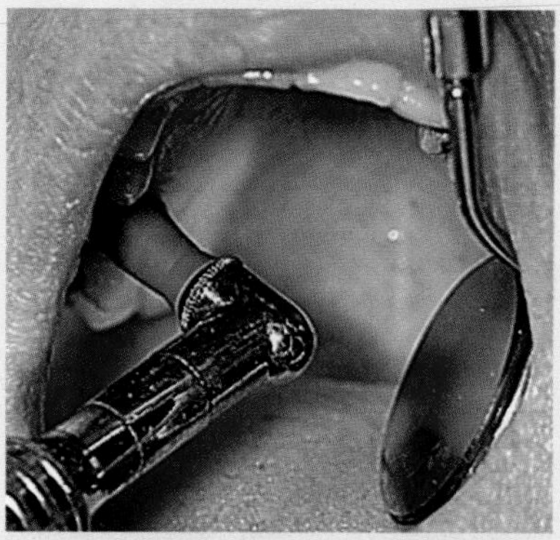

Figure 29-9. Polishing the lingual surfaces of the maxillary right posterior quadrant.

Continued

Procedure 29-1 Rubber-Cup Polishing—cont'd

33. Polish lingual surfaces of mandibular anterior teeth (Figure 29-16). Use mirror for indirect vision and indirect lighting. Avoid resting mirror on sublingual mucosa.
34. Polish lingual surfaces of mandibular left posterior quadrant (Figure 29-17). Use mirror to retract tongue and for indirect vision and lighting. Replace rubber cup with flat or pointed brush and remove occlusal stain.
35. Floss client's teeth with abrasive agent still on teeth, then rinse.
36. Apply topical fluoride therapy (see Chapter 33).
37. Document completion of service in client's record under "Services Rendered" and date the entry (e.g., "Removed tobacco stain with rubber-cup polishing on No. 6-11L, 22-27L; removed client oral biofilm from remaining teeth with a soft toothbrush and fluoride gel toothpaste. Flossed all teeth. APF topical fluoride gel treatment—tray method—provided for 4 minutes. Advised client not to eat, drink, or rinse for 30 minutes").

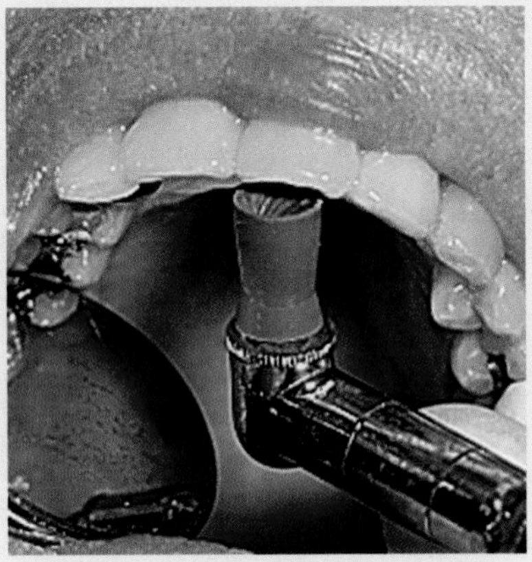

Figure 29-10. Polishing the lingual surfaces of the maxillary anterior teeth.

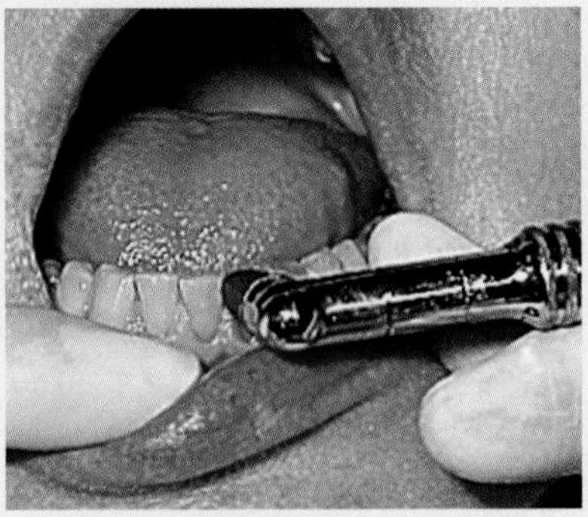

Figure 29-13. Polishing the facial surfaces of the mandibular anterior teeth.

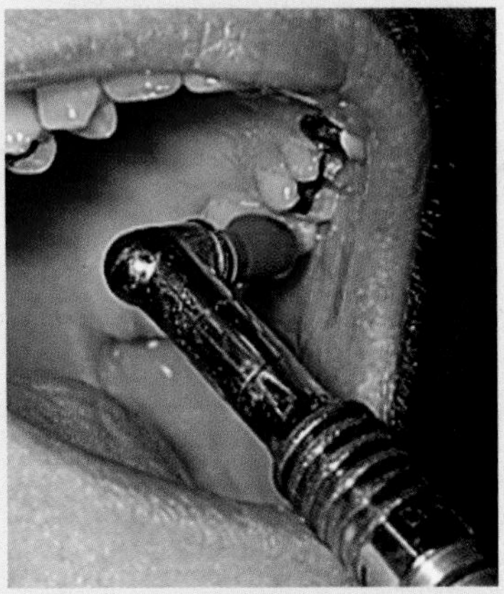

Figure 29-11. Polishing the lingual surfaces of the maxillary left posterior quadrant.

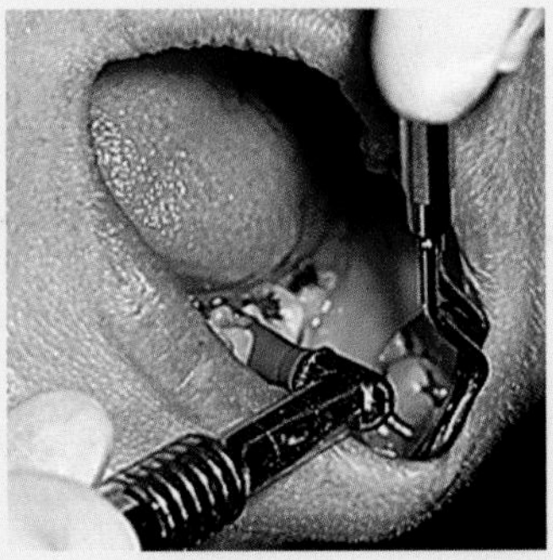

Figure 29-14. Polishing the buccal surfaces of the mandibular left posterior quadrant.

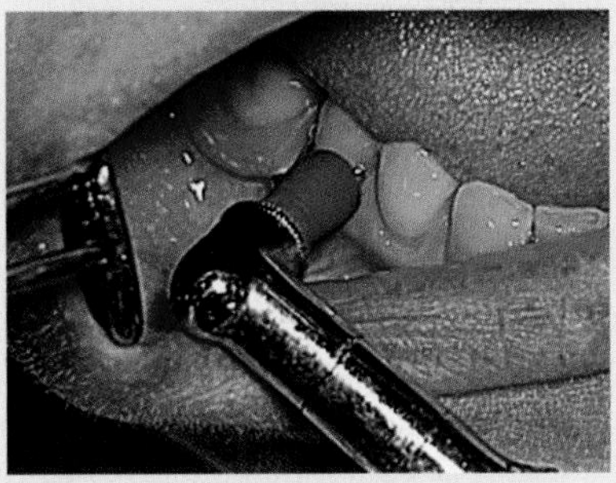

Figure 29-12. Polishing the buccal surfaces of the mandibular right posterior quadrant.

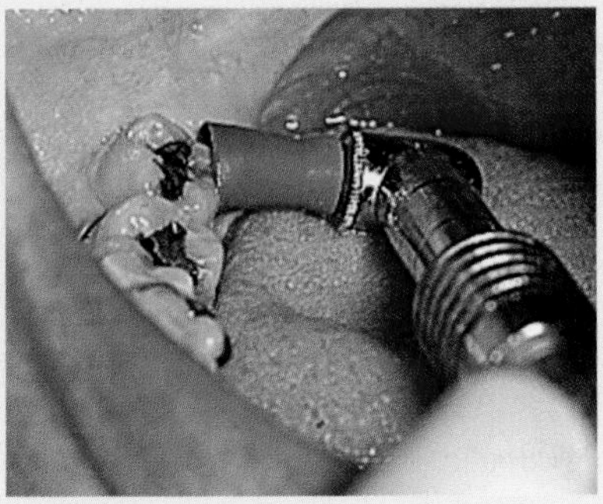

Figure 29-15. Polishing the lingual surfaces of the mandibular right posterior quadrant.

Procedure 29-1 Rubber-Cup Polishing—cont'd

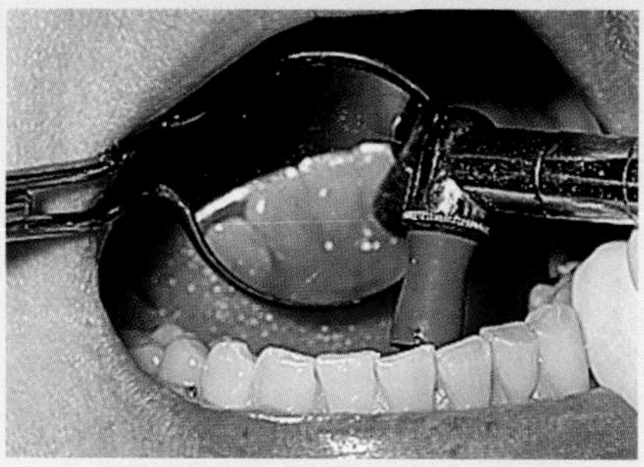

Figure 29-16. Polishing the lingual surfaces of the mandibular anterior teeth.

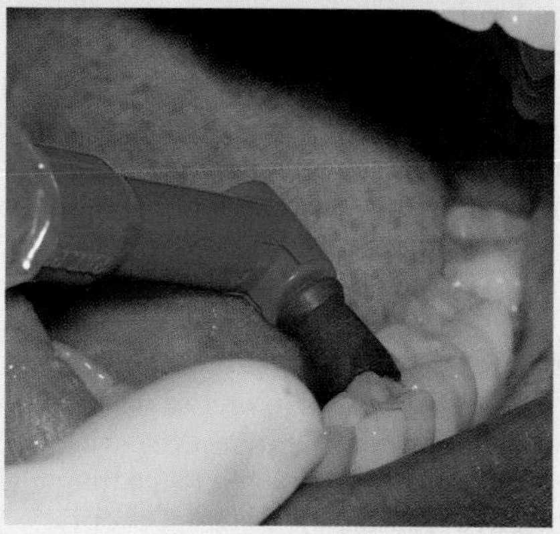

Figure 29-17. Polishing the lingual surfaces of the mandibular left posterior quadrant. (From Bird DL, Robinson DS: *Torres and Ehrlich modern dental assisting,* ed 11, St Louis, 2015, Saunders.)

Photographs courtesy Dr. Margaret Walsh, University of California–San Francisco.

areas of rotated or overlapped teeth. There is usually good client acceptance, and operator fatigue is minimized compared with hand-activated instrumentation. In comparison of the results of studies on the effects of hand-activated instruments versus sonic and ultrasonic instruments on root surface roughness, the findings are ambiguous. Rough cementum and lost tooth structure are encountered with both types of instruments. Using a low power with precision thins tips designed for root debridement is the safest choice when instrumentation is required for stain or calculus removal on exposed root surfaces.

Aerosols are created with sonic and ultrasonic instrumentation and, if used improperly, can generate heat and cause tissue trauma. Aerosols can be minimized with the use of high-volume evacuation.

Air Polishing

Air polishing is a method of stain removal that uses a specially designed device with a handpiece that delivers a spray of warm water and prophy powder (sodium bicarbonate or aluminum trihydroxide) under pressure (see Figures 29-18 and 29-19). An efficient and effective method of stain removal, the air polisher has the following advantages:

- Requires less time than traditional rubber-cup polishing
- Removes stain three times as fast as hand scaling.
- Creates less operator fatigue

Airpolishing also is recommended for cleaning and removing extrinsic stain from pits and fissures before placement of dental sealants. The manufacturer's instructions caution against use in clients with respiratory diseases because of the potential for aspiration.

Effects on Oral and Dental Tissues

Intact enamel surfaces are not damaged when stain removal is accomplished with the air polisher. However, prolonged use of air polishing on cementum and dentin can remove significant tooth structure and should be avoided. Results are inconsistent with regard to which method is ideal for stain removal on root surfaces. Currently it appears that air polishing may be the least damaging and most efficient means of removing stain on enamel, but no polishing method is risk free for cementum.

Gingival bleeding and abrasion are the most common soft-tissue effects of air polishing. These outcomes are temporary, and healing occurs quickly. However, the tip of the air polisher should be pointed away from the gingiva to avoid tissue trauma.

Clients report a salty taste when sodium bicarbonate prophy powder is used in the device, but it is not objectionable if the water-to-powder ratio is adjusted properly. Laying a moist gauze square on the tongue may prevent tongue irritation and an excessively salty taste. Rinsing with water or mouthwash also helps to reduce the salty taste. Another option is the use of mint-flavored or aluminum trihydroxide prophy powder.

Effects on Restorations and Titanium Implants

The effects of air polishing on restorative materials have been researched extensively.

- Extended use of air polishing on all restorative dental materials should be avoided.
- Avoid air polishing on or near the following:
  - Amalgam alloy and other metal restorations, to prevent a matte finish, surface roughness, morphologic changes, and structural alterations
  - Composite restorations to prevent surface roughness or pitting
  - Porcelain, gold alloy, and glass ionomer restorations, to prevent surface roughness, staining, pitting, and loss of marginal integrity
  - Sapphire and pure titanium implants, to prevent surface alteration
  - Dental implants (see Chapter 58)

Safety Issues

Air polishing safety concerns for the client, clinician, and others in the treatment area appear in the literature. Client concerns include the following:

- Systemic problems from absorption of sodium bicarbonate prophy powder; however, aluminum trihydroxide powder is an option for sodium-sensitive clients
- Respiratory difficulties and potential for infection from inhaling contaminated aerosols, especially in clients with respiratory diseases
- Stinging of the lips from the concentrated spray
- Eye problems from spray entering the eyes, especially if contact lenses are worn; therefore safety goggles are recommended

These problems can be managed by coating a client's lips with a protective lubricant, using appropriate technique including safety suction devices, removing contact lenses, wearing safety glasses, and placing a protective drape over the client's nose and eyes.

It is important for the body to maintain a specific balance between acids and bases. Some individuals cannot adjust if this balance is disturbed. Owing to the potential absorption of sodium bicarbonate by the oral mucosa, air polisher manufacturers caution against using the sodium bicarbonate prophy powder during air polishing with such clients. Limited information is available on the systemic effects of sodium bicarbonate or aluminum trihydroxide absorption from air polishing powder.

Because of the marked rise in aerosols generated with air polishing, additional health hazards potentially exist for clients and healthcare professionals present during or after a procedure. To decrease potential risks, clinicians should adhere to standard precautions, including the following:

- Wear a well-fitting face mask with recommended bacterial filtration efficiency (BFE) scores of 74% to 98%.
- Ensure the client rinses with a preprocedural antimicrobial such as 0.12% chlorhexidine gluconate to reduce production of infectious aerosols.
- Use high-volume evacuation, which reduces aerosols better than a saliva ejector.
- Disinfect contaminated surfaces as far away as 6 feet from the immediate treatment area to help prevent cross-contamination between clients. Contaminated surfaces, if not covered with disposable plastic drapes, should be cleaned and disinfected with an approved high-level surface disinfectant (see Chapter 9). To ensure safety of clinicians and clients, the CDC guidelines for infection control as outlined previously for rubber-cup polishing are followed.

Air polishing is included in the dental hygiene care plan only after a careful review of the client's health and dental history and a thorough examination of the oral hard and soft tissues. A synopsis of the medical contraindications to air polishing can be found in Box 29-2. Table 29-2 contains a listing of other contraindications and precautions that should be considered when evaluating appropriateness of air polishing for a particular client.

Air Polishing Technique

Materials and sequence of steps for air polishing are outlined in Procedure 29-2 and the corresponding Competency Form, based on the manufacturer's guidelines for the device (e.g., Cavitron Prophy-Jet, DENTSPLY Preventive Care Division, York, Pennsylvania). Manufacturers' directions should be followed for maintenance and care of equipment.

BOX 29-2

Medical Contraindications and Precautions to Air Polishing

- Low-sodium diet or history of hypertension (for sodium-containing prophy powder only)*
- Respiratory illness that limits swallowing or breathing
- Communicable disease that can be transmitted via contaminated aerosols
- Renal insufficiency or end-stage renal disease
- Addison's disease
- Cushing's disease
- Metabolic alkalosis†
- Medications such as mineralocorticoid steroids, antidiuretics, or potassium supplements†
- High-risk clients needing antibiotic premedication may have to be premedicated for air polishing.
- Clients wearing contact lenses should remove them first and wear safety glasses.

*Air polishing can be performed with sodium-free prophy powder (Cavitron Jet Fresh [blue bottle]).

†Precautions needed, but these are not strict contraindications.

Intrinsic Stain Management

Although intrinsic stains cannot be removed by traditional professional methods (scaling and selective polishing), they may be managed by tooth bleaching with a chemical oxidizing agent to lighten tooth discolorations or by restorative procedures such as veneers and crowns.

Several commonly used oxidizing agents found in professionally applied, professionally dispensed and in over-the-counter (OTC) products include hydrogen peroxide, carbamide peroxide, or papain (an enzyme from papaya fruit) as the active ingredient. A whitening product containing 10% carbimide peroxide is equivalent to another product that contains 3.3% hydrogen peroxide. Recognition of intrinsic staining and referral for appropriate treatment address the client's human need for a wholesome facial image. Intrinsic tooth stain severity and the client's level of concern about tooth color and appearance usually determine which stain management method is recommended. These are discussed later in this chapter.

Tooth Whitening

Tooth whitening is a viable alternative for stain management when tooth stains are intrinsic. It also can be used when a client has a human need for a wholesome facial image that is unmet because of concern about tooth color. Tooth whitening is a cosmetic procedure. Many techniques ranging from OTC products to professionally dispensed whitening to in-office laser systems are available and vary significantly in cost to the client. Whitening procedures must be approached with caution. The dental hygienist has a responsibility to

TABLE 29-2

Dental Contraindications and Precautions Related to Air Polishing

	Specially Processed Sodium Bicarbonate Air-Polishing Powder	Aluminum Trihydroxide Air-Polishing Powder (Sodium Free)
Composite restorations or bonding	No	No
Luting agents	No	No
Porcelain restorations, including crowns, veneers, inlays, onlays	Yes, if margin is avoided; otherwise, no	No
Gold (foil or castings) restorations	Yes, if margin is avoided; otherwise, no	No
Compomer	No	No
Amalgam restorations	Yes	Yes
Microfilled composite restorations	No	No
Glass ionomer restorations	No	No
Hybrid composite restorations	No	No
Absence of stain	No	No
Exposed cementum or dentin	Yes	Yes
Areas of hypersensitivity	No	No
Immediately after deep scaling or root planing when acute gingival or periodontal inflammation is present	Yes	Yes

Procedure 29-2 Air Polishing Technique

EQUIPMENT

Sodium bicarbonate powder or aluminum trihydroxide air-polishing powder and low-abrasive toothpaste (Figure 29-18)
Air-polisher device (Figure 29-19) and toothbrush
Dental floss or tape
Mouth mirror, air-water syringe
Disclosing solution
Lubricant for client's lips
Saliva ejector and high-volume evacuation (HVE) tip
Safety glasses for client
Personal protective equipment (PPE)
Preprocedural antimicrobial mouth rinse

STEPS

Preparation and Positioning

1. Evaluate client's health and pharmacologic history to determine need for antibiotic premedication.
2. Identify tooth surfaces and restorations indicated and contraindicated for polishing and agents to be used.
3. Educate client about selective polishing procedure.
4. Assemble high-speed evacuation and saliva ejector.
5. Verify that slurry exits from device tip when held outside the mouth; adjust saliva ejector as necessary.
6. Use appropriate PPE and provide protective eyewear for client.
7. Clinician, client, and equipment must be in appropriate position for each area.

Grasp

8. Use modified pen grasp.
9. Rest handpiece in V of hand.
10. Have all fingers in contact as a unit.
11. Tuck excess cord around pinkie finger, if desired.

Fulcrum

12. Use external soft-tissue fulcrums.

Adaptation and Stroke

13. Activate foot pedal by pushing halfway down for water and all the way down for combined air-water-powder spray.
14. At about 3 to 4 mm from tooth surface and at correct angulation, use constant circular sweeping motions, from proximal to proximal; pivot nozzle to surface being polished; polish several teeth for 1 to 2 seconds each and rinse (Figure 29-20). Surfaces without stain are cleaned with a toothbrush and low-abrasive toothpaste.

Other

15. Rinse with water; floss all teeth (or have client do so and evaluate their flossing technique).

Continued

Procedure 29-2 Air Polishing Technique—cont'd

16. Evaluate effectiveness with disclosing solution, compressed air, and good lighting.
17. Provide professionally applied topical fluoride treatment.
18. Dispose of single-use items according to federal, state, and local regulations.
19. Properly disinfect and sterilize all other equipment.
20. Document completion of service in client's record under "Services Rendered" and date the entry (e.g., "Removed tobacco stain with air polishing on No. 6-11L, 22-27L; removed client oral biofilm from remaining teeth with a soft toothbrush and fluoride toothpaste. Flossed all teeth. APF topical fluoride gel treatment—tray method—provided for 4 minutes. Advised client not to eat, drink, or rinse for 30 minutes").

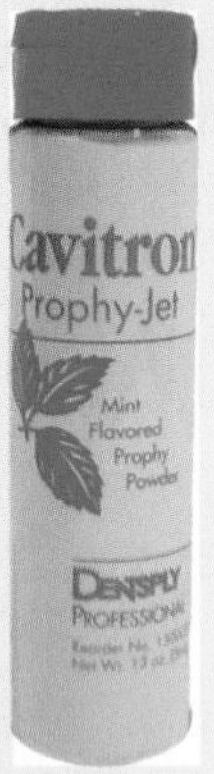

Figure 29-18. Flavored prophy powder for use in air-polishing device. (Courtesy DENTSPLY Preventive Care Division, York, Pennsylvania.)

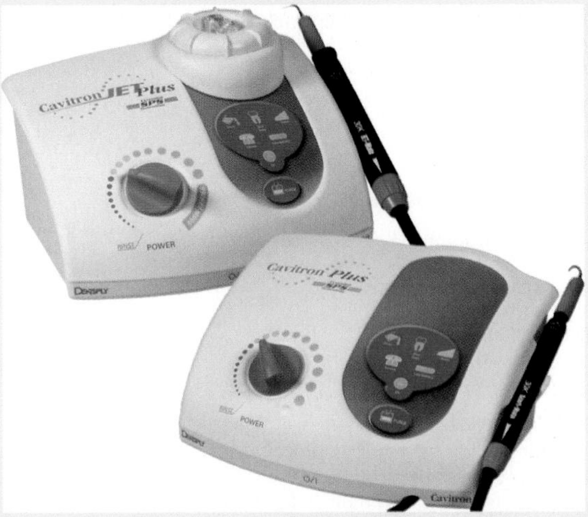

Figure 29-19. Prophy-Jet and ultrasonic scaler combination. (Courtesy DENTSPLY Preventive Care Division, York, Pennsylvania.)

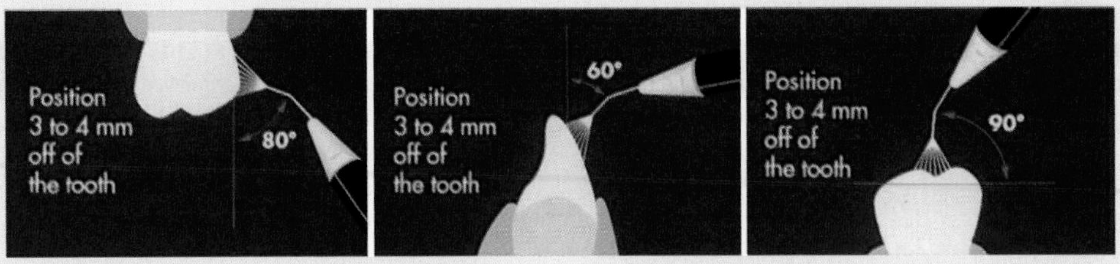

Figure 29-20. Recommended angulations of Prophy-Jet nozzle to tooth surface. (Adapted from DENTSPLY Preventive Care Division, York, Pennsylvania.)

understand the processes involved in tooth whitening. It is also important to ensure that clients understand the ramifications of tooth whitening before its initiation. The dental hygienist's role is summarized in Box 29-3.

Bleaching or Whitening Agents

Over-the-Counter Whitening Products

There are three types of OTC whitening toothpastes:

- Toothpaste containing a mild abrasive to remove extrinsic stains and agents to prevent stain formation. All toothpastes contain some abrasives and are capable of potentially removing stains whether they are labeled "whitening" or not. Toothpastes with a high content of abrasives are not recommended for daily use. These products do not affect intrinsic stains.
- Toothpaste containing a bleaching agent, such as papain, carbamide peroxide, or hydrogen peroxide. Note that the American Dental Association (ADA) Council on Scientific Affairs does not recommend some of these for long-term use.
- Toothpaste containing titanium dioxide. The titanium dioxide covers extrinsic stains like paint covers a wall and does not change the internal tooth color.

Some OTC products are a cause for concern in terms of efficacy and safety owing to the potential for overuse and abuse by uninformed clients. Commercial whitening kits containing an oxidizing agent and materials to form a "boil and fit" mouth tray are available. Oxidizing gel may seep out of improperly fitted trays and harm soft tissues. An acidic prerinse that can damage enamel is found in some kits. Laypersons may not know how to deal with side effects they may encounter. Once removed, extrinsic stain may be prevented by a client's change in self-care practices.

Without a comprehensive oral examination to determine stain cause and the safest, most appropriate method to use in treating the stain, clients may neglect to seek appropriate care for what may be a serious undiagnosed oral problem. For example, a dark area on a tooth may be due to a carious lesion or a tooth in need of a root canal. Whitening would not remedy either situation. Clients should be encouraged to seek professional care to whiten teeth.

BOX 29-3

Dental Hygienist's Role in Tooth Bleaching

- Provide client education on ramifications of bleaching treatment before its initiation. Recommend homecare to reduce dentinal hypersensitivity that may occur with tooth whitening procedures (e.g., use home fluoride therapy, potassium nitrate gels, and/or toothpaste with 5% potassium nitrate and fluoride 2 weeks before procedure, during procedure, and/or after procedure).
- Determine stain cause, allergies to ingredients in bleaching agents, and client expectations.
- Assess for conditions that contraindicate bleaching.
- Assess for any signs of caries or defective restorations that must be addressed before initiation of any bleaching procedure.
- Assess for any tooth sensitivity; clients with extreme tooth sensitivity are poor candidates for tooth bleaching.
- Evaluate translucency of teeth for alternative whitening procedures; highly translucent teeth may appear more gray than white after bleaching.
- Assess presence and extent of gingival recession that may contraindicate bleaching.
- Assess client's oral self-care to guide educational services.
- Assist client in setting realistic short- and long-term expectations (e.g., pretreatment and posttreatment comparisons using a shade guide, intraoral photographs, computer imaging, or an intraoral video camera).
- Use radiograph, percussion, thermal testing, and electrical pulp testing to help determine vitality, size of pulp, and most appropriate method to meet client's needs.
- Assess for tooth cracks using fiberoptics. An intraoral camera also may help to verify and measure enamel cracks. (Deep cracks may be a contraindication to tooth bleaching, depending on their direction.)
- Remove soft and hard deposits before tooth-bleaching procedure.
- Take impressions; fabricate custom bleaching trays for home use; provide instructions.
- If dental practice act permits, provide in-office bleaching.

Professionally Dispensed Whitening Systems for Home Use

Professionally dispensed whitening systems (Table 29-3) involve the in-office fabrication of a custom mouth tray, dispensing of the appropriate whitening agent, and client education on how this is used at home with a prescribed frequency and time period (Figure 29-21). This procedure is also called nightguard vital bleaching (NGVB). The dentist monitors the client until the desired outcome is achieved. Home whitening with a custom-fitted tray and whitening agent is the superior tooth whitening method because of product innovations that control dentinal hypersensitivity and loss of enamel. It is lower in cost to the client than in-office bleaching, and it has the most scientific evidence supporting its effectiveness. It does require client adherence to the protocol for a good outcome. (See Chapter 37 for fabrication of custom-fitted bleaching trays.) In most cases an oxidizing agent, usually 10% to 30% carbamide peroxide, is loaded into a flexible polyvinyl, custom-made tray that the client wears 1 to 2 hours a day or overnight for a 2- to 6-week period. In addition to the oxidizing agent, Carbopol (carboxypolymethylene polymer) may be added to thicken the gel, improve adherence to the tooth surface, and prolong the release of oxygen. This additive keeps the gel contained within the tray and slows the chemical reaction.

Home whitening is effective in producing a lightened tooth surface, but clients should be informed that the degree of change, especially with tetracycline-stained teeth, may be unpredictable. Therefore client expectations must be clarified before any treatment. Clients need to know the following:

- Stains in the yellow to brown range respond better than stains in the blue to gray range.

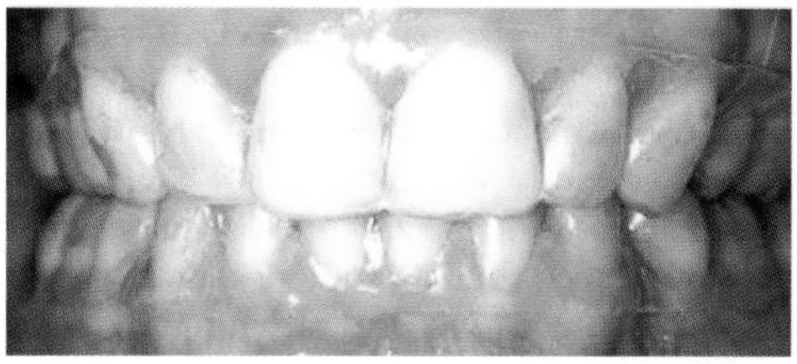

Figure 29-21. Custom-made maxillary and mandibular bleaching trays. (Courtesy Dr. Brent B. Hutson.)

TABLE 29-3

Some Professionally Dispensed Whitening Products

Product	Manufacturer	Active Ingredient	Time Required
Nite White ACP	Discus Dental	10%, 16%, 22% Carbamide peroxide	Overnight (10%), 2-4 hours or overnight (16%), 1 hour once or twice a day (22%)
Opalescence	Ultradent Products	10%, 15%, 20%, 35% Carbamide peroxide	Overnight or 1-3 hours daily
Visible White	Colgate	17%, 23%, 30% Carbamide peroxide	30 minutes once a day
Nupro White Gold	DENTSPLY	10% and 15% Carbamide peroxide	1 hour daily or overnight

Data from Poindexter A, Darby M: Whiter teeth, younger look: how to advise your patients on professionally dispensed, take home whitening methods, *Dimens Dent Hyg* 6:28, 2008.

- Teeth with horizontal bands or striations of various colors, as seen with tetracycline-stained teeth, may bleach at different rates, making enamel defects more noticeable.
- Although the teeth may look lighter, they may not necessarily be whiter, owing to their normal, intrinsic tooth color.
- Tooth-colored restorations subjected to bleaching will not change color and may no longer match the color of the teeth after the bleaching procedure.
- Whitening is temporary, and additional treatments may be necessary in 1 to 3 years, which carry cost and time commitment for the client. Longevity of whitening varies from client to client.
- The tooth surface becomes more porous with whitening and thus daily OTC fluoride toothpaste and mouthrinse or gel is recommended while using bleaching agents.

Side Effects of Tooth Whitening

Short-term side effects are usually minimal and disappear on cessation of treatment. The most common side effects are mild thermal tooth sensitivity and gingival irritation. Tooth sensitivity is attributed to the easy passage of the hydrogen peroxide through the enamel and dentin to the pulp, resulting in a reversible pulpitis. Use of a prescription self-applied fluoride gel or mouth rinse and a shortened bleaching exposure time may decrease sensitivity. Clients with recession should not have bleaching because of the possibility of exposed dentin, which provides the hydrogen peroxide a direct route to the pulp. In 10% of the population there is a gap at the cementoenamel junction (CEJ) between the enamel and the cementum, leaving exposed dentinal tubules that can lead to extreme sensitivity. Gingival irritation may occur if the bleaching tray is overfilled. Use of a syringe dosage system, a highly viscous gel, and a properly fitted tray may prevent any excess from escaping the trays.

Occasionally, sore throats, tooth pain, tingling of tissues, and headaches are reported as side effects of tooth bleaching. Slight morphologic changes in the enamel also have been noted with the vital bleaching gels. A study, however, showed that 10% carbamide peroxide did not significantly alter enamel microhardness. Localized microstructural and chemical changes were seen, but these were not clinically significant. Long-term misuse (overuse) of whitening products can decrease enamel hardness.

Although wide variations in data exist concerning composite restorations, some composites may be more susceptible to alterations, and some higher-concentration bleaching agents are more likely to cause these alterations. These changes, however, are unlikely to be clinically significant. No effects on porcelain or ceramic materials have been reported. Whitening of teeth containing amalgam restorations is not contraindicated but should be approached with caution because some changes in amalgam have been noted. Another possible side effect involves the temporomandibular joint (TMJ). When fabricating the bleaching tray, a thin material should be used to avoid interference with the client's occlusion. No long-term systemic effects have been identified. See Box 29-4 for a complete list of contraindications.

BOX 29-4

Contraindications to Tooth Bleaching

- Pregnant and breast-feeding women*
- Allergy to any of the ingredients
- Medications that cause photosensitivity or hyperpigmentation (important if a light will be used as a catalyst)
- Large, defective restorations (should be replaced before bleaching)
- Gingival, periodontal, or mucosal conditions that could be irritated by use of a bleaching tray or rubber dam
- Recession†
- Cervical erosion†
- Enamel cracks†
- Tooth sensitivity†
- Dental caries†

*No research is available on these population groups because they generally are not used as research participants.

†Tooth sensitivity may increase.

In-Office Whitening Procedures

In-office tooth whitening is any bleaching procedure performed in the office by a dental professional. Techniques may differ based on a number of factors: cause of the stain, tooth vitality, and the number of teeth needing the procedure (single tooth, multiple teeth, one arch, or both arches). Office time involved, client preference and compliance, cost, provider preference, and oral assessment findings are additional factors to consider when selecting the most appropriate procedure.

- Vital tooth whitening is bleaching a tooth that has a vital pulp. In-office techniques for bleaching vital teeth can be classified as professional bleaching, power bleaching, conventional or traditional bleaching, laser bleaching, or combination bleaching. Often the combination of office and home whitening procedures enhances the desired effect.
- Nonvital tooth whitening is bleaching an endodontically treated tooth that has no pulp. For a nonvital tooth or teeth, the procedure is usually intracoronal and also may be combined with one of the procedures indicated for vital teeth.

In-Office Bleaching Procedures for Vital Teeth

Manufacturers of in-office bleaching systems have specific instructions for use of their products, and their instructions always should be followed. In general, the bleaching procedure for vital teeth involves the following:

- Placement of a rubber dam, use of a light-cured paint-on dam, and/or protection of the gingival tissues with a petroleum jelly is necessary.
- Teeth may or may not be etched before placement of the bleaching agent. A gel or liquid bleaching agent, usually 35% hydrogen peroxide, is applied to the enamel surface. If the liquid form is used, gauze squares saturated with the bleaching agent are placed on the facial surfaces. The bleaching agent is allowed to remain on the teeth for about 30 minutes. A heat source, visible light curing lamp (resin curing light), plasma arc, light-emitting diode (LED), xenon-halide light, or laser is applied to catalyze the oxidizing agent and accelerate the chemical reaction. The value of the heat or light source has not been established in the literature (Figure 29-22).

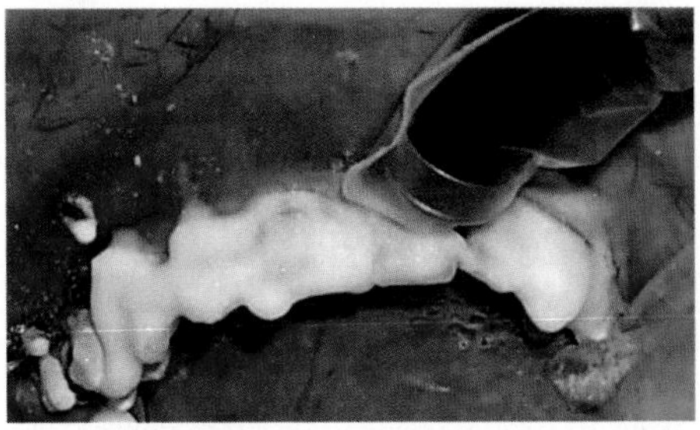

Figure 29-22. In-office bleaching procedure with a rubber dam, bleaching gel, and a resin curing light as the heat source. (Courtesy Dr. Brent B. Hutson.)

- Local anesthesia must never be used during bleaching. Client discomfort is monitored at all times to avoid tissue burns or excess heat buildup in the pulp. Analgesics may be recommended for the first 24 hours postoperatively if tooth sensitivity is experienced.
- At the end of the procedure, all excess bleaching agent should be removed with water before removing the rubber dam. Topical fluoride may be professionally applied or recommended for daily home use.

The in-office bleaching procedure lasts from 30 to 60 minutes and may involve one to three appointments at 2- to 4-week intervals until teeth sufficiently lighten or no further color change is noted. This time interval between appointments allows the pulp to settle down in case irritation develops. Clients should be informed that white spots on the tooth may become whiter and result in a blotchy appearance. If tooth-colored restorations are necessary, it is advisable to wait 2 to 3 weeks to determine the correct color shade. In addition, resin bonds are weakened significantly after tooth bleaching, so this time interval prevents failed restorations owing to inadequate bond strength.

Side Effects of In-Office Bleaching Procedures

Gingival burns and tooth sensitivity can occur. Although rare, more serious side effects such as acute irreversible pulpitis and pulp necrosis may occur after vital bleaching with 35% hydrogen peroxide. Long-term stability is unknown because there are no controlled clinical studies that follow clients for years after bleaching. The use of the light as a catalyst may cause marked photosensitivity and hyperpigmentation in persons taking acne medication, antidepressants, anticancer drugs, antipsychotics, diuretics, hypoglycemics, and nonsteroidal antiinflammatory drugs (NSAIDs). Skin should be shielded.

Laser-Assisted Bleaching

Laser manufacturers claim that laser bleaching is faster, produces fewer side effects, and increases tooth whitening. Lasers are used primarily to accelerate the chemical reaction of the bleaching agent and do not bleach teeth alone. Laser bleaching, however, has not been supported by clinical studies to confirm safety and efficacy. Future research may confirm that lasers are effective for deep stains that conventional bleaching cannot alter. Lasers are more costly and technique sensitive than traditional in-office methods. The U.S. Food and Drug Administration (FDA) granted market clearance to the argon or CO_2 laser for bleaching teeth. The argon laser is approved for use only as a heat source. Clients who desire immediate whitening results may have one in-office procedure to begin the whitening process, followed by 1 or 2 weeks of using home trays to complete the process.

Power and Combination Bleaching

Alternatively, instead of the heat-activated in-office procedure, a high concentration of hydrogen peroxide, 30% to 50%, can be placed in the client's custom-fabricated bleaching trays and worn for about 30 minutes without the application of heat. The client is monitored in the office for color change and discomfort. After the one-time high-concentration office procedure, the client continues the traditional at-home bleaching process with the lower-concentration bleaching agent.

Intracoronal Bleaching

Intracoronal bleaching, a method of in-office bleaching, is used only for bleaching endodontically treated teeth and usually is performed by an endodontist. With both of the following techniques, the bleaching agent is placed within the tooth. Nonvital bleaching techniques usually fall into these two categories:

- Thermocatalytic: The bleaching agent is usually 30% hydrogen peroxide, sodium perborate, or sodium hypochlorite. The agent is placed within the coronal portion of the pulp chamber with a cotton pellet after the cervical portion has been sealed with zinc phosphate or zinc oxide–eugenol cement to prevent penetration of the bleaching agent into the dentinal tubules and the possibility of cervical resorption. Heat (heat lamp, heated instrument, electric heating device, or an ultraviolet light) is applied to hasten the reaction.
- Walking: The walking bleach method is so called because a paste of sodium perborate and hydrogen peroxide is placed in the coronal portion of the pulp chamber, the tooth is sealed, and the client is seen again in a week. At that time, the paste may be reapplied if further alteration in color is necessary. Often only a small amount of color change can be achieved, but it may be sufficient to satisfy the client. This procedure is technique sensitive; failure to follow exact protocols may result in severe pain during or after the procedure. If the cervical area is not sealed well, cervical resorption may occur. To enhance the final effect, both nonvital bleaching methods may be combined with the professional or home bleaching methods for vital teeth.

Microabrasion

Microabrasion is a procedure that removes superficial dark stains or "white spot" decalcified areas of enamel. It is more effective on mild stains than in moderate or severe cases. This procedure involves removal of a thin layer of enamel and uses a paste of abrasives and hydrochloric acid on a specially designed prophy angle attachment. Some commercially prepackaged kits are available. Although considered effective, this procedure is technique sensitive, may require multiple applications of the abrasive paste and hydrochloric acid, and removes some tooth structure.

Side Effects

Burns, sensitivity, pulpal damage, and noticeable removal of the outermost fluoride-rich layer of tooth enamel can occur.

It is sometimes difficult for the dentist to determine the exact amount of enamel to remove, and a restorative procedure may be needed if the stain is deep. Long-term studies are not available. Home bleaching may be recommended after microabrasion to enhance whitening.

Restorative Management of Stained Teeth

Deep stains, mottled or pitted teeth, and grayish-blue stains may need restorative procedures by the dentist, such as composite bonding, veneers, or full crowns to provide the client with a more aesthetic appearance than can be achieved by whitening or microabrasion. All bleaching of teeth should be done before restorative procedures to ensure that crowns, bondings, and veneers will match the new enamel shade. Although not as conservative as bleaching, these procedures may assist the client in achieving a more desirable oral facial image. A dentist performs most restorative procedures, but the dental hygienist should be able to explain all procedures to the client.

Veneers

Veneers are thin, shell-like facings, usually made of composite resin or porcelain, bonded onto anterior facial tooth surfaces.

- Indirect technique: The veneer is fabricated in a dental laboratory on a stone die made from an impression; a small amount of tooth structure must be removed for this restoration.
- Direct technique: Teeth indicated for composite bonding are isolated, polished with pumice, and acid-etched. A bonding agent and an optional opaquer can be added before the composite is molded onto the facial surface. This procedure can change the appearance and shape of the tooth. After curing, the bonded area must be contoured, finished, and polished. Relatively inexpensive, this procedure is done quickly, requires only one visit, is good for young teeth with large pulps, and does not remove much tooth structure. However, it can look bulky and has the potential to chip and stain over time.

Porcelain veneers, although expensive, are ideal for older teeth. Fabrication involves an indirect technique as follows:

- Tooth is prepared by removing a thin layer of enamel, making an impression, and sending the impression to the laboratory for construction of the porcelain veneer.
- A temporary veneer is made and worn.
- On the second visit the temporary veneer is removed and the permanent veneer is checked for proper fit. The tooth is then isolated, polished with pumice, etched, rinsed, and dried. A bonding agent and an optional opaquer are applied. The inside of the veneer is conditioned, and composite is added to bond the veneer to the tooth. The veneer is placed, and excess composite is removed.

If not designed properly, porcelain veneers can be bulky, stain at the margins, and chip. When well designed, they have good aesthetic properties and are more durable than composite veneers.

Full-Coverage Crowns

Full crowns are used when caries, defects, or restorations on the teeth are extensive. In some cases they may be indicated after endodontic treatment to prevent brittle enamel from fracturing. Good aesthetics can be achieved with crowns, but a large amount of tooth structure must be removed. Crowns should not be recommended just to make the teeth appear whiter. More conservative techniques are available and should be discussed with the informed client.

Legal and Ethical Aspects of Extrinsic Stain Removal and Tooth Whitening

State statutes regarding the legality of polishing teeth by allied dental personnel must be followed. Delegation of extrinsic stain removal procedures to dental assistants in states where assistants are not legally allowed to perform them is illegal. An ethical issue arises when delegation to dental assistants is legal, but a lack of background knowledge exists to determine when polishing is contraindicated.

The dental or dental hygiene practice act, rules, and regulations in each jurisdiction determines the extent of the dental hygienist's legal involvement in whitening or restorative services and should be consulted before any clinical whitening service is provided. If the whitening system is defined as a topical medication under the dental practice act, then dental hygienists may, in some states, provide in-office whitening. The exact technique for in-office whitening depends on the specific system used, and manufacturers' directions are followed for maximum safety and efficacy. Protection of the client's gingiva, lips, eyes, and clothing is recommended highly. Some state dental practice acts specifically state that only licensed dentists may provide laser bleaching.

Tooth whitening and stain management options, including risks and benefits of each method that is appropriate, should be discussed with the client. Ethics require that clients be informed and able to make autonomous decisions about their health care.

CLIENT EDUCATION TIPS

- Soft deposits return promptly after professional dental hygiene care. Daily oral self-care using mechanical and chemotherapeutic methods to control oral biofilm and oral infection is critical for long-term oral and systemic health.
- Explain oral self-care interventions to minimize recurrence of extrinsic stains in the context of the client's readiness to change.
- Explain cause, types, prevention, and management of extrinsic and intrinsic stains.
- Explain adverse effects of tooth polishing on tissues, restorative materials, and dental care environment.
- Explain rationale for selective polishing and why teeth should not be polished at each continued-care appointment.
- Teach client to differentiate health from disease, and how clean tooth surfaces look and feel. Use the client's own mouth and a hand mirror.
- Explain tooth bleaching and aesthetic restorative procedures for stain management, including safety, efficacy, side effects, advantages, disadvantages, and indications and contraindications.

LEGAL, ETHICAL, AND SAFETY ISSUES

- Nonmaleficence requires that all recommended guidelines on the safe use of rubber-cup, air polishing, and tooth bleaching systems must be followed to minimize client risk.

- Clients have the right to autonomy and must be informed of and consent to procedures that may harm tooth structure, oral soft tissues, and restorations before the performance of those procedures.
- Risk management strategies for treating medically compromised or immunocompromised clients must be followed.
- State statutes, rules, and regulations regarding the legality of polishing teeth by allied dental personnel must be followed. Delegation of extrinsic stain removal procedures to dental assistants in states where assistants are not legally allowed to perform them is illegal. An ethical issue arises when delegation to dental assistants is legal but a lack of background knowledge exists to determine when polishing is contraindicated.
- The dental hygienist must adhere to laws, rules, and regulations regarding the dental hygienist's role in home or in-office bleaching procedures.
- Client education about advantages, disadvantages, risks, and potential adverse effects of treatment is essential for informed consent to all aesthetic procedures.

KEY CONCEPTS

- Rubber-cup polishing, air polishing, and bleaching are selective procedures that should be included in dental hygiene care plans only after client assessment is complete.
- Although not a pathologic concern, tooth stain is a cosmetic concern.
- Selective polishing is the practice of omitting tooth polishing in areas where there is no stain to avoid removing some of the fluoride-rich outer layer of enamel and other adverse effects on teeth and restorations.
- Knowledge of the indications, contraindications, and various home and in-office techniques for aesthetic management of extrinsic and intrinsic stains is essential for client education.
- For tooth stain removal and stain management, the dental hygienist must use the least abrasive and most effective technique and product to achieve the desired clinical outcome.

CRITICAL THINKING EXERCISES

1. In small groups, read and discuss a current evidence-based published paper on selective polishing, air polishing, tooth bleaching, and/or aesthetic restorative procedures, and report findings to the class.
2. Conduct a mock debate on selective polishing or tooth bleaching. All students should participate, for example, as debate team members, literature reviewers, consumers, expert witnesses (dentists, dental hygienists, clients, parents, insurance company representatives). Half of the class should advocate for the "pro" position; half for the "con" position.
3. Conduct a survey of practicing dentists, dental hygienists, and clients about preferences for or experiences with selective polishing, air polishing, or tooth bleaching. Discuss findings during a designated class session.

ACKNOWLEDGMENT

The author acknowledges Marylou E. Gutmann for her past contributions to this chapter.

EVOLVE RESOURCES

Please visit http://evolve.elsevier.com/Darby/hygiene for additional practice and study support tools.

CHAPTER 30

Decision Making Related to Nonsurgical Periodontal Therapy

Kathleen O. Hodges

COMPETENCIES

1. Discuss basic concepts of nonsurgical periodontal therapy, including:
   - Explain similarities and differences between disease activity and disease severity.
   - Differentiate among nonsurgical periodontal therapy, oral prophylaxis, and periodontal maintenance therapy.
2. Discuss implementation of nonsurgical periodontal therapy.
3. Describe optimal clinical and therapeutic outcomes from nonsurgical periodontal therapy.
4. Explain how dental benefit plans influence nonsurgical periodontal therapy.
5. Explain the rationale for periodontal maintenance therapy and suggest appropriate intervals based on individual client needs.
6. Explain the dental hygienist's role after periodontal surgery.

Basic Concepts in Nonsurgical Periodontal Therapy

Nonsurgical periodontal therapy (NSPT) encompasses "plaque removal, plaque control, supragingival and subgingival scaling, root planing, and the adjunctive use of chemical agents"[1] for the treatment of inflammation, periodontal pockets, and other indications of periodontal disease.

This original definition, which has been transformed into contemporary terms, translates to the removal and control of oral biofilm through self-care and professional periodontal debridement, supplemented by adjunctive therapy with chemotherapeutics or host modulation agents as needed, for the treatment of periodontal disease involving natural teeth and implant replacements. Periodontal health should be attained in the least invasive and most cost-effective manner, and NSPT is often the means used to accomplish that objective. The absence of inflammation—as assessed by no erythema or edema, suppuration, or bleeding on probing—characterizes health.[2]

The goals of periodontal therapy are as follows:

- To preserve, maintain, and improve the natural dentition, implants, periodontium, and peri-implant tissues
- To achieve health, comfort, aesthetics, and function.

Oral biofilm removal alone will not resolve inflammation in all cases. Supragingival biofilm control alone will not control microorganisms in periodontal pockets. Therefore self-care for supragingival and subgingival biofilm control must occur simultaneously with professional therapy to enhance the outcomes of NSPT (oral biofilm control is discussed in Chapters 17, 23, 24, 31, and 58). For more involved cases in which NSPT does not resolve the disease process and achieve health, periodontal surgery is recommended. For this reason, NSPT also is called *phase I of periodontal therapy* or *initial therapy* (see Chapter 22).

The purposes of NSPT are as follows:

- Eliminating or suppressing infectious microorganisms
- Eliminating or controlling infection to prevent reinfection
- Establishing an environment that helps resolve inflammation
- Modifying host and environmental risk factors for periodontal disease
- Employing chemotherapeutic agents when indicated (see Chapter 31)

Scaling—the instrumentation of the crown and root to remove oral biofilm, calculus, and stains—is used for the treatment of clients with healthy gingiva or gingivitis. **Oral prophylaxis** combines both supragingival and subgingival scaling with stain and biofilm removal. This procedure is preventive in nature and not therapeutic like NSPT. The dental hygienist performs the oral prophylaxis when periodontal health or biofilm-induced gingivitis is diagnosed. **Root planing** is a definitive procedure to remove cementum or surface dentin that is rough, impregnated with calculus, or contaminated with toxins or microorganisms. The objective of therapeutic scaling and root planing is to remove as little root structure as possible while returning adjacent tissues to health.

Periodontal debridement is the "removal of all subgingival plaque (oral biofilm) and its by-products (as evidenced by clinical signs of inflammation), clinically detectable biofilm retentive factors (calculus, cement and overhangs), and detectable calculus-embedded cementum to finish the root surface during periodontal instrumentation while preserving as much tooth surface as possible."[3] This intervention focuses on the removal of all plaque retentive factors while preserving tooth structure and using judgment with regard to root roughness; therefore the evaluation of healing 4 to 6 weeks after debridement is critical. Because oral biofilm is a primary causative factor for inflammatory forms of periodontal disease, gingivitis, and periodontitis, subgingival plaque removal is essential. The removal of calculus is important only because of its oral biofilm retentive nature.

Periodontal debridement strives to achieve tissue healing with minimal iatrogenic damage (e.g., damage from professional treatment) to the soft tissue and the cementum. In addition to periodontal debridement, chemotherapeutic agents (via dentifrices, mouth rinses, local controlled delivery, or systemic antibiotics) are used to suppress infectious microorganisms and inflammation (see Chapter 31). **Host modulation therapy** targets the host's role in host–bacteria interactions, which primarily involves the destruction of connective tissue in the gingiva, the periodontal ligament, and the alveolar bone in a periodontal pocket during the development and progression of periodontal disease.

The **therapeutic endpoint** is the restoration of gingival health, a reduction in pocket depth, and a gain in or maintenance of a stable clinical attachment level. These parameters can be expected only after a 4- to 6-week healing interval after periodontal therapy. This appointment, which is called **periodontal reevaluation**, is scheduled to reassess the clinical parameters of health after NSPT. Without a reevaluation visit, the therapeutic endpoint of active therapy is never assessed or documented. The therapeutic endpoint can also be assessed in a segment of the mouth (e.g., a quadrant or half of the mouth) 4 to 6 weeks after therapy during phase I of NSPT while new areas are being treated as part of a complex care plan.

Assessment, Diagnosis, and Care Planning

For a discussion of periodontal assessment, see Chapter 19. A comprehensive evaluation and risk assessment should occur after initial therapy and *at least* annually.[2] Decisions about frequency are based on the assessment of disease extent, the stability or progression of the condition, the client's oral self-care practices, risk factors (e.g., systemic health), and the host response to therapy.

The **periodontal diagnosis** is determined after analyzing information collected during the assessment phase of therapy. The dental hygienist and ultimately the dentist or periodontist must make informed decisions about disease classification, extent, and severity. To accomplish this, the hygienist considers the following:

- The presence or absence of inflammation
- The extent and pattern of clinical attachment loss
- The rate of disease progression
- The presence or absence of additional signs, such as pain, ulceration, and familial aggregation
- The location of plaque biofilm, calculus, and other localized factors (e.g., overhanging margins, cement adjacent to implants)
- The client's risk factors

To classify periodontal disease, the practitioner first differentiates between gingival disease and more advanced forms, such as chronic or aggressive periodontitis. (See Boxes 19-3 through 19-6 in Chapter 19 for the classification of periodontal diseases and conditions.) Clients may simultaneously have areas of health and chronic periodontitis with slight, moderate, and advanced destruction. In addition, other disease states may be detected, such as an acute gingival infection, a periodontal abscess, an atypical form, and systemic-related diseases that often require specific knowledge for appropriate care by the clinician.

The identification of disease includes overall disease severity and disease activity, which can be evaluated as follows:

- **Disease severity** is the measure of the destruction that occurred before the assessment. An important determination is whether the periodontitis is a slowly progressing form, such as chronic periodontitis, or rapidly progressing, such as aggressive periodontitis. This determination is critical when planning the course of nonsurgical care and predicting the prognosis. The clinician considers multiple factors when classifying disease. The rate of disease progression may be determined by the amount of clinical attachment loss at a young age, or it can be determined after multiple periodontal examinations are performed over time and compared with baseline data. Therefore the initial diagnosis may be altered over time as more data become available. For this reason, clinical assessment results in a **preliminary** or **presumptive diagnosis** during initial or active therapy. This type of diagnosis also facilitates decisions that affect **dental hygiene diagnosis** and care planning during initial periodontal therapy. A **dental or periodontal diagnosis** is the result of clinical findings, the client's response to nonsurgical or surgical care at the reevaluation visit, and the need for additional therapy beyond the scope of dental hygiene. The diagnosis may change over time as periodontal maintenance occurs at appropriate time intervals or as clients do not adhere to recommendations for intervals and self-care.
- **Disease activity**, which is more difficult to establish than disease severity, refers to inflammation, connective tissue degeneration, and bone or attachment loss that is ongoing at the time of the examination. Periodontal disease activity involves periods of quiescence (inactivity) and periods of exacerbation (activity) that are evident with active disease. Periods of quiescence are characterized by a reduced host inflammatory response and little or no loss of bone and connective tissue attachment.

Unattached oral biofilm and anaerobic bacteria (i.e., gram-negative and motile) initiate periods of exacerbation that, in conjunction with other risk factors and the host's response, result in the loss of bone and connective tissue attachment, thereby creating deeper periodontal pockets. Periods of exacerbation might last for days, weeks, or months, and eventually quiescence may follow. This description of activity and inactivity explains the episodic nature of periodontal diseases. Clinically disease activity is most commonly measured retrospectively by comparing current examination findings with previous data. Therefore disease activity is routinely assessed during continued-care appointments by closely monitoring and recording probing depths, bleeding with probing, and clinical attachment measurements.

Periodontal diagnosis is different from and yet related to the dental hygiene diagnosis (see Chapter 21). NSPT relates to a variety of unmet human needs, but the clinical parameters of periodontal disease focus on the human need for skin and mucous membrane integrity of the head and neck. Bleeding, gingival inflammation, pocket depth, and attachment loss are all deficits related to this need, and each requires interventions such as NSPT.

The sequencing of therapeutic procedures follows a traditional model of periodontal care planning that involves four phases of periodontal care (see Chapter 22, Table 22-1). NSPT is part of **phase I therapy** (also referred to as *initial therapy, initial preparation,* or *anti-infective therapy*). Much of phase I therapy is the responsibility of the dental hygienist who is working in concert with the general dentist or periodontist. It includes the NSPT and the evaluation of NSPT 4 to 6 weeks after completion. **Active therapy** involves either nonsurgical care, surgical care, or both, depending on the needs of the client. Active therapy includes phase I care, and it can also extend to phase II care, which is periodontal surgery. Phase III involves restorative care. Phase VI, which encompasses periodontal maintenance therapy, is not part of active therapy.

After a series of appointments for NSPT (and surgery, if indicated), the client is moved from active therapy to maintenance therapy. **Periodontal maintenance (PM)**, which is also known as *supportive periodontal therapy, supportive periodontal care,* or *continued care,* is an extension of the periodontal therapy performed at selected intervals to assist the client with the maintenance of oral health. It continues at client-dependent intervals for the life of the dentition or its implant replacements. PM may be discontinued and active therapy reinstituted if recurrent disease is detected. Periodontal disease states that are refractory are indications for bacterial culturing and subsequent systemic antibiotic therapy in addition to mechanical periodontal debridement. The term *refractory* refers to periodontal disease states that continue to progress despite client adherence with recommended oral self-care and professional care that yields successful clinical outcomes for most clients. Care planning approaches to periodontal therapy involve the following variables:

- The classification and diagnosis of the client's periodontitis
- The severity of the client's periodontitis
- The systemic health or disease of the client
- The client's human needs and informed consent
- The practitioner's philosophy of care

When planning care, decisions are made regarding interventions; if such interventions are accepted by the client, they are then scheduled (see Chapter 22). The number, sequence, and length of the appointments are determined to best meet the client's human needs. Although Table 30-1 is not all inclusive, it does outline common periodontal disease features and treatment options in addition to highlighting where surgical intervention may be required.

TABLE 30-1

Clinical Features and Interventions for Common Classifications of Periodontal Diseases (see Chapter 19)

Class	Form	Clinical Features	Interventions
Gingival diseases	Dental plaque induced	Oral biofilm present at gingival margin Disease begins at margin Change in gingival color Sulcular temperature change Increased gingival exudate Bleeding on probing Absence of attachment loss Absence of bone loss Changes reversible with oral biofilm control	Oral self-care education Client removal of biofilm Periodontal debridement or scaling Correction of biofilm retentive factors Home irrigation and/or twice-daily mouth rinsing with effective antimicrobial agent, as needed
Periodontitis	Chronic	Most prevalent in adults; can also occur in children and adolescents Amount of destruction is consistent with presence of local factors Subgingival calculus present Variable microbial pattern Slow to moderate rate of progression; may be periods of rapid progression Further classified on the basis of extent and severity Can be associated with local predisposing factors May be modified by or associated with systemic disease and risk factors, such as type 2 diabetes, smoking, and cardiovascular disease	Elimination, alternation, or control of risk factors Self-care education Periodontal debridement (scaling, root planing) Chemotherapeutics, as needed Locally delivered antimicrobials, as needed Host modulation therapy as needed Reevaluation for surgery needs
Periodontitis	Aggressive	Clients otherwise clinically healthy Rapid attachment loss and bone destruction Familial aggregation Secondary features usually present Amounts of microbial deposits are inconsistent with severity Elevated proportions of *Aggregatibacter actinomycetemcomitans* and *Porphyromonas gingivalis* Phagocyte abnormalities Hyperresponsive macrophage phenotype, including elevated levels of prostaglandin E_2 and interleukin-1β Progression of attachment loss and bone loss may be self-arresting	Oral self-care education Periodontal debridement (scaling, root planing) Control of risk factors Systemic and locally delivered antibiotics Microbial diagnostic testing Host modulating agents Photodynamic disinfection therapy Twice-daily 0.12% chlorhexidine rinses Surgery Genetic susceptibility testing Evaluation and counseling of family members Immunocompetence testing, if indicated

Chronic Disease States[4-7]

Chronic disease states (see Chapter 19, Boxes 19-3, 19-4, and 19-5) that involve dental-plaque–induced gingivitis and periodontitis usually progress slowly and respond in a relatively predictable manner to NSPT directed at reducing disease-causing bacteria, given coinciding self-care. For the treatment of chronic disease states, the main focus of NSPT is oral self-care education and the mechanical removal of oral biofilm and biofilm retentive factors to reduce microbial load and the host's hyperinflammatory response. (Note that it is the chronic hyperinflammatory response of the host that is indirectly responsible for the destruction of collagen and bone.) Oral self-care is ultimately the client's responsibility, whereas instrumentation is the professional's responsibility.

The treatment of gingivitis includes oral self-care education and supragingival and subgingival debridement (scaling) along with antimicrobial and antiplaque agents. The correction of plaque retentive factors is also essential; these include overhanging margins, open margins, overcontoured crowns, narrow embrasure spaces, open contacts, ill-fitting fixed or removable partial dentures, dental caries, and tooth malposition. At times, the surgical correction of gingival deformities that hinder the client's oral self-care is needed to help with the control of the oral biofilm.

Therapy for chronic periodontitis with the slight to moderate loss of periodontal support includes active therapy (i.e., NSPT) and PM. Systemic diseases and other risk factors must be considered in the care plan because of their effect on the therapeutic outcome of NSPT (see Chapters 12, 14, 19, and 20). Diseases and conditions or risk factors that affect the host response also affect the initiation and progression of periodontal disease (e.g., diabetes mellitus, cardiovascular disease, human immunodeficiency virus infection and acquired immunodeficiency syndrome, pregnancy, smoking, substance abuse, and medications). When systemic conditions are present, consultation with the client's physicians may be appropriate to determine the client's current status. Oral self-care and periodontal debridement are the main therapeutic foci, and they are crucial to a successful long-term clinical outcome. Antimicrobial, chemotherapeutic, or host modulation agents or devices are useful adjuncts when treating periodontitis with coexisting gingivitis. Implant therapy can be initiated during the initial phase of care or considered as phase II or III therapy.

Periodontal surgery is also a problem-focused therapy that is aimed at enhancing root debridement and tissue regeneration and reducing gingival recession for clients who have effective self-care practices. Surgery may be indicated for advanced periodontal sites; however, most cases of slight and moderate involvement can be treated nonsurgically, provided access to subgingival deposits and plaque retentive factors is achievable. If the results of initial therapy resolve the periodontal infection and conditions, then PM is scheduled. If the results of initial therapy do not resolve the periodontal condition or if conditions exist that cannot be addressed nonsurgically (e.g., furcation involvement and mobility, deep pockets), then surgery is considered, and referral to a periodontist is indicated (see Referral to a Periodontist).

When advanced periodontitis is present, additional considerations for therapy may be necessary; these include subgingival microbial analysis, antibiotic sensitivity testing, and the extraction of hopeless teeth. In some cases optimal results may not be attainable because of the client's health, age, systemic condition, and extent of disease; initial therapy may in fact be the endpoint of periodontal care.

Aggressive Disease States[8]

Aggressive periodontitis and some uncommon forms of gingivitis will not respond predictably to NSPT. Aggressive periodontitis is seen in clients who otherwise appear healthy, who tend to have a familial aggregation, and in whom the disease progresses rapidly. Traditional NSPT is the basic therapeutic modality for aggressive periodontitis; however, the quantity of oral biofilm and calculus deposits is less important than the host's inflammatory and immune response to specific periodontal pathogens that are present. Initial periodontal therapy alone often is not effective for controlling the host response to specific pathogens. Other care-planning considerations include the following:

- A general medical evaluation to determine if systemic disease is present
- A consultation with a physician to coordinate medical and periodontal care
- The modification of risk factors
- Adjunctive chemotherapeutic therapy, including systemic antibiotics
- Adjunctive host modulation
- Microbiologic identification
- Antibiotic sensitivity testing
- A determination of genetic susceptibility (see Genetic Markers in Chapter 19)

Tooth extraction and occlusal therapy may also be part of the comprehensive care plan. The PM interval should be short (i.e., 1 to 3 months) to slow rapid disease progression. A diagnosis of aggressive periodontitis may occur after active therapy, reevaluation, and several intervals of PM. Referral to a periodontist is most often indicated.

Appointment Planning (see Chapter 22)

One major consideration that affects the appointment plan during NSPT is the use of pain-control or anxiety-management strategies (see Chapters 40 and 41). Need must be established on the basis of assessment data and client-related factors (Table 30-2). Pain-control modalities might require more appointment time, and this time should be considered during care planning. The length of the appointment could vary from 40 to 90 minutes depending on client needs. In general, NSPT takes more time than oral prophylaxis or PM. The most important factor for determining the success of periodontal therapy is the thoroughness of the root surface debridement and the client's oral hygiene care, so appointments should allow ample time and sequencing for thorough periodontal debridement while providing for client comfort and self-care education.

Case Presentation and Informed Consent (see Chapters 22 and 62)

The primary objectives of a case presentation are the following:

- To encourage collaborative treatment between the client and the clinician
- To satisfy legal responsibilities

TABLE 30-2

Determining the Need for Local Anesthetic Agents*

Factor	Comment
Periodontal Assessment Factors	
Pocket depth of >4 mm	Limited accessibility and visibility decrease the chances of complete deposit removal Pain control increases client comfort and operator confidence
Tissue tone	Tight or nonelastic tissue may limit access to deep pockets or challenging root anatomy Local anesthetic may be used to increase the turgor of the gingiva when injected into an edematous interdental papilla
Pocket topography	Cratering at epithelial attachment or narrow intrabony pockets Pain control enhances deposit removal
Furcations	Limited accessibility and visibility decrease the chances of complete deposit removal Pain control increases client comfort and operator confidence
Root anatomy	Anatomic variations may require pain control for nonsurgical periodontal therapy Limited access Unusual longitudinal depressions Deeper pockets with more complex root anatomy Increased sensitivity Overinstrumentated roots Gingival recession Abrasion
Inflammation	Inflamed tissue that is likely to be painful and bleed Incidental curettage will occur inadvertently in some areas Hemostasis may be a concern
Hemorrhage	Use vasoconstrictor when hemostasis is a concern, such as with bleeding on probing or spontaneous hemorrhage
Client-Related Factors	
Pain threshold	If the pain threshold is low, administer a local anesthetic agent to control pain and reduce the anxiety level
Sensitivity	Determine the type of sensitivity (i.e., pulpal or soft tissue) Determine the type of instrumentation (hand-activated vs. mechanized instruments)

From Hodges KO: *Concepts in nonsurgical periodontal therapy,* Albany, NY, 1998, Delmar.

*Always assess the client's health, dental, and pharmacologic histories before the selection and use of pain control agents. Noninjectable anesthetics are also available.

Through case presentation and the gaining of informed consent, the clinician is able to communicate the following to the client:

- The client's periodontal risk and assessment findings that indicate disease, similar to risk factor discussions for other chronic disease states
- How NSPT differs from oral prophylaxis and the need for reevaluation and PM for long-term success
- The extensive nature of periodontal debridement and why the number of appointments and the time involved are critical to the achievement of an optimal outcome
- The need for pain control or conscious sedation/analgesia and an explanation of why this is necessary

Implementation of Nonsurgical Periodontal Therapy

Implementation includes the delivery of preventive and therapeutic procedures identified in the individualized care plan to meet the client's human needs. Preventive and therapeutic entities of NSPT such as self-care education, manual and mechanized instrumentation, chemotherapeutic interventions, pain-control strategies (if indicated), and stain-removal procedures are performed as needed. Supportive interventions for achieving the ultimate goals of NSPT include overhang removal (margination), desensitization, dietary assessment and counseling, smoking cessation counseling, dental caries risk assessment and management, and occlusal therapy. Therapeutic procedures in NSPT may include the following:

- **Mechanical nonsurgical pocket therapy**: scaling and root planing; periodontal debridement with the use of hand-activated or power-driven instruments
- **Chemotherapy for periodontal disease**: the use of systemic, topical, and locally delivered antimicrobials (also known as *anti-infective, chemotherapeutic therapy*) or host modulation agents (e.g., subantimicrobial doses of doxycycline, potential use of nonsteroidal inflammatory agents [NSAIDs], and other such therapies) to selectively target the host–pathogen interaction[9] (see Chapter 31).

Full-mouth disinfection (FMD) involves the scaling and root planing of all pockets within a 24-hour time period. FMD potentially includes the application of 0.12%

chlorhexidine gluconate to all periodontal pockets followed by twice-daily 30-second mouth rinsing with 0.12% chlorhexidine gluconate for 2 months. This treatment may also include additional disinfection of the tongue and tonsils by tongue scraping and chlorhexidine spray for the tonsillar area and subgingival irrigation of the pockets three times within 10 minutes with a 1% chlorhexidine gel repeated for 8 days.[10] The rationale underlying this intervention is that the traditional method of four consecutive appointments for scaling and root planing without proper disinfection may allow for the reinfection of previously disinfected pockets by pathogenic bacteria from an untreated region of the mouth. Limited conclusions can be drawn about the advantages of FMD, although modest improvements in pocket depth and clinical attachment level were noted in moderately deep pockets among clients with chronic periodontitis.[11] Quadrant periodontal debridement, full-mouth debridement, and FMD are all viable approaches. Considerations include client needs and preferences, the practitioner's skills and experience, practice-setting logistics, and cost effectiveness.[10]

Mechanical Nonsurgical Pocket Therapy

The basis of successful NSPT is not the treatment modality but rather the detailed thoroughness of the periodontal debridement and the client's standard of self-care. These principles remain the foundation for NSPT; evidence that supports adjunctive therapies alone is not as strong as evidence that supports meticulous mechanical therapy and client self-care. Advanced hand-activated instrumentation is an extension of basic instrumentation. Instrumentation in pockets of 6 mm or greater that are adjacent to furcations and in which mobility exists is significantly impaired when providing NSPT; therefore subsequent periodontal surgery should be considered. Options for treating areas affected by destructive periodontal disease include standard armamentarium such as ultrasonic instruments with various tips and inserts, periodontal files, universal curets, and area-specific curets (see Chapters 26 and 27) as well as advanced hand instruments such as debridement curets, furcation curets, diamond-coated periodontal instruments, and specialized implant instruments (see Chapter 26 and additional resources for this chapter located on the website at http://evolve.elsevier.com/Darby/hygiene.) The clinician will select instruments on the basis of the following:

- Type of deposit or oral biofilm retentive factor being removed
- Pocket depth
- Inflammation
- Tissue tone
- Access
- Root morphology
- Pocket topography

Deep pockets, furcation involvement, and tooth mobility as a result of clinical attachment loss seriously compromise the prognosis of the tooth; therefore these conditions usually require periodontal surgery for correction. Furcation areas and mobile teeth are treated during initial therapy (i.e., NSPT) preceding surgery, as a compromise when surgery is not feasible, and after surgery (see Chapters 26 and 27 as well as the website http://evolve.elsevier.com/Darby/hygiene for additional information about advanced hand instrumentation in furcation areas and in the presence of mobile teeth.)

A single instrument is not likely to produce the desired clinical and therapeutic endpoints, because multiple clinical factors require a variety of periodontal debridement instruments.

Clinicians are challenged to stay abreast of the most recent developments in hand-activated and power-driven designs and to evaluate their effectiveness for periodontal debridement through clinical use and evidence-based decision making.

Chemotherapeutic Nonsurgical Pocket Therapy

See Chapter 31.

Clinical Outcomes of Periodontal Debridement[11]

Despite documented incomplete calculus and endotoxin removal, nonsurgical instrumentation has been shown to arrest periodontitis (i.e., the host can now manage the microbial challenge). After periodontal debridement, scaling, and root planing, the loss of clinical attachment at sites with initially shallow pockets and a gain in the attachment level at sites with deeper pockets are common. The loss of attachment after NSPT at shallow sites is thought to relate to overinstrumentation and overzealous self-care. In addition, thinner gingival margins experience more loss, and instrumentation at deeper sites adjacent to shallow sites can damage the shallow sites. Clinical attachment loss in shallow sites (1 to 3 mm) is minimal. Conversely, pockets with initial depths of 4 to 6 mm show an attachment level gain of 0.5 to 1 mm. Pockets of 7 mm or greater may have a greater attachment gain, but this is challenging to maintain. Pocket depth reduction is greater initially after surgery than after scaling and root planing; however, over time, the differences become insignificant. These findings highlight the need for clinicians and clients to understand the expected outcomes of mechanical therapy during NSPT, the need for continued care at appropriate PM intervals, and the potential need for additional treatment.

Although clinicians have used bleeding on probing as an indicator of disease activity, there is a poor correlation between bleeding on probing and risk for future clinical attachment loss. The absence of bleeding is a more reliable criterion for stability. Mechanical NSPT predictably reduces the level of inflammation and hence the high levels of proinflammatory mediators (e.g., matrix metalloproteinases, cytokines, and prostaglandins) that cause the breakdown of bone and collagen. After periodontal debridement, scaling, and root planing, several outcomes are expected[11,12]:

- Motile microbes and spirochete microbes are reduced, and cocci and nonmotile microbes increase.
- Microbes that repopulate the subgingival environment after therapy are the result of incomplete instrumentation or the growth of supragingival oral biofilm into the pocket.
- The predictable elimination of periodontal pathogens such as *Aggregatibacter actinomycetemcomitans* associated with aggressive disease does not occur. Likewise, pathogenic anaerobic, subgingival bacteria (e.g., *Porphyromonas gingivalis* and others) are not eradicated, invade the adjacent periodontal tissues.
- Subgingival therapy does not significantly affect other areas that may be a source of reemerging periodontal bacteria, such as the tongue and the tonsillar area.

- Microbial repopulation of subgingival pockets can be slowed or inhibited by effective oral self-care practices. The presence of supragingival oral biofilm facilitates the repopulation of pockets with high percentages of spirochetes and motile rods within 4 to 8 weeks.
- Shifts toward subgingival health are transient; therefore PM at timely intervals is needed to sustain positive effects.
- Hand-activated, ultrasonic, and sonic instrumentation all produce similar clinical and microbiologic results.
- Minimal or no bone repair occurs after scaling and root planing.

As previously discussed, furcations associated with periodontitis present a particularly challenging environment for accomplishing the objectives of mechanical therapy that eventually effect the longevity of these teeth. Problems with mechanical therapy adjacent to furcation involvement typically include the following:

- Identification during the periodontal assessment
- Furcal anatomy (Figure 30-1)
- Lack of access
- Persistence of pathogenic microflora

These same factors affect the client's ability to perform oral self-care.

Aggressive instrumentation to remove endotoxin is unwarranted, because endotoxin is loosely bound to the root surface. In addition, treated root surfaces become recontaminated over short periods of time. Another outcome of mechanical instrumentation to consider is the role that root surface roughness plays in microbial recolonization and in the achievement of the desired clinical endpoint. Both surface free energy and roughness play major roles in the initial adhesion and retention of microbes. These findings are particularly true with regard to supragingival root surfaces; however, they are also important to subgingival root surfaces. Clinicians need to achieve the smoothest root surface in the presence of probable deposits on the root surface without resorting to overinstrumentation.

Clinical and Therapeutic Endpoints

The **clinical endpoint** measures the tooth surface's preparation for the healing of adjacent tissues. This is determined immediately after periodontal therapy by exploring the subgingival environment. To assess the clinical endpoint, a variety of explorers may be used in addition to air and illumination, for example:

- Curved and universal-like designs (Hu-Friedy 2, 2H, or 2R/2L; 3A)
- Pocket feelers (Hu-Friedy 20 F Orban)
- Area-specific–like designs (ODU 11/12, Hu-Friedy EXD 11/12 or 11/12 After-Five)

The area-specific extended shank design is particularly useful during NSPT. Like the extended shank curets, it has a longer terminal shank (3 mm) as compared with the standard design. The 11/12 design is indicated for deep pockets and anterior teeth. A limitation might be midline extension on the posterior proximal surfaces as a result of the short working end (Figure 30-2).

The dental hygiene practitioner is constantly evaluating the clinical endpoint of instrumentation during NSPT to determine if it is sufficient. The topography of the tooth surface is the best criterion for the making of this decision, because the removal of subgingival oral biofilm and its byproducts cannot be measured clinically. The clinical endpoint for the majority of clients is a tooth surface that is devoid of detectable biofilm retentive factors. If subgingival problems remain, the clinician should attempt to remove root roughness. When deciding if instrumentation is complete, the clinician considers the following:

- The self-evaluation of instrumentation technique
- Progress toward the removal of the irregularity
- Probable root anatomy in the areas (see Chapter 28)
- The radiographic appearance of the tooth surfaces
- The extent of gingival inflammation
- The severity of the periodontitis
- The generalized characteristics of the client's calculus and other plaque biofilm retentive factors

If the clinician is in doubt about certain areas, these sites should be recorded in the record of services to ensure their evaluation at the next visit during active therapy or at the reevaluation visit. **Endoscopic therapy** enhances the ability to reassess difficult and refractory areas (see Chapter 26).

The **therapeutic endpoint** of therapy determined at the evaluation visit includes the measurement of critical criteria such as probing depth, clinical attachment level, and gingival inflammation accompanied by bleeding. If bleeding and inflammation are present, site-specific therapy is performed,

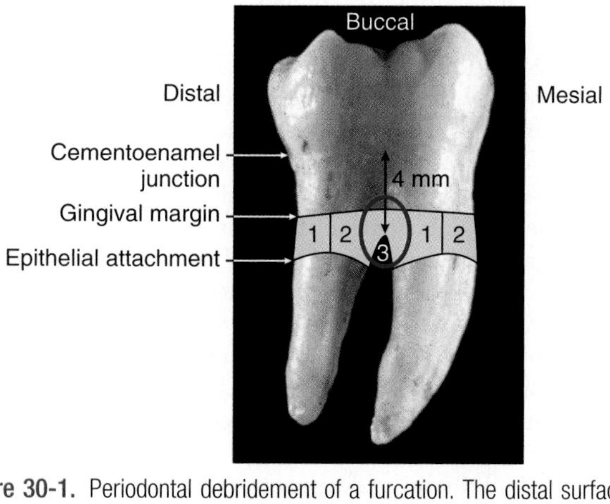

Figure 30-1. Periodontal debridement of a furcation. The distal surface of each root is instrumented *(area 1)*. The buccal, lingual, and mesial surfaces are then treated *(area 2)*. Finally, the concavity is debrided *(area 3)*.

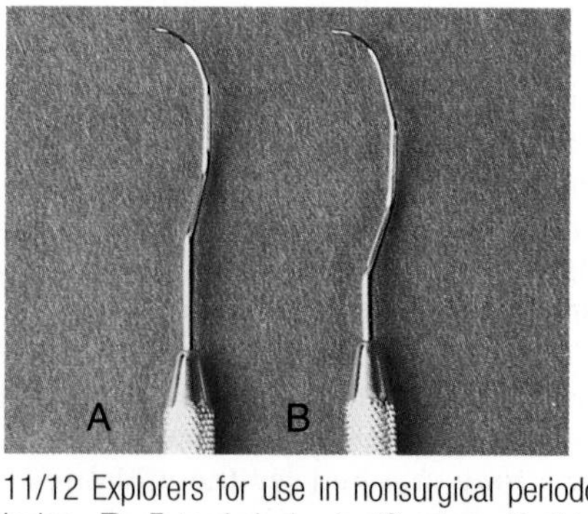

Figure 30-2. 11/12 Explorers for use in nonsurgical periodontal therapy. **A,** Standard design. **B,** Extended shank. (Courtesy Hu-Friedy, Chicago, Illinois.)

including instrumentation, the consideration of chemotherapeutic agents, and further client education regarding self-care practices. Evaluation is the only mechanism for determining if inflammation has been eliminated as evidenced by the absence of bleeding and swelling and by whether the probing depth is reduced and the level of attachment maintained. If the clinical endpoint results in the desired therapeutic endpoint, then the appropriate level of deposit or cementum removal and the elimination of biofilm retentive factors has been attained.

When root roughness and irregularity are not changing despite appropriate detailed instrumentation and the unchanging nature of the tooth surface is not reasonably explained (e.g., tenacious calculus), then the clinician stops instrumentation and waits for the evaluation of the therapeutic endpoint at the 4- to 6-week evaluation appointment. The area is reexamined during the evaluation visit to assess whether the clinical endpoint was appropriate. If the area warrants further instrumentation as a result of persistent inflammation or bleeding, then instrumentation continues. This decision-making process and evaluation build the clinician's experience base and expertise with regard to the provision of NSPT. In addition, the clinician must recognize the client's response during the healing process, so systemic health, other risk factors, and self-care must be evaluated with other clinical parameters.

It is important to note that the basic definition of periodontal debridement includes the removal of all oral biofilm retentive factors, including the removal of detectable calculus until periodontal health is achieved. The removal of 100% of calculus and diseased cementum is not possible or even desirable because of the resulting tooth structure loss and probable dentinal hypersensitivity. Although meticulous periodontal debridement may remove some cementum, aggressive root planing to intentionally remove cementum is not recommended.

By contrast, periodontal debridement requires the complete removal of clinically detectable calculus as determined by the clinical outcome. Calculus removal is critical to the success of periodontal therapy, because calculus retains oral biofilm. There is not one simple standard for assessing the clinical endpoint because the client's systemic health, immune response, and self-care practices influence healing. Sound professional judgment must be practiced to determine the endpoints of NSPT. Intentionally leaving detectable calculus constitutes unethical or substandard care.

Evaluation

Final evaluation of the outcomes of NSPT compares the initial assessment data with client data at the completion of care to determine if therapeutic and client goals were met. Because of the extent of therapy and the multiple visits involved, the clinician has the opportunity to reexamine areas that were previously treated to assess gingival healing via color and shape changes, deposit removal, the client's oral self-care practices, and the results of diagnostic testing or medical screening. Generally the first evaluation of the gingival healing takes place 2 weeks after periodontal debridement of a sextant, quadrant, or half of the mouth. This 2-week period represents the time required for the initial reduction in the clinical signs of inflammation. The assessment of oral biofilm retentive factors also occurs at the next appointment after each segment of periodontal debridement is completed. The care plan is revised to include this new information and to assess client needs.

Comprehensive evaluation occurs at the reevaluation visit 4 to 6 weeks after initial or active therapy. The purposes of reevaluation are as follows:

- To evaluate the client's response to the initial therapy and to recommend additional therapy as needed
- To make a final periodontal diagnosis and prognosis by modifying the presumptive diagnosis, if indicated

The reevaluation visit includes the following:

- Reassessing initial periodontal and risk factor assessment to evaluate host response and self-care practices
- Reeducating and motivating client
- Removing residual deposits or biofilm retentive factors
- Debriding unresponsive areas as indicated by bleeding on probing or gingival inflammation
- Performing any supportive intervention, such as desensitization or antimicrobial therapy
- Reassessing the maintenance interval and adjusting it, if indicated

See Box 30-1 for a reevaluation sequence that can be used in practice.

Clients who were initially diagnosed with plaque-induced gingival disease should demonstrate a reduction in gingival inflammation, stable clinical attachment levels, and a reduction in clinically detectable oral biofilm to a level that is compatible with gingival health. Client factors to be reassessed if

BOX 30-1

Reevaluation Appointment Guide

Assessment
- Probe depth measurements (expected healing is 1 to 2 mm if periodontitis is chronic and not aggressive)
- Bleeding on probing (should be absent)
- Gingival description (should be healthy)
- Soft-tissue assessment information (should be healthy)

Periodontal Diagnosis
- Reevaluation of the presumptive diagnosis

Care Planning: Decision Making for the Appointment
- Localized periodontal debridement
- Need for generalized periodontal debridement; reappointment for re-care visit
- Incorporate adjunctive care; local controlled delivery of antibiotic, antimicrobial rinse, desensitization therapy, and so on
- Referral to periodontist or another specialist
- Set periodontal maintenance or continued-care interval
- Reinforce self-care (teach; focus on skill or management deficiencies)

Implementation
- Delivery of care as planned
- Quality of care

the resolution of their conditions does not occur include the following:
- Self-care practices
- Periodontal disease risk factors
- Systemic disease status
- Residual calculus and oral biofilm
- Oral biofilm retentive factors
- Adherence to the continued-care interval
- Disabilities that may limit self-care

The expected outcomes for clients who were initially diagnosed with chronic periodontitis include reductions of the following:
- The periodontal probing depth (1 to 2 mm)
- Inflammation (or its resolution)
- Bleeding on probing (or its resolution)

If no response is apparent, further evaluation of the affected sites or the client's case is imperative.

Nonresponse does not necessarily imply an aggressive disease state. Retreatment should occur, and another PM visit can be arranged at the appropriate interval. For clients with aggressive periodontitis, the stability and control of the disease are the objectives of reevaluation. If control is not possible, then slowing the progression of disease is the next alternative. The inclusion of reevaluation in a care plan is dependent on multiple factors that are assessed during initial therapy (Box 30-2).

Each client who has completed initial or active NSPT should be reevaluated to assess whether the objectives of NSPT were met. It is critical that individuals with systemic conditions, risk factors, aggressive forms of the disease, pockets of 6 mm or greater, advanced bone loss or attachment loss, furcations, or mobility are evaluated. Adherence on the part of the client requires the discussion of the need for the reevaluation visit as an essential part of the NSPT care plan at the time of case presentation and informed consent. Some practices consider the evaluation visit part of the initial periodontal debridement (i.e., scaling and root planing) fee; other practices believe the reevaluation visit warrants a separate fee. The appointment may also entail other procedures, such as pit and fissure sealants, stain removal, coronal polishing or tooth whitening, and fluoride therapy when indicated to maximize the client's time and the hygienists' productivity.

BOX 30-2

Factors to Consider for Reevaluation

- Gingival inflammation
- Bleeding on probing
- Depth, number, and location of periodontal pockets
- Clinical attachment loss
- Furcations and mobility
- Expected client response to oral self-care recommendations
- Presumptive or preliminary diagnosis and dental hygiene diagnosis
- Other complicating factors, such as restorative needs or occlusion
- Systemic disease and risk factors present
- Client goals for nonsurgical periodontal therapy and degree of adherence to recommendations
- Likelihood of disease progression

In practice, a reevaluation appointment is typically scheduled for 30 minutes; it may be longer if other services are included in the care plan. An additional appointment for retreatment is indicated if more than 30 minutes is needed. Nonresponse is identified as a new problem, and another appointment is scheduled for re-treatment and reeducation, or the client may be referred for a medical evaluation, if indicated. Explanations for the nonresponse focus on the potential reasons for the lack of healing, including incomplete periodontal debridement, systemic disease, inadequate self-care, tobacco use, or the use of inappropriate self-care aids. More than one course of action will be chosen to address the client's nonresponse. The clinician could re-treat the area, reevaluate the self-care aids recommended or used, or use a chemotherapeutic antimicrobial agent (e.g., home oral irrigation, local delivery of antibiotics or antimicrobials) in the area. These additional therapies precipitate the need for more discussion and client decision making (i.e., informed consent).

At the conclusion of the reevaluation visit, the first PM visit is established as follows:
- 8 to 10 weeks after the reevaluation visit if the objectives of care are reached: This interval represents an interval of 3 to 4 months after the last appointment for periodontal debridement.
- 4 weeks after the last appointment at which periodontal debridement was performed if the objectives of care are not reached or if multiple risk factors for continuing periodontal destruction exist: If the objectives of care are not reached and the preliminary diagnosis is mild to moderate periodontitis, then the client is returned to the initial therapy phase of care rather than maintenance. Table 30-3 offers suggested PM intervals.

Referral to a Periodontist

The decision to care for the client in the general dental practice or to refer him or her to a periodontal practice is made on the basis of the following:
- The type and severity of the client's disease
- The dental hygienist's acquired skill level
- The time allotted to maintain periodontally involved clients

For example, if the periodontal diagnosis is advanced periodontitis or an aggressive form of the disease, referral to a periodontist is indicated. A client with moderate chronic periodontitis may also be referred to the periodontist if complicating risk factors exist and if the extent of disease is progressing toward an advanced disease status. Some practitioners use the "5-mm standard" as a factor when referring; this means that a loss of attachment of 5 mm or greater represents a loss of bone support of about one half of the root length of the average tooth. It is then the responsibility of the dental hygienist to strive to maintain the client's periodontal health and to inform the client when that goal is not being achieved.

Some clients decline referral because of geographic constraints, cost, or the fact that they do not want to go to a new office setting. Others may fear or object to surgery. Documentation of the referral to the periodontist and the client's response in the record is imperative.

Most periodontists are willing to alternate visits for PM with the general practitioner. Clients with advanced chronic disease or aggressive disease will probably be maintained at the periodontist's office and be referred to the general dentist

TABLE 30-3

Suggested Periodontal Maintenance Therapy Intervals

Characteristics	Interval
First-year client; routine therapy and healing	3 months
First-year client; difficult case with prosthesis, furcation involvement, poor crown-to-root ratios, and questionable client cooperation	1-2 months
Excellent results well-maintained for 1 year or more	6 months–1 year
Client displays good oral self-care, minimal calculus, no occlusal problems, no complicated prostheses, no remaining pockets, and no teeth with less than 30% of alveolar bone remaining	6 months–1 year
Good results maintained for 1 year or more, but client has some of the following characteristics: • Inconsistent oral self-care (i.e., poor oral hygiene) • Heavy calculus • Systemic disease and risk factors (i.e., a predisposition to disease progression) • Remaining pockets • Occlusal trauma • Complicated prostheses • Ongoing orthodontic therapy • Moderate or high caries risk • Some teeth with <30% of alveolar bone support • Continued smoking or tobacco use • Positive family history or genetic test • >20% of pockets bleed with probing	3-4 months (select the interval on the basis of the number and severity of the negative factors)
Poor results and/or client has some of the following characteristics: • Inconsistent or poor oral hygiene • Heavy calculus formation • Systemic disease (i.e., a predisposition to periodontal breakdown) • Remaining pockets • Occlusal trauma • Complicated prosthesis • Moderate or high caries risk • Periodontal surgery indicated but not performed • Many teeth with <30% of alveolar bone support • Condition too advanced to be improved by periodontal surgery • Smoking • Positive family history or genetic test • >20% of pockets bleed with probing	1-3 months (select the interval on the basis of the number and severity of the negative factors; consider re-treating some areas or extracting severely involved teeth)

Adapted from Newman MG, Takei HH, Klokkevold PR, et al: *Carranza's clinical periodontology,* ed 11, St Louis, 2012, Saunders.

once every 3, 6, 9, or 12 months for restorative examination, depending on the client's caries risk.

Surgical Intervention

Some forms of moderate to advanced periodontitis need to be reevaluated often to determine whether the goals of periodontal therapy are being achieved and maintained. Therapeutic goals for these clients include the following:

- The resolution of gingival inflammation
- A decrease in periodontal probing depths
- The maintenance of or a gain in the attachment level
- The radiologic resolution of osseous defects
- Occlusal stability
- Oral biofilm reduction to a level that is acceptable to the host response

Surgery should be considered when nonsurgical therapy is unsuccessful for reaching these goals. A surgical approach (as opposed to NSPT) is considered in the following circumstances:

- When enhanced access for the removal of causative factors is needed
- When diseased sites with deep periodontal pockets persist
- When the regeneration or reconstruction of the periodontal tissues (e.g., osseous defects) is indicated

Additional Nonsurgical Interventions[10,13]

Systemic antimicrobials or antibiotics are not used for clients with periodontitis unless aggressive periodontitis, severe forms, or progressing periodontitis are present. These treatments are best incorporated as part of NSPT in conjunction with instrumentation of subgingival biofilm, starting on the day of debridement completion and continuing for about a week. Systemic antimicrobials are used discriminately as a result of their side effects, microbiologic adverse effects, and bacterial resistance concerns. Optimal results are achieved when the biofilm is disrupted but not reorganized. To accomplish this, the following time periods are used:

- Debridement occurs within 1 week.
- On the day of completion of debridement, effective levels of the drug should be present.

Laser therapy interventions are being incorporated into some care plans for clients undergoing NSPT. Evidence related to three of the uses in NSPT is as follows[13]:

- *Pocket debridement.* It is accepted that soft-tissue debridement or curettage with and without laser therapy does not provide additional benefits beyond scaling and root planing alone; there is minimal evidence to support the use of laser therapy for this purpose as a monotherapy or as an adjunct to scaling and root planing.
- *Subgingival bacteria reduction.* The use of this treatment is unpredictable and inconsistent with reducing the subgingival bacterial load as compared with scaling and root planing alone; current evidence is lacking or conflicting.
- *Laser-assisted scaling and root planing.* Further study of this method is needed. Some slight benefit has been noted with clinical attachment level changes as compared with scaling and root planing alone in some studies, although no benefit has been noted in other studies. The in vitro removal of calculus and endotoxin has also been noted.

Consensus statements include the following:

- The Er:YAG laser has characteristics that are most suitable for NSPT for chronic periodontitis.
- CO_2, Nd:YAG, Nd:YAP, and diode lasers with different wavelengths do not have efficacy as compared with debridement alone or when added as adjunctive therapy.
- Appropriate radiation parameters, conditions, and techniques must be used to prevent thermal injury to adjacent tissues.

Stronger evidence is needed to make clinical recommendations for laser use with NSPT.

Nonsurgical Periodontal Therapy Insurance Issues (Table 30-4)

Dental benefit plans (dental insurance) influence the NSPT that is provided. The dental hygienist needs to know the following:

- His or her office's philosophy regarding third-party payment
- Common dental terms associated with filing insurance claims for NSPT
- Periodontal insurance codes
- Third-party insurance carriers in the office's geographic area
- Enhanced coverage-of-benefits letters used (if not, letters can be developed)
- Who is responsible for filing insurance claims, explaining insurance-related issues to the client, and communicating with the insurance company
- How to maximize insurance benefits
- That recommendations for optimal dental hygiene care are not dependent on insurance reimbursement

The dental hygienist is a source of information about insurance coverage for periodontal services. The dental hygienist may explain the relationship between the office fees and third-party insurance benefits and the responsibility of the client for the NSPT fee charged. Treatment plans are developed according to professional standards and client needs, not according to the provisions of the client's insurance policy. This philosophy ensures that clients receive appropriate care.

When diagnosing and classifying periodontal disease for insurance claims, the clinician uses the following two considerations:

- Host and microbial parameters (e.g., onset, progression, response to the disease)
- Disease severity (e.g., probing depth, clinical attachment level, furcation involvement)

A specific periodontal diagnosis is used for insurance reporting whenever appropriate; an extensive range of therapies exists for periodontal therapy, and no one treatment is effective for everyone. In fact, one section of the mouth may require one type of therapy while another area requires a different therapy. Therefore the description of disease in one quadrant of the mouth as reported on the insurance claim may differ from that reported for another area.

It is useful to develop a fee-for-service schedule for dental hygienists that includes the following:

- Classifications of periodontal disease
- The American Dental Association procedure codes (updated annually)
- Descriptions of the services
- The fees or ranges of fees charged

This schedule provides standardized fees for service among dental hygienists in the same practice and enhances communication with the office manager. Although there are American Dental Association codes for various supportive services (e.g., local anesthetic, root desensitization), not all dental plans provide reimbursements for these services. In fact, there are variations in insurance coverage by different carriers as well as among different plans from the same carrier with regard to services covered, frequency of payment for services, and maximum fee reimbursed. For example, some insurance plans reimburse for PM every 3 months, whereas others do not. Practice-management computer software programs help staff members and dental hygienists to assess reimbursement rates; however, the ultimate responsibility for the fee rests with the client.

Periodontal Maintenance[14]

PM is planned to occur after the active phase of periodontal care at appropriately timed intervals that are based on client needs. *Periodontal maintenance* is the preferred term for what was formerly referred to as *supportive periodontal therapy* or *periodontal recall.* Although the dentist has ultimate responsibility for PM, the dental hygienist also has the responsibility to provide comprehensive and individually timed PM for clients who have participated in NSPT. PM continues for the life of the dentition or its implant replacements, and this recommendation must be explained to clients who have NSPT. Clients with gingivitis and periodontitis have a chronic disease entity that must be controlled by frequent periodontal care and daily self-care.

Goals of Periodontal Maintenance

- To prevent or minimize the recurrence and progression of periodontal disease among clients who have been treated for gingivitis, periodontitis, and peri-implantitis
- To prevent or reduce the incidence of tooth loss
- To increase the probability of locating and treating other diseases and conditions

TABLE 30-4

Procedure Codes for Nonsurgical Periodontal Therapy

Code	Nomenclature	Descriptor
D0120	Periodic oral evaluation—established patient	An evaluation performed on a patient of record to determine any changes in the patient's dental and medical health status since a previous comprehensive or periodic evaluation. This includes an oral cancer evaluation and periodontal screening where indicated, and may require interpretation of information acquired through additional diagnostic procedures. Report additional diagnostic procedures separately.
D0140	Limited oral evaluation: problem focused	An evaluation limited to a specific oral health problem or complaint. This may require interpretation of information acquired through additional diagnostic procedures. Report additional diagnostic procedures separately. Definitive procedures may be required on the same date as the evaluation. Typically, patients receiving this type of evaluation present with a specific problem and/or dental emergencies, trauma, acute infections, etc.
D0150	Comprehensive oral evaluation—new or established patient	Used by a general dentist and/or a specialist when evaluating a patient comprehensively. This applies to new patients; established patients who have had a significant change in health conditions or other unusual circumstances, by report, or established patients who have been absent from active treatment for 3 or more years. It is a thorough evaluation and recording of the extraoral and intraoral hard and soft tissues. It may require interpretation of information acquired through additional diagnostic procedures. Additional diagnostic procedures should be reported separately. This includes an evaluation for oral cancer where indicated, the evaluation and recording of the patient's dental and medical history and a general health assessment. It may include the evaluation and recording of dental caries, missing or unerupted teeth, restorations, existing prostheses, occlusal relationships, periodontal conditions (including periodontal screening and/or charting), hard and soft tissue anomalies, etc.
D0160	Detailed and extensive oral evaluation: problem focused, by report	A detailed and extensive problem focused evaluation entails extensive diagnostic and cognitive modalities based on the findings of a comprehensive oral evaluation. Integration of more extensive diagnostic modalities to develop a treatment plan for a specific problem is required. The condition requiring this type of evaluation should be described and documented. Examples of conditions requiring this type of evaluation may include dentofacial anomalies, complicated perioprosthetic conditions, complex temporomandibular dysfunction, facial pain of unknown origin, conditions requiring multidisciplinary consultation, etc.
D0180	Comprehensive periodontal evaluation—new or established patient	This procedure is indicated for patients showing signs or symptoms of periodontal disease and for patients with risk factors such as smoking or diabetes. It includes evaluation of periodontal conditions, probing and charting, evaluation and recording of the patient's dental and medical history, and general health assessment. It may include the evaluation and recording of dental caries, missing or unerupted teeth, restorations, occlusal relationships, and oral cancer evaluation.
D0277	Vertical bitewings: 7 to 8 radiographic images	This does not constitute a full mouth intraoral radiographic series.
D0415	Collection of microorganisms for culture and sensitivity	
D0417 (D0418) analysis of the sample	Collection and preparation of saliva sample for laboratory diagnostic testing	May include, but is not limited to, tests for susceptibility to periodontal disease.
D0421	Genetic test for susceptibility to oral diseases	Sample collection for the purpose of certified laboratory analysis to detect specific genetic variations associated with increased susceptibility for oral diseases such as severe periodontal disease.
D1110	Prophylaxis: adult	Removal of plaque, calculus, and stains from the tooth structures in the permanent and transitional dentition. It is intended to control local irritational factors.
D1120	Prophylaxis: child	Removal of plaque, calculus, and stains from the tooth structures in the primary and transitional dentition. It is intended to control local irritational factors.

Continued

TABLE 30-4

Procedure Codes for Nonsurgical Periodontal Therapy—cont'd

Code	Nomenclature	Descriptor
D1310	Nutritional counseling for control of dental disease	Counseling on food selection and dietary habits as a part of treatment and control of periodontal disease and caries.
D1320	Tobacco counseling for the control and prevention of oral disease	Tobacco prevention and cessation services reduce patient risk of developing tobacco-related oral diseases and conditions and improve prognosis for certain dental therapies.
D1330	Oral hygiene instructions	This service may include instructions for home care. Examples include toothbrushing technique, flossing, and use of special oral hygiene aids.
D4341	Periodontal scaling and root planing, four or more teeth per quadrant	This procedure involves instrumentation of the crown and root surfaces of the teeth to remove plaque and calculus from these surfaces. It is indicated for patients with periodontal disease and is therapeutic, not prophylactic, in nature. Root planing is the definitive procedure designed for the removal of cementum and dentin that is rough, and/or permeated by calculus or contaminated with toxins or microorganisms. Some soft tissue removal occurs. This procedure may be used as a definitive treatment in some stages of periodontal disease and/or as a part of presurgical procedures in others.
D4342	Periodontal scaling and root planing, one to three teeth per quadrant	This procedure involves instrumentation of the crown and root surfaces of the teeth to remove plaque and calculus from these surfaces. It is indicated for patients with periodontal disease and is therapeutic, not prophylactic, in nature. Root planing is the definitive procedure designed for the removal of cementum and dentin that is rough, and/or permeated by calculus or contaminated with toxins or microorganisms. Some soft tissue removal occurs. This procedure may be used as a definitive treatment in some stages of periodontal disease and/or as a part of presurgical procedures in others.
D4355	Full-mouth debridement to enable comprehensive periodontal evaluation and diagnosis	The gross removal of plaque and calculus that interfere with the ability of the dentist to perform a comprehensive oral evaluation. This is a preliminary procedure and does not preclude the need for additional procedures.
D4381	Localized delivery of antimicrobial agents via a controlled-release vehicle into diseased crevicular tissue, per tooth, by report	FDA-approved subgingival delivery devices containing antimicrobial medication(s) are inserted into periodontal pockets to suppress the pathogenic microbiota. These devices slowly release the pharmacological agents so they can remain at the intended site of action in a therapeutic concentration for a sufficient length of time.
D4910	Periodontal maintenance	This procedure is instituted following periodontal therapy and continues at varying intervals, determined by the clinical evaluation of the dentist, for the life of the dentition or any implant replacements. It includes removal of the bacterial plaque and calculus from supragingival and subgingival regions, site-specific scaling and root planing where indicated, and polishing the teeth. If new or recurring periodontal disease appears, additional diagnostic and treatment procedures must be considered.
D9910	Application of desensitizing medicament	Includes in-office treatment for root sensitivity. Typically reported on a "per visit" basis for application of topical fluoride. This code is not to be used for bases, liners, or adhesives used under restorations.
D9911	Application of desensitizing resin for cervical and/or root surface, per tooth	Typically reported on a "per tooth" basis for application of adhesive resins. This code is not to be used for bases, liners, or adhesives used under restorations.
D6080	Implant maintenance procedures when prostheses are removed and reinserted, including cleansing of prostheses and abutments	This procedure includes active debriding of the implant(s) and examination of all aspects of the implant system(s), including the occlusion and stability of the superstructure. The patient is also instructed in thorough daily cleansing of the implant(s). This is not a per implant code, and is indicated for implant-supported fixed prostheses.

From the American Dental Association: *CDT 2014: Dental Procedure Coding,* 2013, Chicago, ADA.

Intervals for Periodontal Maintenance

Clients with gingivitis who are in good general health, who do not have a history of attachment loss, and who maintain their oral health status have continued-care appointments every 6 months, usually for oral prophylaxis. For clients with periodontitis, an interval of 3 months or less is ideal for PM. Part of the rationale for 3-month intervals is that, after periodontal pathogens are suppressed, they return to pretreatment levels in 9 to 11 weeks; however, this interval varies significantly among clients. Although 3 months is the ideal interval, the PM interval is customized for the client on the basis of that client's self-care adherence, extent of disease, systemic contributions to disease, risk factors, and consent (see Table 30-3). Factors that influence client consent to a specific interval are cost, third-party benefits, cooperation, personal values, and needs.

Components of Care

The components of PM should be similar at each PM visit; however, the extent of these services may vary depending on client adherence, the length of time in PM, and the extent of periodontitis. Table 30-5 presents a summary of the assessment used for a PM visit to address associated risk factors.

TABLE 30-5

Periodontal Maintenance Assessment Criteria, Procedures, and Associated Risk Factors

Criteria	Procedure	Risk Factors to Evaluate
Health and pharmacologic history	Review and update the following: • Need for prophylactic antibiotics • Making sure medications have been taken • New diseases or medications • Need for medical consultation • Smoking status	Age of client Smoking status Systemic diseases and conditions such as diabetes, cardiovascular disease, osteoporosis, pregnancy, immunosuppression, and so on Stress
Dental history	Review and determine chief complaint	Lack of adherence with the continued-care interval
Extraoral and intraoral soft-tissue assessment	Examine for significant pathology	Dependent on type of pathology
Restorative assessment	Evaluate prostheses (including implants), caries activity and risk, and restorations	Overhangs or ill-fitting restorations Failing implant
Periodontal assessment	Examine gingiva for color, contour, consistency, texture, position, and mucogingival involvement	Inflammation Progressive recession Minimal or no keratinized gingiva
	Probing depth	1- to 2-mm increase Moderate to deep probe depths
	Attachment loss	Extent and severity of disease; type of disease present; 2-mm loss of attachment in 1 year
	Radiographs	Changes in bone levels Vertical bone loss Presence of dental caries
	Bleeding with probing	Presence indicates risk
	Furcation involvement	Presence indicates risk; the more advanced the furcation involvement, the more risk
	Mobility	Presence indicates risk; the more advanced the mobility, the more risk
	Suppuration	Presence indicates risk
Deposit accumulation	Evaluate location and extent of supragingival oral biofilm	Presence of supragingival oral biofilm is strongly correlated with gingivitis
	Supragingival and subgingival deposits	Pathogenicity of microorganisms present in the subgingival environment (i.e., microbiologic monitoring) Lack of adherence with oral self-care Calculus (i.e., biofilm retentive factor)
Radiographic assessment	Evaluate the following: • Risk of advancing disease • Clinical findings, especially progressive attachment loss • Client radiographic history	Advancing radiographic bone loss

Adapted from Hodges KO: *Concepts in nonsurgical periodontal therapy,* Albany, NY, 1998, Delmar.

Appointment Time

The time required for effective PM varies with regard to the following:

- Number of teeth
- Self-care efficacy
- Cooperation
- Systemic health
- Previous frequency of PM
- Instrumentation needs
- Adjunctive therapy needs
- History of periodontal disease
- Practitioner skill

In practice, 60 minutes is probably adequate for a PM visit; however, 45 minutes may suffice in some cases, and others may require 90 minutes. It is challenging in the practice sector to establish a reasonable fee, to work with insurance carriers, and to explain needs to the client. A number of insurance carriers will not cover the four annual PM appointments that the client needs. In this case, the client's out-of-pocket expenses and the consequences of inadequate PM are discussed.

Compliance or Adherence[14]

The less threatening a health problem appears to be to the individual, the less likely he or she is to comply. Compliance is also reduced if therapy is time consuming and no symptoms are present. Other reasons for nonadherence include self-destructive behavior, fear, economics, health beliefs, stress, and perceived professional indifference. The success of long-term PM in university, hospital, and specialist settings is impressive; only 2% to 5% of teeth that are treated for chronic periodontitis are lost over 5 to 10 years.[10] To improve client adherence to professional recommendations, the following are suggested:

- Enhance client education about therapeutic need.
- Discuss the client's risk factors and level of control.
- Keep recommendations simple yet thorough, and have the client implement them in small steps.
- Target recommendations for oral self-care devices and strategies to the client's conditions.
- Minimize the number of aids needed.
- Incorporate adjunctive therapy after meticulous conventional therapy to not burden the client with additional time commitments or costs.
- Pay attention to client questions and needs.
- Remind clients of their appointments.
- Inform clients, in written form, about the disease and appropriate self-care practices.
- Provide positive reinforcement.
- Target potential noncompliers early.
- Ensure dentist, periodontist, and physician involvement as necessary.

Contemporary electronic communication mechanisms can easily send email reminders, text message reminders, and educational information to clients in an attempt to enhance adherence.

Periodontal Surgery

A discussion of periodontal surgical options for clients who need more than NSPT is beyond the scope of this chapter. The reader is referred to any major dental textbook about periodontal therapy. However, after a client has had periodontal surgery, the dental hygienist may be called on to place a periodontal pack. A **periodontal pack** is a puttylike bandage that is positioned over the surgical site to protect the area for about 1 week; it does not have any healing properties. The pack material (Coe-Pak) is prepared as follows:

- Squeeze equal parts of the two pastes (i.e., the accelerator and the base) onto a paper mixing pad.
- Mix these thoroughly for 2 to 3 minutes until the color is uniform. Most clinicians use a wooden tongue depressor for mixing because the material is very tacky and difficult to clean up.

(At this point, antibiotics could be added to create medicinal effects if this is recommended by the dentist or periodontist.)

- When the tackiness is gone, roll the material into two cylinders for placement on the facial and lingual surfaces of the surgical site. The pack material remains workable for about 15 minutes. See Figures 30-3 and 30-4 for pack mixing and placement procedures.

CLIENT EDUCATION TIPS

- Gingivitis is reversible, but periodontitis is not; periodontitis is a chronic infectious disease. The host's response to the microbial challenge determines disease progression or control.
- Oral prophylaxis is not indicated for the treatment of periodontitis.
- Evaluation is an integral aspect of nonsurgical periodontal therapy, especially with regard to the initial therapy phase of care.
- The prevention and successful treatment of periodontal diseases depend on the co-therapy approach in which the client performs adequate oral self-care and complies with the continued-care interval.
- Oral self-care alone will not maintain or prevent the further recurrence of periodontitis. Client risk factors must be assessed and modified.
- The care plan for nonsurgical periodontal therapy and periodontal maintenance is dependent on the client's genetic, systemic, environmental, and oral conditions and not on the client's third-party payment plan benefits.
- Periodontal maintenance at the recommended interval is needed for the long term to control periodontal disease progression.
- Risk factors are associated with the development and progression of periodontitis, and they should be eliminated, reduced, or controlled, depending on the nature of the risk factor itself (see Chapters 19 and 20).
- Treatment plans are developed according to professional standards and client needs and not according to the provisions of the client's insurance policy.

LEGAL, ETHICAL, AND SAFETY ISSUES

- The client needs to be informed about nonsurgical periodontal therapy (including recommendations about how and why to perform self-care, risk factors, and reevaluation) and the PM care plan[2] and to be involved in the decision-making process. Informed consent and informed refusal should be documented in writing.

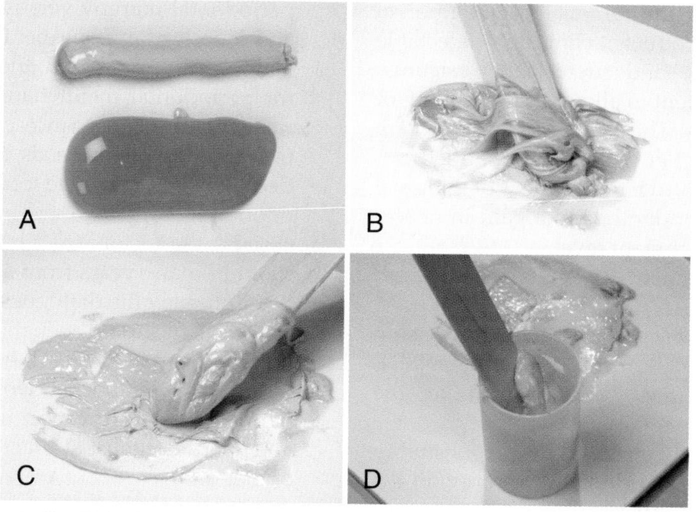

Figure 30-3. Preparing the surgical pack (Coe-Pak). **A,** Equal lengths of the two pastes are placed on a paper pad. **B,** The pastes are mixed with a wooden tongue depressor for 2 to 3 minutes until **(C),** the paste loses its tackiness. **D,** The paste is placed in a paper cup of room-temperature water. With lubricated fingers, the preparer then rolls the paste into cylinders to be placed over the client's surgical wound. (From Newman MG, Takei HH, Klokkevold PR, et al, eds: *Carranza's clinical periodontology,* ed 11, St Louis, 2012, Saunders.)

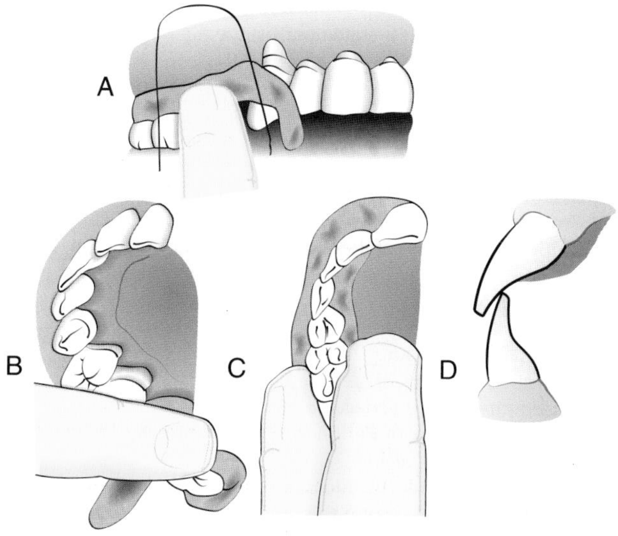

Figure 30-4. Inserting the periodontal pack. **A,** A strip of the pack material is hooked around the last molar and pressed into place anteriorly. **B,** The lingual pack is joined to the facial strip at the distal surface of the last molar and fitted into place anteriorly. **C,** Gentle pressure on the facial and lingual interproximal surfaces joins the pack interproximally. **D,** The periodontal pack should not interfere with occlusion. (From Newman MG, Takei HH, Klokkevold PR, et al, eds: *Carranza's clinical periodontology,* ed 11, St Louis, 2012, Saunders.)

- The client must receive sufficient information to make an informed decision about the care plan.
- Referral to a medical professional or another dental professional (e.g., a periodontist) when indicated is essential. Referral may occur as a result of the clinician's lack of skill or knowledge to treat; advancing disease conditions, despite therapy (i.e., refractory areas or cases); multiple genetic, systemic, or environmental risk factors; or an aggressive form of periodontal disease. A clinician should acquire informed consent if professional consultation related to a medical condition or periodontal disease arises.
- Failure to assess the periodontium adequately is malpractice.
- Negligence may include the dental hygienist's failure to protect a client from harm when the client has a systemic disease and the failure to record information about the assessment, care plan, informed consent, informed refusal, and interventions related to care. Negligence may occur if nonsurgical periodontal therapy or periodontal maintenance is needed by a client and the dental hygienist provides oral prophylaxis instead.
- The hygienist uses evidence-based decision making to select appropriate interventions for care. The dental hygienist must remain current.
- Risks associated with care increase with nonsurgical periodontal therapy that involves subgingival periodontal debridement (i.e., root planing) and local anesthetic agent use during multiple appointments. Clients need to be informed of the consequences of injectable local anesthetic agent use (i.e., hematoma or paresthesia) and the consequences of periodontal debridement (i.e., bleeding, periodontal abscess, and dentinal hypersensitivity).

KEY CONCEPTS

- A disease-free periodontium includes the absence of inflammation and the maintenance of periodontal attachment over time.
- Gingivitis is the presence of inflammation without clinical attachment loss; it is treated with oral prophylaxis (i.e., scaling and stain management).
- Periodontitis is present when there is loss of clinical attachment and supporting bone. It is treated with nonsurgical periodontal therapy (NSPT), surgery, or both.
- NSPT includes oral biofilm removal and control, supragingival and subgingival scaling, root planing (i.e., debridement), and the use of chemotherapeutic agents. The host's response to care must be assessed and his or her risk factors modified. Host modulation may be recommended.

- Periodontal debridement is the removal of subgingival oral biofilm and its by-products, clinically detectable biofilm retentive factors, and detectable calculus-embedded cementum sufficient to allow for the healing of adjacent periodontal tissues. The host's response to care must be assessed and his or her risk factors modified.
- The therapeutic endpoint is the restoration of gingival health, a reduction in pocket depth, and a gain in or stabilization of the clinical attachment level.
- Periodontal infection detrimentally influences overall health.
- Periodontal assessment is the foundation for the provision of successful periodontal care, which includes NSPT, periodontal maintenance (PM), and referral to the periodontist.
- NSPT is phase I periodontal therapy; it is the responsibility of the dental hygienist who is working in concert with the general dentist or the periodontist.
- Chronic disease states of gingivitis and periodontitis usually progress slowly and can respond to NSPT in a predictable manner; however, aggressive disease states progress rapidly and do not respond in a predictable manner.
- Periodontal diagnosis is determined by analyzing information during the assessment phase of therapy; this includes the client's health, dental, and pharmacologic history data as well as disease classification, extent, and severity.
- Mechanical pocket therapy is periodontal debridement that involves manual or power-driven instrumentation. Both methods are efficacious, and a blended approach is recommended.
- Evaluation occurs throughout NSPT. Gingival inflammation is reassessed 2 weeks after the periodontal debridement of an area, the reassessment for oral biofilm retentive factors occurs at each subsequent appointment, and the reevaluation of the full mouth occurs 4 to 6 weeks after the initial therapy of certain areas or of the case.
- PM follows the active phase of therapy, is appropriately timed based on client need, and continues for the life of the dentition or the implant replacements.
- PM prevents or minimizes the recurrence and progression of periodontal disease, prevents or reduces tooth loss, and increases the chances of locating and treating other diseases and conditions.
- Clients with gingivitis can maintain their oral health when PM is performed every 6 months.
- Clients with periodontitis require a 3-month interval or less for PM.

CRITICAL THINKING EXERCISES

1. You are caring for a new client who has not received dental hygiene care for 3 years as a result of "financial constraints"; however, before this 3-year hiatus, she received annual oral prophylaxis. She does not have dental insurance. Dental hygiene assessment findings reveal periodontal pockets that range from 4 to 6 mm, 1- to 2-mm clinical attachment levels, radiographic early bone loss, bleeding on probing, and generalized light to moderate deposits. Develop a dialogue that explains the need for nonsurgical periodontal therapy versus oral prophylaxis, the number and length of appointments estimated, the type of interventions recommended, the need for evaluation, the need for periodontal maintenance, the potential cost, and the relationship of insurance coverage. Include the information that the client needs to know to make an informed decision (i.e., informed consent) about nonsurgical periodontal therapy.
2. Discuss the factors that are considered when referring a client of many years from a general dentist to a periodontist. Role-play the dialogues that you would use to explain why a client should seek the expertise of a periodontist for the treatment of chronic advanced periodontitis associated with 4- to 8-mm pocket depth, clinical attachment levels of 5 mm or more, furcation involvement in multiple areas, and periodontal risk factors of smoking and type 2 diabetes.

REFERENCES

1. Ciancio SG: Non-surgical periodontal treatment. In *Proceedings of the World Workshop in Clinical Periodontics* (Section II), Chicago, 1989, American Academy of Periodontology.
2. American Academy of Periodontology: Comprehensive periodontal therapy: a statement by the American Academy of Periodontology, *J Periodontol* 82:943, 2011.
3. Bowen DM: Introduction to nonsurgical periodontal therapy. In Hodges KO, editor: *Concepts in nonsurgical periodontal therapy*, Albany, NY, 1998, Delmar.
4. American Academy of Periodontology: Parameter on chronic periodontitis with slight to moderate loss of periodontal support, *J Periodontol* 71:853, 2000.
5. American Academy of Periodontology: Parameter on chronic periodontitis with advanced loss of periodontal support, *J Periodontol* 71:856, 2000.
6. Armitage GC: Development of a classification for periodontal diseases and conditions, *Ann Periodontol* 4:1, 1999.
7. American Academy of Periodontology: Parameter on plaque-induced gingivitis, *J Periodontol* 71:851, 2000.
8. American Academy of Periodontology: Parameter on aggressive periodontitis, *J Periodontol* 71:867, 2000.
9. Tonetti MS, Chapple IL: Biological approaches to the development of novel periodontal therapies—consensus of the Seventh European Workshop on Periodontology, *J Clin Periodontol* 38(Suppl 11):114, 2011.
10. Sanz M, Teugheis W: Innovations in non-surgical periodontal therapy: Consensus Report of the Sixth European Workshop in Periodontology, *J Clin Periodontol* 35:3, 2008.
11. Lang NP, Tan WC, Krahenmann MA, et al: A systematic review of the effects of full-mouth debridement with and without antiseptics in clients with chronic periodontitis, *J Clin Periodontol* 35:8, 2008.
12. Cobb CM: Clinical significance of non-surgical periodontal therapy: an evidence-based perspective of scaling and root planing, *J Clin Periodontol* 29:22, 2002.
13. American Academy of Periodontology: Statement on the efficacy of lasers in the nonsurgical treatment of inflammatory periodontal disease, *J Periodontol* 82:513, 2011.
14. American Academy of Periodontology: Position paper: periodontal maintenance, *J Periodontol* 74:1395, 2003.

EVOLVE RESOURCES

Please visit http://evolve.elsevier.com/Darby/hygiene for additional practice and study support tools.

Chemotherapy for the Control of Periodontal Disease

CHAPTER 31

Joanna Asadoorian

COMPETENCIES

1. Discuss indications for chemotherapeutic interventions in the prevention and treatment of inflammatory periodontal disease.
2. Identify the organizations in the United States and Canada that ensure the safety and efficacy of oral chemotherapeutics.
3. Discuss the rationale for chemical therapeutics.
4. Discuss local delivery methods, including:
   - Distinguish between the various modes of delivery available for the client's application of chemotherapeutics.
   - Distinguish between the various modes of delivery available for the clinician's application of chemotherapeutics in professional settings.
   - Make recommendations to clients for product selection for home and professional use of oral chemotherapeutics for periodontitis.
5. Discuss systemic delivery methods.
6. Describe various active ingredients used in oral chemotherapeutic products for periodontal diseases.

Oral Disease and Bacterial Plaque Biofilm

The initiation and progression of periodontal diseases are related to the interaction of a susceptible host, a pathogenic agent, and environmental factors. Therefore the prevention and control of periodontal diseases depend, in part, on controlling bacterial plaque biofilm, which is both the pathogenic agent and a primary contributing factor to these diseases. Mechanical disruption of the plaque biofilm has traditionally occurred through oral self-care (e.g., tooth brushing), and it is supported by professional care. Dental hygienists play a key role in advising clients about performing adequate homecare and providing the necessary preventive and therapeutic professional care. Despite these efforts, it is recognized that a large proportion of the North American population demonstrates some level of oral disease; thus these conventional interventions are not always sufficient. Oral **chemotherapeutic agents**, which refer to the incorporation of an active ingredient within a delivery system for preventing or controlling oral disease, are being increasingly used as an adjunct to traditional mechanical means.

Although the total elimination of bacterial plaque biofilm is unrealistic, a reasonable approach is to prevent disease through methods that reduce bacterial plaque to a level below the individual's threshold for disease. Oral chemotherapeutics contribute to this aim in a number of ways, including reducing the number of pathogenic organisms and altering microorganisms to reduce their pathogenic potential. Dental hygienists are in a key position to recommend and implement various chemotherapeutic therapies in a shared decision-making relationship with clients.

Product Selection and Evaluation

Because chemotherapeutics present a risk of harm and the potential for misbranding, two major organizations in the United States—the U.S. Food and Drug Administration (FDA) and the American Dental Association (ADA) Council on Scientific Affairs—and two in Canada—Health Canada and the Canadian Dental Association (CDA)—contribute to ensuring the safety and efficacy of oral chemotherapeutics. These bodies assist both oral health care providers and their clients with the making of appropriate decisions about oral health products.

The U.S. Food and Drug Administration

The FDA ensures the safety and efficacy of prescription drugs and over-the-counter (OTC) products that make therapeutic claims through federally mandated review and approval processes. For OTC drugs, the FDA reviews active ingredients and labeling within the respective therapeutic class. OTC products are typically marketed using an OTC drug monograph that instructs which active ingredients can be used to treat which conditions without a prescription and that includes appropriate dosages and instructions for use. If an OTC product does not meet the stipulations of an existing monograph, it must be approved in a similar process to prescription drugs. For prescription drugs, a New Drug Application is filed for the FDA to review new pharmaceutical proposals; this process requires appropriate animal studies and human clinical trials.

The American Dental Association Council on Scientific Affairs

The ADA Council on Scientific Affairs assists oral health care providers and the public with the selection and use of chemotherapeutic agents by evaluating new, nonprescription products for safety and efficacy. Products approved by the FDA may apply to receive the **ADA Seal of Acceptance** (Figure 31-1, *A*), which is granted to those products that demonstrate therapeutic efficacy in accordance with published criteria. Specific guidelines for evaluating the effectiveness of oral chemotherapeutics for the reduction of plaque and gingivitis have been developed and are updated regularly (Box 31-1). Approval is granted specifically for one or both of these outcome measures, depending on available research evidence.

Health Canada's Therapeutic Products Directorate

In Canada, similar organizations exist to provide this information. The CDA provides the CDA Seal of Recognition (see Figure 31-1, *B*) program, which aims to assist the public and oral health professionals by identifying products that are of benefit to the oral health of consumers and by helping them to make informed choices about such products. Manufacturers seeking the CDA Seal of Recognition must verify that the product complies with Health Canada's Therapeutic Products Directorate, which is the Canadian federal authority that regulates pharmaceutical drugs and medical devices for human use. To receive market authorization, the manufacturer must present scientific evidence of a product's safety, efficacy, and quality, including laboratory and clinical study data.

BOX 31-1

American Dental Association Council on Scientific Affairs Research Guidelines

- Characteristics of the study population represent typical product users.
- Active product should be used in a normal regimen and compared with a placebo control or, where applicable, an active control.
- Crossover or parallel study designs are acceptable and should be a minimum of 6 months in duration.
- Two studies should be conducted by independent investigators.
- Additional guidelines regarding microbial sampling and evaluation periods are in the guidelines.

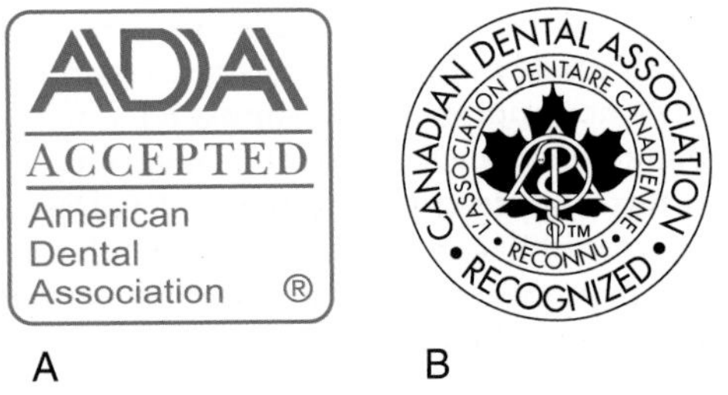

Figure 31-1. A, American Dental Association Seal of Acceptance. **B,** Canadian Dental Association Seal of Recognition.

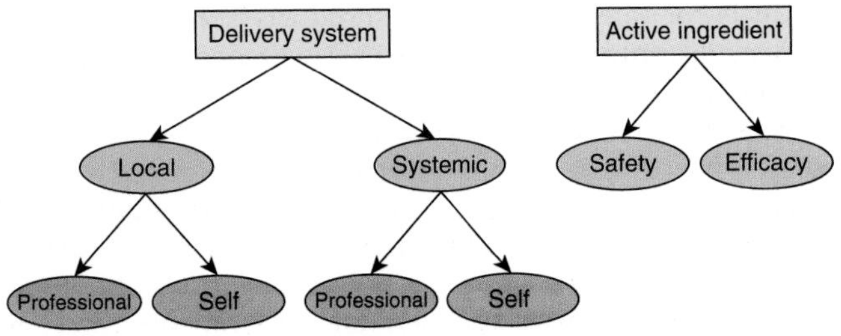

Figure 31-2. Dimensions of oral chemotherapeutics.

A Rationale for Chemical Plaque Control

Despite the widespread use of mechanical plaque removal and technological advances in toothbrushes and interdental tools, difficulties for clients and clinicians remain in the traditional approaches to care, particularly in areas of the mouth that pose access issues. In recent years, research (including a number of systematic reviews) has concluded that some oral chemotherapeutic agents have an adjunctive benefit for reducing plaque biofilm and improving gingival outcomes beyond that accomplished with mechanical means alone.

It is essential for the dental hygienist to access and critically appraise the literature addressing oral chemotherapeutic products on a regular basis, because new studies are continuously being published. Many available products have not demonstrated their efficacy to acceptably high levels over long-term trials to recommend their use. Therefore it is the dental hygienist's role to help clients distinguish between products that have therapeutic benefits and those limited to having cosmetic effects. It is also important to be aware that differences exist between product formulations manufactured in different countries. For example, there are products available in Canada and the United States that have the same name but that contain different active ingredients or concentrations, thus causing some confusion with regard to advertising and research.

To help clarify the literature, dental hygienists can view oral chemotherapeutics as having two dimensions: (1) the delivery system and (2) the active ingredient. For the first dimension, the delivery system can be subcategorized as either being a local or systemic mode of delivery. Local delivery methods are those in which the antimicrobial agent is applied directly to the oral cavity or to a specific location within it for topical application. Systemic delivery methods are those that are ingested and delivered via the bloodstream. Products that fall within one of these two subcategories are usually professionally delivered by the dental hygienist, or they may comprise part of the client's home self-care regimen (Figure 31- 2). Modes of delivery can be thought of as being applied as monotherapy, which means that the intervention is used on its own. Alternatively, these therapies can be used in conjunction with another intervention. Research claims are often based on a specific application mode; therefore the dental hygienist must consider these distinctions when making specific client recommendations.

The second dimension of chemotherapeutics is the active ingredient. The active ingredient refers to the agent, chemical, or drug component within a particular delivery system that is responsible for the therapeutic improvement. Active ingredients may be applied in various ways and found in various delivery systems. For example, the active ingredient fluoride is used in both local delivery systems, such as oral rinses, and systemic vehicles, such as fluoride supplements. Various fluoride formulations may also be available for both home use and professional use. The dental hygienist should not assume that the proven efficacy of a specific active ingredient within a particular delivery system ensures that this same active ingredient is similarly efficacious with other delivery systems or within the same system but in different concentrations.

Active ingredients are effective in that they disable microorganisms or alter the microflora in a number of ways

TABLE 31-1

A Categorization of Active Ingredients in Oral Chemotherapeutics

Category	Description
Antiseptic agents	Usually broad spectrum; kill or prevent propagation of plaque microorganisms
Antibiotics	Broad or narrow spectrum; inhibit or kill specific or groups of bacteria, or modulate host inflammatory response
Modifying agents	Agents that alter the structure and/or metabolic activity of bacteria
Antiadhesives	Products that interfere with the ability of bacteria to attach to the acquired pellicle

(see Table 31-1). They are often referred to as *oral antiseptics.* **Antiseptics** are substances that inhibit the growth and development of microorganisms. They are commonly utilized in oral chemotherapeutics because they demonstrate very little oral or systemic toxicity or microbial resistance, and most have a broad antimicrobial spectrum. They exhibit either **bactericidal** activity, which means that they kill microbes directly, or **bacteriostatic** action, which means that the metabolism or reproduction of the microbe is affected. The term **substantivity** refers to the agent's ability to durably bind with oral tissues and then be released over a period of time, thus aiding in its efficacy. Other active ingredients such as antibiotics, plaque-modifying agents, anti-adherence agents, and host response modulators make varying contributions to reducing plaque accumulations and controlling periodontal disease. Research into these products continues, and some show promising results.

Local Delivery Methods

Self-Applied Modes of Delivery

Oral chemotherapeutics that have been designed to be self-applied within home delivery systems typically have lower concentrations of active ingredients and are used more often as compared with professional delivery systems. One of the most common self-applied delivery modes is dentifrice (see Chapter 25). Commonly known as *toothpaste,* **dentifrice** is available mostly as paste or gel, it is a vehicle for the local delivery of active ingredients. Dentifrice can have both therapeutic and cosmetic effects. From a therapeutic standpoint, the anticariogenic agent **fluoride** (see Chapter 33) is the most well-established active ingredient found in dentifrices.

Other active ingredients in dentifrices are available for the reduction of various oral conditions, including dental caries, plaque accumulation, gingivitis, hypersensitivity, calculus deposits, and remineralization, but some of these products may require additional research to substantiate their therapeutic claims. The incorporation of antimicrobials into dentifrices can sometimes present problems of compatibility with other dentifrice components. The primary motivation for the wide use of dentifrice may be for clients' real or perceived breath-freshening and tooth-whitening benefits.

BOX 31-2

Ideal Properties of an Oral Rinse

- Safe to use over long periods of time
- Palatable to user
- Inexpensive
- Highly soluble and stable in storage
- Effective
- Broad spectrum of effectiveness
- Adequate bioavailability to bacteria
- Minimal side effects
- Adequate retention

Oral rinses, which are often referred to as *mouthwashes,* are available for both cosmetic and therapeutic use, and they are available in prescription and OTC formulations. Therapeutic uses include plaque reduction, the control and reduction of periodontal disease, and caries prevention. Cosmetic uses include breath freshening and whitening. Therapeutic benefits of oral rinses vary depending on the active ingredient and the overall formulation. To date, one OTC antiseptic formulation (Listerine) and one prescription chlorhexidine product (Peridex, Periogard) have received the ADA Seal for therapeutic efficacy for reducing plaque and gingival outcome measures.

Oral rinses are typically recommended as an adjunctive therapy to mechanical methods for the reduction of plaque and gingivitis. Although oral rinses are reportedly well accepted by the public, this has not been well established. It is estimated that approximately half of the population uses some type of oral rinse, but many individuals do not use rinses according to manufacturer directions. For most products, clients should be advised to rinse twice daily for 30 seconds with 1 oz (20 mL) of rinse after mechanical cleansing, but manufacturer instructions should be consulted for specific directions. Oral rinsing is believed to reach the more inaccessible areas of the oral cavity often missed by mechanical means. Although the gel matrix protects the plaque biofilm from penetration by the rinse, certain materials are able to diffuse it. Box 31-2 describes the ideal properties of an oral rinse. Oral rinses, like dentifrices, have a limited effect on subgingival pathogenic microorganisms because of difficulties associated with the penetration of the gingival margin.

In addition to the active ingredients found in oral rinses, these formulations may include water, alcohol, cleansing agents, flavoring ingredients, and coloring agents. Alcohol (10% to 30% by volume) is included in many formulations to emulsify the antimicrobial ingredients within the rinse. It has some antiseptic properties, although this influence is not considered to make an important contribution to overall efficacy. Similar products may also be available in alcohol-free formulations.

Concerns about alcohol's effect on oral tissues and its purported association with oropharyngeal cancer have not been substantiated.[1] According to the FDA, the ADA, and the National Cancer Institute, there is no evidence of a causal relationship between alcohol-containing rinses and oropharyngeal cancer. The risk of oropharyngeal cancer related to alcoholic beverages appears to be associated with other ingredients (e.g., urethane), and this risk is especially pronounced among individuals who are also smokers. Ethanol, which is found in oral rinses, has not been demonstrated to be carcinogenic.[1]

Alcohol in oral rinses has also been implicated with xerostomia, but this relationship remains unsubstantiated. Of the few studies examining this association, alcohol was not significantly associated with either the perception of oral dryness or actual salivary flow.[2] Xerostomic individuals do not appear to have an increased sensitivity to alcohol-containing rinses.[2]

Alcohol-containing oral rinses may be contraindicated for some individuals with other conditions (e.g., recovering alcoholics) and for individuals taking certain antibiotics, in whom gastrointestinal upset may occur. Alcohol-containing rinses can be dangerous if they are ingested, particularly by small children; such ingestion can result in intoxication, illness, or fatalities. It has been traditionally recommended that clients being treated with head and neck radiation and who have mucositis should use bland oral rinses such as sterile water, baking soda in water, or normal saline rinse due to oral sensitivities.

Some mouth rinses also contain substantial amounts of sodium, which can result in sodium absorption through the oral mucosa during rinsing. People on sodium-restricted diets should be aware that some brands of mouthwash may be significant sources of sodium; these clients should consult their physicians about the potential impact of such mouthwashes.

Because most home oral health practices are largely ineffective for the eradication of subgingival microbiota, oral irrigation as a delivery vehicle has been recommended to counteract these organisms. The term **oral irrigation** refers to both powered and manual mechanisms for delivering an active ingredient within a solution via an irrigation tip into the gingival sulcus or a periodontal pocket. This has applications in both the home and professional settings.

Home irrigation typically makes use of standard jet tips (Figure 31-3) that deliver a pulsating stream of fluid (often water) with controlled variable pressure; this has been shown to be effective as an adjunct to toothbrushing for reducing several gingival parameters. Jet irrigation systems for home use have been shown to effectively penetrate subgingivally, and a recent review has demonstrated consistent reductions in gingivitis among users of this technology.[3] Although most of the research conducted has involved water irrigation, home irrigation devices have been shown to have an increased benefit when a chemotherapeutic agent is incorporated. In addition to disrupting microorganisms, research has also demonstrated the selective modulation of inflammatory mediators, including decreases in proinflammatory mediators and increases in anti-inflammatory agents within gingival crevicular fluid (GCF) after the short-term regular use of a home irrigator.

When considering home irrigation, the penetration of the irrigant is dependent on the tip design, the pocket depth, and the individual client's access to the affected sites. Needle-like tips called *cannulas* are available and specially designed to be placed below the gingival margin (Figure 31-4). Although the use of such a tip allows for greater penetration into deep pockets, it is generally reserved for professional use, because these tips require a high level of dexterity and access to the specific disease site. Therefore recommending the use of a cannula with home irrigation for a client's home use should be carefully considered.

Professionally Applied Modes of Delivery

The preprocedural rinse is the professional use of a therapeutic oral rinse before dental hygiene care and other dental procedures. Such rinses are administered with the aim of decreasing the total amount of microorganisms available in the clinical environment during intraoral procedures (e.g., aerosols, spatter). Sprays produced by dental equipment are found at greatest concentration within 2 feet of the client, where the clinician is typically positioned. This is also a concern because some pathogenic organisms can be suspended in aerosols for considerable periods of time. A preprocedural rinse has the potential to significantly reduce the amount of available microorganisms by more than 90%; thus this practice is recommended by the Centers for Disease Control and Prevention in the United States. However, reductions in the cross contamination of the operator or other clients via client microorganisms have not been demonstrated.

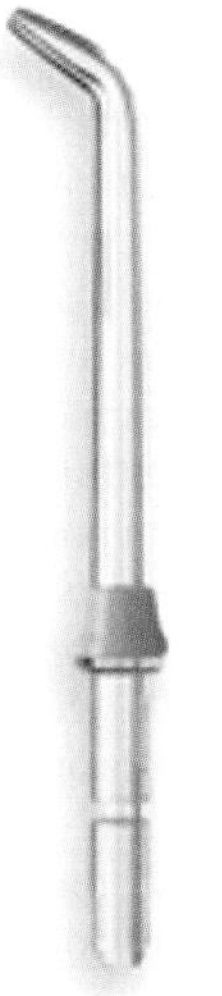

Figure 31-3. Standard jet tips for home irrigation systems.

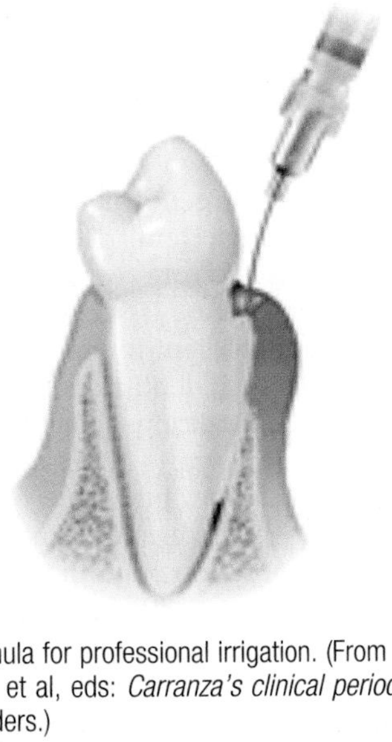

Figure 31-4. Cannula for professional irrigation. (From Newman MG, Takei HH, Klokkevold PR, et al, eds: *Carranza's clinical periodontology*, ed 11, St Louis, 2012, Saunders.)

An additional application for preprocedural rinsing that has gained recent attention is for the reduction of transient bacteremias that result from professional dental hygiene care. A subset of the population appears to be susceptible to bacteremias, and preprocedural rinsing could potentially reduce oral bacteria from reaching the bloodstream and causing subsequent disease (e.g., bacterial endocarditis).[4] Similarly, daily rinsing at home could have an impact on self-induced bacteremias as an outcome of homecare practices. More research into the impact of this intervention is required to substantiate these claims. Either a prescription or OTC product that has been shown to be therapeutically effective can be used for preprocedural rinsing.

Professionally applied subgingival irrigation with various antimicrobials has been investigated, and it has produced equivocal results.[5] Although professionally applied irrigants delivered with a cannula are able to reach the base of the periodontal pocket, they are limited by several factors, including the inability to be retained in adequate concentrations for sufficient duration and the fact that some active ingredients can be deactivated by blood products. The dental hygienist, together with the client, will need to carefully weigh the costs (financial and otherwise) of delivering professionally applied subgingival irrigation in relation to the expected clinical outcomes.

When the professional delivery of subgingival irrigation is indicated, it is not recommended as a monotherapy; it should instead be used in conjunction with periodontal debridement. It is also necessary to irrigate the tooth circumferentially, because the lateral dispersion of chemotherapeutics via a cannula is minimal. However, only minimal pressure is required, because low force has been shown to penetrate the pocket adequately.

Another type of professionally applied vehicle for active ingredients is varnish. Varnishes have received the most attention for use with fluoride applications, particularly as part of public health programs. However, other applications of varnish have been studied, including the application of antimicrobials (e.g., chlorhexidine) directed at periodontal improvements. Other professional applications of active ingredients are available, including rinses, foams, gels, chips, and microspheres. When such products are available for both home and professional use, the professional versions will have higher concentrations. These products may be indicated as a means of reducing plaque, treating periodontal diseases, preventing caries, remineralizing hard dental tissues, reducing sensitivity, and whitening teeth.

Self-care behaviors (e.g., toothbrushing, flossing, mouth rinsing, home irrigation) as well as professional interventions (e.g., mechanical debridement) become less effective as pockets deepen and clinical attachment levels (CALs) worsen. To address the limitations of these conventional therapies, controlled-release drug-delivery methods have been developed. High-level research (including systematic reviews) has been conducted to summarize the benefits of this treatment.[6] **Controlled-release drug delivery** refers to the use of intracrevicular devices that are professionally placed and that provide drug delivery for sustained periods of time.

Typically these intracrevicular devices consist of an antimicrobial active ingredient placed within a reservoir that controls the rate of drug release and that provides a means of sustained administration of the agent directly into the periodontal pocket. In contrast with systemic administration (see Systemic Delivery Methods), controlled-release drug delivery results in 1000 times the concentration of the drug within the GCF at the diseased site, but only one hundredth of the systemic dose reaches the rest of the body. The **minimum inhibitory concentration** (MIC) is a research measurement tool used for these products to describe the lowest concentration of a particular antimicrobial that is able to inhibit microbial growth during incubation. Several of these controlled-release products are available. Selection should be based on the available research, the client's health, the pertinent precautions, the number and severity of sites requiring treatment, the ease of use, and the degree of client-required compliance. Some of the most commonly studied products are discussed in the following paragraphs.

Minocycline in the form of ointment and microspheres has considerable research supporting its benefits for pocket depths and CALs when it is used as an adjunct to scaling and root planing. In one systematic review, minocycline was concluded to be the most promising of all of the controlled-release adjunctive therapies studied.[6] **Minocycline microspheres** (Arestin) include minocycline hydrochloride (1 mg), which is available in North America as a dry powder (Figure 31-5). The product is delivered via a syringe-like handle with a narrow tip that is inserted subgingivally to the base of the pocket and that immediately adheres to the periodontal pocket (Procedure 31-1 and the corresponding Competency Form). The product does not set but rather becomes a sticky paste that is retained within the pocket without periodontal dressing. It well exceeds MIC levels within hours, and it remains effective against predominant periodontal pathogens for more than 20 days while it is slowly resorbed. **Minocycline ointment** has been only

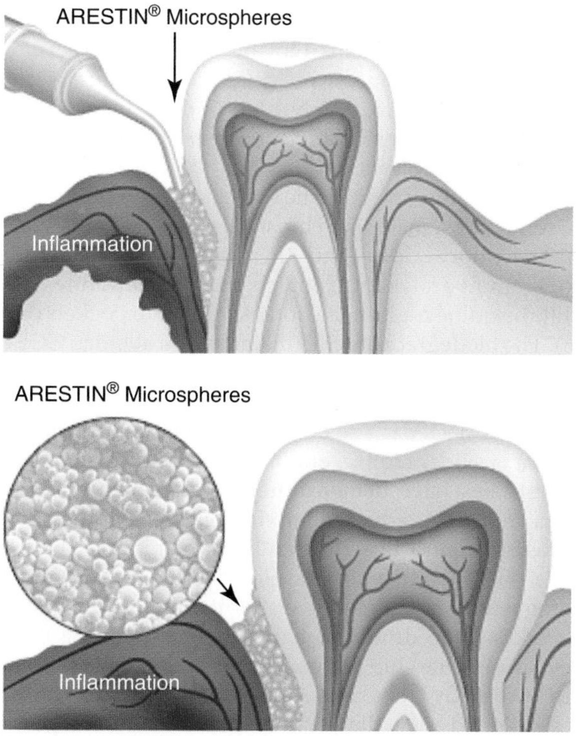

Figure 31-5. Minocycline microspheres. (Courtesy TOLMAR Inc, Fort Collins, Colorado. Atridox is a registered trademark of TOLMAR Inc.)

Procedure 31-1 Placement of Controlled-Release Drug: Minocycline Hydrochloride Microspheres

EQUIPMENT

Personal protective equipment
Mouth mirror
Periodontal probe
Scaler(s)
Unit-dosed cartridges of minocycline hydrochloride product
Dispensing handle

STEP

1. Determine need for controlled-release minocycline microspheres therapy (indicated for the reduction of pocket depth in sites ≥5 mm not responding to mechanical therapy alone in persons with chronic periodontitis).
2. Evaluate contraindications to and precautions for treatment.
3. Explain risks and benefits and alternative to treatment. Obtain informed consent.
4. Remove number of unit-dosed cartridges needed for treatment.
5. Insert cartridge into sterile cartridge handle to administer product, and follow manufacturer instructions.
6. Bend cartridge tip to improve access to diseased sites. Insert tip of cartridge subgingivally to base of pocket; tip should be parallel to long axis of tooth. Press thumb ring to express powder while gradually withdrawing tip from base of pocket. Do not force tip into base of pocket. Withdraw tip further if resistance is felt.
7. No dressing or adhesive is required. Microspheres activate and adhere on contact with moisture in pocket. Discard cartridge and resterilize dispensing handle.
8. Instruct client to delay brushing for first 12 hours after treatment. For 10 days, client should abstain from interdental cleaning in area and from eating hard, crunchy, or sticky foods.
9. Schedule reevaluation and/or reapplication. Reevaluation of pocket depths and clinical attachment levels can coincide with periodontal maintenance visits. Repeat treatment as needed.
10. Document in client record under Services Rendered, and date the entry. For example, "Minocycline microspheres placed in sites not responding to mechanical debridement alone for the reduction of pocket depths: No. 2M, No. 3D, No. 30M, D, No. 31D. Client instructed to delay brushing for first 12 hours after treatment and to abstain from interdental cleaning in area and from eating hard, crunchy, or sticky foods for 10 days."

available in Europe; it consists of 2% minocycline hydrochloride in a hydroxyethyl cellulose matrix. Minocyclines are contraindicated for clients with known sensitivity to minocycline or tetracycline.

One of the first controlled-release devices approved for use for periodontitis was the tetracycline fiber, a monofilament of ethylene/vinyl acetate copolymer that is 0.5 mm in diameter and that contains 12.7 mg of evenly dispersed tetracycline hydrochloride; it provides a continuous release of tetracycline for approximately 10 to 14 days. Its use declined because it was nonresorbable and reportedly had placement and retention problems.

Chlorhexidine, an antiseptic, is found in several controlled-release vehicles, including chips, gels, and irrigants (0.2% to 2%). The **chlorhexidine chip** (PerioChip) is a biodegradable 4- to 5-mm hydrolyzed gelatin chip that incorporates 2.5 mg of chlorhexidine D-gluconate for insertion into pockets (Figure 31-6). The biodegradable chip maintains an average GCF concentration of 125 μg/mL of chlorhexidine over a 7- to 10-day period, thereby exceeding the MIC and inhibiting almost all subgingival bacteria. The suppression of subgingival bacterial flora is evident for several weeks after the drug's release. Some studies have demonstrated improvements in pocket depths and CAL when controlled-release chlorhexidine is used as an adjunct to scaling and root planing.[6]

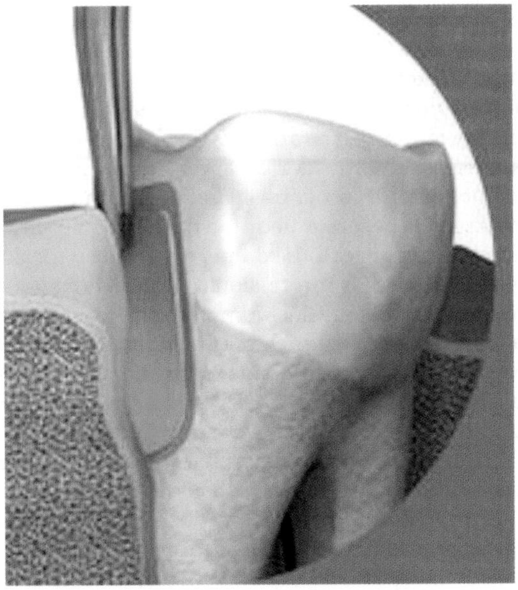

Figure 31-6. Chlorhexidine chip.

The chlorhexidine chip is placed after scaling and root planing, and it is self-retentive after it is exposed to moisture (i.e., GCF) (Procedure 31-2 and the corresponding Competency Form). One chip per pocket site is used and should not be disturbed by homecare regimens for 1 week. The directions included with the product insert should be precisely followed. Because the chip self-resorbs, the need for professional removal is eliminated. The placement of a CHG chip is contraindicated for clients with the rare allergy to chlorhexidine.

Less research is available regarding the antibiotic doxycycline within a controlled-release gel. **Doxycycline gel** (Atridox) consists of 10% doxycycline hyclate in a gel polymer that flows to the pocket base and that solidifies on contact with the moisture of GCF to provide the controlled release of the antibiotic doxycycline for 7 days. The drug reaches GCF concentrations of more than 1500 mg/mL within hours, and these levels remain well above the MIC for most periodontal

Procedure 31-2 Placement of Controlled-Release Drug: Chlorhexidine Chip

EQUIPMENT

Personal protective equipment
Mouth mirror
Periodontal probe
Cotton pliers, cotton rolls, dry angles
Scaler(s)
Chlorhexidine chips

STEPS

1. Determine need for controlled-release chlorhexidine chip therapy (indicated for reduction of pocket depth in sites ≥5 mm not responding to mechanical therapy alone in persons with chronic periodontitis).
2. Evaluate contraindications to and precautions for treatment.
3. Explain risks and benefits and alternatives to treatment. Obtain informed consent.
4. Remove required number of chips from package. Note that product is stored at controlled room temperature of 59° to 77° F (15° to 25° C).
5. Isolate and dry area to prevent wetting chip during placement. Grasp square end of chip with cotton pliers, and insert subgingivally.
6. Use cotton pliers or an instrument of choice to advance chip into deepest part of pocket.
7. Instruct client not to floss area for 10 days and inform him or her that some moderate sensitivity may be experienced for about 1 week in the area of placement. Client should clean other areas of mouth as usual and call the office if any pain, swelling, or problem occurs.
8. Schedule reevaluation and/or reapplication. Reevaluation of probe depths and clinical attachment levels can coincide with periodontal maintenance visit.
9. Document in client's record under Services Rendered, and date the entry. For example, "Chlorhexidine chips placed in sites not responding to mechanical debridement alone for the reduction of pocket depths: No. 2M, No. 3D, No. 30M, D, No. 31D. Client instructed not to brush or floss the area for 10 days and to call if loss of chip occurs."

pathogens for 7 days. This product will biodegrade, which negates the need for professional removal. Although research is limited, it has shown doxycycline gel to decrease pockets and to improve CALs, thereby providing an adjunct to scaling and root planing.[6]

Doxycycline gel is available via a two-syringe system; the product is combined manually and then delivered into the pocket via a cannula (Procedure 31-3 and the corresponding Competency Form). Periodontal dressing can be used and is especially recommended in shallower pockets to ensure continued retention. A known sensitivity to any drug in the tetracycline family is a contraindication to the administration of doxycycline gel.

Metronidazole is an antibiotic that is available as a controlled-release gel (25%). **Metronidazole gel** (Elyzol) is a bioresorbable drug-delivery system that consists of 25% metronidazole benzoate in a readily flowable mixture. It is applied subgingivally via a cannula-fitted syringe. It reaches its peak concentration in the GCF 4 hours after administration, and it maintains levels of more than 100 mg/mL for the first 8 hours. The product maintains concentrations exceeding the MIC for anaerobic pathogens susceptible to metronidazole (1.0 g/mL) for approximately 36 hours. Although several studies conducted on this product have demonstrated improvements in pocket depths and CALs, its efficacy appears to be less than that of minocycline and tetracycline.[6]

A systematic review of controlled-release products found that, overall, adjunctive local antibiotics within controlled-release drug-delivery systems have a positive impact on pocket depths and CALs.[6] Although scaling and root planing alone produce pocket-depth and CAL improvements in the range of 1.5 mm, controlled-release drugs added improvements in the range of 0.25 to 0.5 mm.[6] Although this is statistically significant, the dental hygienist must weigh the clinical relevance of these findings in practice situations.

Photodynamic disinfection therapy (Periowave) is a novel method of inactivating a broad spectrum of subgingival bacteria and potentially damaging enzymes. This two-stage system requires that, first, a photosensitizing solution or dye (i.e., toluidine blue) be placed by the operator within the pocket. This is then followed by the application of a nonthermal diode laser light that illuminates the area for 60 seconds, thereby killing bacteria and inactivating enzymes (Figures 31-7 and 31-8). This therapy acts as a short-term topical disinfectant that eradicates harmful microorganisms that may otherwise remain after debridement. Studies have shown that this system reduces most of the subgingival microbiota and

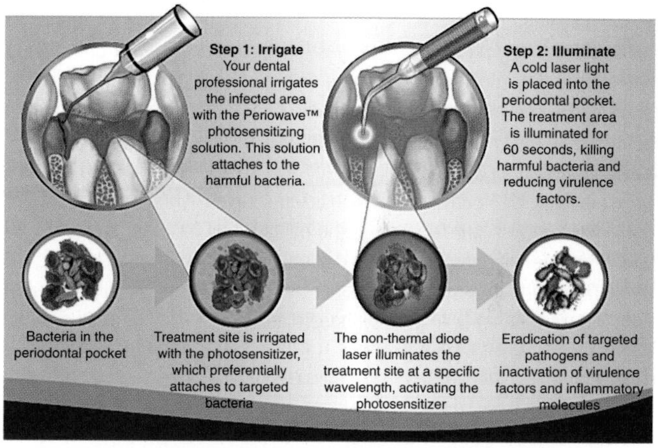

Figure 31-7. Periowave. (Courtesy Periowave Dental Technologies Inc.)

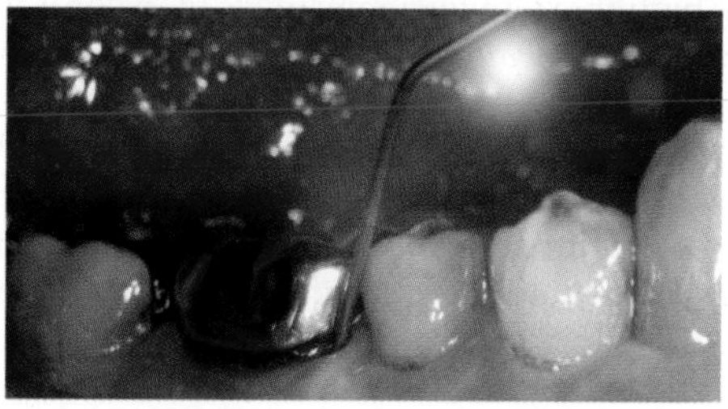

Figure 31-8. Nonthermal diode laser light illuminating the area.

Procedure 31-3 Placement of Controlled-Release Drug: Doxycycline Gel

EQUIPMENT

Personal protective equipment
Mouth mirror
Periodontal probe
Scaler(s) or cord packer instrument
Lubricant
Two unit-dosed syringes for coupling
Blunt-ended cannula
Doxycycline gel product

STEPS

1. Determine need for controlled-release doxycycline therapy (indicated for the reduction of pocket depth and gains in clinical attachment in sites ≥5 mm not responding to mechanical therapy alone in persons with chronic periodontitis).
2. Evaluate contraindications to and precautions for treatment.
3. Explain risks and benefits and alternatives to treatment. Obtain informed consent.
4. Remove syringes for coupling (one containing 10% doxycycline hyclate and one containing liquid polymer) from package. The syringes contain enough material to treat three to four teeth.
5. Hold uncapped syringes with nozzles upright to avoid spilling before coupling.
6. Mix by holding coupled syringes together horizontally in both hands. Inject liquid contents of syringe with purple stripe into syringe with yellow powder, then push contents back into syringe with purple stripe again. This constitutes one mixing cycle and should be repeated for 1½ to 2 minutes for 100 cycles. Finish with contents in syringe with purple stripe by holding coupled syringes vertically, with syringe with purple stripe at the bottom. Pull back on plunger of syringe with purple stripe and allow gel to flow down the barrel. Twist and lock syringes together per manufacturer's instructions. Lock open ends of both syringes together by twisting together until they lock.
7. Uncouple syringes and attach enclosed cannula to syringe by twisting in place. Cannula can be bent at desired angle to resemble a periodontal probe. Product is now ready to use. If product is mixed in advance, refresh mixture with 10 mixing cycles before uncoupling syringes.
8. Insert tip of cannula near base of pocket; express gel into pocket while slowly withdrawing tip coronally until material can be seen at the gingival margin. Gel will begin setting reaction immediately on contact with pocket. Separate tip from newly placed material by using a twisting motion, or cut material by pushing cannula tip against tooth surface or by using a wet blunt instrument.
9. Wipe excess material protruding from pocket with a wet cotton swab, or pack into pocket and interproximal embrasures with back surface of a wet curet or cord packer instrument. Use water or lubricant to prevent sticking. Drip a few drops of water onto the surface of the gel in the pocket to help with coagulation.
10. Secure gel in pocket by applying cyanoacrylate tissue adhesive or noneugenol-type periodontal dressing.
11. Remove retention after 10 days of therapy with cotton pliers.
12. Instruct client to avoid chewing, brushing, and interdental cleaning around area for 7 days; recommend oral rinsing with an effective antimicrobial agent. Client should not be alarmed if small amounts of hardened gel become visible at gum line or are dislodged, because gel is harmless if swallowed.
13. Schedule reevaluation and/or reapplication. Reevaluation of pocket depth and clinical attachment levels can coincide with periodontal maintenance visit.
14. Document in client record under Services Rendered, and date the entry. For example, "Doxycycline gel placed in sites not responding to mechanical debridement alone for the reduction of pocket depths: No. 2M, No. 3D, No. 30M, D, No. 31D. Cyanoacrylate adhesive placed for retention at each site. Client instructed not to brush or floss the area for 7 days and to report any loss of gel to the office."

produces evidence of damaged bacteria as well as thinner and less dense biofilms with fewer channels than control biofilms. This technology may be indicated for localized persistent pockets that have not responded to conventional therapies. Dental hygienists should note that research in this area is limited, particularly with regard to longer-term studies. In addition, not all jurisdictions have approved the use of this technology by dental hygienists or other practitioners.

Systemic Delivery Methods

Systemic delivery methods are those that are ingested and then delivered via the bloodstream. Some of these are self-delivered, such as fluoridated water (see Chapter 33), whereas most require professional administration, such as fluoride supplements and antibiotics. Prescription antibiotics delivered systemically for the treatment of periodontitis travel from the bloodstream to the periodontal tissues and eventually reaching the GCF, where they gain access to the subgingival microflora (albeit in low concentrations). Several antibiotics have been used systemically either singularly or in combination for the treatment of periodontitis, including doxycycline, penicillin, metronidazole, and clindamycin. Recently systematic reviews have been conducted to evaluate the adjunctive benefits of systemic antibiotics; it was concluded that amoxicillin or a combination of amoxicillin and metronidazole, metronidazole alone, or a subantimicrobial dose of doxycycline all provided a benefit over scaling and root planing alone.[7]

Although systemic administration provides a means of delivering antibiotics to deep periodontal pockets, it is also associated with various contraindications, precautions, and side effects (Box 31-3). Successful systemic administration requires ongoing client adherence to the antibiotic protocol; this is a concern, because many clients fail to follow prescriptions. Furthermore, the routine use of antibiotics to treat periodontal diseases is not recommended as a result of concerns about the development of antibiotic-resistant organisms. Therefore the prescribing of systemic antibiotics for periodontal disease must be carefully considered.

As an alternative to studying antimicrobials, researchers are investigating the modulation of the host response as a potential approach to the treatment of periodontal diseases. Host modulation agents can take on several forms, and the use of subantimicrobial systemic doses of antibiotics is

BOX 31-3

Conditions Associated with Antibiotic Therapy

- Gastrointestinal upset
- Sensitivity to sunlight
- Intrinsic staining in developing teeth
- Potential toxicity to pregnant mother and fetus
- Increase in vaginal candidiasis
- Impaired adsorption of some nutrients
- Depressed prothrombin activity
- Potential to render oral contraceptives less effective

one approach. The term subantimicrobial systemic dose refers to the administration of a reduced quantity of a drug for purposes other than the elimination of a pathogenic microorganism: in this case, host modulatory therapy. For example, the antibiotic doxycycline hyclate (Periostat) may be administered in low doses (e.g., 20 mg twice daily) over long periods of time (e.g., 6 to 9 months) to inhibit collagenase and to prevent the breakdown of collagen as part of the periodontal disease process. Although research is limited, studies examining subantimicrobial doses of doxycycline have demonstrated improved periodontal outcomes as compared with scaling and root planing therapy alone.

In subantimicrobial low doses, antibiotics are not antibacterial, and no detrimental shifts in the normal periodontal flora or antibiotic resistance have been observed. Despite the reduced dosages, subantimicrobial doxycycline is contraindicated for clients who are sensitive to tetracycline. In addition, other side effects and potential adverse reactions are possible and should be reviewed before use.

Another approach to modulating the host response is the use of nonsteroidal anti-inflammatory drugs (NSAIDs). NSAIDs are drugs that block enzymes promoting the inflammatory response, thereby reducing inflammation. These drugs have been studied to determine their role in modifying host responses, and some NSAIDs have shown positive outcomes, particularly with regard to alveolar bone preservation. Side effects are a consideration with the long-term use of NSAIDs. Other more novel approaches to modulating the host response include probiotics and vaccines, but research involving oral applications is in its infancy.

Active Ingredients

Dental hygienists need to continuously review the literature related to active ingredients and new products so that they are confident in providing evidence-based information and recommendations to clients. Several key active ingredients for the control of plaque and periodontal diseases have been identified and are available within various delivery systems as discussed previously.

Bisbiguanides

Bisbiguanides are cationic, broad-spectrum antimicrobials effective for both gram-positive and gram-negative bacteria. Of these, chlorhexidine gluconate (CHG or CHX) is one of the most widely investigated and used. For oral applications, it is predominantly used in prescription oral rinses, irrigation solutions, and controlled-release products. CHG strongly binds with the bacterial cell membrane; it causes the cell to leak and disrupts its intracellular components. In addition, CHG can interfere with bacterial colonization and cell attachment. CHG has considerable substantivity binding to oral tissues, and it remains active for 8 to 12 hours. CHG oral rinses (Peridex, Periogard), which are available only through prescription, typically have 0.12% concentration in the United States and Canada, but they may be higher in Europe. Prescription CHG rinses are accepted by the ADA and the CDA for reducing plaque (16% to 45%) and gingivitis (27% to 80%). CHG is considered to be the "gold standard" that provides a benchmark for measurement in studies examining the efficacy of other oral-rinse formulations for plaque and gingivitis reduction.

The primary disadvantage of the use of CHG as an oral rinse is dental and tongue staining. After this brown staining has formed on teeth, it requires professional removal, and this adverse outcome negates the use of CHG for long periods of time. Like many oral rinses, CHG rinses contain alcohol, and therefore necessary precautions must be observed.

The oral-rinse formulation of CHG is typically administered in 18- to 20-mg dosages for 60 seconds twice daily. It is important that clients be advised to allow at least 30 minutes between rinsing with CHG and toothbrushing to avoid an interaction with the detergent sodium lauryl sulfate in toothpaste, which causes the deactivation of CHG. In addition, clients should not rinse with water immediately after CHG use, because this will remove the flavor-masking agents from the oral cavity and increase the medicinal taste of the drug.

Phenolic Compounds

Phenols are a class of chemical compounds with unique properties; some phenols are germicidal and used in the formulation of disinfectants. Essential oils (EOs) are components of plants that contain phenolic compounds that destroy microorganisms by compromising the cell membrane and inhibiting enzyme activity. Listerine is a commercially available EO mouth rinse and toothpaste. This rinse is most well known for its combination of two phenolic-derived EOs, thymol (0.064%) and eucalyptol (0.092%), which are mixed with menthol (0.042%) and other ingredients. It has demonstrated its efficacy in long-term clinical trials. This EO rinse has multidimensional therapeutic effects in that it prevents bacteria from aggregating, slows bacterial multiplication, reduces the bacterial load overall within the oral cavity, prevents the plaque mass from maturation, and reduces the pathogenicity of the plaque mass. This product also has anti-inflammatory properties.

Although EOs have comparatively low substantivity, Listerine Antiseptic has been shown to be highly efficacious for plaque and gingivitis reduction, which approach the levels found with the gold standard CHG. Long-term clinical trials adhering to ADA guidelines have demonstrated plaque reductions of 56% and gingivitis reductions of 35% as compared with negative (placebo) controls. Listerine is the only OTC oral-rinse formulation that has received the ADA Seal of Acceptance for chemotherapeutic control and reduction of bacterial plaque and gingivitis; however, several other brands that have been marketed with the same ingredients and formulation have received approval on that basis. This approval for antiplaque and antigingivitis effectiveness is limited to the antiseptic formulations that contain alcohol.

Because recent trials have shown that Listerine Antiseptic mouth rinse approaches the efficacy of CHG for plaque and gingivitis reductions without the associated stain, that it is considered safe when used as directed, that it produces no changes in bacterial composition, and that it shows no evidence of opportunistic oral pathogens or antimicrobial resistance, it is considered by some to be an ideal OTC adjunctive home mouth rinse.[4,8] Most concern has surrounded the reported "sharp" taste of this product, but recent formulations are reported to be less intense while maintaining effectiveness. The procedure for rinsing with Listerine is similar to that for CHG: clients should rinse with one ounce (20 mL) for 30 seconds after brushing and cleansing interproximally twice daily.

Triclosan, a bisphenol, is considered to be a safe, broad-spectrum antibacterial, and it is not associated with any side effects. It disrupts the cytoplasmic membrane of the cell. Triclosan is predominantly found in dentifrices, but, in short-term trials, commercially available rinses (0.3% triclosan/2.0% copolymer Colgate Total Plax) have demonstrated significant reductions in plaque and gingivitis as compared with negative (placebo) controls. However, studies have shown that triclosan-based rinses are not as effective as those containing CHG. Recently triclosan has been combined with other active ingredients with greater effectiveness (e.g., CHG), which has increased its antiplaque and antigingivitis properties. Combining sources of triclosan, such as toothpaste and rinse, has been shown to increase the drug's overall effectiveness. A commercially available toothpaste formulation (Total) delivers 0.3% triclosan via a 2.0% copolymer that increases triclosan substantivity, and it has demonstrated reductions in plaque and gingivitis.

Quaternary Ammonium Compounds

Quaternary ammonium compounds destroy microorganisms by interacting with the bacterial cell membrane and causing it to become permeable and lose its contents. These compounds affect both gram-positive and gram-negative bacteria, but they are more bactericidal to the former. Like the phenol group, quaternary ammonium compounds bind well with oral tissues, but they have low substantivity as compared with CHG.

Several quaternary ammonium compounds have been available commercially for many years, such as cetylpyridinium chloride (CPC) (Cepacol 0.05%), and they are also available with domiphen bromide (Scope 0.045%) or benzethonium chloride (Colgate 100 0.05%). These formulations are primarily cosmetic in that they have a history of safety, but their efficacy for plaque and gingivitis reduction has not been demonstrated in long-term clinical trials. A more recently introduced CPC rinse (Crest Pro-Health Rinse 0.07%) has demonstrated a small benefit as an adjunct to mechanical homecare for plaque and gingivitis reduction. A recent systematic review that included CPC and positive controls concluded that CPC data were inconsistent and that more long-term clinical trials comparing CPC to positive and placebo controls are required to substantiate its therapeutic use; however, this review was not focused on the higher-concentration formulations that have shown better efficacy than earlier formulations.[9] CPCs have been shown to reduce halitosis. CPCs may cause tooth staining but not to the levels of CHG. In addition, CPC formulations may be inactivated by toothpaste products such as sodium lauryl sulfate.

Sanguinarine is an alcohol extract from the root of the plant *Sanguinaria canadensis*, and it is used in concentrations of 0.03% in both oral rinses and toothpaste (Viadent). Some studies of oral rinses have shown sanguinarine formulations to be more effective than placebo for plaque reduction, but the efficacy of sanguinarine with respect to gingival outcomes has been less positive, thereby limiting recommendations to cosmetic use.

Oxygenating and Oxidizing Agents

Oxygenating agents (i.e., hydrogen peroxide) are mediums that have had oxygen added to them (Amosan); they are antimicrobial as a result of the release of oxygen, which affects both gram-positive and gram-negative microorganisms. Such formulations have been available on the market for years, with no serious side effects. Although some studies have shown a beneficial effect of oxygenating agents on plaque and gingivitis as compared with placebo, a recent systematic review concluded that findings were inconclusive.[10] More long-term studies with positive controls are required in addition to the determination of the ideal strength of the active ingredient within the formulation. Oxygenating agents are sometimes combined with CHG to improve the effectiveness of the former without the stain associated with the latter.

Oxidizing agents (i.e., chlorine dioxide) are products that have had an increase in oxidation number, thereby forming derivatives of oxygen (Oxygene). Oxidizing agents have also been available in mouth rinse and toothpaste formulations for years. Product claims are primarily cosmetic, particularly with regard to the relief of halitosis through the neutralization of volatile sulfur compounds in the oral cavity. To date, there is no evidence to support the use of these products for therapeutic use in the reduction of pathogenic plaque and gingivitis.

Antibiotics

Antibiotics make up an antimicrobial drug group that inhibits or destroys pathogenic microorganisms and that may possess a broad or more narrow spectrum of target organisms. Several antibiotics have been used for the reduction of periodontal diseases, including metronidazole and amoxicillin either alone or in combination. Antibiotics are increasing with regard to their application for the treatment of periodontitis with both systemic and locally delivered vehicles. As discussed previously, locally delivered modes of application have the advantage of being placed—and therefore concentrated—directly at the disease site, without negative systemic side effects. However, known sensitivities to antibiotics need to be avoided with both systemic and locally delivered modes of delivery. Clinicians must weigh the relatively minimal adjunctive benefit of antibiotics with the associated costs and concerns that surround antibiotic resistance.

Halogens/Fluoride

Although the use of fluoride as a caries-preventive agent has been well investigated, its role in the prevention and control of plaque-induced periodontal diseases is less well documented. Stannous fluoride is believed to enter the bacterial cell and impair its metabolism, thereby counteracting its growth and adherence properties. It has had applications within dentifrice (0.454%), with some antiplaque and gingivitis effects. It may be used in combination with other active ingredients (e.g., triclosan); however, as a result of its uncertain clinical value, lack of stability in storage, and increased staining properties, it has had limited acceptance for the prevention of gingival disease. Other fluoride products have been marketed outside of North America for the control of plaque and gingivitis, including a stable amine/stannous fluoride solution (Meridol). The stable amine component, which is only active against caries, stabilizes the stannous fluoride component and does not exhibit side effects. It is absorbed by the bacterial cell surface, thereby inhibiting that surface's metabolism and reducing plaque overall. Some short-term clinical trials have demonstrated positive findings regarding plaque inhibition, but overall the evidence is inconclusive.

Others

Many other agents have shown antimicrobial activity, but this has not been proven in long-term studies with negative controls. Active ingredients including echinacea, goldenseal, povidone–iodine, xylitol, host proteins (lysozyme, lactoferrin, and lactoperoxidase) and probiotics have been used in oral health products and have varying research support to substantiate their use. Xylitol is primarily used as an anticaries agent. Povidone–iodine is used as a professionally applied irrigant (10%), for home irrigation (0.1%), or as an oral rinse (1.0%), and it has a wide spectrum of efficacy. Probiotics are live microorganisms that have health benefits for the host; they can confer an effect by being antimicrobial to pathogens, modulating the host response, or exerting a competitive exclusion mechanism. (Competitive exclusion mechanisms involve situations in which species within the microflora that have a positive effect on the host are favored over those that have a negative effect.) For all of these other active ingredients, long-term studies are lacking or have not demonstrated efficacy for plaque and gingivitis reduction as compared with benchmark controls, thereby largely preventing their recommendation for use.

Oral chemotherapeutics directed at periodontal disease are subject to ongoing research. Therefore dental hygienists must be diligent and stay current in their understanding of these adjunctive interventions. Clients depend on their dental hygienists to help them sift through marketing and product claims and to provide unbiased and evidence-based recommendations. These roles will require a good understanding of oral chemotherapeutic delivery systems and active ingredients as well as the research methodologies used to test them.

CLIENT EDUCATION TIPS

- Explain that the control of bacterial plaque, gingivitis, and periodontitis is primarily addressed by mechanical means through homecare and supported by professional interventions; chemotherapeutic interventions are introduced as an adjunct.
- Discuss that the measurement and evaluation of clinical parameters—such as plaque, bleeding, and gingival scores—will be required after the introduction of chemotherapeutic intervention. If clinical outcomes are improved, chemotherapeutic therapy may no longer be indicated.
- Note that products with effective chemotherapeutic agents have additional costs in terms of both money and time. Therefore, if mechanical plaque control adequately removes soft deposits and controls the plaque biofilm, these resources cannot be justified.
- Discuss both the potential benefits and possible side effects of antimicrobial agents.

LEGAL, ETHICAL, AND SAFETY ISSUES

- Dental hygienists have a legal and ethical obligation to be aware of the current literature surrounding personal and professional chemotherapeutic interventions. Making use of systematic reviews and professional guidelines is helpful for this professional responsibility.
- Client assessment should include the evaluation of the presence and distribution of bacterial plaque and plaque retentive factors. Care plans should include educational, preventive, and therapeutic interventions for the client to address his or her daily personal oral hygiene and periodontal condition, including the consideration of adjunctive chemotherapeutic agents.
- Carefully review the client's health and dental history to be sure that any client selected for oral chemotherapeutic therapy has no potential allergies or drug interactions with the agent being recommended. Instruct all clients to keep antimicrobial agents out of the reach of children.
- Dental hygienists are gaining increasing scopes of practice that include the administration of antibiotics in some jurisdictions. When prescribing systemic subantimicrobial dosages or locally delivered antibiotics, it is important to remember that all of these have special considerations, potential side effects, and contraindications.
- Dental hygienists have a legal and ethical responsibility to ensure that clients are completely informed. The use of evidence-based communication and motivational techniques for changing client behaviors is required.
- Upon completion of the dental hygiene process of care, the legal records of the client should clearly demonstrate that the client has been educated about his or her current disease status and counseled regarding recommendations designed to improve oral status and prevent further deterioration. Records should also include the client's response to the dental hygiene care plan, a description of the implementation of interventions, and notes regarding the monitoring of the client's progress.

KEY CONCEPTS

- Although bacterial plaque biofilm is believed to be the primary etiologic agent in inflammatory periodontal diseases, it is recognized that the host immune response modulates the progression of disease.
- Although the mechanical removal of bacterial plaque biofilm remains the backbone of disease control, oral chemotherapeutics can provide adjunctive benefits to traditional methods.
- Evaluating oral chemotherapeutic products requires supportive evidence from several long-term clinical trials that are conducted in homogeneous population groups with comparable interventions and that include appropriate controls and outcome measures.

- The success of local drug-delivery systems for treating periodontal infections is dependent on the ability of these systems to deliver the antimicrobial agents to the disease site at the minimum inhibitory concentration for a sufficient duration of time.
- Substantivity is the ability of an active ingredient to bond with oral tissues, thus allowing the ingredient to be retained in the oral cavity and to be continually released while maintaining its potency.
- As a homecare adjunct to conventional oral hygiene, supragingival irrigation may be of value for the prevention and control of bacterial plaque and gingivitis. The benefit of professional subgingival irrigation performed in conjunction with scaling and root planing remains inconclusive.
- Controlled drug-delivery devices consist of a drug reservoir that slowly releases the agent directly into the periodontal pocket disease site at high concentrations without the side effects associated with systemic administration. This is an effective adjunct to scaling and root planing in pockets not responding to mechanical therapy alone.
- Alcohol in mouth rinses has not been shown to be carcinogenic or to be linked to real or perceived reductions in salivary flow.
- An essential oil mouth rinse approaches the efficacy of the gold standard (chlorhexidine gluconate) as an adjunct to mechanical methods for plaque control and gingival improvements without undesired side effects.
- New applications for oral chemotherapeutics, including preprocedural rinsing and home rinsing, have the potential to reduce both the contaminants in oral aerosols in the clinical environment and the capacity for the development of bacteremias.

CRITICAL THINKING EXERCISES

1. Develop a case that would support the recommendation of each of the following oral chemotherapeutic interventions:
   - Placement of minocycline microspheres (Arestin)
   - Twice-daily use of over-the-counter therapeutic home oral rinse (Listerine)
   - Professional irrigation with chlorhexidine gluconate
   - Prescription of a subantimicrobial systemic dose of doxycycline hyclate (Periostat)
   - Administration of preprocedural over-the-counter or prescription rinse before dental hygiene care
2. Role-play the following scenario with another student: You and your classmate will play the roles of dental hygiene colleagues in general practice together; your classmate recommends using chlorhexidine gluconate (0.12%) as a subgingival irrigant with all clients who have pockets of 4 mm or greater as a routine intervention. What discussion would you and your colleague have about this intervention?
3. Select a topic or intervention related to oral chemotherapeutics for periodontal disease. Search a scientific database such as PubMed, and determine the level of evidence available for the specific topic or intervention. Distinguish between the evidence provided by a single trial versus that of a systematic review.
4. Visit the website of the American Dental Association at www.ada.org. Find information on the site about the role and publications of the Council on Scientific Affairs. Explain how this resource can contribute to evidence-based decision making in practice.

REFERENCES

1. Gandini S, Negri E, Boffetta P, et al: Mouthwash and oral cancer risk–quantitative meta-analysis of epidemiologic studies, *Ann Agric Environ Med* 19:173, 2012.
2. Kerr AR, Katz RW, Ship JA: A comparison of the effects of 2 commercially available nonprescription mouthrinses on salivary flow rates and xerostomia, *Quintessence Int* 38:440, 2007.
3. Jahn CA: The dental water jet: a historical review of the literature, *J Dent Hygiene* 84:114, 2010.
4. Fine DH: Listerine: past, present and future—a test of thyme, *J Dent* 38(Suppl 1):S2, 2010.
5. Greenstein G: Research, Science and Therapy Committee of the American Academy of Periodontology: Position paper: The role of supra- and subgingival irrigation in the treatment of periodontal diseases, *J Periodontol* 76:2015, 2005.
6. Bonito AJ, Lux L, Lohr KN: Impact of local adjuncts to scaling and root planing in periodontal disease therapy: a systematic review, *J Periodontol* 76:1227, 2005.
7. Moreno Villagrana AP, Gómez Clavel JF: Antimicrobial or subantimicrobial antibiotic therapy as an adjunct to the nonsurgical periodontal treatment: a meta-analysis, *ISRN Dent* 2012:581207, 2012.
8. Gunsolley JC: Clinical efficacy of antimicrobial mouthrinses, *J Dent* 38(Suppl 1):S6, 2010.
9. Haps S, Slot DE, Berchier CE, et al: The effect of cetylpyridinium chloride-containing mouth rinses as adjuncts to toothbrushing on plaque parameters of gingival inflammation: a systemic review, *Int J Dent Hyg* 6:290-303, 2008.
10. Hossainian N, Slot DE, Afennich F, et al: The effects of hydrogen peroxide mouthwashes on the prevention of plaque and gingival inflammation: a systematic review, *Int J Dent Hyg* 9:171-181, 2011.

ACKNOWLEDGMENT

The author acknowledges Kim Krust Bray for her past contributions to this chapter.

EVOLVE RESOURCES

Please visit http://evolve.elsevier.com/Darby/hygiene for additional practice and study support tools.

Acute Gingival and Periodontal Conditions, Lesions of Endodontic Origin, and Avulsed Teeth

CHAPTER 32

Birgitta Söder

COMPETENCIES

1. Explain periodontal abscesses, including the cause, signs and symptoms, and treatment.
2. Discuss lesions of endodontic origin, including the cause, signs and symptoms, and treatment.
3. Explain herpetic infections, including the cause, signs and symptoms, and treatment.
4. Discuss pericoronitis, including signs and symptoms and treatment.
5. Explain necrotizing periodontal diseases, including the causes, signs and symptoms, and treatment.
6. Discuss how to manage the avulsed tooth, including:
   - Collaborate in caring for clients with common periodontal and dental emergencies.
   - Educate clients about the need for immediate treatment of common periodontal and dental emergencies and the expected outcome of emergency care.
   - Follow standard emergency protocol for an avulsed tooth.

The dental hygienist is frequently in a position to identify urgent periodontal conditions in need of treatment. A major part of care provided in these situations is recognizing the disease process. In some situations, the dental hygienist provides therapeutic or palliative care; in other cases, the hygienist's responsibility lies solely with referral for care. Postponement of appropriate care can result in prolonged pain, further periodontal tissue destruction, and tooth loss.

Periodontal Abscess

A **periodontal abscess** is a localized accumulation of pus within the periodontal tissues.[1] Periodontal abscesses are distinguished by location (i.e., either gingival or periodontal) and by the course of the disease (i.e., acute or chronic).

- A **gingival abscess** is a periodontal abscess that is confined to the marginal gingiva and that often occurs in previously healthy gingival areas (Figure 32-1).
- A periodontal abscess is a deeper infection associated with periodontal pockets, furcations, and bone loss (Figure 32-2).
- An **acute periodontal abscess** is a lesion with expressed periodontal breakdown occurring over a limited period of time and with easily detectable clinical symptoms.[1] It is characterized by pain, swelling, and other symptoms that lead the client to seek urgent care (Figure 32-3).
- The **chronic periodontal abscess** is a long-standing infection that often is associated with a sinus tract. This opening permits drainage of the infection and a diminution of acute symptoms such as pain and swelling, thus making the abscess chronic in nature. The sinus tract, which is an abnormal channel that connects the abscess to another space or to the surface, is called a **fistula**[1] (Figure 32-4).

Periodontal abscesses also have been classified by number as either a single abscess or multiple periodontal abscesses.

- A single abscess is caused by local factors that lead to acute or chronic symptoms.
- Multiple abscesses have been related to factors such as medically compromised systemic health, uncontrolled diabetes mellitus, and systemic antibiotic therapy for situations that are not related to oral health.[1]

The importance of recognizing and treating clients with periodontal abscesses cannot be overemphasized. Data show that most abscessed teeth—particularly those receiving regular periodontal maintenance—benefit from treatment and can be preserved. An interesting retrospective study of tooth loss caused by a periodontal abscess demonstrated that 55% of teeth with periodontal abscess were maintained for an average of 12.5 years (range, 5 to 29 years).[1] The importance of recognizing the disease process and encouraging clients to follow through with treatment is significant to one major goal of dental hygiene practice: preserving oral health.

Microbiology of the Periodontal Abscess

All periodontal abscesses share a characteristically complex pathogenic microflora similar to that associated with periodontal diseases. In these pathogenic microflora, the preponderance of bacteria changes from approximately 75% gram-positive facultative rods and cocci associated with gingival health to one harboring approximately 74% gram-negative rods.[2] These are complex mixed infections that vary from person to person and from one site of infection in the mouth to another within the same person.[2]

Those microbial species most associated with abscesses are listed in Box 32-1.

Characteristics and Treatment of Periodontal Abscesses

Acute Periodontal Abscess

The **acute periodontal abscess** is a localized accumulation of pus in the gingival wall of a periodontal pocket. It usually occurs on the lateral aspect of the tooth, and it appears edematous, red, and shiny. It may have a domelike appearance or come to a distinct point. Figure 32-3 presents an example of

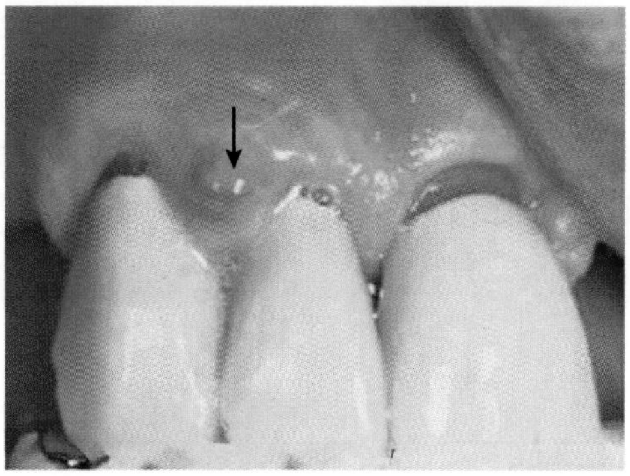

Figure 32-1. Gingival abscess between maxillary lateral incisor and canine.

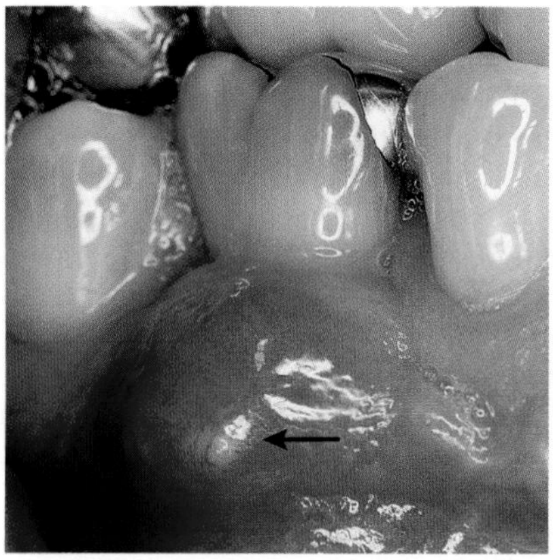

Figure 32-2. Periodontal abscess associated with mandibular right first molar.

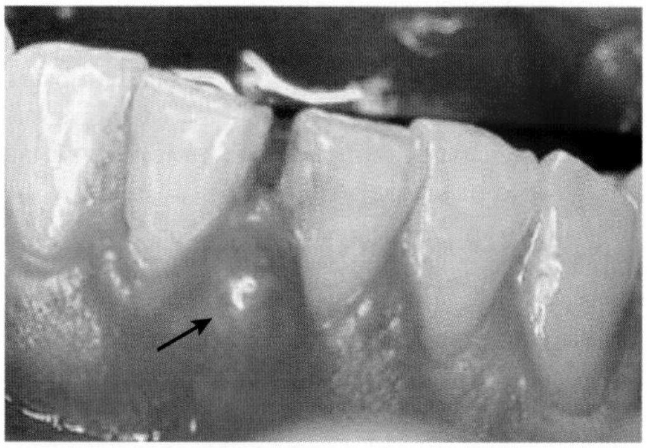

Figure 32-3. An acute periodontal abscess between teeth #24 and #25 shows obvious signs of redness and swelling.

an acute periodontal abscess with these characteristics. Acute abscesses are frequently associated with preexisting periodontal disease. The anatomic features of periodontal pockets—pocket depth of at least 5 mm, furcation involvement, and tortuous pocket anatomy—may predispose the client to occlusion of the pocket orifice. This occlusion permits an exacerbation of infection in the pocket wall as well as pus formation. Pus can often be expressed from the pocket with gentle finger pressure (Figure 32-5).[1]

Abscess formation can also occur when a foreign body becomes lodged in the pocket.[1] An exacerbated inflammatory reaction then occurs. If the pocket continues to drain through the orifice, it can stabilize and become a chronic infection that drains pus to relieve pressure in the tissues. Conversion to the chronic state rarely occurs when foreign objects such as peanut skins and popcorn hulls are embedded in the pocket, thus provoking the acute response.

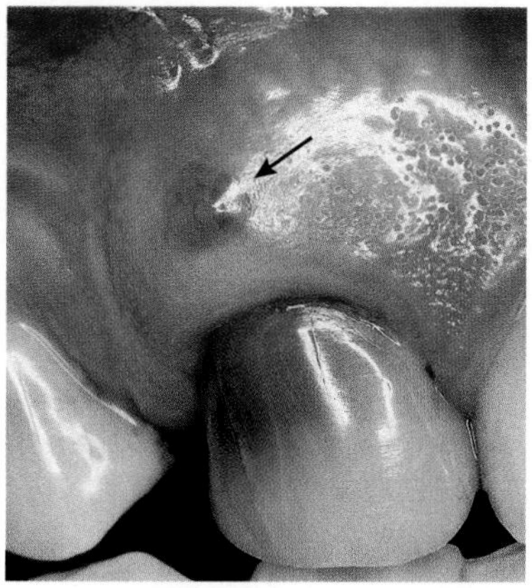

Figure 32-4. Chronic periodontal abscess. Note fistula associated with tooth #6 in attached gingiva.

BOX 32-1

Microbial Species Most Associated with Periodontal Abscess

- *Porphyromonas gingivalis*
- *Prevotella intermedia*
- *Tannerella forsythia* (formerly *Bacteroides forsythus*)
- *Fusobacterium nucleatum*
- *Aggregatibacter (Actinobacillus) actinomycetemcomitans*
- *Capnocytophaga ochracea*
- *Eikenella corrodens*
- *Campylobacter recta*
- *Selenomonas* species
- *Treponema denticola*

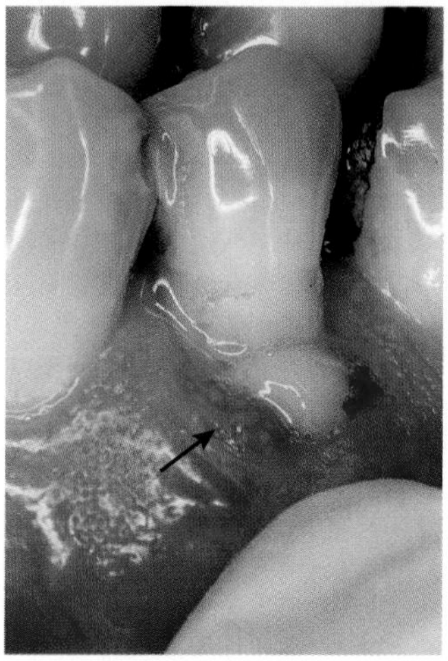

Figure 32-5. Gentle digital pressure may be sufficient to express purulent discharge.

Incomplete scaling and root planing that leaves residual calculus at the base of treated pockets has been suggested as a cause of periodontal abscesses.[1] It is postulated that the pocket orifice tightens from improved gingival health, thereby leaving the calculus and associated plaque to infect the deeper pocket tissues. This perspective is a commonly held belief, but few data support it. In an analysis of 29 persons who sought treatment at a postgraduate periodontics clinic and who had been diagnosed with periodontal abscess, 18 (62%) had untreated periodontal disease, 7 (24%) were on periodontal maintenance, and only 4 (14%) reported a history of recent scaling and root planing. Of these 29 persons, 27 were diagnosed with moderate to severe periodontal disease; the other two had early periodontitis. The mean probing depths of these abscesses were quite deep (i.e., 7.3 mm; range, 3 to 13 mm), and the abscesses were mostly associated with molar teeth.[3]

Given the number of abscesses treated, one would expect to see a much larger proportion of clients returning shortly after scaling and root planing appointments if incomplete treatment were a major cause of acute exacerbation. In another study, four types of periodontal treatment were compared, and abscess rate was noted. Quadrants treated with supragingival scaling alone developed abscesses to a far greater extent than those treated with subgingival scaling and root planing or those treated with periodontal surgery.[1] These data suggest that abscess formation is more associated with deep pockets and untreated disease than with recent scaling and root planing treatment. It is also known that residual calculus and plaque biofilm is often left in pockets after even the most thorough scaling and root planing, especially in deep pockets.[1] This information highlights the following three points:

1. It is extremely difficult to remove all calculus from periodontal pockets.
2. The clinician should scale and root plane as completely as possible with the intention of removing all subgingival deposits.
3. Supragingival scaling alone is totally inadequate for periodontal treatment and may predispose periodontal clients to acute abscess formation.

Signs and Symptoms

Acute periodontal abscess may be associated with any tooth in the mouth. Abscesses appear as shiny, red, raised, and rounded masses on the gingiva or mucosa. Abscesses can point and drain through the tissue or simply drain through the pocket opening. Purulent exudate is usually apparent around the abscess opening, or it can be expressed by finger pressure. Box 32-2 lists the signs of acute periodontal abscesses.

The client also may report that the tooth "feels high," because it may become slightly extruded as a result of swelling.[1] Radiographs may be helpful for locating a preexisting area of bone loss and can suggest the origin of the abscess. However, the infection moves through the tissue in the direction of least resistance, so the external features may appear at some distance from the affected tooth.[1]

Treatment

Treatment consists mainly of drainage and the appropriate use of antimicrobial agents. The acute phase of the disease must be managed to alleviate pain and prevent the spread of infection. The abscess must be drained, either through the pocket opening or through an incision. Drainage through the pocket opening is less invasive; this is commonly performed by the dental hygienist. The tooth or teeth in the affected area are anesthetized and scaled. Postoperative instructions call for rest, fluid intake, and warm saltwater rinses to help reduce swelling. The client is scheduled to return in 24 to 48 hours for reevaluation of the area and to plan for required follow-up treatment (e.g., periodontal surgery to eliminate the problem area).[1]

The dentist often delegates the initial treatment of the acute abscess that does not require surgical intervention to the dental hygienist. However, sometimes treatment requires an incision and reflection of the tissue (i.e., surgical flap procedure) to provide access to perform the debridement. If the client is febrile or if lymphadenopathy is present, the dentist prescribes antibiotic therapy. Figure 32-6 shows an example of debridement therapy for acute periodontal abscess.

Repair potential for acute periodontal abscesses is excellent. After treatment, the gingival appearance returns to normal within 6 to 8 weeks. Bone defect repair requires approximately 9 months. Bone is lost rapidly during the acute phase; however, with immediate problem recognition and proper treatment, the lost tissue can largely be regained.[1] The positive nature of clinical results from healing further emphasizes the importance of the recognition and treatment of acute abscesses by the dental hygienist.

BOX 32-2

Signs and Symptoms of Acute Periodontal Abscess

- Throbbing and radiating pain
- Localized swelling of the gingiva
- Deep-red to bluish color of the affected tissue
- Sensitivity of the tooth and gingiva to palpation
- Tooth mobility
- Cervical lymphadenopathy
- Systemic symptoms of fever and malaise

From Killoy WJ: Treatment of periodontal abscesses. In Genco RJ, Goldman HM, Cohen DW, eds: *Contemporary periodontics*, St Louis, 1990, Mosby.

Chronic Periodontal Abscess

A **chronic periodontal abscess** resembles an acute periodontal abscess in that there is an overgrowth of pathogenic organisms in a periodontal pocket that drains inflammatory exudate.[2] Chronic abscesses have communication with the oral cavity, either through the opening of the pocket or through a sinus tract that permits regular drainage. The chronic periodontal abscess is usually painless, or it may causes dull, intermittent pain; however, the client may recount previous episodes of painful acute infection.[1] Figure 32-7 provides examples of draining chronic periodontal abscesses.

Signs and Symptoms

The signs and symptoms of chronic periodontal abscesses are similar to those of acute periodontal abscesses; however, the pain level can be the distinguishing feature (Box 32-3). The dental hygienist must assess exudate associated with the

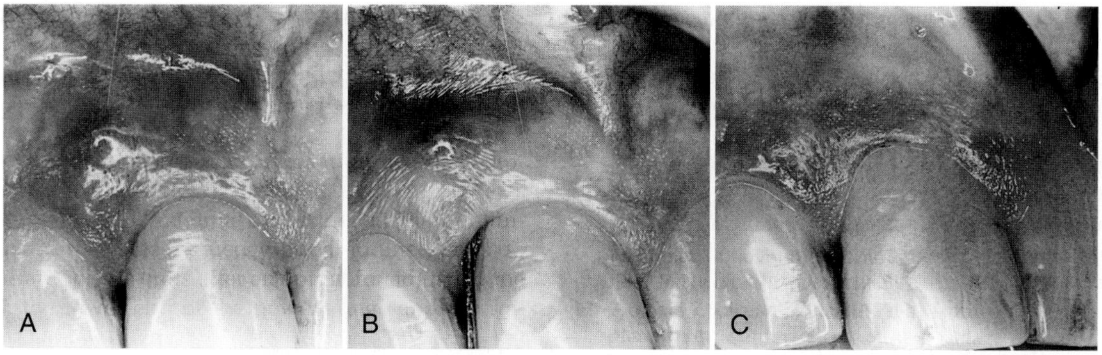

Figure 32-6. Treatment of acute periodontal abscess. Acute abscesses can often be successfully treated without surgical intervention. **A,** Abscess associated with tooth #9 showing swelling and a nondraining fistula. Clinically the tissue appears very red. **B,** Probe in place to show 9-mm pocket depth before scaling, root planing, and curettage. **C,** Healing after 1 month shows normal tissue architecture and little recession. A 7-mm periodontal pocket is still present, but surgical reduction would result in nonaesthetic recession. This situation can continue indefinitely with good homecare and frequent periodontal maintenance. (Courtesy Philip R. Melnick.)

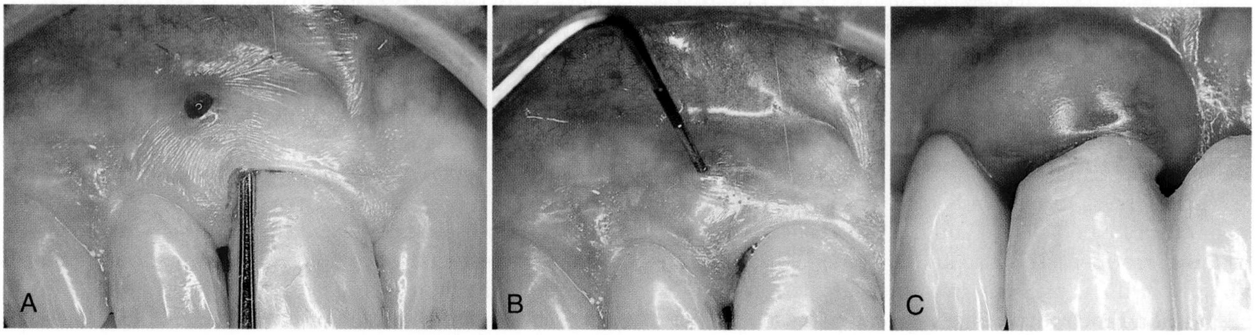

Figure 32-7. Chronic periodontal abscess. **A,** Draining through a sinus tract. **B,** Probe inserted to show communication to periodontal pocket. **C,** Draining through the periodontal pocket. (Courtesy Philip R. Melnick.)

BOX 32-3

Signs and Symptoms of Chronic Periodontal Abscess

- Inflammatory exudate seeping into the oral cavity without inducement or when digital pressure is applied to the pocket or sinus tract
- Reddened and swollen gingival tissue in the area
- Varying degrees of pain (a chronic draining abscess is rarely painful)

periodontium as being indicative of possible chronic abscess to ensure that appropriate dental referral and treatment are provided.

Treatment

Treatment of chronic periodontal abscess is similar to treatment of acute periodontal abscess. Scaling (usually requiring local anesthesia in the abscess area) must be performed. The client returns within 24 to 48 hours for further diagnosis. The dentist must determine the need for more periodontal treatment to reduce pocket depth and to address other periodontal defects. Additional treatment usually includes pocket reduction periodontal surgery, but it also may include tooth extraction and more frequent periodontal maintenance visits. Some chronic periodontal abscesses are better treated initially by gaining surgical access.[10] Figure 32-8 shows the surgical treatment sequence for a chronic periodontal abscess.

The dental hygienist plays a major role in educating the client about the condition's chronic nature. The client is informed of the likelihood of increased bone loss and future acute episodes if no further treatment is performed in addition to the need for frequent maintenance care that includes scaling, root planing, and daily plaque biofilm control. Often the discussion of the risk of rapid bone loss during acute episodes of abscess helps the client value the need to seek further care to better preserve the teeth.[4]

Gingival Abscess

The gingival abscess usually occurs in previously disease-free areas, and it is often related to the forceful inclusion of some foreign body into the area. Gingival abscesses are most frequently found on the marginal gingiva and not associated with deeper tissue pathology.[1]

Signs and Symptoms

The gingival abscess can be observed on the marginal gingiva; Box 32-4 includes a list of signs and symptoms of this condition. A pus-filled lesion that is not associated with the sulcular

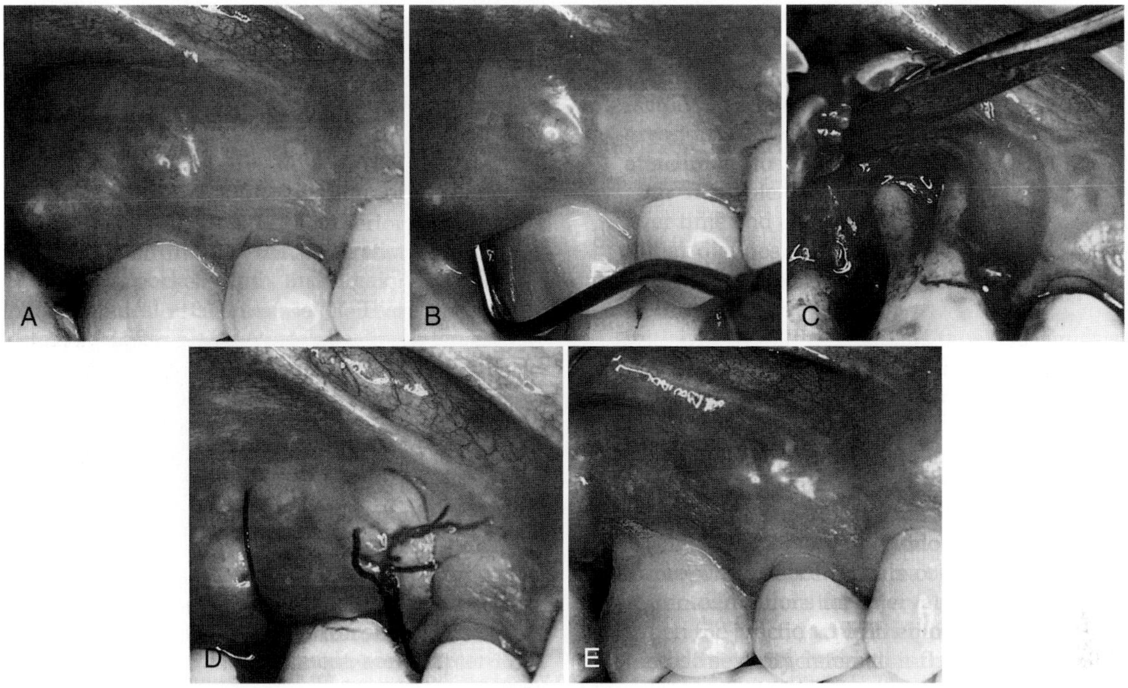

Figure 32-8. Surgical treatment of a chronic periodontal abscess associated with a furcation. **A,** Abscess associated with tooth #3 exhibits swelling and a fistula that is not draining. The tissue is very reddened, and the patient has intermittent severe pain. **B,** Periodontal probe inserted to show the depth of the pocket and determine its association with the buccal furcation. **C,** Flap reflected to permit access for debridement. Note the extent of the bone loss and the depth of the furcation involvement. **D,** After debridement, the flap is sutured in place. **E,** Healing after 1 month shows tissue returned to normal color and consistency and no evidence of the fistula. Note the recession that occurred after surgical treatment. This client must keep the teeth clean and return for frequent periodontal maintenance visits to preserve the tooth. (Courtesy Philip R. Melnick.)

BOX 32-4

Signs and Symptoms of Gingival Abscess

- Reddened tissue (marginal gingiva)
- Swelling (pus-filled lesion)
- Pain

epithelium is often clearly seen. Figure 32-9 shows a gingival abscess in the otherwise healthy periodontium of a teenager.

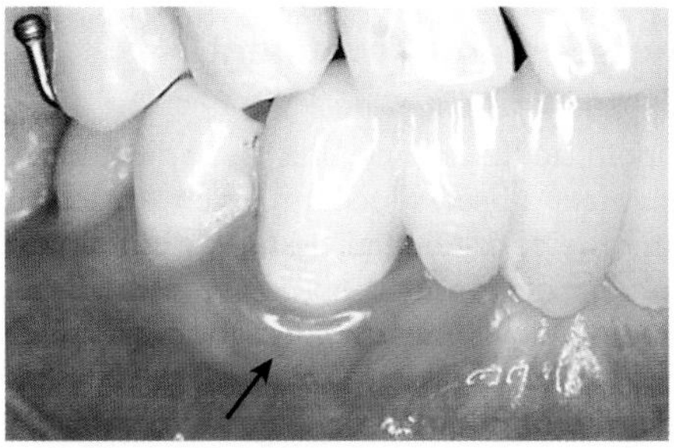

Figure 32-9. Gingival abscess. The gingival abscess is associated with the marginal gingiva and is often the result of inclusion of a foreign body. Note the swelling and color change of the marginal gingiva. (Courtesy Philip R. Melnick.)

Treatment

The gingival abscess must be drained and the foreign object removed by the dentist or periodontist. The acute lesion is incised and irrigated with saline solution. Sutures are not usually required. Warm saltwater rinses are recommended for postoperative therapy at home. The client must return for postoperative observation in about 24 hours, at which time the swelling should be greatly reduced and the acute tenderness subsided.

Lesions of Endodontic Origin

Lesion Types

The lesion of endodontic origin (LEO), which is the most common dental emergency,[1] is also referred to as a *dentoalveolar, apical, periapical,* or **endodontic abscess**.[1] Inflammatory processes in the periodontium associated with necrotic dental pulps have a clear infectious cause. In a LEO, the inflammatory processes are directed toward infectious components released from bacterial growth and bacterial disintegration in the root canal system.[4] It is sometimes difficult to distinguish a LEO from an acute periodontal abscess, because the associated facial pain and tenderness to the tooth are similar. The endodontic abscess commonly results from pulpal tissue infection as a result of caries, traumatic tooth fracture, or dental procedure trauma. Pulpal infection can be spread laterally to a tooth from an adjacent infected tooth, from infected periodontium, or through the lateral canals.[4]

Microbiology

Most commonly, the LEO is caused by microorganisms spreading into the pulp through the dentinal tubules from a carious lesion. However, the inflammatory processes in the periodontium occurring as a result of root canal infection may not only be localized at the apex; they may also appear along the lateral aspects of the root and in furcation areas of multirooted teeth.[4] This lesion type appears to be an infrequent event that does not seem to emerge at a rate that corresponds with the frequency with which lateral canals occur in the teeth.

Dissemination of the microorganisms and their toxic byproducts through the enamel to the dentinal tubules can be very rapid. Although microorganisms are the most common pulpal disease cause, bacterial toxins also can initiate pulpal disease by penetrating through tubules with pores small enough to block bacteria.[4] The toxins affect the odontoblastic cells and then penetrate into the pulp, thus initiating an inflammatory response. The bacterial cells also move toward the pulp by demineralizing the hard tooth structure with acids that they produce along the way. The microorganisms colonize in the pulp and produce a variety of toxins that result in pulp cell death. Bacteria and their metabolic products exit the apical foramen and can cause localized granulation tissue formation; this tissue contains lymphocytes, plasma cells, mast cells, and other immune response elements. If the irritation continues, the granulation tissue gradually replaces the normal bone and periosteum at the tooth apex and gives rise to the common radiographic appearance of the LEO: a defined radiolucency at the apex of the affected tooth called a periapical pathosis (Figure 32-10).[1]

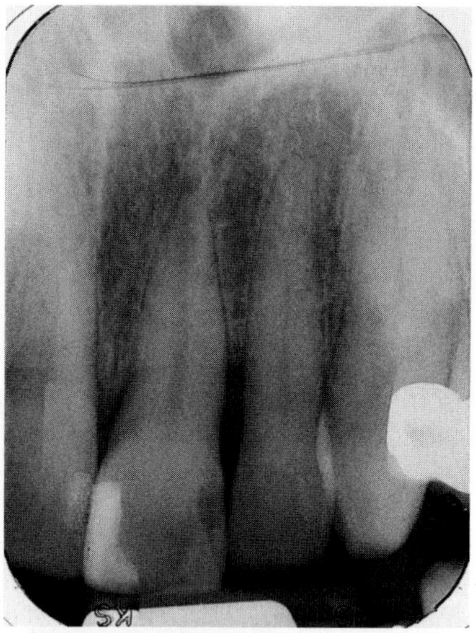

Figure 32-10. Lesions of endodontic origin. The radiographic appearance of an endodontic abscess associated with tooth #9 shows the classic appearance of radiolucency at the root apex. Note that the periodontal ligament does not appear to be intact around the tooth apex. (Courtesy Edward J. Taggert.)

Characteristics and Treatment

Periapical Abscesses

There are both acute and chronic periapical abscesses. The acute periapical abscess occurs when bacteria or toxins rapidly enter the periradicular tissues, usually from the tooth pulp chamber. The confined abscess can cause severe pain. The pain may subside as the infection spreads toward a surface or space to provide relief to the tissues. Clients typically experience pain and swelling and may have systemic symptoms of infection, including osteitis (i.e., inflammation of the bone) or cellulitis (i.e., inflammation of cellular tissue, usually occurring in the loose tissues beneath the skin, in the mucous membranes, around muscle bundles, or around organs, which can be life-threatening). The chronic periapical abscess is associated with a more gradual introduction of irritants from the root canal into the periradicular tissues. The inflammatory response is intense, but the client gets relief from an either constantly or intermittently draining sinus tract.[1] These tracts usually drain into the mouth through a fistula in the bone or through the periodontal ligament, but they can also drain through the facial skin. If a sinus tract through the periodontal ligament is left untreated, it will become a true periodontal pocket.[1]

Signs and Symptoms

The LEO is most identifiable on radiographs as a rounded radiolucency at the apex of the tooth. Figure 32-10 shows the typical appearance. However, early during abscess formation, the radiographic changes are often not obvious. If the LEO drains through a sinus tract in the cortical bone or through the periodontal ligament, it is likely to be much less identifiable on radiographs. LEOs that drain through the periodontal ligament can resemble acute periodontal abscesses, because their symptoms are very similar: both exhibit reddened tissue, swelling, and a sinus tract opening. It is often difficult to determine if the fistula opens into the periodontal pocket or goes to the apex of the tooth (Box 32-5).

When assessing an abscess to determine its origin, it is helpful to know that 85% of tooth pain is pulpal and that 15% is periodontal. In addition, many teeth with endodontic lesions are nonvital, which is a good distinguishing clue. However, some client populations that are likely to be treated by the dental hygienist, such as those treated in the periodontal practice, are much more likely to have periodontal than pulpal abscesses. Pain may be the distinguishing feature for differentiating between periapical and periodontal abscesses. Periapical pain is characterized as sharp, severe, intermittent, and hard to localize. By contrast, periodontal pain tends to be constant, less severe, and localized.[1]

BOX 32-5

Signs and Symptoms of a Lesion of Endodontic Origin

- Sharp pain that is likely to be intermittent
- Sinus tract often present
- Swelling of tissues in a localized area
- Redness of tissues in a localized area
- History of restoration, trauma, or other source of tooth infection
- Rounded radiolucency at tooth apex that appears later in the disease process

TABLE 32-1

Treatment Strategies for Apical Abscesses

Cause	Condition of the Pulp	Treatment
Endodontic	Nonvital	Endodontic
Periodontal	Vital	Periodontal
Endodontic	Nonvital	Endodontic; first observe and then later institute periodontal therapy, if necessary

Treatment

Apical abscess treatment requires either endodontic treatment to remove the tooth pulp and replace it with inert material or tooth extraction. Untreated endodontic abscesses can lead to severe cases of brain abscess or fasciitis of the neck or chest wall that can be life-threatening.[1] The dental hygienist has a responsibility to inform clients with untreated LEOs of the risk of delaying treatment. Clients without acute symptoms caused by abscess draining are likely to have the need for conceptualizing the disease process so that they pursue care and avoid further tissue destruction and ill effects from the infection. Table 32-1 summarizes LEO treatment strategies.

Combination Abscesses

The periodontium is a continuous unit. Pathology at the tooth's apex from infection of the root canal system can extend to the marginal tissues, and infection originating in the periodontal tissues can progress to the pulp through openings at the apex or through lateral canals. A true **combination periodontal and periapical abscess** is present when both of these infectious processes are present. Whatever the route or source of the infection, when both the periodontal and pulpal tissues are involved and the disease has abscess formation, the abscess is considered a combination periapical and periodontal abscess.[1]

Signs and Symptoms

Combination abscesses cause some combination of the signs and symptoms described separately for periapical and periodontal abscesses. They are sometimes difficult to diagnose and can result in extensive damage to the surrounding periodontium, because the intermittent nature of symptoms often causes clients to delay seeking treatment. The dentist diagnoses combination abscesses when symptoms of both pulpal and periodontal infection are identified. Figure 32-11 illustrates a combination abscess.

Treatment

The most common form of treatment for periapical and periodontal abscesses is surgical exposure of the area, including the removal of the granulation tissue.[4] Combination abscesses require the treatment of both sources of infection. Both periodontal and endodontic therapies are indicated to preserve the tooth. In some cases, the periodontal tissue destruction is so severe that the tooth must be extracted even though endodontic therapy could be performed successfully.[5]

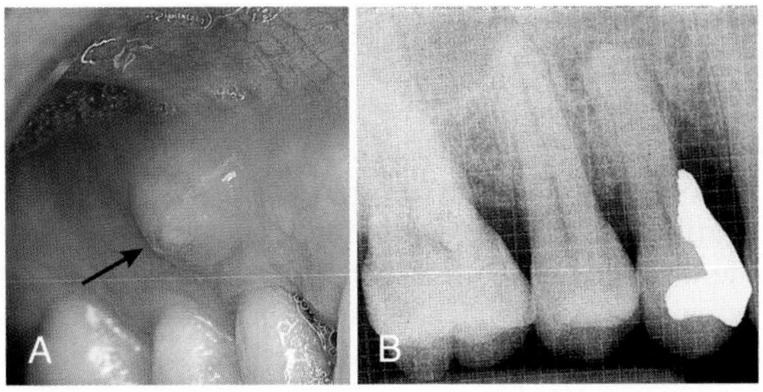

Figure 32-11. Combined periapical and periodontal abscess. The combined abscess is associated with tooth #5. It could have occurred from the spread of pathologic microorganisms from the deep pockets to the tooth pulp, the caries process, or trauma from the placement of the very deep restoration. **A,** The sinus tract (fistula) emerges into the oral cavity. **B,** Radiolucency at the apex and significant bone loss appear on the radiograph. (Courtesy Philip R. Melnick.)

Herpetic Infections

More than 80 herpesviruses have been identified,[6] eight of which are known human pathogens.[1,7]

Herpes simplex viruses (HSVs) belong to the ubiquitous *Herpesviridae* family of viruses, which contains HSV-1, HSV-2, varicella-zoster virus, cytomegalovirus, and Epstein-Barr virus as well as human herpesviruses and Kaposi's sarcoma–associated herpesvirus (type 8).[6]

Herpesvirus infection occurs worldwide, has no seasonal variation, and affects only humans naturally. The prevalence of HSV-1 infection increases gradually from childhood, reaching 60% to 95% prevalence among adults.

Primary HSV-1 infection in oral and perioral sites usually manifests as gingivostomatitis, whereas virus reactivation in the trigeminal sensory ganglion gives rise to mild cutaneous and mucocutaneous disease; this is often called *recurrent herpes labialis.*[6,7]

Primary Herpetic Gingivostomatitis

Irrespective of the viral type, HSV primarily affects the skin and mucous membranes.[7] **Primary herpetic gingivostomatitis (PHGS)** is the most common orofacial manifestation of HSV-1 infection, and it is characterized by oral and perioral vesiculoulcerative lesions.[7] Although herpetic gingivostomatitis is a self-limiting disease, affected individuals may experience severe pain and be unable to eat or drink.

The virus is spread by physical contact, but there is no documentation that it can be spread through the airborne droplet route, contaminated water, or contact with inanimate objects. Most people encounter the virus and never show signs or symptoms of primary infection.[7] It is known that up to 90% of the population has antibodies to HSV-1.

PHGS typically develops after the first-time exposure of seronegative individuals or among those who have not produced an adequate antibody response during a previous infection with either of the two HSVs.[6]

The majority of infections are subclinical. Although PHGS typically affects children between the ages of 1 and 5 years, occasional cases of primary infection affecting adults also occur.[6] Infants are passively protected through maternal immunity for the first 6 months of life. The clinical manifestations of the infection, whether from HSV-1 or HSV-2, may lead to primary oral infection; nearly all are caused by HSV-1.[6,7] The majority of HSV-1–induced primary orofacial infections are subclinical and therefore unrecognized.[6] Symptomatic PHGS is typically preceded or accompanied by a sensation of burning or paresthesia at the inoculation site, cervical and submandibular lymphadenopathy, fever, malaise, myalgia, appetite loss, dysphagia, and headache. The most characteristic signs at presentation are acute, generalized, marginal gingivitis, with the inflamed gingiva appearing erythematous and edematous. Most clients with primary herpetic infections never experience the secondary or recurrent forms. In healthy individuals, primary infection has an excellent prognosis, with recovery expected within 10 to 14 days.[6] Nevertheless, the painful herpetic ulcers in the mouth associated with primary infection often cause a reduction in food and fluid intake, thereby creating a human need for the prevention of the health risks that accompany this disease. Nutritional deficits can be critical in children and infants. Serious dehydration is not uncommon, and this can lead to infant hospitalization.

Signs and Symptoms

Acute herpetic gingivostomatitis is recognized by a set of characteristic systemic and intraoral signs and symptoms (Box 32-6). The vesicular eruptions may occur on the skin, the vermilion border, or the oral mucous membranes. Intraorally, they may appear on any mucosal or gingival surface, the hard palate, and the alveolar mucosa or any other oral soft-tissue area.[6] The discrete grayish vesicles rupture and coalesce within 24 hours to form ulcers. The ulcers have a red, elevated, "halolike" margin with a depressed yellow or gray central area. They are teeming with shedding virus. Figure 32-12 exemplifies the intraoral appearance of primary herpetic infection in a teenager. The disease is commonly associated with systemic symptoms including fever, malaise, headache, and cervical lymphadenopathy.[6]

The recognition of PHGS is based on knowledge of the appearance of the ulcers and the assessment of systemic manifestations. Diagnostic tests, such as culturing for herpesvirus by the client's physician, can be conducted for confirmation of the presence of the virus, but these are not routine. In addition, this is a highly infectious disease; therefore the dental hygienist, the client, and the client's parents (in the case of children), must work together to prevent the transmission of the virus to family members and other members of the oral healthcare team. Figure 32-13 shows a more unusual presentation of primary herpetic infection on the facial skin.

BOX 32-6

Signs and Symptoms of Acute Herpetic Gingivostomatitis

- Ulcers with the characteristic appearance of red halos of tissue immediately surrounding them (extraorally on the skin and the vermilion border of the lip; intraorally on any mucosal surface)
- Generally reddened tissues
- Pain
- Fever
- Malaise
- Headache
- Cervical lymphadenopathy

Treatment

The treatment of gingival inflammation and any other elective dental care should be postponed until the PHGS has run its course. The client is assessed by the dentist to obtain a definitive dental diagnosis. The management of acute herpetic gingivostomatitis is entirely supportive because of the infectious nature of the disease and the fact that it runs its course in 7 to 10 days. The client should be instructed to rest, take fluids, and make every effort to eat a nutritious diet. The client should also try to clean the teeth at home with an extra-soft toothbrush if it can be tolerated.[6,7]

Professional care should not be performed because of the risk of transmission of the virus to other head and neck areas of the client or to the dental hygienist and other workers. Even if the hygienist was previously exposed to the herpesvirus or has had an episode of initial infection with or without recurrent lesions, he or she can still be inoculated with the virus by an inadvertent finger puncture with an HSV-contaminated instrument. This infection could result in the development of herpetic whitlow (Figure 32-14). Herpetic whitlow is a recurrent herpetic finger lesion that can be extremely painful and debilitating. The whitlow can last many weeks longer than the usual 2-week course of herpesvirus infection in the oral tissue.[1]

The dental hygienist educates the client about consuming adequate fluids and soft, nutrient-dense foods; performing oral hygiene as much as possible at home; and using over-the-counter topical anesthetics and systemic nonsteroidal anti-inflammatory agents to minimize discomfort. The client can swab topical anesthetics onto the lesions for controlled local delivery. Topical anesthetics should be used cautiously with children so as not to anesthetize the throat, which can be frightening to them.

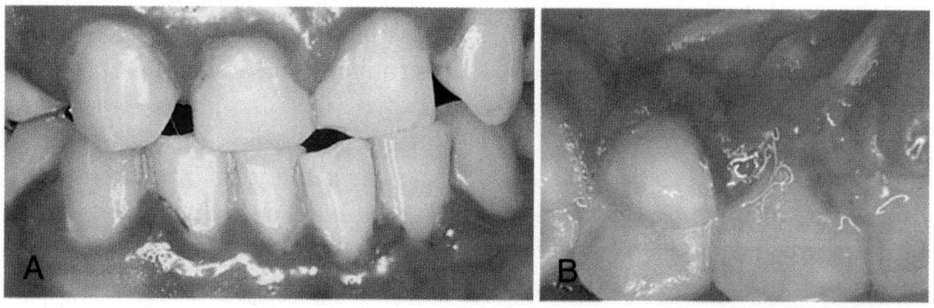

Figure 32-12. Primary herpetic gingivostomatitis. This oral infection of the mouth is characterized by bright red gingiva, vesicles, and pain. **A,** Facial gingiva showing swelling and color change. **B,** Lingual view of the premolar and anterior teeth showing coalesced vesicles. (Courtesy Philip R. Melnick.)

Recurrent Oral Herpes Simplex Infections

After primary infection, latent HSV reactivates periodically, migrating from the sensory ganglia to cause recurrent oral or genital herpes.[6,7] Despite the high prevalence of HSV-1 in the population, only 15% to 40% of seropositive patients ever experience symptomatic mucocutaneous recurrence.[1,6,7] An individual's genetic susceptibility, immune status, age, anatomic site of infection, initial dose of inoculums, and viral subtype appear to influence the frequency of recurrence. As compared with primary infections, recurrent episodes are milder and shorter in duration, with minimal systemic involvement.[7]

Clients often arrive for dental hygiene appointments when they have recurrent herpetic lesions. These lesions are quite common, as previously mentioned, and they do not interfere with activities of daily living, so clients are frequently unaware of the nature of the event. The typical recurrent lesion is on the lip and is referred to as *herpes simplex labialis.* Common names such as *fever blister* and *cold sore* reflect the public's understanding of what precipitates these recurrences. Unfortunately, these are extremely innocuous names for lesions with serious potential effects for the dental hygienist.

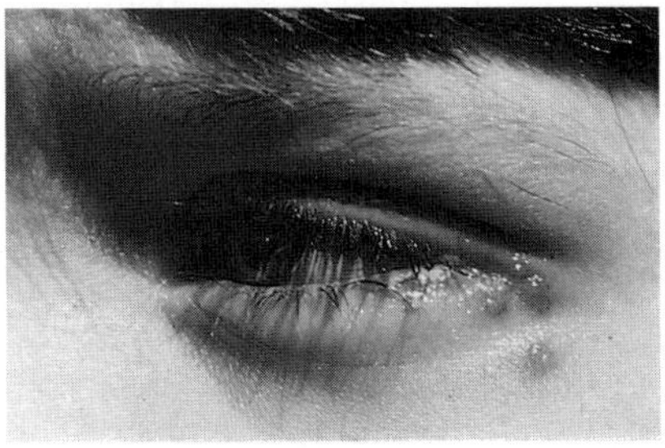

Figure 32-13. Primary herpetic infection on facial skin near the eye. This 8-year-old child had to remain out of school for 3 weeks until the infection ran its course to prevent spread to others.

Signs and Symptoms

Clients often have prodromal symptoms of burning, tingling, or pain at the site where the lesion recurs (Box 32-7). Within hours of the prodromal symptoms, vesicles appear, and these become ulcerated and coalesce into a large ulcer or ulcers. The lesions heal without scarring in about 14 days, and they can recur as often as once per month. Typically lesions will recur in the same place on the vermilion border and on the skin around the face. Figure 32-15 shows an example of a recurrent herpetic lesion.

Treatment

Recurrent lesions shed vast amounts of herpesvirus. For this reason, the dental hygienist must not treat the client while the lesions are present. Sometimes this can be very disconcerting, because it requires reappointing a client who has waited months for an appointment. However, the dental hygienist is placed at great risk of inoculation, just as with primary herpetic infections. Not only are herpetic whitlow lesions a possibility, but the virus is also shed in the saliva, which means that spatter during treatment can be hazardous. Figure 32-16 shows an example of a recurrent herpetic infection of the cornea that was acquired as a result of spatter.

Herpetic lesion treatment is entirely supportive. There are some antiviral agents available by prescription (e.g., acyclovir) that the client may benefit from using. These agents can reduce the extent and duration of the recurrence. The dental

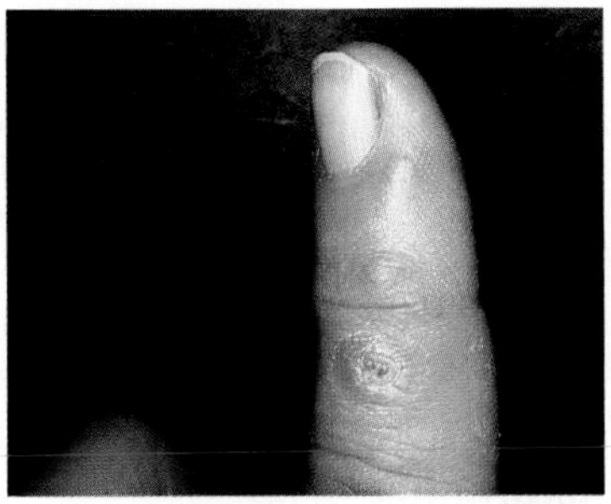

Figure 32-14. Herpetic whitlow.

BOX 32-7

Signs and Symptoms of Recurrent Herpetic Infection

- Prodromal symptoms of burning or tingling at the site
- Ulcer on the lip or the perioral skin
- Pain
- Vesicles early in the course of the infection
- Crusting of the ulcer surface as it heals

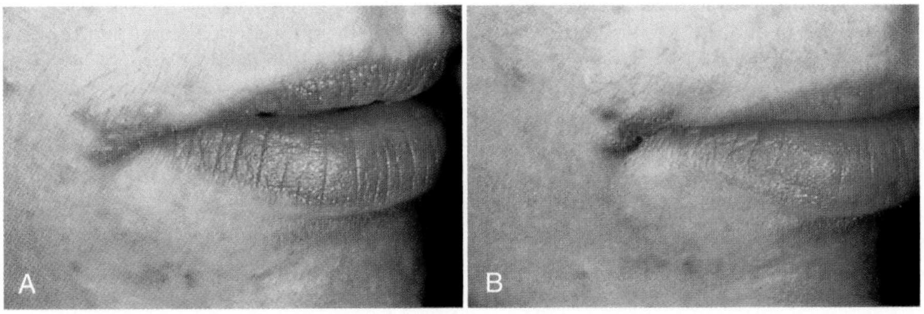

Figure 32-15. Recurrent herpetic infection on the lip, which is also known as a *cold sore.* Clients frequently do not recognize these lesions as recurrent herpetic infections that are highly contagious. **A,** Herpes labialis 12 hours after onset. **B,** Herpes labialis 48 hours after onset. (From Ibsen OAC, Phelan JA: *Oral pathology for the dental hygienist,* ed 6, St Louis, 2013, Saunders.)

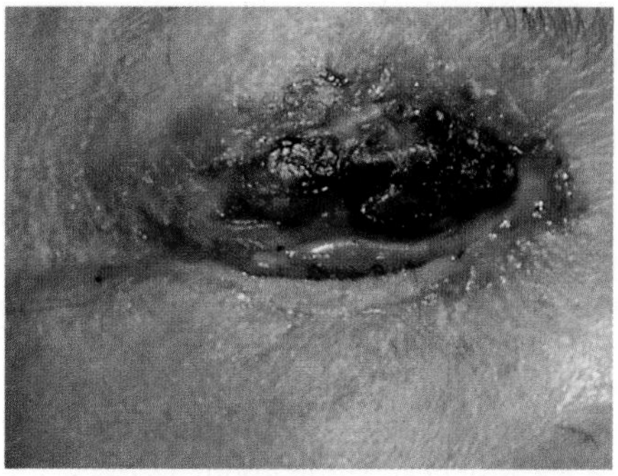

Figure 32-16. Recurrent herpetic infection of the cornea. Without protective eyewear and standard precautions, calculus and other contaminants can enter the eye of the dental hygienist or client and infect the cornea with herpesvirus. Recurrences are extremely painful and last several months. Partial loss of sight and disability can occur. (Courtesy Dr. Sidney Eisig.)

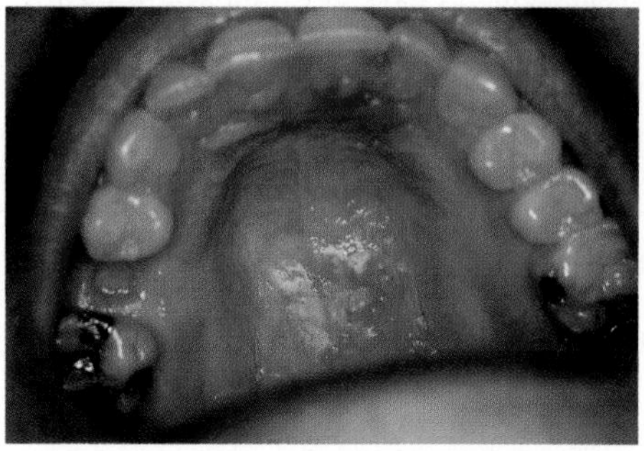

Figure 32-17. Recurrent herpetic infection of the palate. (From Ibsen OAC, Phelan JA: *Oral pathology for the dental hygienist*, ed 6, St Louis, 2013, Saunders.)

hygienist should inform the client of this possibility and refer the client to the physician or dentist for further information.

It is extremely important for the client to be educated about these lesions and about his or her responsibility for preventing the spread of infection. Clients who have common recurrences are often aware of the prodromal symptoms and should be informed to call and reschedule dental appointments until the disease runs its course.

Recurrent herpetic lesions can occur intraorally, and they usually appear on the soft palate.[6] These lesions sometimes erupt after therapeutic scaling and root planing, when repeated palatal injections have been given to the client to achieve anesthesia. The client will either call or return for a subsequent appointment, and the typical oral ulcers will be evident in the area in which the injections were given. Figure 32-17 is an example of recurrent palatal herpes subsequent to periodontal therapy in the maxillary arch. This situation requires the same management as other herpetic episodes. The client should not be treated until the lesions have healed, and the client must be educated about the situation.

Recurrent intraoral herpetic lesions can almost always be easily distinguished from the more commonly occurring **aphthous ulcers**. Reviewing the client history for recent trauma or illness may be helpful, but either lesion can result. The more distinguishing characteristic is that recurrent herpetic lesions almost always occur on the gingiva or the hard palate, and aphthous ulcers almost always appear on the movable mucosa.

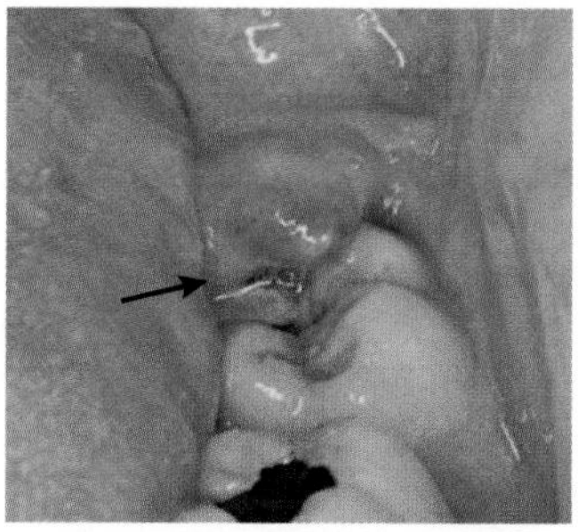

Figure 32-18. Pericoronitis. This condition is most commonly found in the third molar region, and it can be extremely painful. Note the soft-tissue swelling distal to the second molar. Clinically the tissue is intensely red.

Pericoronitis

Pericoronitis is soft-tissue inflammation associated with a partially erupted tooth. It may be acute, subacute, or chronic in nature.[8] The most commonly affected tooth is the mandibular third molar, but maxillary third molars and other teeth that are the most distal in the arch have been associated with the disease. The tissue flap that either completely or partly covers the associated tooth is called an **operculum**. The space between the tissue flap and the tooth is an ideal location for food debris to collect and bacteria to grow. As bacteria increasingly infect the area, the tissue responds by becoming extremely inflamed and painful.[8] There is constant inflammation in the area, so it is always considered subacute or chronically infected, even if the acute symptoms are not present.[8]

Acute pericoronitis involves an extremely high degree of inflammation in the local area. As inflammation increases, the tissue swells, and this can interfere with the complete closing of the jaws. This interference can lead to added trauma, increased inflammation, and severe pain. The tissue becomes quite red, suppuration is evident, and the pain can radiate to the throat and ear.

This disease is a common problem associated with young adults, and it has been considered to be a serious problem for military personnel, most of whom are in the 17- to 26-year-old age group. In fact, 20% of dental emergencies reported by the military during World War II and 16% of those from the Vietnam conflict were acute pericoronitis.[1] Figure 32-18 shows an example of acute pericoronitis.

Signs and Symptoms

Oral areas that have an operculum are predisposed to pericoronitis and typically exhibit chronic signs of the disease, increased redness, and some exudate (Box 32-8).

The tissue may be so swollen that it interferes with mastication, and it is easily traumatized during eating. The infection can extend very deeply into the tissues and cause peritonsillar abscess formation, cellulitis, and Ludwig's angina.[5] These signs are rare sequelae, but they emphasize the importance of recognition and lesion treatment.

A review of military studies documents the extent of symptoms associated with pericoronitis. In a military study of 359 recruits, pain, swelling, and redness were present in every instance. Purulent exudate was reported in half of the cases, few patients bled on palpation, and no individual in that population had a fever. In addition, two thirds of 25 cases in the naval population reported previous episodes of

BOX 32-8

Signs and Symptoms of Acute Pericoronitis

- Extreme pain
- Swelling of the operculum and gingiva associated with the most distal tooth in the arch
- Redness
- Purulent exudate
- Foul taste
- Swelling of the cheek
- Cervical lymphadenopathy
- History of recurrence

pericoronitis, which suggests that pericoronitis is often a recurrent problem.[8]

Treatment

A number of considerations are involved when treating pericoronitis, including the severity of the case, whether it is a recurrence, and possible systemic complications. The dentist may ask the dental hygienist to participate in the care of the client with pericoronitis, which requires multiple visits.

Initial dental management is aimed at treating symptoms with the goal of making the client more comfortable. The infected area is debrided, usually by gentle flushing with warm water or dilute hydrogen peroxide delivered in a disposable irrigating syringe with a blunt needle. Topical anesthetic is applied first. Much tissue manipulation may not be possible, but the tissue needs to be lifted away from the tooth to permit as much debridement as is tolerable at the first treatment appointment.[1] After this initial debridement, the client is instructed to rest at home, use warm saltwater rinses, and drink fluids to avoid dehydration. The dentist may prescribe antibiotics if the client is febrile or if there is cervical lymphadenopathy. The client is asked to return the next day. At the second visit, the area is irrigated again and instrumented if possible, and more thorough homecare is initiated. A marked improvement is usually observed at the second appointment.

After the acute condition has resolved, the client is assessed by the dentist to determine further treatment. Dental treatment may include the extraction of the offending third molar or operculum removal to produce a more normal gingival contour if the tooth is to be retained.[9]

The presence of any operculum is assessed and viewed with suspicion. There is almost always some amount of inflammation present, and the potential for acute exacerbations is likely. The dental hygienist informs clients about the potential issues associated with the condition to permit them to understand the situation and take responsibility for their oral health.

Necrotizing Periodontal Diseases

Acute necrotizing ulcerative gingivitis has been reported widely, and it is not uncommon in developing countries.[10] Classical diagnostic features include ulceration and necrosis of the interdental papillae, pain, and spontaneous gingival bleeding. Necrotizing ulcerative periodontal diseases are clinically recognizable diseases that are distinct from chronic periodontitis. Until 1999, the condition was most commonly called *acute necrotizing ulcerative gingivitis* or just *necrotizing ulcerative gingivitis*. However, the disease is often associated with attachment loss, which makes the term *gingivitis* inaccurate, so the disease is now referred to as *necrotizing ulcerative periodontitis*. It is not certain whether the conditions involving attachment loss are separate diseases from those confined to the gingiva, so the consensus is to use the more general disease name of *necrotizing periodontal diseases.*

Necrotizing ulcerative periodontal diseases are opportunistic gingival infections that are associated with lifestyle risk factors (e.g., stress, tobacco use) as well as with systemic conditions (e.g., blood dyscrasias, acquired immunodeficiency syndrome, Down syndrome).[10]

The disease was first described by Vincent during the late nineteenth century, and it was so common among troops fighting in trenches in Europe during World War I that the name *trench mouth* was adopted. It was primarily seen in young adult individuals, and it was thought to be communicable.[10] However, the disease is not communicable, infectious, or spread through direct contact. Necrotizing ulcerative periodontal diseases are recognized to be recurrent diseases with complex bacteriology consisting of a large proportion of spirochetes and gram-negative organisms. The consistent presence of specific bacteria, fusobacteria, and spirochetes has suggested that the cause could be explained in microbiologic terms. These organisms invade the tissue, which causes the characteristic appearance of the disease. Other contributory factors implicated include poor oral hygiene, mouth breathing, smoking, stress, sepsis, malnutrition, and systemic diseases, including hormonal imbalance and alterations in lymphocyte and neutrophil function.[10]

Signs and Symptoms

Necrotizing ulcerative periodontal diseases have specific clinical characteristics that distinguish them from other forms of acute oral infections. The clinical appearance of the disease is one of cratered or "punched-out" papillae, very reddened gingivae, and pain. There is often a collection of debris, dead cells, and bacteria on the gingival surface that appears gray and that is referred to as the *pseudomembrane*. The gingival lesions may be localized to specific areas or generalized throughout the mouth, and they progressively destroy the gingiva and the underlying periodontal structures. Clients frequently exhibit an extremely offensive and fetid breath odor that can be smelled anywhere in a room that is occupied by the client. They may also complain of a thick or pasty texture to the saliva. In addition, the acute lesions can be extensive and cover parts of the face, as is seen in developing countries in association with malnutrition. Figure 32-19 shows the clinical oral features of necrotizing ulcerative periodontitis.

The three most reliable criteria for recognizing the disease are as follows:

1. Acute necrosis and ulceration of the interproximal papillae
2. Pain
3. Bleeding

Other symptoms have been recognized as being strongly associated with the disease (Box 32-9).

Stress is often related to both the initial occurrence and recurrence of this disease. The role of the psychologic factors

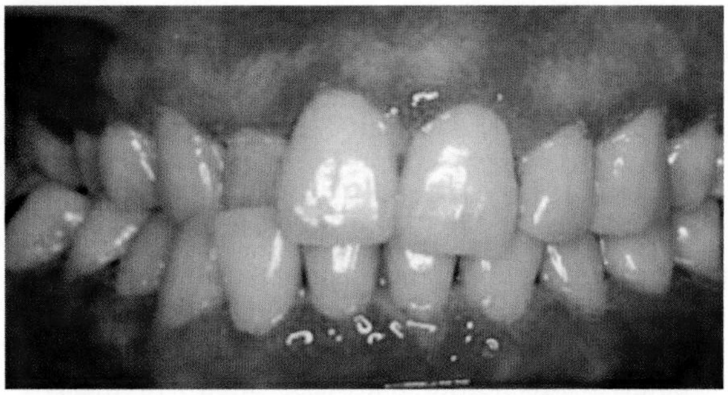

Figure 32-19. Necrotizing ulcerative periodontitis. The classic intraoral signs of this disease—redness, cratered papillae, pseudomembrane, and spontaneous hemorrhage—appear in the anterior areas.

BOX 32-9

Signs and Symptoms of Necrotizing Ulcerative Periodontitis

- Necrosis of interproximal papillae of the gingiva
- Bleeding
- Pain
- Fetid odor
- Pseudomembrane over the gingiva
- Cervical lymphadenopathy
- Fever

TABLE 32-2

Treatment Regimen for Necrotizing Ulcerative Periodontitis

Day 1	First visit: oral therapy	Scale and debride as much as possible. Mechanized (ultrasonic) instruments may be more easily tolerated than hand-activated scalers. Use topical anesthetic as needed. Provide plaque-control instruction. Recommend frequent rinsing at home with a mixture of warm water and 3% hydrogen peroxide to soothe and oxygenate the pseudomembranous plaque.
Day 1	Systemic therapy	Review the client's health history for underlying conditions, and consult with his or her physician as needed. Antibiotic use (e.g., penicillin, erythromycin, metronidazole) is indicated if the client has fever and cervical lymphadenopathy.
Day 2	Second visit	Pain should be reduced considerably. Continue to remove calculus to the limit of the client's tolerance. Oral hygiene instructions should be reinforced. The home rinsing regimen should be continued.
Days 4 to 7	Third visit	Therapeutic scaling and root planing should be completed, taking as many appointments as necessary. Oral hygiene must be reinforced. Hydrogen peroxide rinses can be discontinued. Continue the client on 0.12% chlorhexidine mouth rinse twice daily for 2 to 3 weeks.
Month 1	Reevaluation for continued care	Reinforce oral hygiene. Scale and root plane if necessary. Meticulous and regular debridement by the client and the dental hygienist must occur to control bacterial pathogenicity. Cratering frequently occurs and can result in significant gingival defects that should be evaluated by the dentist for possible surgical correction.
Month 3	Periodontal maintenance therapy	Regular professional mechanical dental hygiene care should be encouraged to minimize the risk of recurrence. Continued-care interval should be 2 to 4 months.

involved with stress is not well understood, but it has been postulated that changes in the immune system that occur at stressful times predispose certain individuals to an exuberant bacterial response that results in necrotizing ulcerative disease.

Treatment

The course of a single episode of necrotizing ulcerative periodontitis is usually short but painful. Clients come to the oral care setting most often as a result of the associated pain. Because of the cyclic and recurring nature of the disease, treatment focuses on microbial control through mechanical debridement by both the client and the clinician. It also requires consultation with the client's physician because of possible predisposing systemic factors, such as human immunodeficiency virus infection.[6] Treatment should progress daily during the acute phase of the disease, because the pain often inhibits thorough cleaning by the client or the dental hygienist at one time. Treatment includes periodontal debridement with ultrasonic scalers, plaque biofilm control, and 0.12% chlorhexidine rinses twice daily. The dentist may prescribe a systemic antibiotic if fever and lymphadenopathy are present. The recommended treatment sequence is described in Table 32-2.

Given the signs and symptoms, most clients with necrotizing periodontal diseases have unmet human needs in the areas of freedom from head and neck pain, skin and mucous membrane integrity of the head and neck, and conceptualization and problem solving. Client health and oral health and well-being are the keys to the successful treatment of these diseases. Clients must be knowledgeable about the roles of stress, bacteria, and nutrition in the disease process and encouraged to take control of their oral health and lifestyle behaviors. Suggestions to identify stress-management techniques and to improve nutrition are necessary components of dental hygiene care (see Chapters 35 and 41).

Avulsed Tooth

Prevalence

The avulsion of permanent teeth is the most serious of all dental injuries. The **avulsed tooth** is one that is separated from the alveolar bone by trauma.[11] Although avulsion is not strictly a periodontal emergency, it does involve traumatized teeth that can be replanted successfully if managed properly. The prognosis depends on the measures taken at the scene of the trauma or immediately after avulsion. In some cases, the dental hygienist may be the first person in the dental profession to meet the patient. In this situation, the dental hygienist may have the opportunity to help the parent of a small child or a student or adult participating in athletic activities to preserve an avulsed tooth through quick action.

Traumas to the oral region occur frequently and comprise 5% of all injuries for which people seek treatment. Among preschool children, the figure is as high as 18% of all injuries. Avulsion is the most common dental injury to children who are less than 15 years old. The situation occurs in as many as 1 in every 200 American children, which results in approximately 2 million occurrences per year. Among all facial injuries, dental injuries are the most common; avulsions occur with 1% to 16% of all dental injuries.[12] Replantation is the treatment of choice, but this cannot always be carried out immediately. To meet the client's need for a biologically sound and functional dentition, it is incumbent on the dental hygienist to respond to this dental emergency. However, the dental hygienist should take responsibility to inform parents, children, students, and adults who are participating in athletic activities to use mouth protectors to prevent oral injuries. In addition, information should be given to teachers and coaches about the risk of oral injuries during certain sports activities. Furthermore, replantation should not be performed when primary teeth have been avulsed because of the risk of injury to the underlying permanent tooth germ.[11,12]

An appropriate treatment plan after an injury is important for a good prognosis. Guidelines are useful for dental hygienists, dentists, and other healthcare professionals to use to deliver the best care possible in an efficient manner. The International Association of Dental Traumatology has developed a consensus statement in response to the dental literature and group discussions. Lost time and improper handling of the avulsed tooth can substantially reduce the long-term success of replantation. Moreover, the dental hygienist should inform parents, teachers, and coaches about the procedure; increased awareness can improve the opportunity for successful tooth replantation when injuries that cause avulsed teeth occur.

Good healing after an injury to the teeth and oral tissues depends, in part, on good oral hygiene. Patients should be advised about how best to care for teeth that have received treatment after injury. Brushing with a soft brush and rinsing with 0.12% chlorhexidine are beneficial to prevent the accumulation of plaque and debris.

The procedure for constructing a custom-made athletic mouth protector is described in Procedure 37-7 of Chapter 37. Athletic mouth protectors are highly recommended to prevent tooth avulsion.

Treatment

The dental hygienist might be present at a sporting event or another venue when a tooth is traumatically avulsed, or he or she may have a child who experiences a traumatically avulsed tooth. The avulsed tooth is quickly separated from the alveolus after a fall or a strike of some kind. Typically a layer of periodontal ligament cells remains on the cemental surface of the avulsed tooth and on the bone in the socket because of the very fast occurrence of the trauma. The successful treatment of avulsed teeth by replantation is dependent on rejoining intact periodontal ligament cells covering the tooth's cementum with those that remain in the socket.

The object of this emergency treatment is to promote periodontal ligament healing after the tooth is replanted in the socket. To maximize the chances of healing, the tooth must be handled only by the crown to prevent damage to the remaining periodontal ligament cells. It is essential that the avulsed tooth not dry out and that it not be debrided in any way. As little as 1 hour of dry storage before replantation negatively affects the procedure success rate.[11,12]

The ideal place to store and transport the avulsed tooth is in the socket, if it can be gently placed and held there while the client is taken to an oral healthcare setting or a hospital emergency department. The socket provides the most nutritious environment for the cells of the periodontal ligament, thereby increasing their survival rate. If it is not possible to replace the tooth temporarily in the socket as a result of other injuries associated with the trauma or emotional upset, physiologic saline is a safe alternative. Unfortunately this substance may not be handy. Milk is also a good medium, because it has physiologic osmolality and relatively few bacteria. Saliva has more bacteria than milk, but the use of milk is a good way to keep the tooth moist. However, the client may be too upset or too young to hold the tooth in the mouth. Warm saltwater can prevent dehydration, but it cannot keep the cells alive for long. Air drying or wrapping the tooth in gauze or other materials, even for a short time, is contraindicated, because such a procedure will kill the periodontal ligament cells.[11,12] Alternatives may have to be thought through quickly and a decision made during a stressful situation to avoid the dehydration and death of cells. The options for the storage and transportation of the avulsed tooth are highlighted in Table 32-3. Box 32-10 discusses the documentation of an avulsed tooth.

At the emergency treatment facility, the tooth is removed from its transport medium, gently rinsed, replanted in the socket after the blood clot is removed, and splinted into place. A 5- to 7-day course of systemic antibiotics typically used for dental infections is prescribed. Endodontic procedures need to be performed at a later time (i.e., about 2 weeks after replantation) to avoid inflammatory root resorption.[12] The

TABLE 32-3

Storage of Avulsed Teeth During Transportation for Treatment

Choice	Transportation Medium
First	Replace in socket.
Second	Store in physiologic saline.
Third	Store in cold, fresh milk.
Fourth	Place in the individual's mouth, either under the tongue or in the cheek.
Fifth	Store in warm saltwater.
Sixth	Store in tap water.

BOX 32-10

General Recommendations for the Documentation of an Avulsed Tooth

Clinical examination
- Soft tissues
- Hard tissues (enamel fracture, dentin or pulp exposures)
- Abnormal mobility, tooth displacement
- Tenderness to percussion, percussion (ankylosis) tone
- Electrometric pulpal sensibility

Radiographic examination
- Soft-tissue examination
- Occlusal radiographic exposure of the traumatized region
- Periapical bisecting angle exposure of each traumatized tooth

Final diagnosis and treatment planning

Procedure 32-1 Emergency Management of the Avulsed Tooth

EQUIPMENT

Clean cup or other container
Transport medium

STEPS	RATIONALE
1. Calm the individual or parent.	1. To gain client cooperation and relieve stress
2. Locate the avulsed tooth.	2. To prepare for reinsertion
3. Handle tooth only by the crown and do not dry the tooth; do not debride the tooth.	
4. Place the tooth in the socket or in the transport medium (see Table 32-3).	
5. Contact the dentist or another emergency facility (e.g., dental clinic, hospital emergency department).	
6. Arrange for transportation of the affected individual to the treatment facility.	
7. Document care rendered in the electronic record. For example, "During a hockey game, an accident occurred, and the first right incisor in the upper jaw was avulsed. After 1 hour, the client with the avulsed tooth replaced in the socket was sent for emergency treatment."	

protocol for the management of the avulsed tooth is presented in Procedure 32-1. A comparative summary of the conditions presented in this chapter can be found in Table 32-4.

CLIENT EDUCATION TIPS

- Educate clients about disease transmission and lifestyle influences, particularly those related to the herpesvirus and necrotizing periodontal diseases.
- Educate clients with painful oral infections to consume adequate fluids and nutrient-dense foods, to perform oral hygiene, and to use over-the-counter topical anesthetics to control their discomfort.
- Review methods to prevent the transmission of an active herpetic infection.
- Teach clients with a history of recurrent herpetic infection to cancel dental appointments when an active oral lesion is present.
- Review methods and treatment to prevent the recurrence of pericoronitis and necrotizing periodontal diseases.
- Teach parents, teachers, and coaches about avulsed teeth and their management to improve the probability of successful tooth replantation.
- Teach clients who are at risk for tooth avulsion about the need for a mouth protector.

LEGAL, ETHICAL, AND SAFETY ISSUES

- Dental hygienists have a legal responsibility to recognize emergency conditions, to make appropriate referrals, and to treat those conditions within the scope of dental hygiene practice.
- Dental hygienists have an ethical responsibility to educate clients about the significance of their diseases and the potential for recurrence and the infection of others.
- Dental hygienists have a responsibility to educate and refer clients in cases of dental trauma and to prevent oral injuries when possible.
- Dental hygienists must consider their own personal safety from infectious diseases when treating clients with acute infectious conditions, such as primary herpetic gingivostomatitis or herpes labialis.

TABLE 32-4

Summary Comparison of Acute Gingival and Periodontal Conditions, Lesions of Endodontic Origin, and Avulsed Teeth

Cause	Risk Factors	Signs and Symptoms	Prevention and Management
Acute Periodontal Abscess			
Periodontal pathogens	Deep pockets Untreated periodontal disease	Swelling Redness Pain Exudate Sinus tract may occur	Education about the disease Scaling and root planing Referral for further treatment
Chronic Periodontal Abscess			
Periodontal pathogens	Deep pockets Untreated periodontal disease	Sinus tract Exudate Pain Swelling Redness Acute episodes	Education about the disease Scaling and root planing Referral for further treatment
Gingival Abscess			
Foreign object	Unknown	Swelling Redness Pain Exudate	Education to prevent recurrences Referral for incision and drainage of abscess
Lesion of Endodontic Origin			
Caries Periodontal disease Tooth fracture Traumatic dental procedures	Dental caries Periodontal disease Traumatic injury	Pain Swelling Sinus tract	Education to reduce likelihood of recurrences Referral for definitive endodontic treatment
Combined Periodontal Abscess			
Caries Periodontal disease Tooth fracture Traumatic dental procedures	Dental caries Periodontal disease	Pain Swelling Bone loss	Education to reduce likelihood of recurrences Referral for definitive endodontic and periodontal treatment
Acute Herpetic Gingivostomatitis			
Herpes simplex virus	Age	Ulcers with halos Pain Systemic symptoms	Reappointment for dental procedures Education to prevent transmission to others Supportive care until the virus has run its course
Recurrent Herpetic Lesions			
Herpes simplex virus	History of recurrences Change in immune status	Ulcer on lip or perioral tissues	Reappointment for dental procedures Supportive treatment Education about antiviral drugs Referral to physician

Continued

TABLE 32-4

Summary Comparison of Acute Gingival and Periodontal Conditions, Lesions of Endodontic Origin, and Avulsed Teeth—cont'd

Cause	Risk Factors	Signs and Symptoms	Prevention and Management
Acute Pericoronitis			
Bacterial plaque	Partially erupted molars Operculum	Pain Swelling Redness Foul odor	Education to pursue treatment and prevent recurrences Debridement and irrigation of area
Necrotizing Ulcerative Periodontitis			
Pathogenic bacteria	Systemic disease Stress Smoking	Pain Bleeding Fetid odor Redness Pseudomembrane Cratered papillae	Education to prevent recurrences Debridement over multiple appointments Definitive scaling as soon as possible Consultation with physician
Avulsed Tooth			
Trauma	Contact sports Accidents	Traumatic separation from alveolus	Preservation of tooth in appropriate transport medium (see Table 32-3) Immediate transport to treatment facility for replantation of tooth Referral for endodontic treatment

KEY CONCEPTS

- Periodontal abscess is a treatable and often preventable disease process.
- A lesion of endodontic origin is a serious infection that requires consultation and referral for immediate treatment. Left untreated, a lesion of endodontic origin could develop into a brain abscess or fasciitis of the neck or chest wall, which can be life-threatening.
- Periodontal abscesses have a pathogenic microflora similar to that associated with periodontal diseases.
- Incomplete subgingival scaling and root planing has been suggested as a cause of periodontal abscesses; however, there are few data to support this assumption.
- Abscesses can point and drain through the tissue or simply drain through the periodontal pocket opening.
- Infection moves through tissue along the pathway of least resistance; therefore clinical features of the infection may appear at a distance from the affected tooth.
- Pain may be the key feature for distinguishing between periapical and periodontal abscesses. Periapical pain is sharp, severe, intermittent, and hard to localize; periodontal pain is constant, less severe, and localized.
- Primary and recurrent herpetic infections are serious but self-limiting conditions that require the postponement of elective dental hygiene and dental treatment. Dental hygiene care should not be performed on a client with a herpetic infection because of the risk of transmission of the virus to the dental hygienist and other workers.
- Pericoronitis at any stage is a serious infection that requires referral and definitive treatment.
- Necrotizing periodontal diseases are complex processes that benefit from the dental hygiene process of care.
- Mouth protectors and their fabrication are significant to comprehensive dental hygiene care.
- Avulsion is the most common dental injury among children who are less than 15 years old. The dental hygienist has a role in the management of avulsed teeth as possibly the most knowledgeable person at the traumatic injury scene.
- The ideal place to store and transport an avulsed tooth is in the victim's tooth socket; if this is not possible, physiologic saline is one alternative.

CRITICAL THINKING EXERCISES

1. A 30-year-old client who has not been treated for several years arrives for a dental hygiene appointment. The client wants to have his "teeth cleaned today" but informs you about some pain and sensitivity in the lower right quadrant and a tooth that feels "high" in that same area. The pain is intermittent but "very bothersome." After taking the client's medical and pharmacologic histories, you determine that he is in good general health with no systemic illnesses, and he is taking no medications. Your intraoral findings indicate that the client has redness and swelling on the buccal surface of tooth #30. The gingival architecture appears normal, and there is no sinus tract, but pus can be elicited from the site by gentle finger pressure.
   A. What condition is most likely causing the client's symptoms?

B. What is the most likely treatment for the condition?
C. What dental hygiene diagnosis should be addressed first for this client?

2. A 20-year-old client comes to the dental office complaining of severe pain in her mouth. You determine that the client has no systemic illnesses, and you examine the oral tissues. The oral findings are extreme redness and swollen gingiva throughout the mouth and small, grayish ulcers on the gingiva and mucosa in several areas.
   A. What condition is most likely causing the client's symptoms?
   B. What is the most likely treatment for the condition?
   C. What dental hygiene diagnosis should be addressed first for this client?
3. A client comes to the dental office without an appointment complaining of exquisite pain in her jaw. In fact, the client can hardly open her mouth. A review of the client's medical and pharmacologic histories shows that the client is in good general health and takes no medications. Intraoral findings reveal extremely reddened and swollen gingiva on the mandibular right posterior area. The client complains of a bad taste in her mouth and says that the condition "comes and goes" but that this is the worst pain she has experienced. The client has many large amalgam restorations and appears to have a partially submerged molar in the quadrant.
   A. What is the most likely emergency condition?
   B. How should the dental hygiene component of the overall dental treatment begin?
   C. What dental hygiene diagnosis should be addressed first for this client?
4. A 45-year-old client arrives at the dental office without an appointment and complains of severe pain. You seat the client and determine that she is in good general health, has no systemic illnesses, and is taking no medications. Intraoral examination reveals a large, pointed fistula on the buccal surface of tooth #3, about one third of the way toward the tooth apex. The client has been treated for periodontal disease in the past, including in some areas that required periodontal surgery, and she has many teeth that have been restored with amalgam and composite restorations. There is a large mesial-occlusal-distal amalgam with a lingual extension on tooth #3. The radiograph you just took shows no obvious apical pathology.
   A. What condition is most likely causing the client's symptoms?
   B. What should the dental hygiene component of overall dental treatment that day include?
   C. What dental hygiene diagnosis should be addressed first for this client?
5. A client arrives for his 4-month continued-care appointment. He is very excited to be leaving tomorrow for a 6-month stay in Europe, and he is anxious to have his dental hygiene maintenance care before he leaves. You notice a round, crusted lesion on his lower lip that is 6 mm in diameter, with some vesicles on the edge. He relates to you that he has never had such a sore before and that it was hurting a few days ago but is fine now. He requests that you cover the lesion with petroleum jelly so that it will not crack while you are treating him.
   A. What condition is most likely present on the client's lip?
   B. What is the dental hygiene care protocol for the client?
   C. What dental hygiene diagnosis should be addressed first for this client?

REFERENCES

1. Newman MG, Takei HH, Klokkevold PR, et al: *Carranza's clinical periodontology, expert consult*, ed 11, St Louis, 2012, Saunders.
2. Socransky SS, Haffajee AD: Periodontal microbial ecology, *Periodontol 2000* 38:135, 2005.
3. Herrera D, Roldán S, Sanz M: The periodontal abscess, a review, *J Clin Periodontol* 377:386, 2000.
4. Gomes BP, Jacinto RC, Pinheiro ET, et al: Molecular analysis of *Filifactor alocis, Tannerella forsythia,* and *Treponema denticola* associated with primary endodontic infections and failed endodontic treatment, *J Endod* 32:937, 2006.
5. Nair PN: Pathogenesis of apical periodontitis and the causes of endodontic failures, *Crit Rev Oral Biol Med* 15:348, 2004.
6. Fatahzadeh M, Schwartz RA: Human herpes simplex virus infections: epidemiology, pathogenesis, symptomatology, diagnosis, and management, *J Am Acad Dermatol* 57:737, 2007.
7. Slots J: Human viruses in periodontitis, *Periodontol 2000* 89:110, 2010.
8. Yamalik K, Bozkaya S: The predictivity of mandibular third molar position as a risk indicator for pericoronitis, *Clin Oral Investig* 12:9, 2008.
9. Dogan N, Orhan K, Gunaydin Y, et al: Unerupted mandibular third molars: symptoms, associated pathologies, and indications for removal in a Turkish population, *Quintessence Int* 38:e497, 2007.
10. Folayan MO: The epidemiology, etiology, and pathophysiology of acute necrotizing ulcerative gingivitis associated with malnutrition, *J Contemp Dent Pract* 5:28, 2004.
11. Flores MT, Andersson L, Andreasen JO, et al; International Association of Dental Traumatology: Guidelines for the management of traumatic dental injuries. II. Avulsion of permanent teeth, *Dent Traumatol* 23:130, 2007.
12. Ram D, Cohenca N: Therapeutic protocols for avulsed permanent teeth: review and clinical update, *Pediatr Dent* 26:251, 2004.

ACKNOWLEDGMENT

The author acknowledges Dorothy A. Perry for her past contributions to this chapter.

Refer to the Procedures Manual where rationales are provided for the steps outlined in the procedure presented in this chapter.

ⓔ EVOLVE RESOURCES

Please visit http://evolve.elsevier.com/Darby/hygiene for additional practice and study support tools.

CHAPTER 33

Caries Management: Fluoride and Nonfluoride Caries-Preventive Agents

Diana Lamoreux

COMPETENCIES

1. Discuss factors involved in caries management.
2. Discuss fluoride therapies, including:
   - Distinguish between the different types of ingested fluorides used for dental caries management and how each type relates to caries risk.
   - Differentiate between acute and chronic fluoride toxicity including causes, signs, symptoms, and management.
   - Identify the methods of delivery for topical fluorides used in dental caries management.
3. Name and describe the self-applied products for clients at risk for caries.
4. Name and describe the professionally applied fluorides for caries management, including product selection and the tray and paint-on techniques.
5. Discuss acute fluoride toxicity including causes, signs, symptoms, emergency management, and prevention.
6. Discuss the evidence-based research and ADA recommendations of nonfluoride caries-preventive agents.
7. Explain why xerostomia places clients at higher risk for caries and address recommendations to manage the symptoms and associated caries risk.
8. Describe the future of caries prevention.
9. Design a caries management plan based on sound clinical judgment and client risk, needs, and preferences.

Caries Risk Assessment

See Chapter 18.

Caries Management[3,7,8,16]

To determine the caries risk for an individual, the number and severity of **pathologic factors** (factors that contribute to the possibility that a client will develop caries) and existing **protective factors** (factors that can improve the chances that a client will not develop caries) are evaluated by the clinician (see Chapter 18, Figure 18-5). Thereafter the integration of evidence-based research, caries risk assessment, clinical observation, radiographic evaluation, professional judgment, and client preferences determine recommendations.

Figures, tables, and boxes marked as "e" are available as supplemental material on the Evolve site. Visit http://evolve.elsevier.com/Darby/hygiene to access these materials.

Caries management is aimed at restoring and maintaining the caries balance, a balance between pathologic factors and protective factors. Remineralization of early carious lesions and/or prevention of future caries can be accomplished by decreasing pathologic factors and increasing protective factors: clients with higher pathologic risk require more protective factors. See Chapter 18 for a discussion of caries management strategies to decrease pathologic factors and increase protective factors.

Caries Management and American Dental Association Recommendations[3,7,8]

The American Dental Association (ADA) Council on Scientific Affairs periodically releases evidence-based clinical recommendations. These recommendations are based on a review of research studies meeting pre-established criteria for inclusion. Randomized controlled clinical trials (RCTs) are considered the gold standard for therapeutic interventions. An RCT is a specific type of scientific experiment designed to test the efficacy or effectiveness of various interventions within a given population; it randomly assigns study participants into one of two or more groups, with one of the interventions being the control. In this review, the ADA panel considered RCTs but also considered nonrandomized trials to formulate its recommendations.[3] These ADA reviews yield product and protocol endorsements.

Apart from product and protocol recommendations, the ADA also released the following guidelines for clinicians: Practitioners first should implement the use of fluorides and sealants in conjunction with dietary counseling before attempting any nonfluoride therapies; recommendations always must be based on a balance of professional judgment and patient preference; and it is standard of care that client compliance with professional recommendations be assessed 3 to 6 months after initial presentation.[3] Recommendations then should be modified or reinforced based on bacterial results and salivary flow assessment, as needed to complete a comprehensive assessment of caries risk and client compliance (see Chapter 18, Boxes 18-2 through 18-5).

Fluoride Therapies[6-9,11,16]

See Chapter 18 for an overview of fluoride therapies.

Fluoride is a naturally occurring nutrient that in the right concentrations can decrease dental caries risk and has a reparative (remineralizing) effect. When fluoride is absorbed by the enamel, along with calcium and phosphate, during the remineralization process, it establishes an improved crystal structure that is more acid resistant. Fluoride also offers a topical antimicrobial action and affects carbohydrate metabolism, acid production, and bacterial adhesive properties.[8]

Fluorides are delivered to teeth in different dosages and in a variety of ways. Fluoride can be **ingested** via drinking water, foods, beverages, and supplements or delivered **topically** by client-applied and professionally applied techniques:

- Community water fluoridation, foods, and beverages containing fluoride and prescription supplements are ingested and delivered via the bloodstream systemically and topically.
- Topical fluoride products (client-applied in a nonprescription or prescription form and professionally applied products) are delivered for prescribed amounts of time to exposed crown and root surfaces and then expectorated.

Ingested Fluoride

Community Water Fluoridation[1,12]

The 2010 Centers for Disease Control and Prevention (CDC) statistics determined that 73.9% of the U.S. population resides in communities where the water supply is fluoridated. The notion of fluoridating the community water supply grew out of a need to address the prevalence of dental caries in the United States in the 1940s and is the most common fluoride delivery system. At that time people were not exposed to the myriad of fluoride-containing products that the population experiences today. One of the 10 great public health achievements of the twentieth century, community water fluoridation, is a nearly ideal public health intervention.

Community water fluoridation systems have the following characteristics and advantages:

- Inexpensive and cost effective
- Systemic effect demonstrated by caries prevalence and severity has decrease of about 50%, statistics vary
- Eminently safe at recommended levels (exhaustive studies conducted since 1951)
- Equitable (benefits all people with access to community water systems)
- Not dependent on client compliance; a cooperative effort
- Beneficial topical effect long-term enhances remineralization, inhibits demineralization
- Instrumental in reducing costs for dental treatment
- Not dependent on professional services of a licensed healthcare provider

As a public health measure, community water fluoridation requires periodic testing of the water supply to determine the naturally occurring level of fluoride. The level of fluoride then is adjusted through fluoridation or defluoridation to the accepted level of 0.7 part per million (ppm) recommended by the Centers for Disease Control (CDC). Upon request city water systems are required to provide customers with an annual "water quality report."[12] Defluoridation is mandatory when the naturally occurring level of fluoride in the water exceeds the recommended level for a given area. Too much fluoride in community water has the potential of causing chronic fluoride toxicity in children.

Community Water Fluoridation and Antifluoridationists[1,3,7,8,12]

Although the benefits of community water fluoridation are well documented, some individuals continue to oppose this public health measure and actively seek, and have succeeded, to prevent or reverse water fluoridation programs. In the 18 months following January 2011, 43 states had faced activities to initiate, retain, or defeat fluoridation, with the city of Milwaukee voting to abolish it.[12]

The opposition acknowledges that fluoride is beneficial in fighting decay but questions whether it is safe for consumption.[12] Some associate fluoride ingestion with an increased risk for certain systemic diseases and conditions (i.e., congenital anomalies, bone fractures, Alzheimer's disease, cancer, skeletal fluorosis, lower IQ) and others view mandated fluoride ingestion as a conspiracy by such entities as the government or the healthcare industry. Antifluoridationists also cite cost, freedom of choice, and a violation of individual and religious rights as reasons for their stance against adding fluoride to community water supplies.

Fluoride in Food and Beverages[1,2,10,11]

Community water fluoridation has a more than 65-year history of success in reducing caries incidence and prevalence. However, the public currently is exposed to a variety of fluoride-containing food, beverages, and additives that have become part of everyone's overall exposure to topical and systemic fluoride. Consequently, there is considerable variation in the amount of fluoride in products routinely ingested. Thorough questioning is necessary to document this information during client assessment procedures, especially in the case of children with developing teeth. Age-appropriate use of fluoride is ideal; daily fluoride exposure should be determined for young clients, monitored, and reassessed often.

Infants primarily ingest breast milk, cow's milk, or milk- and soy-based formulas. Fluoride levels are generally low in human breast milk (<0.01 ppm) and cow's milk (0.05 ppm). When the formula and infant food industry recognized that milk-based formula may be reconstituted with fluoridated water, many voluntarily reduced the fluoride content in powdered formula. Formula packaging should be consulted to determine fluoride levels in prepared powders; for example, soy-based formulas contain more fluoride than do milk-based products.

Beverages prepared from natural ingredients can be a systemic and topical source of fluoride. Raw tea leaves and tea tree oils are high in fluoride content and contain as much as 400 ppm of fluoride. Brewed tea contains an average of 3 ppm of fluoride. Children may be at risk for dental fluorosis (chronic excessive fluoride) in some areas (e.g., England, Australia, India, parts of Asia) where it is customary to drink tea regularly, at a young age, during tooth development.

The fluoride level in processed beverages and bottled waters varies considerably. For example, fluoride content in fruit juices and carbonated beverages ranges from less than 0.1 to 6.7 ppm. Differences in fluoride content in processed beverages are attributed to the variations in the fluoride levels of the water used to prepare these products.[2] Although there is variation in the fluoride content of bottled waters (distilled, drinking, mineral, natural spring), these beverages generally have low fluoride concentration. Given that consumption of tap water among U.S. children has declined and consumption of other beverages, especially bottled water, has grown, it is becoming increasingly difficult to assess clients' fluoride exposure by fluid intake.

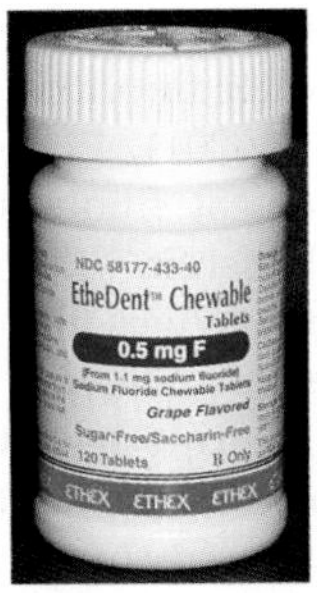

Figure 33-1. Example of a fluoride supplement available by prescription.

TABLE 33-1

Fluoride Supplements Dosage Schedule (Milligrams of Fluoride per Day)*

	LEVEL OF FLUORIDE IN PRIMARY WATER SUPPLY		
Client Age	**<0.3 ppm Fl**	**0.3-0.6 ppm Fl**	**>0.6 ppm Fl†**
Birth to 6 months	None	None	None
6 months to 3 years	0.25 mg	None†	None†
3 years to 6 years	0.50 mg	0.25 mg	None
6 years to at least 16 years	1.0 mg	0.50 mg	None

Data from American Dental Association, Chicago, Illinois; American Academy of Pediatric Dentistry, Chicago, Illinois; and American Academy of Pediatrics, Elk Grove Village, Illinois.

Fl, Fluoride; *ppm*, parts per million.

*2.2 mg of sodium fluoride provides 1 mg of fluoride ions.

†Infants receiving their total diet from breast-feeding need a 0.25-mg supplement.

Other foodstuffs such as shellfish, sardines, fruit juices, carbonated soft drinks, some wines, raisins, cereal, and chicken also may contain substantial levels of fluoride. Prepared foods generally are processed in urban areas with fluoridated water and become additional sources of fluoride for individuals living in fluoridated and nonfluoridated communities. Internationally, other foodstuffs are used as vehicles for delivering fluoride (e.g., in Switzerland, Jamaica, and France) and incorporate fluoride into table salt.[2]

Prescription Fluoride Supplements[1,2,7,8,11,18]

Fluoride supplements in the form of drops, syrups, lozenges, and tablets can provide systemic and topical (if lozenge or tablet is sucked or chewed for 2 minutes) fluoride to children residing in communities without water fluoridation or where well water has low or undetectable levels of fluoride (Figure 33-1).[8] The goal of supplementation is to offer children in nonfluoridated communities a caries reduction advantage similar to children living in fluoridated communities. Clients should be advised to avoid milk products after all fluoride supplements because calcium interferes with the **bioavailability** (dosage available at the site) of fluoride.

Fluoride supplementation recommendations are based on client age, the level of fluoride in the primary water source, and all other sources of fluoride derived from diet (see Chapter 12 and Table 33-1). Fluoride supplementation remains a dilemma, because numerous other sources provide children with fluoride. Dental hygienists can play an important role in analyzing clients' intake and consulting with pediatricians, primary medical care providers, and pediatric dentists. This consultation prevents duplicate prescriptions for supplements and the risk of chronic fluoride toxicity.

In December 2011 the ADA Council on Scientific Affairs issued a statement saying that only children at high risk of developing caries along with deficient primary water supply should receive supplements as follows: ages 6 months to 3 years, 0.25 to 1.00 mg per day; ages 3 to 16, 0.5 to 1.0 mg per day (see ADA Fluoride Supplements Dosage Schedule, Table 33-1).

Regardless of the ADA guidelines, considerable controversy remains regarding dosage because of the following factors:

- Fluoride supplementation increases risk for chronic fluoride toxicity; the risk has increased over the years because of multiple fluoride sources.
- Fluoride supplements can interfere with some medications.[2]
- Prescription fluoride supplements may be inaccurate, and supplements may be prescribed inadvertently by multiple healthcare providers.[2]
- Fluoride supplements may be used unnecessarily in fluoridated communities.
- Fluoride supplements may be recommended erroneously for individuals with untested fluoride levels in well water.
- Compliance of clients or caregivers may be poor.
- Risk of acute toxicity if supplements are not kept sealed and out of reach of small children. (See discussion later in this chapter and Box 33-2 for management protocol.)
- The use of prenatal fluoride supplements is not recommended for pregnant women; permanent teeth do not develop in utero.

The Risk of Chronic Fluoride Toxicity[1,2,7,8,11,12,18]

Dental fluorosis is the hypomineralization of the enamel that results from the chronic ingestion of fluoride that exceeds optimal levels. Dental fluorosis is detected by clinical evaluation and classified by degree (Table 33-2). Mild dental fluorosis is often difficult to identify and requires careful assessment and good lighting. Although some consider fluorosis to be an aesthetic concern only, in its most severe state the enamel is brittle and actually may break down. This alteration in the enamel occurs during tooth formation and is therefore a risk only during the pre-eruptive stages of tooth development (Figure 33-2).

Dental fluorosis is associated with chronic fluoride toxicity and can occur only as a result of systemic ingestion of fluoride during tooth development, that is, children 8 years of age and younger. An increase in the prevalence of enamel fluorosis the past two decades may stem from an increase in the

TABLE 33-2
Classification of Degree of Dental Fluorosis

Grade of Fluorosis	Description
Normal	None
Questionable	A few white flecks or white spots
Very mild	Small, opaque, paper-white areas involving less than 25% of the surface
Mild	White opacities are more extensive but do not involve as much as 50% of the surface
Moderate	All enamel surfaces affected; frequent brown staining
Severe	Discrete or confluent pitting; brown stains are widespread; all enamel surfaces affected

Adapted from Newburn E: *Fluorides and dental caries*, Springfield, IL, 1986, Charles C Thomas.

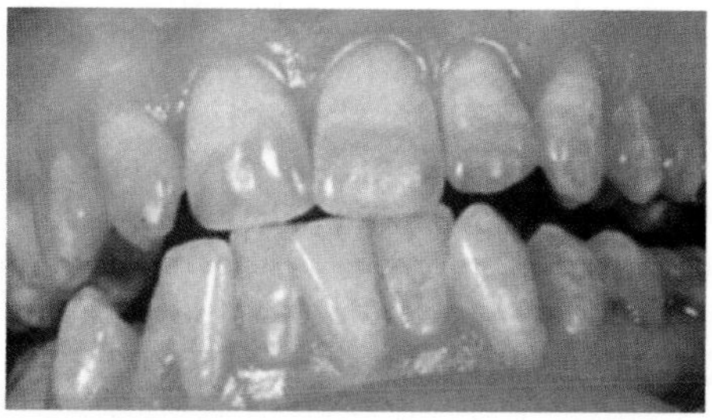

Figure 33-2. Moderate dental fluorosis. (From Ibsen OAC, Phelan JA: *Oral pathology for the dental hygienist*, ed 6, St Louis, 2013, Saunders.)

number of sources of exposure to fluoride. Studies have shown a correlation between fluorosis and individuals who develop hypothyroidism and brittle bones.[2]

People cannot develop fluorosis as a result of topical fluoride exposure, even if the topical exposure is excessive (high-concentration fluoride at frequent intervals). The only way an individual can develop dental fluorosis from topical fluoride is by chronic swallowing of the product during periods of tooth development, which would change the mechanism of fluoride action from topical to systemic.

Fluorosis risk increases with chronic ingestion of low-concentration fluoride products such as fluoride-containing dentifrices or mouth rinses. These products are concerning because they are sometimes used unsupervised by young children, have an appealing taste and appearance, are often swallowed, and sometimes are stored within reach of small children. Careful observation of children during oral care prevents this risk.

Although the administration of professionally applied, high-concentration fluoride products initially may appear to be a risk factor for dental fluorosis, scientific evidence confirms that some fluoride ingestion occurs as the result of topical treatments and that plasma levels of fluoride are elevated slightly after the treatment. Even though fluoride concentration in professionally administered products is high, the infrequent application of these products poses little to no risk and does not result in clinically evident enamel disturbances.

Ingested Fluoride—Issues for Consideration[1,2,7,8,11,18]

- Ingested fluoride delivery, especially community water fluoridation, has an impressive history of success in reducing caries incidence and prevalence.
- Community water fluoridation remains a successful public health approach and is the cornerstone of a fluoride protocol and caries management program. This systemic fluoride vehicle is available to all individuals residing in fluoridated communities, regardless of socioeconomic background or ability to access other fluoride therapies. (Clinicians can direct clients to the U.S. Department of Health and Human Services, Centers for Disease Control and Prevention website, "My Water's Fluoride," for their community's statistics.)
- Debate continues regarding the need for additional systemic supplementation. Need should be based on the multiple sources of fluoride children receive from processed foodstuffs, prepared beverages, and naturally occurring fluoride.
- Bottled waters often have low fluoride concentrations and sometimes do not reveal fluoride content. Many households use bottled water as their primary water source. Increased numbers of manufacturers do identify fluoride content on product labels. Other companies are adding fluoride as a marketing tool (e.g., "nursery water with fluoride").
- Water filtration systems often remove significant amounts of fluoride from water.
- Individuals commonly attach water filtration devices (reverse osmosis, bubbling ozone, activated charcoal, and so on) to household water taps.
- Persons who use well water as their primary water source should have the water tested to determine fluoride level. Without this information, it is impossible to prescribe fluoride supplements accurately. Dental hygienists can facilitate by providing clients with contact information, testing kits, and specimen submission guidelines.
- Well water may contain water from multiple sources with varying fluoride concentrations.
- Some water supplies are monitored poorly for optimal fluoride levels.
- There may be a systemic effect from topical fluoride preparations. Some topical preparations, especially fluoride-containing dentifrices and oral rinses, may be swallowed, causing the client to receive a topical and systemic exposure to fluoride. Children using fluoride products must be monitored to decrease risk of acute and chronic fluoride toxicity. (See Box 33-2 for management protocol.)

Topical Fluoride

Topical fluoride is delivered into the oral cavity in three primary forms (see Chapter 18):

- Self-applied by clients in the form of nonprescription products available over the counter (OTC) applied frequently, or low (potency) fluoride concentration (Note: Products that carry the ADA Seal of Acceptance or the

Canadian Dental Association [CDA] Seal of Recognition should be recommended first to clients.)
- Self-applied by clients in the form of prescription products; higher concentration of fluoride than OTC products for higher caries risk
- Professionally applied prescription products, high (potency) fluoride concentration, used less frequently, every 3 to 6 months (Note: The ADA suggests that clients who are low caries risk may not receive additional benefit from professional fluoride applications.[7])

The myriad product types and concentrations offered OTC and by prescription can be confusing. It is important to focus on the fluoride concentration/parts per million and client risk level when choosing and recommending products for clients. Typically, OTC self-applied topical fluoride agents for at-home use are lower in fluoride concentration (fewer parts per million) than those that are applied in office.

The action of high-potency fluorides is similar to low-potency fluorides; repeated exposure is necessary for both to maintain a high concentration on tooth surfaces. The difference is that exposure is needed less often with high-concentration fluorides. A low fluoride level maintained in saliva, biofilm, and enamel can prevent or help control caries throughout life. Because fermentable carbohydrate exposures create daily opportunities for enamel demineralization, the frequent use of topical, low-potency fluoride products is recommended for the daily management of areas of demineralization and prevention of dental caries (Table 33-3). See the website for information on dentifrices/toothpastes and eFig 33-3.

Fluoride and Children

Special consideration must be given when recommending fluoridated dentifrices for children under 6 years of age. The primary concern is that young children swallow toothpastes because they enjoy the taste and/or are not capable of (or efficient at) expectorating dentifrice from their mouths. Only 5% of children younger than 2½ years of age expectorate after brushing and only 32% of 2½- to 4-year-olds expectorate.[11] This inability to expectorate results in the ingestion of an agent designed for topical use and increases dental fluorosis risk. When recommending dentifrices for young children, dental professionals must involve the client's parent or caregiver and emphasize the following:
- The importance of supervising children when brushing their teeth until more than 6 years of age
- Involving parents and caregivers in decisions about use of fluoride
- Delaying introduction of fluoridated toothpaste until some children are 2 years of age if the ability to refrain from swallowing is not anticipated
- Limiting toothpaste to a smear from 6 months until the age of 2; a pea-sized amount after the age of 2 (These ADA-recommended amounts provide adequate dosage and little risk when supervised.)
- Stressing the importance of fully expectorating and not rinsing after brushing with a fluoridated dentifrice
- Avoiding higher-concentration fluoride in toothpastes and refraining from use of other fluoride products (rinses) with children under 6 years of age
- Storing fluoridated products out of the reach of children

TABLE 33-3

Topical Fluorides: Self-Applied Pastes, Rinses, and Gels

Fluoride Agent	Fluoride Concentration	Frequency of Application	Method of Delivery	Availability and Examples of Products
0.1% sodium fluoride (NaF) or 0.1% sodium monofluorophosphate (MFP) dentifrices	1000-1500 ppm Some countries manufacture children's toothpaste at 50-550 ppm	Twice daily	Brush-on	OTC: Crest, Colgate, Arm & Hammer
0.05% NaF rinse	230 ppm	Once daily	Rinse	OTC examples: Act, Fluorigard
0.2% neutral NaF rinse	910 ppm	Once weekly	Rinse; typically in a school-based program	Prescription examples: Fluorinse, PreviDent
0.4% stable stannous fluoride (SnF_2) gel	1000 ppm	Once daily	Brush-on after brushing with conventional dentifrice	OTC example: Gel-Kam
1.1% neutral NaF gel	5000 ppm	Once daily	Custom tray or brush-on after using conventional dentifrice	Prescription examples: PreviDent, NeutraCare
1.1% NaF and acidulated phosphate fluoride	5000 ppm	Once daily	Custom tray or brush-on after using conventional dentifrice	Prescription example: PreviDent, Clinpro5000

Adapted from Warren DP, Chan JT: Topical fluorides: efficacy, administration, and safety, *Gen Dent* 45:134, 1997.
OTC, Over-the-counter; *ppm*, parts per million.

Self-Applied Products for Clients at Risk for Caries: Rinses, Gels, and Pastes[1,7-9,11,12,16]

Over-the-Counter Daily Client-Applied Fluoride Mouth Rinses

Low-potency, high-frequency fluoride rinses, usually 0.02% or 0.05% NaF (sodium fluoride) compounds with at least 230 ppm (e.g., Act by Chattem Inc., Listerine Total Care by Johnson & Johnson, Crest Pro Health by Oral-B), can be used daily as an adjunct to brushing with a fluoridated dentifrice to manage dental caries (see Table 33-3). Research suggests that daily fluoride rinsing reduces caries 30% to 35%. Clients should be instructed specifically to use 1 to 2 teaspoons of the rinse, to swish vigorously for 60 seconds, and then to expectorate thoroughly. Because there is a risk for young children to swallow fluoride rinses, this product is not recommended for children under 6 years of age and should be stored out of reach. Older children with a moderate-to-high caries risk should use alcohol-free fluoride rinses. Parents and caregivers should check labels carefully.

Prescription Client-Applied Fluoride Mouth Rinses

Low-potency, high-frequency 0.044% NaF in an acidulated/APF solution (e.g., OrthoWash Daily Rinse by 3M ESPE) (phosphoric acid added to fluoride lowers the pH and enhances the rate of reaction between fluoride and hydroxyapatite) used daily and 0.2% neutral NaF rinses (Prevident by Colgate, Nupro by Dentsply, Fluorinse by Oral-B, Cavi-Rinse by 3M) that equate to 1000 ppm used weekly are available by prescription only (see Figure 33-4). Clients must rinse for a full 60 seconds to achieve maximum results with fluoride rinses. Prescription rinses generally are indicated for the following:

- Caries, white spot lesions/demineralized areas, caries prevention
- Dentinal hypersensitivity
- Orthodontic clients
- Clients with xerostomia
- Moderate caries risk
- Exposed roots

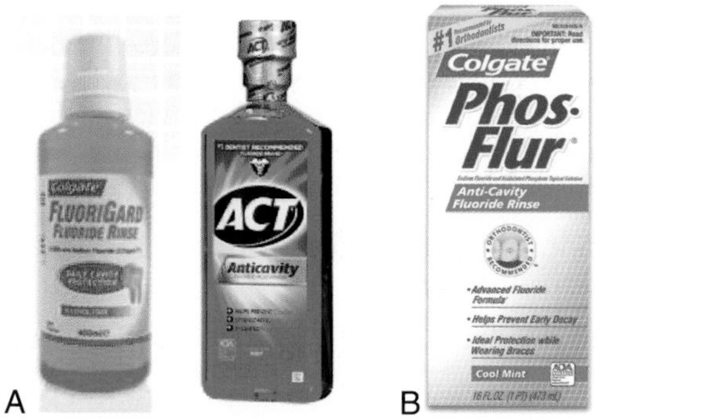

Figure 33-4. **A** and **B,** Sample of over-the-counter 0.05% sodium fluoride rinses with the American Dental Association Seal of Acceptance. (**A** and **B,** Courtesy Colgate Oral Pharmaceuticals, New York, New York; and Chattem, Inc, Chattanooga, Tennessee.)

A prescription 0.63% SnF_2 (stannous fluoride) rinse (PerioMed by 3M ESPE, Fluoridex by Philips, Oral Rinse by Oral Science offers 5% xylitol added) is diluted per manufacturer's directions and can be used twice daily for up to 4 weeks after nonsurgical periodontal therapy as an antimicrobial (stannous fluoride has demonstrated antimicrobial activity against periodontal pathogens and *S. mutans*), to manage dentinal hypersensitivity, and to protect against root caries. Evidence is not as strong, however, supporting this option in comparison to stannous fluoride dentifrices.

Prescription Weekly Fluoride Mouth Rinses in School-Based Programs

High-potency, low-frequency NaF rinses (0.2%), 910 to 1000 ppm, also are used weekly in school-based programs for children who do not reside in communities with water fluoridation (e.g., Fluorinse by Oral-B, PreviDent by Colgate, Nupro by Dentsply, Cavi-Rinse by 3M). School-based programs are effective because they are administered by school personnel, closely supervised, performed as part of a class schedule, and result in good compliance. Young children rinse with 1 teaspoon; older children and adults rinse with 2 teaspoons. After 60 seconds of brisk rinsing, the product is expectorated. Up to 55% caries reduction has been reported with regular weekly use. Weekly fluoride rinses are the highest concentration allowed for individual use and may be administered at home with strict supervision.

Over-the-Counter and Prescription Daily Fluoride Gels and Pastes

These products (available in prescription strength higher concentrations of acidulated phosphorus fluoride (APF) and neutral sodium fluoride) also can reduce caries 30% to 35% and are designed for daily use by clients with high or extreme caries risk, for example, rampant caries, xerostomia, head and neck radiation exposure, dentinal hypersensitivity, or special needs. Careful client, parent, and caregiver education is required when these products are recommended and used at home. The products should be used as directed in a custom tray or brushed on the teeth for 1 minute and then expectorated. Clients may prefer the convenience of brushing when feasible. Most manufacturer tray instructions are as follows:

- Remove oral biofilm with toothbrush, floss, interdental aid, and tongue cleaner
- Load tray with fluoride gel or paste, per product directions
- Dry teeth with cloth or gauze
- Place loaded tray over the desired arch; hold head upright and avoid swallowing product and saliva; suggest clients frequently expectorate during tray placement
- Leave tray on arch for 4 minutes; remove tray and expectorate several times
- Repeat steps for the other arch
- Do not eat or drink for 30 minutes to maintain level of ambient fluoride
- Rinse, clean, and air-dry trays

OTC fluoride gels are marketed as a 0.4% SnF_2/1000 ppm OTC product (Gel-Kam) and 1.1% neutral NaF prescription gel (PreviDent by Colgate, NeutraCare by Oral-B) (see Figure 33-5).

Prescription toothpastes are available as 1.1% NaF with 5% potassium nitrate (e.g., PreviDent5000 Sensitive) and 1.1%

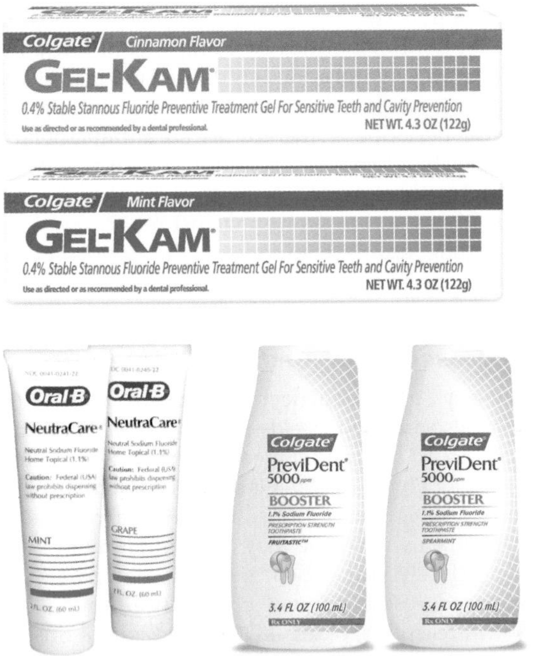

Figure 33-5. Examples of 0.4% stable stannous fluoride gels and pastes, and 1.1% sodium fluoride prescription toothpaste. (Colgate products courtesy Colgate Oral Pharmaceuticals, New York, New York; Oral-B products courtesy Procter & Gamble, Cincinnati, Ohio.)

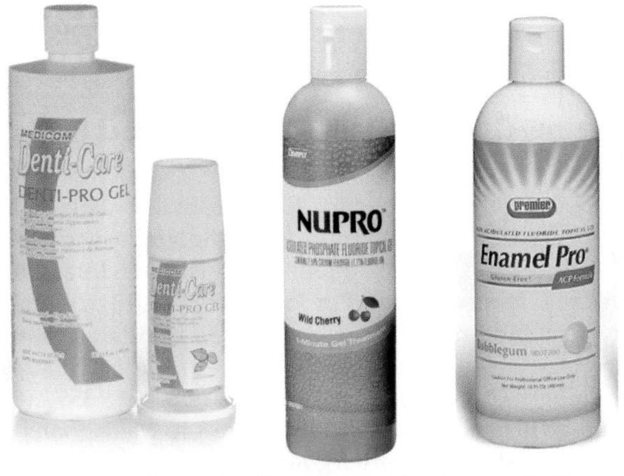

Figure 33-6. Topical fluoride gels for professional applications.

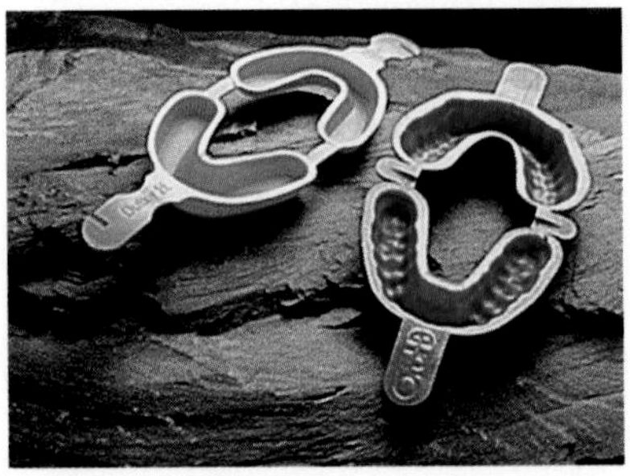

Figure 33-7. Dual-arch trays. (Courtesy *Dental Hygienist News*, funded by an educational grant from Procter & Gamble, Cincinnati, Ohio, and published by Harfst Associates, Inc, Troy, Michigan.)

NaF/5000 ppm (e.g., PreviDent, Clinpro 5000 with tricalcium phosphate, by 3M ESPE, Figure 33-5). Some gels and pastes have varied degrees of abrasives and others do not. Pastes and gels with high fluoride content should not be used in custom trays overnight.[9]

These products recently have gained widespread use for clients with special needs. Clinicians should be diligent about educating clients and caregivers that some of these products do not contain cleaning ingredients or abrasives. When this is the case, clients must be instructed to use such gels and pastes *after* toothbrushing with a conventional OTC fluoride dentifrice. Furthermore, clients should be reminded that these products are available by prescription owing to their moderate levels of fluoride and therefore should be stored carefully out of the reach of children.

Because young children may swallow fluoride gels and pastes, such products are not recommended for children under 6 years of age or those who have difficulties controlling swallowing. Although a very limited number of studies document their efficacy, the ADA Council on Scientific Affairs has approved OTC SnF_2 gels (Gel-Kam by Colgate). In addition, the U.S. Food and Drug Administration (FDA) approved SnF_2 gels for sale OTC because they contain the same fluoride concentration as conventional dentifrices.

Professionally Applied Fluorides: Gel, Foam, Rinse, and Varnish[6,7,9,11,14,16]

Fluoride "treatments" are one of the last procedures performed in the appointment sequence and are administered solely by licensed or certified dental professionals. (Fluoride-containing prophylaxis pastes should not be used in place of this service.) Professionally applied topical fluoride products, gels, and varnishes have been used successfully (Figures 33-6 and 33-19). Although fluoride foams (not ADA-endorsed) and in-office rinses (not FDA-approved) also are used, few data support their efficacy. More research is needed before foams and rinses can be used with the same confidence as gels and varnishes.[7]

Gel (and foam) fluoride products typically are delivered using a 4-minute disposable tray (Procedure 33-1, Figure 33-7); varnishes are applied using a paint-on technique (Procedure 33-2). Considerable data on caries reduction and prevention with 4-minute tray placement are plentiful. (Data regarding caries prevention with regular varnish application are pending.) One-minute gels and foams in trays and 2-minute rinses are used widely, but research is needed to document their effectiveness in comparison with other delivery mechanisms; the ADA does not endorse them. Clinicians and clients often prefer these fluoride delivery systems because they are quicker and easier. However, contemporary standards of practice require that dental hygienists make client care decisions based on scientific evidence.

Professionally Applied Fluoride Products: Evolution and Types

Professionally applied fluoride evolved from solutions to gels to thixotropic gels (gels that flow under pressure, remain viscous when not under pressure) to foams. Gels initially were developed for ease of application and use with fluoride trays. However, cellulose added to gels to increase viscosity inhibited the fluoride to flow into critical areas. To overcome this problem, thixotropic gels were devised.

Procedure 33-1 Professionally Applied Topical Fluoride Using the Tray Technique for In-Office Fluoride Treatment (Gel or Foam)

EQUIPMENT

Mouth mirror
Cotton forceps
Fluoride tray(s)
Cotton rolls
1.23% acidulated phosphate fluoride (APF) or 2.0% sodium fluoride gel
Air syringe
Timer
Saliva ejector
2 × 2 gauze
Tissues
2-oz cup
Personal protective barriers and equipment barriers

STEPS

1. Assemble equipment (Figure 33-8).
2. Seat client in upright position. Reiterate benefits and obtain informed consent (Figure 33-9).
3. Try tray of appropriate size. Complete dentition must be covered, including areas of recession (Figure 33-10).

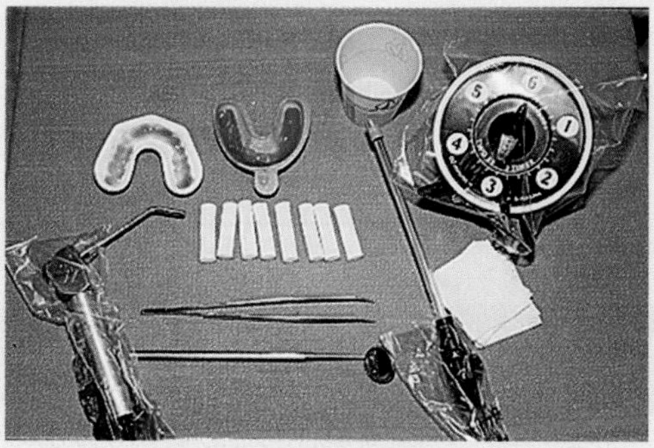

Figure 33-8.

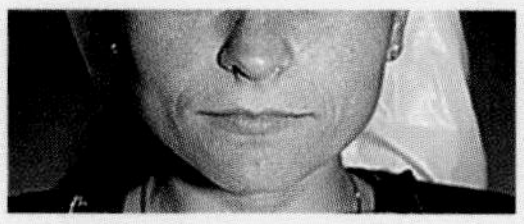

Figure 33-9.

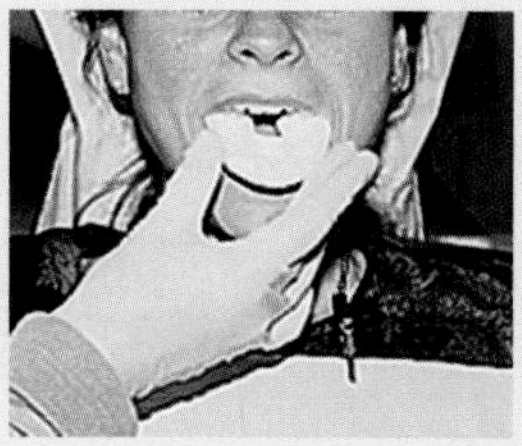

Figure 33-10.

4. Load fluoride gel into trays: 2 mL maximum per tray for small children; 4 mL maximum per tray for large children (>44 lb), 2.5 mL maximum per tray for adults (Figure 33-11).
5. Isolate teeth with cotton rolls. Dry with air syringe (Figure 33-12).

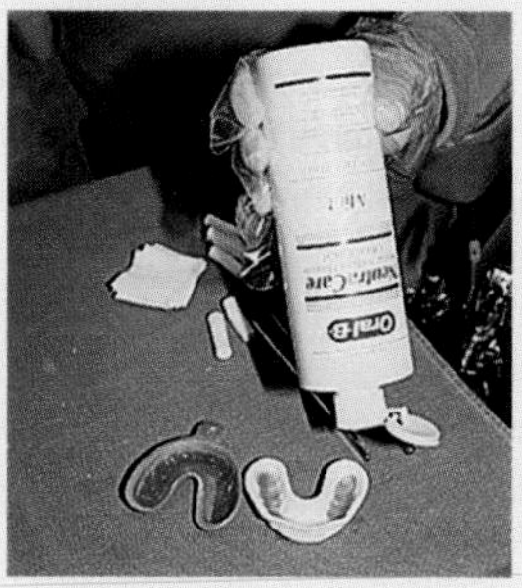

Figure 33-11.

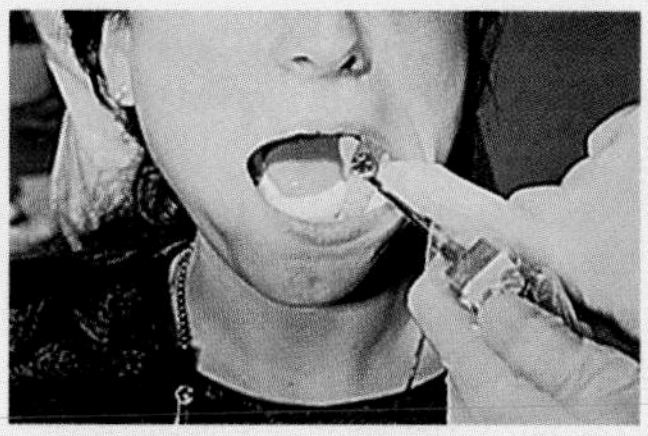

Figure 33-12.

6. Insert both trays or a dual arch tray in mouth (Figures 33-7, 33-13, and 33-14).
7. Press tray against teeth and ask client to close mouth and bite gently on trays or cotton rolls (Figure 33-15).

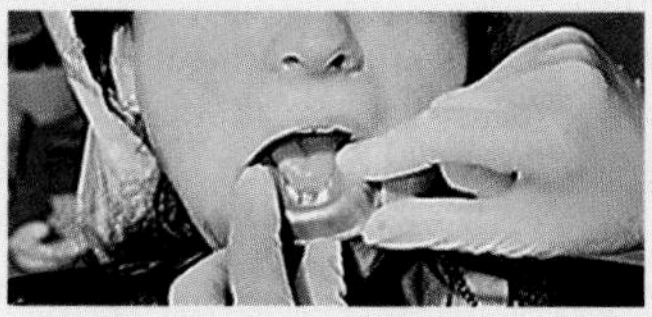

Figure 33-13.

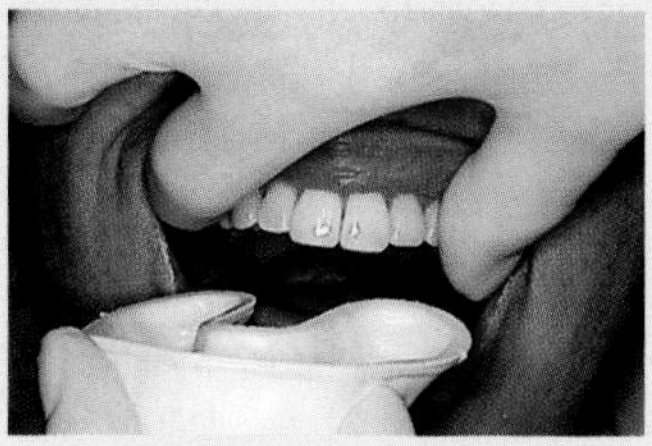

Figure 33-14.

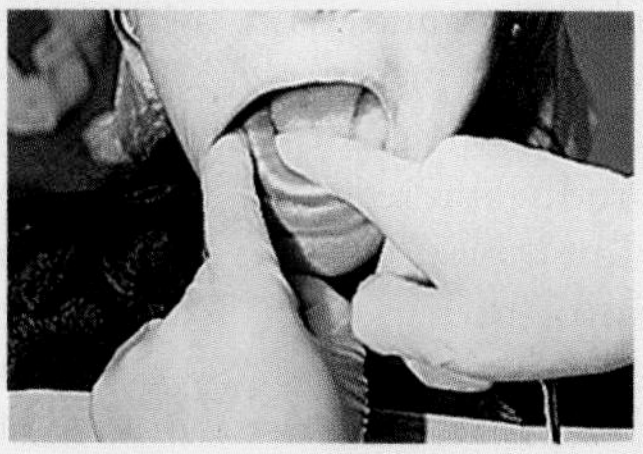

Figure 33-15.

Continued

Procedure 33-1 Professionally Applied Topical Fluoride Using the Tray Technique for In-Office Fluoride Treatment (Gel or Foam)—cont'd

8. Place saliva ejector over mandibular tray. Set timer for 4 minutes. Never leave client unattended during procedure (Figure 33-16).
9. Tilt chin down to remove trays (Figure 33-17).
10. Ask client to expectorate; suction excess fluoride from the mouth with saliva ejector (Figure 33-18).

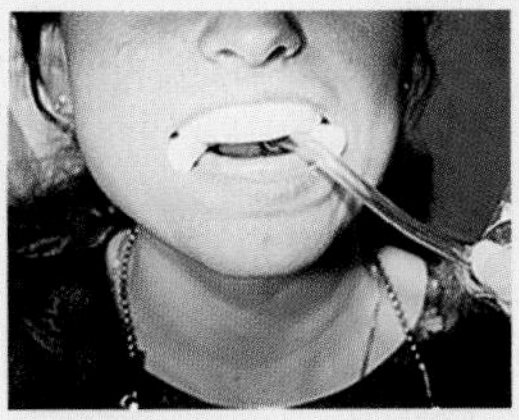

Figure 33-16.

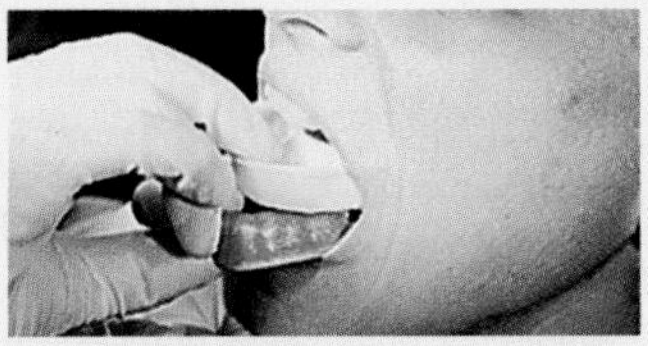

Figure 33-17.

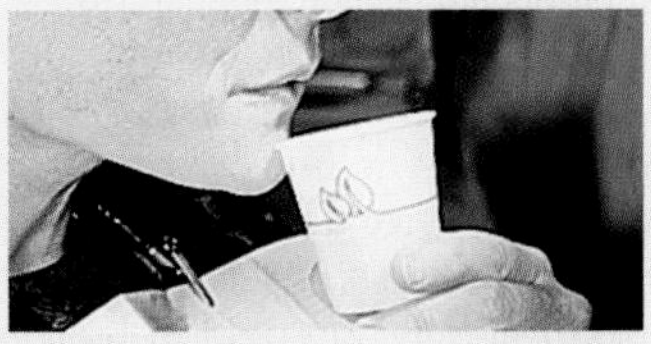

Figure 33-18.

11. Instruct client not to eat, drink, or rinse for 30 minutes.
12. Record service in client's chart under "services rendered"; for example, "Applied topical APF fluoride gel to existing teeth for 4 minutes. Used stock trays to apply approx. 2 to 2.5 mL of 1.23% APF (insert brand name). Client consented to procedure; no complications or adverse reactions during treatment. Client instructed not to eat or drink for 30 minutes."

Procedure 33-2 Professionally Applied Sodium Fluoride Varnish Using the Paint-on Technique

EQUIPMENT

Mouth mirror
5% sodium fluoride varnish (unit dosage)
Cotton-tip applicators or syringe applicator
Personal protective barriers and equipment barriers

STEPS

1. Select unit-dose fluoride varnish product; gather equipment and supplies for application.
2. Provide client with information about procedure; reiterate benefits. Obtain informed consent.
3. Unless an oral prophylaxis has been performed at the same appointment, have client cleanse teeth with toothbrush.
4. Recline client for ergonomic access to oral cavity.
5. Wipe application area with gauze or cotton rolls and insert a saliva ejector. Can be applied in the presence of saliva and without a saliva ejector.
6. Using a cotton-tip, brush, or syringe-style applicator, apply 0.3 to 0.5 mL of varnish (unit dose) to clinical crown of teeth: application time is 1 to 3 minutes. Figure 33-19 shows a colored varnish for tracking coverage; white varnishes also are available.
7. Dental floss may be used to draw the varnish interproximally.
8. Allow client to rinse on completion of procedure.
9. Remind client to avoid eating hard foods, drinking hot or alcoholic beverages, brushing, and flossing until the next day or at least for 4 to 6 hours after application.
10. Record service in client's record under "Services Rendered," e.g., "Applied 0.3 mL of 5% (22,600 ppm) sodium fluoride varnish (insert brand name) per tooth. Client consented to this procedure; no complications or adverse reactions during treatment. Client instructed to keep varnish on the teeth for at least 4 to 6 hours or preferably until the next day. Client told to drink through a straw and avoid hard foods, alcoholic and hot beverages, brushing, and flossing until preferably the next day to prolong the varnish treatment. Varnish can be removed the next day with toothbrushing and interdental cleaning."

Foam-based fluoride was developed to address the ingestion risk associated with using high-potency fluoride products. With foam products, 75% less fluoride is used, dramatically reducing the risk of acute fluoride toxicity and cost. APF foam products release the same fluoride concentration as APF gels, but limited research has demonstrated less retention with foam and few clinical trials have evaluated caries prevention with foam products.[7] Regardless, professionally applied APF and neutral NaF are available as foam-based products and thixotropic gels.

Four high-potency, low-frequency, professionally applied topical fluoride systems have been approved by the FDA for in-office use. These products are manufactured as gels and foams (acidulated and neutral) or varnishes and have a caries reduction rate of approximately 30%:

- 1.23%, 12,300 ppm APF (used for most patients; gluten-free now available)
- 2.0%, 9050 ppm neutral NaF (used for composite, porcelain, titanium, sealants, sensitivity)
- 8.0% SnF_2 (rarely used, see later)
- 5% NaF/2.26% or 22,600 ppm varnish (lacquer in a rosin base) (FDA-approved for root sensitivity control and cavity liners only[7])

The 1.23% APF gel system is used widely and is a choice for clients without tooth-colored restorations or sealants. APF is a lower pH product as a result of added phosphoric acid and may cause etching of some dental materials. APF products were developed because of the discovery that the lower the pH of fluoride compounds, the more enhanced the rate of reaction between the fluoride and hydroxyapatite.

The 2.0% neutral NaF gel is another common professionally applied fluoride product. Neutral fluoride is selected by the clinician when it is inappropriate to use an acidulated (APF) product, when clients present with composite, porcelain, titanium, sealants, or sensitivity. If a neutral fluoride product is not available, at-risk dental materials should be protected with a nonpetroleum gel.

The 8.0% SnF_2 system is rarely used owing to its limited availability and lack of stability in aqueous solution. In addition, this product has poor client acceptance because of bitter taste, tissue irritation, gingival sloughing, and extrinsic tooth staining. It is, however, an effective decay-preventive agent.

Varnishes have been used in Europe for years and more recently have been used widely in the United States. This type of fluoride delivery quickly has become standard of care for certain populations. See varnish discussion in the next section, eTable 33-4, and Procedure 33-2.

Professionally Applied Tray Technique: Client and Product Selection

Key issues to consider when selecting the clients who benefit from professionally applied fluoride therapy and the appropriate products for each client are the following (see Box 33-1 for factors affecting client selection and Chapter 18, Table 18-1, for CAMBRA clinical recommendations):

- The client's fluoride history should include fluoride level in primary water plus food and beverage intake. Risk factors should be reassessed and updated periodically.
- Caries risk factors that make children and adults candidates for professionally applied topical fluoride treatments are summarized in Box 33-1. As a general rule, moderate-risk patients should receive 4-minute gel applications or fluoride varnish at 6-month intervals; high-risk patients at 3- to 6-month intervals. (Decrease re-care intervals when clients present with new areas of mineralization or are at higher risk.)
- The client's type of restorations guide fluoride type (e.g., choose a neutral fluoride product for clients with tooth-colored restorations, implants, and sensitivity).
- Clinicians frequently must review evidence-based research on products.
- The presence of newly erupted teeth must be considered, because studies indicate that teeth are most susceptible to caries formation during the first 2 years after eruption.
- The client's ability to tolerate a 4-minute topical fluoride application:
    - Extreme care should be used when in-office fluoride treatments are administered to a child under 6 years of age or elderly clients. Four minutes is a long time to sit with fluoride trays. Inadvertent swallowing of fluoride and the inability to effectively expectorate or use a saliva ejector places clients at risk for ingesting high-potency fluoride. This could result in vomiting or acute fluoride toxicity (see Box 33-2). (Fluoride varnish therapy is often a better choice for young children and older clients.)
    - Physical or cognitive disabilities: Clients with an inability to expectorate or understand the importance of refraining from swallowing, with severe gag reflex, or those who cannot sit for 4 minutes are not candidates for fluoride trays.

BOX 33-1

Client Selection for Professionally Applied Fluoride Treatments—Risk Factors*

- Caries risk factors that may indicate a need for a professionally applied topical fluoride include the following: new carious lesions on previously sound surfaces, dental caries experience in the previous 2 to 3 years
- Secondary lesions associated with restoration margins
- High levels of cariogenic bacteria
- Poor family oral health status
- Irregular professional dental care
- Enamel defects, white spots, exposed roots
- Cariogenic diet
- Wearing of orthodontic appliances
- Compromised salivary flow (e.g., from medical conditions, stress, medications)
- Radiation therapy
- Age-related conditions (e.g., hypersensitivity)
- Medical conditions (e.g., Sjögren's syndrome, eating disorders); physical or cognitive disabilities
- For children and infants, poor dental caries status of the caregiver and siblings and low socioeconomic status

*Individuals who are at low risk for dental caries may have no additional benefit from professionally applied fluoride therapy, particularly if they use a fluoride toothpaste and drink fluoridated water.

Professionally Applied Fluoride Tray Technique: Features and Advantages

The following are features and advantages of the professionally applied fluoride tray technique (see Procedure 33-1):

- Entire dentition can be treated simultaneously with optimal fluoride exposure
- Minimal soft-tissue contact; tray design and fit enhances client comfort
- Less dilution and contamination of fluoride with saliva; time and cost effective
- Reduced potential for fluoride ingestion (maximized with use of foam products)
- Diversity of tray designs and sizes, S-M-L-XL*

Professionally Applied Fluoride Tray Technique: Procedure

The procedural steps for professionally applied topical fluoride begin with client and product selection as outlined in the previous section. Sequence for administration using the tray technique is described in Procedure 33-1.

*Choosing the correct size optimizes anticaries efficacy and prevents ingestion. Trays should create a distal dam to prevent flow past the posterior border of the tray, anatomically fit the arches and allow for anterior and posterior vertical coverage.

Varnish[6,7,9,11,14,18]

Fluoride varnish is a lacquer containing the highest available concentration of 5% sodium fluoride (in the United States), often 22,600 ppm, alone or in combination with other bioavailable anticaries agents (xylitol, thymol) in a rosin (transparent saps derived from trees) base. Varnish hardens on the tooth upon contact with saliva. The varnish system offers clients a prolonged (1 to 7 days), temporary exposure of a high concentration of fluoride (Figures 33-19 and 33-20). Varnish holds fluoride in close proximity to teeth surfaces for longer periods of time than other concentrated fluoride products.[6] These products may slow, arrest, and/or reverse the progression of caries. Teeth are dried with gauze a quadrant at a time, and a thin coat of the varnish is applied with a tiny brush (see Procedure 33-2). Clients should be instructed to avoid hot, hard, or crunchy foods and brushing and flossing for 4 to 6 hours after placement. Refer to the manufacturer's instructions, which often are provided for clients. Varnish has the following practical advantages over gels (and foams):

- Ease of application with short delivery time, especially good choice for young children
- Minimal risk of ingestion and discomfort
- Inoffensive taste
- Cost effective/small amount of material needed (7 mg versus 30 mg for gel in trays)
- Eating soft foods and drinking immediately after is acceptable

In the United States, thus far, the FDA has approved varnish for use only as cavity liners and the treatment of hypersensitive teeth, *not* as a caries-preventive agent, because the FDA considers caries prevention a drug claim. For the FDA to approve varnish as a caries-preventive agent, manufacturers would need to conduct additional clinical trials with convincing results despite the existing evidence supporting effectiveness of fluoride varnish in caries prevention, especially in children, adolescence, and the elderly.

Expert opinion regarding varnish application varies. Some recommend application of the product every 3 to 6 months based on caries risk. The ADA endorses fluoride varnish application in some cases and issued the following comments in their 2006 report: "Fluoride varnish applied every 6 months is effective in preventing caries in the dentitions of children and adolescents and two or more varnish applications per year are effective in preventing caries in high-risk clients"[7] (see Table 33-9). Procedure 33-2 outlines the steps for fluoride varnish therapy, the paint-on technique.

Because of numerous clinical studies and successful use of fluoride varnishes in other countries, fluoride varnish dispensed in unit doses recently has become a standard of care, albeit off-label (ADA limited endorsement but not FDA-approved), in the following situations:

- For infants, toddlers, children, elderly, and adults at moderate-to-high risk for dental caries
- For reversing demineralization and white spot areas
- When longer fluoride contact is desired
- For control of dentinal hypersensitivity
- For clients with physical or cognitive disabilities or severe gag reflexes or people who cannot tolerate 4-minute tray techniques

The following are some of the fluoride varnishes available in the United States:

- 5% NaF/2.26% fluoride or 22,600 ppm (Duraphat, Duraflor, Vanish, Fluoridex, X-Pur White) (see Figure 33-19)

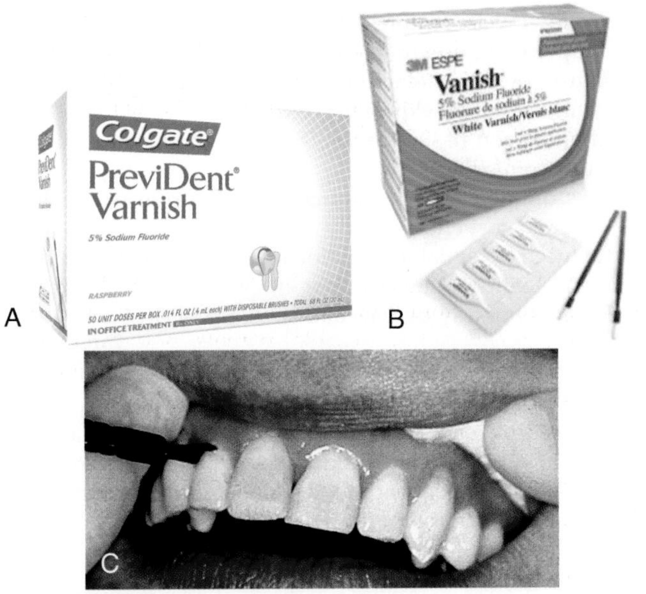

Figure 33-19. **A** and **B,** Examples of unit-dose 5% sodium fluoride varnish. **C,** Fluoride varnish being applied to teeth. (**A,** Courtesy Colgate Oral Pharmaceuticals, New York, New York. **B,** Courtesy 3M ESPE, St Paul, Minnesota.)

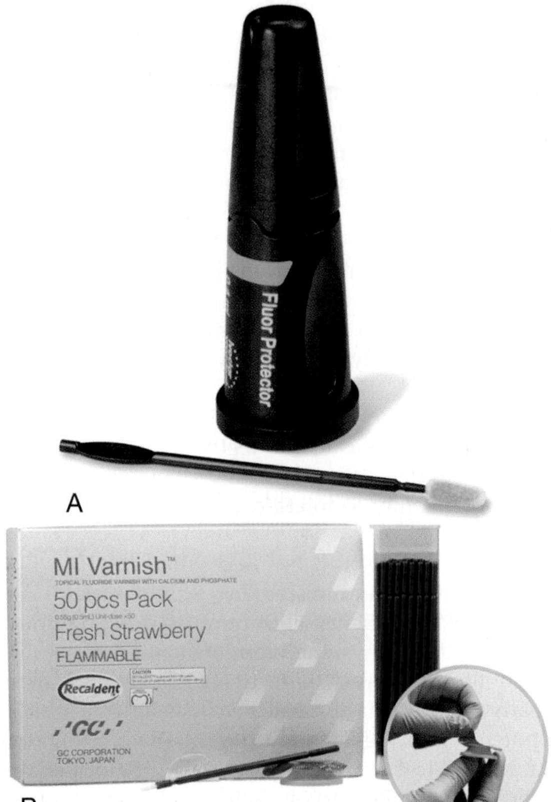

Figure 33-20. Fluoride varnish. (**A,** Courtesy Ivoclar Vivadent, Inc, Amherst, New York. **B,** Courtesy GC America, Inc, Alsip, Illinois.)

- 1% difluorosilane/0.1% fluoride or 1000 ppm (Fluor Protector)
- Cervitec Plus/1:1chlorhexidine/thymol—This combination reduces pathogen levels and is the only ADA-endorsed varnish for root caries (see Figure 33-20)
- Embrace/5% fluoride with xylitol-coated calcium and phosphate
- MI varnish/NaF plus RECALDENT (CPP-ACP) (see Figure 33-20)
- Enamel Pro varnish with fluoride and ACP

Safety of Fluoride Varnish

No incidents of acute or chronic fluoride toxicity as a result of using fluoride varnish have been documented. The rapid setting characteristic of fluoride varnish seems to prevent ingestion and to minimize risk for a toxic dose, especially important for children, the elderly, and the disabled. The release of fluoride after placement peaks early and then drops dramatically. Plasma levels of fluoride after varnish applications are similar to those experienced after the use of an OTC fluoridated toothpaste. The varnish breaks down over a period of several days, so ingestion occurs slowly over a period of time, reducing the likelihood of acute fluoride toxicity. Because varnish contains rosin, it should not be used on persons with a known sensitivity to this material or with clients who present with ulcerative gingivitis, stomatitis, or large, open lesions.[6]

Acute Fluoride Toxicity[1,2,7,11,18]

The amount of fluoride that causes a toxic reaction or results in a lethal dose is based on a variety of factors. Terms used to describe how much fluoride can be tolerated by a client are the safely tolerated dose (STD) and the certainly lethal dose (CLD):

- STD is the amount of fluoride that can be ingested without causing serious acute toxicity; it is approximately one quarter of the CLD.
- The CLD is the amount of fluoride that results in client death; 5 to 10 g of sodium fluoride is considered a CLD for a 70-kg or 154-lb adult.

Acute toxicity from the rapid ingestion of a topical fluoride agent within a short period of time may yield a mild systemic reaction (stomach upset or vomiting) to death. Many factors influence the toxicity of fluoride compounds: route of administration, client age and weight, and rate of absorption. When fluoride is swallowed, it reacts with stomach acids; the reaction product is hydrogen fluoride (HF). HF is very irritating to the stomach lining. Abdominal distress can occur after a relatively small amount of higher-concentration product is swallowed.

Initial symptoms of acute fluoride toxicity are nausea, gastrointestinal pain, and vomiting. If sufficient quantities of fluoride are ingested, these first symptoms may be followed by muscular weakness and spasms that occur as a result of fluoride combining with blood calcium ions. Toxic doses of fluoride affect major body systems as follows:

- Gastrointestinal: abdominal pain and cramps, nausea, vomiting, diarrhea
- Neurologic: paresthesia, tetany, central nervous system depression, coma
- Cardiovascular: weak pulse, pallor, hypotension, shock, cardiac irregularities, cardiac failure
- Cases of acute toxic doses of fluoride in children have been documented

BOX 33-2

Management of Acute Fluoride Toxicity

1. Induce vomiting by administering an emetic, such as ipecac syrup (this should occur only if the client has a gag reflex, is conscious, and is not convulsing).
2. Administer a fluoride-binding liquid orally: 1% calcium chloride or calcium gluconate, milk of magnesia, or milk.
3. While client is receiving attention, second person should activate emergency medical services (EMS); client should be transported to hospital as soon as possible.
4. Support respiration and circulation if necessary. Response by emergency personnel is dependent on severity of symptoms.
5. Supportive therapies include the following:
   - Calcium gluconate for muscle tremors or tetany
   - Endotracheal intubation, followed by gastric lavage with a calcium-containing solution or activated charcoal
   - Establishing an airway
   - Intravenous feeding to restore blood volume and electrolytes and reverse effects of vomiting and diarrhea and to maintain urine flow
   - Maintaining cardiovascular circulation and monitoring
   - Blood monitoring for plasma fluoride levels, hyperkalemia, hypocalcemia, pH
   - Intravenous calcium replacement, glucose administration, oxygen, artificial respiration, or other supportive therapies
6. If the client responds favorably, supportive therapies are continued until normal mental alertness, vital signs, and serum chemistry profile are achieved.

Emergency Management of Acute Toxicity

The initial treatment goal for acute fluoride toxicity is to reduce the amount of fluoride available for absorption from the gastrointestinal tract. Depending on the amount of fluoride ingested, initial emergency response in the dental office should be followed by medical treatment. Box 33-2 outlines emergency treatment.

Prevention of Acute and Chronic Fluoride Toxicity

Although fluoride products have evident therapeutic benefits, their use and storage must be monitored. Oral care professionals should educate clients, parents, and caregivers regarding the safe use and storage of even low-dosage fluorides. Furthermore, dental professionals always should exercise extreme caution when using high-potency prescription agents. To use safely professional-strength fluoride products, the hygienist must select carefully the clients for this therapy and understand the following:

- Fluoride concentration and amount of product in unit packaging
- Whether the client can well tolerate fluoride application (especially 4-minute trays)
- Accurate amount used in the treatment (infant, child, or adult dose)

- How the amount provided relates to the CLD
- ***Never leave a client alone during treatment.***

Nonfluoride Caries-Preventive Agents: Evidence-Based Research and American Dental Association Recommendations[3,4-7,9-17,19]

The prevalence of dental caries has led to focused research and product development aimed at prevention and control.[3] Studies have been challenging because of the need for long-term clinical trials, which are expensive, and the numerous variables that contribute to caries formation (e.g., placing something in the mouth stimulates salivary flow and alters pH). However, research has resulted in several promising nonfluoride products. The ADA conducted a systematic review of current evidence-based research regarding these products in 2010, reported in 2011.

After exhaustive study by the ADA Council on Scientific Affairs, a panel of experts conveyed their findings and offered guarded recommendations to clinicians. The experts' findings regarding nonfluoride caries-preventive agents are addressed in the following sections of this chapter: fluoride use for caries prevention is well documented, whereas nonfluoride agents have less history, less evidence.

Regardless of research findings and the array of OTC and prescription nonfluoride agents available, it is important for the clinician to remember that the use of fluoridated agents, professionally applied fluorides, fluoridated municipal water, sealants, and carbohydrate intake control remain the modalities of choice for caries management. The American Dental Association currently recommends using nonfluoride agents as adjuncts only; the first line of defense for caries control remains fluoride.[7] (Note: An ADA product report of insufficient evidence does not mean that an intervention is ineffective, rather that the panel did not find enough evidence to support a recommendation.[3,7] This consideration is important when analyzing research or using professional judgment to formulate a caries management plan for clients.)

Chlorhexidine Products and Claims

Chlorhexidine has been shown to reduce *S. mutans* levels, but chlorhexidine use as a caries-preventive agent remains controversial. The ADA found sufficient evidence to recommend a chlorhexidine/**thymol** (a broad-spectrum biocide) combination varnish for the control of root caries (CervitecPlus Varnish by Ivoclar Vivadent, see Figure 33-20). Other chlorhexidine-containing products need further research with evidence to be recognized fully as caries-preventive agents by the ADA and FDA.

Chlorhexidine as an Agent to Control Dental Caries

Chlorhexidine gluconate has been used as an antibacterial for the management of dental caries and periodontal diseases (see Chapters 18 and 31). See the website for eFig. 33-21 and more information.

For high-risk and extreme-risk individuals, use of 0.12% chlorhexidine gluconate rinse for 1 minute daily for 1 week each month is recommended to reduce mutans streptococci and lactobacilli levels in the plaque biofilm (see Table 18-1). This regimen was shown in a 3-year clinical trial to reduce caries incidence by 24% as compared to a conventional treatment control group.[12] It is important to note the regimen, because this was developed during the trial and shown to be effective compared to other less-frequent doses that have been proposed by previous authors. Chlorhexidine therapy reduces the bacterial challenge but must be used in conjunction with fluoride for remineralization as described in detail previously. Rinsing once daily for 1 week markedly reduces the mutans streptococci levels, but this begin to return quickly. Therefore the regimen must be repeated each month, thereby driving the bacterial levels down to safe regions over a period of 6 months.[12] Minimal staining occurs with this regimen.

Clinicians should inform clients that chlorhexidine is neutralized by two toothpaste additives: sodium lauryl sulfate (SLS) and sodium monofluorophosphate (MFP). Therefore chlorhexidine rinses should be used 2 hours after brushing with dentifrices containing these ingredients.

Xylitol Products and Claims

The 2011 American Dental Association's Systematic Review of Nonfluoride Caries-Preventive Agents yielded the following guarded (meaning that future research is needed, professional judgment exercised and client needs considered) evidence-based recommendations regarding products containing xylitol:

- Children's use of xylitol or **polyol** (sugar alcohol)-combination chewing gum for 10 to 20 minutes after meals *may* reduce the incidence of coronal caries.
- Adult use of xylitol or polyol-combination chewing gum for 10 to 20 minutes after meals may reduce the incidence of coronal caries.
- Children's use of lozenges or candy/mints containing xylitol dissolved after meals may reduce the incidence of coronal caries.
- Insufficient evidence exists that xylitol in dentifrices prevents caries.
- Insufficient evidence exists that xylitol reduces vertical transmission from mother-to-child or that xylitol use helps reduce horizontal transmission among siblings.

Furthermore, the ADA review panel highlighted the fact that it is biologically plausible that the act of using xylitol-containing products itself increases saliva production and neutralizes acids, thereby potentially lowering the incidence and progression of caries, not necessarily the pure action of the xylitol.[3] (Note: The FDA recently approved the use of the limited claim "Does not promote tooth decay"; the ADA position statement reads "sugar-free foods do not promote decay" regarding products containing polyols.)

Xylitol as a Nonfluoride Agent to Control Dental Caries

Xylitol is a noncariogenic sweetener that looks and tastes like sucrose, is derived mainly from birch trees, and is one of many polyols, or "sugar alcohols." Other polyols, such as sorbitol, mannitol, maltitol, and sucralose, also are used widely to sweeten foods and beverages but are considered low cariogenic, not noncariogenic, like xylitol. Because *S. mutans* cannot ferment xylitol, the replication, and therefore the acid production, is reduced. Furthermore, any remaining acidogenic bacteria in oral biofilm has less adhesion capability, thus reducing the amount of attached biofilm.[9]

Xylitol can be delivered through chewing gum, mints, breath (and nasal) sprays, toothpaste, lozenges, or syrup as an effective way to control acid production, along with fluoride use and limiting carbohydrates (Figures 33-22 and 33-23). Ideally, clinicians should recommend products with xylitol listed as the first and only sweetening agent. Manufacturers often use a combination of polyols because it is cheaper. Some of the Trident (Cadbury Adams USA) and Icebreakers (Hershey, Inc.) OTC chewing gums contain xylitol as their first ingredient and only polyol; X-Pur gum and mints by Oral Science contain 100% xylitol (see Figure 33-23).

For a **therapeutic dose** (dose required to produce the desired result), chewing gum, lozenges, or mints must contain 1.55 g (two pieces of Orbit contain 3 g) of xylitol and be used at least four to five times daily: 6 to 10 g/day, three to eight pieces, depending on the product choice.

Lozenges with xylitol can be located on the Internet or at health food stores; candy with xylitol can be ordered on the Internet or where sugar-free candy is sold; gum with xylitol and fluoride is available in Europe. Availability is limited because of lack of authorization by agencies. All clients should be forewarned that excess xylitol (more than 20 g/day) can cause diarrhea. Persons with diabetes should be cautioned that xylitol can interfere with glucose control.

The 2011 ADA Systematic Review of Nonfluoride Caries-Preventive Agents decided that insufficient evidence exists to support the following protocol—xylitol (or chlorhexidine) use as a convincing means of reducing vertical transmission of *S. mutans* from mother-to-child.[3] Many studies have been conducted to investigate this practice. The most optimistic conclusions have stated that "mothers with high *S. mutans* counts using chlorhexidine or xylitol is better than basic prevention alone and may delay *S. mutans* transmission. Timing, dose, frequency, and duration for maximum benefit remains elusive."[17] Given that caries is a multifactorial process, this regimen remains difficult to prove and is unsubstantiated today.

Also, pregnant women who were infected with *S. mutans* used to be encouraged aggressively to use xylitol during the last months of pregnancy and during the first 3 months postpartum to reduce the risk of vertical caries transmission to their infants. That course of therapy is no longer considered standard practice. As with other nonfluoride agents, further randomized controlled clinical trials are needed to prove worthiness.

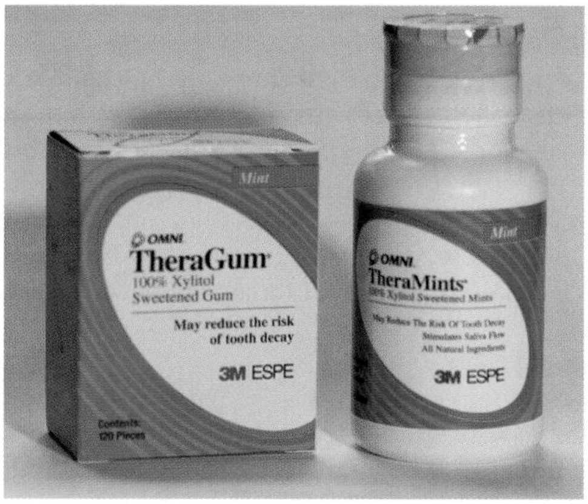

Figure 33-22. Examples of xylitol-containing mints and gum. (Courtesy 3M ESPE, St Paul, Minnesota.)

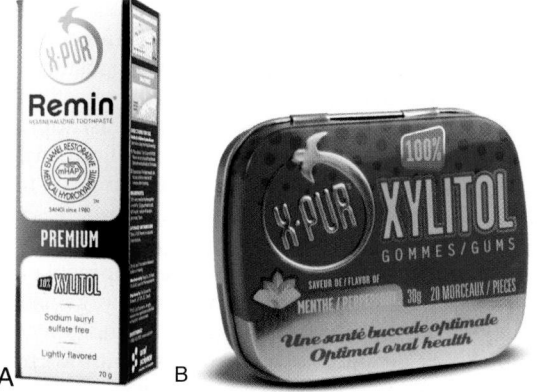

A B

Figure 33-23. Examples of xylitol-containing toothpaste and mints. (Courtesy Oral Science, Inc, Brossard, Quebec City, Canada.)

Calcium- and Phosphorus-Based Products and Claims

Although much research has been conducted and the companies who manufacture OTC and prescription products that contain calcium, phosphates, and casein protein have made substantial claims, the ADA panel found that these agents could not be recommended with confidence at that time. After a systematic review of the available evidence-based research, the ADA determined that there is insufficient evidence to show that use of ACP- and CPP-ACP–containing products lowers the incidence of either coronal or root caries.[3] Nevertheless, calcium- and phosphorus-based technologies and products are selected as adjuncts to fluoride products for caries control. Research regarding effectiveness continues and additional findings are needed to document effectiveness.

Amorphous Calcium Phosphate

Amorphous calcium phosphate (ACP) contains the same minerals as the hydroxyapatite crystals of tooth enamel and is the first commercial compound of its kind. Scientists discovered that calcium and phosphate ions in ACP have an affinity for areas of demineralization upon contact with salivary ions and protease enzymes. Claims of products with amorphous calcium phosphate include the following:

- Can help prevent demineralization and slow caries progression
- Can stimulate remineralization via bioavailability of calcium and phosphate
- May increase fluoride uptake—calcium and phosphate ions have an affinity for fluoride
- Occlude dentinal tubules to reduce dentinal hypersensitivity
- Form a new hydroxyapatite coating with larger crystals—This action renders teeth more resistant to acid penetration and demineralization than the original enamel crystals.

OTC client-applied ACP products include Enamel Care with Liquid Calcium, Age Defying and Mentadent Replenishing White dentifrices (Arm and Hammer). Professionally applied products with ACP include tooth-whitening agents Zoom! Day White (Philips) and Nite White with ACP (Smilox), the prophylaxis paste Enamel Pro, 5% NaF with ACP varnish, and Enamel Pro Varnish (Premier Dental).

ACP-containing products are not a substitute for fluoride therapy, but clinicians can use ACP products during treatment and recommend to clients at risk for caries.

Casein Phosphopeptides–Amorphous Calcium Phosphate

Shortly after the discovery of ACP, researchers realized that if they combined casein phosphopeptides (CPP) with ACP (CPP-ACP), the compound had greater affinity for bacterial biofilm because the presence of CPP stabilizes ACP and allows for more ions to reach the enamel.[9] This stabilization provides for a larger calcium reservoir within biofilm and slows the diffusion of free calcium from tooth structure.[10] CPP is an ingredient derived from casein, part of the protein found in cow's milk; therefore it is contraindicated in people with milk protein allergies.

CPP-ACP products (e.g., RECALDENT, GC America, Inc., [Figure 33-24]) help maintain essential minerals (calcium and phosphate) in a soluble form that binds to and penetrates tooth structure. Products with CPP-ACP make the following claims:

- Can improve salivary flow, xerostomia symptoms, fluoride uptake, and enamel luster
- Provide a supersaturated environment of "free" calcium and phosphate for remineralization and microscopic enamel defect repair
- Can reduce dentinal hypersensitivity
- Buffer acids, reduce acid levels, and raise oral pH

This compound also is found in Trident Xtra Care Gum (Cadbury Adams USA) and prescription-only MI Paste, MI Paste Plus with fluoride (GC America, Inc.), and MI Varnish (see Figure 33-20). MI Paste (see Figure 33-24) should be applied directly to the teeth without a brush, and overnight use in custom trays is well tolerated because of lack of fluoride content (not so with MI Paste Plus). Similar to products with only ACP, CPP-ACP–containing products are not a substitute for fluoride therapy either but can be used in tandem with fluoride for clients at risk for caries. Additional long-term clinical trials are needed to document effectiveness in caries reduction.

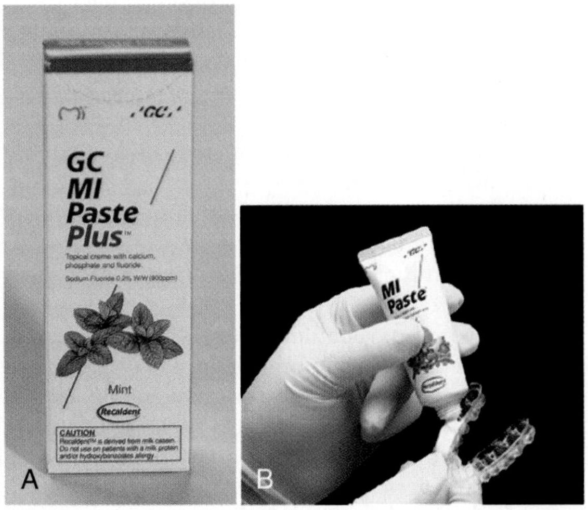

Figure 33-24. A, Example of professionally administered casein phosphopeptide–amorphous calcium phosphate product. **B,** Product can be delivered as a prophylaxis paste or via a tray. (**B,** Courtesy GC America, Inc, Alsip, Illinois.)

Other Nonfluoride Products and Claims[3-5,9]

The ADA has not yet conducted a systematic review of evidence-based research for calcium sodium phosphosilicate, sodium bicarbonate, or probiotics. The ADA Council on Scientific Affairs did issue a statement regarding triclosan and povidone-iodine in dental products and found insufficient evidence that these agents lower the incidence of caries.[3]

Calcium Sodium Phosphosilicate

NovaMin is the brand name of the bioactive glass, calcium sodium phosphosilicate (CSD). This inorganic chemical binds to tooth surfaces and delivers calcium, phosphorus, sodium, and silica to replace lost minerals. When the glass particles come in contact with saliva, calcium and phosphate ions are released. A calcium-phosphate layer forms and crystallizes as new hydroxyapatite. Dentinal tubules are occluded in the process.

NovaMin is available in products OTC and on the Internet: for example, Sensodyne Repair and Protect (GlaxoSmithKline) and X-Pur (Oral Science) toothpaste (can be used in overnight trays because of lack of fluoride content), mints, and gum (see Figure 33-23), NUPRO Prophylaxis Paste (Dentsply), and by prescription, Sensodyne NUPRO Toothpaste with NovaMin plus 5000 ppm fluoride or SootheRx (3M ESPE). Limited availability is due to lack of complete validation by the FDA of nonfluoride caries-preventive agents.

Tricalcium Phosphate

Another calcium phosphate technology on the market is tricalcium phosphate (TCP). TCP protects calcium ions and frees phosphate ions; this material prohibits calcium from reacting prematurely with fluoride before reaching tooth surfaces. Once TCP is exposed to saliva on tooth structure, calcium, phosphate, and fluoride ions are released. TCP is an ingredient in Clinpro 5000 toothpaste and Vanish varnish.

Sodium Bicarbonate

Sodium bicarbonate ($NaHCO_3$, or baking soda) neutralizes acids produced by acidogenic bacteria and is bactericidal. It is mildly abrasive, can be mixed with water for brushing or rinsing (a good choice for clients with hyposalivation), and is available in combination with other ingredients in many dental products on the market, such as Orbit White (Wrigley) gum and Arm & Hammer and Tom's of Maine dentifrices.

Probiotics

Use of probiotics to replace and displace cariogenic bacteria with noncariogenic bacteria has shown promising preliminary results; however, evidence regarding effectiveness in reduction of caries incidence is lacking. This approach to caries control creates a balance between beneficial and pathogenic bacteria in the oral cavity. Probiotics are live microorganisms, which, when administered in adequate amounts, award a health benefit on the host.[4] Research has focused on identifying which bacteria prevent the development of pathogenic oral biofilm: low acid-producing microorganisms such as *Streptococcus rattus, Streptococcus oralis,* and *Streptococcus uberis* quickly replicate and colonize to inhibit the growth of pathogenic varieties.[5] The most extensively studied probiotic, *Lactobacillus rhamnosus,* was found to inhibit *S. mutans* aggressively.[4]

The long-range treatment goal of probiotic therapy is to choose the appropriate probiotic, supplement the oral environment with beneficial bacteria, and promote healthier plaque ecologies.[3] The hope is that in the future the clinician will be able to target specific bacteria based on singular needs, altering biofilm on an individualized basis to prevent dental disease, whether caries or periodontal disease. Probiotics (GUM PerioBalance by Butler, EvoraPro and ProBiora3 by Oragenics, Figure 33-25) are available in health food stores, drug stores, and on the Internet, but the effectiveness has not been tested rigorously.

Caries Control for Clients with Xerostomia[3,7,9,16]

There are growing numbers of clients who present with xerostomia because of a longer life span, radiation treatment, and numerous medications that cause a dry mouth. Patients with xerostomia are at higher risk for developing caries because of less saliva and its benefits. Loss of saliva decreases pH, acidophilic bacteria thrive, acids are not buffered as effectively, and mineral availability is reduced.[9] Given all these deleterious effects, clinicians must make a commitment to educating these patients and recommending anticaries and palliative products.

The major causes of salivary hypofunction are more than 700 medications, autoimmune and systemic diseases, radiation to head/neck, stress, and depression. Lack of salivary function causes any or all of the following symptoms: viscous, sticky saliva; difficulty speaking and swallowing; halitosis; altered sense of smell and taste; burning mouth and lips; cracking, fissuring, and increased biofilm formation on the tongue. Some patients become so uncomfortable they resort to electrical stimulation of the glands and acupuncture.

Besides diet counseling, diligent home care, regular prophylaxis, and application of a chlorhexidine-thymol varnish on root surfaces of patients with xerostomia, numerous products are available that can substitute for the functions of saliva, counteract damage, and compensate for a less-than-favorable oral environment:

- Prescription fluoridated dentifrices such as PreviDent or Clinpro 5000
- OTC/Internet dentifrices containing higher amounts of xylitol, 10% to 36% (e.g., Tom's of Maine, Spry by Xlear and Epic Dental)
- OTC fluoride and/or xylitol mouth rinses (Spry offers a xylitol rinse on the Internet)
- Regular use of 100% xylitol-containing products that mechanically stimulate salivary flow[9] (e.g., TheraGum by 3M ESPE and X-Pur mints, gum)
  - Gels that neutralize oral pH (e.g., GC America), lozenges with citric acid that chemically stimulate salivary flow (available on the Internet, several manufacturers)
  - OTC products that stimulate, moisten, and lubricate (e.g., Biotene products by GlaxoSmithKline; Figure 33-26)
  - Customized night trays with remineralizing agents
  - Adhesive tablets applied to the palate (e.g., OraMoist by Quantum Health, Figure 33-27 and Xylimelts by OralHealth). Such products contain xylitol, a lubricant, oral enzymes, buffering compounds, and saliva secretion inducers.
  - OTC and prescription artificial saliva (e.g., Salivart, NeutraSal)
  - Prescription salivary-stimulating drugs such as pilocarpine (Salagen), cevimeline HCl (Evoxac), anethole trithione (Sialor), bethanechol (Urecholine)*

*The ADA currently does not recommend the use of sialogogues (medications that increase the flow rate of saliva) because of a lack of quality evidence-based research on such medications.[3] Often such products are palliative only.

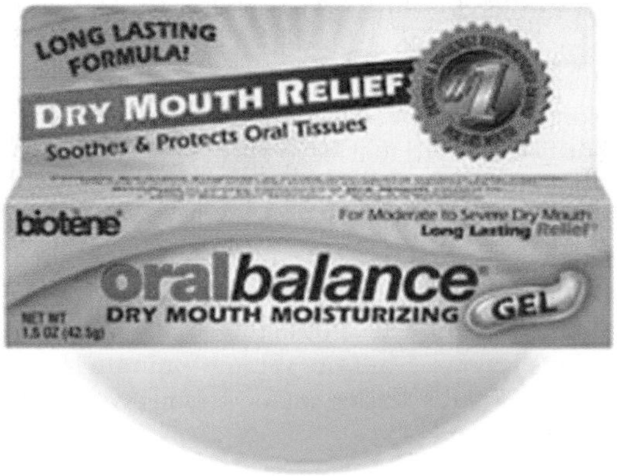

Figure 33-26. Example of Biotene products for xerostomia treatment. (Courtesy GlaxoSmithKline, Moon Township, Pennsylvania.)

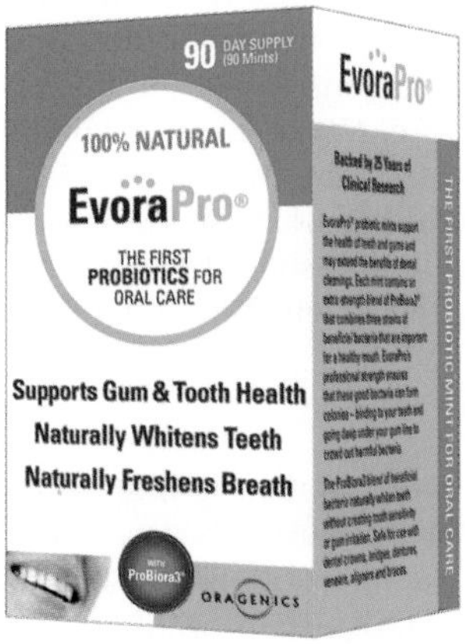

Figure 33-25. Example of a probiotic. (Courtesy Oragenics, Inc, Tampa, Florida.)

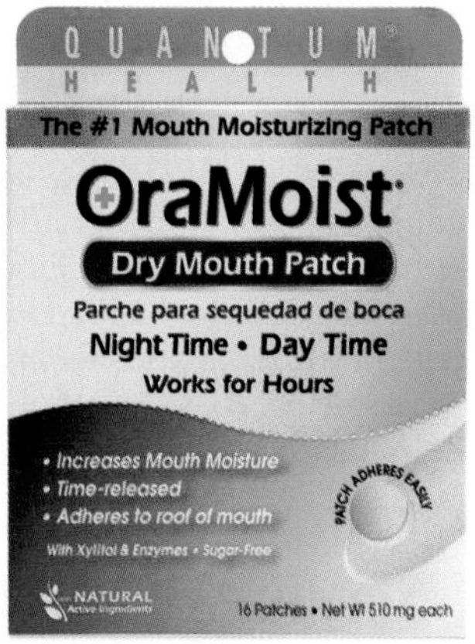

Figure 33-27. Example of palatal tablets to alleviate xerostomia symptoms. (Courtesy Quantum, Inc, Eugene, Oregon.)

- Clients with xerostomia should not use dentifrices containing SLS because it increases dryness.

The Future of Caries Prevention[3,4,5,9,10,12,14,15,17]

Caries prevention research has increased during the last decade because of an expanding elderly population, more medications that cause xerostomia, and a renewed focus on the underserved.

Research has been costly, subject retention has been challenging, and most studies have focused on various combinations of ingredients in varnish. Other investigations have yielded the following promising insights into the fight against dental caries: polyvinylpyrrolidone iodine with fluoride varnish, arginine, diamine silver fluoride, and xylitol lozenges. Natural compounds including tea extracts, grape seed extracts, coconut oil, Chinese herbs, and bioactive flavonoids (or plant pigments) also have been examined for their effect on the inhibition of oral bacterial activity.[3] Research has been hopeful but inconclusive for all of the above.

New advances also have been made recently by an American/Chilean team of scientists with the development of biomolecules. Biomolecules are "smart molecules" that preferentially eradicate specific bacteria. One of these, "Keep 32," kills *S. mutans* quickly, and its effects last for hours. Human trials are ongoing, and pending results of testing, the scientists are optimistic that products containing this biomolecule will be on the market 18 months after trial completion. Various groups of scientists also are investigating the possibility of a vaccine for caries. DMG America released a demineralization repair resin infiltrant, ICON, in February 2013, which demonstrates hope for yet another approach to caries prevention. Last, a new infectious agent, *Scardovia wiggsiae*, was identified in 2011 that may play a more important role than *S. mutans* or *L. acidophilus* in the caries process.

In 2011 the ADA identified the following priorities for future evidence-based research: varnish and gel for the prevention of root caries, ideal intervals for fluoride and varnish applications in high-risk populations, remineralization of early carious lesions, 1-minute versus 4-minute tray applications, fluoride foams, caries risk assessment, and chewable fluoride supplements.

Caries Management Planning[2,3,6-13,16]

First and foremost, hygienists should suggest that all clients have a "dental home" by the age of 12 months. Thereafter careful consideration must be given to the information gathered during risk assessment (see Chapter 18) at *every* appointment. This information yields pathologic and protective factors and level of client risk for dental caries. Preventive strategies that address client needs can be recommended based on the obtained information (see Chapter 18, Tables 18-1 and 18-2, Boxes 18-2 to 18-10, and Figures 18-5 to 18-7 and sealant discussion in Chapter 34).

Caries management must be an ongoing, dynamic data collection and reassessment process. It involves careful attention and planning by the dental hygienist and adherence by the client.

CLIENT EDUCATION TIPS

- Explain the caries process, including carbohydrate frequency and role of acidophilic bacteria.
- When well water is a client's primary water source, address the rationale for fluoride level testing.
- Present products and services available to prevent and control future caries.
- Address the significance of using daily, multiple therapeutic doses of xylitol to control the bacteria that can initiate caries and how to best select xylitol-containing products.
- Explain that it is possible to transmit the infectious agent *Streptococcus mutans*.
- Emphasize how fluoride and nonfluoride caries-preventive agents can repair demineralized tooth structure or suppress infectious pathogens and how to use and store the products safely.
- Describe how a reduced salivary flow can increase dental caries risk. Recommend products to help counteract xerostomia symptoms and combat caries.
- Explain how dental caries management is a lifelong issue that requires periodic reassessment as clients age and health status and diet change.
- Advise parents and caregivers that they are critical partners in the management of dental caries, especially for children under 6 years of age.

LEGAL, ETHICAL, AND SAFETY ISSUES

- It is the dental hygienist's ethical responsibility always to document accurately chemotherapeutic agents used during treatment and product recommendations made.
- It is the dental hygienist's ethical obligation to read current scientific literature. This commitment will lead to solid evidence-based decisions that substantiate treatment and recommendations.
- Never insist a client accept fluoride therapy when refused.
- Offer professionally applied fluoride to patients who warrant it.
- Take comprehensive fluoride histories; analyze overall fluoride exposure for clients.
- Make recommendations based on *all* client assessments, including caries risk.
- Emphasize safe use, storage, and supervision of self-applied products around children.
- It is the hygienist's duty to explain the risks, benefits, and after-treatment instructions pertaining to fluoride and nonfluoride agents to all clients.
- Safely store, monitor expiration dates, and manage professional-strength fluorides in the dental setting.
- Work in collaboration with other oral care providers to develop a response plan in the event of an acute fluoride overdose. ***Never leave children unattended in the office.***
- Have a clear understanding of the amount of professional-strength fluoride that should be administered and how it relates to a certainly lethal dose (CLD) and a safely tolerated dose (STD).

KEY CONCEPTS

To effectively assist clients with caries management, lifelong learning is essential to sustain professional judgment.

- Caries management is aimed at restoring and maintaining a balance between pathologic and protective factors.

Dental hygienists help clients maintain this balance via caries risk assessments (number and severity of risk factors), diet counseling (reduction of carbohydrate frequency), educating clients about the caries process, oral hygiene care, and individualized fluoride and nonfluoride product recommendations.

- Chlorhexidine does reduce the number of *S. mutans* but research evidence, regimen recommendations, and professional opinion vary regarding use for caries control.
- An ongoing challenge for clients and clinicians, demineralization and remineralization occur continuously in the oral cavity. Saliva, fluoride, and nonfluoride caries-preventive agents are instrumental in the remineralization process. Hygienists should guide clients with timely product selections based on current caries risk level and preferences.
- Ingested and topical fluoride delivery systems are proven caries-preventive agents.
- Community water fluoridation is the cornerstone of ingested and topical fluoride delivery.
- The incidence of dental fluorosis has increased; it is the dental hygienist's responsibility to assess regularly systemic fluoride exposure for young clients.
- Use of professionally applied fluoride gels and varnishes has been well documented in the literature; in-office product selection is based on client caries risk and demineralized areas.
- Acute fluoride toxicity is a risk, especially during the administration of professional-strength fluorides. The dental hygienist has a primary role in the prevention of acute toxicity.
- Dental hygienists should pay special attention to oral hygiene instruction and product recommendations for clients with xerostomia, because caries risk is usually higher.

CRITICAL THINKING EXERCISES

1. Individually research the definition of evidence-based research. Locate an example of evidence-based research and share with peers.
2. Divide the group into the following subgroups: chlorhexidine gluconate, xylitol products, amorphous calcium phosphate (ACP) and CPP-ACP products, probiotics, xerostomia products, and fluoride dentifrices and mouth rinses. The groups should visit a drug store to collect information about over-the-counter products available, active and inactive ingredients in the products, manufacturer's instructions, and which products have been awarded the ADA Seal of Acceptance or CDA Seal of Recognition. Report back to other subgroups.
3. Have members of the group conduct an Internet search on the fluoride and nonfluoride caries-preventive agents reviewed by the ADA Council on Scientific Affairs. Include the evidence base that supports (or fails to support) these agents.
4. On the CDC website, research the specific fluoride statistics for various cities in your area.

REFERENCES

1. Department of Health and Human Services, Centers for Disease Control and Prevention: *Water fluoridation statistics and dental fluorosis*. Available at: http://www.cdc.gov/fluoridation/safety/statistics.htm. Accessed June 22, 2012. http://www.cdc.gov/fluoridation/safety/dental_fluorosis.htm. Accessed July 17, 2012.
2. USDA National Fluoride Database of Selected Foods and Beverages. United States Department of Agriculture, Agricultural Research Service. Available at: http://www.nal.usda.gov/fnic/foodcomp/Data/Fluoride/fluoride.pdf. Accessed June 30, 2012.
3. American Dental Association Council on Scientific Affairs: Nonfluoride caries preventive agents—a systematic review and evidence-based recommendations. *J Am Dent Assoc* 142(9):1065, 2011.
4. Bhushan J, Chachra S: Probiotics: their role in prevention of dental caries, *J Oral Health Comm Dent* 4(3):78, 2010.
5. Cannon ML: Clinical application of probiotic therapy—new adjunctive therapies offer new alternatives for treatment. Available at: http://www.dentalaegis.com/id/2011/06/clinical-application-of-probiotic-therapy. Accessed July 10, 2012.
6. Association of State and Territorial Dental Directors: Fluoride varnish: an evidence-based approach. Available at: http://www.kdheks.gov/ohi/download/Flvarnishpaper.pdf. Accessed August 22, 2012.
7. American Dental Association Council on Scientific Affairs: Professionally-applied topical fluoride: evidence-based clinical recommendations. *J Am Dent Assoc* 137(8):1151, 2006.
8. American Dental Association Council on Scientific Affairs: Evidence-based recommendations on the prescription of dietary fluoride supplements for caries prevention. *J Am Dent Assoc* 141(12):1480, 2010.
9. Su N, Marek C, Ching V: Caries prevention for patients with dry mouth. *J Can Dent Assoc* 77:b85, 2011.
10. Zhao J, Liu Y, Sun W, et al: Amorphous calcium phosphate and its application in dentistry. *Chem Cent J* 5:40, 2011.
11. Larsen C, Daronch M, Moursi A: *Topical fluoride therapy*, 2012, American Academy of Pediatric Dentistry Special Continuing Education Supplement.
12. Crozier S: The state of fluoridation. *ADA News* 43(13):22, 2012.
13. The decay-preventive sweetener. Available at: http://www.cda.org/popup/xylitol. Accessed June 21, 2012.
14. Papas AS, Vollmer WM, Gullion CM: Efficacy of chlorhexidine varnish for the prevention of adult caries. *J Dent Res* 91(2):150, 2012.
15. *Researchers discover promising anti-caries molecule*. Available at: http://www.dimensionsofdentalhygiene.com/ddhright.aspx?id=14047. Accessed July 20, 2012.
16. Domejean-Orliaguet S, Gansky SA, Featherstone JD: Caries risk assessment in an educational environment. *J Dent Educ* 70:1346, 2006.
17. O'Connell A: Use of xylitol chewing gum in mothers may delay transmission of mutans streptococci to their infants. *J Evid-Bas Dent Prac* 11(1):62, 2011.
18. Whitford GM: Acute toxicity of ingested fluoride. *Monogr Oral Sci* 22:66, 2011.
19. Autio-Gold J: The role of chlorhexidine in caries prevention. *J Oper Dent* 33(6):710, 2008.

ACKNOWLEDGMENT

The author acknowledges Michele Darby, Jeanne Maloney and Anne Miller for their past contributions to this chapter.

EVOLVE RESOURCES

Please visit http://evolve.elsevier.com/Darby/hygiene for additional practice and study support tools.

CHAPTER

34

Pit and Fissure Sealants

Judy Yamamoto, Maureen E. Fannon

COMPETENCIES

1. Discuss sealant placement, including:
   - Identify the role of pit and fissure sealants in a caries management program.
   - Explain the role of sealants in primary and secondary prevention.
   - Define pit and fissure sealants.
   - Explain indications and contraindications for sealant placement.
2. Explain how sealants are classified and describe each type.
3. Do the following regarding the procedure for sealant placement:
   - Describe the procedure for sealant placement.
   - Select the appropriate sealant material and apply it to the tooth.
   - Assess the retention of sealants at each re-care visit.

The dental hygienist plays an important role in the detection, recognition, and management of dental caries. The placement of pit and fissure sealants is an integral part of a comprehensive caries management program. As part of the dental hygiene process of care, the hygienist should assess the client's tooth morphology (pit and fissures) and caries risk. Once these have been identified, an appropriate intervention plan can be developed to include fluoride therapy, dietary counseling, xylitol use, and the application of pit and fissure sealants.

Deep pits and fissures in teeth are risk factors for dental caries.[1] Topically applied fluorides are most effective in preventing dental caries formation on the smooth surfaces of the teeth and least effective in preventing pits and fissure caries. Although the overall rate of smooth surface caries has decreased, the caries rate in pit and fissure surfaces of permanent posterior teeth is approximately 90%.[2] Adolescence can be a time of increased caries activity because of increased consumption of cariogenic substances and reduced self-care measures.[2] Retained dental sealants are effective in preventing dental caries.[3] Research indicates that dental sealant placement reduces caries 86% after 1 year, 79% after 2 years, and 59% after 3 years.[3,4] Therefore it is important to consider the placement of pit and fissure sealants in planning dental hygiene care for the maximum prevention and control of dental caries throughout the lifetime of the client.

Sealants are placed on an individual basis or as part of a public health program to prevent the initiation and progression of dental caries. They can be placed in caries-free teeth of at-risk individuals as a primary prevention strategy, or over early noncavitated lesions as part of a secondary preventive strategy.

A pit and fissure sealant is a thin plastic coating of an organic polymer (resin) placed in the pits and fissures of teeth (Figure 34-1). The sealant acts as a physical barrier to oral bacteria and carbohydrates, thereby preventing dental caries (Figure 34-2). The sealant bonds mainly by mechanical retention to the enamel tooth surface, forming a protective layer so that caries-producing bacteria cannot colonize within pits and fissures. Pit and fissure sealants along with radiographic monitoring of caries progression, fluoride therapy, xylitol use, dietary counseling, and active surveillance of incipient carious lesions are integral components of an effective caries management protocol (Box 34-1).

Indications for Sealant Placement

Caries Risk Assessment

Determining an individual's risk for dental caries involves identifying the age of the client and assessing biologic factors, protective factors, and clinical findings that contribute to or protect from dental caries (see Chapter 18). Dental caries is an infectious disease that occurs over the lifetime of an individual. Therefore it is important to assess continually a client's risk for developing dental caries. During the assessment phase of the dental hygiene process the dental hygienist identifies the caries risk of each client including pit and fissure morphology and makes a recommendation for sealant placement. Dental sealant placement for the reduction and/or progression of dental caries is indicated for low, moderate, or high-risk individuals age 3 years and older with deep fissure anatomy or developmental defects.[5]

Tooth Assessment

Pit and Fissure Anatomy

Tooth assessment to determine the need for sealant placement involves identifying the pit and fissure morphology of the tooth. If the occlusal contour shows deep and irregular pits and fissures, and there is no radiographic evidence that the tooth has proximal dental caries, then a sealant should be placed[5] (Figure 34-3). Figure 34-4 outlines the guidelines for making critical decisions about sealant placement. Sealant placement targets teeth with anatomy most at risk for pit and fissure caries and is not directed at teeth with well-coalesced pits and fissures. Tooth surfaces most at risk for dental caries in young children are occlusal surfaces of permanent first and second molars, followed by buccal surfaces of lower molars and lingual surfaces of upper molars.[6] Primary teeth that demonstrate deep pits and fissures also should be treatment

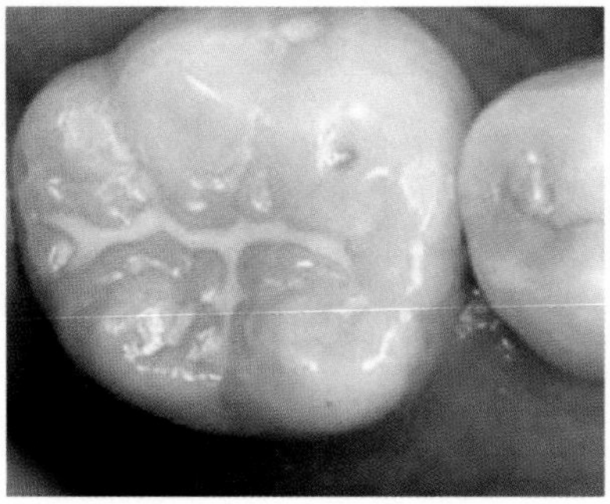

Figure 34-1. A dental sealant.

BOX 34-1

Integral Components for Caries Management

- Caries risk assessment
- Occlusal morphology/developmental defect assessment
- Fluoride, xylitol
- Pit and fissure sealants
- Diet counseling
  - Monitoring of incipient carious lesions
  - Parent involvement

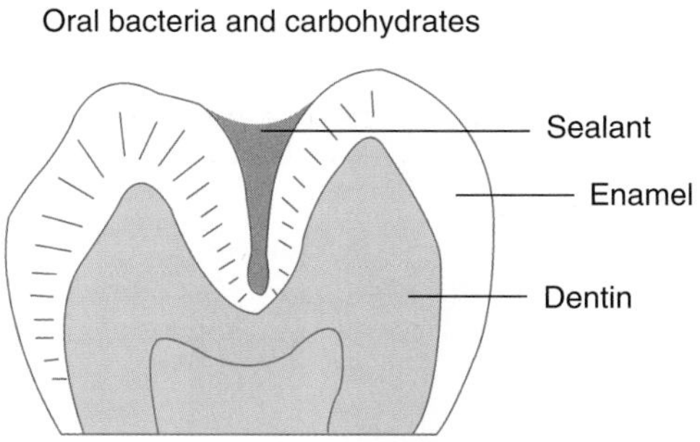

Figure 34-2. Sealant acts as a physical barrier to oral bacteria and carbohydrates. (From *Preventing pit and fissure caries: a guide to sealant use,* Boston, 1986, Massachusetts Department of Public Health and Massachusetts Health Research Institute.)

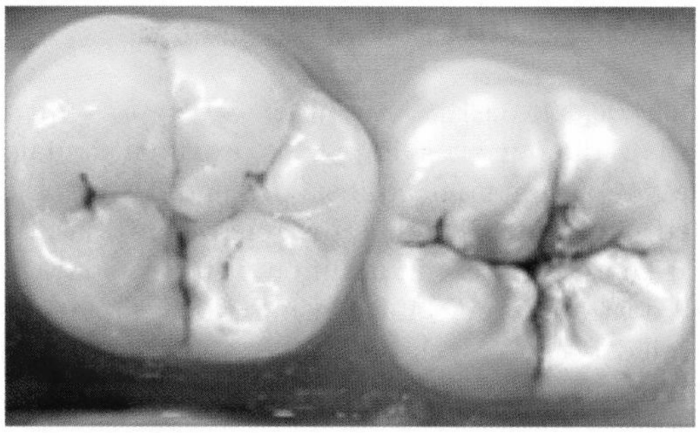

Figure 34-3. The tooth on the left should be sealed. The tooth on the right should be restored. (Courtesy Steve Eakle, University of California–San Francisco School of Dentistry.)

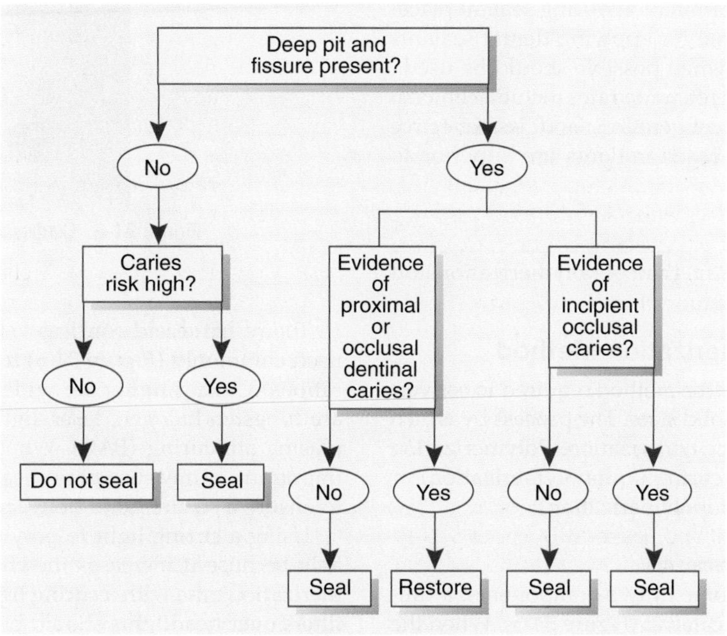

Figure 34-4. Guidelines for sealant placement decision making.

planned for dental sealants.[5] Newly erupted teeth must be sealed as soon as they are fully erupted since retention rates of dental sealants are higher for fully erupted teeth than for partially erupted teeth. The pits and fissures of molars remain susceptible to dental caries into adolescence and adulthood; therefore posteruptive age of teeth should not be used as the sole criterion for sealant placement.[5]

Noncavitated Lesions

Clients with **noncavitated lesions** can benefit from having dental sealants placed. These incipient lesions are demineralized areas confined to the enamel. Clinically they appear as white demineralized lines or spots, or areas of yellowish brownish discoloration around the pit and fissures of teeth. Sealants placed over these lesions can stop the caries from progressing into the dentin for as long as 5 years after sealant placement compared with unsealed teeth.[7]

Pit and fissure morphology makes it difficult to evaluate whether occlusal surfaces are capable of remineralization. In addition, occlusal decay is not apparent on dental radiographs until the carious lesions are advanced. As discussed in Chapter 18, current research does not support the process of pressing a sharp explorer into the pits and fissures of teeth to identify incipient carious lesions. The resistance of the explorer against the tooth can be simply the physical wedging of the instrument in the pit or fissure and not a carious lesion. Moreover, the explorer's force can cause an incipient lesion to cavitate. This cavitation allows bacteria to penetrate deeper into the tooth and ultimately accelerates the caries process. Visual inspection of the tooth surface after cleaning and drying is effective in detecting noncavitated lesions in pits and fissures.

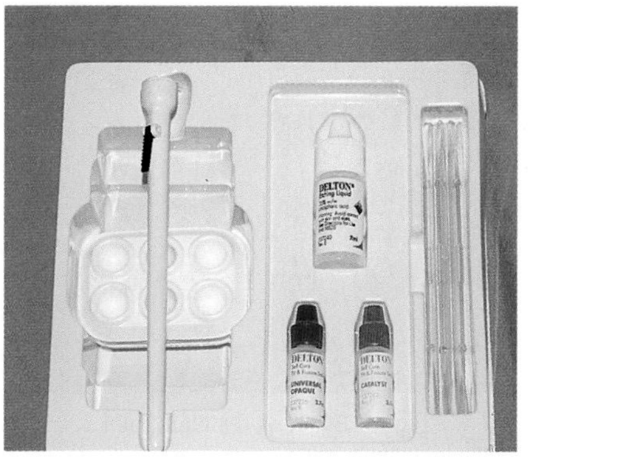

Figure 34-5. Universal liquid and catalyst vials shown with mixing wells and a mixing stick.

Contraindications to Sealant Placement

If there is radiographic evidence of proximal dental caries, then sealant placement in occlusal pits and fissures is contraindicated, and the client must be referred to the dentist to have the tooth restored. In addition, if the pits and fissures are well coalesced and self-cleansing, then sealants are contraindicated because such occlusal contours are at low risk for developing caries.

Retention Rates

The ability of a pit and fissure sealant to prevent dental caries is highly dependent on its ability to be retained on the tooth surface (**sealant retention**). The most common reason for sealant failure is salivary contamination during sealant placement. A four-handed technique for applying dental sealants enhances their integrity and when possible should be used.[8] Other factors affecting sealant retention rates include clinician inexperience, lack of client cooperation, and less-effective sealant material used (resin-based sealants are superior to glass ionomer sealants).[8]

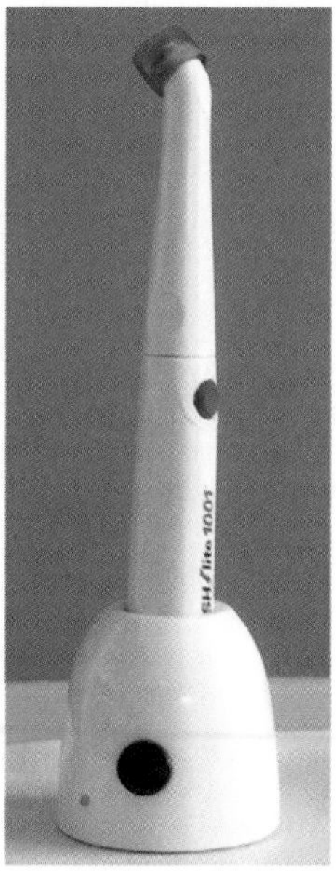

Figure 34-6. Cordless dental curing light.

Types of Sealants

Sealants are classified by their method of polymerization and their filler content.

Classification by Polymerization Method

Sealants can be categorized by the method required to convert them from a liquid state to a solid state. The process by which sealants harden is known as polymerization. Polymerization can be accomplished by self-curing (autopolymerization) or with a curing light unit (photopolymerization).

Self-Curing or Autopolymerized Sealants

Autopolymerized sealants come in two components: a universal liquid monomer and a catalyst (Figure 34-5). When the two components are mixed together, they harden (polymerize). Polymerization starts as soon as mixing begins, and the material hardens within 60 to 90 seconds. Self-curing sealants are used in community health or school-based programs because there is no special equipment required.

Photopolymerized or Visible Light–Cured Sealants

Photopolymerized sealants harden when exposed to a restorative curing light. Because no mixing time is required, the clinician controls the start of polymerization.

Today, handheld cordless visible lights (curing lights) are used commonly (Figure 34-6) for curing tooth-colored restorations. **Curing lights** are widely available. Various models are tungsten halogen, laser, light-emitting diode (LED), and plasma arc curing (PAC). Whatever light unit is used, it is important to measure periodically the light intensity output to ensure a secure bond between the sealant and enamel.

Using a curing light to polymerize sealants is seen favorably because it increases the clinician's working time. Polymerization time with a curing light is 10 to 20 seconds. Special filters over headlights should be used to protect the clinician from potential retinal damage (Figure 34-7). Dental loupes with protective shield often are used by clinicians. Unlike self-cured sealant methods, the photopolymerized sealant method requires additional time for infection control. The curing light tip, a semicritical item, is most likely to be in contact with mucous membranes and therefore requires sterilization of the tip or the use of a plastic barrier. Plastic barriers, however, must not decrease the intensity of the light beam. If the output intensity of the curing light is less than 280 mW/cm^2, the polymerization process of the monomer

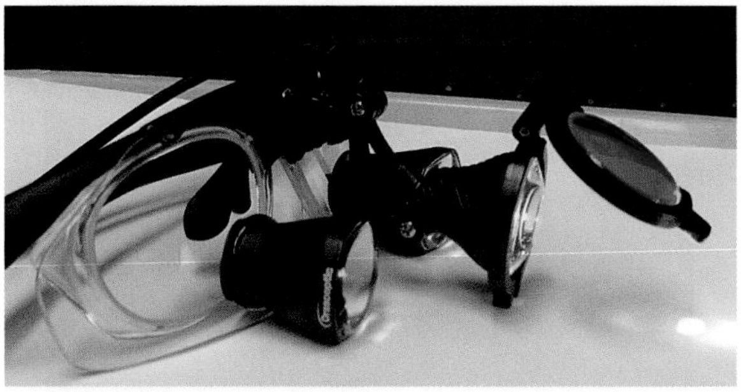

Figure 34-7. Protective shield attached to the headlamp for operator's eye protection from the curing light.

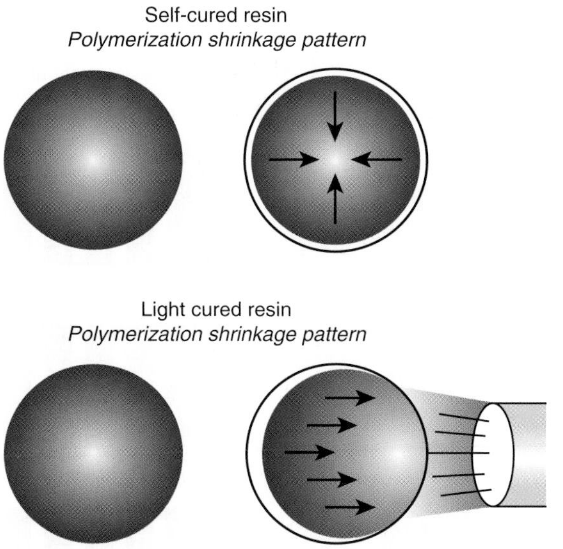

Figure 34-8. Polymerization shrinkage patterns. (From Albers HF: *Tooth-colored restoratives*, ed 9, Hamilton, Ontario, Canada, 2002, BC Decker.)

will be incomplete and early loss of the sealant may occur. Research indicates the Sani-Shield barrier (DW Technology, Las Vegas, Nevada) to be the least likely to interfere with light output intensity. The intensity of the curing light can be measured with a dental radiometer.

Comparison of Shrinkage Patterns

Autopolymerized sealants cure or shrink toward the center of the material and provide good sealant-to-tooth margins. However, photopolymerized sealants shrink toward the source of initiation or towards the *high-intensity* light. Therefore *light-cured sealants* may be *slightly* compromised and prone to marginal leakage (Figure 34-8).

Classification by Sealant Content

The American Dental Association (ADA) evaluates the effectiveness and safety of sealant materials. The type of sealants available based on content are filled and unfilled sealants. After placement of resin sealants, trace amounts of bisphenol-A (BPA) may be found in the saliva. Systemic BPA has not been detected as a result of the use of resin sealants. Any residual sealant material can be rinsed with water or blotted with a cotton roll.[9]

Filled Sealants

Filled sealants are a mixture of resins, chemicals, and fillers. The resins contain monomers and chemicals to hold the filler particles together. The purpose of the filler is to increase bonding strength and resist occlusal forces and wear. In addition, fillers increase the rate of flow (viscosity) of the sealant, promoting easy and thorough flow into the depths of pits and fissures. The monomers are liquid at room temperature and are activated or hardened by either chemical reactions or exposure to a curing light.

The fillers are usually glass and quartz particles of high hardness. Ground quartz (silicon dioxide) particles are categorized as large particle–sized fillers, which give strength and hardness to the material. Silica particles are considered small particle–sized fillers (microfill) and are less able to handle strong abrasive or occlusal forces. The ultimate combination of durability and strength in a composite sealant is with hybrid materials. This is a mixture of small and midsize particles that make up 50% to 70% of the total weight of the composite, and each filler particle is coated with saline to provide greater bonding strength between fillers and resins.

Research indicates that filled sealants are twice as wear-resistant as unfilled sealants and that a 10- to 20-second light cure is all that is needed for the filled sealant to have adequate bonding to the enamel surface. However, up to 75% of filler material can be added to sealants. The higher the filler content, the longer the polymerization time. It is best to check with each manufacturer's recommendation for optimal light curing time. Because of hardness and wear resistance, filled sealants must be checked after placement with articulating paper for occlusal high spots and adjusted with a slow-speed handpiece and round burr.

Unfilled Sealants

Unfilled sealants are clear, making it difficult to see during placement. Because unfilled sealants do not contain particles, they are less resistant to wear over the long term. Unfilled sealants are best used when the "high spots" in the occlusion cannot be adjusted with a dental handpiece. These sealants are most useful in school-based settings.

Fluoride-Releasing Sealants (Glass Ionomer Material)

In restorative dentistry, glass ionomers are used as cavity liners or intermediary bases to occupy a small space between the tooth and the restoration. Glass ionomer material also is used as a sealant because of its ability to flow easily into pits and fissures. Benefits to glass ionomer sealants is that this material can be purchased with a slow-releasing fluoride, which enhances the caries resistance of the tooth. This can be seen as a beneficial component with the bonding of the sealant margins with enamel, particularly when shrinkage patterns are of concern.

When glass ionomer sets, water is a by-product. Therefore glass ionomer is hydrophilic and not of great concern with moisture, particularly when used on partially erupted teeth or teeth under operculums.

However, studies show that glass ionomer sealants may be brittle and show high rates of occlusal wear.

Classification of Sealants by Color

Clear, tinted, and opaque sealants are available. The addition of color to the sealant material enhances the visibility of the

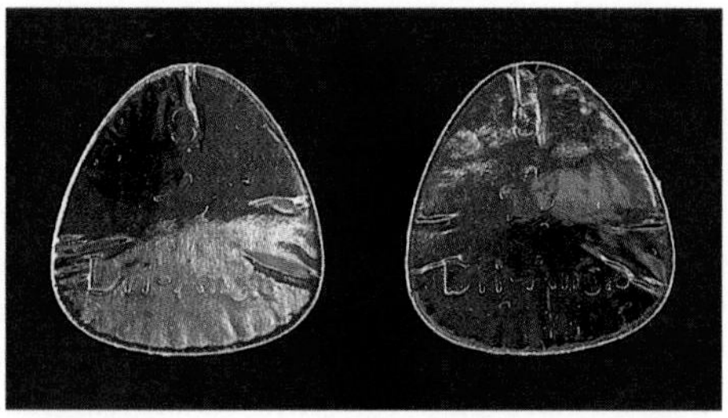

Figure 34-9. Dri-Angles for placement over Stensen's duct for isolation and moisture control.

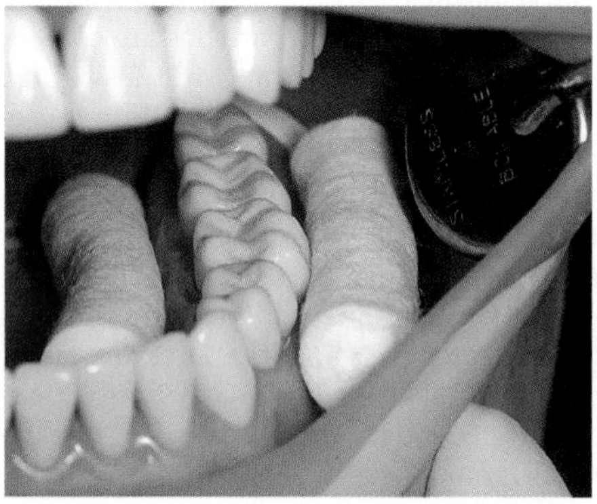

Figure 34-10. Isolation of site with cotton rolls. (Courtesy Cara Miyasaki.)

sealant for the operator and aids in monitoring retention. Color does not affect sealant retention.

Procedure for Sealant Placement

The proper placement of a sealant requires that the newly erupted tooth or teeth considered to be of high risk is isolated properly and dry to ensure that the treatment site is visible and accessible. Teeth can be cleaned using a dry toothbrush or prophy cup/brush to remove debris. A rubber dam is effective for isolation when several teeth in the quadrant are worked on; however, bibulous pads (e.g., Dri-Angles) placed over Stensen's duct and proper placement of cotton rolls in the vestibules and at the sides of the tongue are effective in promoting moisture control (Figures 34-9 and 34-10).

It is critical to keep the working site free of water and saliva. The saliva ejector should be used to aid in moisture control, and the teeth should be dried thoroughly with compressed air. The use of hydrophilic primers aids in drying the enamel surface, which enhances the sealant attachment to the etched surface. Other critical factors that influence sealant retention are surface cleanliness and the successful creation of etched micropores on the enamel surface.

Once isolated, cleaned, and dried, the enamel surface is ready for acid etching. An acid etching solution is applied to the tooth. The acid supplied by most manufacturers is concentrated to a level of 35% to 38% phosphoric acid in either liquid or gel form. The acid etching creates microscopic pores on the enamel to increase surface irregularities for sealant retention. The liquid acid is applied with a fine plastic-bristled brush, using a continuous dabbing motion. The gel is placed on the tooth surface with a special syringe and left undisturbed (Figure 34-11). Many dental hygienists prefer to use gels because they are colored, making it easy to tell where the

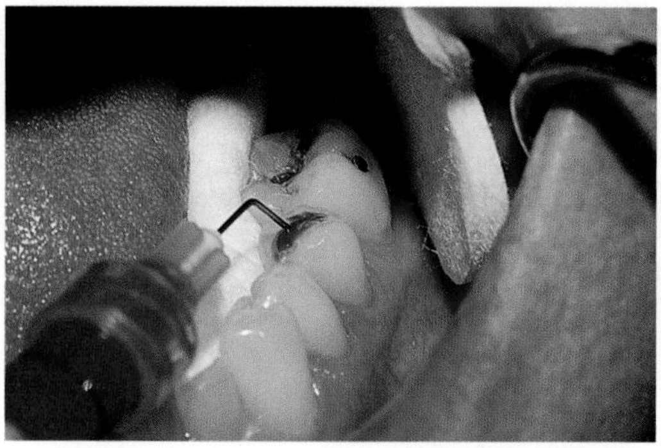

Figure 34-11. Acid etching solution in gel form.

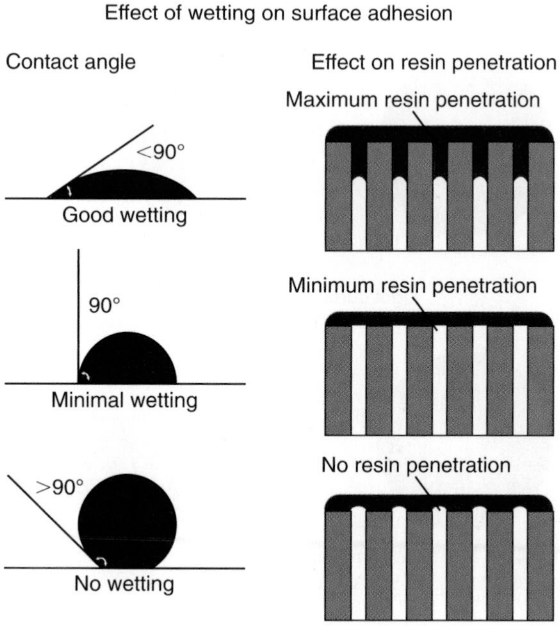

Figure 34-12. Acid etching solution in gel form.

gel has been applied. Care should be taken that the acid does not come in contact with mucosal surfaces.

The sealant brush should approach the etched tooth with a low contact angle of less than 90 degrees. With a small contact angle there is a greater ability of the liquid sealant to penetrate into the newly created enamel micropores on the tooth surface. This process is known as *wetting* when there is maximum penetration of a liquid (sealant) to a solid structure (tooth). Wetting plays a significant role in determining the penetration, adhesion, and ultimately retention of sealants (Figure 34-12). Detailed methods for placement of light-cured and self-cured sealants are described in Procedures 34-1 and 34-2.

CLIENT EDUCATION TIPS

- Explain the rationale for placing a sealant.
- Explain that sealants prevent the initiation and progression of dental caries. Sealants are not permanent, may become partially lost, and therefore may have to be replaced.

Procedure 34-1 Applying Light-Cured (Photopolymerized) Sealants

EQUIPMENT
Mouth mirror
Explorer
Cotton forceps
Saliva ejector
Sealant kit
Cotton rolls and rubber dam
Air-water syringe tip
Dri-Angles
High-speed evacuation tube
Low-speed handpiece or air-polishing device
Bristled brush
Pumice
Floss
Light protective shield
Client protective eyewear
Personal protective equipment
Light cure unit
Round finishing burr
Articulating paper

STEPS

1. Assemble sealant armamentarium (Figure 34-13).

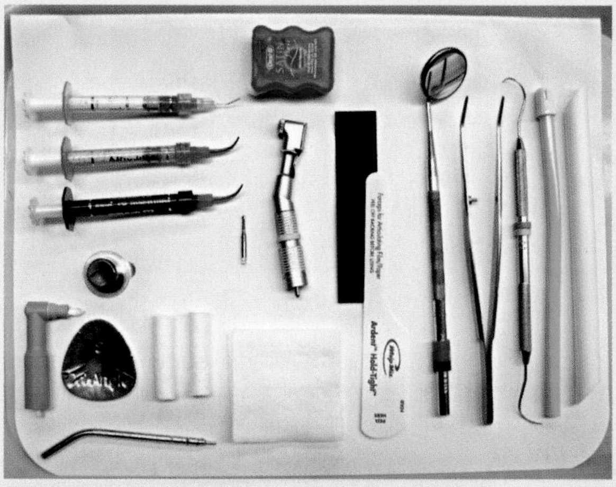

Figure 34-13. Armamentarium for pit and fissure sealant in addition to the client protective shield and clinician protective lenses. (Courtesy Lisa Hoang.)

2. Provide client with protective eyewear with filter. Wear personal protective equipment.
3. Identify tooth or teeth to be sealed.
4. Polish the intended surface with a slurry of pumice and water. Use air polishing or a bristled brush attached to a low-speed handpiece. Rinse with water (Figures 34-14 and 34-15).

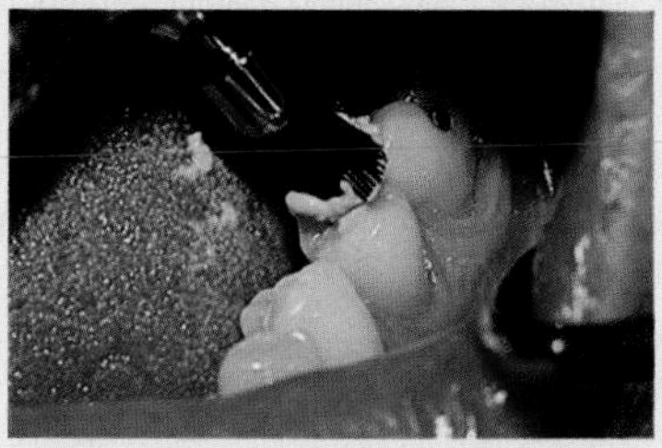

Figure 34-14.

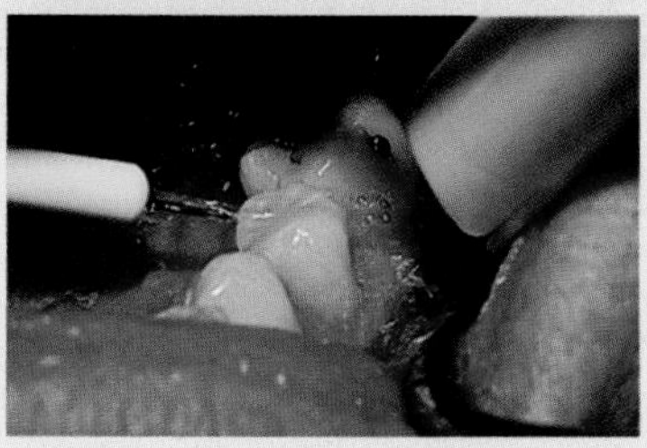

Figure 34-15.

5. Isolate teeth with a rubber dam, or place Dri-Angle over Stensen's duct and insert cotton rolls. Place saliva ejector into client's mouth.
6. Dry the site to be sealed with compressed air that is free of oil and moisture (Figure 34-16).

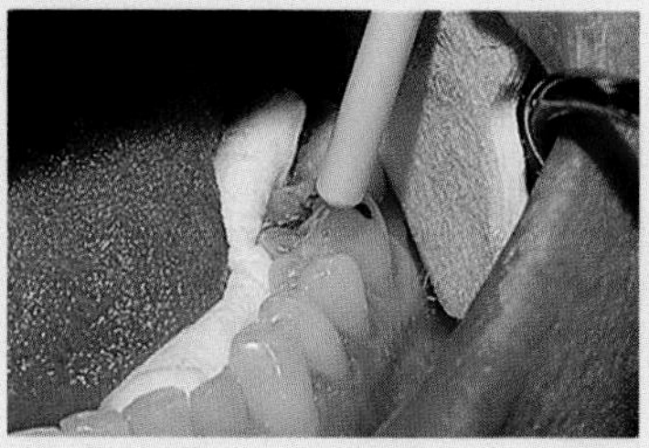

Figure 34-16.

7. Apply phosphoric acid to the clean, dry tooth surface. Etch the tooth for 10 to 20 seconds. If using a liquid etch, apply it with a brush. If using a gel etch, apply it and leave undisturbed.
8. Rinse etched surfaces for 30 to 60 seconds using a water syringe and high-speed evacuation. If gel etch is used, rinse for an additional 30 seconds (Figure 34-17).

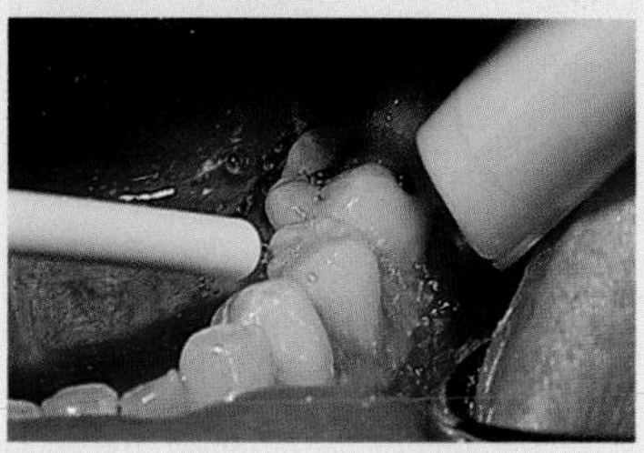

Figure 34-17.

9. Using cotton forceps, replace cotton rolls and Dri-Angles as they become wet (Figure 34-18).

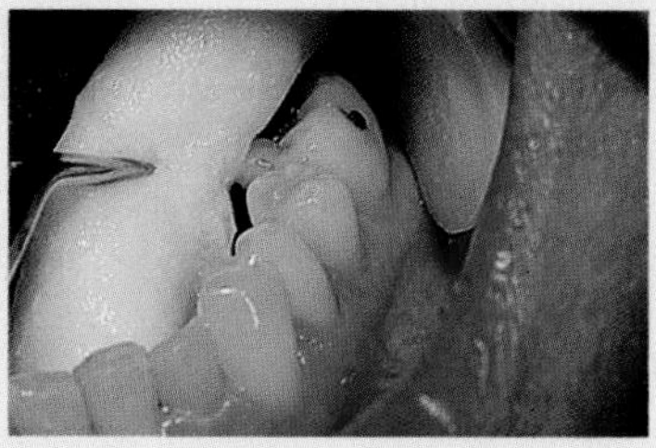

Figure 34-18.

Continued

Procedure 34-1 Applying Light-Cured (Photopolymerized) Sealants—cont'd

10. Dry the treatment site with compressed air for 10 seconds. Evaluate etched surface (Figure 34-19).

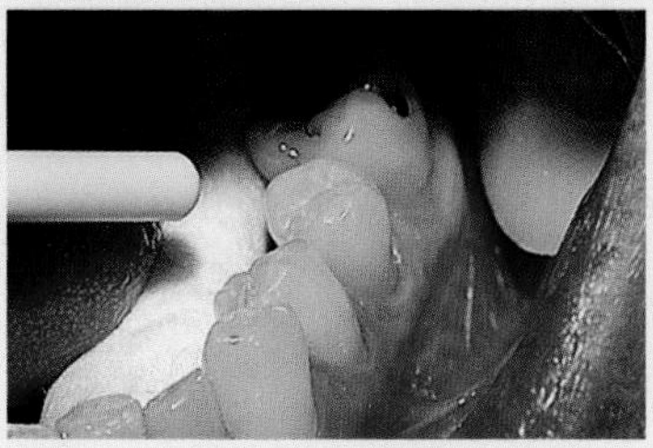

Figure 34-19.

11. Apply hydrophilic primer and dry with compressed air.
12. Apply liquid sealant over the pits and fissures at less than 90 degrees. Allow the sealant to flow into the etched surfaces (Figure 34-20).

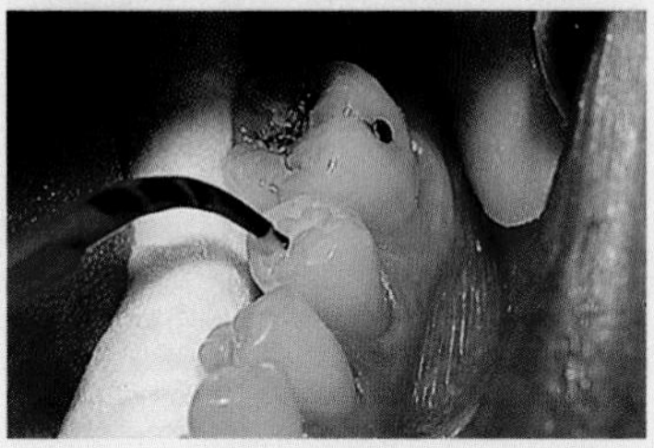

Figure 34-20.

13. Apply light-cure tip to sealant. Place tip of light source 2 mm from sealant. Check manufacturer's instructions for time before advancing the light to another area (Figure 34-21).

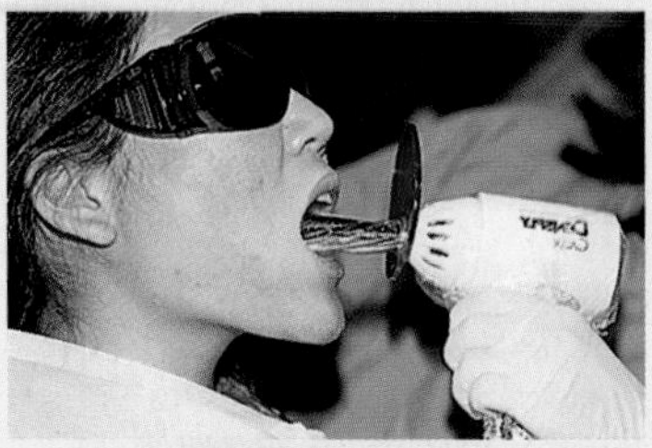

Figure 34-21.

14. After the polymerization process, evaluate the sealant with an explorer and check for hard, smooth surface and retention. Set sealant appears as a thin, polymerized film.
15. If imperfections are noted (e.g., incomplete coverage, air bubbles), re-etch tooth for 10 seconds; wash and dry teeth and apply additional sealant (Figures 34-22 and 34-23).

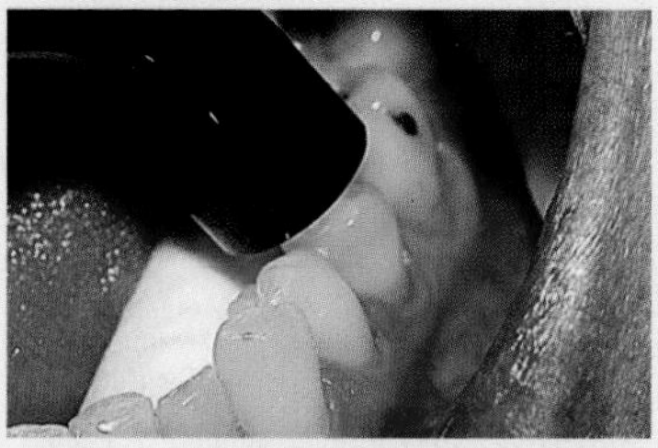

Figure 34-22.

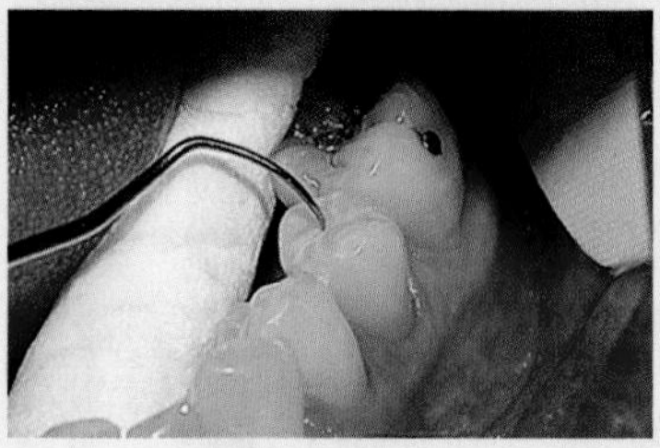

Figure 34-23.

16. Check occlusion with articulating paper to detect high spot areas. Remove excess filled sealant material with a finishing burr (Figure 34-24).

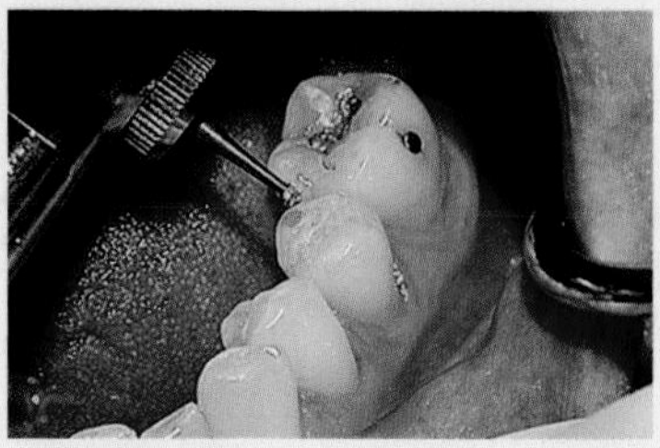

Figure 34-24.

17. Remove any residual unsealed liquid sealant with dry gauze. Floss treated teeth.
18. Apply topical fluoride.
19. Record type of sealant and teeth sealed in client's dental record.
20. Evaluate sealants 3 months after application and at every continued-care appointment.

Photographs courtesy Catrin Backlund.

Procedure 34-2 Applying Self-Cured (Autopolymerizing) Sealants

EQUIPMENT

Mouth mirror
Explorer
Saliva ejector
Self-cure sealant kit
Gauze
Cotton rolls and rubber dam
Air-water syringe tip
Dri-Angles
High-speed evacuation tube
Low-speed handpiece or air-polishing device
Bristled brush
Pumice
Floss
Personal protective equipment
Protective barriers

Procedure 34-2 Applying Self-Cured (Autopolymerizing) Sealants—cont'd

STEPS

1. Follow steps 1 to 10 as described for light-cured sealants in Procedure 34-1.
2. Mix one drop of universal liquid and one drop of catalyst liquid in mixing well. Follow manufacturer's directions, especially when sealing more than two teeth (Figure 34-25).

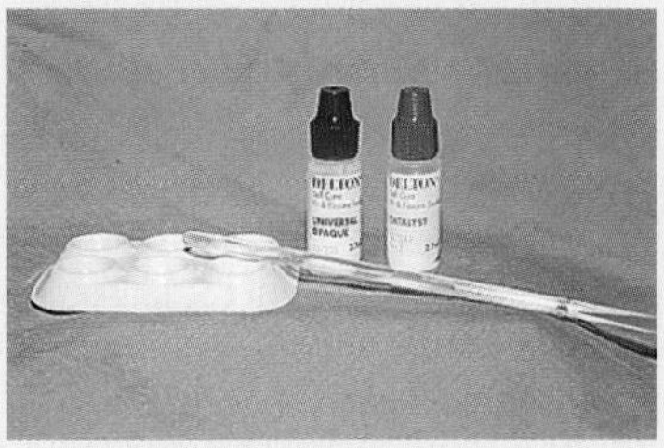

Figure 34-25.

3. Mix for 10 to 15 seconds or as specified by manufacturer's directions.
4. Apply sealant with brush over pits and fissures. Working time: 45 seconds.
5. Allow sealant to set for 60 to 90 seconds or according to manufacturer's instructions.
6. Follow steps 14 to 20 as described for light-cured sealants in Procedure 34-1.

- Explain that sealant placement does not eliminate the need for topical fluoride application, oral hygiene instruction, use of antimicrobials, or modification of caries risk factors. Sealants in combination with these other strategies are part of a total caries management program.
- Ask client if sealant feels "high" when biting, and explain the need to adjust occlusion.
- Explain the need for client cooperation for optimal sealant placement.

LEGAL, ETHICAL, AND SAFETY ISSUES

- Care must be taken when using the acid-etch solution to avoid contact with any oral tissues other than the tooth surface to be sealed.
- Clients must wear protective glasses as a barrier to the sealant chemicals and curing light.
- Clients must be told not to look at the curing light tip
- Clients must understand that sealants are not permanent and may have to be replaced for continued protection against pit and fissure caries.
- It is legal for dental hygienists to place dental sealants in all 50 states. Supervision requirements and clinical setting vary from state to state. The American Dental Hygienists' Association Office of Governmental Affairs has the most recent information concerning setting and supervision requirements for each of the 50 states.
- Always follow sealant manufacturers' instructions.
- Systemic bisphenol-A (BPA) has not been detected with the use of dental sealants.

KEY CONCEPTS

- Dental sealants can be a preventive and/or therapeutic treatment for caries control.
- Epidemiologic data reveal that dental caries are concentrated more on the occlusal surfaces than on smooth surfaces of the teeth.
- Clients' risk for developing dental caries is determined by identifying their prior caries experience, fluoride history, tooth morphology, and plaque load. This information is integral to assessing their need for dental sealants.
- Sealant placement should be targeted to the most susceptible surfaces of the most susceptible teeth.
- Sealants are indicated for clients at any age at risk for developing dental caries.
- A dental hygiene diagnosis related to dental sealants is based on the client's deficits in the human needs for a biologically sound dentition, conceptualization and problem solving, and responsibility for oral health.
- Resin sealants can be either filled or unfilled.
- Glass ionomer sealants release fluoride to provide a benefit to the high caries risk client.
- Filler particles in dental sealants enhance their wear resistance.
- Before a dental sealant is placed, the tooth surface must be cleaned, dried, etched, rinsed, and then dried again.
- The use of a primer aids in tooth surface dryness.
- When placing a dental sealant, the clinician must allow the material to flow into the grooves of the tooth surface. This minimizes the presence of air bubbles.
- Use of the "wetting" technique during the sealant placement maximizes the penetration of the sealant into the enamel micropores.
- The process by which the sealant material hardens is called *polymerization.*
- Autopolymerization causes the sealant material to harden chemically by mixing an activator with a catalyst.
- Photopolymerization causes the sealant material to harden by use of a high-intensity curing light.
- Shrinkage patterns differ between autopolymerization and photopolymerization.
- The retention rate of dental sealants is enhanced by keeping the working area free from salivary contaminants, using a hydrophilic primer to dry the tooth surface, and thoroughly cleaning the tooth surface to be sealed.
- Chart documentation should include the type of sealant used and the teeth that were sealed.
- The integrity of the dental sealant should be evaluated at each continued-care visit.

CRITICAL THINKING EXERCISES

Patient Profile: Julia is a 14-year-old Hispanic female who visits the office every 6 months for an examination and oral prophylaxis. She has been a patient at this practice for 10 years.

Chief Complaint: "I am here today because I noticed some white spots on the chewing surfaces of my lower back teeth."

Health History: Noncontributory

Dental History: Julia has occlusal composite fillings on Nos. 3, 14, 19, and 30.

Social History: She is single and lives at home with her parents. Julia states that she is snacking more frequently since she started high school. She drinks approximately three soft drinks a day and buys snacks from the vending machines during her breaks at school.

Oral Self-Care Assessment: The client states that she brushes her teeth with a fluoride toothpaste two times a day. However, her technique reveals that when brushing she covers only the facial surfaces of her maxillary and mandibular teeth. She uses no interdental aids.

Supplemental Notes: Client has deep fissures in all her posterior teeth.

1. Use this information in planning dental hygiene care to meet the client's need for a biologically sound and functional dentition. What interventions would you plan, and why?
2. Would pit and fissure sealants be beneficial for her? Where? Explain your response.
3. What would you say in educating Julia about her caries risk prevention and treatment options during her dental hygiene care appointment?

Patient Profile: Henry is 7 years old. He is treatment planned to receive dental sealants on all his permanent first molars.

Chief Complaint: Henry's mom has read that sealants contain bisphenol A and does not want her son exposed to a carcinogen.

Health History: Henry is allergic to latex and suffers from eczema and asthma. His asthma is well controlled and is brought on by exercise.

Dental History: Henry had three of his primary first molars extracted because of dental decay. He has deep grooves in all his posterior teeth.

Social History: Henry is in second grade and lives with his parents.

Oral Self-Care Assessment: Henry's mom brushes his teeth once a day with water only.

Supplemental Notes: Henry has just started to brush his teeth on his own once a day without toothpaste.

1. How would you alleviate Henry's mom's concerns about the bisphenol A in sealants?
2. Would you recommend that additional sealants be placed in Henry's mouth? If so, where?
3. How might fluoride toothpaste benefit Henry?

REFERENCES

1. Featherstone JD, Domejean-Orliaguet S, Jenson L, et al: Caries risk assessment in practice for age 6 through adult, *J Calif Dent Assoc* 35:703, 2007.
2. National Center for Health Statistics, Centers for Disease Control and Prevention: National Health and Nutrition Examination Surveys, 1999-2004.
3. Ahovuo-Salorante A, Hiiri A, Nordblad A, et al: Pit and fissure sealants for preventing decay in the permanent teeth of children and adolescents, *Cochrane Database Syst Rev* (3):CD001830, 2004.
4. Llodra JC, Bravo M, Delgado-Rodriquez M, et al: Factors influencing the effectiveness of sealants, a metanalysis, *Commun Dent Oral Epidemiol* 21(5):261, 1993.
5. American Academy of Pediatric Dentistry Council on Clinical Affairs: *Guideline on caries-risk assessment and management for infants, children, and adolescents*, Chicago, 2011, American Academy of Pediatric Dentistry.
6. Feigal RJ, Donly KJ: The use of pit and fissure sealants, *Pediatr Dent* 28:143, 2006.
7. Griffin SO, Oong E, Kohn W, et al: The effectiveness of sealants in managing carious lesions, *J Dent Res* 87(2):169, 2008.
8. Beauchamp J, Caufield P, Crall J, et al: Evidence-based clinical recommendations for the use of pit-and-fissure sealants. A report of the American Dental Association Council on Scientific Affairs, *J Am Dent Assoc* (139):257, 2008.
9. Anusavice KJ: Biocompatibility, *Phillips' science of dental materials*, ed 12, St Louis, 2013, Saunders.

EVOLVE RESOURCES

Please visit http://evolve.elsevier.com/Darby/hygiene for additional practice and study support tools.

CHAPTER 35

Nutritional Counseling

Lisa F. Harper Mallonee

COMPETENCIES

1. **Discuss nutrition assessment, including:**
   - **Identify individuals in need of nutritional counseling to control dental caries, promote postsurgical healing and tissue regeneration, reduce bone loss due to osteoporosis and osteopenia, or achieve optimal health.**
   - **Calculate ideal body mass index, waist circumference, and ideal body weight.**
2. **Discuss dietary assessment, including:**
   - **Determine client compliance with U.S. Dietary Guidelines.**
   - **Evaluate a client's diet for adequacy of intake using the U.S. Department of Agriculture Food Guidance System (MyPlate).**
3. **Identify methods for conducting successful nutritional counseling.**
4. **Discuss the nutritional needs of different client populations, including the differences in nutritional requirements throughout the life span.**

Diet and nutrition are vital oral health components. **Nutritional counseling** is a process that can be used in the oral healthcare setting to help clients maintain optimum oral health and develop healthful behaviors that promote overall health. When providing nutritional counseling, clinicians must consider individual factors such as age, gender, culture, economics, lifestyle, dental health, chronic disease, medications, allergies, and food avoidances.

Nutritional deficiency or metabolic disease diagnosis is made by a physician after extensive data collection. Much of this information is outside of the scope of dental hygiene and therefore precludes the dental hygienist from functioning in the role of nutrition professional. As a health professional who sees clients on an ongoing basis, however, the dental hygienist must be knowledgeable about nutrition (Figure 35-1), oral manifestations of nutritional deficiencies (Figure 35-2), and oral health.[1,2] For nutritional concerns outside the scope of dental hygiene practice, referral to a registered dietitian is indicated.

Nutrition Assessment

Nutrition assessment is the systematic collection of information to identify the need for nutritional counseling and make the appropriate recommendations and referrals. The client's personal history can reveal information regarding educational, cultural, financial, and environmental influences on food intake. The health and pharmacologic histories identify health factors and medications that interfere with an individual's ability to eat or the body's ability to absorb nutrients. The dental history provides information about caries susceptibility, fluoride use, and dentition concerns that may affect food intake; the extraoral and intraoral examination may reveal the physical results of any nutritional excesses or deficiencies as well as salivary concerns that may affect food clearance. These findings, along with a dietary assessment, direct the dental hygienist in the role of dietary counselor. Determining which clients need nutritional counseling involves analyzing information collected during the assessment phase of care.

Every client could benefit from nutritional counseling, but those most often targeted include clients with the following characteristics:
- At risk for osteoporosis
- Diagnosed with osteopenia
- Undergoing periodontal or oral maxillofacial surgery
- Evidence of dental caries or periodontal disease
- Oral manifestations of a possible nutritional deficiency

Health and Pharmacologic Histories

Questions normally included in a comprehensive health history provide clues to nutritional status, lifestyle behaviors, and overall health (see Chapter 12, Figure 12-2, and Table 12-2). The health history must include weight and height measurements and space to note conditions and medications that interfere with food digestion, absorption, and metabolism. The dental hygienist must ask about dietary supplements, vitamins, and herbal preparations if not specified on the health history and question clients about recent illnesses, changes in health behaviors, or modifications to their diets.

Height and Weight

Height and weight can be used to determine the client's body mass index. **Body mass index (BMI)** reflects weight in relation to height (Table 35-1); it is not a measure of lean body mass.
- A BMI of 18.5 to 24.9 is considered within the normal range.
- A BMI less than 18.5 is an indication of being underweight.
- A BMI of 25 to 29.9 is in the overweight category.
- A BMI of 30 and above is considered obese.

Although a BMI measurement does not reflect how much of the weight is fat, it does give a measurement associated

Figures, tables, and boxes marked as "e" are available as supplemental material on the Evolve site. Visit http://evolve.elsevier.com/Darby/hygiene to access these materials.

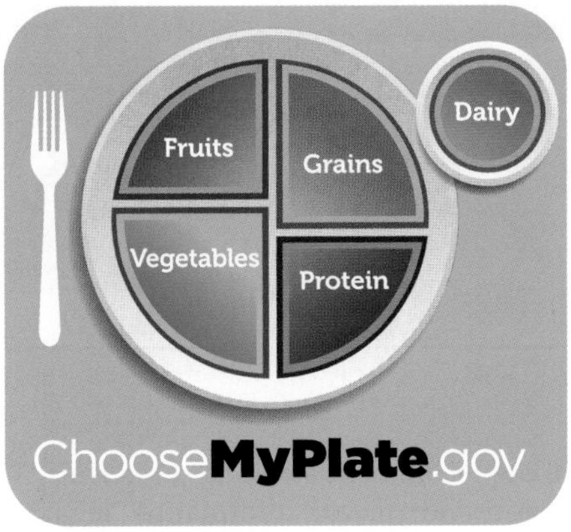

Balancing Calories

- Enjoy your food, but eat less.
- Avoid oversized portions.

Foods to Increase

- Make half your plate fruits and vegetables.
- Make at least half your grains whole grains.
- Switch to fat-free or low-fat (1%) milk.

Foods to Reduce

- Compare sodium in foods like soup, bread, and frozen meals – and choose the foods with lower numbers.
- Drink water instead of sugary drinks.

Figure 35-1. MyPlate Food Guidance System. (From USDA, Center for Nutrition Policy and Promotion, 2010 [http://www.choosemyplate.gov].)

with health risks such as heart disease, hypertension, diabetes, and cancer. Waist circumference (see Table 35-1) also can be used to indicate health risk. Waist circumference is a numeric measurement of the waist. It is used most effectively in those clients who are categorized as normal or overweight on the BMI scale. A female with a waist measurement of 35 inches and a male with a waist measurement of 40 inches is associated with upper body obesity. Upper body obesity is correlated strongly with heart disease and type 2 diabetes. Another useful and simple calculation is ideal body weight. Although commonly used, it is not the most accurate method because it does not take age, race, or frame size into consideration. Calculation of BMI is the most practical method to integrate into client care, making use of the client's reported height and weight during the health history interview. The U.S. Department of Health and Human Services National Heart, Lung and Blood Institute has an online BMI calculation tool that can be accessed at http://nhlbisupport.com/bmi.

Exercise Patterns

Activity levels ascertained during the health history interview may be used to determine more accurately daily calorie needs (see eFigure 35-7). An approximate daily caloric expenditure can be useful in planning for weight loss or weight gain. However, the primary goal in the dental setting is to identify nutrition concerns that may contribute to oral disease risk—not modify weight. Nonetheless, activity level, along with anthropometric measures such as height and weight can be plugged into one of the interactive tools on MyPlate to determine an individual's caloric needs and provide clients with recommendations for a healthy lifestyle.

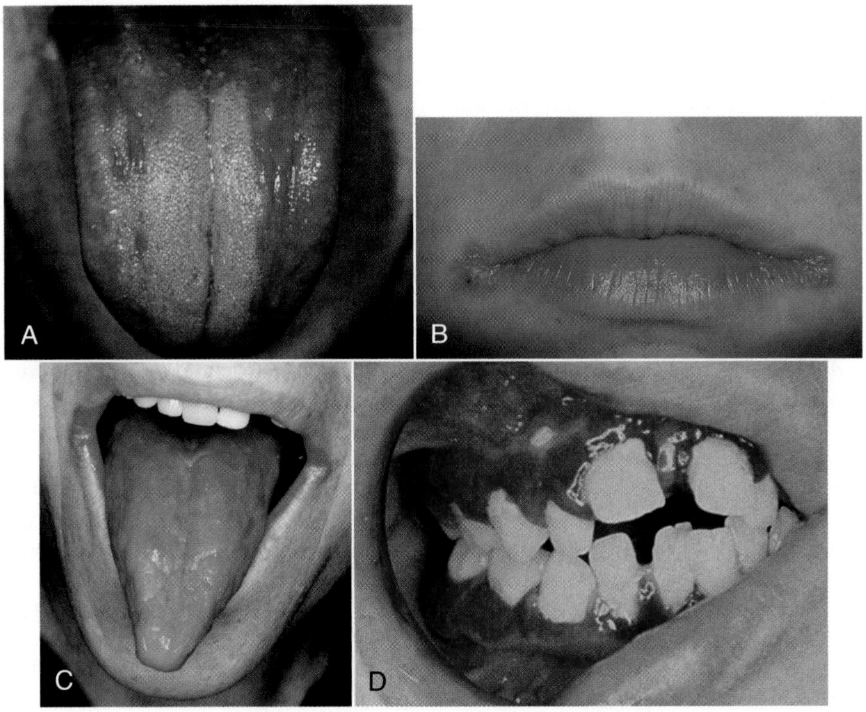

Figure 35-2. Some oral manifestations of nutritional deficiencies. **A,** Atrophy of the filiform and fungiform papillae on the dorsum of the tongue associated with iron deficiency anemia. **B,** Riboflavin deficiency characterized by erythema, maceration, and soggy white debris at the commissures of the mouth. **C,** Pernicious anemia. **D,** Severe gingivitis associated with scurvy. (**A** and **D,** From Eisen D, Lynch DP: *The mouth: diagnosis and treatment,* St Louis, 1998, Mosby. **B** and **C,** From Ibsen OAC, Phelan JA: *Oral pathology for the dental hygienist,* ed 6, St. Louis, 2014, Saunders.)

TABLE 35-1
Nutrition-Related Formulas and Calculations

Formula or Calculation	Definition	Use	Disadvantage
Body Mass Index (BMI)			
Weight in lb × 703 ÷ Height in inches^2	Measurement of weight in relation to height	Useful in determining if client is underweight or overweight	Does not measure lean tissue in relation to fat (i.e., bodybuilders may have a higher BMI owing to a larger amount of lean tissue but are not overweight or obese)
Waist Circumference			
For men, 40 inches; for women, 35 inches	Measurement of waist used to determine central obesity.	Useful in determining health risks if a client is overweight or obese.	Incorrect placement of tape measure could produce inaccurate result
Ideal Body Weight (Hamwi Equation)			
For men, 106 lb for the first 5' of height and 5 lb for each inch above 5'; or 6 lb subtracted for each inch under 5 feet. For women, 100 lb for the first 5' and 5 lb for each inch above 5'; or 5 lb subtracted for each inch under 5 feet.	Determines ideal body for height of individual	Useful in determining if client is underweight or overweight	Does not measure lean tissue in relation to fat. A client may be considered underweight but may still be "overfat"

Prescription Medications and Dietary Supplement Intake

Assessment of the ingestion of prescription medications as well as vitamin and mineral supplements provides insight about such oral manifestations as xerostomia, lichenoid reactions, candidiasis, cheilitis, and glossitis. Dietary supplements and herbal products are used routinely by dental clients. Many of these products have effects on the oral tissues that may interfere with dental care, so it is essential that the dental hygienist update and review these nonprescription medications before treatment. Increased bleeding, elevated blood pressure, and delayed wound healing are potential effects that may occur.[3]

Dietary Assessment

Dietary assessment is the identification of current dietary practices and dietary requirements of the client. Dietary assessment includes frequency of food intake, methods of food preparation, cultural or religious dietary considerations, and exercise or activity levels; it reflects the Dietary Guidelines for Americans based on the U.S. Department of Agriculture (USDA) updated food guidance system titled "MyPlate."[2] Types of dietary assessments include the dietary history, a food frequency questionnaire, and a computer dietary analysis.

Dietary History

A **dietary history** may consist of a 24-hour food record (Figure 35-3), a food frequency questionnaire (eFigure 35-4), or a 3-, 5-, or 7-day dietary history (Figure 35-5), in which the client records all foods and drinks consumed within the defined period. The dietary history determines a client's usual intake over a period of time and is a screening tool to identify persons in need of nutritional counseling. A dietary history is obtained by interview or self-administered questionnaire.

Although not practical in the dental hygiene care setting, food models such as measuring cups and spoons help the client recall the amount of food consumed and should be used when possible. A 24-hour dietary history usually requires 10 to 15 minutes for the dental hygienist to complete and does not require the client to possess a long memory. This requires asking the client about all foods eaten in the previous 24 hours. If taken unannounced or with no prior indication, it minimizes the likelihood that the client will alter his or her diet. However, the 24-hour dietary recall may not be representative of the person's usual food intake. For most people, workdays, weekends, and holidays influence food intake considerably.

An advantage of the 24-hour dietary recall is that it serves as a teaching session. Accuracy as well as content can be discussed during the session, and the technique can be applied to a 3-, 5-, or 7-day dietary recall. The client and the dental hygienist determine the length of time the diet will be documented. The shorter the period, the less likely it is that the record will reveal usual eating patterns. A 24-hour dietary recall in combination with a food frequency questionnaire or a 3-, 5-, or 7-day dietary recall provides a more accurate account of the client's regular intake.

Food Frequency Questionnaire

A **food frequency questionnaire** (see eFigure 35-4) is similar to a 24-hour dietary recall but specifically asks the client to record foods most frequently eaten within a stated timeframe (e.g., as short as a day or as long as a month). The 24-hour

24-HOUR FOOD RECORD

Was yesterday a typical day? Write down everything you ate or drank yesterday from the time you got up in the morning until you went to bed. Also include how much of each food you ate and approximately the time you ate or drank it.

Example:

AM meal Time: 6:00 AM
½ cup orange juice
¾ cup corn flakes and ½ cup whole milk
1 cup coffee with 2 teaspoons sugar

MORNING MEAL TIME:	MORNING SNACK TIME:	MIDDAY MEAL TIME:
AFTERNOON SNACK TIME:	**EVENING MEAL TIME:**	**EVENING SNACK TIME:**

List any vitamin or herbal supplements (including the amounts of each). Record all oral hygiene habits/regimens, if any, after meals: i.e., brushing, flossing, chew gum with xylitol

Figure 35-3. Twenty-four–hour food record. (Courtesy Dr. L. Boyd. Adapted from C. Palmer, Tufts University School of Dental Medicine, 1998.)

dietary recall, 3-, 5-, or 7-day dietary recall, and food frequency questionnaire can be useful in assessing the cariogenic potential of the diet.

Computer Dietary Analysis

All dietary records have the potential for computer analysis. There are various programs available, and often the choice depends on the information obtained, its purpose, and the type of computer hardware available. Some programs are designed for research and provide everything from bar graphs to merging data for community-based programs. Most computer programs provide information on caloric intake as well as deficient or excess nutrient amounts. Some programs analyze sugar intake, including percentage of sugars in the diet (e.g., simple versus complex carbohydrates). SuperTracker is a simple, inexpensive option that can be used to assess the general nutrition of a client in the dental setting (see http://www.choosemyplate.gov/supertracker-tools/supertracker.html).

Dietary Evaluation

A simple and practical client assessment includes the following:

- Daily sugar exposures
- Adequacy of food intake based on the five food groups and MyPlate (see http://www.choosemyplate.gov)

Evaluation of the Cariogenic Potential of the Diet

To assess the cariogenic potential of the diet, a 24-hour dietary recall (see Figure 35-3) is best used in the dental setting. However, this may not represent the client's typical eating patterns, so a 3-, 5-, or 7-day food record (see Figure 35-5) may be indicated for a more accurate account of the client's diet. Type and amount of each food eaten, food preparation, and time of day the food was eaten are reported. In the dental hygiene care setting, including the client's daily oral hygiene regimen also is suggested. The 24-hour dietary recall then is used to calculate the diet's cariogenic potential. The foods ingested are reported on the 24-hour dietary form and categorized according to the physical form of carbohydrate: liquids, solid and sticky, and slowly dissolving foods. The frequency with which each form is ingested is tallied and multiplied by 1, 2, or 3, depending on the source (Figure 35-6). A dietary caries risk score of 9 or more indicates that the individual is in need of nutritional counseling to reduce the cariogenic potential of his or her diet.

Evaluation of Diet Adequacy Using MyPlate

The same 24-hour dietary form used to calculate the cariogenic potential can be used to calculate diet adequacy using the USDA MyPlate (see Figure 35-6). Individual caloric needs are determined based on age, gender, and activity level (eFigure 35-7). Once energy needs are established, the dental hygienist can compare an individual's intake to the specified amount recommended by MyPlate and the previous food guidance system, MyPyramid (eFigure 35-8) to assess the client's dietary adequacy. Foods reported on the 24-hour dietary survey are placed into one of the MyPlate food groups on the form. This information is useful in identifying individuals in need of general nutritional counseling. Nutritional requirements vary depending on the age, gender, and activity level of the individual.

Evaluation of the 3-, 5-, or 7-Day Food Diary

Once an individual is identified for nutritional counseling, a more comprehensive dietary assessment must be completed. This assessment is accomplished by instructing the client to keep a 3-, 5-, or 7-day food diary (Procedure 35-1) and then evaluating the diary.

A food diary that includes a weekend is more likely to represent the individual's normal eating habits. All foods consumed in a 24-hour period are recorded, including type of food eaten, manner in which it was prepared, exact amount of each food eaten, and time of day in which it was eaten (see Figure 35-3). Clients are encouraged to adhere to their normal dietary regimen during the assessment period.

If the client's 24-hour caries risk score based on the physical form of carbohydrates consumed indicates the need for nutritional counseling, the dental hygienist may ask the client to complete a 3-, 5-, or 7-day food diary. On completion, the dental hygienist and client evaluate the diet for intake adequacy from the five food groups (see Figure 35-6). With the USDA MyPlate, foods consumed are categorized into each of the five food groups. The average number of servings for a

Five-Day Food Diary Form

Instructions: please record everything you eat or drink for a 5-day period, which includes one weekend day. Don't forget to include all snacks, gum, candies, soft drinks, etc.

Be specific! It is very important to write down the following:

Amount
- 1/2 cup string beans
- 1 tablespoon butter
- 6 ounces steak

What was added to the food/drink
- 1 cup coffee—1 tsp milk
- 1/2 grapefruit—1 tsp sugar

How food was prepared
- 1/2 cup string beans—boiled
- 6 ounces steak—fried
- 1 orange—fresh
- 1 peach—canned

Time of day
- Lunch-12:30 P.M.
- Snack-3:00 P.M.

Include the order that foods/beverages are consumed. Indicate if beverage was consumed at end of meal, or sipped on continously after meal or snack.

Client name ___________________________

First day			Second day			Third day		
	Food	Quantity prepared		Food	Quantity prepared		Food	Quantity prepared
Breakfast			Breakfast			Breakfast		
Snack			Snack			Snack		
Lunch			Lunch			Lunch		
Snack			Snack			Snack		
Dinner			Dinner			Dinner		
Extras			Extras			Extras		

Fourth day			Fifth day			
	Food	Quantity prepared		Food	Quantity prepared	
Breakfast			Breakfast			
Snack			Snack			
Lunch			Lunch			
Snack			Snack			
Dinner			Dinner			
Extras			Extras			

Figure 35-5. Five-day food diary form. (Adapted from form created by Lynn Tolle Watts, Gene W. Hirschfield School of Dental Hygiene, Old Dominion University and from Nizel AE, Papas AS: *Nutrition in clinical dentistry,* ed 3, St Louis, 1989, Saunders.)

COMPARE YOUR DIET TO MYPYRAMID: STEPS TO A HEALTHIER YOU

GRAINS

1 serving =
1 slice bread
1 cup dry cereal
1/2 cup pasta or rice

A						
B						

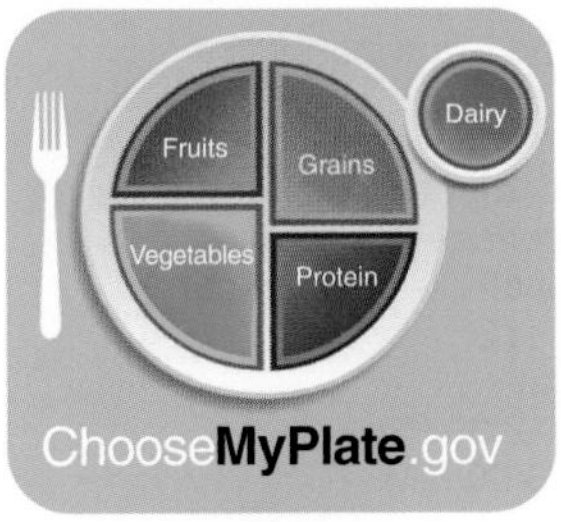

MEAT AND BEANS

1 serving =
1 ounce lean beef, fish, poultry
1/2 cup cooked beans
1/2 ounce nuts or seeds
1 tablespoon peanut butter

A					
B					

VEGETABLES

1 serving =
1/2 cup cooked veggies
1 cup raw veggies
3/4 cup juice

A			
B			

FRUITS

1 serving =
1 medium piece
1 cup raw
1/2 cup juice

A					B		

MILK

1 serving =
1 cup milk or yogurt
1 1/2 ounces cheese
1 1/2 cups frozen yogurt, cottage cheese

A				B			

How much do you need?
Sedentary, female, or older adults: Check off only the "A" boxes for each food group
Teenage boy or active male: Check off all the "A" and "B" boxes for each food group

DETERMINE YOUR CARIES RISK

Using the list of what you eat on a typical weekday:
1. CIRCLE all the sweets, crackers, soda, juice, etc.
2. In the table below, put a CHECKMARK by the appropriate category for each of the items you circled that was consumed at the end of a meal or between meals.
3. ADD up the number of checks in each frequency box and multiply by the caries risk.

FOOD	No. times consumed per day (put checkmarks for each food)	Caries risk
Liquid Soft drinks, fruit juice, fruit-flavored drinks, energy drinks, sports drinks, mochas, lattes, sugar, honey, nondairy creamer, ice cream, sherbert, gelatin, flavored yogurt, pudding, custard, popsicles		_____ × 1 =
Solid and sticky Cake, cupcakes, donuts, sweet rolls, pastry, canned fruit in syrup, bananas, cookies, crackers, pretzels, potato chips, dry cereal, fat free and regular cereal/granola bars, chocolate candy, caramel, toffee, jelly beans, chewing gum, jelly, marshmallows, jam, raisins, and fruit leather		_____ × 2 =
Slowly dissolving Hard candies, breath mints, antacid tablets, cough drops, Altoids, Tums		_____ × 3 =
	TOTAL SCORE	_________

PUT YOUR SCORE ON THE CARIES RISK LINE BELOW

LOW RISK 0-1 2-4 5-7 8-9 >9 HIGH RISK

Figure 35-6. Form to assess adequacy of the diet and calculate the cariogenic potential of the diet from a 24-hour food diary. (Courtesy Dr. L. Boyd. Adapted from C. Palmer, Tufts University School of Dental Medicine, 1998.)

Procedure 35-1 Food Record Instructions for Dental Patients

STEPS

1. Record everything you eat or drink for the suggested period of time (3, 5, or 7 days) on a specific form such as the one shown in Figure 35-5; in a notebook or on a single piece of paper
2. Include 1 weekend day.
3. Try to record as soon after eating as possible; indicate if foods are consumed as meals and those consumed between meals. Record time consumed.
4. Indicate any oral hygiene regimens incorporated throughout day (e.g., brush teeth after meal, chew gum with xylitol, rinse with antiseptic mouth rinse)
5. Exclude days that you are sick, dieting, or fasting for medical/religious purposes.
6. Be as specific as possible when recording the amounts consumed; when possible use measuring terms to indicate sizes of servings, such as cup (C), tablespoon (T), teaspoons (tsp), ounces (oz). Also try to include all ingredients when consuming a dish with multiple ingredients.
7. Record all added sauces, gravies, condiments, and extras such as sugar or cream.
8. Indicate food preparation method (e.g., baked, fried, grilled, or broiled).
9. All gum, hard candies, cough drops, or mints should be recorded; indicate if sugar free.
10. Use brand names whenever possible and include restaurant name if food is consumed outside the home.
11. Record all liquids consumed; indicate if sugar free.

Form of Sugar	When Eaten	1st Day	2nd Day	3rd Day	4th Day	5th Day	Total
Liquid (e.g., soda, sugar in coffee)	With meals						
	Between meals						
Solid (e.g., cookie, candy)	With meals						
	Between meals						

Grand total = ______ (Sugar in liquid form)

Grand total = ______ (Sugar in solid form)

______ (Liquid Exposure) × 20 minutes (pH below 5.5) = ______ (Acid Production) ÷ 5 DAYS = ______ (Daily liquid acid production)

______ (Solid Exposure) × 40 minutes (pH below 5.5) = ______ (Acid Production) ÷ 5 DAYS = ______ (Daily liquid acid production)

Total daily acid production = ______ (Liquid acid production total) + ______ (Solid acid production total) = ______ (Total time tooth is exposed to acid daily (demineralization))

Figure 35-9. Form to calculate the cariogenic potential of the diet from a 5-day food diary. (Adapted from Nizel AE, Papas AS: *Nutrition in clinical dentistry,* ed 3, St Louis, 1989, Saunders.)

client's diet based on a 3-, 5-, or 7-day period is compared with the recommended servings on MyPlate (see eFigure 35-8).

In addition, the cariogenic potential of the diet also may be analyzed further by calculating the amount of acid produced in the diet (Figure 35-9). Each **sugar exposure**, defined as any sweet or sugar-sweetened solid food or liquid, is circled in red. The total number of liquid and solid sugar exposures ingested over a 3-, 5-, or 7-day period is tallied and multiplied by the appropriate time interval. The number of liquid sugar exposures ingested over the period is multiplied by 20 minutes, and the number of solid sugar exposures ingested over the period is multiplied by 40 minutes. This resulting figure is divided by the number of days assessed to determine the amount of time daily that the teeth are subjected to an acid exposure. The **total daily acid production** is calculated by adding the daily acid production from liquid and solid sugars. Sugars consumed at the same time are considered one acid exposure (e.g., ice cream and cake eaten for dessert equals one acid exposure). Sweet foods or liquids eaten 20 minutes apart are recorded as two acid exposures. Calculating the number of acid exposures further illustrates the cariogenic potential of the client's diet.

Nutritional Counseling

Using the information obtained from the health history and dietary assessment, the dental hygiene clinician and client

BOX 35-1

Suggestions for Nutritional Counseling in the Oral Care Setting

- Maintain a separate space in the office for discussion of diet. This space ensures that infection control is maintained and provides a more casual and relaxed atmosphere for discussion of nutrition issues.
- Use plastic examples of foods to help client conceptualize size of portion.
- Keep a set of measuring spoons and cups handy to help determine portion size.
- Laminate an 11 × 14 picture of MyPlate to use as a teaching tool. With a wipe-away marker, checkmarks can be placed in the appropriate section to illustrate dietary choices from a dietary recall. The laminated picture also makes it easy to maintain infection control.
- Have available brochures and information about the U.S. Dietary Guidelines, MyPlate and the dietary recommendations from the American Diabetes Association, American Heart Association, and American Cancer Society.

formulate a plan. Box 35-1 contains suggestions for nutritional counseling in the oral care setting.

Cultural Sensitivity

Culture should be a part of every assessment and counseling session (see Chapter 6). Different beliefs and lifestyles exist in society, and each should be accorded respect. The challenge for healthcare providers is to be culturally adaptable, to display cross-cultural communication skills, and to remain aware of nonverbal cues that are culturally based to establish a trusting relationship. There are many different population subgroups. These groups often have specific cultural, ethnic, or religious beliefs and practices to consider. Hindus and Buddhists advance a vegetarian lifestyle, and other religions adhere to different dietary restrictions. The Jewish religion includes dietary laws (the Kashrut) about the source, fitness, and preparation of foods and describes what types of foods may or may not be consumed together. Similarly, Muslims may follow Halal. Vegetarianism is a component of many cultural and religious philosophies but it is also a personal choice for many based on a desire for a healthier lifestyle.

Different ethnic groups also have dietary preferences and aversions. Although many internationals become acculturated, some still follow traditional dietary customs (Box 35-2). The culturally competent dental hygienist maintains knowledge of different cultures and remains sensitive to their beliefs and practices.

Identifying Nutritional Deficiencies

Nutritional problems manifest themselves both orally and systemically. A **primary nutritional deficiency** is caused by inadequate dietary intake of a nutrient (Table 35-2).

Once identified, this type of deficiency can be corrected after dietary assessment followed by nutritional counseling that promotes proper selection and intake of nutrients. A **secondary nutritional deficiency** is caused by a systemic disorder that interferes with the ingestion, absorption, digestion, transport, and use of nutrients. This type of deficiency is more complex, and referrals to a physician and a registered dietitian are necessary for treatment.

After potential dietary deficiencies and excesses are identified, the dental hygienist and client develop a dietary program to promote optimum oral health. When dietary modifications are made, the following should be kept in mind:

- The overall nutritional adequacy should be maintained by conforming to the USDA MyPlate for at least the recommended number of servings from each of the food groups.
- The diet should vary as little as possible from the normal dietary pattern.
- The diet should meet the body's requirements for essential nutrients as generously as the diseased condition can tolerate.
- The diet should accommodate the individual's cultural and religious beliefs and practices, likes and dislikes, food habits, and other environmental factors, as long as they do not interfere with the objectives.

The use of the **Dietary Guidelines for Americans** in conjunction with the USDA MyPlate guides the necessary dietary modifications. The **USDA MyPlate** in conjunction with previous recommendations stresses balance among all the food groups (see Figures 35-7 and 35-8). Serving sizes shown in eBox 35-3 can assist the client in recording a detailed food diary.

The dental hygienist also tailors recommendations to the client's lifestyle. Although most healthy clients have similar nutrient needs, stages within the life cycle may require special consideration, including pregnancy, infancy, childhood, and old age. Moreover, the dental hygienist should consider clients' special nutritional needs related to their risk for caries, periodontal disease, oral surgery, and osteoporosis.

Nutritional Needs of Different Client Populations

Nutritional Needs During Pregnancy

All stages of pregnancy require an increase in nutrients and energy intake, but the most relevant to fetal oral health may be the first and second trimesters when the development and calcification of teeth occur. Bone growth, which is equally important, occurs mainly in the second and third trimesters when most of the calcium essential for this process is transferred from mother to child. In most cases, the exception being an underweight or teenage pregnancy, the woman's energy requirement increases by approximately 350 to 450 kilocalories a day. Unlike energy needs, however, vitamin and mineral requirements nearly double. During pregnancy the woman may experience changes in taste and smell, food cravings, and food aversions that do not necessarily reflect real

BOX 35-2

Examples of Dietary Preferences According to Some Cultural and Religious Beliefs

African American
- Diet varies greatly according to region of country and lifestyle.
- High incidence of lactose intolerance; low consumption of dairy products.
- Most popular meat dishes include pork (variety cuts), fish, small game, poultry.
- Frying and boiling are the most common preparation methods.
- Primary grain product is corn.
- Green leafy vegetables most popular, cooked with ham, bacon, lemon, broth.
- Intake of fresh fruits and vegetables often low.
- Dishes frequently seasoned with hot-pepper sauces. Onions and green pepper are common for flavoring.
- Honey, molasses, and sugar products are preferred as snacks.

Asian
- High incidence of lactose intolerance; traditional alternative sources of calcium include tofu, soy milk, small bones in fish and poultry.
- Variety of protein-rich foods, often preserved by salting and drying.
- Pastes of shrimp and legumes.
- Wheat and rice are primary grain products.
- Fresh fruits and vegetables, also pickled, dried, or preserved.

Buddhism
- Vegetarianism with five pungent foods excluded: garlic, leek, scallion, chives, and onion.

Hinduism
- Mostly vegetarian except in northern India where meat is eaten (except for beef).

Islam
- No consumption of unclean foods (carrion or dead animals, swine).
- No consumption of animals slaughtered without pronouncing the name of Allah or killed in manner that prohibits the complete draining of blood from their bodies.
- No consumption of carnivorous animals with fangs, birds of prey, and land animals without ears (frogs, snakes).
- Pork and pork products such as gelatin are prohibited.
- Alcoholic beverages and alcohol products are prohibited.

Latino
- High incidence of lactose intolerance; low consumption of dairy products.
- Vegetable protein is more common in countries with large rural and urban poor populations.
- Pork, goat, and poultry are common meats. Much of it is marinated, chopped, or ground. Often mixed with vegetables and cereals.
- Principal bread is tortilla.
- Foods are often heavily spiced.
- Common fruits and vegetables include avocados, tomatoes, cactus, chiles, corn, jicama, guava, lemons, limes, banana, oranges, plantains.

Native American
- High incidence of lactose intolerance; low consumption of dairy products.
- High incidence of diabetes owing to consumption of the modern American diet
- Meat highly valued, mostly grilled, stewed, or preserved through drying and smoking.
- Primary grain used is corn; wild rice also popular.
- Preferred fruits and vegetables include indigenous plants, gathered, or cultivated.

Alaskan Natives
- Obesity and diabetes mellitus are common in this group.
- Diet is high in protein and fat.
- Seaweed, willow leaves, and sour dock are some of edible plants consumed.

Orthodox Judaism
- Prohibits consumption of swine, shellfish, and carrion eaters.
- Kosher foods are consumed.
- Ritual breaking of bread.
- Meat and milk are prepared in separate dishes with separate utensils and containers and are not cooked, served, or eaten together.
- Fish with fins and scales (i.e., no shellfish or eel) and eggs can be eaten with milk.
- Fruits, vegetables, cereal products can be consumed with no restrictions.

Vegetarianism
- Often motivated by philosophic, religious, or desire for healthier lifestyle.
- Lactovegetarians do not eat meat, fish, poultry, or eggs but do consume milk, cheese, and other dairy products.
- Lacto-ovovegetarians also consume eggs.
- Vegans do not consume any food of animal origin.
- Megaloblastic anemia is often a concern in vegans owing to deficiency of vitamin B_{12}, which is only found in animal products.
- On the whole, vegetarians should pay special attention to ensure they get adequate calcium, iron, zinc, and vitamins B_{12} and D.

From Food and nutrient delivery: planning the diet with cultural competence. In Mahan LK, Raymond JL, Escott-Stump S, eds: *Krause's food and the nutrition care process,* ed 13, St Louis, 2012, Saunders.

physiologic needs. These pregnancy-related experiences, along with varying levels of nausea, create a potential for nutrient imbalance. Fortunately, the developing fetus is usually not at risk during these short episodes because a healthy mother provides the essential nutrients from her own nutrient stores. However, a prolonged nutrient deficiency poses a problem.

The dental hygienist treating a pregnant woman reinforces the recommendations of the obstetrician. Reinforcement of the importance of eating nutrient-dense foods along with

TABLE 35-2

Vitamins and Minerals Grouped According to Function, Including Sources, Human Deficiency and Excess Syndromes, and Oral Implications

Nutrient	Dietary Source	Deficiency Syndrome	Oral Implications of Deficiency	Excess or Other
Functions: Structure and Calcification				
Vitamin A (fat soluble)	Vitamin A is present only in animal foods; beef liver is an excellent source Beta carotene: carrots, melon, squash, sweet potato, spinach	Growth failure, xerosis, keratomalacia	Enamel hypoplasia and defective dentin formation	Excess may cause headache, vomiting, severe liver damage, defect in long bone formation.
Vitamin D (fat soluble)	Synthesized in skin exposed to sunlight	Rickets, osteomalacia	Enamel hypoplasia and loss of lamina dura	Excess may cause vomiting and diarrhea, hypercalcemia.
Vitamins E (fat soluble)	Vegetable seed oils, widely distributed in foods	Anemia, neuropathy, myopathy	Loss of resistance to inflammation in periodontium	Excess may inhibit vitamin K functions, causing problems with blood clotting.
Vitamin K (fat soluble)	Synthesized by intestinal bacteria: green leafy vegetables, soybeans, beef liver	Defective blood clotting	May be involved in bone formation	High doses of synthetic form may cause oxidation of membrane lipids, severe jaundice in infants.
Vitamin C (water soluble)	Citrus fruits, papaya, cantaloupe, broccoli, potato, strawberries	Scurvy	Inhibition of formation of fibroblasts, osteoblasts, and odontoblasts	Can cause gastrointestinal (GI) distress and interfere with vitamin B_{12} absorption.
Calcium	Milk and milk products, sardines, clams, turnip and mustard greens, broccoli	Rickets, osteomalacia, osteoporosis, stunted growth	Tooth exfoliation due to osteoporosis in alveolar bone	Excess may cause constipation.
Phosphorus	Meat, poultry, fish, eggs, milk products, chocolate	Rickets, osteomalacia	Possible failure of reparative dentin formation	Symptoms associated with excess are rare; problems appear to occur only when calcium to phosphorus ratios are altered significantly in infants.
Magnesium	Nuts, legumes, cereal grains, chocolate, blackstrap molasses, spinach	Growth failure, neuromuscular dysfunction, personality changes, muscle spasms	Reduced formation of alveolar bone, hypoplasia of enamel, widening of periodontal ligament space, and gingival hyperplasia	Acute toxicity from excessive intravenous administration results in nausea, depression, and paralysis.
Fluoride	Mackerel, salmon, shrimp, meat, potatoes, wheat, sardines	Osteoporosis, osteosclerosis	Dental caries	Excess results in fluorosis.
Function: Soft Tissue, Including Oral, Salivary, and Taste Function				
Vitamin B_1, thiamine (water soluble)	Pork, sunflower seeds, legumes	Beriberi, muscle weakness, tachycardia, enlarged heart, edema, anemia, neuropathy, myopathy	Glossitis, gingival tissue discoloration	Excessive doses may cause headache, convulsion, cardiac arrhythmia, anaphylactic shock.

TABLE 35-2

Vitamins and Minerals Grouped According to Function, Including Sources, Human Deficiency and Excess Syndromes, and Oral Implications—cont'd

Nutrient	Dietary Source	Deficiency Syndrome	Oral Implications of Deficiency	Excess or Other
Vitamin B_2, riboflavin (water soluble)	Beef liver, lean steak, mushroom, ricotta cheese, milk	Photophobia, dermatitis, anemia	Cheilosis, glossitis, edema of pharyngeal and oral mucous membranes, angular stomatitis	No toxicity symptoms reported.
Vitamin B_6, pyridoxine (water soluble)	Sirloin steak, navy beans, potato, banana	Dermatitis, neurologic symptoms of confusion, drowsiness, neuropathy	Glossitis	Excess causes sensory and peripheral neuropathy. Minimal dosage at which toxicity occurs is not defined.
Vitamin B_{12} (water soluble)	Meat, fish, shellfish, poultry, milk	Megaloblastic anemia (pernicious anemia), degeneration of peripheral nerves, skin hypersensitivity	Glossitis, eventual disappearance of the filiform and fungiform papillae; glossopyrosis	No effects from excessive doses have been reported.
Niacin (water-soluble B vitamin)	Tuna, beef liver, chicken breast, mushrooms	Pellagra, diarrhea, dermatitis, dementia	Stomatitis, atrophic changes of filiform and fungiform papillae, tongue smooth and shiny	Large doses used in the treatment of hypercholesterolemia. Excess may cause facial flushing, release of histamines, which may be detrimental to asthmatics.
Folate (water-soluble B vitamin)	Brewer's yeast, spinach, asparagus, turnip greens, lima beans, beef liver	Megaloblastic anemia, increased risk of spina bifida and neural tube defects during pregnancy	Glossitis, chronic periodontitis, *Candida* infection; cleft lip and cleft palate	Large doses may cause kidney damage; may mask symptoms of vitamin B_{12} deficiency and may provoke seizures in patients taking anticonvulsants.
Pantothenic acid (water-soluble B vitamin)	Widespread in foods, egg yolk, liver, kidney	Deficiency very rare, numbness and tingling of hands and feet	May impair healing of oral tissue	Diarrhea is the only reported effect from excessive doses.
Biotin (water-soluble B vitamin)	Synthesized in intestinal tract	Deficiency very rare, anorexia, nausea, depression, dermatitis	Glossitis, lingual and mucous pallor, patchy atrophy of lingual papilla	No effects from excessive doses reported.
Vitamin C (water soluble)	See above	Scurvy	Weakened collagen formation, leading to gingivitis and poor oral wound healing	Overdose may cause diarrhea, kidney stones.
Vitamin A (fat soluble)	See above	Xerosis, keratomalacia	Decreased salivary secretion and xerostomia; delayed or impaired wound healing	Excess may cause fetal birth defects, headache, vomiting, severe liver damage, defect in long-bone formation.
Vitamin E (fat soluble)	See above	Anemia, neuropathy	Loss of integrity in cell membranes of mucosa	Can act as an anticoagulant and may increase the risk of bleeding problems.
Sodium	Table salt, meat, seafood, cheese, milk, bread, vegetables	Muscle atrophy, poor growth, weight loss	Thirst, dry, sticky tongue and mouth	High sodium intake may affect calcium excretion.

Continued

TABLE 35-2

Vitamins and Minerals Grouped According to Function, Including Sources, Human Deficiency and Excess Syndromes, and Oral Implications—cont'd

Nutrient	Dietary Source	Deficiency Syndrome	Oral Implications of Deficiency	Excess or Other
Potassium	Avocado, banana, dried fruits, wheat bran, eggs, dairy products	Muscular weakness, mental apathy, cardiac arrhythmias, paralysis, adrenal hypertrophy, decreased growth rate	None	Hyperkalemia is toxic, resulting in severe cardiac failure.
Chloride	Table salt, seafood, eggs, meat, milk	Failure to thrive in infants, muscle weakness, hypokalemia, metabolic acidosis	None	No excess effects have been noted.
Iron	Organ meats, clams, oysters, legumes, enriched and/or whole grain cereals and breads	Fatigue, palpitations on exertion, anemia, decreased resistance to infection	Pallor of lips and oral mucosa, angular cheilitis, atrophy of filiform papillae, and glossitis	Excess causes damage to tissues including liver and other organs.
Zinc	Wheat germ, oysters, beef liver, dark meat of poultry	Poor wound healing, subnormal growth, skin inflammation, anemia, retarded development of reproductive organs	Abnormal taste and smell; increased susceptibility to periodontal disease; flattened filiform papillae; congenital defect cleft lip and palate	Acute toxicity produces metallic taste, nausea, vomiting, epigastric pain, abdominal cramps. Can result in renal damage, pancreatitis, and even death.
Iodine	Iodized salt, saltwater shellfish, spinach, pumpkin, broccoli, chocolate	Hypothyroidism or Graves' disease, cretinism, increase in blood lipids	Delayed eruption of primary and secondary teeth, an enlarged tongue, and malocclusion commonly occur in cretinism. Craniofacial growth and development is also altered	Enlargement of thyroid gland; toxicity symptoms are similar to deficiency symptoms.

From Dietary Guidelines Advisory Committee: *Dietary guidelines for Americans,* Washington, DC, 2010, U.S. Department of Agriculture, U.S. Department of Health and Human Services; National Institutes of Health Office of Dietary Supplements: *Dietary supplement fact sheets.* Available at: http://ods.od.nih.gov/factsheets/list-all. Accessed November 19, 2012; Stegeman CA, Davis JR: *The dental hygienist's guide to nutritional care,* ed 3, St Louis, 2010, Saunders.

meticulous oral hygiene minimizes the occurrence of pregnancy-associated gingivitis, pregnancy granulomas, and giving birth to premature, low-birthweight infants. Prenatal nutrient supplements recommended by the client's obstetrician ensure that the developing fetus receives adequate vitamins and minerals to promote healthy bone and tooth development.

Nutritional Needs During Infancy and Childhood

Nutrient intake and food choices during infancy and childhood influence growth patterns. Undernutrition, overnutrition, and improper nutrient amounts can set the pattern for a lifelong struggle with weight, developmental delays, or social discrimination.

Children often grow in spurts. Children are born with an innate sense of how much food they require. Parents who advocate completely finishing an entire meal may be causing their children to override their internal sense of satiety. The simplest advice is the provision of nutrient-dense foods, regular meal times, and the achievement of a balanced diet by offering a variety of foods from all of the food groups.

Unless a child has extenuating medical circumstances, children should not ingest significant amounts of alternative sweeteners. Children need calories for growth and development. Artificial sweeteners should not be part of the diet of infants or children under 2 years of age. Although the anticariogenicity of alternative sweeteners may offer a desirable choice to most parents, good oral hygiene care, fluoridation, and healthy snack choices can reduce dental caries risk. Examples of appropriate snacks for children are listed in Box 35-4.

The focus of nutritional counseling for children in the oral care setting is primarily caries control. In addition, the importance of vitamins and minerals responsible for bone growth

BOX 35-4

Healthy Snack Ideas for Children and Adults

Breads, Crackers, Grains
Unsweetened cereal
Plain crackers
Toast (whole wheat)
Unbuttered popcorn
Tortillas
Dried rice and corn cakes
Baked tortilla chips
Pizza

Vegetables
Raw and cut-up carrots, celery, broccoli, cauliflower, cucumbers, tomatoes
Low-sodium vegetable juice, 6- to 8-ounce serving

Fruits
Apples, peaches, pears, plums, oranges, tangerines
Bananas (with peanut butter)
Cut-up watermelon, cantaloupe, or other melon
Berries
Unsweetened fruit juice, 4- to 6-oz serving
Canned fruit in natural juice

Meat and Protein
Sliced chicken or turkey or deli meat
Tuna on crackers
Bean and legumes
Hummus on crackers
Nuts (not recommended for young children because of choking hazard)

Dairy
Milk
Yogurt
Cheese
Cottage cheese
Sugar-free pudding

Other
Sugar-free ice pops
Sugar-free candy and chewing gum
Sugar-free gelatin

Adapted from U.S. Department of Health and Human Services, National Institutes of Health, National Institute of Dental and Craniofacial Research: *Snack smart for healthy teeth.* Available at: http://www2.nidcr.nih.gov/health/pubs/snaksmrt/main.htm. Accessed November 16, 2012.

should be included in a discussion with the child and caregiver. As children age, their preference for beverages often changes from milk and juices to carbonated beverages. Dairy products, some of the best sources of calcium, phosphorus, and magnesium, are essential for adequate bone and tooth formation. Replacing dairy products with carbonated beverages eliminates the main source of these nutrients. This change may affect adversely the bone growth and tooth development of children and teenagers.[4]

Nutritional Needs of Elderly Clients

Significant nutritional issues in the elderly include a reduced energy requirement, a possible need for increased protein in a segment of the population, and an increased need for certain vitamins and minerals such as vitamins D, E, B_6, B_{12}, folate, and minerals such as calcium, magnesium, iron, and zinc (see Chapter 55). Most elderly people are not as active as younger people and therefore do not require the same amount of energy intake. The decrease in energy and increase in nutrient needs means that the elderly client may need guidance in choosing nutrient-dense foods such as whole grains, breads, and pastas. Along with complex carbohydrates, fruits and vegetables are a natural source of the vitamins and minerals that promote tissue growth and regeneration. Because of a decrease in lean body mass per kilogram of body weight, elderly adults have a higher protein requirement. Also, certain chronic disease conditions can decrease protein absorption. The current recommended dietary allowance (RDA) for protein for adults is 0.8 g/kg of body weight.[5,6] Because of a decline in kidney function as humans age, a general recommendation to increase protein consumption is not indicated for the elderly. Based on the recommendation of a physician or registered dietitian, need should be determined on an individual basis.

An indirect factor that could affect nutrient intake is lack of dental insurance. Many elderly people may be unable to afford dental care. Periodontal disease and carious teeth can be painful and restrict the elderly individual's ability to chew and swallow food. Hot or cold foods can aggravate oral disease conditions. In addition, crisp or fibrous foods that require significant force when biting or chewing also can cause pain. The aging process results in increased vulnerability to oral injury because of thinning of the oral tissues. For convenience, older adults may choose cakes, cookies, and breakfast cereals, which contribute to dental decay. Xerostomia also contributes to root caries and an inability to chew and swallow food adequately.

The consumption of nutrient-dense foods is essential to the elderly diet. Sources of high-quality protein such as eggs, dairy products, and well-cooked meats, chicken, and fish should be promoted as an important part of the diet. Protein also provides a good source of vitamin B_{12}, often deficient in the elderly. The decrease of intrinsic factor, a protein that aids in the absorption of vitamin B_{12} in the stomach, often makes intramuscular injections of the vitamin necessary.[5] Pernicious anemia and burning mouth syndrome commonly are noted in elderly clients with a diagnosed deficiency of vitamin B_{12}. Vitamins A, C, and B_6 can be obtained from a diet rich in cooked green vegetables and potatoes. Fresh fruit is also a good source of vitamins and minerals and can be tolerated if the fruit is ripe or peeled. Table 35-3 lists oral signs and symptoms of possible nutrient deficiencies in the elderly.

Finally, guidance should be given to the elderly to achieve optimum nutrition. Referral to a registered dietitian may be indicated. Community-based services such as Meals on Wheels, congregate meal sites, and shopping assistance provide an opportunity for socialization and assistance for those who are disabled or who lack transportation. Also, modifications applied to oral hygiene aids for people with manual dexterity problems can be applied to eating

TABLE 35-3

Signs of Nutritional Deficiencies in the Elderly

Clinical Signs	Possible Deficiency	Comments
Skin		
Edema	Protein, thiamine	Common in protein-calorie malnutrition as a result of aging
Poor tissue turgor	Water	Pellagra or hemochromatosis
Dermatitis	Protein	None
Keratosis	Vitamin A, essential fatty acids	None
Pigmentation	Niacin	Loss of lubrication or dryness of skin
Petechiae	Vitamin A, vitamin C	None
Xerosis	Essential fatty acids	None
Eyes		
Dull, dry conjunctiva	Vitamin A	Can lead to other eye problems including blindness
Keratomalacia	Vitamin A	Usually results in blindness
Bitot's spot	Vitamin A	Associated with night blindness
Corneal vascularization	Vitamin A	None
Photophobia	Riboflavin Zinc	Extreme sensitivity to light; individuals who suffer with migraines may experience this condition. Other eye problems such as night blindness may be present
Tongue		
Magenta tongue	Riboflavin	None
Fissuring, raw	Niacin	May also be caused by food irritants, antibiotic administration, uremia
Glossitis	Pyridoxine, folacin, iron, vitamin B_{12}	Seen if anemia is not pronounced
Fiery red tongue	Folacin, vitamin B_{12}	None
Pale tongue	Iron, vitamin B_{12}	Seen in severe cases
Atrophic papillae	Riboflavin, niacin, iron	Also seen with ill-fitting dentures, food irritants, aging
Lips and Oral Structures		
Angular fissures, scars, or stomatitis	B-complex, iron, protein, riboflavin	Also seen with ill-fitting dentures
Cheilosis	B_6, iron, niacin, riboflavin, protein	Could also be a result of fungal infections
Ageusia, dysgeusia	Zinc	Certain conditions and medications can contribute; also seen with ill-fitting dentures
Swollen, spongy, bleeding gums	Vitamin C	Also associated with altered sense of smell, if not edentulous

utensils to increase the likelihood of adequate nutritional intake.

Nutritional Needs of Clients with Dental Caries Risk

Nutritional counseling for dental caries prevention must emphasize decreasing the frequency with which sugar is consumed and replacing cariogenic foods with nutritionally sound foods. Although sugar consumption is an important factor in caries risk assessment[7,8] (see Chapter 18), the following factors are involved in the development of dental caries:

- Acid-producing microorganisms *(Lactobacillus, Streptococcus mutans)*
- Cariogenic diet
- A susceptible tooth surface
- Salivary factors

Nutritional counseling for dental caries prevention targets the elimination or reduction of fermentable carbohydrates from the diet. Dissolving foods that sit on the teeth for extended periods of time and solid, sticky foods that don't clear readily from the mouth contribute the greatest risk. Frequent consumption of fermentable carbohydrates and acidic beverages subjects the tooth enamel to repeated acid exposures. The demineralization process weakens the tooth and leads to the formation of dental caries. (See Chapter 16 for types of caries and Chapter 18 for a review of the caries process.[9]) Healthy alternatives can contribute to demineralization and subsequent caries formation. Consumption of low-calorie carbonated beverages, sticky foods such as baked chips, pretzels, granola, and dried fruit that do not clear readily from the mouth and trends such as juicing are examples. Box 35-5 includes recommendations and strategies for reducing the cariogenic potential of an individual's diet.

Nutritional Needs of Clients Undergoing Surgery

Periodontal and oral and maxillofacial surgical clients are often unable to consume an adequate amount of recommended nutrients owing to loss of function.[9] In a healthy adult, creation of new proteins and breakdown of existing

BOX 35-5

Dietary Recommendations for the Reduction of Dental Caries

- Limit the use of fermentable carbohydrates to mealtime. Consume foods higher in protein and fat to help buffer and neutralize plaque acids.
- Reduce the frequency of cariogenic and acidogenic foods if susceptible to caries.
- Between-meal snacks should consist of protective, noncariogenic foods such as raw vegetables. Raw, unrefined foods in the vegetable and fruit group require chewing. The chewing action increases the salivary flow, thus aiding in the removal and dilution of sugars and their harmful by-products.
- Use as few concentrated sweets as possible in the preparation of foods.
- Do not eat sweets before bedtime unless the teeth are brushed afterward. Salivary flow decreases at night and foods are not cleared as readily from the mouth as they are during waking hours. Acid left undisturbed remains in the mouth for 1½ to 2 hours.
- Limit natural sugars: they are as detrimental to the tooth surface as refined sugars.
- Avoid sticky foods because they are retained in the mouth longer than nonsticky foods.
- Encourage consumption of sugar-free gum with xylitol after meals if brushing is not an option.

proteins closely balance one another. Typically, well-nourished, healthy individuals experience very few complications and require minimal dietary modifications. However, some clients such as chronic alcoholics, extremely underweight individuals, or those taking steroids or immunosuppressants may have depleted stores of nutrients. These individuals may need to postpone surgical procedures 1 to 2 weeks or until more favorable nutrition levels are achieved. To optimize immune function to promote healing and overall health, clients should be instructed in proper postsurgical nutritional rehabilitation. Immunocompromised individuals, as well as those with complex medical histories, should be referred to a registered dietitian for more in-depth analysis and guidance before surgery. A team effort between the dental hygienist and a registered dietitian ensures a more positive client outcome. Presurgical nutrition education provided by the dental hygienist includes the following:

- Discussion of the client's present food intake pattern and recommended caloric needs based on height, weight, and activity level using MyPlate as a guide
- Review of adequate nutrients to enhance and facilitate the healing process
- Extent of surgery, potential discomfort, and client's ability to eat after the surgery should be considered; food preferences and dislikes also should be taken into account

In addition to caloric and protein requirement increases, there also may be an increase in select nutrient needs because of blood loss, increased catabolism, and tissue regeneration that occurs after surgery. The first 1 to 3 days after surgery, high-calorie, high-protein, full-liquid diets consisting of choices such as powdered skim milk that can be used to fortify milk, soups, puddings, milkshakes, broth, and fruit or vegetable juices may be necessary. Clients then may progress to a **mechanical soft diet**. This is a regular diet that is modified to a consistency that makes foods easier to consume. A mechanical soft diet consists of soft, ripened, chopped, ground, mashed, and pureed foods. This type of diet may be recommended for 3 to 7 days or until the client is able to consume a regular diet. Small, frequent meals ensure adequate intake. Raw fruits and vegetables and foods with seeds or nuts should be avoided; bland foods should be encouraged to avoid irritating tissue. Eight glasses of fluid also is recommended. It is always preferable to obtain nutrients through a food source, but in cases in which the client is unable to ingest the required nutrients adequately, a liquid form of supplemental nutrition such as Ensure or Boost may be acceptable. If supplemental liquid nutrition is indicated, clients should be educated on the high sugar content and the need for meticulous oral hygiene. Liquid and soft diets are not indicated for simple procedures such as tooth extractions. These diets are recommended more commonly for clients who require periodontal surgery, jaw surgery, intermaxillary fixation, or temporomandibular joint surgery.[9]

A practical client education program is accomplished using the USDA MyPlate and Dietary Guidelines for Americans. Quick calculations and charts provided by MyPlate can be used as visual aids for client education. Individualized meal plans that incorporate caloric, protein, and other suggested nutrient needs postsurgically are an excellent resource in the dental setting. Often it is easier to obtain compliance when clients are presented with an actual list of foods or meal plans to follow. The dental hygiene clinician can provide only basic recommendations. Referral to a registered dietitian is indicated to develop a comprehensive meal plan that meets individual needs. The Academy of Nutrition and Dietetics is an exceptional resource for examples of full liquid and mechanical soft diets designed to provide optimum calories and nutrients for surgical patients. It is also a great source for locating a local registered dietitian for referrals (see http://www.eatright.org).

Nutritional Needs of Clients with Osteoporosis

Many factors affect bone mineralization in the human body, including metabolic and dietary interactions and certain disease states. Improper bone mineralization can affect the dentition. Although several vitamins and minerals ultimately contribute to bone and tooth formation and preservation, calcium, phosphorus, and vitamin D directly support these processes. Calcium can be found throughout the body in bone, serum, and tissues. Approximately 98% of the calcium present in the human body is contained in bone and teeth. The balance of serum calcium is important in that it often causes the release or deposit of calcium from hard body tissues.

Phosphorus is equally important to bone growth and preservation. Approximately 85% of the phosphorus in the human body is found in combination with calcium in hydroxyapatite crystals of bones and teeth. Calcium and phosphorus are important components of bones and teeth, but vitamin D directs the use of these minerals in the body. The interaction of calcium, phosphorus, and vitamin D is required for adequate maintenance of bone growth and mineralization.

Osteopenia, a loss of mineralized bone tissue, regardless of its cause, is considered a precursor to osteoporosis. Osteoporosis is a disease characterized by low bone mass, microarchitectural deterioration of bone tissue leading to enhanced bone fragility, and consequent increase in fracture risk. Osteoporosis has become significant as a disease owing to its relationship to mortality, morbidity, quality of life, and medical expense worldwide. Osteoporosis causes more than 1.5 million fractures annually in the United States alone. Vertebral, wrist, and hip fractures are responsible for much of the mortality and morbidity of osteoporosis. Osteoporosis is a leading cause of disability in the elderly. Box 35-6 identifies risk factors associated with osteoporosis. Osteoporosis may be a risk factor or risk indicator for periodontal disease, for tooth loss preceding dental implants, and in the prognosis of periodontal therapy (see Chapter 54).

When the control of osteoporosis is discussed, the nutrient mentioned most often is calcium. Although important throughout the life cycle, this nutrient is especially crucial during the peak bone-forming years. The RDA for calcium is 1000 mg for young adults 19 to 50 years of age. It increases to 1200 mg for individuals 51 and older.[6] It has been found that a calcium intake of at least the RDA can slow or prevent age-related bone loss and reduce the risk of fractures in postmenopausal women and the elderly.

A thorough health history, oral screening (intraoral exam, periodontal charting, radiographs), and dietary analysis help to identify clients at risk for osteoporosis[10,11] (see Chapter 54). These individuals must be encouraged to consume at least 3 cups of calcium food sources daily. The preferred calcium source is dairy products and foods fortified with calcium. Calcium bioavailability from dairy foods is excellent, especially when consumed with a meal (see Table 35-2 and eBox 35-7). Emphasis also needs to be on vitamin D to promote optimal calcium absorption. eTable 35-4 provides a list of the minerals and vitamins essential for calcified structures. For individuals who have inadequate intake of dairy, a calcium supplement may be indicated. The dose should be taken in halves to ensure proper absorption (e.g., 500 to 600 mg taken twice daily). For an individual diagnosed with osteoporosis or at risk, referral to a physician or a registered dietitian may be recommended to make sure calcium needs are being met.

BOX 35-6

Risk Factors Associated with Osteoporosis

Dietary Constituents

Alcohol abuse
Excessive antacid use
Low-calcium diet
Lactose intolerance
Vitamin D deficiency
Caffeine use
High-sodium diet
High-protein diet
Excessive carbonated drink intake
Foods with high amounts of phytate such as whole-grain bread, beans, seeds, nuts, grains
Foods with high amounts of oxylate such as spinach, collard greens, and sweet potatoes
100% wheat bran
Vegan diet

Hormones

Estrogen deficiency
Low testosterone
Chronic thyroid hormone use
Early menopause

Drugs

Chronic steroid use
Anticonvulsants
Mineral oil or stimulant laxatives
Aluminum- or magnesium-containing antacids

Genetic Factors

Caucasian
Asian
Thinness
Family history of osteoporosis

Gender

Female

Other

Advanced age
Anorexia nervosa
Lack of weight-bearing exercise
Cigarette smoking

Nutritional Concerns of the Overweight and Obese Client

Obesity is a growing concern in children, adolescents, and adults. Currently, more than one third of U.S. adults and approximately 17% of children and adolescents aged 2 to 19 years are obese.[12,13] Obesity is defined as having a body mass index (BMI) greater than or equal to 30 (see Table 35-1). Obesity is associated with many chronic diseases including periodontal disease. It is beyond the role of the dental hygienist to create diet plans for use in weight loss. However, as health care providers, it is the dental hygienist's responsibility to educate clients on health promotion, disease prevention techniques, and habits that benefit oral health as well as overall health. Clients may be educated on positive lifestyle changes as they relate to healthy eating habits and exercise, the link between obesity, diabetes, and periodontal health as well as the impact of systemic health on oral health. Referral to a physician and/or a registered dietitian is indicated for those clients interested in weight loss.

Bariatric surgery is common in this population. After surgery, it is recommended that these individuals eat small meals throughout the day, and beverages should be consumed separate from meals. Although this method of consuming foods and beverages optimizes the digestion process for the bariatric surgery patient, the frequency and timing of foods and beverages can increase risk of caries. In addition, nutrient deficiencies may occur as a result of surgical alterations to the

GI tract, thus healing after periodontal therapy or surgery may be affected. Collaboration with the medical team to ensure the most favorable client outcome is recommended.

CLIENT EDUCATION TIPS

- Explain that a diet rich in nutrient-dense foods promotes oral health and overall health and prevents osteopenia and osteoporosis in later life.
- Emphasize that decreasing the amount and frequency of simple sugars consumed promotes oral health, weight management, and systemic health.
- Explain that nutrient needs change during the life cycle and at times of stress such as periodontal and oral surgery.
- Explain recommended dietary allowances (RDAs), nutrition labels on foods purchased, Dietary Guidelines for Americans, and the U.S. Department of Agriculture MyPlate as the basis for appropriate food choices.
- Discuss how healthy, nutrient-dense snack foods can be substituted for dental caries–promoting snacks.
- For clients undergoing oral and maxillofacial surgery, discuss present nutritional status and recommendations for prevention of loss of lean body mass; review foods that promote healing. Refer to a registered dietitian if more detailed assessment is indicated.
- Explain how positive lifestyle changes in regard to healthy eating habits and exercise can benefit overall health as well as periodontal health.

KEY CONCEPTS

- Client nutritional status assessment is part of comprehensive dental hygiene care.
- Nutritional counseling helps clients develop healthful eating behaviors.
- Dietary assessment is the identification of the client's current dietary practices and dietary requirements. Dietary assessment includes a dietary history that may be gathered through a 1-, 3-, 5-, or 7-day recording of food intake. Dietary assessment may provide clues to overall health through analysis of nutrient content.
- Key factors influence an individual's food selection, including age, gender, ethnicity and culture, income, educational level, and lifestyle.
- Cultural sensitivity is an essential part of dietary assessment and nutritional counseling.
- Pregnancy, infancy, childhood, and aging require special consideration when the dental hygienist counsels clients or their caregivers on nutrition as it relates to dental health.
- The elderly often require increased amounts of protein but not calories.
- Dietary assessment and nutritional counseling promote healing postoperatively in clients undergoing periodontal or oral and maxillofacial surgery.
- Minimizing the amount of sugar consumed and replacing cariogenic foods with nutrient-dense foods decrease dental caries risk.

LEGAL, ETHICAL, AND SAFETY ISSUES

- Dental hygienists should refrain from practicing nutrition assessment or counseling that is beyond the scope of their practice (e.g., weight management, development of comprehensive dietary plans, metabolic disease control, eating disorders).
- Refer signs of nutrition-related diseases or deficiencies to a physician or licensed nutrition professional.
- Alert clients to potential signs and symptoms of nutritional deficiencies and refer to a physician for diagnosis.
- In the client's record, document information provided to the client during nutritional counseling for oral disease prevention and health promotion.

CRITICAL THINKING EXERCISES

Three scenarios present clients with specific nutritional needs. Read each case and prepare a complete dental hygiene care plan for each (see useful calculations for nutrition assessment at the end of the scenario). Do you agree or disagree with the nutritional plans presented? Is there anything you would do differently?

SCENARIO 35-1

CLIENT WITH OSTEOPOROSIS

Client: Ms. Xi Tsing
Age: 50 years
Gender: Female
Height: 5′2″
Weight: 85 lb (38.6 kg)
Race: Asian American

Health History: Client underwent early menopause, is lactose intolerant, and currently us being treated for irritable bowel disease.

Pharmacologic History: Medications include steroid treatment for her bowel problems and estrogen replacement therapy.

Dental History: Several carious areas. Radiologic examination shows moderate bone loss of the supporting structures and within her jaws. Suspect osteoporosis. Will discuss this with the dentist. After dental treatment Ms. Tsing will be referred to her physician for evaluation and treatment of suspected osteoporosis.

Chief Complaint: "My teeth are hurting me."

Dietary Assessment: Food frequency questionnaire shows that Ms. Tsing follows a typical Asian dietary pattern with fish and tofu as the main sources of protein. Eats a variety of vegetables including green leafy

Continued

SCENARIO 35-1

CLIENT WITH OSTEOPOROSIS—cont'd

vegetables such as spinach and green leaf lettuce, bean sprouts, bok choy, broccoli, and carrots. Does not consume any dairy products owing to her lactose intolerance. Drinks tea. Loves sweets and desserts and consumes candy regularly. Diet consists of approximately 20% fat, 10% protein, and 70% carbohydrate.

Social History: Client does not exercise and rarely goes outside during the day in an effort to avoid the sun and its damaging effects. Worked as a seamstress for many years but is now retired. Belongs to an informal social women's group and occasionally has the opportunity to meet for walks at the local mall.

Nutritional Risk Factors:

Asian descent
Underweight and of small stature
Long-term steroid treatment
Early menopause
Low exercise level

Nutritional Counseling Plan:

1. Using MyPlate, discuss the positive aspects of the client's diet including the following:
   Calcium-rich foods such as bok choy, broccoli, and tofu
   Herbal tea, no caffeine
   Fish such as salmon or sardines that have a high level of calcium
2. Find solutions collaboratively with the client regarding the following:
   Lack of dairy products
   Large amount of simple sugars
   Lack of weight-bearing exercise
   No sun exposure for vitamin D
3. Recommendation of a vitamin D supplement or 5 to 10 minutes per day of early morning sunshine exposure.
4. A regular exercise plan can be recommended, starting with increasing walks at the mall.
5. Alternative sources of calcium or over-the-counter lactase enzymes or commercially available supplements such as Ensure or Boost. A dietitian should be consulted for the best sources of well-absorbed supplements.

Dental Hygiene Diagnoses:

Unmet need for protection from health risks due to lack of calcium-containing foods in diet as evidenced by suspected osteoporosis (radiographic jaw bone loss)

Unmet need for biologically sound and functional dentition due to a combination of diet and oral hygiene care as evidenced by chief complaint of tooth pain

Goals:

Increase amount of foods containing calcium in diet and daily vitamin D supplements.

Increase nutrient values in diet to prevent osteoporosis and educate patient in proper oral hygiene care.

SCENARIO 35-2

CLIENT WITH RAMPANT DENTAL CARIES

Client: Kathleen Mulvaney
Age: 8 years
Gender: Female
Height: 3′10″
Weight: 55 lb (25 kg)
Race: Caucasian

Health History: Client has experienced several childhood illnesses, including chickenpox, measles, and mumps, and frequent sore throats and common cold symptoms. Client was injured on the school playground at age 6 years and underwent treatment for fractures of the right leg and arm.

Pharmacologic History: Because of frequent cold symptoms and sore throats, client regularly ingests over-the-counter cough drops. Her favorite flavors are cherry and honey lemon. These cough drops are not sugar free.

Dental History: Because of her health history and subsequent treatment for illness and injury, Kathleen's parents have not taken her to the dentist often in an effort to avoid "overtraumatizing" her. Intraoral examination reveals rampant caries of remaining primary teeth with the largest lesions in the molar area. Radiographic examination shows decay throughout the mouth. Permanent tooth development appears to be normal. Erupted molars have incipient lesions with some surfaces requiring Class I restorations at this time.

Chief Complaint: "My friends at school make fun of my teeth because they are black. Sometimes it's hard to chew." Client does not appear to be experiencing pain at this time.

Dietary History: Food frequency questionnaire indicates that client has a high intake of foods containing added sugars and appearing in the moderate- to high-cariogenic potential category. Using MyPlate SuperTracker, client can point out most foods in her diet. Client indicates that she adds sugar to her breakfast cereals and on top of the fruit she eats with lunch. Client loves raisins and dried fruit as a snack. She keeps a little bag in her desk at school in case she gets hungry during the day. Client's favorite snack is a

SCENARIO 35-2

CLIENT WITH RAMPANT DENTAL CARIES—cont'd

bowl of chocolate ice cream, which she has every night before bed. Client drinks regular Coca Cola with each meal except breakfast. Friends eat candy bars, but Kathleen prefers gummy bears, Dots, Sour Patch Kids, and other sticky fruit candies.

Social History: Client is the youngest child in a family of six. Parents both work outside the home. Family status is middle class with occasional financial challenges because of large family. Client stays after school until picked up by older siblings. Because of work and social obligations, parents have left most of the childcare responsibilities to older siblings. Previous injuries and chronic illnesses have promoted special reward system at home of sweet desserts and ice cream before bed. Limited parental supervision has caused client to adopt diet and habits of older siblings who enjoy regular Coca Cola with meals instead of milk. Client appears to understand the importance of a healthy diet and appears receptive to adjusting habits "as long as my parents say it's OK."

Nutritional Risk Factors:

Preferred snack foods have high concentration of added sugars and limited nutritional value.

Snack habits (e.g., dried fruits available throughout the day) promote caries.

Choice of beverage with meals unsatisfactory for promoting growth and development.

Limited parental supervision allows for poor food choices.

Dental Hygiene Diagnoses:

Deficit in the need for biologically sound and functional dentition due to poor dietary choices and poor oral hygiene care as evidenced by rampant decay

Deficit in the need for responsibility for oral health due to lack of parental supervision and infrequency of dental visits as evidenced by parental self-reports

1. Given the history and dental hygiene diagnosis, develop a comprehensive overall dental hygiene care plan including client goals, nutritional counseling plan, interventions, and evaluative measures. What factors would you use as motivators to change behavior? Share your approach to care with your peers.
2. Access the Internet. Find at least three sites that you could recommend for nutritional information appropriate for children, teens, adults, and senior citizens.
3. How might your nutritional counseling plan change if the client were Asian? Native American? Hispanic? African American?
4. Generate a list of healthy snacks that might be culture specific. Consider the culture represented in your community.

SCENARIO 35-3

ELDERLY CLIENT

Client: Mr. Conrad Farmer
Age: 71-year-old
Gender: male
Height: 5′11″
Weight: 160 lb
Race: African American

Health History: Has high blood pressure, rheumatoid arthritis, and depression

Pharmacologic History: Currently taking atenolol and amlodipine (Norvasc) for blood pressure, trazodone for depression, and celecoxib (Celebrex) for rheumatoid arthritis.

Dental History: Presents to the dental clinic with carious lesions on the facials of #3, 14, 15, 18 and the mesial of tooth #24. He has moderate supragingival calculus and slight to moderate subgingival deposits. He has generalized bleeding with 5-mm pockets noted on the mesial and distal of all posterior teeth.

Chief Complaint: "My mouth is really dry and I have a few teeth that kinda ache."

Social History: Retired widower; lost his wife to cancer a year ago. He and his wife never had children. He does not have any extended family in the local area.

Dietary Assessment: Mr. Farmer frequently keeps cinnamon hard candies in his mouth to stimulate his saliva. He also sips on Dr. Pepper throughout the day to keep his mouth moist.

Since Mr. Farmer's wife died, he cooks for himself. His cooking skills are minimal. Breakfast usually consists of a whole-grain bagel or muffin. Lunch is usually a sandwich of some sort with a bowl of soup. Dinner is often a frozen dinner. However, he often skips the evening meal because he doesn't like eating alone at night. He snacks frequently throughout the day on pretzels, trail mix, and Cheez-It snack crackers. To take the edge off his hunger before he goes to bed, Mr. Farmer often snacks on peanut butter crackers or his personal favorite—a bowl of chunky chocolate banana ice cream. He drinks coffee continuously throughout the day. He likes it with 3 T sugar and lots of cream.

Continued

SCENARIO 35-3

ELDERLY CLIENT

Nutritional Risk Factors:

Snack choices are sticky consistency and contribute to caries risk

Frequency of acidic beverages

Lack of variety and balance in his diet

Slow-dissolving candies promote caries

Cariogenic food choices couples with decreased salivary function

Dental Hygiene Diagnosis:

Unmet need for responsibility for oral health due to inadequate homecare and dietary habits as indicated by presence of carious lesions, bleeding points, and bone loss.

Unmet need for protection from health risks due to lack of nutrient-dense foods in the diet and skipping meals.

1. Do you have any recommended interventions for Mr. Farmer's dietary practices?
2. What snacks would you suggest to replace some of the cariogenic choices? What questions would you ask Mr. Farmer prior to suggesting alternative foods to him?
3. Access the Internet to find some community nutrition services that you may recommend to Mr. Farmer.

REFERENCES

1. U.S. Department of Agriculture, U.S. Department of Health and Human Services: *Dietary guidelines for Americans 2010*, ed 7, Washington, DC, December 2010, U.S. Government Printing Office. Available at: http://www.cnpp.usda.gov/dgas2010-policydocument.htm. Accessed November 11, 2012.
2. U.S. Department of Agriculture: *MyPlate*. Available at: http://www.choosemyplate.gov. Accessed November 11, 2012.
3. Abdollahi M, Rahimi R, Radfar M: Current opinion on drug-induced oral reactions: a comprehensive review, *J Contemp Dent Pract* 9(3):1, 2008. Available at: http://www.jaypeejournals.com/eJournals/ShowText.aspx?ID=1859&Type=FREE&TYP=TOP&IN=~/eJournals/images/JPLOGO.gif&IID=159&isPDF=YES.
4. Da Fonseca M: Osteoporosis: an increasing concern in pediatric dentistry. *Pediatric Dentistry* [serial online]. 33(3):241, 2011. Available at: Food and Science Source, Ipswich, MA. http://www.ingentaconnect.com/content/aapd/pd/2011/00000033/00000003/art00010. Accessed September 24, 2013.
5. Mahan LK, Raymond JL, Escott-Stump S, editors: *Krause's food and the nutrition care process*, ed 13, St Louis, 2012, Saunders.
6. Committee on Dietary Allowances: *Recommended dietary allowances*, ed 10, Washington, DC, 1989, National Academy Press.
7. Gustafsson BE, Quensel CE, Lanke LS, et al: The Vipeholm dental caries study: the effects of different levels of carbohydrate intake on caries activity in 436 individuals observed for five years, *Acta Odontol Scand* 11:232, 1954.
8. Screenby LM: Sugar availability, sugar consumption and dental caries, *Community Dent Oral Epidemiol* 10:1, 1982.
9. American Association of Oral and Maxiollofacial Sureons: *Oral surgery and nutrition*. Available at: http://www.aaoms.org/nutrition.php. Accessed November 19, 2012.
10. Kaye EK: Bone health and oral health, *J Am Dent Assoc* 138:616, 2007.
11. Devlin H: Identification of the risk for osteoporosis in dental patients, *Dent Clin North Am* 56(4):847, 2012.
12. Ogden CL, Carroll MD, Kit BK, et al: *Prevalence of obesity in the United States, 2010*. NCHS Data Brief No. 82, January 2012. Available at: http://www.cdc.gov/nchs/data/databriefs/db82.pdf. Accessed November 20, 2012.
13. Ogden CL, Carroll M: *Prevalence of obesity among children and adolescents: United States, trends 1963-1965 through 2007-2008*. Available at: http://www.cdc.gov/nchs/data/hestat/obesity_child_07_08/obesity_child_07_08.pdf. Accessed November 20, 2012.

ACKNOWLEDGEMENT

The author acknowledges Stacy Long for her past contributions to this chapter.

EVOLVE RESOURCES

Please visit http://evolve.elsevier.com/Darby/hygiene for additional practice and study support tools.

Tobacco Cessation

Margaret M. Walsh, Kirsten A. Jarvi

CHAPTER 36

COMPETENCIES

1. Describe systemic effects and oral health effects of tobacco use.
2. Explain the challenges to successful tobacco cessation.
3. Discuss the different aspects of nicotine addiction.
4. Discuss how to help clients to become tobacco-free, including:
   - Apply the National Cancer Institute's Five A's approach to tobacco cessation.
   - Assist clients with tobacco cessation based on their readiness to quit.
   - Describe three characteristics of patient-centered communication.
5. For clients who are not ready to quit, describe the following:
   - The brief intervention.
   - Motivational interviewing and its four "opening strategies" to elicit change talk.
6. For clients who are ready to quit, describe the following:
   - The initial Elicit-Provide-Elicit Model for brief assistance.
   - The Ask, Advise, Refer (AAR) approach to tobacco cessation.
7. Discuss the key elements of intensive tobacco cessation treatment programs, including coping strategies to prevent relapse.
8. Name the U.S. Food and Drug Administration–approved pharmacologic products to facilitate tobacco cessation.
9. Explain the key elements of an intensive, multiple-session tobacco cessation program.
10. Explain the dental hygienist's role related to tobacco in the community.

Tobacco is the chief avoidable cause of preventable illness and death in the United States. Each year, more than 450,000 people die as a result of tobacco-related diseases.[1] It is imperative that all healthcare providers assess and treat tobacco use to increase the likelihood of tobacco cessation. Tobacco cessation occurs when a person stops tobacco use with the goal of achieving permanent abstinence. Although some tobacco users achieve permanent abstinence during an initial quit attempt, the majority persist in tobacco use and typically cycle through multiple periods of abstinence and relapse (i.e., reverting to regular tobacco use). All tobacco contains nicotine, a highly addictive drug that creates physical and psychologic dependence on tobacco. Tobacco dependence makes it difficult for individuals to stop tobacco use even if they have health problems. Tobacco dependence is a chronic disorder characterized by a vulnerability to relapse that persists for months and even years. Relapse is likely because of the chronic nature of tobacco dependence; it is not a result of a clinician's personal failure, and it is not a failure on the part of the client. The relapsing nature of tobacco dependence requires the need for ongoing rather than just acute care.[2] As with other chronic disorders (e.g., periodontal disease, hypertension, diabetes), dental hygienists who encounter tobacco-dependent clients are encouraged to provide ongoing advice, counseling, and referral. Despite the potential for relapse, however, numerous effective treatments are available to promote tobacco cessation.

Systemic Health Effects

All tobacco products contain cancer-causing chemicals such as *N*-nitrosamines, aromatic hydrocarbons, and polonium 210. In addition, smoking produces tar, carbon monoxide, and other chemically destructive by-products that are present in tobacco smoke. During the inhalation process, smokers absorb nicotine, cancer-causing chemicals contained in tobacco, and the toxic by-products of burning tobacco through the lungs. These toxins enter the bloodstream and are distributed to tissues throughout the body. This exposure to toxic chemicals threatens the health of smokers. Smoked tobacco is responsible for 87% of lung cancers, and, on average, half of smokers lose 20 to 25 years of their life expectancies.[3] Box 36-1 lists numerous adverse systemic effects associated with tobacco use.

Oral snuff and chewing tobacco, which are also known as spit (smokeless) tobacco, are associated with cancer and cardiovascular disease. Oral snuff (known as *snus* in Sweden and some other countries) is a finely ground tobacco leaf, packaged either loose or in a tea-bag–like sachet (Figure 36-1). Snuff users place a small amount of oral snuff between the cheek and gum. Chewing tobacco is a more coarsely shredded tobacco leaf. Tobacco chewers place a "chaw" of loose leaf tobacco or a "plug" of compressed tobacco in the cheek (Figure 36-2). Oral snuff and chewing tobacco users generally spit out the tobacco juices and saliva that are generated, but sometimes such users swallow them.

Most spit tobacco products contain much larger amounts of nitrosamines (cancer-causing chemicals) than those legally allowed in other consumable products. Moreover, manufacturers control the amount of free nicotine available for uptake into the body by controlling the pH of their products. Free nicotine is ionized nicotine that passes rapidly through the oral mucosa into the bloodstream and into the brain. Because

BOX 36-1

Systemic Effects of Tobacco Use

- Cancer (mouth, pharynx, esophagus, stomach, bladder, lung, breast, uterine)
- Cardiovascular disease (aortic aneurysm, atherosclerosis, chronic obstructive heart disease, coronary artery disease)
- Hypertension, stroke
- Respiratory disease (emphysema, bronchitis, chronic obstructive lung disease, upper respiratory infection)
- Reproductive problems (miscarriage, preterm birth, low-birthweight babies, infants with cleft lip and palate, growth retardation, tooth malformation, early menopause, sudden infant death syndrome)
- Impotence
- Ulcers
- Osteoporosis
- Facial wrinkling
- Nicotine addiction

BOX 36-2

Oral Effects of Tobacco Use

- Oral and pharyngeal cancers
- Chronic periodontitis
- Failure of periodontal therapy
- Failure of dental implants
- Dental caries
- Oral pain
- Biofilm increase of red complex bacteria
- Tooth abrasion
- Stain
- Calculus
- Halitosis
- Impaired taste and smell
- Attrition
- Delayed wound healing or dry socket
- Hairy or coated tongue
- Nicotine stomatitis
- Oral leukoplakia
- Tooth loss
- Xerostomia

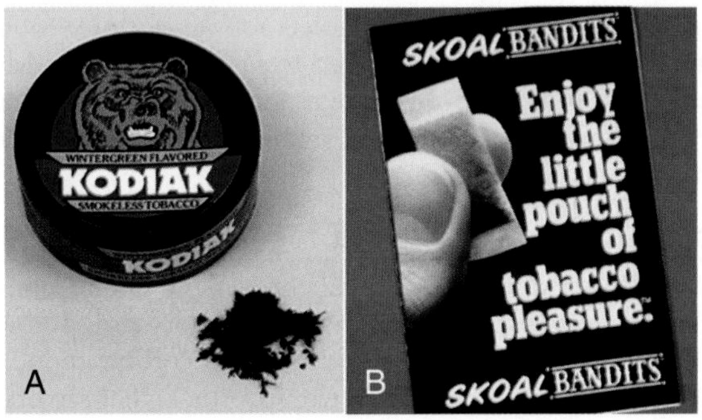

Figure 36-1. Example of oral snuff products. **A,** Packaged loose. **B,** In a tea-bag–like sachet.

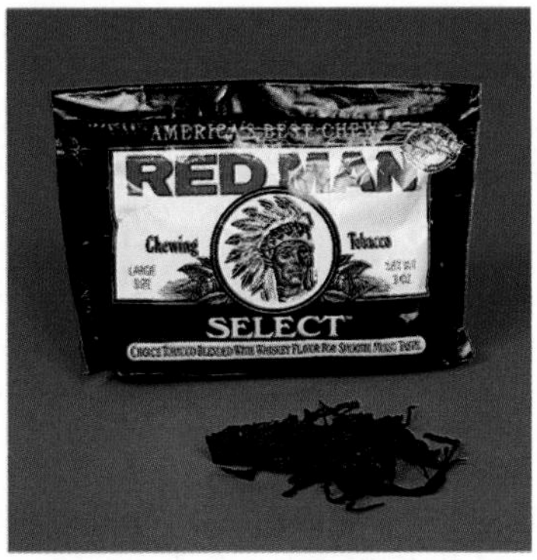

Figure 36-2. Example of a chewing tobacco product.

TABLE 36-1

The pH and Percentage of Free Nicotine in Oral Snuff Brands

Brand	pH	Percentage of Available Free Nicotine
Copenhagen	8.0	57%
Skoal Fine Cut	7.5	29%
Skoal Long Cut (varying brands)	7.2	23%
Skoal Bandits	5.4	<1%

From Djordjevic MV, Hoffmann D, Glynn T, Connolly GN: US commercial brands of moist snuff, 1994, I: assessment of nicotine, moisture, and pH, *Tob Control* 4:62, 1995.

free nicotine is formed in an alkaline environment, the higher the pH of a spit tobacco product, the more available free nicotine. For example, at a neutral pH of 7.0, there is no free nicotine available; however, at a pH of 8.0, about 60% of the nicotine is ionized and available for use by the body to create dependence. The amount of free nicotine available in spit tobacco products is controlled by manufacturers through the addition of alkaline buffering agents. Usually new users start with products with low amounts of free nicotine to avoid the unpleasant side effects of nicotine toxicity (e.g., nausea, vomiting). Eventually, however, as a result of nicotine dependence, many individuals need to use products with higher amounts of free nicotine. Table 36-1 shows the pH of popular oral snuff brands and the percentage of free nicotine available in each. Brands with high levels of available free nicotine are very addictive, thereby making it difficult for individuals to quit using them.

Oral Health Effects

The oral effects of tobacco use[3] are listed in Box 36-2. The dental hygienist points out and discusses with clients the visible effects of their tobacco use and documents all relevant findings. For example, a smoker may have nicotine stomatitis (Figure 36-3) on the palate, and smokers are three to six times more likely than nonsmokers to develop periodontal disease.[4]

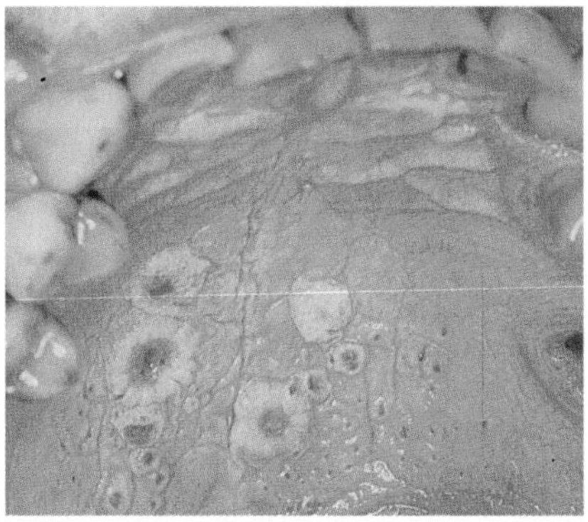

Figure 36-3. Nicotine stomatitis on the palate of a smoker.

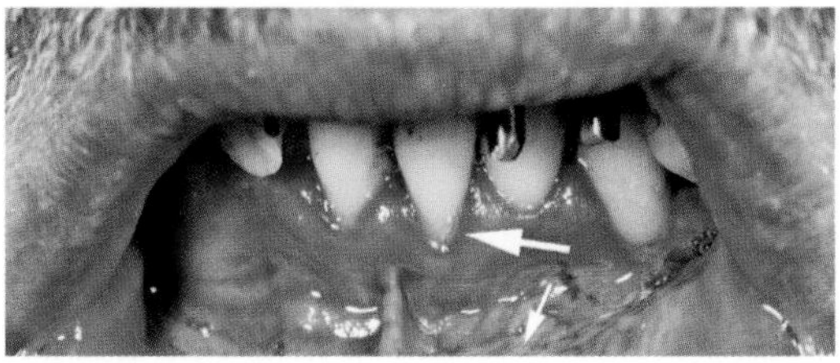

Figure 36-4. Gingival recession and hyperkeratosis of the vestibular mucosa that developed after the use of chewing tobacco. (From Newman MG, Takei HH, Klokkevold PR, et al: *Carranza's clinical periodontology*, ed 11, St Louis, 2012, Saunders.)

In addition, almost half of spit tobacco users have oral mucosal lesions and gingival recession associated with use (Figure 36-4). The oral mucosal lesions are typically characterized as being white, hyperkeratinized, and wrinkled; they often disappear if tobacco use is terminated at an early enough stage.

Table 36-2 lists actual or potential unmet human needs related to tobacco use. In addition, the clinical manifestations of tobacco-induced periodontal disease and their biologic bases are presented in Table 36-3. All forms of tobacco are associated with oral, pharyngeal, and esophageal cancer.[3] The long-standing relationship between oral cancer and tobacco use is well documented (see Chapter 45). Concomitant use of alcohol with tobacco increases the risk of oral cancer tenfold. Seventy-five percent of oral and pharyngeal cancers are attributed to tobacco use with or without heavy alcohol use.[3] Consequently, during a health history assessment, clients are questioned about alcohol use, tobacco use, and sun exposure, all of which are risk factors for head, neck, skin, and lip cancers. The extraoral and intraoral examination must be thorough, and all tissue changes must be noted in the client's chart.

Challenges to Successful Tobacco Cessation

Findings from a national survey report that 70% of smokers want to quit. Each year, approximately 46% try to quit, but less than 10% achieve abstinence. Among smokers who attempt to quit, 60% relapse within the first 7 days of quitting, and 70% relapse within the first month. Most tobacco users require multiple attempts at stopping their tobacco use before they are ultimately successful.[2] Addiction to nicotine makes it very difficult to quit.

TABLE 36-2

The Tobacco-Using Client and the Human Needs Model

Human Needs	Actual or Potential Deficits*
Wholesome facial image	Tooth staining, halitosis, periodontal disease, missing teeth, facial wrinkling
Protection from health risks	Tobacco-related illness (e.g., heart disease, high blood pressure, cancer); delayed wound healing
Biologically sound and functional dentition	Missing teeth, abrasion, erosion, chewing difficulties, abscesses
Freedom from fear and stress	Withdrawal as a result of nicotine addiction
Responsibility for oral health	Inadequate ownership of personal oral health and hygiene
Conceptualization and problem solving	Misconceptions and lack of knowledge about systemic and oral effects of tobacco use

*All unmet human needs can be addressed by efficient and effective tobacco interventions.

Nicotine Addiction

The hallmarks of nicotine addiction are as follows:
- Compulsive use
- Use despite harmful effects
- Pleasant (euphoric) effects
- Difficulty with quitting or controlling use
- Recurrent drug cravings
- Tolerance
- Physical dependence
- Relapse after abstinence

Helping a tobacco-using client achieve abstinence requires an understanding of nicotine addiction. Aspects of nicotine addiction can be categorized as physical, psychologic, sensory, behavioral, and social.

Physical Aspects

The physical aspects of nicotine addiction include reinforcing effects, tolerance, and physical dependence.[5]

Reinforcing Effects

Nicotine causes the brain to release chemicals such as dopamine, norepinephrine, acetylcholine, vasopressin, serotonin, and beta-endorphins. These chemicals produce effects in the brain that cause the user to experience pleasure, anxiety and tension reduction, a sense of well-being when one feels down, arousal (perks one up when tired), short-term memory improvement, and appetite suppression. These neurochemical rewards that nicotine provides a tobacco user are called **reinforcing effects**.[5] These reinforcing effects reward tobacco users and increase their desire to continue using tobacco (Table 36-4).

Tolerance

With chronic exposure to nicotine, brain cells adapt to compensate for the actions of nicotine. This process is called

TABLE 36-3

Tobacco-Induced Periodontal Tissue Changes

TISSUE		
Changes with Use	**Biologic Bases for Changes**	**Tissue Changes with Abstinence**
Paler tissue color	Increased vasoconstriction	Increased blood flow
Decreased bleeding	Oxygen depletion	Initially more bleeding and erythema
Thickened fibrotic consistency; minimal erythema relative to extent of disease	Compromised immune response • Fewer and impaired polymorphonuclear neutrophils • Reduced immunoglobulin G antibody	Healthier consistency and anatomy
Gingival recession around anterior sextants	Increased collagenase production	
Greater probing depths, bone and attachment loss, furcation invasion	Reduction of bone mineral; impaired fibroblast function	Stabilization of attachment levels
Refractory status: continued use	Impaired wound healing	

TABLE 36-4

Effects of Chemicals Released by the Brain with Exposure to Nicotine

Chemical	Effect
Dopamine	Pleasure
Serotonin	Mood modulation
Beta-endorphin	Anxiety reduction
Acetylcholine	Cognitive enhancement (i.e., perks one up if tired)
Vasopressin	Short-term memory enhancement
Norepinephrine	Appetite suppression

neuroadaptation. **Tolerance** results from neuroadaptation so that, over time, a given level of nicotine eventually has less of an effect on the brain and a larger dose is needed to produce the rewarding effects that lower doses formerly produced. Thus the longer clients use tobacco, the more nicotine they need to achieve the desired reinforcing effects.[5]

Physical Dependence

Although the brain adapts to function normally in the presence of nicotine, it also becomes **physically dependent** on nicotine for that normal functioning. When nicotine is not available, the brain function becomes disturbed, which results in **withdrawal symptoms** (Table 36-5). Symptoms peak within 12 to 24 hours and last 2 to 4 weeks if tobacco use is discontinued. Not all individuals experience withdrawal symptoms, and the degree of discomfort from withdrawal also varies. In general, however, the nicotine withdrawal symptoms produced by nicotine abstinence require clients to continue to increase their tobacco use to prevent those withdrawal symptoms going forward. Therefore, although initially individuals use tobacco for the reinforcing effects of pleasure, enhanced short-term memory, and mood modulation, tobacco use often ends up dominating their lives. Because tobacco use produces tolerance and physical dependence, it results in addiction and the loss of control over use. This loss of control is the result of the individual's intense need to use tobacco to self-medicate to prevent withdrawal symptoms.[5] In general, the highly dependent tobacco user poses the greatest challenge to cessation efforts; this type of client usually requires pharmacotherapy in combination with intense behavioral counseling.

Psychologic, Behavioral, Sensory, and Sociocultural Aspects

Psychologic, behavioral, sensory, and sociocultural aspects of nicotine addiction also sustain tobacco use.[5]

Psychologic Aspects

Psychologic aspects of nicotine addiction relate to a tobacco-using client's need to use tobacco to cope with stress or depression. Many tobacco users perceive their tobacco as "a friend" that is always with them, providing a sense of comfort and security. Tobacco use also initially may be used as passive entertainment to decrease boredom or as a diversion from a strife-filled existence.

Behavioral Aspects

Behavioral aspects of nicotine addiction relate to learned anticipatory responses that tobacco users develop from having experienced various forms of gratification from tobacco use in certain previous situations.[5] When a tobacco user encounters these environmental cues, they serve as situational reminders of tobacco use (e.g., after a meal, when drinking alcohol) and its associated pleasure or other reinforcing effects. These cues or stimuli then generate a strong urge to use tobacco; this is known as a **learned anticipatory response**. Such learned anticipatory responses can last 6 months or longer after physical dependence has been overcome, and they are often responsible for relapse that occurs beyond the first 2 to 4 weeks of cessation. For successful cessation, tobacco users have to learn to anticipate situational

TABLE 36-5
Nicotine Withdrawal Symptoms and Suggested Behavioral Coping Strategies

Symptoms	Mechanisms for Coping
Cravings	Realizing that cravings last only 3 to 5 minutes; "waiting them out" Thinking responses (e.g., "I can do this and I will") Distraction techniques: carrying and reading a list of reasons for stopping or inspirational poems Considering non-nicotine aspects of craving and using substitutions (e.g., oral stimulation: chewing gum; hand usage: doodling) Avoiding triggers (e.g., people, places, or things associated with former habit) Getting exercise
Irritability, frustration, anger, depression	Professional counseling Support groups Exercise Deep breathing with slow exhalation Self-reward for abstinence
Anxiety	Deep breathing Positive imaging Relaxation exercises Aerobic exercise
Depression, sad mood	Physician referral Professional counseling Support groups Exercise Self-reward for abstinence
Insomnia	Relaxation exercises Going to bed later Getting up and moving around Avoiding caffeine Deep breathing Aerobic exercise (but not within 2 hours of bedtime)
Difficulty concentrating	Recognition that symptom is short-lived Relaxation exercises Patience Deep breathing
Stomach or intestinal problems	Mild over-the-counter medications High-fiber diet Drinking water Relaxation exercises
Hunger or weight gain	Aerobic exercise Healthy eating Drinking water Chewing xylitol gum or eating xylitol hard candy Support groups (e.g., Overeaters Anonymous, Weight Watchers) Restrictive dieting is not recommended; too much deprivation may be overwhelming

Modified from Severson H: *Enough snuff: a guide to quitting smokeless tobacco,* Point Richmond, Calif, 1997, Applied Behavior Science.

cues that will trigger the desire to use tobacco and to plan ahead to identify alternative rewards and ways to cope with these trigger situations so that they can remain tobacco-free.

Sensory Aspects

Puffing on a cigarette or having a dip of a specific size and texture in one's mouth provides oral gratification, which relates to the sensory aspect of nicotine addiction. Because of the sense of well-being this oral gratification provides, the use of nontobacco oral substitutes (e.g., chewing gum, sunflower seeds) is important to the quitting process.[5] In addition, because nicotine is an appetite suppressant, individuals often increase their food intake when they reduce their nicotine exposures. Individuals who successfully stop their tobacco use on average gain 10 pounds. Drinking a lot of water, getting exercise, and eating a balanced low-fat diet can help these individuals to avoid this weight gain.[6]

Sociocultural Aspects

Sociocultural aspects of nicotine addiction that pose challenges to cessation include peer pressure, the influence of family members and significant others who use tobacco, and a social network that supports and accepts tobacco use. Tobacco users who are trying to stop their tobacco use often need to avoid situations in which they will be tempted to use until they are sure that they can refrain from using tobacco in these situations.

Helping Clients Become Tobacco-Free

When one assists clients with their efforts to stop using tobacco, all aspects of nicotine addiction must be confronted and alternative coping strategies identified. Being supportive and assisting the client with problem solving are critical to the promotion of tobacco cessation.

The Five A's Approach

A general framework for helping clients in the healthcare setting to become tobacco-free is the **Five A's approach**, a strategy developed by the National Cancer Institute and the Agency for Healthcare Research and Quality.[2] The Five A's approach to tobacco cessation involves *asking* clients about tobacco use, *advising* users to quit, *assessing* their readiness to quit, *assisting* with the quitting process, and *arranging* follow-up. Table 36-6 provides sample language for the dental hygienist to use while performing components of the five A's. The Five A's approach serves as a model for brief, effective interventions that have been successfully implemented in both medical and dental care environments.[2,7] Each component of the Five A's approach is described briefly in the following sections. A team approach that involves all office staff facilitates the Five A's approach.

Ask

It is important to identify all tobacco users systematically at every visit. This identification occurs by using an in-office system, such as including an item on the health history form that asks about tobacco use and having all tobacco users complete a separate Tobacco Use Assessment Form, such as the one presented in Figure 36-5, for inclusion in the client-care record. In addition, the dental hygienist verbally asks each client about tobacco use (see Table 36-6 for suggested language). Cues or prompts, such as chart stickers or codes on the client schedule, are recommended to remind the hygienist to ask each client.

Advise

The dental hygienist advises all tobacco users to stop their tobacco use to protect their current and future health. Such advice should be clear, unequivocal, nonjudgmental, and related to something immediately relevant to the client (see Table 36-6 for suggested language). For example, if clients have oral mucosal tissue changes as a result of tobacco use (see Figure 36-4), the dental hygienist points out the tissue changes to the clients in their own mouths and incorporates this information to personalize advice to stop using tobacco. Personalizing cessation advice with findings visible to the client provides a "teachable moment" that can motivate the client to decide to make a quit attempt.[2] During the advice

TABLE 36-6

The Five A's Approach to Tobacco Cessation: Ask, Advise, Assess, Assist, Arrange[2]

Approach	Suggested Actions and/or Language
Ask	"Do you ever smoke or use any type of tobacco?" "I take time to ask all of our clients about tobacco use because it is important."
Advise	*Personalize (connect with oral findings):* "There have been some tissue changes in your mouth, and your periodontal disease is getting worse since your last visit. Smoking is affecting your health." *Clear but nonjudgmental:* "The best thing that I can do for you today to protect your current and future health is to advise you to stop smoking."
Assess (readiness to quit)	"Would you like to try to quit smoking in the next month? If so, we can help."
Assist	*For clients who are not ready to quit:* Provide a brief intervention or a motivational interview *For clients who are ready to quit:* Perform Elicit-Provide-Elicit strategy
Arrange	*For clients not ready to quit, state:* "If it is okay with you, I'd like to check in with you at your next dental hygiene care appointment to see where you are in your decision making." (Document in chart.) *For clients who are ready to quit:* Refer to 1-800-QUIT-NOW and provide information about a community-based tobacco cessation program in the area. Make a note in the chart to check on the client's quitting progress at the next dental hygiene care appointment. *For clients who are ready to quit who have elected to participate in a cessation program in the dental office:* Schedule one to four separate appointments, each 45 to 60 minutes in length, to begin tobacco cessation counseling.

From the U.S. Department of Health and Human Services: *Treating tobacco use and dependence*, U.S. Department of Health and Human Services Publication No. 69-0692, Washington, DC, 2000, U.S. Government Printing Office.

Tobacco Use Assessment Form

Name ______________________________

Date ______________

1. Do you use tobacco in any form? ☐ Yes ☐ No

1A. If no, have you ever used tobacco in the past? ☐ Yes ☐ No

How long did you use tobacco? _____ years _____ months

How long ago did you stop? _____ years _____ months

If you are not currently a tobacco user, no other questions should be answered. Thank you for completing this form.

Questions 2-10 are for current tobacco users only.

2. If you smoke, what type? (Check) How many? (Number)
☐ Cigarettes _____ Cigarettes per day
☐ Cigars _____ Cigars per day
☐ Pipe _____ Bowls per day

3. If you chew/use snuff, what type? How much?
☐ Snuff _____ Days a can lasts
☐ Chewing _____ Pouches per week
☐ Other (describe) ______________________
Amount __________ per ______________________

3A. How long do you keep a chew in your mouth?
_______minutes

4. How many days of the week do you use tobacco?
7 6 5 4 3 2 1

5. How soon after you wake up do you first use tobacco?
☐ within 30 minutes ☐ more than 30 minutes

6. Does the person closest to you use tobacco?
☐ Yes ☐ No

7. How interested are you in stopping your use of tobacco?
☐ not at all ☐ a little ☐ somewhat ☐ yes ☐ very much

8. Have you tried to stop using tobacco before? ☐ Yes ☐ No

8A. How long ago was your last attempt to quit?
_____ years _____ months

9. Have you discussed stopping with another physician, dentist, or dental hygienist? ☐ Yes ☐ No

10. If you decided to stop using tobacco completely during the next two weeks, how confident are you that you would succeed?
☐ not at all ☐ a little ☐ somewhat ☐ very confident

Thank you for completing this form

Client Tobacco Use Assessment Form

Contact Record

Date client contacted	Client asked Y/N	Advice given Y/N	Assist describe service

Figure 36-5. Tobacco use assessment form. (Adapted from the U.S. Department of Health and Human Services: *Tobacco effects in the mouth,* National Institutes of Health Publication No. 94-3330, Bethesda, Md, 1992, U.S. Government Printing Office.)

component of the Five A's approach, it is very appropriate to discuss actual and potential adverse health effects associated with tobacco use. After the advice component, however, the dental hygienist replaces the discussion of negative health effects with discussions about the benefits of quitting to enhance the client's motivation to stop tobacco use (Box 36-3).

Assess

For all clients who report tobacco use, the dental hygienist determines which tobacco users are willing to make a quit attempt by assessing their readiness to quit.[8] To assess readiness to quit, the dental hygienist simply asks clients if they would like to stop their tobacco use in the next month. Whether clients respond "yes" or "no" will determine the appropriate strategy for assisting them with the quitting process.

As individuals attempt to stop tobacco use, **relapse** (i.e., reverting to regular tobacco use) often occurs. The dental hygienist encourages clients to view relapse as a learning opportunity, because what is learned from relapse can be applied to the next quit attempt. See Table 36-7 for a summary and suggested dental hygiene interventions.

BOX 36-3

Benefits of Stopping Tobacco Use

- I won't have the smell of tobacco on my breath or stains on my teeth.
- I will save money.
- It will reduce my chances of getting mouth cancer.
- My friends and family want me to quit.
- I'll be setting a good example for my children.
- I'll feel more in control of my life.
- I'll feel more liberated and self-assured that I can set goals and accomplish them.
- It will reduce my chances of heart trouble.
- It will reduce my chances of gum disease.
- It will reduce my chances of hypertension and circulatory problems.
- It will increase my chances of being around to support my family and of seeing my children grow up.
- Two weeks to 3 months after quitting smoking, circulation improves, walking becomes easier, and lung function increases up to 30%.
- One year after quitting smoking, the risk of coronary heart disease decreases to half that of a smoker.
- Five years after quitting smoking, the risk of stroke is reduced to that of people who have never smoked.
- Fifteen years after quitting smoking, the risk of coronary heart disease is similar to that of people who have never smoked.

Adapted from the U.S. Department of Health and Human Services: *Surgeon General report on the health benefits of smoking cessation,* DHHS Publication No. (CDC) 90-8416, United States. Public Health Service, Office on Smoking and Health, 1990.

Assist

The manner in which the dental hygienist assists a client with quitting tobacco use depends on the client's readiness to quit (see Figure 36-6 for a tobacco intervention flow chart and the detailed discussion that follows). Whether or not clients are ready to quit, it is critical that the dental hygienist engage them by applying **patient-centered communication**.[9,10]

Characteristics of patient-centered communication include the following[7,9]:

- *Collaborating, not persuading:* The dental hygienist–client relationship involves a partnership that honors the client's experience and perspectives. The dental hygienist seeks to create a positive interpersonal atmosphere that is conducive to change while not being coercive.
- *Eliciting information, not imparting information:* The dental hygienist's tone is not one of imparting information but rather of drawing out motivation for change from the person. Clients do most of the talking, and dental hygienists listen carefully.
- *Emphasizing the client's autonomy, not the authority of the expert:* Responsibility for change is left with the client.

Arrange

Arranging a follow-up contact is the fifth A, and it is comparable to the evaluation phase of the dental hygiene process of care. During follow-up contacts, the dental hygienist checks in on where clients are in their thinking process about quitting or on their progress with regard to coping with the quitting process. For those clients who have made an unsuccessful quit attempt, modifications (e.g., new quit date, other

TABLE 36-7

Client Tobacco Use Status and Recommended Interventions Related to Readiness to Quit, Maintenance, and Relapse[8]

Client Status	Client Characteristics and Behavior	Dental Hygiene Intervention
Ready to quit? No*	No thought of quitting in the next 6 months	Dispense educational material about reasons for quitting. Client may be defensive when confronted with the information.
Ready to quit? No*	Thinking about quitting within the next 6 months	Dispense educational material, and discuss pros and cons of quitting. Ambivalence may be present, but clients will more likely accept information as they are developing more belief in the value of change.
Ready to quit? Yes*	Willing to set a quit date in the next month and to make small changes in preparation for quitting in the next month	Client believes advantages outweigh disadvantages of behavior change. May need assistance with planning for the change. Implement cessation counseling.
Ready to quit? Yes*	Actively engaged in strategies to change behavior. This stage may last up to 6 months. May have stopped using tobacco, but less than 6 months ago.	Praise. Identify barriers to and facilitators of change. Discuss relapse prevention.
Already has quit: Maintenance	Has stopped using tobacco for more than 6 months. Sustained change over time. This stage begins 6 months after action has started and continues indefinitely.	Praise. Discuss relapse prevention. Changes need to be integrated into the client's lifestyle.
Relapse	Using tobacco again and may reach higher levels than before.	Set new quit date and begin cycle again.

*Client response to the following question: "Would you like to make a quit attempt in the next month?"Adapted from Prochaska JO, DiClemente CC: Stages of change in the modification of problem behaviors, *Prog Behav Modif* 28:184, 1992.

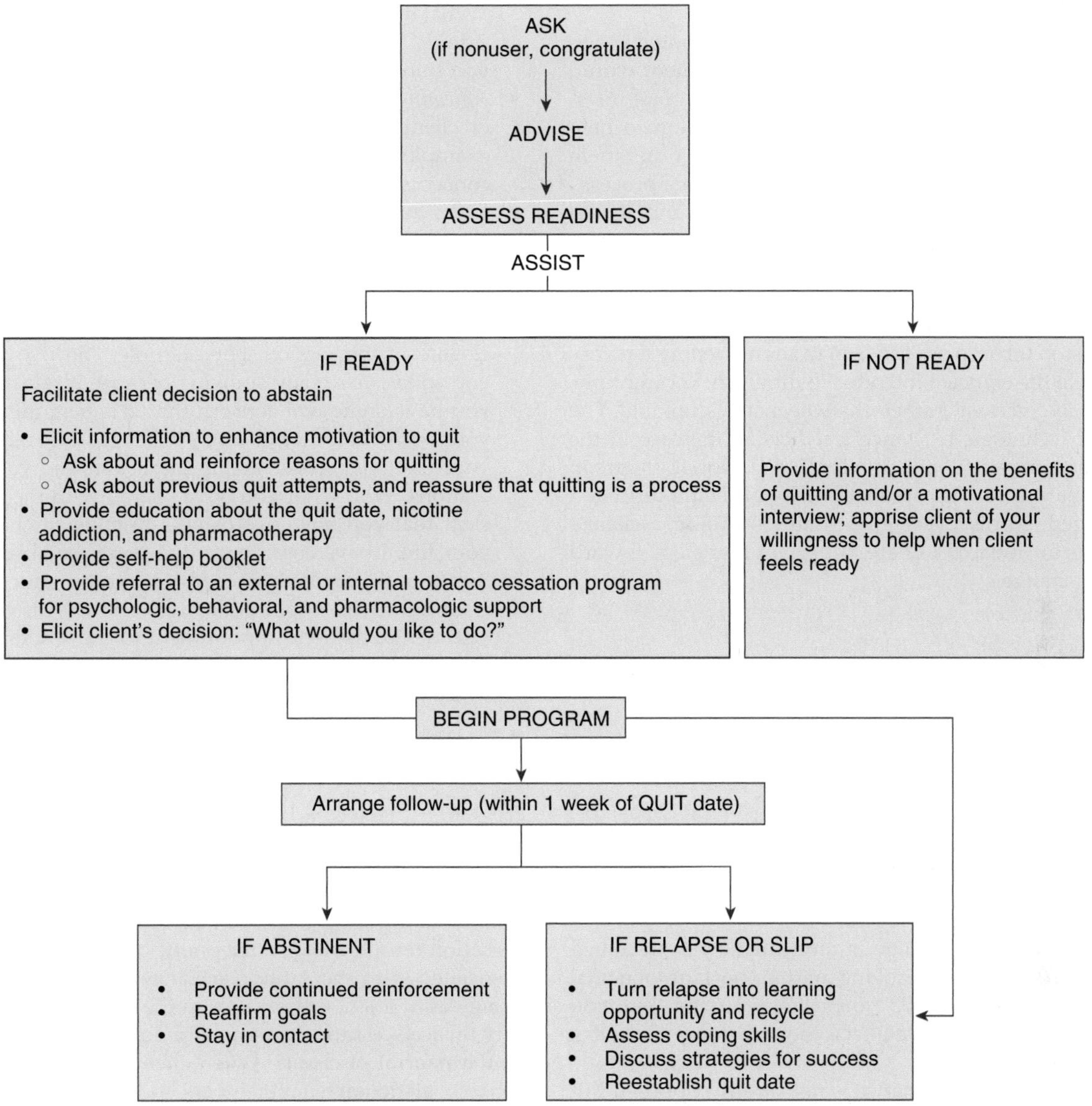

Figure 36-6. Tobacco intervention flow chart.

pharmacologic adjuncts, and different coping mechanisms, as described in later sections) may be introduced. New goals may need to be set.[2,10]

Assisting Clients Who Are Not Ready to Quit

For clients who are not ready to stop their tobacco use within the next month, the primary goal is to help them to think about the benefits of using tobacco versus the benefits of stopping tobacco use. When the benefits of stopping outweigh the benefits of using, the client will make a decision to quit. For this goal to be accomplished, a brief intervention or a motivational interview is recommended.

The Brief Intervention

The brief intervention takes less than 3 minutes to perform. The goal is to communicate acceptance of the client's decision not to make a quit attempt at this time and to provide information about the benefits of stopping tobacco use.[10] When a client refuses an offer of help to stop tobacco use during the brief intervention, the dental hygienist does the following[10]:

- States, "I understand that you are not ready to stop smoking now, but if you don't mind, I would like to give you some information on the benefits of stopping for you to consider" (see Box 36-3). This statement communicates to clients that they have been heard and that the dental hygienist understands that they are not ready to stop now. In addition, the dental hygienist offers information about the benefits of quitting to help move clients in the direction of making a decision to quit someday.
- Reassures clients by stating, "When you decide to try to stop, if you wish, we can help you."
- Asks permission to check in again at the next visit to see where clients are in the decision-making process by stating, "Would it be all right if I check in with you at your next dental hygiene care appointment regarding your thinking about all this?"
- Makes a note in the chart to check in again at the next continued-care visit.

The Motivational Interview

In addition to applying the brief intervention as noted previously, the dental hygienist may judge that the client would be open to a motivational interview.[9] The **motivational interview** is a form of patient-centered communication to help clients get "unstuck" from the ambivalence that traps them in their tobacco use so that they can start the change process.[9] Ambivalence is a common human experience, and it is a normal stage in the quitting process. After ambivalence is resolved, little else may be required for the client to decide to stop tobacco use. It is interesting to note, however, that attempts to force the resolution of ambivalence by direct persuasion to stop tobacco use can lead to strengthening the very behavior that the clinician intended to diminish. For example, nagging may increase rather than decrease smoking. The theory of psychologic reactance[9] predicts an increase in the rate and attractiveness of "problem" behavior if a person perceives that his or her personal freedom is being infringed or challenged, so discovering and understanding a client's motivations for tobacco use are important first steps toward promoting change.

Principles

The four general principles that underlie motivational interviewing are as follows[9]:

1. *Express empathy:* The attitude is one of acceptance. The dental hygienist respectfully listens to the client with a desire to understand his or her perspectives without judging, criticizing, or blaming. The client's perspectives are responded to as understandable and valid. Paradoxically, the acceptance of people "as they are" seems to free them to change, whereas insistent nonacceptance tends to immobilize the change process.
2. *Develop discrepancy:* Change is motivated by a perceived discrepancy between smoking and important personal goals or values (e.g., "So you enjoy smoking, but you worry about the negative effect your smoking may have on your teenage son").
3. *Roll with resistance:* Resistance is not directly opposed but is acknowledged as being natural and understandable. The dental hygienist avoids arguing for change.
4. *Support self-efficacy (self-confidence):* The dental hygienist enhances clients' confidence in their capabilities to cope with obstacles and to succeed in change. The hygienist's own expectations about a client's likelihood of stopping tobacco use can have a powerful effect on outcome.

Tools

The goal of motivational interviewing is to have the client voice the arguments for change; this is known as ***change talk***. Change talk includes reasons for concern and the advantages of change (i.e., the good things to be gained). Tools for eliciting change talk include four strategies referred to by the acronym ***OARS***.[9,10] These tools are as follows:

- *Open-ended questions:* Open-ended questions are questions that cannot be answered by a simple "yes" or "no" response. Open-ended questions begin with asking "What," "How," or "Why" and require the client to explain the response. During the motivational interview, the dental hygienist allows the client to express himself or herself and explores both sides of the client's ambivalence about tobacco use by asking open-ended questions. For example, "What do you like about tobacco use?" "What is the downside?" "So what kind of roadblocks come to mind when you think about stopping smoking?"
- *Affirming change talk:* This strategy reinforces and focuses on client comments that support stopping tobacco use. For example, "That's a good point. Do you have any other concerns?"
- *Reflective responding:* This technique acknowledges to the client, "Here is what I heard you say." For example, "So one of the most important considerations for you is how your smoking may affect your daughter."
- *Summarizing results of the dialogue:* This strategy brings closure to the session. For example, "So if I understand you so far, you enjoy smoking because it relaxes you, but you have some real concern that it is beginning to affect your health and that you may be a negative role model for your daughter. These are all important and valid considerations. With what you have shared with me today, it is clear that you have overcome a number of challenges in your life. I have confidence that you'll be able to resolve this issue of smoking once you make up your mind. If it is all right with you, I'd like to check in with you at your next dental hygiene appointment to see where you are in your thinking about all of this. Just know that if you decide to try to stop smoking, we can help."

Assisting Clients Who Are Ready to Stop Tobacco Use

For clients who state that they are ready to quit during the next month, the dental hygienist provides brief assistance with referral for more intensive assistance. Such referral may be either to an internal tobacco cessation program in the dental setting or to an external, community-based tobacco cessation resource (e.g., a telephone quitline; support groups associated with the American Cancer Society, the American Lung Association, or hospitals in the area). A list of community tobacco cessation programs should be developed for use in the referral of clients. When clients choose to stop using tobacco, all dental team members lend support to the tobacco user's goal of abstinence by providing positive reinforcement and by caring.

The Elicit-Provide-Elicit Model

A recommended model for tobacco cessation assistance with referral is the **Elicit-Provide-Elicit model** promoted by the Mayo Clinic.[7] Using this model, the dental hygienist does the following:

- *Elicits* information to enhance the client's motivation to quit
  - Asks about the client's reasons for quitting and reinforces them (e.g., "That's a great reason!")
  - Asks about past quit attempts and reassures client
    - States that most individuals have to try multiple times to quit before they are successful and that each time they try to quit, they learn something new about the quitting process that better prepares them to quit the next time they try
    - Concludes that, as long as individuals are trying to quit, they are not failing
- *Provides* the following:
  - Education about the concept of a **quit date** (i.e., the date clients select that is 2 to 4 weeks from the time

BOX 36-4

Basic Nicotine Information that Clients Need

- Tobacco contains nicotine.
- Nicotine is an addicting drug that changes brain chemistry.
- Nicotine withdrawal lasts 2 to 4 weeks; it is the brain's way of healing.
- Medications can minimize the discomfort of nicotine withdrawal and the associated cravings.
- Untreated nicotine withdrawal symptoms may include cravings, irritability, frustration, anger, anxiety, difficulty concentrating, increased appetite, depression or sad mood, insomnia, and gastrointestinal problems.

they decide to quit and on which they will be tobacco-free)
  - Education about nicotine addiction and withdrawal (Box 36-4)
  - Education about the types of pharmacotherapy
  - A self-help booklet about stopping tobacco use and printed materials about the benefits of quitting (see Box 36-3)
  - Encouragement to seek social support from family and friends
  - Referral to an external or internal tobacco cessation treatment program
- *Elicits* the client's decision about cessation treatment (e.g., "What would you like to do?")

The American Dental Hygienists' Association Ask. Advise. Refer. Model

The American Dental Hygienists' Association, in partnership with the Smoking Cessation Leadership Center at the University of California, promotes a public health action plan for dental hygienists that simplifies tobacco cessation to a three-step process. The three-step process promotes *asking* about tobacco use at every visit, *advising* those who use tobacco to quit, and *referring* tobacco users to a state or national tobacco quitline by distributing a card with a national number: 1-800-QUIT-NOW. This model addresses time constraints expressed by dental hygienists related to tobacco cessation counseling. To enhance understanding of the Ask. Advise. Refer. tobacco cessation model, the American Dental Hygienists' Association has developed a website (www.askadviserefer.org) with resources to download for use during chairside communications.

Statewide Tobacco Use Quitlines

Excellent external resources for referral for tobacco cessation assistance are tobacco use telephone quitlines that can be accessed from any state in the United States. They offer easy access at no cost to the client, and they address ethnic and geographic disparities. Many tobacco users prefer quitlines to face-to-face programs, because telephone counseling is more convenient and provides anonymity. Key factors that increase quitline effectiveness include the use of trained counselors, a proactive format in which staff initiates contact and follow-up, and the combination of the quitline with client self-help materials and approved pharmacotherapy.[5]

BOX 36-5

Key Elements of Intensive Tobacco Cessation Treatment Programs

- Assessing the following:
  - Motivation to quit
  - Reasons for quitting
  - Previous quit attempts
  - Nicotine dependence
  - Patterns of tobacco use
  - History of mood disorders
  - Contraindications for pharmacotherapy
- Setting a quit date
- Establishing a plan for quitting
- Offering coping skills training
- Encouraging the enlistment of support from others
- Recommending pharmacologic agents
- Preventing relapse
- Following up

Key Elements of Intensive Tobacco Cessation Treatment Programs

Whether the dental hygienist refers the client to an intensive (i.e., multiple appointment) tobacco cessation treatment program within the dental setting or within the community, key elements shared by high-quality tobacco cessation programs are listed in Box 36-5 and discussed in detail in the following sections.[10]

Assessment

Initially the tobacco cessation counselor assesses clients' motivation to quit, reasons for quitting, previous quit attempts, nicotine dependence level, tobacco use patterns in a typical day (i.e., the number of dips, chews, or cigarettes used per day and associated cravings and mood states), mood disorder history, and pharmacotherapy contraindications. These assessment data are used to tailor client quit plans on the basis of individual needs. The following information relates to this assessment process.

Motivation to Quit

Motivation is fundamental to changing behavior. A client's level of motivation to stop tobacco use is often a good predictor of outcome.[9] To enhance clients' motivation and to measure motivation to quit, the counselor reads the following question and asks clients to circle an answer[7]:

On a scale of 0 to 10, how important would you say it is for you to stop your tobacco use?

0	1	2	3	4	5	6	7	8	9	10
Not at all important										Extremely important

The number circled then serves to measure clients' initial motivation, and it is used to monitor motivation to stop tobacco use at subsequent appointments.[7] The number circled also serves as the basis for a discussion to increase clients' motivation to quit. For example, if a client circles the number 5, the counselor might say, "Great! But why did you circle a 5 rather than a 3?" This open-ended question requires clients to talk positively about their motivation to quit, which serves to enhance their motivation. In general, asking clients why they circled a *higher* number rather than a lower number on the importance of quitting scale triggers clients to respond positively about their motivation to quit. Alternatively, asking clients why they circled a lower number rather than a higher number requires clients to talk negatively about their motivation to quit, which can become discouraging for them and decrease their motivation to make a quit attempt.

Reasons for Quitting

To enhance motivation to quit, the counselor also asks clients about their reasons for wanting to stop their tobacco use. The counselor may suggest that clients write these reasons down, because motivation may be high initially but may wane somewhat with time. Remembering one's reasons for quitting enhances motivation and provides incentive to get through tough times during the quitting process. Strong motivation is essential for tobacco users who are trying to quit, and success is unlikely without it.[9]

Previous Quit Attempts

The counselor assesses clients' previous experience with quit attempts by asking them if they have tried to quit before and, if so, what problems were encountered.[6,7,10] If nicotine replacement or other pharmacologic adjuncts were used, it is important to find out what happened. When discussing quit attempts, the counselor promotes clients' positive self-images by telling clients something along the lines of the following: "Quitting tobacco is a process that takes most people several tries before they are able to quit for good, but most people who persist eventually do quit."[10]

Nicotine Dependence

There are many ways to assess nicotine dependence. Recommended evidence-based questions to ask clients include the following:

- "Do you smoke every day?"
- "Do you use tobacco within 30 minutes of waking?"
- "Do you use tobacco most of the day?"
- "Do you crave tobacco when you have not used it for 2 hours?"

Clients who respond "yes" to any of these questions, especially with regard to using tobacco within 30 minutes of waking, are determined to be nicotine-dependent.[6]

Nicotine dependence also can be assessed by asking the question, "When you smoke, how many cigarettes per day do you usually have?" Clients who report that they smoke 1 to 15 cigarettes per day are considered to be lighter nicotine-dependent smokers as compared with those who report that they smoke more than 15 cigarettes per day. To minimize discomfort from nicotine withdrawal, it is important for nicotine-dependent tobacco users to wean themselves off of nicotine before the quit date rather than to stop abruptly (i.e., "cold turkey"). Strategies that combine behavioral and adjunctive pharmacologic support approved by the U.S. Food and Drug Administration (FDA) achieve the best outcomes for nicotine-dependent clients.[2,5]

Patterns of Tobacco Use

To assess patterns of use in a typical day, clients are asked to recall each cigarette, chew, or dip that they have during a typical day.[6] By focusing on a typical day, the counselor helps the client to fill out the form shown in Figure 36-7. Beginning with the first dip, chew, or cigarette of the day, the time of day that tobacco is usually used and the situation in which the use occurs are recorded.[6] Clients are then asked to do the following:

- Rate their desire or craving for each recorded tobacco use on a scale of 1 to 10, where a score of 1 represents "do not crave it at all" (the lowest craving) and a score of 10 indicates "have to have it" (the strongest craving). The tobacco uses with lower craving scores are the easiest to eliminate, and it is recommended that clients give them up first during the weaning process.
- Describe their mood at each recorded tobacco use by indicating a number between 1 and 10, where 1 = relaxed; 2 = bored; 3 = angry; 4 = happy; 5 = stressed; 6 = excited; 7 = tired; 8 = sad; 9 = hungry; and 10 = irritable.

Understanding the level of craving and the client's mood when tobacco is used helps to establish a quit plan and to identify coping strategies to prevent relapse after the client quits. After working with the client to monitor tobacco use in a typical day, the counselor may say something like the following:

"To help you to prepare for quitting, I would like you to continue to monitor your tobacco use over the next week. To accomplish this, I will give you a diary to assess the number of cigarettes you have each day during the next week, the time of day you smoke, the intensity of cravings you have for each cigarette, the place where you are when you use your tobacco, the activity you are doing at the time, and your associated mood state. I would like you to complete the diary I am going to give you and bring it to your next appointment so we can review it together. The craving scores will help us understand which cigarettes might be the easiest to give up first. The mood scores will help us to understand why you use, and that knowledge will help identify ways to help you cope with not using. For example, if you smoke to relieve stress, then we need to find other ways for you to manage your stress so you won't need to use tobacco for that purpose."[10]

History of Mood Disorders

Because nicotine is a mood elevator, some clients may be using tobacco to self-medicate for depression or anxiety. If this is the case, then there is the potential that stopping tobacco use abruptly may trigger the mood disorder. To assess the history of mood disorder, clients are asked if they have ever been treated for depression or anxiety. Clients who have a history of a mood disorder are asked how they currently manage their negative moods. After determining their coping strategies, the client's physician is contacted to determine the best way to manage the mood disorder during and after the tobacco cessation process.[10]

Contraindications to Pharmacotherapy

Clinical practice guidelines[2] for treating tobacco use and dependence state the following: "All patients attempting to quit should be encouraged to use effective pharmacotherapies for cessation except in the presence of special circumstances."

Monitoring Tobacco Use Form

Please record during the next 7 days the number of cigarettes/dips/chews you have each day and the associated cravings (scale 1-10)* and mood state for each.

Time	Craving	Place/Activity	Mood+

*Score on a scale of 1-10 where 1 = lowest craving.

+Indicate how you feel at the time you take tobacco using the following numerical system.

1 = relaxed	2 = bored	3 = angry	4 = happy
5 = stressed	6 = excited	7 = tired	8 = sad
9 = hungry	10 = irritable		

Figure 36-7. Diary for monitoring patterns of tobacco use. (From Jensen J, Hatsukami D: *Tough enough to quit using snuff: a self-help manual for quitting spit tobacco,* Minneapolis, 1994, University of Minnesota Tobacco Research Laboratory.)

To identify special circumstances that would contraindicate certain types of pharmacologic agents that have been approved for the treatment of smoking cessation, the cessation counselor assesses the presence of any contraindications to FDA-approved medications. Tables 36-8 and 36-9 list contraindications for specific pharmacologic agents.

Setting a Quit Date

Counselors encourage clients to set a quit date 2 to 4 weeks from the time that they decide to quit.[5] Then, between the time clients decide to quit and their actual quit date, they can get ready to quit. There is no "ideal" time to quit, but some times are better than others. Low-stress times are best, such as a day when there are no work deadlines. Some clients will select a date of particular significance to them, such as a birthday, anniversary, or new car purchase. On the quit date, total abstinence is essential. The goal is not even a single puff or dip after the quit date.

Choosing a Method

After a quit date is set, the counselor helps clients establish a method to get ready to quit and to cope with the quitting process. The two basic methods of quitting tobacco use are "cold turkey" and gradual nicotine reduction. **Cold turkey** is the approach of quitting tobacco use abruptly on one's quit date (Box 36-6).[5] **Gradual nicotine reduction** is the approach that slowly and systematically reduces the amount of nicotine clients use so that they will have fewer symptoms of withdrawal on their quit date. Nicotine reduction can be accomplished either by brand switching or by gradually tapering down use of the original brand.[6]

Brand switching involves changing to another brand of tobacco with a lower level of available nicotine to gradually reduce exposure to nicotine. For example, Table 36-1 lists some brands of spit tobacco according to their levels of bioavailable nicotine. The counselor emphasizes to clients that, if they switch to a brand of tobacco with a lower nicotine content, they must be careful not to increase the amount of tobacco they use in an effort to maintain the same level of nicotine.[6]

Tapering down use is a method of systematically reducing the number of tobacco uses by a set amount, such as one to two every few days; tapering may also be accomplished with

BOX 36-6

Preparing to Quit "Cold Turkey"

- Have a positive attitude that the quit date will be the last day tobacco will ever be used.
- Tell others and ask for their support.
- Practice going without tobacco at a time when use would be common or enjoyable, and use coping skills.
- Plan rewards.

TABLE 36-8

Over-the-Counter Pharmacotherapies for Tobacco Cessation*

Pharmacotherapy	Contraindications	Dose	Duration	Side Effects	Cost per Day‡
Nicotine gum	Recent myocardial infarction Life-threatening arrhythmias Severe or worsening angina Pregnancy† Lactation Stomach ulcer Active temporomandibular joint disease Dentures, fixed dental bridges, or loose teeth	1 to 20 cigarettes/day: 2 mg gum (≤24 pieces/day) ≥20 cigarettes/day: 4 mg gum (≤24 pieces/day)	≤12 weeks	Mouth soreness Aphthous ulcers Jaw muscle ache Improper use: Dyspepsia Hiccups Gastrointestinal disturbances	2 mg: $3.28 to $6.58 (9 pieces) 4 mg: $4.31 to $6.58 (9 pieces)
Nicotine lozenge	Recent myocardial infarction Life-threatening arrhythmias Severe or worsening angina Pregnancy† Lactation Stomach ulcer	Initial dose based on time to first cigarette: within 30 minutes of waking, begin with 4-mg lozenge; after 30 minutes of waking, begin with 2-mg lozenge; ≥9 lozenges/day, ≤20 lozenges/day	≤12 weeks	Sore mouth and jaw Improper use: Nausea Hiccups Flatulence	2 mg: $3.66 to $5.26 (9 pieces) 4 mg: $3.66 to $5.26 (9 pieces)
Nicotine patch§	Recent myocardial infarction Life-threatening arrhythmias Severe or worsening angina Pregnancy† Lactation Stomach ulcer Psoriasis or eczema	21 mg/24 hours 14 mg/24 hours 7 mg/24 hours 15 mg/16 hours	4 weeks then 2 weeks then 2 weeks	Local skin reaction Insomnia During the first hour, mild itching, burning, and tingling After patch removal, the skin may appear red for the next 24 hours If the skin stays red more than 4 days or swells or if a rash appears, contact healthcare provider and do not put on a new patch Improper use: Nightmares (dose is too high) Insomnia or headache (dose is too low)	$1.90 to $3.89 (1 patch)

Adapted from Fiore MC, Bailey WC, Cohen SJ, et al: *Treating tobacco use and dependence: quick reference guide for clinicians,* Rockville, Md, 2000, U.S. Department of Health and Human Services, Public Health Service.

*The information contained within this table is not comprehensive. Please see package inserts for additional information.

†Controversy surrounds pregnant women's use of the patch. However, some feel that nicotine replacement poses less risk to the mother and fetus than smoking because it is not inhaled and mainstream smoke effects are eliminated.

‡Average wholesale price from Wolters Kluwer Health: Medi-Span Electronic Drug File, Indianapolis, September 2008.

§Generic brands of the nicotine patch recently became available and may be less expensive.

TABLE 36-9

Prescription Pharmacotherapies for Tobacco Cessation*

Pharmacotherapy	Contraindications	Dose	Duration	Side Effects	Cost per Day‡
Bupropion SR†	History of seizure, eating disorder, head injury, bipolar disorder, or anxiety disorder Use of Wellbutrin, monoamine oxidase inhibitors, sedatives, stimulants, excess alcohol Alcohol or sedative withdrawal	150 mg every morning for 3 days then 150 mg twice daily (begin treatment 1 to 2 weeks before quit date)	7 to 12 weeks; maintenance ≤6 months	Insomnia Dry mouth	\$3.62 to \$7.40 (2 tablets)
Chantix† (varenicline)	<18 years old Pregnant Breast-feeding Kidney problems (may prescribe a lower dose)	Days 1 through 3: white tablet (0.5 mg), one tablet each day Days 4 through 7: white tablet (0.5 mg) twice a day (one in the morning and one in the evening) Day 8 until the end of treatment: blue tablet (1 mg) twice a day (one in the morning and one in the evening)	12 weeks	Nausea Changes in dreaming Constipation Gas Vomiting	\$4.49 to \$4.75 (2 tablets)
Nicotine inhaler†	Recent myocardial infarction Life-threatening arrhythmias Severe or worsening angina Pregnancy§ Lactation Stomach ulcer	6 to 16 cartridges/day	≤6 months	Local irritation of mouth and throat Dyspepsia Rhinitis Hiccups Headaches Unpleasant taste in mouth Cough	\$5.29 (6 cartridges)
Nicotine nasal spray†	Recent myocardial infarction Life-threatening arrhythmias Severe or worsening angina Pregnancy§ Lactation Stomach ulcer	8 to 40 doses/day	3 to 6 months	What to expect during the first week: Sneezing Coughing Watery eyes Runny nose Hot peppery feeling in back of throat or nose Side effects lessen over a few days	\$3.72 (8 doses)

Adapted from Fiore MC, Bailey WC, Cohen SJ, et al: *Treating tobacco use and dependence: quick reference guide for clinicians,* Rockville, Md, 2000, U.S. Department of Health and Human Services, Public Health Service.

*The information contained within this table is not comprehensive. Please see package inserts for additional information.

†First-line pharmacotherapies (approved for use for smoking cessation by the U.S. Food and Drug Administration).

‡Average wholesale price from Wolters Kluwer Health: Medi-Span Electronic Drug File, Indianapolis, September 2008.

§Controversy surrounds pregnant women's use of the patch. However, some feel that nicotine replacement poses less risk to the mother and fetus than smoking because it is not inhaled and mainstream smoke effects are eliminated.

nontobacco oral substitutes. When clients get to the point at which they are using half of their original amount of tobacco, they can try to quit cold turkey. For clients who choose to taper down their tobacco use, the counselor refers to their pattern of use in a "typical day" diary collected during the assessment phase of counseling. On the basis of the diary information, the counselor suggests that clients start cutting back on those cigarettes or dips with the lowest craving scores.[6] Table 36-6 lists some helpful suggestions for behavioral strategies to cope with nicotine withdrawal and the temptation to use tobacco. Specific coping strategies that clients decide to use and the rewards they plan for themselves on their quit day and for the first week without tobacco use are recorded in the client record.

Coping Skills Training

Coping skills training involves helping clients to identify action responses (i.e., things they can do) and thinking responses (i.e., things they can say to themselves) to avoid tobacco use[6] when tempted (Box 36-7).

Action Responses

The following strategies are suggested action responses to cope with the temptation to use tobacco.[6]

Avoidance. During the first 2 weeks of being tobacco-free, many clients avoid situations in which their potential for using tobacco is high, such as socializing with other tobacco users. During these high-risk situations, cravings and temptations may be strong, and the motivation to stop using tobacco may waver.

Distraction. Because a craving disappears after 3 to 5 minutes whether the client uses tobacco or not, teaching clients to focus their attention on doing something else can help them to cope with cravings. For example, when a craving arises, clients could have a glass of water, do a crossword puzzle, doodle, call a friend, brush their teeth, take a walk, or do any number of other activities.

Use of Oral Substitutes. The counselor helps clients make a list of nontobacco oral substitutes to use when they have a strong craving for tobacco. Clients are counseled to stock up on these substitutes in advance and to put them where they normally keep their tobacco. Examples of nontobacco substitutes include sugarless chewing gum, sunflower seeds in the shell, popcorn, fruits, raw vegetables, flavored toothpicks, hard candy, and herbal substitutes. Clients are instructed to throw out all tobacco and to stock up on nontobacco substitutes the night before they quit.[6]

On the Quit Date. Clients are encouraged to change their daily routine on the quit date to break away from tobacco triggers and to decrease temptation to use tobacco (e.g., get right up from the table after meals). It is important for clients to make plans to keep busy. For example, aerobic exercise helps clients to relax and boosts energy and stamina. In addition, a dental hygiene care appointment is a good action strategy that promotes health and provides a fresh clean feeling in the mouth.

BOX 36-7

Strategies to Cope with Cravings and Temptation to Use Tobacco

Action Responses
- Avoidance—Get away
- Distraction—Do something
- Alternatives—Have some sunflower seeds
- Relaxation—Deep breathing

Thinking Responses
- Positive Thinking—I can do it!
- Imagery—Kissing your honey
- Delay—I'll decide later
- Rewards—I am proud of myself

From Jensen J, Hatsukami D: *Tough enough to quit using snuff: a self-help manual for quitting spit tobacco*, Minneapolis, 1994, University of Minnesota Tobacco Research Laboratory.

Thinking Responses

Thinking responses are the client's thoughts about quitting tobacco use.[6] Some thinking responses that the client can use to cope with temptation to use tobacco are listed in the following paragraphs.

Positive Thinking. Counselors encourage clients to be as supportive of themselves as they would be of their best friends. It is important for clients to tell themselves, "I will succeed." When a negative thought or self-doubt comes to mind (e.g., "I can't do this"), counselors instruct clients to substitute a positive thought such as, "I know it's difficult, but I *can* do this, and I will. I just need to get through today or the next hour." In addition, clients need to be encouraged to think in terms of "getting rid of" an addiction rather than "giving up" cigarettes or dip.

Delay. If clients can delay satisfying a craving, it will go away in 3 to 5 minutes. Therefore counselors encourage clients to tell themselves, "I won't have a cigarette now, I'll decide again in an hour." In the meantime, if clients find something else to do to get their mind off of the craving, by the time an hour passes, they may have forgotten all about it.

Rewards. Helping clients to plan a reward system for attempting to stop their tobacco use is another important strategy. Rewards are important to the quitting process, because they help avoid the feeling of deprivation while quitting tobacco. Clients are encouraged to choose rewards for themselves every day for the first week that they are tobacco-free and to reward themselves on anniversaries. For example, they could buy a new CD, get a magazine, or go to a movie with a friend. With the money that they save by not buying tobacco, they could plan to buy something for themselves that they really want. Rewards also can be free, such as sleeping late on the weekend or getting a massage from a friend.

Support from Others

Clients are encouraged to tell family, friends, and co-workers that they are trying to quit tobacco use and to request understanding and support.[5,6] Stopping tobacco use requires a great deal of effort and energy. Having the support of others is very important. If clients who are trying to quit are feeling irritable, spouses or partners, family members, and friends will be more understanding if they are informed about the situation. These individuals can help clients by not offering clients tobacco, by giving clients a pat on the back to reinforce clients

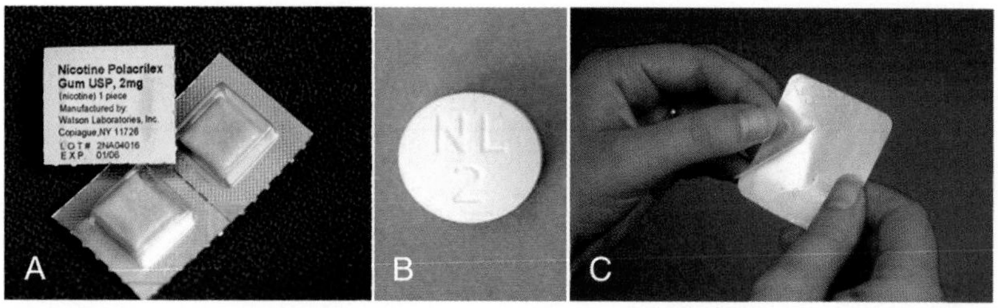

Figure 36-8. U.S. Food and Drug Administration–approved over-the-counter nicotine replacement therapies for smoking cessation. **A,** Nicotine gum. **B,** Nicotine lozenge. **C,** Transdermal nicotine patch.

refraining from tobacco use, and by giving clients encouragement if things are not going well.

Relapse Prevention

Although nicotine withdrawal lasts only 2 to 4 weeks, the temptation to use can last for years. To prevent relapse, it is critical for clients to identify at least three tough situations in which they know they will be tempted most to use tobacco and then to plan ahead regarding what they will do instead to remain tobacco-free. Planning for these high-risk situations helps clients to out-think their tobacco habit and to avoid relapse.[6] In addition, because drinking alcohol is highly associated with relapse, counselors often encourage clients to review their alcohol use and to consider limiting their alcohol consumption or abstaining from alcohol during the quit process.

Follow-Up Contact

Follow-up contact is arranged and scheduled either in person or via telephone. Initial follow-up occurs on the quit date, during the first week after the quit date, and within the first month of the quit date. Additional follow-up contacts are scheduled as needed. During follow-up, the counselor congratulates the client on his or her success. For clients who have experienced a slip (i.e., the use of tobacco but not a resumption of regular tobacco use), it is important to transform the event into a learning situation. For example, clients may have learned that they really cannot be around friends who smoke or that they need to focus on nontobacco stress-reduction techniques. The cessation counselor helps clients to identify what caused the slip or relapse and to think about what they can do to prevent a recurrence. If a full relapse has occurred, a new quit date needs to be set. Ongoing support is critical. For some clients seeking cessation assistance in the dental setting, referral to a more specialized intensive tobacco cessation program may be appropriate.[5,10]

U.S. Food and Drug Administration–Approved Pharmacologic Adjuncts

Nicotine-dependent clients usually need pharmacologic support to facilitate their quitting process.[2,5] The extent of support the client needs, whether behavioral or pharmacologic, drives the tobacco cessation care plan. Although prescribing pharmacologic adjuncts is the dentist's legal responsibility, the dental hygienist may recommend over-the-counter (OTC) nicotine replacement therapies and other prescription FDA-approved adjuncts. Clients often ask for advice about particular products. The different types of FDA-approved OTC nicotine replacement therapies for smoking

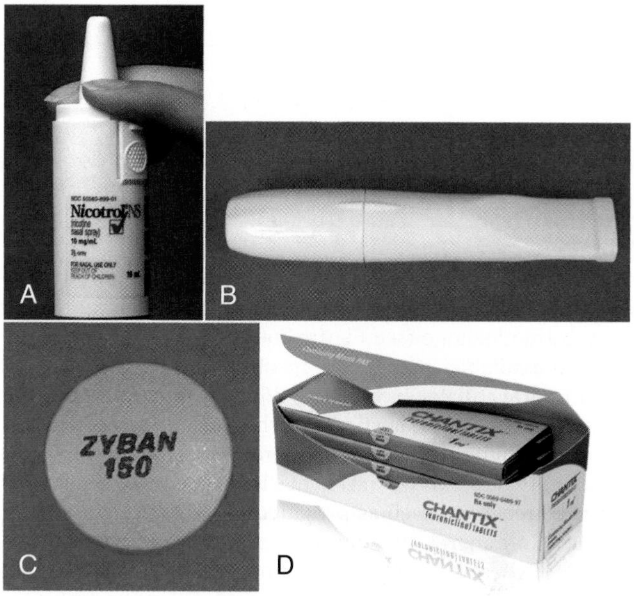

Figure 36-9. U.S. Food and Drug Administration–approved nicotine and non-nicotine prescription pharmacologic therapies for smoking cessation. **A,** Nicotine nasal spray. **B,** Nicotine oral inhaler. **C,** Bupropion (Zyban). **D,** Varenicline (Chantix).

cessation are shown in Figure 36-8, and their use and related contraindications and side effects are summarized in Table 36-8. Figure 36-9 shows the FDA-approved nicotine and non-nicotine prescription pharmacologic therapies for smoking cessation, and Table 36-9 summarizes their use and related contraindications and side effects. Clients need to be cautioned that no pharmacologic adjunct is a magic bullet. Such adjuncts are helpful for diminishing cravings and other withdrawal symptoms, which allows clients to concentrate on action and thinking coping strategies to resist the temptation to use.

Nicotine Replacement Therapy

The purpose of nicotine replacement therapy is to provide some blood concentration of nicotine to reduce or eliminate withdrawal symptoms so clients can focus on the psychosocial and behavioral changes necessary to stop their tobacco use.[5,10] However, there may be a period of trial and error to determine the optimum dose of nicotine replacement to avoid nicotine withdrawal symptoms while at the same time avoiding nicotine toxicity (i.e., nicotine overdose). Nicotine replacement products must be used according to manufacturers'

BOX 36-8

Management of Nicotine Toxicity (Overdose)

SIGNS AND SYMPTOMS OF OVERDOSE	MANAGEMENT
• Nausea • Vomiting • Diarrhea • Dizziness • Headaches • Disorientation • Weakness in limbs • Nightmares	If the client is using tobacco with nicotine replacement, tell the client to discontinue either the use of tobacco or the use of the nicotine replacement product. Instruct the client that all tobacco use must be discontinued before nicotine replacement is used to avoid an overdose of nicotine. If the client is not using tobacco, reduce the dose of nicotine replacement; if symptoms are severe, the client should discontinue use of the nicotine replacement and call a physician.

instructions. Clients must discontinue all tobacco use before starting nicotine replacement therapy to prevent nicotine toxicity, which can cause serious adverse health effects (Box 36-8).

Current OTC nicotine replacement products are the nicotine transdermal patch system, nicotine polacrilex gum, and the nicotine lozenge (see Figure 36-8). Prescription products that are available include the nicotine nasal spray and the nicotine oral inhaler (see Figure 36-9). All types of nicotine replacement enhance abstinence when used properly and in conjunction with cognitive behavioral counseling.[2] The choice of modality depends on the client's history, contraindications, and preferences as well as provider experience with a given product. In general, nicotine replacement products are contraindicated for clients with underlying cardiovascular disease, especially those who have experienced recent myocardial infarction, life-threatening arrhythmias, or severe or worsening angina. Other contraindications related to specific products are listed in Tables 36-8 and 36-9. Nicotine toxicity can also result if clients overuse nicotine replacement products. See Box 36-8 for the symptoms and management of nicotine toxicity.[6]

Transdermal Nicotine Replacement Therapy (Patch)

Transdermal nicotine patches are marketed for 24-hour use. One advantage of the patch is that it delivers a constant dose of nicotine across the skin throughout its use. A small percentage of clients who have used the 24-hour patch have reported sleep interrupted by nightmares, which is an indication of nicotine toxicity. If this occurs, the dose of nicotine should be reduced either by removing the patch during sleeping hours or by using a lower-dose patch. Clients may also experience dermatitis as a side effect of using the patch (see Table 36-8). Directions for use require the client to place a new patch each day on a nonhairy site of the upper trunk. No one site should be used again until more than a week has passed. Used patches should be disposed of carefully, because residual nicotine could harm small children and animals. Patches work on a dosing-down principle, and the aim is to gradually discontinue use over the course of 12 weeks (e.g., 21 mg for weeks 1 to 8; 14 mg for weeks 8 to 10; and 7 mg for weeks 10 to 12). The client is eventually weaned off of nicotine completely. Each patch dose is generally of a 2- to 4-week duration, depending on client response. Small-framed or obese clients may require dose modification. Triage with the client's physician is advised, particularly if the client has systemic disease. In general, client compliance is easier to achieve with the patch than with other forms of nicotine replacement that require more behavior modification. After the patch is placed, the client does nothing more until the next day.[10]

Nicotine Polacrilex (Gum)

Nicotine gum is available OTC in 2- or 4-mg doses. The dose is based on the client's smoking pattern. For clients who smoke less than 25 cigarettes per day, 2-mg gum is recommended. For those who smoke more than 25 cigarettes per day, 4-mg gum is recommended. The aim is to discontinue gum use gradually over 10 to 12 weeks. The recommended schedule is one piece of gum every 1 to 2 hours per day for weeks 1 through 6; one piece of gum every 2 to 4 hours for weeks 7 through 9; and one piece of gum every 4 to 8 hours for weeks 10 through 12. Proper gum use requires clients to chew the gum very slowly, because the nicotine is absorbed through the oral mucosa (in an alkaline environment) and not the gut (in an acidic environment). The client should stop chewing at the first sign of a peppery, minty, or citrus taste or tingle and then "park" the gum between the cheek and the gingiva. Overchewing can result in nicotine toxicity, during which the client may experience stomach upset, nausea, or vomiting. Success with nicotine gum is greater when the client has a fixed dosage schedule throughout the day to prevent craving. Often if clients wait until a craving arises before using a piece of gum, they will relapse to tobacco use, because a cigarette or dip provides more rapid absorption of nicotine into the blood as compared with the gum. To avoid withdrawal and relapse, nicotine gum is sometimes used in the morning in combination with the patch when the patch is first placed. This action enables the client to receive a quick boost of nicotine with the addition of the gum to prevent breakthrough craving (see Combination Nicotine Replacement Therapy). The nicotine patch provides nicotine to the bloodstream at a constant rate and dosage. (See Table 36-8 for contraindications and side effects.)

Nicotine Lozenge

The nicotine lozenge is available OTC in 2- or 4-mg doses. The lozenge provides 25% more nicotine than the equivalent nicotine gum dose, because the lozenge dissolves in the mouth completely in 20 to 30 minutes. Like the gum, it is used on a regular schedule (every 1 to 2 hours) throughout the day to prevent cravings. The initial dose is based on the time of first cigarette use after waking. Those who have a history of having their first cigarette within 30 minutes of waking begin with the 4-mg lozenge. The aim is to discontinue use gradually over 12 weeks on a schedule similar to that used for the gum. The lozenge is meant to be parked next to the oral mucosa. The client should not chew or swallow the lozenge for maximum effectiveness and to avoid adverse side effects similar to those reported with the improper use of the gum.[5] (See Table 36-8 for contraindications and side effects.)

Nicotine Spray

The nicotine nasal spray is available by prescription only as a result of the rapid absorption of its nicotine through the nasal membranes into the blood and therefore its potential for abuse. Of all of the nicotine replacement products, the nicotine spray provides the fastest nicotine delivery system (i.e., nicotine is absorbed into the blood the fastest). Each dose spray is metered to deliver 0.5 mg of nicotine in each nostril. It is used on a daily fixed schedule that begins with one or two doses per hour. For best results, at least eight doses are recommended daily for the first 6 to 8 weeks. Dosage should never exceed five doses in 1 hour or 40 doses in 24 hours. The aim is to gradually discontinue use over an additional 4 to 6 weeks. (See Table 36-9 for contraindications and side effects.)

Nicotine Oral Inhaler

The nicotine oral inhaler is available by prescription only (see Figure 36-9). It consists of a mouthpiece and a plastic cartridge that deliver 4 mg of nicotine vapor. The client inhales into the back of the throat by puffing in short breaths. The nicotine is absorbed across the oropharyngeal mucosa. In general, the use of 6 to 16 cartridges per day for 3 to 12 weeks is recommended. However, use depends on the client's individual smoking history. The inhaler is most effective if it is puffed frequently for 20 minutes at a time. The aim is to discontinue use gradually over an additional 6 to 12 weeks. (See Table 36-9 for contraindications and side effects.)

Combination Nicotine Replacement Therapy

The nicotine patch is a long-acting formulation that produces relatively constant levels of nicotine. Short-acting, rapidly absorbed formulations such as the nicotine gum, lozenge, inhaler, and spray are often used to augment the patch to prevent or control breakthrough cravings or withdrawal symptoms. These short-acting formulations allow for acute dose titration as needed for severely nicotine-dependent tobacco users who are trying to stop their tobacco use.[5,10]

Sustained-Release Bupropion (Zyban)

Some tobacco users achieve successful abstinence from tobacco by using sustained-release bupropion, a non-nicotine prescription antidepressant drug (see Figure 36-9). Bupropion increases the levels of dopamine and norepinephrine released from the brain. Clients can continue their tobacco use for 7 to 14 days after they start the medication. Initially clients take one tablet (150 mg) in the morning for 3 days. If the drug is tolerated, the dosage is increased to two tablets per day 8 hours apart (300 mg per day) for 7 to 8 weeks. A history of head injury, seizure disorder, eating disorder, or use of monoamine oxidase inhibitors during the previous 14 days contraindicates the use of bupropion. (See Table 36-9 for other contraindications and side effects.)

BOX 36-9

Key Steps for Implementing Tobacco Intervention Programs

- Provide staff members with in-service training about the adverse health effects of tobacco use and the Five A's.
- Suggest mechanisms for program incorporation.
- Designate a program coordinator to do the following:
  - Facilitate team involvement.
  - Publicize the program to clients.
  - Order literature.
  - Implement an office-wide system that ensures client tobacco use status is queried and documented.
  - Ensure client follow-up.
  - Reinforce chart documentation.
- Create a tobacco-free environment by posting signs and ordering magazines that do not advertise tobacco products.
- Address reimbursement issues of the practices chosen for the provision of intensive interventions. Code 01320 is designated for "Tobacco Counseling for the Prevention and Control of Oral Disease."

Varenicline (Chantix)

Varenicline, a prescription drug, binds to nicotine receptors to block the neurochemical effects of nicotine (see Figure 36-9). Clients can continue their tobacco use for 7 days after they start the medication. Initially clients take one white tablet (0.5 mg) in the morning for 3 days. If the drug is tolerated, the dose is increased to two tablets per day 8 hours apart (1 mg per day) for days 4 through 7. At the end of the first week, clients quit their tobacco use. Starting on day 8 and for up to 12 weeks, clients take one blue tablet (1.0 mg) twice a day with 8 ounces of water after eating. (See Table 36-9 for contraindications and side effects.)

Implementing a Tobacco Intervention Program in the Oral Healthcare Setting[7]

Dental hygienists are often the strongest proponents of tobacco intervention activities in their employment settings. Four key steps are necessary to ensure the successful incorporation of tobacco intervention programs into clinical settings: generating team support, designating a coordinator, creating a tobacco-free environment, and addressing reimbursement issues (Box 36-9).

The Dental Hygienist's Role in the Community

The dental hygienist's role related to tobacco extends beyond the immediate clinical environment. Given its magnitude as a public health issue, tobacco use commands dental hygienists' action at both the professional and societal levels. Ethically dental hygienists are committed to the health and well-being of society. Involvement with tobacco-related issues helps with the achievement of that goal. Professional and societal activities that dental hygienists can pursue within their professional associations and communities include the following:

- Endorsing tobacco intervention policies within local, state, national, and international associations
- Ensuring that continuing education related to tobacco issues is on the agenda for professional conferences
- Reinforcing peer awareness of key tobacco information
- Volunteering organizational support for tobacco-related events
- Supporting existing policies that promote a tobacco-free society
- Advocating for tobacco-free children
- Lobbying for ordinances that encourage tobacco-free environments
- Providing tobacco use education to children, sports teams, parent–teacher associations, and other relevant community groups

CLIENT EDUCATION TIPS

- Explain that medications can minimize the discomfort of nicotine withdrawal and the associated cravings.
- Inform that most tobacco users who successfully quit establish a quit date that is 2 to 4 weeks from the time that they decide to quit. Then, between the time that they decide to quit and their actual quit date, they get ready to quit.
- Explain that most tobacco users have to try multiple times to stop their tobacco use. However, each time they try, they learn something new about the quitting process that makes them better prepared to quit the next time. As long as they are trying, they are not failing.
- Explain that telephone quitlines are an excellent source of assistance during the quitting process (e.g., 1-800-QUIT-NOW).

LEGAL, ETHICAL, AND SAFETY ISSUES

- As oral healthcare providers, dental hygienists are ethically obligated to address clients' tobacco use and its relationship to their oral health and overall well-being.
- Because tobacco use is a life-threatening habit, all tobacco-using clients must be informed of its deleterious effects and educated and guided toward abstinence.
- The links among tobacco use, oral cancer, and periodontal disease are undisputed. Clients who are diagnosed with oral cancer and periodontal disease could potentially sue providers who have not informed them of the relationship among tobacco use, oral cancer, and periodontal disease.
- With the current emphases on prevention, health promotion, and litigation, tobacco use interventions are a standard of care and are therefore expected behaviors of oral health professionals.

KEY CONCEPTS

- Tobacco use is the number one cause of preventable disability and death.
- There are numerous adverse systemic and oral health effects of tobacco use.
- Nicotine addiction is a physical, psychologic, behavioral, and sensory dependence that makes it very difficult for one to stop tobacco use.
- The Five A's approach, which is an evidence-based approach that involves a brief and effective tobacco cessation intervention, is a methodology endorsed by the Agency for Healthcare Research and Quality and the National Cancer Institute for implementation by oral health and medical care teams in private practice and community settings.
- The Five A's approach requires healthcare providers to ask all clients about tobacco use; to advise tobacco users to quit and to show them the visible effects of tobacco use in their own mouths; to assess their readiness to quit; to assist with the quitting process; and to arrange follow-up regarding their cessation progress.
- The type of assistance provided to promote tobacco cessation is determined by the client's readiness to quit.
- Explain the health benefits associated with quitting tobacco use.
- Explain that tobacco contains nicotine, an addicting drug that changes the brain's chemistry.
- Explain that nicotine withdrawal lasts 2 to 4 weeks and is the brain's way of healing.
- Characteristics of patient-centered communication are collaboration, not persuasion; elicitation of information, not imparting information; and emphasis on client autonomy, not the authority of the expert.
- The motivational interview is a form of patient-centered communication to help clients get unstuck from the ambivalence that traps them in their tobacco use.
- When the benefits of quitting tobacco use outweigh the benefits of continuing tobacco use, a client will make a decision to quit.
- Motivation is fundamental to changing behavior. Asking clients why they circled a higher number rather than a lower number on a 1-to-10 scale rating the importance of reasons to quit (where 10 indicates the highest motivation) requires clients to talk positively about their motivation to quit and serves to enhance their motivation.
- Pharmacologic adjuncts help to reduce or eliminate nicotine withdrawal symptoms so that clients can concentrate on developing behavioral and psychologic factors that support abstinence from tobacco use.
- There are key elements associated with high-quality intensive tobacco cessation treatment programs.
- The dental hygienist's role related to tobacco issues extends beyond the immediate clinic environment and commands action on both professional and societal levels.

CRITICAL THINKING EXERCISES

Scenario 1

Client: Mr. Z

Profile: A 45-year-old white male visits the dental hygiene clinic. He has been dipping snuff for 18 years. He drinks approximately three beers per day.

Chief Complaint: "My tooth hurts on the upper left back."

Dental History: The client seeks care erratically. He has not seen a dentist or a dental hygienist in more than 5 years.

Social History: The client is divorced and lives alone. He frequently travels abroad for business reasons. He is a full-time employee for a computer company.

Health History: The client reports no use of medications. He broke his arm in a skiing accident 2 years ago. He reports no systemic disease.

Oral Health Behaviors Assessment: The client reports brushing one time per day with a hard brush. He does not rinse or floss. He uses no aids.

Supplemental Notes: On clinical examination, a 10-mm × 20-mm mixed leukoplakic and erythroplakic lesion is found on the vestibular right labial mucosa of the maxilla; it extends to the surrounding alveolar mucosa and the attached gingiva. The client places his oral snuff in that area. He was unaware of the lesion, and the lesion was asymptomatic.

1. Will Mr. Z's lesion disappear if he abstains?
2. When assessing Mr. Z's tobacco use, he reports that oral gratification is a key factor in his dependence. On the basis of this finding, what pharmacologic adjunct that has been approved by the U.S. Food and Drug Administration may be the most beneficial for him?
3. Mr. Z states that snuff use is safer than cigarette smoking. How would you respond?
4. Mr. Z also reports daily alcohol use. How would you use this information when educating Mr. Z?

Scenario 2

Client: Ms. J

Profile: A 35-year-old female visits for a 3-month recall appointment. The client reports smoking three packs of cigarettes per day.

Chief Complaint: "I am unhappy about the stains on my front teeth and the color of the fillings on my front teeth."

Dental History: The client makes regular dental visits, although she is 9 months overdue for her dental hygiene visit. She has consistently reported interest in tobacco cessation but has rejected the use of nicotine replacement. She states, "I want to do it on my own."

Social History: The client has been smoking for 25 years. She drinks six to eight cups of coffee per day. She is a recovering alcoholic. She is unmarried and lives with her father. Ms. J is weight conscious.

Health History: The client has a history of depression. She takes ibuprofen as needed for back pain from an injury that was sustained 10 years ago.

Oral Health Behaviors Assessment: The client reports brushing three times per day with a power toothbrush, flossing one time per day, and using a mouth rinse several times per day. She rarely exercises.

Supplemental Notes: The client has thick, heavy, generalized black stains. She reports the presence of xerostomia.

1. Which pharmacologic adjuncts that have been approved by the U.S. Food and Drug Administration may be most acceptable to Ms. J?
2. What message would best motivate Ms. J to stop smoking?
3. If Ms. J worries about weight gain with cessation, how should you advise her?

REFERENCES

1. National Cancer Institute: *Tobacco research implementation plan: priorities for tobacco research beyond year 2000*, Bethesda, Md, 1998, National Cancer Institute.
2. Fiore MC, Bailey WC, Cohen SJ, et al: *Treating tobacco use and dependence: clinical practice guideline*, Rockville, Md, 2000, U.S. Department of Health and Human Services, Public Health Service.
3. U.S. Department of Health and Human Services: *The health consequences of smoking: what it means to you*, Bethesda, Md, 2004, U.S. Department of Health and Human Services, Centers for Disease Control and Prevention, National Center for Chronic Disease Prevention and Health Promotion, Office of Smoking and Health.
4. American Academy of Periodontology, Research, Science and Therapy Committee: Position paper: Tobacco use and the periodontal patient. Available at: www.perio.org/practitioner/tobacco.htm. Accessed November 15, 2007.
5. Walsh MM, Ellison J: Treatment of tobacco use and dependence: the role of the dental professional, *J Dent Educ* 69:521, 2005.
6. Jensen J, Hatsukami D: *Tough enough to quit using snuff: a self-help manual for quitting spit tobacco*, Minneapolis, 1994, University of Minnesota Tobacco Research Laboratory.
7. Mayo Clinic, University of Minnesota: Stop smoking services. Available at: www.mayoclinic.org/stop-smoking. Accessed November 15, 2007.
8. Prochaska JO, Norcross JC, DiClemente CC: *Changing for good: the revolutionary program that explains the six stages of change and teaches you how to free yourself from bad habits*, New York, 1994, William Morrow.
9. Miller W, Rollnick S: *Motivational interviewing: preparing people for change*, New York, 2002, Guilford Press.
10. Walsh MM, Heckman B, Murray J, et al: *UCSF School of Dentistry translating clinical guidelines for treating tobacco use and dependence*, San Francisco, 2006, University of California–San Francisco.

ACKNOWLEDGMENT

The authors acknowledge Jacquelyn Fried for her past contributions to this chapter.

EVOLVE RESOURCES

Please visit http://evolve.elsevier.com/Darby/hygiene for additional practice and study support tools.

CHAPTER 37

Impressions, Study Casts, and Oral Appliances

Carol Dixon Hatrick

COMPETENCIES

1. Discuss dental impressions, including:
   - Describe the uses of preliminary impressions.
   - List and describe the supplies required to take an alginate impression.
   - List the criteria for an acceptable alginate impression.
   - Describe the criteria for the proper handling of an alginate impression.
2. Discuss dental casts, including:
   - List the various gypsum products and their uses.
   - Describe the procedure for mixing and handling gypsum products for constructing a dental cast.
   - List the criteria for properly trimmed and finished study model/diagnostic cast.
3. Discuss custom-made removable oral appliances, including:
   - Differentiate between the various custom-made oral appliances used for dental procedures.
   - List and describe the uses and benefits of each type of custom-made oral appliance.
4. Identify the types of oral surgical splints and stents and explain their uses.
5. Explain the dental hygienist's role in working with clients with custom-made oral appliances.

A **dental impression** is a negative imprint of the teeth and the surrounding tissues; it is used to create an accurate or exact three-dimensional reproduction of these structures. This positive reproduction is called a *study model*, a *diagnostic cast*, or a *die*. There are three main types of dental impressions used in dentistry: a preliminary impression, a final impression, and a bite registration. **Preliminary impressions** are accurate reproductions of clients' mouths that are used to construct study models for diagnosing, documenting the dental arches as part of the permanent record, and enhancing client education as a visual aid. Preliminary impressions may also be used to construct diagnostic casts for the construction of removable oral appliances. **Final impressions** are used to make casts and dies with exact details of the tooth structures and their surrounding tissues. Casts and dies are used by dental laboratory technicians for the construction of crowns, bridges, partial or full dentures, and restorations that are placed on titanium implants. A **bite registration** is used to record the occlusal relationship between arches. This relationship is essential when establishing the articulation of maxillary and mandibular casts. The responsibilities of the dental hygienist often include creating preliminary dental impressions and related bite registrations, constructing casts, trimming models, and fabricating custom-made oral appliances. In some states, dental hygienists are licensed to perform extended functions that include the taking of final impressions.

Custom-made oral appliances are trays or stints that are used for the targeted delivery of materials (e.g., tooth-whitening products, home fluoride application); for the fabrication of provisional restorations, orthodontic retainers, and aligners; and for the protection of oral structures from bruxism and contact sports. Oral **surgical stents** are guides that provide communication between the surgeon and the restoring dentist so that an implant is placed at the ideal prosthetic position and angulation. This chapter provides an overview of concepts related to making dental impressions, study models, diagnostic casts, bite registrations, and custom-made oral appliances. The reader is advised to consult a text about dental materials for complete information about properties and the manipulation of the different types of dental materials.

Dental Impressions

Impression Trays

Impression material is placed into the mouth in an impression tray. Because dental impressions are used in oral healthcare for many purposes, there are various types of impression trays. Impression trays are designed for different areas of the mouth and include quadrant trays, which cover half an arch, and full trays, which cover the complete maxillary or mandibular arch (Figure 37-1). Tray selection depends on the purpose of the impression. Metal, plastic, or disposable Styrofoam trays are available in standard small, medium, and large sizes for children and adults. They may be perforated to promote a mechanical lock with the impression material (Box 37-1). Procedure 37-1 and the corresponding Competency Form describes the details of selecting the correct size tray and preparing it for use.

Traditional Alginate Impression Material

The impression material that is most widely used in dentistry for preliminary impressions is irreversible hydrocolloid (*hydro,* meaning "water," and *colloid,* meaning "gelatin"). Because hydrocolloid is in a water suspension, the product is considered **hydrophilic**, a term that means "loves water." Hydrocolloids can exist in a sol (solution) or a gel (solid) state. Depending on the type of hydrocolloid used, the physical change from sol to gel is either reversible (changed by thermal factors) or irreversible (changed by chemical factors). Gelation is the transformation from sol to gel.[1,2]

Irreversible hydrocolloids do not change their physical state after gelation. **Alginate** is an irreversible hydrocolloid

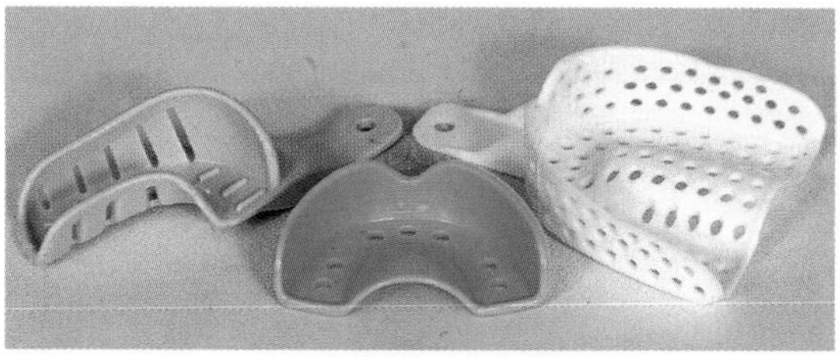

Figure 37-1. Types of impression trays. (From Bird DL, Robinson DS: *Modern dental assisting,* ed 11, St Louis, 2015, Elsevier.)

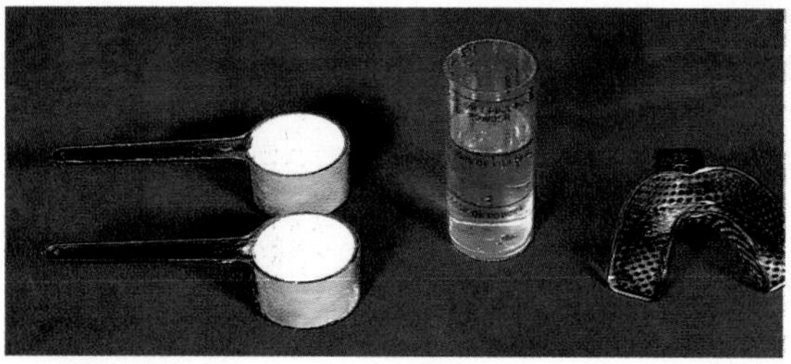

Figure 37-2. A plastic scoop and a plastic cylinder are supplied with alginate. (From Bird DL, Robinson DS: *Modern dental assisting,* ed 11, St Louis, 2015, Elsevier.)

BOX 37-1

Guidelines for Proper Impression Tray Selections

- Tray should feel comfortable to the client.
- Tray should extend slightly beyond the facial surfaces of the teeth and the alveolar process to enclose all teeth, the musculature, and the vestibule.
- Tray should extend 2 to 3 mm beyond the most posterior tooth in the arch and include the retromolar or maxillary tuberosity area.
- Apply wax to customize the tray length or the height of the palatal vault.
- Tray should allow for a 2- to 3-mm depth of material beyond the biting surfaces or edges of the teeth.
- Tray should be comfortable and minimize tissue trauma during insertion and removal.

powder and water impression material that changes from a sol to a gel state by means of a chemical reaction. Cool water is added to the potassium alginate powder and mixed to produce a sol. The impression material reaches the gel state after the chemical setting reaction in the client's mouth. After reaching the gel state, the impression is removed from the mouth. Alginate materials are ideal for preliminary impressions in which accurate detail is important. However, these materials are not appropriate for final impressions that require exact fine detail for the precise fabrication and fit of a restoration.[1,2]

Packaging and Storage

Alginate impression material is available either in premeasured packages or in bulk canisters. The premeasured packages are more expensive, but they save time by eliminating the need to measure the powder. Because the powder deteriorates when it is exposed to elevated temperatures or water, it is important to store the powder in a tightly closed container in a cool, nonrefrigerated place. The individual premeasured packages should be used immediately upon opening to avoid water condensing on the powder from humidity in the air. Properly stored alginate impression material has a shelf life of about 1 year.

Although an alginate impression does not change its physical state after gelation, it is subject to distortion as a result of slight changes in its physical surroundings. Thus alginate impressions must be "poured up" within an hour of having been made. The potential for dimensional change is due to the fact that so much of the material is made of water. For example, if left exposed to the room environment uncovered, the impression may shrink in response to **syneresis** (i.e., the loss of water) from evaporation. **Imbibition** is the uptake of water in the presence of moisture. It is recommended that a disinfected impression be wrapped in a slightly moistened towel and placed in a plastic biohazard bag or unwrapped in a **humidor** (i.e., a covered container with a moist environment) to cause the least amount of distortion. As a result of the loss of water and the resultant dimensional changes that occur upon pouring with gypsum products, alginate impressions can only be poured once.[1,2]

Water-to-Powder Ratio

When alginate powder that has been stored in canisters is used, a plastic scoop for dispensing the powder and a calibrated plastic cylinder for measuring the water are supplied (Figure 37-2). Caution should be taken when dispensing and mixing the product; a mask should be worn to protect the clinician from inhaling potentially hazardous particles contained within the powder. Mandibular alginate impressions generally require two scoops of powder and two measure lines of water. A large mandible may require three scoops of powder to three measure lines of water. A maxillary impression generally takes three scoops of powder and three measure lines of water.[1,2]

Setting Time

The time needed to mix the impression material, load the tray, and seat it in the client's mouth is called the **working time**. The time required for gelation, after which the impression tray is removed from the client's mouth, is called **setting time**. Alginate impression material is available in regular-set powder (with a working time of 2 minutes and a setting time of up to 4.5 minutes) and fast-set powder (with a working time of 1.25 minutes and a setting time of 1 to 2 minutes). Currently there are several brands of color-changing alginate available. The color-coded handling sequence guides the clinician during the mixing, loading, and setting of the material. When the alginate powder is mixed with water, its color changes to purple; its color changes to pink when it is time to load the tray and place it into the mouth, and its color changes to white at gelation.

The alginate powder is mixed with room-temperature water (68° to 70° F or 20° to 21° C). Altering the temperature of the water is the best method for controlling the working and setting time of the material. Cooler water increases the working and setting time, and warmer water decreases these times. Powder is incorporated into the water to wet the powder completely and then vigorously spatulated against the sides of the mixing bowl until a smooth, creamy

Procedure 37-1 Selecting the Correct Tray Size and Preparing It for Use

EQUIPMENT (FIGURE 37-3)

Personal protective equipment
Antimicrobial mouth rinse
Lubricating gel
Maxillary and mandibular impression trays
Mouth mirror
Utility wax

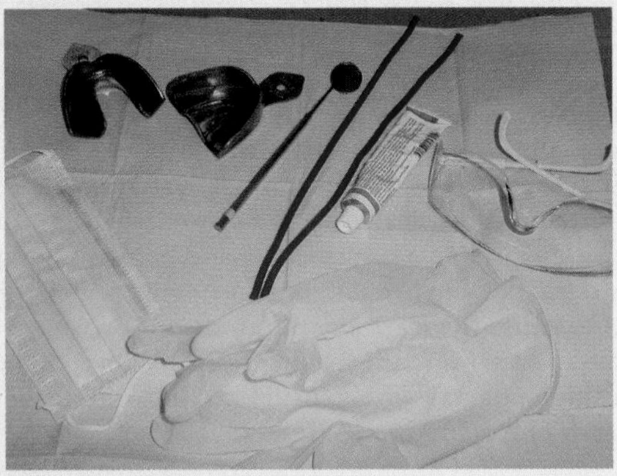

Figure 37-3. Equipment for selecting and preparing an impression tray. (Courtesy Gwen Essex.)

STEPS

Preparation

1. Gather all necessary supplies.
2. Position yourself at the side and in front of client, and seat the client in an upright position.
3. Explain the procedure to the client. Have the client remove any removable oral appliances.
4. Place protective eyewear on the client.
5. Provide preprocedural antimicrobial mouth rinse.
6. Don personal protective equipment. Disinfect hands and don gloves.
7. Lubricate the client's lips with a small amount of lubricating gel.

Mandibular Tray Selection

8. Inspect the client's mouth to estimate tray size. Note any teeth that are out of alignment, any tori or exostosis, and the presence of a dental arch of such a length that may require additional tray adaptation for client comfort.
9. Instruct the client to tilt the chin down. Retract the client's lip and cheek with the index and middle fingers of the nondominant hand and at the same time turn the tray sideways and distend the lip and cheek on the opposite side of the mouth with the side of the tray to gain entry into the client's mouth. Insert the tray with a rotary motion (Figure 37-4).
10. Make sure that the tray is centered over the lower teeth by placing the handle at the midline, usually between the central incisors and in line with the center of the chin.
11. Instruct the client to raise the tongue. Lower the tray and at the same time retract the cheek to make sure that the buccal mucosa is not caught under the rim of the tray.

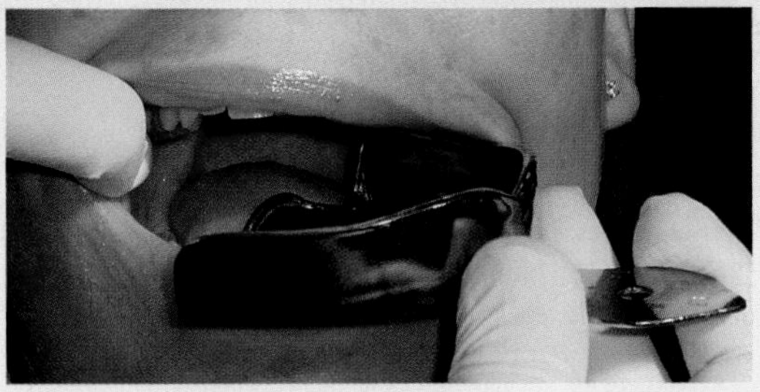

Figure 37-4. Inserting impression tray. (Courtesy Gwen Essex.)

12. Check to be sure that the tray covers the teeth and the soft tissue. Lift the front of the tray to be sure that the area posterior to the retromolar pad is covered and that there is enough room to allow for 2 to 3 mm of impression material at the facial and lingual surfaces of the teeth. If necessary, adapt the tray borders with utility (beading) wax to extend into the depth of the vestibule or to extend to the posterior length of the tray (Figure 37-5).
13. Reselect a larger or smaller tray as needed.

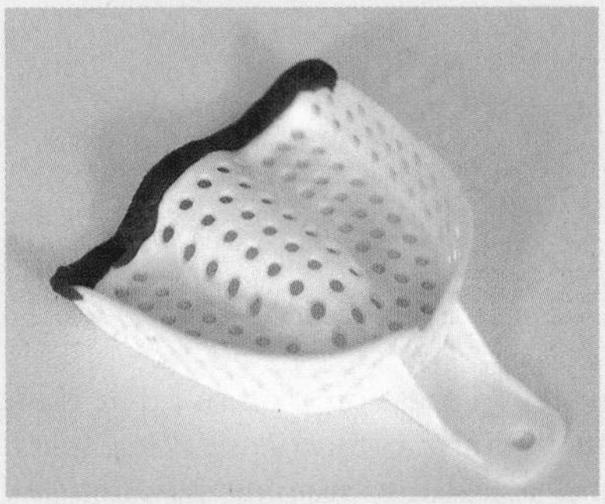

Figure 37-5. Extending impression tray with utility wax. (From Bird DL, Robinson DS: *Modern dental assisting,* ed 11, St Louis, 2015, Elsevier.)

Maxillary Tray Selection

14. Repeat steps 8 and 9, and include an evaluation of the height of the palatal vault.
15. Center the tray by placing the handle between the central incisors in line with the center of the nose.
16. Bring the front of the tray about 2 to 3 mm anterior to the incisors.
17. Seat the tray first by lowering the handle toward the mandibular teeth.
18. Make sure that all of the posterior teeth and soft tissue, including the maxillary tuberosity, are covered. Check that laterally there is enough room to allow for 2 to 3 mm of space between the inside of the tray and the facial and lingual surfaces of the teeth.
19. Retract the client's lip and raise the anterior portion of the tray into place. The tray should fit to the depth of the vestibule and not impinge on the soft tissue.
20. Reselect a larger or smaller tray as needed.

Tray Preparation

21. Spray or coat nonperforated trays with adhesive. Wait 15 minutes before use.

TABLE 37-1

Factors That Affect Gelation

Factor	Comments
Ratio of water to alginate powder	The manufacturer's directions must be followed carefully, and the water-to-powder ratio must be exact. Too much water in the mix will make a weak impression that will tear easily during removal from the mouth as a result of tension. Too little water creates a grainy impression that will cause an inaccurate reproduction of the hard and soft tissues. If the container holding the alginate is not fluffed before measuring, too much powder will be dispensed, which will result in a grainy impression.
Water temperature	Water temperature affects gelation time. If the water is too warm, the product will gel at a faster rate, thereby resulting in poor detail in the impression. If the water is cool, the product will gel at a slower rate, and the final impression will be more accurate in detail. In hot, humid climates, it is recommended to use cooler water and to refrigerate the bowl and spatula.
Spatulation technique	Proper mixing (spatulation) will determine setting time. A mechanical device that automatically mixes the material can be used. Too much spatulation will decrease the strength of the impression material, because the gel will be broken as it forms. Too little spatulation decreases strength up to 50% and will cause a grainy impression that is inaccurate with regard to the details of the mouth.
Tray movement	Movement of the tray during gelation causes an inaccurate impression. It is important to hold the impression tray steady in the mouth during gelation.
Removal of impression	Premature removal of the impression from the mouth creates an inaccurate impression because the material has not fully gelled. The most frequent result of premature removal is the inaccuracy of the incisor teeth. The elasticity of alginate increases with time. A better impression results from being patient. Rocking the tray back and forth to release it from the client's mouth may cause distortion of the impression.
Improper storage of impression	The impression should be poured within 1 hour. Leaving the impression unprotected to the environment can result in imbibition or syneresis. After disinfection, maintain the integrity of the impression (if it cannot be poured with a gypsum product) by immediately wrapping it in a damp towel or storing it in a humidor. A humidor is a closed plastic container with a moist bottom layer of paper towels that creates a humid environment. Before taking the maxillary impression, wrap the mandibular impression in a wet towel.

consistency is achieved. To allow the chemical reaction to proceed effectively, the manufacturer's instructions with regard to mixing time should be followed. Loading the tray and inserting it should take no more than 1 minute. The objective is for the impression material to reach the gel state in the client's mouth. Procedure 37-2 and the corresponding Competency Form describes the details for mixing alginate impression material. Table 37-1 presents factors that affect gelation and therefore the success of the impression.[1]

New Silicone Alginate-Alternative Materials

New alginate-alternative materials are becoming increasingly popular for the fabrication of preliminary impressions. These materials have the elasticity of alginate and the dimensional stability of polyvinyl siloxane impression materials, thus enabling the pouring and re-pouring of models at any time from immediately after disinfection to up to several weeks later. This option of delayed or repeated pours enhances the flexibility of this product, especially for multiple molds and when time constraints do not allow for the immediate pouring of the impression.

The materials are available in smaller automix cartridges for extruder mixing guns with mixing tips and in 380-mL volume cartridges for automatic mixing machines. The extruder tips eliminate the need for mixing and the resultant cleanup. The convenience and flexibility of these products comes with a price, however: they are roughly eight times more expensive than traditional alginate products.

BOX 37-2

Mouth Areas to Precoat with Alginate

Precoat the following areas with a small amount of alginate to prevent excessive air bubbles on the tooth surfaces and to customize areas that are not adequately covered by the insertion of the impression tray:

- Occlusal surfaces
- Tooth surfaces adjacent to edentulous areas
- Areas of erosion, abfraction, or abrasion
- Vestibular areas
- A high palatal vault

Impression Taking

Before the impression is taken, the procedure is explained to the client to enhance the client's comfort and cooperation. Specifically, clients should be informed of the following:

- That the material will feel cool, that it has a specific flavor, and that it will gel quickly
- That breathing deeply through the nose during the procedure will help them to relax
- That they need to refrain from talking after the tray has been placed
- That, if he or she needs to communicate during the procedure, raising a hand is best

Box 37-2 lists areas to precoat with alginate before placing the tray. Box 37-3 lists criteria for a quality impression.

Procedure 37-2 Mixing Alginate

EQUIPMENT (FIGURE 37-6)

Personal protective equipment
Alginate powder
Water
Measuring scoop
Vial for measuring water
Wide-blade spatula
Rubber mixing bowl
Timer
Thermometer

STEPS

1. Read the manufacturer's directions for the dispensing and manipulation of the alginate.
2. Place one measure of room-temperature water into the mixing bowl for each scoop of alginate. Check the temperature of the water; room-temperature water is recommended. Use warmer water to accelerate the mix and cooler water to retard the mix.
3. Shake or fluff the alginate by tipping the container two or three times.
4. Overfill the correct scoop with powder, and then tap the scoop with the side of the spatula. Scrape the excess from the scoop with the spatula.
5. Sift the powder into the water, and stir this with the spatula until all of the powder has been moistened.
6. Cup the rubber bowl in your hand with the mouth of the bowl next to your wrist. Firmly spread the alginate between the spatula and the side of the rubber bowl. Spatulate the mixture vigorously using a back-and-forth hand motion, spreading the material against the sides of the bowl. Use both sides of the spatula, and turn the bowl with your fingers during spatulation (Figure 37-7).
7. Spatulate vigorously for 30 seconds for fast-set products, and gather the material together. Use the spatula to crush the mixture and spread it out again. Repeat until a smooth, creamy consistency is achieved within the designated mixing time for either the normal-set or fast-set alginate.
8. Gather the material into one mass, and wipe it on the inside edge of the mixing bowl.

Figure 37-6. Equipment for mixing alginate impression material. (From Hatrick CD, Eakle WS, Bird WF: *Dental materials: clinical applications for the dental assistant and dental hygienist,* ed 2, St Louis, 2011, Elsevier.)

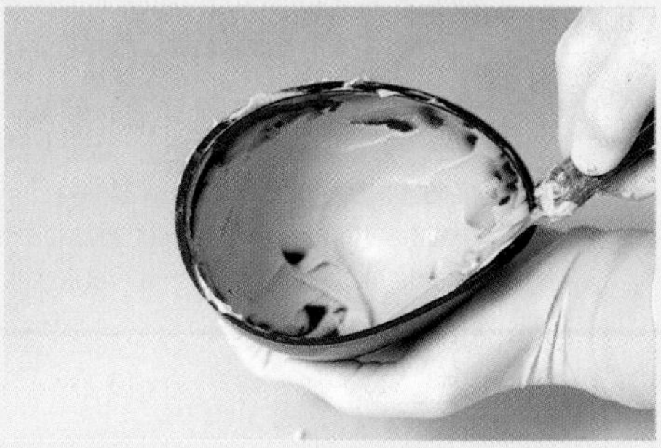

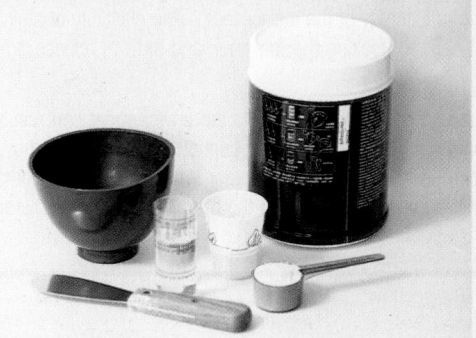

Figure 37-7. Proper consistency of mixed alginate impression material. (From Hatrick CD, Eakle WS, Bird WF: *Dental materials: clinical applications for the dental assistant and dental hygienist,* ed 2, St Louis, 2011, Elsevier.)

BOX 37-3

Criteria for a High-Quality Alginate Impression

- No visible voids, tears, or debris
- Clear and distinct detail of desired structures
- All teeth and alveolar process recorded
- Retromolar area or maxillary tuberosity present
- Alginate material firmly attached to tray
- Adequate peripheral roll

Procedures 37-3 and 37-4 and their corresponding Competency Forms illustrate details for making mandibular and maxillary dental impressions, respectively. Mandibular teeth impressions should be taken first, because gagging is less likely in the mandibular area and enhances trust in the clinician (see Box 37-4 for additional suggestions to minimize gagging).

Disinfecting Impressions

Dental impressions are considered contaminated and must be disinfected before handing them into the office laboratory or sending them to a commercial laboratory. Impressions should be rinsed first with water to remove saliva, blood, and debris. The excess water is then shaken from the impression, and an appropriate spray is used to adequately cover all surfaces of the impression. After the required period of time, the impression must be rinsed thoroughly to remove all disinfectant before the gypsum is poured into the mold.

Bite Registration

When an impression is made of both dental arches, the clinician and the laboratory technician need an accurate registration of the normal centric occlusion (i.e., the interocclusal record). **Centric occlusion** is the maximal stable contact between the occluding surfaces of the maxillary and mandibular arches when the jaws are closed. This relationship is often recorded with a wax-bite registration. Silicone impression materials are also used as bite registration materials for their accuracy and dimensional stability. The bite registration is made at the time that the impression is taken. The bite registration is used to articulate the models or diagnostic casts after the client has left the office. Articulated models can then be trimmed to ensure accurate articulation.

When a wax-bite registration is used, **baseplate wax** and **wax wafers** are used to record the client's bite registration

Procedure 37-3 Making a Mandibular Preliminary Impression

EQUIPMENT (FIGURE 37-8)

Personal protective equipment
Antimicrobial rinse
Occupational Safety and Health Administration–approved disinfectant
Alginate powder
Measuring scoop
Vial for measuring water
Wide-blade spatula
Rubber mixing bowl
Selected and adapted mandibular impression tray
Saliva ejector

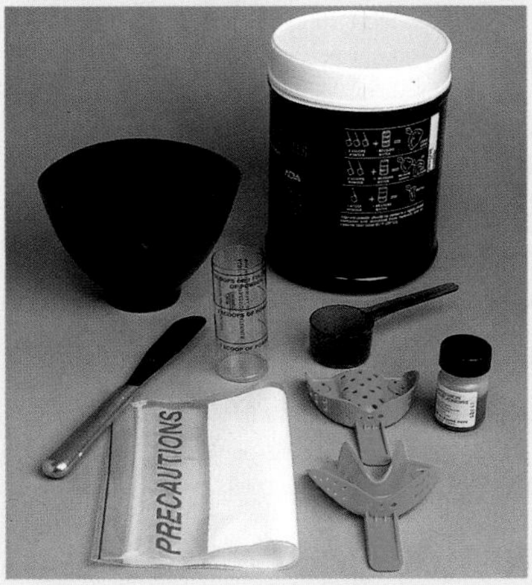

Figure 37-8. Scoop for alginate powder, water dispensers, mixing bowl, spatula, and stock impression tray. (From Bird DL, Robinson DS: *Modern dental assisting,* ed 11, St Louis, 2015, Elsevier.)

STEPS

Preparation

1. Gather all necessary supplies. Seat the client upright, and explain the procedure. Have the client remove any removable oral appliances.
2. Check the client's health history to determine the presence of any risk factors that may complicate the procedure.
3. Place protective eyewear on the client.
4. Provide preprocedural antimicrobial mouth rinse.
5. Don personal protective equipment, safety glasses, mask, and bonnet. Disinfect hands and don gloves.
6. Lubricate the client's lips with a small amount of moisturizer.
7. Dry the teeth with compressed air.
8. Combine two measures of room-temperature water with two scoops of alginate, and mix the alginate.

Loading the Tray

9. Quickly gather half of the alginate in the bowl onto the spatula. Wipe the alginate into one side of the tray from the lingual side, working from the posterior toward the anterior edge of the tray. Fill the tray to an area just below the rim. Quickly press the material down to the base of the tray.
10. Gather the remaining half of the alginate in the bowl onto the spatula and load the other side of the tray in the same way.
11. Moisten your fingers with cold water and smooth over the alginate. Make a slight indentation where the teeth will insert (Figure 37-9).

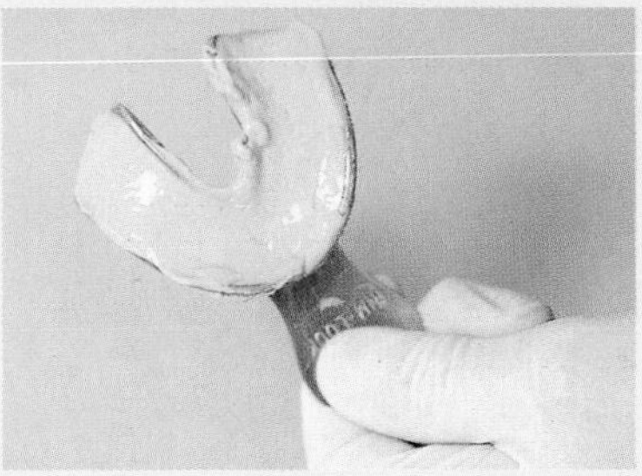

Figure 37-9. The mandibular impression tray is filled with alginate and smoothed. (From Hatrick CD, Eakle WS, Bird WF: *Dental materials: clinical applications for the dental assistant and dental hygienist,* ed 2, St Louis, 2011, Elsevier.)

12. Take a small amount of impression mixture from the spatula and quickly apply it to the occlusal surfaces of the teeth, the undercut areas, and the vestibular areas.

Seating the Tray

13. Place yourself at the 8-o'clock position (or the 4-o'clock position if you are left-handed), and ask the client to tilt his or her chin down to make the occlusal plane parallel to the floor.
14. Turn the impression tray sideways.
15. Retract the client's lip and cheek with the fingers of the nondominant hand. Turn the tray sideways when placing it in the client's mouth, and distending the client's lip and cheek on the opposite side of the mouth with the side of the tray.
16. Center the tray over the teeth, and center the handle in line with the center of the client's chin.
17. Align the tray 2 to 3 mm anterior to the incisors. Press down the posterior portion of the tray first, and then seat the anterior portion of the tray directly down. Instruct the client to raise the tongue (Figure 37-10).

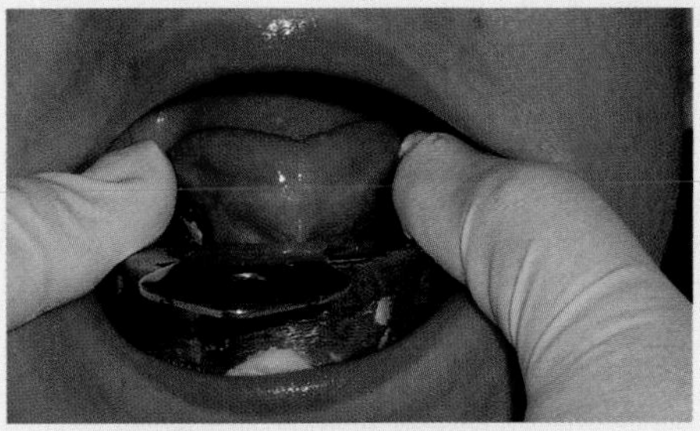

Figure 37-10. The mandibular impression tray is seated in the arch with the tongue out of the way. (Courtesy Gwen Essex.)

18. Instruct the client to move his or her lips and to breathe normally.
19. Hold the tray steady in place until the material has gelled. Apply firm bilateral pressure with the middle fingers, and use the thumbs to support the jaw (Figure 37-11).

Continued

Procedure 37-3 Making a Mandibular Preliminary Impression—cont'd

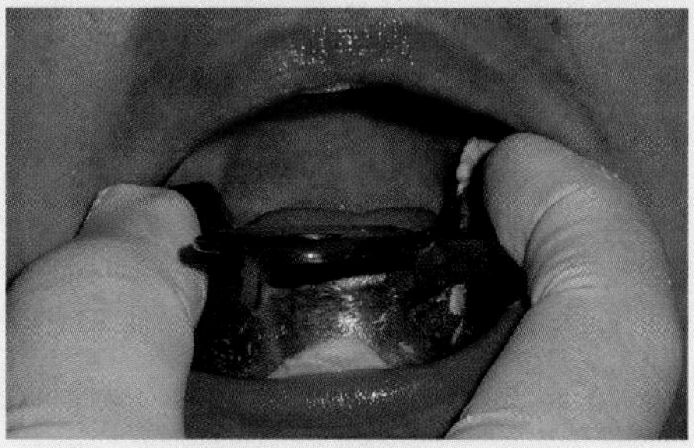

Figure 37-11. Holding the mandibular tray. (Courtesy Gwen Essex.)

Removing the Impression

20. Place the fingers of the nondominant hand on top of the tray. The index finger of the nondominant hand rests on the incisal surface of the maxillary anterior teeth.
21. Move the index finger of other hand along the buccal mucosa posteriorly between the impression and the peripheral tissues. The index finger is placed under the posterior facial portion of the tray to lift the tray and break the seal between the impression and the teeth. Grasp the handle of the tray with the thumb and the index finger of the dominant hand, and use a firm lifting motion.
22. Remove the tray by turning it sideways to take it out of the client's mouth.
23. Evaluate the impression for accuracy (Figure 37-12).

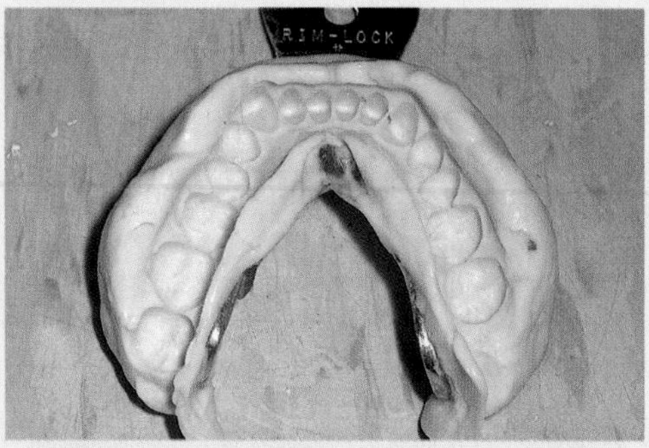

Figure 37-12. How a mandibular impression must look. (From Hatrick CD, Eakle WS, Bird WF: *Dental materials: clinical applications for the dental assistant and dental hygienist,* ed 2, St Louis, 2011, Elsevier.)

Postimpression Care

24. Give the client water to rinse his or her mouth.
25. Gently rinse debris from the impression under a stream of cold water (Figure 37-13).
26. Spray the impression with an approved disinfectant (e.g., 1:213 iodophor or 1:10 sodium hypochlorite) within 10 to 15 minutes. Follow the manufacturer's recommended procedure (Figure 37-14).
27. Wrap the impression in a moist paper towel, and place it in a biohazard bag before pouring it up (Figure 37-15) or placing it in a humidor; label it with the client's name. Prepare the laboratory prescription if you are sending the impressions to the dental laboratory.
28. Remove any remaining alginate from the client's mouth with floss, a scaler, or an explorer.
29. Remove any alginate from the client's face and lips with a warm cloth.
30. Return any removable oral appliances to the client.
31. Document the completion of this service in the client's electronic record under Services Rendered, and date the entry. For example, "9-1-12 Alginate impression for diagnostic casts."

Rationale

This ensures the integrity of the client's record for both the client's health and the protection of the legal practitioner.

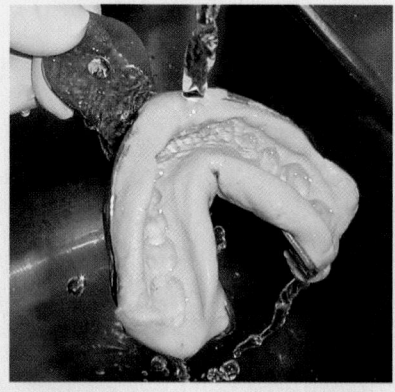

Figure 37-13. Rinsing the impression. (From Bird DL, Robinson DS: *Modern dental assisting,* ed 11, St Louis, 2015, Elsevier.)

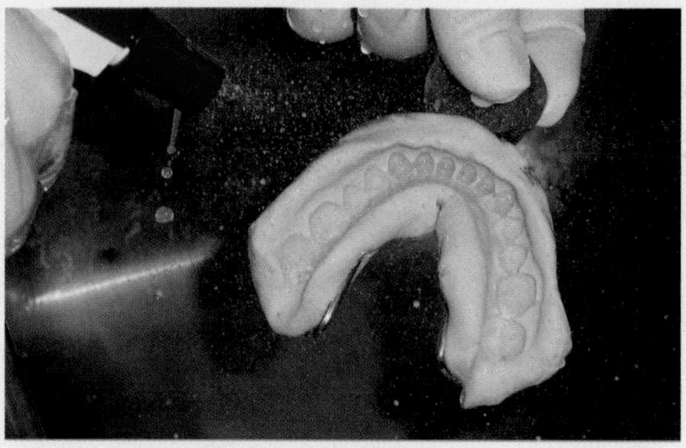

Figure 37-14. Spraying the impression. (Courtesy Gwen Essex.)

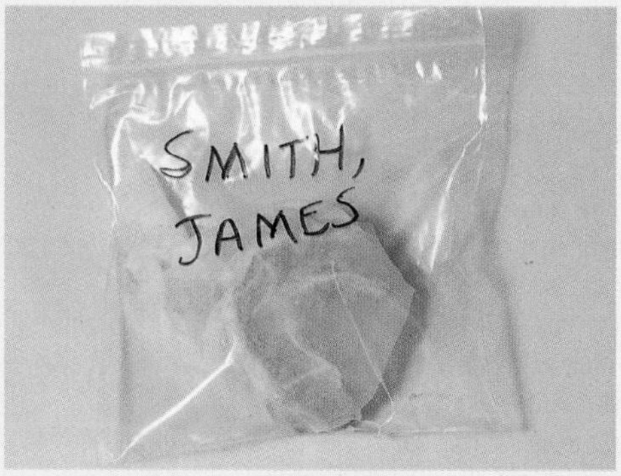

Figure 37-15. Impression in precaution bag with client name. (From Hatrick CD, Eakle WS, Bird WF: *Dental materials: clinical applications for the dental assistant and dental hygienist,* ed 2, St Louis, 2011, Elsevier.)

Procedure 37-4 Making a Maxillary Preliminary Impression

EQUIPMENT

Personal protective equipment
Antimicrobial rinse
Occupational Safety and Health Administration–approved disinfecting solution
Alginate powder
Powder measuring scoop
Vial for measuring water
Wide-blade spatula*
Rubber mixing bowl*
Selected and adapted maxillary impression tray
Saliva ejector

STEPS

Preparation

1. Gather all necessary supplies. Seat and prepare the client.
2. Combine three units of room-temperature water and three scoops of alginate, and mix the alginate.

Loading the Tray

3. Load the maxillary tray in one large increment. Load from the posterior end of tray. Use a wiping motion to bring the material forward with the spatula, being careful to place the bulk of the material in the anterior palatal area of the tray. Fill the tray to an area just below the edge of the wax rim.
4. Be careful not to overfill the posterior portion of the tray that rests against the palate.
5. Moisten your fingers with water, and smooth the surface of the alginate (Figure 37-16).

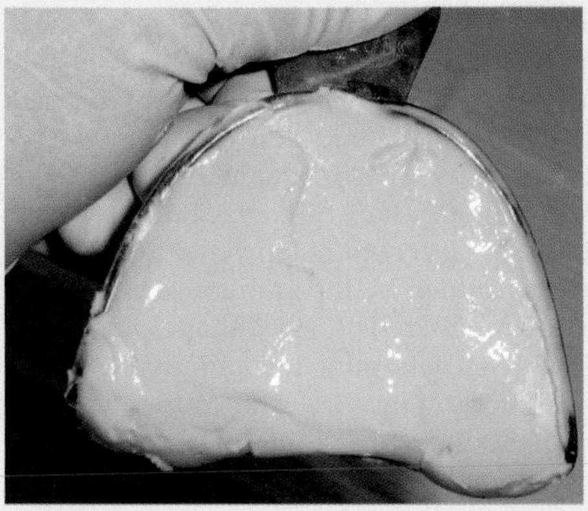

Figure 37-16. The maxillary impression tray is filled with alginate. The filled tray is smoothed on the alginate surface. (Courtesy Gwen Essex.)

Seating the Tray

6. Position yourself at the 11-o'clock position (or the 1-o'clock position if you are left-handed), and ask the client to tilt his or her head forward and chin down to make the occlusal plane parallel to the floor.
7. Retract the client's lips and cheek with the fingers of the nondominant hand. With the dominant hand, turn the impression tray sideways and at the same time distend the lip and cheek on the opposite side of the mouth with the side of the tray.
8. Center the tray over the client's teeth, and center the handle at the midline in line with the center of the client's nose.
9. Seat the back of the tray against the posterior border of the hard palate to form a seal. Place the tray $\frac{1}{4}$ inch or 6 mm anterior to the incisors, and seat it in a posterior to anterior direction with a slight vibratory motion.
10. Gently move the client's lips up and over the tray as it is seated (Figure 37-17).
11. Place your middle fingers over the premolar areas, and hold the client's lip out with your index finger and thumb.
12. Instruct the client to breathe slowly through the nose and to form an "O" with his or her lips.
13. Hold the tray in place until the material has gelled.

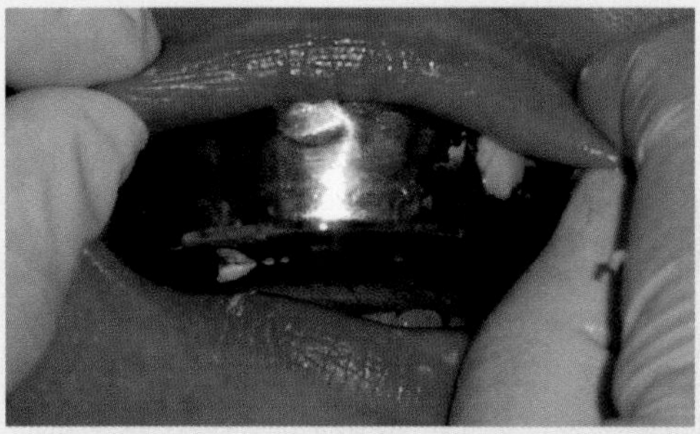

Figure 37-17. A maxillary alginate impression is placed in the arch. The maxillary lip is lifted and positioned outside of the tray. (Courtesy Gwen Essex.)

Removing the Impression

14. Place an index finger under the posterior facial portion of the tray to break the seal between the impression and the teeth.
15. Place the index finger of the nondominant hand on the incisal surface of the mandibular anterior teeth.
16. Move the index finger of the other hand along the buccal mucosa posteriorly between the impression and the peripheral tissues. The index finger is placed under the rim of the tray to lift and break the seal between the impression and the teeth. Grasp the handle of the tray with the thumb and the index finger of the dominant hand to lower it from the maxillary teeth.
17. Remove the tray by turning it sideways to take it out of the client's mouth.
18. Evaluate the impression for accuracy (Figure 37-18).

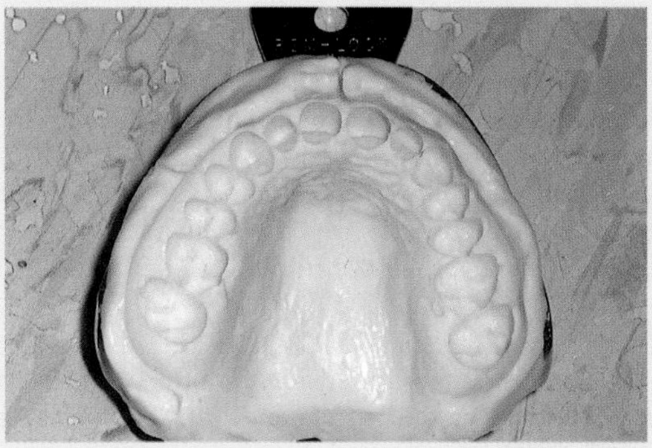

Figure 37-18. How a maxillary impression must look. (From Hatrick CD, Eakle WS, Bird WF: *Dental materials: clinical applications for the dental assistant and dental hygienist,* ed 2, St Louis, 2011, Elsevier.)

Continued

Procedure 37-4 Making a Maxillary Preliminary Impression—cont'd

Postimpression Care

19. Give the client water to rinse his or her mouth.
20. Gently rinse debris from the impression under a stream of cold water (see Figure 37-13).
21. Spray the impression with an approved disinfectant (e.g., 1:213 iodophor or 1:10 sodium hypochlorite) within 10 to 15 minutes. Follow the manufacturer's recommended procedure (see Figure 37-14).
22. Wrap the impression in a moist paper towel and place it in a biohazard bag before pouring it up (see Figure 37-15) or placing it in a humidor; label it with the client's name. Prepare the laboratory prescription if sending the impressions to the dental laboratory.
23. Remove any remaining alginate from the client's mouth with floss, a scaler, or an explorer.
24. Remove any alginate from the client's face and lips with a warm cloth.
25. Return any removable oral appliances to the client.
26. Document the completion of this service in the client's electronic record under Services Rendered, and date the entry. For example, "9-1-12 Alginate impression for diagnostic casts."

Rationale

This ensures the integrity of the client's record for both the client's health and the protection of the legal practitioner.

*If the same bowl and spatula are used that were used for the mandibular impression, they must be thoroughly cleaned and dried to prevent contamination of the maxillary mix (see Figure 37-8).

BOX 37-4

Guidelines to Minimize Gagging During Impression Taking

- The gag reflex is located on the posterior third of the tongue. It is important to keep material from flowing onto this area.
- Seat the maxillary tray from posterior to anterior to direct the flow of impression material anteriorly away from the soft palate.
- Place a wax dam on the posterior border of the maxillary tray to help contain the material.
- Avoid overfilling the tray with impression material. Fill to the level just below the wax beading of the tray rim.
- Seat the client upright. During the insertion of the tray, instruct the client to bend the head forward with the chin tilting down.
- Avoid using too small of a tray, because the material will flow out of the confines of a tray that is too small to accommodate the needs of the arch.
- Use a calm, confident, yet gentle approach, and work efficiently.
- Instruct clients to breathe slowly and deeply through the nose, to point their toes, and to pinch the skin between the index finger and the thumb.

(Procedure 37-5 and the corresponding Competency Form). Baseplate wax and wax wafers are pliable at room temperature. Baseplate wax is supplied in 1- to 2-mm–thick red or pink sheets, and wax-bite wafers are shaped like horseshoes. The most common technique used to obtain a bite registration is to have clients close their teeth into softened wax.

Dental Cast

A cast is an accurate three-dimensional model of the teeth and the surrounding tissues of the client's maxillary and mandibular arches that is created from a dental impression. Gypsum products are used to make dental casts. A diagnostic cast is frequently constructed of plaster or stone and used for treatment planning, the tracking of treatment progress, patient education, and the construction of custom-made oral appliances (e.g., trays, splints, stents). These casts are also referred to as study models. A working cast is frequently constructed of stone that is strong enough for the fabrication of indirect restorations or prostheses. These casts also are referred to as master casts. A die is a replica of a prepared tooth that is constructed from the densest of the gypsum products. Dental laboratories use these exact replicas for the construction of cast restorations.

Gypsum Products

Gypsum is a powdered hemihydrate, which means that it is made from one part water to one part calcium sulfate. When mixed with water, the hemihydrate crystals form clusters that grow during the setting process. The interlinking of the crystals results in a stronger and harder final product. There are three types of gypsum products used when pouring casts: model plaster, dental stone, and high-strength stone. These materials consist of hemihydrate crystals that vary in size, shape, and porosity. These differences determine the physical properties of the product. Strength, hardness, abrasion resistance, dimensional accuracy, reproduction of detail, and solubility are determined by the amount of water needed to mix the gypsum product. The size, shape, and porosity of the gypsum particles determine the amount of water required to mix the product. An increase in the amount of water needed to mix the product will result in a weaker final product. Working casts and dies require the most resistance to stresses and thus need higher properties of strength, abrasion resistance, and accuracy.

Plaster, which is a beta calcium sulfate hemihydrate (plaster of Paris), has very porous crystals that are large and that vary in shape. Because of its porosity, plaster requires the most water when mixing as compared with the other types of gypsum products. It is used for pouring preliminary impressions to construct models when strength is not critical but a detailed reproduction of the mouth is required (e.g., study models).[1,2]

Dental stone, which is an alpha calcium sulfate hemihydrate, is stronger than plaster. Its crystals are uniform in shape, and they are smaller and less porous than plaster. Dental stone is used when a stronger working diagnostic cast is needed to make oral appliances, orthodontic retainers and aligners, custom trays, and provisional restorations. High-strength stone has very dense crystals and requires the least

Procedure 37-5 Making a Wax-Bite Registration

EQUIPMENT (FIGURE 37-19)

Protective barriers (safety glasses, mask, gloves, hair bonnet)
Antimicrobial rinse
Bite registration wax (baseplate wax or wax wafer)
Wide-blade laboratory knife
Heat source (warm water, Bunsen burner, or torch)
Occupational Safety and Health Administration–approved disinfectant

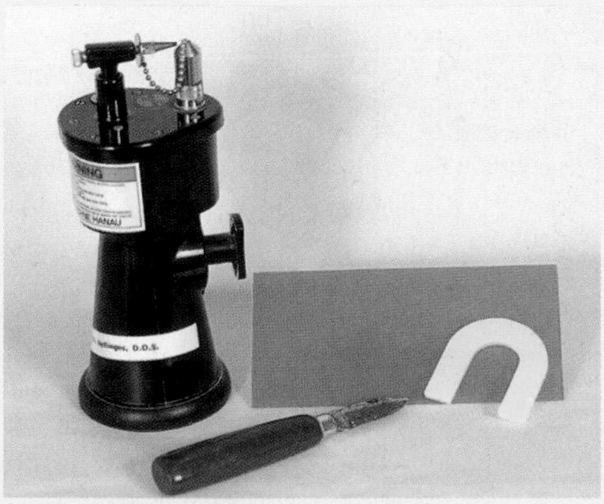

Figure 37-19. Supplies for taking a wax-bite registration. (From Hatrick CD, Eakle WS, Bird WF: *Dental materials: clinical applications for the dental assistant and dental hygienist,* ed 2, St Louis, 2011, Elsevier.)

STEPS

Preparation

1. Gather all necessary supplies. Seat the client upright, and explain the procedure.
2. Reassure the client that the wax will be warm and not hot.
3. Measure the length of the wax needed by placing the wax over the biting surfaces of the client's teeth. If the wax extends past the last tooth, use the laboratory knife to shorten its length after removing the wax from the client's mouth.
4. Soften the bite registration wax in hot water or with another heat source (e.g., Bunsen burner, torch).

Seating

5. Place the softened warm wax over the maxillary occlusal surfaces. Instruct the client to bite together on the posterior teeth gently and naturally into the wax (Figure 37-20).
6. Allow the wax bite to cool in the mouth. If necessary, air from the air-water syringe can cool the wax.

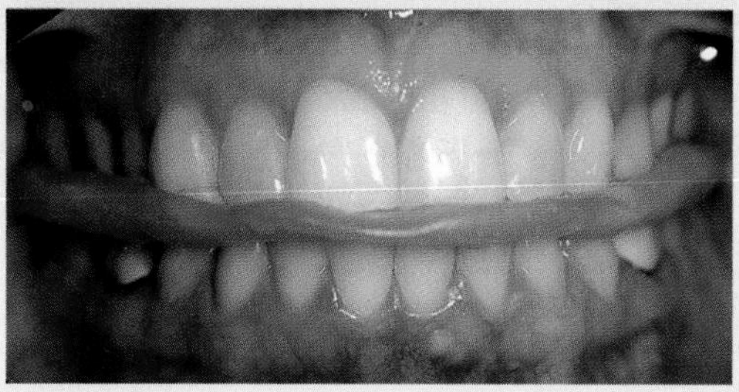

Figure 37-20. Wax-bite registration in client's mouth. (From Hatrick CD, Eakle WS, Bird WF: *Dental materials: clinical applications for the dental assistant and dental hygienist,* ed 2, St Louis, 2011, Elsevier.)

Removal

7. Remove the wax carefully when it has cooled.

Post–Wax-Bite Care

8. Inspect the wax to be sure it represents the client's bite (Figure 37-21). Chill the wax in cold water until it is firm.
9. Write the client's name on a piece of paper, and keep it with the wax-bite registration.
10. Disinfect the wax-bite registration with the disinfectant.
11. Store the wax-bite registration with the impressions or casts until it is needed for the trimming of the casts.
12. Document the completion of this service in the client's electronic record under Services Rendered, and date the entry. For example, "9-1-12 Bite Registration for diagnostic casts."

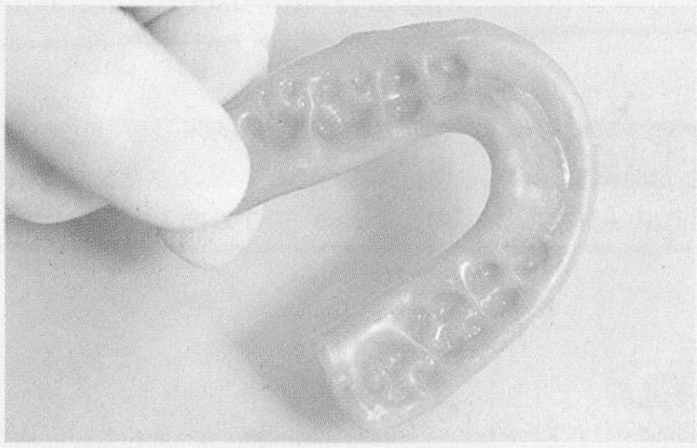

Figure 37-21. Wax-bite registration on a wax wafer. (From Hatrick CD, Eakle WS, Bird WF: *Dental materials: clinical applications for the dental assistant and dental hygienist,* ed 2, St Louis, 2011, Elsevier.)

Rationale

This ensures the integrity of the client's record for both the client's health and the protection of the legal practitioner.

amount of water for mixing. High-strength stone has a hardness that makes it ideal to create the casts and dies used for the production of crowns, bridges, and indirect restoration. Both plaster and stone are mixed by hand with a spatula or mechanically with a vacuum mixer, which eliminates the trapping of air into the mix.[1,2]

Water-to-Powder Ratio

Each gypsum product has an optimal water-to-powder ratio that is specified by the manufacturer. The water-to-powder ratio affects the setting time and the product strength. For one preliminary impression and its base, the commonly used water-to-powder ratio for plaster is 50 mL of water to 100 g of powder; for dental stone, it is 30 mL water to 100 g of powder; and for high-strength stone, it is 24 mL of water to 100 g of powder.[1,2]

Setting Time

Time is another critical factor in the setting reaction of plaster and stone. There is working time, which occurs immediately after mixing, when the mixture will flow into the alginate impression. Initial setting time occurs when a semihard mass forms and is the point at which the mixture can no longer be poured into the impressions. For plaster, the initial setting time is 12 to 14 minutes; final setting time is 45 to 60 minutes. For stone, the initial setting time is 8 to 10 minutes; final setting time is 45 to 60 minutes. Final setting time occurs after the exothermic reaction (a chemical change accompanied by the liberation of heat) and the final product can no longer be manipulated without fracture. After the final setting time (i.e., 45 to 60 minutes), the preliminary alginate impression can be removed from the model or cast. Table 37-2 presents factors that affect the setting times of plaster and stone.[1]

Pouring the Cast

The cast consists of the anatomic portion and the art portion. The **anatomic portion** includes the teeth, the oral mucosa, and the muscle attachments. The **art portion** forms the base (Figure 37-22). The procedure for pouring the cast from a preliminary impression consists of two components: filling the impression with the mixed gypsum material to form the anatomic portion of the cast and then forming its base by mounding mixed gypsum on a smooth, nonabsorbent surface. These two parts are then connected by inverting the poured impression and seating it on the base. Procedure 37-6 and the corresponding Competency Form provides details for pouring the cast from a preliminary alginate impression using dental plaster.

Trimming and Finishing Casts

After the casts have set and the impression trays have been separated from them, the casts are trimmed to a geometric standard with the use of a model trimmer. The purpose of trimming is to produce attractive and useful diagnostic casts for the fabrication of removable oral appliances, for case presentation, or for use as part of the client's permanent record. A **model trimmer** is a laboratory machine that has a circular abrasive wheel that is set to be 90 degrees perpendicular to the cast (Figure 37-32). The bite registration is used to ensure

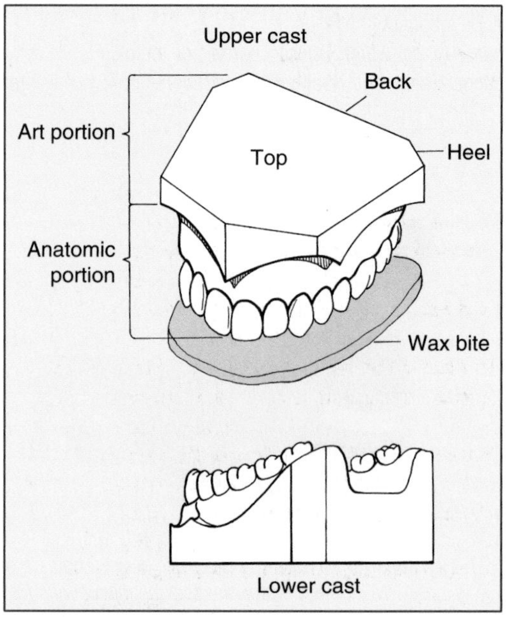

Figure 37-22. Anatomic and art portion of the diagnostic cast. (From Bird DL, Robinson DS: *Modern dental assisting,* ed 11, St Louis, 2015, Elsevier.)

TABLE 37-2

Factors That Affect Setting Time and the Quality of the Cast

Factor	Comment
Setting Time	
Type of gypsum	Dental stone sets more slowly than dental plaster.
Water-to-powder ratio	The less water used, the faster the set. Follow the manufacturer's proportions exactly. Too much water increases setting time and decreases strength; the resultant cast is smooth in appearance. Too little water decreases setting time and decreases strength; the resultant cast is grainy in appearance.
Water temperature	The warmer the water, the faster the set. Water that is too warm creates a cast that sets too fast, and water that is too cool creates a cast that sets too slowly. In general, water should be at room temperature and no warmer than 70° F (21.1° C). Cool water increases setting time, and warm water decreases setting time. On a humid day, the powder can absorb water, which results in a slower set.
Mixing time	The longer and faster the spatulation, the faster the set. Prolonged and very rapid mixing shortens the setting time by increasing the chemical reaction and decreases the strength of the study model as a result of the breakage of the crystals that are forming. Too little mixing also decreases strength and makes the study model grainy.
Improper storage of gypsum	The stone and the scoop dispenser need to be kept clean and dry. The stone should be stored in a tight container that is closed immediately after use to eliminate exposure to humidity and problems with moisture (see Procedure 37-2). Purchase gypsum products only as needed to avoid possible contamination with moisture.
Quality of Cast	
Factors that affect setting time	See above.
Removal of the impression	Premature or improper removal of the alginate impression from the cast will break teeth or crack the cast.
Movement of the tray or cast	Movement of the alginate impression or cast during the setting process will create a thin, flat base.

Procedure 37-6 Pouring the Cast and the Base

EQUIPMENT (FIGURE 37-23)

Personal protective equipment
Rubber bowl
Gypsum laboratory spatula
Scale
Room-temperature water
Dental plaster
Two Plexiglas squares or ceramic tiles
Laboratory spatula
Disinfected alginate impressions
Water-measuring device
Plaster knife
Vibrator covered with plastic
Occupational Safety and Health Administration–approved disinfectant

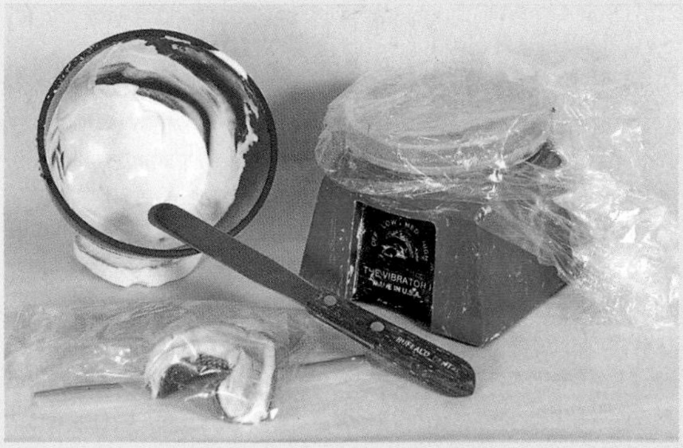

Figure 37-23. Supplies needed for pouring dental casts. (From Hatrick CD, Eakle WS, Bird WF: *Dental materials: clinical applications for the dental assistant and dental hygienist,* ed 2, St Louis, 2011, Elsevier.)

Figure 37-24. Smooth, creamy mix. (From Hatrick CD, Eakle WS, Bird WF: *Dental materials: clinical applications for the dental assistant and dental hygienist,* ed 2, St Louis, 2011, Elsevier.)

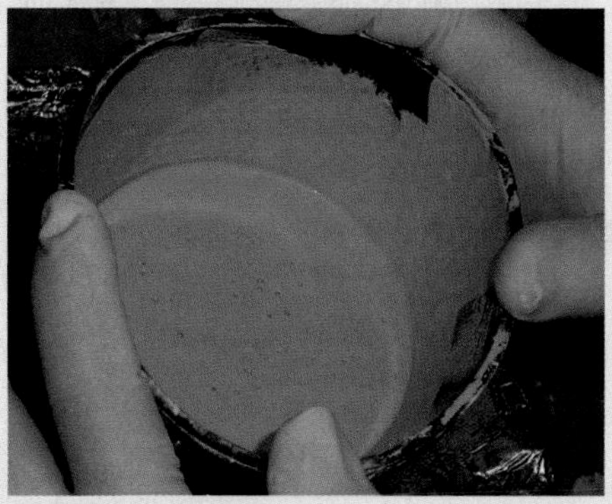

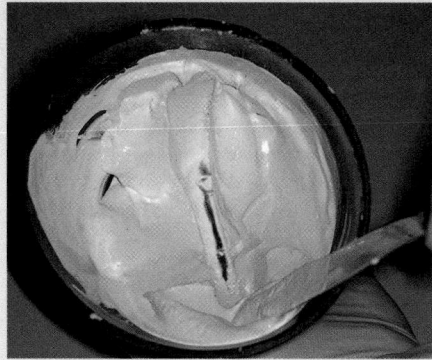

Figure 37-25. Mixing bowl on vibrator. (Courtesy Gwen Essex.)

STEPS

Preparation

1. Don personal protective equipment.
2. Disinfect the alginate impression in accordance with the manufacturer's instructions. Rinse it with cool running water, shake the excess water off in the sink, and gently dry it with compressed air.
3. Use the laboratory knife to remove any excess impression material that will interfere with the pouring of the model (i.e., impression material past the end of the tray or excess material from the tongue area).

Pouring the Mandibular Impression

4. Measure 50 mL of room-temperature water, and place it into a clean mixing bowl.
5. Place a paper towel on a scale, and make necessary adjustments. Obtain a measure of 100 g of dental plaster.
6. Add the powder into the water in steady increments to allow the powder to settle.
7. Use the spatula to incorporate the powder into the water. Use a wiping motion against the sides of the bowl. Spatulate the mixture for 20 seconds to achieve a smooth, creamy mix (Figure 37-24).
8. Set the vibrator at low speed. Place the bowl on the vibrator, and vibrate the material for 10 to 15 seconds. Lightly press and rotate the bowl on the vibrator.
9. Gather the gypsum as a mass in the bowl. Remove the bowl from the vibrator (Figure 37-25).
10. Hold the impression tray by the handle, and press the handle against the vibrator.
11. Use the end of the spatula to pick up about a ½ teaspoon of mixed material. Allow the mix to flow into the impression at the distal end of the most posterior tooth while the impression is vibrated so that the material flows toward the anterior teeth. Turn the tray on its side to provide the continuous flow of material forward into each tooth. Tip the impression forward to make the gypsum mixture flow into the bottom of the alginate impression. Continue to add the gypsum product in small increments at the same place until the occlusal and incisal surfaces are filled. Vibrate continually (Figure 37-26).

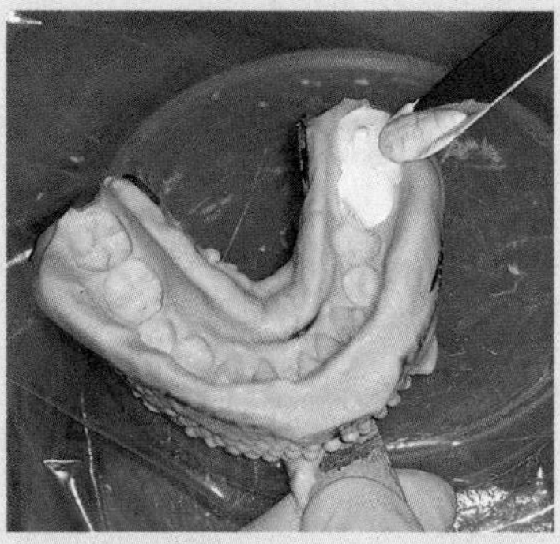

Figure 37-26. Initial placement of material in distal area of most posterior tooth. (From Hatrick CD, Eakle WS, Bird WF: *Dental materials: clinical applications for the dental assistant and dental hygienist,* ed 2, St Louis, 2011, Elsevier.)

Continued

Procedure 37-6 Pouring the Cast and the Base—cont'd

12. When all tooth indentations are filled, use the spatula to add larger amounts of gypsum to fill the impression. Continue to vibrate until the entire impression is filled (Figure 37-27), and then set the poured impression aside.

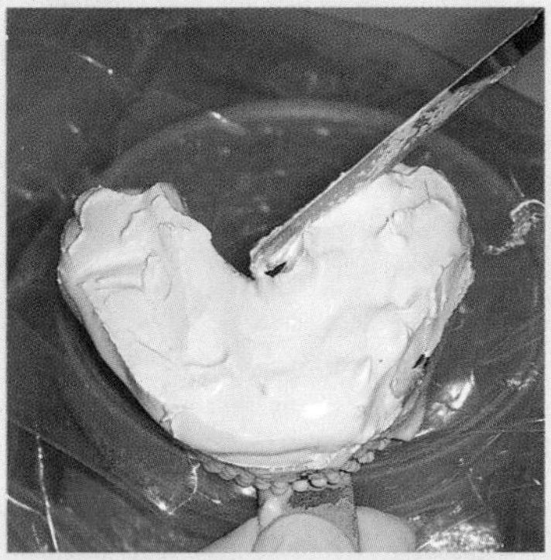

Figure 37-27. Impression filled with large amounts of gypsum. (From Hatrick CD, Eakle WS, Bird WF: *Dental materials: clinical applications for the dental assistant and dental hygienist,* ed 2, St Louis, 2011, Elsevier.)

Pouring the Base for the Mandibular Cast

13. Gather the remaining amount of mixed material together in the bowl.
14. Place the mix in a mound on a Plexiglas square or ceramic tile. Shape the base to be approximately 2 × 2 inches wide and 1 inch thick (Figure 37-28).

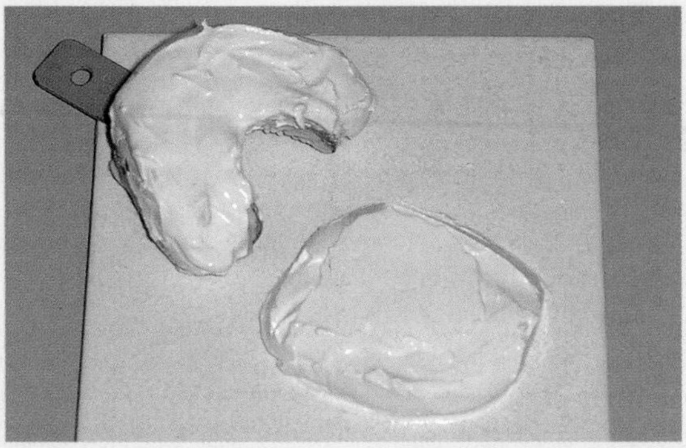

Figure 37-28. Filled impression tray and base on Plexiglas. (From Hatrick CD, Eakle WS, Bird WF: *Dental materials: clinical applications for the dental assistant and dental hygienist,* ed 2, St Louis, 2011, Elsevier.)

15. Invert the firm, poured impression onto the firm base. Do not push the impression into the base.
16. Position the impression tray on the center of the mound to provide a uniform thickness all around it. Position the occlusal plane of the posterior teeth parallel with the tabletop as judged by the handle of the tray.
17. Hold the tray steady. With the laboratory spatula or a moistened finger, smooth the sides around the base onto the margins of the impression tray (Figure 37-29).
18. Remove any excess stone or plaster above the edge of the tray rim.
19. Allow the gypsum to reach the initial set before moving the Plexiglas square or ceramic tile.

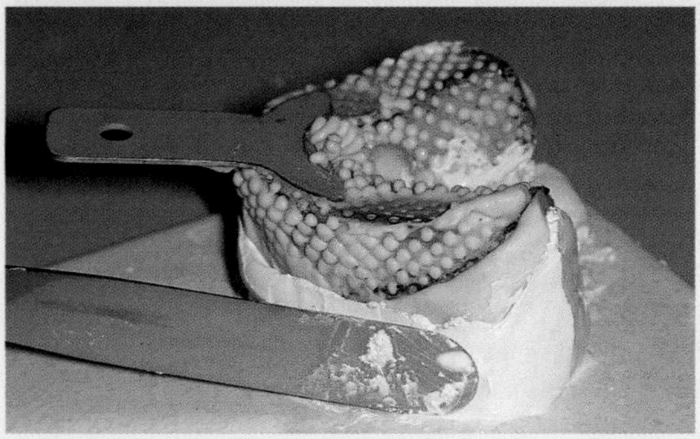

Figure 37-29. Smoothing the plaster base mix up into the margins of the tray. (From Hatrick CD, Eakle WS, Bird WF: *Dental materials: clinical applications for the dental assistant and dental hygienist,* ed 2, St Louis, 2011, Elsevier.)

Pouring the Maxillary Impression and Base

20. Repeat steps 2 through 19 for the maxillary impression to create an anatomic and art portion of a dental cast. Use clean equipment for the fresh mix of plaster.

Separating the Impressions from the Casts

21. Wait 45 to 60 minutes after the base has been poured before attempting to separate the impression from the cast.
22. Use a plaster knife to remove excess material from the edges of the impression tray and to gently separate the margins of the tray from the cast (Figure 37-30).

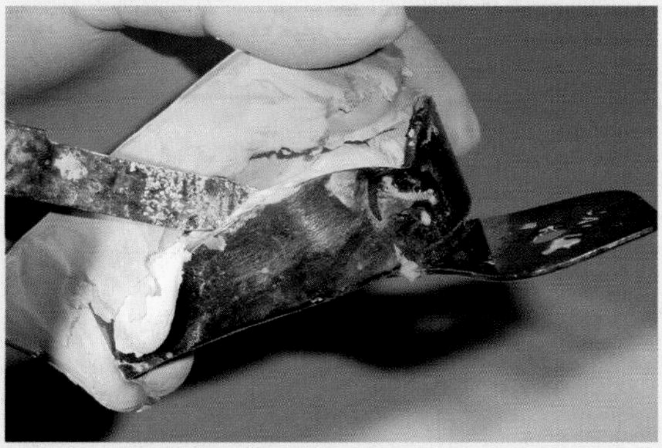

Figure 37-30. Plaster knife used to free tray from stone. (Courtesy Gwen Essex.)

23. If the teeth are in good alignment, remove the tray and impression material together. First release the anterior portion by gently pulling downward and forward one time. Next, make a firm, straight pull upward. Do not apply lateral pressure or rock the tray (Figure 37-31).
24. If the tray does not separate, check to see where the tray may be locked by the gypsum. Use the plaster knife to free the tray from the gypsum.
25. If teeth are misaligned, remove the tray first, and then cut the impression material carefully along the occlusal line and gently peel it off.

Procedure 37-6 Pouring the Cast and the Base—cont'd

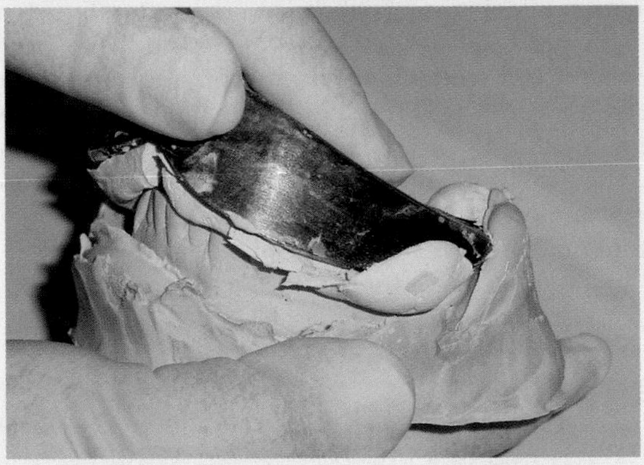

Figure 37-31. Removing impression from cast. (Courtesy Gwen Essex.)

Postseparation Procedures

26. Use a pencil or permanent marker to label the base (bottom) of the model or cast with the client's name. Keep the wax bite with the gypsum models and casts.
27. Store the casts until they can be trimmed.
28. Remove the gypsum material from the vibrator, the spatula, and the mixing bowl, and clean all supplies with cool water.

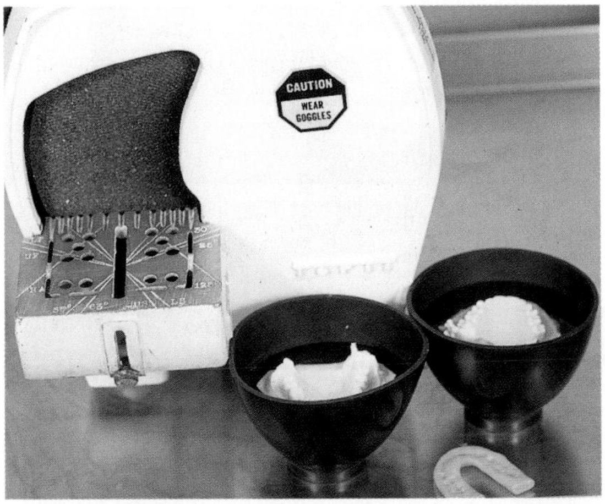

Figure 37-32. Model trimmer. (From Hatrick CD, Eakle WS, Bird WF: *Dental materials: clinical applications for dental assistants and dental hygienists*, ed 2, St Louis, 2011, Elsevier.)

that the teeth of the casts are in proper occlusion during the trimming process. The desired trimming outcomes are to make the bases parallel to themselves and to the occlusal plane, to make the base one third of the cast height, and to make the anatomic portion two thirds of the cast height (see Figure 37-22 and Box 37-5). The reader is advised to refer to a standard dental materials textbook for specific information about the trimming procedure and the care of the trimming equipment.

Custom-Made Removable Oral Appliances

A removable oral appliance is a tray or device that is used for a variety of dental and medical procedures. Custom-made oral appliances are also referred to as *trays, guards, aligners, splints,* and *stents.* In dentistry, these appliances are most frequently placed intraorally for the targeted delivery of materials, the protection of oral structures, the movement of teeth, and the determination of implant placement.

Wearing the appliance is useful for the following purposes:

- The application of fluoride and tooth-whitening products
- The protection of the teeth, mucosa, and bone
- Orthodontic alignment for tooth movement
- The control of obstructive sleep apnea
- The containment of radon seeds as part of radiation treatment for head and neck cancer
- The protection of the teeth during endotracheal anesthesia, bronchoscopy, tonsillectomy, and electric shock therapy
- The protection of the palate during the long-term intubation of premature infants and palatal skin graft donor sites

BOX 37-5

Criteria for the Evaluation of Study Models and Diagnostic Casts

- No visible voids, air bubbles, excess material, or fractures are present.
- The surface is smooth and hard.
- The anatomic structures are visible and account for two thirds of the cast.
- The base accounts for one third of the cast; the tops and bottoms of the bases are parallel to the floor.
- The angles and cuts of the base are accurate and symmetric.
- The cast remains in occlusion when placed on each trimmed side.
- All oral landmarks are present.

Home Fluoride Trays

Home fluoride trays are constructed for the target delivery of topical fluoride for clients with high caries risk, such as individuals who have xerostomia.

Tooth-Whitening Trays

Clients often seek oral healthcare to improve their appearance. A focus on self-image is predominant in the media. Because the smile speaks a thousand words, the appearance of the teeth dominates our image-conscious society, and it is an important factor for meeting a person's human need for a wholesome facial image. Consequently, tooth discoloration and its removal are often the reasons that individuals seek oral healthcare.

Many tooth-whitening procedures require the use of a whitening tray by the client. (See Chapter 29 for dentist-dispensed home-use and in-office tooth whiteners that carry the American Dental Association Seal of Acceptance.) This tooth-whitening tray is a custom-made device constructed in the same manner as a mouth guard with the use of an acrylic material. Tooth-whitening trays are filled with carbamide or hydrogen peroxide gels for tooth bleaching.

However, not all teeth will respond similarly to whitening procedures. Yellow teeth whiten the best, brown teeth whiten less well, and gray teeth may not bleach well at all. Tetracycline stain and fluorosis may be treated with a combination of tooth whitening, microabrasion, and restorative dentistry cosmetic procedures.

Some tooth-whitening systems on the market do not require a tray for delivery. Tooth-whitening strips are a viable option for clients with temporomandibular joint (TMJ) disorder who cannot tolerate trays. Procedure 37-7 and the corresponding Competency Form describes the construction of a custom-made tray. See Chapter 29 for descriptions of in-office tooth whitening procedures.

Procedure 37-7 Constructing a Custom-Made Oral Appliance (A Single-Layer Mouth Guard, a Fluoride Tray, or a Tooth-Whitening Tray)

EQUIPMENT (FIGURE 37-33)

Personal protective equipment
Silicone lubricant
Polyurethane
Mouth guard, 4 × 4 square
Long-shank acrylic burr in a laboratory engine
Matches
Diagnostic casts
Crown and collar scissors
Hanau torch
Vacuum-forming machine
Laboratory knife

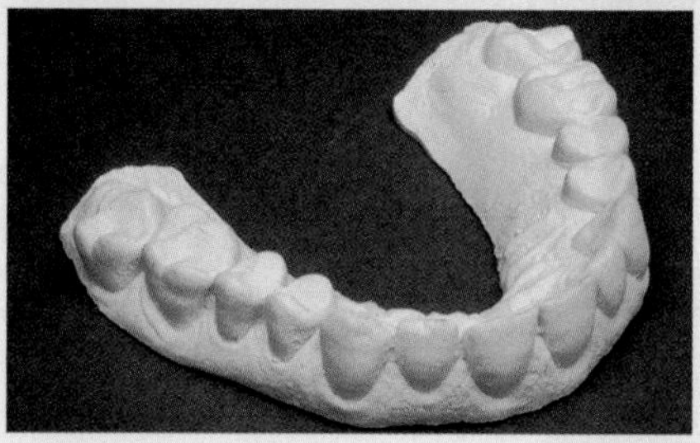

Figure 37-34. Trimmed diagnostic cast. (Courtesy Ultradent Products, Inc, South Jordan, Utah.)

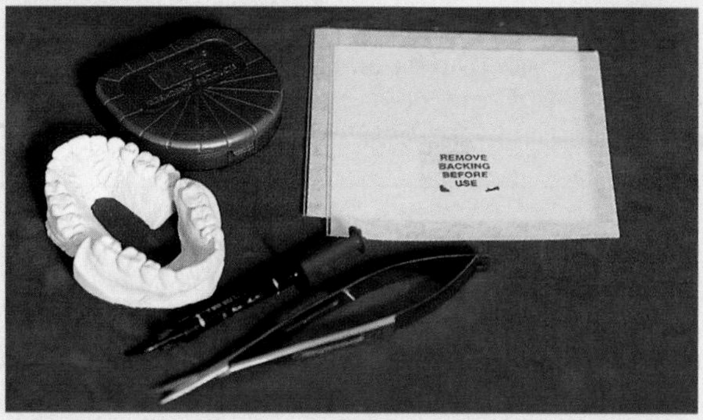

Figure 37-33. Supplies for constructing a custom-made stent. (From Hatrick CD, Eakle WS, Bird WF: *Dental materials: clinical applications for the dental assistant and dental hygienist*, ed 2, St Louis, 2011, Elsevier.)

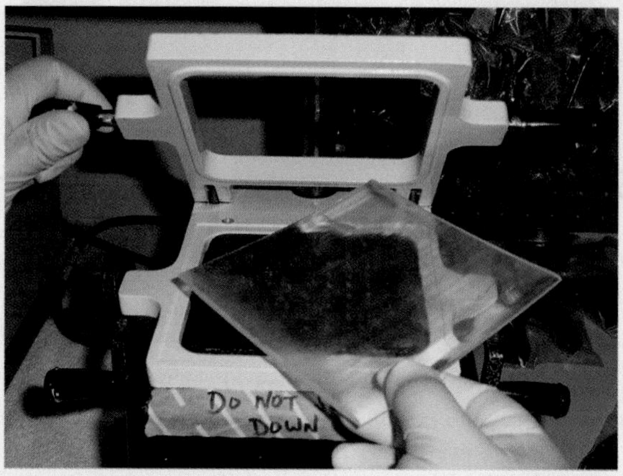

Figure 37-35. Opening hinge and placing mouth guard material. (Courtesy Gwen Essex.)

STEPS

1. Don personal protective equipment.
2. Trim the diagnostic cast so that the base extends 3 to 4 mm past the gingival border and the vertical height is minimal. Spray the cast with the silicone lubricant (Figure 37-34).
3. Place the vacuum-forming machine under a hood fan to control organic emissions.
4. Prepare the machine. The perforated vacuum plate and the sides of the hinged frame must be lightly sprayed with the silicone lubricant.
5. Open the hinged frame, and center the polyurethane material onto the lower frame (Figure 37-35).
6. Close the frame, and secure the frame with the latch knob.
7. Grasp both handles of the locked, hinged frame, and lift it until it clicks into position approximately 3 inches above the vacuum plate.
8. Swing the heating unit to the center position, and turn on the heating element switch at the base of the unit.
9. Center the cast on the vacuum plate. Some units have extra holes at the front and back of the machine; place the cast between these holes.
10. Do not leave the machine unattended. Watch the material as it heats for 1 to 2 minutes and until it sags a ½ inch below the hinged frame (Figure 37-36).
11. Grasp both handles of the hinged frame, and pull it down over the vacuum plate. The material will be draped over the cast (Figure 37-37).
12. Turn on the vacuum motor for 10 seconds.
13. Swing the heating unit out of the way, and turn the switch off.

Procedure 37-7 Constructing a Custom-Made Oral Appliance (A Single-Layer Mouth Guard, a Fluoride Tray, or a Tooth-Whitening Tray)—cont'd

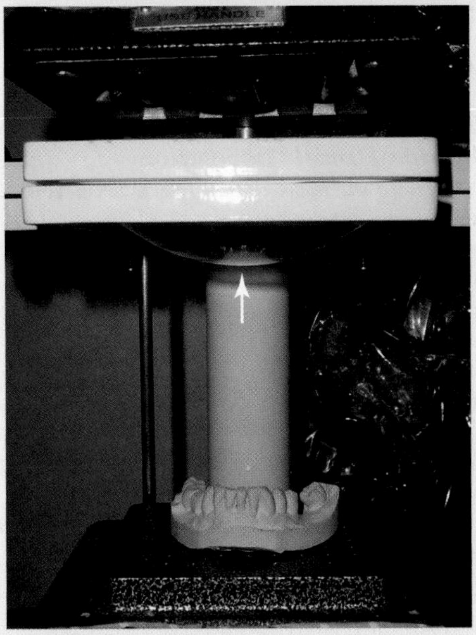

Figure 37-36. Sagging mouth guard material. (Courtesy Gwen Essex.)

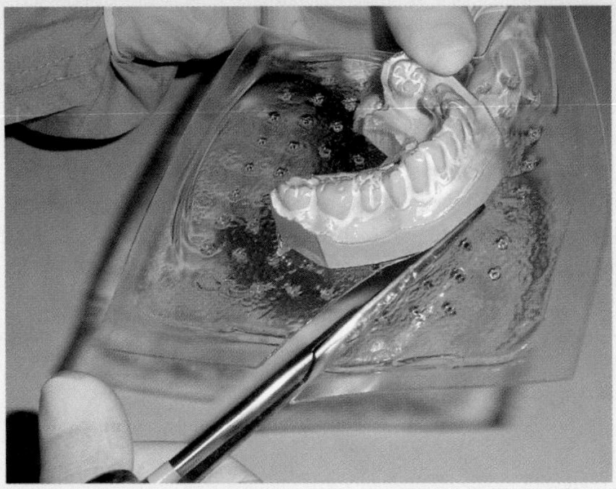

Figure 37-38. Cutting away gross excess material. (From Bird DL, Robinson DS: *Modern dental assisting,* ed 11, St Louis, 2015, Elsevier.)

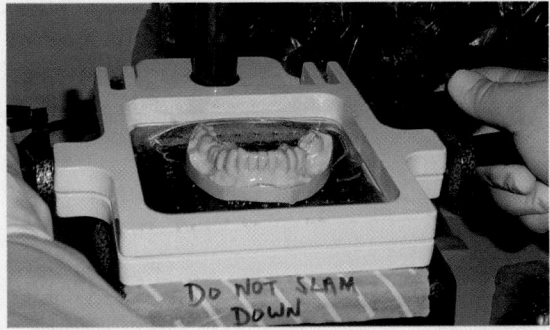

Figure 37-37. Hinged frame pulled over vacuum plate. (Courtesy Gwen Essex.)

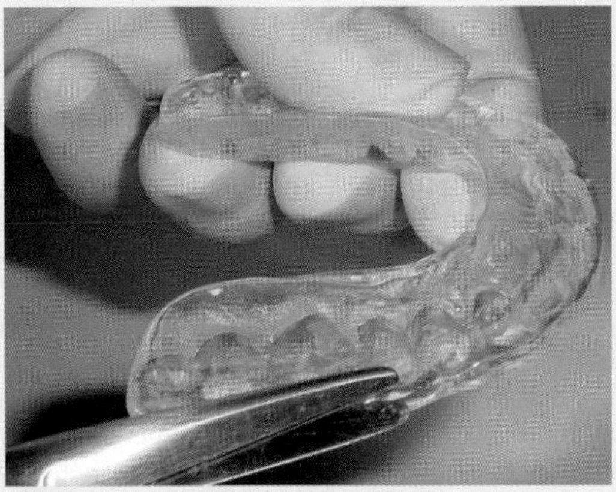

Figure 37-39. Trimming material away from the gingival margin. (Courtesy Gwen Essex.)

14. Turn off the vacuum switch. Release the hinged frame knob, open the frame, and then hold it by the edges to remove it from the vacuum plate.
15. Hold the splint and cast under running cold water for at least 30 seconds.
16. Cut excess material just below the depth of the periphery to remove it from the cast (Figure 37-38).
17. Use small, sharp crown and collar scissors to trim approximately 0.5 mm away from the gingival margin (Figure 37-39).
18. Place the mouth guard back on the cast.
19. If necessary, place a thin coat of petroleum jelly on the facial surfaces. Use a low flame to gently readapt the margins so that they cover the entire tooth, but do not overlap the gingivae.
20. While wearing a mask and safety goggles, trim the mouth guard with an acrylic burr in a laboratory engine (Figure 37-40).
21. Use the Hanau torch to smooth the edges from the peripheral border of the mouth guard.

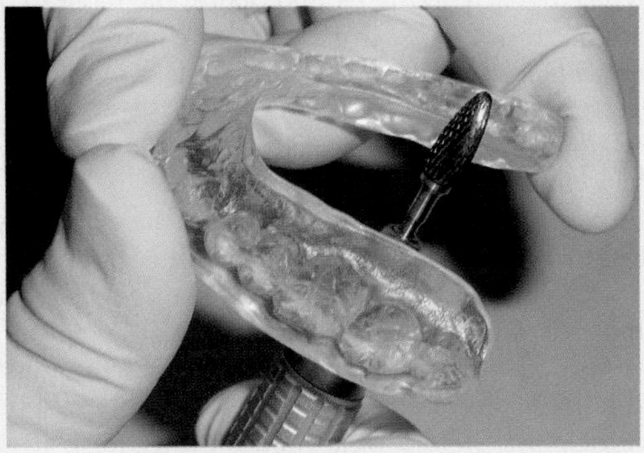

Figure 37-40. Trimming mouth guard with an acrylic burr. (Courtesy Gwen Essex.)

BOX 37-6

Sports Dentistry Facts

Facts from the National Youth Sports Foundation for Safety

- Dental injuries are the most common type of orofacial injury sustained during participation in sports; the majority of these dental injuries are preventable.
- An athlete is 60 times more likely to sustain damage to the teeth when not wearing a protective mouth guard.
- The cost of a fractured tooth is many times greater than the cost of a dentist-recommended and professionally made mouth guard.
- Every athlete involved in contact sports has about a 10% chance per season of sustaining an orofacial injury and a 33% to 56% chance of sustaining such an injury during an athletic career.
- It is estimated that face guards and mouth guards prevent approximately 200,000 injuries each year in high school and college football.
- A stock mouth guard that can be bought at a sports store without any individual fitting provides only a low level of protection, if any. If the wearer is rendered unconscious, there is a risk that the mouth guard may lodge in his or her throat, potentially causing an airway obstruction.

Facts from the American Dental Association and the California Dental Association

- A properly fitted mouth guard reduces the chances of sustaining a concussion from a blow to the jaw.
- Mouth guards should be worn at all times during competition, both during practice and during games.
- Contact your local dental society and association for information about dentists and mouth-guard programs in your area.
- The American Dental Association recommends wearing custom mouth guards for the following sports: acrobatics, basketball, boxing, field hockey, football, gymnastics, handball, ice hockey, lacrosse, martial arts, racquetball, roller hockey, rugby, shot putting, skateboarding, skiing, skydiving, soccer, squash, surfing, volleyball, water polo, weightlifting, and wrestling.

Data from Sports Dentistry Online: Home page. Available at: http://www.sportsdentistry.com. Accessed October 12, 2012.

Athletic Mouth Guards

A **mouth guard** is a protective appliance that covers the teeth and palate and that fits to the depth of the vestibule to stabilize the mandible. Mouth guards help meet the client's human need for protection from health risks.

The wearing of a mouth guard serves the following purposes:

- *The protection of the teeth, the oral tissues, the maxilla, the mandible, the TMJ, and the head and neck from intracranial pressure changes and bone deformation during contact sports.*[2] Blows transmitted to the TMJ during athletic competition can be absorbed and distributed throughout the mouth guard.
- *The protection of the brainstem from shear stress during contact sports.* A properly fitting mouth guard separates the mandible from the maxilla and thus reduces the force transmitted to the base of the brain at the TMJ.
- *The prevention of tooth avulsion.* More than 5 million teeth are avulsed yearly in the United States; the most frequent injuries occur among 8- to 15-year-old children.
- *The prevention of facial bone fractures, TMJ injury, and head injuries.*
- *The provision of an occlusal cushion for protection from bruxism and clenching.*

The American Dental Association and the Academy for Sports Dentistry suggest that a properly fitted mouth guard be worn while individuals play contact sports or participate in nonimpact sports. Nonimpact sports (e.g., weightlifting) require mouth protectors as a result of the clenching of teeth involved in these strenuous sports (see Box 37-6 for sports in which participants should wear mouth protection).[2,3]

Box 37-7 summarizes the types of athletic mouth guards available. The following are guidelines that apply to mouth guards:

BOX 37-7

Types of Athletic Mouth Guards Available

Stock Type

"One size fits all," purchased over the counter, inexpensive, offers the least protection

Boil and Bite

User formed, purchased over the counter, inexpensive, offers little protection

Custom Vacuum-Formed Single-Layer Mouth Guard

Fabricated in the dental office, custom fit, moderately expensive, provides good protection

Pressure-Laminated Multiple-Layer Mouth Guard

Fabricated in the dental laboratory, custom fit, expensive, provides the best protection

- They should be of adequate thickness in all areas to reduce impact forces.
- They should have a fit that is retentive so that the device does not dislodge on impact.
- They should offer full palatal coverage that equals the demands of the playing status of the athlete.
- They should be constructed with U.S. Food and Drug Administration–approved materials.
- The life of the mouth guard should be limited to one season of play.

In addition to preventing tooth avulsion, a full palatal coverage mouth guard worn during sports participation helps to prevent or moderate a variety of head injuries. Concussion is the alteration of consciousness or the disturbance in vision and equilibrium caused by a direct blow to the head, the rapid acceleration or deceleration of the head, or a direct blow to the base of the skull from a vertical impact to the mandible.

Single-Layer Mouth Guards

Vacuum-formed thermoplastic polymers are used to make single-layer mouth guards. These guards are fabricated from one sheet of polyurethane or soft ethylene vinyl acetate (EVA) acrylic; they are custom fitted, they allow for breathing and speech, and they do not deform with time and use. In dental offices, they are the most commonly prescribed mouth guards. These vacuum-formed mouth guards, which are custom fabricated by dental staff or laboratory technicians, are superior to the store-bought stock or boil-and-bite mouth guards. Strap attachments for helmets are easily adapted to custom-made single-layer mouth guards, and the client can select the color and decorative pattern of the mouth guard (see Procedure 37-7).

Multiple-Layer Mouth Guards (Pressure Laminated)

Multiple-layer mouth guards made of EVA are recommended for participants in full-contact sports. Dental technicians in a dental laboratory setting fabricate pressure-laminated mouth guards, which maintain their shape better than single-layer mouth guards. Two or three layers of EVA material are fused to achieve the necessary thickness. At a minimum, mouth guards should have a labial thickness of 3 mm, a palatal thickness of 2 mm, and an occlusal thickness of 3 mm. The mouth guard material should be biocompatible and last 1 to 2 years; however, mouth guard replacement is recommended after one season of play.

Several commercial laboratories fabricate pressure-laminated mouth guards in the United States and Canada. PlaySafe Mouthguards from Glidewell Dental Labs are pressure-laminated mouth guards made from EVA material. One of the following four types of pressure-laminated mouth guards is recommended on the basis of the client's degree of risk:

- Light (two layers, approximately 2 mm thick)
- Medium (two layers, approximately 5 mm thick)
- Heavy (two layers, approximately 5 mm thick, with power-dispersion strips)
- Heavy Pro (three layers, approximately 5 mm thick, with a hard support)

Parafunctional Occlusal Forces

Parafunctional occlusal forces result when there is tooth-to-tooth contact made when the client is not in the act of eating. **Clenching** is the continuous or intermittent forceful closure of the maxillary teeth against the mandibular teeth. **Bruxism** is the forceful grinding of the teeth. Bruxism and clenching are often subconscious habits that usually occur during sleep. Studies indicate that 5% to 20% of the adult population experiences nocturnal teeth grinding. Occlusion discrepancy between centric occlusion and centric relation is thought to be one cause of nocturnal bruxism and clenching. Stress is a major contributing factor to both clenching and bruxism, and it may increase the frequency and intensity of both. Central nervous system disorders such as Parkinson's disease and Huntington's disease can contribute to nocturnal bruxism. Many individuals experience clenching and bruxism, but the degree of either condition determines the sequelae. Box 37-8 lists the possible sequelae of bruxism and clenching.

BOX 37-8

Sequelae of Bruxism and Clenching

- Abfraction lesions
- Exostosis to support the teeth
- Gingival recession
- Headaches
- Impaired hearing
- Limited range of motion of mandible
- Linea alba
- Pain
- Periodontal pockets
- Tenderness of muscles of mastication
- Tinnitus
- Temporomandibular joint disorders
- Temporomandibular joint noise with movement
- Tooth fracture
- Tooth mobility
- Tooth sensitivity
- Tooth wear facets (attrition)

Treatment of Parafunctional Occlusal Forces

The treatment of parafunctional occlusal forces is categorized as reversible or irreversible. Reversible treatment is conservative and noninvasive, and it causes no permanent changes in the structure or position of the jaw or teeth. Most therapies start with reversible interventions, but treatment may progress to irreversible procedures. Irreversible treatment is invasive, and it causes permanent changes in the structure or position of the jaw or teeth.

Reversible Procedures

Appliance therapy is the use of removable oral appliances in a variety of situations. Dental appliances such as night guards and day guards treat bruxism and clenching. Evidence suggests that wearing a night guard during sleep to reduce bruxism and clenching will decrease damage to the teeth and relax strained muscles.[4]

Biofeedback is the use of electromyography to record muscle activity to help the patient recognize when he or she is overusing the muscles of the head and neck. During treatment, the client wears pairs of electrodes attached to the surface of the skin that is in contact with the muscles of mastication. The electrodes transmit muscle activity information to a computer monitor that the client can see to allow the client to consciously reduce muscle tension. Sleep biofeedback therapy involves electromyography-activated alarms, which sound during sleep to awaken the client to stop the habit. Sleep biofeedback can also use electrical stimulation to produce pain during nocturnal bruxism to awaken the patient, thus stopping the bruxism.

Drug therapy is the use of antianxiety, sedative, anti-inflammatory, and muscle-relaxing drugs to control bruxism. When the overuse of the mastication muscles produces muscle fiber changes, methocarbamol (Robaxin) can be injected into muscle trigger points to provide pain relief. Over-the-counter medications such as ibuprofen and naproxen are recommended as nonsteroidal anti-inflammatory agents.

Exercise therapy using isokinetics and the stretching of the mastication muscles can be performed by the client. Reflex and relaxation exercises may also be useful.

Physical therapy procedures may be effective for restoring normal muscle function. Heat and cold therapy using moist heat or ethylene chloride spray may end the muscle spasm and thus the pain cycle. Mandibular relearning therapy helps the client to work on the opening and closing of the mouth.

Psychotherapy from an appropriate mental health professional may be indicated to reduce stress via relaxation, medication, and guided imagery. The antidepressant amitriptyline can be prescribed by a mental health professional. Other stress-reduction strategies may also be recommended for the client to perform before sleep.

Irreversible Procedures

Equilibration therapy is used to adjust the occlusion of the teeth by recontouring occlusal enamel with dental burs. The objective is to create a centric occlusion that coincides with the centric relation. Orthognathic surgery can be employed to improve a skeletal malocclusion. Splint therapy must first be used to reconfirm the effectiveness of equilibration therapy for relieving the client's symptoms. Surgery is recommended only after preliminary orthodontics has eliminated the dental compensations of the malocclusion.

Night Guards and Day Guards

A **night guard** or **day guard** is a hard acrylic appliance that fits over the maxillary or mandibular teeth to protect the teeth from clenching and bruxism. If this appliance is worn during sleep, it is referred to as a *night guard.* If the appliance is to be worn throughout the day, it is called a *day guard.* The purposes of these appliances are to do the following:

- Reduce the clenching or grinding of the teeth
- Minimize the loss of tooth structure (attrition)
- Ease muscle hyperactivity
- Reduce pressure on the TMJ

There are several night guard and day guard designs:

- Full occlusal coverage night guards and day guards are fabricated in acrylic to cover the occlusal surfaces. A night guard or day guard that fully covers either the maxillary or mandibular teeth is the most appropriate design, because the dentist can adjust the occlusion on the appliance. The life span for full occlusal coverage night guards and day guards varies from 3 to 10 years.
- A single-layer athletic mouth guard may be used as an inexpensive night guard or day guard to temporarily change the neuromuscular behavior and produce muscle relaxation in a client with mild clenching and bruxism. This appliance usually lasts less than 1 year. However, the occlusion cannot be adjusted, and the mouth guard can create increased parafunctional clenching and related temporomandibular disorders.

The fabrication of night guards and day guards usually requires two dental appointments. During the first appointment, accurate alginate impressions are made. The alginate impressions are poured in Class I dental stone to create diagnostic casts. A centric relation bite registration is made to enable the placement of the casts on an anatomic articulator that simulates tooth occlusion and TMJ positioning. The articulated models are sent to the dental laboratory for fabrication of the appliance by a dental technician.

Sleep Guards for Sleeping Disorders

Sleep disorders comprise a group of medical conditions. Snoring and obstructive sleep apnea are two sleep disorders that are recognized by the dental hygienist for referral. Snoring and obstructive sleep apnea are treated intraorally with a sleep guard oral splint, which is also called a **snore guard**. Snoring is successfully managed via the wearing of a snore guard appliance. Clients with mild to moderate obstructive sleep apnea have the choice of a snore guard appliance as one of several treatment options. The snore guard is constructed from hard acrylic resin, and it is designed to fit over the maxillary dentition to reposition the mandible. It repositions the mandible to prevent the tongue from obstructing the oropharynx, thereby making it a splint, because it stabilizes the mandible.

Orthodontic Aligners

Many children and adults seek orthodontic treatment to straighten their teeth for cosmetic reasons. Properly aligned teeth and a proper occlusion are beneficial to the client's overall periodontal health. Tooth malposition often compromises the client's ability to clean and maintain the dentition. Malocclusion may cause trauma to the periodontium as it attempts to accommodate the forces exerted on the crown of the tooth. Correcting these malocclusions is important to prevent and minimize the tissue injury associated with trauma from occlusion. The movement of teeth that have drifted can provide improved adjacent tooth positioning before implant placement or tooth replacement.

A new approach to the traditional bracket and arch-wire type of orthodontic movement uses aligners to straighten the teeth. A series of custom-made soft plastic aligners will gradually and gently shift the teeth into place using the movements that the dentist has planned. There are no brackets or arch wires to adjust. The client inserts a new set of aligners approximately every 2 weeks, thereby advancing himself or herself to the next stage of treatment until the treatment is complete. Aligners are worn for 20 to 22 hours per day and removed for eating and home care.

The treatment typically takes approximately 12 to 18 months for adults, and it is comparable in time to that of traditional bonded appliances for teens. This system is not recommended for severe crowding or spacing or when client compliance is a concern. Generally speaking, this system is best suited for adults and responsible teens.

Because the aligners are removed for homecare, the client is able to brush and floss normally for better periodontal health. The smooth plastic aligner eliminates the gingival irritation that is often caused by sharp metal or plastic brackets and arch wires. Orthodontic aligners may be an acceptable orthodontic treatment for adults who are seeking a subtle method to align their teeth and who feel that traditional orthodontic treatment is too embarrassing or disruptive.

Oral Surgical Splints and Stents

Periodontal Splints

Periodontal splints are used for the stabilization of mobile teeth to prolong their presence in the mouth.

Surgical Splints

Surgical splints are orthopedic devices that are used to cover the graft donor site for the protection of the palate after the harvesting of soft tissue for periodontal soft-tissue graft surgery.

Oral Surgical Stents

Oral surgical stents provide communication between the surgeon and the restoring dentist so that an implant is placed at the ideal prosthetic position and angulation.

Custom-Made Oral Appliances and Dental Hygiene Treatment Planning

Factors that contribute to the development of periodontal diseases include those risk factors that cause direct damage to the periodontium as a result of occlusal forces as well as those that increase plaque biofilm retention. The dental hygienist must identify these contributing factors during a clinical assessment so that they can be eliminated or minimized. When these contributing factors are identified, the clinician is able to recommend the appropriate treatment. The recommendation of a custom-made oral appliance may be a valuable component of this treatment.

After identifying the damages that result from parafunctional occlusal forces, the clinician will be able to recommend a custom-made oral appliance that is appropriate for mediating the excessive forces placed on the teeth and the periodontium. Malpositioned teeth increase plaque biofilm retention. The correction of these malpositions with the appropriate appliance will greatly improve the ability of clients to maintain their periodontal health.

CLIENT EDUCATION TIPS

- Explain the purposes of study casts and models and why they are necessary.
- Explain the purposes of mouth guards and why they are recommended for use during contact sports.
- Describe the differences between custom-made and over-the-counter mouth guards.
- Explain the use of a multiple-layer mouth guard to reduce concussion injury.
- Describe the factors that contribute to bruxism and the differences between the reversible and irreversible treatments of bruxism.
- Describe sleeping disorder treatment and appliance care.
- Describe the use of removable oral appliances that are used for the alignment of teeth in orthodontic cases.

LEGAL, ETHICAL, AND SAFETY ISSUES

- In most states, dental hygienists can legally make preliminary dental impressions. In some states, dental hygienists with special advanced function licenses can legally make final impressions. It is the dental hygienist's responsibility to practice within the scope authorized by state law.
- Impression trays can be a source of cross-contamination. They are classified as semicritical instruments, because they become contaminated by saliva. They must be either discarded if disposable or sterilized for reuse.
- Impression trays that are tested for size in the client's mouth but not used for the impression are either discarded if disposable or sterilized for reuse.
- Anything that comes into contact with contaminated impression trays must be appropriately disinfected or sterilized (e.g., spatulas, bowls, measuring devices used for mixing alginate).
- Countertops and other contaminated treatment areas must be disinfected with the use of an Occupational Safety and Health Administration–approved surface disinfectant after the impression procedure has been completed and the client has been dismissed (see Chapter 9).
- After an alginate impression is removed from the mouth, it is biohazardous material. Because such impressions are contaminated with the client's blood and saliva, they must be disinfected according to the manufacturer's recommendations and labeled as biohazardous material before being sent to a dental laboratory.
- The manufacturer's protocol for the disinfection of a dental impression needs to be followed.
- According to Occupational Safety and Health Administration laws, product manufacturers are required to provide written handling instructions called *material safety data sheets*. The warnings listed on such sheets for alginate include eye irritation, congestion, and irritation of the throat, the nasal passages, and the upper respiratory system. Unnecessary exposure to alginate powder should be avoided.
- The hygienist is advised to always read the manufacturer's directions and the material safety data sheets about the gypsum materials used in his or her office.
- Health conditions aggravated by exposure to alginate powder include the lung diseases bronchitis, emphysema, asthma, and silicosis. Long-term exposure to alginate may produce silicosis because of the crystalline silica element of the diatomaceous earth ingredient. Dustless alginate powder is now available. Clinicians must wear a mask when dispensing and mixing the material to protect themselves from inhaling these potentially harmful particles.
- Study models and diagnostic casts are retained as part of the client's permanent record.

KEY CONCEPTS

- A dental impression is used to create an accurate three-dimensional reproduction of the teeth and the surrounding tissues called a *diagnostic cast*, a *study model*, or a *study cast*.
- There are three main types of dental impressions used in dentistry: a preliminary impression, a final impression, and a bite registration.
- Loading and inserting the impression tray should take no more than 1 minute. The objective is for the impression material to reach the gel state in the client's mouth.
- A maxillary impression tray is seated in a posterior to anterior direction to avoid triggering the gag reflex, to prevent the excess material from going toward the back of the mouth, and to move the impression material forward, thereby ensuring complete alginate coverage of the oral structures.
- Stone casts and plaster models are made of gypsum products; stone casts are stronger than plaster models.

- Safety precautions must be used when handling alginate and gypsum materials.
- Baseplate wax and wax wafers are used for bite-registration procedures (i.e., interocclusal records).
- Mouth guards should be recommended to clients who are at risk for sports-related dentofacial injuries. Tooth avulsion, facial bone fractures, temporomandibular joint injuries, and concussions can be reduced by using properly fitted, professionally manufactured mouth guards.
- Signs and symptoms of bruxism include abfraction lesions, exostosis, gingival recession, headaches, impaired hearing, temporomandibular joint noise with movement, limited range of jaw motion, linea alba, tenderness of the muscles of mastication, pain, periodontal pockets, tinnitus, temporomandibular joint disorders, tooth fracture, tooth mobility, tooth sensitivity, and tooth wear facets (attrition).
- Bruxism and clenching are treated with reversible and irreversible therapies. Reversible therapies include biofeedback, drug therapy, appliance therapy, exercise therapy, physical therapy, heat and cold therapy, mandibular relearning therapy, and psychotherapy. Irreversible therapies include orthognathic surgery and occlusal equilibration.
- Sleep disorders are treated in the dental practice with the use of a snore guard. Snoring is reduced while a snore guard is worn as a result of the repositioning of the mandible and the tongue. Mild to moderate obstructive sleep apnea can be treated with the use of a snore guard, which repositions the mandible and the tongue.

CRITICAL THINKING EXERCISES

1. Visit a local pharmacy and an athletic store. Review the types of athletic mouth protectors available over the counter. What would you say to a client about these products?
2. Review the factors that affect alginate and gypsum materials. Manipulate the alginate and gypsum materials by purposefully using the factors in your procedure. What is the outcome in terms of quality?
3. What signs and symptoms are commonly associated with bruxism? Compare these signs and symptoms with those of students in your class who experience bruxism.
4. Joseph is a healthy 27-year-old man who works in an urban setting as an attorney. He has just been diagnosed with bruxism. To prevent any further tooth damage, he was informed about tooth attrition, tooth breakage, and tooth loss. He has opted to have a custom-made night guard constructed. During the procedure setup, he informs you that he is a "gagger." The clinical evaluation of this client reveals that he has an average-sized mouth with maxillary and mandibular exostoses. How would you factor this information into your dental hygiene care plan? Write a care plan for Joseph that includes a diagnosis, client goals, interventions, and methods of evaluation.

REFERENCES

1. Anusavice KJ: *Phillips' science of dental materials*, ed 12, St Louis, 2012, Elsevier.
2. Hatrick CD, Eakle WS, Bird WF: *Dental materials: clinical applications for dental assistants and dental hygienists*, ed 2, St Louis, 2011, Elsevier.
3. Sports Dentistry Online: Home page. Available at: http://www.sportsdentistry.com. Accessed October 12, 2012.

EVOLVE RESOURCES

Please visit http://evolve.elsevier.com/Darby/hygiene for additional practice and study support tools.

CHAPTER 38

Restorative Therapy

Brigette R. Cooper

COMPETENCIES

1. Describe the rationale for restorative therapy.
2. Discuss the collaborative role of the dental hygienist in restorative therapy.
3. Discuss rubber dam isolation.
4. Discuss permanent restorations, including:
   - Compare the characteristics of the different types of permanent restorative materials.
   - Describe placement techniques of permanent restorative materials.
5. Define liners, sealers, and bases.
6. Explain gingival retraction.
7. Delineate the various temporary or interim restorative materials and techniques.
8. Discuss the evaluation, documentation, and maintenance of restorative therapy.

Restorative therapy requires diagnosis and treatment planning by a licensed dentist. Each state's or province's laws delineate the services dental hygienists may deliver, the settings in which they can practice, and the level(s) of supervision required. Typically restorative services provided by dental hygienists and dental assistants are limited to supportive services, in which the dentist prepares a tooth for restoration and the dental hygienist or dental assistant places and finishes the restorative material.[1] At times a special endorsement or licensure may be required for dental hygienists wanting to provide restorative expanded functions creating a recognized subgroup of providers such as a **Restorative Function Endorsement Dental Hygienists, Expanded Functions Dental Auxiliaries (EFDAs)**. In others restorative services are required for entry-level practice for all dental hygienists, or any function not forbidden may be delegated by the dentist to the dental hygienist. Advanced practice dental hygienists and advanced dental therapists also provide restorative care in some settings. The numbers of dental hygienists delivering restorative services are increasing to address access to care issues. Wide variability exists in the extent of delegation of restorative functions to dental hygienists. In some jurisdictions, dental hygienists are permitted to perform a broad range of restorative therapies that includes, but is not limited to, placement and removal of rubber dams; placement and removal of matrices and wedges; fabrication, placement, and removal of temporary restorations; placement of retraction cords; placement of cavity liners and bases; amalgam polishing; placement, carving, and finishing of permanent restorations; and placement of stainless steel crowns.

Dental hygienists provide educational information about restorative therapies. Therefore it is important for dental hygienists to understand the rationale and goals of restorative therapy, the types of restorations, maintenance of restorative dental materials, and the procedures involved in the restorative process.

Rationale for Restorative Therapy

When a client's need for a biologically sound and functional dentition is deficient, the optimal course of action would be to intervene and restore the dentition to a state of health, support the maintenance of health and function, and provide esthetic modification. Restorative therapy includes the restoration of damaged tooth structure, defective restorations, esthetic modifications, and anatomic and physiologic abnormalities. In many cases, restorative therapy prevents tooth loss by halting disease progression. It is used in conjunction with antimicrobial therapy to eliminate the bacterial infection that causes dental caries and caries prevention therapies, such as fluoride, xylitol, sealants, amorphous calcium phosphate, dietary counseling, and salivary aids.

Defective Restorations

Defective restorations no longer restore the dentition to an acceptable state of form and function. Although restorations can be either temporary or permanent, no restoration can be considered truly permanent. Physical properties of restorative materials make them susceptible to alteration and deterioration. Certain materials, however, have withstood the test of time and are recognized more readily for their longevity. When used properly, gold restorations are durable and compatible in the oral environment. Their resistance to corrosion, nonirritating chemistry, and similarity to enamel in texture and wear resistance are qualities that other materials often lack. Amalgam is still a commonly used restorative material in dentistry because of its cost effectiveness, versatility, workability, and clinical longevity. However, masticatory forces and tooth-to-tooth contact eventually could wear the occlusal margins of the amalgam restorations (Figure 38-1). Tooth-colored composite restorations are a popular choice for esthetic reasons, but they shrink slightly during the curing process and require careful technique to obtain desired long-lasting results. Cement materials dissolve in the oral environment, which could result in secondary decay.

Defective restorations, however, may not always be related to the restorative material. Defective restorations also can be caused by the placement techniques of the clinician. For example, overhangs, open margins, poor contours, and open proximal contacts are the result of improper technique, poor

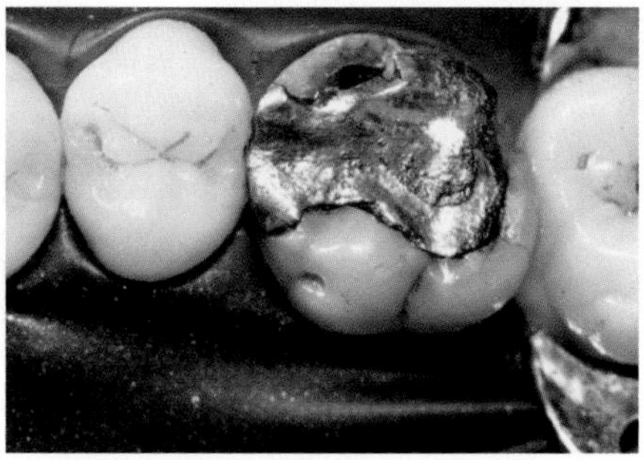

Figure 38-1. Large amalgam restoration, which has served for many years despite its poor design, exhibits defective margins.

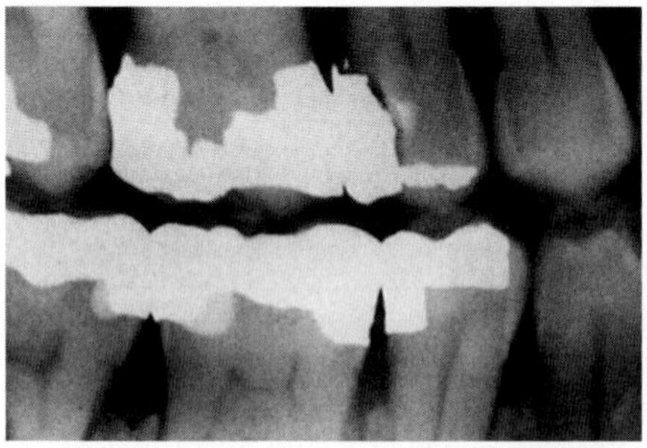

Figure 38-2. This radiograph shows poor proximal contour and a gingival overhang on the distal surface of the maxillary first molar. The maxillary second premolar exhibits amalgam fractures and dislodgement.

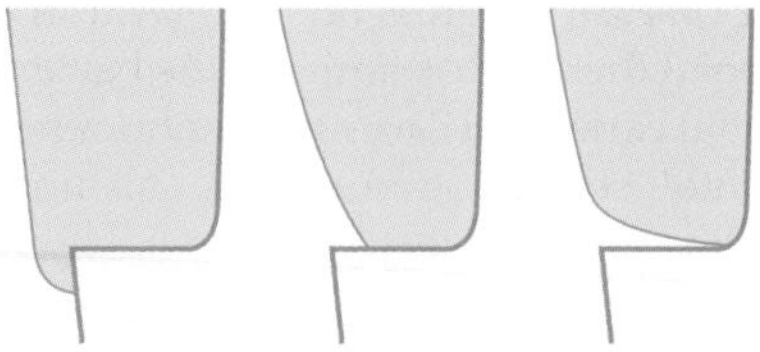

Figure 38-3. Note possible defects at the gingival margins of restorations. It may be possible to remove an overhang without replacing the restoration; however, restorations with short and open margins require replacement.

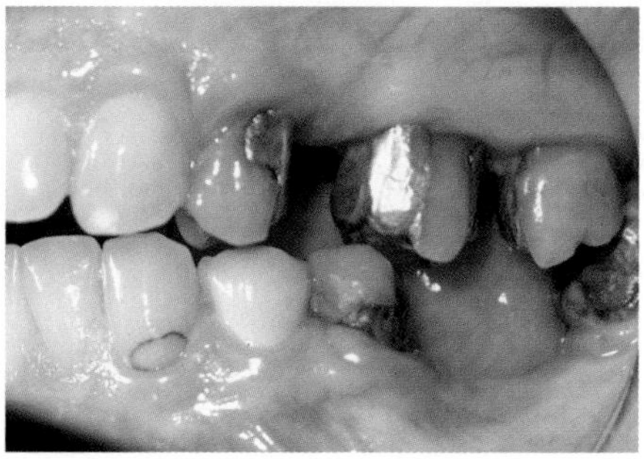

Figure 38-4. Tooth darkening resulting from the amalgam restorations and associated internal staining.

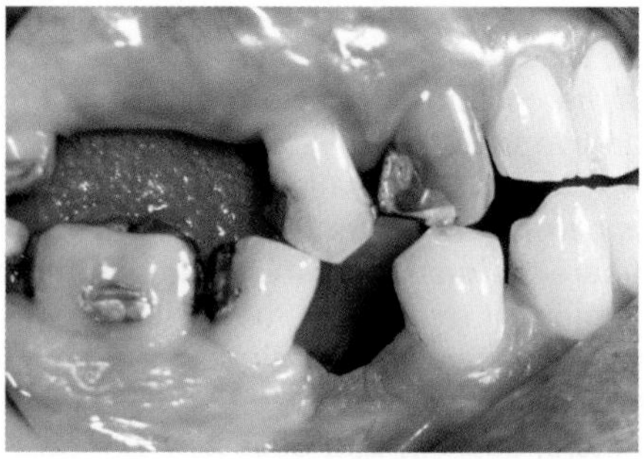

Figure 38-5. Tooth loss has resulted in pathologic occlusion from tooth movement (tip, drift, and extrusion).

judgment, and lack of attention to detail (Figures 38-2 and 38-3). These are avoidable defects and an unacceptable standard of care.

Esthetic Appearance

Restorative therapy is an important factor in meeting a client's need for a satisfactory facial image. Missing, broken, or obviously decayed teeth are often the reasons individuals seek dental treatment. Dental anomalies such as diastemas, mottled enamel, congenital tooth defects, and intrinsic tooth discolorations such as tetracycline staining also may require restorative treatment to improve appearance. One main disadvantage of metallic restorations has been esthetics (Figure 38-4). Many clients are opting for tooth-colored restorations, such as composite, glass ionomer, porcelain, or ceramic, because they have the appearance of natural teeth.

Occlusion

The occlusal relationship influences the function and health of the dentition. Restorative treatment can be provided to improve a client's occlusion. Occlusal adjustment, the selective reduction of enamel, may be indicated to improve occlusion. This is especially true when previous restorations have been contoured poorly. When teeth become misaligned because of the loss of adjacent or opposing teeth, it may be necessary to replace or recontour them to establish a stable, functional occlusion by realigning the occlusal forces to be more parallel to the long axis of the teeth (Figure 38-5). More complex restorations are indicated if the recontouring results in substantial tooth removal. Crown and bridge restorative work may be necessary to restore occlusion in dentitions with extensive damage.

Mastication

The most basic function of teeth is to chew food and thus begin the process of digestion. A significant number of clients indicate inadequate chewing as their chief complaint. Often, frustration exists because certain foods are difficult to chew. Therefore a missing tooth, defective restoration, or carious lesion can compromise an individual's nutrition.

Types of Restorations

Direct Restorations

Restorations are categorized by the technique required for placement of the restorative material. These placement techniques have been classified as direct and indirect. Direct restorations are placed and formed directly in the cavity preparation. These restorations typically are placed in increments, adapted closely to the cavity walls, and shaped to the desired contours. Shaping is completed with carvers when the materials are still in a soft or unset state, and with rotating instruments such as burs and discs when the restorative materials are in a hard or set state. Materials commonly used

TABLE 38-1
Direct Restorations

Material	Primary Area of Use	Main Advantages	Main Disadvantages
Amalgam	Posterior	Ease of placement Minimal leakage over time	Marginal breakdown Tarnish Color
Composite	All	Color Relative ease of placement	Maintaining proximal contact for Class II restorations
Resin-modified glass ionomer	Class V Restorations in primary teeth	Ease of placement Bonds to enamel and dentin Fair color Releases fluoride	Easily abraded Color
Preformed stainless steel crowns	Primary molars Where amalgam may fail Extensive decay or fracture Permanent molars	Longevity Low cost Access to care	Esthetics Temporary for permanent teeth

in direct restorations include moldable substances such as **amalgam**, **composite (resin)**, and **resin-modified glass ionomer**. In addition, **preformed stainless steel crowns** that are adapted to prepared teeth using trimming techniques and crimping pliers are considered direct restorations. Restorative procedures that have been delegated legally to REF dental hygienists fall within the direct restoration category. Table 38-1 outlines the uses, advantages, and disadvantages of direct restorative materials.

Indirect Restorations

Gold and porcelain crowns, inlays, and onlays are typical indirect restorations. Indirect restorations fall within the scope of practice of dentists rather than dental hygienists; however, dental hygienists provide education to clients regarding these procedures, especially when recommended in their dental treatment plan. One technique for fabrication of indirect restorations is to form it on reproductions (dies) of prepared teeth. The restoration is shaped by preparing the desired form in wax and then casting this form in metal or ceramic. Porcelain restorations are formed by building the restoration to shape with porcelain powder and then solidifying the mass in a special "firing" oven. Because indirect restorations are rigid, solid objects, the cavity preparation must be designed specifically to allow for complete seating of the restoration at the time of permanent cementation. Another technique for fabrication of indirect restorations is by computer-aided design and computer-aided manufacture (CAD-CAM), which are prepared chairside using a computer. With a small intraoral camera, the dental professional makes a digital picture of the tooth before and after the preparation. This digital image contains three-dimensional information about the size of the tooth, the defect being restored, and the adjacent teeth. The dental professional then designs the desired restoration directly on a computer screen using CAD-CAM software. Once the pertinent information has been entered, a tooth-colored block of ceramic material is machined by the computer.

Table 38-2 outlines the uses, advantages, and disadvantages of indirect restorative materials.

Cavity Preparation

Black's Classification System and the Complexity Classification System, presented in Chapter 16, are used to describe the type and location of dental caries and dental restorations. These systems expedite communication among those involved in the delivery of dental services.

A critical step in restoring the dentition is the preparation of the cavity. The intent of this section is to present the fundamentals of cavity preparation essential to each member of the dental team. A basic understanding of the principles and instrumentation of cavity preparation supports the dental hygienist as a collaborative member of the team.

(Please visit the website at http://evolve.elsevier.com/Darby/hygiene for additional nomenclature and diagrams related to cavity preparations.)

Principles of Cavity Preparation

Although the dental hygienist is not responsible for cavity preparation in the majority of jurisdictions without an advanced degree or credential, there is value in understanding the systematic procedure of cavity preparation based on biomechanical principles. Cavity preparation typically follows these steps:

1. Establish outline form.
2. Obtain resistance and retention form.
3. Obtain convenience form.
4. Remove caries.
5. Finish enamel.
6. Debride cavity.

Outline Form

Establishment of an outline form provides the framework from which the remainder of the cavity preparation develops and includes removal of weak or undermined enamel and existing defective restorative materials. The preparation

TABLE 38-2
Indirect Restorations

Material	Primary Area of Use	Main Advantages	Main Disadvantages
Gold alloy	Posterior (inlays, onlays, and crowns)	Durability Contours	Color
Porcelain	All (inlays, onlays, and crowns)	Esthetics	Abrades opposing teeth Marginal seal
Porcelain fused to metal	All (crowns)	Esthetics Strength	Abrades opposing teeth Marginal seal
CAD-CAM restorations	All (inlays, onlays, and crowns)	Esthetics Completed in one appointment	Expensive equipment

CAD-CAM, Computer-aided design and manufacturing.

margins should extend laterally beyond the decay or defect into cleansable and sound tooth structure.

Resistance and Retention Form

Obtaining the resistance and retention form involves the shaping of the internal aspects of the preparation to protect the tooth and restoration from forces that result in breakage or displacement. Primary concerns in this step are the extension and direction of cavity walls and the refinement of internal features. The retention form deals with the ability of the cavity preparation to retain the restoration, and the resistance form is important for preventing lateral displacement in more complex restorations. The need for retention and resistance form for composite restorations is decreased because of the bond between enamel and composite material.

Convenience Form

In obtaining the convenience form, the operator enlarges and extends the cavity preparation to enable proper instrumentation for decay removal, thereby providing an optimal final result.

Caries Removal

Depending on the severity of the carious lesion, caries may have been removed in the previous steps. However, if carious dentin remains, it is removed to establish a disease-free environment.

Finish Enamel

At this stage the operator smoothes the walls, sharpens the margins, and removes any unsupported enamel from the margins. This process supports the desired marginal seal between the tooth structure and the restorative material.

Debridement

The final step in cavity preparation is the removal of debris and moisture that compromise the restoration, typically accomplished with the air-water syringe. Each tooth and cavity presents a unique challenge. The severity of the carious lesion influences the complexity of the cavity preparation process. However, these fundamental steps in cavity preparation result in a preparation ready for restoration.

Collaborative Role of the Dental Hygienist

Participation of the dental hygienist in the delivery of restorative therapy affords a unique collaborative opportunity for the dentist and dental hygienist in oral healthcare delivery. The efficient use of the dentist, dental hygienist, and dental assistant allows all members of the team to contribute their expertise, ensuring high-quality, cost-effective restorative treatment. Figure 38-6 illustrates the restorative care cycle that integrates the roles of the dentist and dental hygienist throughout the delivery of restorative care.

The dental hygienist collaborates with the dentist to achieve effective restoration of the dentition. During the assessment phase of dental hygiene care, tooth damage and its cause may be identified and communicated to the dentist. In addition, based on assessment of the client's oral hygiene status and oral health behaviors, the dental hygienist plans, implements, and evaluates oral disease prevention and health promotion strategies for the client.

Delivery of Restorative Therapies and the Dental Hygienist

Originally, the dental hygienist was chiefly responsible for the prevention of oral disease, which explains why today the dental hygienist is recognized as an oral disease preventive and health promotion specialist. However, in the 1960s and 1970s the dental hygienist role began to encompass the delivery of restorative therapies. The primary focus of the dental profession became improving the oral health of the public through the elimination and treatment of dental caries. Therefore the rationale for the initial delegation of restorative services was to provide a mechanism to respond to an expanding need and demand for dental care, broadening dental hygienists' responsibilities.

Because the scope of dental hygiene practice varies dramatically among states, provinces, and territories, not all educational programs prepare dental hygienists to practice in all locations. The dental hygienist has the legal and ethical responsibility to practice within the scope of the law at all times.[2]

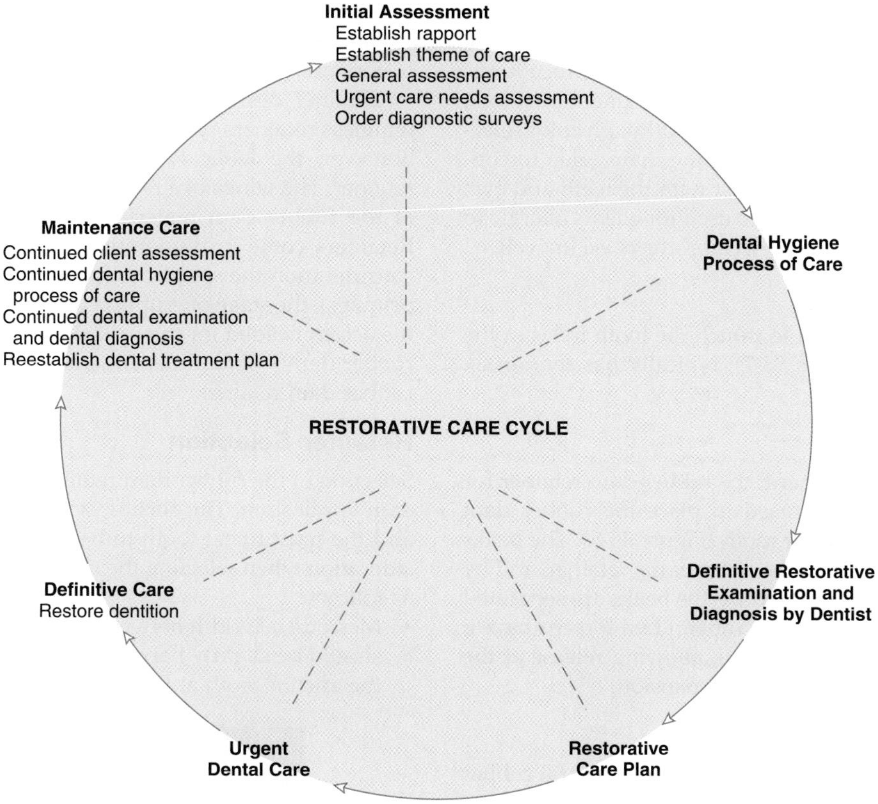

Figure 38-6. Comprehensive restorative care cycle.

Rubber Dam Isolation

Rationale

The purpose of the rubber dam is to improve the quality of restorative dental treatment via the following:

- Moisture control
- Accessibility and visibility
- Client and operator protection

Moisture Control

The moisture-control property of the rubber dam ensures the essential dryness of the operating field. Some restorative materials also are affected negatively when exposed to moisture during placement. The bond of composite resin to the tooth especially is affected by moisture contamination and cleanliness of the prepared surface. Amalgam can undergo delayed expansion beyond the tooth preparation after placement and finishing.

Accessibility and Visibility

The rubber dam provides accessibility and visibility by retracting the gingival tissue surrounding the site of restoration and by retracting the cheeks, lips, and tongue from the field of operation. The background of a dark rubber dam provides excellent contrast with the tooth structure and reduces glare from the moist surfaces of the oral tissues.

Client and Practitioner Protection

The client is protected by the rubber dam because it limits the possibility of aspirating or swallowing debris and materials associated with restorative care. The rubber dam also protects oral tissues from instruments and medications that may cause injury.

Disadvantages

The disadvantages of the rubber dam most often cited are time consumption and client objection. The efficient practitioner overcomes the perception of the procedure as time consuming. The quality of restorations completed with the rubber dam should outweigh perceived inconvenience.[3] Client objections usually can be minimized with education.

Contraindications

Rubber dam application may be contraindicated because of cracks or fissures of the commissures, herpetic lesions, respiratory congestion, claustrophobia, asthma, and latex allergy, although latex-free rubber dam material is widely available.

Rubber Dam Material

Features considered in the selection of rubber dam material are as follows:

- Size (in inches)
- Weight
- Color
- Latex versus nonlatex

The rubber dam material typically is marketed as a 5- × 5-inch child size or a 6- × 6-inch adult size latex sheet. Weights of rubber dam material are light, medium, heavy, extra heavy, and special heavy. The lighter-weight, thinner dams are easier to apply because of flexibility and client comfort, whereas the heavier-weight, thicker dams provide better retraction of tissues and protection from instruments. Medium and heavy weights are used most commonly for restorative procedures. Rubber dam material is available in an assortment of colors, such as green, purple, gray, and pastels. Although color selection is based on operator preference, the main issue to consider in color selection is the contrast with the teeth and eye. Nonlatex rubber dam materials are used for clients allergic to latex or for offices that use latex-free products exclusively.

Rubber Dam Punch

The rubber dam punch, used to punch the tooth holes in the rubber dam material (Figure 38-7), typically has five or six hole sizes.

Rubber Dam Forceps

Rubber dam forceps that expand the rubber dam retainer for placement on the tooth are used to place the rubber dam retainer (clamp) on the anchor tooth (Figure 38-8). The beaks of the forceps are placed into the holes of the retainer, and by squeezing the handles of the forceps, the beaks are separated and the retainer is expanded. The rubber dam forceps have a locking device that may be engaged, allowing release at the handles without loss of the desired expansion.

Rubber Dam Frame

The rubber dam frame is used to secure the extraoral rubber dam material during the procedure (Figure 38-9). Several styles of frames are available to accommodate operator preference; however, the frame must be sterilizable or disposable. The most commonly used rubber dam frame is a U-shaped stainless steel frame with small projections for securing the edges of the rubber dam sheet.

Rubber Dam Retainer

The rubber dam retainer provides intraoral stabilization of the rubber dam material by anchoring the material securely in place. The rubber dam retainer is produced in winged and wingless designs. The parts of the rubber dam retainer include the jaws, prongs, bow, and forceps holes, as follows (Figure 38-10):

- The prongs contact the clamped tooth.
- The bow joins the two retainer jaws.

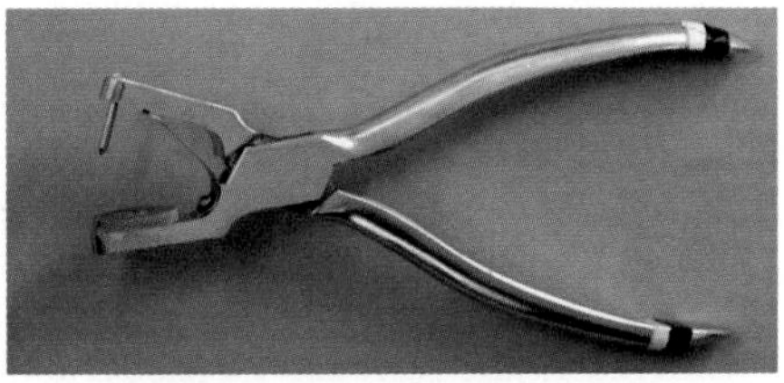

Figure 38-7. Rubber dam punch.

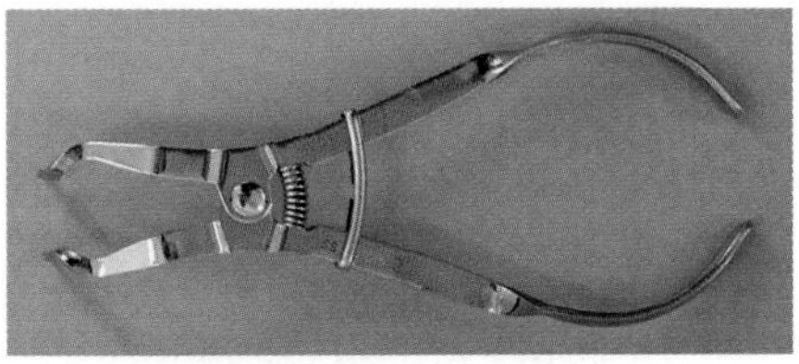

Figure 38-8. Rubber dam forceps.

- The forceps holes are the insertion point for the rubber dam forceps during the placement and removal of the retainer.

Retainer designs are identified by number. Winged and wingless retainers of the same number are identical in shape; however, the letter *W* is used to designate the wingless retainer. The wings of a retainer provide additional retraction of the rubber dam material away from the retainer tooth. Retainers come in numerous shapes and sizes to take into consideration the specific tooth to be retained (permanent or primary), the stage of eruption of the tooth to be retained, and the access needed for the operation (Figure 38-11). Success of rubber dam isolation depends largely on the stability of the rubber dam retainer.

Retainer Selection

Selection of the rubber dam retainer is the next step in rubber dam application. The anchor tooth is the tooth to be retained and the most distal tooth to be isolated. Four points of consideration when selecting the retainer for the anchor tooth are as follows:

- Mesiodistal width between the prongs of the retainer jaws should be slightly narrower than the mesiodistal width of the anchor tooth at the cementoenamel junction (CEJ).

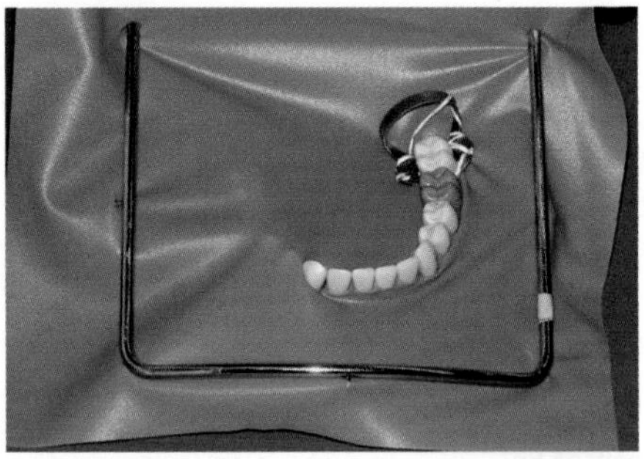

Figure 38-9. The rubber dam frame is used to secure the edges of the rubber dam.

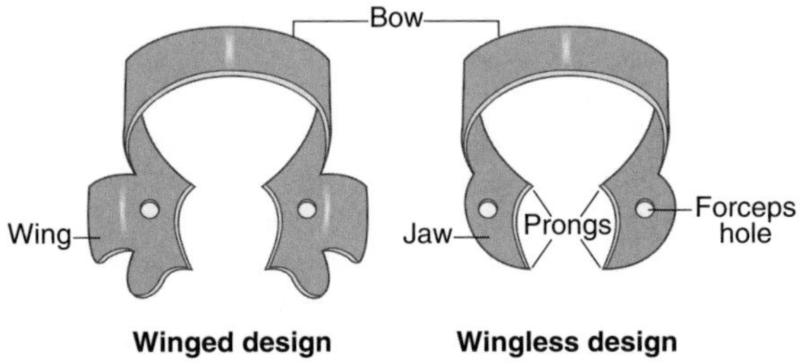

Figure 38-10. Rubber dam retainer design and parts.

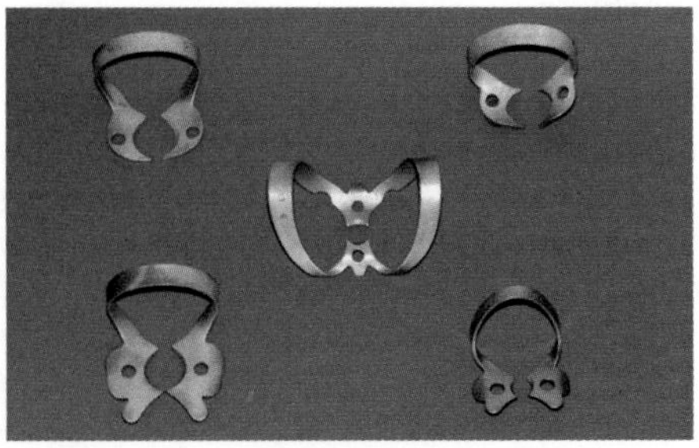

Figure 38-11. Rubber dam retainer variations: wingless molar retainers *(upper left and right)*, winged premolar retainer *(lower right)*, winged molar retainer *(lower left)*, and anterior retainer *(center)*.

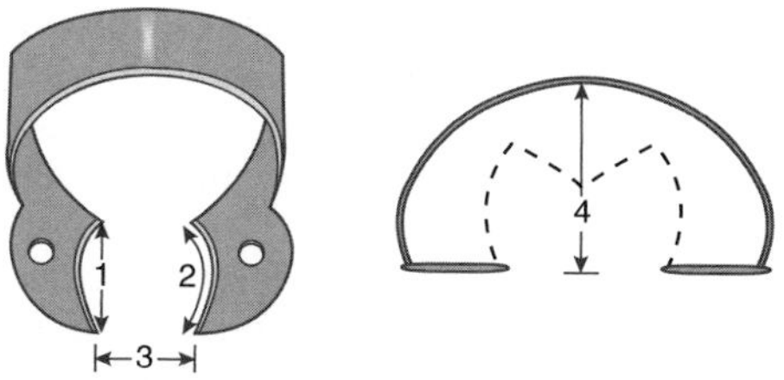

Figure 38-12. Retainer selection criteria: mesiodistal width of the retainer *(1)*; mesiodistal curvature of the retainer *(2)*; faciolingual width of the retainer *(3)*; and height of the retainer *(4)*.

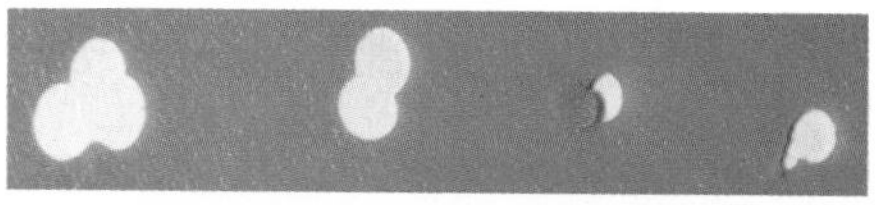

Figure 38-13. As pictured left to right, triple hole, double hole, tag, and tear.

- Mesiodistal curvature of the retainer jaws must be greater than the mesiodistal curvature of the anchor tooth at the CEJ.
- Faciolingual width between the prongs of the retainer jaws should be narrower than the faciolingual width of the anchor tooth at the CEJ.
- Bow of the retainer must arch high enough to clear the occlusal surface of the anchor tooth when the retainer is appropriately seated.

Each of these criteria (illustrated in Figure 38-12) permits the correct and stable seating of the jaw prongs on the anchor tooth. Usually in the anterior aspects of the arches, the rubber dam can be retained successfully without the use of a retainer. Small pieces of rubber dam, or other devices such as wooden wedges and/or floss, can be inserted between teeth to hold the dam in position.

Rubber Dam Material Preparation

Several techniques are used to determine hole placement on the rubber dam. A rubber stamp or cardboard template can be used as a guide for marking the placement of holes for primary and permanent dentition (i.e., marks correspond to the teeth to be punched). As the operator becomes proficient, the template may no longer be needed. The tooth to receive the retainer may require a double or triple hole. The holes must be punched precisely without tags and tears, as the weakened area facilitates further tearing when the dam is stretched over the tooth (Figure 38-13). For clean holes to be punched, the rubber dam punch must be well maintained and free of lodged rubber dam material. In addition, the action of punching the dam must be sharp and determined to avoid tears or tags.

When the dentition is normally spaced and aligned, 3 to 4 mm should be left between holes. Holes punched too closely together cause stretching and inadequate seal around the tooth, whereas holes punched too far apart result in excess material and bunching (Figure 38-14).

Rubber Dam Placement Technique

Two techniques for placement of retainer and rubber dam material are as follows:

- The two-step process of placing the retainer and then the rubber dam material (Figure 38-15)

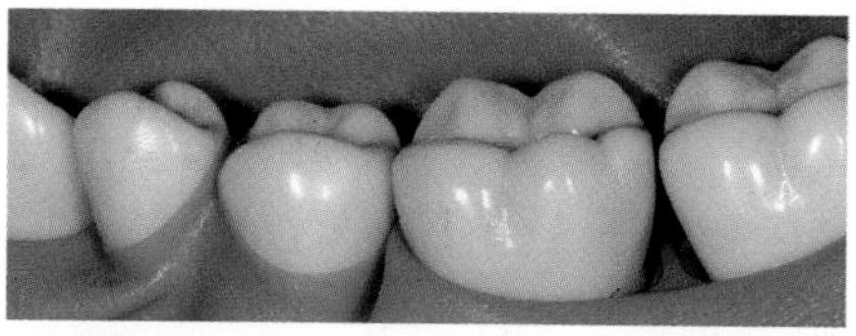

Figure 38-14. Rubber dam problems: dam not through proximal contact between teeth 20 and 21; bunching of the dam between teeth 19 and 20; and stretching of the dam, exposing the gingiva between teeth 18 and 19.

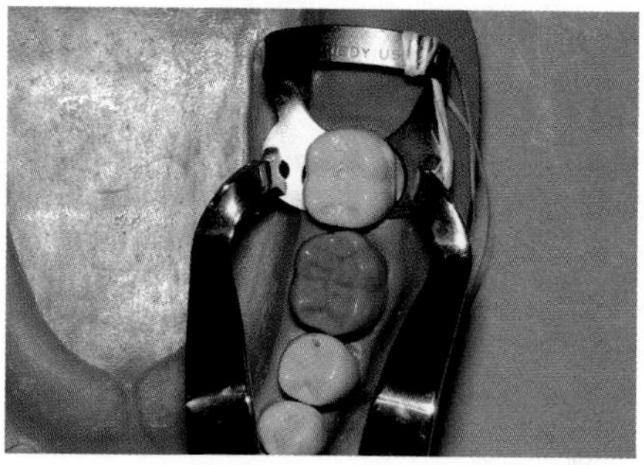

Figure 38-15. The retainer is positioned with rubber dam forceps.

- The placement of retainer and rubber dam material in a single step, which requires that the rubber dam material be placed over the bow of the retainer and then carried to its desired intraoral location

Selection of a technique is best left to operator preference. The remaining steps are identical for both techniques. In a posterior application, the bow of the retainer is positioned toward the distal aspect of the anchor tooth. The anchor tooth is the tooth the retainer is placed on, ideally located two teeth distal to the tooth being restored. The beaks of the rubber dam forceps are placed in the forceps holes, and using a palm grasp, the handles of the forceps are squeezed to separate the jaws of the retainer. The lingual jaw of the retainer is seated first, ensuring that both prongs are in contact with the tooth below the height of contour. While continuing to squeeze the forceps to separate the jaws of the retainer, the clinician rotates the facial jaw over the occlusal surface of the anchor tooth. The jaw then is seated below the height of contour on the facial surface by releasing the pressure on the forceps handles. There should be no rocking or shifting of the retainer when pressure is applied to check for stability, because that would indicate the four prongs of the retainer jaws are not in proper contact with the tooth.

The punched hole in the rubber dam material then is stretched to the lingual side and spread over the lingual jaw; the procedure is repeated for the facial side. The anchor tooth is now the only tooth isolated in the rubber dam (Figure 38-16). A piece of dental floss is tied to the jaw of the retainer to facilitate retrieval should the retainer break or become dislodged (Procedures 38-1 and 38-2 and their corresponding Competency Forms).

Permanent Restorations

Amalgam

Amalgam remains an acceptable restorative material for posterior teeth; this reputation is based on decades of clinical

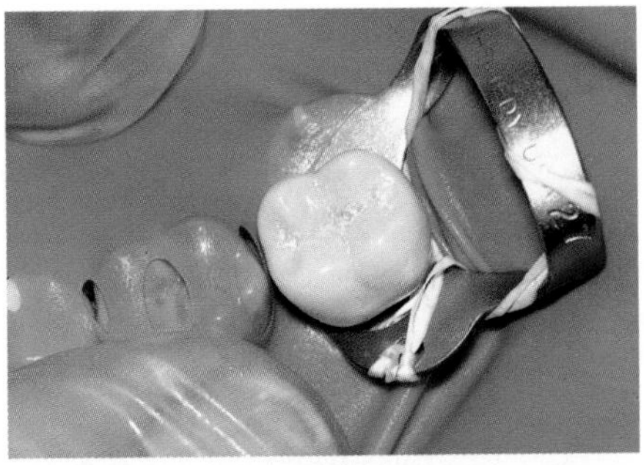

Figure 38-16. The rubber dam hole is stretched to enclose and isolate the retainer and anchor tooth.

evaluation during which it has proven to be a durable material even when placed in compromised circumstances.[4] Its longevity is related directly to proper cavity preparation, attention to basic principles of manipulation, and condensation in a moisture-free environment. Some countries have discontinued use due to environmental or health concerns (e.g., Denmark and Norway). Scientific studies have not verified these concerns without question, and its use is permitted in the United States and Canada.

Material

Amalgam is a compound of an alloy—a mixture of metals, mainly silver, copper, and tin—with mercury. Mercury, which

Procedure 38-1 Applying a Rubber Dam

EQUIPMENT

Personal protective equipment
Protective eyewear for client
Rubber dam material
Dental floss or tape
Rubber dam punch
Petrolatum
Rubber dam retainers
Water-soluble lubricant
Rubber dam forceps
Spoon excavator
Rubber dam frame
Air-water syringe
Mouth mirror

STEPS

1. Explain procedure to client. Instruct client to breathe through the nose after application of the rubber dam and to maintain an open mouth after placement of the rubber dam retainer.
2. Put on protective eyewear and mask; wash hands and put on gloves.
3. Place protective eyewear on client.
4. Lubricate client's lips with petrolatum, especially corners of mouth.
5. Use a bite block to maintain an open mouth position when individuals are unable to do this unassisted.
6. Assess client's dentition and soft tissues. Confirm tooth or teeth to be restored.
7. Remove oral biofilm, debris, and supragingival calculus.
8. If determined to be necessary, infiltrate a small amount of anesthetic solution adjacent to area of retainer placement.
9. Select correct size, color, and weight of rubber dam material for the procedure.
10. Mark holes on the rubber dam.
11. Punch holes as marked with sharp, determined punching action.
12. Select appropriate rubber dam retainer for anchor tooth (see Figure 38-11).
13. Tie approximately 18 inches of dental floss to retainer (Figure 38-17). Tie floss through lingual forceps hole, wrap it around the bow, and then tie it through facial forceps hole.
14. If using the "one-step" placement technique, fixate the anchor tooth hole over the retainer bow before placement in the oral cavity.
15. Seat the rubber dam and retainer on the anchor tooth with the rubber dam forceps.
16. Place rubber dam frame.
17. Isolate remainder of teeth, working from front to back, through the holes; tease small amount of rubber dam at a time through tight contacts.
18. Pass floss through contacts using double floss technique to assist in sliding rubber dam material through proximal contacts.
19. Invert rubber dam material when all teeth are isolated completely and rubber dam is between all contacts. (Any instrument can be used to invert, or tuck, the dam.) Use an air stream to support the inversion process. When the teeth are isolated properly, secure the floss safety ligature to the frame or remove (Figures 38-18 and 38-19).
20. Center rubber dam frame on client's face, with the upper lip covered and nose revealed. If the nose is covered inadvertently, fold or cut the rubber dam at the top of frame to expose the nose. If the client is experiencing nasal congestion or difficulty in breathing through the nasal passage, cut an incision in the rubber dam away from the surgical site to allow air passage.
21. Place saliva ejector under the rubber dam if client reports or exhibits signs of difficulty in swallowing.

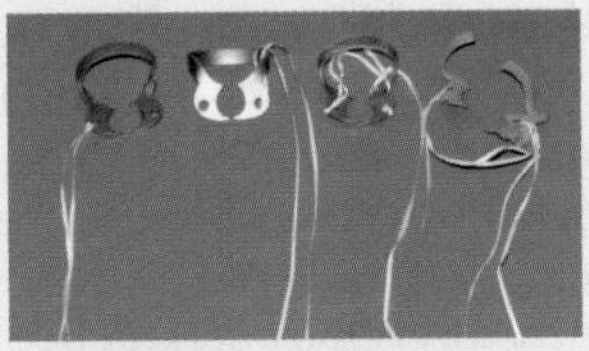

Figure 38-17. Retainer ligation progressing from lingual *(left)* to facial *(right)*, and a broken ligated retainer at far right.

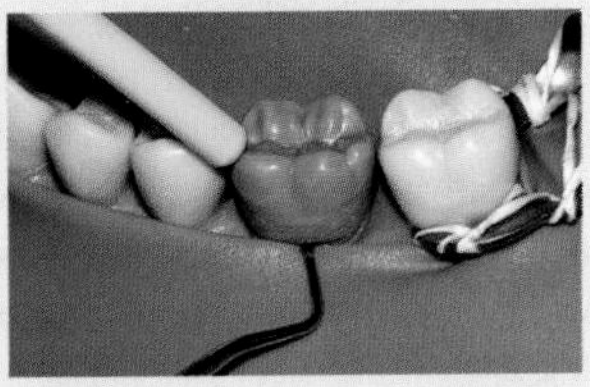

Figure 38-18. The spoon excavator is supported by an air stream to invert the dam and create a seal.

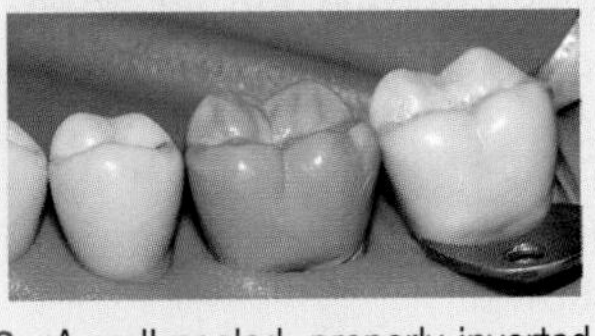

Figure 38-19. A well-sealed, properly inverted rubber dam.

Procedure 38-2 Removing a Rubber Dam

EQUIPMENT

Personal protective equipment
Protective eyewear for client
Scissors
Rubber dam forceps
Dental floss or tape

STEPS

1. Cut safety ligature, if still present. Replace beaks of the rubber dam forceps in the retainer forceps holes, and spread jaws of rubber dam retainer. Raise the facial jaw of the retainer over the contour of the tooth, then raise the lingual jaw to remove the retainer.
2. Cut each septum between teeth with sharp, blunt scissors. On mandibular arch, stretch septa facially to improve access for cutting: place a finger under dam to protect oral tissues (Figure 38-20). On maxillary arch, stretch rubber dam lingually to improve access for cutting.
3. Remove dam and frame together.
4. Wipe client's lips to remove excess saliva and debris; rinse and evacuate the mouth.
5. Briefly massage client's facial muscles.
6. Examine rubber dam to ensure removal of all rubber dam fragments and septa (Figure 38-21).
7. Floss dental contacts to remove any dam fragments as necessary.

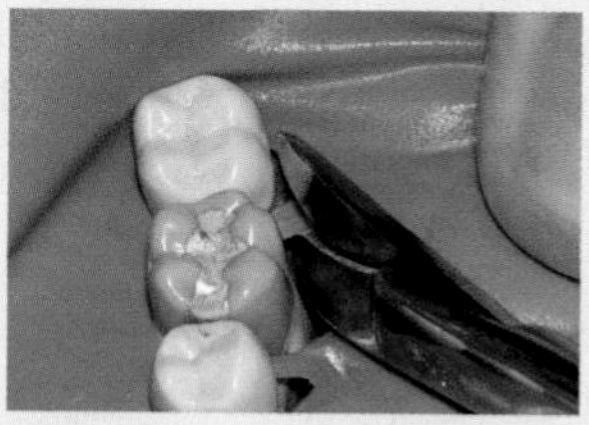

Figure 38-20. Rubber dam is stretched, and septa are cut with scissors.

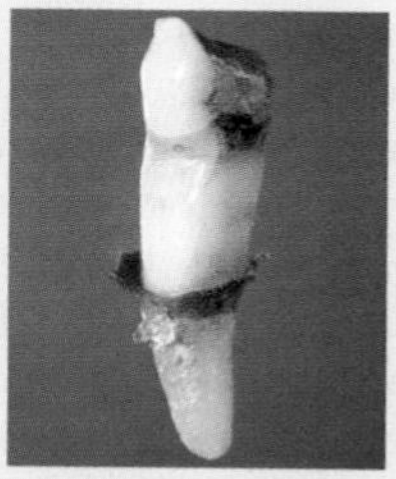

Figure 38-21. Tooth lost to undetected band of rubber dam left after dental treatment.

makes up approximately half of the amalgam mixture, functions to wet the alloy particles, causing the mass to undergo metallurgical changes and hardening. Early amalgams were unpredictable in their clinical longevity and particularly subject to delayed expansion (creep), corrosion, and margin deterioration. New amalgam materials show marked improvement in stability, strength, and margin integrity. Amalgam alloy powders are available with spheric particle shapes for ease of condensation, lathe-cut particles for additional strength, or with a blend of spheric and lathe-cut particles (dispersed) that provides both advantages. Selection of particle type is a matter of personal preference.

Armamentarium

The following equipment is needed for placement of an amalgam restoration.

Triturator (Amalgamator)

The triturator is a mechanical device used to mix the encapsulated alloy and mercury (Figure 38-22). The speed and time of trituration is adjustable to achieve the correct amalgam mix.

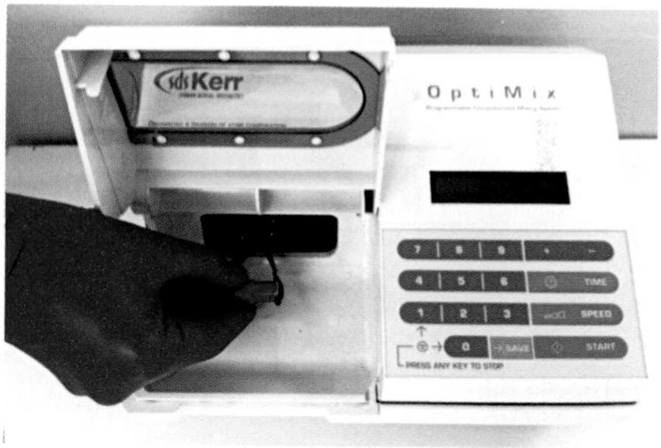

Figure 38-22. Amalgam capsule is placed in the triturator. Mixing time is set according to manufacturer's instructions.

Amalgam Well

The amalgam well is a small, heavy, stainless steel dish with a cuplike recess that confines the mixed amalgam to facilitate pickup with the amalgam carrier (Figure 38-23). Mixed amalgam is transferred immediately from the amalgam capsule to the amalgam well after trituration.

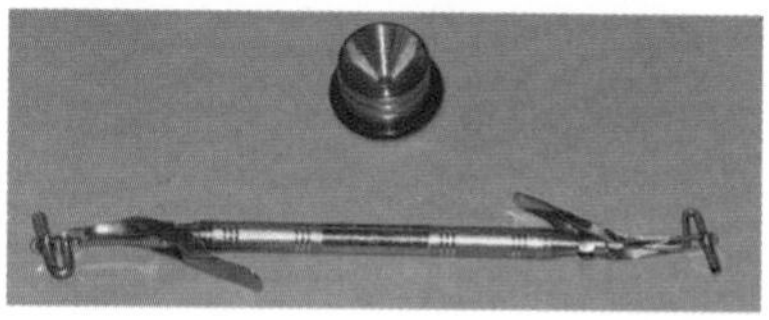

Figure 38-23. Amalgam well and carrier.

Amalgam Carrier

The instrument used to carry and dispense amalgam into the cavity preparation is the amalgam carrier (see Figure 38-23). The operator loads amalgam into the barrel (cylinder) by pressing the barrel tip into the amalgam mass contained in the amalgam well. When pushed, the instrument lever forces a plunger to dislodge the contained restorative material from the barrel.

Condensing Instruments

Condensing instruments are used to pack amalgam and other restorative materials firmly into a cavity preparation. There are numerous shapes and sizes of condensers (Figure 38-24). Selection is based on size and configuration of the cavity preparation and amount of material to be condensed.

Carving and Burnishing Instruments

Carving and burnishing instruments are used to remove excess restorative material and refine the margins of the restoration. All carvers are sharp cutting instruments. Numerous blade shapes and sizes are selected for use based on carving action to be completed and personal preference (Figure 38-25). Burnishing instruments can be ball-, egg-, or acorn-shaped instruments that give a smooth surface to the setting amalgam (Figure 38-26).

Tofflemire Matrix System

The Tofflemire matrix system is a device that reproduces proximal wall(s) removed during the preparation of the tooth. Numerous matrix techniques are available, but by far the most popular and versatile for amalgams is the Tofflemire matrix system. This system is composed of a Tofflemire retainer, matrix bands, and wedges (Figure 38-27). The Tofflemire retainer is a stainless steel mechanical device used to hold the matrix band. After preparation of Class II, III, or IV cavity prep, the matrix does the following:

- Confines the restorative material during insertion, thereby allowing adequate condensation pressure
- Provides a framework for reconstruction and contouring of missing tooth anatomy

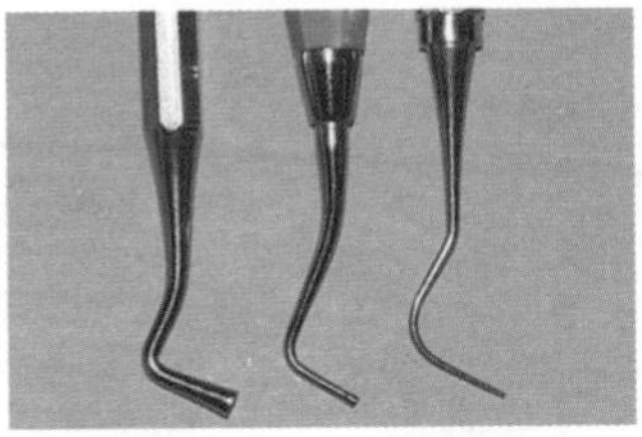

Figure 38-24. Large and small amalgam condensers.

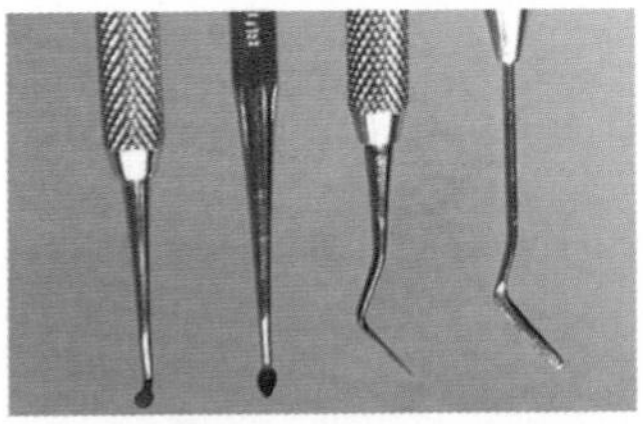

Figure 38-25. Common amalgam carvers. As pictured left to right, cleoid, discoid, 1/2 Hollenback, and Baum interproximal carver.

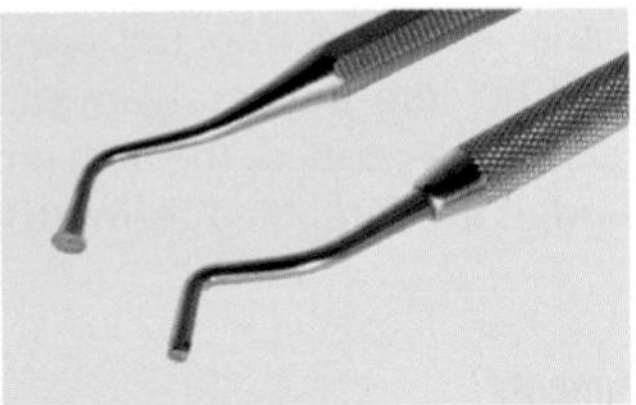

Figure 38-26. Burnishing instruments. (From Boyd LB: *Dental instruments: a pocket guide*, ed 5, St Louis, 2015, Saunders.)

- Supports establishment of proper proximal contacts
- Prevents overhangs

Wedges

Wedges are typically triangular (in cross-section) pieces of wood or plastic that are available in numerous sizes and adaptations. They usually are placed from the lingual side because the lingual embrasure is larger than the facial embrasure, thereby allowing a more complete wedge placement (see Procedure 38-3 and the corresponding Competency Form). A properly shaped and positioned wedge does the following:

- Gently displaces rubber dam and gingival papilla in an apical direction
- Supports the matrix band in the proximal space without encroaching on the contact area
- Adapts the band to the gingival cavity margin
- Provides slight tooth separation that supports the attainment of a positive proximal contact after removal of the matrix band

Trituration

Amalgam materials are pre-encapsulated to prevent mercury spills and provide consistent quality of mixes. Capsules contain small and large quantities for selection according to the cavity size. Within each capsule, a plastic diaphragm separates the mercury from the alloy. At the start of trituration the diaphragm ruptures, allowing amalgamation (trituration) to begin. Thorough mixing occurs within a few seconds, according to the metallurgy of the mass and the speed of the amalgamator. The operator determines the proper setting of the instrument based on the manufacturer's recommendation, the amalgam material, and the desired mix. After amalgamation, the mass is transferred to the amalgam well. Generally, a proper mix of amalgam is shiny, homogeneous, and easily manipulated with the amalgam carrier and condensers (Figure 38-33).

Condensing, Carving, and Burnishing Amalgam

Condensation is the process of packing the amalgam into the prepared cavity. Adequate pressure is approximately 8 lb/inch^3 for lathe-cut alloys and slightly less for spheric alloys. Carving and burnishing is the process of using hand instruments to shape the freshly placed amalgam into the anatomic form that will restore tooth function (see Procedure 38-4 and the corresponding Competency Form).

Finishing and Polishing Amalgams

The purpose of finishing and polishing amalgams is to produce a restoration that can be cleaned easily by the patient,

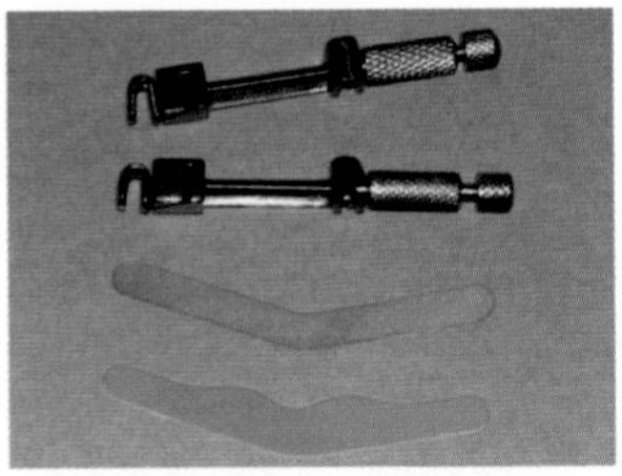

Figure 38-27. Tofflemire retainers and bands. As pictured top to bottom, straight retainer, and modified bands that fit either retainer.

Procedure 38-3 Placing a Tofflemire Matrix System

EQUIPMENT

Personal protective equipment
Protective eyewear for client
Tofflemire retainer
Matrix bands
Wooden wedges
Metal-cutting scissors
Cotton forceps
Modeling compound
Burnishing instrument
Tofflemire matrix system

STEPS

1. Evaluate the prepared tooth.
2. Select a matrix band that best encloses all lateral aspects of the cavity and extends 1 to 2 mm above the adjacent marginal ridge and 1 mm beyond the gingival margin.
3. Select a matrix retainer.
4. Loop band in fingers so that ends match. The convergent opening (smaller) of the loop should be positioned next to the gingiva (rubber dam).
5. Position locking vise approximately $\frac{1}{4}$ inch from end of retainer and free locking screw (spindle) from band slot in the locking vise (Figure 38-28).
6. Position loop in retainer (leading with the occlusal edge of the band); insert matched ends into the slots in the locking vise and the loop into the appropriate guide channel. When positioned, the guide channels of the retainer open toward the gingiva. The loop of band should exit guide channel to allow the loop to be positioned from the preferred side of the tooth (usually the facial side).

   When inserting band into the retainer, first insert the wider occlusal aspect of the band so that the retainer is seated with the slots of the retainer toward the gingiva (Figure 38-29).
7. Secure matrix band by advancing the locking screw (smaller nut).
8. Shape matrix loop into a rounded form: (1) insert an instrument handle through the loop, (2) pinch the band between the instrument handle and your thumb, and (3) rotate your wrist as you pinch the band.
9. Position loop around tooth with slots of the Tofflemire and narrow aspect of band toward the gingiva (Figure 38-30); brace lingual aspect of loop with thumb of opposite hand; gently tighten band by rotating the adjusting nut (larger nut).

   Examine placement of band to ensure that band extends occlusally 1 to 2 mm beyond the adjacent marginal ridge; it also should extend apically approximately 1 mm beyond the gingival margin without impinging on soft tissue.
10. Moisten wedge(s) and place into the lingual embrasure between band and adjacent tooth, slightly beyond the gingival margin. Apply steady pressure on base of the wedge to move it in a facial direction to desired position (Figure 38-31). Numerous pretrimmed wedges are available for selection.
11. Burnish internal aspect of band against the adjacent tooth (or teeth) with a thin, rigid instrument.
12. Conduct a final evaluation of cavity preparation with matrix system in place (Figure 38-32).

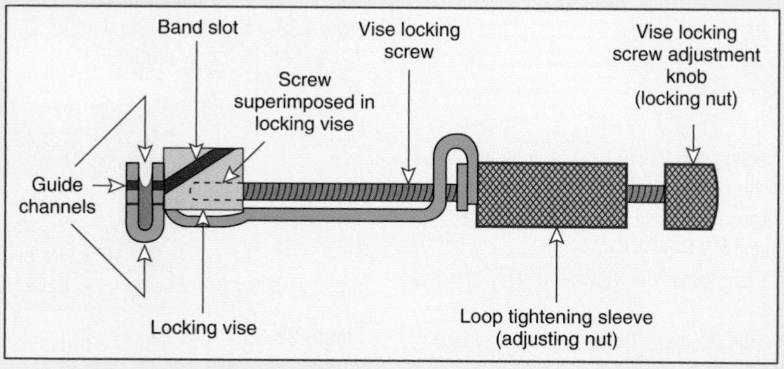

Figure 38-28. Diagram of the Tofflemire retainer.

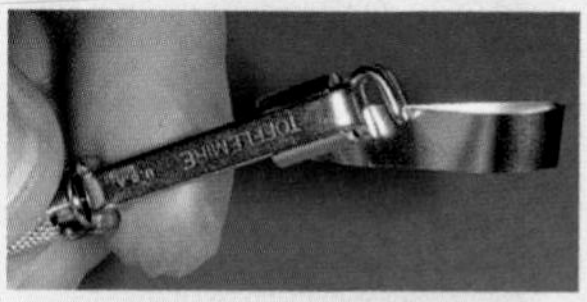

Figure 38-29. Initial placement of band in retainer slot with occlusal aspect of loop being inserted first, followed by tightening of the locking nut.

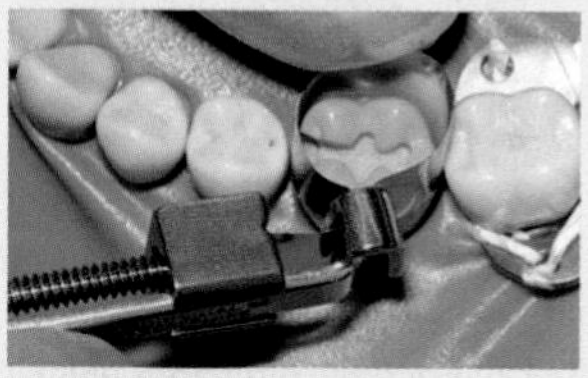

Figure 38-30. Initial placement of band after it has been rounded over prepared tooth. Finger pressure supports lingual aspect of band.

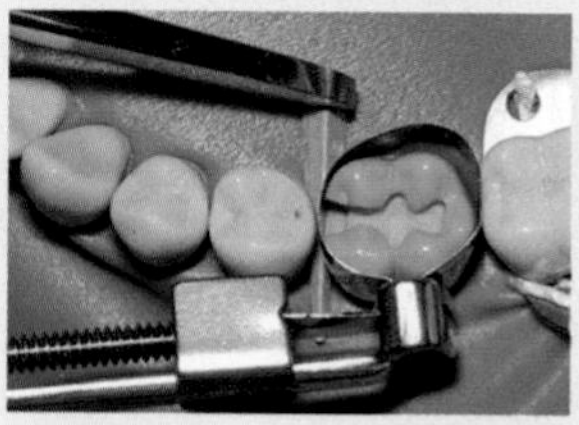

Figure 38-31. After insertion, the handle of the cotton forceps is used to position the wedge firmly.

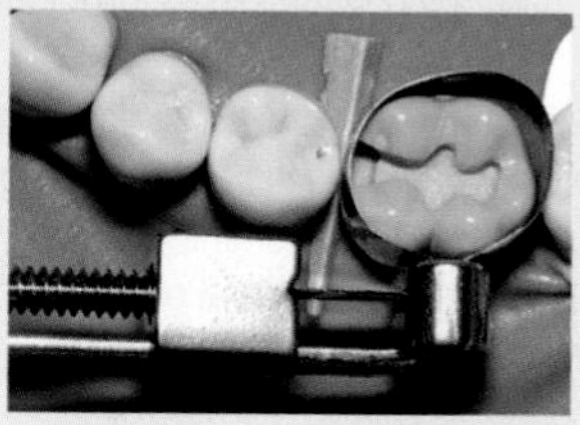

Figure 38-32. Final preparation and matrix system.

decreasing plaque retention. Polished amalgam retains less oral biofilm and resists tarnish and corrosion better than unpolished amalgam. Finishing refers to producing the final shape and contour of a restoration, and polishing refers to abrading the surface to reduce scratches to make a shiny surface.[5] Over time, the amalgam hardens completely and can be polished to a high degree of smoothness; amalgam restorations must be allowed to set for at least 24 hours before rotary finishing or polishing.

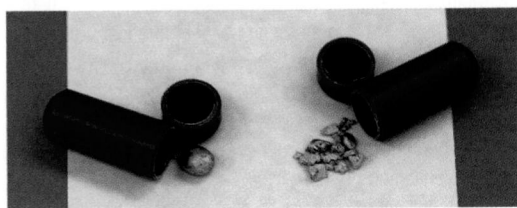

Figure 38-33. Soft, shiny proper amalgam mix *(left)* and dry, crumbly overtriturated mix *(right)*.

In the polishing procedures excess heat must not be generated from rotating rubber cups and points as they contact the amalgam. Such heat can harm the pulp, leaving the tooth very sensitive. The metallurgy of the amalgam also can be affected adversely. A wet field should be maintained whenever heat generation is occurring.

During amalgam finishing, marginal irregularities are removed, and areas of roughness are smoothed. During amalgam polishing, the surface is smoothed to a high luster using a sequence of abrasives from coarse to fine grit. When an amalgam restoration is finished, it must be followed by polishing. If finishing is not indicated, polishing can be done

Procedure 38-4 Placing an Amalgam Restoration

EQUIPMENT

Personal protective equipment
Protective eyewear for client
Isolation materials
Triturator
Amalgam well
Amalgam carrier
Amalgam capsules
Condensing instruments
Tofflemire matrix system
Carving and burnishing instruments
Articulating paper

STEPS

1. Pretest access to cavity by holding condenser nibs in confined areas of preparation to verify accurate condenser selection.
2. Adjust triturator settings for speed and time of mix, according to manufacturer's recommendations.
3. Secure amalgam capsule in triturator locking device; close protective lid.
4. Mix amalgam, then remove capsule; open it over a catch tray and dispense mix into the amalgam well.
5. Examine mixed amalgam; note time, or set a timer for 3 minutes.
6. Load small end of amalgam carrier; dispense a portion into the most confined area of the preparation (Figure 38-34).
7. Using small condensers and a stable hand position, firmly adapt the amalgam into all internal cavity features and over margins (Figure 38-35).
8. Continue to add increments; gradually increase condenser size; remove any "mercury-rich" surface by lateral scooping motions of the condenser nib.
9. Triturate fresh amalgam as needed; continue to add increments and condense, to build a moderate excess over cavity margins (Figure 38-36).
10. Rub and grossly shape the occlusal surface with a few firm strokes using a large ball or egg-shaped burnisher (Figure 38-37).
11. Carve and suction away excess amalgam.
12. Establish marginal ridge height and outer contours next to matrix band by carving with an explorer or similar fine, sharp instrument. Carve excess amalgam away rapidly and recover occlusal margins (Figures 38-38 to 38-39).
13. Release matrix band from retainer by loosening band tightener and locking nut; remove wedges (Figure 38-40).

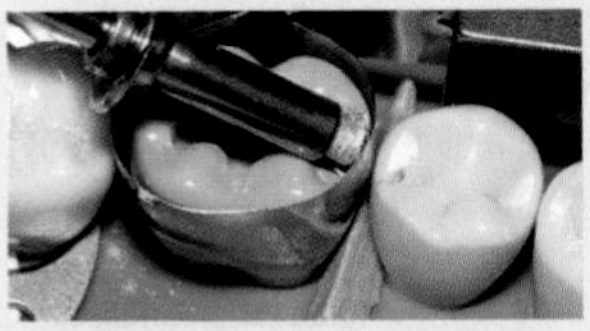

Figure 38-34. Small increments of amalgam is expressed into the proximal box of the cavity preparation.

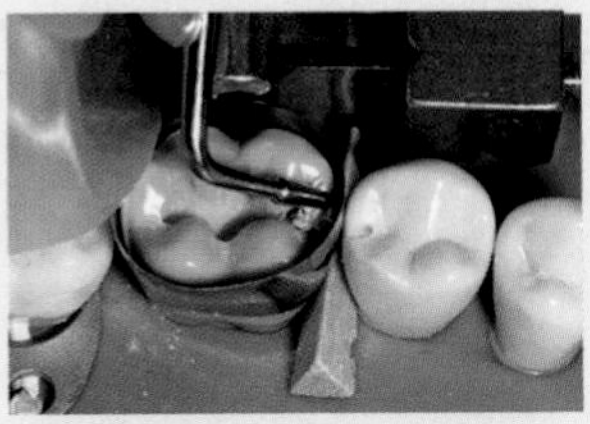

Figure 38-35. Initial condensation is begun with a small condenser in the proximal box.

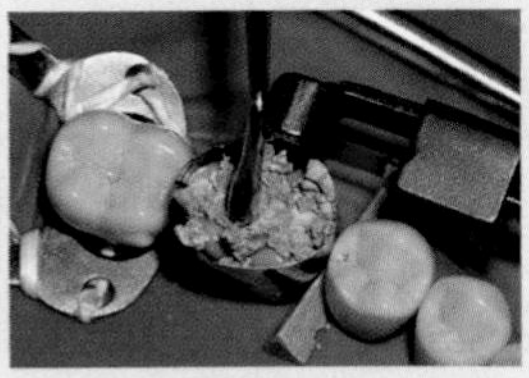

Figure 38-36. The cavity is overfilled with amalgam, and a large condenser is used to complete condensation.

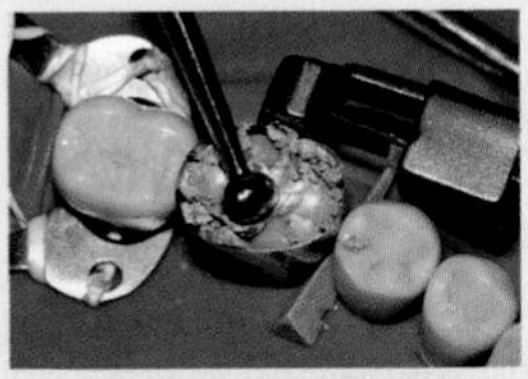

Figure 38-37. Burnishing of the overpacked amalgam.

Procedure 38-4 Placing an Amalgam Restoration—cont'd

14. While maintaining gentle pressure on marginal ridge with a large amalgam condenser, lift matrix band from unrestored proximal area first, then finally from the restored area (Figure 38-41).
15. Explore gingival margin for excess (overhang); carve away excess with a fine-bladed instrument (an interproximal carver) (Figures 38-42 and 38-43).
16. Carve proximal and outer contours to final form. Recover all margins. At margins, all cutting strokes should be directed parallel to margins to maintain a seal and avoid overcarving. Tooth surface is used as a guide by resting the carving edge on it as shaving strokes are made. Carve occlusal anatomy to general form, keeping pits and grooves shallow.
17. Remove rubber dam; caution client against biting at this time.
18. Wipe client's lips; suction mouth to remove saliva; isolate operating site with cotton rolls.
19. Insert articulating paper over area and have client "gently tap back teeth together."
20. Carve away marking spots on the amalgam until centric occlusion is reestablished as it was before the procedure; re-mark the occlusion as necessary, carving away high spots each time with a carver or round bur, if the amalgam has set up (Figure 38-44).
21. Insert ribbon and have client gently grind the back teeth; make sure the client moves teeth in all functional directions. Remove markings until presurgical contacts are restored.
22. Finalize carving and burnish carved amalgam to create smooth finish. Rinse and suction away all debris; caution client to avoid chewing on restored tooth for 24 hours.
23. After putting client in an upright position, have client "tap-tap-tap" again, then look at the new restoration for shiny spots. Repeat procedure; have client grind the teeth for lateral movement. Adjust high spots as necessary.
24. Caution client that discernable high spots should be adjusted to avoid fracture.

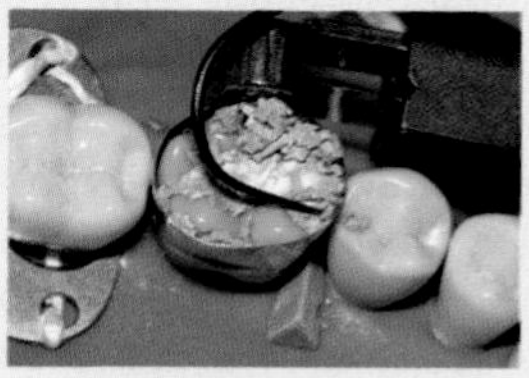

Figure 38-38. Marginal ridge height and outer contours are established with an explorer.

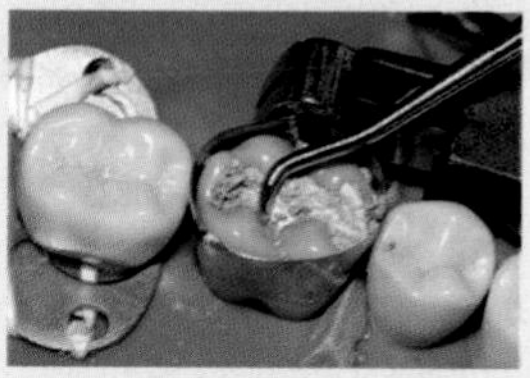

Figure 38-39. Excess amalgam is removed and occlusal margins are recovered with a carver.

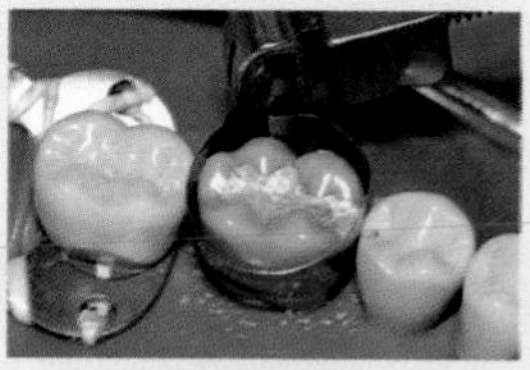

Figure 38-40. The wedge has been removed, and the retainer loosened from the band.

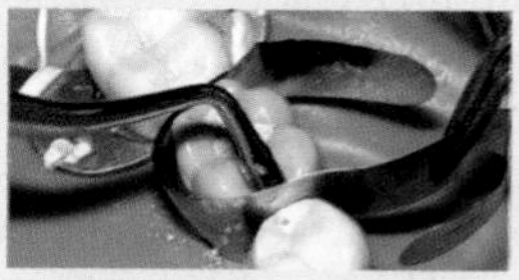

Figure 38-41. An amalgam condenser is used to stabilize the marginal ridge during the removal of the band.

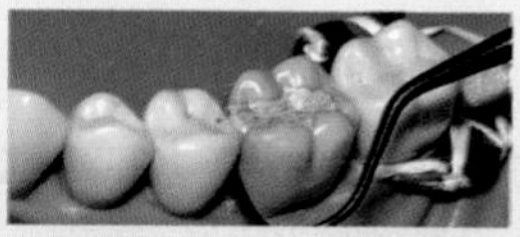

Figure 38-42. Gingival margin is checked for excess amalgam with an explorer.

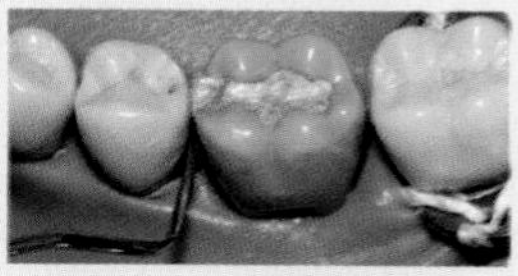

Figure 38-43. Excess amalgam at the gingival margin is carved away.

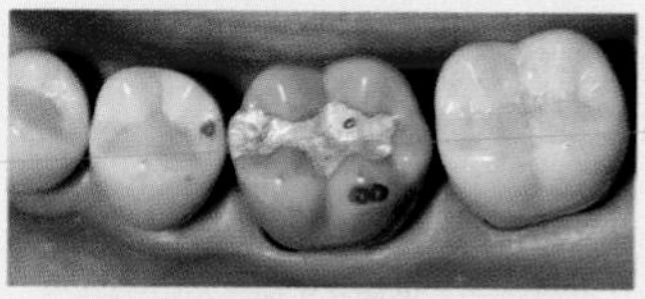

Figure 38-44. The occlusal markings show that the contact on amalgam, although present, is lighter than that on the natural tooth. As a result the operator does not need to further reduce the occlusal contact.

alone. Abrasives used during finishing are coarser than abrasives used during polishing.

Finishing and polishing procedures vary in materials and technique. Finishing the proximal surface may be done with hand instruments or finishing burs, discs, and strips. Hand instruments include dental files, gold knives, and amalgam knives. Finishing disks come in a variety of sizes and grits and are used in a sequence of more abrasive to less abrasive. Finishing strips with fine or medium grit may be used after discs, burs, files, or knives. Finishing the buccal and lingual surfaces also is accomplished by flame-shaped finishing burs or discs. Finishing the occlusal surface may be done with a round finishing bur or rubber cups and points. Moderate pressure is indicated to define the occlusal anatomy and/or remove occlusal excess by beginning at the center of the restoration and working toward the margins. The restoration should appear smooth and shiny. Evaluation of the finishing procedure is necessary before moving on to polishing, because polishing will not accomplish a smooth surface unless the finishing process is complete. Excess amalgam must be removed from the cavosurface margins, occlusion must be adjusted properly with articulating paper, anatomy should be well defined, and the contour of the restoration approximates the original contour of the tooth.

Polishing the amalgam may be accomplished by using a pumice and tin oxide slurry. The slurry mix of pumice and water is prepared in a dappen dish, and using a brush or rubber cup, the amalgam is polished to a smooth, satin appearance. The tooth is rinsed and dried, and a mix of tin oxide and water is prepared. The amalgam is polished with the slurry using a clean brush or rubber cup. The tooth is rinsed and dried, and the restoration should be evaluated for a smooth, shiny finish.

Polishing the amalgam also may be accomplished using rubber cups and points incorporated with abrasive particles. They are available in three colors: brown, green, and yellow-banded green. Each color identifies a different degree of abrasiveness. Some practitioners refer to them as "brownies," "greenies," and "super greenies." The cups are designed to be used on the proximal surfaces and the points are used on the occlusal surfaces. Using a light intermittent touch and low-to-moderate rotary speeds, they polish restorations quickly and are a less messy alternative to the slurry mixes. Brown abrasive cups and points, the most abrasive of the three, are used first to polish the occlusal, proximal, and then the facial and lingual surfaces, followed by decreasing abrasiveness as polishing continues. The green cups and points are used next in the same manner. The final step is polishing with the yellow-banded green cup or point, and then evaluating the restoration for a smooth, shiny finish (see Procedure 38-5 and the corresponding Competency Form).

Mercury Hygiene

Care exercised in preventing bodily harm from mercury ingestion or inhalation is termed **mercury hygiene**. Disregard for mercury's toxic potential may produce injury and disease. However, in decades of use, careful handling of mercury has made its usage in dental amalgam safe. Pre-encapsulated amalgam alloys also have reduced the potential for exposure to mercury.

Mercury Hygiene and Dental Personnel

Individuals primarily at risk from mercury exposure are dental personnel; however, common sense provides a more-than-adequate margin of safety. Safety begins with well-ventilated work and storage spaces and special filters and detectors to monitor mercury vapors. All handling of amalgam mixes should be done over a deep tray to contain loose particles and promote easy cleanup of scrap amalgam. Carpeting in the work area is not recommended because

Procedure 38-5 Finishing and Polishing Amalgam Restorations

EQUIPMENT

Personal protective barriers
Isolation materials
Finishing burs
Carving instruments
Handpiece
Rubber polishing cups and points (or flour of pumice and polishing powders)

STEPS

1. Question client regarding occlusion and tooth sensitivity since restoration was placed.
2. Explain value of polished versus unpolished restoration to the client.
3. Examine amalgam for burnish marks; adjust occlusion as necessary with a round finishing bur.
4. Refine occlusal margins with a sharp discoid carver, drawn in shaving strokes parallel to margins (Figure 38-45).
5. Using low to moderate speeds and intermittent brief strokes, polish amalgam with abrasive-impregnated rubber cups and points (Figures 38-46 and 38-47). Begin with most abrasive, end with least abrasive. Maintain wet field during polishing procedures; avoid overpolishing established occlusal contacts.
6. Rinse mouth of debris.
7. Show client polished restorations (Figure 38-48).

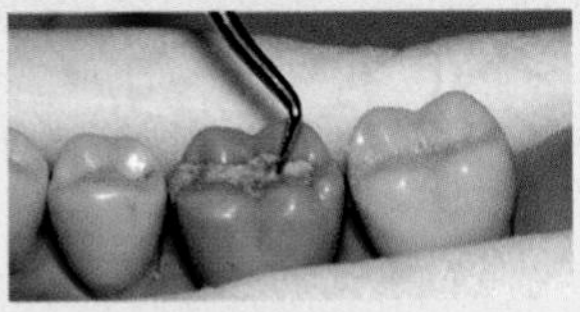

Figure 38-45. Using a stroke parallel to the margin, a sharp carver refines occlusal margins of the amalgam.

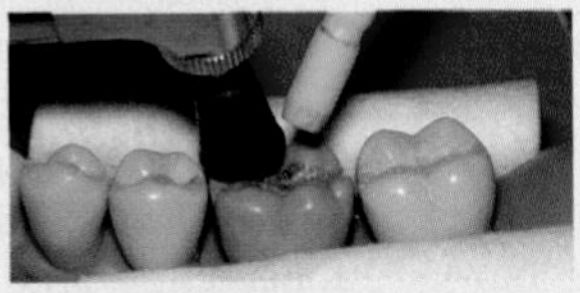

Figure 38-46. A rubber polishing cup is used to polish the marginal ridge and cusp slopes. An air stream is used as a coolant.

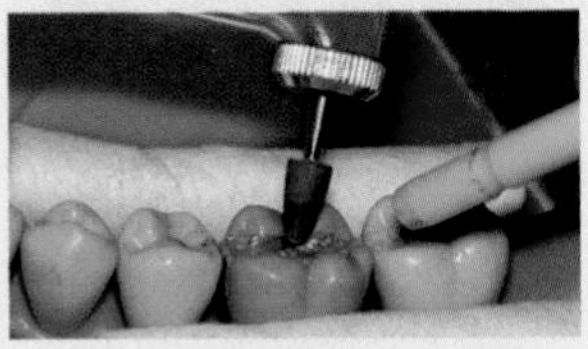

Figure 38-47. A rubber polishing point is used to polish pits and grooves.

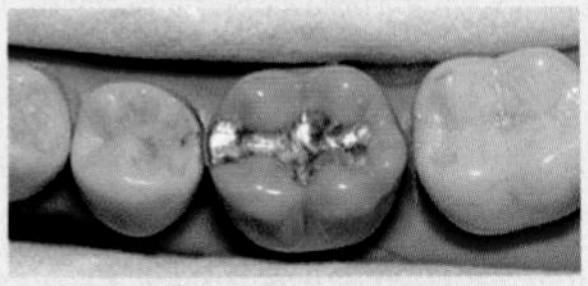

Figure 38-48. A polished amalgam.

vacuuming of scrap amalgam may release mercury vapors. Scrap amalgam should be stored in airtight containers. Disposal of amalgam capsules and other contaminated materials should be done in compliance with state and local environmental and safety policies. Careful examination and cleaning of trays, amalgam wells, chair seams, and other susceptible areas may reveal small scrap particles that should be recovered safely and stored. In addition, evacuation traps should be cleaned routinely and amalgam scrap properly stored. Amalgam carriers should be checked for residual amalgam. The practice of heating a carrier over a flame to soften and remove clogged amalgam should be avoided because the released mercury fumes are toxic.

Mercury Hygiene and the Client

Significant client exposure to mercury is negated by the brevity of the dental appointment and by controlled placement of the amalgam. Rubber dam isolation provides the best control of the working area. All scrap is removed readily when the dam is in place and thorough suctioning of particles is recommended. The combining of the mercury with the alloy prevents the release of mercury in a significant quantity.

Practitioners routinely may restore teeth with amalgam with the assurance that if they exercise reasonable care, no harm will come to the professional staff or their clients. Motivated by myths or half-truths, some individuals have attempted to discredit the benefits of amalgam and the virtues of dentists who recommend amalgam. Claims that dentists are poisoning their clients have not been demonstrated or proven scientifically.[6] Except in the rare case of client allergy to mercury, dental professionals may continue to provide restorative care using amalgam.

Composite Restorations

Composite is a tooth-colored restorative material composed of resin matrix and filler particles. It is a popular choice for many clients and the most widely used esthetic material because many prefer the esthetics of tooth-colored restorations.

Material

The matrix of a dental composite resin is a polymer, usually bis-GMA or a similar monomer. Polymerization, the chemical reaction that links the monomers together, is activated by a chemical reaction or light energy, which is the most common.[7] The matrix forms a solid mass and bonds to tooth structure, but is soft, weak, and prone to wear. It also absorbs water and can stain and discolor. To make a stronger material, manufacturers minimize the matrix content and maximize the filler content. Filler particles are coated with silane for adhesion and coupling, which include barium silicate glass, quartz, or zirconium silicate. They usually are combined with very small-sized particles of colloidal silica. Light-cured composites include a photopolymerizable synthetic organic resin matrix. Radiopaque fillers are added to make the composite restorations visible on radiographs. There are several types of composite materials, most of which are classified by the size and/or type of filler particle such as microfilled, hybrid, and nanofilled composites. Composite resin often is provided by manufacturers in convenient dispensing devices (Figure 38-49).

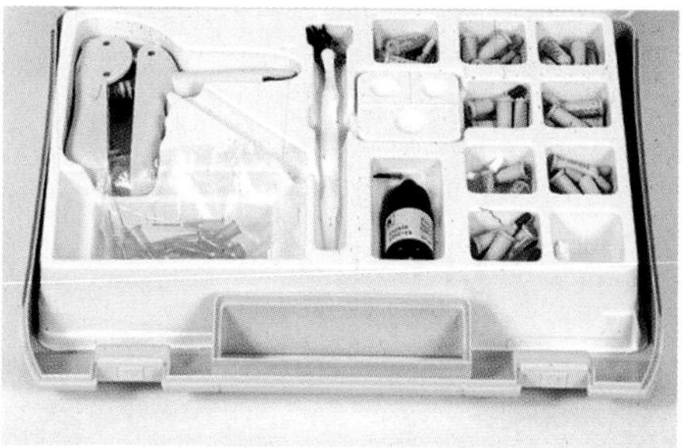

Figure 38-49. Composite kit includes applicator, etchant and bonding agents, and various shades of composite material. (From Bird DL, Robinson DS: *Modern dental assisting*, ed 11, St Louis, 2015, Saunders.)

Preparation

Composite placement procedures and cavity design are unique. Cavity preparations can be very conservative in the tooth structure because retention and resistance form for composites can be created on enamel. This concept, known as micromechanical or enamel bonding, has become the basis for the routine placement of direct composite restorations and for popular procedures such as pit and fissure sealants and bonded veneers. As long as the prepared tooth presents an adequate enamel surface area, significant retention can be achieved. The enamel surface is shaped with instruments such as rotary burs or diamonds to establish the desired design. Application of an acidic conditioning agent to the prepared enamel roughens the surface, known as acid etching. Thorough rinsing and forced-air drying displays the etched enamel as a frosty appearance, which is ready to receive a primer and/or bonding resin and thereby retain a composite restoration.

Compared with enamel bonding, dentin bonding is far less predictable. Most cavities extend into dentin, so the treatment of this tissue surface is in question. Lack of inorganic structure results in a weaker bond to organic collagen fibrils. The composition of dentin presents special challenges for those attempting to bond to it. Dentin is more organic than enamel and when instrumented leaves a surface covered with microscopically observable debris called the smear layer. This smear layer may interfere with strong bonding at the dentin-composite interface. In addition, a trace amount of moisture from the vital pulp is present on the dentin surface. Because restorative resins are incompatible with moisture (hydrophobic), numerous adhesive systems (hydrophilic) have been developed to unite chemically the composite with the moist dentin surface. Hybridization bonding is the bond between the dentin and the composite, and success in this area continues to be made.

Armamentarium

The following equipment is needed to place a composite.

Curing Light

A curing light is required to initiate polymerization of the resin matrix. Types of curing lights include quartz tungsten halogen, plasma arc, argon laser, and light-emission diode (LED). The light is in the blue range and is transmitted from its electrical source via a fiberoptic bundle to the tip of a small wand that is positioned on the tooth surface (Figure 38-50).

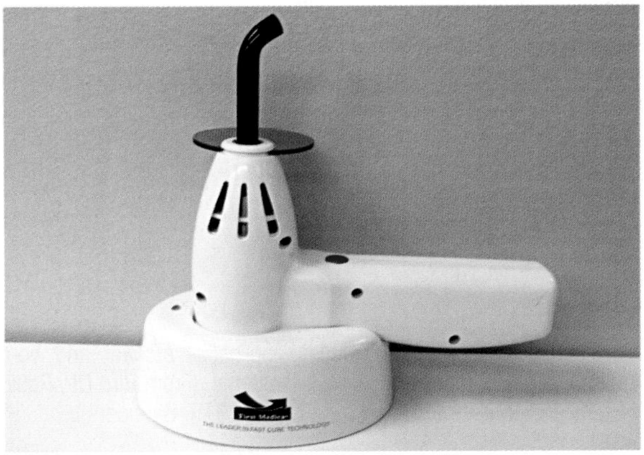

Figure 38-50. A light source for polymerization.

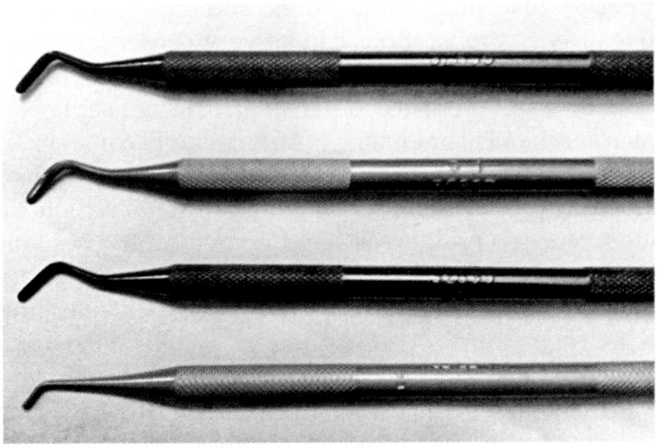

Figure 38-51. Common plastic instruments.

An intensity of 400 mW/cm^2 or higher is considered adequate. The wavelengths produced by the curing light have been shown to damage the retina and must be screened to protect the operator and assistant. Protective shields for screening typically are attached to the wand.

Plastic Instruments

Plastic instruments are designed conveniently to carry, shape, and mold soft (plastic) materials. They may be blunt-ended instruments or flat blades not intended for firm condensation or cutting (Figure 38-51). Selection of instruments is based on the location of the cavity preparation and personal preference. Anodized instruments have been developed specifically to facilitate placement of sticky, tooth-colored materials without adherence to the instrument.

Tofflemire Matrix and Wedge or Ring System

For Class II composite restorations, like amalgam restorations, a matrix and wedge are needed to restore anatomic proximal contours and contact areas. Composite materials differ from amalgam in relation to their ability to establish a proximal contact. Amalgam can be condensed against a metal matrix and maintain its shape to create a proximal contact. If a traditional Tofflemire retainer is used, a thinner matrix band (Ho band or dead soft band) is preferred for enhanced flexibility and malleability (0.001 mm rather than 0.002 mm or 0.015 mm used for amalgam) to restore contour and contact. Alternatively a sectional matrix system designed for

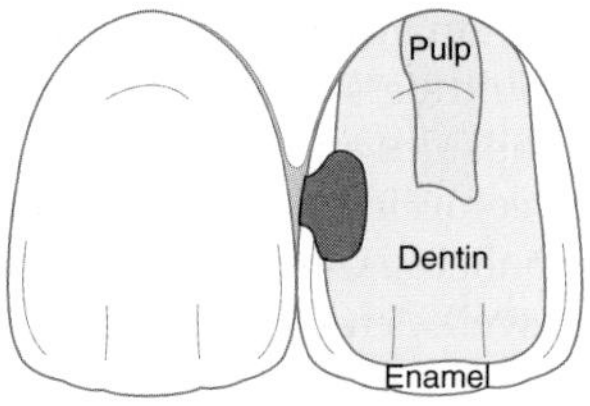

Figure 38-52. Class III carious lesion depicted. Caries is shown invading the dentin, but the cavity does not endanger the incisal corner.

composites may be used in combination with a ring. The ring establishes additional tooth separation during placement of the composite resin material in the proximal area. Proximal contacts with a sectional matrix system and separation rings result in tighter proximal contacts.[8] Several companies make posterior composite matrix band systems.

Composite Restoration Placement

Client demands for natural-looking teeth have resulted in use of composites for restoring anterior and posterior teeth. Placing composite restorations is extremely technique sensitive. In addition to the need for careful isolation and moisture control, accurate manipulation of the matrix band for Class II, III, and IV restorations, and preferably a sectional matrix band with a ring system for Class II restorations, is critical.[9] Establishing a proximal contact that is contoured physiologically is one of the biggest challenges facing the clinician. To place a composite, the clinician must first select the desired shade of composite and then place a rubber dam for optimal moisture control. After etching, rinsing, and drying the prepared cavity following the manufacturer's instructions, the practitioner covers the preparation with one or more coats of a priming agent and lightly air dries it. Next, the bonding resin is spread gently over the internal surface, lightly air dried, and cured for 15 to 20 seconds. This is followed by incremental placement and curing of the composite. Contour can be developed by pressing the final increments into place with an instrument tip that has been dipped in bonding resin to prevent adhesion to the composite. This procedure produces a smooth, contoured surface that requires a minimum of finishing. After the final curing, shaping and polishing are accomplished with finishing burs and discs, if necessary.

A typical Class III carious lesion is illustrated in Figure 38-52. The preparation is made with emphasis on conservatism in outline form. The plastic nature of the composite material allows it to be placed under virtually no force, and specifically designed instruments are available for placement and finishing. In the maxillary anteriors, access is usually from the lingual direction, and care is taken to preserve the marginal ridge whenever possible. In deep restorations, dentin coverage with glass ionomer helps decrease microleakage and the possibility of sensitivity by bacterial invasion (Figure 38-53; see Procedure 38-6 and the corresponding Competency Form). Class II carious lesions usually are detected on radiographs because of their proximal location. Although Class II composite restorations are challenging to place and technique sensitive, clients frequently prefer them because they are tooth colored and more esthetic than other types of direct restorations. Procedure 38-7 outline placement and finishing techniques for Class II composite restorations.

A challenging problem in restorative dentistry is the treatment of decay at the gingival margin. Abrasion, erosion, dental caries, or combinations of these can create defects that are difficult to restore properly and often require isolation with special rubber dam retainers, because they frequently extend into the gingival sulcus.

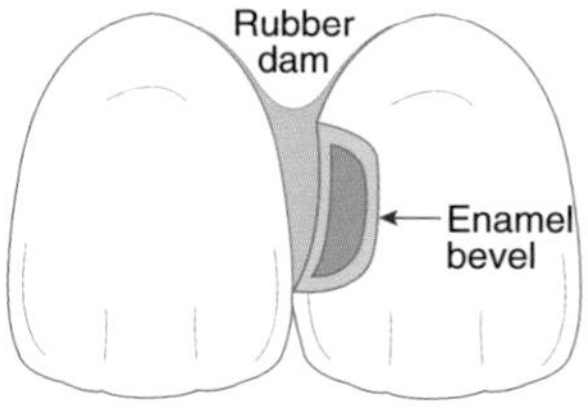

Figure 38-53. Lingual view of the completed Class III cavity preparation. The dentin is protected by a cavity liner, an enamel bevel has been placed, and the rubber dam retracts the gingiva to provide access.

Finishing and Polishing Composite Restorations

The purpose of finishing and polishing composite restorations is to create a smooth, plaque-resistant surface with optimal esthetics and contours. Unlike amalgam restorations, composites can be finished and polished immediately after placement. The finishing procedure involves removal of flash (overextension of composite material), occlusal adjustment, and recontouring of the anatomy. Polishing refers to producing a smooth, shiny finish. Many products are available, including burs, finishing strips and discs, points, cups, pastes, and brushes.[10] The process is the same as other finishing and polishing procedures, which involves progressing from coarse to fine abrasives.

Finishing the occlusal surface of a composite includes smoothing the margins, defining anatomy, and removal of flash. This is best accomplished with an egg- or football-shaped finishing bur, using smooth, intermittent strokes on

Procedure 38-6 Placing and Finishing a Class III Composite Restoration

EQUIPMENT

Personal protective equipment
Protective eyewear for client
Isolation materials
Glass ionomer cavity liner or sealer as needed
Conditioning agent (acid gel)
Priming agent
Bonding resin
Composite
Resin surface coating
Matrix system
Dispensing syringe
Curing light and protective shields
Plastic instruments
Finishing burs and discs
Articulating paper

STEPS

1. Question client regarding expectations; explain nature of composites.
2. Select composite shade, place small amount of material on the tooth near the lesion and cure it; involve client in shade selection.
3. Place rubber dam.
4. After cavity preparation, apply cavity liner, sealer, and/or base as needed.
5. Position a clear, plastic matrix strip between the preparation and the adjacent tooth.
6. Dry tooth and apply etchant to the entire cavity surface according to manufacturer's instructions. Rinse with an air-water spray for at least 15 seconds; dry with forced-air drying. Reposition matrix as necessary; position a wedge interproximally.
7. Inspect the peripheral etched pattern.
8. Apply thin coats of primer to etched surfaces according to manufacturer's instructions and lightly dry.
9. Apply a thin coat of bonding resin to primed surface; spread resin over etched enamel with a small brush or sponge and a gentle stream of air (Figure 38-54).
10. Polymerize bonding resin with curing light for 15 to 20 seconds; light wand should be as close as possible without direct contact.

    Careful inspection of cured bonding resin will reveal a slightly tacky surface. This very thin layer of resin is unable to polymerize completely because of the influence of air. It will polymerize rapidly once covered by composite or a matrix strip and re-exposed to the curing light.
11. Remove cap from composite dispensing device; express small amount of selected composite onto a small paper pad; replace cap. Many systems are pre-encapsulated.
12. With a plastic instrument, or pre-encapsulated mixture placed in dispensing gun, place increment of composite (no more than 2 mm thick) in preparation; adapt to walls and margins; cure this first increment for 20 to 30 seconds (Figure 38-55).

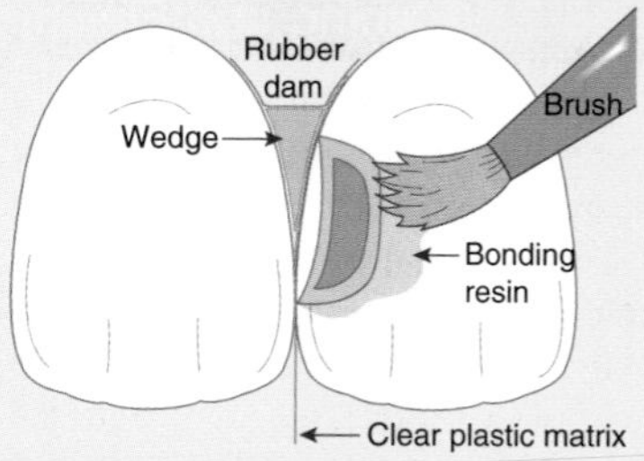

Figure 38-54. The etched enamel receiving a coating of bonding resin. A matrix separates the cavity from the adjacent tooth and is contoured and stabilized by a wedge placed interproximally.

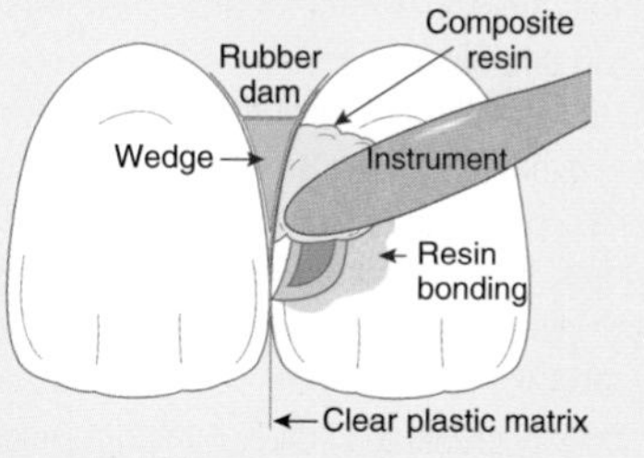

Figure 38-55. Placement of increments of composite into the preparation. The composite must be adapted into the recesses of the cavity and built against the matrix and cavity walls.

Continued

Procedure 38-6 Placing and Finishing a Class III Composite Restoration—cont'd

13. Continue to add and cure increments, building form to a slight excess in contour. In small cavities final form may be achieved by firmly wrapping clear matrix against tooth and curing through it (Figure 38-56); remove wedge and matrix.
14. Contour restoration with finishing burs and discs, exercising care to avoid tooth damage (Figures 38-57 and 38-58).
15. Remove rubber dam and check for occlusal prematurities on restoration. Lingual high spots can be reduced carefully with a large, round finishing bur or a football-shaped fine diamond.
16. Polish accessible parts of restoration with polishing discs; examine gingival sulcus and remove debris.
17. Condition restoration surface with conditioning agent.
18. Apply resin surface coating with a cotton pellet or foam applicator; cure for 10 seconds.
19. Show client finished restoration (Figure 38-59).

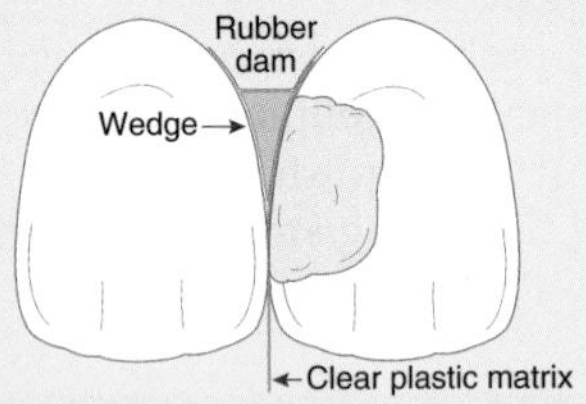

Figure 38-56. Cavity filled to slight excess, cured, and prepared for finishing.

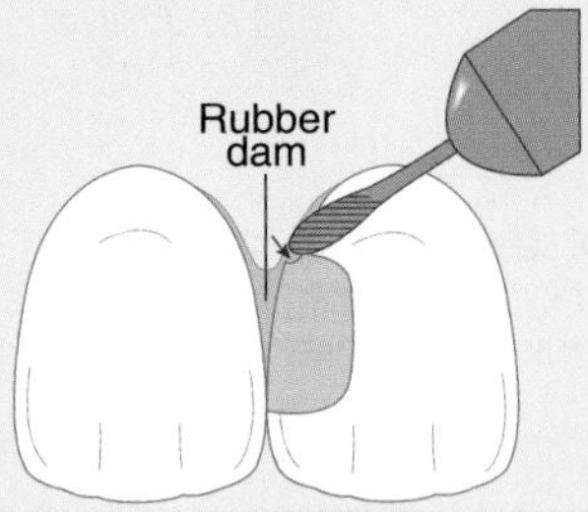

Figure 38-58. Damage to the tooth structure occurs if due caution is not exercised with the use of a bur in the finishing procedure.

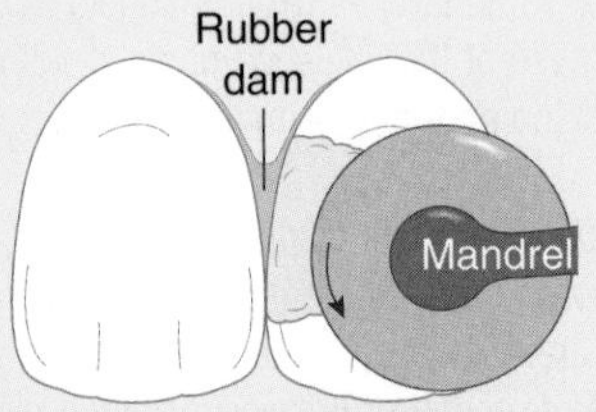

Figure 38-57. Contouring the composite with a disc to achieve the final form. The wedge and matrix have been removed.

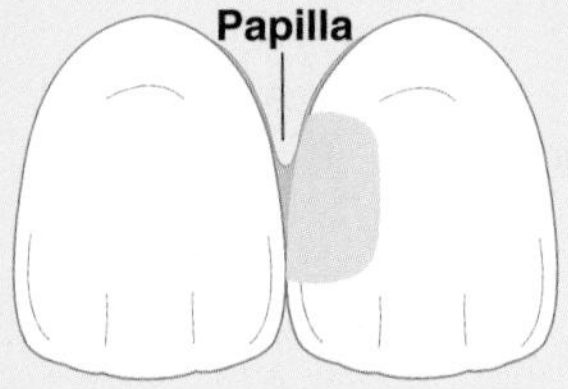

Figure 38-59. Finished Class III composite restoration.

Procedure 38-7 Placing and Finishing a Class II Composite Restoration

EQUIPMENT

See equipment list for Class III composite restorations PLUS:

- Sectional ring matrix system OR
- Tofflemire retainer with dead soft or Ho (0.001 mm) matrix band
- Composite placement and carving instruments

STEPS

1-4. Repeat steps 1 through 4 listed for Class III composite restorations.

5. Place matrix and wedge to obtain tight seal at gingival margin. If using a Tofflemire retainer with dead soft or Ho band refer to Procedure 38-3. To use a sectional ring matrix system, select an appropriate-sized contoured band. Place the band between the preparation and the adjacent tooth. Place wedge from lingual (Figures 38-60 and 38-61).
6. Use forceps to place the bi-tine ring. Ring forceps are designed for and supplied with ring kit. Rubber dam forceps also may be used. The ring can be placed on either side of the wedge, depending on size of the prep. The tines of the ring should be positioned as close as possible to the cavosurface margin to ensure a tight seal (Figures 38-62 and 38-63).
7. Examine the cavity preparation carefully and develop a mental picture of the outline form of the preparation as well as the anatomy of the adjacent tooth surface. An overfilled restoration can be difficult to finish if you do not remember the location of the cavosurface margins.

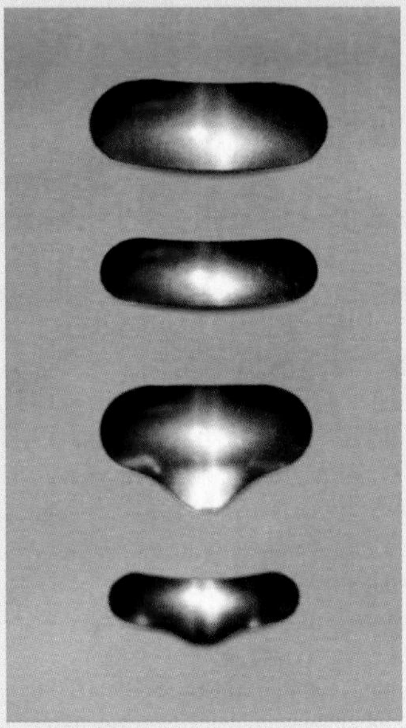

Figure 38-60. Sectional bands are available in a variety of sizes and shapes to fit different restorations (e.g., premolars, molars, deep cervical preps, primary molars).

Procedure 38-7 Placing and Finishing a Class II Composite Restoration—cont'd

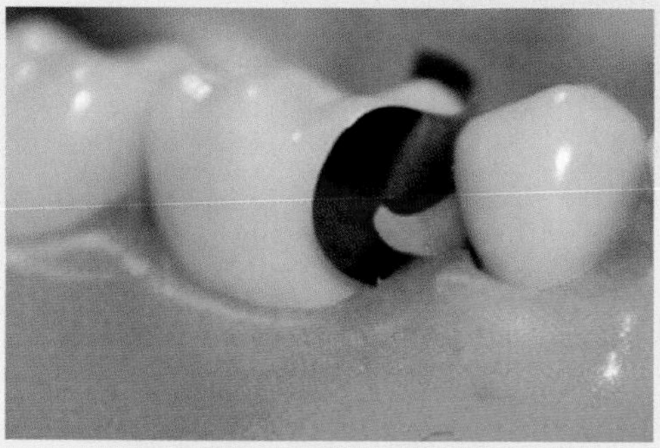

Figure 38-61. The band should extend from 0.5 to 1 mm below gingival cavosurface margin to the height of marginal ridge.

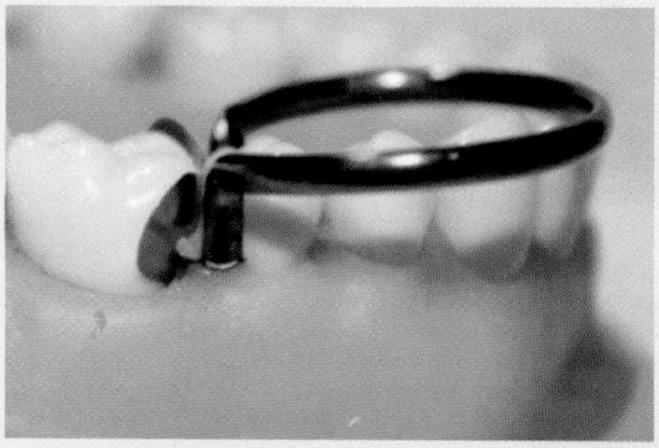

Figure 38-62. Using ring placement forceps, spread the ring and place as close as possible to the cavosurface margin, forcing the band tight against the tooth to provide a tight seal.

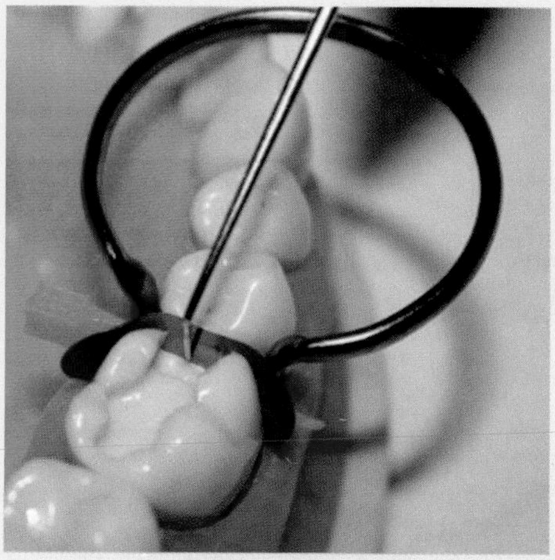

Figure 38-63. Use an explorer to check the seal of the band at the gingival floor. Also check the height of the band and the contact with the adjacent tooth.

8. Etch, prime, and bond the tooth preparation. Before placement of composite restorative materials, the clinician must etch, prime, and bond the tooth preparation (collectively called *adhesives*). The proper use of adhesives is critical to the success of composite restorations. There are different types, systems, and manufacturers of adhesives (e.g., total etch, prime and bond, all-in-one). Because they are applied in different manners, it is important to follow the directions from the respective manufacturer (Figures 38-64 and 38-65).

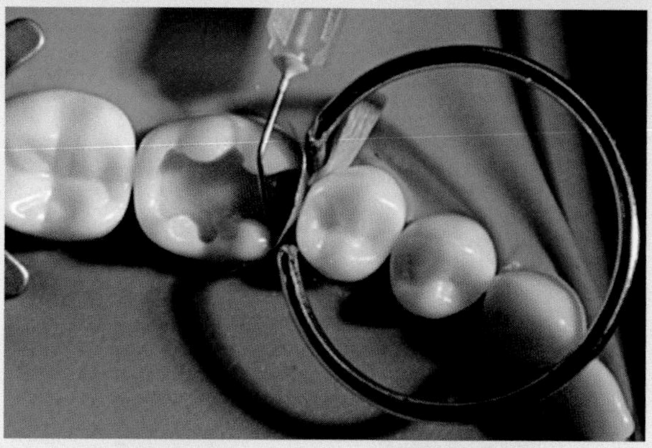

Figure 38-64. A conditioner/etchant (phosphoric acid) is placed, rinsed, and dried in accordance with manufacturer's recommendation.

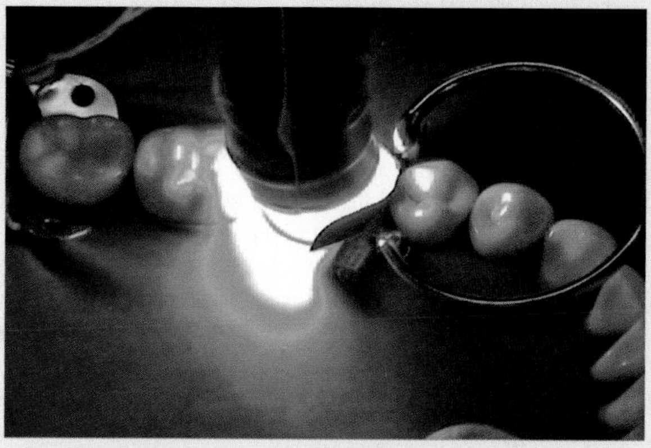

Figure 38-65. Primer and bonding agent are applied and light cured according to package directions.

9. Many clinicians promote the application of a flowable resin to line the floor of the proximal box. There is some evidence that it improves the adaptation of this area and minimizes the potential for voids. The flowable composite is applied by ejecting a small amount across the gingival floor of the preparation. A thickness of only 0.5 mm is needed. After light curing for 20 seconds, the next step is to layer the composite material into the preparation.
10. Incrementally fill: Composite is added in incremental layers because the light emitted from a curing light can penetrate through only a certain thickness of material. Most curing lights cure to a maximum depth of 2 mm, so small increments are required. Another reason composite is added in thin increments is as composite material sets, it shrinks on a microscopic level. Keeping each layer of composite thin means that the cumulative effects of this distortion will be less problematic than if the composite were placed and cured as a single thick mass. Each layer should be cured for 20 seconds (Figure 38-65).

    Using a composite placement instrument, pat/tamp the material into the proximal box of the preparation. Angle the instrument so that the composite will be pushed into the line angles and point angles of the cavity preparation and against the matrix band (Figure 38-66).

Procedure 38-7 Placing and Finishing a Class II Composite Restoration—cont'd

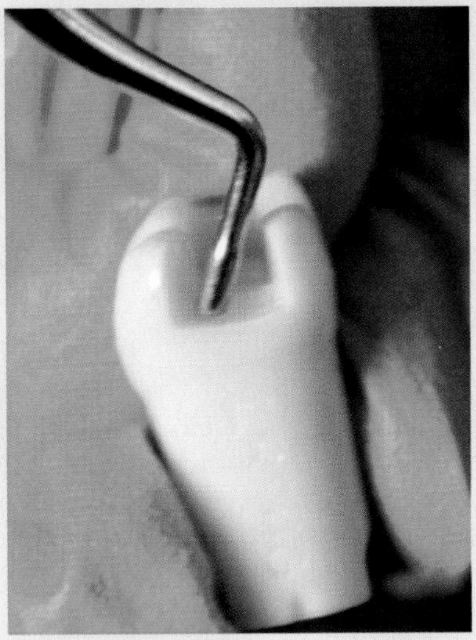

Figure 38-66. A critical element of composite placement is the elimination of any voids. Note the angle of the proximal box: to compact composite completely into the line angles and point angles, an instrument must be angled obliquely to adapt to the walls, gingival floor, and matrix band.

11. Place subsequent layers and shape the anatomy. Depending on the depth of the preparation a third layer or even a fourth layer may be required. The anatomy is shaped by using appropriate composite instruments. Keeping the tip in the central groove and angling the instrument up to the cavosurface margin, pat/tamp the material in place. Excess material is wiped up and over the cavosurface margin (Figures 38-67 and 38-68).
12. Round and contour the height of the marginal ridge (Figure 38-69). An explorer or paddle-shaped blade can be used to remove excess composite from and around the matrix band. Again, cure the composite for 20 seconds.
13. Remove the matrix/wedge. After removing the metal matrix band, cure the interproximal area from the buccal and lingual aspects for 20 seconds each. This provides a final cure to ensure that those areas previously shielded by the metal matrix band are cured fully.
14. Finishing and polishing posterior composite resins can be accomplished immediately after polymerization of composite restorations using any of the variety of composite supplies available. Check the proximal area for overhangs, proper contour, and contact. Using light shaving strokes, a gold knife or Bard Parker blade can be used to remove minor overhangs that may remain.

    A flame-shaped finishing bur or composite disc can be used to correct overcontoured areas and remove flash in other areas. Polish the entire surface of the restoration with composite polishing points followed by a composite polishing paste in a rubber cup (Figures 38-70 through 38-73).
15. Check the proximal contact with floss. If it is too tight, a finishing strip or tapered bur can be used to correct it.
16. After assessing the restoration, remove the rubber dam (Figure 38-74).
17. Evaluate the occlusion with articulating paper and adjust as required. If occlusal adjustment is required, re-polish the areas that were adjusted.
18. In addition to the Clinic Education Issues listed at the end of this chapter, the clinician should inform the patient of the following:

    They may experience some minor discomfort of the tissues around the restored tooth because of irritation of the gingival wedge and the finishing of the gingival margin area.

    Desiccation of the tooth may make the tooth look lighter, resulting in a temporary mismatch of the composite shade selection. After a few hours the tooth will rehydrate and the composite color will blend with the natural tooth.

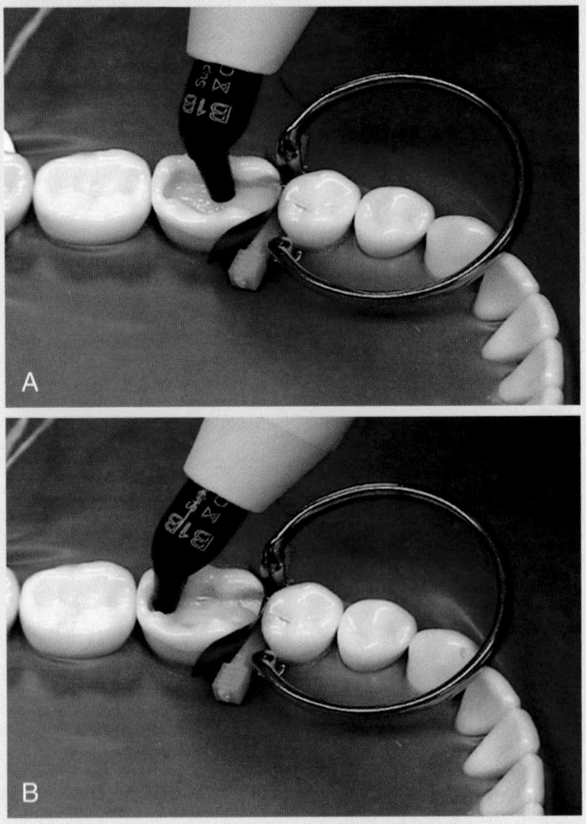

Figure 38-67. After the proximal box has been filled and cured up to the level of the AB pulpal floor, the remainder of the prep is filled incrementally and cured along the pulpal floor. Incremental layers should be no thicker than 2 mm for the light to cure the composite completely. The size of the preparation will determine the number of layers needed.

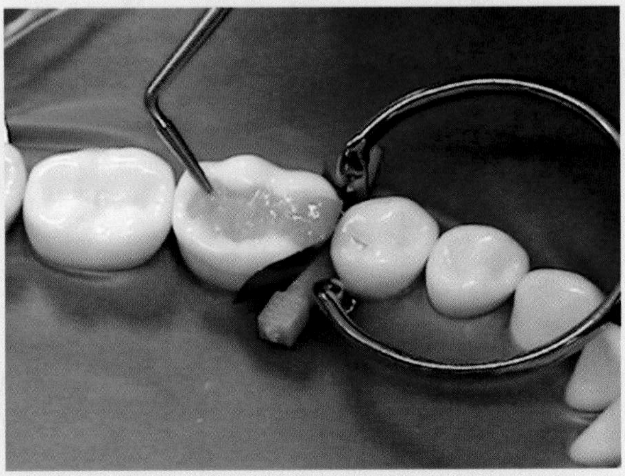

Figure 38-68. There is a variety of instruments that can be used to help shape the anatomy when approaching the occlusal layer.

Procedure 38-7 Placing and Finishing a Class II Composite Restoration—cont'd

19. Document procedure.
(Figures courtesy Carlene Paarmann, Anita Herzog, and Carole Christie, Professors, Idaho State University Department of Dental Hygiene; and Ardean Nickerson, Professor, Eastern Washington University Department of Dental Hygiene.)

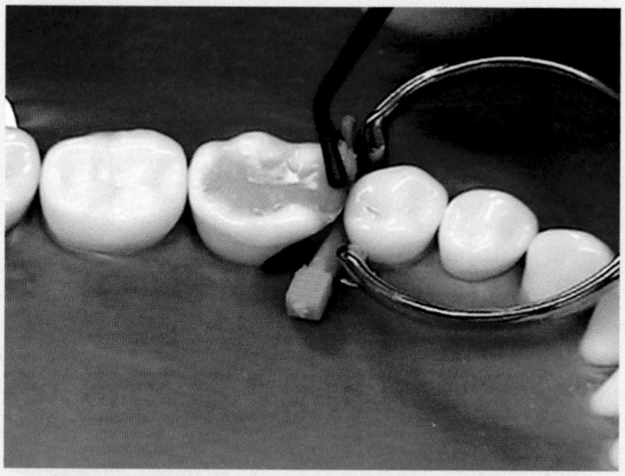

Figure 38-69. Developing the height and shape of the marginal ridge before curing.

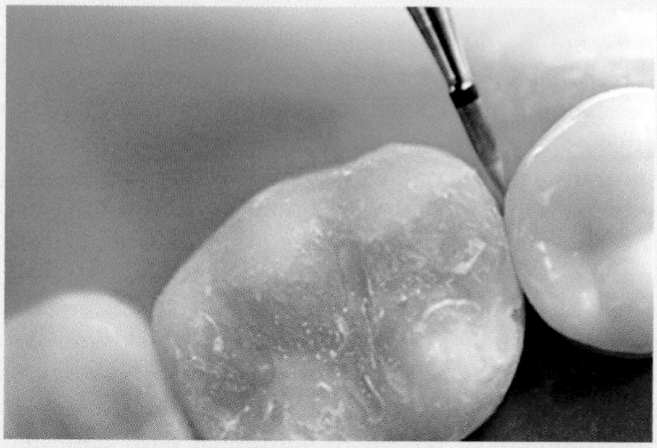

Figure 38-70. A flame shaped finishing bur is used here to shape the marginal ridge, embrasures, and proximal contact areas.

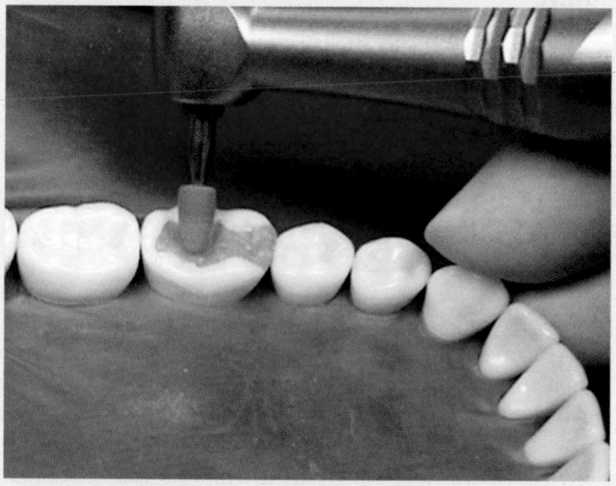

Figure 38-71. Many excellent polishing points, cups, and discs are available for finishing and polishing composite resin. As with all polishing abrasives, begin with most abrasive graduating to least abrasive, taking care not to generate excessive heat.

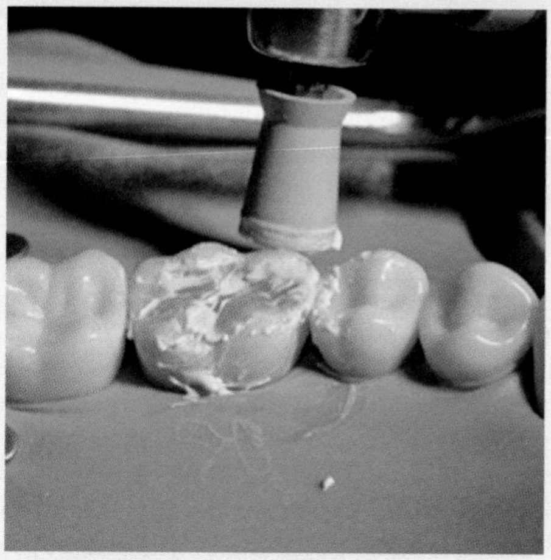

Figure 38-72. Polishing paste designed specifically for composite resin is shown here as the final step in polishing.

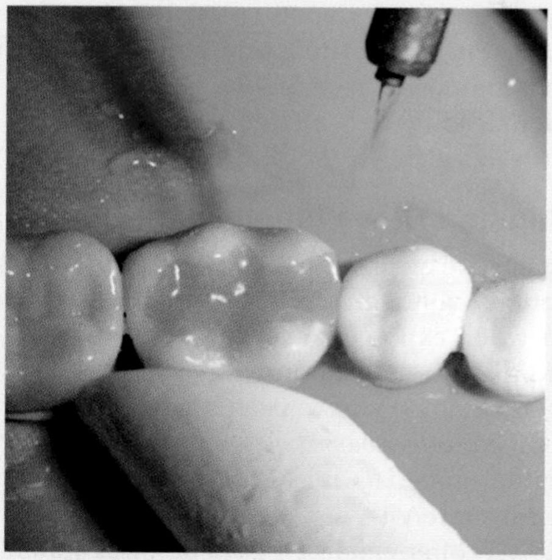

Figure 38-73. Thoroughly rinse and dry the area before assessing the restoration.

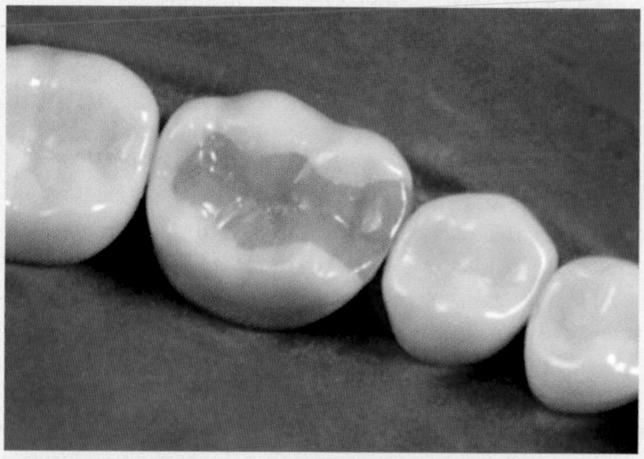

Figure 38-74. Check the restoration for any excess or deficiencies, proper proximal contour and contact, no voids, smooth surface finish. Remove the rubber dam and check occlusion.

the composite material. Finishing cups or points can be used to smooth the surface or grooves. Finishing the facial and lingual surfaces of composite restorations is done best with a flame-shaped bur to contour the surfaces, smooth margins, and remove flash. An egg- or football-shaped finishing bur, points, and cups can be used on the lingual surfaces of anterior teeth. Finishing discs and cups are used on the facial surfaces of anterior teeth. Discs, cups, and points are indicated on posterior teeth. The finishing procedure is evaluated before moving on to polishing. The composite restoration should be smooth, flash removed, occlusion registered correctly with articulating paper, and occlusal anatomy well defined.

Polishing composite restorations is similar to finishing, except finer abrasives are used, less material is removed, and it results in a high shine. Polishing points or cups specifically designed for use with composite resins are used on the occlusal surface, and the same polishing points and cups, as well as composite polishing discs are used on the facial and lingual surfaces and proximal line angles. Some clinicians use polishing paste with a rubber cup as an optional final step. Evaluation of the polished composite restoration is important, including checking for a smooth, scratch-free surface with a shiny surface. Proper finishing and polishing enhances the esthetics of composite restorations and decreases plaque accumulation, leading to healthier tissues.

Resin-Modified Glass Ionomer

Glass ionomers are available as cavity liners as well as definitive restorations, although one disadvantage is they undergo dissolution when exposed to saliva. To compensate for the tendency to dissolve and improve their use as a restorative material, glass ionomers have been modified. The improved product is called *resin-modified glass ionomer (RMGI)*. All glass ionomer dental materials release fluoride ions. As a result, recurrent caries rarely is seen at the margin of an RMGI restoration. RMGIs offer enhanced esthetics, less solubility, and greater strength than regular glass ionomer but retain some of their fluoride-release characteristics. RMGIs are an important class of materials for restoration of primary teeth.

Materials

Glass ionomers are composed of aluminosilicate glass (powder) and polyalkenoic acid (liquid) that set through an acid-base reaction between the filler and the resin. A great benefit is that this material truly adheres (chemical bonding) to prepared tooth structure.

Indications for RMGI Restorations

Indications include root caries, Class V abrasion and erosion (gingival margin) lesions in permanent teeth, and Class I, II, III, and IV restorations in primary teeth (see Procedure 38-8 and the corresponding Competency Form).

Preformed Stainless Steel Crowns

Stainless steel crowns are used to restore primary molars with large areas needing restoration.[11] In some jurisdictions dental hygienists are able to place stainless steel crowns because this procedure falls within their scope of practice (see Procedure 38-9 and the corresponding Competency Form).

Indications

Stainless steel preformed crowns are indicated for primary molars where an amalgam is likely to fail, for extensive caries damage involving multiple surfaces of the tooth, and after pulp or endodontic therapy.[12] Stainless steel crowns provide a suitable intermediate option when financial considerations prevent use of a permanent cast restoration in permanent molars.

Materials and Armamentarium

Materials needed include the following:
- Preformed crowns
- Trimming scissors
- Crimping pliers
- Glass ionomer cement

Liners, Sealer, and Bases

Preserving and protecting the dental pulp are concerns in every restorative procedure on vital teeth.

Vital dentin is a dynamic tissue. At a microscopic level, it is easy to understand how a gentle stream of air may cause injury to a delicate pulp that is covered by a paper-thin thickness of dentin. Deep cavities in particular must be treated to protect the pulp from further insult; liners and bases provide such protection.

Liners

Liners are liquid-like materials applied in thin coatings (thinner than 0.5 mm) that act as cavity sealers and provide beneficial functions such as fluoride release, adhesion to tooth structure, and/or antibacterial action that promotes the health of the pulp. Calcium hydroxide preparations are used commonly to protect the pulp in deep cavity preparations, and in situations when the pulp has been exposed, to stimulate the vital pulp to heal if the wound is small and clean. These liners are prepared easily. Equal amounts of agents are dispensed onto a small pad, quickly mixed, and then placed specifically on the dentin or over the pulp exposure (Figure 38-83). Because these materials typically do not resist compressive forces, an additional hard base material often is used for protection.

Sealers

Cavity sealers are used to seal dentinal tubules to protect the pulp from chemical irritation. Sealing of dentinal tubules is accomplished by using bonding resins or liners. Dentin bonding agents provide a hybridization bond formed between the restorative material and the tooth structure (hybrid layer) that has been found to better seal tubules and provide some retentive strength for resin composites when used.

Bases

Bases, materials placed to provide thermal insulation and support under restorations, must be strong enough to resist occlusal forces and, in the case of amalgam, resist firm condensation. This category includes zinc phosphate and glass ionomer cements. Bases of zinc phosphate cement have served dentistry well, providing dependable support and insulation under metallic restorations. The rationale for its use in preventing sensitivity, however, is questionable. Sealing the dentinal tubules to prevent microleakage is believed to be far more important in controlling postoperative sensitivity

Procedure 38-8 Placing a Resin-Modified Glass Ionomer (RMGI) Restoration of Class V Abrasion Lesions

EQUIPMENT

Personal protective equipment
Protective eyewear for client
Isolation materials
RMGI
Polyacrylic acid/conditioner
Pumice
Polishing cup
Plastic instruments
Carving instrument
Bonding resin
Special protective varnish
Curing light and protective shields
Matrix system

STEPS

1. Examine lesions; assess need for local anesthetic agent.
2. Select shade of restorative material to be used; involve client in selection.
3. Place rubber dam.
4. Briefly, debride cavity and adjacent tooth structure with pumice and water slurry in a rubber polishing cup; rinse thoroughly and dry.
5. According to manufacturer's instructions, apply conditioner to abrasion lesion (approximately 15 seconds); rinse thoroughly for 15 seconds with a strong air-water spray, and dry lightly, ensuring a moist surface.
6. Mix glass ionomer according to manufacturer's directions or triturate pre-encapsulated RMGI.
7. Rapidly fill cavity to slight excess, using a plastic instrument to place material (Figure 38-75); position cervical matrix over cavity to hold cement against tooth (Figure 38-76); light-cure per directions using protective shield.
8. Remove matrix.
9. Contour restoration with finishing burs and discs (Figure 38-77); take care to avoid damage to tooth root (Figure 38-78).
10. Apply thin coat of bonding resin to cement restoration surface and cure resin for 15 to 20 seconds.
11. Remove rubber dam; examine gingival sulcus and remove debris.
12. Show final result to client.

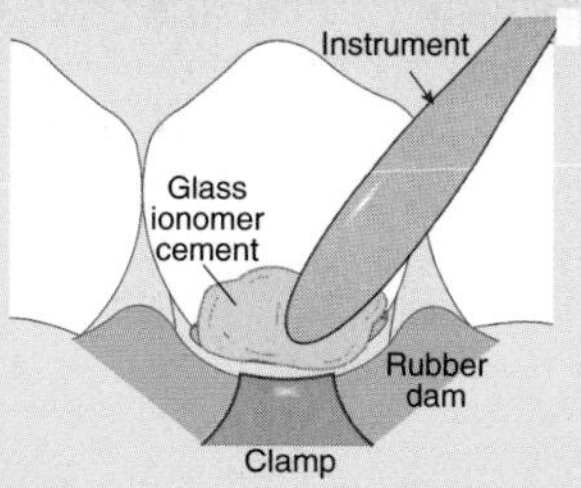

Figure 38-75. Placement of the resin-modified glass ionomer to overfill the cavity slightly.

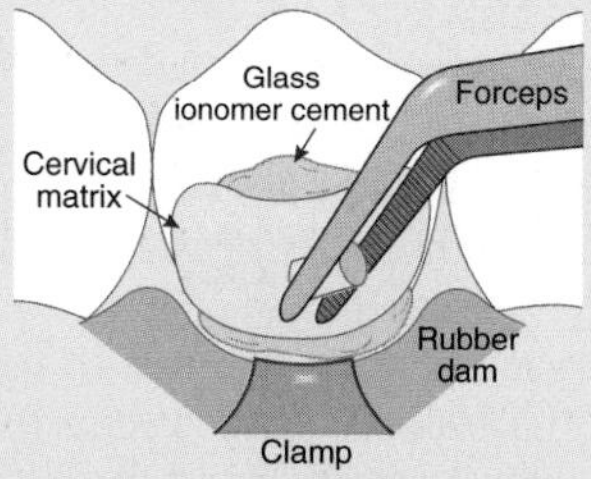

Figure 38-76. Positioning the clear cervical matrix over the cavity and expressing excess resin-modified glass ionomer at the edges of the matrix.

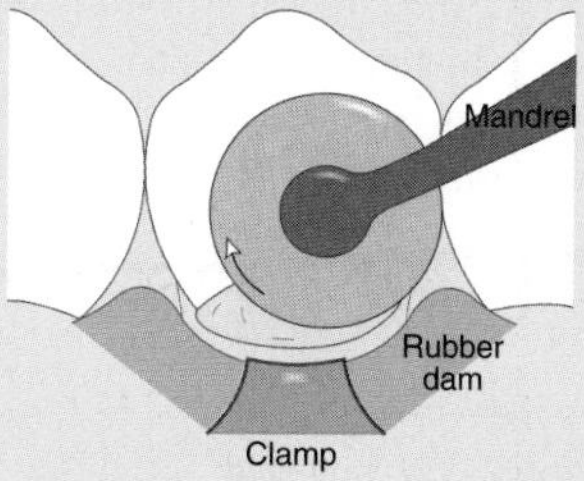

Figure 38-77. Final contouring of the restoration with a disc.

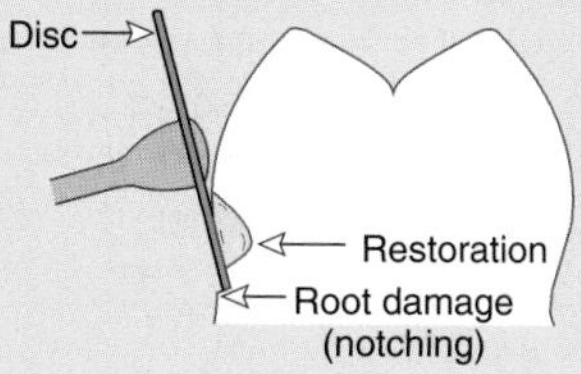

Figure 38-78. Root damage from improper disc use.

than is physical insulation. When zinc phosphate cement is used, its preparation requires attention to detail.

Compared with zinc phosphate cement, glass ionomer cements require less time to prepare and bond to dentin, achieving a desirable seal. Most glass ionomer cements are available in a self-dispensing form and do not require manual mixing. However, when these cements are prepared manually, mixing and manipulation times are critical.

Gingival Retraction

The essential first step for the fabrication of an indirect restoration is the making of an accurate impression. Although dental hygienists may in some jurisdictions place gingival retraction cord, indirect restorations are placed by the dentist or dental specialist. Gingival tissue management ensures that the margins of the preparation are captured appropriately in the impression. Gingival retraction, through the use of retraction cord around the preparation, is a critical step in achieving the desired impression. Retraction cord relaxes the gingival tissue, thereby "opening" the gingival sulcus and allowing impression material into the gingival crevice to capture the gingival margins of the preparation. Please visit http://evolve.elsevier.com/Darby/hygiene for additional information about the procedure for placing gingival retraction cord, eFigures 38-84 through 38-87, and eProcedure 38-10.

Procedure 38-9 Placing a Stainless Steel Crown

EQUIPMENT

Personal protective equipment
Protective eyewear for client
Isolation materials
Stainless steel preformed crowns
Crown trimming scissors
Crimping pliers
Resin-modified glass ionomer cement
Floss
Articulating paper

STEPS

1. Evaluate prepared tooth for size.
2. Correct size is selected by measuring the mesiodistal width between contact points of a matching tooth in mouth.
3. Choose smallest crown that will fit.
4. To seat, place crown lingually and adapt it over the occlusal and buccal aspects of prepared tooth.
5. Use firm pressure to seat crown. May hear an audible click as it springs over gingival undercut area of preparation.
6. To evaluate fit, observe marginal gingiva. It will blanch somewhat with a well-fitting crown. If excess blanching is observed, crown will have to be trimmed.
7. In a properly seated crown, margin should extend approximately 1 mm subgingivally. To trim crown, scribe a line where marginal gingival hits crown with an explorer.
8. Trim crown 1 mm below scribed line. Use crown scissors or an abrasive wheel to trim crown (Figure 38-79).
9. Use crimping pliers to adapt edge of crown for a tighter fit (Figure 38-80).
10. Seat crown once more to evaluate fit.
11. Crown is now ready to be cemented.
12. Use resin-modified glass ionomer cement. Fill entire crown with cement (Figure 38-81).
13. Excess cement will flow out from margins as crown is seated.
14. Use an explorer, a scaler, and knotted floss to remove excess cement (Figure 38-82).
15. Check occlusion using articulating paper.

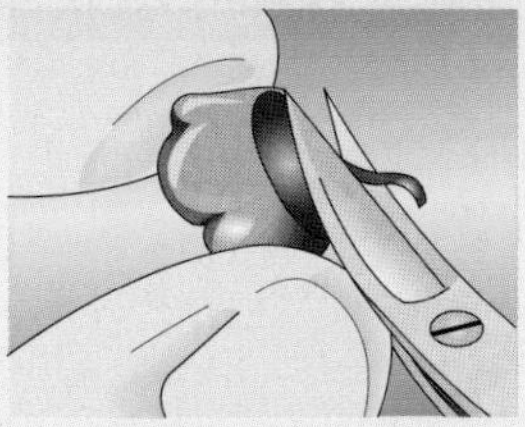

Figure 38-79. Trim the margin of the crown with crown scissors.

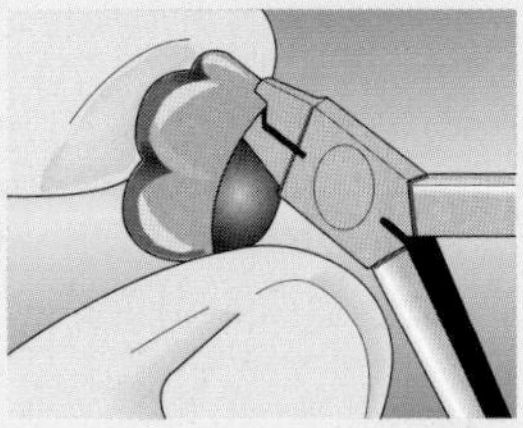

Figure 38-80. Crimping pliers are used to adapt the margin of the crown.

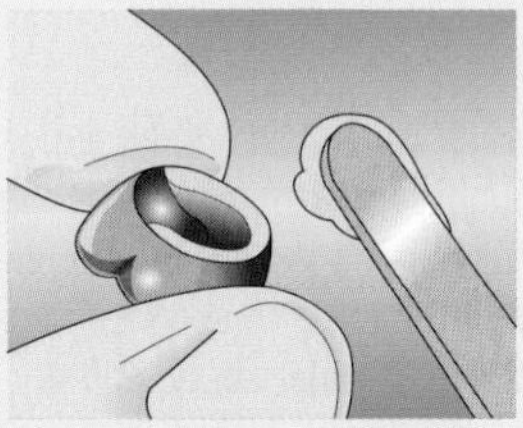

Figure 38-81. Overfill the crown with cement.

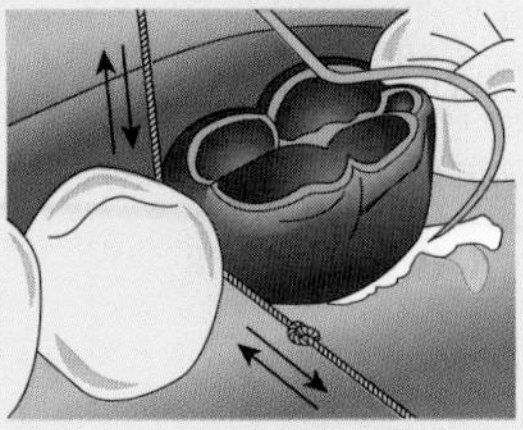

Figure 38-82. Use knotted floss and a scaler or explorer to remove excess cement after seating the crown.

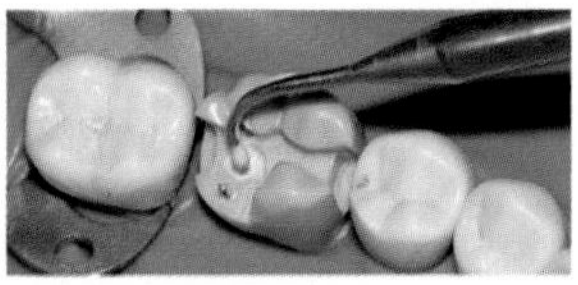

Figure 38-83. Placement of mixed calcium hydroxide in the deeper areas of the cavity preparation.

Temporary or Interim Restorations

Rationale for Use

Temporary restorations offer client comfort and tooth protection while a client waits for delivery of a permanent restoration by providing the following:

- Coverage of exposed dentin to prevent tooth sensitivity, plaque biofilm accumulation, caries and pulpal involvement
- Prevention of unwanted tooth movement
- Ability of clients to eat and speak normally
- Maintenance of the health and contours of the adjacent gingival tissue
- Means of addressing cosmetic or functional preferences and concerns of the client

Temporary Materials and Placement Techniques

Reinforced Zinc Oxide with Eugenol

Reinforced zinc oxide with eugenol readily restores intermediate-size cavities that require a more durable material; it is prepared with a mixture of zinc oxide powder and eugenol liquid. The insulating properties of the hardened zinc oxide mass and the obtundent effect of the eugenol result in a material that protects the vital pulp against chemical and thermal insults. Reinforced zinc oxide with eugenol is relatively easy to prepare and place and is reliable for interim periods of a few months.

The powder and liquid are mixed on a nonabsorbent pad according to the manufacturer's instructions. Firm pressure on the spatula is needed to mix the material thoroughly. Properly mixed, the material is thick and clay-like. The material then is rolled with the fingertips (on the pad) into a cylindric form. Increments can be pinched off the end of the mass with a placing instrument and firmly packed into the preparation until it is full (see Procedure 38-11 and the corresponding Competency Form).

Custom-Made Acrylic Resin

The custom-made acrylic resin temporary restoration is recommended for complex restorations such as inlays, onlays, veneers, and crowns; the technique permits the reproduction of the tooth anatomy. A limitation of this technique is that the tooth restored must be intact enough to allow adequate retention of the temporary restoration. However, the final product is durable, smooth, and comfortable and can serve for several months.

Preformed Stock Crown (Metal or Polycarbonate)

Preformed stock crowns make useful temporary crowns. These crown forms are trimmed readily, modified for fit, and provide a satisfactory alternative to the custom-made acrylic crown previously discussed. The final product is extremely durable; however, it is a compromise in form and shape. These temporary crowns are usually comfortable for the client.

Luting Agents

Indirect restorations are fabricated in the dental laboratory on dies made from impressions of prepared teeth. These restorations include crowns and inlays made of rigid materials such as metal, ceramic, or porcelain. When these restorations are seated completely, all margins should be smooth with no gaps between tooth and restoration. However, a very small space exists between the restoration and the tooth that is filled with a **luting agent** (cement) that, when set, prevents the indirect restoration from loosening.[14] Dislodging forces of occlusion and mastication are resisted by this firm interface of cement. Without a proper luting agent, restorations leak, loosen, and fail.

Zinc Phosphate Cement

Zinc phosphate, the oldest of the luting agents, can be used for cementation of most indirect restorations. Because zinc phosphate is acidic, vital pulps often are protected by a varnish barrier between the cement and dentin.

Procedure 38-11 Preparing Reinforced Zinc Oxide and Eugenol Temporary Restorations (Class II Cavity Preparation)

EQUIPMENT

Personal protective equipment
Protective eyewear for client
Isolation materials
Tofflemire matrix system
Petrolatum
Reinforced zinc oxide and eugenol
Nonabsorbent mixing pad
Plastic instruments
Cotton pellets and rolls, dry aids
Finishing burs
Carving instruments
Articulating paper

STEPS

1. Isolate operating site as appropriate.
2. Prepare Tofflemire matrix system. Apply thin coat of petrolatum on the inside of the matrix band; position matrix, secure it, and place interproximal wedges as needed.
3. Use manufacturer's instructions for measuring and mixing.
4. Prepare mix; when material reaches consistency of firm clay, carry an ample amount to cavity with a plastic instrument. Firmly adapt rubbery material to all walls of cavity with a placement instrument (Figures 38-88 and 38-89).
5. Fill cavity to slight excess; shape occlusal anatomy by using a moist cotton pellet in cotton forceps to create a general anatomic form.
6. When material has hardened, remove wedge(s), retainer, and matrix band; apply pressure apically on the temporary restoration to counteract removal of band.
7. Check proximal and gingival margins for excess material and remove with sharp, narrow-bladed carving instrument.
8. Remove isolation materials; evaluate premature occlusion on temporary restoration with articulating paper and adjust as necessary with large, round bur and carving instruments (Figure 38-90).
9. Examine gingival sulcus for debris and remove as necessary; excess material at gingival margin can be removed using a bladed instrument such as the ½ Hollenbeck or IPC carver.

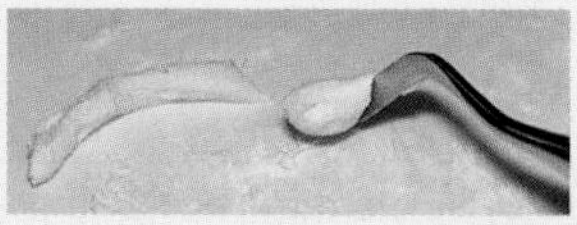

Figure 38-88. Properly mixed reinforced zinc oxide with eugenol ready for placement.

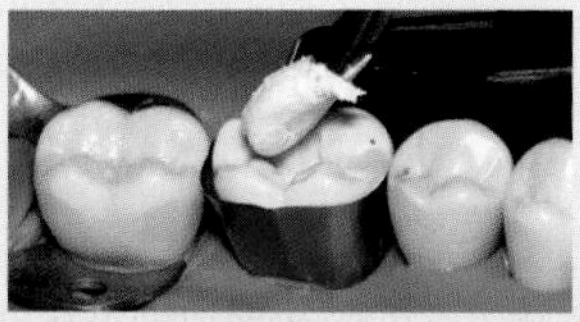

Figure 38-89. Reinforced zinc oxide with eugenol being placed in cavity preparation.

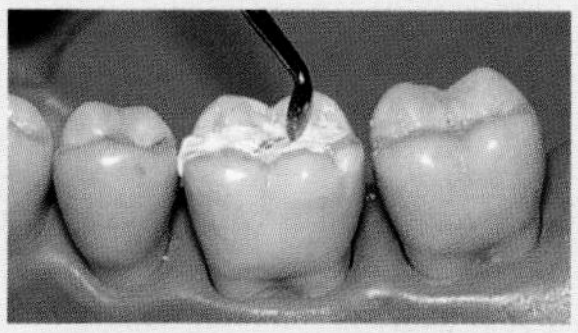

Figure 38-90. Final adjustment to the occlusal aspect of the temporary restoration with a carver.

Glass Ionomer Cement

The chemical adhesion of this material to the tooth surface and relative ease in handling has led to its popularity as a luting agent. When compared with zinc phosphate, it is less acidic and more compatible with the dental pulp. It inhibits recurrent caries through the slow release of fluoride. The mixing and working times for the chemical-cured glass ionomer cement are short, so the dental team must be efficient when luting restorations with glass ionomer cement. Most cements of this type can be prepared on a nonabsorbent paper pad, in accordance with the manufacturer's instructions. The luting cement is mixed to a much less viscous state than the glass ionomer cement base material or restorative material previously described.

Resin Cements

Chemical-cured resin cements are used when strength of bonding is needed and light activation is not possible (e.g., cementation of cast post and cores and Maryland bridges). The bond strength of resin cements is much greater than that of other cements, but handling characteristics are more sensitive and the working time is shorter. The modified resin cements are also useful for cementation of complete metal or metal-ceramic crowns to be placed on tooth preparations with minimal retentive features.

Zinc Oxide and Eugenol

Primary materials for temporary cementation of restorations are preparations of zinc oxide with eugenol. These materials vary in hardness and retaining abilities and are selected accordingly. Temporary cements are contained most commonly in small tubes and have a fluid-paste consistency. Equal amounts of base and catalyst are expressed onto a small pad and rapidly mixed. The cement is applied to cover the inside of the restoration (usually a temporary restoration), which is then seated and held in place until the cement has hardened. Excess, hardened cement is removed with an instrument such as a scaler or curette.

Evaluation

The restorative care cycle demands ongoing assessment and evaluation. Appropriateness of treatment must be judged from the perspectives of the professional and the client. The professional must be responsible for proper manipulation and technical quality of the restoration, and the client should be prepared to address issues such as comfort, function, and appearance.

Documentation

Restorative treatment must be documented accurately in the client's record, including all procedures involved in the restorative treatment. Documentation may include, but is not limited to, the tooth number, surfaces, and location of the restoration, anesthetic agents and medications, tooth isolation procedures, restorative materials, complications, and client education. When restorative treatment dictates special precautions for future treatment, specific details should be recorded.

Maintenance or Continued Care

Assessment is an ongoing component of restorative therapy. During continued-care appointments, the dental hygienist thoroughly reviews the medical and dental histories of the client, assesses the outcomes of preventive and restorative care, and evaluates the client's current oral health status. Assessments at the continued-care appointment that include evaluation and maintenance of existing restorations provide optimal restorative care for the client.

CLIENT EDUCATION TIPS

- Advise clients of importance of oral plaque control in maintaining the integrity of dental restorations.
- Explain advantages and disadvantages of various dental restorations.
- Emphasize that restorations treat signs of dental caries but not the bacterial cause of caries.
- Discuss that a restored mouth takes additional time and effort to maintain.
- Explain that professional maintenance care, on a regular basis, is necessary to monitor status of restorations and oral health.
- Discuss that poor oral hygiene contributes to necessary replacement and extension of existing restorations.
- Explain that the maximum strength of amalgam occurs many hours after placement; care is required when chewing with force on newly placed amalgam restorations.
- Discuss that for best esthetics, whitening of teeth should be done before restoration placement because tooth-colored restorations are not affected by the whitening products.
- Emphasize that use of stannous fluoride can stain tooth-colored restorations.
- Discuss that food and other substances will stain tooth-colored restorations. (e.g., coffee, tea, red wine, fruit juices, medications, and tobacco).
- Emphasize that temporary restorations are placed for short-term, interim comfort of the client and protection of the cavity preparation. Permanent follow-up treatment is necessary.
- Explain that temporary restorations are easily broken or removed and do not fit as well as permanent restorations; therefore special care is required. Caution should be taken with regard to sticky and hard food consumption (e.g., caramels and peanuts) and oral habits (e.g., gum chewing).
- Explain that any change in the client's occlusion (e.g., high spots) after dental treatment should be reported immediately to the dentist for follow-up assessment.

LEGAL, ETHICAL, AND SAFETY ISSUES

- The dental hygienist must practice legally within the scope authorized by state law. Check statutes carefully to determine scope of practice in restorative dental procedures.
- Overhangs, open margins, poor contours, and open proximal contacts are avoidable defects and not acceptable standards of care.
- The final plan of restorative dental treatment must reflect agreement between the dentist and an educated, informed client. When the dentist is unable to render the restorative service of choice, there is an ethical obligation to refer the client to a dentist who has the necessary skills and expertise.

- All restorative plans are subject to change as a result of unknowns; the principle of informed consent should be applied, and clients should be informed about possible modifications to the care plan.

KEY CONCEPTS

- Restorative therapies restore the dentition to a state of health, support the maintenance of health, and provide esthetic modifications to the dentition.
- The dental hygienist's role in restorative therapies continues to expand.
- Black's Classification System is a system for communicating the characteristics of a cavity preparation.
- The rubber dam is an isolation technique used to control moisture, improve accessibility and visibility, and protect the client and operator.
- Amalgam is a durable and safe restorative material to restore teeth.
- Composite is a popular tooth-colored restorative material used for restorations.
- Glass ionomers and resin-modified glass ionomers release fluoride ions and are indicated for restoration of root caries, Class V abrasion and erosion lesions, and Class I and II caries on primary teeth.
- Stainless steel preformed crowns are the most durable restoration for primary molars with multisurface caries.
- Gingival retraction is essential for making an accurate impression of gingival margins of an indirect restoration.
- Temporary restorations ensure client comfort, provide tooth and gingival protection, and prevent tooth movement during the period between initial and final tooth preparation and restoration placement.
- Luting agents are used to cement indirect restorations and prevent the restoration from leaking and loosening.

CRITICAL THINKING EXERCISES

Profile: A very well-groomed 53-year-old professional woman, Ms. G, has signs of root caries on teeth 29, 28, 8, 9, and 27. She has lost an MOD amalgam on tooth 30 and an MO amalgam on tooth 20. She states she has some concerns about putting any more mercury in her mouth and wonders if the new tooth-colored fillings are as good as silver fillings.

Chief Complaint: "My teeth have become very sensitive, and I have lost two fillings. I can't decide if I should have silver fillings put back in or if I should go with white fillings."

Health and Dental History: Client is in excellent general health, is single, and lives alone. She currently takes no medications, and her blood pressure is within normal limits. Radiographic and clinical findings reveal no additional dental caries; however, generalized gingivitis, moderate plaque, calculus, and tobacco stain are present.

Oral Health Behavior Assessment: Client states that she brushes her teeth once a day, does not use floss, and visits the dentist once every 2 years.

Supplemental Notes: She has dental insurance and demonstrates a sincere interest and motivation to maintain her teeth but states she would prefer to not wear that piece of rubber when the dentist fills her teeth.

1. Use the assessment data to formulate a dental hygiene diagnosis, set client goals, and plan dental hygiene interventions.
2. From an evidence-based perspective, how would you respond to Ms. G's question about the relative benefits of amalgam restorations versus tooth-colored restorations? How would you respond to Ms. G's concern about mercury exposure associated with dental amalgam? How would you respond to Ms. G's desire not to wear a rubber dam during restorative care?

REFERENCES

1. American Dental Hygienists' Association, Governmental Affairs Division: *Overview of restorative services provided by dental hygienists and other non-dentist practitioners,* June 2012.
2. American Dental Hygienists' Association (ADHA): ADHA website. Available at: www.adha.org. Accessed October 2012.
3. Gilbert G, Litaker M, Pihlstrom D, et al: Rubber dam use during routine operative dentistry procedures, *Oper Dentistry* 35:491, 2010.
4. American Dental Association (ADA): Statement on dental amalgam. Available at: http://www.ada.org. Accessed October 2012.
5. Gladwin M, Bagby M: *Clinical aspects of dental materials,* ed 4, Philadelphia, 2013, Lippincott Williams & Wilkins.
6. Rathore M, Singh A, Pant VA: The dental amalgam toxicity fear: a myth or actuality, *Toxicol Int* 19:81, 2012.
7. Malhotra N, Kundabala M, Shashirashmi A: Strategies to overcome polymerization shrinkage—materials and techniques. A review, *Dent Update* 37:115, 2010.
8. Strassler HE: Meeting the challenge of the class II composite resin proximal contact, *Oralhealth,* August 2010, p 60. Available at: http://www.oralhealthjournal.com. Accessed May 2013.
9. Simos S: Direct composite resin restorations: placement strategies. *Dentistry Today.* Available at: http://www.dentistrytoday.com/restorative/5980. Accessed October 2012.
10. Barnes C: Polishing esthetic restorative materials, *Dimens Dent Hygiene* 8:24, 26, 2010.
11. Larson T: The clinical significance of marginal fit, *Northwest Dent* 91:22, 2010.
12. Seraj B, Shahrabi M, Motahari P, et al: Microleakage of stainless steel crowns placed on intact and extensively destroyed primary first molars: an in-vitro study, *Prevent Dent* 33:525, 2011.
13. Prasad KD, Hegde C, Agrawal G, et al: Gingival displacement in prosthodontics: a critical review of existing methods, *J Interdiscip Dent* 80, 2011.
14. Raghunath Reddy MH, Subba Reddy VV, Basappa N: A comparative study of retentive strengths of zinc phosphate, polycarboxylate and glass ionomer cements with stainless steel crowns—an in vitro study, *J Indian Soc Pedod Prev Dent* 28:245, 2010.

ACKNOWLEDGMENTS

The author acknowledges Cheryl A. Cameron and Richard B. McCoy for their past contributions to this chapter. The authors also wish to acknowledge James R. Clark and Carlene S. Paarmann for the photography provided for this chapter and Carlene S. Paarmann for the chapter review.

EVOLVE RESOURCES

Please visit http://evolve.elsevier.com/Darby/hygiene for additional practice and study support tools.

CHAPTER 39

Dentinal Hypersensitivity Management

Juliana J. Kim

COMPETENCIES

1. Discuss dentinal hypersensitivity, including:
   - Describe dentinal hypersensitivity and its etiology.
   - Explain the hydrodynamic theory.
   - Explain the prevalence of dentinal hypersensitivity and list teeth most likely to experience it.
   - Distinguish between dentinal hypersensitivity and other sources of tooth pain.
2. Discuss the management of dentinal hypersensitivity, including:
   - Identify risk factors contributing to dentinal hypersensitivity.
   - Explain factors that reduce dentinal hypersensitivity.
   - Describe active ingredients available to treat hypersensitivity and mechanisms of action.
   - Identify self-applied and professional (in-office) interventions for dentinal hypersensitivity.

Dentinal Hypersensitivity

Tooth pain and sensitivity are common client complaints in the oral care environment. Several conditions may elicit a pain response; the nature and extent of pain vary substantially individually and among persons. Therefore assessment of oral sites of sensitivity using a standardized approach is critical to identify an appropriate cause and thus manage the problem correctly. **Dentinal hypersensitivity** is characterized by short, sharp pain arising from exposed dentin that occurs in response to stimuli, typically thermal (both hot and cold), evaporative, tactile, osmotic, or chemical, and that cannot be ascribed to any other form of dental defect or pathology.

Etiology and Nature of Dentinal Hypersensitivity

Tooth development results in the following cementum-to-enamel relationships:

- Cementum overlaps the enamel (14% of time)
- Cementum and enamel meet without overlap (76% of time)
- Cementum and enamel do not meet (10% of time) but with no exposed dentin

Histologically, dentin is composed of numerous thin tubules that transverse from the pulp to the outer dentinal surface. Three types of sensory nerve fibers, known as A-delta fibers, A-beta fibers, and C-fibers, are found to extend 10% to 15% of the distance from the pulpal side of the dentinal tubule to the dentinoenamel junction. Stimulation of these sensory nerve fibers manifests as tooth pain. **A-delta fibers** are composed of small myelinated fibers that evoke a sensation of well-localized sharp pain and are thought to be responsible for dentinal hypersensitivity. Similarly, **A-beta fibers** are susceptible to the same types of stimuli but respond more sensitively to electrical stimulation. In contrast to the A-delta and A-beta fibers, stimulation of the **unmyelinated C-fibers** results in a dull, poorly localized, aching type of pain usually associated with pulpal pain. Thus the activation of specific fibers results in different types of tooth pain.

Hypersensitive dentin has the following characteristics:

- Dentinal tubules open to the oral cavity
- Large and numerous dentinal tubules
- Thin, poorly calcified or breached **smear layer** (a deposit of salivary proteins, debris from dentifrices and/or other calcified matter that occludes dentinal tubules)

In nonsensitive dentin, the smear layer covers the opening of the dentinal tubules, or mineral compounds occlude the tubules, thereby reducing the ability of stimuli to induce fluid flow (see section on hydrodynamic theory) and thus stimulate nerve conduction to the pulp. Therefore the loss or removal of a smear layer may result in exposed tubular nerve fibers, leading to a pain response. Nonsensitive dentin also is found to have fewer dentinal tubules present at the surface than sensitive dentin.[1] Scanning electron photomicrographs verify that hypersensitive dentin has eight times as many open dentinal tubules and twice the diameter of open tubules as nonsensitive dentin. These findings serve as the basis for treatment options.

Hydrodynamic Theory

Brannstrom was the first to provide evidence to support the widely accepted hydrodynamic theory explaining the pain of dentinal hypersensitivity.[2] The hydrodynamic theory proposes that stimuli (e.g., thermal, tactile, or chemical) are transmitted to the pulp surface via movement of fluid or semifluid materials found within the dentinal tubules. This fluid movement acts as a transducing medium that conveys peripheral stimuli to free A-delta nerve endings near the odontoblastic layer of the pulp-dentin interface. Subsequently, this reaction is interpreted as tooth pain by the client (Figure 39-1).

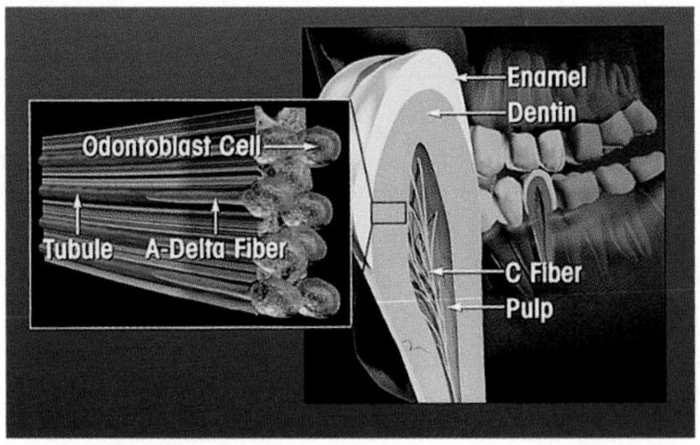

Figure 39-1. Structure of dentinal tubules. (Courtesy Osprey Communications, Stamford, Connecticut.)

For dentinal hypersensitivity, an open dentinal tubule channel must traverse from the exposed dentin surface to a vital pulp. The exposed dentin necessary for such hypersensitivity is most commonly the result of gingival recession or enamel loss along with other causes. When gingival recession occurs, cementum is exposed. This exposed layer of cementum is thin and labile and is easily abraded or eroded away, thus offering little protection against sensitivity.

Causes of Gingival Recession

Gingival recession is considered an enigma and causes are largely unknown.[3] It may be caused by the following:

- *The anatomy of the alveolar bone.* A thin, fenestrated, or absent labial alveolar bone is a predisposing factor to recession. Tooth anatomy and tooth position also may affect the thickness of the labial plate. For example, orthodontic treatment may move the tooth through the buccal plate, predisposing it to recession.
- *Poor oral hygiene status.* Poor oral self-care results in plaque-induced gingival disease, which can progress to attachment loss and result in recession. However, research reveals that even greater recession occurs with aggressive oral hygiene.
- *Trauma from abrasion.*[3] Gingival trauma caused by toothbrushing and/or injury from abrasive dentifrices or a combination may be risk factors. The technique, frequency, duration, and force of brushing and toothbrush filaments have been implicated in recession.
- *Frenal attachment at the gingival margin.* Progressive recession may occur when the fibers of the frenum insert near the gingival margin and cause a tight frenal pull on the gingival tissues during function. Tissue movement resulting from speech and mastication pulls the gingiva from the cementoenamel junction (CEJ), resulting in gingival recession.
- *Occlusal trauma.* A number of studies performed on human subjects have concluded that occlusal discrepancies appear to be a significant risk factor for attachment loss in subjects with active periodontal disease.[4] Occlusal forces may exceed the resistance threshold of a compromised attachment apparatus, thereby exacerbating a pre-existing periodontal lesion and thus possibly leading to further recession.

Causes of Enamel Loss[3]

See Chapters 16 and 25.

- *Attrition.* Sites of tooth structure wear are found commonly on the incisal or occlusal surfaces of teeth caused by masticatory forces. Unless malocclusion is involved, it is highly unlikely that attrition is observed at the buccal sites.
- *Abrasion.* Toothbrush variation (stiffness and configuration of the bristles), together with force, method, frequency, abrasiveness of toothpaste, and duration of brushing, results in tooth structure loss. When the teeth are brushed, enamel has been found to abrade much more slowly than dentin or cementum. For example, dentin abrades 25 times and cementum 35 times faster than enamel.
- *Erosion.* Tooth structure loss caused by a chemical process is most responsible for enamel loss. Intrinsic erosion is caused by acid regurgitation associated with medical and psychologic disorders (e.g., bulimia, acid reflux disease, morning sickness). Extrinsic erosion also may result from dietary factors that contribute to a highly acidic oral environment (e.g., the frequent consumption of acidic, carbonated, or fruit drinks or frequent sugar consumption).
- *Abfraction.* The ongoing flexion, tension, and compression forces exerted in the cervical area of a tooth from mastication and occlusal trauma can result in cracking and eventual loss of cervical tooth structure.

Additional Causes

Aggressive scaling and root planing, especially after periodontal surgery, can remove layers of protective cementum and dentin, thus exposing tubular dentin and causing sensitivity. One study reported an estimated 73% to 98% prevalence of dentinal sensitivity in periodontal patients, as opposed to 36% in the general population.[5]

Vital teeth bleaching procedures using peroxides to enhance the esthetic appearance of teeth have become popular over the years. The most common side effect associated with bleaching is tooth sensitivity.[6] Whether the sensitivity is caused by the penetration of the bleach through the enamel and dentin to the pulp resulting in reversible pulpitis, or the mechanical pressure exerted by the bleaching tray, or some other factor, the sensitivity tends to be transient in nature. The degree of sensitivity can be affected by the frequency of application/concentration of bleaching agents. Although it is difficult for the clinician to predict which clients will experience sensitivity, there are preventive measures that have been recommended based on studies. For example, before initiating the bleaching procedure, clients can be instructed to brush with a 5% potassium nitrate toothpaste for 2 weeks.[7]

Prevalence and Distribution of Dentinal Hypersensitivity

Reports of dentinal hypersensitivity range among all ages of clients. However, as an individual ages, the prevalence of dentinal hypersensitivity decreases because of an increase in reparative dentin formation; reduction in pulpal chamber size, vascularity, and pulpal nerve fibers; and dentinal sclerosis (reduction of the dentinal tubule lumen as a result of the deposition of intratubular dentin). Dentinal hypersensitivity is most prevalent on the buccal cervical regions of teeth. Similarly, these same sites have a predilection for gingival recession and are the areas where the enamel is the thinnest. Thus gingival recession and loss of enamel appear to be related to the initiation of dentinal hypersensitivity.

BOX 39-1

Characteristics of Hypersensitive Versus Nonsensitive Dentin

Hypersensitive Dentin
- Ends of dentinal tubules open to the oral cavity
- Tubules larger and more numerous than in nonsensitive dentin
- Smear layer is thin, poorly calcified, or breached

Nonsensitive Dentin
- Fewer dentinal tubules at tooth surface are present than in sensitive dentin
- Either a smear layer is present or tubules are occluded by mineral compounds

Persons with moderate to severe sensitivity exhibit hypersensitivity at the same tooth sites, and there is a greater frequency of left-sided tooth sensitivity in comparison with their right contralateral tooth types. Therefore individuals who are right-handed tend to clean their left-sided teeth more vigorously than their right-sided teeth, contributing to unilateral hypersensitivity.

Diagnosis

Many oral conditions exhibit symptoms similar to dentinal hypersensitivity. Conditions such as chipped or fractured teeth, dental caries, pulpal pathology, or leaking, fractured, or failing restorations require completely different treatment from dentinal hypersensitivity. It is vitally important for the treating practitioner to understand that dentinal hypersensitivity is a diagnosis of exclusion. Therefore a thorough clinical and radiographic examination must be conducted to exclude these conditions and arrive at a differential diagnosis of dentinal hypersensitivity (Box 39-1). For a diagnosis of dentinal hypersensitivity to be made, specific clinical and radiographic criteria must be present.

Clinical Criteria

- Sensitivity or pain when a stimulus is applied (either hot, cold, or tactile)
- Exposed dentin at the site of sensitivity
- No clinical signs of dental caries
- No evidence of fracture lines in tooth structure
- Restoration margins flush with tooth structure

Radiographic Criteria

- Radiolucency may be present at the cervical third of the tooth where pain is reported (indicating possible abrasion, erosion, abfraction, or radiolucent restorative material), but one or more of these findings must be confirmed clinically to exclude dental caries
- No pulpal inflammation or apical pathology
- Absence of distinct fracture lines
- No radiolucent areas under restorations

Additional Testing

Salivary tests for flow and buffering capacity can be done to evaluate the client's ability to flush and neutralize acids and promote remineralization necessary to occlude tubules.

BOX 39-2

Factors That Contribute to Dentinal Hypersensitivity

Factors that may expose dentin or opening tubules that are already blocked or sealed:
- Gingival recession
- Loss of enamel
- Toothbrush abrasion
- Erosion
- Abfraction
- Acidic foods
- Periodontal surgery
- Occlusal hyperfunction
- Cusp grinding
- Instrumentation (root planing, scaling, extrinsic stain removal)
- Cosmetic tooth whitening (see Chapter 29)

TABLE 39-1

Desensitizing Agents and Their Mode of Action

Mode of Action	Desensitizing Agent
Nerve inactivator	Potassium nitrate
Tubule obtundents	Fluorides Oxalates Calcium compounds (including CPP-ACP) Sodium citrate Strontium chloride
Protein precipitants	Strontium chloride Silver nitrate Formaldehyde Glutaraldehyde

CPP-ACP, Casein phosphopeptide–amorphous calcium phosphate complex.

Management of Dentinal Hypersensitivity

Managing dentinal hypersensitivity requires identification of the condition's cause and risk factors (Box 39-2). Failure to address these conditions can result in inadequate and/or unnecessary therapy.

After a cause is established, the client needs to be educated about behaviors that exacerbate symptoms of dentinal hypersensitivity. If necessary, behavior modification may be discussed (e.g., dietary choices such as avoiding carbonated beverages, acidic foods, and extremes in hot and cold foods; use of a daily fluoride mouth rinse and a low-abrasive, fluoride dentifrice for sensitive teeth) to arrest the hypersensitivity.

Treatment options include self-applied (at-home) desensitizing agents and professionally applied (in-office) desensitizing procedures and surgeries. Desensitizing agents used in treatment are classified by mode of action (Table 39-1): inactivation of the nerve membrane (hyperpolarization) or occlusion of the open dentinal tubules.

- *Nerve hyperpolarization.* Intradental nerves are hyperpolarized by raising their extracellular potassium ion concentration. The sustained hyperpolarized state reduces nerve excitation, and the nerves become insensitive to further stimulation for a finite duration of time. A common example of an agent to use is potassium nitrate.
- *Dentinal tubule occlusion.* Examples of agents to use include oxalate compounds, strontium chloride, calcium phosphate–based compounds, fluorides, silver nitrate, and hydroxyethyl methacrylate (HEMA).

Without effective daily oral biofilm control, the desensitizing effects of these agents are limited.

Self-Applied Desensitizing Agents

Self-applied desensitizing agents should be recommended to manage mild dentinal hypersensitivity (Table 39-2 and Figure 39-2; see Chapter 25). These agents are cost effective, safe, noninvasive, and simple to use and can be applied at home for convenience. Clients must be informed that regular and continuous application is necessary to manage sensitivity and that the time required to decrease the level of sensitivity is variable. Clients may apply a range of desensitizing agents in the form of dentifrices, gels, or rinses as part of their daily self-care regimen at home.

Potassium nitrate is the most common desensitizing agent in over-the-counter dentifrices. A concentration of 5% potassium nitrate (in conjunction with sodium or monofluorophosphate fluoride) significantly reduces symptoms within 2 weeks of daily use. Potassium ions penetrate the length of the dentinal tubule and block repolarization of the nerve ending. Increasing the extracellular potassium ion concentration depolarizes nerve fiber membranes and renders them unable

TABLE 39-2
Desensitizing Dentifrices

Brand	Variations	Manufacturer	Active Ingredients	Comments
Arm and Hammer	Sensitive Whitening Freshening Multiprotection	Arm and Hammer	Amorphous calcium phosphate	
Colgate	Sensitive Multi-Protection Enamel Protection Whitening	Colgate-Palmolive	5% potassium nitrate	
	Sensitive Pro-Relief Original Gentle Whitening Enamel Repair		8% arginine and calcium carbonate	
	PreviDent 5000 Sensitive	Colgate-Palmolive	5% potassium nitrate, 1.1% sodium fluoride	Prescription-strength toothpaste for sensitive teeth (Rx)
	PreviDent 5000 Enamel Protect	Colgate-Palmolive	5% potassium nitrate, 1.1% sodium fluoride	Prescription-strength toothpaste for sensitive teeth (Rx)
Crest	Sensitivity Clinical Sensitivity Relief Extra Whitening Whitening Plus Scope Toothpaste Minty Fresh	Procter & Gamble	Potassium nitrate	
	Pro-Health Sensitive + Enamel Shield Toothpaste	Procter & Gamble	0.4% stannous fluoride	
Sensodyne	Original Repair and Protect Extra Whitening Full Protection Plus Whitening Tartar Control Plus Whitening Fresh Impact Fresh Mint Cool Gel	GlaxoSmithKline	5% potassium nitrate	Original is sodium lauryl sulfate–free
Tom's of Maine	Maximum Strength Sensitive Fluoride Toothpaste Fluoride-Free Sensitive Toothpaste	Colgate-Palmolive	5% potassium nitrate	Sodium lauryl sulfate–free

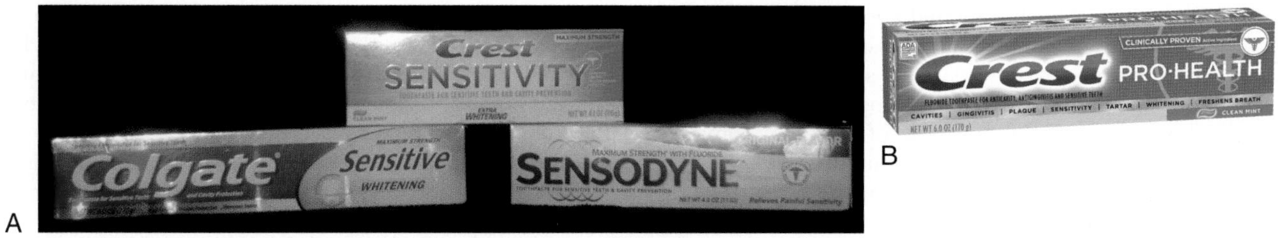

Figure 39-2. Some commonly used desensitizing dentifrices with active ingredients supported by the evidence: **A,** Examples with potassium nitrate. **B,** Example of 0.454% stannous fluoride dentifrice. (**B,** Courtesy Proctor & Gamble.)

to repolarize (i.e., they are hyperpolarized). Frequent and regular application of a potassium nitrate dentifrice is necessary to avoid recurrence of symptoms, maintain a high abundance of extracellular potassium ions, and maintain the intradental nerves in a hyperpolarized state. Therefore application via a dentifrice is ideal. Moreover, clients can be instructed to dab very small amounts of sensitivity-protection dentifrice on the sensitive area of the tooth at bedtime, which is left overnight.

Stannous fluoride (0.4% or 0.454%), a known antihypersensitivity ingredient, has been formulated into gels and toothpastes for daily use in controlling pain associated with dentinal hypersensitivity. Stannous fluoride produces the rapid onset or formation of a protective smear layer and the precipitation of calcium fluoride crystals, which physically block exposed dentinal tubules and hence act as a desensitizing agent against acidic or other environmental challenges.[8] Clinical studies have shown that when subjects brushed twice daily with a 0.454% stannous fluoride dentifrice for 8 weeks reduced hypersensitivity.[9]

Dentifrices containing 8.0% arginine and calcium carbonate also have been shown to relieve dentinal hypersensitivity by occluding the dentinal tubules. This occurs when the arginine component triggers physical adherence of the calcium carbonate to the exposed dentin surface and to the inner surfaces of dentin tubules, thereby inducing deposition of calcium and phosphate-rich materials on the dentin surface and occluding the dentin tubules. Studies demonstrate that toothpastes containing 8.0% arginine and calcium carbonate are effective in the everyday treatment of dentin hypersensitivity when used twice daily during routine brushing.[10]

Self-applied desensitizing agents also are marketed as gels and rinses. The active agents for these products are various fluoride compounds, such as sodium fluoride, sodium silicofluoride, and stannous fluoride. Some dentifrices have the American Dental Association (ADA) Seal of Acceptance for treatment of dentinal hypersensitivity. Application of fluoride to exposed dentin leads to the formation of calcium fluoride and other precipitates, reducing the functional radius of the dentinal tubules or blocking the dentinal tubules. Therefore relief can be achieved via the use of fluoride-containing gels and rinses; however, extended periods of use are necessary. It is important for the treating practitioner to inform the client that using products containing potassium nitrate provides only immediate, short-term relief from dentinal hypersensitivity. Long-term relief requires continued use of fluoride-containing substances to permanently seal off the exposed tubules with calcium fluoride particles.

Professionally Applied Desensitizing Agents

(See Procedure 39-1 and the corresponding Competency Form, Table 39-3, and Figure 39-3.) Although mild hypersensitivity may be managed by using a sensitivity-protection toothpaste twice daily, moderate to severe dentinal hypersensitivity must be treated professionally. Professionally applied agents include varnishes and precipitants, primers containing HEMA, and polymerizing agents. In severe cases, loss of cervical tooth structure often requires restoration with glass ionomer and/or composite resin materials to control hypersensitivity.

Before any desensitizing treatment, hard and soft deposits should be removed from the tooth surfaces. Therapeutic scaling may cause considerable discomfort, in which case teeth should be anesthetized before mechanical treatment.

Varnishes

- *5% sodium fluoride varnish.* Fluoride varnishes temporarily occlude dentinal tubules because the material is lost over time. This desensitizing agent is effective for relief of dentinal hypersensitivity and is sold in a tube and single unit dose packages. The single dose packaging facilitates application (see Figure 39-3; and Chapter 33, discussion of topical fluorides, professionally applied varnishes).

Precipitants

- *8% arginine and calcium carbonate.* After scaling, application of an in-office desensitizing paste containing arginine–calcium carbonate to teeth exhibiting sensitivity has been demonstrated to be effective in providing immediate relief.[9] As with polishing teeth, the paste should be applied using a prophylaxis cup on a prophy angle and using low speed and a moderate amount of pressure; the paste is burnished into the exposed tubules to occlude them.

Procedure 39-1 Administration of Desensitizing Agents

EQUIPMENT

Isolating materials (cotton rolls, gauze, or dry angles)
Cotton applicators
Dappen dish
Personal protective equipment
Desensitizing agent

STEPS

1. Assemble armamentarium for desensitization.
2. Explain rationale, procedure, and limitations of desensitizing agent to client.
3. Identify sensitive sites requiring desensitization treatment.
4. Remove oral biofilm and debris from tooth surfaces before desensitizing agent is applied.
5. Isolate area with cotton rolls, and dry dentin surface by blotting with gauze.
6. Dispense desensitizing agent and apply according to manufacturer's instructions.
7. Evaluate treated areas for success; reapply if necessary.
8. Discard materials according to infection-control procedures.
9. Record treatment in services-rendered section of client record, including tooth number, region of treatment, agent used, and client response.
10. Educate client about supplementary procedures for controlling sensitivity.

TABLE 39-3

Some Professionally Applied Desensitizing Agents

Brand	Manufacturer	Active Agent	Mechanism of Action	Comments
Colgate Duraphat Single unit-dose application of 0.05% fluoride varnish	Colgate-Palmolive	5% sodium fluoride		Indicated for caries prevention FDA approved as a treatment for dentinal hypersensitivity
Colgate PreviDent Varnish	Colgate-Palmolive	5% sodium fluoride		Indicated for caries prevention
Colgate Gel-Kam Preventive Treatment Gel	Colgate-Palmolive	0.4% stannous fluoride	Blocks dentinal tubules	
Colgate Sensitive Pro-Relief Paste	Colgate-Palmolive	8% arginine and calcium carbonate	Obturation of dentinal tubules	Post scaling and root planing; use as polishing paste on hypersensitive sites
Zarosen Desensitizing	Cetylite Industries	6.9% copal resin, 0.146% strontium chloride	Seals dentinal tubules, cavity varnish	After scaling, before and after extrinsic stain removal, after cavity preparation, before crown and bridge cementation, and before pin and after seating
HemaSeal G Desensitizing Solution	Germiphene Corporation	35% HEMA, 5% glutaraldehyde	Binds with proteins to seal dentinal tubules	
HurriSeal	Beutlich	Benzalkonium chloride, HEMA, 0.5% sodium fluoride, water	HEMA seals the dentinal tubules to produce a physiologic barrier for densensitizing, and benzalkonium chloride acts as an antibacterial	Used in conjunction with bonding adhesive systems and crown and bridge luting agents
Gluma Desensitizer	Heraeus Kulzer	HEMA, glutaraldehyde, water	Seals dentinal tubules	No mixing or curing involved, strong smell and taste
MI Paste	GC America	Casein phosphopeptide–amorphous calcium phosphate complex	Thought to seal dentinal tubules through release of soluble calcium and phosphate precipitate during acid challenge	Current evidence regarding ability to reduce sensitivity is weak
NUPRO NUSolutions	DENTSPLY	NovaMin (calcium sodium phosphosilicate)	Seals dentinal tubules	Prophylaxis paste that cleans, occludes tubules, and desensitizes

HEMA, Hydroxyethyl methacrylate.

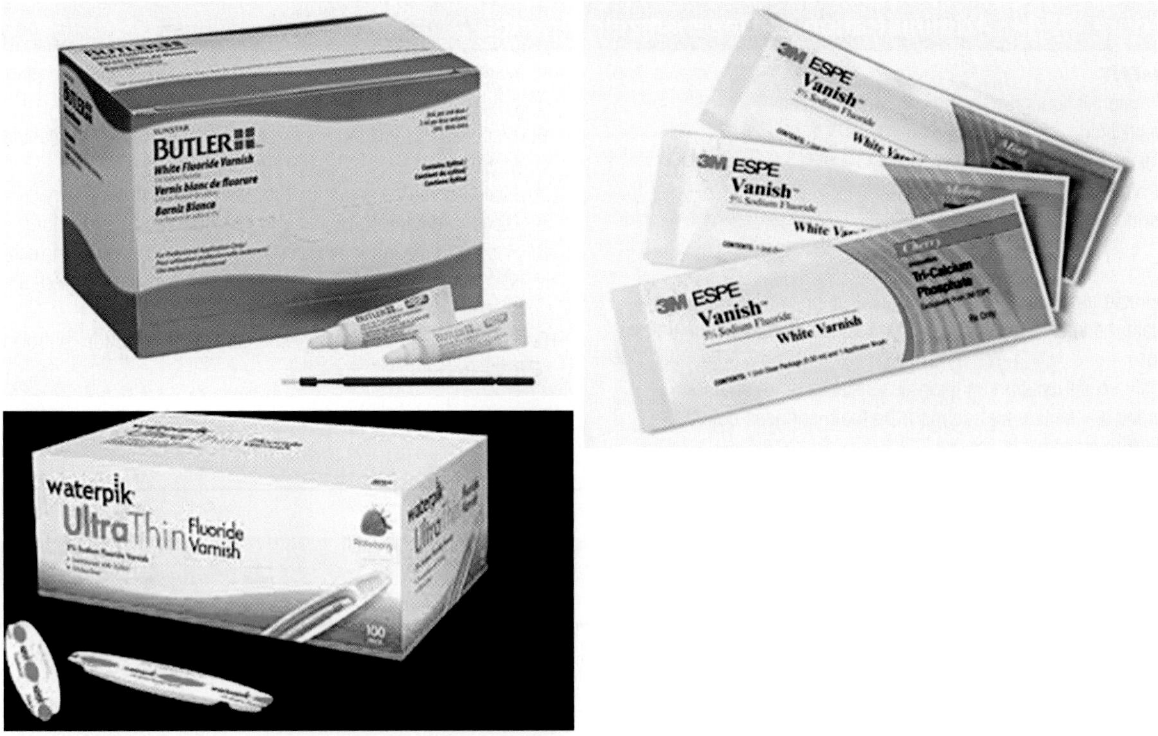

Figure 39-3. Unit-dose packaging of 5% sodium fluoride varnish. (**A,** Courtesy Sunstar Americas, Inc., Chicago, IL; **B,** Courtesy 3M ESPE, St. Paul, MN; **C,** Courtesy Water Pik, Inc, Fort Collins, CO.)

Calcium phosphates have been shown to occlude dentinal tubules.[11] For furcations and other sites that are difficult to access, the paste also can be applied with a cotton-tipped applicator or a microbrush.

- *Oxalates.* The efficacy of oxalate-containing agents is unclear. Comparison of the clinical evidence fails to objectively demonstrate the efficacy of oxalate-containing agents because of various experimental designs.
- *Calcium phosphate compounds.* Burnishing of calcium phosphate into areas of sensitive dentin significantly relieves discomfort. There are several formulations of calcium phosphate compounds that can be used as desensitizing agents and the formulations are improving over time. The mechanism of action involves the occlusion of dentinal tubules by forming a calcium phosphate precipitate.[11,12]
  - *Calcium hydroxide.* This desensitizing agent has been used to block dentinal tubules and promote peritubular dentin formation. It also has been used to reduce the permeability of acid-etched dentin and smear layers.
  - *Casein phosphopeptide–amorphous calcium phosphate (CPP-ACP).* Shortly after the discovery of ACP, researchers realized that if they combined CPP with ACP, the compound had greater affinity for bacterial biofilm because the presence of CPP is a protein found in cow's milk and has the ability to stabilize and bind calcium and phosphate ions, thus making them soluble and bioavailable. When applied orally, this nanocomplex has been found to bind to soft tissues, pellicle, oral biofilm, and hydroxyapatite and subsequently releases calcium and phosphate ions when challenged by acid attack. It is thought that this ion release leads to a precipitate which plugs open dentinal tubules.[11] CPP-ACP formulations in prophylaxis pastes are approved for desensitization claims by the FDA (e.g., MI Paste prophylaxis paste; see Figure 39-4). Because of its origins, this product should not be used in clients with a milk protein allergy and/or with a sensitivity or allergy to benzoate preservatives.
- *Calcium sodium phosphosilicate (CSP).* NovaMin is the brand name of the bioactive glass CSP. This inorganic chemical binds to tooth surfaces and delivers calcium, phosphorus, sodium, and silica to replace lost minerals. When the glass particles come in contact with saliva, calcium and phosphate ions are released. A calcium-phosphate layer forms and crystallizes as new hydroxyapatite. Dentinal tubules are occluded in the process and desensitization is effective.[13] This agent is approved by the FDA for desensitization claims (see examples of professional products in Figure 39-4).
- *Tricalcium phosphate (TCP).* A new calcium phosphate technology on the market is TCP, so research is needed to substantiate effectiveness; however, it shares properties with the other products in this category. TCP protects calcium ions and frees phosphate ions—this material prohibits calcium from prematurely reacting with fluoride before reaching tooth surfaces. Once TCP is exposed to saliva on tooth structure, calcium, phosphate, and fluoride ions are released. TCP is an ingredient in Enamel Pro 5% Sodium Fluoride Vanish, for example (see Figure 39-4).

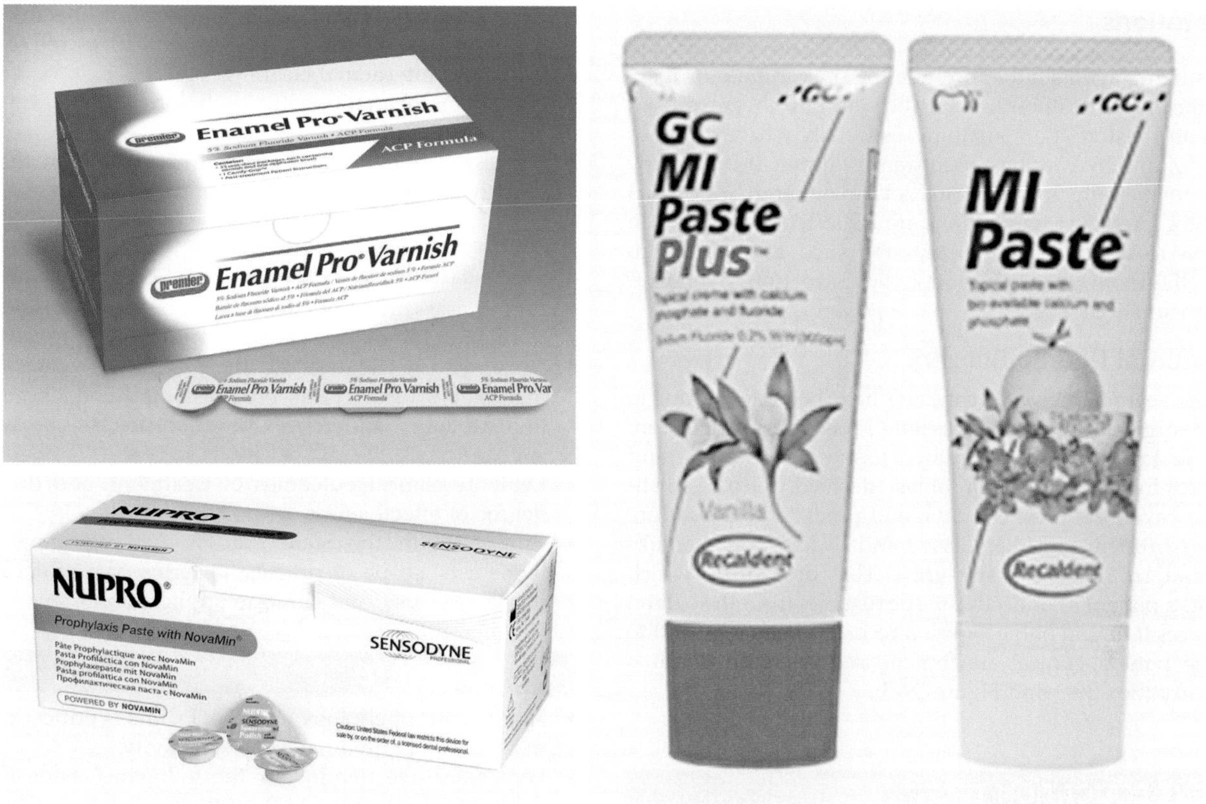

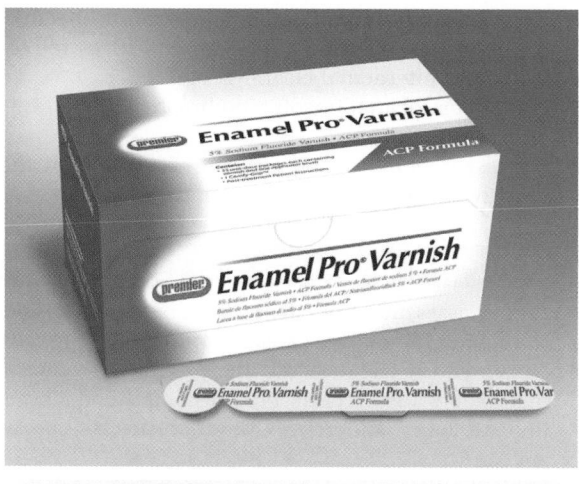

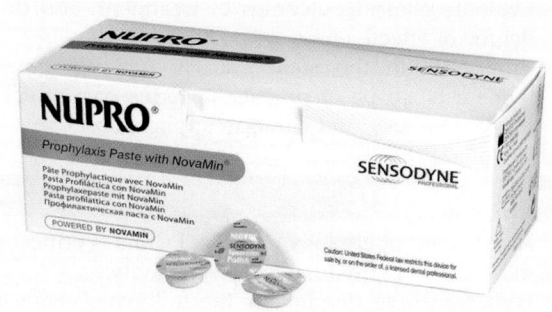

Figure 39-4. Example of desensitizing calcium and phosphorus products with FDA approval for treatment of dentinal hypersensitivity. (Courtesy Premier Dental Group, Plymouth, MN; GlaxoSmithKline, Brentford, Middlesex, UK; GC America, Alsip, IL.)

Primers Containing Hydroxyethyl Methacrylate (HEMA)

Although few controlled clinical trials have been conducted on the efficacy of HEMA-containing primers, desensitizing agents containing either 5% glutaraldehyde and 35% HEMA in water or 35% HEMA in water alone are popular.

- *5% Glutaraldehyde, 35% HEMA in water.* Studies regarding a primer containing 5% glutaraldehyde and 35% HEMA in water (e.g., Gluma and Gluma 2000) have shown mixed results regarding effectiveness in reducing dentinal hypersensitivity long term. More evidence is needed to document effectiveness of this formulation.

Polymerizing Agents

- *Glass ionomer cements (GICs).* GICs are used in cervical abrasions and abfractions for the treatment of dentinal hypersensitivity. The cervical areas of a tooth are etched with 50% citric acid for 30 to 45 seconds, rinsed with water, and dried before GIC placement. GICs are effective in treating hypersensitivity if they cover the affected area.
- *Adhesive resin primers.* Adhesive resin primers decrease dentin permeability by occluding the open dentinal tubules. Resin primers come in either a two- or one-bottle system. The product is gently rubbed on the hypersensitive dentin for approximately 30 seconds and air dried, and the procedure possibly is repeated.

Iontophoresis

Iontophoresis involves the delivery of sodium fluoride by passing an electrical current through the cervical dentin. This procedure is based on the principle that similar electromagnetic charges repel each other. When the negative fluorine ions contact the negatively charged electrode and a current is passed through the tooth to the other electrode (which is held by the client, completing the circuit), fluoride ions are pushed into the dentinal tubules, where they react with ions in the hydroxyapatite. Fluorapatite precipitate, an insoluble compound, is formed, thus occluding the tubules.

Use of this technique-sensitive procedure to treat hypersensitive dentin has proponents. Lack of efficacy reported by others may be the result of the inadvertent passage of current through adjacent gingival tissue rather than through cervical dentin. Mild cases of dentinal hypersensitivity may require only a single treatment, whereas in more severe cases, two or three applications 1 week apart may be necessary. The procedure requires a special apparatus.

Lasers

Laser therapy is relatively quick, and one treatment drastically reduces or eliminates sensitivity by sealing the dentinal tubules. Dentin treated with laser is harder than untreated dentin. Studies of lasers used for dentinal hypersensitivity, such as the neodymium:yttrium-aluminum-garnet (Nd:YAG) laser, have shown varying results, so the evidence is inconclusive. Evidence is more promising with low-level laser treatment or photodynamic therapy, which appears to be effective in reducing dentinal hypersensitivity when compared with placebo for desensitization.[12,14] The current high cost of equipment precludes widespread clinical use.

Restorations

Desensitizing agents either occlude the open tubule or inactivate the nerve. Restorations may be placed to cover exposed dentin and restore tooth anatomy, especially where esthetics are important. In extreme circumstances, it may be necessary to remove the pulp and perform root canal therapy or extract the tooth. These last two options are indicated for reasons in addition to dentinal hypersensitivity, such as inability to restore the tooth, severe periodontal destruction, overeruption, or esthetics.

Periodontal Plastic Surgery

Over the years numerous techniques have been developed to correct surgically gingival recession. Procedures range from use of juxtaposed gingiva, guided tissue regeneration, and tissue engineered human fibroblast–derived dermal substitute; however, the most common and predictable procedure for the treatment of Miller Class I and II defects is the **subepithelial connective tissue graft**. This procedure, which harvests a patient's connective tissue (usually from the palate) and places it on top of the exposed root, has been reported to increase patient clinical attachment and decrease dentinal sensitivity (Box 39-3 and Figure 39-5).

CLIENT EDUCATION TIPS

- Explain multifaceted causes of dentinal hypersensitivity and modifiable risk factors.
- Discuss dietary information, and monitor acidic and sugary fruits and beverages that may contribute to hypersensitivity.
- Explain significance of oral biofilm control; effective toothbrushing; low-abrasive, fluoride dentifrices for sensitive teeth; and interdental cleaning.
- Explain use of an ultrasoft toothbrush without the application of a toothpaste.
- Suggest dabbing a desensitizing dentifrice on the most sensitive areas of the tooth at bedtime.

LEGAL, ETHICAL, AND SAFETY ISSUES

- Proper assessment of client's hypersensitivity is essential to rule out alternative causes of pain.
- Document in client record the problem, product recommendation, instructions provided, and client's response to care (e.g., adherence, product success, or adverse effects).
- Evaluate clinical outcomes of treatment, and document degree of effectiveness.
- Comply with the State Practice Act regarding dental hygienists' scope of practice in terms of product recommendation, use, and clinician application.

KEY CONCEPTS

- Assessment of etiology and risk factors is critical to identify accurately dentinal hypersensitivity.
- Hypersensitive dentin has the following characteristics: dentinal tubules open to the oral cavity, large and numerous dentinal tubules, and thin, poorly calcified, or breached smear layer (a deposit of salivary proteins, debris from dentifrices, and other calcified matter).
- Abfraction is damage resulting from the ongoing flexion, tension, and compression forces exerted in the cervical

BOX 39-3

Case Study of Client Treated with a Connective Tissue Graft to Control Dentinal Hypersensitivity

CM came to the practice complaining of severe sensitivity to cold air and fluids around teeth 28 and 29 over the past 5 months, and as a result had avoided toothbrushing or flossing in that area. Periodontal assessment revealed localized erythema, oral biofilm accumulation, and recession of 3 mm and 1 mm on teeth 28 and 29, respectively. In addition, tooth 28 had minimal keratinized tissue (1 mm), extrinsic staining, and cervical abrasion. CM acknowledged a history of aggressive tooth brushing.

CM's care plan included oral self-care instructions, with emphasis on the modified Bass brushing technique with a sensitivity toothpaste, scaling and root planing under a local anesthetic, and use of a soft-bristled toothbrush to improve gingival health before periodontal surgery.

A connective tissue graft procedure was performed to provide a thicker gingival biotype buccal to tooth 28 and to achieve root coverage over both premolars. Before surgery, CM reported a Visual Analog Scale (VAS) value of 10 when tooth 28 was subjected to a cold air blast from an air-water syringe.

Six weeks after the surgical procedure was performed, the client's reported VAS value improved to 5.

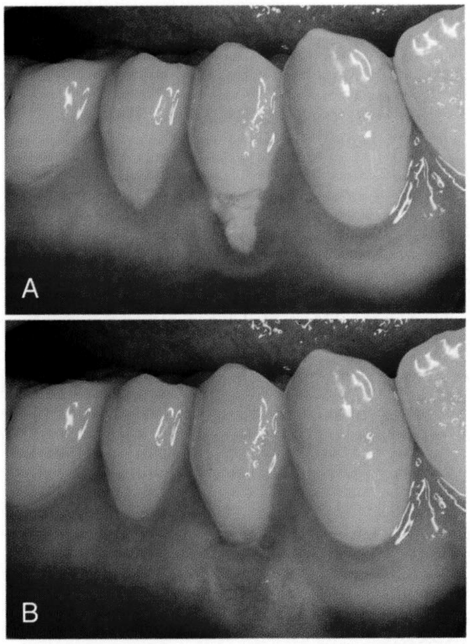

Figure 39-5. Client with severe dentinal hypersensitivity of teeth No. 28 and 29. **A,** Before connective tissue graft surgery. **B,** After connective tissue graft surgery. (Courtesy Dr. Angela Demeter, The University of British Columbia.)

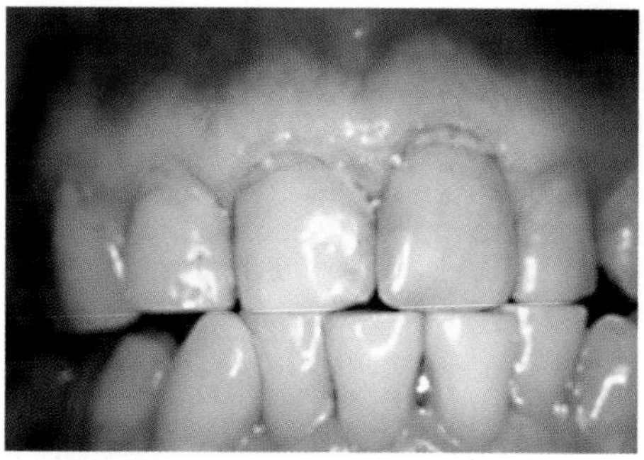

Figure 39-6. Intraoral photo of a young woman. Note accumulation of oral biofilm, gingival recession, cervical abrasion, and attrition.

area of a tooth as a result of mastication and occlusal trauma. These forces result in cracking and eventual loss of cervical tooth structure.

- Dentinal hypersensitivity is characterized by short, sharp pain, arising from exposed dentin, that occurs in response to stimuli, typically thermal (both hot and cold), evaporative, tactile, osmotic, or chemical, and that cannot be ascribed to any other form of dental defect or pathology.
- The hydrodynamic theory proposes that stimuli (i.e., thermal, tactile, or chemical) are transmitted to the pulp surface via movement of the fluid or semifluid materials in the dentinal tubules.
- Desensitization measures are incorporated into the client's care plan and daily self-care regimen.
- Most persons experiencing dentinal hypersensitivity can be treated with self-applied desensitizing dentifrices; however, if the sensitivity persists, professionally applied tubule-occluding desensitizing agents and restorative interventions can reduce sensitivity.
- Dental hygienists have a role in the management of dentinal hypersensitivity. This includes staying informed of current research and new products, selecting treatments that meet the patient's needs, and educating patients about effective self-care habits.

CRITICAL THINKING EXERCISES

Use Figure 39-6 and the following information to answer the questions about this case.

Client Profile: This 32-year-old female, a single mother of two boys (ages 2 and 4), is an emergency care nurse.

Chief Complaint: "My teeth are very sensitive when I eat or drink cold foods and beverages."

Health History: No significant findings

Pharmacologic History: The client takes the following medications:

- Ortho Tri-Cyclen (norgestimate/ethinyl estradiol)
- Wellbutrin SR (bupropion HCl 100 mg)
- Imitrex (sumatriptan succinate 50 mg)

Dental History:

- Regular 6-month continued-care appointments
- History of frequent aphthous ulcers
- Brushes twice daily
- Flosses once daily

Clinical Examination Findings:

- Absence of soft-tissue pathology
- Absence of clinical carious lesions
- Light to moderate calculus
- Localized attrition along anterior incisal and canine surfaces
- Localized recession and cervical abrasion evident on teeth 6, 7, 8, 9, 22, 23, 24, 25, 26, 27, 28, and 29
- There appears to be a hairline fracture on the labial of tooth 9

Radiographic Findings:

- Incipient enamel lesions (distal aspect of 3, mesial aspect of 15, distal aspect of 19)
- Linear radiolucent areas along the CEJ of 28 and 29 premolar teeth, consistent with the clinically observed posterior cervical abrasion

Given the client profile, chief complaint, and examination findings, answer the following questions:

1. What client characteristics indicate that she is at risk for dentinal hypersensitivity?
2. What are some common explanations for gingival recession?
3. What dental conditions must be considered to arrive at a differential diagnosis?
4. Based on the differential diagnosis determined by you and the dentist, what are the treatment options?
5. What special self-care instructions will relieve the client's symptoms of sensitive teeth? What specific products may reduce the occurrence of aphthous ulcers?
6. Explain the potential significance of the hairline fracture on tooth No. 9.

REFERENCES

1. Absi EG, Addy M, Adams D: Dentine hypersensitivity. A study of the patency of dentinal tubules in sensitive and non-sensitive cervical dentine, *J Clin Periodontol* 14(5):280, 1987.
2. Brannstrom M: A hydrodynamic mechanism in the transmission of pain-produced stimuli through dentine. In Anderson D, editor: *Sensory mechanisms in dentine*, Oxford, 1963, Pergamon.
3. Canadian Advisory Board on Dentin Hypersensitivity: Consensus-based recommendations for the diagnosis and management of dentin hypersensitivity, *J Can Dent Assoc* 69(4):221, 2003.
4. Hallmon WW, Harrel SK: Occlusal analysis, diagnosis and management in the practice of periodontics, *Periodontology 2000* 34: 151, 2004.
5. Drisko CH: Dentin hypersensitivity—dental hygiene and periodontal considerations, *Int Dent J* 52:385, 2002.
6. Leonard RH, Jr, Bentley C, Eagle JC, et al: Nightguard vital bleaching: a long-term study on efficacy, shade retention, side effects, and patients' perceptions, *J Esthet Restor Dent* 13(6):357, 2001.
7. Haywood VB: Treating sensitivity during tooth whitening, *Compend Contin Educ Dent*, 26(9 suppl 3):11, 2005.
8. Thrash WJ, Dodds MW, Jones DL: The effect of stannous fluoride on dentinal hypersensitivity, *Int Dent J* 44(1 suppl 1):107, 1994.
9. Walters PA: Dentinal hypersensitivity: a review, *J Contemp Dent Pract* 2(6):107–117, 2005.
10. Docimo R, Montesani L, Maturo P, et al: Comparing the efficacy in reducing dentin hypersensitivity of a new toothpaste containing 8.0% arginine, calcium carbonate, and 1450 ppm fluoride to a benchmark commercial desensitizing toothpaste containing 2%

potassium ion: an eight-week clinical study in Rome, Italy, *J Clin Dent* 20(4):137–143, 2009.
11. Lin PY, Cheng YW, Chu CY, et al: In-office treatment for dentin hypersensitivity: a systematic review and network meta-analysis, *J Clin Periodontol* 40(1):532, 2012.
12. Orchardson R, Gillam DG: Managing dentinal hypersensitivity, *J Am Dent Assoc* 137(7):990, 2006.
13. Gendreau L, Barlow AP, Mason SC: Overview of the clinical evidence for the use of NovaMin in providing relief from the pain of dentin hypersensitivity, *J Clin Dent* 22(3):90, 2011.
14. Sgolastra F, Petrucci A, Gatto R, et al: Effectiveness of laser in dentinal hypersensitivity treatment: a systematic review, *J Endo* 37(3):297, 2011.

ACKNOWLEDGMENT

The author acknowledges Dr. Dimitrios Karastathis and Ms. Nancy Zinser for their past contributions to this chapter.

ⓔ EVOLVE RESOURCES

Please visit http://evolve.elsevier.com/Darby/hygiene for additional practice and study support tools.

Local Anesthesia

CHAPTER 40

Elena Ortega

COMPETENCIES

1. Describe the physiologic mechanism of nerve conduction.
2. Discuss local anesthetic agents and vasoconstrictors used in dentistry, including:
   - Explain the rationale for using a particular agent.
   - Calculate the maximal safe dose of each local anesthetic agent and vasoconstrictor for each client.
3. Assess clients' health and pharmacologic history to determine their suitability to receive local anesthetics or vasoconstrictors.
4. Identify the equipment used for the administration of a local anesthetic agent.
5. Assemble, disassemble, and properly maintain the armamentarium required for local anesthetic administration.
6. Discuss the trigeminal nerve.
7. Describe the three types of injections: local infiltration, field block, and nerve block.
8. Discuss the procedures necessary for a successful injection.
9. Discuss injection techniques for the maxillary teeth and facial hard and soft tissues, including:
   - Identify the anatomic landmarks on both a skull and a client for the following injections: supraperiosteal, anterior superior alveolar nerve block, middle superior alveolar nerve block, infraorbital nerve block, and posterior superior alveolar nerve block.
   - Identify which nerves, teeth, and soft-tissue structures are anesthetized with each injection.
10. Discuss injection techniques for the palatal hard and soft tissues, including:
    - Identify the anatomic landmarks on both a skull and a client for the following injections: greater palatine nerve block and nasopalatine nerve block.
    - Identify which nerves, teeth, and soft-tissue structures are anesthetized with each injection.
11. Discuss injection techniques for the mandibular teeth and facial hard and soft tissues, including:
    - Identify the anatomic landmarks on both a skull and a client for the following injections: inferior alveolar nerve block, lingual nerve block, buccal nerve block, mental nerve block, and incisive nerve block.
    - Identify which nerves, teeth, and soft-tissue structures are anesthetized with each injection.
12. Identify the local complications that may result from local anesthetic administration and their proper management.
13. Identify the systemic complications that may result from local anesthetic administration and their proper management.
14. Discuss trends in pain management.

The administration of intraoral local anesthetic when needed during dental hygiene care allows the dental hygienist to provide local anesthesia to meet the client's human needs for freedom from pain and freedom from fear and stress. **Local anesthesia** involves sensation loss in a circumscribed body area as a result of the depression of excitation in nerve endings or the inhibition of the conduction process in peripheral nerves.[1] Local anesthetic agents used in clinical practice today prevent both the generation and conduction of nerve impulses. The local anesthetic agent essentially provides a chemical roadblock between the source of the impulse (e.g., a periodontal abscess) and the brain. The impulse is unable to reach the brain and is therefore not interpreted as pain or discomfort by the client. Local anesthesia differs dramatically from general anesthesia in that local anesthesia produces a loss of sensation without inducing a loss of consciousness.[1]

Not all dental hygiene clients require local anesthesia. Those receiving preventive oral prophylaxis or even periodontal maintenance care may experience little or no discomfort; however, local anesthetic administration is usually required if the dental hygiene care plan includes therapeutic scaling and root planing or if a client is simply experiencing undue tooth or soft-tissue sensitivity. In addition, a dental hygienist working in collaboration with a dentist may be called on to anesthetize individuals for the dentist in preparation for restorative or surgical periodontal therapy.

Physiology of Nerve Conduction

To understand how local anesthetic agents work, the dental hygienist needs to be familiar with the physiology of nerve conduction. Two principal ions are needed for nerve conduction: potassium (K^+) and sodium (Na^+). Because these two molecules are positively charged, they normally exist in equal concentrations across a membrane; however, in a nerve cell, this equilibrium does not exist (Figure 40-1, *Phase 1*). As a result of a sodium pump located within the cell membrane, the positively charged sodium molecules are forced outside the nerve cell. As the sodium leaves the intracellular fluid, a state of negativity is created inside the nerve cell. At the same time, the extracellular fluid, which has received the sodium,

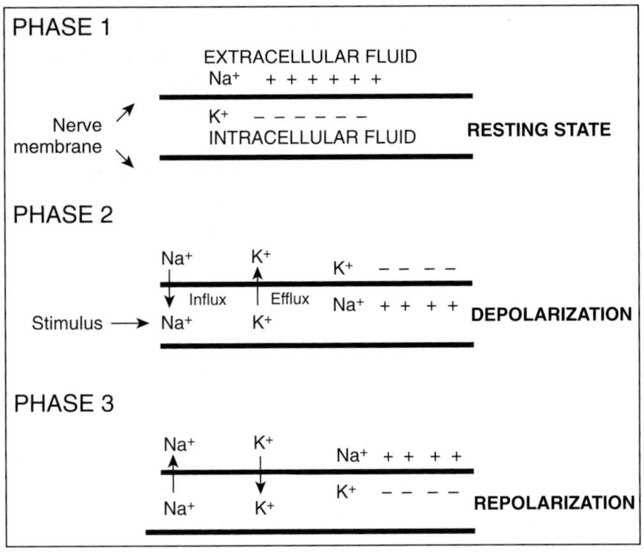

Figure 40-1. A rapid sequence of changes that involves depolarization and repolarization is called *action potential.*

becomes positive. After the sodium ion is transported out of the cell, it is not able to diffuse back into the intracellular fluids because of the relative impermeability of the nerve membrane to this ion. Although the nerve membrane is freely permeable to the potassium, this ion remains within the nerve cell, because the negative charge of the nerve membrane restrains the positively charged ion by electrostatic attraction. The nerve is polarized or in a resting state or at **resting potential** when this balance exists between positive sodium ions on the outside of the nerve membrane and negative potassium ions on the inside of the membrane. Polarization of the membrane continues as long as the nerve remains undisturbed.

A stimulus—which may be chemical, thermal, mechanical, or electrical in nature (e.g., pain)—produces excitation of the nerve fiber and therefore a change in the ion balance (see Figure 40-1, *Phase* 2). During this phase, which is referred to as **depolarization**, the nerve membrane becomes more permeable to the sodium ion. Consequently, the positive sodium ions move rapidly across the nerve membrane to the inside of the nerve cell. During this influx of sodium, the potassium ions diffuse from the inside to the outside of the nerve membrane.

Thus, during depolarization, the ion balance of the nerve cell reverses. On the interior of the nerve membrane are the positive sodium ions, whereas on the exterior of the nerve cell are the potassium ions. The inside of the nerve is now electrically positive as compared with the outside of the nerve.

Immediately after depolarization, the permeability of the membrane to the sodium ion once again decreases (see Figure 40-1, *Phase* 3). This situation is referred to as *repolarization.* During this phase, the sodium pump actively transports the sodium ion out of the nerve cell, whereas potassium ions diffuse and are pumped to the inside of the nerve cell. Thus, the nerve's resting potential is reestablished: the interior of the nerve cell is negative, and the exterior of the nerve cell consists of the positive sodium ions. This rapid sequence of changes from depolarization to repolarization is called the **action potential**.

When the resting potential of the nerve membrane is disrupted by a stimulus (e.g., pain) and depolarization occurs, the impulse must be transmitted along the nerve fiber. This impulse propagation is achieved when the ion changes during depolarization produce a new electrical equilibrium (i.e., the interior of the cell changes from negative to positive, the exterior of the cell changes from positive to negative). These ion changes in turn produce local currents that flow from the depolarized segment of the nerve to the adjacent resting area. As a result of this electrical current flow, depolarization begins in this previously resting area and continues propagating itself along the entire length of the nerve fiber. The depolarization step thus begins a chain reaction that continues the action potential along the nerve. In this manner, the impulse is propelled along the nerve fiber to the central nervous system.[1]

TABLE 40-1
Amide Local Anesthetics

Generic Name	Proprietary Name
Articaine	Septocaine
Bupivacaine	Marcaine
Lidocaine	Xylocaine, Alphacaine, Octocaine
Mepivacaine	Carbocaine, Arestocaine, Isocaine, Polocaine
Prilocaine	Citanest

Mechanism of Action of Local Anesthetic Agents

Although there are several theories regarding how local anesthetics work, it is commonly accepted that the primary action of these drugs is in reducing the permeability of the nerve membrane to the sodium ions (Na^+). The nerve membrane remains impermeable to the sodium ions despite the introduction of a stimulus to the nerve. Because the sodium ions remain on the outside of the nerve cell and are unable to enter the nerve membrane, an action potential never occurs. The nerve cell remains in a polarized state (i.e., a resting state) because the ionic movements responsible for the action potential do not develop. The action of depolarization that is required to initiate or to continue nerve impulse transmission (propagation) is thus blocked. An impulse that arrives at the blocked nerve segment is unable to be transmitted to the brain and is therefore not interpreted as pain or discomfort by the client.

Local Anesthetic Agents

Although many drugs are classified as local anesthetics, only a few are used in dentistry. Ester-type local anesthetics continue to be used as topical anesthetics (primarily benzocaine), but the injectable ester-type local anesthetics have been taken off the market. Currently the injectable local anesthetic agents employed in North America consist exclusively of amides[1] (Table 40-1).

Metabolism (Biotransformation) and Excretion

The mechanism by which local anesthetic agents are metabolized is important, because the overall toxicity of an agent depends on the balance between the agent's rate of absorption into the bloodstream at the injection site and the rate of the agent's removal from the blood through the processes of tissue uptake and metabolism.

Amide local anesthetics undergo biotransformation in the liver with the help of microsomal enzymes. Therefore the liver function of a client influences the rate of biotransformation of an amide drug. Those clients with impaired liver function are unable to metabolize amide local anesthetics at a normal rate, thereby leading to excessive levels of the agent in the blood, which increases the potential for toxic overdose (see Preanesthetic Client Assessment; Systemic Complications).

The metabolic products of amide local anesthetics are almost entirely excreted by the kidneys. In addition, a small amount of a given dose of local anesthetic agent is excreted unchanged in the urine. Amides are usually excreted in their original form in small concentrations in the urine. Clients with significant renal impairment or those undergoing renal dialysis may be unable to efficiently remove the unchanged form of the local anesthetic compound or its breakdown products from their blood. This renal impairment leads to elevated local anesthetic blood levels and an increased potential for toxicity (see Preanesthetic Client Assessment; Systemic Complications).[1]

Vasoconstrictors

All local anesthetic agents presently used in dentistry produce some degree of vasodilation (i.e., the relaxation of the blood vessel wall resulting in increased blood flow to the injection site). After local anesthetic injection into the tissues, the following reactions occur[1]:

- Increased blood flow to the injection site as the local anesthetic agents dilate the blood vessels
- Accelerated local anesthetic absorption into the bloodstream, thereby causing the anesthetic to be carried away from the injection site
- Higher amounts of local anesthetic in the blood, with the attendant greater risk for an overdose reaction
- Decreased duration of action and decreased local anesthetic effectiveness because the medication diffuses away from the administration site more rapidly
- Increased bleeding at the injection site because of the increased blood flow to the area

To counteract the vasodilating properties of local anesthetic agents, vasoconstrictors are added to the local anesthetic solution. Vasoconstrictors are drugs that constrict the blood vessels and thus control blood flow in the area of the injection. Vasoconstrictors are important additions to a local anesthetic solution, because vasoconstriction leads to the following[1]:

- Decreased blood flow to the injection site
- Slowed rate of local anesthetic absorption into the bloodstream, thus keeping it at the injection site longer and producing lower levels in the bloodstream
- Lower local anesthetic amounts in the blood, thereby decreasing the risk for an overdose reaction (or reducing the potential for systemic toxicity)
- Increased duration of action and increased local anesthetic effectiveness as higher concentrations of the agent remain in and around the nerve for a longer period
- Decreased bleeding at the injection site (i.e., hemostasis) as a result of the decreased blood flow to the area

Vasoconstrictors are an important addition to a local anesthetic solution because they decrease the potential toxicity of the anesthetic solution while increasing the duration and effectiveness of pain control. For example, the addition of 1:100,000 or 1:200,000 epinephrine to 2% lidocaine increases the duration of pulpal and hard-tissue anesthesia from approximately 10 minutes to 60 minutes. Dental hygiene appointments are frequently 60 minutes in length, and therefore vasoconstrictors are necessary to provide a pain-free state for clients during the completion of dental hygiene care.

Moreover, dental hygiene care often involves soft-tissue manipulation, and hemorrhage is a frequent result, especially when inflammation is present. Local anesthetic use without vasoconstrictors is problematic because the vasodilating properties of the anesthetic actually increase bleeding at the site of the injection. Vasoconstrictors are added to the anesthetic solution to counteract this unwanted action by preventing or minimizing bleeding during dental hygiene care.

For pain control when providing dental hygiene care, nerve blocks (e.g., posterior superior alveolar [PSA] nerve block, inferior alveolar nerve block) are frequently the techniques of choice. To derive the bleeding control benefits from the vasoconstrictor, however, the drug must be administered via local infiltration directly into the area where the bleeding is occurring or is expected to occur. For example, to provide pain control to the maxillary molars and the buccal tissue over these teeth, a PSA nerve block is administered. The anesthetic agent is deposited posterior and superior to the posterior border of the maxilla, some distance from the area being anesthetized. If hemostasis is needed on the buccal tissue over any of the molars, however, the administration of a local infiltration into the area is necessary, even though the anesthesia may be profound. Fortunately, only small volumes of solution are required (approximately 1 mL) for hemostatic purposes.[1]

Mechanism of Action

In addition to performing other functions, the sympathetic nervous system component of the autonomic nervous system controls the dilation and constriction of various blood vessels throughout the body. Adrenalin, which is also known as epinephrine, is one of the naturally occurring agents responsible for sympathetic nervous system activity.[1] The local anesthetic vasoconstrictors used are chemically identical to or very similar to the adrenalin that is produced naturally during sympathetic nervous system stimulation. Therefore, because the actions of the vasoconstrictors so closely mimic the action of the sympathetic autonomic nervous system, they are referred to as *sympathomimetic* or *adrenergic agents.*

Throughout the body tissues, adrenergic receptors are found that are stimulated by the chemicals released by the sympathetic nervous system or a sympathomimetic agent (i.e., a drug). These receptor sites are divided into two major categories: alpha and beta. Activation of the alpha receptors by a sympathomimetic agent (drug) results in smooth muscle contraction in blood vessels. This contraction produces a constriction of the vessels that is referred to as vasoconstriction.

TABLE 40-2

Vasoconstrictors Used in Dental Local Anesthetic Solutions

Generic Name	Proprietary Name	Concentrations
Epinephrine	Adrenalin	1:50,000 1:100,000 1:200,000
Levonordefrin	Neo-Cobefrin	1:20,000
Norepinephrine (levarterenol)*	Levophed	1:30,000

*No longer available in the United States and Canada.

TABLE 40-3

Recommended Maximum Doses of Epinephrine

	CARTRIDGES (ROUNDED OFF)	
Epinephrine Concentration (mcg/cartridge)	Normal, Healthy Patient (ASA I)*	Patient with Clinically Significant Cardiovascular Disease (ASA III or IV)†
1:50,000 (36)	5.5	1
1:100,000 (18)	11‡	2
1:200,000 (9)	22‡	4

From Malamed SF: *Handbook of local anesthesia*, ed 6, St Louis, 2013, Mosby.

ASA, American Society of Anesthesiologists Classes I, III, IV.

*Maximum epinephrine dose of 0.2 mg or 200 mcg per appointment.

†Maximum recommended dose of 0.04 or 40 mcg per appointment.

‡Actual maximum volume of administration is limited by the dose of the local anesthetic drug.

The primary reason that sympathomimetic agents are added to local anesthetic solutions is to produce this desirable vasoconstriction.

The activation of the beta receptors by a sympathomimetic agent (drug) produces smooth muscle relaxation and cardiac stimulation. Beta receptors have been further characterized as $beta_1$ and $beta_2$ receptors. The activation of $beta_1$ receptors increases cardiac rate and force, whereas $beta_2$ receptors are responsible for bronchodilation and vasodilation. Those changes that result from beta-receptor stimulation are the undesirable side effects of sympathomimetic drug incorporation into local anesthetic solutions. These beta effects are potentially hazardous.[2]

Concentrations

Vasoconstrictor concentrations are most often expressed as a ratio, such as one part per 100,000. This ratio appears as "1:100,000" in a written format. Table 40-2 lists the vasoconstrictors and their concentrations that are incorporated into dental local anesthetic solutions in the United States and Canada. The least concentrated solution that produces effective pain control should be used.[1]

Epinephrine

Epinephrine is available as a synthetic preparation, and it can also be obtained from the adrenal medulla of animals. Whereas a variety of vasoconstrictors are presently used for oral healthcare, epinephrine is the most potent and widely employed, and it is the standard by which all other vasoconstrictors are measured. Epinephrine 1:100,000 is the most commonly used concentration; however, it is thought that the optimal concentration for prolongation of pain control is 1:200,000 or even 1:250,000. The use of 1:50,000 epinephrine for pain control is neither necessary nor recommended. The 1:50,000 dilution contains twice the epinephrine per milliliter as a 1:100,000 dilution and four times that contained in a 1:200,000 concentration, and it does not increase the quality or duration of pain control. Although the 1:50,000 dilution may be more effective for the control of bleeding, effective hemostasis may also be obtained with concentrations of 1:100,000 epinephrine.

There are few contraindications to vasoconstrictor administration at the concentrations in which they are found in dental local anesthetics. Because there is always concern about the systemic effects, however, it is recommended that the less-concentrated solution be used, particularly with clients who are known to be cardiovascularly compromised.[3] For all clients, however, the benefits and risks of including a vasoconstrictor in the local anesthetic solution must be weighed against the benefits and risks of using an anesthetic solution without a vasoconstrictor (see Preanesthetic Client Assessment and Systemic Complications).

Side Effects and Overdose

Epinephrine overdose, which is caused by high amounts of this substance in the blood, is related to central nervous system stimulation. Clinical manifestations include increasing fear and anxiety, tension, restlessness, throbbing headache, tremor, weakness, dizziness, pallor, respiratory difficulty, and palpitation. With increasing epinephrine levels in the blood, cardiac dysrhythmias, ventricular fibrillation, dramatic increases in blood pressure, and stroke are rare but possible. Because of epinephrine's rapid inactivation, overdose reactions are usually brief. Nevertheless, in cardiovascularly compromised clients, it is prudent to limit or avoid exposure to vasoconstrictors if possible. Table 40-3 lists the maximum doses of epinephrine recommended by Malamed.[1]

Norepinephrine (Levarterenol)

Norepinephrine (levarterenol) is one fourth as potent as epinephrine; it is used clinically in a 1:30,000 dilution. Norepinephrine's clinical manifestations of overdose are similar to those of epinephrine, but they occur less frequently. The extravascular injection of norepinephrine, however, produces necrosis and sloughing (Figure 40-2). In the United States, norepinephrine is no longer available in the local anesthetic solutions used in dentistry.[1]

Levonordefrin

Levonordefrin is approximately one sixth (15%) as potent a vasoconstrictor as epinephrine; therefore, it is used in a greater concentration of 1:20,000. It is similar to using epinephrine in 1:50,000 or 1:100,000 concentrations. In the

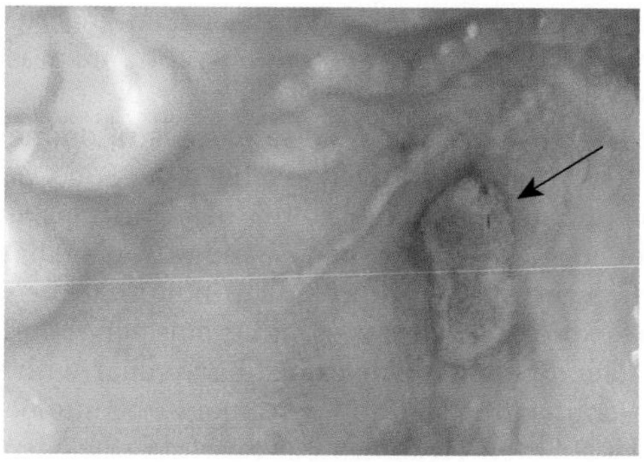

Figure 40-2. Sterile abscess on the palate produced by excessive norepinephrine vasoconstrictor use. (From Malamed SF: *Handbook of local anesthesia,* ed 6, St Louis, 2013, Mosby.)

United States, it is available with mepivacaine in a 1:20,000 dilution.[1]

Selection of a Local Anesthetic Agent

Table 40-4 lists the local anesthetics and the combinations of vasoconstrictors that are currently available in the United States and Canada. The dental hygienist must weigh the following factors when determining the appropriate anesthetic agent to use during dental hygiene care:

- The duration of action of the local anesthetic agent and the length of time that pain control is needed
- The need for pain control after treatment
- The client's health status
- The current medications being taken by the client
- Any allergy to local anesthetics

TABLE 40-4

Duration of Pulpal and Soft-Tissue Anesthesia with Available Local Anesthetics

	DURATION (APPROXIMATE NO. OF MINUTES)	
Drug Formulation	**Pulpal**	**Soft Tissue**
Mepivacaine 3% (infiltration)	5-10	90-120
Prilocaine 4% (infiltration)	10-15	60-120
Prilocaine 4% (nerve block)	40-60	120-240
Articaine 4% + epinephrine 1:200,000	45-60	180-240
Lidocaine 2% + epinephrine 1:50,000	60	180-300
Lidocaine 2% + epinephrine 1:100,000	60	180-300
Mepivacaine 2% + levonordefrin 1:20,000	60	180-300
Articaine 4% + epinephrine 1:100,000	60-75	180-300
Prilocaine 4% + epinephrine 1:200,000	60-90	180-480
Bupivacaine 0.5% + epinephrine 1:200,000	>90	240-720

From Malamed SF: *Handbook of local Anesthesia,* ed 6, St. Louis, 2013, Mosby.

Duration of Action and Length of Time That Pain Control Is Needed

An important consideration when selecting a local anesthetic agent for pain control during dental hygiene care is the local anesthetic agent's approximate duration of action in combination with the length of time that pain control is needed. Table 40-4 lists the local anesthetic agents and their approximate durations of pulpal and soft-tissue anesthesia.

In addition to the presence or absence of a vasoconstrictor, several other factors described in the following sections may affect both the duration and depth of the anesthetic agent's action by either increasing or, more commonly, decreasing the drug's effectiveness.[4]

Variation in Response to the Agent Administered

Although most individuals respond predictably to an anesthetic agent (e.g., the duration of pulpal anesthesia after the administration of 2% lidocaine with epinephrine 1:100,000 is approximately 60 minutes), some clients exhibit either a longer or a shorter duration of action than anticipated. This variation in response is normal and is simply a variation in the individual's reaction to the anesthetic agent.

Accuracy of the Administration of the Agent

Accuracy becomes significant when a substantial amount of soft tissue must be penetrated to reach the nerve to be anesthetized. For example, the inferior alveolar nerve block involves advancing through 20 to 25 mm of soft tissue before reaching the nerve, thereby influencing the accuracy of the injection. When injecting where it is not necessary to penetrate a large amount of tissue to block the nerve (e.g., with an infiltration), accuracy is seldom a problem.

Condition of the Soft Tissues at the Site of Drug Deposition

Anesthetic duration is increased in areas of decreased vascularity. Conversely, the presence of inflammation or infection increases vascularity and often decreases the anesthetic agent's duration of action as a result of more rapid absorption.

Anatomic Variation

The injection techniques described in this chapter are based on a "normal" anatomy. Of course, anatomic variations from this "norm" exist and can decrease the duration of local anesthetic action. Anatomic variations in the maxilla that may account for failed effectiveness and shortened duration include the following:

- Extra dense alveolar bone
- Palatal roots of maxillary molars that flare more than normal to the midline of the palate, thereby affecting the anesthetic's action on these roots
- An unusually low zygomatic arch, which is common in children and which prevents anesthesia or lessens its duration in the first and second molars

Anatomic variations in the mandible that are cause for concern include the following[1,4]:

- The height of the mandibular foramen
- A wide, flaring mandible
- A wide ramus in the anterior-posterior direction
- A long ramus in the superior-inferior direction
- Bulky musculature or excess adipose tissue
- Accessory innervation to the mandibular teeth

Suggestions for overcoming these variations in anatomy when administering anesthetic solution are discussed later in this chapter in Injection Techniques for the Maxillary Teeth and Facial Hard and Soft Tissues.

Type of Injection Administered

For any anesthetic solution administered, both pulpal and soft-tissue anesthesia are sustained for a longer period when a nerve block rather than a supraperiosteal infiltration injection is administered. For example, if 2% lidocaine with 1:100,000 epinephrine is administered, a PSA nerve block provides approximately 60 minutes of pulpal anesthesia, whereas a supraperiosteal injection (i.e., an infiltration) allows only 40 minutes of anesthesia. To achieve the desired duration, the recommended minimal volume of anesthetic must be administered.

Need for Pain Control after Treatment

Although the need for pain control after dental hygiene care may be limited, long-duration agents may be administered if post-treatment discomfort is a factor. Anesthetic agents such as 4% prilocaine with 1:200,000 epinephrine can provide 5 to 8 hours of soft-tissue anesthesia, whereas 0.5% bupivacaine or 1.5% etidocaine with 1:200,000 epinephrine can alleviate posttreatment discomfort for 8 to 12 hours. These agents can be administered before dental hygiene care is begun or even at the end of care to allow for maximal post-treatment anesthesia. These drugs should not be given to children or to people who are mentally or physically disabled, because these individuals may lack the ability to refrain from chewing or biting their lips, cheeks, or tongues.

Maximal Safe Doses of Local Anesthetics

All drugs, if administered in excess, can produce an overdose reaction. The exact dose or the blood level at which a toxic reaction occurs is impossible to predict, because biologic variability greatly influences how individuals respond to a drug. However, recommended maximal doses can be calculated to serve as a guideline for the dental hygienist. A **maximal safe dose** is the maximal amount of drug that can be safely administered to a healthy individual. Maximal doses of injectable local anesthetics should be determined after consideration of the following factors[1]:

- *Client's age.* Individuals on both ends of the age spectrum (i.e., the young child and the elderly adult) may be unable to tolerate normal doses. The dose of local anesthetic should thus be decreased accordingly.
- *Client's physical status.* The calculated dose must be adjusted for clients with compromised health. For example, a client with significant liver or renal dysfunction needs to be given a reduced dose of local anesthetics.
- *Client's weight.* The larger the individual (within limits), the greater the drug distribution. When administering a normal local anesthetic dose to a large individual, the blood drug level is lower than that of a small person, so a larger dose can be safely given. Although this rule is generally true, there may be exceptions, and care must always be exercised.

Table 40-5 lists the maximal safe doses recommended by manufacturers and approved by the U.S. Food and Drug Administration (FDA). Table 40-5 also includes the milligrams of local anesthetic per cartridge for available local anesthetic agents. It is important to note that the maximal doses are expressed in terms of milligrams per pound of body weight. The dental hygienist must be familiar with the relationships among the solution percentage, the number of milligrams of solution contained per cartridge, the client's body weight, and the maximum recommended dose per pound. With this information, the hygienist can calculate the maximum dose and the number of cartridges that can safely be administered.

Box 40-1 provides examples of how to calculate maximum doses and numbers of local anesthetic cartridges to be administered to various clients when only one local anesthetic is used. Box 40-2 provides similar calculation examples when multiple drugs are used.[1]

Fortunately maximum doses are unlikely to be reached for most dental hygiene procedures. If the dental hygiene care plan involves scaling and root planing a quadrant, the administration of one to two cartridges often suffices. There is seldom a need to administer more than four cartridges during any appointment involving dental hygiene care.

In addition to considering the recommended maximal safe doses, the dental hygienist must follow other procedural guidelines to increase safety during local anesthetic

BOX 40-1

Calculation of Maximum Doses and Number of Cartridges (Single Drug)

Patient: 22 Years Old, Healthy, Female, 110 lb

Local Anesthetic: Lidocaine HCl + Epinephrine 1:100,000
Lidocaine 2% = 36 mg/cartridge
Lidocaine: 3 mg/lb = 330 mg (MRD-m)
No. of cartridges: Manufacturer: 330/36 = approximately 9

Patient: 40 Years Old, Healthy, Male, 200 lb

Local Anesthetic: Prilocaine HCl + Epinephrine 1:200,000
Prilocaine 4% = 72 mg/cartridge
Prilocaine: 2.7 mg/lb = 540 mg (MRD-m)
Absolute maximum = 400 mg
No. of cartridges: Manufacturer: 400/72 = 5.5

Patient: 6 Years Old, Healthy, Male, 40 lb

Local Anesthetic: Mepivacaine HCl, No Vasoconstrictor
Mepivacaine 3% = 54 mg/cartridge
Mepivacaine: 3 mg/lb = 120 mg (MRD-m)
Absolute maximum = 400 mg
No. of cartridges: Manufacturer: 120/54 = 2

From Malamed SF: *Handbook of local anesthesia*, ed 6, St Louis, 2013, Mosby.
HCl, Hydrochloride; *MRD-m*, manufacturer's maximum recommended dose.

TABLE 40-5

Maximum Recommended Doses of Local Anesthetics Available in North America

	MANUFACTURER'S AND U.S. FOOD AND DRUG ADMINISTRATION MAXIMUM RECOMMENDED DOSE		
Local Anesthetic	**mg/kg**	**mg/lb**	**Maximum Recommended Dose (mg)**
Articaine			None listed
With vasoconstrictor	7.0	3.2	
Bupivacaine			
With vasoconstrictor	None listed	None listed	90
With vasoconstrictor (Canada)	2.0	0.9	90
Lidocaine	7.0	3.2	500
With vasoconstrictor			
Mepivacaine			
No vasoconstrictor	6.6	3.0	400
With vasoconstrictor	6.6	3.0	400
Prilocaine			
No vasoconstrictor	8.0	3.6	600
With vasoconstrictor	8.0	3.6	600
	CALCULATION OF MILLIGRAMS OF LOCAL ANESTHETIC PER DENTAL CARTRIDGE (1.8-mL CARTRIDGE)		
Local Anesthetic	**Percent Concentration**	**mg/mL**	**× 1.8 mL = mg/cartridge**
Articaine	4	40	72*
Bupivacaine	0.5	5	9
Lidocaine	2	20	36
Mepivacaine	2	20	36
	3	30	54
Prilocaine	4	40	72

From Malamed SF: *Handbook of local anesthesia,* ed 6, St Louis, 2013, Mosby.

*Cartridges of articaine hydrochloride in the United States are printed with the following statement: "Minimum content of each cartridge is 1.7 mL."

BOX 40-2

Calculation of Maximum Doses and Number of Cartridges (Multiple Drugs)

Patient: 100-lb Female, Healthy

Local Anesthetic: Prilocaine 4% + Epinephrine 1:200,000

Prilocaine 4% = 72 mg/cartridge

Prilocaine: 2.7 mg/lb = 270 mg (MRD-m)

Patient receives 2 cartridges = 144 mg, but anesthesia is inadequate

Doctor wishes to change to lidocaine 2% + epinephrine 1:100,000

How Much Lidocaine Can This Patient Receive?

Lidocaine 2% = 36 mg/cartridge

Lidocaine: 2 mg/lb = 200 mg

Total dose of both local anesthetics should not exceed the lower of the two calculated doses (in this case, 200 mg)

Patient has received 144 mg (prilocaine); can still receive 56 mg of lidocaine

Therefore 56 mg/36 mg per cartridge = 1.5 cartridges of lidocaine 2% + epinephrine 1:100,000

From Malamed SF: *Handbook of local anesthesia,* ed 5, St Louis, 2004, Mosby.

MRD-m, Manufacturer's maximum recommended dose.

administration and to prevent an overdose reaction. These guidelines include the following:

- A careful evaluation of the client's health history
- The use of a vasoconstrictor whenever possible
- Aspiration before local anesthetic deposition
- Slow injection
- The use of the smallest amount of drug necessary

A more detailed discussion of these guidelines can be found in the Procedures for a Successful Injection section later in this chapter.

Preanesthetic Client Assessment

To meet the human need for protection from health risks, an evaluation of the client's health history and his or her current health status is an essential prerequisite to dental hygiene care. The dental hygienist must ascertain whether any conditions represent contraindications or require alterations to the dental hygiene care plan to eliminate or decrease client risk. The administration of local anesthetic and vasoconstricting agents provides an additional rationale for a thorough health history and health status review. Local anesthetics and vasoconstrictors, like all drugs, exert actions on multiple body systems. It is important to evaluate, through the health history, the client's ability to physically tolerate them, to determine the client's history of allergic responses, and to identify the client's current medications. The collection of these data helps the dental hygienist to determine the appropriateness of administering a local anesthetic or a vasoconstrictor, of seeking medical consultation, and of modifying the dental hygiene care plan. A thorough preanesthetic client assessment helps to prevent or minimize complications and emergencies.[2]

Contraindications to local anesthetics and vasoconstrictors are divided into two categories: absolute and relative. **Absolute contraindications** require that the drug in question not be administered to the individual under any circumstances.[1] The administration of such a drug is contraindicated in all situations because it substantially increases the possibility of a life-threatening risk for the client. An example is a documented local anesthetic allergic reaction.

A **relative contraindication** means that the drug in question may be administered to the client after careful weighing of the risk of using the drug against its potential benefit if an acceptable alternative drug is not available. The smallest clinically effective dose should always be used in these situations.

Client Health Status

Although local anesthetics and vasoconstrictors are considered relatively safe drugs when administered properly, certain health conditions require limiting or eliminating their use. Table 40-6 summarizes those health conditions that affect the selection of a local anesthetic or vasoconstrictor and the appropriate actions that the dental hygienist may follow.[1]

Few health conditions, such as documented allergy, are absolute contraindications to vasoconstrictors in the concentrations found in the local anesthetic solutions used in oral healthcare; however, the dental hygienist must carefully consider the benefits versus the risks of administering a vasoconstrictor to clients with a history of hypertension, cardiovascular disease, or hyperthyroidism, because often the risks outweigh the benefits.

Current Client Medications

A drug interaction occurs when one drug modifies the action of another drug. A drug may potentiate or diminish the action of another drug, or it may alter the way in which another drug is absorbed, metabolized, or eliminated from the body.[1,2] Although local anesthetics and vasoconstrictors exhibit few interactions with other drugs, the dental hygienist should consult the *Physicians' Desk Reference* or a comparable reference when a client reports being treated with any medication.

TABLE 40-6

Health Conditions That Require Special Consideration When Local Anesthetics Are Administered

Health Condition	Reason for Modification	Recommended Action
Hyperthyroidism	Possible exaggerated response to vasoconstrictors	Avoid or limit (uncontrolled) use of vasoconstrictors; use 3% mepivacaine or 4% prilocaine.
Atypical plasma cholinesterase	Toxic overdose to esters	Use amide anesthetic agents.
Methemoglobinemia	Potential for cyanosis-like state, respiratory distress, and lethargy in response to prilocaine and articaine	Use other anesthetic agents.
Malignant hyperthermia	Life-threatening syndrome caused by administration of certain drugs in combination with amide agents	Use amides or esters in normal doses; seek medical consultation.
Significant liver dysfunction	Difficulty metabolizing amide agents, potential for overdose	Seek medical consultation; use amide agents judiciously.
Significant renal dysfunction	Difficulty excreting local anesthetic agents, potential for overdose	Seek medical consultation; use anesthetic agents judiciously.
Pregnancy	Potential for complications with pregnancy	Avoid elective treatment during first trimester; use local anesthetics judiciously.

This practice enables the clinician to assess both the drug's activity and the drug-to-drug interactions between the local anesthetic and vasoconstrictor and the prescribed medication. In doing so, the dental hygienist meets the client's human need for protection from health risks. If further questions remain regarding the use of a local anesthetic or vasoconstrictor while a prescribed medication is being taken, the dentist or the individual's physician should be consulted.

Table 40-7 summarizes those medications that may affect the selection of a local anesthetic or vasoconstrictor and the appropriate actions that the dental hygienist may choose.

Local anesthetics have few interactions with other prescribed drugs. Procaine has been cited as interfering with the action of antiinfective sulfonamide drugs. When central nervous system depressants or cardiovascular system depressants are being taken by an individual, it is recommended that doses of local anesthetics be kept to a minimum, because they may cause further depression.[1,2]

There are many conflicting reports of drug-to-drug interactions between vasoconstrictors and prescribed medications, but it is recommended that the dental hygienist proceed cautiously when administering a vasopressor to a person who is being treated with any of the following groups of drugs:

- Tricyclic antidepressants
- Phenothiazines
- Beta-receptor blockers
- Adrenergic neuron blockers

Currently none of the drugs described in the following paragraphs poses an absolute contraindication to the administration of a vasoconstrictor; however, it is recommended that the dental hygienist exercise caution by administering the smallest dose that is clinically effective (e.g., the dose recommended for persons at cardiovascular risk) or eliminating the vasopressor entirely. If the dental hygienist is uncertain about the inclusion of a vasoconstrictor in the local anesthetic solution, consultation with the client's physician is advisable.

Tricyclic Antidepressants

Tricyclic antidepressant medications (e.g., amitriptyline, clomipramine, imipramine) have been cited as possibly potentiating the action of epinephrine and norepinephrine and resulting in an increase in blood pressure.[2] Phenothiazines such as prochlorperazine are categorized as antipsychotic drugs, but they are also often prescribed for the treatment of nausea. There is concern that these drugs, when combined with vasoconstrictors, may cause an exaggerated response to the vasopressor.

Beta-Receptor Blockers

Beta-receptor blockers such as propranolol, nadolol, timolol, pindolol, and penbutolol decrease the systolic and diastolic blood pressures.[3] (Note that these generic drugs end in *-olol.*) When these drugs are combined with epinephrine from a local anesthetic injection, however, significant increases in blood pressure may result.

Adrenergic Neuron Blockers

Adrenergic neuron blockers such as guanethidine and reserpine are also used to lower blood pressure through interference with the normal release of norepinephrine.[1] When these drugs are combined with a vasoconstrictor, the effects of the vasopressor may be exaggerated, thereby resulting in an increase in blood pressure.

TABLE 40-7

Medications That Affect the Selection of Local Anesthetic Agents or Vasoconstrictors

Medication	Type of Contraindications	Drugs to Avoid	Potential Problems	Action or Alternative Drug
Cardiovascular system depressants, central nervous system depressants	Relative	Large doses of local anesthetics	Increased depression of the cardiovascular system or the central nervous system	Minimize dose of local anesthetic
Tricyclic antidepressants	Relative	Large doses of vasoconstrictors	Potentiate the action of epinephrine and increase blood pressure	Epinephrine concentrations of 1 : 200,000 or 1 : 100,000 used judiciously or mepivacaine 3% or prilocaine 4%
Phenothiazines	Relative	Large doses of vasoconstrictors	Potentiate the action of epinephrine and increase blood pressure	Epinephrine concentrations of 1 : 200,000 or 1 : 100,000 used judiciously or mepivacaine 3% or prilocaine 4%
Beta-receptor blockers	Relative	Large doses of vasoconstrictors	Potentiate the action of epinephrine and increase blood pressure	Epinephrine concentrations of 1 : 200,000 or 1 : 100,000 used judiciously or mepivacaine 3% or prilocaine 4%
Adrenergic neuron blockers	Relative	Large doses of vasoconstrictors	Potentiate the action of epinephrine and increase blood pressure	Epinephrine concentrations of 1 : 200,000 or 1 : 100,000 used judiciously or mepivacaine 3% or prilocaine 4%
Sulfonamides	Relative	Esters	Esters inhibit the action of sulfonamides	Amides

TABLE 40-8

Allergies That Affect the Selection of Local Anesthetic Agents or Vasoconstrictors

Reported Allergy	Type of Contraindication	Drugs to Avoid	Potential Problems	Alternative Drug
Local anesthetic allergy, documented	Absolute	All local anesthetics in same chemical class (i.e., esters vs. amides)	Allergic response, mild (e.g., dermatitis, bronchospasm) to life-threatening reactions	Local anesthetics in different chemical class (i.e., esters vs. amides)
Sulfa	Absolute	Articaine	Allergic response	Non–sulfur-containing local anesthetic
Sodium bisulfate or metabisulfite	Absolute	Local anesthetics that contain a vasoconstrictor	Severe bronchospasm, usually in asthmatic clients	Local anesthetic without a vasoconstrictor

Allergies

An allergy is a hypersensitive reaction that is acquired through exposure to a specific substance known as an *allergen;* reexposure to the allergen increases one's potential to react. Approximately 1% of all reactions that occur during local anesthetic administration are true allergic reactions.[1] However, a documented local anesthetic allergy represents an absolute contraindication and must be investigated for authenticity. Table 40-8 summarizes allergies that affect the selection of a local anesthetic agent or vasoconstrictor and lists appropriate alternative drugs from which the dental hygienist may choose. A true allergic response to a pure amide drug is extremely rare. A true allergy to amides may exist, but a verifiable occurrence is virtually nonexistent.

Allergic reactions to various dental cartridge contents have been documented. Sodium bisulfite and metabisulfite are antioxidants that are incorporated into local anesthetic solutions to act as preservatives for the vasoconstrictor. In addition to their use in local anesthetic cartridges, these agents are often sprayed on fruits and vegetables to keep them appearing fresh, and they are also included in a variety of canned foods. Allergy to bisulfites has been reported.[5-8] Clients with a history of asthma may be particularly susceptible to an allergic response. The FDA estimates that 5% of the 9 million allergy sufferers in the United States may be hypersensitive to sulfites[1] and thus has enacted regulations limiting the use of bisulfites on food. If a client reports a history of sulfite sensitivity, the dental hygienist should be alerted to the possibility of a similar response if a sulfite is included in the dental cartridge. Although sodium bisulfite or metabisulfite is found in all dental cartridges that contain a vasoconstrictor, these agents are not included in solutions in which there is no vasopressor. Therefore it is recommended that the dental hygienist administer local anesthetics that contain no vasoconstrictor to clients with a history of sulfite sensitivity.[1]

Armamentarium

The equipment essential for the administration of a local anesthetic agent includes the following:
- Syringe
- Needle
- Cartridge of local anesthetic agent
- Supplementary armamentarium

Syringe

The syringe is the component of the local anesthetic armamentarium that holds the needle and the cartridge of anesthetic, thus allowing the solution to be delivered to the client. Several types of syringes may be used for local anesthetic administration, including the following[1]:

1. Reusable
   a. Breech-loading metallic cartridge-type aspirating syringe
      - Aspirating
      - Nonaspirating
      - Self-aspirating
   b. Computer-controlled anesthetic delivery system
   c. Pressure-type syringe
   d. Jet injector syringe
2. Disposable

The syringes that are most often employed in oral healthcare are the reusable aspirating syringe and the self-aspirating syringe.

Reusable Breech-Loading Metallic Cartridge-Type Aspirating Syringe

The reusable breech-loading metallic cartridge-type aspirating syringe is the most commonly used syringe for the administration of an intraoral local anesthetic agent (Figure 40-3).

The needle is affixed to the threaded portion (or needle adaptor) at one end of the syringe. At the other end, a thumb ring and a finger rest provide the dental hygienist with a means to grasp and control the syringe. The body of the syringe holds the cartridge of anesthetic solution. The aspirating syringe is characterized by a barbed piston that is also referred to as a **harpoon**. The harpoon engages the rubber or silicone stopper of the cartridge of anesthetic. It also allows the dental hygienist to exert negative pressure on the thumb ring to assess the location of the lumen of the needle during a procedure referred to as **aspiration**. If the needle lumen rests within a blood vessel, blood appears in the cartridge after negative pressure is applied to the thumb ring. If this occurs, the dental hygienist needs to withdraw the needle, replace the cartridge of anesthetic solution and the needle, and repeat the procedure. Positive pressure on the thumb ring injects the anesthetic solution into the tissues. Advantages and disadvantages are listed in

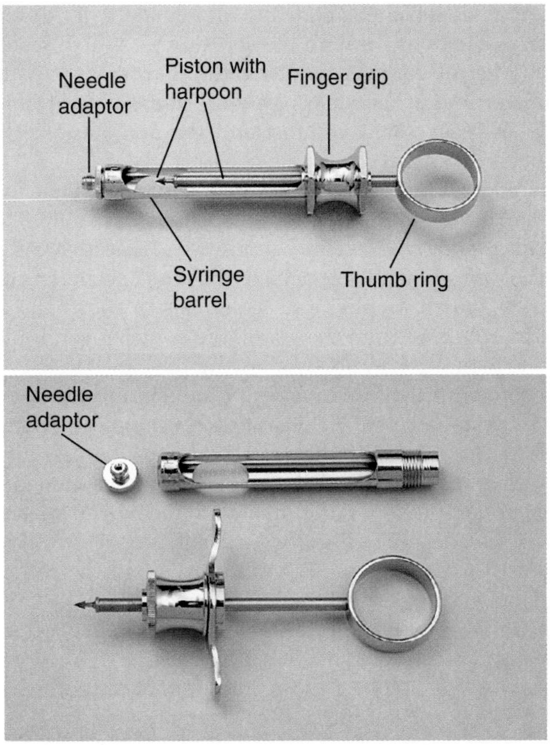

Figure 40-3. Breech-loading metallic cartridge-type syringe. (From Malamed SF: *Handbook of local anesthesia,* ed 6, St Louis, 2013, Mosby.)

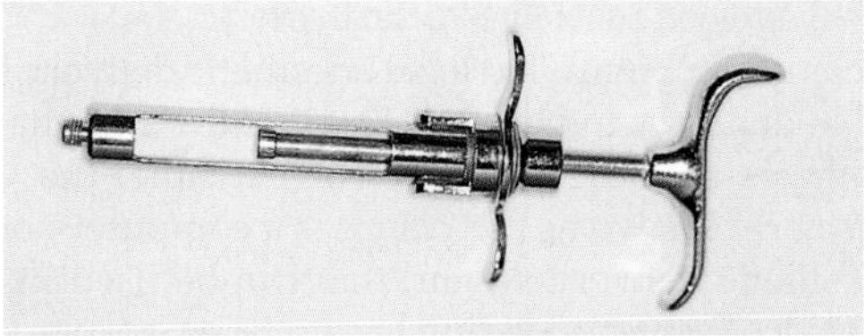

Figure 40-4. Nonaspirating syringe. This type is not to be used for local dental anesthesia.

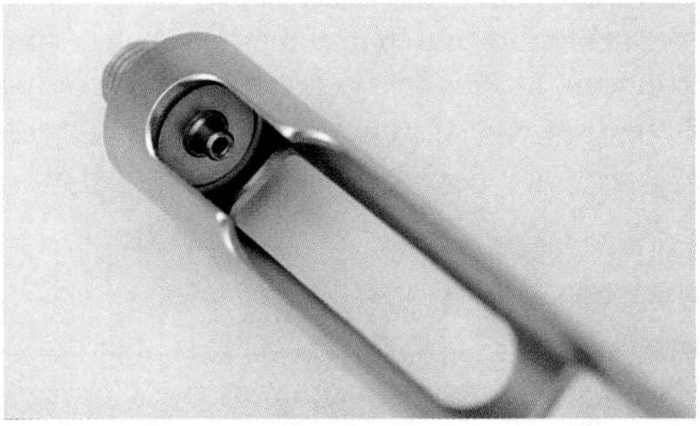

Figure 40-5. A metal projection within the barrel depresses the diaphragm of the local anesthetic cartridge. (From Malamed SF: *Handbook of local anesthesia,* ed 6, St Louis, 2013, Mosby.)

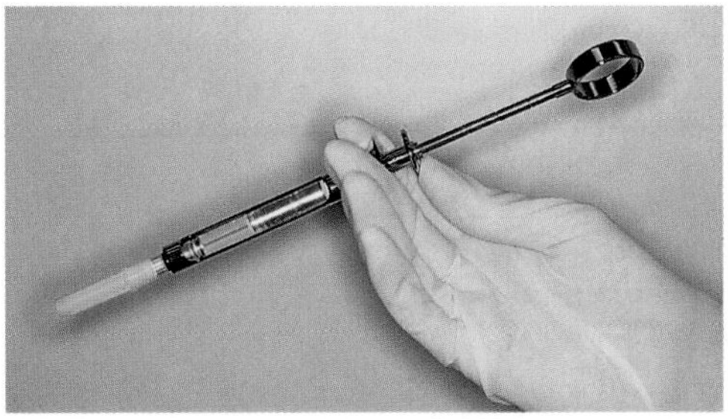

Figure 40-6. Pressure exerted on the thumb disc (as shown in the figure) or the thumb ring increases pressure within the cartridge. Aspiration occurs when the pressure is released.

BOX 40-3

Advantages and Disadvantages of the Metallic Breech-Loading Aspirating Syringe

ADVANTAGES	DISADVANTAGES
• Visible cartridge	• Weight (heavier than plastic syringe)
• Aspiration with one hand	• Syringe may be too big for small operators
• Autoclavable	• Possibility of infection with improper care
• Rust resistant	
• Long lasting with proper maintenance	

From Malamed SF: *Handbook of local anesthesia,* ed 6, St Louis, 2013, Mosby.

Box 40-3. A plastic, autoclavable, nonrusting model is also available.[1]

Reusable Breech-Loading Metallic Cartridge-Type Nonaspirating Syringe

The reusable breech-loading metallic cartridge-type nonaspirating syringe does not have a harpoon on the end of the piston; therefore the dental hygienist is unable to aspirate before depositing the anesthetic solution (Figure 40-4).

It is impossible for the dental hygienist to ascertain the precise location of the needle tip with a nonaspirating syringe, so this type of instrument should never be employed when a local anesthetic is administered during dental hygiene care.

Reusable Breech-Loading Metallic Cartridge-Type Self-Aspirating Syringe

The importance of aspirating before injecting an anesthetic solution is widely accepted, and the self-aspirating syringe was developed to help the oral healthcare provider to complete this important step. This type of syringe achieves the negative pressure necessary for aspiration via the elasticity of the rubber diaphragm in the anesthetic cartridge. When the cartridge is placed in the syringe, the diaphragm rests against a metal projection inside the syringe; this projection also directs the needle into the cartridge (Figure 40-5).

Pressure exerted by the dental hygienist on the thumb disc (Figure 40-6) or on the plunger by way of the thumb ring moves the cartridge slightly toward the metal projection, thereby stretching the rubber diaphragm. When the pressure is released, the cartridge rebounds slightly, thus producing enough negative pressure within the cartridge to achieve aspiration. Therefore the dental hygienist does not need to pull back on the thumb ring to aspirate, as is necessary with an aspirating syringe.

Computer-Controlled Local Anesthetic Delivery

Several computer-controlled local anesthetic delivery systems are used in dentistry today.[1] Box 40-4 lists the advantages and disadvantages of these systems. For example, the CompuDent (formerly known as the Wand) is a computer-controlled local anesthetic delivery system that can be used instead of the traditional breech-loading aspirating syringe (Figure 40-7). The CompuDent has several unique features. The handpiece is light and ergonomic; it is held with a pen grasp instead of a palm grasp, thereby allowing for a higher level of comfort and control for the clinician. The handpiece is also good for use with fearful clients, because it looks nothing like the traditional syringe and therefore is much less threatening. The local anesthetic delivery is controlled by a computer that regulates the flow rate of the agent and the pressure of the deposition. The computer-controlled rate allows for the creation of an anesthetic pathway immediately in front of the needle as it moves through the soft tissues, which results in a high level of comfort for the client. Particularly with the administration of palatal injections, the CompuDent can greatly increase client comfort and the acceptance of local anesthetic procedures.

To initiate anesthetic delivery and aspiration, the clinician controls the computer via a foot pedal (Figure 40-8). The pedal allows for two levels of deposition: (1) a slow rate, with 1 drop of anesthetic being delivered every 2 seconds; and (2) a fast rate, which supplies a steady stream of anesthetic. After removing the foot from the pedal, the clinician can initiate a 5-second aspiration cycle. By allowing the clinician to control the needle with the fine muscles of the hand rather than the large muscles required to operate a traditional syringe, the clinician can penetrate the soft tissues by gently rotating the needle back and forth between the thumb and fingers (bidirectional rotation) rather than with the typical linear penetration. This technique has two advantages: (1) by allowing the bevel to cut into the tissues via rotation, the technique causes no tearing of the tissue on penetration; and (2) the bidirectional rotation results in less needle deflection as the tissue is penetrated. The lessened needle deflection can increase the effectiveness of the injection, because the needle is more likely to be at the desired deposition site.[1]

Another type of computer-controlled local anesthetic delivery system is the Comfort Control Syringe (Figure 40-9) delivery system. This system is similar to the CompuDent, but it offers handpiece control rather than foot-activated control. Although the handpiece is bulkier than a regular syringe, the advantages of this system include the similarities that it has to a manual syringe, a lower price point than other computer delivery systems, and the choice of delivery rate that can be matched to the user's technique.

BOX 40-4

Advantages and Disadvantages of the Computer-Controlled Local Anesthetic Delivery Systems

ADVANTAGES	DISADVANTAGES
• Precise control of flow rate and pressure produces a more comfortable injection, even in tissues with low elasticity (e.g., palate, attached gingiva, periodontal ligament) • Increased tactile "feel" and ergonomics from the lightweight handpiece • Nonthreatening • Automatic aspiration • Rotational insertion technique minimizes needle deflection	• Requires additional armamentarium • Cost

From Malamed SF: *Handbook of local anesthesia*, ed 6, St Louis, 2013, Mosby.

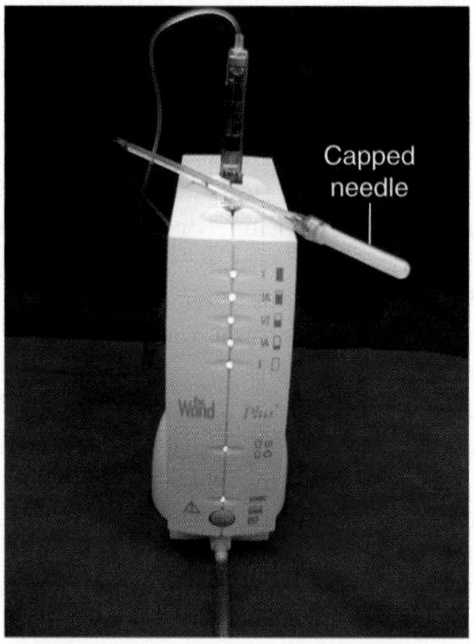

Figure 40-7. Computer-controlled local anesthetic delivery system with lightweight handpiece: the Wand or CompuDent. (From Malamed SF: *Handbook of local anesthesia*, ed 6, St Louis, 2013, Mosby.)

Pressure-Type Syringe

Another type of syringe that the dental hygienist may encounter is a pressure-type syringe (Figure 40-10).

This type of instrument is used for the administration of a periodontal ligament injection or an intraligamentary injection, which provides pulpal anesthesia to one tooth on the mandible. A standard aspirating syringe can be used for this type of injection, but the pressure-type syringe is equipped

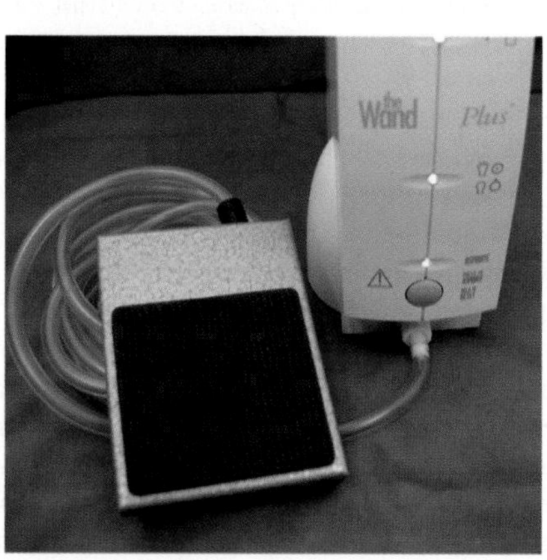

Figure 40-8. Foot-activated control. (From Malamed SF: *Handbook of local anesthesia*, ed 6, St Louis, 2013, Mosby.)

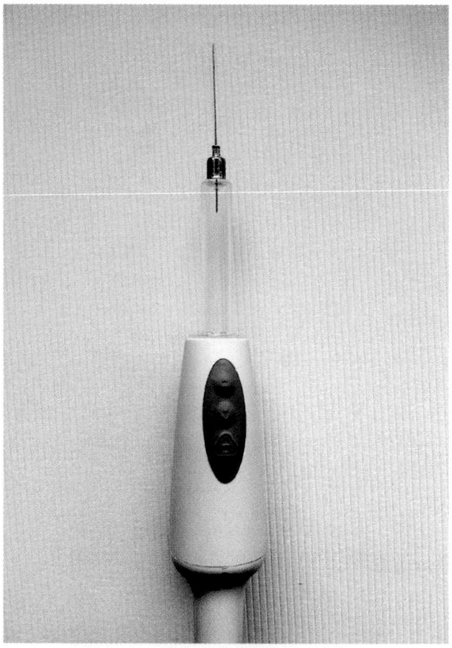

Figure 40-9. Comfort Control Syringe handpiece. (From Malamed SF: *Handbook of local anesthesia,* ed 6, St Louis, 2013, Mosby.)

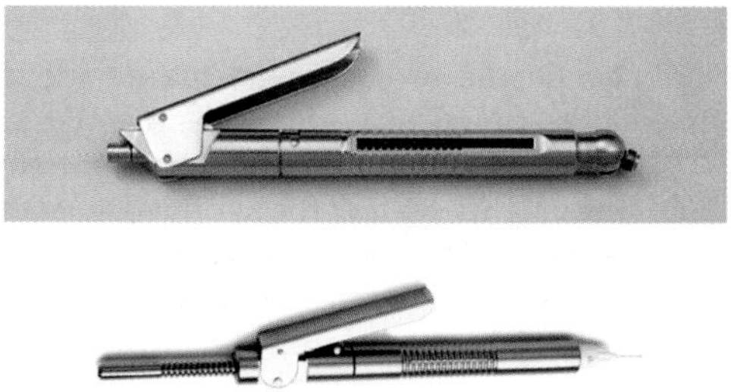

Figure 40-10. Second-generation pressure syringes for periodontal ligament injection. (From Malamed SF: *Handbook of local anesthesia,* ed 6, St Louis, 2013, Mosby.)

with a trigger mechanism that delivers a measured dose (0.2 mL) of anesthetic solution and that allows the administrator to more easily express the solution despite significant tissue resistance. This type of syringe allows for the easy administration of the solution; however, the dental hygienist must take care to slowly inject even this small measured dose of anesthetic agent. If agent deposition is done too rapidly, client discomfort may ensue during the injection and after the anesthesia has worn off. See Box 40-5 for advantages and disadvantages of the pressure-type syringe.[1]

Jet Injector Syringe

The jet injector syringe delivers 0.05 to 0.2 mL of anesthetic agent to the mucous membranes at a high pressure (2000 psi) via small openings called *jets* (Figure 40-11). The jet injector is used primarily to obtain topical anesthesia before the insertion of a needle or to achieve palatal soft-tissue anesthesia. To acquire complete anesthesia, nerve blocks or supraperiosteal injections must also be administered with a conventional syringe and needle. With the jet injector, the anesthetic solution is delivered without the use of a needle; therefore it becomes a needleless injection. Clients may dislike the jolt of the jet injection, however, and post-injection discomfort may follow. Properly applied topical anesthetics accomplish the same objectives as the jet injector.[1]

See Box 40-6 for advantages and disadvantages of the jet injector.

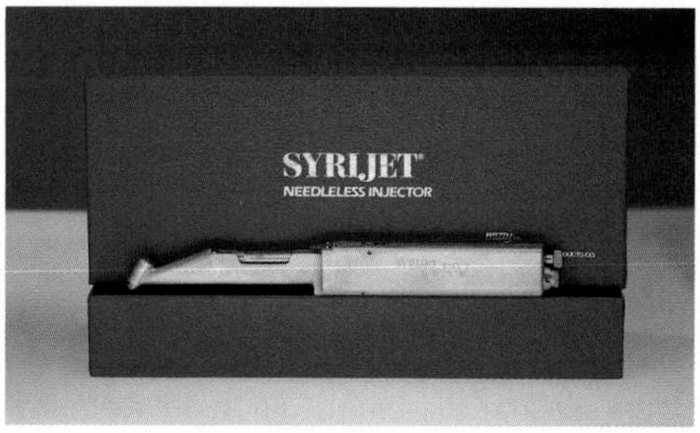

Figure 40-11. Jet injector syringe (needleless). (From Malamed SF: *Handbook of local anesthesia,* ed 6, St Louis, 2013, Mosby.)

BOX 40-5

Advantages and Disadvantages of the Pressure Syringe

ADVANTAGES	DISADVANTAGES
• Measured dose	• Cost
• Overcomes tissue resistance	• Easy to inject too rapidly
• Nonthreatening (new devices)	• Threatening (original devices)
• Cartridges protected	

From Malamed SF: *Handbook of local anesthesia,* ed 6, St Louis, 2013, Mosby.

BOX 40-6

Advantages and Disadvantages of the Jet Injector

ADVANTAGES	DISADVANTAGES
• Does not require use of needle (recommended for needle-phobic individuals)	• Inadequate for pulpal anesthesia or for regional block
• Delivers very small volumes of local anesthetic (0.01 to 0.2 mL)	• Some patients are disturbed by the "jolt" of the injection
• Used in lieu of topical anesthetics	• Cost
	• May damage periodontal tissues

From Malamed SF: *Handbook of local anesthesia,* ed 6, St Louis, 2013, Mosby.

Disposable Syringe

Disposable plastic syringes are most often used for intramuscular or intravenous drug administration, but they may be employed during intraoral injections. These syringes do not accept standard dental cartridges, and therefore it is necessary to insert the attached needle into a vial or cartridge of local anesthetic drug and then eject the appropriate amount of solution. Furthermore, because these syringes have no thumb ring, aspiration is difficult and may require two hands. Because the disadvantages of the disposable syringe far outweigh the advantages, this type of syringe is not recommended for routine use.

Care and Handling of the Syringe

Recommendations for the care of reusable syringes that are used for local anesthetic administration are as follows[1]:

- The syringe should be sterilized after each use by following the appropriate infection-control protocol. Deposits that resemble rust may accumulate on the syringe and interfere with function and appearance. Such deposits may be removed with ultrasonic cleaning or scrubbing (see Chapter 9).
- After several autoclavings, the hygienist should dismantle the syringe and lubricate all of the threaded joints.
- The piston and harpoon may be replaced if the harpoon loses its sharpness and fails to engage the rubber stopper of the cartridge.

Problems with the Syringe

- *Bent harpoon.* The syringe harpoon must be sharp and straight to embed the cartridge's rubber stopper. If the harpoon becomes bent, it may fail to engage the rubber stopper accurately. Consequently, aspiration may be unreliable.
- *Disengagement of the harpoon from the rubber stopper of the cartridge during aspiration.* Disengagement may ensue if the harpoon is dull or if the dental hygienist applies excessive pressure to the thumb ring during aspiration. With regard to aspiration, only a gentle retraction of the thumb ring is needed; forceful action is not required.
- *Difficulty aspirating because of practitioner's hand size.* When using an aspirating syringe, the dental hygienist must be able to stretch his or her fingers and thumb to retract the syringe thumb ring. If this cannot be done effectively, reliable aspiration does not occur. Therefore it is important that the syringe fit the practitioner's hand. Most syringes are similar with regard to their dimensions, but variations do exist. When selecting an aspirating syringe, it is beneficial to hold the syringe and test your ability to aspirate efficiently. If this is not possible, a self-aspirating syringe should be selected.

Needle

The **needle** is the component of the armamentarium that delivers the anesthetic agent from the cartridge to the tissues surrounding the needle tip. Virtually all needles used in oral healthcare today are made of stainless steel, presterilized by the manufacturer, and disposable.

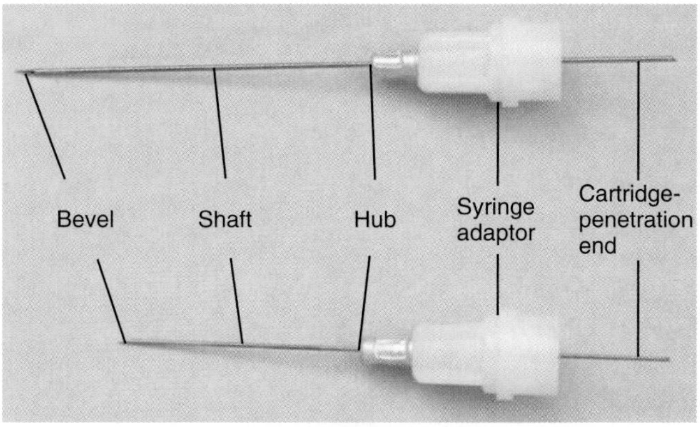

Figure 40-12. Parts of the dental local anesthetic needle. Long needle *(top)*; short needle *(bottom)*. (From Malamed SF: *Handbook of local anesthesia*, ed 6, St Louis, 2013, Mosby.)

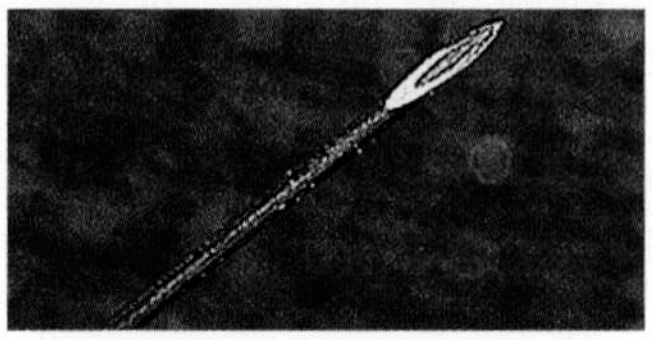

Figure 40-13. Bevel of the needle.

Parts of the Needle

Needles used for local anesthetic administration have several components (Figure 40-12). The bevel (Figure 40-13) is the angled surface of the needle point that is directed into the tissues. The shank is the length of the needle from the point to the hub. The hub or syringe adaptor is a plastic or metal piece that attaches the needle onto the syringe. The interior surface of metallic syringe adaptors is prethreaded. Plastic syringe adaptors are not prethreaded. Consequently, to attach a plastic-hubbed needle to a syringe, the dental hygienist must concurrently push and screw the needle onto the syringe. The syringe or cartridge-penetrating end enters the needle adaptor component of the syringe and engages the rubber diaphragm of the local anesthetic cartridge. This sterile needle is packaged in a plastic encasement that consists of two protective shields. A colored shield protects the part of the needle that is inserted into the tissues, and a clear or white shield covers the syringe and cartridge end of the needle.

Gauge

The gauge is the diameter of the lumen of the needle. The higher the gauge number, the smaller the lumen diameter; for example, a 30-gauge needle has a smaller internal diameter than a 27-gauge needle. The most commonly employed needles in oral healthcare are the 25-, 27-, and 30-gauge needles.

A common assumption is that a larger-diameter needle (e.g., a 25-gauge needle) is more uncomfortable for the client during insertion than a smaller-diameter needle (e.g., a 30-gauge needle); however, this assumption is untrue. Research suggests that people cannot distinguish among a 25-, a 27-, and a 30-gauge needle when injected with each.[1]

Larger-gauge needles (e.g., 25-gauge needles) actually have several advantages over smaller-gauge needles. Less deflection occurs when the larger-gauge needle passes through the tissues. Because it is larger and more rigid, this type of needle can be guided to the deposition site with minimal deviation, thus ensuring greater accuracy and a higher rate of injection success. The rigidity of this needle is particularly important for injections that require significant penetration of the soft tissues, such as the inferior alveolar nerve block. Although needle breakage is uncommon with

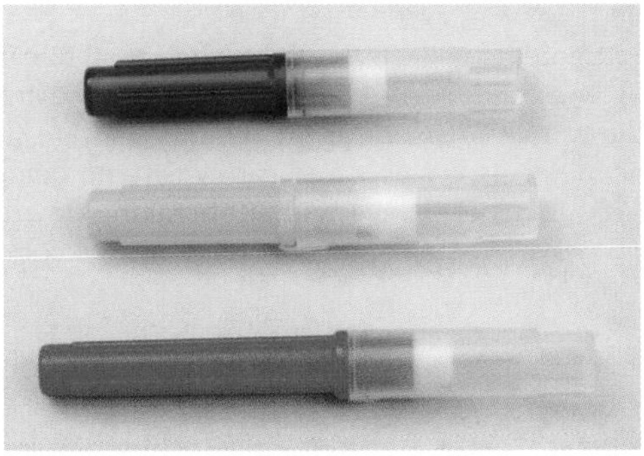

Figure 40-14. Color-coding by needle gauge: 25 gauge, red; 27 gauge, yellow; 30 gauge, blue. (From Malamed SF: *Handbook of local anesthesia*, ed 6, St Louis, 2013, Mosby.)

disposable needles, it is less likely to occur with larger-gauge needles. Another advantage of larger-gauge needles is the ability to aspirate and thereby reduce the possibility of intravascular injections.

Opinions vary, but many authorities conclude that aspiration is easier and more reliable with a larger lumen, and smaller-gauge needles (e.g., 30-gauge needles) have diameters that are too narrow for adequate aspiration.[1] Blood may be aspirated through a 25-, 27-, or 30-gauge needle, but more pressure is required when a smaller-gauge needle is employed. This difficulty with aspiration may decrease the reliability of the procedure and increase the likelihood of the harpoon of the aspirating syringe becoming disengaged from the rubber stopper. Therefore it is recommended that the dental hygienist use a 25-gauge needle for those injections that pose a high risk for aspiration or when a significant depth of soft tissue must be penetrated (e.g., inferior alveolar, PSA, or mental or incisive nerve blocks). The 27-gauge needle may be used for all other injections as long as the possibility of aspiration and the depth of tissue penetration are minimal. The 30-gauge needle is not recommended. In the United States, needles are color-coded by gauge (Figure 40-14).

Length

The most common needle lengths used in oral healthcare are the short (i.e., approximately 1 inch or 25 mm) and the long (i.e., approximately 1⅝ inches or 40 mm) as measured from the hub to the needle tip. The choice of needle length depends on the accessibility of the area to be anesthetized. Long needles are preferred for those injections that require the penetration of a significant thickness of soft tissue (e.g., inferior alveolar nerve block). Short needles are indicated for injections in which smaller amounts of tissue are to be entered (see Figure 40-12).

Care and Handling of the Needle

Recommendations for the care and handling of the disposable needles used for local anesthetic administration include the following[1]:

- Never use a needle for more than one client.
- Change the needle after the administration of approximately three or four injections on the same client. Some clinicians recommend changing the needle even more often. The stainless steel becomes dull after several injections, thereby causing each succeeding tissue penetration to be potentially traumatic and to result in postinjection soreness.
- Cover the needle with a protective sheath when it is not being used, both before the injection and immediately after the completion of the injection.
- Watch the position of the uncovered needle tip at all times to prevent needle injury to both the client and the operator.
- Dispose of needles in an approved sharps container. These rigid, puncture-proof, leak-resistant containers need to be disposed of in accordance with federal, state, and local regulations (see Chapter 9).

Problems with the Needle

The following are problems that the dental hygienist may encounter with the needle when administering local anesthetic agents:

- *Pain on insertion.* Clients may experience tissue discomfort during insertion if the needle is dull; to avoid this pain, the clinician needs to change the needle after three or four insertions.
- *Pain on withdrawal.* Client discomfort may occur when the needle is being withdrawn from the tissues if any barbs are on the needle tip. Barbs may be a result of the manufacturing process; they are more likely to occur if the needle tip contacts bone or any hard surface with too much force. To check for needle sharpness during armamentarium preparation, the practitioner may draw the needle tip backward across a sterile piece of gauze. A needle barb will snag the gauze, thus indicating the need for replacement with a new needle. In addition, a needle should never be pushed forcefully against bone.
- *Needle stick exposure of the clinician.* To prevent an accidental needle stick injury, the needle remains capped with a protective shield before use and immediately after the completion of the injection. Should a needle stick exposure occur, follow the percutaneous exposure protocol and postexposure evaluation procedure outlined in Chapter 9.
- *Needle breakage.* See Local Complications later in this chapter.

Cartridge

The cartridge is the component of the armamentarium that contains the local anesthetic drug in addition to other ingredients. The local anesthetic cartridge is often referred to as a *carpule* by oral health professionals; however, this term is a registered trademark name for the anesthetic cartridge manufactured by Cook-Waite Laboratories.[1]

Parts of the Cartridge

The cartridges that are used for local anesthetic administration have four components (Figure 40-15):

1. The rubber stopper or plunger is located on one end of the cartridge and is the part in which the harpoon of an aspirating syringe is embedded. This component is pushed into the glass cylinder via pressure on the syringe thumb ring, thereby ejecting the local anesthetic solution through the needle. During manufacturing, the rubber stopper is often treated with silicone to allow it to transverse the glass cylinder without sticking. In an unused local anesthetic cartridge, the rubber stopper end is slightly indented from

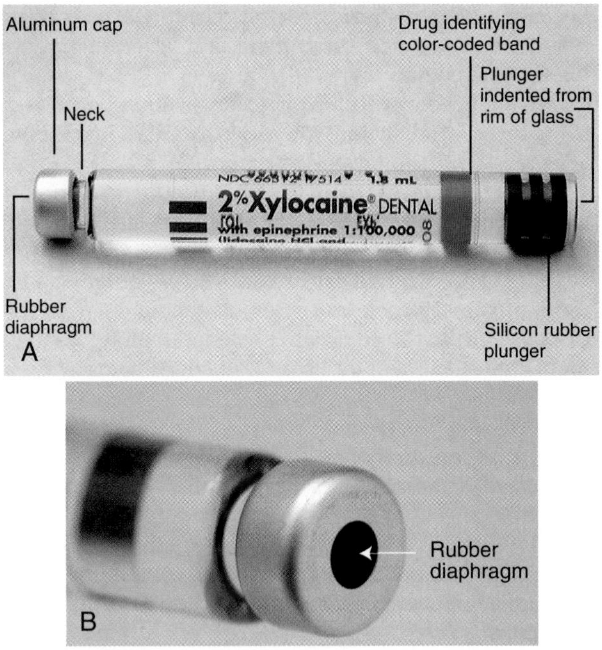

Figure 40-15. **A,** Components of the local anesthetic cartridge. **B,** Aluminum cap and rubber diaphragm *(arrow)*. (From Malamed SF: *Handbook of local anesthesia*, ed 6, St Louis, 2013, Mosby.)

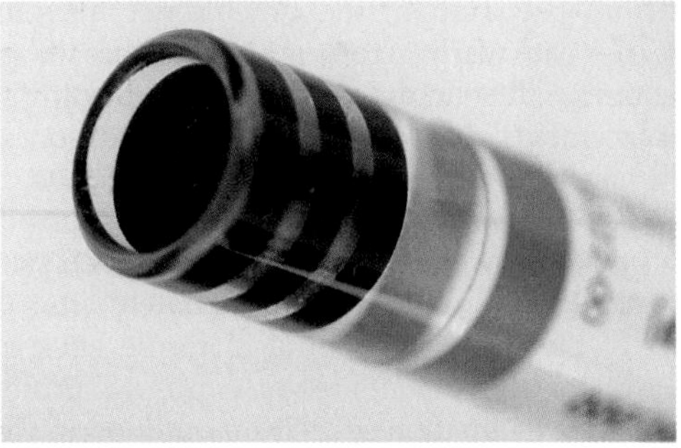

Figure 40-16. The rubber plunger is slightly indented from the rim of the glass. (From Malamed SF: *Handbook of local anesthesia*, ed 6, St Louis, 2013, Mosby.)

the glass cylinder rim (Figure 40-16). Cartridges that do not exhibit this characteristic should not be used, because it is an indication that the solution has been contaminated. This topic is discussed more fully in the later section on problems.

2. On the opposite end of the cartridge is a diaphragm into which the needle penetrates. The diaphragm is made of a semipermeable material, usually rubber, that allows solutions to diffuse into the cartridge if the cartridge is stored improperly (see Figure 40-15, *B*).
3. An aluminum cap fits securely around the cartridge neck to hold the diaphragm in place.
4. The glass cylinder makes up the cartridge body, on which the cartridge contents, the solution amount, and the manufacturer's name are imprinted. In addition, several manufacturers now place a color-coding band around the glass cylinder to help with drug identification.

Ingredients

Several ingredients collectively form the anesthetic solution. The local anesthetic drug or combination of drugs is, of course, the primary reason for the dental cartridge. The local anesthetic molecule is stable and can withstand being boiled or processed in an autoclave without breaking down. Unfortunately, other ingredients and dental cartridge components are more fragile.

A vasoconstricting drug in any of various concentrations is included in some anesthetic cartridges. This component increases safety as well as the duration of action of the local anesthetic agent. Those cartridges that include a vasoconstrictor also contain a preservative for the vasoconstrictor. The agent that is most often employed is sodium bisulfite, which prevents the biodegradation of the vasoconstrictor by oxygen.

Sodium chloride is added to the dental cartridge to make the solution isotonic with the body tissues. Finally, distilled water is incorporated into the anesthetic solution to produce a sufficient volume of solution in the cartridge. Cartridges available in the United States contain a total of 1.8 mL of solution.

Cartridge Care and Handling

Local anesthetic cartridges are packaged either in a vacuum-sealed metal canister that contains 50 cartridges or in boxes that include 10 sealed units of 10 cartridges each, which are referred to as *blister packs*. Regardless of how the cartridges are packaged, it is recommended that they be stored in their original containers at room temperature in a dark place. Exposure to prolonged heat or direct sunlight results in accelerated solution deterioration, particularly of the vasoconstrictor. In addition, if they are kept in these original containers, the cartridges remain clean and uncontaminated.

It is not necessary to prepare a cartridge before use. The local anesthetic solution is sterilized during the manufacturing process, and bacterial cultures taken from exterior cartridge surfaces immediately after opening a container usually fail to produce bacterial growth.[1] If the oral healthcare provider is concerned about the cartridge exterior, however, all components may be wiped with a disinfectant approved by the American Dental Association and the Environmental Protection Agency. Plastic cartridge dispensers are also available to help with the disinfecting of cartridges. They can hold a single day's supply of cartridges with the diaphragm or aluminum cap placed downward. Gauze that has been moistened with a disinfectant is placed in the center. When assembling the armamentarium for local anesthetic administration, the oral healthcare provider may wipe the diaphragm end of the cartridge against the moistened gauze.

Cartridges should never be immersed in liquid disinfectant or sterilant. These solutions may diffuse through the semipermeable material of the diaphragm and contaminate the cartridge contents, or they may corrode the aluminum cap. In addition, local anesthetic cartridges should not be processed in the autoclave. Neither the labile vasoconstrictor nor the seals of the cartridge can withstand the extreme temperatures.

Cartridge warmers that bring the local anesthetic solution to body temperature to promote client comfort during administration are commercially available; however, they are neither necessary nor recommended. Local anesthetics that are stored and injected at room temperature are not uncomfortable to clients. Indeed, an overheated cartridge may cause a burning sensation during the injection and may destroy the heat-sensitive vasoconstrictor, thereby producing a shorter duration of anesthesia.

Each box or canister is marked with an expiration date by the manufacturer. This expiration date also appears on the individual cartridges. Cartridges should not be used beyond the expiration date, because injection with an outdated local anesthetic solution may result in client discomfort and unreliable anesthesia.

A product identification package insert is placed in all local anesthetic containers. It includes important information about the local anesthetic agent, including dosages, contraindications, warnings, care and handling specifics, and more. It is imperative that the dental hygienist be familiar with this material to ensure client safety and comfort.

Problems

Problems are seldom encountered with cartridges, but the following may occur[1]:

- *Bubble in the cartridge.* Small bubbles (i.e., 1 to 2 mm in diameter) may at times be seen in a cartridge. These bubbles consist of nitrogen gas that was bubbled into the anesthetic solution during the manufacturing process to preclude oxygen, which destroys the vasoconstrictor, from being trapped in the cartridge. The bubbles are harmless and may be ignored. A larger bubble (i.e., >2 mm) in the cartridge, however, is an indication that the solution has been frozen. In this case, the stopper may also extend beyond the cartridge end (i.e., it may be extruded). Because solution sterility is no longer guaranteed, the cartridge should not be used.
- *Extruded stopper.* As noted previously, an extruded rubber stopper accompanied by a large bubble in the cartridge is an indication that the solution has been frozen. Having a stopper that extends beyond the rim of the glass cylinder with no bubble present is often a sign that the cartridge was stored in a disinfectant and that the solution has diffused through the diaphragm and into the cartridge. When this occurs, the contents are contaminated, and the cartridge should be discarded.
- *Sticky stopper.* A sticky stopper does not advance smoothly through the glass cylinder when pressure is applied to the syringe thumb ring. Because rubber stoppers are more frequently being treated with silicone during manufacturing, this has become less of a problem. However, if paraffin is being employed by the manufacturer, difficulty may be encountered. To minimize the sticky stopper problem, cartridges should be stored at room temperature. If the problem persists, the healthcare provider should consider using only cartridges that have a silicone-treated stopper to facilitate a smooth, even depositing of solution.
- *Corroded cap.* Aluminum cap corrosion may be observed if the cap has been immersed in quaternary compounds such as benzalkonium chloride. If disinfecting the cartridge is necessary, a disinfectant that has been approved by the American Dental Association and the Environmental Protective Agency is recommended. Cartridges that exhibit corrosion should not be used.
- *Rust on the aluminum cap.* The presence of rust signifies that a cartridge has broken or leaked in the metal container. The metal container rusts, and deposits appear on the cartridge cap. A cartridge that has a rust deposit should not be used, and each cartridge in the container should be carefully inspected.
- *Broken cartridge.* Cartridge breakage may occur if the cartridge has been fractured during handling. Damaged containers should be returned to the supplier. Before being used, each cartridge is checked for signs of cracked or chipped glass. The area surrounding the stopper and the cylinder–cap interface need to be carefully examined. If a fractured cartridge is subjected to the pressure of an injection, it may shatter. Fortunately, the introduction of the color-coding band around the glass cylinder has minimized such occurrences by reinforcing the glass.
  - A broken cartridge may result if excessive force is used when the dental hygienist engages the harpoon of an aspirating syringe. The harpoon is engaged by gently pressing the thumb ring and piston into the rubber stopper. If it is necessary to use more pressure to embed the harpoon, the dental hygienist should use one hand to cover the glass cartridge.
  - Pressure on the syringe thumb ring may cause the cartridge to break if the syringe harpoon is bent or if the needle is bent and not perforating the cartridge diaphragm. Thorough examination and proper armamentarium preparation before use prevent cartridge breakage from occurring. One should never apply excessive pressure on the dental cartridge if significant resistance is met.
- *Leakage during injection.* An off-center perforation of the needle into the cartridge diaphragm produces an oval-shaped puncture. When positive pressure is applied to the plunger, anesthetic solution may leak through the perforation. It is important to carefully insert the needle into the cartridge diaphragm so that a centric perforation occurs and to prevent leakage during the injection.
- *Burning on injection.* See Local Complications later in this chapter.

Supplementary Armamentarium

In addition to the syringe, needle, and cartridge, other items are needed to effectively administer local anesthetics. These include topical antiseptic, topical anesthetic, applicator sticks, gauze, and a hemostat or cotton pliers.

Topical Antiseptics

Topical antiseptics may be applied to the mucosa surface at the injection site to reduce the risk of introducing surface microorganisms into the tissue, which could result in inflammation and infection. Betadine (povidone–iodine) and Merthiolate (thimerosal) are agents that are commonly used for this purpose.[1] A small quantity of the agent is placed at the injection site for 15 to 30 seconds before the topical anesthetic placement and the initial needle penetration. The use of sterile gauze for wiping the surface is considered an adequate alternative, with topical antiseptic application as an option for further microbe reduction. Because postinjection infections may occur, however, the use of a topical antiseptic should be considered, especially when local anesthetic agents are administered to individuals who may be immunosuppressed.[1]

Topical Anesthetic Agents

Topical anesthetic agents are applied to the mucous membrane before the initial needle penetration to anesthetize the

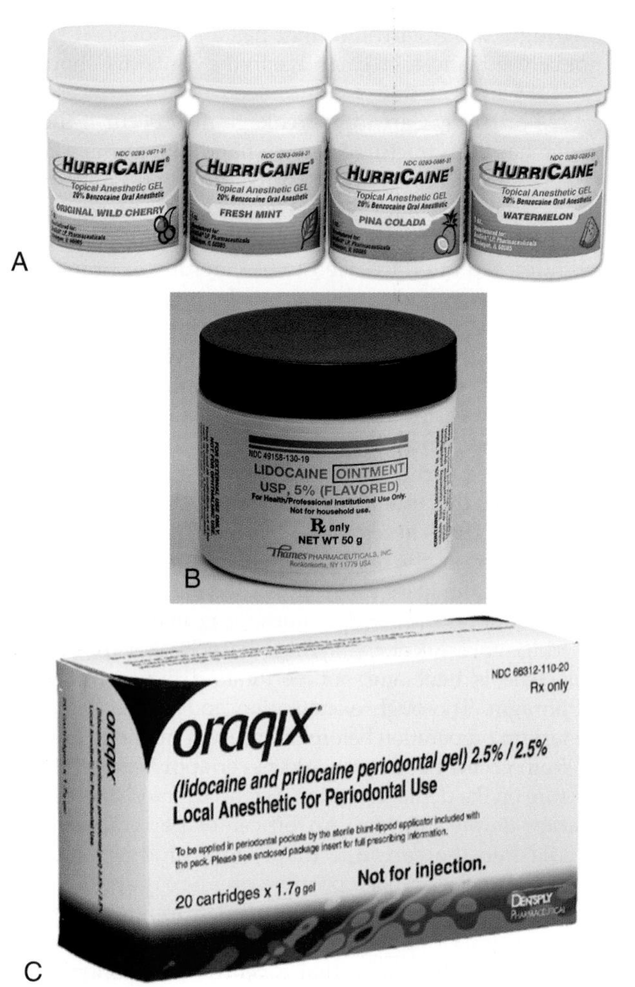

Figure 40-17. **A,** Example of a topical anesthetic that contains benzocaine. **B,** Example of a topical anesthetic that contains lidocaine (DentiPatch). **C,** Example of Oraqix, which contains lidocaine and prilocaine. (**A,** Courtesy Beautlich LP Pharmaceuticals, Waukegan, Illinois. **B,** Courtesy Septodont, New Castle, Delaware. **C,** Courtesy DENTSPLY Pharmaceutical.)

terminal nerve endings and thus promote client comfort during the injection procedures (Figure 40-17). For maximal effectiveness, the topical anesthetic agent is placed at the penetration site on dried tissue for 1 to 2 minutes.

The concentration of agents used for topical application is high to facilitate diffusion of the drug through the mucous membranes (i.e., usually 2 to 3 mm). Therefore only small amounts applied to a limited area are used to avoid toxicity. Both ester and amide topical anesthetic agents are available; these are prepared in the form of gels, ointments, solutions, and sprays. Topical anesthetic sprays that, when activated, deliver a continuous stream until deactivated may potentially deliver a very high anesthetic agent dose and are therefore not recommended. Those sprays that deliver a measured dose limit the amount that can be expelled and are much preferred.

Oraqix is an amide topical anesthetic that contains 2.5% lidocaine and 2.5% prilocaine (see Figure 40-17, *C*). Oraqix is a periodontal gel that has been approved by the FDA for intraoral use and that is available by prescription. It is indicated for adults who require localized anesthesia subgingivally during scaling or root planing. Oraqix comes in a cartridge that is inserted into a specially designed dispenser for administration. The cartridge has a safety collar that prevents loading of the product into a standard dental syringe. **Oraqix is not for injection.** This product has unique thermosetting properties. It is fluid at room temperature, which ensures delivery subgingivally, but it becomes a gel at body temperature, which keeps it at the site. Oraqix contains no epinephrine; it has a 30-second onset, and the anesthetic benefits will last an average of 20 minutes. A maximum dose of five cartridges per hygiene appointment is advised, and caution is advised when administering this product to nursing mothers[10] (see Procedure 40-1 and the corresponding Competency Form).

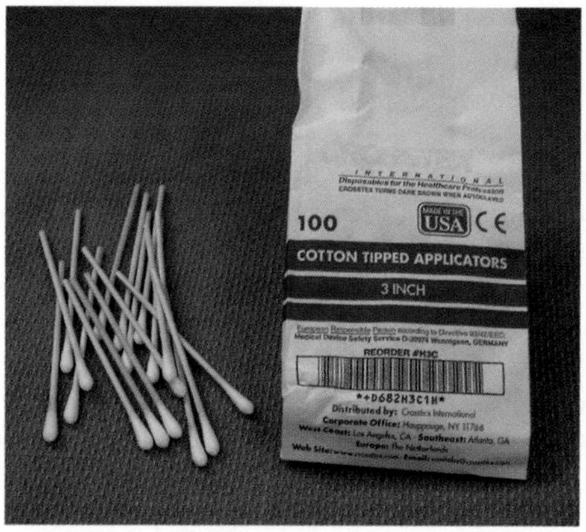

Figure 40-18. Cotton-tipped applicator sticks. (From Malamed SF: *Handbook of local anesthesia,* ed 6, St Louis, 2013, Mosby.)

Cotton-Tipped Applicator Sticks

Cotton-tipped applicator sticks are needed for topical antiseptic and anesthetic agent application. They also may be used to apply pressure to the tissue before and during palatal injections (Figure 40-18).

Gauze

Gauze is used to wipe the tissue at the injection site before application of the topical antiseptic and anesthetic agents and again before the insertion of the needle. This procedure removes the saliva and debris from the injection site. It may also serve as a suitable—although not as effective—replacement for the topical antiseptic (see Topical Antiseptics earlier in this chapter). In addition, the gauze helps with retraction, visibility, and stability during the injection procedures (Figure 40-19).

Hemostats, Forceps, and Cotton Pliers

Hemostats, forceps, and cotton pliers are armamentarium components to have on hand in the unlikely event that a needle breaks during administration and must be retrieved from the soft tissues (Figure 40-20).

Preparation of Armamentarium

Loading and Unloading the Metallic or Plastic Cartridge-Type Syringe

Proper loading of the syringe is essential to prevent complications associated with the syringe, cartridge, and needle and

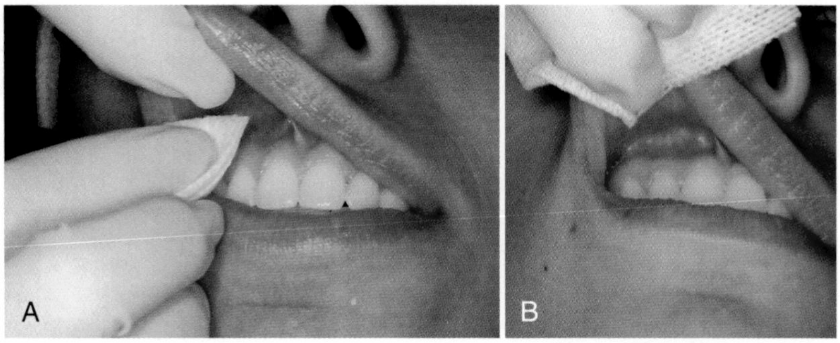

Figure 40-19. Sterile gauze is used **(A)** to wipe the mucous membrane at the site of needle penetration and **(B)** to help with tissue retraction, if necessary. (From Malamed SF: *Handbook of local anesthesia,* ed 6, St Louis, 2013, Mosby.)

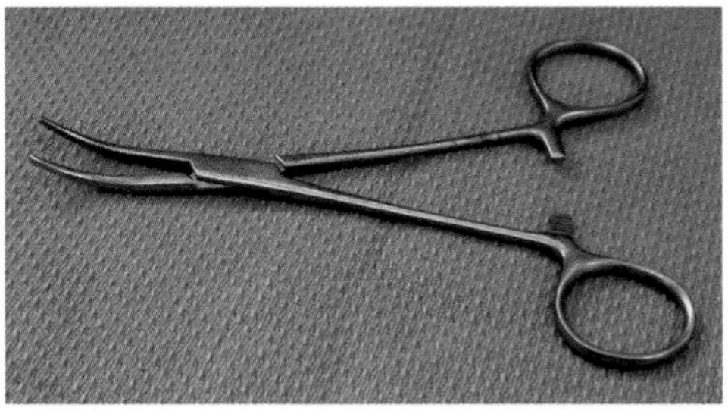

Figure 40-20. Hemostat. (From Malamed SF: Handbook of local anesthesia, ed 6, St Louis, 2013, Mosby.)

to ensure client safety and comfort during local anesthetic administration (see Procedure 40-2 and the corresponding Competency Form).

Unsheathing and Resheathing the Needle

A needle should be covered with a colored protective shield when it is not being used. Concerns regarding the possibility of a needle stick exposure have led to the formulation of guidelines for resheathing needles. Oral healthcare providers are most often injured with needles when the needle is being resheathed after an injection.[1] At this time in the procedure,

Procedure 40-1 Oraqix Topical Anesthetic Application for Use During Scaling and Root Planing

EQUIPMENT

Personal protective equipment
2.5% lidocaine and 2.5% prilocaine cartridge
Oraqix dispenser
Blunt-tip applicator
Hemostat or cotton pliers
2 × 2 gauze

STEPS

1. Assemble the armamentarium (Figure 40-21).
2. Place the blunt-tip applicator into the tip of the Oraqix dispenser, and turn it to lock it in place (Figure 40-22).
3. Press the reset button on the body of the handle (Figure 40-23).
4. Load the cartridge stopper-end first into the body of the handle, join the tip to the applicator body, and twist to lock it in place (Figure 40-24, *A* and *B*).

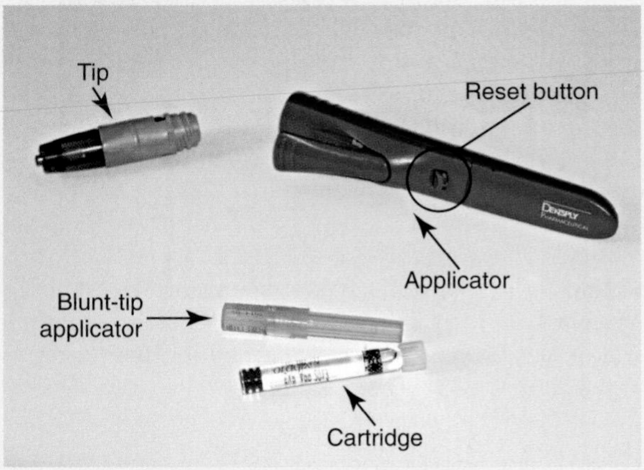

Figure 40-21. Oraqix armamentarium. From the top left: applicator tip, applicator body, blunt-tip applicator in blue cap, and cartridge of Oraqix topical gel. (Courtesy F. O'Brien Photography.)

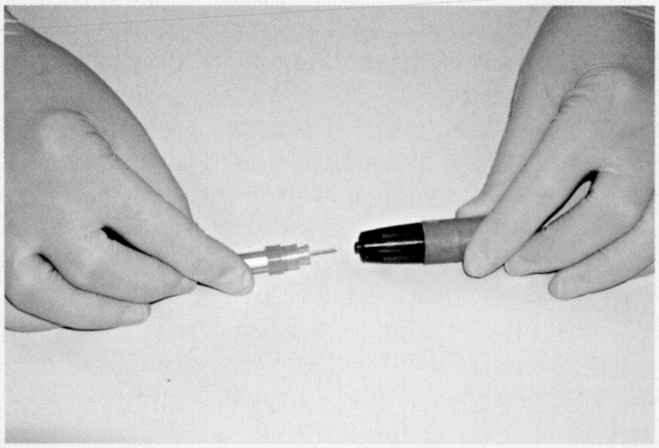

Figure 40-22. Connect the blunt-tip applicator with the applicator tip. (Courtesy F. O'Brien Photography.)

Continued

Procedure 40-1 Oraqix Topical Anesthetic Application for Use During Scaling and Root Planing—cont'd

5. Partially remove the blunt-tip applicator cap to bend the tip into a shape to suit individual client or clinician needs (Figure 40-25).
6. Select three to four teeth, apply the Oraqix gel by tracing the gingival margin, and wait 30 seconds (Figure 40-26).
7. Move the blunt-tip applicator directly into the periodontal pocket, and fill the pocket with the Oraqix gel (Figure 40-27).
8. For a detailed demonstration, go to www.oraqix.com to view a video of the application process.

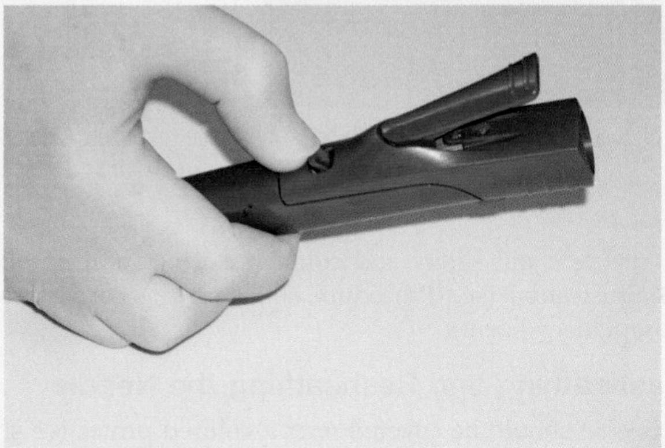

Figure 40-23. Press the reset button on the body of the handle. (Courtesy F. O'Brien Photography.)

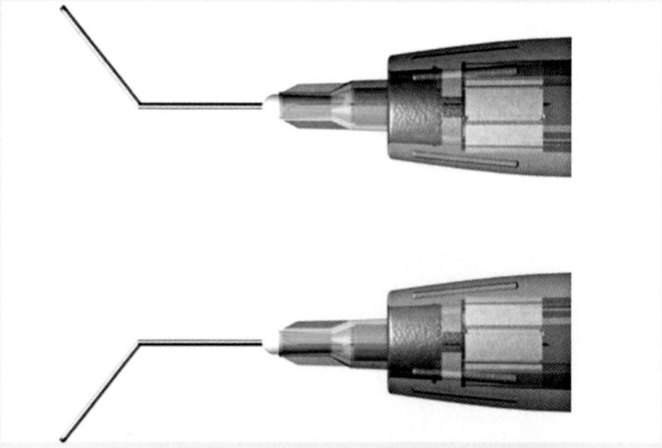

Figure 40-25. Partially remove the cap on the blunt-tip applicator and bend it to suit the client's and clinician's needs. (From Oraqix: Product information available from Dentsply Pharmaceuticals, York, PA. Available at: www.dentsplydental.com.)

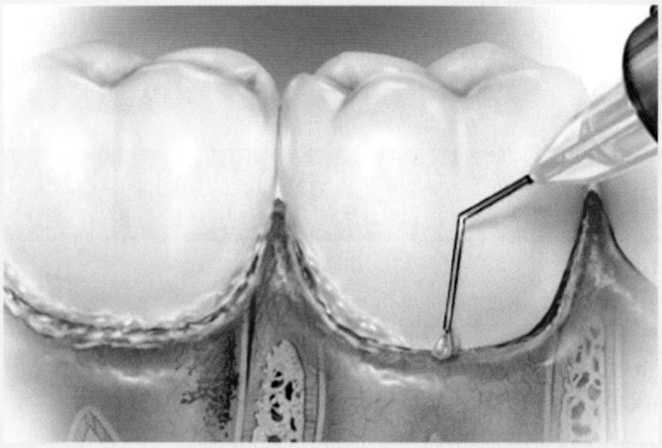

Figure 40-26. Apply the gel by tracing the gingival margin. (From Oraqix: Product information available from Dentsply Pharmaceuticals, York, PA. Available at: www.dentsplydental.com.)

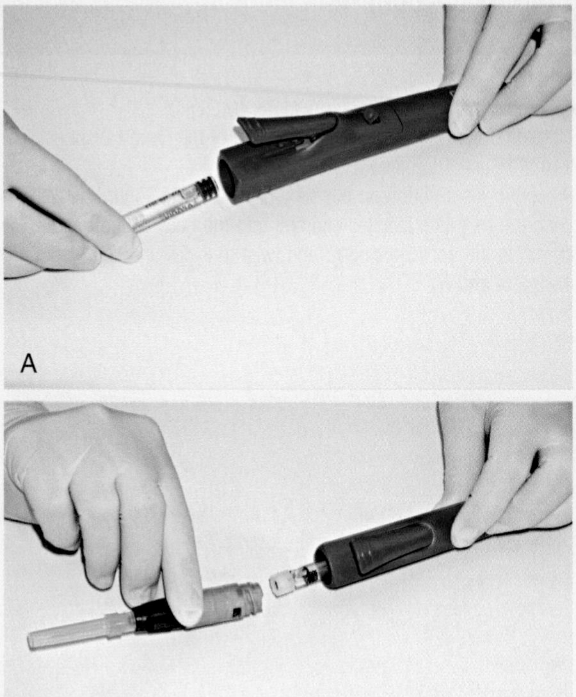

Figure 40-24. A, Load the cartridge stopper-end first into the main applicator body. **B,** Join the tip to the applicator. Twist to lock in place. (Courtesy F. O'Brien Photography.)

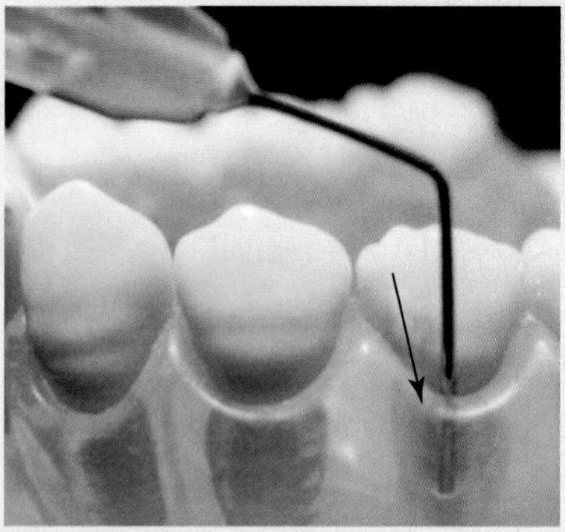

Figure 40-27. Move the blunt-tip applicator directly into the periodontal pocket, and fill it with the gel. (From Oraqix: Product information available from Dentsply Pharmaceuticals, York, PA. Available at: www.dentsplydental.com.)

Procedure 40-2 Loading the Metallic or Plastic Cartridge-Type Syringe

EQUIPMENT

Personal protective equipment
Syringe
Needle
Gauze
Anesthetic cartridge
Topical anesthetic
Cotton-tipped applicator
Hemostat or cotton pliers

STEPS

1. Assemble the armamentarium (Figure 40-28).

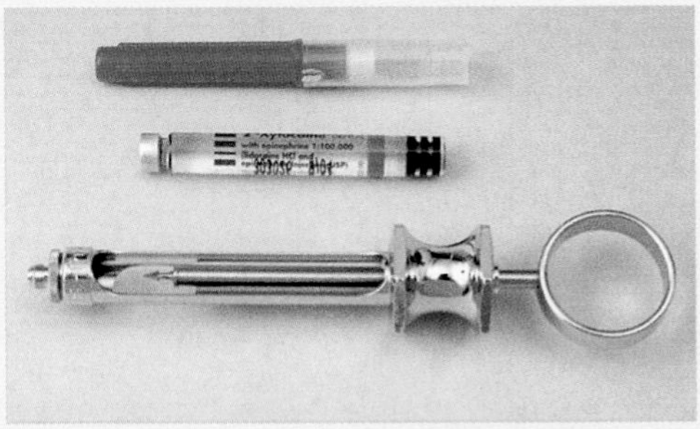

Figure 40-28. Armamentarium. From the top: needle, cartridge, and syringe. (From Malamed SF: *Handbook of local anesthesia,* ed 6, St Louis, 2013, Mosby.)

2. Remove the sterilized syringe from its container, and inspect it to ensure that the harpoon is sharp and straight.
3. Retract the piston (Figure 40-29).

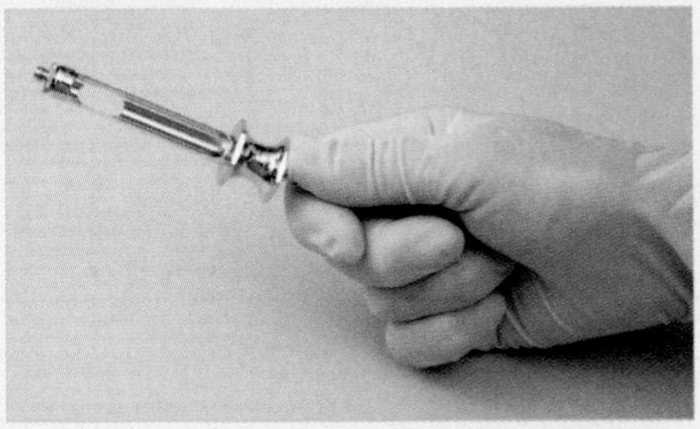

Figure 40-29. Retract the piston. (From Malamed SF: *Handbook of local anesthesia,* ed 6, St Louis, 2013, Mosby.)

4. Insert the cartridge (Figure 40-30).

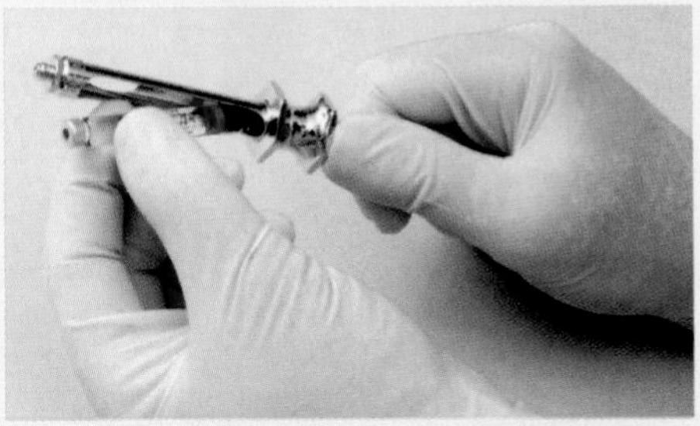

Figure 40-30. Insert the cartridge. (From Malamed SF: *Handbook of local anesthesia,* ed 6, St Louis, 2013, Mosby.)

5. Engage the harpoon in the plunger with gentle finger pressure (Figure 40-31).

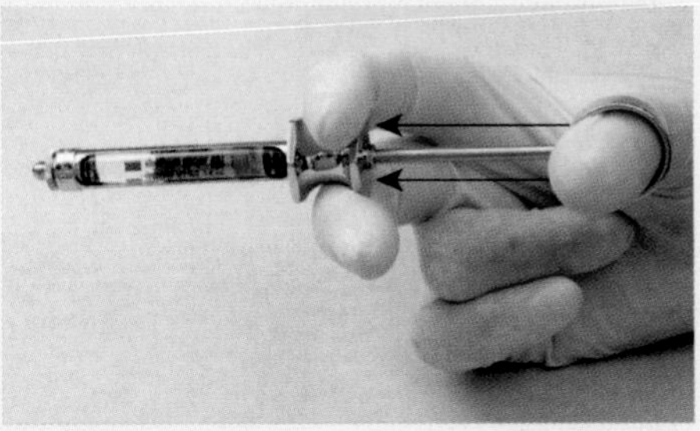

Figure 40-31. Engage the harpoon in the plunger with gentle finger pressure. (From Malamed SF: *Handbook of local anesthesia,* ed 6, St Louis, 2013, Mosby.)

6. Do not exert force on the plunger, because the glass may crack (Figure 40-32).

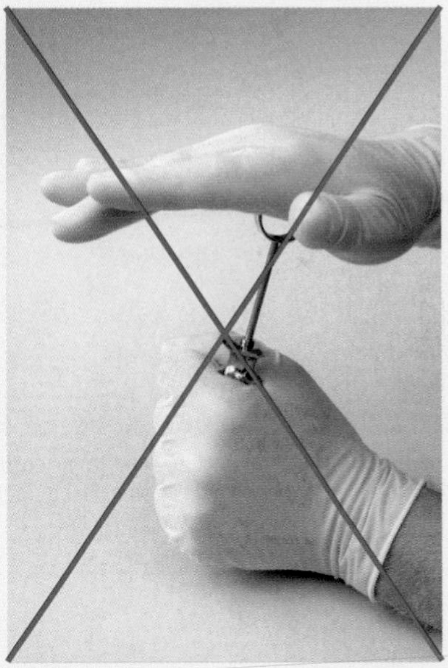

Figure 40-32. Do not exert force on the plunger. (From Malamed SF: *Handbook of local anesthesia,* ed 6, St Louis, 2013, Mosby.)

7. Remove the clear or white plastic protective shield that covers the syringe and cartridge end of the needle (Figure 40-33).

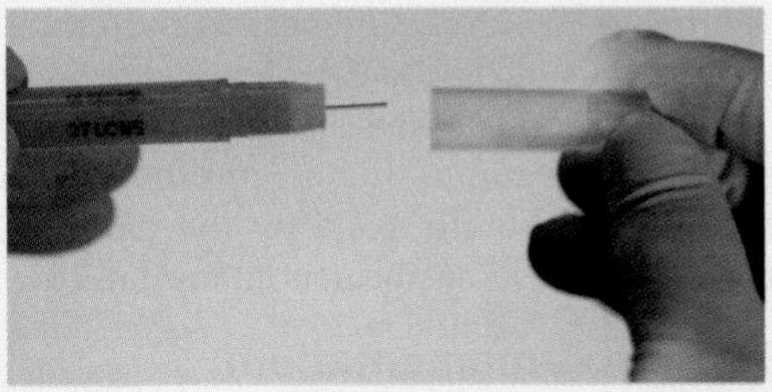

Figure 40-33. Remove the clear plastic protective cap from the opposite end of the colored plastic cap that hubs the needle.

Continued

Procedure 40-2 Loading the Metallic or Plastic Cartridge-Type Syringe—cont'd

8. Screw the colored plastic-hubbed needle onto the syringe while simultaneously pushing it into the metal needle adapter of the syringe (Figure 40-34).

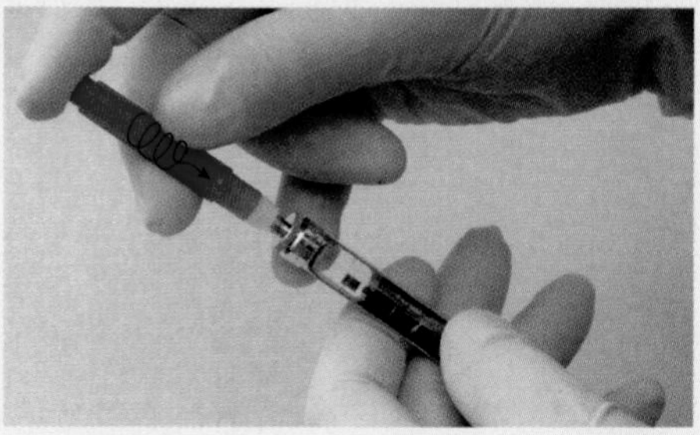

Figure 40-34. A plastic-hubbed needle must be screwed onto the syringe while simultaneously being pushed into the metal needle adaptor of the syringe *(arrow).* (From Malamed SF: *Handbook of local anesthesia,* ed 6, St Louis, 2013, Mosby.)

9. While directing the needle away from the body, keep the hand at the needle hub, and loosen the colored plastic protective cap from the needle (Figure 40-35).

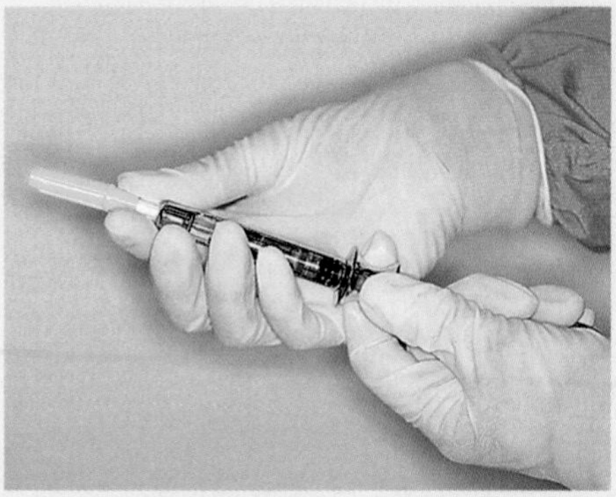

Figure 40-35. While directing the needle away from the body, keep the hand at the needle hub, and loosen the colored plastic protective cap from the needle.

10. Let the cap slide off of the needle and onto a piece of sterile gauze (Figure 40-36).
11. Expel a few drops of solution to test for proper flow, and then recap the needle using the scoop technique (Figure 40-37).
    a. Hold the syringe with one hand, and glide the needle into the colored plastic cap lying on the instrument tray. Never attempt to hold the cap with the other hand, because this may lead to an accidental needle stick exposure.
    b. Tilt the syringe upward to allow the cap to slide down to the hub and cover the needle. If the cap starts to slip off of the needle, do not attempt to stop it with the other hand. Instead, let the cap fall on the instrument tray, and begin the process again.
12. The syringe is now ready for use.

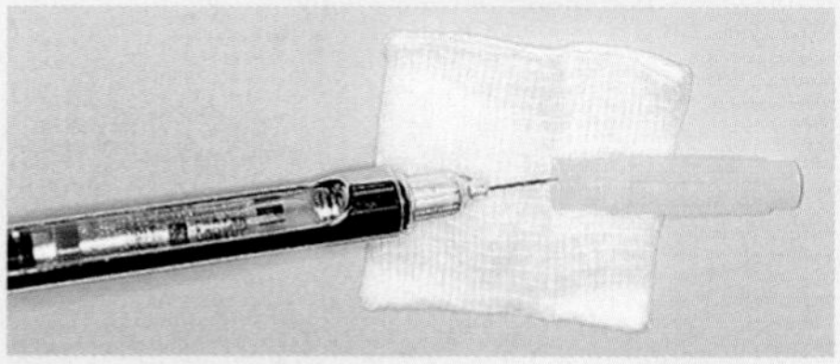

Figure 40-36. Let the cap slide off of the needle and onto a piece of sterile gauze.

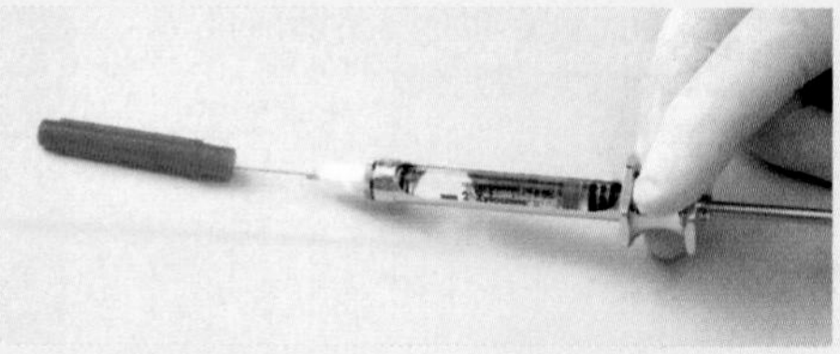

Figure 40-37. "Scoop" technique for recapping the needle after use. (From Malamed SF: *Handbook of local anesthesia,* ed 6, St Louis, 2013, Mosby.)

the needle is contaminated with blood, saliva, and debris, and the potential for disease transmission exists. A variety of techniques have been suggested, but currently a one-handed "scoop" technique for sheathing the needle is recommended and described in Procedure 40-2.

Mechanical devices such as shields and needle sheath props are available to help prevent accidental needle stick exposures (Figure 40-38). Dental hygienists should be familiar with the devices available and determine which technique or mechanical device is most acceptable to them. The one-handed resheathing technique or an approved mechanical device should be consistently used by the dental hygienist whether or not the needle has been contaminated.

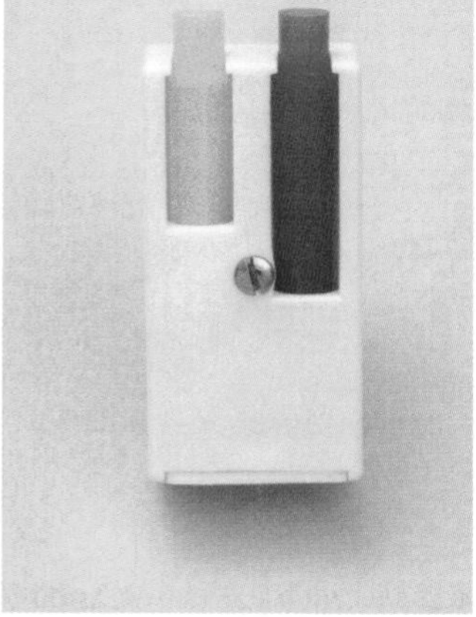

Figure 40-38. Plastic needle cap holders. (From Malamed SF: *Handbook of local anesthesia,* ed 6, St Louis, 2013, Mosby.)

Dismantling the Armamentarium

At the completion of the dental hygiene care appointment, the local anesthesia armamentarium needs to be dismantled. Procedure 40-3 and the corresponding Competency

Procedure 40-3 Unloading the Breech-Loading Metallic or Plastic Cartridge-Type Syringe

EQUIPMENT

See Procedure 40-2.

STEPS

1. Pull the cartridge away from the needle with your thumb and forefinger as you retract the piston, until the harpoon disengages from the plunger (Figure 40-39).
2. Remove the cartridge from the syringe by inverting the syringe, and permit the cartridge to fall free (Figure 40-40).
3. Carefully unscrew the recapped needle; be careful to not accidentally discard the metal needle adaptor (Figure 40-41).
4. Place the needle in a sharps container (Figure 40-42) and the cartridge in a separate sealed container or in the sharps container (Figure 40-43).

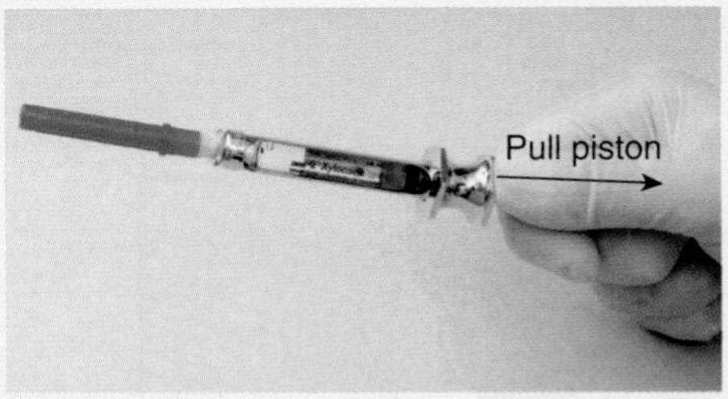

Figure 40-39. Retract the piston. (From Malamed SF: *Handbook of local anesthesia,* ed 6, St Louis, 2013, Mosby.)

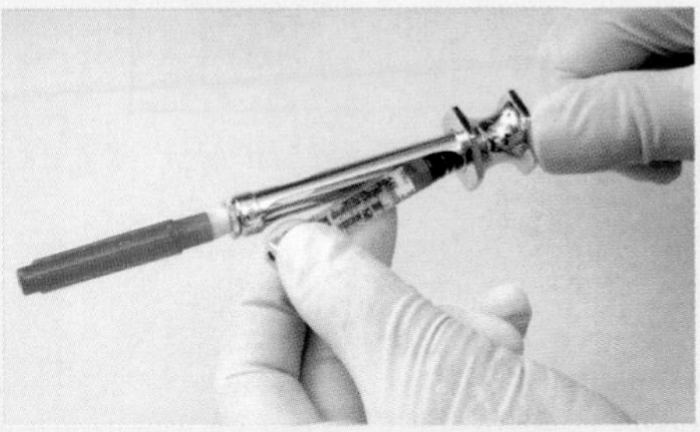

Figure 40-40. Remove the used cartridge. (From Malamed SF: *Handbook of local anesthesia,* ed 6, St Louis, 2013, Mosby.)

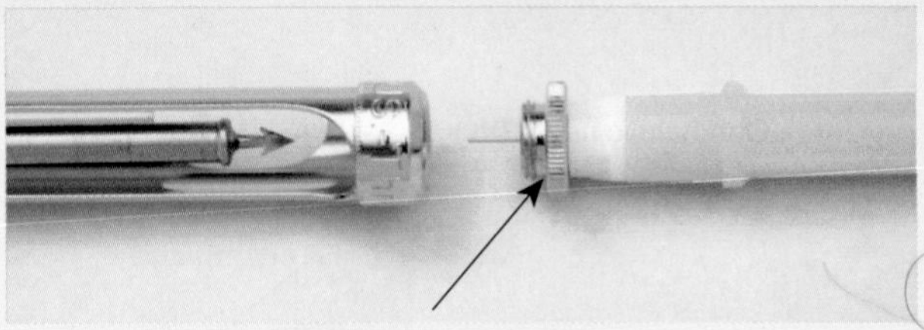

Figure 40-41. When discarding the needle, check to be sure that the metal needle adaptor from the syringe is not inadvertently discarded as well *(arrow).* (From Malamed SF: *Handbook of local anesthesia,* ed 6, St Louis, 2013, Mosby.)

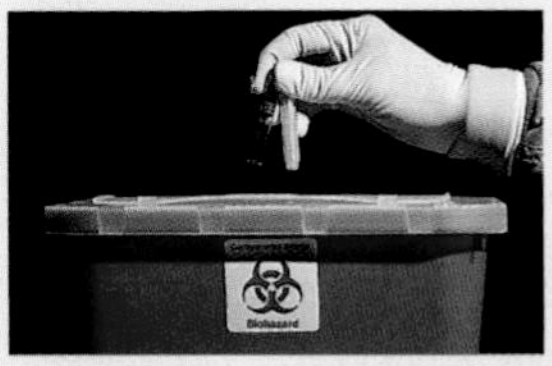

Figure 40-42. Used needles and cartridges are considered infectious. Sharps must be discarded in a rigid, puncture-proof, leak-resistant container.

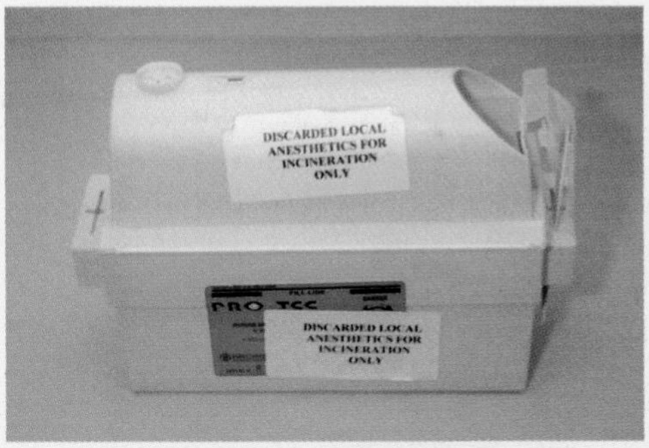

Figure 40-43. Separate sealed container. (From Malamed SF: *Handbook of local anesthesia,* ed 6, St Louis, 2013, Mosby.)

Form describe the sequence for properly unloading the syringe.

Trigeminal Nerve

The trigeminal nerve is the fifth and largest of the 12 cranial nerves (Figure 40-44). The three divisions of the trigeminal nerve include the ophthalmic (V_1), maxillary (V_2), and mandibular (V_3) divisions. The ophthalmic and maxillary divisions are completely sensory; the mandibular division is sensory and also carries the motor root to the mandibular muscles.

Ophthalmic Division (V_1)

The ophthalmic nerve, which is the first and smallest division of the trigeminal nerve, branches off the trigeminal (semilunar or gasserian) ganglion and forms three branches: the nasociliary nerve, the frontal nerve, and the lacrimal nerve. This division of the trigeminal nerve innervates tissues superior to the oral structures, including the eye, the nose, and the frontal cutaneous tissues. It has only sensory function. Of the three divisions of the trigeminal nerve, the ophthalmic is the least important to intraoral local anesthetic administration.

Maxillary Division (V_2)

The maxillary division of the trigeminal nerve, which is entirely sensory in function, arises from the trigeminal (semilunar or Gasserian) ganglion, exits the cranium via the foramen rotundum, and then passes into the pterygopalatine fossa, where it gives off several branches (Figure 40-45). Only those branches pertinent to intraoral local anesthesia are discussed here.

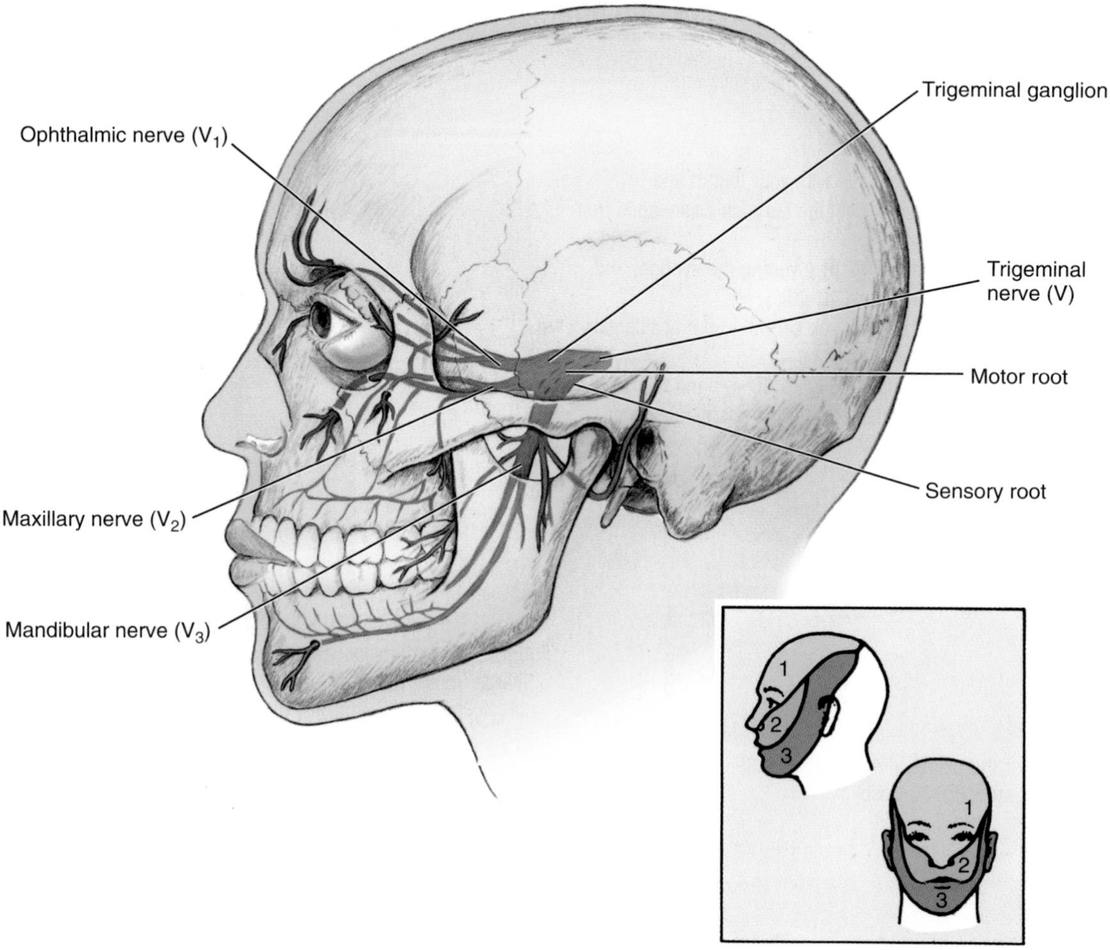

Figure 40-44. Trigeminal nerve distribution. (From Fehrenbach MJ, Herring SW: *Illustrated anatomy of the head and neck,* ed 4, St Louis, 2012, Saunders.)

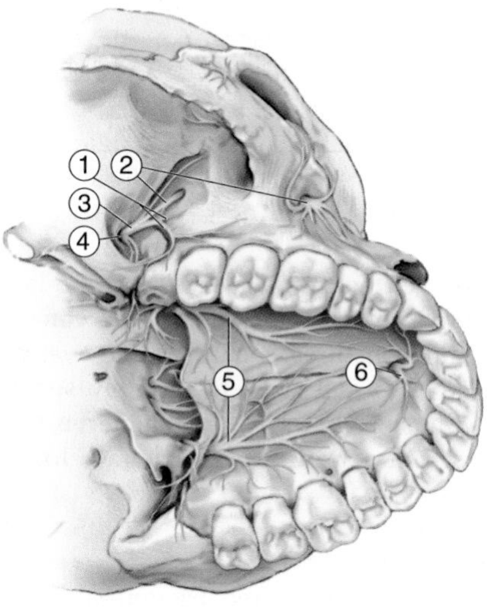

Figure 40-45. Distribution of the maxillary division (V_2). *1,* Posterior superior alveolar branches; *2,* infraorbital nerve; *3,* maxillary nerve; *4,* foramen rotundum; *5,* greater palatine nerve; *6,* nasopalatine nerve. (Data from Haglund J, Evers H: *Local anaesthesia in dentistry,* ed 2, Södertälje, Sweden, 1975, Astra Läkemedel.)

Pterygopalatine Nerves

Two branches pass through the pterygopalatine ganglion and form the greater (anterior) palatine nerve and the nasopalatine nerve (see Figure 40-45). The greater palatine nerve enters the oral cavity on the hard palate via the greater palatine foramen and innervates the palatal soft tissues and bone of the posterior teeth. The nasopalatine nerve leaves the pterygopalatine ganglion and passes forward and downward, entering the oral cavity through the incisive foramen. This nerve provides sensory innervation to the lingual bone and soft tissues in the premaxilla (i.e., canine to canine).

Posterior Superior Alveolar Nerve

The PSA nerve (Figure 40-46) descends from the main trunk of the maxillary nerve just before it enters the infraorbital canal. Most often there are two PSA branches that pass downward on the posterior surface of the maxilla. An internal branch enters the PSA foramen located on the superior portion of the maxillary tuberosity. This branch provides sensory innervation to the pulpal and osseous tissues and the periodontal ligaments of the maxillary third, second, and first molars (usually with the exception of the mesiobuccal root of the first molar). An external branch of the PSA nerve remains on the outer surface of the maxilla and continues downward

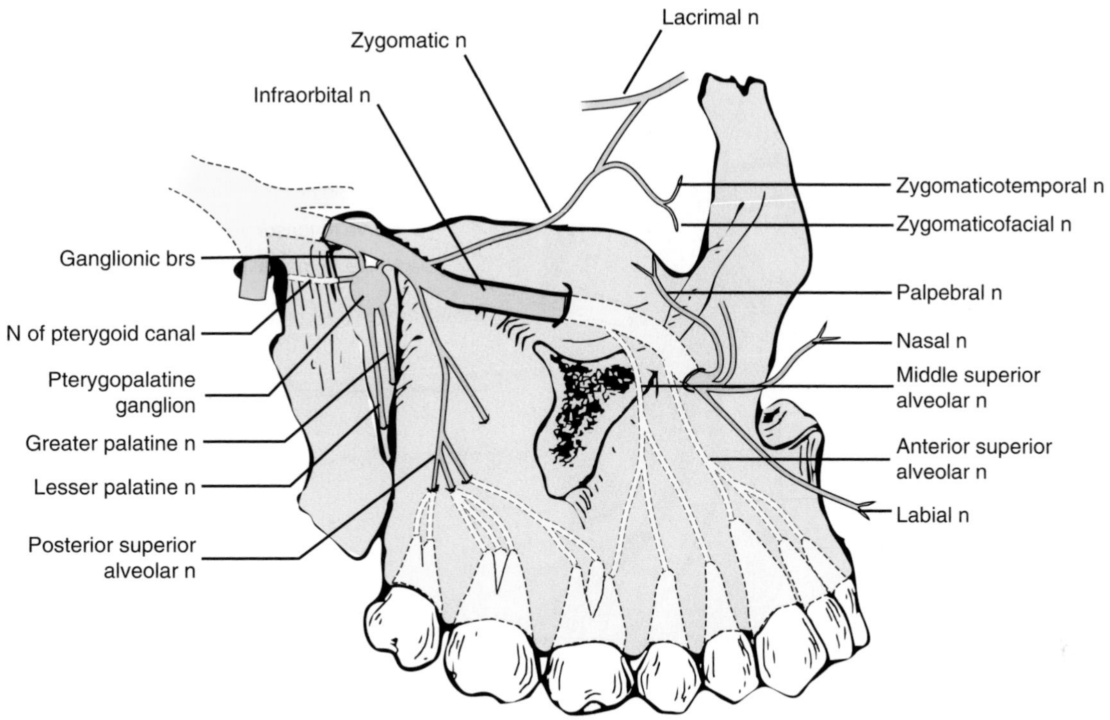

Figure 40-46. Maxillary nerve and its branches. *brs,* Branches; *n,* nerve. (From Liebgott B: *The anatomical basis of dentistry,* ed 3, St Louis, 2011, Mosby.)

to innervate the facial gingiva of the maxillary molars and the adjacent vestibular mucosa.

Branches of the Infraorbital Nerve

The maxillary nerve continues anteriorly after having given off the PSA nerve and enters the infraorbital canal. At this point, the maxillary nerve is referred to as the *infraorbital nerve* (see Figure 40-46). Two branches may descend from the infraorbital nerve: the middle superior alveolar (MSA) and the anterior superior alveolar (ASA) nerves.

The MSA nerve branches off of the infraorbital nerve within the infraorbital canal. This nerve provides sensory innervation to the maxillary premolars, the mesiofacial root of the first molar, the periodontal tissues, and the facial soft tissue and bone in the premolar area. The MSA nerve is not present in approximately 60% of individuals.[9] In its absence, these areas are innervated by the PSA nerve or, more commonly, the ASA nerve.

The ASA nerve descends from the infraorbital nerve just before the latter's exit from the infraorbital foramen. The ASA nerve provides innervation to the central and lateral incisors, the canine, the periodontal tissues, and the facial soft tissue and bone over these teeth. In those individuals without an MSA nerve, the ASA nerve most often provides innervation to the premolars and possibly the mesiofacial root of the first molar.

Mandibular Division (V_3)

The mandibular nerve, which is the third and largest division of the trigeminal nerve, has a sensory root in addition to carrying the motor root of the trigeminal nerve (Figure 40-47). The sensory root arises from the trigeminal ganglion, after which it is joined by the motor root. Both roots emerge from the cranium via the foramen ovale, and, at this point, they unite to form the main trunk of the mandibular nerve.

The trunk then divides into an anterior branch and a posterior branch. The nerves arising from these branches that relate to intraoral local anesthesia are described in the following paragraphs.

Branches of the Anterior Division

The anterior division is smaller than its posterior counterpart and contains primarily motor fibers. The motor component innervates the muscles of mastication: the masseter, the temporalis, and the lateral and medial pterygoid. The sensory component of the anterior division is the buccal nerve. At the level of the occlusal plane of the mandibular molars, it crosses the anterior border of the ramus and branches to innervate the buccal gingiva of the mandibular molars.

Branches of the Posterior Division

The posterior division of the mandibular nerve is primarily sensory, but it also has a small motor component. The posterior division branches related to mandibular anesthesia are the lingual and inferior alveolar nerves (Figure 40-48).

The lingual nerve emerges between the lower head of the lateral pterygoid and medial pterygoid muscles; it lies between the ramus and the medial pterygoid muscle in the pterygomandibular space. It turns anteriorly, where it enters the oral cavity and innervates the anterior two thirds of the tongue, the mucous membranes of the floor of the mouth, and the lingual gingiva of the mandible.

The inferior alveolar nerve runs posterior and parallel to the lingual nerve within the pterygomandibular space, where it enters the mandibular foramen. Within the mandible, the inferior alveolar nerve travels in the mandibular canal and

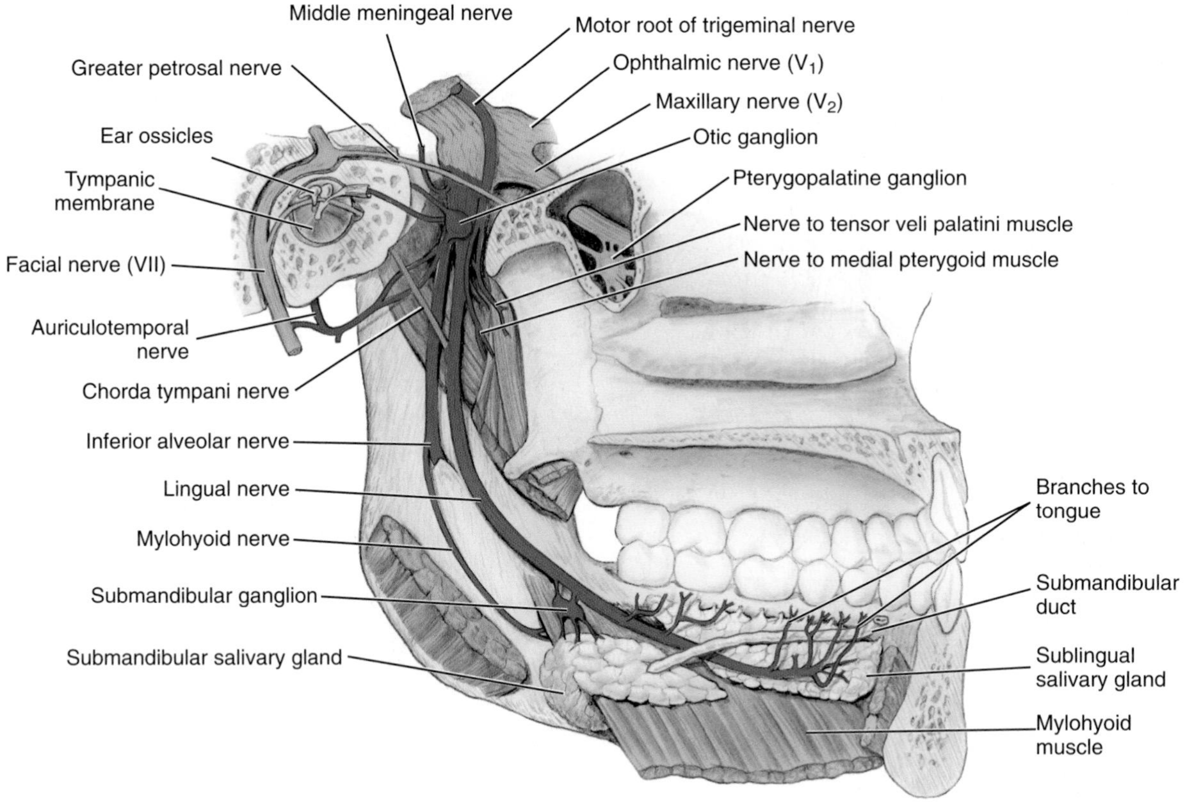

Figure 40-47. Medial view of the mandible showing the motor and sensory branches of the mandibular nerve. (From Fehrenbach MJ, Herring SW: *Illustrated anatomy of the head and neck,* ed 4, St Louis, 2012, Saunders.)

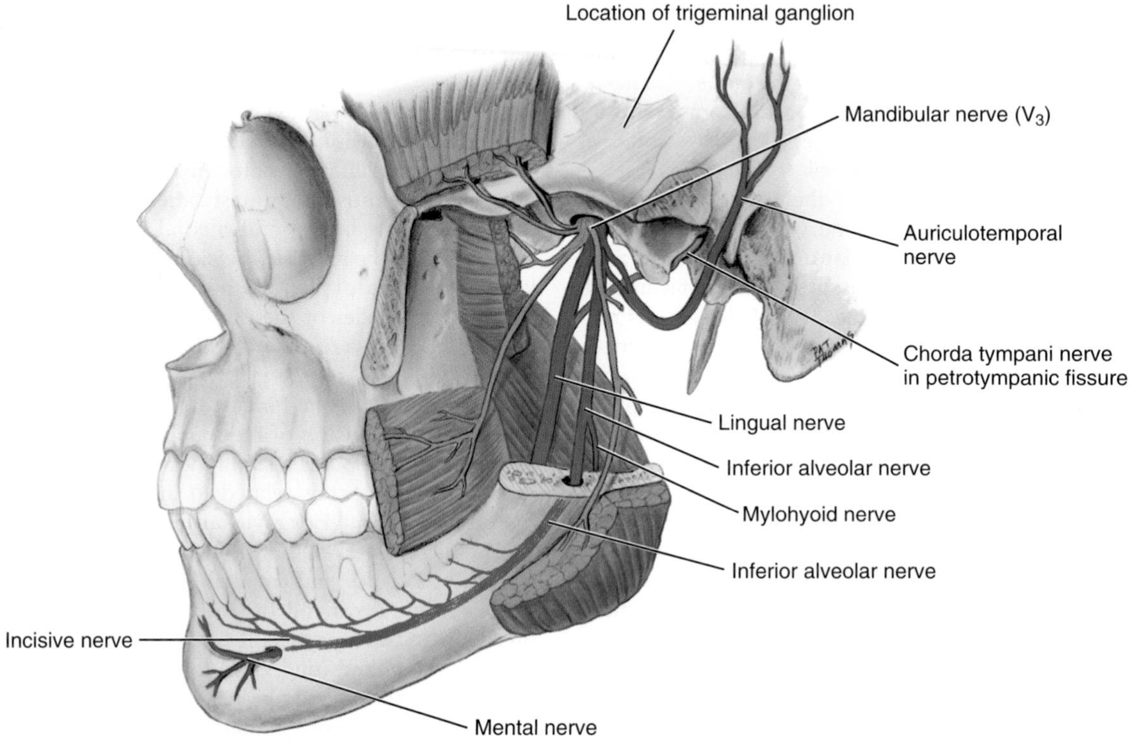

Figure 40-48. The pathway of the posterior trunk of the mandibular division of the trigeminal nerve. (From Fehrenbach MJ, Herring SW: *Illustrated anatomy of the head and neck,* ed 4, St Louis, 2012, Saunders.)

innervates the pulpal and osseous tissues of the mandibular teeth in the quadrant and the facial soft tissues anterior to the first molar. Throughout its course, the inferior alveolar nerve is accompanied by the inferior alveolar artery and vein.

As the inferior alveolar nerve reaches the mental foramen, it divides into two terminal branches. The incisive nerve is a direct extension of the inferior alveolar nerve, continuing anteriorly within the mandibular canal. It innervates the pulpal and osseous tissues of the mandibular first premolar, the canine, and the lateral and central incisors as well as the facial periodontal tissues of the teeth.

The mental nerve branches from the inferior alveolar nerve, exits the mandible via the mental foramen, and provides sensory innervation to the mucous membranes and skin of the lower lip and chin.

The mylohyoid nerve branches from the inferior alveolar nerve before the latter enters into the mandibular foramen. It advances downward and forward in the mylohyoid groove on the medial side of the ramus and provides motor innervation to the mylohyoid and anterior digastric muscles. In some individuals, the mylohyoid nerve may supply accessory sensory innervation to the mandible in the premolar and molar areas.

Local Anesthesia Techniques

When choosing the appropriate injection to be administered, the dental hygienist needs to consider the area to be treated, the procedure to be performed, the extent of anesthesia necessary, and the client's needs and comfort. In oral healthcare, there are three major types of injections that are used to obtain local anesthesia:

1. Local infiltration
2. Field block
3. Nerve block

These types are differentiated by the site of anesthetic solution deposition relative to the area that will be receiving treatment.

Local Infiltration

A local infiltration injection involves placement of the anesthetic solution close to the smaller terminal endings of the nerve fibers in the immediate area to be treated (Figure 40-49). An example would be the injection of anesthetic solution into an interproximal papilla before therapeutic scaling and root planing.

Field Block

The field block method of obtaining anesthesia involves the deposition of solution near large terminal nerve branches (Figure 40-50). The resulting anesthesia is more circumscribed, most often involving one tooth and the tissues that surround that tooth. Treatment occurs away from the site of the injection. The deposition of anesthetic solution above the apex of a maxillary tooth, such as the maxillary right central incisor, is an example of a field block. In oral healthcare, a field block is often incorrectly referred to as a *local infiltration*.

Nerve Block

The nerve block involves the deposition of anesthetic solution close to a main nerve trunk, often at some distance from the treatment area (Figure 40-51). This injection type most often anesthetizes a larger area than that of a field block. Examples include a PSA nerve block and an inferior alveolar nerve block.

When dental hygiene care is to be performed in a small, isolated area, infiltration anesthesia may be the best choice, whereas a field block is the injection of choice when one or two teeth are to be treated. When the dental hygiene care plan involves a sextant or quadrant, nerve block anesthesia is recommended.

The term *anesthesia* is often preceded by either *local* or *regional*. Either phrase is correct; each indicates that a specific area is anesthetized and that the client is conscious; this differs from general anesthesia, with which the client is unconscious. The use of either term is therefore appropriate, and the terms can be used interchangeably, although *local anesthesia* appears to be more commonly used.

Procedures for a Successful Injection

The goal for each local anesthetic administration is, of course, to provide a safe and comfortable injection for the control and

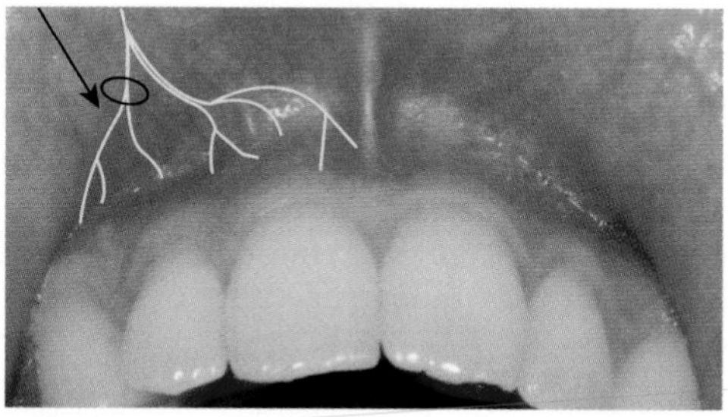

Figure 40-50. Field block. Local anesthetic is deposited near the larger terminal nerve endings *(arrow)*. An injection is made away from the site of injection. (From Malamed SF: *Handbook of local anesthesia*, ed 6, St Louis, 2013, Mosby.)

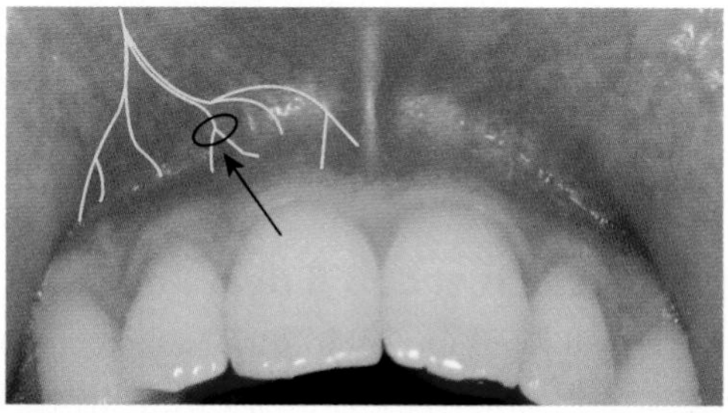

Figure 40-49. Local infiltration. The area of treatment is flooded with local anesthetic. An injection is made into the same area *(arrow)*. (From Malamed SF: *Handbook of local anesthesia*, ed 6, St Louis, 2013, Mosby.)

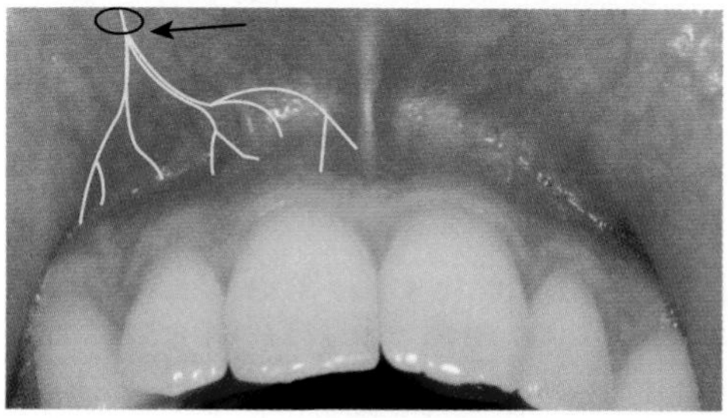

Figure 40-51. Nerve block. Local anesthetic is deposited close to the main nerve trunk and located at a distance from the site of injection. (From Malamed SF: *Handbook of local anesthesia*, ed 6, St Louis, 2013, Mosby.)

elimination of painful sensations during and after dental hygiene care. It is ironic, however, that a procedure meant to control pain for clients is often reported to be the most dreaded. Although the prospect of receiving an intraoral injection provokes fear and apprehension in many individuals, local anesthetic agent administration need not be painful. There are technical and communication components to an atraumatic injection.

Technical Aspects

Technical strategies include using a topical anesthetic before needle insertion, depositing a few drops of anesthetic solution, waiting 5 seconds before cautiously advancing the needle, and slowly depositing the anesthetic solution; these techniques help to minimize or eliminate client discomfort. In addition, it is essential to maintain complete control over the syringe at all times so that tissue penetration may be accomplished readily, accurately, and without the inadvertent nicking of tissues. Figure 40-52 presents hand positions to use when giving injections.

Figures 40-53 and 40-54 illustrate some hand rests and finger rests that can be used to stabilize syringes.

Figure 40-55 presents incorrect techniques that are to be avoided.

Communication Aspects

Communication aspects include keeping clients informed of the procedures in a calm manner and using nonthreatening language to minimize apprehension and to promote trust and cooperation. For example, telling clients that you're "applying the topical anesthetic to the tissue so that the remainder of the procedure is more comfortable" uses words with less-threatening (i.e., more positive) connotations to place a positive idea in the client's mind about the impending procedure. Saying "administer the local anesthetic" in place of "give an injection" or "give a shot" and using the word *discomfort* rather than the word *pain* are recommended. Avoid saying "This will not hurt," because clients often only hear the word *hurt* and ignore the rest of the statement.[2] Taking the extra time to communicate in a less-threatening manner produces less fear and results in a more comfortable procedure for the client, thus meeting the human needs for freedom from pain, fear, and stress.

Procedure 40-4 and the corresponding Competency Form present steps that can be used to ensure comfort, safety, and success that are common to all injections. Although each injection is unique with regard to anatomic considerations, these steps should be employed no matter what injection is being administered. Not every injection is successful and totally free of discomfort, because the clients' reactions and the hygienists' skills vary; however, if the steps in Procedure 40-4 are followed, the client and the dental hygienist will enjoy the benefit of the safest and least traumatic injection possible.

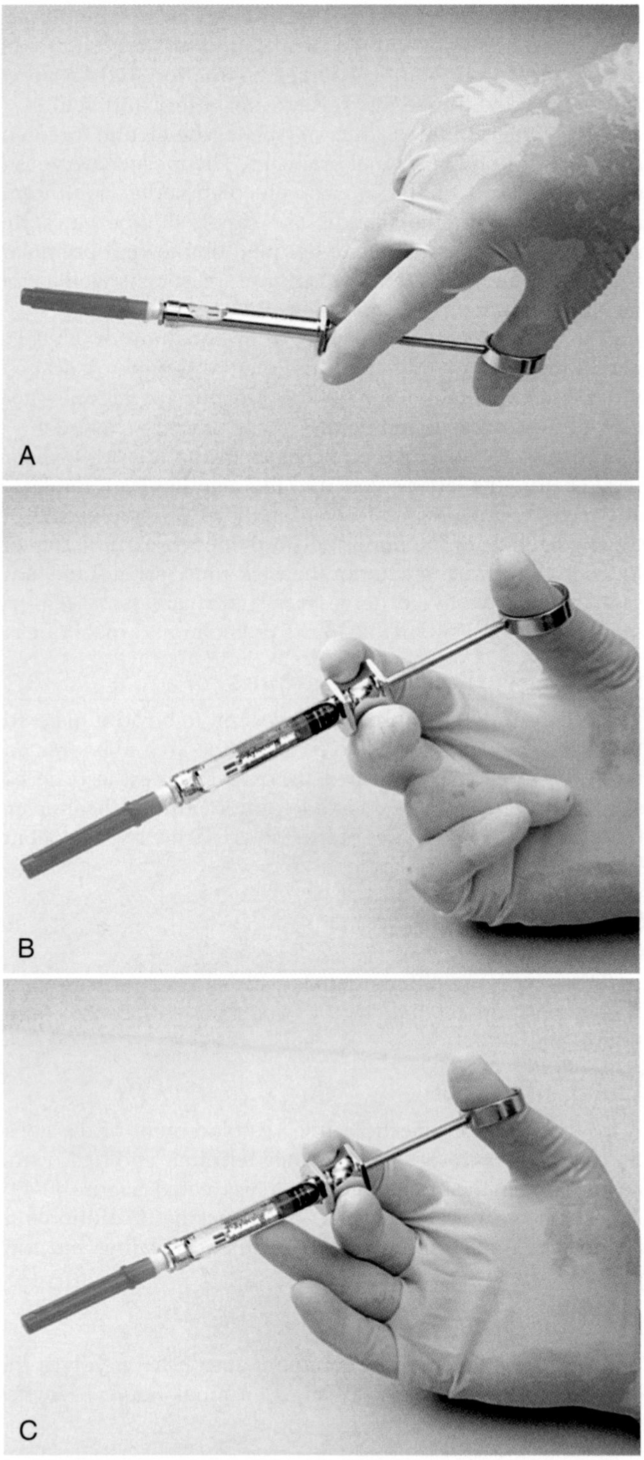

Figure 40-52. Hand positions for injections. **A,** Palm down: poor control over the syringe; not recommended. **B,** Palm up: better control over the syringe because it is supported by the wrist; recommended. **C,** Palm up and finger support: greatest stabilization; highly recommended. (From Malamed SF: *Handbook of local anesthesia*, ed 6, St Louis, 2013, Mosby.)

Injection Techniques for the Maxillary Teeth and Facial Hard and Soft Tissues

The injection techniques available to anesthetize the maxillary teeth and the facial hard and soft tissues include supraperiosteal injection, ASA nerve block, MSA nerve block, infraorbital nerve block, and PSA nerve block.

Supraperiosteal Injection (Local Infiltration)

A supraperiosteal injection (Table 40-9), which is more commonly referred to as a *local infiltration,* involves depositing anesthetic solution near the apex of a single tooth, thus providing anesthesia of the tooth and the immediate surrounding area (Figure 40-62). This injection is most often used to

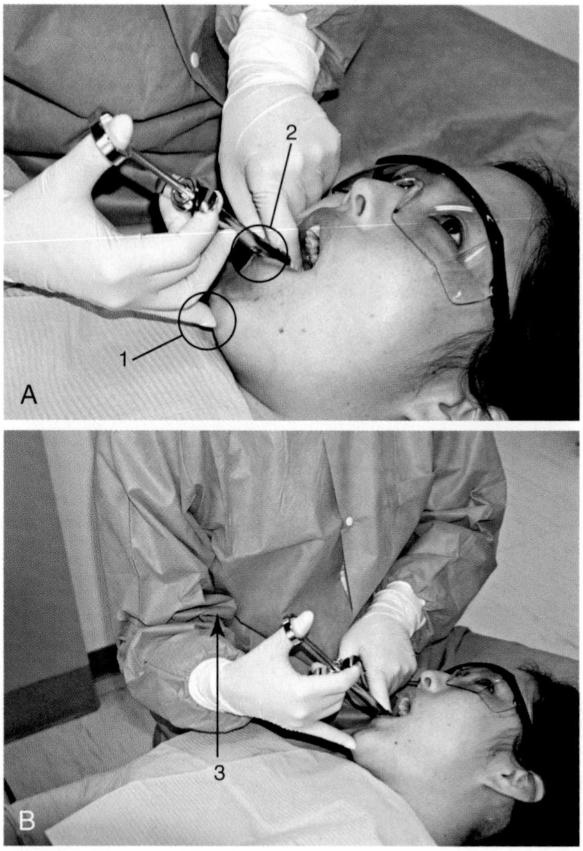

Figure 40-53. A, Use of the chin *(1)* as a finger rest, with the syringe barrel stabilized by the client's lip *(2)* during a right inferior alveolar nerve block. **B,** When necessary, stabilization may be increased by drawing the clinician's arm in against his or her chest *(3)*. (Courtesy F. O'Brien Photography.)

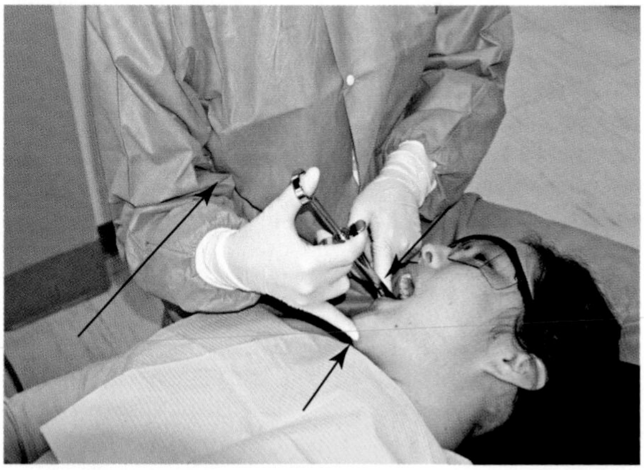

Figure 40-54. Syringe stabilization of a right posterior superior alveolar nerve block. The syringe barrel is placed on the client's lip, with one finger resting on the chin and one on the syringe barrel *(arrows)*. The upper arm is kept close to the clinician's chest to maximize stability. (Courtesy F. O'Brien Photography.)

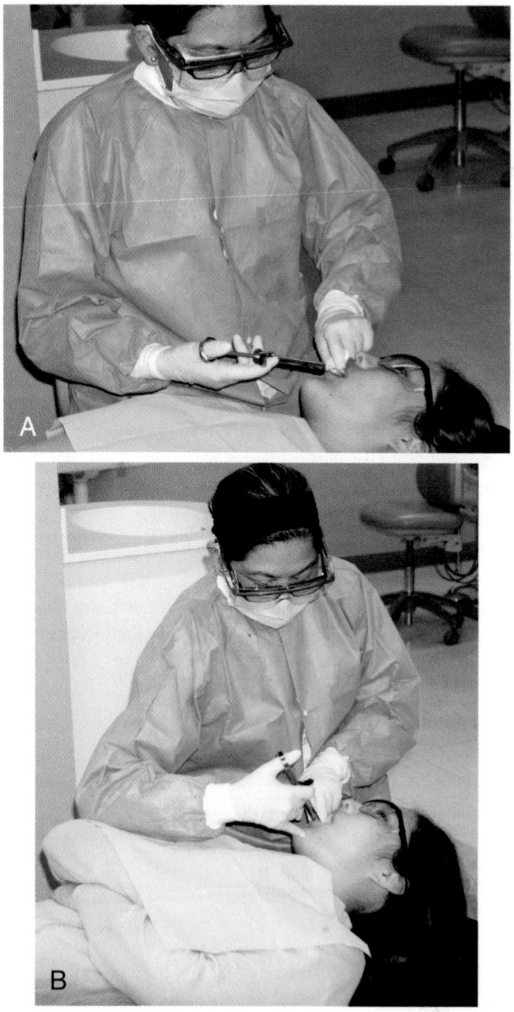

Figure 40-55. A, Incorrect position: no hand or finger rest for stabilization of the syringe. **B,** Incorrect: clinician resting the elbow on the client's arm. (Courtesy F. O'Brien Photography.)

anesthetize maxillary teeth. The rather thin, porous nature of the bone in the maxilla facilitates diffusion of the anesthetic solution from the deposition site to the apex of the tooth to be treated.

By contrast, the mandible consists of much denser bone, which prevents diffusion of the anesthetic agent to the apices of the posterior teeth, therefore precluding the supraperiosteal injection in this area. A supraperiosteal injection may be used to anesthetize the central and lateral teeth in the mandible, because the bone in this area is thinner and nutrient canals may be present. Figure 40-63 shows hand rests that may be used for a maxillary supraperiosteal injections and ASA and MSA nerve blocks.

Indications for this injection include the need for pulpal anesthesia of the maxillary teeth when only a limited number of teeth are to be treated and for soft-tissue procedures to be performed on a circumscribed area. Because the anesthetic and the vasoconstrictor are deposited so near the area to be treated, this injection provides effective hemostasis, which is often needed during dental hygiene care. Conversely, if there is infection or severe inflammation in the area, the administration of the anesthetic solution at a distance from the area of inflammation (i.e., nerve block) provides better and safer pain control as a result of the presence of more normal tissue conditions at the deposition site. Furthermore, if a large area involving several teeth needs to be treated, the supraperiosteal injection is not suitable because of the need for multiple

Procedure 40-4 Basic Techniques for a Successful Injection

EQUIPMENT

See Procedure 40-2.

STEPS

1. Assess the individual's health history, and obtain his or her vital signs (include blood pressure, heart rate, and respiratory rate at a minimum).
2. Confirm the care plan.
3. Check the armamentarium.
4. Load the syringe, and determine the syringe window and needle bevel orientation. The window of the cartridge should face the clinician, and the bevel of the needle should face the bone.
5. Check that the needle is sharp and that it has no fishhook-type barbs on the tip by placing the needle against a sterile 2 × 2 gauze square. If the gauze is snagged, which indicates that a barb is present, discard the needle.
6. Expel a few drops of the anesthetic solution to determine if a free flow of solution exists.
7. Position the client in a supine position (i.e., with the head and heart parallel to the floor) with his or her feet elevated slightly (Figure 40-56).

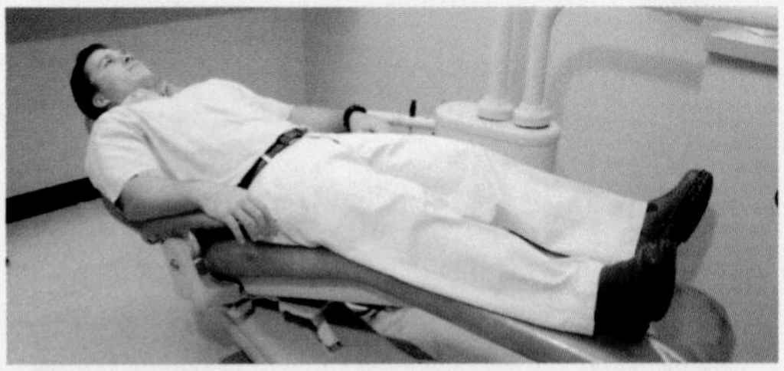

Figure 40-56. Physiologic position of patient for receipt of local anesthetic injection. (From Malamed SF: *Handbook of local anesthesia,* ed 6, St Louis, 2013, Mosby.)

8. Communicate with the client to place positive ideas in the client's mind about the injection. Tell the client about the reasons for the use of the topical anesthetic (e.g., "I am applying a topical anesthetic to the tissue so that the remainder of the procedure will be much more comfortable.") Do not use words with a negative connotation, such as *injection, shot, pain,* or *hurt.* Instead, use less-threatening terms, such as *administer the local anesthetic.*
9. Visualize or palpate to locate the penetration site.
10. Dry the needle penetration site with gauze (Figure 40-57).

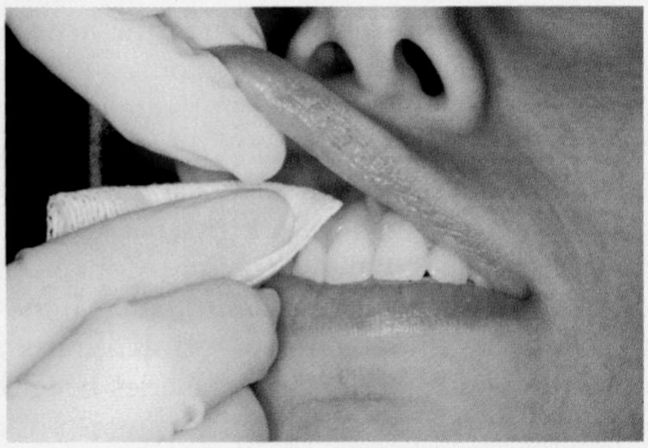

Figure 40-57. Sterilized gauze is used to gently wipe the tissue at the site of the needle. (From Malamed SF: *Handbook of local anesthesia,* ed 6, St Louis, 2013, Mosby.)

11. Apply topical anesthetic to the needle penetration site for 1 to 2 minutes (Figure 40-58).

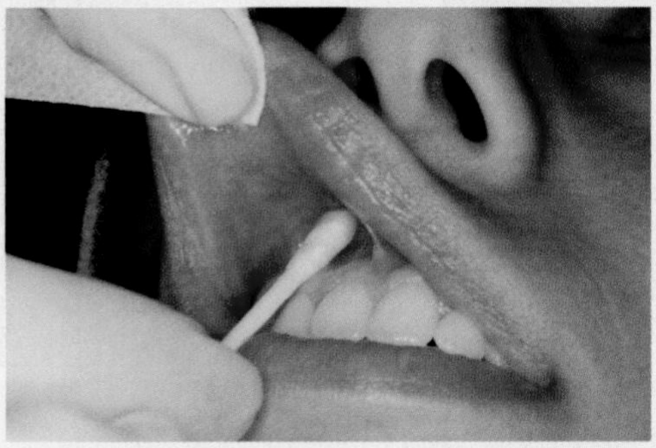

Figure 40-58. A small quantity of topical anesthetic is placed at the site of needle penetration and kept in place for at least 1 minute. (From Malamed SF: *Handbook of local anesthesia,* ed 6, St Louis, 2013, Mosby.)

12. In the case of palatal injections, when placing topical anesthetic on the injection site, apply considerable pressure with the cotton swab for a minimum of 1 minute before the injection. Move the swab immediately adjacent to the penetration site, and maintain pressure at this site during the injection (see Figures 40-82 and 40-83).
13. After the topical anesthetic swab is removed from the tissue, dry the penetration site.
14. Pick up the prepared local anesthetic syringe, and establish a firm hand rest. Never place the arm holding the syringe directly on the client's arm or shoulder.
15. Make the tissue taut at the penetration site by retracting it (except on the palate) using sterile gauze; this helps with both visibility and atraumatic needle insertion (Figure 40-59).
16. Keep the syringe and the needle out of the client's line of vision.
17. Gently insert the needle into the mucosa until the bevel is completely under the tissue (see Figure 40-59).

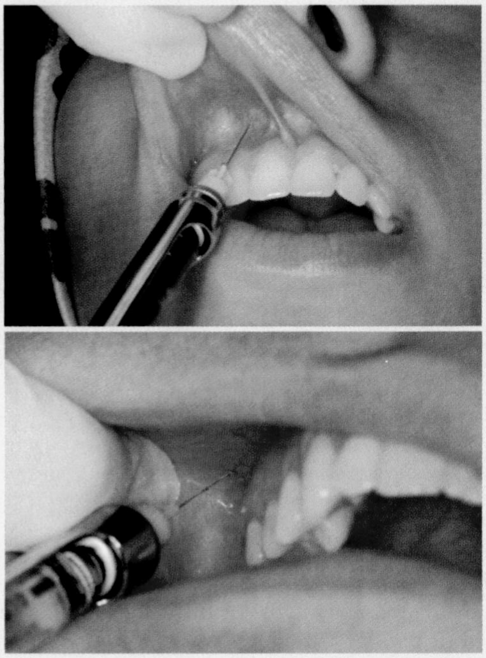

Figure 40-59. Tissue at the needle penetration site is pulled taut to promote both visibility and atraumatic needle insertion. (From Malamed SF: *Handbook of local anesthesia,* ed 6, St Louis, 2013, Mosby.)

Procedure 40-4 Basic Techniques for a Successful Injection—cont'd

18. Observe and communicate with the client. Watch for any signs of discomfort or distress.
19. Deposit a few drops of anesthetic solution, pause for 5 seconds, and then advance the needle a few millimeters. Repeat the process as you slowly advance to the deposition site. Communicate with the client by saying, "To make you more comfortable, I will deposit a little anesthetic as I advance toward the target."
20. Aspirate on arrival at the deposition site by pulling the thumb ring back gently. Movement of only 1 or 2 mm is needed. The tip of the needle must remain unmoved.
21. Rotate the barrel of the syringe about 45 degrees, and aspirate a second time to ensure that the needle is not located inside a blood vessel and abutting against the wall of the vessel, thereby providing a false-negative aspiration (Figures 40-60 and 40-61, *B*).

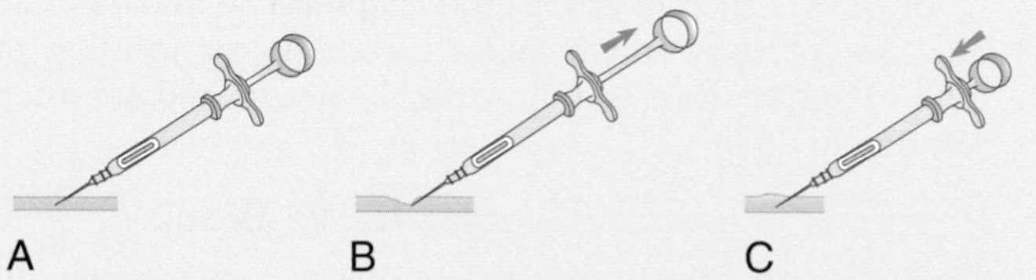

Figure 40-60. Intravascular injection of local anesthetic. **A,** The needle is inserted into the lumen of a blood vessel. **B,** An aspiration test is performed. Negative pressure pulls the vessel wall against the bevel of needle, so no blood enters the syringe (i.e., negative aspiration). **C,** Drug is injected. Positive pressure on the plunger of the syringe forces local anesthetic solution out through the needle. The wall of the vessel is forced away from the bevel, and anesthetic solution is deposited directly into the lumen of the blood vessel. (From Malamed SF: *Handbook of local anesthesia,* ed 6, St Louis, 2013, Mosby.)

22. If no blood appears (i.e., negative aspiration), slowly deposit the local anesthetic solution at a rate of 1 mL/min for approximately 2 minutes for a full cartridge.
23. Observe and communicate with the client. Watch for any signs of discomfort or distress. Reassure the client with statements such as, "I am depositing the solution slowly so this procedure will be comfortable for you."
24. Slowly withdraw the needle when the indicated amount of anesthetic has been deposited.
25. Replace the needle sheath using the scoop technique (see Figure 40-37).
26. Observe the client.
27. Rinse the client's mouth.
28. Massage the tissue over the injection site when indicated.
29. Test for anesthesia by first touching the rounded back of an explorer to an area that is not anesthetized and then secondly to the area that is anesthetized. The client should have little or no sensation in the anesthetized area.
30. Reassure the client that numbness, tingling, and a sense of swelling or of the tooth feeling different are normal responses.
31. Record the injection(s) in the client's chart, and include the following information:
    a. The area anesthetized and the specific injection(s) given
    b. The type of anesthetic used and the type of vasoconstrictor used and its concentration (ratio)
    c. The type(s) of needle(s) used
    d. The total amount of solution administered in milliliters and/or total cartridges
    e. The client's reaction

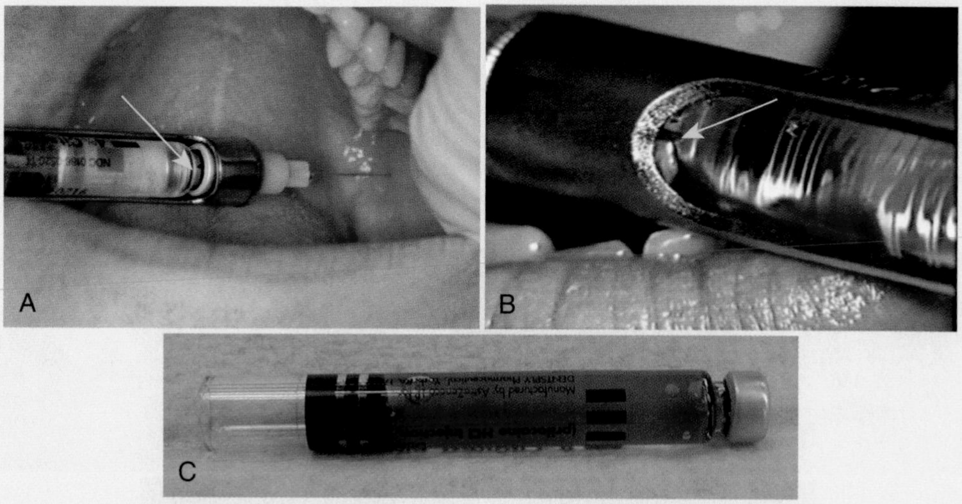

Figure 40-61. A, Negative aspiration. With the needle in position at the injection site, the administrator pulls the thumb ring of the harpoon aspirator syringe 1 or 2 mm. The needle tip should not move. Check the cartridge at the site where the needle penetrates the diaphragm *(arrow)* for bubbling or blood. **B,** Positive aspiration. A slight reddish discoloration at the diaphragm end of the cartridge *(arrow)* on the aspiration usually indicates venous penetration. Reposition the needle and reaspirate; if negative, deposit the solution. **C,** Positive aspiration. Bright red blood rapidly filling the cartridge usually indicates arterial penetration. Remove the syringe from the mouth, change the cartridge, and repeat the procedure. (From Malamed SF: *Handbook of local anesthesia,* ed 6, St Louis, 2013, Mosby.)

needle insertions and the necessity of administering large volumes of anesthetic solution.

Table 40-9 summarizes the criteria that are pertinent to a supraperiosteal injection and provides tips for success.

Anterior Superior Alveolar Field Block

The ASA nerve block is recommended for pain management when treatment is to be done only on the maxillary anterior teeth. Table 40-10 describes the criteria specific to the ASA nerve block.

Middle Superior Alveolar Field Block

The MSA nerve block is the injection of choice when treatment involves only the premolars or if the infraorbital nerve block fails to provide pain control distal to the maxillary canine (Table 40-11).

Research indicates that the MSA nerve is present in only 28% to 40% of the population; for those without the MSA nerve, the area is most often innervated by the ASA nerve.[1] Regardless of the MSA nerve's presence or absence, this area can be anesthetized easily by means of the MSA technique described in Table 40-11, which provides guidelines for administering an MSA nerve block and suggestions to ensure success.

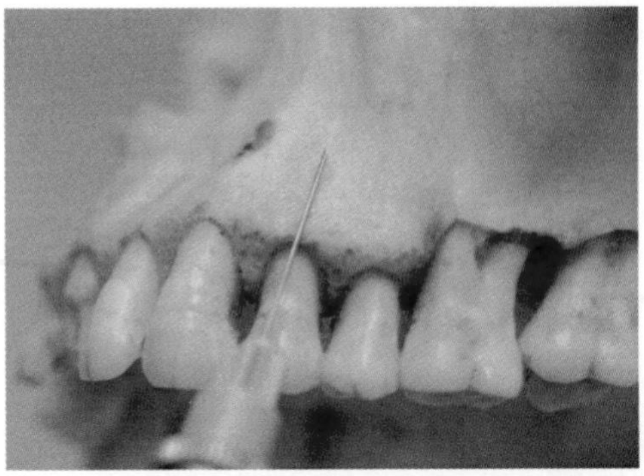

Figure 40-62. The syringe should be held parallel with the long axis of the tooth and inserted at the height of the mucobuccal fold over the tooth. (From Malamed SF: *Handbook of local anesthesia,* ed 6, St Louis, 2013, Mosby.)

Infraorbital Nerve Block

Whereas the ASA (see Table 40-10) and MSA (see Table 40-11) nerve blocks can be employed by oral healthcare professionals when they are anesthetizing the maxillary anterior and premolar teeth, the infraorbital nerve block is the injection of choice for many authorities when pain control is provided to this area.[1] The infraorbital nerve block provides both pulpal and facial soft-tissue anesthesia of the maxillary central incisor through the premolars in approximately 60% of individuals.[1] One injection of 0.9 to 1.2 mL of solution provides pain control in a relatively large area, effectively minimizing needle penetrations and the volume of solution administered. Despite these advantages, this injection is not used as often as indicated, because many operators are fearful of injuring the client's eye. However, this fear is unfounded. When the appropriate procedures are followed, this injection is highly effective and safe (Figures 40-72, 40-73, and 40-74).

Table 40-12 describes the criteria applicable to the infraorbital nerve block and includes directions for locating the infraorbital foramen and directing the needle and anesthetic solution to the nerve.

Posterior Superior Alveolar Nerve Block

The PSA nerve block, which is employed to anesthetize the maxillary molars, is preferred to supraperiosteal (infiltration) injections because it minimizes both the number of injections required and the volume of anesthetic solution administered. In addition, because the anesthetic solution is deposited into an area of soft tissue with no bony landmarks (and hence no bone contact), it is a comfortable injection for the client (Figures 40-77 and 40-78).

Complete pulpal anesthesia is obtained in the first, second, and third molars in at least 77% of individuals.[1] However, dissection studies reveal that, when the MSA nerve is present, it may supply sensory innervation to the mesiobuccal root of the first molar, thereby necessitating either a supraperiosteal injection, an MSA nerve block, or an infraorbital nerve block to anesthetize the remainder of this tooth. If access is difficult or if the third molar is missing and treatment is limited to only the first and second molars, supraperiosteal injections may be substituted.

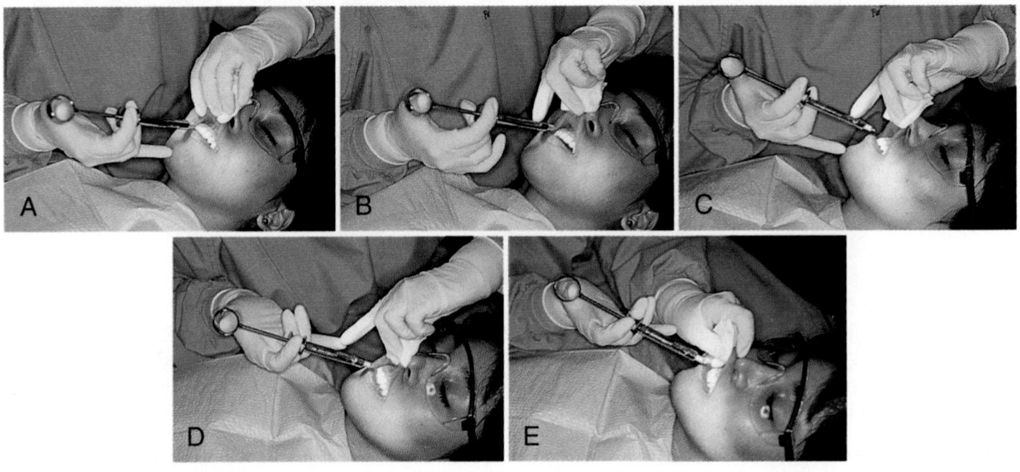

Figure 40-63. A through **E,** Syringe orientation, hand rests, and finger rests that may be used for a maxillary supraperiosteal injection and for anterior superior alveolar and middle superior alveolar nerve blocks. (From Malamed SF: *Handbook of local anesthesia,* ed 5, St Louis, 2004, Mosby.)

TABLE 40-9

Supraperiosteal Injection (Local Infiltration)

Nerves anesthetized	Large terminal branches of dental plexus
Areas anesthetized	Entire region innervated by the large terminal branches of the plexus: Pulp of the tooth Facial periosteum Connective tissue Mucous membranes overlying the tooth (Figure 40-64)
Needle gauge and length	25- or 27-gauge short
Operator position	8 or 9 o'clock
Penetration site	Height of the mucobuccal fold above the apex of the target tooth (Figure 40-65)
Landmarks	Mucobuccal fold Crown of tooth Root contour of tooth
Syringe orientation	Parallel to the long axis of the tooth (see Figure 40-62)
Hand rests	Client's chin Forefinger or wrist of operator's opposite hand (see Figure 40-55)
Deposition site	Apical region of the target tooth
Penetration depth	Usually only a few millimeters; no more than 5 mm or one quarter of a short needle
Amount of anesthetic to be deposited	0.6 mL or one third of a cartridge
Length of time to deposit	Approximately 30-60 seconds

Potential Problems	***Technique Tips***
Anesthetic deposition below apex of target tooth, resulting in insufficient pulpal anesthesia	Increase depth of penetration so that the needle is at the apical region of the target tooth.
Needle too far from bone, so solution deposited into buccal tissue	Redirect needle closer to the periosteum.
Dense bone may cover apices; most often occurs on permanent maxillary first molars in children, because the apex is located under the dense zygomatic bone; may occur on central incisors where the apex lies beneath the nose	Administer a nerve block.
Pain on insertion with the needle against the periosteum	Withdraw the needle and reinsert it farther away laterally from the periosteum.

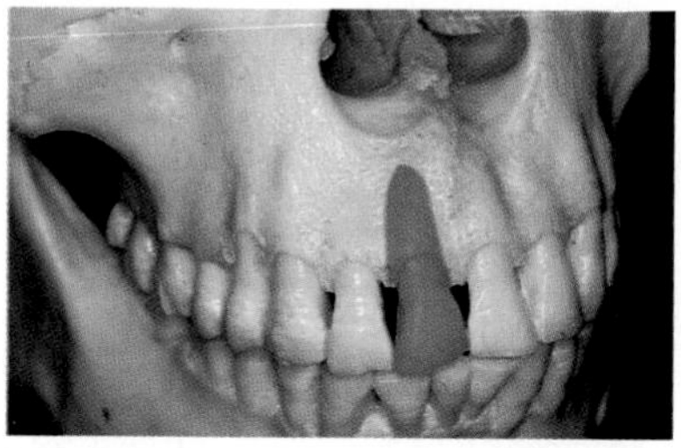

Figure 40-64. Areas anesthetized with a local infiltration of a maxillary central incisor. The deposition site is at the apical region of the target tooth.

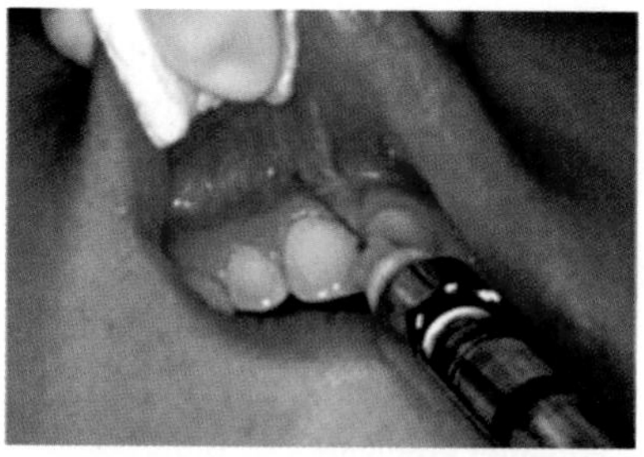

Figure 40-65. Penetration site for a supraperiosteal injection of the maxillary right central incisor.

Other considerations involve safety and needle length. A long 25-gauge needle is often recommended for this injection. Problems associated with needle length, however, may result in an increased risk of hematoma formation. There are no anatomic safety features to prevent inadvertently inserting the needle too far posteriorly into the pterygoid plexus of veins and the facial artery, thereby causing a hematoma. To minimize the risk of hematoma formation after the PSA nerve block, a short 25- or 27-gauge needle is recommended. Although the depth of insertion with the long needle is 16 mm or one half of its length, the short needle is inserted three fourths of its length. Thus, the risk of overinsertion and hematoma formation decreases when a short needle is used. Regardless of the needle length used, multiple aspirations

TABLE 40-10

Anterior Superior Alveolar Field Block

Nerves anesthetized	Anterior superior alveolar
Areas anesthetized	Pulpal tissue of the following maxillary teeth unilaterally: Central incisor Lateral incisor Canine Facial periodontal tissues and bones of these same teeth (see Figure 40-66)
Needle gauge and length	25- or 27-gauge short
Operator position	8 or 9 o'clock
Penetration site	Height of the mucobuccal fold just mesial to the canine (Figure 40-67)
Landmarks	Mucobuccal fold Canine and canine eminence
Syringe orientation	Parallel to the long axis of the canine (Figure 40-68)
Hand rests	Client's chin Forefinger or wrist of operator's opposite hand (see Figure 40-63)
Deposition site	Apical region of the canine
Penetration depth	Usually only a few millimeters; no more than 5 mm or one quarter of a short needle
Amount of anesthetic to be deposited	0.6-0.9 mL or one third to one half of a cartridge
Length of time to deposit	Approximately 30-60 seconds

Potential Problems	**Technique Tips**
Anesthetic deposition below apex of target tooth, resulting in insufficient pulpal anesthesia	Increase the depth of the penetration so that the needle is at the apical region of the canine.
Needle too far from bone, so solution deposited into buccal tissue	Redirect the needle closer to the periosteum.
Pain on insertion with the needle against the periosteum	Withdraw the needle and reinsert it farther away laterally from the periosteum.
Persistent sensitivity at mesial surface of central incisor as a result of cross-innervation	Infiltrate contralateral to the central incisor.

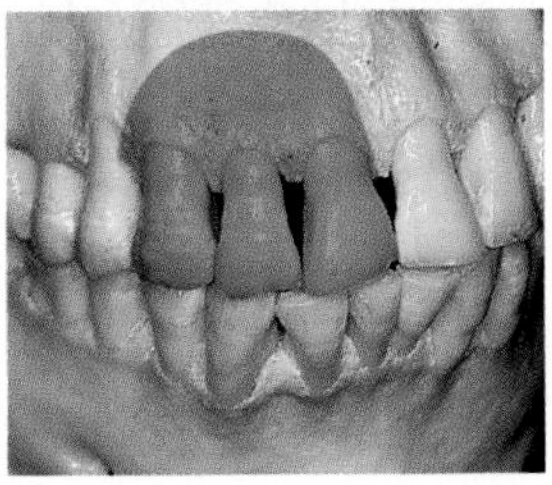

Figure 40-66. Areas anesthetized with the anterior superior nerve block.

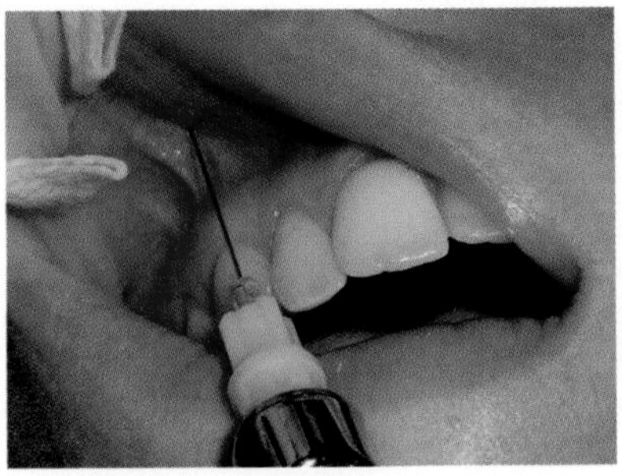

Figure 40-67. Penetration site for the anterior superior nerve block.

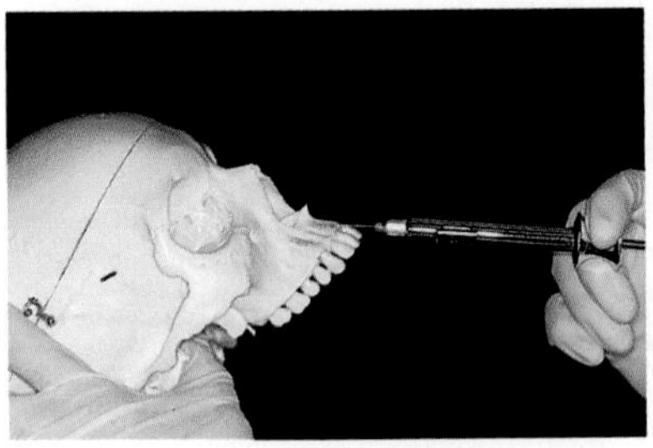

Figure 40-68. Syringe orientation for the anterior superior nerve block.

TABLE 40-11

Middle Superior Alveolar Nerve Block

Nerves anesthetized	Middle superior alveolar
Areas anesthetized	Pulpal tissue of the following maxillary teeth unilaterally: First premolar Second premolar Mesial root of first molar Buccal periodontal tissues and bones of these same teeth (Figure 40-69)

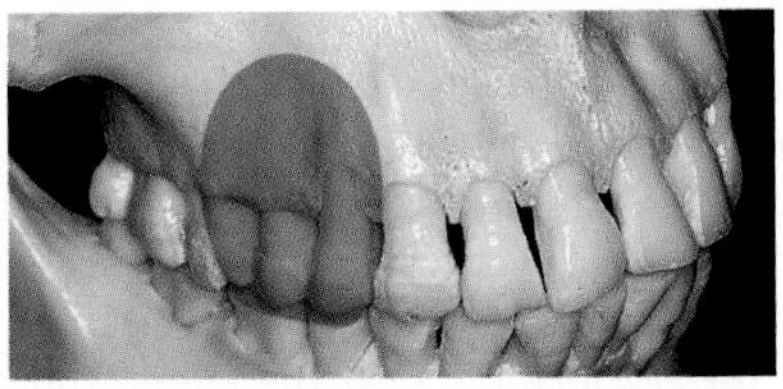

Figure 40-69. Area anesthetized by a middle superior alveolar nerve block.

TABLE 40-11
Middle Superior Alveolar Nerve Block—cont'd

Needle gauge and length	25- or 27-gauge short
Operator position	8 or 9 o'clock
Penetration site	Height of the mucobuccal fold above the second premolar (Figure 40-70) 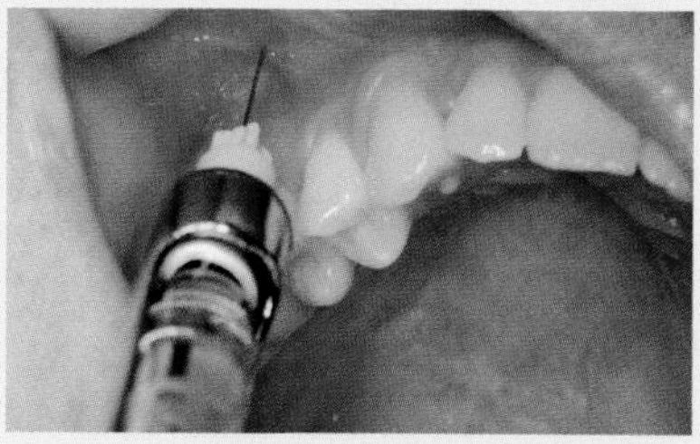 **Figure 40-70.** Needle penetration for a middle superior alveolar nerve block. (From Malamed SF: *Handbook of local anesthesia,* ed 6, St Louis, 2013, Mosby.)
Landmarks	Mucobuccal fold Second premolar
Syringe orientation	Parallel to the long axis of the second premolar, closer to vertical than in the anterior maxilla (Figure 40-71) 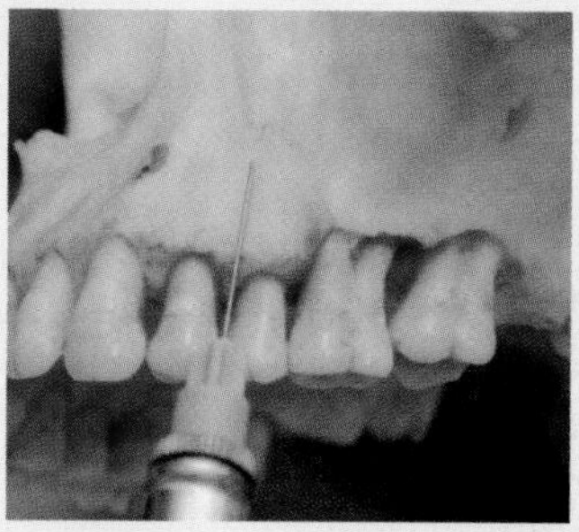 **Figure 40-71.** Position of the needle between the maxillary premolars for a middle superior alveolar nerve block. (From Malamed SF: *Handbook of local anesthesia,* ed 6, St Louis, 2013, Mosby.)
Hand rests	Client's chin Client's cheek Forefinger or wrist of operator's opposite hand (see Figure 40-63)
Deposition site	Above the apical region of the second premolar
Penetration depth	Usually only a few millimeters; no more than 5 mm or one quarter of a short needle
Amount of anesthetic to be deposited	0.9-1.2 mL or one half to two thirds of a cartridge
Length of time to deposit	Approximately 60-90 seconds
Potential Problems	**Technique Tips**
Anesthetic deposition below the apex of target tooth, resulting in insufficient pulpal anesthesia	Increase the depth of penetration so that the needle is at the apical region of the second premolar.
Needle too far from bone, so solution deposited into buccal tissue	Redirect the needle closer to the periosteum.
Pain on insertion with the needle against the periosteum	Withdraw the needle and reinsert it farther away laterally from the periosteum.
Dense bone of the zygomatic arch at the injection site prevents diffusion of anesthetic solution	Administer an infraorbital block instead of the middle superior alveolar block.
Buccal frenum present at preferred penetration site	Penetrate slightly mesial to the frenum.

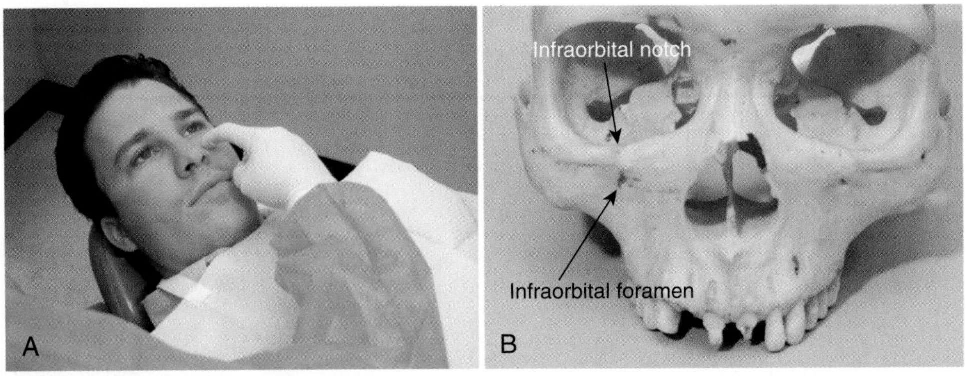

Figure 40-72. **A,** Palpation of the infraorbital notch. **B,** Location of the infraorbital foramen in relation to the infraorbital notch. (From Malamed SF: *Handbook of local anesthesia,* ed 6, St Louis, 2013, Mosby.)

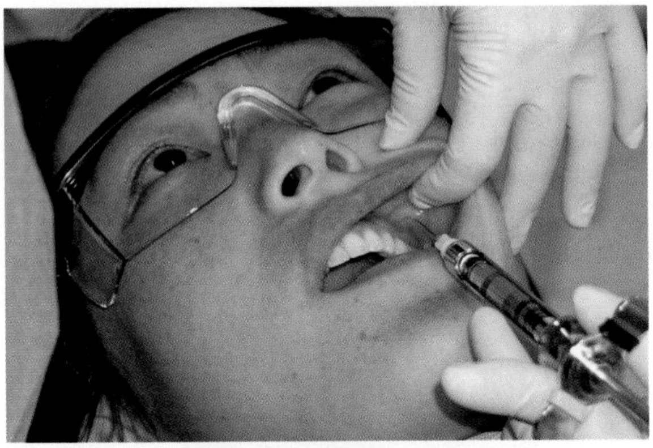

Figure 40-73. With a finger placed over the foramen, lift the lip, and hold the tissues in the mucobuccal fold taut. (Courtesy F. O'Brien Photography.)

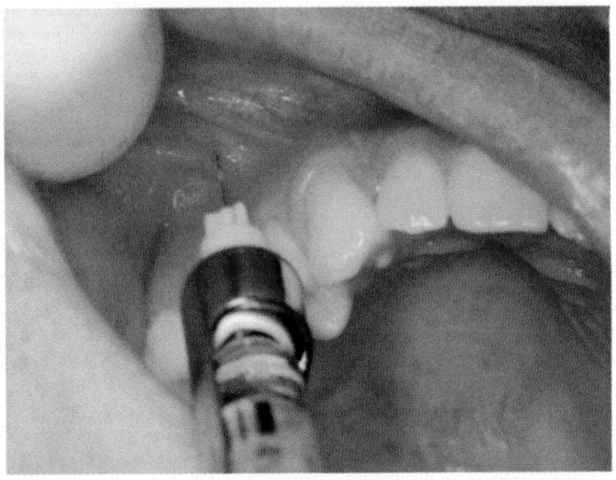

Figure 40-74. Insert the needle for an infraorbital nerve block in the mucobuccal fold over the maxillary first premolar. (From Malamed SF: *Handbook of local anesthesia,* ed 6, St Louis, 2013, Mosby.)

and slow anesthetic deposition are imperative to ensure a safe injection.

Table 40-13 provides the essential criteria for a PSA nerve block. Of particular significance to this injection is the syringe orientation of 45 degrees to the maxillary occlusal plane and 45 degrees to the midsagittal plane. This angulation, which is maintained throughout the injection, advances the needle around the maxillary tuberosity to reach the deposition site.

Injection Techniques for the Palatal Hard and Soft Tissues

When dental hygiene care involves the hard and soft tissues of the palate (e.g., during therapeutic scaling, root planing, and soft-tissue curettage procedures), anesthesia of the palatal tissue may be needed. Unfortunately, for many clients, these injections are traumatic, but palatal injections need not be painful if appropriate techniques are followed. The following tasks are especially important for facilitating comfort during palatal injections:

- Provide pressure anesthesia with a cotton swab at the penetration site both before (Figure 40-81) and during (Figure 40-82) the injection, because topical anesthetics have limited value on keratinized tissues such as the palate.
- Deposit the solution slowly to avoid tearing the palatal tissue, which is dense and firmly attached to the bone.
- Be confident that you, the dental hygienist, will administer the injection with minimal client discomfort.
- Use a triple injection technique whenever possible when administering the nasopalatine nerve block to minimize client discomfort (see Nasopalatine Nerve Block and Figure 40-86).

The injection techniques that are used to anesthetize the palatal hard and soft tissues are the greater palatine nerve block and the nasopalatine nerve block.

Greater Palatine Nerve Block

The greater palatine nerve block is used to anesthetize the hard and soft palatal tissues overlying the molars and premolars; no pulpal anesthesia is obtained (see Figure 40-81). This nerve block provides anesthesia to a large area, thereby minimizing the number of needle penetrations and the total amount of anesthetic solution needed; however, the greater palatine nerve can be blocked at any point after it emerges from the foramen and passes anteriorly between the hard and soft tissues. As a result, anesthesia is obtained only anterior to the injection site. For example, if treatment is limited to the first molar and the premolars, the injection site should be slightly posterior to the first molar along the greater palatine nerve path. This practice ensures that the areas to be treated are anesthetized but that the posterior region of the palate is not unnecessarily anesthetized.

TABLE 40-12
Infraorbital Nerve Block

Nerves anesthetized	Infraorbital Anterior superior alveolar Middle superior alveolar Inferior palpebral Lateral nasal Superior labial
Areas anesthetized	Pulpal tissue of the following maxillary teeth unilaterally: Central incisor Lateral incisor Canine First premolar Second premolar Mesial root of first molar Buccal periodontal tissues and bone of these same teeth Lower eyelid Lateral aspect of the nose Upper lip (Figure 40-75)
Needle gauge and length	25- or 27-gauge short; in rare instances, a long needle may be preferred
Operator position	8 or 9 o'clock (see Figure 40-73)
Penetration site	Height of the mucobuccal fold above the first premolar (see Figure 40-74)
Landmarks	Infraorbital notch Infraorbital ridge Infraorbital foramen Mucobuccal fold First premolar (see Figure 40-72, *B*)
Syringe orientation	Parallel to the long axis of the first premolar; follow the angle (see Figures 40-73 and 40-74)
Hand rests	Client's chin Client's cheek Forefinger or wrist of operator's opposite hand (see Figure 40-63)
Deposition site	Upper rim of the infraorbital foramen; the needle should gently contact bone before deposition (Figure 40-76)
Penetration depth	16 mm or three quarters of a short needle
Amount of anesthetic to be deposited	0.9-1.2 mL or one half to two thirds of a cartridge
Length of time to deposit	Approximately 60-90 seconds

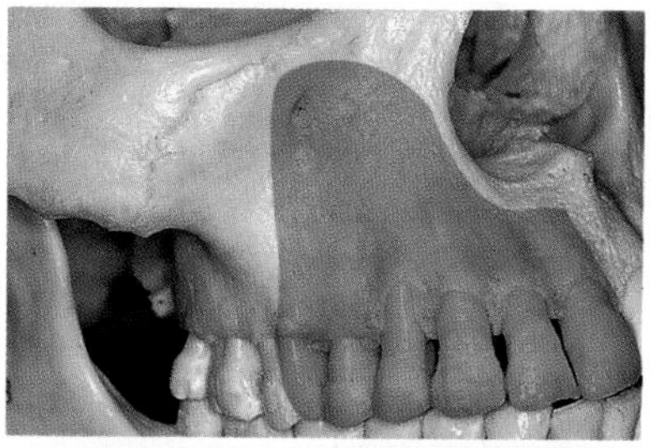

Figure 40-75. Area anesthetized by an infraorbital nerve block in approximately 60% of individuals.

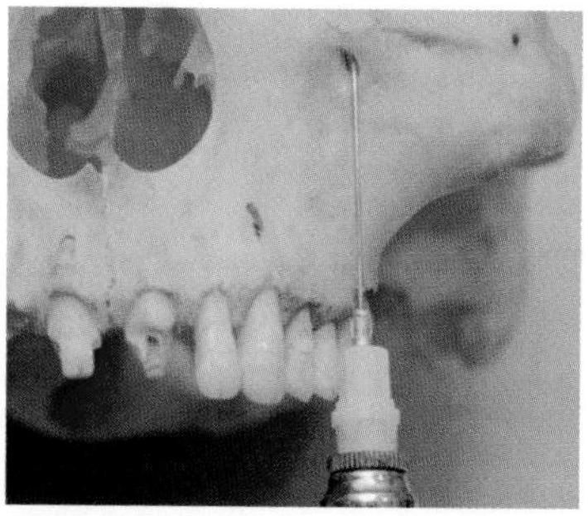

Figure 40-76. Position of the needle tip before the deposition of local anesthetic at the infraorbital foramen. (From Malamed SF: *Handbook of local anesthesia,* ed 6, St Louis, 2013, Mosby.)

Technique Notes

1. Locate the infraorbital foramen: With your forefinger, palpate across the zygomatic arch. The foramen lies at the area of concavity directly below the medial border of the client's iris when the client gazes straight ahead.
2. Maintain finger pressure over the foramen throughout the injection and for 1 to 2 minutes after deposition. This will aid in directing the needle to the foramen and assist with directing the anesthetic solution to the foramen.

Potential Problems

Needle contacting bone below the infraorbital foramen; anesthesia of the lower eyelid, the nose, or the upper lip with little or no pulpal anesthesia

Technique Tips

Keep the needle in line with the infraorbital foramen during penetration; line the syringe up with your finger over the foramen.

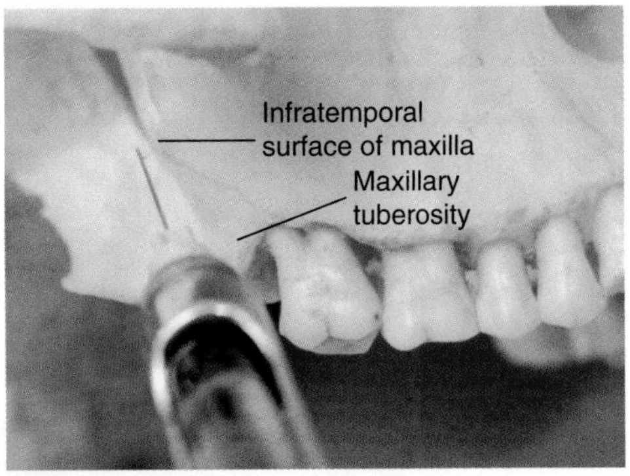

Figure 40-77. Needle at the target area for a posterior superior alveolar nerve block. (From Malamed SF: *Handbook of local anesthesia,* ed 6, St Louis, 2013, Mosby.)

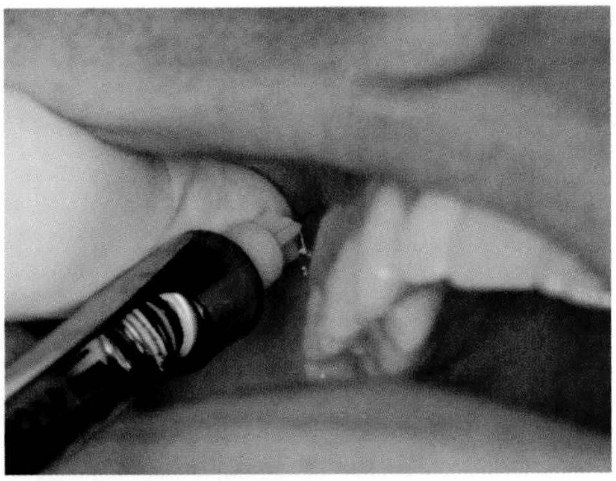

Figure 40-78. Posterior superior alveolar nerve block using a "short" dental needle approximately 20 mm in length. (From Malamed SF: *Handbook of local anesthesia,* ed 6, St Louis, 2013, Mosby.)

TABLE 40-13
Posterior Superior Alveolar Nerve Block

Nerves anesthetized	Posterior superior alveolar
Areas anesthetized	(Figure 40-79)
Needle gauge and length	25- or 27-gauge short; in rare instances, a long needle may be preferred
Operator position	8 or 9 o'clock
Penetration site	Height of the mucobuccal fold posterior and superior to the second molar (see Figure 40-78)
Landmarks	Mucobuccal fold Maxillary tuberosity Maxillary occlusal plane Midsagittal plane Maxillary molars
Syringe orientation	45 degrees to the maxillary occlusal plane and 45 degrees to the midsagittal plane (Figure 40-80)
Hand rests	Forefinger or thumb of opposite hand as it retracts client's buccal tissue
Deposition site	Posterior and superior to the posterior border of the maxilla at the posterior superior alveolar nerve foramina (see Figure 40-77)

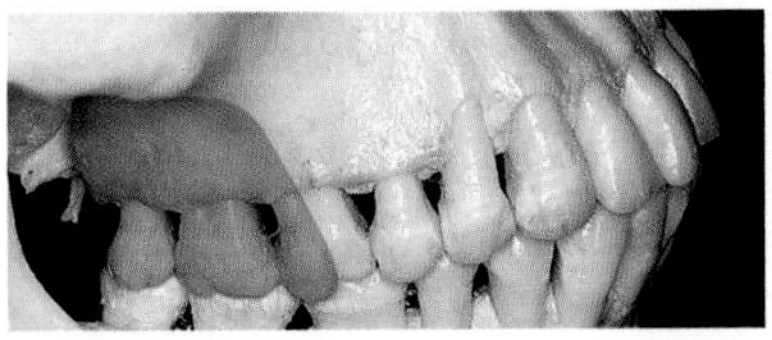

Figure 40-79. Area anesthetized by the posterior superior alveolar nerve block.

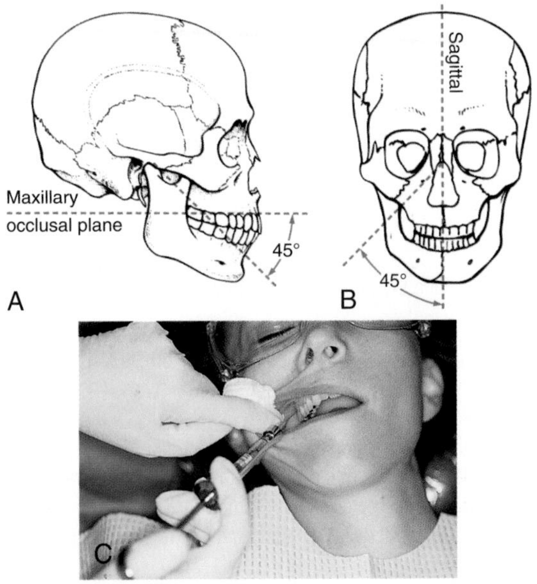

Figure 40-80. **A,** Forty-five degrees to the maxillary occlusal plane. **B,** Forty-five degrees to the midsagittal plane. **C,** Orientation of the syringe during the posterior superior alveolar nerve block.

TABLE 40-13

Posterior Superior Alveolar Nerve Block—cont'd

Penetration depth	16 mm or three quarters of a short needle
Amount of anesthetic to be deposited	0.9-1.8 mL or one half to one cartridge
Length of time to deposit	Approximately 60-120 seconds

Technique Notes

Owing to the high vascularity of the deposition site for the posterior superior alveolar nerve block, a triple aspiration is recommended to ensure that the needle bevel is not against the interior wall of a vessel, which would provide a false-negative aspiration (see Figure 40-60). To aspirate in multiple planes, perform a single aspiration as usual, then rotate the body of the syringe toward you slightly, reaspirate, rotate the body of the syringe back to the original position, and perform a final aspiration. If all three aspiration tests are negative, it is safe to administer the anesthetic solution.

Potential Problems	*Technique Tips*
Bone is contacted when the angle of the needle is too great in reference to the midsagittal plane	Withdraw the needle and bring the syringe closer to the midline.
Mandibular anesthesia: the mandibular division of the trigeminal nerve is lateral to the posterior superior alveolar nerves	Review the landmarks and the syringe orientation so that you do not deposit lateral to the posterior superior alveolar nerves.

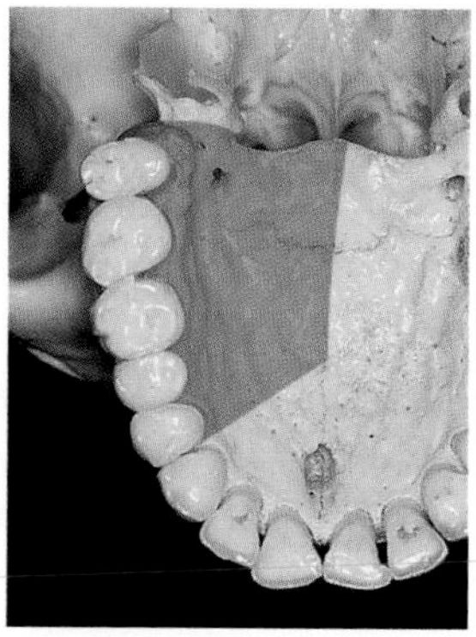

Figure 40-81. Area anesthetized with the greater palatine nerve block.

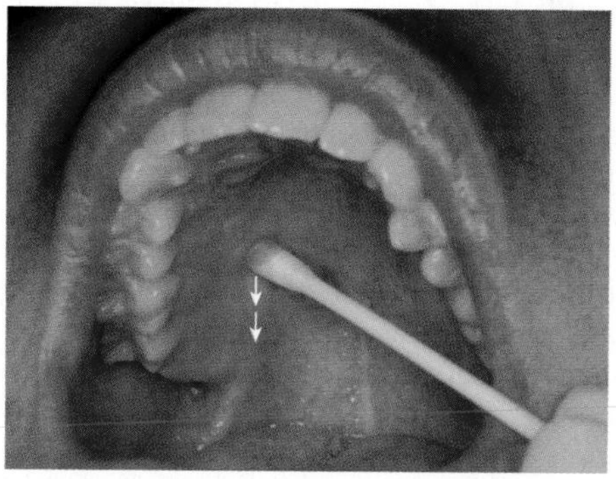

Figure 40-82. A cotton swab is pressed against the hard palate at the junction of the maxillary alveolar process and the palatal bone. The swab is slowly moved distally *(arrows)* until a depression in the tissue is felt; this is the greater (anterior) palatine foramen. Apply pressure for a minimum of 30 seconds. (From Malamed SF: *Handbook of local anesthesia,* ed 6, St Louis, 2013, Mosby.)

Table 40-14 provides the criteria that are pertinent for the administration of a greater palatine nerve block and includes suggestions for locating the greater palatine foramen and maximizing client comfort.

Nasopalatine Nerve Block

The nasopalatine nerve block anesthetizes the palatal hard and soft tissues from the mesial aspect of the right premolar to the mesial aspect of the left premolar. As with the greater palatine nerve block, a minimal number of needle penetrations and a small amount of anesthetic solution are needed to anesthetize a wide area. Because the soft tissue is dense, firmly attached to the bone, and very sensitive, however, this nerve block is potentially the most painful of all of the injections, unless the protocol for an atraumatic injection is closely followed.

Two techniques are available for giving this injection. The first involves only one needle penetration on the lateral side of the incisive papilla (Figure 40-85, *D*). The second technique includes giving two or three sequential injections: one between the maxillary central incisors followed by a second penetration into the papilla between the maxillary central incisors. In some cases, these two injections provide sufficient pain control for dental hygiene care. If not, an injection is made into the partially anesthetized palatal tissues on the lateral side of the incisive papilla to complete the nasopalatine nerve block (see Figure 40-85, *A* through *D*).

Each approach is acceptable, and dental hygienists should select the procedure that they feel most comfortable with and that provides the most atraumatic injection possible for the client (Table 40-15).

Injection Techniques for the Mandibular Teeth and the Hard and Soft Tissues

The dense bone of the mandible that covers the apices of the teeth eliminates the possibility of supraperiosteal injections into the posterior teeth. In addition, as a result of mandibular bone density, anesthetic solution must be deposited within 1 mm of the target nerve to obtain pulpal anesthesia.

The injection techniques available to anesthetize the mandibular teeth and the hard and soft tissues include the inferior alveolar, lingual, buccal, mental, and incisive nerve blocks. Of these, only the inferior alveolar and incisive nerve blocks cause pulpal anesthesia.

Inferior Alveolar Nerve Block and Lingual Nerve Block

The inferior alveolar and lingual nerve blocks are often employed when dental hygiene care involves the mandible. The biggest advantage is that one penetration anesthetizes the entire quadrant, with the exception of the facial soft tissue over the molars. The disadvantages, however, are formidable, and the success rate of the inferior alveolar nerve block is considerably lower than that of many other injections. The reasons for the lack of success include the following:

- Anatomic variations with regard to the height of the mandibular foramen on the medial side of the ramus
- Accessory innervation by means of the mylohyoid nerve or a bifid inferior alveolar nerve
- The considerable depth of soft-tissue penetration needed to reach the nerve

In addition, the inferior alveolar nerve block has the highest rate of positive aspiration of all of the intraoral injections.[1] Table 40-16 describes the criteria that are essential for administering the inferior alveolar and lingual nerve blocks. It is important to carefully follow the guidelines regarding the landmarks for the penetration and deposition sites to ensure a successful injection and to minimize or eliminate complications. To determine the height of the injection, place the index finger or thumb of your nondominant hand in the coronoid notch (Figure 40-88). An imaginary line extends posteriorly from the fingertip in the coronoid notch to the deepest part of the pterygomandibular raphe, thereby determining the height of injection. This imaginary line should be parallel with the occlusal plane of the mandibular molar teeth; it usually lies 6 to 10 mm above the occlusal plane (Figure 40-89).

To locate the pterygomandibular triangle, roll the index finger or thumb of your nondominant hand from the coronoid notch to locate the internal oblique ridge (see Figure 40-89). The point of needle penetration is between the internal oblique ridge and the pterygomandibular raphe in the pterygomandibular triangle. The syringe barrel is placed in the corner of the mouth on the contralateral side (Figures 40-90 and 40-91).

Appropriate care planning is important when the mandible is anesthetized. Bilateral inferior alveolar and lingual nerve blocks should be avoided. Such procedures produce anesthesia of the client's entire tongue and lingual soft tissues, thereby resulting in the inability to swallow and enunciate as well as a lack of sensation. Anesthetizing the entire mandible thereby creates a high risk of client self-injury to the soft tissues and is not recommended. The optimal care plan is to anesthetize only the right side or only the left side at one appointment. Another alternative is to administer the inferior alveolar nerve block to the side that requires the most treatment (particularly involving lingual tissue) or that has the greatest number of teeth and to then administer the incisive nerve block (see Table 40-19) on the opposite side. Because the incisive nerve block does not provide pain control to the lingual tissues, a lingual infiltration may be given, if necessary.

In many instances, the deliberate deposition of anesthetic solution to anesthetize the lingual nerve is unnecessary, because solution deposited for the inferior alveolar nerve block diffuses and anesthetizes the lingual nerve. However, a separate technique for a lingual nerve block is described in Table 40-16 in the event that deliberate anesthetic solution deposition is needed.

Buccal Nerve Block

The buccal nerve block provides pain control to the soft tissues buccal to the mandibular molars. This injection, along with the inferior alveolar and lingual nerve blocks, anesthetizes the entire quadrant in which it is given. If dental hygiene care involves the manipulation of the buccal tissues of the molars (e.g., therapeutic scaling, root planing, and soft-tissue curettage), this injection is indicated. If treatment does not include these tissues, however, the dental hygienist may simply forgo this injection. Unlike the other injections needed to anesthetize the mandible, the buccal nerve block is easy to administer (Figure 40-97) and has a high success rate. Table 40-17 describes the technique for the buccal nerve block.

Mental Nerve Block

At or near the premolar apices, the mental nerve exits the mental foramen and innervates the facial soft tissues anterior to the foramen, the lower lip, and the chin on the side of the injection. Because of the easy access of the anatomic landmarks, the mental nerve block is simple to administer, has a high success rate, and is usually atraumatic (Figure 40-100).

Although this injection has limited applications for restorative dentistry, it may be used more commonly by dental hygienists who are performing gingival curettage in the anterior portion of the mandible. Because the mental nerve block does not provide pain control to the lingual tissues, a lingual infiltration may be needed.

Table 40-18 presents essential criteria for the administration of the mental nerve block, including suggestions for locating the mental foramen.

Incisive Nerve Block

The incisive nerve originates at the mental foramen and innervates the teeth anterior to the foramen. As a terminal

Text continued on p. 752

TABLE 40-14
Greater (Anterior) Palatine Nerve Block

Nerves anesthetized	Greater palatine
Areas anesthetized	Hard palate and overlying soft tissue unilaterally from the maxillary third molar to the first premolar (see Figure 40-81)
Needle gauge and length	25- or 27-gauge short
Operator position	8 or 9 o'clock
Penetration site	Just anterior to the greater palatine foramen (see Figure 40-82)
Landmarks	Greater palatine foramen Junction of alveolar process and palatine bone Maxillary second molar
Syringe orientation	Approach from the opposite side that is being injected with the needle at a right angle to the penetration site (Figure 40-83)
Hand rests	Back of opposite hand Corner of client's mouth (Figure 40-84)
Deposition site	Just anterior to the greater palatine nerve foramen
Penetration depth	3-6 mm; often only the bevel is inserted
Amount of anesthetic to be deposited	0.45 mL or one quarter of a cartridge; determined by development of blanching of palatal tissues
Length of time to deposit	Approximately 20-30 seconds

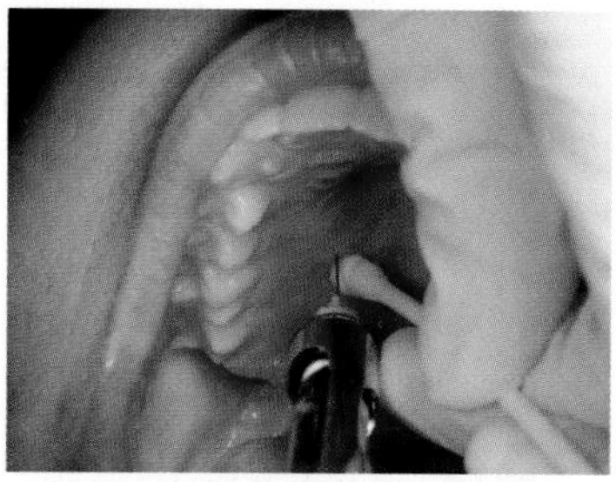

Figure 40-83. Notice the angle of needle entry into the mouth. The insertion is made into ischemic tissues slightly anterior to the applicator stick. The barrel of the syringe is stabilized by the corner of the mouth and the teeth. (From Malamed SF: *Handbook of local anesthesia,* ed 6, St Louis, 2013, Mosby.)

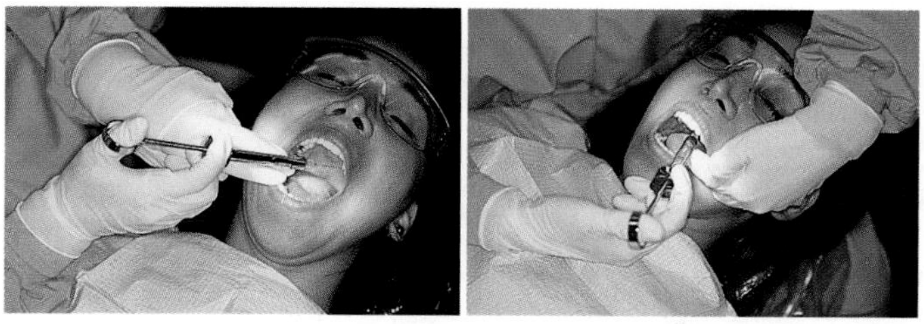

Figure 40-84. Hand rests for a greater palatine nerve block.

Technique Notes

1. To locate the greater palatine foramen, palpate the posterior palate with a cotton-tipped applicator or your forefinger at the junction of the hard palate and the alveolar process near the second molar until a depression is felt.
2. Topical anesthetics have very limited action on keratinized tissue such as the palate. To ensure client comfort, pressure anesthesia with a cotton-tipped applicator is recommended for a minimum of 1 minute before injection and throughout deposition (see Figure 40-82).

Potential Problems	***Technique Tips***
Deposition of the anesthetic solution too far anterior to the foramen, resulting in inadequate anesthesia	Move the needle posteriorly.
Inadequate anesthesia of the first molar as a result of cross-innervation from the nasopalatine nerve	Infiltrate the palate in the area of the first molar.

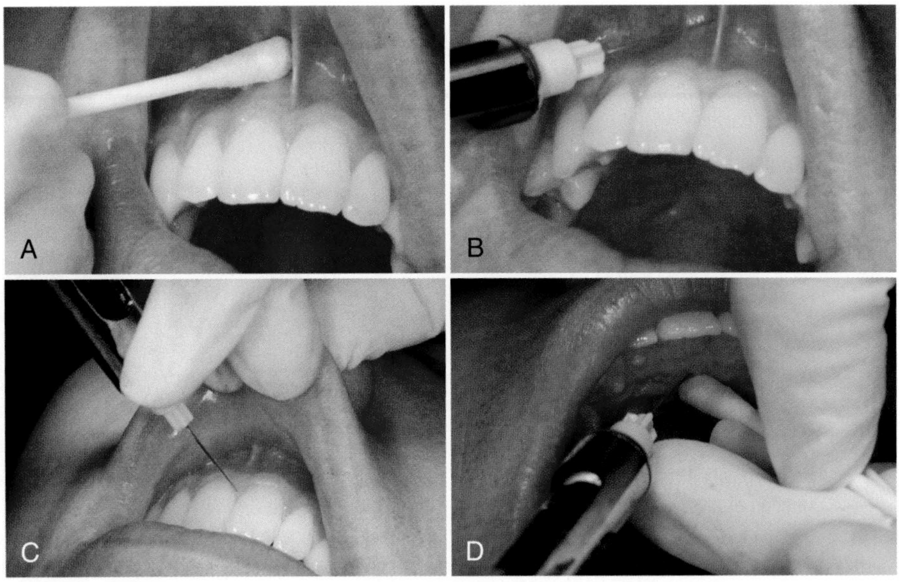

Figure 40-85. **A,** Topical anesthetic is applied to the mucosa of the frenum. **B,** First injection into the labial frenum. **C,** Use a finger of the opposite hand to stabilize the syringe during the second injection into the intended papilla between the central incisors. **D,** Pressure is maintained until the deposition of solution is completed. Needle penetration occurs just lateral to the incisive papilla. (From Malamed SF: *Handbook of local anesthesia,* ed 6, St Louis, 2013, Mosby.)

TABLE 40-15

Nasopalatine Nerve Block

Nerves anesthetized	Nasopalatine	
Areas anesthetized	Hard palate and overlying soft tissue bilaterally from the maxillary canine to the canine (Figure 40-86)	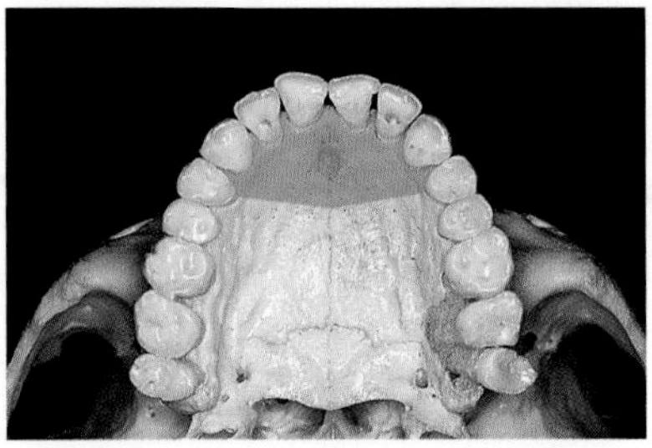 **Figure 40-86.** Area anesthetized with the nasopalatine nerve block.
Needle gauge and length	25- or 27-gauge short	
Operator position	8 or 9 o'clock	
Penetration site	Just lateral to the posterior portion of the incisive papilla (Figure 40-87; see Figure 40-85, *D*)	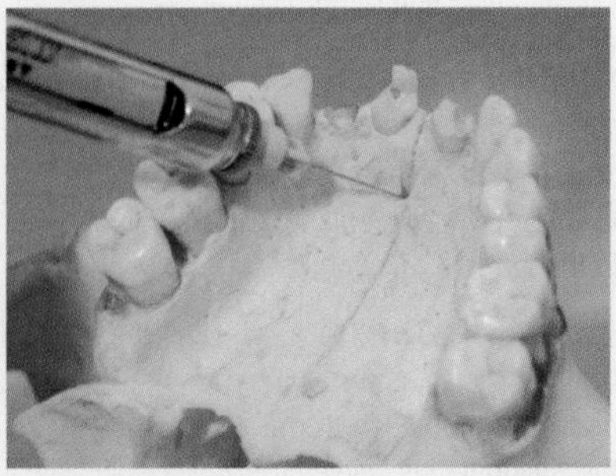 **Figure 40-87.** Target area for a nasopalatine nerve block. (From Malamed SF: *Handbook of local anesthesia,* ed 6, St Louis, 2013, Mosby.)
Landmarks	Central incisors Incisive papilla	

TABLE 40-15

Nasopalatine Nerve Block—cont'd

Syringe orientation	Approach from the canine or premolar region at a 45-degree angle to the incisive papilla (see Figure 40-85, *D*)
Hand rests	Finger of opposite hand Syringe can be stabilized against the corner of the client's mouth (see Figure 40-84)
Deposition site	Incisive foramen, beneath the incisive papilla
Penetration depth	3-6 mm; often only the bevel is inserted
Amount of anesthetic to be deposited	0.45 mL or one quarter of a cartridge; determined by development of blanching of palatal tissues
Length of time to deposit	Approximately 20-30 seconds

Technique Notes

1. Topical anesthetics have very limited action on keratinized tissue such as the palate. To ensure client comfort, pressure anesthesia with a cotton-tipped applicator is recommended for a minimum of 1 minute before injection and throughout deposition (see Figure 40-85, *D*).
2. For greatest client comfort, the nasopalatine nerve block is best administered in a triple injection sequence as follows: infiltration of a central incisor, papillary infiltration of teeth nos. 8 and 9, and then infiltration of the nasopalatine. Each injection anesthetizes the area of the subsequent injection, thereby resulting in an atraumatic procedure for the client (see Figure 40-85).

Potential Problems	Technique Tips
Unilateral anesthesia as a result of the deposition of anesthetic solution to one side of the incisive foramen	Reinsert the needle until it is directly over the incisive foramen.
Inadequate anesthesia of the canine or first premolar as a result of cross-innervation from the greater palatine nerve	Infiltrate the palate at the area of the canine or the first premolar.

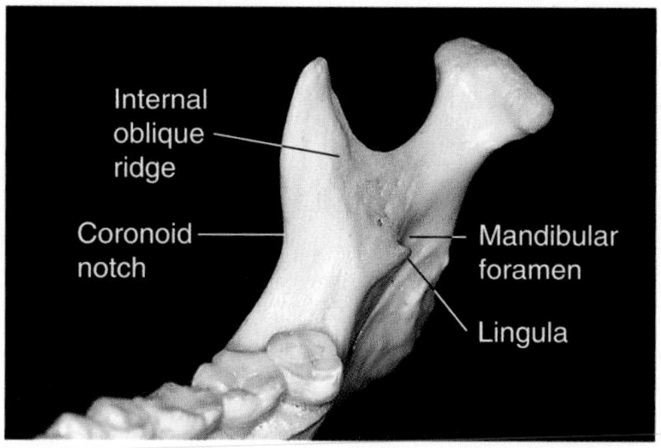

Figure 40-88. Landmarks on the mandible for the inferior alveolar and lingual nerve blocks.

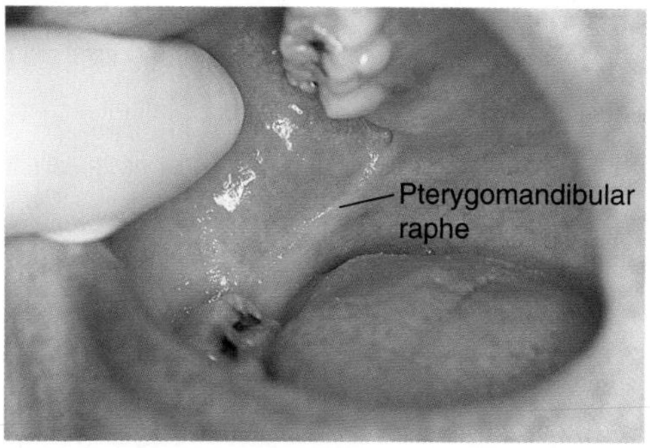

Figure 40-90. The posterior border of the mandibular ramus can be approximated intraorally by using the pterygomandibular raphe as it turns superiorly toward the maxilla.

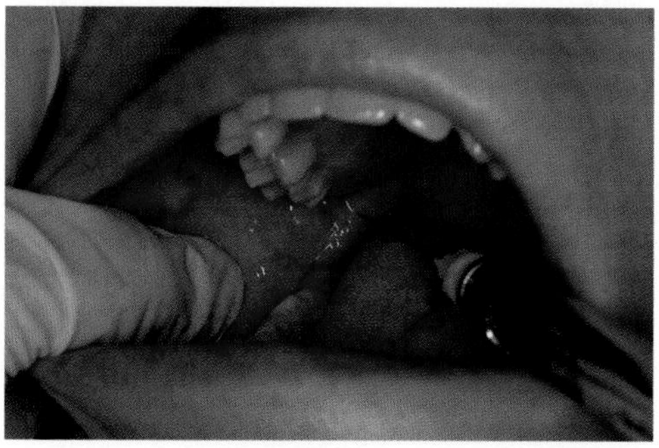

Figure 40-89. Notice the placement of the syringe barrel at the corner of the mouth, which usually corresponds with the premolars. The needle tip gently touches the most distal end of the pterygomandibular raphe. (From Malamed SF: *Handbook of local anesthesia,* ed 6, St Louis, 2013, Mosby.)

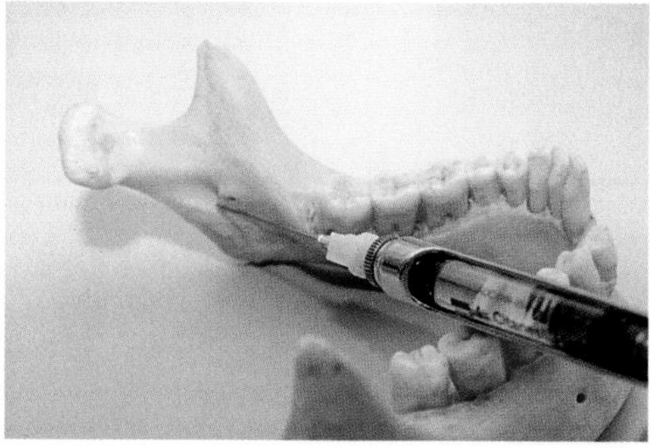

Figure 40-91. Placement of the needle and syringe for an inferior alveolar nerve block. (From Malamed SF: *Handbook of local anesthesia,* ed 6, St Louis, 2013, Mosby.)

TABLE 40-16
Inferior Alveolar and Lingual Nerve Blocks

Nerves anesthetized	*Inferior alveolar:* Inferior alveolar Incisive Mental *Lingual:* Lingual
Areas anesthetized	*Inferior alveolar:* Mandibular teeth unilaterally to midline Body of mandible Inferior portion of the ramus Facial tissue anterior to the first molar Lower lip to midline *Lingual:* All lingual gingival tissue unilaterally to midline Anterior two thirds of the tongue Floor of the mouth unilaterally (Figure 40-92)
Needle gauge and length	25- or 27-gauge long
Operator position	8 or 9 o'clock
Penetration site	Middle of the pterygomandibular triangle (formed by the pterygomandibular raphe medially and the internal oblique ridge laterally) at the height of the coronoid notch, 6-10 mm above the mandibular occlusal plane (see Figure 40-90)
Landmarks	Anterior border of the ramus External oblique ridge Coronoid notch Internal oblique ridge Pterygomandibular raphe Pterygomandibular triangle Mandibular occlusal plane (see Figures 40-89 and 40-90)
Syringe orientation	Approach from the contralateral premolar area, parallel to the occlusal plane
Hand rests	Small finger on the client's chin
Deposition site	*Inferior alveolar:* Superior to the mandibular foramen *Lingual:* Withdraw the needle halfway after deposition for the inferior alveolar block
Penetration depth	*Inferior alveolar:* Until bone is gently contacted (see Figure 40-91) Approximately 20-25 mm or two thirds to three quarters of needle (withdraw 1 mm before deposition) *Lingual:* Withdraw needle halfway after deposition for inferior alveolar block
Amount of anesthetic to be deposited	*Inferior alveolar:* 0.9-1.8 mL or one half to one cartridge *Lingual:* 0.45 mL, or one quarter of a cartridge
Length of time to deposit	*Inferior alveolar:* 60-120 seconds *Lingual:* 10-15 seconds

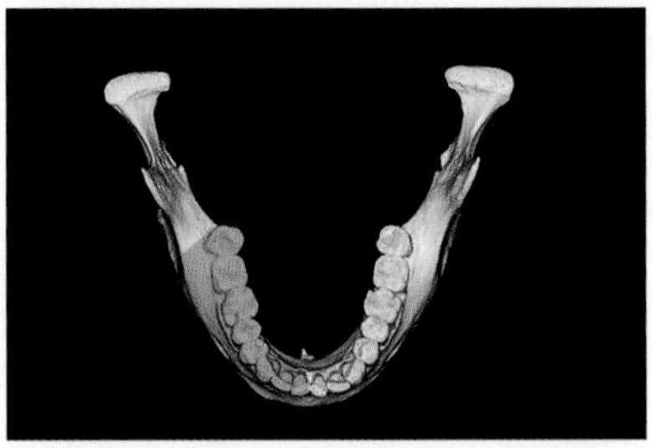

Figure 40-92. Area anesthetized with the inferior alveolar and lingual nerve blocks.

TABLE 40-16

Inferior Alveolar and Lingual Nerve Blocks—cont'd

Technique Notes

1. To locate the pterygomandibular triangle, place your thumb or index finger on the greatest depression on the anterior border of the ramus; this is the coronoid notch. Roll your finger medially to locate the internal oblique ridge. The point of penetration is between the internal oblique ridge and the pterygomandibular raphe in the pterygomandibular triangle, 6-10 mm above the mandibular occlusal plane (see Figures 40-88 and 40-89). While inserting, advancing, and withdrawing the needle, it is important to place the thumb or index finger on the internal oblique ridge and at the same time to grasp the posterior border of the mandible with the remainder of the hand. This technique provides stabilization and control in the event that the client moves unexpectedly during the procedure.
2. As a result of the high vascularity of the deposition site for the inferior alveolar block, a triple aspiration is recommended to ensure that the needle bevel is not against the interior wall of a vessel, thus providing a false-negative aspiration (see Figure 40-60). To aspirate in multiple planes, perform a single aspiration as usual, rotate the body of the syringe toward you slightly, reaspirate, rotate the body of the syringe back to the original position, and then perform a final aspiration. If all three aspiration tests are negative, it is safe to administer the anesthetic solution.
3. If bone is contacted prematurely, before half of the needle length has entered the tissues, it is likely that the needle is too far anterior and has contacted the lingula, which covers the mandibular foramen (Figure 40-93, *A*). To correct this, withdraw the needle halfway, but do not remove it from the tissues. Bring the body of the syringe over the mandibular anterior teeth, and reinsert it past the depth previously penetrated. Redirect the body of the syringe back over the contralateral premolars, and continue to penetrate until bone is contacted (Figure 40-93, *B*).

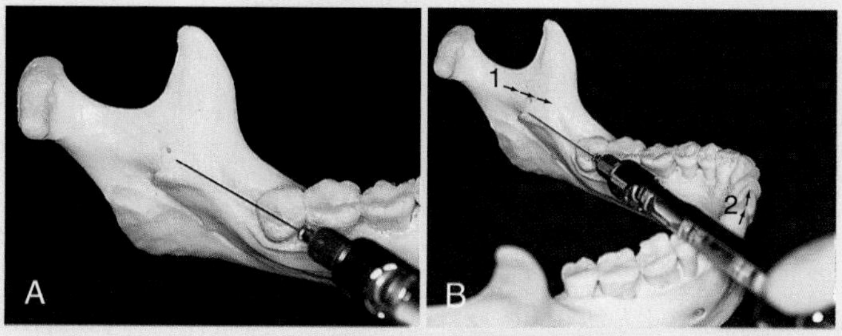

Figure 40-93. **A,** Premature bone contact on the lingula. **B,** Path of syringe orientation to correct for premature contact with bone.

4. If bone is not contacted and the penetration depth is nearing the hub of the needle, it is likely that the needle is too far posterior (Figure 40-94, *A*). To correct this, withdraw the needle halfway, but do not remove it from the tissues. Redirect the syringe further over the contralateral molars, and continue insertion until bone is contacted (Figure 40-94, *B*).

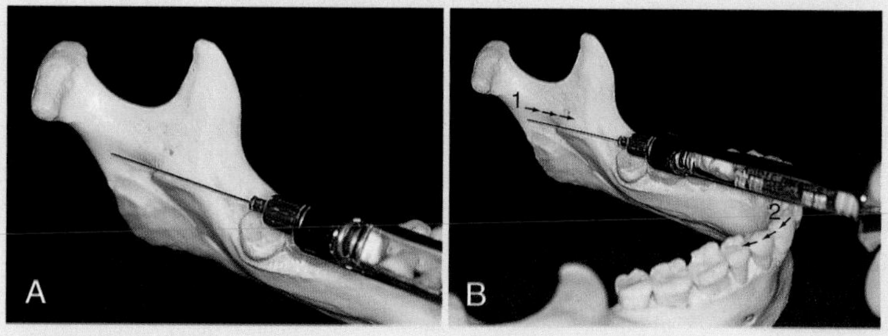

Figure 40-94. **A,** The needle is too far posterior; no bone is contacted. **B,** Path of syringe orientation to correct the needle position.

5. At the deposition site, deposit two thirds of the solution. Withdraw the needle halfway, and deposit the remaining one third of the solution to anesthetize the lingual nerve.

Potential Problems	*Technique Tips*
Deposition of anesthetic below the mandibular foramen	Reinject at a higher penetration site.
Deposition of anesthetic too far anterior on the ramus as indicated by early bone contact with less than one half of the needle length inserted	See Technique Note 3.

Continued

TABLE 40-16
Inferior Alveolar and Lingual Nerve Blocks—cont'd

Incomplete pulpal anesthesia of the molars (often mesial root of the first molar) or premolars; it has been theorized that the mylohyoid nerve, which is not blocked by the inferior alveolar block, provides accessory innervations to these areas	Using a 27-gauge long needle, direct the syringe from the opposite corner of the client's mouth, and penetrate the apical region of the tooth just distal to the unanesthetized tooth. Advance 3-5 mm and deposit 0.6 mL or one third of a cartridge over 20 seconds (Figure 40-95). 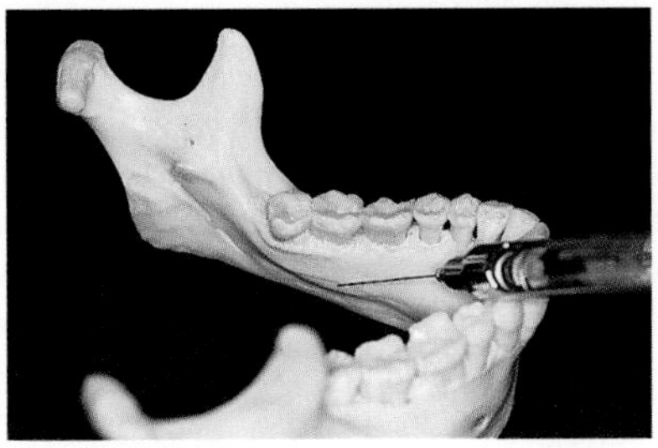 Figure 40-95. Direct the needle tip below the apical region of the tooth immediately posterior to the tooth in question.
Incomplete anesthesia of the central or lateral incisors; may be a result of the cross-innervation of the opposite side's inferior alveolar nerve	Using a 27-gauge short needle, infiltrate the mucobuccal fold, and advance to the apical region of the unanesthetized tooth. Deposit 0.6 mL or one third of a cartridge over 20 seconds (Figure 40-96). 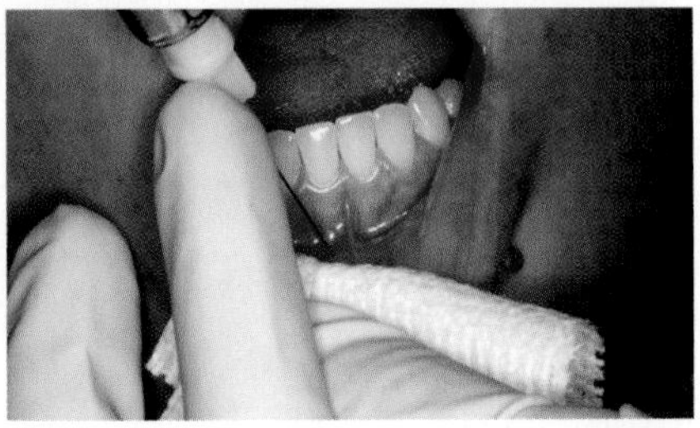 Figure 40-96. Local infiltration of the mandibular incisors.

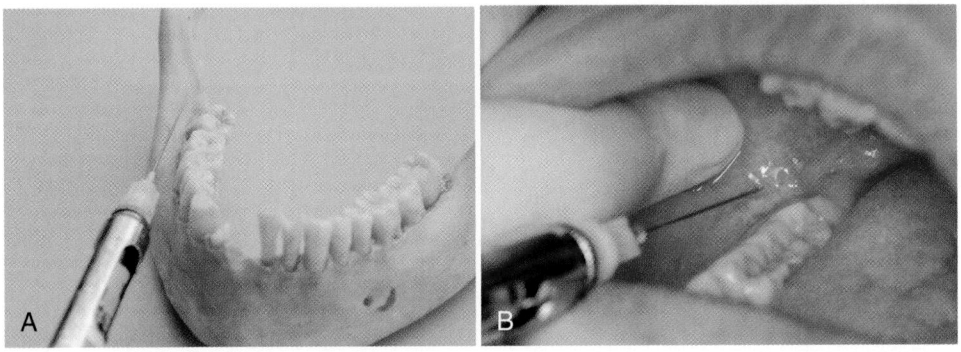

Figure 40-97. Syringe alignment. **A,** Parallel with the occlusal plane on the side of injection but buccal to it. **B,** Distal and buccal to the last molar. (From Malamed SF: *Handbook of local anesthesia,* ed 6, St Louis, 2013, Mosby.)

branch of the inferior alveolar nerve, the incisive nerve is anesthetized when an inferior alveolar nerve block is successfully given. The incisive nerve block, however, may be the injection of choice in several instances. Because bilateral inferior alveolar and lingual nerve blocks are contraindicated as a result of associated client discomfort and function, an alternative may be to administer the inferior alveolar and lingual nerve blocks to the side that needs the most treatment or that has the greatest number of teeth and to then administer the incisive nerve block on the other side. The incisive nerve block may also be used concurrently on both the right and left sides when dental hygiene care requires the incisive nerve block. If lingual soft tissues in isolated areas require anesthesia, local infiltration can be accomplished readily by inserting a 27-gauge short needle through the interdental papilla on both the mesial and distal aspects of the tooth being treated. Because the incisive nerve block already anesthetized the buccal soft tissues, the needle penetration is atraumatic. Local anesthetic solution is deposited as the needle is advanced through the tissue toward the lingual aspect.

TABLE 40-17

Buccal Nerve Block (Long Buccal)

Nerves anesthetized	Buccal
Areas anesthetized	Soft tissues buccal to the mandibular molars unilaterally (Figure 40-98)
Needle gauge and length	25- or 27-gauge long
Operator position	8 or 9 o'clock
Penetration site	In the vestibule, distal and buccal to the most distal molar at the height of the occlusal plane (see Figure 40-97, *B*)
Landmarks	Mandibular molars Buccal vestibule Mucobuccal fold
Syringe orientation	Parallel to the mandibular occlusal plane on the buccal side of the teeth (see Figure 40-97)
Hand rests	Client's cheek or chin Back of operator's opposite hand (Figure 40-99)
Deposition site	Buccal nerve as it passes over the anterior border of the ramus
Penetration depth	1-4 mm; often only the bevel is inserted
Amount of anesthetic to be deposited	0.3-0.45 mL or one eighth to one quarter of a cartridge
Length of time to deposit	Approximately 10-20 seconds

Technique Notes

The buccal nerve block can be administered immediately after the inferior alveolar/lingual block. Therefore the penetration sites can be prepared simultaneously with topical anesthetic.

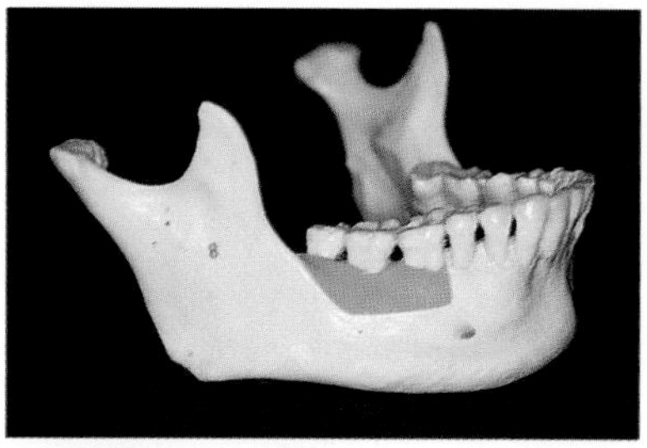

Figure 40-98. Area anesthetized with the buccal nerve block.

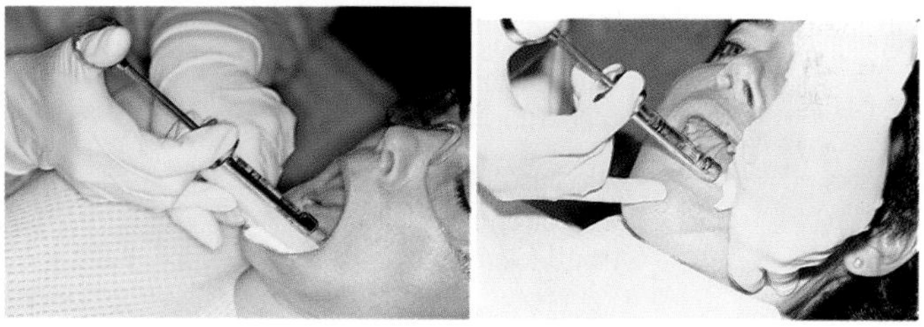

Figure 40-99. Hand rests for the buccal nerve block.

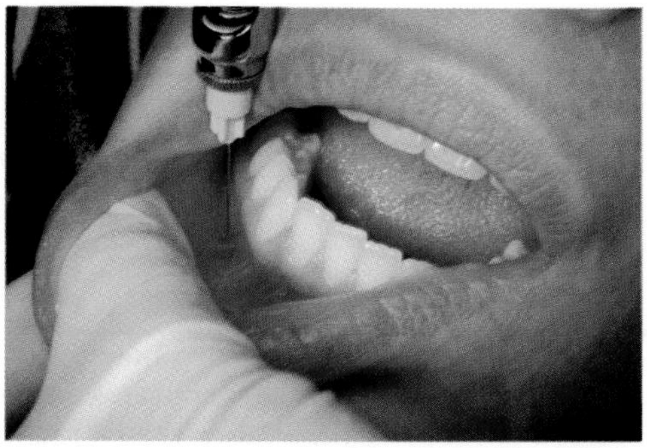

Figure 40-100. Mental nerve block needle penetration site. (From Malamed SF: *Handbook of local anesthesia*, ed 6, St Louis, 2013, Mosby.)

Table 40-19 presents the criteria that are necessary for the administration of the incisive nerve block and offers suggestions for locating the mental foramen. Although some authorities recommend penetrating the needle into the mental foramen to reach the incisive nerve, anesthesia can be obtained much more easily and safely by depositing the solution outside the foramen and using digital pressure over the site to direct the anesthetic into the foramen.

Local Complications

Despite careful preanesthetic client assessment and adherence to the recommended procedures for local anesthetic administration, the following local complications may develop.

TABLE 40-18
Mental Nerve Block

Nerves anesthetized	Mental (terminal branch of inferior alveolar nerve)
Areas anesthetized	Facial soft tissues unilaterally from the mental foramen anterior to midline Lower lip Skin of chin (Figure 40-101)
Needle gauge and length	25- or 27-gauge short
Operator position	8 or 9 o'clock or 11 or 1 o'clock
Penetration site	Mucobuccal fold directly over the mental foramen (see Figure 40-100)
Landmarks	Mucobuccal fold Mandibular premolars Mental foramen
Syringe orientation	Directed toward the mental foramen
Hand rests	Client's chin Back of operator's opposite hand or wrist (Figure 40-102)
Deposition site	Directly over the mental foramen, between the apices of the premolars
Penetration depth	5-6 mm or one quarter the needle length; do not enter the mental foramen
Amount of anesthetic to be deposited	0.6 mL or one third of a cartridge
Length of time to deposit	Approximately 30-60 seconds

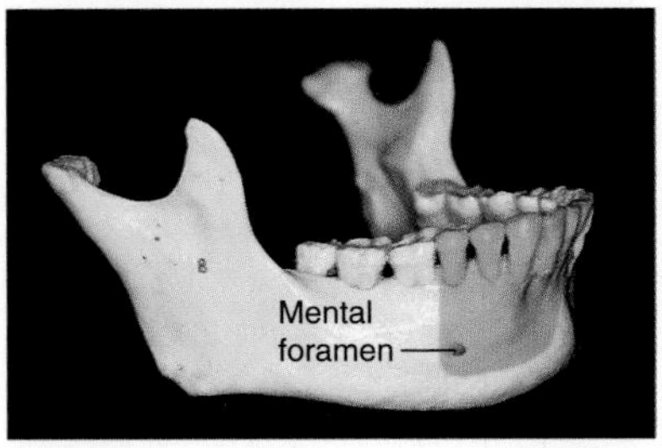

Figure 40-101. Area anesthetized with the mental nerve block.

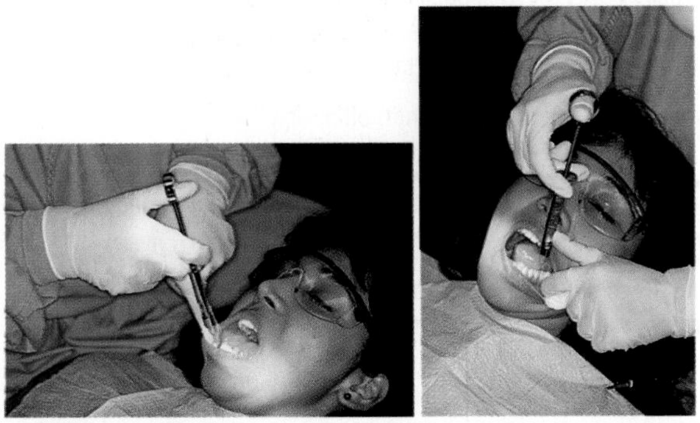

Figure 40-102. Hand rests for the mental and incisive nerve blocks. When possible, hold the arms close to the body to increase stabilization.

TABLE 40-18
Mental Nerve Block—cont'd

Technique Notes

1. To locate the mental foramen, place your forefinger in the mucobuccal fold against the body of the mandible near the first molar. Palpate anteriorly until a depression is felt or the bone feels irregular. This is the mental foramen, which is most often found between the apices of the first and second premolars (Figure 40-103).

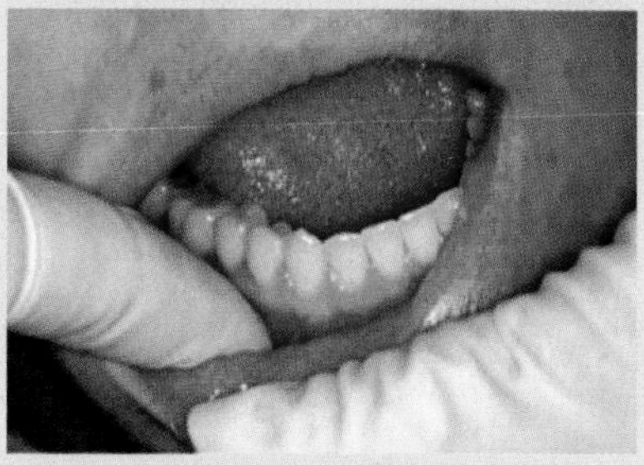

Figure 40-103. Locate the mental nerve foramen by palpating the vestibule at the premolars.

2. Use radiographs to assist you with finding the mental foramen (Figure 40-104).

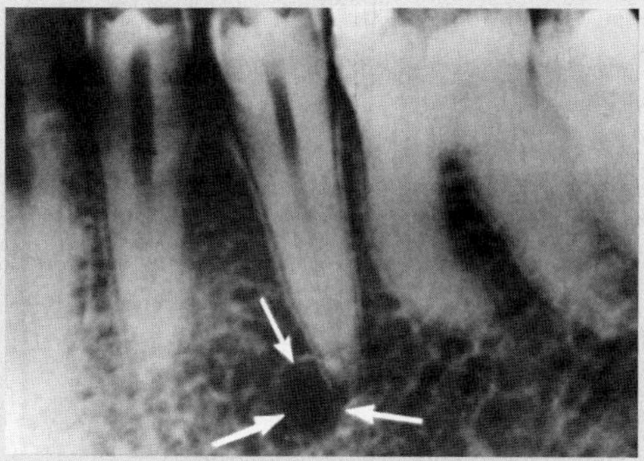

Figure 40-104. Radiographs can assist with locating the mental foramen.

TABLE 40-19
Incisive Nerve Block

Nerves anesthetized	Incisive Mental (terminal branch of inferior alveolar)
Areas anesthetized	Mandibular second premolar to central incisor unilaterally Facial soft tissues unilaterally from the mental foramen anterior to midline Lower lip Skin of chin (Figure 40-105)
Needle gauge and length	25- or 27-gauge short
Operator position	8 or 9 o'clock or 11 or 1 o'clock
Penetration site	Mucobuccal fold directly over the mental foramen
Landmarks	Mucobuccal fold Mandibular premolars Mental foramen

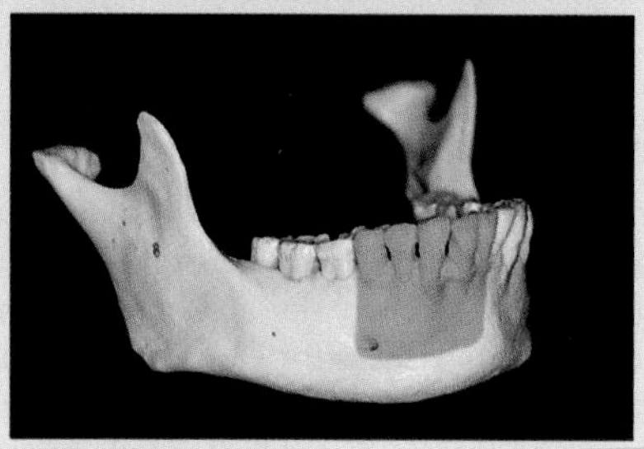

Figure 40-105. Area anesthetized with the incisive nerve block.

Continued

TABLE 40-19
Incisive Nerve Block—cont'd

Syringe orientation	Directed toward the mental foramen
Hand rests	Client's chin Back of operator's opposite hand or wrist (see Figure 40-104)
Deposition site	Directly over the mental foramen, between the apices of the premolars
Penetration depth	5-6 mm or one quarter of the needle length; do not enter the mental foramen
Amount of anesthetic to be deposited	0.6-0.9 mL or one third to one half of a cartridge
Length of time to deposit	Approximately 30-60 seconds

Technique Notes

1. The incisive nerve block is administered in the same manner as the mental nerve block, differing only in the application of pressure over the deposition site to direct the anesthetic solution into the mental foramen, thereby resulting in pulpal anesthesia.
2. To locate the mental foramen, place your forefinger in the mucobuccal fold against the body of the mandible near the first molar. Palpate anteriorly until a depression is felt or the bone feels irregular. This is the mental foramen, which is most often found between the apices of the first and second premolars (see Figure 40-102).
3. Use radiographs to assist you with finding the mental foramen (see Figure 40-104).
4. Maintain pressure over the mental foramen with your finger for 1-2 minutes after the injection. This aids the flow of solution into the foramen, thus providing the pulpal anesthesia.

Potential Problems	***Technique Tips***
Incomplete anesthesia of the central or lateral incisors; may be the result of cross-innervation from the opposite side's inferior alveolar nerve	Using a 27-gauge short needle, infiltrate the mucobuccal fold, and advance to the apical region of the unanesthetized tooth. Deposit 0.6 mL or one third of a cartridge over 20 seconds (see Figure 40-100).
Incomplete pulpal anesthesia	Redirect needle toward the mental foramen, and maintain pressure over the deposition site.

Needle Breakage

The introduction of disposable stainless steel needles has significantly reduced the incidence of needle breakage; however, virtually all needle breaks are preventable. When breakage does occur, it is primarily caused by a sudden, unexpected movement by the client during needle insertion or by poor injection technique.[1] If a needle does break during insertion and can be retrieved without surgical intervention, no emergency exists. Those needles that are not retrieved most often remain in place and become encased by scar tissue. Leaving the needle in the tissue often produces fewer difficulties than the surgery required for its removal.

To prevent needle breakage, do the following:

- Inform the client about the local anesthetic procedure both before and during the injection. Effective communication helps the client to anticipate the dental hygienist's actions and to control anxiety.
- Use long, large-gauge needles (e.g., 25-gauge) when penetrating significant tissue depth. These are less likely to break than smaller needles.
- Never bend the needle, because bending weakens the metal.
- Advance the needle slowly. A forceful contact with bone may break the needle or precipitate a quick movement by the client in response to associated pain.
- Never force a needle against firm resistance such as bone.
- Do not change the direction of the needle when it is almost completely within the tissues. If it is necessary to redirect the needle, first withdraw it almost completely out of the tissue, and then modify the direction.
- A needle should not be inserted into the tissues all the way to the hub. This juncture at the needle shaft and hub is the weakest part of the needle, and it is vulnerable to breakage. If needle breakage occurs at this point, a portion of the shaft must be exposed for the needle to be retrieved without surgery.

When a needle breaks, do the following:

- Remain calm; do not panic.
- Tell the client not to move. Do not remove your hand from the client's mouth, and keep the client's mouth open. If possible, place a bite block in the client's mouth.
- If the needle fragment is protruding, attempt to remove it with cotton pliers or a hemostat.

If the needle fragment is not visible and cannot be readily retrieved, do the following:

- Calmly inform the client about the situation. Attempt to alleviate his or her fears and apprehension.
- Refer the client to an oral and maxillofacial surgeon for consultation.

- Document the incident and the client's response in the client's chart. Keep the remaining needle fragment. Inform your insurance carrier immediately.

When a needle breaks, surgical removal should be considered as follows:

- If the needle fragment is superficial and easily located through radiologic and clinical examination, removal by an oral and maxillofacial surgeon is possible.
- If, despite the superficial location, retrieval is unsuccessful, it is prudent to abandon the attempt and allow the needle fragment to remain in the tissue.
- If the needle is located in deeper tissues or is difficult to locate, permit it to remain without an attempt at removal. There is considerable precedent to justify the retention of a fragment of a broken needle if removal appears difficult.

Pain During the Injection

Pain during local anesthetic agent administration may be attributed to several factors: a careless injection technique and callous attitude toward the client; a dull needle as a result of multiple injections; a barbed needle caused by the hitting of bone; or rapid deposition of the anesthetic solution. It is not possible to ensure that every injection is totally free from discomfort, because clients' reactions vary; however, the dental hygienist should take every precaution to prevent pain during the injection or to prevent its recurrence.

To prevent pain during injection, do the following:

- Adhere to the proper techniques of administration as described in Procedure 40-4 and Tables 40-9 through 40-19.
- Deposit a few drops and then wait 5 seconds before advancing the needle 2 to 3 mm. Repeat the process until the deposition site is reached.
- Use sharp, disposable needles.
- Apply topical anesthetic before needle insertion.
- Use sterile anesthetic agents.
- Inject the anesthetic agent slowly.
- Store anesthetic solutions at room temperature; avoid using cartridge warmers.

Burning During the Injection

A burning sensation reported by the client during deposition of the local anesthetic agent may be caused by a local anesthetic with a vasopressor that is more acidic than the tissue in which it is deposited. The burning sensation, which lasts only a few seconds, disappears as anesthesia develops and is unapparent when the anesthesia fades. A more acute burning sensation may occur, however, if the local anesthetic solution is contaminated via improper storage of the cartridge in a chemical disinfectant; if the cartridge is overheated in a cartridge warmer; if the expiration date of the solution has lapsed; or if the solution is deposited too rapidly, particularly on the palate. When burning occurs as a result of these factors, the tissue is damaged, and subsequent postanesthetic trismus, edema, or possible paresthesia may develop.

To prevent burning during the injection, do the following:

- Store the cartridges in a dark place at room temperature in the original container. Avoid storing cartridges in chemical disinfectants or using cartridge warmers.

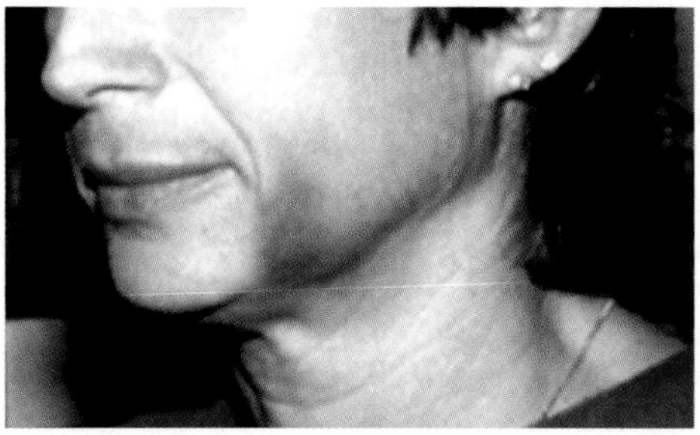

Figure 40-106. Hematoma as a result of the administration of a left mental block.

- Check the expiration date of each cartridge before use. Anesthetic solution that has exceeded the expiration date should be discarded.
- Inject the anesthetic solution slowly.

Most often, burning during an injection is a temporary condition that requires no specific treatment.

Hematoma

A hematoma is a swelling and discoloration of tissue that results from the effusion of blood into the extravascular spaces (Figure 40-106). Hematomas occur after an inadvertent puncture of a blood vessel (particularly an artery) during local anesthetic administration. They appear most often after the administration of a PSA or inferior alveolar nerve block, because the tissues associated with these injections are less dense and readily accommodate large volumes of blood. Bleeding continues until extravascular pressure exceeds intravascular pressure or until clotting occurs. A hematoma is less likely to develop after a palatal injection because of the density of the tissue in this area.

A hematoma that ensues after a PSA nerve block is the largest and most visible. The bleeding occurs in the infratemporal fossa, and swelling and discoloration appear on the side of the face. Clinical manifestations of a hematoma after an inferior alveolar nerve block include intraoral tissue discoloration and swelling on the lingual aspect of the ramus. In addition to the bruise, which may or may not be visible extraorally, a hematoma may be accompanied by trismus and pain.

To prevent a hematoma, do the following:

- Be attentive to anatomic details involved with each injection.
- Modify the injection technique as indicated by the client's anatomy. For example, the depth of needle penetration for a PSA nerve block may be shallower for a client with small anatomic features.
- Use a short needle for the PSA nerve block to minimize the risk of overinsertion and the potential for hematoma formation.
- Minimize the number of needle insertions.
- Observe the appropriate techniques for local anesthetic administration.

Management includes the following:

- If swelling appears, immediately apply direct pressure to the site of the bleeding for at least 2 minutes. For an inferior alveolar nerve block, the pressure point is the medial side of the ramus. For the mental or incisive nerve block, pressure is applied over the mental foramen. If

hematoma formation follows an infraorbital nerve block, the pressure point is the skin over the infraorbital foramen. Unfortunately, it is difficult to apply pressure directly to the site of bleeding after a PSA nerve block, because the vessels are located posterior, superior, and medial to the maxillary tuberosity. Pressure may be applied to the tissues of the mucofacial fold as far distally as the client can tolerate.
- Apply ice to the region when hematoma formation begins. Ice constricts the blood vessels, thereby minimizing the size of the hematoma, and it also acts as an analgesic.
- Inform the client about the possibility of soreness and movement limitation. If soreness develops, analgesics may be taken. Beginning the next day, warm, moist towels may be applied to the affected region for 20 minutes every hour. This application provides comfort and helps with blood resorption. Heat therapy should not commence for at least 4 to 6 hours after hematoma formation, however. Before this time, heat may produce further vasodilation and an even larger hematoma.
- Advise the client that the swelling and discoloration will gradually disappear over 7 to 14 days.
- Dismiss the client when the bleeding has stopped. Avoid further dental hygiene care in the area until signs and symptoms of the hematoma have disappeared. Document the incident and the client's response in the client's chart.

Facial Nerve Paralysis

Facial paralysis is a loss of motor function of the facial expression muscles. Unilateral facial nerve paralysis occurs when the local anesthetic solution is inadvertently deposited into the parotid gland, which is located on the posterior border of the ramus, during an inferior alveolar nerve block.

Motor function loss is temporary and subsides after a few hours; however, during this time, the client is unable to control these muscles, and the face appears lopsided. It also may be impossible for the client to voluntarily close the eye on the affected side. Fortunately, the corneal reflex is functional, and tears continue to lubricate the eye.

To prevent facial nerve paralysis, do the following:
- Adhere to the techniques recommended for the inferior alveolar nerve block.
- Make sure that the needle contacts bone (i.e., the medial aspect of the ramus) before deposition of the local anesthetic solution.
- If bone is not contacted, withdraw the needle almost entirely out of the tissue, bring the barrel of the syringe more posterior (thereby directing the needle more anterior), and readvance the needle until bone is contacted.

Following these steps precludes solution deposition into the parotid gland.

Within a short time after anesthetic solution deposition into the parotid gland, the client senses a weakening of the facial muscles on the affected side. The inferior alveolar nerve is not anesthetized. Management includes the following[1]:
- Reassure the client. Explain that the paralysis lasts only a few hours and that it resolves with no residual effects.
- Instruct the client to remove his or her contact lenses.
- Ask the client to close the eyelid manually to keep the cornea lubricated.
- There are no contraindications to proceeding with treatment at this time, but it may be advisable to reschedule the client.
- Document the incident and the client's response in the client's chart.

Paresthesia

Prolonged anesthesia or paresthesia is a condition with which the client experiences numbness for many hours or days after a local anesthetic injection. Paresthesia may be the result of irritation of the nerve after the injection of an anesthetic agent that has been contaminated with alcohol or a disinfectant. The ensuing edema places pressure on the nerve, which leads to paresthesia. Persistent anesthesia may also result from trauma to the nerve sheath caused by the needle contacting the nerve during an injection. Clients often report the sensation of an electric shock when this occurs. Finally, hemorrhage into or around the neural sheath may create pressure and subsequent paresthesia.

A complication of paresthesia is the client inadvertently precipitating a biting, thermal, or chemical injury as a result of the diminished sensation in the area.

To prevent paresthesia, do the following:
- Store dental cartridges properly. Avoid placing cartridges in disinfectants.
- Follow the proper injection protocol as recommended in Procedure 40-4 and Tables 40-9 through 40-19.

Most often paresthesia involves the lingual nerve or the inferior alveolar nerve. The sensory deficit is usually minimal, and it is rarely accompanied by permanent nerve damage. Fortunately, most incidents resolve within 8 weeks. Recommendations for the management of a client with paresthesia are as follows[1]:
- Reassure the client. The client usually contacts the dental office the day after treatment to report continuing numbness. Explain that paresthesia after local anesthetic administration is not uncommon.
- Arrange for an examination of the client by the dentist, who will determine the location and extent of paresthesia. Explain to the client that paresthesia often continues for 2 months and may last longer.
- Arrange to have the client examined every 2 months until cessation of the paresthesia. Consultation with an oral and maxillofacial surgeon is advisable if paresthesia persists after 12 months or sooner if the client and dentist consider it appropriate.
- Record the incident, conversations with the client, and all clinical findings in the client's chart. Inform your liability carrier of the circumstances.
- Dental and dental hygiene care may continue. Avoid injecting into the area of the traumatized nerve, and employ alternative pain-control techniques.

Trismus

Trismus, which is a spasm of the mastication muscles that results in soreness and difficulty opening the mouth, most often occurs as a result of trauma to the muscles in the infratemporal space after intraoral injections. This trauma may be the result of multiple needle insertions, the administration of an anesthetic solution contaminated with a disinfectant, the injection of large amounts of local anesthetic solution into a restricted area that causes distention of the tissues, hemorrhage that leads to muscle dysfunction as the blood is resorbed, or a low-grade infection.

To prevent trismus, do the following:

- Store the local anesthetic cartridges properly. Avoid immersing the cartridges in a disinfectant.
- Use sharp, sterile, disposable needles.
- Follow appropriate infection-control protocols. Needles that become contaminated should be replaced.
- Use minimal effective amounts of local anesthetic solution, and deposit the solution slowly.
- Adhere to the recommended techniques of local anesthetic administration as outlined in Procedure 40-4 and Tables 40-9 through 40-19. Observe anatomic landmarks, and strive to improve administration techniques. Each of these recommendations facilitates atraumatic injections and prevents repeated needle insertions.

Clients often complain of soreness and difficulty when opening the mouth the day after the administration of an inferior alveolar or a posterior superior nerve block. Recommendations for the management of clients with trismus follow[1]:

- Arrange for an examination of the client by the dentist.
- Start heat therapy immediately. Place moist, hot towels on the affected area for 20 minutes every hour. Analgesics may be recommended to manage the discomfort. Codeine and muscle relaxants may be prescribed by the dentist if needed.
- Direct the client to open and close and to move the mandible from side to side (laterally) for 5 minutes every 3 to 4 hours. These exercises may be accomplished by chewing gum.
- Continue heat therapy, the administration of analgesics, and exercise until the client is symptom free. Improvement is often reported within 48 hours, and symptoms diminish gradually over several days.
- If symptoms continue after 48 hours, the possibility of an infection exists. Antibiotic therapy, which can be prescribed by the dentist, should be added to the recommended care regimen.
- If severe pain and dysfunction continue despite therapy, refer the client to an oral and maxillofacial surgeon for consultation.
- Record the incident, conversations with the client, the results of clinical examinations, and care recommended in the client's chart.
- Avoid elective dental hygiene care until symptoms resolve and the client is more comfortable.

Infection

Infection as a result of local anesthetic administration occurs rarely with the introduction of sterile disposable needles and glass cartridges; however, post-injection infection may be precipitated by the contamination of the needle before the injection, improper handling of the local anesthesia armamentarium, or improper tissue preparation before the injection. When a contaminated needle or local anesthetic solution is introduced into the deeper tissues, infection may occur. If infection is not recognized and treated, trismus may ensue.

To prevent infection, do the following:

- Use sterile, disposable needles.
- Sheath the needle before use and resheath it after use to prevent it from coming into contact with nonsterile surfaces.
- Use appropriate infection-control protocols when handling the anesthetic cartridges. Store the cartridges in their original containers, and, if necessary, wipe the cartridge diaphragm with a disinfectant before syringe assembly.
- To reduce microorganisms at the penetration site, wipe the tissue with gauze, and apply a topical antiseptic before the initial needle insertion.

When infection occurs, the client often reports pain and dysfunction similar to those associated with trismus a few days after dental hygiene care. At this point, signs and symptoms of infection are often not obvious, and immediate treatment includes procedures for managing trismus (e.g., heat therapy, physiotherapy, analgesics, muscle relaxants). If the client does not respond to therapy within 3 days, an infection most likely exists, and antibiotic therapy should be prescribed by the dentist or physician. Document the recommended therapy and client progress in the client record.

Edema

Edema, which is a swelling of the tissues, is a clinical sign of a complication. It may be caused by trauma during the injection, the administration of contaminated solutions, hemorrhage, an infection, or an allergic response. Most often edema manifests as localized pain and dysfunction. In the most severe case, edema precipitated by an allergic response may produce airway obstruction and represent a life-threatening emergency.

To prevent edema, do the following:

- Follow appropriate infection-control protocols when storing and handling components of the local anesthesia armamentarium.
- Observe the guidelines for administering atraumatic injections as described in Procedure 40-4.
- Conduct an adequate preanesthetic client assessment before local anesthetic administration.

The course and treatment of edema depend on its cause.[1] When produced by the administration of a contaminated anesthetic solution or traumatic injection, edema usually subsides after 1 to 3 days without treatment. Analgesics may be recommended. If edema is caused by hemorrhage, the tissue appears discolored and should be managed in the same manner as a hematoma. Resolution of the edema may take 7 to 14 days as the blood is resorbed into the tissues. Edema produced by infection often becomes progressively worse. If the pain and dysfunction do not subside within 3 days, antibiotic therapy may be instituted by the dentist or physician. The treatment of edema caused by an allergic reaction depends on the degree and location of the tissue swelling. If there is no airway obstruction, treatment involves the administration of intramuscular and oral antihistamines and consultation with an allergist or physician. If the edema occurs in an area in which it compromises the airway, the recommendations outlined in the Systemic Complications section later in this chapter should be followed.

Tissue Sloughing

Surface layers of epithelium may be lost as a result of tissue irritation caused by the application of topical anesthetic for an extended period or a client's heightened sensitivity to the local anesthetic. A sterile abscess, which is the form of tissue sloughing that most frequently occurs on the hard palate, may develop after prolonged ischemia induced by the inclusion of a vasoconstrictor in the local anesthetic agent.

To prevent tissue sloughing, do the following:

- Use topical anesthetics appropriately. Apply a limited amount of topical anesthetic to the tissue for 1 to 2 minutes to minimize irritation and maximize effectiveness.
- When using vasoconstrictors for hemostasis, avoid using high concentrations. Epinephrine 1:50,000 and norepinephrine (Levophed) 1:30,000 are the agents that are most likely to cause prolonged ischemia and lead to a sterile abscess.

Tissue sloughing usually requires no treatment and disappears within a few days. A sterile abscess resolves in 7 to 10 days. Analgesics may be recommended for discomfort, and topical ointment can be applied to minimize irritation. Document the progress and the response of the client in the client's record.

Soft-Tissue Trauma

Lip, tongue, or cheek trauma results when the client inadvertently chews or bites these tissues while they are still anesthetized. Trauma, which is most often observed in children or in mentally or physically disabled individuals, may lead to swelling and significant discomfort when the anesthesia subsides.

To prevent soft-tissue trauma, do the following:

- Select a local anesthetic agent with appropriate duration for the length of the dental hygiene appointment.
- Warn the client not to eat, drink, or test the anesthetized area by biting until normal sensation has returned. The client's guardian should also be advised about the potential for injury.
- If anesthesia is still present on dismissal, place a cotton roll between the client's teeth and soft tissues. The cotton roll can be held in position with dental floss that is then wrapped around the teeth.
- Warning stickers may be placed on children to serve as a reminder to the child and the guardian to be careful.

The management of soft-tissue trauma includes the following:

- Coat the lip with petrolatum to minimize irritation and discomfort.
- Recommend warm saline rinses to help decrease swelling.
- Recommend analgesics for pain.
- If infection occurs, the dentist or physician may prescribe antibiotic therapy.

Postanesthetic Intraoral Lesions

Intraoral lesions, such as those that occur with aphthous stomatitis or herpes simplex virus, may develop after the administration of local anesthesia or trauma to the intraoral tissues. Aphthous stomatitis occurs on tissue that is not attached to bone, such as the mucofacial fold or the inner lip. Herpes simplex virus lesions may develop intraorally on tissues that are attached to bone, such as the hard palate, or extraorally. Trauma to the area by a needle or any equipment used during the dental hygiene care appointment may activate herpetic recurrence.

Preventing the development of postanesthetic intraoral lesions is impossible in susceptible clients; however, minimizing trauma during procedures for local anesthetic administration is advisable.

Approximately 2 days after the dental hygiene care appointment, the client reports ulcerations and intense pain, usually near the injection sites. If the discomfort is tolerable, no management is necessary. If the pain is acute, topical anesthetic solutions or protective pastes (e.g., Orabase) may provide relief. The lesions last for 7 to 10 days. Reassure the client, and document the occurrence of the lesion in the client's record.

Systemic Complications

Client assessment is a key factor in the prevention of systemic complications associated with local anesthetic administration. It is estimated that a comprehensive health assessment will prevent approximately 90% of potential life-threatening situations.[2] The remaining 10% occur despite all preventive efforts.

The dental hygienist should be able to recognize the signs and symptoms of an adverse drug reaction and to properly manage the emergency that may develop. To be adequately prepared for an emergency, the dental hygienist—as well as all members of the oral healthcare team—should be able to recognize and manage medical emergencies, monitor vital signs, administer oxygen, and perform basic life support procedures. By establishing an airway and performing basic cardiopulmonary resuscitation, the dental hygienist administers care to reverse the emergency or to sustain the client until advanced life support systems arrive (see Chapter 10).

Local Anesthetic Overdose

A drug overdose reaction or a toxic reaction involves those signs and symptoms that result from overly high blood levels of a drug in various organs and tissues.[1] Normally the drug is continually absorbed from its site of administration into the circulation while at the same time being removed from the blood as it undergoes redistribution and biotransformation. When this equilibrium exists, high blood levels of the drug seldom occur. If this equilibrium is altered, however, the elevation of the blood level of the drug may be sufficient to produce an overdose reaction.

Many factors influence the rate at which a local anesthetic drug level is elevated and the length of time it remains elevated. The presence of one or more of these factors predisposes the client to the development of an overdose reaction. These factors are divided into predisposing client factors and drug factors. Client factors modify the response of an individual to the usual drug dosage. Drug factors involve the drug and its site of administration. Table 40-20 describes how each of these factors influences the potential for an overdose reaction.

Causes and Prevention

High blood levels of local anesthetics may occur in one or more of the following ways[1]:

- Biotransformation of the anesthetic is unusually slow.
- Elimination of the anesthetic from the body through the kidneys is unusually slow.
- The total dose administered is too large.
- Absorption of the anesthetic from the site of injection is unusually rapid.
- The anesthetic is inadvertently administered intravascularly.

TABLE 40-20
Predisposing Factors to Local Anesthetic Overdose Reaction

Predisposing Factors	Causative Factors
Client Factors	
Age	Biotransformation may not be fully developed in younger age groups and may be diminished in older age groups
Body weight	Lower body weight increases risk.
Genetics	Genetic deficiencies may alter response to certain drugs (e.g., atypical plasma cholinesterase)
Disease	Presence of disease may affect the ability of the body to biotransform the drug into an inactive substance (e.g., hepatic or renal dysfunction, cardiovascular disease)
Mental attitude and environment	Psychologic attitude affects response to stimulation; anxiety decreases seizure threshold
Gender	Very slight risk increases during pregnancy
Drug Factors	
Vasoactivity	Vasodilation increases risk
Drug dose	Higher dose increases risk
Route of administration	Intravascular route increases risk
Rate of injection	Rapid injection increases risk
Vascularity of injection site	Increased vascularity increases risk
Presence of vasoconstrictors	Presence decreases risk
Other medications	Concomitant medications may influence local anesthetic drug levels

Adapted from Malamed SF: *Medical emergencies in the dental office*, ed 6, St Louis, 2007, Mosby.

The first two potential causes of an overdose—delayed biotransformation and the elimination of the anesthetic agent—relate to the health of the client. Therefore it is imperative that the dental hygienist carefully assess the client's health status, obtain medical consultation if necessary, and modify the dental hygiene care plan as indicated to prevent drug-related complications.

The three remaining causes of an overdose reaction—excessive dose, rapid absorption, and intravascular injection—may be prevented through adherence to the proper technique for local anesthetic agent administration. Thus careful assessment of the client before dental hygiene care and proper administration technique minimize the risk of a local anesthetic overdose.

Biotransformation and Elimination of the Anesthetic

Ester anesthetics are biotransformed primarily in the blood by the enzyme pseudocholinesterase, which causes the drug to undergo hydrolysis to para-aminobenzoic acid. Clients with a familial history of atypical pseudocholinesterase may be unable to detoxify ester anesthetic agents at the usual rate. As a result, high blood levels of anesthetic may develop. Amide anesthetics may be administered to these individuals without an increased risk of overdose.

Biotransformation of amide anesthetics occurs in the liver. A history of liver disease may indicate some hepatic dysfunction, and the ability of the liver to biotransform amide anesthetics may be compromised. Clients with a history of liver disease who are ambulatory may still receive amide local anesthetics; however, only small amounts should be injected, because average amounts may produce an overdose reaction.

Both ester and amide anesthetics are eliminated to some degree through the kidneys. Renal dysfunction may delay the elimination of the local anesthetic from the blood, thereby precipitating accumulated levels of local anesthetic and increasing the potential for an overdose. Those clients who have significant renal impairment or who require renal dialysis should receive the minimal amount of local anesthetic needed for effective pain control.

Excessive Total Dose of Anesthetic

If an excessive total dose of local anesthetic is administered to a client, toxic effects develop. Responses to drugs vary considerably, but guidelines exist that the dental hygienist can use to calculate maximal safe doses of local anesthetic agents on the basis of the client's body weight. The dental hygienist also needs to factor in the client's age and physical status and adjust the dose accordingly. A more detailed discussion can be found earlier in this chapter in Maximal Safe Doses of Local Anesthetics.

Rapid Absorption of Anesthetic into the Circulation

The addition of a vasoconstricting drug to the local anesthetic solution reduces the systemic toxicity of the anesthetic agent by slowing its absorption into the cardiovascular system. Therefore, unless specifically contraindicated as a result of the client's health status or a limited duration of dental hygiene care, local anesthetic solutions that contain a vasoconstrictor should be employed. A vasoconstrictor minimizes the potential for an overdose reaction and subsequently increases client safety.

Topical anesthetic agents applied to the oral mucosa are absorbed rapidly into the circulation. The concentrations of these topical agents are much greater than those of injectable anesthetic solutions. When small amounts are used in a localized area, there is little chance of complications developing. If topical anesthetic agents are applied over a large area, such as a quadrant or the entire arch, a significant increase in blood level may occur and precipitate an overdose reaction.[1] To prevent complications with topical anesthetics, it is recommended to limit the area of application and to avoid topical anesthetic aerosol sprays because of the associated lack of dosage control and sterility concerns.

Intravascular Injection

The introduction of a local anesthetic solution directly into the bloodstream via an intravascular injection (i.e., intravenous or intra-arterial) may produce an overdose response. An intravascular injection may result with any intraoral injection; however, it is more likely to occur during a nerve block and particularly during an inferior alveolar, mental, incisive, or PSA nerve block.

Fortunately, an overdose reaction from an intravascular injection can be prevented by having complete knowledge of the anatomic features of the area to be anesthetized and by adhering to careful injection technique. This includes using an aspirating syringe, using a 25- or 27-gauge needle, aspirating in two planes before deposition, and slowly administering the anesthetic agent.

Clinical Manifestations and Management

The onset, intensity, and duration of a local anesthetic toxic reaction may vary, depending on the original cause of the overdose. Table 40-21 compares the various patterns of local anesthetic overdose reactions.

Table 40-22 describes the clinical signs and symptoms that may occur during an overdose reaction (with minimal to moderate and moderate to high blood levels of anesthetic) and the procedures for managing a local anesthetic overdose response. The management of an overdose response depends on the severity of the reaction. Most often the reaction is mild and transitory, with little or no specific treatment need.[1] A severe or longer-duration reaction necessitates prompt recognition and immediate care.

Epinephrine Overdose

Although several vasoconstrictors are currently used in oral healthcare (Table 40-23), epinephrine is the most potent and the most widely employed. Consequently, overdose reactions occur more often with epinephrine than with other vasopressor agents because the latter agents are weaker and are used less frequently.

Causes and Prevention

An epinephrine overdose reaction is more likely to develop if concentrations of epinephrine of more than 1:100,000 are administered. Some authorities state that an epinephrine concentration of 1:250,000 provides an adequate duration of action for dental procedures in addition to having minimal toxicity. Therefore the use of a 1:50,000 concentration of epinephrine for pain control is unwarranted. The only benefit that this concentration may have over lesser concentrations is its ability to control bleeding. If epinephrine is to be used for hemostasis, only small quantities of solution need be infiltrated into the immediate area. Overdose reactions under these circumstances are rare. Therefore, to avoid an epinephrine overdose reaction, it is recommended that the dental hygienist use the lowest effective concentration of

TABLE 40-21
Comparison of Patterns of Local Anesthetic Overdose

Factors Related to Overdose	Rapid Intravascular	Too Large a Total Dose	Rapid Absorption	Slow Biotransformation	Slow Elimination
Likelihood of occurrence	Common	Most common	Likely with "high normal" doses if no vasoconstrictors are used	Uncommon	Least common
Onset of signs and symptoms	Most rapid (seconds); intra-arterial faster than intravenous	3-5 minutes	3-5 minutes	10-30 minutes	10 minutes to several hours
Intensity of signs and symptoms	Usually most intense	Gradual onset with increased intensity; may prove quite severe		Gradual onset with slow increase in intensity of symptoms	
Duration of signs and symptoms	2-3 minutes	Usually 5-30 minutes; depends on dose and ability to metabolize or excrete		Potentially longest duration because of inability to metabolize or excrete agents	
Primary prevention	Aspirate, slow injection	Administer minimal doses	Use vasoconstrictor; limit topical anesthetic use or use nonabsorbed type (base)	Adequate pretreatment physical assessment of client	
Drug groups	Amides and esters	Amides; esters only rarely	Amides; esters only rarely	Amides and esters	Amides and esters

From Malamed SF: *Medical emergencies in the dental office,* ed 6, St Louis, 2007, Mosby.

TABLE 40-22

Clinical Manifestations and Management of a Local Anesthetic Overdose Reaction

Signs and Symptoms	Management
Minimal to Moderate Blood Levels (Mild Overdose Reaction)	
Confusion Talkativeness Apprehension Excitedness Lightheadedness Dizziness Ringing in ears (tinnitus) Headache Slurred speech Generalized stutter Muscular twitching and tremor of face and extremities Blurred vision, inability to focus Numbness of perioral tissues Flushed or chilled feeling Drowsiness, disorientation Elevated blood pressure Elevated heart rate Elevated respiratory rate Loss of consciousness	Terminate procedure. Reassure client. Position client comfortably. Administer oxygen. Provide basic life support as indicated. Monitor vital signs. Summon medical assistance if needed. Allow client to recover. Discharge client.
Moderate to High Blood Levels (Severe Overdose Reaction)	
Tonic-clonic seizure, followed by one or more of the following: Central nervous system depression Depressed blood pressure, heart rate, and respiratory rate Unconsciousness	Terminate procedure. Position client supine with the legs elevated. Summon medical assistance. Manage seizure; protect client from injury. Provide basic life support as indicated. Administer oxygen. Monitor vital signs. Administer an anticonvulsant if seizure is prolonged. Transport client to hospital after stabilization.

Some data from Malamed SF: *Medical emergencies in the dental office*, ed 6, St Louis, 2007, Mosby.

epinephrine needed to produce the desired effect and carefully observe dosage guidelines (Table 40-24).

Clients with cardiovascular disease have a greater potential for epinephrine overdose. An increased workload may precipitate further cardiac distress in an already compromised cardiovascular system. The total dose of vasoconstrictor must thus be reduced to avoid systemic complications (see Table 40-3).

An intravascular injection may also produce an epinephrine overdose reaction.[1] Recommendations for the prevention of an intravascular injection may be found in the Local Anesthetic Overdose section earlier in this chapter.

TABLE 40-23

Clinical Manifestations and Management of a Client with an Epinephrine Overdose Reaction

Signs and Symptoms	Management
Fear, anxiety Tenseness Restlessness Throbbing headache Tremor Perspiration Weakness Dizziness Pallor Respiratory difficulty Palpitations Sharp elevation in blood pressure, primarily systolic Elevated heart rate Cardiac dysrhythmias	Terminate procedure. Position client upright. Reassure client. Provide basic life support as indicated. Monitor vital signs. Summon medical assistance if needed. Administer oxygen if needed. Allow client to recover. Discharge client.

Some data from Malamed SF: *Medical emergencies in the dental office*, ed 6, St Louis, 2007, Mosby.

Clinical Manifestations and Management

Clinically the signs and symptoms of epinephrine toxicity resemble the fight-or-flight response. Table 40-23 identifies the signs and symptoms of an epinephrine overdose reaction and the procedures for its management. Most cases of epinephrine overdose are of short duration and need little or no definitive management. If a prolonged reaction occurs, however, the dental hygienist must be prepared to respond accordingly.

Allergy

Allergic reactions are the result of an antigen–antibody response to a specific agent. Exposure to an initial dose of a medication causes an immunologic response. The drug acts as an antigen, which prompts antibodies to be produced. As a result, the administration of a subsequent dose causes the client to develop an allergic response to the drug, its chemical preservative, or a metabolite. After a client manifests a specific drug allergy, he or she remains allergic to that drug indefinitely.

Causes

Allergic reactions to amide-type local anesthetics are extremely rare (see Table 40-1). As a result of their nonallergenic nature, amides are now used almost exclusively for pain control during dental and dental hygiene procedures.

Allergic responses to other contents of the dental cartridge have been demonstrated. Reports of allergy to sodium bisulfite and metabisulfite are numerous.[5-8] Bisulfites are incorporated in all dental cartridges that contain a vasoconstrictor; however, they are not included in cartridges

TABLE 40-24

Clinical Manifestations and Management of an Allergic Reaction

Type of Allergic Response	Signs and Symptoms	Management
Delayed		
Skin	Erythema Urticaria (hives) Pruritus (itching) Angioedema (localized swelling of extremities, lips, tongue, pharynx, and larynx)	Administer antihistamine. Obtain medical consultation.
Respiratory	Bronchospasm Distress Dyspnea Wheezing Perspiration Flushing Cyanosis Tachycardia Anxiety	Terminate procedure. Position client semi-erect. Reassure client. Provide basic life support as indicated. Summon medical assistance if needed. Administer epinephrine. Monitor vital signs. Administer antihistamine. Allow client to recover. Discharge client.
Laryngeal edema	Swelling of vocal apparatus and subsequent obstruction of airway Respiratory distress Exaggerated chest movements High-pitched sound to no sound Cyanosis Loss of consciousness	Terminate procedure. Position client supine. Summon medical assistance. Administer epinephrine. Maintain airway. Administer oxygen. Administer additional drugs (e.g., antihistamine, corticosteroid). Perform cricothyrotomy if needed. Transfer client to hospital.
Immediate Anaphylaxis		
Skin	Pruritus (itching) Flushing Urticaria (face and upper chest) Feeling of hair standing on end Conjunctivitis Vasomotor rhinitis	Terminate procedure. Position client supine with the legs elevated. Provide basic life support as indicated. Summon medical assistance. Administer epinephrine. Administer oxygen. Monitor vital signs. Administer additional drugs (e.g., antihistamine, corticosteroid). Transport client to hospital.
Gastrointestinal or genitourinary	Abdominal cramps Nausea, vomiting Diarrhea	Same as management of anaphylaxis related to skin.
Respiratory	Substernal tightness or chest pain Cough, wheezing Dyspnea Cyanosis of mucous membranes and nail beds Laryngeal edema	Same as management of anaphylaxis related to skin.
Cardiovascular	Pallor Lightheadedness Palpitations, tachycardia Hypotension Cardiac dysrhythmias Unconsciousness Cardiac arrest	Same as management of anaphylaxis related to skin.

that contain no vasopressor. These agents are also sprayed on fruits and vegetables to prevent discoloration. A client with a history of bisulfite allergy (e.g., an asthmatic client) should alert the dental hygienist to the possibility of a similar reaction if a local anesthetic that contains a vasoconstrictor is administered. See the earlier sections entitled Preanesthetic Client Assessment and Allergies for further discussion.

Prevention

The preanesthetic client assessment is the primary measure for the prevention of an allergic reaction. A client who has multiple allergies (e.g., asthma, hay fever, allergy to foods) has an increased potential for allergic reactions to medications.[2] Thus the dental hygienist must proceed cautiously when considering the administration of local anesthetics to these clients.

If the client reports that he or she has experienced an allergic reaction to local anesthetics, it is important that the dental hygienist assume that the client is truly allergic to the local anesthetic in question until proven otherwise. Unfortunately, any adverse drug reaction is often labeled an allergy by clients when in fact overdose reactions occur much more frequently than allergic reactions.[2] Thus it is imperative for the dental hygienist to seek as much information as possible from the client so that the exact nature of the reaction can be determined. A dialogue history is used, whereby the dental hygienist asks the client a series of questions to ascertain the validity of the allergy[2] (Box 40-7). It is important that the anesthetic agent or any closely related agent to which the client claims to be allergic not be used until the allergy is disproved.

If, after the dialogue history, questions remain about the cause of the reaction, the dental hygienist should consult with the dentist and the client's physician, and referral for allergy testing should be considered. Dental hygiene care that requires local anesthetics, whether topical or injectable, should be delayed until an evaluation of the client is complete. Dental hygiene procedures that do not require anesthesia may be performed during the interim.

For clients who have a confirmed allergy to local anesthetics, management varies according to the nature of the allergy.

BOX 40-7

Dialogue with Patient to Evaluate an Alleged Allergic Reaction to a Local Anesthetic

- Describe exactly what occurred.
- What treatment was given?
- What position were you in during the injection?
- What was the time sequence of events?
- What drug was used?
- What amount of drug was administered?
- Did the drug contain a vasoconstrictor?
- Were you taking any other medications at the time of the incident?
- What is the name and address of the doctor/dentist/physician/hospital who was treating you when the reaction occurred?

Adapted from Malamed SF: *Handbook of local anesthesia*, ed 6, St Louis, 2013, Mosby.

Table 40-8 describes alternative drugs that may be employed in place of agents that cause an allergic response.

Clinical Manifestations and Management

The amount of time that elapses between exposure to an allergenic agent and the manifestation of signs and symptoms is important. As a rule, the more rapid the onset of signs and symptoms after exposure, the more severe the ultimate reaction.[2] Conversely, the greater the time between exposure and onset of signs and symptoms, the less severe the reaction. This time factor helps the dental hygienist to determine the appropriate management of the reaction.

The most common allergic reaction associated with local anesthetics is a dermatologic reaction. A skin reaction that appears alone or after a considerable lapse of time (i.e., ≥60 minutes) is usually not life-threatening; however, if a skin reaction develops rapidly, it may be the first indication of an ensuing generalized reaction.

An allergic reaction may manifest solely in the respiratory tract, or it may accompany other systemic responses. In slowly evolving generalized allergic reactions, respiratory distress follows skin and gastrointestinal reactions but occurs before cardiovascular signs and symptoms.

Generalized anaphylaxis is the most life-threatening allergic reaction. Most reactions develop quickly and reach their maximum intensity within 5 to 30 minutes of exposure, although delayed responses have been reported.[2]

Table 40-24 describes the signs, symptoms, and management of clients with dermatologic and respiratory reactions as well as generalized anaphylaxis. Reaction types are further defined as delayed or immediate.

Other Trends That Promote Client's Freedom from Pain

Clients will often comment that receiving an intraoral injection stings or burns. This happens as a result of the acidic nature of the anesthetic solution. For example, a local anesthetic with a vasoconstrictor has a pH of approximately 3.5.[1] The body's pH is approximately 7.4. Before this acidic solution can cross the nerve membrane to block the nerve conduction, it must buffer itself to a level of more than 7.35, which can take up to 10 minutes.[1] Adding a buffering solution to the cartridge before depositing the solution has two clinical benefits: (1) it takes less time for the anesthetic to take effect; and (2) the client does not feel the sting of the acidic solution as it is being deposited into the tissue.[1] A buffering agent (e.g., sodium bicarbonate) cannot be added to the anesthetic cartridge during manufacturing; it would shorten the shelf life of the product, and, with time, carbon dioxide would form in the cartridge.[1] A device called a *mixing pen* has been developed to be used chairside to allow an anesthetic cartridge to be mixed with a buffering solution before the administration of a local anesthetic injection. This creates a more comfortable and faster-acting anesthetic experience for the client.

Another issue that concerns clients is the long duration of soft-tissue anesthesia, which is manifested as numbness of the lips, cheeks, and tongue. Soft-tissue anesthesia can last long after the client has left the dental office; it can interrupt normal daily activities such as eating, drinking, and speaking. For certain clients, this lack of sensation is awkward or embarrassing, and, in some instances, it causes self-inflicted injury. The vasodilator phentolamine mesylate can be used to reverse the soft-tissue effects of local anesthetic by increasing the blood flow at the injection site, thereby causing the local anesthetic to leave the nerve and diffuse into the bloodstream more rapidly. It is given at the same location using the same injection technique as the previous local anesthetic that was given to the client. The dose is based on an equal ratio to the amount of local anesthetic plus vasoconstrictor that was given to the client; however, the maximum dosage is 2 cartridges.[1] Study trials show that, for adults and adolescents who had received maxillary injections, 50 minutes was the median time to regain feeling in the upper lip. For mandibular injections, the median time to regain feeling in the tongue was 60 minutes when using phentolamine mesylate.[1] The use of this reverse anesthetic solution has the potential to reduce the time of soft-tissue anesthesia significantly, thereby meeting the client's needs for a wholesome facial image, freedom from stress and anxiety, and freedom from head and neck discomfort.

It is predicted that a new drug delivery system via nasal spray will be in use in the near future. This system will provide soft-tissue anesthesia and pulpal anesthesia to maxillary teeth #4 through #13. This type of anesthesia is particularly useful in pediatric dentistry. In addition, 3% tetracaine solution, which is an ester-type anesthetic solution, can be used with the vasoconstrictor oxymetazoline to provide a needleless application that offers client comfort during maxillary anterior dental procedures.[1]

CLIENT EDUCATION TIPS

- Explain the advantages of receiving a local anesthetic agent during dental hygiene procedures that may produce discomfort.
- Explain measures that can be taken to ensure comfortable local anesthetic delivery.
- Explain the normal, anticipated sensations associated with local anesthesia, including areas that will be anesthetized and the anticipated duration of the anesthesia.
- Explain the importance of following postoperative instructions to minimize the possibility of self-inflicted soft-tissue injury.

LEGAL, ETHICAL, AND SAFETY ISSUES

- It is the legal responsibility of the dental hygienist to practice within the scope authorized by state law with regard to the delivery of a local anesthetic agent.
- It is imperative that the dental hygienist carefully evaluate the client's health history to determine the suitability of local anesthetic procedures.
- The client treatment record must accurately reflect any local anesthetic procedure completed, including the complete drug name and the amount of agent delivered.

KEY CONCEPTS

- Local anesthesia is the temporary loss of sensation in a circumscribed area brought about by the reduction of nerve membrane permeability to sodium ions. When sodium ions are blocked, the nerve cell cannot depolarize, thereby stopping the transmission of a stimulus to the brain.
- Local anesthetic agents are classified chemically as either amides or esters, which differ with regard to how they are metabolized: esters are metabolized in the blood by pseudocholinesterase, and amides are metabolized in the liver.
- Local anesthetic agents produce vasodilation. For the maximum anesthetic effect, vasoconstrictors are often combined with local anesthetics to slow down absorption, reduce hemorrhage, and increase the length of time that the anesthesia is effective.
- Many local anesthetic drugs are available. The clinician must choose the best agent for the circumstances and consider each of the following: the health of the client, medications taken by the client, possible client allergies, the amount of time that anesthesia is desired, the areas being anesthetized, the planned procedure and injections, the client's previous responses to anesthesia, and the possible need for hemostasis.
- There is a maximum amount of local anesthetic agent and vasoconstrictor that can safely be administered to a client at one time. This amount varies with the client's weight, health status, age, and the specific agent administered.
- A thorough health history evaluation before local anesthetic delivery is crucial. Many medications influence a client's response to local anesthesia. There are also several systemic conditions that require modifications of local anesthetic delivery, such as pregnancy, hyperthyroidism, liver dysfunction, renal dysfunction, allergies to sulfa or bisulfite, atypical plasma cholinesterase, methemoglobinemia, and malignant hyperthermia.
- Medications that are excreted renally may be retained in the body of the diabetic client with kidney disease, thereby causing toxic effects. When local anesthetic agents are administered, the minimal use of vasoconstrictors is required, because epinephrine is capable of raising blood glucose levels.
- The local anesthetic armamentarium includes a syringe, a needle, a local anesthetic agent, a topical anesthetic agent, cotton-tipped applicators, gauze, cotton forceps or a hemostat, and a mouth mirror.
- Oral anesthetic procedures involve the maxillary and mandibular branches of cranial nerve V, which is the trigeminal nerve.
- There are three categories of local anesthetic procedures: local infiltration, field block, and nerve block. These differ with regard to the relationship between the area anesthetized and the area of delivery of the anesthetic agent and in the scope of the area anesthetized; nerve blocks are delivered further from the treatment site and anesthetize a larger area as compared with local infiltrations, which are delivered directly at the apex of the target tooth and anesthetize only one or two teeth.
- The attitude and demeanor of the clinician have a significant impact on the comfort of the client and the overall success of the local anesthetic injection.
- Local anesthetic procedures for maxillary anesthesia include local infiltration, anterior superior alveolar field block, middle superior alveolar field block, infraorbital nerve block, posterior superior alveolar nerve block, greater palatine nerve block, and nasopalatine nerve block.
- Local anesthetic procedures for mandibular anesthesia include inferior alveolar nerve block, lingual nerve block, buccal nerve block, mental nerve block, and incisive nerve block.

- Local anesthetic delivery has the potential to cause both local and systemic complications. Potential local complications include needle breakage, pain during injection, burning during injection, hematoma, facial nerve paralysis, paresthesia, trismus, infection, edema, tissue sloughing, soft-tissue trauma, and postanesthetic intraoral lesions. Potential systemic complications include local anesthetic overdose, epinephrine overdose, and allergy. Most of these potential complications can be avoided with proper preanesthetic client assessment, the careful selection of the anesthetic agent, conscientious delivery techniques, and proper postoperative instructions.

CRITICAL THINKING EXERCISES

Scenario: Ms. S

Client Profile: 45-year-old woman who lives alone

Chief Complaint: "I want my periodontal maintenance scheduled at 4-month intervals. I have experienced discomfort during previous scaling throughout my upper jaw."

Dental History: Past history of orthodontic treatment. Received four quadrants of scaling and root planing 3 years ago with very good results. Third molars removed. Low caries rate. Clinically client exhibits extensive maxillary buccal recession.

Social History: Limited social drinking, nonsmoker, exercises regularly

Health History: Noncontributory; weighs 123 lb

Oral Health Behaviors: Client is compliant with the homecare regimen and maintains appropriate re-care schedule.

Assessment: Client requires local anesthetics to allow for comfortable periodontal maintenance.

Review the previous client profile and make the following determinations:

- Client suitability for local anesthetic agent administration
- Preferred local anesthetic agent
- Preferred injection(s)
- Maximum dose of local anesthetic agent

REFERENCES

1. Malamed SF: *Handbook of local anesthesia*, ed 6, St Louis, 2013, Mosby.
2. Malamed SF: *Medical emergencies in the dental office*, ed 6, St Louis, 2007, Mosby.
3. Goulet JP, Pérusse R, Turcotte JY: Contraindications to vasoconstrictors in dentistry: Part III. Pharmacologic interactions, *Oral Surg Oral Med Oral Pathol* 74:692, 1992.
4. Wong M, Jacobsen PL: Reasons for local anesthesia failures, *J Am Dent Assoc* 123:69, 1992.
5. Schwartz HJ: Sensitivity to ingested metabisulfites: variations in clinical presentation, *J Allergy Clin Immunol* 71:487, 1983.
6. Simon RA, Green L, Stevenson DD: The incidence of ingested metabisulfite sensitivity in an asthmatic population, *J Allergy Clin Immunol* 69:118, 1982.
7. Twarog FJ, Leung DYM: Anaphylaxis to a component of isoetharine (sodium bisulfite), *J Am Med Assoc* 248:2030, 1982.
8. Seng GF, Gay AJ: Dangers of sulfites in dental local anesthetic solutions: warning and recommendations, *J Am Dent Assoc* 113:769, 1986.
9. DuBrul EL: *Sischer and DuBrul's oral anatomy*, ed 8, St Louis, 1988, Ishiyaku EuroAmerican.
10. Oraqix: Product information available from Dentsply Pharmaceuticals, York, PA. Available at: www.dentsplydental.com. Accessed November 12, 2012.

ACKNOWLEDGMENT

The author acknowledges Renee Hannebrink, Gwen Essex, Michele Darby, and Margaret Walsh for their past contributions to this chapter.

EVOLVE RESOURCES

Please visit http://evolve.elsevier.com/Darby/hygiene for additional practice and study support tools.

CHAPTER

41

Nitrous Oxide–Oxygen Analgesia

Margaret M. Walsh

COMPETENCIES

1. **Discuss the chemistry, pharmacology, and physiology of nitrous oxide-oxygen (N_2O-O_2).**
2. **Explain the stages of anesthesia.**
3. **Discuss the indications and contraindications for use of N_2O-O_2 sedation.**
4. **Discuss the advantages and disadvantages associated with nitrous oxide-oxygen sedation.**
5. **Discuss the signs and symptoms of baseline level N_2O-O_2 sedation.**
6. **List and define the equipment used in N_2O-O_2 sedation.**
7. **Explain the safety features associated with equipment used in N_2O-O_2 sedation.**
8. **Discuss the administration of N_2O-O_2 sedation, including:**
   - **Calculate the percentage of N_2O and the percentage of O_2 from the tidal volume.**
   - **Safely administer N_2O-O_2 sedation by using titration to induce the proper level of sedation, monitoring the client during analgesia, and oxygenating the client at the completion of the sedation period.**
9. **Describe potential complications that may arise as a result of N_2O-O_2 sedation.**

Delivery of nitrous oxide (N_2O) in combination with oxygen (O_2) is an inhalation method of conscious sedation known as *nitrous oxide–oxygen analgesia.* This conscious sedation method can enhance the clinician's ability significantly to meet the client's need for freedom from pain, stress, and fear in a safe and effective way. When used as the sole sedative, N_2O-O_2 relaxes individuals who are mildly apprehensive about the dental or dental hygiene experience and provides pain control for procedures that are only slightly or moderately painful. Such procedures include scaling hypersensitive root surfaces, removing periodontal sutures, cementing crowns or inlays, irrigating under an inflamed operculum, or administering a local anesthetic agent. If significant pain is anticipated during a dental or dental hygiene procedure, then N_2O-O_2 is accompanied by local anesthesia. N_2O-O_2 is used in combination with other general anesthetics, such as halothane and meperidine (Demerol), by oral surgeons to achieve surgical anesthesia. When used alone, N_2O-O_2 is a weak anesthetic but an intense analgesic.[1] This pharmacologic property of N_2O-O_2 makes it ideal for use in dental hygiene care because clients often are mildly apprehensive and require minor pain control but also must remain conscious and responsive.

Several synonyms refer to N_2O-O_2 analgesia, including the following[1]:

- Conscious sedation
- Inhalation sedation
- N_2O psychosedation
- Relative analgesia

Conscious sedation refers to the fact that during the administration of N_2O-O_2 the client is always awake and able to respond to verbal commands, breathe automatically, and cough so that aspiration is avoided.[2] **Inhalation sedation** reflects that the N_2O and O_2 gases are inhaled through the nose. N_2O **psychosedation** refers to the fact that N_2O acts on the psyche or the central nervous system in such a way that pain impulses are not relayed to the cerebral cortex or their interpretation is altered. **Relative analgesia** refers to the state of sedation produced—mood is altered and pain reaction threshold is increased, but pain sensations are not blocked completely.

Chemistry

Nitrous Oxide

Nitrous oxide is a colorless, tasteless, sweet-smelling agent that supports combustion. It is stored in the liquid and gaseous states in a blue compressed-gas cylinder (Figure 41-1). The pressure of the N_2O vapor floating above the liquid N_2O is approximately 700 to 750 pounds per square inch (psi) (Figure 41-2). Although it is stored as a liquid and vapor (gas) in equilibrium, N_2O is delivered as a gas to the client. The pressure within the cylinder, indicated by the needle reading on the pressure gauge, reflects the pressure created by the N_2O gas in the cylinder (see Figure 41-2). As the client inhales the gaseous N_2O from the cylinder, liquid N_2O vaporizes to replace it. The pressure of this "new" gas is 700 to 750 psi, until no more liquid remains to replace the gas. The pressure gauge for N_2O therefore cannot be used as an accurate measurement of the contents of the cylinder (Figure 41-3). Once all of the liquid N_2O is gone and only gaseous N_2O remains, the pressure gauge falls in relation to the pressure of gas remaining.

Consequently, clinicians use their N_2O for a considerable amount of time before the pressure gauge reads 500 psi. Once the pressure reading drops to 500 psi, the pressure gauge precipitously drops, indicating that the cylinder is empty. Because the amount of N_2O in the cylinder cannot be determined by the pressure gauge reading until the cylinder is almost empty, it is important for the operator to keep a close eye on the N_2O pressure gauge of portable gas machines. This monitoring allows the clinician to detect when the pressure

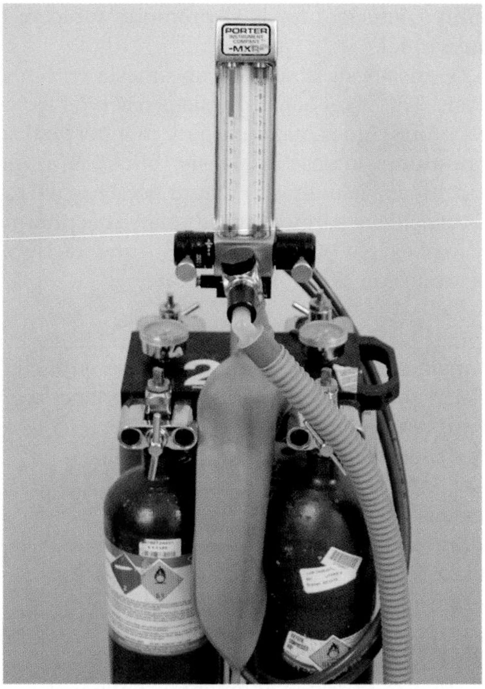

Figure 41-1. A portable gas machine with a green cylinder containing O_2 and a blue cylinder containing N_2O, stored directly on the gas machine. (Courtesy Dr. Mark Dellinges.)

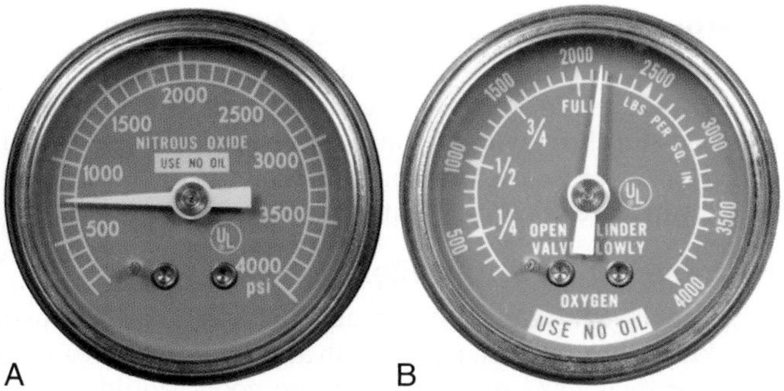

A B

Figure 41-2. Pressure gauges on inhalation sedation unit. **A,** N_2O pressure gauge for N_2O cylinder. **B,** O_2 pressure gauge for O_2 cylinder. Note color-coding of blue for N_2O and green for O_2. (Courtesy Dr. Mark Dellinges and Cory Price.)

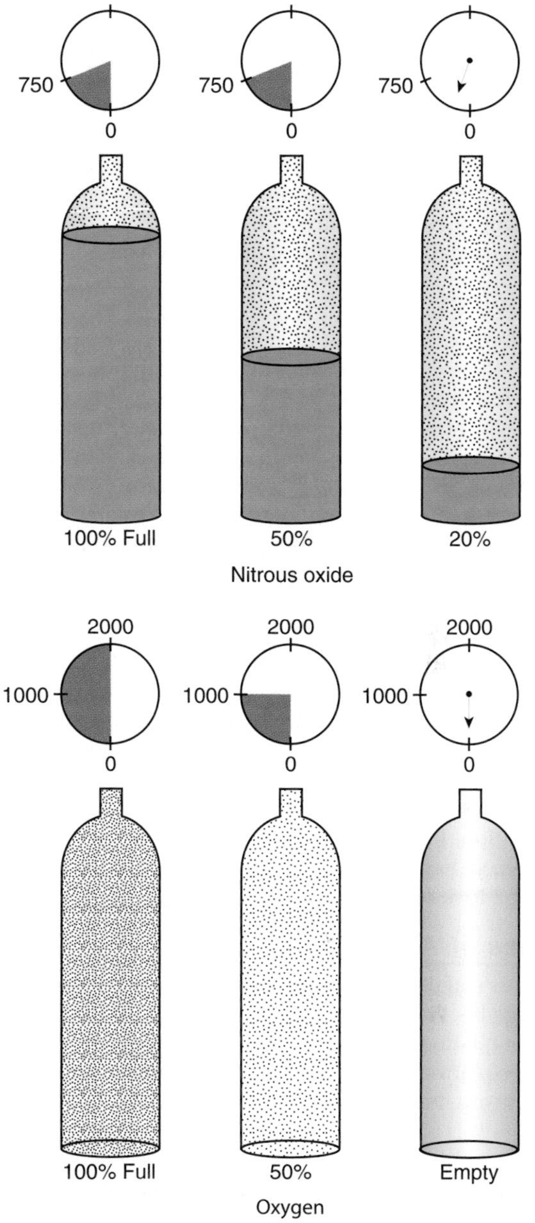

Figure 41-3. Pressure gauge readings for N_2O and O_2 cylinders. (From Clark MS, Brunick AL: *Handbook of nitrous oxide and oxygen sedation,* ed 4, St Louis, 2015, Mosby.)

begins to fall and to substitute a full N_2O cylinder before the original cylinder is empty. In addition, each N_2O cylinder should be marked with the date the full tank was opened and the dates and lengths of subsequent use to facilitate the monitoring process and to prevent the clinician from running out of N_2O before the client care procedure is completed.

The blood-gas solubility coefficient of N_2O is 0.47, meaning that 100 mL of blood dissolves 47 mL of N_2O. This blood-gas solubility coefficient accounts for the rapid onset and rapid recovery from the analgesic effects of N_2O sedation. Because N_2O is 15 times more soluble in blood than nitrogen, it displaces nitrogen in the blood. It does not compete with O_2 and carbon dioxide for combination with the hemoglobin molecule.[1]

Oxygen

O_2 is stored as a gas in green compressed-gas cylinders and is delivered as a gas (see Figure 41-1). The contents of the O_2 cylinder can be determined by the reading on the pressure gauge. A full tank of O_2 is reflected by a pressure gauge reading of 2100 psi (see Figure 41-2). As the O_2 is depleted in the cylinder as a result of use, the pressure falls correspondingly, as indicated by the needle position on the O_2 pressure gauge (see Figure 41-3). This allows an accurate assessment of how much O_2 is left in the cylinder at all times.

Pharmacology

N_2O has no effect on the heart rate, blood pressure, liver, or kidney as long as an adequate amount of O_2 is delivered concurrently.[2] It does, however, have an effect on all sensations, such as hearing, touch, pain, and warmth. With regard to hearing, clients report that they can hear distant sounds better than close sounds. Consequently, clients under the influence of N_2O may focus on background sounds such as music or the conversation in the next room rather than to what the clinician is saying. In addition, N_2O reduces the gag reflex but does not eliminate it. Therefore if a client tends to gag, this sedation modality should be considered for use.[1]

Physiology

N_2O depresses the central nervous system. Specifically, it affects the cerebral cortex, thalamus, hypothalamus, and reticular activating system. The exact mechanism of action is unknown; however, it results in either altering the relay of nerve impulses to the cerebral cortex or causing them to be interpreted differently.[2] As a result, the individual experiences reduced anxiety and increased pain tolerance. Pain perception is not blocked, however, and N_2O-O_2 must be used in combination with a local anesthetic for many procedures. N_2O does not combine with any body tissues, and it is the only anesthetic used that is not metabolized. The N_2O molecule enters the blood through the lungs, where it displaces nitrogen, and eventually exits unchanged through the lungs.[1]

Nevertheless toxic reactions are associated with oversedation with N_2O. **Hypoxia** (lack of O_2 to the tissues), characterized by a headache and nausea, is associated with receiving too much N_2O and lack of a subsequent oxygenation period. In addition, bone marrow depression and white blood cell depression have been reported after prolonged administration of 2 to 4 days.

Stages of Anesthesia

The four stages of anesthesia are depicted in Figure 41-4.

- Stage I is the analgesia stage. In **analgesia** the person feels pain but does not care. The analgesia stage of anesthesia has three planes. The first two planes are relative analgesia, and these are the planes appropriate for dental hygiene care.
- Stage II is the delirium or **excitement phase** of light anesthesia. This stage of anesthesia is characterized by hyperresponsiveness to stimuli, exaggerated inspirations, and loss of consciousness. For individuals receiving dental hygiene care, the immediate treatment of entry into the excitement stage of anesthesia is to increase the percentage of O_2 immediately to 100% and to turn the N_2O off.
- Stage III is **surgical anesthesia**, and it has four planes. Oral and maxillofacial surgeons take their patients to this level of anesthesia, and it is acceptable; dental hygienists never need to provide this level of anesthesia for their clients. Loss of consciousness by an individual receiving dental hygiene care indicates oversedation, and the immediate treatment is to increase the percentage of O_2 immediately to 100% and to turn the N_2O off. The 0.47 blood-gas solubility coefficient for N_2O promotes rapid recovery of the individual.
- Stage IV anesthesia is surgical anesthesia with respiratory paralysis. This level of anesthesia is reserved for use when a person undergoes major surgery in a hospital setting.

N_2O produces intense analgesia, but it is a very weak anesthetic. In fact, usually one would need to give more than 80% N_2O to achieve surgical anesthesia.[1] This pharmacologic property makes N_2O-O_2 a good pain and anxiety control modality for use in dental hygiene care.

Indications for Use

N_2O-O_2 analgesia is recommended for use with clients who have at least one of the following characteristics[1,2]:

- Mild apprehension
- Allergy to local anesthetics
- Refusal of local and general anesthesia
- Hypersensitive gag reflex
- Intolerance for long appointments
- Cardiac conditions
- Hypertension
- Asthma
- Cerebral palsy
- Intellectual and/or developmental challenges

Mild Apprehension

Individuals who are fearful of, or mildly anxious about, the oral healthcare experience are good candidates for N_2O-O_2 because it relaxes them and takes the edge off their apprehension.

Allergy to or Refusal of Other Anesthetics

Individuals who are allergic to all types of local anesthetics, those who refuse a local or general anesthetic for other reasons, and those who are unable to experience good local anesthesia because use of a vasoconstrictor is medically contraindicated are good candidates for N_2O-O_2 analgesia.

Hypersensitive Gag Reflex

Individuals who are prone to gagging easily during oral healthcare procedures, such as those having impressions taken or their third molars scaled, are good candidates for N_2O-O_2 because this analgesic reduces the gag response.

Inability to Tolerate Sitting for Long Periods

N_2O-O_2 analgesia is recommended for persons with back problems or other conditions that make them unable to tolerate sitting in the dental chair for long periods. N_2O-O_2 creates the perception that time is passing quickly.

Cardiovascular Disease and Hypertension

Individuals who have cardiovascular disease or hypertension are good candidates for N_2O-O_2 because it decreases stress

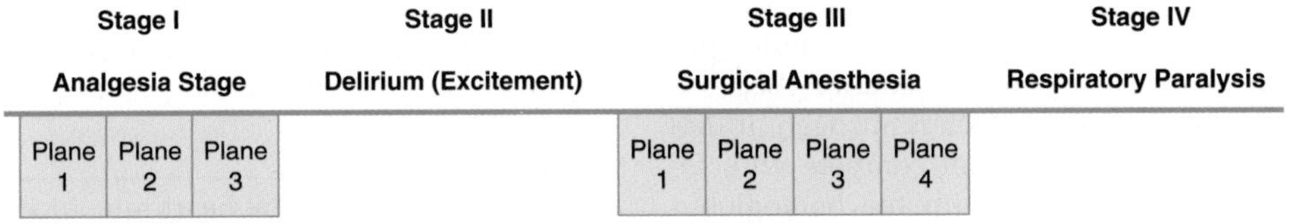

Figure 41-4. Stages of anesthesia.

and exposes the individual to more O_2 than is normally available. For example, even at a gas ratio of 50:50, the client is receiving 50% O_2 compared with the 22% O_2 available in room air. This O_2 enrichment coupled with stress reduction is a major advantage of N_2O-O_2 sedation for these medically complex clients.

Asthma

Individuals who have asthma are candidates for N_2O-O_2 because during sedation they receive more O_2 than normally is available to them. This O_2 enrichment facilitates breathing and decreases stress.

Cerebral Palsy and Intellectually and Developmentally Challenged Persons

Persons with cerebral palsy and who are challenged developmentally or cognitively are candidates for N_2O-O_2 because they are sometimes difficult to manage in the oral healthcare setting, and this analgesic relaxes them. The client, however, must be able to communicate with the operator, breathe through the nose, and cooperate by leaving the mask in place.

Relative Contraindications to Use

There are no absolute medical contraindications to use of N_2O-O_2 analgesia, but there are some relative contraindications that make it a poor choice for certain clients. The following conditions contraindicate the use of N_2O-O_2 sedation[1,2]:

- Pregnancy
- Communication difficulty
- Nasal obstruction
- Chronic obstructive pulmonary disease
- Emotional instability
- Epilepsy
- Negative past experience or fear of sedation

Pregnancy

N_2O-O_2 analgesia is not recommended for individuals who are pregnant. Although there is no evidence that sufficient N_2O crosses the placenta to produce depression of the fetal central nervous system, it is better to err on the side of caution with pregnant women given that long-term exposure to N_2O is associated with spontaneous abortion.[1] In general, all unnecessary drugs are avoided during pregnancy, especially during the first trimester.

Communication Barrier

Individuals who have a language barrier or with whom communication is difficult should not be given N_2O-O_2 because communication between the client and the operator is essential for success with conscious sedation. The operator must question the client during the administration of N_2O-O_2 to determine the appropriate level of sedation and the client's response to the drug. Communication barriers make it difficult or impossible for this monitoring to occur.

Nasal Obstructions

Individuals who have a cold, allergy, or other type of nasal obstruction are not good candidates for N_2O-O_2 because the gas is inhaled. Nasal obstruction prevents the client from obtaining the benefit of the drug. Also, respiratory infections contaminate the tubing and reservoir bag.

Chronic Obstructive Pulmonary Disease

The respiratory systems of persons with emphysema or chronic bronchitis function on less O_2 than those of healthy individuals because these diseases affect the lung's capacity to exchange air. Consequently, they depend on a lowered blood O_2 level to stimulate respiration. The increased blood O_2 saturation made available with N_2O-O_2 removes the stimulus of the lowered O_2 blood level and may indicate to the brain that the individual need not perform as many inspirations, thus producing apnea.[2]

Emotional Instability

N_2O-O_2 is contraindicated for individuals who are emotionally unstable. Because this type of sedation causes a distortion of one's perception of reality, it can precipitate problems for clients with a history of schizophrenia or alcoholism. Moreover, individuals who have experienced the death of a loved one recently or who are going through a painful divorce often go through a period of emotional instability. Therefore it is not recommended to use N_2O-O_2 sedation because unpleasant feelings may surface under the influence of this drug and cause the client to cry uncontrollably.

Epilepsy

N_2O-O_2 analgesia may trigger epileptic seizures in individuals with epilepsy. Therefore its use is not recommended for clients with a history of epilepsy.

Fear of Nitrous Oxide–Oxygen Sedation

Individuals who are fearful of having N_2O-O_2 or those with compulsive personalities who must be always in control may tear off the sedation mask suddenly from fear of the unknown or of becoming unconscious. In the dental hygiene care setting, a good rule of thumb is never to talk someone into being sedated with N_2O-O_2. Individuals should be willing to and want to try this sedation method.

Advantages of Use

The following are advantages associated with N_2O-O_2 analgesia:

- It is an excellent choice of sedation for the high-risk person with a history of cardiovascular disease.
- It is a simple, relatively safe procedure to perform and does not require the services of special personnel such as an anesthetist.
- Equipment is not cumbersome and requires little maintenance.
- Restraining straps and pharyngeal airways are not required.
- Individual is awake and responsive at all times, and the depth of sedation can be controlled moment to moment.
- Onset and recovery are nearly always rapid.
- Most adults being sedated do not have to be accompanied to their appointment by another responsible adult.
- There is no need for preoperative laboratory tests or for food intake to be restricted before sedation, as is the case before having general anesthesia.
- A special recovery room is unnecessary, as is monitoring the person for a long time after recovery.

Disadvantages of Use

The following are disadvantages associated with N_2O-O_2 analgesia:

- Production of vertigo, nausea, or vomiting may occur if too much N_2O is given or if the operator fluctuates the levels of N_2O too much during administration of the agent. Aspiration is not a problem, however, because the client is awake and the gag reflex is not eliminated (Figures 41-5 and 41-6).
- Individuals with extremely difficult behavioral problems cannot always be managed.
- When instrumenting teeth in the maxillary anterior region, the mask gets in the way.

Signs and Symptoms of Nitrous Oxide–Oxygen Sedation

A **sign** is something that can be observed directly. A **symptom** is something that must be reported to one person by another. Thus signs of N_2O-O_2 sedation are observed objectively by the operator, and symptoms of N_2O-O_2 sedation are reported subjectively by the client. Based on this information, the dental hygienist determines when an appropriate level of sedation has been achieved to relax the client sufficiently to begin treatment.

Signs

Objective signs that clients have reached a desirable level of N_2O-O_2 sedation are that they are awake but drowsy and relaxed in appearance (e.g., feet pointing out and hands limp; Figure 41-7). They have reduced reaction to painful stimuli, and respiration is normal and smooth. In contrast, if a client demonstrates hyperresponsiveness to stimuli and exaggerated inspirations, these are signs of oversedation (i.e., entry into the excitement stage of anesthesia) and of the need to give 100% O_2 to the person and discontinue the N_2O altogether.

Other signs that clients have reached a desirable level of N_2O-O_2 sedation are that their blood pressure and pulse, eye reaction, and pupil size are observed to be normal.[2] Little or no gagging or coughing is observed. The client's speech is slow and tends to be guttural.[1] There may be some perspiration and lacrimation (tearing). Heavy perspiration and lacrimation, although possibly reflecting appropriate sedation for oral surgery treatment, are inappropriate for dental hygiene care and indicate a need to turn down the N_2O by about 2 L and increase O_2 by 2 L. Likewise, uncontrollable laughing by the client indicates a need to turn down the N_2O level (by about 2 L) and increase the O_2 level by an amount equal to the N_2O reduction (Box 41-1).

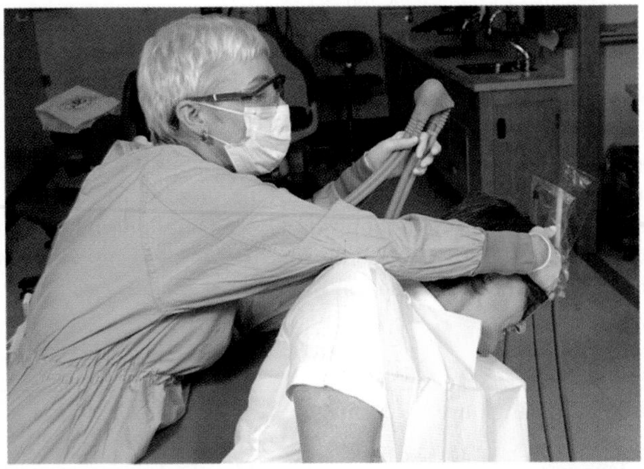

Figure 41-5. If vomiting occurs, turn the client's head and body to the side away from the operator. (Courtesy Dr. Mark Dellinges.)

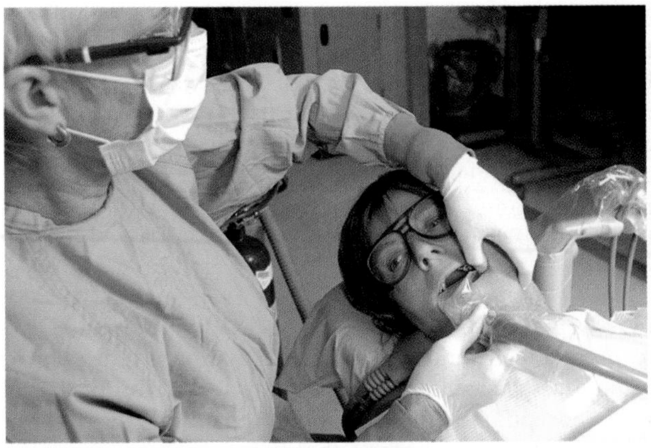

Figure 41-6. Vomitus is removed with suction or finger. Treatment is discontinued, and the client should receive 100% O_2. (Courtesy Dr. Mark Dellinges.)

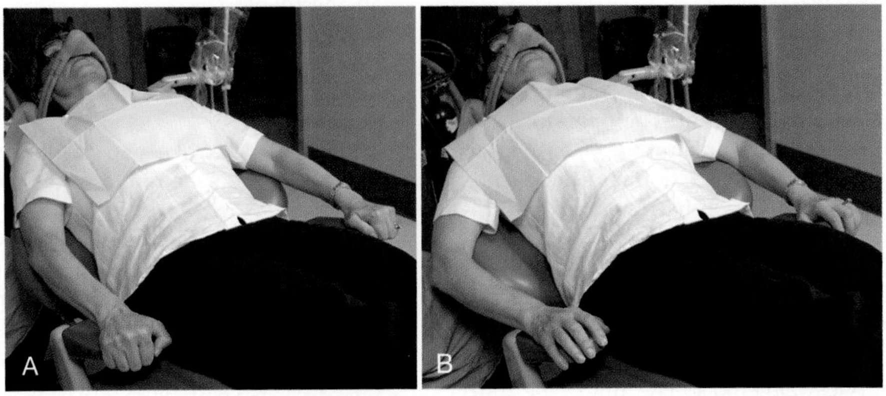

Figure 41-7. **A,** White-knuckle syndrome exhibited by apprehensive client at start of procedure. **B,** Relaxation of hands commonly is observed when client becomes sedated. (Courtesy Dr. Mark Dellinges.)

BOX 41-1

Signs of Nitrous Oxide–Oxygen Analgesia Appropriate for Dental Hygiene Care

- Client awake
- Lessened pain reaction
- Drowsy, relaxed appearance
- Eye reaction and pupil size normal
- Respiration normal
- Blood pressure and pulse normal
- Minimal movement of limbs
- Flushing of skin
- Perspiration
- Lacrimation
- Little or no gagging or coughing
- Speech infrequent and slow

Symptoms

Subjective symptoms of N_2O-O_2 sedation can be determined by direct questioning of the client as well as by observation. For example, asking, "How do you feel?" or "Do you feel relaxed?" elicits desired information. If clients report that they are relaxed or that sounds seem distant and if they indicate an indifference to their surroundings, these are symptoms that the desired level of sedation for dental hygiene care has been achieved. For instance, if the operator says to the client, "Shall I go ahead and numb up this area?" and the client replies, "I don't care," indifference is apparent. Other desirable symptoms are client reports of lessened pain awareness, for example, during probing of a previously sensitive tooth, and of feeling tingling, lightheadedness, a floating sensation, or waves of warmth over the entire body. A tingling sensation in the fingers and toes and then in the arms and the legs is usually one of the first symptoms reported, indicating a desirable level of sedation. The operator may begin by asking the client, "Do you feel any tingling in your fingers or toes or in your arms and legs?"

The point at which the client reports a relaxed pleasant floating sensation can be taken as the baseline level of sedation. **Baseline** is the term used to designate the ideal minimal amount of N_2O-O_2 needed to relax the client (Box 41-2). Once baseline sedation is obtained, the client should be maintained at a slightly reduced N_2O level by decreasing the N_2O level by 1 to 2 L and increasing the O_2 level by 1 to 2 L.

Reported feelings of heaviness in the chest or of vibration or spinning, although reflecting appropriate sedation for oral surgery treatment, are not symptoms of appropriate sedation levels for dental hygiene care. Instead, they indicate a need to turn down the N_2O level (e.g., by 2 L) and to increase the O_2 level by a similar amount. If the client does not respond to questioning, this indicates that he or she has sunk below the desirable level of sedation. The operator should decrease immediately the liter flow of N_2O and increase the O_2 by 2 L. If this does not produce a client response, 100% O_2 should be given and N_2O discontinued.

The percentage of N_2O delivered to the lungs determines the sedative effect on the central nervous system. Although individual reactions at any given concentration of N_2O may vary greatly from individual to individual, a range of responses may occur at given concentrations, as summarized in Table 41-1.

BOX 41-2

Symptoms of Baseline Level of Nitrous Oxide–Oxygen Analgesia

- Mental and physical relaxation
- Indifference to surroundings and passage of time
- Lessened pain awareness
- Floating sensation
- Drowsiness
- Warmth
- Tingling or numbness
- Sounds seem distant

TABLE 41-1

Signs and Symptoms in Response to Nitrous Oxide and Oxygen Conscious Sedation

Concentration N_2O	Response
10%-20%	Body warmth Tingling of hands and feet
20%-30%	Circumoral numbness Numbness of thighs
20%-40%	Numbness of tongue Numbness of hands and feet Droning sounds present Hearing distinct but distant Dissociation begins and reaches peak Mild sleepiness Analgesia (maximum at 30%) Euphoria Feeling of heaviness or lightness of body
30%-50%	Sweating Nausea Amnesia Increased sleepiness
40%-60%	Dreaming, laughing, giddiness Further increased sleepiness, tending toward unconsciousness Increased nausea and vomiting
50% and over	Unconsciousness and light general anesthesia

From Bennett CR: *Conscious sedation in dental practice,* ed 2, St Louis, 1978, Mosby.

Equipment

The armamentarium for the delivery of N_2O-O_2 inhalation sedation consists of a supply of the gases stored in containers called *cylinders,* an apparatus for their delivery to the client, called a *gas machine,* and a *nasal inhaler* or mask through which the client breathes the N_2O-O_2 analgesic. The modern gas machine or *inhalation sedation unit* is a compact, continuous-flow machine used for the administration of compressed gases under controlled conditions. The N_2O-O_2 inhalation sedation unit is altered to deliver only two gases: N_2O and O_2.

Cylinders

N_2O and O_2 are dispensed in steel containers called **cylinders**, which are colored green for O_2 and blue for N_2O (see Figure 41-1). Compressed-gas cylinders are manufactured in a variety of sizes. In inhalation sedation with N_2O-O_2, the cylinder size used commonly in portable units for N_2O and O_2 is the E size, whereas larger cylinders are used in central storage systems, specifically G cylinders for N_2O and H cylinders for O_2.

Cylinders always should be returned to the appropriate vendor for refilling. Refilling a small cylinder from a larger one is hazardous; this should not be attempted by oral healthcare personnel. For quality control, the Hazardous Materials regulations of the U.S. Department of Transportation require that cylinders be tested every 5 years by the manufacturer to ensure their integrity. The date of the test is stamped permanently on the cylinder.

Cylinders should be stored in an upright position, away from a heat source, and chained to the wall to prevent them from falling on their cylinder valve stem, which could cause the cylinder to explode. In addition, at high pressures O_2 and N_2O can form an explosive mixture in the presence of grease or oil. Therefore grease or oil never should be used on cylinder valves or gauges on the gas machine. Box 41-3 lists important considerations for handling compressed-gas cylinders.

Cylinders may be stored directly on the gas machine (see Figure 41-1) or in an area away from the gas machine (Figure 41-8). When cylinders are stored in an area away from the gas machine, regulation copper tubing with a ⅜-inch outside diameter is fed through drilled holes in the wall to a quick-coupling type of outlet. A **quick-coupling outlet** on the wall of the treatment room is ideal because it permits rapid hookup and disengagement of the gas machine (Figure 41-9).

Continuous-Flow Gas Machines

N_2O-O_2 continuous-flow gas machines are available as a portable system (Figure 41-10; see Figure 41-1) or as a central storage system (see Figure 41-8). Although each is the same basic unit, the differences between them are the manner in which compressed gases are delivered to the unit and their portability. In the portable system (see Figure 41-10) compressed-gas cylinders are attached to the gas machine at

BOX 41-3

Handling Compressed-Gas Cylinders

- Use no grease, oil, or lubricant of any type to lubricate any part of the gas machine that may come into contact with gases. *This is extremely dangerous.*
- Store full cylinders in the vertical position.
- Store cylinders in an area in which the temperature does not fluctuate; heat should be avoided.
- Handle cylinders with care. Avoid dropping them.
- Open cylinder valves slowly in a counterclockwise direction. Valves must be opened fully to prevent gas leakage from the valve stems.
- Close all cylinder valves tightly when cylinder is not in use, to prevent contamination from water or dirt, regardless of whether the cylinder contains gas or is empty.
- Cylinders should be opened just slightly, allowing some gas to escape, thereby blowing out any particles of dust that may have lodged in the cylinder orifice.

Adapted from Malamed SF, editor: *Sedation: a guide to patient management*, ed 4, St Louis, 2003, Mosby.

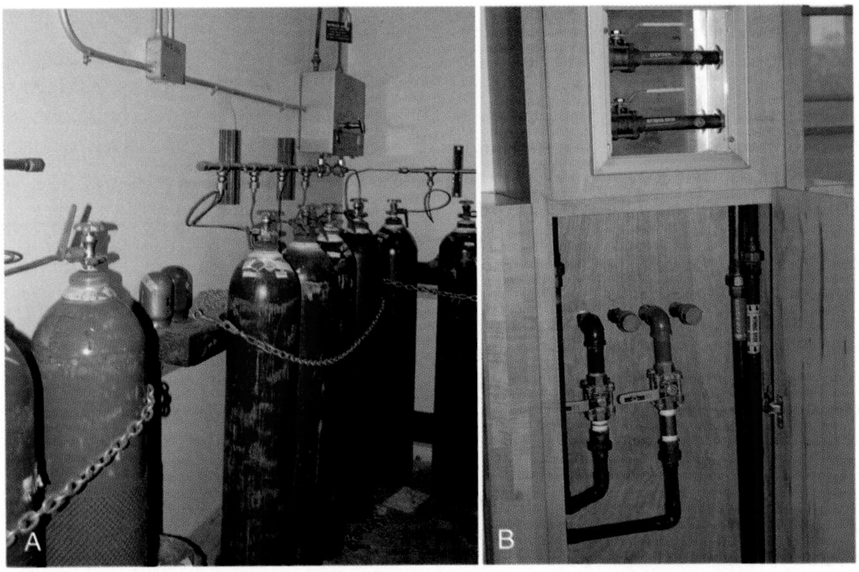

Figure 41-8. **A**, N_2O and O_2 cylinders stored in an area away from the gas machine. **B**, Gas is carried under low pressure to each station outlet in the individual operatories through specially designed wall plumbing. (Courtesy Dr. Mark Dellinges and Cory Price.)

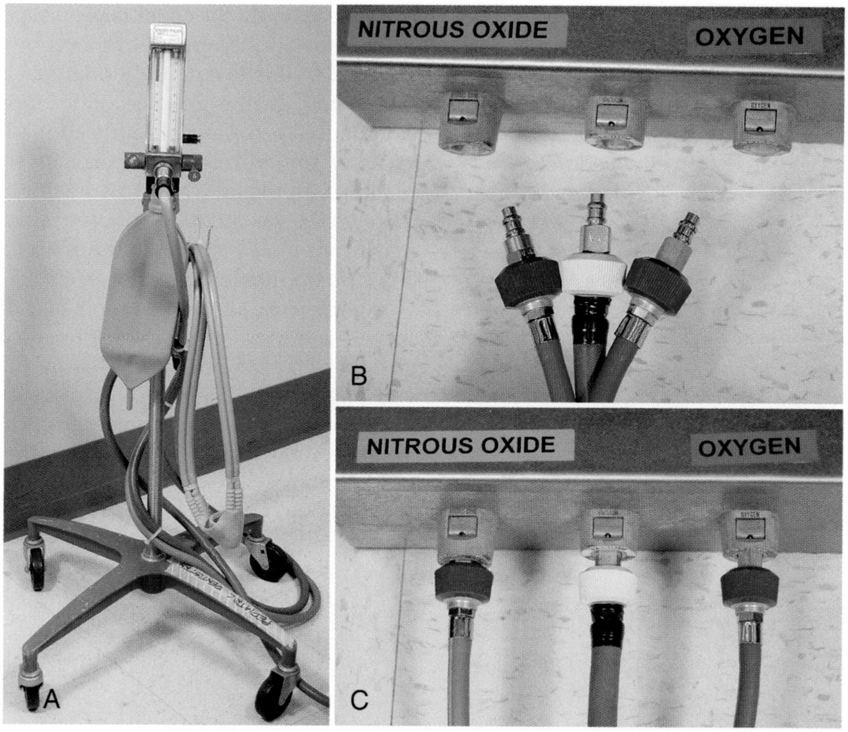

Figure 41-9. A, Quick-coupling gas machine (cylinders are stored in an area away from the gas machine). **B**, Quick-coupling outlets at base of unit or wall. Note different shapes of coupling plugs for N_2O and O_2 as a safety mechanism. **C,** Quick-coupling plug plugged into base of chair. (Courtesy Dr. Mark Dellinges and Cory Price.)

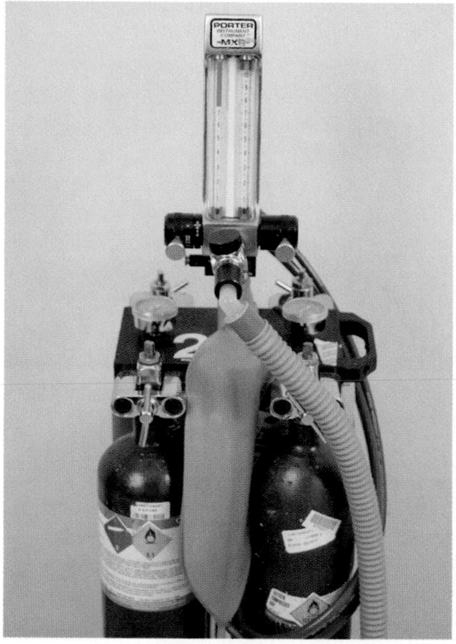

Figure 41-10. Portable gas machine. Compressed gases are attached to the unit at the yoke assembly. (Courtesy Dr. Mark Dellinges.)

the yoke assembly. This system is used in offices where the frequency of N_2O-O_2 use is low or in situations in which the expense of a central storage system is prohibitive.

Components of portable continuous-flow gas machines are yokes, control valves, flowmeters, pressure gauges, a reservoir bag, and a gas hose (Figure 41-11). These major components are discussed in depth below.

Yokes

In the portable continuous-flow gas machine, yokes hold the cylinders in contact with the gas machine (Figure 41-12). From each yoke, gas goes through an automatic pressure-reducing valve and then to a fine-control valve that allows the gas to be delivered to the client at 50 psi.

Flowmeters

The flowmeter indicates the rate of flow of the gas. A small ball floats in the stream of gas that flows upward through a tapered tube. The greater the flow of volume of the gas used, the higher the ball rises. Separate color-coded flowmeters are used for N_2O and O_2, and each is calibrated to measure the volume of gas delivered in liters per minute (L/min) (Figure 41-13). In the United States the O_2 control knob is green, whereas the N_2O control knob is blue. In North America the O_2 flowmeter is positioned on the right side of the bank of flowmeters. Flowmeters show the exact volume and proportions of gas output from the gas machine.

Pressure Gauge

The pressure gauge indicates the pressure of the cylinder contents (see Figures 41-2 and 41-3).

Reservoir Bag

Reservoir bags are bladder-type bags made of rubber or silicone and ranging in size from 1 to 8 L. The 3-L reservoir bag is the most frequently used in dentistry. The reservoir bag is attached to the gas machine. A portion of the gases being delivered through the unit to the client is diverted into the reservoir bag, where it is mixed and stored for use if the respiratory demands of the client exceed the gas flow being delivered from the machine. During normal respiration the client receives only gases delivered from the sedation unit, with little or none being taken from the reservoir bag. However, should the client take an especially deep breath, the machine will be unable to accommodate the necessary volume. In this event, additional gas is drawn from the reservoir bag. In the absence of the reservoir bag, the client experiences a feeling of suffocation. The reservoir bag prevents or minimizes this occurrence so that the client has a plentiful supply on which to draw for breathing. The gas hose delivers the gas mixture from the reservoir bag to the client's mask continually at the volumes and proportions set by the clinician on the flowmeter.

Another use of the reservoir bag during conscious sedation is as a monitoring device for respiration. Assuming an airtight seal of the mask and no mouth breathing, the reservoir bag inflates slightly with every exhalation and deflates slightly with each inspiration, permitting the dental hygienist to observe the respiratory rate (Figure 41-14).

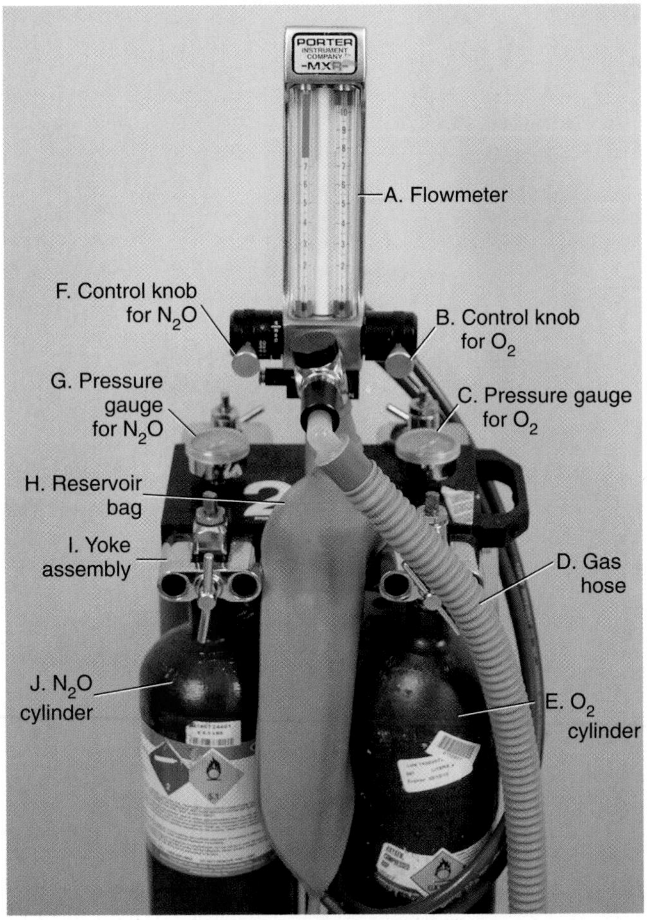

Figure 41-11. Continuous-flow inhalation sedation unit (portable, front view). **A**, Flowmeter. **B**, Control knob for O_2. **C**, Pressure gauge for O_2. **D**, Gas hose. **E**, O_2 cylinder. **F**, Control knob for N_2O. **G**, Pressure gauge for N_2O. **H**, Reservoir bag. **I**, Yoke assembly. **J**, N_2O cylinder. (Courtesy Dr. Mark Dellinges.)

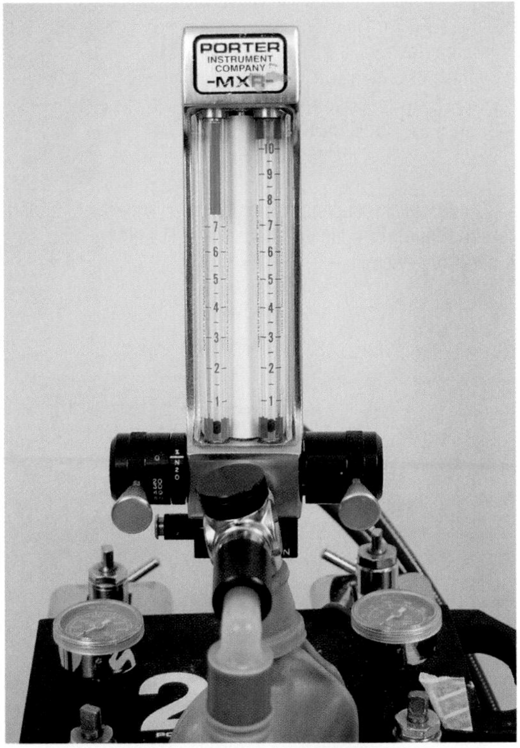

Figure 41-13. Flowmeter. (Courtesy Dr. Mark Dellinges.)

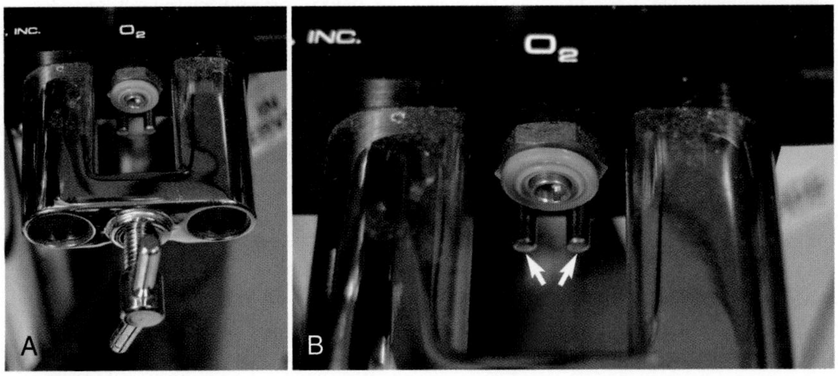

Figure 41-12. **A**, Yoke assembly to hold cylinder in contact with gas machine. Note prongs that will insert into the valve stem of the O_2 cylinder. **B**, Close-up of prongs. (Courtesy Dr. Mark Dellinges and Cory Price.)

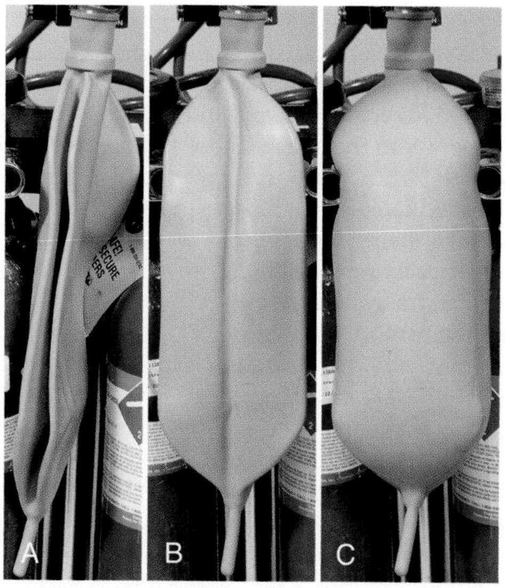

Figure 41-14. **A**, Deflated reservoir bag usually indicates either a leak around the mask or a deficient tidal volume. **B,** Partially inflated reservoir bag usually indicates adequate seal and tidal volume. **C**, Distended reservoir bag indicates either an overly large minute volume or occluded breathing tubes. (Courtesy Dr. Mark Dellinges and Cory Price.)

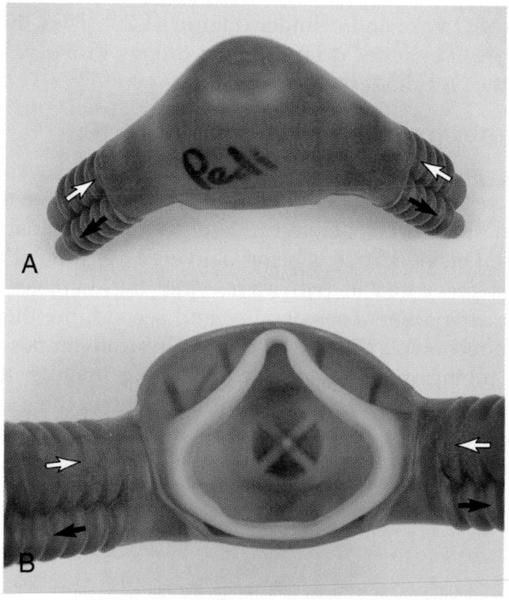

Figure 41-15. **A**, An exterior view of a nasal mask. Gas intake *(white arrows)*, waste gas removal *(black arrows)*. **B,** An interior view of a Brown mask revealing the double-mask construction and gas flow. (Courtesy Dr. Mark Dellinges.)

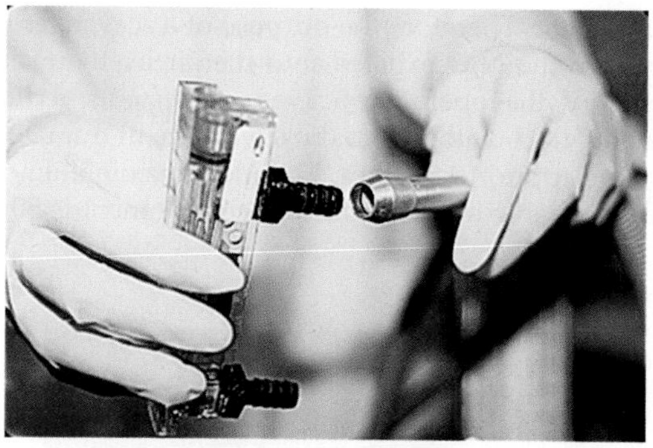

Figure 41-16. The suction calibrator is attached to the high-speed vacuum and adjusted to obtain the optimal level of suction for the scavenger system.

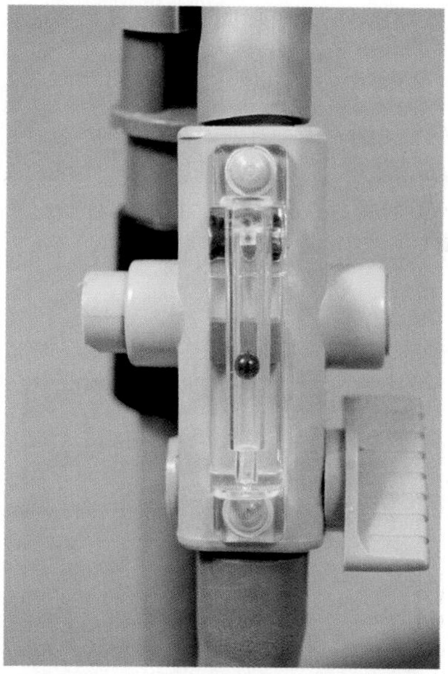

Figure 41-17. Suction calibrator. (Courtesy Dr. Mark Dellinges and Cory Price.)

Nasal Mask

The nasal mask is the nasal inhaler through which the client breathes the N_2O-O_2 analgesic. Masks come with and without a scavenger system. With concern over the possible long-term effects of trace levels of N_2O on chairside personnel, the scavenging nasal mask has been developed. The scavenging mask is the most effective means of minimizing N_2O contamination in the oral healthcare treatment area.[1,2]

Although a number of scavenging nasal masks are available, the principle behind their effectiveness is similar. The Brown nosepiece was one of the earliest scavenging devices and serves as the example in Figure 41-15. In general, scavenging nasal masks have a double nosepiece that consists of a smaller inner mask receiving anesthetic gases from the machine and a slightly larger outer mask that sits directly over the first, which removes exhaled gases from the treatment area. The outer nosepiece is connected to the suction device in the dental unit, permitting exhaled gases to be vented from the treatment area through the vacuum system.[1,2] The instrument used to calibrate the degree of suction in the high-suction vacuum system is a suction calibrator; it ensures that the suction removes the exhaled N_2O-O_2 at an appropriate rate—not so fast that gas is removed before air has been inhaled, and not so slow that gas overaccumulates in the mask and leaks into the breathing zone of the clinician. The suction calibrator is attached to the high-speed vacuum system (Figure 41-16), and the suction is adjusted until the steel ball in the calibrator is made to float in the green zone of the calibrator window (Figure 41-17). If there is no scavenger system in place, the mask will have only one hose coming off each side of it (Figure 41-18). These hoses carry the N_2O-O_2 to the client. However, if there is a scavenger system in place, the mask has two hoses coming off each side of it (Figure 41-19). One pair of hoses delivers the N_2O-O_2 to the client, and the other pair carries away the exhaled N_2O-O_2 into the suction system. Therefore the purpose of a scavenger system is to reduce the N_2O exhaled into the air by the client and breathed by the operator. Scavenger systems reduce the amount of N_2O breathed into the environment from 900 parts per million (ppm) to 30 ppm. The ideal maximal amount of N_2O-O_2 allowable in the healthcare environment is 50 ppm.

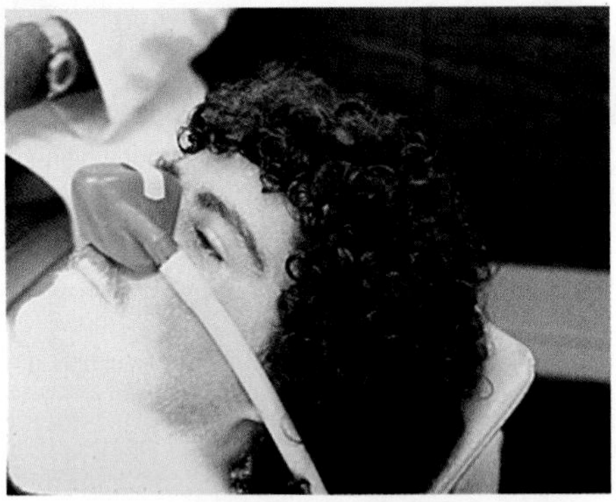

Figure 41-18. Nasal mask with only one hose coming off each side of it, indicating there is no scavenger system in place.

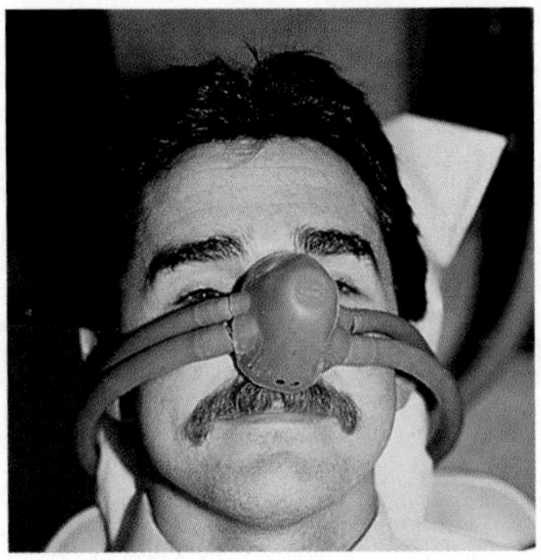

Figure 41-19. Nasal mask with two hoses coming off each side of it, indicating that there is a scavenging system in place.

Safety Measures

Safety features are built into cylinders and gas machines to prevent the inadvertent delivery of N_2O when one is intending to deliver O_2 to the client. These failsafe mechanisms are as follows[1,2]:

- Color-coded tanks
- Pin index system
- Diameter index system
- Audible alarm system
- Automatic turnoff
- O_2 automatically maintained at 2 to 3 L
- O_2 flush

Color-Coding

Cylinders, quick-coupling tubing, outlets, flowmeters, and pressure gauges are color-coded according to the gas they contain and monitor. Green indicates O_2 and blue indicates N_2O.

Pin Indexing System

The pin indexing safety system consists of prongs (pins) on the yoke that hold the O_2 cylinder and the corresponding holes on the O_2 cylinder head that are placed a specific distance apart, which is different from that of their counterparts on the N_2O yoke and cylinder (Figure 41-20). Thus the holes on the N_2O cylinder do not fit the prongs in the yoke that holds the O_2 cylinder and vice versa.

Diameter Indexing System

The diameter index safety system is designed to ensure that the correct medical gas enters the correct part of the gas machine to prevent delivering N_2O to an individual in the mistaken belief that O_2 is being delivered. Accidental attachment is prevented in two ways. First, the diameter of the attachments differs considerably, and second, the threading of the attachments differs, making it physically impossible to attach tubing inadvertently to the wrong inlet on the gas machine (Figure 41-21). Once in the machine, the gases are directed to the appropriate flowmeters, where precise volumes may be delivered to the client.[1,2]

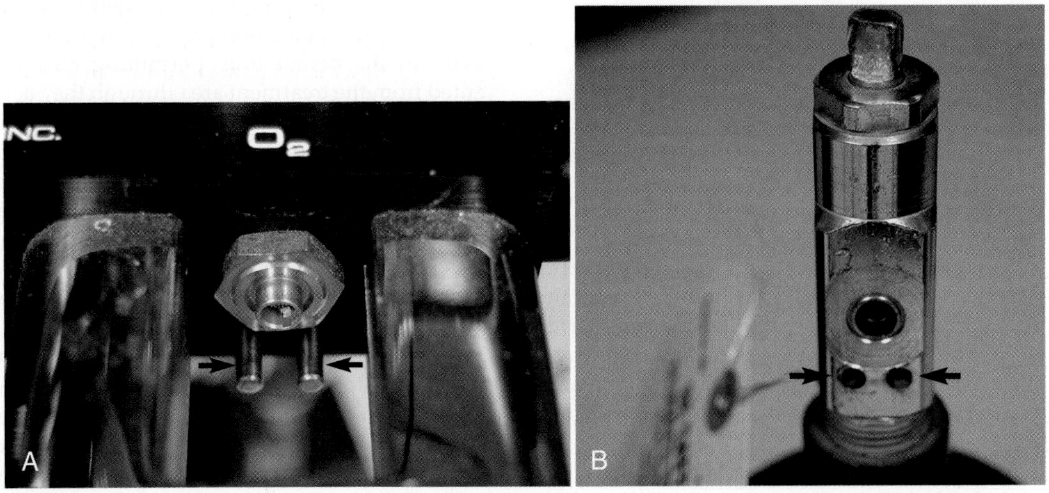

Figure 41-20. **A,** Pins *(arrows)* that are located on the yoke of the gas machine are aligned to permit attachment of only one specific type of compressed gas, either O_2 or NO_2 but not both. **B,** O_2 cylinder head with holes *(arrows)* placed at a specific distance apart to fit the prongs on the yoke designed to hold O_2 cylinder. (Courtesy Dr. Mark Dellinges.)

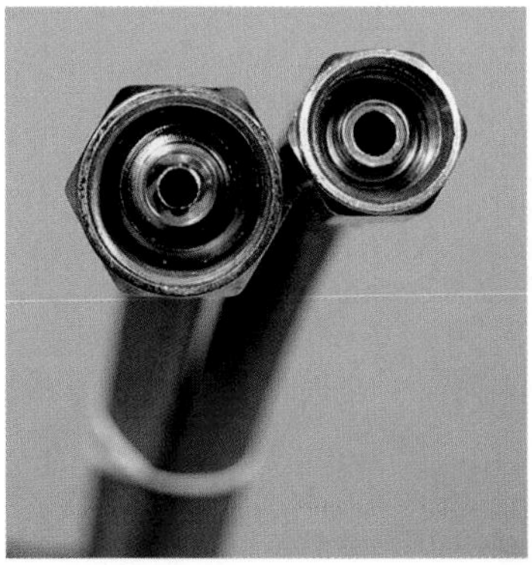

Figure 41-21. Diameter index safety system. Diameter and threading of N_2O coupling *(left)* differ from those of O_2 coupling *(right)*, thus preventing accidental attachments to wrong side of inhalation unit. (Courtesy Dr. Mark Dellinges and Cory Price.)

Indicators That Oxygen Is Depleted

Many gas machines have an alarm that goes off when the O_2 runs out. Other machines simply turn off automatically when the O_2 is depleted. These features prevent the operator from administering 100% N_2O to the client.

Automatic Maintenance of Minimal O_2 Levels

On most gas machines the O_2 flowmeter cannot go below 2 to 3 L of O_2. When the machine is turned on, the O_2 volume automatically goes to 2 to 3 L. This constant flow of O_2 is provided at all times when the gas machine is on, thus preventing the possibility of providing 100% N_2O to the client.

Oxygen Flush Button

All machines have an O_2 flush button that, when pushed, fills the reservoir bag with 100% O_2 and enables O_2 at a high flow rate to be administered to the client very quickly, if needed.

Administration

Administration of N_2O-O_2 includes the following:

- Inducing the appropriate level of analgesia
- Monitoring the individual during the sedation period
- Oxygenating the individual for the appropriate amount of time on completion of treatment

Although a step-by-step approach to N_2O-O_2 administration is explained in Procedure 41-1 and the corresponding Competency Form, the general points are highlighted for emphasis in the following sections.

Preparation

The office should have a quiet atmosphere throughout the sedation period. All oral healthcare personnel who interact with clients should experience the sensations produced by N_2O-O_2 sedation. This experience allows them to relate their feelings to clients. In addition, the dental hygienist prepares the N_2O-O_2 armamentaria before seating clients scheduled to receive the sedation procedure. On seating, clients are asked if they need to visit the restroom. Those who wear contact lenses also are asked to remove them because sometimes gas escaping from the mask can dry out the cornea and increase the risk of corneal abrasion.

After reviewing the health history and vital signs, the dental hygienist explains to the client what is about to happen and describes the sensations of warmth and tingling that will be experienced. For example, clients are told that they will feel very relaxed, as if they have had a couple of alcoholic drinks. The dental hygienist assures clients that they are in complete control throughout the sedation procedure in the sense that if they feel they are receiving too much N_2O-O_2 sedation, they just need to inform the operator, who will turn down the N_2O and turn up the O_2, which will increase the feeling of normalcy. The client then is positioned in a comfortable, reclined position in the dental chair. The partially reclined position may be used for client comfort and clinician convenience during the procedure (Figure 41-22).

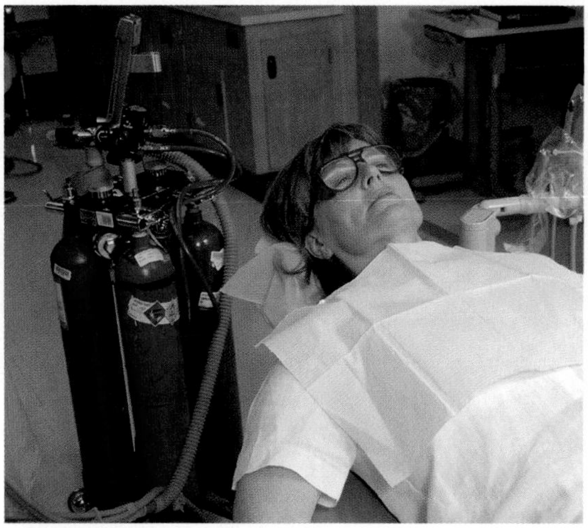

Figure 41-22. Client is in a comfortable reclined position. (Courtesy Dr. Mark Dellinges.)

Estimate Tidal Volume, Start Flow of Oxygen, Secure Nasal Mask Over Client's Nose

Starting the flow of O_2 before placing the nasal mask on the client prevents the client from feeling suffocated when breathing through the nose. The client's tidal volume is estimated. **Tidal volume** is the amount of air a person needs for one respiration cycle. For an average adult, it could be from 6 to 8 L, depending on the size and metabolic rate of the individual. A flow of O_2 is introduced based on the estimated tidal volume. For example, if the tidal volume is estimated to be 6 L, the O_2 flowmeter is set to a 6 L/min flow of 100% O_2, and the nose mask is placed over the nose and centered on the face snugly to prevent leakage at the edges of the mask. The nasal mask should have two pairs of hoses on each side of it. These are placed around the sides of the dental chair, and the nasal mask is secured by adjusting the slip ring behind the back of the chair (Figure 41-23). The client may be asked to hold the nasal mask in a comfortable position as this is being done. If the mask is too big and gas is escaping at its edges, a gauze square may be used to contour around the mask to adapt it to the client's nose and plug some of the leakage spaces (Figure 41-24). After mask adjustment, clients are asked if they have enough air to breathe comfortably. If not, the tidal volume of 100% O_2 is increased. If the air is reported to be blowing up the client's nose, the tidal volume of O_2 is decreased. The client must be able to breathe comfortably before the start of N_2O flow to be comfortable throughout the procedure.[1]

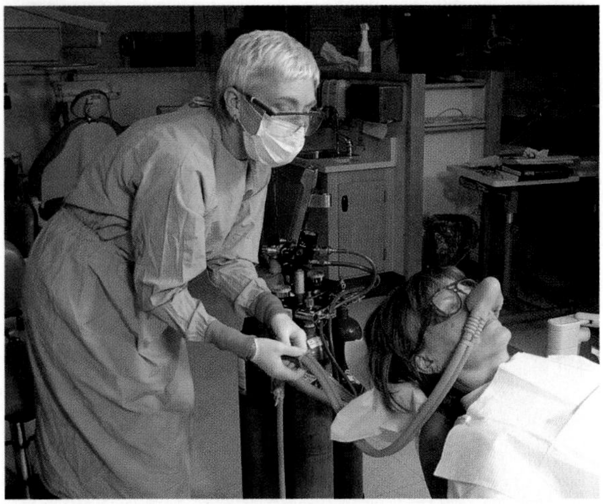

Figure 41-23. Nasal mask is secured by adjusting slip ring behind back of chair. (Courtesy Dr. Mark Dellinges.)

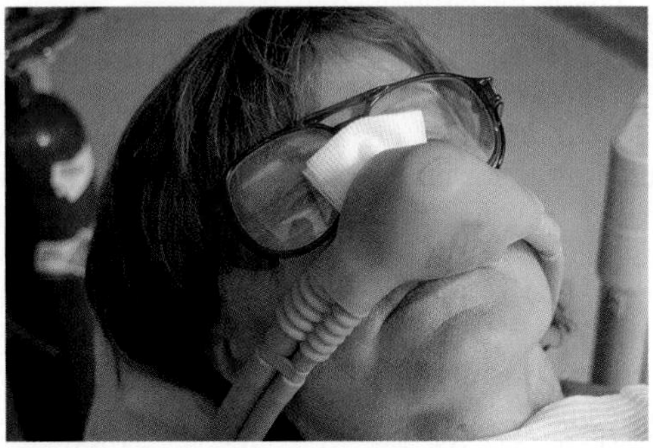

Figure 41-24. Folded 2- × 2-inch gauze on bridge of nose prevents leaks. (Courtesy Dr. Mark Dellinges.)

Titration of Nitrous Oxide–Oxygen

Titration is the process of adjusting the percentage of gases (N_2O and O_2) to the desired concentration of N_2O and O_2 gases while keeping the total liter flow of gases (tidal volume) constant. The goal of titration is to produce baseline sedation signs and symptoms in the client. Once the correct tidal volume has been established with 100% O_2 and documented in the client's record, a **constant liter flow technique** is used to introduce N_2O at the rate of 0.5 to 1 L/min while decreasing the O_2 flow at a similar rate. This constant liter flow technique keeps the total liter flow of gases (N_2O and O_2) per minute constant throughout the procedure. For example, given a tidal volume of 6 L/min, the dental hygienist increases the N_2O flow to 1 L/min and then decreases the O_2 flow rate to 5 L/min. A 1- to 2-minute pause is made after each adjustment, during which the dental hygienist observes the client for signs of baseline. After the pause the hygienist asks the client how he or she is feeling, to evaluate responses for symptoms indicating the client has reached baseline. This process is repeated until the baseline state is reached. Generally for dental hygiene care, 50% N_2O or less is effective for achieving baseline. Once baseline is reached, the operator should drop back on the N_2O flow about 0.5 to 1 L, because with time the intensity of the sedation increases. This titration technique minimizes the risk of overshooting baseline and causing a problem by carrying the person too deeply into the excitement stage of general anesthesia.

Once baseline is reached, the dental hygienist works efficiently and quietly, asking clients periodically how they are doing. Unnecessary talking is avoided to allow clients to relate to the sedation and because their talking expels N_2O into the immediate environment of the practitioner.

Health history and vital signs WNL; TV = 7 L; N_2O = 2 L (29%); O_2 = 5 L (71%) for 45 minutes. Oxygenation period = 15 minutes. Client did well. Probing WNL, scaled and polished. Excellent oral hygiene, no gingival inflammation observed throughout. Continued-care interval 6 months.

Figure 41-25. Sample entry in client's record.

BOX 41-4

Calculating the Percentage of Gas Being Delivered

$$\text{Percentage of } N_2O = \frac{L/min\ N_2O}{L/min\ O_2 + L/min\ N_2O}$$

$$\text{Percentage of } O_2 = \frac{L/min\ O_2}{L/min\ O_2 + L/min\ N_2O}$$

Oxygenation, Client Discharge, and Documentation

When scaling and root planing are completed, the N_2O is turned off and the O_2 increased to maintain the tidal volume. For every 15 minutes of exposure to N_2O, the client must receive 5 minutes of 100% O_2. Therefore, if clients receive 45 minutes of N_2O-O_2 sedation, they should receive 15 minutes of 100% O_2 at the end of the sedation procedure. If clients are sedated for less than 5 minutes, they still are oxygenated for a minimum of 5 minutes. This oxygenation period is essential to prevent tissue hypoxia, characterized by headache and upset stomach, on completion of the sedation procedure.

The tidal volume, the time baseline was reached, and the amount or percentage of gases administered should be recorded in the client's chart. To calculate the percentage of gases administered, the flow rate of a specific gas is divided by the tidal volume and multiplied by 100 (Box 41-4). For example, if the client's tidal volume (TV) is 7 L/min, the O_2 flow is 5 L/min, and the N_2O flow rate is 2 L/min, the percentage of N_2O delivered is $2/7 \times 100$, which is 29% of total flow, and the percentage of O_2 delivered is $5/7 \times 100$, which is 71%. Notation for documentation would be as follows:

TV = 7 L
N_2O = $2/7$ or 29%
O_2 = $5/7$ or 71%

In addition to the tidal volume and the percentages of gases used, the duration of sedation, the length of the oxygenation period, the client's response, and the dental hygiene care delivered should be documented in the client's chart (Figure 41-25).

Procedure 41-1 Administration of Nitrous Oxide–Oxygen Analgesic Using the Constant Liter Flow Technique

EQUIPMENT

Personal protective barriers
Gas machine
Sterilized nasal mask
2 × 2 gauze
Saliva ejector
Suction calibrator

STEPS

Prepare Equipment

1. Prepare the gas machine and related armamentaria before seating the client. Select appropriate sterilized nasal mask for size and attach it to mask tubing.
2. Open gas cylinder valves and check gas supply. Open oxygen (O_2) tank slowly, then the nitrous oxide (N_2O) cylinder. (Centralized systems are turned on at the beginning of the day.) (See Figure 41-26.)
3. Obtain suction calibrator, attach it to the high-speed vacuum system, and adjust the suction until the steel ball in the calibrator is made to float in the green zone of the calibrator's window (Figure 41-27).
4. Remove the suction calibrator from the high-speed suction system, and tape in place the button used to adjust the suction.
5. Connect the sterilized nose mask to two hoses coming off each side of it (Figure 41-28). Each pair of hoses is joined by an adaptor.

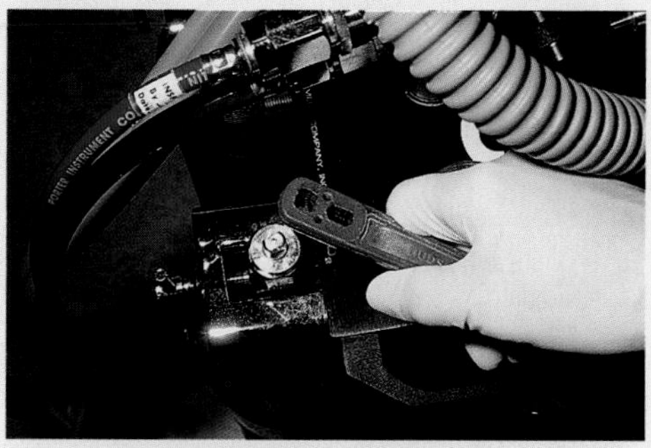

Figure 41-26. Opening gas cylinder valves.

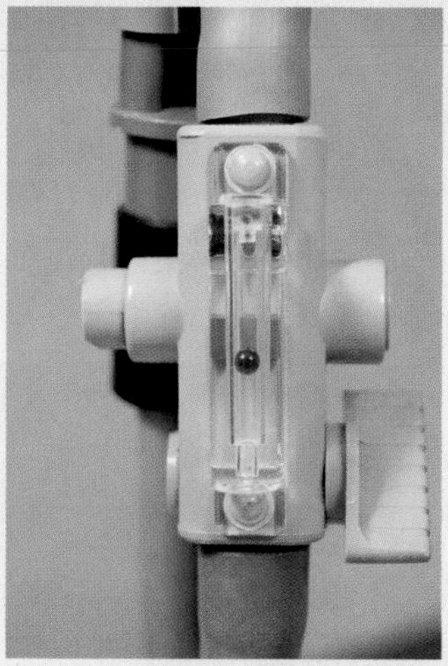

Figure 41-27. Suction calibration. (Courtesy Dr. Mark Dellinges and Cory Price.)

6. Connect the larger adaptor on the nasal mask to the gas machine (Figure 41-29).
7. Connect the smaller adaptor on the nasal mask to the calibrated high-speed suction system (Figure 41-30).
8. Turn on the gas machine.

Prepare the Client

9. Seat the client; check and record the health history, blood pressure, and pulse (Figure 41-31).
10. Request that the client visit the restroom if necessary.
11. If client wears contact lenses, request that they be removed before the start of the sedation procedure.
12. Familiarize client with procedures; discuss nasal breathing and nose mask, and describe sensations of warmth and tingling that will be experienced. Reaffirm the relaxing, comfortable feeling the client will experience. Assure clients that they will be aware of and in control of their actions (Figure 41-32).
13. Position client in comfortable, reclined position in dental chair.
14. Start O_2 flow at an estimated tidal volume of 6 L/min (Figure 41-33).
15. Activate O_2 flush valve to fill the reservoir bag with O_2.

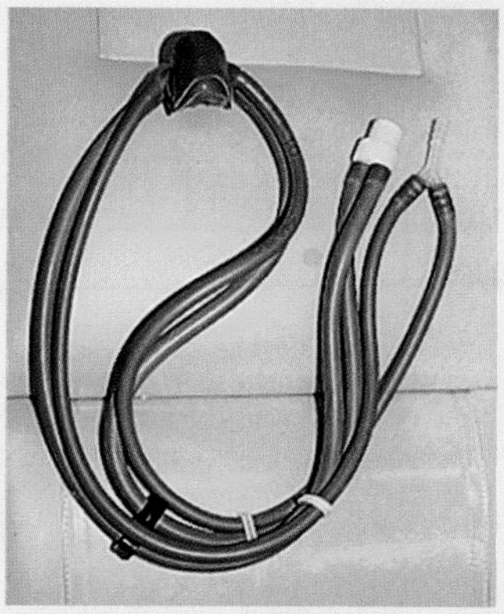

Figure 41-28. Nasal mask with two pairs of hoses.

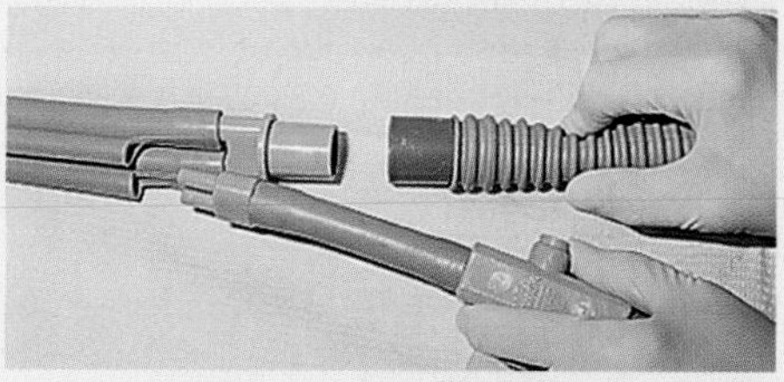

Figure 41-29. Attaching the larger adaptor of the sterilized nasal mask to the gas machine gas hose (held in right hand).

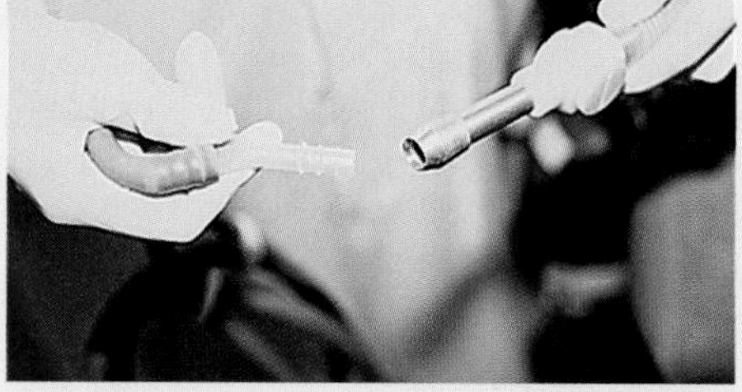

Figure 41-30. Attaching the smaller adaptor on the sterilized nasal mask to calibrated high-speed suction to provide for the scavenging system.

Continued

Procedure 41-1 Administration of Nitrous Oxide–Oxygen Analgesic Using the Constant Liter Flow Technique—cont'd

16. Seat the nasal mask and have client hold the mask in a comfortable position while you adjust the slip ring to hold the mask in place (Figure 41-34).
17. Confirm comfortable mask fit with the client. If mask is impinging on a sensitive area on the face or if mask is too big, place a gauze square under the edge of the mask (Figure 41-35).

Determine Exact Tidal Volume

18. Remind the client to breathe through the nose.
19. Ask the client if he or she has enough air to breathe comfortably. Adjust volume of O_2 as per client response. If client requests a greater volume, increase the O_2 by 1 L, wait a minute, and then ask the same question. This process is repeated until the client becomes comfortable and the exact tidal volume is established (Figure 41-36).

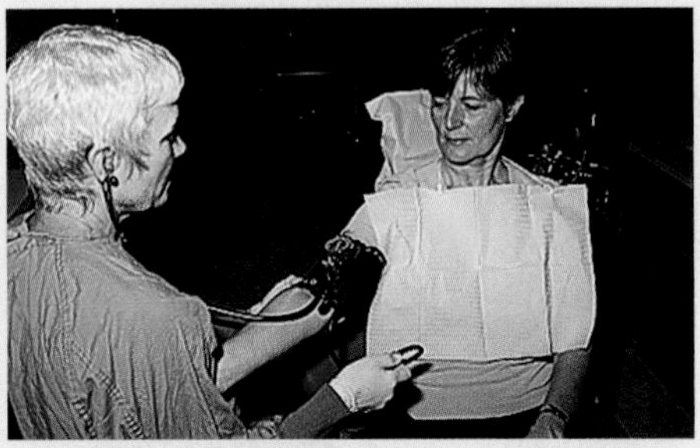

Figure 41-31. Checking client's vital signs.

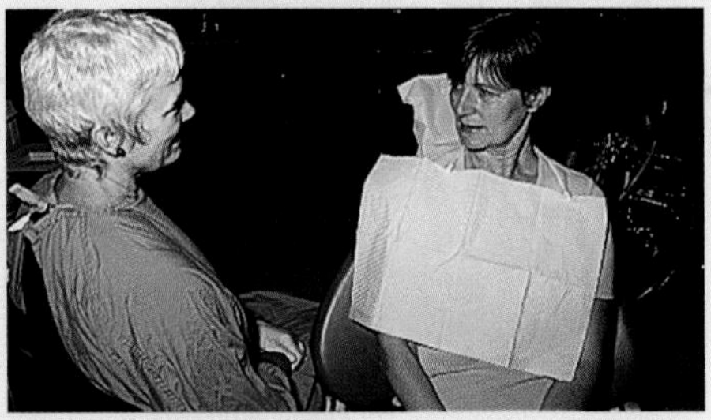

Figure 41-32. Familiarizing client with procedure.

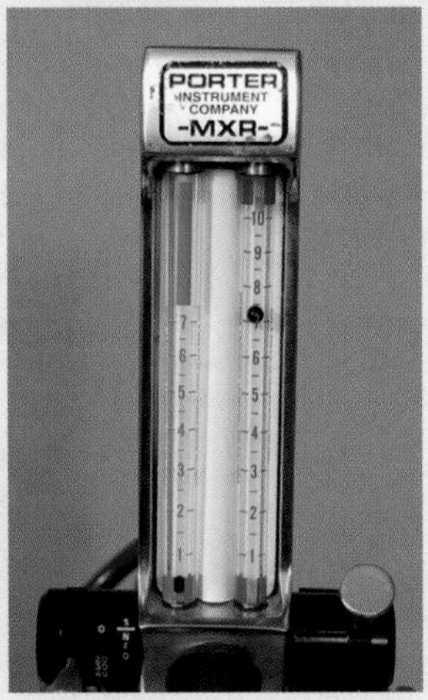

Figure 41-33. Start O_2 flow at estimated tidal volume. (Courtesy Dr. Mark Dellinges.)

20. Observe the reservoir bag as an indicator of appropriate flow rate.
21. Write the established tidal volume in the client record.

Begin Titration of N_2O

22. Decrease O_2 by 0.5 L, and introduce 0.5 L/min of N_2O (Figure 41-37). Wait 60 to 90 seconds and observe the client for signs of sedation. At the end of the 60- to 90-second waiting period, ask the client, "What are you feeling?" It is important to ask an open-ended question that requires the client to respond with more than a simple "yes" or "no."
23. Continue titration of N_2O. If the initial concentration of N_2O proves inadequate, decrease the level of O_2 again by 0.5 to 1 L and increase N_2O by 0.5 to 1 L. Again wait 60 to 90 seconds, observing the client, then question the client to elicit signs and symptoms of baseline.
24. Continue titration (i.e., decreasing O_2 by 0.5 to 1 L and increasing N_2O by 0.5 to 1 L and waiting 60 to 90 seconds to observe for signs, then questioning to elicit symptoms) until observation and questioning elicit positive indications of baseline.
25. Record the time the baseline was reached and the associated percentages of N_2O and O_2 in the client's chart.
26. Monitor client and reassure as necessary; comment on how comfortable and relaxed the client seems.

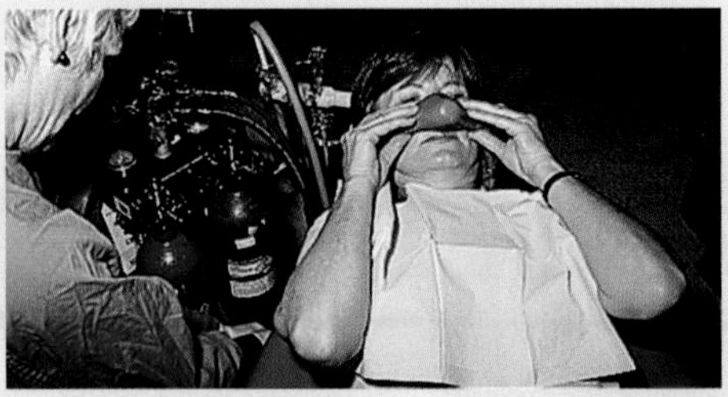

Figure 41-34. Client holding nasal mask in a comfortable position while dental hygienist adjusts the mask tubes to hold the mask in place.

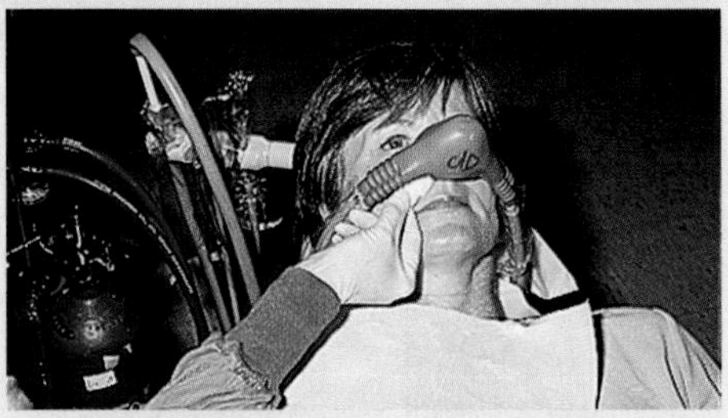

Figure 41-35. Placing gauze square under the edge of the mask.

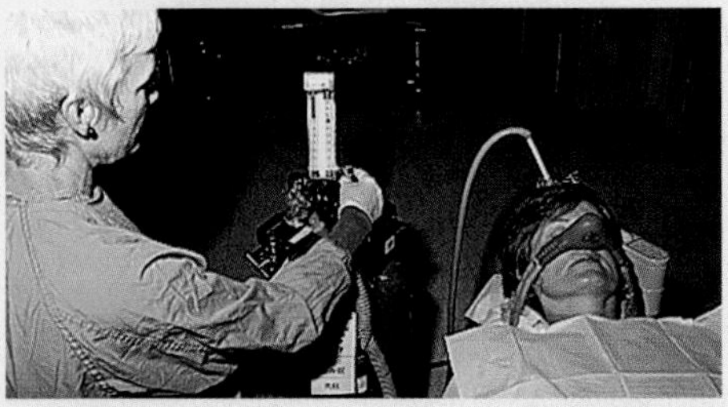

Figure 41-36. Determining the tidal volume.

Procedure 41-1 Administration of Nitrous Oxide–Oxygen Analgesic Using the Constant Liter Flow Technique—cont'd

27. Begin dental hygiene care and continue to observe the client and gas machine during the procedure.

Terminate the Flow of N_2O and Begin Oxygenation

28. Near the end of the appointment (e.g., during tooth polishing), discontinue the N_2O, and increase the O_2 concentration to 100%.
29. Oxygenate 5 minutes for every 15 minutes of exposure to N_2O-O_2.

Discharge the Client and Document Procedure in Chart

30. Remove the nose mask and slowly bring the client to an upright position (Figure 41-38).
31. If the client feels normal, discharge him or her (Figure 41-39).
32. Document the experience in the client's record. Note vital signs, concentrations of N_2O and O_2 administered, length of time of sedation and oxygenation, the care provided, and the client's response to the sedation (Figure 41-40).

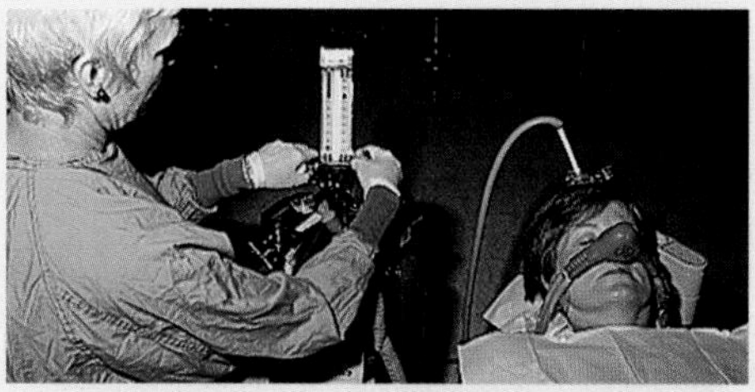

Figure 41-37. Initiating titration of N_2O.

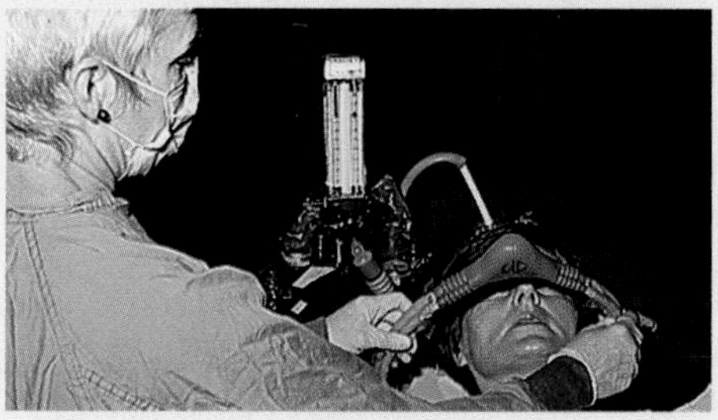

Figure 41-38. Removing nasal mask.

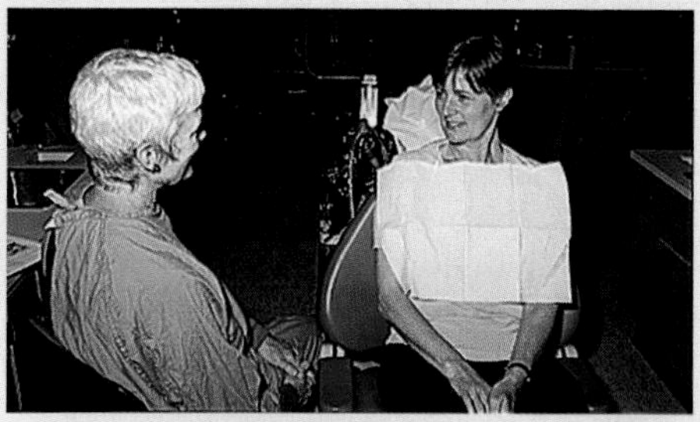

Figure 41-39. Assessing client before discharge.

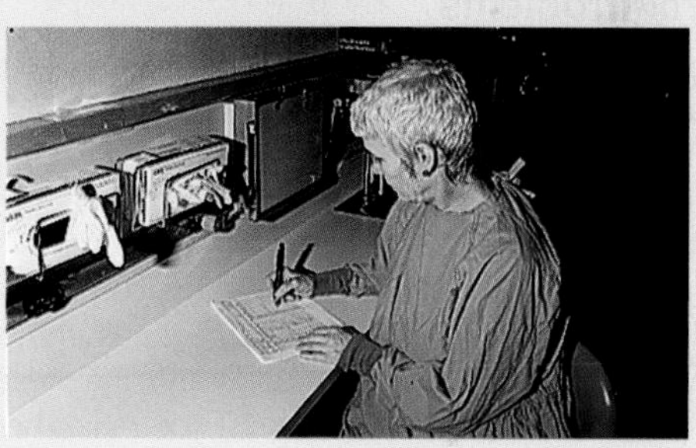

Figure 41-40. Documenting care rendered.

The specific techniques for N_2O-O_2 administration are presented in Procedure 41-1.

Potential Complications

Complications[1] associated with N_2O-O_2 can be mitigated by carefully selecting candidates based on their health and personal history, and by adopting the technique described in Procedure 41-1 for the administration of this sedation modality. Specifically, inducing clients to an individualized baseline level by the process of titration and oxygenating them for an appropriate amount of time facilitate the avoidance of some complications with this somewhat innocuous agent. The possible complications associated with N_2O-O_2 sedation are as follows[1]:

- Diffusion hypoxia
- Head injury during expectoration
- Nausea
- Vomiting
- Corneal irritation
- Behavior problems
- Airway obstruction
- Repeated closing of the mouth
- Rigid mandible
- Reluctance to awaken
- Emotional reaction
- Excessive perspiration

Diffusion Hypoxia

Diffusion hypoxia, a lack of O_2 to the tissues, is characterized by headache, grogginess, nausea, and what generally may be described as a "hungover" feeling after exposure to N_2O-O_2 analgesia. This complication is related to not being oxygenated for an appropriate period after the completion of the sedation procedure.

Head Injury During Expectoration

Sedated clients are at risk for bumping their heads on the cuspidor if they attempt to expectorate while under sedation. Consequently, a saliva ejector or high-vacuum suction should be used in place of allowing the client to rinse or expectorate into a cuspidor. If such expectoration cannot be avoided, however, the clinician should place her or his hand on the client's forehead to guide the client to the cuspidor and prevent possible injury.

Nausea and Vomiting

Nausea and vomiting are associated with giving the client too much N_2O-O_2 sedation, although it also may occur when the client consumes a heavy meal before the dental hygiene care appointment. In addition, nausea can be brought on by fluctuating the N_2O levels back and forth during the titration process. For example, giving a client 3 L of N_2O then increasing the amount to 5 L and decreasing it back down to

4 L and then back up to 6 L in a short period can produce nausea. If a client indicates nausea (either verbally by self-report or nonverbally by holding the stomach), the N_2O should be turned down by 2 L and O_2 increased by 2 L. If the nausea persists, N_2O should be discontinued and the client should be given 100% O_2 for an appropriate oxygenation period.

If vomiting occurs, the N_2O must be turned off immediately, the mask removed, and the client's head turned to the side away from the operator to facilitate emesis (see Figure 41-5). A high-vacuum suction may be used to facilitate removal of vomitus (see Figure 41-6). The client is given a cool, wet towel to clean up, and the treatment area cleaned as quickly as possible. The individual is reassured that he or she will feel better after breathing 100% O_2.

Corneal Irritation

Leakage of gas from the mask can dry out the eyes and cause corneal abrasion in individuals wearing contact lenses. This problem can be prevented by having clients remove their contact lenses before the N_2O-O_2 sedation is administered to them.

Behavioral Problems

Several types of behavioral problems can be associated with N_2O-O_2 sedation. Repeated closing of the mouth and a rigidity of the mandible are usually signs of too much N_2O. Turning the N_2O down by 2 L and increasing the O_2 by 2 L eliminate the problem.

Individuals who do not like to give up control often are threatened by the tingling and floating feelings characteristic of this mode of sedation. As a result, they may respond by suddenly sitting forward and taking off the mask because of fear of the unknown or of becoming unconscious. This problem can be prevented by carefully screening candidates for this sedation method, thoroughly explaining what they can expect to experience, and never talking clients into having N_2O-O_2.

Individuals who are going through a period of emotional instability may be prone to crying under the influence of N_2O-O_2 sedation. If this occurs, the N_2O should be discontinued and 100% O_2 should be given for an appropriate oxygenation period. Careful screening of candidates before offering this sedation modality prevents this problem, which can be embarrassing to client and clinician.

Sexual fantasies and attempts at amorous behavior have been reported in individuals who have been given N_2O concentration greater than 50% and who were sedated without an assistant as a witness in the room. Decreasing the amount of N_2O by at least 2 L and increasing the O_2 by a corresponding amount may solve the problem. If not, the N_2O should be discontinued and 100% O_2 given to the client for an appropriate amount of time. Individuals who respond with this type of behavior problem should not be judged harshly because they have placed themselves in the care of the clinician and have allowed their sense of reality to be altered based on the trust and confidence they have in the clinician. It is the responsibility of the clinician to protect the client while the client is under the clinician's care.

Equipment Malfunction

Contaminated N_2O cylinders can contain nitrogen dioxide and on administration may produce nitric acid with serious consequences to a client. Valves on the N_2O cylinders must be kept closed when not in use to prevent this dire circumstance from occurring.[1]

Hazards to Personnel

The effects of chronic exposure to N_2O (1000 to 15,000 ppm) reported in animal and human studies of operating room personnel and of oral surgeons and others who used N_2O in their practice include the following:

- Spontaneous abortion
- Birth defects
- Bone marrow depression
- Anemia
- Hepatic and renal diseases
- Cancer

Hazardous concentrations of N_2O in the oral healthcare setting can be reduced from 900 ppm to 30 ppm using a combination of the following methods:

- Using an N_2O scavenging system
- Fitting the nasal mask to the client as well as possible
- Discouraging client conversation and mouth breathing
- Venting the suction machine containing the exhaled gases outside the building
- Using a fan to direct the N_2O away from the breathing zone of the operator
- Maintaining the anesthetic equipment, testing for leakage, and inspecting the connectors at frequent intervals
- Monitoring N_2O in the oral healthcare environment; a badge can be worn to detect N_2O levels in the operator's breathing zone
- Opening a window in the treatment area to improve air circulation or using a nonrecycling air-conditioning system
- Limiting the duration of N_2O exposure for clients
- Shutting off and securing the equipment at the end of each day that it is used

CLIENT EDUCATION TIPS

- Explain what nitrous oxide–oxygen (N_2O-O_2) analgesia is and what it does.
- Explain the sensations that will be experienced, and describe them in positive terms (e.g., warmth, tingling).
- Explain that clients are in control and responsive at all times. If they feel they are receiving too much sedation, they just need to say so and the hygienist will turn down the N_2O and turn up the O_2.
- Advise no heavy meals, alcohol, or fasting before the appointment.
- Explain the importance of contact lens removal to avoid extreme drying of the eyes resulting from gas leaks around the mask, which could lead to corneal abrasion.

LEGAL, ETHICAL, AND SAFETY ISSUES

- The dental hygienist has the legal responsibility to practice within the scope authorized by state law concerning nitrous oxide–oxygen (N_2O-O_2) analgesia administration.
- It is important to gain informed consent.
- The dental hygienist must evaluate carefully the client's health history to determine suitability for N_2O-O_2 sedation.
- The dental hygienist is responsible for protecting the client while the client is under the influence of N_2O-O_2 sedation during dental hygiene care.

- The dental hygienist must document completely the provision of N_2O-O_2 sedation in the client's record, including the client's condition on leaving the dental hygiene care setting.

KEY CONCEPTS

- Delivery of nitrous oxide (N_2O) in combination with oxygen (O_2) is an inhalation method of conscious sedation known as *N_2O-O_2 analgesia.* It relaxes individuals who are mildly apprehensive about the dental or dental hygiene experience and provides pain control for procedures that are only slightly or moderately painful.
- O_2 is present in a compressed-gas cylinder in a gaseous state.
- N_2O is present in a compressed-gas cylinder in a liquid and gaseous state.
- The treatment of entry into the excitement stage of analgesia is increasing the percentage of O_2 immediately to 100%.
- Light anesthesia rather than relative analgesia may be indicated by the patient becoming hyperresponsive to stimuli and producing exaggerated inspiration.
- Subjective symptoms of relative analgesia include heaviness of limbs, floating sensation, tingling, decreased fear, decreased pain memory, desire to maintain that state, feeling of warmth, and decreased awareness of time.
- Objective signs of a desired level of sedation are normal eye reaction and pupil size, normal blood pressure and pulse, ability to answer questions, and relaxation of hands, fingers, and mandible.
- Headache, grogginess, and a "hangover" feeling after N_2O-O_2 are symptoms of diffusion hypoxia.
- Relative contraindications to N_2O-O_2 include breathing difficulties, communication difficulties, epilepsy, pregnancy, nasal obstruction, chronic obstructive pulmonary disease, multiple sclerosis, negative past experience, fear of sedation, and emotional instability.
- N_2O-O_2 sedation may be particularly useful for clients with a history of hypertension, asthma, and cardiovascular disease.
- Nausea after N_2O-O_2 exposure may be induced easily by fluctuating the N_2O delivery.
- Oversedation with N_2O may be manifested by nausea and/or loss of consciousness.
- After the administration of N_2O-O_2 analgesia, O_2 alone should be given for a minimum of 5 minutes for each 15 minutes of use before the client is released.
- When adjusting the proportions of N_2O and O_2 to achieve the desired level of analgesia, the clinician should ensure each adjustment should be at the rate of ½ to 1 L N_2O for at least 1 minute.
- A scavenger system incorporated into the N_2O-O_2 units takes out N_2O that is exhaled through the mask.
- The ideal maximum room air concentration of N_2O is 50 parts per million.
- The effects of chronic exposure to N_2O may include spontaneous abortion, birth defects, bone marrow depression, anemia, hepatic and renal diseases, and cancer.
- To reduce N_2O exposure, the dental hygienist uses a scavenging mask system, discourages unnecessary client talking, and has all the equipment leak-tested regularly.
- Before the mask is placed on the client, a predetermined mixture of N_2O and O_2 never should be established.
- The N_2O blood-gas solubility coefficient of 0.47 accounts for rapid onset of and rapid recovery from N_2O sedation.
- The ideal minimal amount of N_2O needed for a client is referred to as the *baseline.*

CRITICAL THINKING EXERCISES

1. You administer 3 L of N_2O and 3 L of O_2 for 30 minutes to a client. Just as you are finishing the scaling procedure, the client complains of nausea. You oxygenate the client for 15 minutes and after determining the client is fine, dismiss him. What exactly would you write in the treatment record?
2. List five client symptoms that would indicate to you, the operator, to decrease the amount of N_2O at least 2 L and increase the O_2 by the same amount?
3. The flowmeters indicate that the client is receiving 4 L of N_2O and 6 L of O_2. What are the tidal volume and the proportion of N_2O that is being delivered?
4. Scenario:

   Client: Ms. G

   Profile: A 35-year-old woman arrives for dental hygiene care. She wears contact lenses.

   Chief Complaint: "My teeth really need to be cleaned. I have finally got up my courage to come in and have it done."

   Dental History: Client makes regular dental visits, but she is 12 months overdue for her dental hygiene care appointment. She reports her teeth are sensitive.

   Social History: Client is single and lives with her mother.

   Health History: Client's blood pressure is 140/90 mm Hg. She reports she is trying to control it with diet and exercise and is under the care of her physician.

   Oral Self-Care Assessment: Client reports brushing once a day but does not floss or use any other interdental cleaning device.

   Supplemental Notes: Client presents with moderate subgingival calculus and gingival inflammation throughout. Mesial and distal probing depths of 4 to 5 mm are in all posterior teeth.

   A. How would you use this information in planning dental hygiene care to meet the client's need for freedom from fear and stress? What interventions would you plan and why?

   B. Would N_2O-O_2 be beneficial for her? Explain your response.

   C. What would you say in educating Ms. G about her stress-control options during her dental hygiene care appointment?

REFERENCES

1. Malamed SF: *Sedation: a guide to patient management,* ed 4, St Louis, 2003, Mosby.
2. Clark MS, Brunick A: *Handbook of nitrous oxide and oxygen sedation,* ed 3, St Louis, 2008, Mosby.

EVOLVE RESOURCES

Please visit http://evolve.elsevier.com/Darby/hygiene for additional practice and study support tools.

CHAPTER 42

Persons with Disabilities

Kathleen B. Muzzin

COMPETENCIES

1. **Name key legislative policies that benefit disabled persons.**
2. **Identify barriers for clients with special healthcare needs.**
3. **Discuss the value of personal self-worth, including how stereotypes and attitudes affect the acceptance of persons with disabilities.**
4. **Explain the classifications of disabilities, including:**
   - **Distinguish among developmental, acquired, and age-associated disabilities.**
   - **Identify portrayal issues associated with persons with special healthcare needs.**
5. **Describe assistive devices for activities of daily living.**
6. **Describe oral self-care devices.**
7. **Discuss client positioning and stabilization.**
8. **Explain how to stabilize a client during wheelchair transfers and professional care.**
9. **Discuss the opportunities for the dental hygienist in health promotion and advocacy for clients with disabilities.**

Special healthcare needs include a broad spectrum of "physical, developmental, mental, sensory, behavioral, cognitive, and emotional impairments that require medical management, healthcare interventions, and/or use of specialized services or programs."[1] According to the 2010 United States Census Bureau, 56.7 million Americans are considered disabled and have special healthcare needs (Figure 42-1).[2] Over the next 20 years, this figure is expected to increase significantly, especially as the baby boomer generation ages. Medical advancements have reduced the incidence of developmental disorders, childhood illnesses, infectious diseases, and chronic health conditions that can occur among the disabled population. Many disabled people are now living longer, which has created an overwhelming demand for health and rehabilitation services.

Disabilities often are associated with elderly people; however, an individual can be disabled at any time during the life span. Common misconceptions about individuals with disabilities are that they are sick, are dependent on others, are mentally and physically debilitated, or live in institutions. In reality, most of these individuals are capable of living within the community either alone or with assistance. The trend has been to transition these individuals into the local community[3]; **normalization** is a process that enables challenged individuals to engage in normal patterns of everyday life. The outcome is **mainstreaming**, which means incorporating individuals with special needs into conventional activities. This concept promotes **deinstitutionalization** of challenged persons and allows them to live and function independently with little or no assistance from a caregiver.[4] Mainstreaming is the goal of long-term care providers and educators assisting people with disabilities.

Mainstreaming disabled people creates a host of problems—problems that demand attention and resources. Disabled individuals encounter obstacles to healthcare, education, and employment opportunities. Access to these services is essential for persons to function at an acceptable level of health and wellness and to maintain independence. Nationwide networks and organizations are instrumental in influencing standards to achieve equal opportunities for the disabled.

Legislation for Disabled Persons

Numerous legislative policies enable disabled individuals access to goods and services as well as healthcare; for example, the Rehabilitation Act of 1973, the Americans with Disabilities Act (ADA) of 1990, the Olmstead Decision of 1999, the New Freedom Initiative of 2001, and the Affordable Care Act of 2010 (see Disability Legislation Table in Online Resources for Chapter 42 at http://evolve.elsevier.com/Darby/hygiene). Section 504 of the Rehabilitation Act of 1973 and the ADA achieved the most significant outcomes in removing barriers for the disabled by guaranteeing that no qualified person shall be discriminated against from acquiring education, employment, social services, or healthcare because of his or her handicap. The Affordable Care Act of 2010 created a Patient Bill of Rights which provides protection against discriminatory practices by insurance companies. Disabled individuals with pre-existing medical conditions can no longer be denied coverage, and lifetime dollar limits will be phased out by 2014.

The most significant policy statements regarding healthcare for individuals with disabilities are in *Healthy People 2020* and the *Call to Action to Improve the Health and Wellness of Persons with Disabilities.* (Please visit the Web Resources section of the website at http://evolve.elsevier.com/Darby/hygiene.) These initiatives promote the health and well-being of children and adults with disabilities and ensure that they have access to comprehensive healthcare, enabling them to live full and productive lives. Even though statutes, regulations, court decisions, and programs provide equal opportunity for persons with disabilities, they alone cannot ensure quality of life.

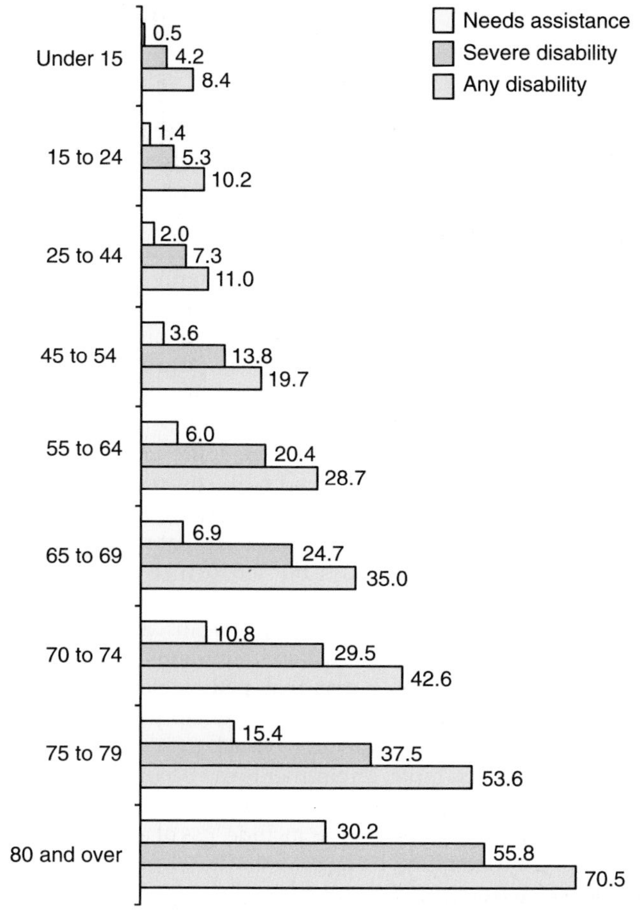

Figure 42-1. Disability prevalence and the need for assistance by age: 2010.

Barriers to Healthcare

Financial Barriers

Cost remains the primary barrier to oral healthcare services.[5] Financial resources are needed to obtain an education, participate in rehabilitative programs, train for a job, find adequate housing, use basic transportation, and survive. State and federal funds fail to cover the costs of everyone's needs, forcing many disabled people to prioritize their spending, often at the expense of basic needs. Most disabled people rely on state and federal support (e.g., Social Security payments) to cover daily expenses. Individuals who are able to work earn low wages, and unemployment rates remain relatively high.

Without adequate funds for daily expenses, healthcare often is neglected. Most cannot afford private healthcare insurance and rely on Medicare and Medicaid reimbursement for financial assistance. For those on a limited income without health insurance, money for healthcare is an out-of-pocket expense; healthcare often is sought on a crisis basis, for emergencies or pain control. Disabled individuals with health insurance often have policies that either do not meet their healthcare needs or lack coverage for the costs associated with their disability.[6] Oral healthcare often is denied and is considered by most health care plans as an unnecessary medical service.

For disabled individuals living in an institution, medical and limited dental services may be provided, but high fees are associated with these services, the cost of which is passed on to the family or state. If a severely disabled person needs to be institutionalized, costs to the family may drain their financial resources. Eligibility requirements for Medicare and Medicaid limit access of mainstreamed residents to oral care services that otherwise would have been provided in an institutional setting. Many families choose to care for a severely disabled individual at home because long-term care is too great a financial burden.

Architectural Barriers

The ADA mandates that all public facilities contain a **barrier-free design**. This law requires that all structural and communication barriers be removed from public areas of existing facilities (e.g., in hotels, restaurants, theaters, museums, retail stores, schools, banks, and healthcare facilities, including dental offices and clinics) when their removal is readily achievable. In addition, people who own, lease, sublet, or operate places of public accommodation in existing buildings are responsible for ensuring that all barriers are removed. Often, removal of the barrier can be made by making minor physical modifications to the facility. A facility that is barrier free enables a person to function independently within and outside of the home environment. For example, a building that contains elevators and accessible restrooms is not considered truly barrier-free if there are no ramps or electronically operated doors to gain entrance. Specific building codes and architectural standards for a barrier-free facility are available from federal and state resources (please see the Web resources section of the Evolve website at http://evolve.elsevier.com/Darby/hygiene).

Transportation Barriers

One frequently overlooked barrier is transportation. All too often, clients with disabilities have long distances to travel to a healthcare facility that is qualified and willing to treat them.[7] Public transportation such as subways, buses, rail systems, and airplanes provide limited assistance to the disabled, despite federal regulations that require modifications for greater access. Interpreting the schedule, finding the exact fare, waiting at a boarding stop during inclement weather, boarding the right vehicle, and tracking the number of stops can be extremely difficult for someone with impairments. As a result, many disabled individuals choose not to use mass transportation and would rather stay home than risk traveling.

Many stations and transportation vehicles also remain inaccessible, partly because the ratio of disabled persons to nondisabled persons is low and renovations are costly. When renovations are made, expenses are passed along to passengers, escalating transportation costs. Traveling expense then becomes an additional barrier to disabled people, who are usually on fixed incomes and unable to afford transportation services. Reliance on others for transportation to and from the home may not be convenient for the disabled or for the driver. This reliance on others places an added burden on family members or caregivers who accompany disabled persons.

Attitude of Healthcare Professionals

Healthcare practitioners pose a significant barrier to care. More disabled persons live outside of institutional settings;

therefore more of them need to be treated within the private sector. A major complaint that disabled individuals have is finding practitioners willing to treat them.[8] Some practitioners choose not to treat disabled individuals because Medicare and Medicaid reimbursements are often not equivalent to the fee schedules typically charged.[9] In addition, extra time often is needed to treat these individuals, so time for and income from treating others is lost. Fear of interacting with disabled people and conflicting personal values about the disabled may make a practitioner avoid treating them.[8] Advanced training and education on the healthcare needs of persons with disabilities is limited and lacks support from state and federal funding. As a result, many practitioners do not feel qualified to treat these individuals.

Many healthcare providers are unaware of the relationship between the mouth and the body (see Chapter 20) and fail to recognize oral diseases as infections that need immediate attention. Nurses and aides who work in institutions for the severely disabled may view oral care as a low priority and an unpleasant task and many times do not include this service in the client's care plan.

Attitudes of Disabled Clients

Oral care holds significance as the lifeline for the disabled client. For example, the mouth is important for mastication, speaking, expressing personality, using telecommunication devices, working at a job, and portraying a positive self-image. However, many disabled individuals and/or their caregivers do not recognize the importance of maintaining good oral health. Often, medical treatment consumes the majority of their time and money; dental care becomes a low priority. Some disabled individuals, unaware of oral health, lack the motivation to keep the mouth disease free. Others feel that dentists do not understand their impairment, which can lead to a negative dental experience. Dental hygienists must reach out to disabled individuals and establish a **dental home** for them. A dental home provides disabled individuals access to continuous, coordinated, comprehensive, patient-centered dental care and enables them access to specialized oral healthcare services.[10]

Personal Self-Worth

A healthy, functioning mouth implies that the individual values health and physical appearance. This positive portrayal of the mouth contributes to the client's acceptance into society, self-worth, self-esteem, self-concept, and self-image. All people have achievements that build confidence and disappointments that lower confidence. The disabled client copes with life events with the same behaviors as the nondisabled individual; however, disabled people's physical appearance may interfere with how others view them, which in turn affects how they view themselves.

Positioning of the disabled person may cause intimidation or self-consciousness in proximity to others. For example, people in wheelchairs are physically lower than those who do not use wheelchairs; hence others look down on them while conversing. People who use assistive devices (canes, braces, or walkers) may be viewed as inept or unable to ambulate on their own. People who are hearing or visually impaired may have difficulty following a conversation and therefore may be excluded from the group. People with tremors or other muscular disorders may take a longer time to speak and may be viewed as mentally impaired by those unwilling to listen.

Disabled clients are individuals who have their own personal capabilities and limitations and adapt to life in much the same way as others. Therefore clients should be viewed as individuals who contribute to society despite their disabilities and who have needs similar to those of others.

Defining Disabilities

According to the ADA Act of 1990, the term "disability" is associated with a limitation in a major life activity. **Major life activities** are those that the an average person can perform with little or no difficulty (e.g., self-care, walking, hearing, seeing, breathing, standing, speaking, sitting, learning, thinking, and interacting with others). The ADA Amendment Act of 2008 broadened the definition of major life activities to also include the operation of major bodily functions (e.g., the immune system, normal cell growth, and all major organ functions). This is an age-related measure that takes into consideration the activities that are normal for a given age group.

The World Health Organization (WHO) defines disability as an all-encompassing term for impairments, activity limitations, participation restrictions, and environmental factors.[11] **Impairments** occur as a result of pathology, accident, or disease and include any loss or abnormality—physiologic, anatomic, or mental—in function, which may or may not be permanent; for example, impairments can occur as a result of a stroke, which can cause sensory loss, aphasia, and paresis. Other examples of impairments include loss of a limb or body organ or a broken limb or hip. An **activity limitation** is difficulty in performing activities (e.g., having difficulty with basic activities of daily living because of a medical condition). A **participation restriction** is the inability to engage in everyday life circumstances for reasons that may not be under the client's control; for example, a working-age person with a severe health condition may have a hard time finding work because of the environment within the workplace (e.g., lack of reasonable accommodations by the employer) or may be denied access to employment because of discrimination (social environment). WHO's definition includes the society's viewpoint on disability and does not limit disability to just a medical or biologic abnormality. Including social factors further defines the impact that the environment has on the client's ability to function in society.[11]

Classification of Disabilities

Several methods are used to categorize individuals with disabilities. Government classification standards are based on criteria delineated in the ADA, that is, an individual with a disability is one who meets the following criteria:

- Has a physical or mental impairment that substantially limits one or more major life activities
- Has a record of such an impairment that limits major life activities
- Is regarded as having an impairment[12]

These criteria are used to determine eligibility for federal assistance.

Disabilities (i.e., disabling conditions) also are categorized as follows:

- **Developmental disabilities** occur congenitally or during the developmental period of the child, a period that lasts from birth to age 22 years.[13] Developmental disabilities are generally chronic in nature; continue throughout the life of the person; and appear as mental, physical, or combined impairments. Individuals with developmental disabilities may experience difficulties with many functions and may be limited in their abilities to care for themselves, communicate effectively, learn new concepts, ambulate, or live independently.

- **Acquired disabilities** occur after the age of 22 years or are caused by a disease, trauma, or injury to the body.[13] Common acquired disabilities include spinal cord paralysis from sports or motorcycle accidents, limb amputation because of disease, and limitations in range of motion from arthritis.
- **Age-associated disabilities** occur later in life, typically over the age of 65. As people age, they are at higher risk for developing chronic disease, which in turn may result in disability.[14] Chronic diseases include cancer, diabetes, cardiovascular disease, arthritis, osteoporosis, and chronic obstructive pulmonary disease. Cognitive impairments, such as dementia and Alzheimer's disease, and physical deterioration also can cause an elderly individual to become disabled.

Another classification groups disabilities into several major categories, clustering impairments with similar manifestations together (Table 42-1). These categories are useful when studying a group of disorders or when attempting to classify the condition of a client with oral pathology associated with a known disorder. This system categorizes a person mainly according to medical status and provides little information about how well an individual can compensate for limitations in daily function.

Functional status is perhaps the most useful method for categorizing disabilities because each disabled person has different abilities and limitations, regardless of medical

TABLE 42-1

Classifications of Disabilities

Disability	Characteristics
Developmental Disabilities	
Intellectual disabilities	Includes Down syndrome; reflects difficulties with learning, critical thinking, and skill development
Cerebral palsy	Nonprogressive disorder caused by brain damage either at birth or before the central nervous system (CNS) reaches maturity
Epilepsy	Caused by a chemical imbalance in the brain; associated with head injury, infection, and developmental disorders
Autism spectrum disorders	Lifelong neurologic disability with limitations in communication and social interactions
Sensory Impairments	
Visual impairments	Range from changes in visual acuity to blindness
Hearing impairments	Varying degrees of hearing loss to deafness
Orthopedic Disorders	
Paralysis	Most commonly associated with stroke
Spinal cord injury	Most commonly associated with accidents or injury
Missing extremities	Most commonly associated with injury or diabetes
Medical Disabilities	
Cardiovascular diseases	Hypertension, congestive heart disease, angina, valvular disease
Autoimmune diseases	Systemic lupus erythematosus, gout, Sjögren syndrome, scleroderma, rheumatoid arthritis, and osteoarthritis
Human immunodeficiency virus (HIV) infection and acquired immunodeficiency syndrome (AIDS)	Infection that destroys white blood cells, resulting in breakdown of the immune system
Cancer	Oral and systemic cancer
Diabetes	Type 1 or type 2
Respiratory disease	Tuberculosis, chronic obstructive pulmonary disease
Renal disease	End-stage renal disease
Blood disorders	Bleeding disorders, platelet disorders, sickle cell anemia, other anemias

TABLE 42-1

Classifications of Disabilities—cont'd

Disability	Characteristics
Cognitive Impairments and Psychiatric Disorders	
Anorexia and bulimia	Eating disorders; characterized by self-starvation or massive food binges followed by self-induced vomiting or excessive use of diuretics
Mood disorders	Major depression, bipolar disorder, schizophrenia
Dementia	Alzheimer's disease, vascular dementia, Pick's disease
Cerebrovascular accident (CVA, stroke)	Blockage of blood flow to the brain that can cause sudden partial or complete loss of function on one side of the body or death
Substance use disorder	Abuse of alcohol and/or psychoactive drugs
Degenerative Nervous System Disorders	
Alzheimer's disease	Neuronal degeneration in the cerebral cortex, resulting in loss of memory, critical thinking, and reasoning ability
Parkinson's disease	Degeneration of deep cerebral nuclei, resulting in loss of control of voluntary movements; tremors, slowness of movement (bradykinesia); gradual onset of dementia
Huntington's disease	Autosomal-dominant disorder that causes degeneration of the deep nuclei, cauda, and putamen; behavioral problems and constant muscle movement (chorea)
Cerebellar ataxias	Normal mental status; changes in gait and coordination
Motor neuron disease and amyotrophic lateral sclerosis (ALS)	Cell death in the motor neurons of the spinal cord and cerebral cortex; progressive muscle atrophy leading to respiratory failure; no loss of mental or sensory functions
Multiple sclerosis (MS)	Muscle weakness characterized by cyclic nature of progression
Myasthenia gravis	Muscle weakness around the eyes and throat; difficulty in swallowing
Neurofibromatosis	Genetic autosomal-dominant disease; multiple benign tumors
Creutzfeldt-Jakob disease	Mutation of prion protein gene; degeneration of neurons; neuronal loss, amyloid plaque formation and rapidly progressive dementia
Communication Disorders	
Dysarthria	Speech disorder from muscle weakness caused by damage to central or peripheral nervous system or both; slurred speech patterns
Apraxia	Speech disorder caused by a lesion within the CNS; impaired capacity to position muscles to form speech; stuttering
Aphasia	Language disorder caused by neurologic damage; inability to put thoughts into words or to comprehend words

diagnosis or degree of system involvement. Functional status describes how well the client can conduct basic and instrumental activities of daily living.

- Basic activities of daily living (BADLs) include activities required for personal care such as feeding, dressing, grooming, bathing, and toileting.[15]
- Instrumental activities of daily living (IADLs) encompass more complex tasks required for independent living (e.g., using a telephone, preparing meals, cleaning the house, driving a car, or using public transportation).[15]

Every individual values the ability to live independently. Functional independence enables individuals to participate in life situations that are meaningful and purposeful; participation in BADLs and IADLs is essential to health and well-being. The dental hygienist who is able to improve the client's functional abilities and oral health behaviors also increases the client's functional status and quality of life.

Impairments can affect five aspects of function: communication, movement, mental ability, medical health, and sensory perception. These aspects of function are limited; they do not address the degree of severity or extent of involvement of impairments, which may cause varying degrees of functional limitations. Table 42-2 illustrates how functional limitations are related to the severity of impairment according to four levels of involvement.

TABLE 42-2

Functional Levels for Categorizing Disabilities Based on Ability to Conduct Basic Activities of Daily Living

Level of Impairment	Communication	Movement	Mental Ability
Level I			
Near-normal function	Practitioner may have difficulty understanding client and vice versa.	Client may walk more slowly than normal.	Extra effort is required for explanations and reassurance to client.
Level II			
Simulation of normal function with adaptive equipment, medication, or methods	Client may use communication board, writing, or gesturing instead of speech.	Setting must be wheelchair accessible; have furniture rearranged to allow room for movement. Client may need special arrangements for transportation. Possible assistance getting into treatment chair.	Client may be using medications to maintain emotional equilibrium or may need special approach to accept dental and dental hygiene care.
Level III			
Simulation of normal function with aid of third party	Deaf person may need interpreter. Client may bring friend, parent, or attendant to assist in communication. Client consent needed to give information to third party.	Attendant or other caregiver may be responsible for dental hygiene. Obtain client consent to give information to third party. Will need assistance getting into treatment chair.	Client may have legal guardian. If so, practitioner should have guardian's consent and proof of guardianship.
Level IV			
Simulation of normal function not possible	Client will have legal guardian. Practitioner should have guardian's consent and proof of guardianship for care. Residential caregiver responsible for dental hygiene should be given information and education.	Home visit required for routine dental and dental hygiene care. If practitioner cannot make one, refer to appropriate resource.	Client will have legal guardian. Must have guardian's consent and proof of guardianship for care.

Adapted from Shaffer S, Margon C, Stiefel DJ: *Principles of rehabilitation (Project DECOD),* Seattle, 1985, University of Washington School of Dentistry.

Interaction with People with Disabilities[16]

Key points when describing or interacting with persons who have disabilities are as follows:

- Avoid the term "handicap." This term is no longer used owing to its negative connotations.
- A person is not a disability; rather a person has an impairment. Therefore it is inappropriate to say, "She is my multiple sclerosis case." It is more appropriate to say, "This is my client, Mrs. Jones. She has multiple sclerosis."
- An impairment does not override other client characteristics; therefore the impairment should be addressed only when necessary or relevant to the situation. Emphasizing the impairment without reason should be avoided.
- Clients with disabilities are not superhuman; learning to function as a person despite the impairment is survival, not a unique act that requires special talents. Sensationalizing goal attainment by impaired people is a common reaction, such as by saying, "He triumphed over his inability to walk," implying that the client was a victim of the impairment.
- Sensationalizing terms that draw on emotions, such as "relies on a cane" or "bound to a wheelchair," are inappropriate and imply a false level of dependency on the part of the client.
- People with disabilities are not necessarily sick, regardless of whether the impairment was caused by an illness. It is inappropriate to describe an impaired client as a "patient" or a "case" unless that person is actively under medical care.
- Don't assume that all disabled clients need help. Instead ask the client, "How can I assist you?" Disabled individuals should be able to direct their care and inform the dental clinician what type of assistance they will need.
- Clinicians should position themselves at eye level when talking to clients in a wheelchair.
- When greeting clients who have a disability, offer to shake their hand. If they are unable to extend their hand, they will greet you in another way.

Negative portrayal issues are encountered through personal contact or the mass media. For example, people may express pity for a disabled person without knowing the individual, or disbelief when seeing a disabled person enjoying himself "despite his impairment." Healthcare professionals who work with disabled clients often are viewed as having special motivation or as "truly patient." Television portrayals often treat the disabled adult like a child or an inferior. A disabled adult may be addressed by first name or with a surname when the situation dictates a more formal title. Other examples include speaking for a disabled person as if they were not there and assuming that they cannot make decisions independently. Negative portrayals should be avoided for a positive therapeutic relationship.

Assistive Devices

Many clients have complex oral needs associated directly with their conditions or with medications taken to stabilize or control the symptoms of their conditions. Clients may require special assistance in accomplishing self-care behaviors necessary for oral health and awareness.

The client's impairment may dictate the need for tools used to achieve independence in daily functions and communication. Many devices are available through area pharmacies and agencies; others are tailored specifically for the client. Digital technology devices, such as computer tablets and video games, also are being incorporated into educational and rehabilitation programs for individuals with disabilities.[17] Dental hygienists must be familiar with these devices because their use may affect client goals and decisions in care.

Walking Devices

Various devices are available for the client who has difficulty with ambulation. Canes, leg braces, crutches, and walkers are devices that assist the client by bearing the weight of the body during motion (Figure 42-2). These devices replace function either unilaterally or bilaterally, greatly increase mobility for ambulation, and support individuals while they move from bed to chair. The walking device should remain close to the client. For example, if the dental hygienist moves the device, the client must be informed of its location to avoid feeling trapped. The dental hygienist retrieves the device when needed or at the client's request and hands the device directly to the client for use. Anxious clients may prefer to hold the device as a measure of security. Although not ideal, this behavior may be tolerable as long as the device does not interfere with care.

Wheelchairs are devices that assist clients who have limited or no mobility in the legs for ambulation. Wheelchairs increase mobility for those who may otherwise be confined to bed or chair. Because of improvements in building design, many facilities are completely accessible to wheelchairs, thus enabling clients to move freely without being inhibited by physical limitations in ambulation. Clients may be treated in the wheelchair or transferred to the dental chair for care (see section and procedures on wheelchair transfer techniques in this chapter). Most clients prefer to operate the wheelchair themselves; assistance should be provided only at their request.

Prosthetic Devices

Prosthetic devices enhance client appearance and improve function. Fitted after amputation, prosthetic legs improve ambulation, prosthetic arms increase reach and range of motion, and prosthetic hands improve grasp. Other devices may replace structures or organs because of congenital anomalies or that were removed because of pathology or trauma. Prosthetic devices may be fitted permanently through surgical implantation or may be removable and worn only when needed for functional or cosmetic purposes. Clients with removable devices such as those designed for loss of facial structure may feel more comfortable when the prosthesis is in place; therefore, removal should occur only during assessment or when indicated during care. All devices should be replaced immediately after completion of the procedure to ensure client comfort and ease. Privacy must be maintained when the prosthetic device is removed, preferably in a closed area or examination room. Prophylactic antibiotic premedication is indicated before dental hygiene care can begin for the client with a prosthetic joint replacement (see Chapter 12).

Assistive Listening Devices

Assistive listening devices for clients with hearing deficits detect sounds and assist with understanding speech. Hearing

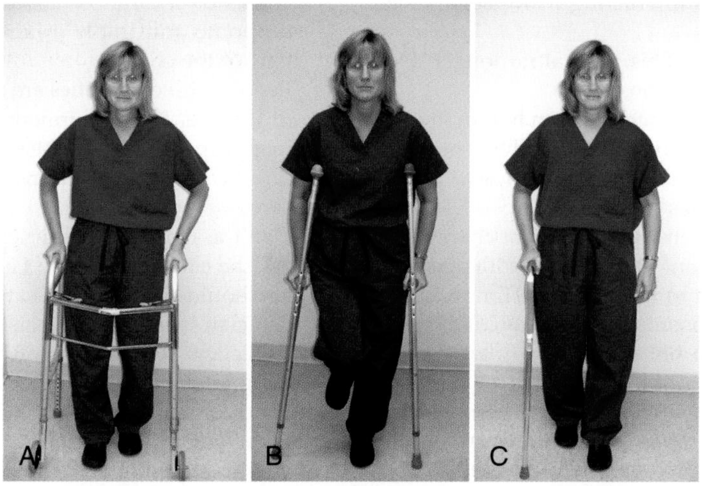

Figure 42-2. Walking devices. **A,** Use of walker greatly increases client's mobility. **B,** Crutches assist client by bearing the weight of the body during motion. **C,** Canes assist the client with balance and decrease weight bearing on the leg opposite the side on which the cane is held. (Courtesy Kathleen Muzzin, Texas A&M University, Baylor College of Dentistry, Caruth School of Dental Hygiene, Dallas, Texas.)

aids amplify sounds and are effective only when some hearing capacity exists. Hearing aids may be worn in the outer ear to improve sound conduction (e.g., conventional hearing aids) or surgically implanted under the skin or in the bone behind the ear for inner ear conduction (e.g., cochlear implants or bone anchor hearing aids). Because many people deny hearing loss, some may own a hearing aid but choose not to wear the device out of self-consciousness or embarrassment. These clients may appear unresponsive to questions or conversation. Such behaviors should alert the dental hygienist to possible hearing impairment, and the client should be asked about the use of a hearing device.

The oral environment can create annoyances for persons with hearing aids. Close operator proximity or incorrect placement of the hearing aid may cause it to squeal; high-pitched noises from dental handpieces or ultrasonic devices initiate this reaction. The client should be instructed to turn off or remove the hearing aid during dental care. Clients adapting to a new hearing aid often turn down the aid because "everything seems so noisy." Because all sounds are amplified, these clients may become aware of sounds they never heard before or have not heard in a long time, especially if the hearing loss was gradual and untreated. Most environments contain background noise, and clients may turn off the hearing aid before coming for their appointment.

Other assistive listening devices are available. Amplifiers can be used on telephones, televisions, and radios to increase sound volume for those with partial hearing loss. Closed-captioned television programs assist the hearing-impaired client with lip reading. Telecommunication devices for telephones reproduce sounds from a caller and convert them into written type that can be read from a monitor. A typed response transmits a message back to the caller.

Aids for the Visually Impaired

Clients who are visually impaired usually wear corrective lenses to improve vision and augment communication. If oral care instructions are given to clients who have forgotten their glasses, written material can be provided to read after the appointment. These materials should contain large print with adequate contrast. Clients who are blind frequently wear dark glasses to protect the eyes from light sensitivity. Blind clients require guidance, especially in an unfamiliar environment, and depend on tactile stimulation to understand the environment, as follows:

- A blind client can be greeted by the grasping hands of the hygienist.
- To accompany the client to the treatment area, the client's nondominant hand should be placed under the elbow of the hygienist, and the client should be asked to stand next to but slightly behind the hygienist.
- Specific directions guide the client (e.g., "Take three steps forward, and then turn right. We're going to step down onto a smooth floor. There is only one step.").
- When arriving in the treatment area, the client should be told the location of objects in the room (e.g., "The chair is directly in front of you, about one foot away from where you are standing now.") Allow the client to feel the location and direction of the chair by placing the client's hands onto the chair while giving verbal instructions. Remaining close with a hand resting on the client's shoulder conveys comfort and concern while the client is getting settled into the chair.

Blind clients may use a cane or a guide dog during ambulation and prefer to use these aids to assistance by another individual. Guide dogs are permitted to remain in the treatment area and should be directed by the client to sit close and within clear view of the client. The clinician should not attempt to pet the guide dog, because such dogs may feel threatened and may attack anyone who approaches them. In addition, guide dogs should never be left alone in another area; they may become anxious in the absence of their owners.

Assistive Speaking Devices

Assistive speaking devices recreate sounds that mimic normal speech patterns for persons who have had surgical removal of the larynx and cannot make sounds from the throat. Electronic speech devices held against the throat detect vibrations of air passing through the throat as the person mimics normal speech. The device reproduces a noise that resembles an automated, robotlike speech. Use of this device enhances verbal communication. Speech therapists train clients with laryngectomies to expel air from the esophagus for sound formation to produce altered speech.

Augmentative and alternative communication (AAC) is a method of communication used by clients with severe speech and language impairment (e.g., amyotrophic lateral sclerosis, aphasia, apraxia, traumatic brain injury, cerebral palsy). AAC is used for clients who are unable to use verbal speech yet are cognitively able, or when speech is extremely difficult to understand. The client will use, alone or in combination, gestures, communication boards, pictures, computer tablets, symbols, or drawings.[18] For example, if the client is hungry, he or she will point to the picture on the ACC of someone eating. Clients who use an electronic communication board have it programmed by a speech-language pathologist based on their functioning level (Figure 42-3).

When treating this type of client, the dental hygienist must listen carefully and repeat the message given by the client to ensure accuracy in understanding. It is also important to allow enough response time when communicating with a client who uses AAC. With practice, it becomes relatively easy to understand and communicate with these clients.

Assistive Devices for Paralyzed Persons

Elimination Devices

Clients paralyzed below the waist experience difficulty with normal waste elimination and may use a catheter for

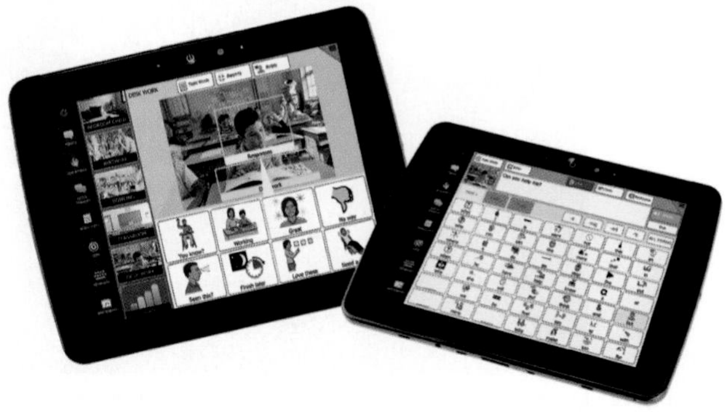

Figure 42-3. Augmentative and alternative communication device used for clients with severe speech and language impairment. (Courtesy DynaVox Technologies, Pittsburgh, Pennsylvania.)

assistance with urination. Care must be taken when moving a client with a catheter so that it does not become kinked or dislodged. Also, clients may have a bowel and bladder routine to regulate waste elimination. Clients should be questioned regarding their elimination schedules and instructed to complete their bowel and bladder routine before appointments.

Communication Devices

Clients paralyzed below the neck use a variety of devices to accomplish BADLs, most of which are designed by occupational or speech therapists. The mouth is needed to operate many of these devices, which alters the health and function of oral structures. The most common device used by tetraplegic clients is the **mouthstick**, a simple plastic or balsa wood rod with a rubber tip held in place by the teeth and lips (Figure 42-4).

Mouthsticks can be used for communication, such as typing on a keyboard or pressing the buttons on a telephone. Mouthsticks also are used to turn book pages, operate a computer, and use appliances such as microwave ovens and remote-control televisions.

Teeth may be subjected to occlusal trauma from the mouthstick, which, in the presence of inflammation and risk factors, may result in rapid periodontal destruction and tooth loss. A biologically sound dentition and skin and mucous membrane integrity are of great significance to these clients. Without healthy teeth and supporting structures, they may not be able to hold the stick and therefore lose the ability to communicate and function independently.

Mouthsticks may contribute to muscle fatigue, oral tissue trauma from inserting the stick, difficulty with insertion without the assistance of a caregiver, unpleasant taste, temporomandibular joint (TMJ) discomfort, and gagging. Considerations in the fabrication of mouthstick appliances are listed in Box 42-1.

Fabrication of a mouthstick begins with an alginate impression of the client's maxillary and mandibular arch. Stone dental casts are made and can be used to create the two types of mouthsticks that are currently available:

- *Mouthstick with an acrylic mouth guard.* The mouth guard is designed over the mandibular stone cast then adjusted in the client's mouth for fit and occlusal stability. A hole is made in the appliance and adapted for the mouthstick. The occupational or speech therapist assists the prosthodontist with final evaluation of the length and design of the stick based on client needs.
- *Mouthstick with moving parts between the maxillary and mandibular arches.* This device is used by persons who cannot move the head or neck. It contains a telescoping mouthstick that is held in a ball-and-socket joint at the anterior portion of the appliance and a rack-and-pinion device that is fitted into the joint. Muscles of mastication are used to produce vertical movements of the mouthstick; the tongue controls lateral movement and the telescoping function.[19]

BOX 42-1

Mouthstick Appliance: Key Considerations

- Does not cause tooth movement
- Is stable when held in place
- Is lightweight and comfortable
- Does not inhibit speech or swallowing
- Is not in the client's line of vision
- Has a neutral color and acceptable taste
- Holds a variety of implements to best meet client's needs
- Ensures that biting forces are distributed equally across as many teeth within the arch as possible to decrease periodontal destruction and muscle fatigue

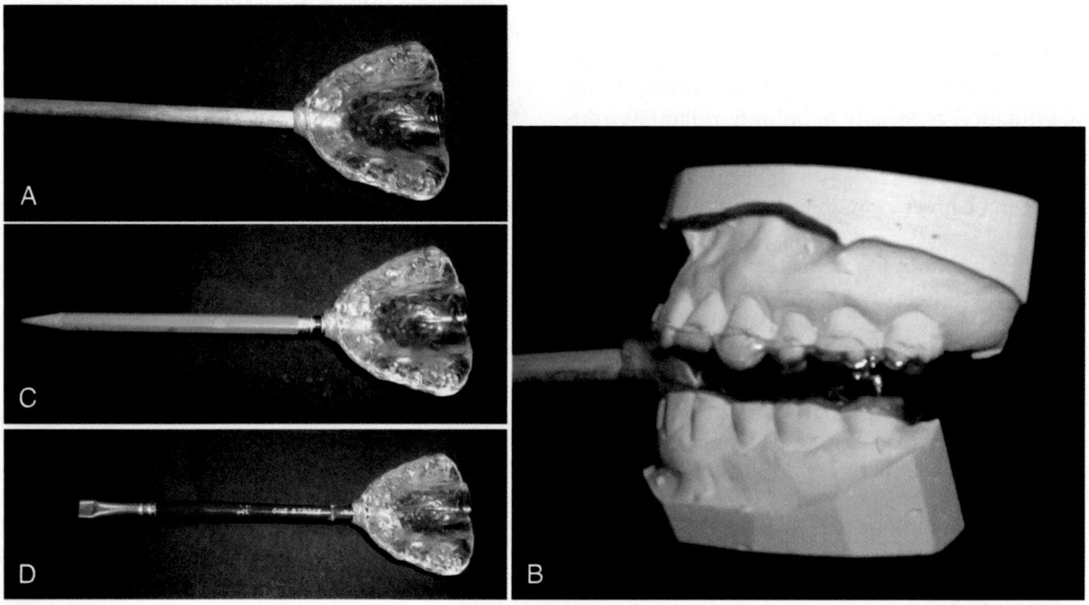

Figure 42-4. Mouthstick. **A,** Custom-fabricated mouthstick for persons with tetraplegia. **B,** Mouthstick is fabricated so that the biting forces are equally distributed across the maxillary arch. **C** and **D,** Hole on anterior surface of mouth guard can also hold a pencil or a paintbrush. (Courtesy Kathleen Muzzin, Texas A&M University, Baylor College of Dentistry, Caruth School of Dental Hygiene, Dallas, Texas.)

Before insertion of either appliance, oral inflammation should be eliminated. Careful monitoring of the fit and use of the appliance minimizes periodontal trauma and ensures optimal benefit for the client.

Assistive Devices for Protection and Oral Function

Assistive devices for protection and oral function (e.g., custom mouth protectors) are used to prevent self-inflicted trauma by clients with behavioral problems or who are comatose. The custom mouth protector does the following:

- Prevents neuropathologic chewing and self-inflicted trauma to the lips, tongue, and buccal mucosa
- Protects traumatized tissues so they can heal without further injury
- Trains clients to stop injuring oral tissues

The devices should be used only in consultation with a behavioral specialist.

Clients with neuromuscular disorders such as Parkinson's disease and/or stroke or clients who have had surgery in which a portion of the throat or palate has been removed may experience difficulty in speaking and swallowing and require a device to assist with oral function. Palatal lifts, palatal augmentation devices, and obturators are devices that improve function by recreating normal physiologic movement of the oral tissues. The dental hygienist caring for the client with this type of device must monitor changes in speaking patterns, swallowing ability, and device cleanliness. If adjustment of the device is needed, the client should be referred to a prosthodontist.

Oral Self-Care Devices

Although many devices facilitate BADLs, few existing devices help the client carry out oral self-care behaviors independently. Creative alternatives to traditional oral hygiene devices are designed for those with limitations in function. These devices should adapt to the client's needs, skill level, and functional status.

Client Assessment

The dental hygienist assesses the client's physical and mental limitations that affect how the client adapts to using a device.

- **Range of motion.** The client's ability to reach the oral cavity with the arms and hands is determined. Extent of range of motion dictates the length of the device required to accommodate physical limitations in reaching the mouth. For example, clients with a muscular impairment may be able to reach halfway across their body yet elevate the arm only to heart level. Such clients need an extended length to compensate for the limited motion of reaching above heart level. Similarly, clients who are unable to bend at the elbows or wrists may have difficulty reaching certain areas of the oral cavity and may need an angled device for improved reach to fit in all areas of the mouth.
- **Grip strength.** Clients with arthritis or neuromuscular disorders experience difficulty holding a device that is too narrow or too small (Figure 42-5). To assess grip strength, the client is asked to grasp various sizes of foam cylinders. These are more functional than having the client grip tennis balls or softballs. Another measure of grip strength includes assessing the client's ability to retain finger closure for an extended length of time. The hygienist should grasp the client's hand gently, ask the client to squeeze with as much force as possible, and hold this position for 1 minute. This assessment determines the strength needed to hold the device for a given length of time. If the client is unable to keep the fingers closed for 1 minute, a universal cuff, such as a palmar Velcro strap, may be needed for holding the device.

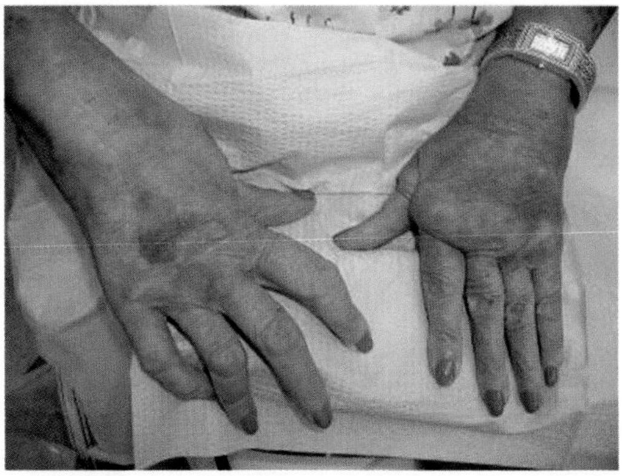

Figure 42-5. Persons with arthritis may have difficulty holding an oral self-care aid such as a toothbrush or interdental cleaner. A modified oral self-care aid or power toothbrush or interdental cleaner is indicated. Right hand of client has been repaired surgically to allow more range of motion. At time of photo, left hand had not been treated. (Courtesy Kathleen Muzzin, Texas A&M University, Baylor College of Dentistry, Caruth School of Dental Hygiene, Dallas, Texas.)

- **Skill level.** Watching clients simulate the motion used to brush their teeth, or watching them actually brush their teeth with their current technique, is used to assess skill level. Clients should be prompted to perform skills such as reaching into the upper right quadrant, brushing the tongue, cleaning the lingual surfaces, and brushing the facial surfaces of anterior teeth. It is important to note what the client is capable of performing with relative ease and which behaviors present difficulty or confusion.
- *Ability to understand and follow directions.* This ability is evaluated during the grip strength assessment. The hygienist asks a sufficient number of questions to determine whether the client is capable of responding accurately to verbal commands and instructions. For example, the client who is cognitively impaired may have difficulty in producing a response on command and may require a device such as a power toothbrush that accomplishes the task with little effort.
- *Perception about what seems easy or difficult.* Direct client feedback is essential for a complete assessment, in that clients' perceptions may influence compliance with any device, whether well adapted for their needs or not. The client should understand their role in the use of the device—a motivational strategy that promotes ownership of the responsibility for oral self-care behaviors.
- *Current oral status and oral self-care techniques, the range of opening of the mouth, and the activity of the oral musculature, especially the tongue.* Intraoral assessment provides information about existing oral conditions that may dictate the need for certain device design characteristics. Widening of the oral cavity can be accomplished through the use of cones or tongue depressors (adding one on top each day to extend the opening of the mouth).

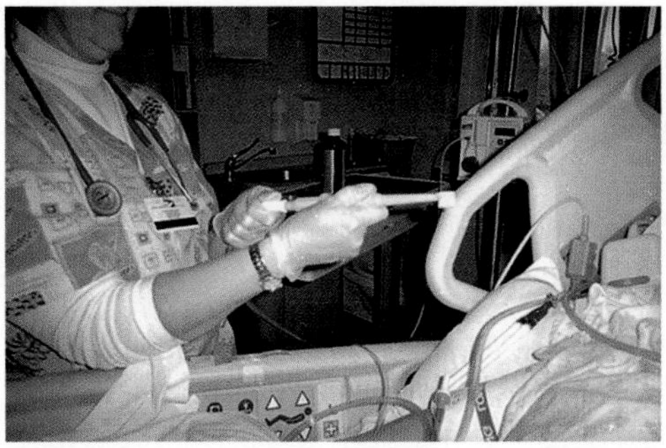

Figure 42-6. Plak-Vac Oral Suction Brush being connected to the bedside suction device in a critical care unit. (Courtesy Michelle Bopp, Gene W. Hirschfield School of Dental Hygiene, Old Dominion University, Norfolk, Virginia.)

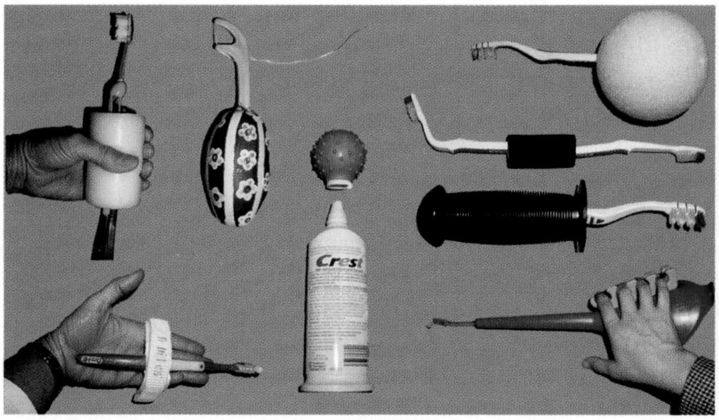

Figure 42-7. Customized oral care aids for persons with physical disabilities. (Courtesy Kathleen Muzzin, Texas A&M University, Baylor College of Dentistry, Caruth School of Dental Hygiene, Dallas, Texas.)

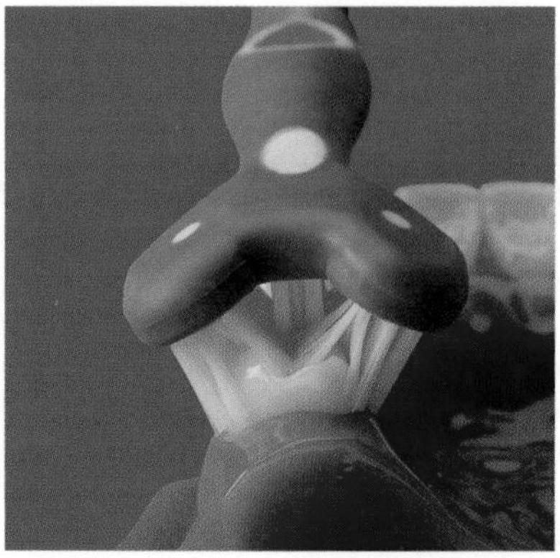

Figure 42-8. The Surround Toothbrush is designed to clean lingual, facial, and occlusal surfaces at the same time. (Courtesy Specialized Care Co, Hampton, New Hampshire.)

A comatose or semicomatose person in a hospital or extended care facility may benefit from toothbrushes such as the Plak-Vac Oral Suction Brush (Trademark Medical Corporation), which is a specially designed toothbrush that can be connected to a bedside suction device (Figure 42-6).

These assessment measures work well with clients who are mentally and physically capable of learning self-care techniques; however, some clients may not move their upper extremities at all and therefore rely on a primary caregiver to perform daily care. Caregiver interviews are important to assess willingness to provide daily oral care, determine the existing skill level of the caregiver, and identify concerns.

Customizing Oral Self-Care Devices

For clients with a limited range of motion, adaptations to oral self-care aids may be needed.[20] Plastic rulers and rods, available from most hardware stores, can be attached to toothbrushes and floss holders with heavy electrical tape. The added length of the handle facilitates reach but may make placement of the working end of the self-care device in the mouth difficult. To compensate, a toothbrush with a compact head size may be used for better intraoral fit. The existing plastic handle of the toothbrush can be bent to angle the brush bristles against the curve of the arches. To bend the toothbrush handle, the handle is held above a flame or under hot tap water until pliable.

To assist the client with weak grip strength, the device handle can be built up with a variety of materials to fit the client's finger closure capability. For the client with limited finger closure, a wide bulky handle is needed to assist with grip. Bicycle grips, Styrofoam molds, and arts-and-crafts compounds as alternative handles greatly improve the client's ability to hold the device (Figure 42-7). Toothbrushes and floss holders can be inserted into these items and changed when necessary. Clients who have difficulties with coordination may find that a lightweight handle is hard to manage and that a weighted end may be easier to find and hold. Plastic bicycle grips are preferred because they are available in a variety of sizes, textures, and weights, are inexpensive, and are cleaned easily after use.

The occupational therapist or dental hygienist is responsible for making these devices initially, but the caregiver should be trained to construct them thereafter. Custom-made devices should be brought to every appointment to assess design, usage, and need for replacement.

Clients with poor dexterity and coordination, and/or limited gripping ability, benefit from power toothbrushes with large handles that are used easily on the client by a caregiver.

Several manufacturers market manual toothbrushes that can be bent by hand without heating to promote better angulation and mouth access. Floss holders and toothbrushes with wide handles or with specific handle designs promote improved grasping ability by the client. Other manufacturers of manual toothbrushes have reconfigured the head of the brush—for example, with brush bristles that surround the tooth, enabling the client and/or caregiver to brush the entire tooth surface at one time (Figure 42-8). Toothpaste containers with alternative dispensers, such as flip-top lids and levers, should be recommended to clients with limited finger motion because grip strength is needed to dispense the toothpaste. Oral irrigation devices are excellent supplemental aids for self-care and local delivery of antimicrobial agents.

For clients who are unable to hold devices on their own, a **universal cuff** may be used for assistance. The strap, with Velcro adhesive on which various adaptive devices can be attached, fits around the arm or wrist and acts as a splint for stabilization. Universal cuffs may be adapted for use with oral physiotherapy aids. The dental hygienist should consult with an occupational therapist when treating a client who may benefit from a universal cuff for self-care devices.

Several design characteristics of the device include the following:

- Made of a lightweight, readily available, inexpensive material and easily constructed; plastics are preferred because they resist water damage and can be cleaned, rinsed, and dried easily
- Interchangeable parts (e.g., a constructed alternative handle on a device should adapt easily, so that worn-out toothbrushes can be changed without having to replace the handle)
- Ease of use and minimal setup time

Client Positioning and Stabilization

Physically challenged clients frequently have problems with support and balance; therefore a physical assessment before care determines whether adaptations are needed to treat the client safely. A list of client stabilization and supportive devices can be found online at the Special Care Dentistry Association website (http://www.scdaonline.org). Click on the link to Publications and Resources and scroll down to SCDA Product Guide.

Clients with neuromuscular problems, such as tremors, muscle spasms, or hyperflexive responses, may require a stabilization device, such as a seatbelt, to help remain in an upright and secure position. Other medical immobilization devices, such as papoose boards (Figure 42-9), are available to use with clients who have extreme spasticity or severe behavioral problems. Routine use of immobilization should be limited because it can promote client distrust and may decrease the possibility of future cooperation.[21] In addition, physical restraints have been associated with bruising, respiratory compromise, aspiration pneumonia, and cellulitis from limb restraint. Immobilization or support devices also should be used with caution with a seizure-prone client because these devices must be removed quickly in the event of a seizure. However, in certain individuals in whom cooperation is near impossible, it may be necessary to use these devices at every visit to render care. The risks and benefits of using any form of immobilization must be explained to the client, parent, and/or caregiver, and informed consent must be obtained and documented in the client's medical record.[21]

Pillows or rolled towels also may be placed underneath the knees and the neck of the client to prevent muscle spasms and to provide additional support during care.

To prevent injuries during care, a dental assistant or caregiver may hold the client's arms and legs in a comfortable position. Dental assistants easily can rest their arm closest to the client across the client's chest, with the client's arms tucked underneath. With this technique, the client's arms are prevented from moving into the working area in the event of a muscular reflex. In the case of a child who is difficult to keep still in the dental chair, the child may lie on top of the parent, with the parent's arms around the child's body. This practice should be discontinued early in the course of care after behavioral guidance techniques and trust exercises have been conducted with the child (Table 42-3). If a client is uncooperative and resists sitting in a chair, parents and caregivers can have the client lie on the floor with the client's head in the caregiver's lap so that improved access into the mouth is obtained. Clients who are extremely combative and unable to remain still may need sedation.

The dental hygienist may find the need for additional head support and stabilization for the client during care. Sitting at the 12-o'clock position, the dental hygienist wraps her or his nondominant arm around the client's head and firmly under the chin for stabilization. Small pillows, neck rolls, or a rolled bath sheet also may be placed on either side of the client's head for additional support. Beanbag chairs placed in the dental chair can provide additional support for physically challenged children with unstable joints and limbs (Figure 42-10).

Headrests, solid backrests, seatbelts, chest straps, lateral trunk supports, and hip guides are used commonly on wheelchairs to help keep the client positioned correctly in the chair. Cushions are helpful with paralyzed clients to provide additional support and to minimize the occurrence of pressure sores (decubitus ulcers or decubiti).

To reduce aspiration risk, caregivers must not apply dentifrice or topical agents when the client is supine. The client with a neuromuscular or behavioral problem may use ingestible toothpaste as a safe alternative.

During care the practitioner should place the client in a sitting or semi-inclined position to prevent aspiration of materials, fluids, or instruments. Rubber dam isolation also prevents aspiration of dental materials; however, routine use is not recommended for impaired clients, especially those

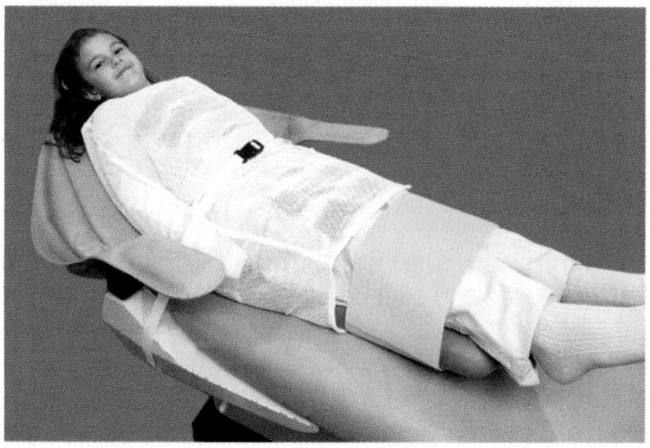

Figure 42-9. Physical restraint used to maintain the disabled client in a stable, safe position. (Courtesy Specialized Care Co, Hampton, New Hampshire.)

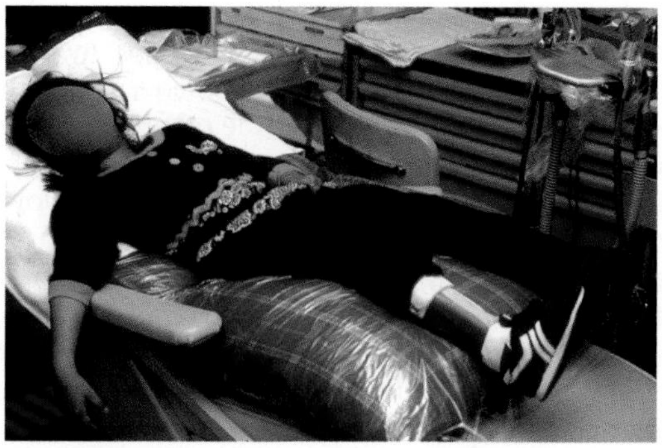

Figure 42-10. Beanbag chairs help support limbs of physically challenged children during dental treatment.

TABLE 42-3

Behavioral Guidance Techniques

Technique	Description
Desensitization (explanation and exposure)	Graduated exposure to the oral healthcare setting instills familiarity with the environment.
Familiarization visit	Introducing client to the oral healthcare environment before initiation of care reduces fear and stress.
Tell-show-do	Demonstrations reinforce verbal instructions.
Modeling	Live or videotaped model aids in skill development by demonstrating desired behavior or technique.
Feedback	Immediate feedback improves client learning and skill development through evaluation of progress and performance.
Contingent escape	Offers brief breaks in treatment and/or gives a positive reward based on a set time period of good behavior (e.g., after counting to ten, the hygienist informs the client that they are allowed to close their mouth and rest).
Positive reinforcement	Rewards strengthen behavior and encourage the repetition of a behavior; rewards include praise, special privileges, token systems, and material goods.
Distraction	Audiovisual stimuli (e.g., listening to music through headphones or watching a videotape), decrease uncooperative behavior by providing stimuli on which client can focus during care.
Communication	Words and phrasing that reflect empathy, respect, and warmth enhance client-provider interaction and trust.
Hand signals	Allow fearful client to raise a hand as a sign to stop treatment; promotes the client's feelings of safety and security.
Nonverbal communication (touch)	Disabled clients have a heightened awareness to a person's body language and facial expression. Reassuring touch displays warmth and understanding toward anxious client.
Relaxation, hypnosis, sedation	Clients who exhibit mild to moderate anxiety may benefit from deep breathing, meditation, or guided imagery. Medication may be needed for clients with extreme anxiety, fear, or uncooperative behavior.
Voice control	Alteration in volume, pace, and tone can be used to gain the client's attention and influence their behavior. This refers to the manner in which the message is delivered to the client.
Social stories	Describes a social situation, skill, or concept and the expected behavior that must be displayed by the client. Stories can be read by the clients or by their caretakers or presented via audio or video players or computer software.

Data from Lyons RA: Understanding basic behavioral support techniques as an alternative to sedation and anesthesia, *Spec Care Dentist* 29(1):39, 2009. Quirmbach LM, Lincoln AJ, Feinberg-Gizzo MJ, et al: Social stories: mechanisms of effectiveness in increasing game play skills in children diagnosed with autism spectrum disorder using a pretest-posttest repeated measures randomized control group design, *J Autism Dev Disord* 39(2):299, 2009.

who have a compromised airway, are aggressive or uncooperative, or have swallowing difficulties. During dental treatment, it is essential to use good evacuation with the aid of a dental assistant, especially when increased salivation is present.

To prevent closure of the mandible onto the operator's fingers, use of a **mouth prop** is recommended for treating impaired clients who are seizure prone, have muscle weakness, or experience muscle spasms. Standard mouth props should have one end of the dental floss tied through the hole at the base of the mouth prop and the other end attached to the client's napkin clip. This allows the mouth prop to be pulled quickly from the mouth and prevents swallowing in the event of an emergency. Larger hand-held mouth props also can be used during assisted oral self-care (Figure 42-11).

The client is usually the best source of advice on how to approach positioning and movement. Ideally, all clients should be treated in the dental chair, but on occasion a client in a wheelchair may be too weak to transfer into the dental chair or may require positioning that only the wheelchair can provide. Some power wheelchairs have seat functions that recline or tilt for adequate positioning, and this may be more comfortable for the client. The client may be treated in the wheelchair if the treatment area is wide enough for positioning the client either alongside or behind the dental chair. Clients who remain in the wheelchair need additional head support during care, which can be obtained by using a

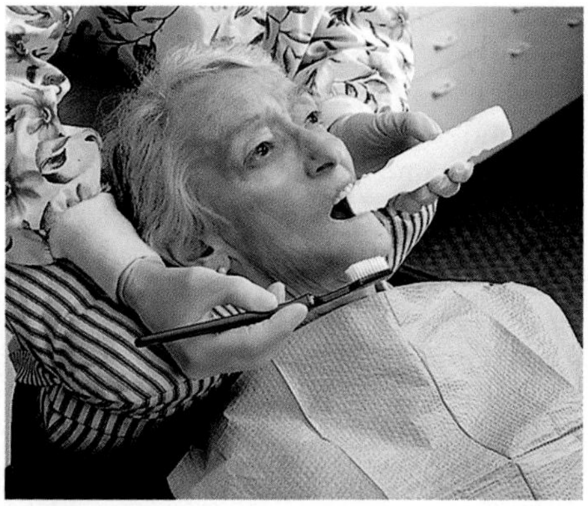

Figure 42-11. Clinician using the Open Wide disposable mouth prop on an adult. (Courtesy Specialized Care Co, Hampton, New Hampshire.)

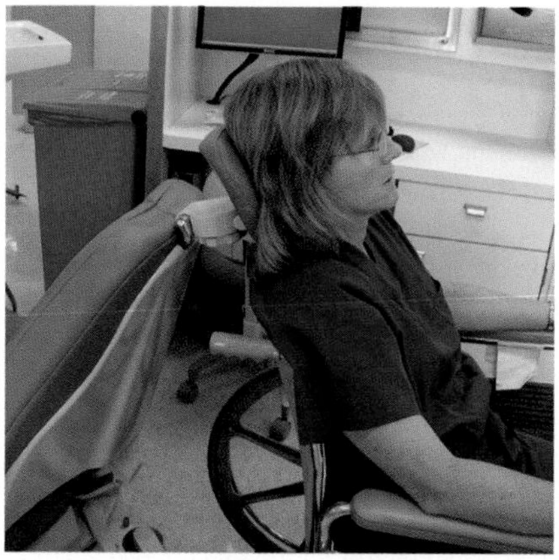

Figure 42-12. Wheelchair positioned so that the head is leaning against the back of the dental chair's headrest. (Courtesy Kathleen Muzzin, Texas A&M University, Baylor College of Dentistry, Caruth School of Dental Hygiene, Dallas, Texas.)

portable headrest or by turning the wheelchair around so that the client's head is leaning against the back of the dental chair's headrest (Figure 42-12). Treating multiple clients from this position may cause musculoskeletal problems for the clinician; therefore clients who cannot be transferred should be treated early in the day while the hygienist is well rested. After providing care from a compromised operator position, the hygienist should break for adequate rest and muscle stretching before treating another client (see Chapter 11).

Wheelchair Transfer Techniques

Transferring from Wheelchair to Dental Chair

Procedure 42-1 and the corresponding Competency Form describes transferring the client from the wheelchair to the dental chair using a one-person lift. Before making the transfer, however, the health history must be assessed carefully to determine the client's current health status, nature of the condition that dictates wheelchair use, existing physical strength, risk of inducing muscle spasms, and areas of the body that could be injured if the client is moved incorrectly. In addition, the client should be questioned regarding use of urinary appliances (catheters and collecting bags) that may become dislodged during a transfer. A kinked catheter results in inadequate bladder drainage, causing toxic waste accumulation, and could trigger an emergency situation. The client must be asked about use of waste elimination appliances so that proper care can be taken during the transfer. The client's physician should be consulted about specific medical concerns identified on the health history assessment before any transfer is attempted.

The client's physical ability to participate with the transfer is assessed. Many clients who have undergone physical therapy for their condition may be accustomed to transfer techniques, especially if they have been taught to transfer at home by themselves. Some clients have the ability to assist with the transfer, although they may be unfamiliar with the actual procedural steps involved. Others may perceive that they have the physical strength and skills needed to assist with the transfer when actually they do not possess these abilities. Misconceptions may be dangerous if the transfer is attempted without verifying whether the client's perceptions and abilities are realistic. Also, the client's willingness to transfer is essential for the dental hygienist to know; in any transfer procedure the client depends on the practitioner to some extent, especially during lifting from the wheelchair. An uncooperative client who overestimates or underestimates his or her abilities or a client who resists transfer attempts poses significant management challenges, as well as increased risks for injury to the client and dental hygienist.

The client's level of coordination and balance determines need for assistance with the transfer process. Assistance may be required from another operator (see Procedure 42-2 and the corresponding Competency Form) or may be obtained with the use of a transfer belt or sliding board.

- **Transfer belts** are straps secured around the client's waist to provide a place to hold the client in the event that the person begins to fall during the transfer process. These are especially useful with clients who have little to no upper body strength, such as tetraplegics.
- **Sliding boards** are used to assist the client with fair to good upper body strength by helping the client slide out of the wheelchair, across the board, and into the dental chair. The wheelchair must be positioned beside the dental chair, and the arms to both chairs must be removed to accommodate the board. One end of the board is placed underneath the client, and the other end is laid across the dental chair. The client uses upper arm and body strength to move across the board while the board provides support from underneath the client's legs. Sliding boards also are useful with clients who are overweight or are otherwise too difficult for one person to safely move alone. Transfer belts may be used as an added precaution during a sliding board transfer.

Operator safety also must be ensured as follows:

- The operator should never attempt to transfer a client alone. Although the one-person transfer technique requires only one individual to maneuver the client, an additional person must be available to provide assistance if needed. The additional person reduces the risk of falling or injury to the client during a transfer.
- One operator never should attempt to transfer a client who is very tall or heavy, especially clients who have no upper body strength. These clients have a much greater chance of falling because of their lack of coordination and balance, and they may injure themselves and the operator.
- All transfer movements performed by the operator should be done with feet separated for good balance and knees bent to protect against back strain.
- All lifting procedures should be performed with the legs, while keeping the back straight and slightly bent forward at the waist to prevent muscular back injury to the operator.
- While lifting the client from the wheelchair, the operator should never twist his or her back; twisting may cause severe muscular back strain and injury. Instead, the operator should move with small steps or pivot to position the client.

Preparation for a Wheelchair Transfer

Before beginning the transfer procedure, the hygienist explains the steps to reduce client fear. If the client is expected to assist with the transfer, the client is informed of how and when assistance is needed. A simulation is helpful before the actual procedure is performed, especially for clients who

Procedure 42-1 Transferring Client from Wheelchair to Dental Chair Using a One-Person Lift

STEPS

1. Position transfer belt around client's waist just below ribcage (Figure 42-13).
2. Insert your hands underneath client's thighs, and gently slide client forward in wheelchair seat so that client's buttocks are positioned on front portion of seat. Place sliding board under client so that one end of board is underneath client's thighs and other end is laid across the dental chair (Figure 42-14).
3. Place client's feet together and hold them in place on either side by your feet. Close your knees or thighs on the client's knees, thus supporting and stabilizing client's leg, which allows client to bear some of own weight during the lift.
4. Place client's arms on his or her lap or on the side of wheelchair; instruct client to rest the head over your shoulder so as to look in the opposite direction of the transfer (Figure 42-15).
5. Grasp client around waist and hold transfer belt securely between both hands. If there is no transfer belt available, use an overlapping wrist grasp for greater stability.
6. Rock gently backward onto your heels and, using your leg muscles, lift client off seat. Client is now resting against you, the operator (Figure 42-16).
7. Pivot on your foot closer to the dental chair, and maneuver client over seat of dental chair. This should be done in a smooth motion.
8. Lower client onto dental chair by bending at your knees. Do not release transfer belt around client until client is securely placed into chair.
9. Release one hand to lift client's legs onto chair while still supporting client with the other hand. Reposition armrest of dental chair for client safety.

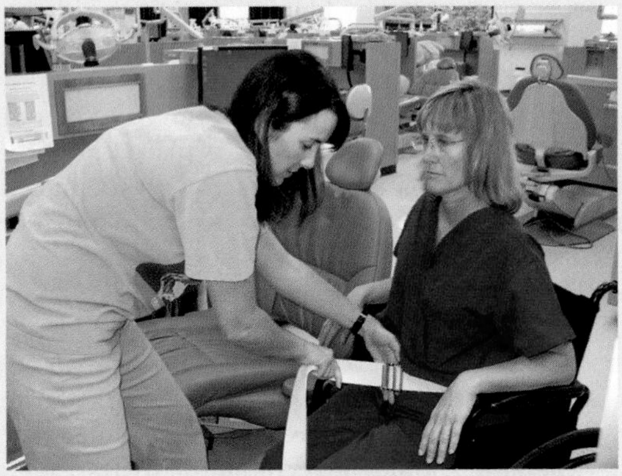

Figure 42-13. Transfer belt is placed around the client's waist and below the ribcage. (Courtesy Kathleen Muzzin, Texas A&M University, Baylor College of Dentistry, Caruth School of Dental Hygiene; and Bobi Robles, Baylor Institute for Rehabilitation, Dallas, Texas.)

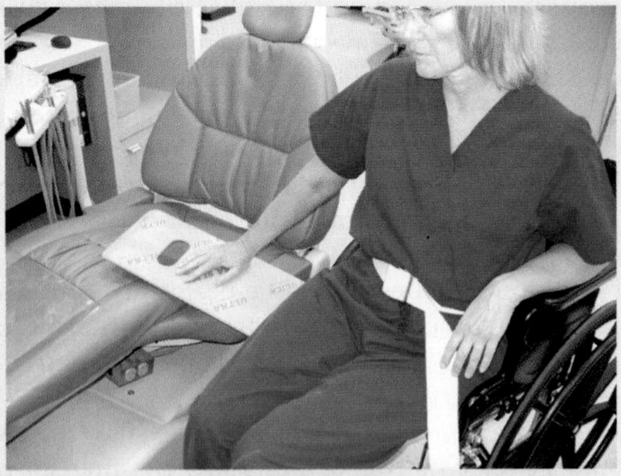

Figure 42-14. One end of the sliding board is placed underneath the client, and the other end is laid across the dental chair. (Courtesy Kathleen Muzzin, Texas A&M University, Baylor College of Dentistry, Caruth School of Dental Hygiene; and Bobi Robles, Baylor Institute for Rehabilitation, Dallas, Texas.)

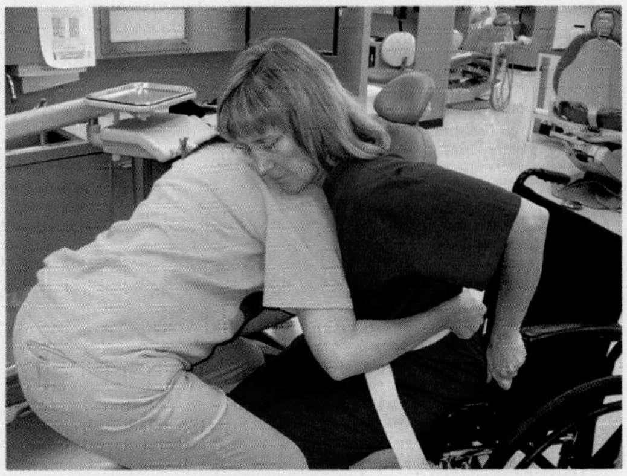

Figure 42-15. Client's hands are placed on side of wheelchair, and head is positioned on the operator's shoulder opposite the direction of the transfer. (Courtesy Kathleen Muzzin, Texas A&M University, Baylor College of Dentistry, Caruth School of Dental Hygiene; and Bobi Robles, Baylor Institute for Rehabilitation, Dallas, Texas.)

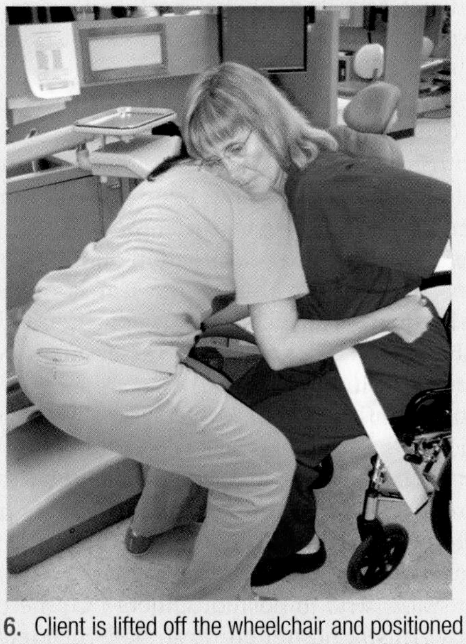

Figure 42-16. Client is lifted off the wheelchair and positioned for transfer to the dental chair. (Courtesy Kathleen Muzzin, Texas A&M University, Baylor College of Dentistry, Caruth School of Dental Hygiene; and Bobi Robles, Baylor Institute for Rehabilitation, Dallas, Texas.)

Procedure 42-2 Transferring Client from Wheelchair to Dental Chair Using a Two-Person Lift

STEPS

1. First operator stands behind client and reaches around client's torso underneath armpits. Operator crosses her or his arms in front of client and grasps client's hands at the wrists with opposite hands (right over left, left over right). Operator then slides her or his arms down so that arms are positioned under the client's ribcage on the abdomen. Stronger and/or taller of two operators is placed behind client.
2. Second operator is positioned on the far side of the wheelchair at the client's knees or thighs. Bending at the knees, operator slides one arm underneath the client's thighs (approximately midway point) while other arm is placed slightly above the knees (Figure 42-17).
3. Client is lifted by both operators at a prearranged signal ("1, 2, 3, lift"). One person coordinates the lift, preferably the operator who is supporting the client's torso (the operator who is lifting the most weight) (Figure 42-18).
4. Client is lifted in one smooth motion and placed into dental chair (Figure 42-19).
5. Operator holding the legs releases the grasp on the client and repositions client in chair. Other operator does not release client until the client is stabilized and arm of dental chair is replaced.

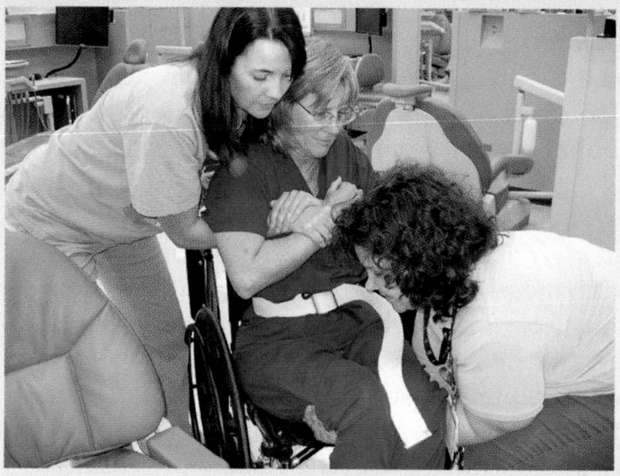

Figure 42-18. The operator who is supporting the client's torso coordinates the lift. (Courtesy Kathleen Muzzin, Texas A&M University, Baylor College of Dentistry, Caruth School of Dental Hygiene; and Bobi Robles, Baylor Institute for Rehabilitation, Dallas, Texas.)

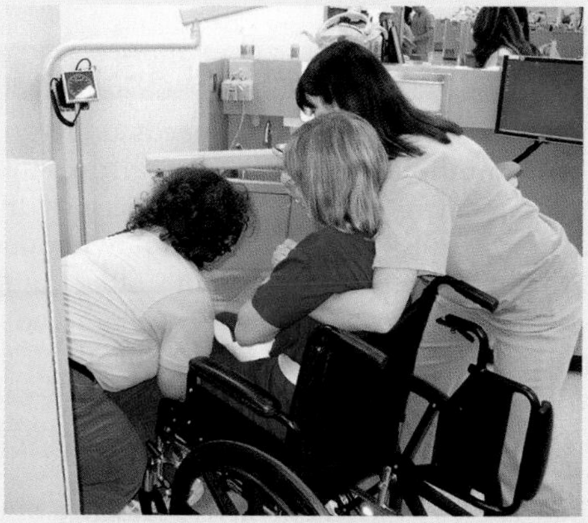

Figure 42-17. During the two-person transfer, the first operator stands behind the wheelchair and the second operator positions herself at the client's thighs. (Courtesy Kathleen Muzzin, Texas A&M University, Baylor College of Dentistry, Caruth School of Dental Hygiene; and Bobi Robles, Baylor Institute for Rehabilitation, Dallas, Texas.)

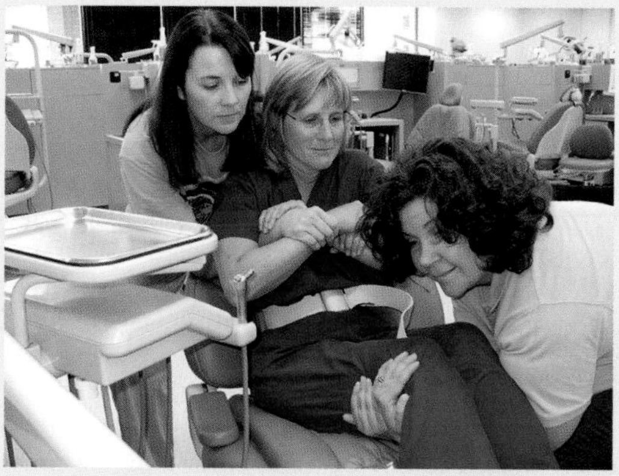

Figure 42-19. Client is lifted in one smooth motion and placed in the dental chair. (Courtesy Kathleen Muzzin, Texas A&M University, Baylor College of Dentistry, Caruth School of Dental Hygiene; and Bobi Robles, Baylor Institute for Rehabilitation, Dallas, Texas.)

have never been transferred. When preparing for a wheelchair transfer, the hygienist does the following:

- Positions the wheelchair at a slight angle to the dental chair. The dental chair should be slightly lower than the wheelchair.
- Positions the wheelchair wheels facing forward and locks the wheels. This stabilizes the chair and prevents tipping or slipping during the transfer.
- Places the transfer belt around the client's waist.
- Removes footrests from the chair or folds them back so that the client's feet do not become caught during the transfer. The client's feet are placed gently on the floor to prevent spasm and to position the feet for the transfer.
- Removes arms of both wheelchair and dental chair. If the arm of dental chair is not removable, then the hygienist positions it as far back as possible so that it does not interfere with the transfer.
- Checks area for any sharp edges, hazards, obstacles, or cords that could cause injury during transfer.
- Unfastens the client's safety belt. After the belt is removed, the operator must support the client to prevent falling.
- Transfers any special padding underneath the client to the dental chair. The hygienist gently rocks the client forward while an assistant removes padding from wheelchair and places it onto the dental chair.

Complications in Wheelchair Transfer

Muscle Spasms

Movement may stimulate muscle spasms, and the hygienist must be prepared to protect the client from injury if spasms occur. Continuous spasms are reduced by massaging the affected area or waiting until the muscle relaxes. Use of supportive pillows reduces the incidence of spasms induced by movement. Anxiety also can contribute to spasms; therefore fear and stress reduction strategies are used before a transfer is initiated.

Decubitus Ulcers (Pressure Sores)

Individuals who use wheelchairs are prone to decubitus ulcers. Decubiti form in areas that lack blood flow, such as on the buttocks and on the backs of thighs. Decubiti can be extremely painful and become infected easily. The dental hygienist questions the impaired client during the health history review about the presence of decubiti. To relieve pressure from the skin and prevent decubiti from occurring, clients must perform weight shifts every 20 minutes. When clients are transferred into the dental chair, supportive devices and weight shifts must be incorporated into the client's appointment plan. Changes in skin integrity are monitored carefully and discussed with the client's physician.

Bowel and Bladder Elimination Schedules

Clients who are transferred into the dental chair need to adhere to their bowel and bladder elimination program. Adequate time must be allotted to transfer the client back into the wheelchair if the client needs to use the restroom during an appointment. The elimination schedule should be documented in the client's record.

Autonomic Dysreflexia

Any of the aforementioned complications poses a significant risk for the development of autonomic dysreflexia, a severe condition that can be fatal if untreated. Noxious stimuli, such as urinary backflow or pain from decubitus ulcers, leads to the development of dysreflexia, manifested by a variety of signs and symptoms. The client may appear disorientated and flushed and exhibit profuse sweating, severe headache, anxiety, and shortness of breath.[22] The most characteristic dysreflexia manifestation is an extremely elevated blood pressure, which ultimately results in stroke (see Chapter 47). The practitioner, alerted to any of these clinical signs, must stop work immediately, check the client's blood pressure, and identify the cause of the reaction. Usually, eliminating the cause (such as when a kinked catheter is straightened) produces an immediate, favorable response. Suspicion of dysreflexia is treated as a severe medical emergency, and assistance must be summoned immediately. The client should be placed in an upright position. This position helps facilitate a drop in blood pressure. Because of the nature of this risk, it is imperative that no client who is transferred to the dental chair be left unattended.

Transferring from Dental Chair to Wheelchair

When the appointment is completed, the client must be transferred from the dental chair back into the wheelchair. The same procedures are conducted to move the client, with special attention given to replacing the padding and supports underneath the client before seating him or her in the wheelchair. The chair wheels always must be locked when the client is transferred back into the wheelchair.

Transfer techniques require practice. Practicing these techniques, especially for those who conduct client transfers infrequently, ensures competence in performing transfer procedures. Physical therapists can help hygienists who are unfamiliar with providing dental care for clients in wheelchairs. Transfer techniques enable hygienists to treat special needs clients who may otherwise not receive oral care.

Health Promotion and Advocacy

The hygienist supports clients with special healthcare needs in the healthcare arena and by promoting these clients as contributing members of society. Opportunities abound to work to improve access to dental hygiene services (e.g., participating on councils, on local boards, and in area support groups; holding leadership positions in organizations; initiating community programs; and contributing to lay and professional communities via speaking engagements and publications).

CLIENT EDUCATION TIPS

- Work with caregivers; physicians; nurses; dietitians; and speech, physical, and occupational therapists to identify needs, set goals, and plan client care.
- Provide other healthcare providers with information on the oral health–systemic health link.
- Clarify information and maximize roles of family and caregivers as healthcare providers for the special needs client.
- Demonstrate methods for modifying and using oral self-care devices to achieve optimal oral health.

LEGAL, ETHICAL, AND SAFETY ISSUES

- Clients with special healthcare needs undergo long-term care with multiple providers, so oral care interventions must complement other health services. If the client is ambulatory, fully functional, and without cognitive impairment, consent to speak with other caregivers and providers, as well as permission to proceed with care, must be obtained directly from the client.
- If client is under the care of a legal guardian, the guardian must provide informed consent for planned care and consultations with other providers.
- Original copies of written correspondence and information from other care providers are maintained in the client's dental record.
- Care is taken to ensure client stability during positioning and transfer; clients never should be left unattended.
- Client is an active participant in all conversations with caregivers who attend the appointment.
- Some individuals with special needs may become victims of violence, abuse, or neglect. The hygienist is obliged ethically to report suspected cases of abuse and neglect to the proper authorities (see Chapter 60).

KEY CONCEPTS

- Access to healthcare, education, and employment opportunities is essential to achieve an acceptable level of health and wellness and to maintain as much independence as possible.
- Oral care is significant for special needs clients because the mouth is used for mastication, speaking, expressing personality, using telecommunication devices, working at a job, and portraying a positive self-image.
- Disability is an all-encompassing term for impairments, activity limitations, participation restrictions, and environmental factors.

- Impairments occur as a result of pathology, accident, or disease and includes any loss or abnormality of physiologic, anatomic, or mental function.
- The term "handicap" is no longer used because of its negative connotations.
- Developmental disabilities occur congenitally or during the developmental period of the child and are generally chronic in nature, continue throughout the life of the individual, and appear as mental, physical, or combined impairments.
- Acquired disabilities occur in early adulthood, from disease or some type of trauma or injury to the body.
- Age-associated disabilities occur later in life, typically after the age of 65.
- Assistive devices are used to achieve independence in daily functions and communication.
- The dental hygienist assesses the client's cognitive awareness, ability to ambulate with or without an assistive device, ability to communicate and interpret information, and need for caregiver assistance.
- The dental hygienist develops specialized self-care devices to promote oral health among those with functional limitations.
- Caregiver interviews assess willingness to provide daily oral care for the client, determine the existing skill level of the caregiver, and identify concerns in performing oral care procedures.
- Most impaired clients can be transferred safely and easily into the dental chair with proper procedures.
- Autonomic dysreflexia, a life-threatening medical emergency, can be prevented.
- Dental hygienists work with lay and professional communities to improve quality of life for citizens with special needs.

CRITICAL THINKING EXERCISES

1. Form groups of three to practice wheelchair transfers and client positioning and stabilization techniques. Students should alternate roles as clients and practitioners. Practical exercises should include one-person and two-person lifts and, when possible, a sliding board. Consider consulting a physical therapist or physical therapy students for collaborative learning.
2. Assume the role of an impaired person for several hours, and complete a set of exercises designed to enhance one's appreciation of the difficulties associated with conducting BADLs. Randomly draw from a list that includes hearing and visual impairment, inability to speak, blindness, and limited mobility (arm, leg, both legs). Assemble equipment and assistive devices for use during these activities (e.g., canes, dark glasses, safety glasses coated with petroleum jelly, ear plugs, crutches, wheelchairs, splints, slings, shoe lifts). Consult a physical therapist or physical therapy students for assistance. While "impaired," students should complete a health history form in the clinical setting, ride in elevators, visit another building to retrieve a newspaper or beverage, obtain signatures from faculty in other departments, or purchase supplies from the campus bookstore. After the exercises, discuss the experiences. (Extreme caution and care must be taken to plan activities that will not place the student in danger while "impaired." Students should not be permitted to cross roadways or other high-traffic areas, to prevent accidental injury. Consideration should be given to severely "impaired" students who may benefit from pairing with a buddy for assistance or safety. Always inform campus officials when students will be completing this exercise, to help ensure student safety and participation by others.)
3. Select a medical condition associated with impairment, and prepare a dental hygiene care plan tailored to meeting client needs. Use the care plan approach presented in Chapter 22. Include information on population affected, age of onset, rate of onset, rate of change or disease progression, need for assistive devices, related medical conditions, medications used to manage this condition, oral manifestations, and special clinical considerations for providing dental hygiene care. Prepare oral presentations about the care plans, and provide copies of all care plans to peers as a guide.
4. Design oral self-care devices for the following client conditions: inability to grasp and hold; inability to raise hand; inability to move forearm in a back-and-forth motion.

REFERENCES

1. American Academy of Pediatric Dentistry, Council on Clinical Affairs: Definition of special health care needs. Available at: http://www.aapd.org. Accessed November 26, 2012.
2. United States Census Bureau: Americans with disabilities: 2010 household economic studies current population reports. Available at: http://www.census.gov/prod/2012pubs/p70-131.pdf. Accessed November 26, 2012.
3. Salmi P, Scott N, Webster A, et al: Residential services for people with intellectual or developmental disabilities at the 20th anniversary of the Americans with Disabilities Act, the 10th anniversary of *olmstead*, and in the year of community living, *Intellect Dev Disabil* 48(2):s168, 2010.
4. Kozma A, Mansell J, Beadle-Brown J: Outcomes in different residential settings for people with intellectual disability: a systematic review, *Am J Intellect Dev Disabil* 114(3):193, 2009.
5. Rapalo DM, Davis JL, Burtner P, et al: Cost as a barrier to dental care among people with disabilities: a report from the Florida behavioral risk factor surveillance system, *Spec Care Dentist* 30(4):133, 2010.
6. Szilagyi PG: Health insurance and children with disabilities, *Future Child* 22(1):123, 2012.
7. Kagihara LE, Huebner CE, Mouradian WE, et al: Parent's perspective on a dental home for children with special health care needs, *Spec Care Dentist* 31(5):170, 2011.
8. Nelson LP, Getzin A, Graham D, et al: Unmet dental needs and barriers to care for children with significant special health care needs, *Pediatr Dent* 33(1):29, 2011.
9. Rouleau T, Harrington A, Brennan M, et al: Receipt of dental care and barriers encountered by persons with disabilities, *Spec Care Dentist* 31(2):63, 2011.
10. Nowak AJ, Casamassimo PS: The dental home. A primary care oral health concept, *J Am Dent Assoc* 133(1):93, 2002.
11. World Health Organization (WHO): International classification of functioning, disability, and health (ICF). Available at: http://www.who.int/topics/disabilities/en/. Accessed November 26, 2012.
12. United States Department of Justice ADA Home Page. Available at: http://www.ada.gov. Accessed November 26, 2012.
13. Stiefel DJ: Dental care considerations for disabled adults, *Spec Care Dentist* 22(3):26S, 2002.
14. Smeltzer SC: Improving the health and wellness of persons with disabilities: a call to action too important for nursing to ignore, *Nurs Outlook* 55(4):189, 2007.

15. Gold DA: An examination of instrumental activities of daily living assessment in older adults and mild cognitive impairment, *J Clin Exp Neuropsychol* 34(1):11, 2012.
16. People First Language. Available at: http://www.disabilityisnatural.com/explore/language-communication. Accessed November 26, 2012.
17. Kagohara DM, van der Meer L, Ramdoss S, et al: Using iPods and iPads in teaching programs for individuals with developmental disabilities: a systematic review, *Res Dev Disabil* 34(1):147, 2012.
18. Clarke M, Price K: Augmentative and alternative communication for children with cerebral palsy, *Paediatric Child Health* 22(9):367, 2012.
19. Scott LK, Ranalli D: Adaptations of mouth guards for patients with special needs, *Spec Care Dentist* 5(6):296, 2005.
20. Brownstone E: Handicapped dental patients: mechanical methods and modifications for oral hygiene care, *Can Dent Hyg* 24(1):32, 1990.
21. Romer M: Consent, restraint, and people with special needs: a review, *Spec Care Dentist* 29(1):58, 2009.
22. Milligan J, Lee J, McMillan C, et al: Autonomic dysreflexia. Recognizing a common serious condition in patients with spinal cord injury, *Can Fam Physician* 58(8):831, 2012.

ACKNOWLEDGMENT

The author acknowledges Ann Eshenaur Spolarich for her past contributions to this chapter.

Refer to the *Procedures Manual* where rationales are provided for the steps outlined in the procedures presented in this chapter.

EVOLVE RESOURCES

Please visit http://evolve.elsevier.com/Darby/hygiene for additional practice and study support tools.

CHAPTER 43

Cardiovascular Disease

Laura Mueller-Joseph

COMPETENCIES

1. **Discuss cardiovascular disease, including:**
   - **Discuss cardiovascular disease risk factors.**
   - **Critically evaluate the relationship between cardiovascular disease and periodontal disease.**
   - **Identify signs and symptoms of rheumatic heart disease, infective endocarditis, valvular heart defects, hypertension, coronary heart disease, cardiac arrhythmias, congestive heart failure, and congenital heart disease.**
2. **Identify the types of cardiovascular surgery.**
3. **Discuss oral manifestations of cardiovascular medications.**
4. **Discuss the prevention and management of cardiac emergencies, including:**
   - **Determine the need for emergency medical care in clients with coronary heart disease.**
   - **Develop a dental hygiene diagnosis and care plan for a client with cardiovascular disease.**

Cardiovascular Disease

Clients presenting with cardiovascular disease have a unique set of health concerns that may or may not influence dental hygiene care directly. These clients are considered individuals with special needs and, depending on their situation, dental hygiene care plans may have to be altered to ensure optimal treatment outcomes. Normal cardiovascular structure and physiology establish the baseline for discussion of cardiac pathology (Figure 43-1).

Cardiovascular disease (CVD), an alteration of the heart and/or blood vessels that impairs function, is the leading cause of death, responsible for 30% of all deaths or 17.3 million people worldwide.[1] Projected statistics indicate that by 2030, 236 million people will develop some form of CVD. Prevention through management of CVD risk factors remains important. Risk factors associated with poor cardiovascular health are listed in Table 43-1.

The American Heart Association notes that periodontal disease and heart disease share common risk factors such as diabetes, smoking, and age; however, the association between these two diseases appears to go beyond their common risk factors.[2,3] Research suggests that chronic infections, such as periodontitis, may increase one's risk for CVD.[4,5] In recent reports, the American Dental Association and the American Heart Association have acknowledged this association and believe more evidence is needed to establish an indisputable causative relationship.[2,3,6] Changing risk-related behaviors assists in decreasing the risk and prevalence of heart disease in the population (see Table 43-1).

Rheumatic Heart Disease

Rheumatic heart disease (RHD) is the cardiac manifestation of rheumatic fever. Persons with a history of rheumatic fever often have valvular heart damage that is affected detrimentally by bacteremia (microorganisms in the bloodstream), often occurring during dental hygiene care. Persons with a history of RHD are not at high risk for infective endocarditis (IE), and prophylactic antibiotic premedication before dental hygiene care is not required.

Etiology

Rheumatic fever is an acute or chronic systemic inflammatory process characterized by attacks of fever, polyarthritis, and carditis. The latter eventually may result in permanent valvular heart damage.

Risk Factors

Persons who have had a beta-hemolytic streptococcal pharyngeal infection (strep throat) may develop rheumatic fever within 2 to 3 weeks after initial infection. People with a history of rheumatic fever are predisposed to RHD because of the involvement of the heart muscles, resulting in cardiac valve damage.

Disease Process

The most destructive effect of rheumatic fever is carditis, an inflammation of the cardiac muscle that is found in most individuals exhibiting signs and symptoms of rheumatic fever. Carditis may affect the endocardium, myocardium, pericardium, or heart valves. Valvular damage is responsible for the familiar organic (nonfunctional) heart murmur associated with rheumatic fever and RHD. The heart murmur is an irregularity of the auditory heartbeat caused by a turbulent flow of blood through a valve that has failed to close. Valves most commonly affected are the mitral valve and the aortic valve. Damaged valves are susceptible to infection that may lead to IE. Severe rheumatic carditis may cause difficulty in breathing, elevation of diastolic blood pressure, and increasing signs of heart failure.

Prevention

RHD prevention requires early diagnosis and treatment of streptococcal pharyngeal infections that may lead to rheumatic fever. Clients need to be informed of the importance of early medical diagnosis and treatment for prevention of this disease.

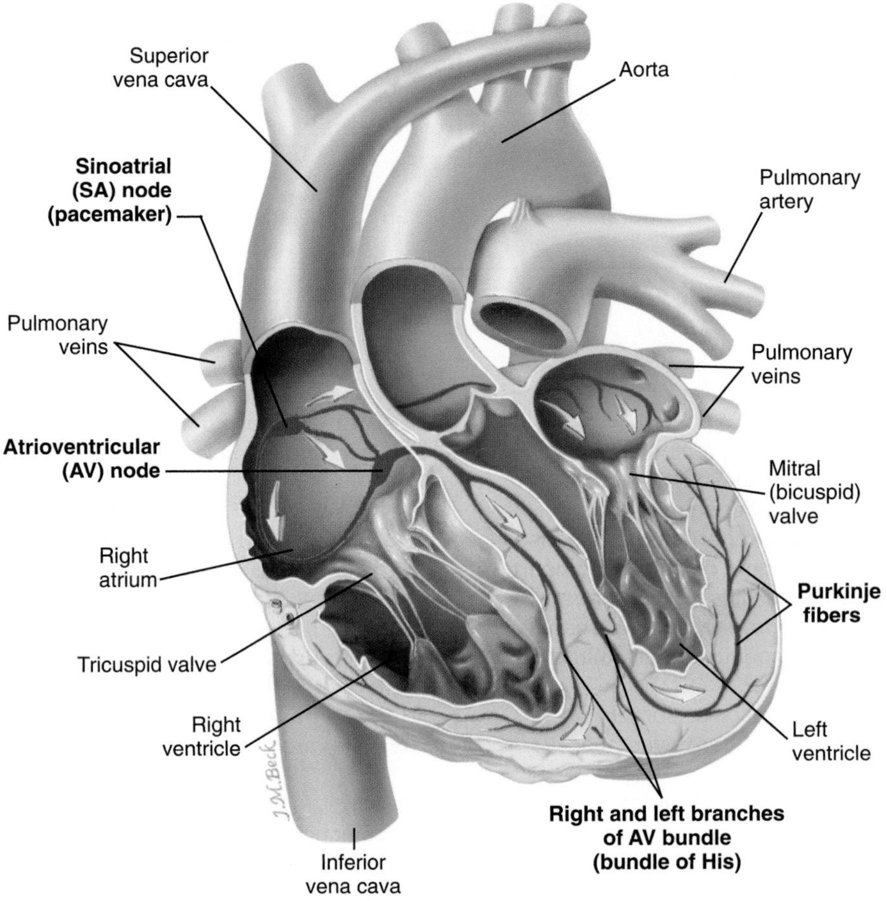

Figure 43-1. Diagram of the heart. (From Patton KT, Thibodeau GA: *Anatomy and physiology*, ed 8, St Louis, 2013, Mosby.)

Dental Hygiene Care

According to the American Heart Association's Guidelines for the Prevention of Infective Endocarditis, prophylactic antibiotic premedication is not required for clients with RHD.[7] To protect clients from health risks, the care plan must include meticulous oral biofilm control. Good oral health maintenance by the client reduces the possibility of developing a self-inflicted bacteremia during toothbrushing or interdental cleaning.

Appointment Guidelines

- Frequent continued-care intervals to maintain good oral health
- Client-centered homecare instruction to maintain optimal oral health practices
- Preprocedural antimicrobial rinse before tissue manipulation to reduce severity of bacteremia

Infective Endocarditis

Infective or bacterial endocarditis is an infection of the endocardium, heart valves, or cardiac prosthesis resulting from microbial invasion.

Etiology

IE, caused by the formation of a bacteremia (microorganisms in the bloodstream), is characterized in most cases by vegetative growths of *Staphylococcus aureus, Staphylococcus epidermidis, Streptococcus viridans,* and, the most prevalent, alpha-hemolytic streptococci on heart valves or endocardial lining. Although staphylococci and streptococci are found in the majority of cases, yeast, fungi, and viruses also have been identified, hence the term *infective* rather than *bacterial.* If untreated, endocarditis is usually fatal; with proper antibiotic treatment, recovery is possible.

Risk Factors

During invasive dental or dental hygiene therapy (defined as procedures that involve manipulation of oral soft tissues, manipulation of the periapical area of teeth, or oral mucosa perforation), a transient bacteremia is produced. Tissue trauma from instrumentation coupled with periodontal disease status determines the severity of infection. In addition, a client may create a self-induced bacteremia via mastication and daily oral hygiene care. Risk factors for IE include clients with a previous history of endocarditis, artificial heart valves, or serious congenital heart conditions and heart transplant patients who develop a problem with a heart valve.[7] Box 12-4 in Chapter 12 delineates risk conditions with the highest risk for adverse effects of IE for which antibiotic prophylaxis is recommended.

Disease Process

There are two types of IE, as follows:

- Acute bacterial endocarditis (ABE) is a severe infection with a rapid course of action usually caused by pathogenic microorganisms, such as *S. aureus* and *S. epidermidis,* that are capable of producing widespread disease.

TABLE 43-1
Risk Factors for Cardiovascular Disease

Factors	Examples
Nonmodifiable Risk Factors	
Personal Factors	
Genetic predisposition or family history	Family members have cardiovascular disease; congenital abnormality
Age	Pathologic changes within coronary arteries severe enough to cause symptoms appear predominantly in persons >40 years of age
Race	Blacks and Hispanics are more likely to have cardiovascular disease than whites or Pacific Islanders
Gender	Men are four times as likely to have coronary heart disease as women up to age 40 years
Disease Patterns	
History of anorexia nervosa or bulimia	Women <40 years old are at increased risk of developing coronary heart disease if they have (had) an eating disorder
Past use of fen-phen (fenfluramine and phentermine)	May damage heart valves if used longer than 2 months
Modifiable Risk Factors	
Personality traits (type A personality)	Hard-driving, competitive individuals who worry excessively about deadlines and consistently overwork
Professional stresses	Occupations that impose tremendous responsibility
Oral contraceptive use	Women <40 years of age who take oral contraceptives
Tobacco use	Smoking and use of smokeless tobacco increase risk of coronary heart disease
Sedentary occupation and lifestyle	Lack of exercise promotes mental depression and obesity
Diet high in calories, cholesterol, fat, and sodium	Overeating and consuming fatty foods promote obesity, lipid abnormalities, diabetes, metabolic syndrome; high-sodium diet promotes hypertension
Hypertension	Individuals with sustained blood pressure of 160/95 mm Hg or higher double their risk of myocardial infarction
Obesity	Weight 30% or more above that considered standard for an individual of a certain height and build
Lipid abnormalities	Serum cholesterol >200 mg/100 mL or a fasting triglyceride of >250 mg/100 mL; abnormal level of C-reactive protein
Diabetes mellitus	Fasting blood sugar of >120 mg/dL, or a routine blood sugar level of ≥180 mg/dL increases risk
Periodontal disease	Periodontal disease increases chronic systemic inflammation, possibly increasing risk of fatal cardiovascular disease

- Subacute bacterial endocarditis (SBE) is a slow-moving infection with nonspecific clinical features. Affected persons usually exhibit a continuous low-grade fever, marked weakness, fatigue, weight loss, and joint pain. Dental and dental hygiene procedures that manipulate soft tissue may be responsible for the development of SBE. As endocarditis progresses, the circulating microorganisms attach to the damaged heart valves or other susceptible areas and proliferate in colonies. This invasion results in cardiac failure from continued valvular damage and embolization (vessel obstruction) owing to fragmentation the colonized microorganisms.

Prevention

Clients with conditions that increase their susceptibility to IE, such as previous IE, unrepaired cyanotic congenital heart disease (CHD), completely repaired congenital heart defect with prosthetic material or device within the first 6 months after the procedure, repaired CHD with residual defects at the site, or adjacent to the site, of a prosthetic patch or prosthetic device (which inhibits endothelialization), cardiac valvulopathy in cardiovascular transplantation recipients, and prosthetic cardiac valves, all require preventive antibiotic therapy before procedures that produce bacteremias (see Chapter 12, Box 12-4 and Tables 12-4 and 12-5).[7]

BOX 43-1

Sample Dental Hygiene Care Plan: Client Needs Prophylactic Antibiotic Premedication

Dental Hygiene Diagnosis
- Protection from health risks: Potential for developing a resistance to prescribed antibiotic if taken over a period of time
- Skin and mucous membrane integrity of the head and neck

Client Goals
- Schedule invasive procedures so that appointments are 9 to 14 days apart
- Reduce gingival bleeding by 80% by last appointment
- Reduce periodontal probing depths by 1 mm by last appointment

Expected Outcomes
- Complete chart of periodontal probing depths
- Dentition and periodontium free from soft and hard deposits
- Root surfaces debrided and tissue healing observed
- Bleeding index score reduced by 80%
- Periodontal probing depths reduced by at least 1 mm

Dental Hygiene Interventions
- Schedule treatment into three appointments.

Appointment 1
- Probe entire mouth, scale and debride maxilla; oral biofilm control with toothbrush, interdental cleaning device, and ADA-accepted antibacterial mouth rinse.
- Plan for host response time; no treatment for 9 to 14 days.

Appointment 2
- Evaluate tissue on maxillary arch; scale and debride mandibular arch; oral biofilm control continued; evaluate and modify self-care regimen as needed.
- Plan for host response time; no treatment for 9 to 14 days.

Appointment 3
- One month after treatment, reassess; evaluate overall outcome; repeat periodontal probing, measure gingival bleeding, reevaluate and modify self-care regimen as needed.

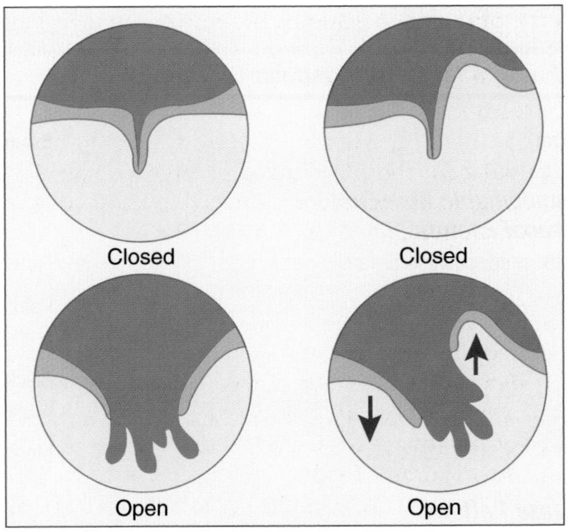

Figure 43-2. Diagram of a normal and a prolapsed mitral valve. (Courtesy Mid-Island Hospital, Bethpage, New York.)

Dental Hygiene Care

The following steps help prevent IE:
- Identify high-risk individuals via the health history and client questioning.
- Ensure that preventive antibiotic is administered 1 hour before procedures that produce bacteremias so that optimal blood levels are established.
- Direct client to use a preprocedural antimicrobial rinse before tissue manipulation.
- Prevent unnecessary trauma during intraoral procedures to reduce severity of bacteremia.
- Help client maintain optimal oral health and daily oral biofilm control to minimize self-induced bacteremias.
- Encourage client to schedule continued-care visits as needed.

Appointment Guidelines

When a client is taking the prescribed prophylactic antibiotic regimen, appointment scheduling is affected. (See Chapter 12, Table 12-5.) It is not in the client's best interest to prolong treatment procedures. If therapeutic scaling and root planing are necessary, appointments should be scheduled in longer periods and as close together as possible. The interval between antibiotic coverage should be 9 to 14 days. If a client has periodontitis, a care plan may divide invasive procedures (therapeutic scaling and root planing) into an organized sequence that allows for 9 to 14 day periods between prophylactic antibiotic premedication. The client's human need for protection from health risks is met by dividing the invasive treatment appointments into two separate intervals with a lag time between the appointments. See Box 43-1.

Valvular Heart Defects

Valvular heart defects (VHDs) result in cardiovascular damage from malfunctioning heart valves such as the mitral valve, the aortic valve, or the tricuspid valve (see Figure 43-1). **Mitral valve prolapse** (MVP) is one of the most frequently occurring VHDs. When the left ventricle pumps blood to the aorta, the mitral valve flops backward (prolapses) into the left atrium, resulting in MVP. Other names for MVP are "floppy mitral valve syndrome" and the "click murmur syndrome," referring to the sound the valve makes when it flops backward (Figure 43-2).

Etiology

VHDs commonly are associated with rheumatic fever but also may be caused by congenital abnormalities or may develop after IE.

Disease Process

Valvular malfunction can occur by **stenosis,** an incomplete opening of the valve, or regurgitation, a backflow of blood through the valve because of incomplete closure. When malfunction occurs, the left ventricle hypertrophies to compensate for the increased amount of blood. This, in turn, causes the left atrium to hypertrophy, leading to pulmonary congestion and right ventricular failure. If the condition is left untreated, the person ultimately develops congestive heart failure (CHF).

Echocardiography uses ultrasonic waves to detect heart size, valvular function, and other structural deformities. The echocardiogram is the record produced by the evaluation and used by the physician to diagnosis VHD.

Medical Treatment

Corrective surgery is done for most VHDs. If the valve cannot be repaired, in most cases prosthetic valves are available to replace defective valves. For clients with MVP, surgical treatment (not always necessary) is aimed at alleviating symptoms such as palpitations, chest pain, nervousness, shortness of breath, and dizziness. Medications are given to control chest pain, slow the heart rate, reduce palpitations, and/or lower anxiety.

Dental Hygiene Care

To protect the client from health risks, frequent continued care appointments and meticulous daily oral biofilm control are necessary. Good oral health maintenance reduces the possibility of developing a self-induced bacteremia from toothbrushing or interdental cleaning. In cases in which defective valves are replaced with prosthetic valves, prophylactic antibiotic premedication is required before dental hygiene care (see Chapter 12, Boxes 12-4 and 12-5, and Tables 12-4 and 12-5).

Appointment Guidelines

VHDs require care plan modifications if the client has an underlying cardiovascular condition or is on anticoagulant drug therapy. The frequently prescribed anticoagulants—heparin, warfarin (Coumadin), and indanedione derivatives—affect the dental hygiene care plan if scaling or root planing procedures are indicated or if the gingiva bleeds spontaneously.

Consultation with the client's physician is recommended to validate the client's current health and medication status. When the client is taking anticoagulant medication, the dental hygienist in collaboration with the dentist consults with the client's physician to determine if a dose reduction should be made or if it is safer to maintain the prescribed dosage and use treatment precautions to minimize hemorrhage.

- Reduction in medication dosage should increase the prothrombin time by 2 seconds.
    - Normal prothrombin time varies between 11 and 14 seconds.
- Optimal prothrombin time for dental hygiene therapy in persons taking anticoagulants should be less than 20 seconds on the day of the scheduled procedure.[8]

For laboratory consistency, the International Normalization Ratio (INR) is used to document bleeding time. When the INR value is used, normal range is less than 1.5, and routine care can be performed when the INR is 2 to 3.[8] Treatment of a client on anticoagulant medication includes the following steps:

- Consult client's physician to verify prothrombin time.
- Scale one area at a time to manage bleeding.
- Begin in the least inflamed area so that bleeding will be minimal.
- Periodically check for clotting; discontinue therapy if there is a long delay in clotting.
- Emphasize importance of daily oral biofilm control for reduction of disease and associated bleeding during professional treatment.

Hypertensive Cardiovascular Disease

Hypertensive cardiovascular disease (HCD) or hypertension is a persistent elevation of the systolic and diastolic blood pressures at or above 140 mm Hg and 90 mm Hg, respectively (see Chapter 13). Half of the 60 million hypertensive people in the United States are undiagnosed. Many individuals with diagnosed hypertension are not treated or are treated inadequately, leaving the client's condition uncontrolled and the client at risk for other serious diseases.

Etiology

Hypertension is not considered a disease but rather a physical finding or symptom. A sustained, elevated blood pressure affects the heart and leads to HCD, resulting in heart failure, myocardial infarction (MI), cerebrovascular accident (stroke), and kidney failure.

Risk Factors

Risk factors for hypertension include family history, race, stress, obesity, a high dietary intake of saturated fats or sodium, use of tobacco or oral contraceptives, fast-paced lifestyle, and age (over age 40). Hypertension is three times more common in obese persons than in normal-weight persons. There is a higher incidence of hypertension among African Americans than American whites.

Disease Process

The two major types of hypertension are as follows:

- Primary hypertension (essential idiopathic hypertension), with cause unknown, is the most common type, characterized by a gradual onset or an abrupt onset of short duration.
- Secondary hypertension is the result of an existing disease of the cardiovascular system, renal system, adrenal glands, or neurologic system. Because hypertension usually follows a chronic course, the client may be asymptomatic. Early clinical signs and symptoms are occipital headaches, vision changes, ringing ears, dizziness, and weakness of the hands and feet. As the condition persists, advanced signs and symptoms can include hemorrhages, enlargement of the left ventricle, CHF, angina pectoris, and renal failure. The dental hygienist refers clients for medical diagnosis if a hypertensive disorder is suspected.

Prevention

Blood pressure measurement identifies individuals with elevated readings possibly indicating undiagnosed heart disease or hypertensive heart disease (see Chapter 13). Early identification of hypertensive clients minimizes the occurrence of medical emergencies, helps meet the client's human need for protection from health risks, and may be lifesaving for undiagnosed individuals.

Medical Treatment

Treatment of hypertension aims at lifestyle changes to reduce risk factors, antihypertensive drug therapy, and/or correction of the underlying medical condition in the case of secondary hypertension. The goal is to reduce and maintain the diastolic pressure level at 90 mm Hg or lower. Some clients need only to watch their dietary consumption of sodium and saturated fats; others must reduce daily stress level and alter their lifestyle (see Table 43-1). When a client needs drug therapy, periodic monitoring is essential. Some drugs may stabilize the condition temporarily and then an elevation can occur, indicating that an alternative drug is needed.

Drugs used for hypertension vary in their method of action as follows:

- Diuretics—promote renal excretion of water and sodium ions
- Sympatholytic agents—modify sympathetic nerve activity
- Vasodilators—increase blood vessel size and facilitate blood flow

Clients receiving hypertensive drug therapy may experience fatigue, gastrointestinal disturbances, nausea, diarrhea, cramps, xerostomia, orthostatic hypotension with dizziness, and/or depression (Table 43-2).

Dental Hygiene Care

If the individual's hypertension is uncontrolled, treatment is postponed until the disorder is regulated. If the client is being treated with antihypertensive agents and if clinical blood pressure evaluations are within normal limits, care can continue; however, stress and anxiety reduction strategies and local anesthetic drug modification will reduce the risk for medical emergencies. Drug considerations for local anesthetic use in clients with hypertensive heart disease are based on the careful use of vasopressors (such as epinephrine), which constrict blood vessels, concentrate the anesthetic in the desired area, and prevent its dissipation. A vasopressor side effect is elevation in blood pressure. In normal persons a slight elevation in blood pressure is harmless; however, with vasopressors, hypertensive individuals have increased risk of cerebrovascular accident, MI, and CHF. Therefore anesthetic agents with vasopressors are relative contraindications in persons with a history of hypertension (see Chapter 40). The risk versus the benefit of using a low concentration of epinephrine to local anesthetic agent is considered, and the physician of record should be consulted.

Appointment Guidelines

Care plan considerations for individuals with controlled hypertension focus on stress reduction strategies (see Chapters 10 and 41) and local anesthetic drug modification to reduce potential for medical emergencies (as discussed in previous section). Box 43-2 displays cases based on initial blood pressure measurement and family history information. Each situation demonstrates appropriate dental hygiene care modifications to meet a specific human need.

BOX 43-2

Clients with Various Hypertensive Conditions and Appropriate Dental Hygiene Actions

Client with No History of Hypertension, Elevated Blood Pressure

During assessment, the client reports no history or symptoms of hypertension; however, a blood pressure reading of 160/100 mm Hg was obtained. One dental hygiene diagnosis may be an unmet need for protection from health risks caused by a potential for heart attack or stroke as evidenced by an elevated blood pressure of 160/100 mm Hg. The dental hygienist should repeat blood pressure measurements during the assessment phase, approximately 5 to 10 minutes apart. If after repeated measurements the diastolic pressure is still more than 100 mm Hg, the appointment should be limited to assessment and planning; no treatment is implemented. The client must be referred to the physician of record for medical consultation and diagnosis. If the client is diagnosed as nonhypertensive by the physician, it can be inferred that dental care anxiety causes the elevated blood pressure. Blood pressure must be monitored at each appointment thereafter and strategies implemented to minimize stress.

Client Under Treatment for Hypertension

During assessment, the client indicates that he is hypertensive and under a physician's care. At each visit the hygienist obtains information on the client's medications and verifies that the prescribed medication has been taken. Client may have an unmet need for freedom from fear and stress; therefore the care plan may include the administration of nitrous oxide–oxygen analgesia to reduce client anxiety. At each visit the client's blood pressure is monitored, periodically remeasured, and recorded.

Client Noncompliant with Hypertension Treatment

Client indicates that she is hypertensive and has discontinued her recommended medication because it is too expensive. Rather, she takes the medication irregularly based on her symptoms. This client has uncontrolled hypertension and a need for protection from health risks. Dental hygiene care is stopped after assessment and should not resume until her hypertension is stabilized. Client is referred to her physician for further medical evaluation and treatment. Although dental hygiene care is postponed, the remaining appointment time can facilitate the client's need for protection from health risks via educational strategies directed toward the importance of controlling hypertension, information about the oral inflammation and systemic inflammation link, and possible lethal effects if hypertension is uncontrolled. Throughout the appointment the client's blood pressure is monitored and recorded periodically.

Client with Hypertension and Acute Symptoms

During assessment, the client demonstrates hypertension with diastolic readings greater than 110 mm Hg and symptoms (e.g., headache, dizziness, restlessness, decreased level of consciousness, blurred vision, palpitations) indicative of hypertensive cardiovascular disease (HCD). To meet the client's need for protection from health risks, the client is referred to his physician for immediate medical consultation and evaluation. Dental hygiene care is delayed until the HCD is controlled. Because hypertension can be related to anxiety and stress, the dental hygienist must determine if the client needs stress management and, if affirmative, can reduce apprehension associated with therapy (e.g., encourage client to express fears and concerns, involve client in goal setting and care planning, explain procedures completely, obtain informed consent, demonstrate humanistic behaviors, and discuss apprehensions directly).

TABLE 43-2
Commonly Prescribed Cardiovascular Medication

Brand Name	Generic Name	Indications for Use	Oral Implications
Glycosides			
Lanoxin	Digoxin	Congestive heart failure (CHF), atrial fibrillation	Excessive salivation, sensitive gag reflex
Diuretics			
Diuril	Chlorothiazide	CHF, hypertension	Decreased salivary flow
Midamor	Amiloride		
Lasix	Furosemide		
Beta Blockers			
Tenormin	Atenolol	Hypertension, angina	Xerostomia
Inderal	Propranolol		
Lopressor	Metoprolol		
Calcium Channel Blockers			
Cardizem	Diltiazem	Hypertension, angina	Decreased salivary flow, gingival enlargement
Procardia	Nifedipine		
Calan	Verapamil		
Vascor	Bepridil		
ACE (Angiotensin-Converting Enzyme) Inhibitors			
Capoten	Captopril	Hypertension	Xerostomia, taste impairment, oral ulceration
Vasotec	Enalapril		
Zestril	Lisinopril		
Vasodilators			
Nitroglycerin	Nitroglycerin	Angina	Burning under tongue
Angiotensin II Receptor Inhibitors			
Avapro	Irbesartan	Hypertension	Xerostomia, taste impairment, oral ulceration
Losartan	Cozaar		
Diovan	Valsartan		
Anticoagulants			
Lovenox	Enoxaparin	Angina, stent placement, after MI	Increased bleeding
Coumadin	Warfarin		
Calciparine	Heparin		
Antiplatelet Agents			
Aspirin	Acetylsalicylic acid	Angina, after MI	Decreases blood clotting
Ticlopidine	Ticlid		
Clopidogrel	Plavix		

Coronary Heart Disease

Coronary heart disease (coronary artery disease or ischemic heart disease) results from insufficient blood flow from the coronary arteries into the heart or myocardium. Disorders associated with this condition are arteriosclerotic heart disease, angina pectoris, coronary insufficiency, and MI.

Etiology

The major cause of coronary heart disease is **atherosclerosis,** a narrowing of the lumen of the coronary arteries, thereby reducing blood flow volume. Narrowing of the lumen occurs by deposition of fibro-fatty substances containing lipids and cholesterol. Deposits thicken with time and eventually

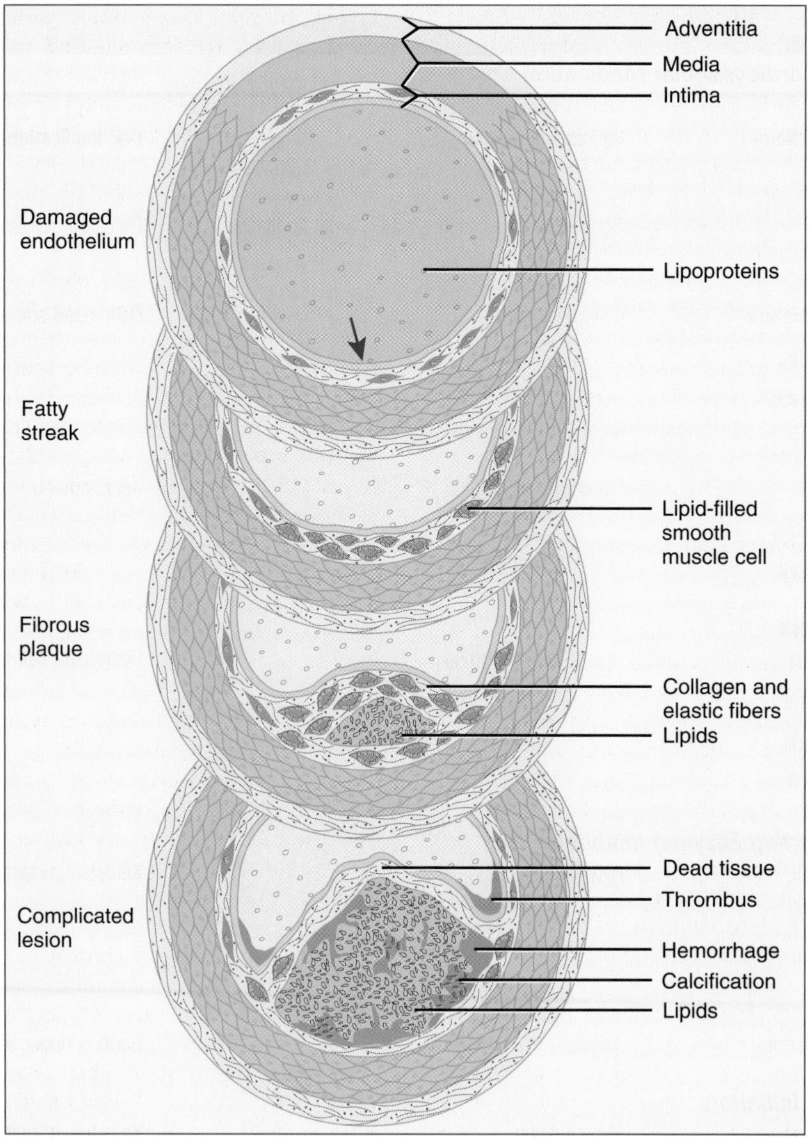

Figure 43-3. Types of atherosclerotic lesions. (From Debakey M, Grotto A: *The living heart*, New York, 1977, David McKay.)

occlude the vessel (Figure 43-3). Atherosclerosis usually develops in high-flow, high-pressure arteries and has been linked to many risk factors. Other coronary heart disease causes are congenital abnormalities of the arteries and changes in the arteries because of infection, autoimmune disorders, and coronary embolism (blood clot).

Risk Factors

Coronary heart disease is influenced by systemic risk factors such as age, gender, race, diet, lifestyle, and environment. Individuals who are obese, anorectic, bulimic, or physically inactive or who smoke increase their coronary heart disease risk (see Table 43-1).

- Age. Being older than 40 is associated with coronary heart disease. Pathologic changes in the arteries are noticeable with age, usually producing disease symptoms.
- Gender. Men are four times more likely to suffer from coronary heart disease than women up to age 40; after age 40, prevalence of coronary heart disease among women and men is the same. Women younger than 40 years old are at an increased risk for developing coronary heart disease if they are taking oral contraceptives or have a history of anorexia nervosa or bulimia.
- Race. White men and nonwhite women are at a higher risk for coronary heart disease than nonwhite men and white women. Researchers are trying to determine the genetic factors involved; however, a familial connection is suspected.
- Diet. Populations in which a low-cholesterol, low-fat diet is consumed have little coronary heart disease; populations in which the diet consists of foods rich in cholesterol and saturated fat have a very high rate of coronary heart disease.
- Environment. Coronary heart disease is seven times more prevalent in North America than in South America, and urban populations are at a higher risk than rural dwellers. Stressful life situations increase an individual's chance of developing coronary heart disease at an early age.

- Tobacco use. Cigarette smoking and use of smokeless tobacco increase an individual's chance of developing coronary heart disease at an early age.

In addition, research supports an association between inflammation in the body and coronary heart disease. C-reactive protein (CRP) levels are used to determine systemic inflammation associated with disease including an individual's risk for cardiovascular disease. Elevated levels of CRP are key markers of atherosclerosis. Studies have correlated increased CRP levels with the presence of periodontitis.[4,5,9] This finding supports other studies that suggest the presence of periodontis increases one's risk for CVD.[10,11] Although the exact link is unclear, evidence suggests that a relationship exists. Further research is needed to determine a causal relationship whereby periodontal disease would be considered a direct risk factor.

Disease Process

Basic manifestations of coronary heart disease are angina pectoris, MI, and sudden death.

Angina Pectoris

Angina pectoris is the direct result of inadequate oxygen flow to the myocardium, manifested clinically as a burning, squeezing, or crushing tightness in the chest that radiates to the left arm, neck, and shoulder blade. The person typically clenches a fist over the chest or rubs the left arm when describing the pain. When sudden attacks of angina pectoris follow physical exertion, emotional excitement, or exposure to cold, and the symptoms are relieved by administration of nitroglycerin, they are classified as stable angina. Conversely, unstable angina may occur at rest or during sleep, and pain is of longer duration and not relieved readily with nitroglycerin.

Medical treatment for angina pectoris has two goals: reduce myocardial oxygen demand and increase oxygen supply. Therapy consists primarily of physical rest to decrease oxygen demand and the administration of nitrates, such as nitroglycerin, to provide more oxygen. Nitroglycerin (glyceryl trinitrate) is a vasodilator that increases blood flow (oxygen supply) by expanding the arteries. Administration can be sublingual for immediate absorption, or by nitroglycerin pads and patches for time-released medication absorbed by the skin and into the bloodstream; an overdose can cause headache. Obstructive lesions that do not respond to drug therapy may necessitate surgery.

Myocardial Infarction

Myocardial infarction (MI), the second manifestation of coronary heart disease, is a reduction of blood flow through one of the coronary arteries, resulting in an infarct. An infarct is an area of tissue that undergoes necrosis because of the elimination of blood flow. An MI is also known as a heart attack, coronary occlusion, and coronary thrombosis.

Symptoms associated with MI are similar to those experienced with angina pectoris; however, the pain usually persists for 12 or more hours and begins as a feeling of indigestion. Other manifestations include a feeling of fatigue, nausea, vomiting, and shortness of breath.

Medical treatment includes combination therapy to reduce cardiac workloads and increase cardiac output. Cardiac workload reduction therapies include bed rest, morphine for pain reduction and sedation, and oxygen if necessary. To increase cardiac output, therapy for the control and reduction of cardiac dysrhythmias is recommended (e.g., antiarrhythmic drugs, possibly a cardiac pacemaker). Nitroglycerin can relieve chest pain and increase cardiac output by intensifying the blood flow and redistributing blood to the affected myocardial tissue. Anticoagulants may be used to thin the blood in an effort to increase blood flow and reduce the possibility of another MI.

Sudden Death

Sudden death, the last manifestation of coronary heart disease, occurs during the first 24 to 48 hours after the onset of symptoms. Most sudden cardiovascular deaths are caused by ventricular fibrillation. For example, ventricular fibrillation results in ventricular standstill (cardiac arrest) if insufficient blood is pumped into the coronary arteries to supply the myocardium with oxygen. Biologic death results when oxygen delivery to the brain is inadequate for 4 to 6 minutes. Therefore the use of an automated external defibrillator (AED) (also known as *precordial shock*) is followed by cardiopulmonary resuscitation (CPR) to maintain enough blood oxygen to sustain life. Transportation to the hospital for emergency medical care is necessary.

Prevention

Lifestyle behaviors associated with the prevention of coronary heart disease are as follows:

- Regular medical checkups
- Healthy diet (e.g., reduction in saturated fat and cholesterol; increases in whole grains, fruits, and vegetables)
- Regular physical exercise
- Stress management
- Avoidance of tobacco
- High blood pressure control
- Prevention of periodontal disease
- Knowledge of the warning signs of a heart attack

Factors associated with coronary heart disease must be taken into consideration when providing nutritional counseling to improve a client's oral health. In facilitating the client's human need for protection from health risks, the dental hygienist recognizes the importance of dietary choices related to coronary heart disease and incorporates that knowledge into the nutritional education session (see Chapter 35).

Given that periodontal disease is a risk factor for coronary heart disease, clients need this information to make sound decisions about their oral health. Therefore client education should emphasize the link between oral disease and systemic disease. By stressing the importance of oral disease prevention, the dental hygienist promotes active self-care by the client—for example, teaching self-care behaviors to maintain oral wellness, encouraging active participation in formulating goals for care, and facilitating choices and client decision making.

Dental Hygiene Care

Clients with coronary heart disease are susceptible to angina pectoris and MI.

Angina Pectoris

The client with angina pectoris should be treated in a stress-free environment to meet the client's need for protection from health risks and freedom from stress. Considerations associated with angina pectoris include identification of the client's condition and frequency of angina attacks. Health history

interview questions to ascertain the stability of the client's angina are as follows:
1. Do you have chest pain on exertion? At rest?
2. How frequent are your attacks?
3. Is your chest pain relieved promptly with nitroglycerin?
4. How long are your periods of discomfort?

If clients report that their angina has worsened and that the painful episodes occur more frequently and not only during exertion, their condition is classified as unstable angina. These clients should be referred to their physician of record, and dental hygiene care postponed.

For clients with stable angina, appointments should be short and preferably scheduled for the morning. The atmosphere should be friendly and conducive to relaxation. If the client becomes fatigued or develops significant changes in pulse rate or rhythm, termination of the appointment is suggested.

Before care for a client with a history of angina pectoris is initiated, the client's supply of nitroglycerin should be placed within reach of the dental hygienist. Potency of nitroglycerin is lost after 6 months outside of a sealed container; consequently, fresh supplies should be available in the oral care environment. If an emergency develops, dental hygiene treatment is stopped; the client is placed in an upright position, reassured, and given nitroglycerin sublingually. Emergency medical services (EMS) should be activated if the client continues to experience pain after administration of nitroglycerin (see Chapter 10). Vital signs must be monitored and recorded on the client's record.

Myocardial Infarction

Clients who have a history of MI with no complications do not require care plan modifications. However, if the MI has occurred within the past 30 days, dental hygiene therapy should be postponed until the individual is 30 days or more postinfarction with no complications and no other risk factors or ischemic symptoms such as chest pain, shortness of breath, dizziness, or fatigue. The client's medical status and dental hygiene treatment plan require medical consultations if symptoms, risk factors, or complications persist after 30 days.

Drugs used to treat MI are anticoagulants, digitalis, and antihypertensive agents. These drugs necessitate care plan alterations. Anticoagulant drugs increase bleeding time and may have to be stopped several days before care that involves tissue manipulation. Some cardiologists believe that it is more dangerous to take the individual off the anticoagulant than it is to keep the individual on the drug and provide care; therefore confirmation from the client's cardiologist is recommended.

Digitalis, a glycoside, is a drug that increases the contractility of the heart. Improvement in force makes the heart more efficient as a pump, increasing its volume in relation to cardiac output. The most commonly prescribed digitalis drug is digoxin (Lanoxin).

Oral health professionals may detect early signs of digitalis toxicity in clients (i.e., anorexia, nausea, vomiting, neurologic abnormalities, and facial pain). If digitalis toxicity is not detected early, cardiac irregularities can develop (e.g., arrhythmias can progress to ventricular fibrillation and sudden death).

Antihypertensive agents used to control MIs are similar to those used to control hypertension. These agents do not influence the care plan unless the underlying condition is uncontrolled.

Clients with coronary heart disease may experience fear, depression, and disturbances in body image, associated with a change in lifestyle (e.g., dietary restrictions, exercise, and maintaining low stress). The client's psychologic condition also may influence oral health.

Emergency situations associated with MI should be managed by an emergency medical team. Oral health professionals are responsible for monitoring vital signs, administering nitroglycerin, and performing AED and CPR if the client experiences cardiac arrest. Certification in Basic Life Support (BLS) should be maintained by all oral health professionals (see Chapter 10).

Appointment Guidelines

The following steps should be taken for an individual with coronary heart disease:
- Clarify the stability of the client's angina or symptoms after 30 days following MI. If uncontrolled, do not treat. If stable, continue treatment with caution.
- Schedule short morning appointments to help control environmental stress.
- Use of adequate pain control modalities including nitrous oxide–oxygen analgesia to reduce stress if no contraindications exist.
- Select interventions that address the client's lifestyle changes and periodontal disease status.

Cardiac Dysrhythmias and Arrhythmias

Cardiac dysrhythmias and arrhythmias, terms used interchangeably, are dysfunctions of heart rate and rhythm that manifest as heart palpitations. Dysrhythmias may develop in normal and diseased hearts. In healthy hearts, arrhythmia may be associated with physical and emotional stresses (e.g., exercise, emotional shock) and usually subsides in direct response to stimulus reduction. Diseased hearts develop dysrhythmias directly associated with the CVD present, most commonly RHD, arteriosclerotic heart disease, or coronary artery disease. In some cases a cardiac dysrhythmia may develop in response to drug toxicities and electrolyte imbalances.

Etiology

Dysfunction of heart rate and rhythm arises from disturbances in nerve impulse formation or nerve impulse conduction and is categorized according to the part of the heart in which it originates. Common dysrhythmias include bradycardia, tachycardia, atrial fibrillation, premature ventricular contractions (PVCs), ventricular fibrillation, and heart block.

Cardiac dysrhythmias are medically diagnosed using an electrocardiogram (ECG) and/or a Holter monitoring system. Electrocardiography, a graphic tracing of the heart's electrical activity, determines heart rate, rhythm, and size. Each dysrhythmia is associated with a specific graphic pattern indicating a definitive medical diagnosis.

Risk Factors

See Table 43-1.

Disease Process

Bradycardia.

Bradycardia is defined as slowness of the heartbeat as evidenced by a decline in the pulse rate to less than 60 beats per minute (BPM). This normally occurs during sleeping; however, severe bradycardia can lead to fainting and convulsions. If a client has an episode of bradycardia following a normal pulse rate of 80 BPM, emergency medical treatment is necessary. This individual may be encountering the initial symptoms of an acute MI. Emergency medical treatment would include discontinuance of the dental hygiene appointment, oxygen administration, and activation of EMS.

Tachycardia.

Increased heartbeat, termed tachycardia, is associated with an abnormally high heart rate, usually greater than 100 BPM. Tachycardia can increase risk of developing angina pectoris, acute heart failure, pulmonary edema, and MI if not controlled. These conditions are related directly to the amount of work the heart is doing and decreased cardiac output. Treatment consists of antiarrhythmic drug therapy to control tachycardia and reduce potential of recurrence.

Atrial Fibrillation.

Atrial fibrillation, a condition of rapid, uneven contractions in the upper chambers of the heart (atrium), is the result of inconsistent impulses through the atrioventricular (AV) node transmitted to the ventricles at irregular intervals. The lower chambers (ventricles) cannot contract in response to the impulses, the contractions become irregular, with a decreased amount of blood pumped through the body.

During assessment the pulse rate may appear consistent with periods of irregular beats. Medical treatment targets the causative factors, not the condition itself. CHF, mitral valve stenosis, and hyperthyroidism may be linked to atrial fibrillation.

Premature Ventricular Contractions

PVCs are identified easily as pauses in an otherwise normal heart rhythm. The pause develops from an abnormal focus of the ventricle, allowing the ventricle to be at a refractory (resting) period when the impulse for contraction arrives. The feeling of the heart skipping a beat is PVC; these increase with age and are associated with fatigue, emotional stress, and excessive use of coffee, alcohol, or tobacco.

Recognition of PVCs has significance in the client with CVD. If five or more PVCs are detected during a 60-second pulse examination, medical consultation is recommended strongly. Individuals who are distressed and have five or more detectable PVCs per minute may be undergoing an acute MI or ventricular fibrillation. The following steps can protect the client from health risks:

- Terminate dental hygiene care.
- Place client on oxygen.
- Activate EMS.

Ventricular Fibrillation

Ventricular fibrillation, one of the most lethal dysrhythmias, is characterized as an advanced stage of ventricular tachycardia with rapid impulse formation and irregular impulse transmission. The heart rate is rapid and disordered and contains no rhythm. Immediate medical treatment for ventricular fibrillation is the use of an AED (precordial shock) to halt the dysrhythmia, followed by CPR. Electric current at the time of shock depolarizes the entire myocardium, allowing the cardiac impulses to gain control of the heart rate and rhythm. This depolarization should reestablish cardiac regulation. The person then is placed on drug therapy to maintain regulation of cardiac rate and rhythm. Without immediate medical attention (advanced cardiac life support), blood pressure falls to zero, resulting in unconsciousness; death may occur within 4 minutes.

Heart Block

Heart block is a dysrhythmia caused by the blocking of impulses from the atria to the ventricles at the AV node; it is an interference with the electrical impulses controlling the heart muscle. Each of the three forms of heart block is dangerous; however, third-degree heart block presents the greatest danger of cardiac arrest. The three forms are as follows:

- First-degree heart block—usually associated with coronary artery disease or digitalis drug therapy. The individual usually is asymptomatic with a normal heart rate and rhythm.
- Second-degree heart block—atrial and ventricular rates are disordered; impulses from the AV node are fully blocked in irregular patterns.
- Third-degree heart block—blocking of all impulses from the atria at the AV node, resulting in atrial and ventricular dissociation. The ventricles begin beating in response to their biologic pacemaker cells, producing an independent heartbeat from the atrium.

Medical Treatment

The cardiac pacemaker, an intracardiac device, is an electronic stimulator used to send electrical currents to the myocardium to control or maintain heart rate. Two types of pacemakers that control one or both of the heart chambers are as follows:

- Temporary pacemaker—used in emergency situations to correct ventricular standstill or arrhythmias that are not responding to other forms of treatment.
- Permanent pacemaker—inserted into the body; electrodes are transvenously placed in the endocardium and function for 5 to 10 years before battery replacement is necessary. Two general systems of cardiac pacing for the permanent pacemaker are as follows:
  - Fixed-rate pacing—based on a preset or fixed impulse
  - Demand or standby pacing—operates only when needed to stimulate ventricular contraction; pacemaker contains mechanisms that sense when the client has an independent heartbeat and stimulates the heart only when the rate deviates from normal (most commonly used because of its increased sensitivity to the body's natural metabolic requirements)

Pacemakers vary in their sensitivity to electrical interference that may alter or cease their function. Newer models, bipolar and shielded to protect against interference, do not require any special consideration during dental hygiene care. The older unipolar pacemaker models are less protected from electrical interference and can be affected negatively by dental devices and equipment that applies an electric current. When in doubt, consult the client's cardiologist.

Dental Hygiene Care

During assessment, the dental hygienist determines the type of pacemaker a client has and whether it is shielded from electrical interference. Dental devices that apply an electrical current directly to the client (e.g., ultrasonic scaling systems, electrodesensitizing equipment, pulp testers, power toothbrushes, and electrosurgery equipment) are likely to cause interference in unshielded pacemakers. Use of such equipment even in the proximity of the client with an unshielded pacemaker is contraindicated. Instead, nonelectrical alternatives to avoid functional interference are used (e.g., hand-activated instruments, tooth desensitization with a nonelectronic technique, and pulp testing performed by tooth percussion). Additional pacemaker protection can be accomplished by placing a lead apron on the client as a barrier to interrupt electrical interference generated by dental equipment such as the air-abrasive system, low- or high-speed handpiece, and computerized periodontal probe. Care should be taken in an open clinical setting where electrical dental equipment may be used for an adjacent client.

Prophylactic antibiotic premedication before dental hygiene care is not recommended after pacemaker implantation to prevent IE.

Care plan development for the individual with a cardiac pacemaker also can be affected by the drugs used to treat the underlying medical condition—anticoagulants and antihypertensive agents. Monitoring and assessment of drug therapy provide information necessary to modify treatment.

If the cardiac pacemaker fails or malfunctions during the dental hygiene appointment, the client may experience difficulty breathing; dizziness; a change in the pulse rate; swelling of the legs, ankles, arms, and wrists; and/or chest pain. When this situation arises, do the following:

1. Turn off all sources of electrical interference.
2. Activate EMS.
3. Prepare to administer basic life support (BLS) (see Chapter 10, Procedure 10-1).

Appointment Guidelines

Although uncommon, the older, unshielded pacemaker can be affected by electrical interference in the oral healthcare setting.

- Use a lead apron to interrupt electrical interference generated by dental equipment.
- Use manual rather than mechanized procedures to avoid electrical interference created by dental equipment.
- Monitor client and be prepared to administer BLS (see Chapter 10).

Congestive Heart Failure

Congestive heart failure is a syndrome characterized by myocardial dysfunction that leads to diminished cardiac output or abnormal circulatory congestion. The weakened heart develops compensatory mechanisms to continue to function (i.e., tachycardia, ventricular dilation, and enlargement of the heart muscle).

CHF can occur as two independent failures (left-sided and right-sided heart failure); however, because the heart functions as a closed unit, both pumps must be functioning properly or the heart's efficiency is diminished.

Etiology

Causative factors associated with CHF are arteriosclerotic heart disease, hypertensive CVD, valvular heart disease, pericarditis, circulatory overload, and coronary heart disease. These factors contribute to the gradual failure of the heart by reducing the inflow of blood to the heart, increasing the inflow to the lungs, obstructing the outflow of blood from the heart, or damaging the heart muscle itself.

Risk Factors

See Table 43-1.

Disease Process

Clients who have left-sided heart failure have difficulty receiving oxygenated blood from the lungs, resulting in increased fluid and blood in the lungs, causing dyspnea on exertion, shortness of breath on lying supine, cough, and expectoration. These clients tend to require extra pillows to sleep and cannot be placed in a supine position.

Right-sided heart failure is associated with the blood return from the body, resulting in systemic venous congestion and peripheral edema. Clients with right-sided heart failure have feet and ankle edema and often complain of cold hands and feet.

Medical Treatment

CHF treatment is related directly to the removal of the cause. Usually the corrective therapy associated with the underlying disease eliminates the presence of CHF. Some patients require additional methods of rehabilitation, such as dietary control, reduced physical activity, and drug therapy (e.g., diuretics to reduce salt and water retention and digitalis to strengthen myocardial contractility).

Dental Hygiene Care

Individuals with CHF who are monitored closely by a physician do not require a change in conventional dental hygiene care; however, factors associated with the cause of CHF should be considered in the care plan. Alterations are based on the causative factors (e.g., hypertension, valvular heart disease, coronary heart disease, and MI) in association with the individual's current medical status.

Clients taking digitalis are prone to nausea and vomiting during dental procedures. Therefore procedures that may promote gagging should be performed with extra care. In addition, the dental hygienist should be aware of any underlying heart conditions that are responsible for CHF. These conditions must be evaluated and appropriate precautions taken.

Alterations in the care plan for a client with left-sided CHF are related to the human needs for protection from health risks and for freedom from fear and stress. Client positioning must be upright to support breathing. Actions should be taken to minimize distress, and instructions should reinforce the need for a reduced-sodium diet to alleviate fluid retention.

If an emergency arises, medical assistance should be obtained. The client is usually conscious with difficulty breathing. The following treatment is recommended:

1. Position the person upright to facilitate breathing.
2. Administer oxygen if necessary.
3. Monitor vital signs.

Appointment Guidelines

The following steps should be taken when treating clients with CHF:

- Position client upright to decrease collection of fluid in the lungs.

- Limit ultrasonic instrumentation use so that unnecessary fluid does not back up in the oral cavity. This fluid reduction minimizes client anxiety and facilitate breathing.
- Recommend nutritional counseling to decrease sodium intake and alleviate fluid retention.

Congenital Heart Disease

Congenital heart disease is an abnormality of the heart's structure and function caused by abnormal or disordered heart development before birth. Commonly observed congenital heart malformations are ventricular septal defect, atrial septal defect, and patent ductus arteriosus.

Etiology

The cause of congenital heart disease is generally unknown; however, genetic and environmental factors have been attributed to poor intrauterine development. Genetic conditions, related to heredity, are apparent in some situations. Environmental factors are based on the mother's health—for example, rubella (German measles) and drug addiction have produced delayed fetal development and growth retardation associated with the cardiovascular structure.

Disease Process and Medical Treatment

Congenital heart disease is the result of various heart defects that dictate the disease process:

Ventricular Septal Defect

A ventricular septal defect—a shunt (opening) in the septum between the ventricles—allows oxygenated blood from the left ventricle to flow into the right ventricle (Figure 43-4). Small defects that close spontaneously or are correctable by surgery have a good prognosis. Larger defects that are left untreated or are irreparable usually result in death from secondary cardiovascular complications. The ventricular septal defect can be detected by a characteristic heart murmur audible at birth.

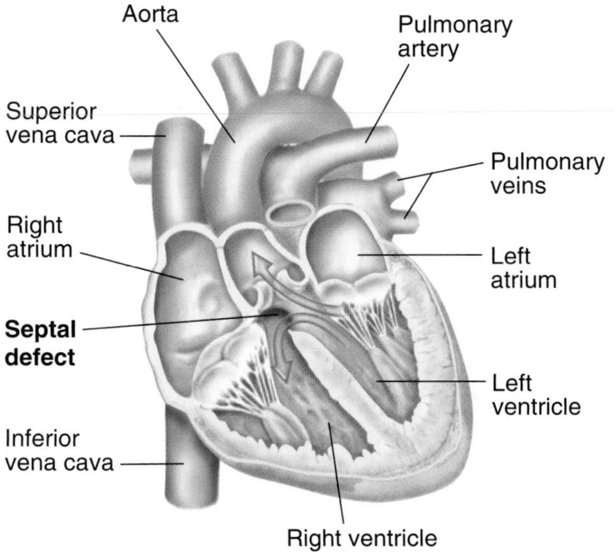

Figure 43-4. Ventricular septal defect. (From Bleck E, Nagel D: *Physically handicapped children: a medical atlas for teachers,* ed 2, Needham Heights, Mass, 1982, Allyn and Bacon.)

Clinical manifestations vary with size of defect, infant age, and the effect of the deviated blood passage on the cardiovascular structure. Large ventricular septal defects cause hypertrophy of the ventricles, resulting in CHF.

Atrial Septal Defect

The atrial septal defect—a shunt (opening) between the left and right atria—is responsible for approximately 10% of congenital heart defects. The blood volume overload eventually causes the right atrium to enlarge and the right ventricle to dilate (Figure 43-5).

Usually the client is asymptomatic and the defect goes undetected; however, in adults, clinical symptoms become more pronounced. The client is fatigued easily and short of breath after mild exertion. Treatment includes cardiovascular repair surgery, observance of developing atrial arrhythmias, and monitoring of vital signs.

Patent Ductus Arteriosus

Patent ductus arteriosus is the most common congenital heart defect found in adults. During development the fetal heart contains a blood vessel called the *ductus arteriosus.* This vessel connects the pulmonary artery to the descending aorta. Normally after birth the vessel closes. If the vessel fails to close, a congenital heart defect forms. Failure to close is associated with premature births and therefore failure of the vessel's contracture necessary for closure. Patent ductus arteriosus has been linked to rubella syndrome.

Shunting of blood in a patent ductus arteriosus defect is from the aorta to the pulmonary artery (Figure 43-6). This type of blood flow results in the recirculation of oxygenated blood through the lungs. Thus the left atrium and ventricle have an increased workload from increased pulmonary blood return, which can result in CHF. If the condition is left untreated, severe obstructive pulmonary vascular disease may develop.

Clinical manifestations include respiratory distress, susceptibility to respiratory tract infections, and slow motor development. Treatment consists of surgical correction and elimination of symptoms associated with secondary complications.

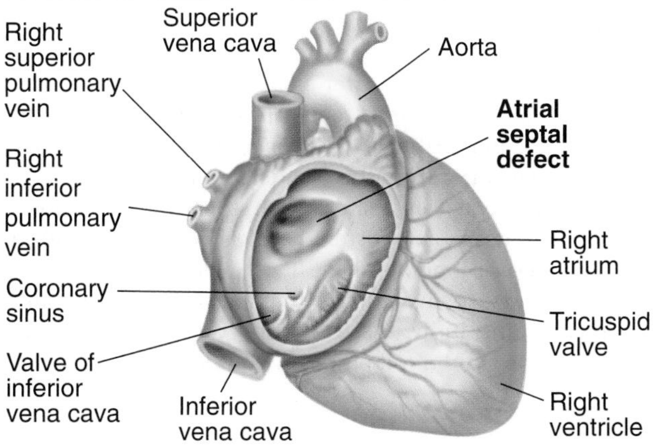

Figure 43-5. Atrial septal defect. (From Bleck E, Nagel D: *Physically handicapped children: a medical atlas for teachers,* ed 2, Needham Heights, Mass, 1982, Allyn and Bacon.)

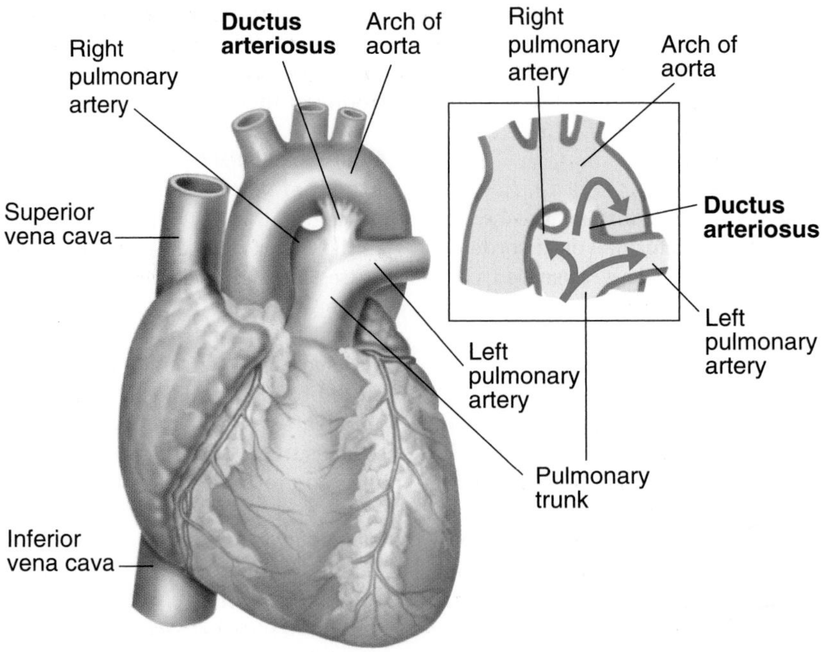

Figure 43-6. Patent ductus arteriosus defect. (From Bleck E, Nagel D: *Physically handicapped children: a medical atlas for teachers,* ed 2, Needham Heights, Mass, 1982, Allyn and Bacon.)

Tetralogy of Fallot

Tetralogy of Fallot is a rare and complex congenital heart defect generally associated with cyanosis. The defect is composed of four congenital abnormalities: ventricular septal defect, pulmonary stenosis, right ventricular hypertrophy, and malposition of the aorta. The blood shunts right to left through the ventricular septal defect, permitting unoxygenated blood to mix with oxygenated blood, resulting in cyanosis. Treatment includes measures to relieve cyanosis and palliative and corrective surgery.

Dental Hygiene Care

The individual with congenital heart disease does not require extensive alterations in care. However, the American Heart Association recommends antibiotic premedication before dental hygiene procedures to prevent IE in persons with residual defects following repair, with unrepaired cyanotic congenital heart defects including palliative shunts, and during the first 6 months after surgery to correct congenital defects. Secondary concerns focus on the management of cardiovascular complications, such as CHF and cardiac dysrhythmias, resulting from the congenital defect.

Dental hygiene care includes physician consultation to confirm drug usage and current medical status, prophylactic antibiotic medication to prevent IE, and assessment of symptoms secondary to the disease that may require treatment alteration. If the individual develops CHF, then care plan considerations should follow those outlined.

Cardiovascular Surgery

Open-heart surgery is necessary for complex procedures that need direct visualization of the heart while being performed (e.g., heart transplants, some heart valve replacements, and coronary bypass surgery). Open-heart surgery always is performed with the use of a heart-lung machine that completely controls cardiopulmonary function, enabling surgeons to operate for long periods without interfering with the individual's metabolic needs. Closed-heart surgery usually is associated with cardiac catheterization.

Types of Cardiovascular Surgery

Angioplasty

The most common type of closed-heart surgery, **angioplasty** (also known as *percutaneous coronary intervention* [PCI]), involves the use of a catheter (a long, slender tube) with a tiny balloon at the end that is inserted into the coronary artery. Specifically, the balloon is inserted into places where the artery narrows, is inflated to flatten fatty deposits, and is deflated to allow the increased blood flow to compress and redistribute the atherosclerotic lesion. This procedure is used in individuals who have a small atherosclerotic lesion constricting blood flow. If the lesion cannot be corrected by the angioplasty procedure, bypass surgery may be necessary.

Coronary Stent

The coronary stent is a mesh-like metal used to open narrow arteries. Placed in conjunction with PCI procedures, the stent maintains the lumen opening in the arteries, allowing blood to flow freely, thereby reducing angina and potential myocardial infarctions.

Coronary Bypass Surgery

Coronary bypass surgery, a common procedure to replace blocked arteries, is performed by removing part of the leg vein or chest artery and then grafting it onto the coronary artery, thereby creating a new passageway for the blood. This type of surgery can be done for more than one artery at a time and is named accordingly (double-bypass, triple-bypass). The benefits of coronary bypass surgery include relief from angina, increased tolerance to exercise, improved quality of life, and extended life span. A person who has had bypass surgery has no contraindications to dental hygiene therapy.

Valvular Defect Repair

Valvular defect repair or replacement is performed frequently. Persons with artificial cardiac valves are at high risk for infections and IE and must be premedicated with an antibiotic before dental hygiene care (see Box 43-1 and Chapter 12, Tables 12-4 and 12-5, and Boxes 12-4, 12-5, and 12-6).

Heart Transplantation

Heart transplantation is a viable option for individuals with end-stage heart disease in which no other therapeutic intervention is considered effective. Although many hospitals perform cardiac transplantation, the dilemma is finding donors.

Future goals and implications of heart transplantation include the development of a safe, reliable, permanent, totally implantable artificial heart device that allows a recipient to carry out normal activities. The development of such a device may increase availability of this life-saving procedure for eligible recipients who at this time await donors.

Dental Hygiene Care

Client Who Has Had Closed-Heart Surgery

No contraindications are associated with dental or dental hygiene treatment unless the individual is taking anticoagulant medication. As in all cardiac-associated situations, consultation with the client's cardiologist is recommended.

Client After Open-Heart Surgery

No dental hygiene procedures relate uniquely to the individual who has had cardiovascular surgery. When in doubt, the cardiologist is consulted; however, prosthetic valvular heart replacements and those cardiac surgeries that make the client susceptible to infection require prophylactic antibiotic premedication.

Complications from dental hygiene care observed in clients who have had cardiovascular surgery are associated with the drug therapy used rather than the surgery itself. Most postsurgical clients are placed on medication to increase healing, suppress immune response, reduce infection, and/or decrease clot formation. Careful evaluation of drug contraindications and reactions is necessary.

Client Who Has Had a Heart Transplant

A major concern of the heart transplant patient is infection and transplant rejection. Before care, consultation with the client's cardiologist is recommended highly to determine if additional premedication is indicated. Most transplant patients are on long-term preventive antibiotic therapy to control systemic bacteremias. They also are placed on immunosuppressant medications such as cyclosporine (Sandimmune) to reduce the possibility of rejection.

Oral Manifestations of Cardiovascular Medications

Some medications used in CVD therapy have a profound effect on the oral cavity. (See Chapter 14 and Table 43-2.) These medications typically include those that treat hypertension, heart transplant stabilization, and CHD. Persons taking cardiovascular medications should seek regular dental hygiene care and maintain excellent oral biofilm control to balance their increased vulnerability to dental and periodontal diseases.

Most medications for the treatment of hypertension cause xerostomia, increasing the individual's risk for dental caries and periodontal disease. Individuals with exposed root surfaces are at risk for root surface caries and dentinal hypersensitivity. Self-administered fluoride therapy, ACP therapy, and use of saliva substitutes and xylitol products should be part of the individual's daily self-care regimen to meet the client's needs. Some calcium channel blockers alter taste perception, cause drug-influenced gingival enlargement, and create salivary gland pain. Immunosuppressants used for the stabilization of heart transplants increase the individual's risk for developing periodontal disease or may exaggerate a preexisting condition, leading to an unmet need in skin and mucous membrane integrity.

Another dental hygiene diagnosis to consider is a need for protection from health risks because immunosuppressants increase risk for developing opportunistic infections such as candidiasis, herpes simplex, herpes zoster, necrotizing ulcerative gingivitis, and drug-influenced gingival enlargement. In addition to regular professional dental hygiene care, these individuals should use an antimicrobial mouth rinse for 30 seconds twice daily as part of their self-care regimen to reduce oral disease risk.

Persons with a history of heart attack or cerebrovascular accident are placed on blood thinners (anticoagulants) to increase blood flow. The side effects are prolonged bleeding and spontaneous oral bleeding in the presence of infection. These individuals must maintain a healthy periodontium to reduce periodontal disease risk.

Preventing and Managing Cardiac Emergencies

The individual with a CVD or cardiovascular symptom or defect is considered high risk—one whose life may be threatened by daily activities. These clients have a need for protection from health risks because of their increased potential for an emergency. The most common physical pain encountered is chest pain accompanied by difficulty breathing. If the client complains of physical pain that cannot be alleviated, EMS should be activated or 911 called.

For individuals with angina pectoris, hypertension, previous MI, and CHF, the risk for life-threatening medical emergencies rises as a result of an increase in fear and stress.

Assessing past responses in oral healthcare situations and monitoring the client's reactions to dental hygiene procedures are important. Muscular tenseness, perspiration, and verbal cues indicate a potential emergency, and the client's need for protection from health risks must be met.

Individuals with CVD may not take responsibility for their oral health. Understandably, these individuals fail to relate their life-threatening medical condition with oral disease; however, by increasing a client's awareness that periodontal disease and the systemic condition are linked, the dental hygienist may change the client's value system and oral health behavior and improve systemic health. Accurate assessment of the client's personal beliefs, behaviors, and values can identify motivators (needs) that may lead to the client's commitment to therapeutic goals and priorities.

Table 43-3 illustrates sample dental hygiene diagnoses for a client with coronary heart disease.

Planning prevents emergencies and ensures that client needs are the focus of therapeutic interventions. When a care plan is developed, attention is given to drug therapies to ensure that no contraindications are present and that side effects are identified (see Table 43-2). Tables 43-4 and 43-5 can be used when developing care plans for clients with a CVD.

Implementation of care takes into consideration the possibility of a medical emergency (see Chapter 10). The most life-threatening emergency situation is cardiac arrest. Emergency situations require the following steps:

1. Contact EMS or call 911.
2. Monitor vital signs and state of consciousness.
3. Administer oxygen.
4. Provide BLS.

Other medical emergencies associated with CVD are attacks of angina pectoris and MI. Box 43-3 lists actions to be taken.

Oral care professionals evaluate the client's current health status in light of the established client goals. By reviewing assessment data, dental hygiene diagnoses, care plan, and interventions used, practitioners can determine where less-than-desirable outcomes occurred and modify care as necessary. Table 43-6 illustrates an evaluation of dental hygiene interventions for the care plan in Box 43-1.

TABLE 43-3

Sample Dental Hygiene Diagnoses—Client with Coronary Heart Disease

Dental Hygiene Diagnosis	Related to	As Evidenced by
Protection from health risks: potential for myocardial infarction	Stress Anxiety Recent life-threatening medical diagnosis	Chest, jaw, neck, throat, interscapular area, and left arm pain Agitation
Responsibility for oral health	Low value ascribed to oral health	Lack of interest in performing daily oral self-care
Potential for health risks: potential for infection	History of infective endocarditis	Condition indicated on health history questionnaire
Biologically sound and functional dentition	Drug therapy (diuretics) taken by client	Xerostomia Root caries
Biologically sound and functional dentition (nutrition)	Dietary restrictions of cholesterol, saturated fat, and sodium	Obesity, high LDL cholesterol or lipid blood values

TABLE 43-4

Quick Reference—Signs, Symptoms, and Treatment of Individuals with Cardiovascular Disease

Disease	Signs and Symptoms	Medical and Surgical Treatment
Rheumatic heart disease	Carditis, polyarthritis, chorea, erythema marginatum, subcutaneous nodules, fever	Bedrest and medications associated with manifestations
Infective endocarditis	Initial high fever, cardiac decompensation, heart murmur	Antibiotic therapy
Valvular heart defects	Fatigue, shortness of breath, and pulmonary edema If defects are left untreated, congestive heart failure will develop	Valvular repair or replacement with prosthetic heart valve
Mitral valve prolapse	Palpitations, chest pain, nervousness, shortness of breath, dizziness	Treatment is not always necessary; aimed at alleviating symptoms
Cardiac dysrhythmias and arrhythmias	Bradycardia: pulse rate <60 beats per minute (BPM) Tachycardia: pulse rate >150 BPM	Antiarrhythmic drug therapy or cardiac pacemaker
Hypertension	Headache, fatigue, diminished exercise tolerance, shortness of breath	Antihypertension drug therapy; dietary control of sodium
Coronary (ischemic) heart disease	Angina pectoris, discomfort in jaw, neck, throat, interscapular area, and left arm	Bedrest; administration of nitroglycerin
Congestive heart failure	Fatigue, weakness, dyspnea, cough, anorexia	Treatment directed at the underlying cause
Congenital heart disease	Dependent on type of defect	Surgery to correct defect

TABLE 43-5

Quick Reference—Dental Hygiene Care Implications for Individuals with Cardiovascular Disease

Disease	Implications for Dental Hygiene Care	Dental Hygiene Actions
Rheumatic heart disease	Special attention to oral self-care practices; self-inflicted bacteremias may occur when oral disease is present.	Careful manipulation of soft tissues during instrumentation; ADA-accepted antibacterial mouth rinse to reduce transient bacteremia
Infective endocarditis	Client susceptible to reinfection with transient bacteremia. Prophylactic antibiotic premedication is indicated for invasive dental hygiene procedures.	Careful manipulation of soft tissue; antibacterial mouth rinse to reduce transient bacteremia
Valvular heart defects	Infective endocarditis may occur after dental hygiene procedures that cause transient bacteremias. Clients receiving anticoagulant medication may have a prolonged bleeding time.	If anticoagulant medication is being used and scaling procedures are planned, dosage of anticoagulant medication should be discussed with client's cardiologist
Mitral valve prolapse	Special attention to oral self-care practices because self-inflicted bacteremias may occur when oral disease is present.	Careful manipulation of soft tissues during instrumentation and preprocedural antimicrobial rinsing to reduce transient bacteremia
Cardiac dysrhythmias and arrhythmias	Electrical interference can cause unshielded pacemaker to malfunction.	Use of electrical dental equipment is contraindicated
Hypertension	Stress and anxiety about treatment may increase blood pressure.	Use stress reduction strategies; if blood pressure is uncontrolled, dental hygiene care is contraindicated
Coronary (ischemic) heart disease	Stress and anxiety about treatment may precipitate angina.	Have nitroglycerin available during treatment. Implement stress reduction strategies; create atmosphere conducive to relaxation
Congestive heart failure	None if person is under appropriate medical care.	Keep client in upright position to decrease lung fluid

TABLE 43-6

Sample Evaluation of Dental Hygiene Interventions

Client Goals	Evaluation Measures	Expected Outcomes
Complete invasive dental hygiene therapy (scaling and root debridement) so that antibiotic coverage occurs with a 9- to 14-day interval between coverage	Appointments scheduled 9-14 days apart	No drug resistance occurring Hard and soft deposits removed
By 9/13, reduce gingival bleeding by 90%	Document clinical outcomes using bleeding on probing	Minimal to no gingival bleeding on probing
By 12/13, reduce periodontal probing depths	Document clinical outcomes using periodontal probing depths and clinical attachment levels	Periodontal probing depths reduced by at least 1 mm Clinical attachment levels stable

BOX 43-3

Basic Steps in a Cardiac Emergency Situation

Make certain client is comfortable; loosen restricting garments, elevate head slightly, provide reassurance.

Angina Pectoris

- Immediately administer nitroglycerin sublingually and 100% oxygen with a face mask or nasal cannula to prevent disease transmission.*
- Monitor vital signs.

Myocardial Infarction

- Have client transferred to an emergency facility as soon as possible.
- Apply automated external defibrillator and/or administer cardiopulmonary resuscitation if necessary.
- Stay with the client until the physician or emergency medical technician takes over.

*Note: An overdose of nitroglycerin can cause headache.

Finally, it is important to document in the client record all components of the dental hygiene process of care. This documentation includes the objective, complete, concise, and accurate recording of all collected data, treatment planned and provided, consultations sought, recommendations made, and all other information relevant to client care and treatment. Doing so meets ethical and legal standards and ensures continuity of care by subsequent healthcare providers.

CLIENT EDUCATION TIPS

- Explain that prophylactic antibiotic premedication must be taken 1 hour before the scheduled appointment to achieve optimal blood levels and to reduce the possibility of infective endocarditis (IE) in persons with the highest categories of risk for IE (see Chapter 12, Box 12-4).
- Explain that oral health maintenance reduces self-induced and professionally induced transient bacteremias (prevention of IE).
- Explain that reducing gingival inflammation and oral biofilm is important when taking anticoagulant medication.
- Explain that periodontal disease may increase one's risk for coronary heart disease.
- Discuss how some forms of cardiovascular disease are preventable by lifestyle changes such as following a low-sodium, low-fat, low-cholesterol diet that is rich in fruits, vegetables, and whole grains; getting daily exercise; performing stress management; and not using tobacco.

LEGAL, ETHICAL, AND SAFETY ISSUES

- The client with cardiovascular disease (CVD) poses a malpractice risk if treatment procedures fail to follow the standard of care. Legal issues as a result of a medical emergency include the following[12]:
  - The original "incident" may subject the practitioner to liability for causing additional harm (even death) resulting from (1) later negligent care and treatment of the original injury, (2) later care and treatment (not negligent), or (3) later care and treatment when an inherent risk (e.g., infection) is the aftermath.
  - If a client with CVD develops chest pain and begins to feel nauseous and sweat profusely, the provider should (1) stop dental hygiene care; (2) alert the dentist; and (3) together with the dentist manage the immediate emergency situation, which may include use of the automated external defibrillator and Basic Life Support.
  - If dental hygiene care is continued and the client experiences a myocardial infarction, liability charges may be brought against the practitioner.
  - If dental care is performed on a client who was not appropriately assessed and his or her status is not documented on an acceptable health history form, the practitioner could be held responsible for any damage resulting from care.
  - If a client reports a cardiac condition that requires antibiotic premedication to prevent infective endocarditis (per American Heart Association guidelines) and he or she is not premedicated, the practitioner may be liable for morbidity and mortality that develops after treatment.
  - Medical emergency situations must be prevented and properly managed or a malpractice suit could arise.

KEY CONCEPTS

- Review health history, dental history, cultural history, pharmacologic history, and risk factors for systemic and oral disease as a standard of care; consult with client's physician or cardiologist as required.
- Periodontal disease may contribute to one's risk for developing cardiovascular disease (CVD) (e.g., the inflammatory process increases risk for thrombosis development).
- The practitioner must follow the *Prevention of Infective Endocarditis* guidelines from the American Heart Association and strive to maintain the oral health of clients with cardiovascular disease.
- Hypertension can be detected by measuring blood pressure as part of the dental hygiene assessment.
- Unstable angina pectoris indicates that a client has increasing chest pain at rest and during sleep. Clients with unstable angina are at risk for a possible medical emergency and should not be treated in the dental setting until medical clearance is obtained.
- The drug of choice for a client experiencing angina is nitroglycerin, usually administered sublingually. Too much nitroglycerin can cause headache.
- Dental hygiene care should be postponed if a client has had a myocardial infarction within 30 days of the scheduled appointment or if ischemic symptoms persist.
- Cardiac dysrhythmias and arrhythmias are dysfunctions of the heart rate and rhythm and may be detected when assessing the client's pulse rate.
- Unshielded cardiac pacemakers may be susceptible to interference generated by some dental equipment (e.g., ultrasonic scalers, pulp testers, electrodesensitizing equipment, air-abrasion systems, computerized periodontal probes, low- or high-speed handpieces).
- Clients with congestive heart failure have difficulty breathing in a supine position.
- Clients with a history of CVD can be given local anesthetic agents that contain epinephrine at the minimally safe dose.
- Anticoagulant medications increase bleeding time. Clients taking such medications need a medical consultation and prothrombin time values within the range of normal before dental hygiene care is performed.
- Clients taking immunosuppressant medication for a heart transplant and calcium channel blockers for hypertension are at risk for drug-influenced gingival enlargement.
- Prevention of CVD requires healthy lifestyles (i.e., reduction in saturated fat, cholesterol, and sodium intake; increased exercise; decreased stress; no tobacco use; and control of hypertension).

CRITICAL THINKING EXERCISES

Case 1: Client with History of MI on Anticoagulant Therapy

During assessment, the client reports that he had an MI 2 years ago and is taking Coumadin twice daily. The client has early periodontitis.

1. Cite implications of MI and anticoagulant medication on dental hygiene care.
2. What unmet human needs does this client have?
3. Should this client receive dental hygiene care? Why or why not?

4. If client is treated, should the dental hygiene care plan be altered?
5. What client education topics need to be addressed?

Case 2: Documentation of Health History—Client with Coronary Heart Disease

Medical Profile: Mrs. J, age 56, was last examined by her physician in September. On completion of the health history, you note that Mrs. J has responded "yes" to some questions concerning coronary heart disease, experiences chest pain, and carries nitroglycerin. Although the nitroglycerin usually helps, she sometimes needs to take two doses.

1. What additional questions should the dental hygienist ask Mrs. J?
2. What unmet human needs does this client have?
3. Cite implications for dental hygiene care. Explain.
4. Should the dental hygiene care plan be altered? Explain.
5. The client is at risk for what medical emergency?

REFERENCES

1. World Health Organization (WHO): *World health statistics: annual report*, Washington, DC, 2012, WHO.
2. Lockhart P, Bolger A, Papapanou P, et al: Periodontal disease and atherosclerotic vascular disease: Dose the evidence support an independent association? AHA Scientific Statement, *Circulation* 125:2520, 2012.
3. Bolger A, Papanou P, Osinbowale O: Periodontal disease and atherosclerotic vascular disease: Dose the evidence support an independent association? AHA Scientific Statement, *Circulation* 125:2520, 2012. Update available at: http://newsroom.heart.org/pr/aha/periodontal-disease-and-atherosclerotic-234243.aspx. Accessed May 15, 2012.
4. Dorn J, Genco R, Grossi S, et al: Periodontal disease and recurrent cardiovascular events in survivors of myocardial infarction: the Western New York Acute MI Study, *J Periodontol* 81:502-511, 2010.
5. Tonetti M: Periodontitis and risk for atheroscelerosis: an update on intervention trials, *J Clin Periodontol* 36:15, 2009.
6. Berry J: Setting the record straight, ADA News Release. Available at: http://www.ada.org/news/7275.aspx. Accessed July 16, 2012.
7. Wilson W, Taubert KA, Gewitz M, et al: Prevention of infective endocarditis. Guidelines from the American Heart Association, *Circulation* 116:1736, 2007.
8. Pickett F, Gurenlian J: *The medical history: clinical implications and emergency prevention in dental settings*, Baltimore, 2007, Lippincott Williams and Wilkins.
9. Kaptoge S, Di Angelantonio E, Lowe G, et al: Emerging risk factors collaboration; C-reactive protein concentration and risk of coronary heart disease, stroke, and mortality: an individual participant meta-analysis, *Lancet* 375:132, 2010.
10. Chopra R, Sudhir P, Shivani M: Comparison of cardiovascular disease risk in two main forms of periodontitis, *J Dental Res* 9:74, 2012.
11. Frisbee S, Chambers C, Frisbee J, et al: Association between dental hygiene, CVD risk factors and systemic inflammation in rural adults, *J Dental Hygiene* 84:177, 2010.
12. McCarthy F: *Essentials of safe dentistry for the medically compromised patient*, Philadelphia, 1989, Saunders.

EVOLVE RESOURCES

Please visit http://evolve.elsevier.com/Darby/hygiene for additional practice and study support tools.

CHAPTER 44

Diabetes Mellitus

Deborah Blythe Bauman

COMPETENCIES

1. Define diabetes and prediabetes, and explain the role of the dental hygienist in the care of a person with diabetes.
2. Discuss the classification of diabetes, including:
   - Differentiate between type 1 and type 2 diabetes mellitus in terms of prevalence, characteristics, and potential complications.
   - Explain gestational diabetes and its potential complications.
   - Identify other specific types of diabetes mellitus.
3. Recognize the pathophysiology of diabetes, including the signs, symptoms, and oral and systemic complications.
4. Recognize a diabetic emergency, and take appropriate action for management.
5. Appreciate lifestyle adjustments required by the individual with diabetes.
6. Explain the dental hygiene process of care for clients with diabetes mellitus, including:
   - Plan appropriate dental hygiene care for an individual with diabetes mellitus.
   - Assist the client in preventing diabetes when risk factors are present and recommend referral for screening.

Diabetes mellitus, which is one of the most widespread diseases, affects approximately 25.8 million adults and children in the United States or about 8.3% of the population. Of these individuals, more than 7 million are unaware of their diabetes. These numbers are increasing substantially with increasing obesity. As many as one in three people born in 2000 will develop diabetes.[1] Individuals with diabetes face shortened life spans and the probability of developing acute and chronic health complications.

Diabetes mellitus is actually a group of disorders characterized by **hyperglycemia** (abnormally increased blood glucose) that results from defective insulin secretion, defective insulin action, or a combination of both. Chronic hyperglycemia damages the eyes, kidneys, nerves (**neuropathy**), heart, and blood vessels (**microangiopathy**). The dental hygienist plays a key role in managing oral disease in persons with diabetes (Box 44-1).

Prediabetes

Prediabetes is a condition that precedes type 2 diabetes. People with prediabetes have blood glucose levels that are higher than normal but below diagnostic levels. Approximately 10% to 15% of the U.S. population has prediabetes. Prediabetes is also called **impaired glucose tolerance** and **impaired fasting glucose**, all of which refer to metabolic stages that are somewhere between normal glucose homeostasis and diabetes (Figure 44-1). People with prediabetes are at high risk for developing diabetes and cardiovascular disease. Impaired glucose tolerance and impaired fasting glucose are associated with abdominal obesity; high triglyceride levels, low high-density lipoprotein (i.e., "good cholesterol") levels, or both; and hypertension. Individuals who are at high risk for developing diabetes can use a variety of interventions that can delay and often prevent diabetes. Interventions that have been shown to reduce the development of type 2 diabetes by 58% to 71%, include the following:

- Increasing physical activity to include 150 minutes per week of moderate activity, such as walking
- Targeting a 7% weight reduction
- Reinforcing behaviors with follow-up counseling
- Adding metformin therapy for those with body mass indices of more than 35 kg/m^2 who are less than 60 years old and for those women with prior gestational diabetes mellitus; see Oral Hypoglycemic Agents later in this chapter for more information.
- Obtaining annual monitoring

Prediabetes has no symptoms, so it is important for the dental hygienist to know the risk factors, to ask questions, to refer clients for screening, and to encourage clients to make healthy changes.

Classification of Diabetes (Table 44-1 and Box 44-2)

The four major clinical types of diabetes mellitus are as follows[2]:

- Type 1 diabetes mellitus
- Type 2 diabetes mellitus
- Gestational diabetes mellitus
- Other specific types

Type 1 (Insulin Deficient) Diabetes Mellitus

Type 1 diabetes mellitus, which involves about 5% of the adult diabetic population, commonly presents during childhood and adolescence, but it can strike at any age. In individuals with type 1 diabetes, the body does not produce insulin. People who develop type 1 diabetes mellitus are rarely obese. To survive, people with type 1 diabetes require the regular lifelong administration of insulin via injection or pump. The disease results from the destruction of the pancreatic beta cells by the body's immune system. Genetic predisposition related to the presence of certain human leukocyte antigens that influence immune activity directed against islet cells is essential for type 1 diabetes. Research studies suggest a genetic origin associated with type 1 and type 2 diabetes. The role of genetics is weaker in type 1 diabetes than in type 2 diabetes. Environmental factors, which are still poorly defined, have been postulated to play a causative role in genetically predisposed individuals. Autoimmune reactions and environmental factors (e.g., viral infections) have been demonstrated in research. Twin studies reveal that, if one twin develops type 1 diabetes, the other twin will develop the disease in approximately 50% of cases.[3]

Type 2 (Insulin Resistant) Diabetes Mellitus

Type 2 diabetes mellitus, which is the most common form of diabetes, results from insulin resistance and is preventable. Most individuals with type 2 diabetes are obese, and obesity itself causes some degree of insulin resistance. Individuals who are not obese by traditional weight criteria may have an increased percentage of body fat distributed in the abdominal region. People with type 2 diabetes constitute approximately 90% to 95% of the diabetic population. Of the undiagnosed, the vast majority have type 2 diabetes. The risk of developing type 2 diabetes increases with obesity, age, lack of physical activity, history of gestational diabetes mellitus, hypertension, and **dyslipidemia** (i.e., abnormal amounts of blood

BOX 44-1

The Dental Hygienist's Role in the Care of a Person with Diabetes

- Conduct periodontal risk assessment.
- Determine the need for co-management.
- Monitor the pharmacologic history for drug interactions with insulin.
- Minimize potential risks for emergencies.
- Detect undiagnosed and uncontrolled diabetes and refer.
- Modify dental hygiene care plan on the basis of client needs.
- Monitor the outcomes of dental hygiene care (evaluation).

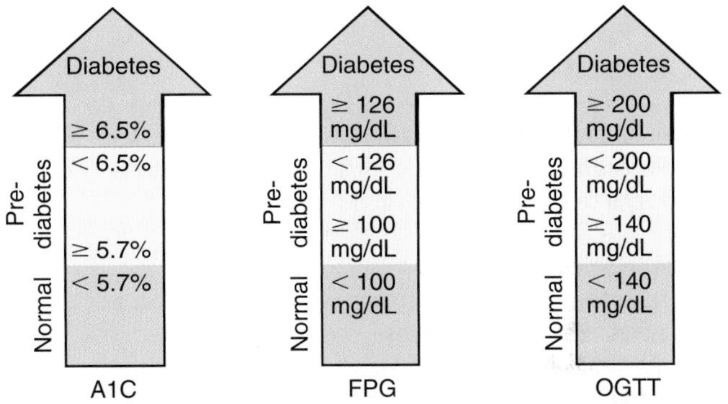

Figure 44-1. The arrows demonstrate the progression from normal to a diagnosis of prediabetes and from prediabetes to a diagnosis of diabetes. Prediabetes and diabetes can be identified using any one of three tests: glycosylated hemoglobin A_{1c} *(A1C)*, fasting plasma glucose *(FPG)*, or oral glucose tolerance test *(OGTT)*. These tests each have distinct diagnostic thresholds for the diagnosis. (From the American Diabetes Association. Available at: http://www.diabetes.org/diabetes-basics/prevention/pre-diabetes/diagnosis.html. Accessed April 30, 2013.)

TABLE 44-1

Characteristics of Type 1 and Type 2 Diabetes Mellitus

Factor	Type 1	Type 2
Age at onset	Usually young, but may occur at any age	Usually in persons >40 years old, but may occur at any age
Type of onset	Usually abrupt	Gradual and subtle
Genetic susceptibility	Human leukocyte antigen–related DR3, DR4, and others	Frequent genetic background; not related to human leukocyte antigen
Environmental factors	Viruses, toxins, autoimmune stimulation	Obesity
Islet-cell antibody	Present at outset	Not observed
Endogenous insulin	Minimal or absent	Stimulated response is adequate but with delayed secretion or reduced but not absent
Nutritional status	Thin, catabolic state	Obese or may be normal
Symptoms	Thirst, polyuria, polyphagia, fatigue	Frequently none or mild
Ketosis	Prone at onset or during insulin deficiency	Resistant except during infection or stress
Control of diabetes	Often difficult, with wide glucose fluctuation	Variable; helped by dietary adherence
Dietary management	Essential	Essential; may suffice for glycemic control
Insulin	Required for all	Required for about 40%
Sulfonylurea	Not efficacious	Efficacious
Vascular and neurologic complications	Seen in majority after ≥5 years of diabetes	Frequent

BOX 44-2

Diabetes Mellitus

Prediabetes

- Metabolic stage intermediate between normal glucose homeostasis and diabetes; indicates relatively high risk for development of diabetes

Type 1 Diabetes Mellitus

- Results from beta-cell destruction, usually leading to absolute insulin deficiency
  A. Immune mediated
  B. Idiopathic

Type 2 Diabetes Mellitus

- Ranges from insulin resistance with relative insulin deficiency to insulin secretion defect with insulin resistance

Other Specific Types

- Other types of diabetes associated with certain conditions or syndromes: pancreatic disease, endocrinopathies, infections, chemical- or drug-induced disease, genetic defects, genetic syndromes, insulin-receptor abnormalities, and others

Gestational Diabetes Mellitus

- Any degree of glucose intolerance with onset or first recognition during pregnancy

TABLE 44-2

Complications of Diabetes Mellitus

Affected Area	Complications and Results
Eyes	Retinopathy Blindness Cataracts Glaucoma
Kidneys	Glomerulonephritis Chronic dialysis Nephrosclerosis Kidney transplant Pyelonephritis
Mouth	Gingivitis Dental caries Periodontitis
Reproductive system	Sexual dysfunction Stillbirths Miscarriages Babies with high birth weights Congenital defects Neonatal deaths
Skin	Xanthoma diabeticorum Pruritus Furunculosis Limited joint mobility
Vascular system	Atherosclerosis Stroke Microangiopathy Heart disease Large-vessel disease Hypertension Myocardial infarction
Peripheral nerves	Earliest recognized complication Erectile dysfunction Somatic neuropathy Autonomic neuropathy Slowed digestion in stomach Impaired sensation in feet and hands Carpal tunnel syndrome Lower-extremity amputations

lipids). The frequency of type 2 diabetes varies with racial and ethnic groups. Ketoacidosis seldom occurs in clients with type 2 diabetes, but, when it is present, it is associated with infection. Type 2 diabetes usually goes undiagnosed for years because hyperglycemia develops gradually without classic symptoms. It is estimated that people have type 2 diabetes for 10 years before they are clinically diagnosed. Nevertheless, the risk of developing macrovascular and microvascular complications (i.e., problems in the large and small blood vessels) is high. Symptoms may be gradual, and weight loss is uncommon (Table 44-2).

Persons with type 2 diabetes often respond to weight reduction, dietary management, exercise, and oral hypoglycemic medications. Persons with type 2 diabetes may require insulin therapy to achieve good control or during illness, which is an important distinction between insulin-dependent and insulin-treated individuals.

Type 2 diabetes is recognized as a heterogeneous disorder that results from insulin resistance and insulin secretory defects. Type 2 diabetes is predominantly genetically inherited, and it has no association with autoimmune beta-cell destruction. In studies, if one twin develops type 2 diabetes, the other twin has a 100% chance of developing the disease.[3] Obesity has a major role in the development of type 2 diabetes, but more research is needed.

Gestational Diabetes Mellitus

Gestational diabetes mellitus (GDM) occurs in 4% of pregnancies in the United States.[4] Clinical characteristics include glucose intolerance that has its onset or recognition during pregnancy. Therefore diabetic women who become pregnant do not fall into the GDM classification. High-risk individuals include women with the following conditions:

- Marked obesity
- Previous GDM
- Strong family history of diabetes
- Glucosuria (i.e., glucose in the urine)

Even in the nondiabetic individual, normal pregnancy affects both fetal and maternal metabolism and exerts a diabetogenic effect. GDM generally reverts after birth because the condition is a consequence of the normal anti-insulin effects of pregnancy hormones and the diversion of natural glucose to the fetus.

GDM increases the risk of perinatal morbidity and mortality. Maternal complications include an increased rate of cesarean delivery and chronic hypertension. Furthermore, women with a history of GDM have a 35% to 60% chance of developing diabetes during the next 10 to 20 years. Six weeks or more after pregnancy ends, the woman with GDM should be reclassified as having one of the following:

- Diabetes
- Prediabetes
- Normal glucose regulation

Other Specific Types of Diabetes Mellitus

The category of other specific types of diabetes mellitus is heterogeneous in nature and includes diabetes in which the causative relationship is known, such as diabetes mellitus associated with certain conditions and syndromes (e.g., genetic defects of the beta cells, pancreatic disease, endocrine disease, chemical-induced agents, genetic syndromes).

Pathophysiology of Diabetes

To use glucose, the body must produce insulin. A person with diabetes produces too little insulin or has an inability to use insulin. **Insulin**, which is an anabolic hormone (i.e., it is used to build up the body), stimulates the entry of glucose into the cell and enhances fat storage. Without insulin, glucose remains in the bloodstream (hyperglycemia) rather than being stored or used by cells to produce energy.

Insulin Deprivation

The net effect of insulin deficiency is that blood glucose concentration rises (**hyperglycemia**). Without insulin, the glucose derived from a meal cannot be used or stored. When the blood glucose level rises to more than 150 mg/dL, the kidney tubules become incapable of resorption. Glucose appears in the urine (**glucosuria**), taking with it a large amount of fluid, thereby raising the volume of urine (**polyuria**) and necessitating frequent urination. Dehydration follows, leading to excessive thirst (**polydipsia**). **Ketoacidosis** may follow hyperglycemia when blood glucose levels rise to more than 400 mg/dL (Box 44-3). Impaired carbohydrate metabolism, which the body interprets as energy starvation, causes the excessive ingestion of food (**polyphagia**) and necessitates the use of fats and proteins (hyperglycemia progressively glycates body proteins) to satisfy energy requirements. Keto acids and ketone bodies (acetone) are produced as a result of the catabolism of fatty acids (**lipolysis**). Ketones accumulate in the tissues; they are excreted in the urine (**ketonuria**) and circulated in the blood (**ketonemia**), thereby causing a drop in the pH of the blood and leading to seizures and diabetic coma.

Clinical Signs and Symptoms

Diabetes is characterized by hyperglycemia. In type 1 diabetes mellitus, the predominant problem is impaired insulin production; in type 2 diabetes mellitus, the predominant problem is the inability to use the insulin produced by the body. However, a considerable overlap exists with regard to the clinical features of the two forms of diabetes. The deficiency of insulin action leads to defects in the metabolism of carbohydrates, protein, and lipids. In clinical practice, the suspicion of diabetes is gleaned from the client's history and physical findings (Box 44-4).

BOX 44-3

Signs and Symptoms of Ketoacidosis

Common Cardinal Symptoms

"Fruity" acetone breath
Frequent urination
Excessive thirst
Unusual hunger
Weight loss
Weakness
Nausea
Dry skin and mucous membranes
Flushed facial appearance
Abdominal tenderness
Rapid, deep breathing
Depressed sensory perception

Other Symptoms

Recurrence of bedwetting
Repeated skin infections
Malaise
Drowsiness
Headache
Marked irritability

BOX 44-4

Warning Signs of Diabetes

Type 1 diabetes mellitus is characterized by the sudden appearance of the following:

- Frequent urination
- Unusual thirst
- Extreme hunger
- Unusual weight loss
- Irritability
- Extreme fatigue

Type 2 diabetes mellitus is characterized by its slow onset; it includes any of the type 1 symptoms in addition to the following:

- Frequent infections
- Blurred vision
- Cuts and bruises that are slow to heal
- Tingling or numbness in the hands and feet
- Recurring or hard-to-heal skin, gingival, or bladder infections

Adapted from the American Diabetes Association: *Diabetes symptoms.* Available at: http://www.diabetes.org/diabetes-basics/symptoms/?loc=DropDownDB-symptoms. Accessed November 1, 2012.

Indicators of probable diabetes mellitus (i.e., the cardinal signs of diabetes) include the following:

- Polydipsia
- Polyuria
- Polyphagia
- Unexplained weight loss
- Weakness

Symptoms of marked hyperglycemia also include **polyphagia** (eating extreme amounts of food) and blurred vision.

Impairment of growth and susceptibility to certain infections may also accompany chronic hyperglycemia. A family history of diabetes, obesity, GDM, premature atherosclerosis, and neuropathic disorders also are indications of probable diabetes mellitus. Dental hygienists aware of indications and risk factors can refer potentially undiagnosed clients for testing (see Figure 44-4 and Boxes 44-5 and 44-6).

Chronic Complications

People with both types of diabetes mellitus show a tendency for severe, multisystem, long-term complications (see Table 44-2), including the following:

- Microvascular and macrovascular disease
- Diabetic retinopathy with potential vision loss
- Nephropathy leading to renal failure
- Peripheral neuropathy with risk of foot ulcers, amputation, and neuropathic joint disease
- Autonomic neuropathy causing gastrointestinal, genitourinary, and cardiovascular symptoms as well as sexual dysfunction
- Periodontal disease

Mechanisms thought to cause tissue damage in diabetics involve alterations in the host immunoinflammatory response, including altered function of immune cells (i.e., neutrophils, monocytes, and macrophages); elevated levels of tumor necrosis factor-alpha; alterations in connective tissue metabolism; and the glycation of tissue proteins forming advanced glycation end products[5] and advanced glycation end product–modified collagen.[5] Individuals with diabetes have an increased incidence of atherosclerotic, cardiovascular, peripheral vascular, and cerebrovascular disease. Hypertension, abnormalities in lipoprotein metabolism, and periodontal disease are found in people with diabetes. The emotional and social impact of diabetes and the demands of therapy cause significant unmet human needs in individuals with diabetes and their families (Table 44-3). All complications affect clients with both type 1 and type 2 diabetes, although clinical consequences differ greatly. Generally, kidney and eye diseases predominate with type 1 diabetes, atherosclerotic disease predominates with type 2 disease, and neuropathy occurs with both types (see Table 44-2).

Diabetes and Periodontal Disease: A Two-Way Relationship

For more information about this topic, see Modifiable Risk Factors in Chapter 19 and all of Chapter 20.

Periodontal disease is the sixth most common complication of diabetes. Young adults with diabetes have twice the periodontal disease risk of those without diabetes. One third of individuals with diabetes have severe periodontal disease[6] with attachment loss of 5 mm or more.[6] Several meta-analyses confirm that periodontal therapy can result in reduced glycated hemoglobin (A_{1c}) levels. Reduced systemic inflammation seems to be an important determinant in the relationship.[7]

Diabetic Emergencies (see Chapter 10)

Individuals with uncontrolled diabetes increase their risk of the following medical emergencies:

- Coma
- Hypoglycemia
- Ketoacidotic hyperglycemia

TABLE 44-3

Some Unmet Human Needs of Persons with Diabetes and Their Effect on Outcomes of Self-Monitoring of Blood Glucose

Unmet Human Need	Client's Feeling	Example of Client's Behavioral Response
Protection from health risks	I want to be 100% okay.	Seeking perfection; therefore records results as 100% okay.
Responsibility for oral health	I want you to be pleased/proud. I want to be in charge. I don't want you to punish me. I don't want you to question or accuse me.	Seeking approval; therefore "I'll give you information that makes you pleased or proud" Seeking independence; therefore "I'll give you records that show what I want you to see" Avoiding punishment; therefore "I'll give you records so that you think I don't deserve punishment" Avoiding confrontation and criticism; therefore "I'll give you records that encourage you to leave me alone"
Conceptualization and problem solving	I don't want to hear if I'm good or bad. I don't have diabetes.	Avoiding judgment; therefore "I'll give you records that you won't have to comment about" Expressing denial; therefore "I'll need no test"
Freedom from fear and stress	I don't want to pay attention to diabetes and feel sad. I hate diabetes/I hate how you make me deal with diabetes. I cheated.	Avoiding depression; therefore "I won't test so that I won't have to face sadness" Expressing resentment or anger; therefore "I won't do what you ask me to do" Expressing guilt; therefore "I'll hide it"

Adapted from Skyler JS, Reeves ML: Intensive treatment of type I diabetes mellitus. In Olefsky JM, Sherwin RS, eds: *Diabetes mellitus: management and complications*, New York, 1985, Churchill Livingstone.

- Nonketotic hyperosmolar hyperglycemia
- Lactic acidosis
- Uremia
- Nondiabetic coma
- Infection
- Myocardial infarction
- Stroke
- Emergency surgery

The occurrence of stupor or coma in clients with diabetes may be the result of several causes. For example, the diabetic condition may be undiagnosed, or the person with type 1 disease may not have followed the required insulin regimen. Stress, infection, and an increased level of activity contribute to an emergency situation.

Hypoglycemia (Box 44-7; Tables 44-4 and 44-5)

Hypoglycemia (i.e., a blood glucose concentration of <70 mg/dL) is the most common metabolic emergency in persons with type 1 diabetes mellitus; it results from an excess of insulin and a glucose deficiency in the body. (A blood glucose concentration of 80 to 120 mg/dL is normal.) Each year, severe episodes affect approximately 20% of diabetic individuals; minor episodes occur every 2 weeks on average in each insulin-treated person. In clients with type 2 disease who are treated with sulfonylurea agents, hypoglycemia is more common than is generally recognized, and it may be severe, especially among older persons treated with longer-acting agents. Hypoglycemia signs and symptoms result from a lack of glucose in the brain and compensation by the nervous system for this lack (see Box 44-7). Main causes of hypoglycemia in persons with type 1 disease are listed in Table 44-4.

Individuals with diabetes can manage mild hypoglycemia themselves by ingesting glucose, sweet drinks, or milk. Between 10 and 20 g of glucose (i.e., about the amount in an 8-ounce glass of 2% fat milk, a 4-ounce glass of orange juice, three pieces of hard candy, or eight Life Savers candies) is generally adequate, although many persons take considerably more because they fear prolonged hypoglycemia. More severe hypoglycemia can also be treated via the oral ingestion of carbohydrates, but another person may have to administer the carbohydrates. If the victim is unconscious, treatment requires intravenous dextrose solution or an intramuscular injection of 0.5 mg to 1.0 mg glucagon; this should be followed on awakening by oral complex carbohydrates with a protein source (e.g., a small meat or cheese sandwich, cottage cheese and fruit).

Hyperglycemic Ketoacidotic Coma (Diabetic Coma) (see Table 44-6 and Box 44-8)

Although the percentage of all diabetic deaths caused by hyperglycemia ketoacidotic coma has decreased dramatically from more than 60% during the preinsulin days to 1% at present, it is still considerable, especially among younger individuals. Prevention is the best treatment; however, emergency treatment requires hospitalization to correct fluid and electrolyte imbalances.

Coma that results from absolute insulin deficiency is found in persons with acute-onset type 1 diabetes in whom diagnosis was unknown or delayed and in individuals with known diabetes who discontinued or decreased their insulin dose for some reason. Coma from a temporary insulin deficiency may be caused by infection or stressful situations in which there is an increase in the secretion of anti-insulin hormones (i.e., glucagon, cortisol, and catecholamines; see Box 44-8). Infection is the most common precipitating factor, and it is present in more than 50% of all persons with diabetic ketoacidotic coma.

A series of biochemical events explains the basis of severe ketoacidosis, the signs and symptoms of which are presented in Table 44-6. Clear guidelines for maintaining control should be provided to the diabetic client with infection to resolve the infection early (Box 44-9).

TABLE 44-4

Causes of Hypoglycemia in Individuals with Type 1 Diabetes Mellitus

Factor	Cause
Insulin	Inappropriate insulin regimens Day-to-day variability in absorption Insulin antibodies Inappropriate site rotation Factitious hypoglycemia Renal failure
Food	Delayed intake Decreased intake
Exercise	Increased energy requirements Increased insulin absorption
Other	Impaired counterregulation Liver disease Hypoendocrine states Alcohol Potentiating drugs Hypoglycemic unawareness (absence of signs and symptoms, long-standing diabetes, autonomic neuropathy)

TABLE 44-5

Hypoglycemia Compared with Hyperglycemia

Signs and Symptoms	Hypoglycemia (<70 mg/dL)	Hyperglycemia (400-600 mg/dL)
Onset	Rapid (minutes)	Slow (days to weeks)
Thirst	Absent	Increased
Nausea and vomiting	Absent	Frequent
Vision	Double	Dim
Respirations	Normal	Difficult; hyperventilation
Skin	Moist, pale	Hot, dry, flushed
Tremors	Frequent	Absent
Blood pressure	Normal	Hypotension

TABLE 44-6

Features of Severe Diabetic Ketoacidosis

Features	Possible Causes
Symptoms	
Thirst	Dehydration
Polyuria	Hyperglycemia, osmotic dieresis
Fatigue	Dehydration, protein loss
Weight loss	Dehydration, protein loss, catabolism*
Anorexia	Depression*
Nausea, vomiting	Ketones,* gastric stasis, ileus
Abdominal pain	Gastric stasis,* ileus, electrolyte deficiency*
Muscle cramps	Potassium deficiency*
Signs	
Hyperventilation	Acidemia
Dehydration	Osmotic diuresis, vomiting
Tachycardia	Dehydration
Hypotension	Dehydration, acidemia
Warm, dry skin	Acidemia (peripheral vasodilation)
Hypothermia	Acidemia-induced peripheral vasodilation (when infection is present)
Impaired consciousness or coma	Hyperosmolality
Ketotic breath	Hyperketonemia (acetone)

*Indicates speculated or unknown cause.

Diabetic ketoacidosis treatment requires hospitalization to restore the disturbed metabolic fluid and electrolyte state to normal. Fluid rehydration (i.e., salt and water), insulin, potassium, broad-spectrum antibiotic therapy, and the treatment of precipitating factors are the main elements of diabetic coma treatment.

Disease Management

Glycemic Control: Self-Monitoring of Blood Glucose and A_{1C}

The most important aspect of the control of diabetes mellitus is the self-monitoring of blood glucose with small automated devices. The frequency of self-monitoring is highly individualized. Monitoring is done by placing a small drop of blood on a reagent strip, which is then inserted into a meter. The meter measures glucose concentration and displays a value of glucose in millimeters per deciliter (mm/dL) of blood.

The hemoglobin A_{1c} laboratory test (also known as *A1C*) is used by the physician to monitor overall glycemic control. Hemoglobin A is made during the 120-day life span of a red blood cell. Blood glucose attaches to hemoglobin A and is used as a record of blood glucose levels over the prior 3 months. In addition, the A_{1c} test is the preferred test for prediabetes. An A_{1c} level between 5.9% and 6.4% indicates prediabetes; 6.5% or greater indicated diabetes. Abnormal A_{1c} levels correlate with glucose intolerance and the development of diabetic complications. Each 1% reduction in A_{1c} is associated with significant reductions (i.e., 14% to 37%) in the risk of diabetic complications.[2] Thus early diagnosis and good control are very important. Recommendations for A_{1c} levels and blood measurements in clients with diabetes are presented in Box 44-10.

Medical Nutrition Therapy

Diet remains the hallmark of diabetes therapy, despite advances in insulin formulations, insulin delivery systems, and oral medications. Diabetic diets are designed to provide appropriate quantities of food at regular intervals, to supply daily caloric requirements to help with achieving or maintaining desirable body weight, and to reduce fat intake to correct an unfavorable lipid profile that is conducive to atherosclerosis.

With type 2 diabetes, a reduction in hyperglycemia is correlated with weight loss. With type 1 diabetes mellitus, nutritional strategies involve monitoring the percentages of carbohydrate (i.e., 55% to 60% of total calories) and protein (i.e., 12% to 20% of total calories) intake. Meal planning for diabetics is based on the food exchange list system of the American Diabetes Association.

Insulin Therapy

More than 20 different insulins are sold in the United States. Approximately 12% of people with diabetes (either type 1 or type 2) use insulin only to control hyperglycemia; 58% use oral medications only, 14% use a combination of insulin and oral medications, and 16% do not take either insulin or oral medication. Persons with type 1 diabetes have essentially no pancreatic insulin, they are unresponsive to oral sulfonylurea hypoglycemic agents, and they are prone to ketosis; they are therefore dependent on lifelong exogenous insulin administration.

Human insulin and insulin analogues are categorized by their speed of onset, their peak effect, and their duration; they are also available in mixture preparations as follows:

- Rapid-acting
- Short-acting
- Intermediate-acting
- Long-acting

Insulin may be injected subcutaneously with an insulin syringe or a penlike device. Insulin pumps are widely used to deliver a programmed steady drip of insulin (i.e., a basal rate) under the skin 24 hours a day. The push of a button on the pump delivers a bolus dose to respond to the number of carbohydrate grams consumed at a meal. Numerous new products are awaiting approval from the U.S. Food and Drug Administration. Table 44-7 illustrates insulin types that may be used alone or in combination. Dosages, frequency, and times of administration are highly individualized.

Oral Hypoglycemic Agents

When the control of hyperglycemia in clients with type 2 diabetes is not achieved with diet and exercise, oral hypoglycemic agents are prescribed by an endocrinologist. Generally oral hypoglycemic agents stimulate the pancreas to secrete more insulin (insulin secretagogues), to increase the body's

TABLE 44-7
Types of Insulin

Type	Onset of Action	Peak Effect (hr)	Duration (hr)
Rapid-acting			
Insulin lispro Insulin aspart Insulin glulisine	5 minutes	1	2 to 4
Short-acting			
Regular	30 minutes	2 to 3	3 to 6
Intermediate-acting			
Neutral protamine Hagedorn	2 to 4 hours	4 to 12	12 to 18
Long-acting			
Ultralente	6 to 10 hours	16 to 18	20 to 24
Glargine and detemir	1 to 2 hours	None	24

response to insulin (insulin sensitizers), to slow glucose digestion, or to decrease glucose production by the liver as follows:

- Biguanides (metformin [Glucophage]) decrease the amount of glucose secreted by the liver, decrease intestinal glucose absorption, and increase insulin action. Hypoglycemia is not a side effect. Metformin is contraindicated for people with reduced kidney function.
- Sulfonylureas (glyburide [Glynase, Micronase, Diabeta]; glipizide [Glucotrol]; glimepiride [Amaryl]) increase insulin secretion. Hypoglycemia and weight gain are disadvantages.
- Meglitinides (repaglinide [Prandin]; nateglinide [Starlix]) increase insulin secretion in the presence of glucose. These drugs are taken before each meal.
- Thiazolidinediones (pioglitazone [Actos]; rosiglitazone [Avandia]) make the body more sensitive to insulin. The target cell response to insulin is improved, thereby reducing insulin doses.
- Alpha-glucosidase inhibitors (acarbose [Precose]; miglitol [Glyset]) inhibit enzymes in the small intestines that are responsible for the digestion of starchy food, thus delaying carbohydrate metabolism.
- Dipeptidyl peptidase-4 inhibitors (sitagliptin [Januvia]; saxagliptin [Onglyza]) prevent the breakdown of glucagon-like peptide-1 (a naturally occurring hypoglycemic in the body), thus allowing it to be active longer.

Injectable Agents for Type 2 Diabetes

The following are injectable agents for the treatment of type 2 diabetes:

- Exenatide (Byetta), which is derived from the saliva of the Gila monster, stimulates the incretin effect (increased insulin response), which is diminished in clients with type 2 diabetes.
- Amylinomimetics (pramlintide [Symlin]) are an analogue of human amylin, which modulates gastric emptying. Pramlintide is also approved for clients with type 1 diabetes, but it requires an additional injection.

Dental Hygiene Process of Care

Well-controlled diabetes occurs when the client's blood glucose is within the normal range as a result of a careful balance of medication, diet, and exercise. (A blood glucose concentration of 80 to 120 mg/dL is normal.) Clients with well-controlled diabetes can be treated safely, provided that their daily routine is not affected. Diabetics with well-controlled disease have a reduced incidence of dental caries. It is important for dental hygienists to know that only 37% of people with type 2 diabetes attain an A_{1c} level of less than 7%.[8]

Infections of any type can cause a profound disturbance of glycemic control that potentially leads to ketoacidosis and diabetic coma. When infection is present, counterregulatory hormone secretion increases (specifically cortisol and glucagon), thereby leading to hyperglycemia and increased ketogenesis. Infection is the most common precipitating factor for severe ketoacidosis. In the client with poorly controlled diabetes, phagocytic function is impaired, and resistance to infection is decreased. The prevention of oral diseases and infections is critical to the client's diabetic control, and poor diabetic control may aggravate the oral disease status.

Several unmet human needs relate to dental hygiene care for individuals with diabetes. For example, emotional stress induced by a dental appointment causes the release of epinephrine, which mobilizes glucose from glycogen stored in the liver. Stress, therefore, can contribute to a hyperglycemic condition becoming ketoacidotic. Periods of waiting and treatment time should be minimized to meet the client's need for freedom from stress.

Diabetes among people who undertake intensive regimens of multiple insulin injections and the daily self-monitoring of blood glucose may abruptly become uncontrolled as a result of an active periodontal infection. When this is unrecognized, the periodontal infection may cause the human needs for skin and mucous membrane integrity and protection from health risks to become compromised. Table 44-3 reflects some unmet human needs and their effect on outcomes of blood glucose self-monitoring. Figures 44-2 and 44-3 show clinical examples of periodontal disease in diabetics.

Assessment

Health History

When obtaining a client's health history, the dental hygienist questions the client about the signs and symptoms of ketoacidosis (see Boxes 44-3 and 44-4) to determine whether an undiagnosed diabetic condition is present[9] or if the client is at high risk for diabetes (see Boxes 44-5 and 44-6). The administration of the American Diabetes Association's Diabetes Risk Test is recommended to assist with early diagnosis. In addition, the Centers for Disease Control and Prevention recommend that dental offices administer the A_{1c} test or use a blood glucose self-monitoring device to screen clients who are at risk for prediabetes and to refer them to a physician when their results confirm higher than normal ranges.[14] Among the aging population, classic symptoms do not usually manifest. Rather, clinical findings are related to chronic complications of the disease, such as vascular disorders or neuropathic syndromes.

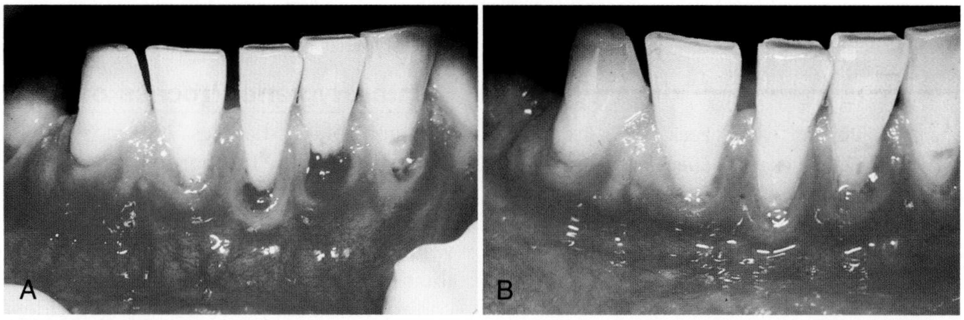

Figure 44-2. Diabetes and periodontal disease. **A,** An adult with diabetes (blood glucose level of 400 mg/100 mL). Note the gingival inflammation, spontaneous bleeding, and edema. **B,** The same person after 4 days of insulin therapy (glucose level of <100 mg/100 mL). The gingival tissues have improved in the absence of professional mechanical therapy. (From Newman MG, Takei HH, Klokkevold PR, Carranza FA, eds: *Carranza's clinical periodontology,* ed 11, St Louis, 2012, Saunders.)

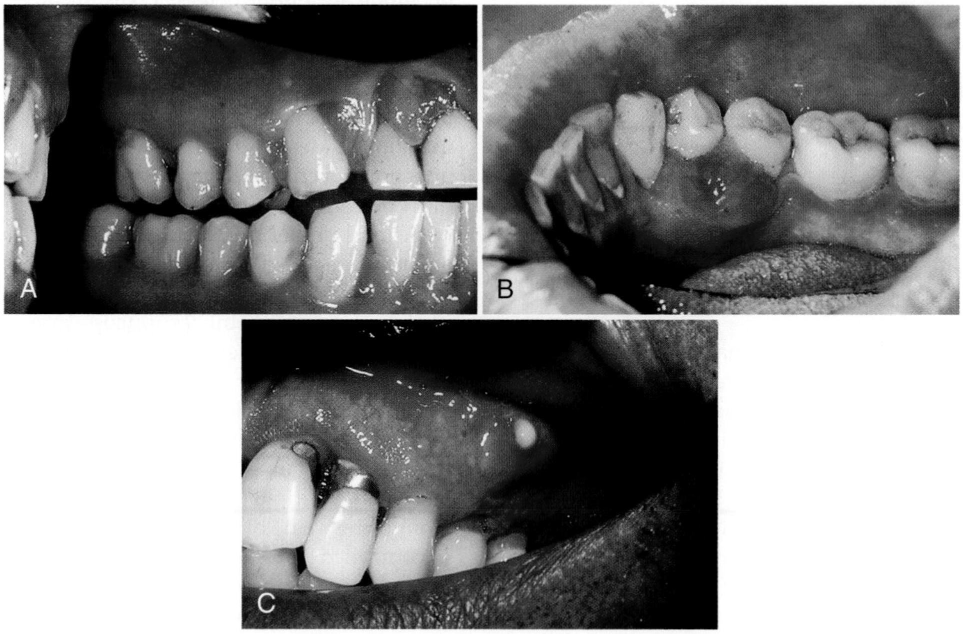

Figure 44-3. Uncontrolled diabetes and periodontal therapy. **A,** An adult with uncontrolled diabetes. Note the enlarged, smooth, red gingiva with initial enlargement in the anterior area. **B,** The same person. Note the inflamed, enlarged area around teeth #27 to #30. **C,** Suppurating abscess and facial or maxillary cleft area in a person with uncontrolled diabetes. (From Newman MG, Takei HH, Klokkevold PR, Carranza FA, eds: *Carranza's clinical periodontology,* ed 11, St Louis, 2012, Saunders.)

When the person is a known diabetic, the client and health history interview should address the following:

- The type of diabetes
- The methods used to control diabetes (e.g., medications, diet, exercise, weight loss)
- The medication schedule and dosages
- The date and results of the last A_{1c} test
- The frequency of self-monitoring of blood glucose
- The fasting blood glucose levels
- The results of self-monitoring (i.e., trends as well as those of the day of the appointment)
- The blood glucose levels 2 hours after meals
- The date of the last hypoglycemia episode
- The date of onset of diabetes
- The regularity of appointments with a physician
- The six complications of diabetes

The decision to continue the assessment, consult with a physician, or defer treatment and refer the client to a physician should be made on the basis of the client's responses to questions during the health history and pharmacologic assessment (Boxes 44-11, 44-12, and 44-13).

Oral Assessment

Intraoral findings may reveal the following conditions that are common in clients with poorly controlled diabetes (Table 44-8):

- Cheilosis
- Xerostomia
- Glossodynia
- Enlarged salivary glands
- Increased glucose in the saliva
- Fungal infections such as candidiasis (thrush)
- Dental caries
- Periodontal disease

Diabetes is an important risk factor for periodontal disease. The American Academy of Periodontology published a

TABLE 44-8

Oral Complications of Diabetes Mellitus

Clinical Signs and Symptoms	Pathophysiology
Salivary and Oral Changes	
Xerostomia	Increased fluid loss
Bilateral asymptomatic parotid gland swelling with increased salivary viscosity	Increased fatty acid deposition Increased salivary glucose levels Compensatory hypertrophy as a result of a decrease in saliva production
Increased dental caries, especially in the cervical region	Secondary to xerostomia and salivary glucose levels
Unexplained odontalgia and percussion sensitivity (acute pulpitis)	Pulpal arteritis from microangiopathies
Lingual erosion of anterior teeth*	Complications of anorexia nervosa and bulimia
Periodontal Changes	
Periodontal disease†	Induction and accumulation of advanced glycation end products
Tooth mobility	Loss of attachment associated with poor glycemic control
Rapidly progressive pocket formation	Degenerative vascular changes
Gingival bleeding	Microangiopathies Local factors
Subgingival polyps	Cause unknown
Infection and Wound Healing	
Slow wound healing (including periapical lesions after endodontics) and increased susceptibility to infection	Hyperglycemia reduces phagocytic activity Ketoacidosis may delay chemotaxis of granulocytes Vascular changes lead to decreased blood flow Abnormal collagen production
Oral ulcers refractory to therapy, especially in association with a prosthesis	Microangiopathies Neuropathies
Irritation fibromas	Altered wound healing
Increased incidence and prolonged healing of dry socket	Degenerative vascular changes Post-extraction infection
Tongue Changes	
Glossodynia	Neuropathic complications Xerostomia Candidiasis
Median rhomboid glossitis (glossal central papillary atrophy)	*Candida albicans*
Other Changes	
Opportunistic infections: *Candida albicans* and mucormycosis	Repeated use of antibiotics Compromised immune system
Acetone or diabetic breath (seen when the person is close to a diabetic coma)	Ketoacidotic state
Increased incidence of lichen planus (as high as 30%)	Compromised immune system

Adapted from Lalla RV, D'Ambrosio JA: Dental management considerations for the patient with diabetes mellitus, *J Am Dent Assoc* 132:1425, 2001.

*Although this is not a complication of diabetes per se, this pattern is seen when the person wants to maintain the weight-loss aspect of diabetes while ignoring or tolerating the hyperglycemic side effects. The client may not be taking proper insulin doses and may not be truthful when asked about this.

†Periodontal disease is more common among people with diabetes. Among young adults, those with diabetes have about twice the risk of those without diabetes. Adults who were 45 years old or older with poorly controlled diabetes (i.e., $A_{1c} > 9\%$) were 2.9 times more likely to have severe periodontitis than those without diabetes. The likelihood was even greater (i.e., 4.6 times greater) among smokers with poorly controlled diabetes. About one third of people with diabetes have severe periodontal disease that consists of a loss of attachment (≥5 mm).

BOX 44-5

Type 2 Diabetes: Risk Factors and Criteria for the Testing of Asymptomatic Undiagnosed Adults[2]

Testing for diabetes should be considered in the following situations:
- Beginning at age 45 years for all adults who are overweight (i.e., body mass index of ≥25 kg/m^2*); if results are normal, testing should be repeated at 3-year intervals.
- At a younger age or more frequently for adults who are overweight (i.e., body mass index of ≥25 kg/m^2*) with additional risk factors:
  - Physical inactivity
  - First-degree relative with diabetes
  - Member of a high-risk ethnic population (e.g., African American, Latino, Native American, Asian American, Pacific Islander)
  - Delivered a baby weighing >9 lb or diagnosed with gestational diabetes mellitus
  - Hypertensive (≥140/90 mm Hg or receiving therapy for hypertension)
  - High-density lipoprotein cholesterol level of ≤35 mg/dL (0.90 mmol/L) and/or triglyceride level of ≥250 mg/dL (2.82 mmol/L)
  - Polycystic ovary syndrome
  - A_{1c} level of ≥5.7%, impaired glucose tolerance, or impaired fasting glucose on previous testing
  - Another clinical condition associated with insulin resistance (e.g., severe obesity, acanthosis nigricans [see Figure 44-4])
  - History of cardiovascular disease
- Those with prediabetes should be tested annually.

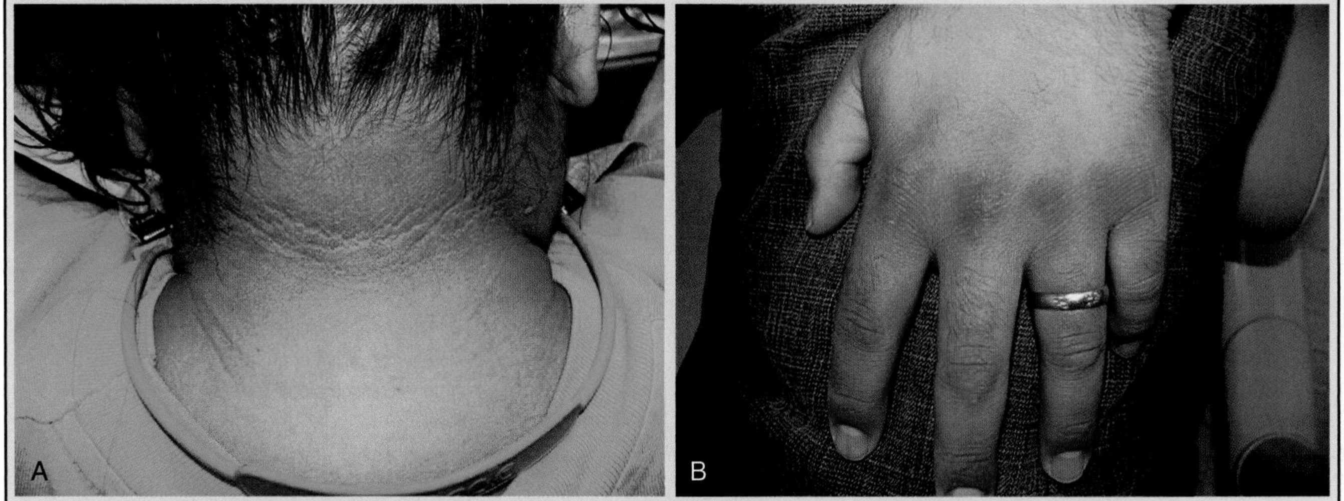

Figure 44-4. **A,** Acanthosis nigricans affecting the back of the neck. **B,** Acanthosis nigricans affecting the hand. (Courtesy Lana Crawford.)

*At-risk body mass index may be lower in some ethnic groups.

BOX 44-6

Type 2 Diabetes in Children: Risk Factors and Criteria for Testing[2]

- Overweight (body mass index of >85th percentile for age and sex, weight for height >85th percentile, or weight >120% of ideal for height) plus any two of the following risk factors:
  - Family history of type 2 diabetes in first- or second-degree relative
  - Native American, African American, Latino, Asian American, or Pacific Islander race or ethnicity
  - Signs of insulin resistance or conditions associated with insulin resistance (e.g., acanthosis nigricans, hypertension, dyslipidemia, polycystic ovary syndrome, birth weight low for gestational age)
  - Maternal history of diabetes or gestational diabetes mellitus during the child's gestation
- Age at initiation of testing: 10 years or at onset of puberty, if puberty occurs at a younger age
- Frequency of testing: every 3 years

comprehensive review of diabetes mellitus and periodontal disease.[5] The prevalence and severity of periodontal disease increase in individuals with both type 1 (insulin deficient) and type 2 (insulin resistant) forms of diabetes as compared with individuals without diabetes. Clients with diabetes with A_{1c} levels of more than 8% have a greater increase in periodontal inflammation, attachment loss, and bone loss than clients with diabetes with A_{1c} levels of less than 8%.[10] The presence of hyperglycemia contributes to enhanced periodontal inflammation and alveolar bone loss in clients with diabetes. Hyperglycemia progressively leads to an increase of proinflammatory cytokines such as tumor necrosis factor-alpha, interleukin 6, and others that destroy connective tissue and bone. The chronic increased cytokine levels augment inflammatory tissue destruction. The control of hyperglycemia reduces the level of proinflammatory cytokines. Glycemic control is an integral part of the control of periodontal disease in individuals with diabetes (see Figure 44-2).[5]

Uncontrolled diabetes increases dental caries risk as a result of reduced saliva secretion and increased glucose in saliva. Other oral complications associated with diabetes may

BOX 44-7

Identification and Treatment of Hypoglycemia in the Dental Office

Symptoms of Hypoglycemia

Shakiness
Anxiety
Palpitations
Increased sweating
Hunger

Signs of Hypoglycemia

Tremors
Tachycardia
Altered consciousness (lethargy and obtundation or personality change)
Blood glucose level of less than 60 mg/dL

General Principles

Treatment should be initiated as soon as possible, and staff members should not wait for laboratory results or for a response from a physician.

If the blood glucose levels are extremely low (e.g., less than 40 mg/dL), a transfer for medical evaluation may be needed as blood should be drawn and sent to the laboratory for accurate blood glucose level measurement because the precision of glucometers is low at extremely low blood glucose levels.

Conscious Hypoglycemic Patient

Treat with 15 grams of simple carbohydrates

- One-half can of regular soda
- 4 ounces of regular fruit juice
- 3 to 4 glucose tablets

Repeat finger-stick glucose test in 15 minutes.

If the blood glucose level is more than 60 mg/dL, the patient should be asked to eat a meal if it is close to mealtime. If it is not close to mealtime, a mixed snack that includes carbohydrates, proteins, and fat (e.g., peanut butter and jelly sandwich or graham crackers with peanut butter, or milk and crackers) should be given to maintain the blood glucose level. A pure carbohydrate snack will cause the patient to revert back to hypoglycemia quickly. Proteins and carbohydrates in the snack provide sustained glucose release.

If the blood glucose level is less than 60 mg/dL, repeat treatment of 15 g of simple carbohydrates and check the blood glucose level in 15 minutes. Continue this protocol until the blood glucose level is higher than 60 mg/dL and then follow with a mixed snack.

Ask the patient to discuss the hypoglycemia with his or her physician who is managing his or her diabetes mellitus.

Unconscious Hypoglycemic Patient or Patient Unable to Consume Oral Carbohydrate

With Intravenous Access

Administer 5 to 25 g of 50% dextrose immediately; it will be followed by quick recovery.

Notify patient's physician immediately.

Without Intravenous Access

Apply glucose gel inside the mouth in a semiobtund patient or treat with 1 mg of glucagon intramuscularly or subcutaneously; the patient should regain consciousness in 15 to 20 minutes.

Repeat the blood glucose test in 15 minutes.

Establish intravenous access and notify the patient's physician immediately.

Adapted from Alamo SM, Soriano YJ, Perez MGS: Dental considerations for the patient with diabetes, J Clin Exp Dent 3(1):e25-30, 2011.

BOX 44-8

Causes of Hyperglycemic Ketoacidotic Coma

Absolute Insulin Deficiency

- Newly diagnosed type 1 diabetes with beta-cell depletion
- Incorrect insulin dose (omitted or decreased)

Relative Insulin Deficiency

- Stress states
- Infection
- Myocardial infarction
- Trauma
- Cerebrovascular accident

Drugs and Endocrine Disorders

- Steroids
- Adrenergic agonists
- Hyperthyroidism
- Pheochromocytoma
- Thiazide diuretics

BOX 44-9

Guidelines for Maintaining Glycemic Control in Persons with Diabetes Mellitus

- Perform frequent self-monitoring of blood glucose.
- Obtain a regular A_{1c} test twice a year if glycemic control is good, four times a year if treatment or control has changed.
- If not eating normally, replace carbohydrate content of meals and snacks with sugar-containing drinks or milk; ensure adequate fluid intake (2 to 3 L/day).
- If two preceding blood tests show a glucose level of >200 mg/dL (11.1 mmol/L), contact the physician.
- Test for urine ketones if the blood glucose level is >300 mg/dL.
- If vomiting occurs or if the blood glucose level is >300 mg/dL in the presence of positive ketones for >24 hours, call for urgent medical advice.

BOX 44-10

Glycemic Control: Summary of Recommendations for Adults with Diabetes[2]

A_{1c}	<7.0%*
Preprandial capillary plasma glucose	70 to 130 mg/dL
Peak postprandial capillary plasma glucose†	<180 mg/dL

Key Concepts for Setting Glycemic Goals
- Goals should be individualized.
- Children, pregnant women, and elderly clients require special considerations.
- More or less intense glycemic goals may be appropriate for certain individuals.
- Postprandial glucose may be targeted if A_{1c} goals are not met despite preprandial glucose goals being reached.

*American Diabetes Association: Standards of medical care in diabetes – 2012. Position statement, *Diabetes Care* 35(Suppl):4, 2012.

†Postprandial glucose measurements should be made 1 to 2 hours after the beginning of the meal, which is generally when the peak level occurs in persons with diabetes.

BOX 44-11

Levels of Blood Glucose for Care Planning

- <70 mg/dL: Too low; hypoglycemia. Provide 15 mg of carbohydrates and wait 15 minutes. If condition continues, check with a physician. Risk for emergency situations.*
- 70 to 79 mg/dL: Monitor at least once during dental hygiene care appointment to prevent an emergency.
- 80 to 149 mg/dL: Normal levels.
- 150 to 200 mg/dL: Higher levels. Monitor infections, insulin intake, stress, and food intake.
- >200 mg/dL: Too high; tendency toward hyperglycemia. Check with physician. Risk for emergency situations.*

*Indicates that dental hygiene care should not be provided at these blood glucose levels.

BOX 44-12

When to Refer to a Physician

Refer the client to a physician for diagnosis and treatment when the client has the following:
- Cardinal signs of diabetes (see Box 44-3)
- Symptoms that suggest diabetes
- Estimated fasting blood glucose level of ≥126 mg/mL
- 2-hour postprandial blood glucose level of ≥200 mg/mL
- Long period since client was last seen by a physician
- Frequent episodes of hypoglycemia
- Diagnosed diabetes plus signs and symptoms of diabetes (not controlled)
- Type 1 diabetes with extreme hyperglycemia and hypoglycemia
- An infection anywhere in the body

Adapted from Little JW, Falace DA, Miller CS, Rhodus NL: *Dental management of the medically compromised patient,* ed 8, St Louis, 2013, Elsevier.

BOX 44-13

When to Consult with the Client's Physician

- Client has type 1 or 2 diabetes; determine level of control
- Client has complications such as renal disease or cardiovascular disease
- Client takes insulin
- Client is not under good medical management
- Client is undergoing extensive periodontal or oral–maxillofacial surgery

Adapted from Little JW, Falace DA, Miller CS, Rhodus NL: *Dental management of the medically compromised patient,* ed 8, St Louis, 2013, Elsevier.

affect nutrition by causing the person to select foods that are easy to chew but nutritionally inadequate.

Diagnosis and Planning

A dental hygiene care plan focuses on the client's unmet human needs and allows the clinician to manage risks of potential diabetic emergencies, thereby protecting the client from health risks. Persons with diabetes may not be under good glycemic control. In a study of 97 patients who entered a dental clinic, 28 patients were found to be hyperglycemic (i.e., >130 mg/100 mL), and 2 were noted to be hypoglycemic (i.e., <70 mg/100 mL)[11] (see Box 44-11). Appointments should be brief to minimize anxiety and stress and to avoid interference with medication and eating schedules. Morning appointments are ideal because most people with diabetes are best controlled at this time. An hour to an hour and a half after breakfast is best for appointments to avoid the peak action time of medication. Regular (short-acting) insulin, which is often taken in the morning or at each meal, peaks within 2 to 3 hours after the injection. Oral hypoglycemic agents do not cause peaks.

Therapeutic scaling and periodontal debridement are contraindicated for people with uncontrolled diabetes (i.e., blood glucose levels of <70 mg/dL or >200 mg/dL)[12] (see Box 44-11 and Figure 44-3). Clients should be treated in consultation and referred to the physician of record for systemic evaluation. Dental hygiene care should not begin until the diabetic condition is controlled. The short-term risk for infections in persons with diabetes has been shown to increase with average blood glucose levels of 200 to 230 mg/100 mL.[12] When care is planned, interventions are likely to include the following:
- Emphasis on oral biofilm control
- Health status monitoring
- Nutritional and dietary analysis (see Chapter 35)
- Fluoride and chlorhexidine therapies and the use of xylitol-containing and amorphous calcium phosphate-containing products (see Chapter 33)
- Salivary replacement therapy
- A longer initial appointment, a re-evaluation appointment and frequent periodontal maintenance intervals[13]
- Collaboration with a physician and a certified diabetes educator

A sample dental hygiene care plan is shown in the Critical Thinking Exercises section. Other management concerns are shown in Box 44-14.

Implementation

Therapeutic Scaling and Periodontal Debridement

Gingival and periodontal diseases associated with systemic factors, which are often found in persons with diabetes, may not respond well to subgingival scaling, periodontal debridement, and oral biofilm control. However, the removal of hard and soft deposits and bacterial toxins from tooth crown and root surfaces is critical to the prevention of periodontal infection in people with diabetes. Unnecessary tissue manipulation and trauma are avoided to minimize the risk of postoperative infection and poor healing.

Severe periodontitis is associated with an increased risk of poor glycemic control; therefore severe periodontitis may be a risk factor in the progression of diabetes. Thorough periodontal therapy is indicated in clients with diabetes and periodontitis to enhance control of both diseases. Evidence also suggests that antimicrobial treatment (specifically systemic subantimicrobial doses of doxycycline [20 mg twice daily]) has the potential to improve glycemic control after scaling and root debridement in clients with diabetes.[15]

Increased glucose in gingival crevicular fluid may result in the proliferation of oral microflora, thus increasing periodontal disease and dental caries risk. The short-term (i.e., 3 to 4 months) response in the clinical parameters (i.e., probing depths, bleeding on probing, attachment levels, subgingival microbiota) of clients with diabetes to nonsurgical periodontal therapy appears to be equivalent to the response seen in clients without diabetes; however, clients with poorly controlled diabetes have more rapid clinical attachment loss and a compromised long-term response. At 5 years after nonsurgical periodontal therapy and surgical periodontal treatment in combination with regular periodontal maintenance therapy, clients with diabetes who were well controlled had clinical attachment levels similar to those of clients without diabetes.[5]

A client with well-controlled diabetes with no evidence of infection does not require prophylactic antibiotic premedication.[10] In fact, antibiotic use in clients with diabetes may lead to oral or systemic fungal infections. If an infection is present either preoperatively or postoperatively, antibiotic therapy is mandatory. Prophylactic antibiotic premedication before periodontal instrumentation should be considered for the client with uncontrolled diabetes after consultation with the client's physician.

Diabetic microangiopathy causes blindness and kidney disease. Therefore a client who is exhibiting eye disorders may also have kidney disease. Medications that are excreted renally may be retained in the body of the client with diabetes who also has kidney disease, thereby causing toxic effects. When local anesthetic agents are administered, the minimal use of vasoconstrictors is required, because epinephrine is capable of raising blood glucose.

BOX 44-14

Alterations in the Dental Hygiene Care of Older Adults with Diabetes

Potential Risks Related to Dental Hygiene Care

In older adult with controlled diabetes:
- Infection
- Poor wound healing

In older adult being treated with insulin:
- Insulin reaction

In older adult with poorly controlled diabetes:
- Early onset of complications related to cardiovascular system, eyes, kidneys, nervous system, angina, myocardial infarction, cerebrovascular accident, renal failure, peripheral neuropathy, blindness, hypertension, or congestive heart failure

Prevention of Medical Complications

Detection via the following:
- Health history
- Clinical findings
- Screening blood sugar
- Referral for medical diagnosis

Older adult receiving insulin:
- Prevent insulin reaction.
- Advise older adults to eat normal meals before appointments.
- Schedule appointments in the morning or the midmorning.
- Advise older adults to inform you of any symptoms of insulin reactions when they first occur.
- Have sugar in some form to give if an insulin reaction occurs.
- Older adults with diabetes who are being treated with insulin and who develop oral infections may require an increase in insulin dosage; consult with a physician in addition to performing local and systemic aggressive management of infection.

Drug considerations:
- Insulin: insulin reaction
- Hypoglycemic agents: on rare occasions, aplastic anemia and similar conditions may occur
- In severe diabetics, avoid general anesthesia

Dental Hygiene Care Plan Modifications

For older clients with well-controlled diabetes, no alteration of dental hygiene care plan is indicated unless complications of diabetes are present, such as the following:
- Hypertension
- Congestive heart failure
- Myocardial infarction
- Angina
- Renal failure

Oral Complications

- Accelerated periodontal disease
- Periodontal abscesses
- Oral ulcerations and opportunistic infections
- Numbness, burning, or pain in the oral tissues
- Xerostomia
- Glossodynia
- Prolonged healing

Data from Little JW, Falace DA: *Dental management of the medically compromised patient,* ed 8, St Louis, 2013, Mosby. Table prepared by Pamela P. Brangan.

Evaluation and Documentation

The periodontal tissues of the client with well-controlled diabetes respond positively to nonsurgical periodontal therapy. However, delayed healing may indicate hyperglycemia, which decreases the normal healing actions of leukocyte phagocytosis, chemotaxis, and adherence properties. Frequent oral assessments, periodontal maintenance, the evaluation of the client's response to dental hygiene care, and the monitoring of diabetic control with current hemoglobin A_{1c} test results are recommended.

It is important to accurately record all data that are collected, the treatment that is planned and provided, and recommendations and other information that are relevant to client care and treatment. All relevant information and interactions between the client and the practitioner need to be recorded objectively to enhance interprofessional communication and to promote risk management.

CLIENT EDUCATION TIPS

- Relate the client with diabetes' greater risk of infection and increased healing times to the need for oral biofilm control.
- Teach the use of daily subgingival irrigation for the target delivery of an antimicrobial agent or the twice-daily use of an American Dental Association–accepted antimicrobial mouth rinse; the use of an antiplaque and antigingivitis dentifrice; the use of caries-control products (e.g., fluoride mouth rinse, xylitol mints and chewing gum, calcium- and phosphorus-based products); and the use of saliva replacement therapy (e.g., artificial saliva, sucking on ice chips, xylitol gum and mints).
- Discuss the maintenance of dentition for chewing healthy foods and the fact that diet and nutrition are essential to diabetes control.
- Emphasize that individuals with diabetes may not tolerate dentures because of their oral conditions.
- Stress meticulous daily oral biofilm removal as a method to control oral disease progression and diabetes. Oral health contributes significantly to long-term systemic health in the client with diabetes.

LEGAL, ETHICAL, AND SAFETY ISSUES

- Collaborate with the physician when healing is delayed after periodontal instrumentation.
- Collaborate with a certified diabetes educator, a health education consultant, or staff at hospital-based diabetes management centers.
- Dental hygienists can collaborate with diabetes management centers, for example, by sharing their expertise in the area of oral disease prevention and by providing client education, oral health screenings, and referrals.

KEY CONCEPTS

- Many people with diabetes do not know that they have the condition.
- Type 2 diabetes can be prevented or delayed with actions taken by the individual who is at risk. Dental hygienists can make a difference, and resources are available to help.
- Type 1 diabetes involves about 5% of the diabetic population. These individuals need to take insulin injections or use an insulin pump.
- The presence of certain human leukocyte antigens creates a genetic predisposition for the autoimmune cause of type 1 diabetes mellitus.
- Type 2 diabetes affects about 90% to 95% of clients with diabetes. These individuals usually respond well to weight reduction, dietary management, exercise, and oral medications.
- Insulin resistance or a defect in insulin secretion is the cause of type 2 diabetes. The risk of developing type 2 diabetes increases with obesity, age, inactivity, history of gestational diabetes mellitus (GDM), hypertension, and dyslipidemia.
- GDM occurs in 4% of pregnancies. Those who are at high risk include women with obesity, a family history of diabetes, and previous GDM.
- GDM usually disappears after birth because the condition is a consequence of the normal anti-insulin effects of pregnancy hormones and the diversion of natural glucose to the fetus.
- Without insulin, glucose remains in the blood (hyperglycemia) rather than being stored or used by the cells to produce energy. The suspicion of diabetes is gleaned from a history of symptoms: glucosuria, polyuria, polydipsia, weight loss, polyphagia, and blurred vision.
- Diabetes mellitus causes severe multisystem, long-term complications. Kidney and eye diseases predominate with type 1 diabetes mellitus; atherosclerosis predominates with type 2; peripheral nerve disease occurs with both.
- Hypoglycemia, which is the most common emergency in persons with type 1 diabetes mellitus, results from insulin excess and glucose deficiency.
- Hyperglycemic ketoacidosis requires hospitalization to correct fluid and electrolyte imbalances.
- Infection is the most common precipitating factor of hyperglycemic ketoacidosis.
- Well-controlled diabetes occurs when the individual's blood glucose level is within the normal range as a result of a careful balance of medication, diet, and exercise.
- Emotional stress (which can be induced in the oral healthcare setting) causes a release of epinephrine, which mobilizes glucose in the body, thereby contributing to a hyperglycemic condition becoming ketoacidotic.
- The strict application of oral care protocols increases the chances of achieving good clinical outcomes for individuals with diabetes.
- Dental hygiene care should not be provided when blood glucose levels are less than 70 mg/dL or more than 200 mg/dL.
- When administering local anesthetics, it is recommended to use the lowest dose and lowest concentration of a vasoconstrictor that produces the desired effect, because epinephrine is an insulin antagonist that is capable of raising the blood glucose level. Monitor the client for signs of hyperglycemia.
- A client with well-controlled diabetes with no evidence of infection does not require prophylactic antibiotic premedication.

CRITICAL THINKING EXERCISES

1. Find evidence-based information on the Internet about periodontal disease and diabetes that can be used to educate clients.
2. Review the office emergency kit. What in the emergency kit would be used if the diabetic client were to become disoriented and confused and was reporting that he or she took his or her insulin but did not have time to eat breakfast?
3. At the local pharmacy, purchase glucose tablets that can be kept in the treatment areas. When would these glucose tablets be indicated?
4. Read the following scenario and dental hygiene care plan, and then answer the questions that follow.

Client with Diabetes

Bettie Douman is a 40-year-old professional secretary who is employed full-time at a large university. She has had type 1 diabetes mellitus for 20 years. Bettie has been using an insulin pump for 2 years, and this has greatly lowered her blood glucose levels. Her 24-hour blood sugar test results average 180 mL/dL, and her 3-month A_{1c} level was 8%. Bettie walks the family dog at a fast pace every evening for 30 minutes. She is embarrassed that she has not been careful about eating a nutritionally balanced diet for the last year and a half. During Bettie's examination, the dental hygienist notes a low risk for dental caries and generalized moderate gingival bleeding on probing, with localized 4- and 5-mm pocket depths in the molar areas.

- What changes would you make, if any, to the following dental hygiene care plan?
- What emergency would you prepare for when treating this client? What steps would you take to prevent this emergency?
- Develop a detailed self-care plan for this client.

DENTAL HYGIENE DIAGNOSIS	GOAL OR EXPECTED BEHAVIOR
Unmet need for conceptualization and problem solving	By 12/1, client explains the role of oral biofilm in causing periodontal disease.
Unmet need for responsibility for oral health	By 12/1, client verbalizes the role of oral infection in glycemic control.
Unmet need for skin and mucous membrane integrity	By 1/1, client decreases bleeding points by 75%. By 1/1, client reports improvement in hyperglycemia through the control of periodontal disease.

Dental Hygiene Interventions

1. Present "bleeding gums" as an indicator of a bacterial infection that further complicates glycemic control; explain diabetes as a risk factor for periodontal disease.
2. Demonstrate oral biofilm control measures.
3. Discuss antimicrobial agents for the control of plaque and inflammation and the technique for their application.
4. Scale and root debride with ultrasonic and hand instrumentation.
5. Consult with the dentist regarding possible systemic doxycycline therapy.
6. Monitor the client's oral health behavior through frequent evaluation.
7. Schedule follow-up evaluation.

Evaluative Statements

1. Client explains the two-way relationship of diabetic control and periodontal infection. Goal met.
2. Client demonstrates oral health behavior congruent with the maintenance of glycemic control. Goal met.
3. Client decreases gingival bleeding by 75% to enhance glycemic control. Goal met.

DENTAL HYGIENE DIAGNOSIS	GOAL OR EXPECTED BEHAVIOR
Unmet need for skin and mucous membrane integrity of the head and neck (undernutrition and increased frequency of carbohydrate consumption)	By 2/1, client verbalizes the need for adequate nutrition. By 2/1, client participates in dietary counseling. By 4/1, client increases nutrients in the diet.

Dental Hygiene Interventions

1. Relate nutritional needs for diabetes control and integrity of the periodontium.
2. Relate the frequency of eating to the need for oral biofilm control.
3. Relate the importance of a healthy dentition and periodontium to optimal diet consumption and glycemic control.
4. Design oral biofilm control measures that are consistent with the client's frequency of carbohydrate consumption.
5. Refer the client to a certified diabetes educator for dietary prescription and meal planning.

Evaluative Statements

1. Client reports normal blood glucose levels and 1% point reduction in A_{1c} level. Goal met.
2. Client indicates compliance with individual dietary prescription and meal plan. Goal met.

REFERENCES

1. Centers for Disease Control and Prevention: *Diabetes data and trends, 2012.* Available at: http://www.cdc.gov/diabetes/statistics/diabetes_slides.htm. Accessed November 1, 2012.
2. American Diabetes Association: Executive summary: Standards of medical care in diabetes—2012, *Diabetes Care* 35(Suppl 1):4, 2012.
3. Inzucchi SE, Sherwin RS: Type 2 diabetes mellitus. In Goldman L, Schafer A, eds: *Cecil medicine*, ed 24, Philadelphia, 2011, Saunders.
4. Centers for Disease Control and Prevention: *National diabetes fact sheet, national estimates and general information on diabetes and prediabetes in the United States, 2011.* Available at: http://www.cdc.gov/diabetes/pubs/pdf/ndfs_2011.pdf. Accessed October 3, 2012.
5. Mealey BL, Oates TW; American Academy of Periodontology: Diabetes mellitus and periodontal diseases, *J Periodontol* 77:1289, 2006.
6. Kidambi S, Patel S: Diabetes mellitus: considerations for dentistry, *J Am Dent Assoc* 139(Suppl):8S, 2008.

7. Preshaw PM, Alba AL, Herrera D, et al: Periodontitis and diabetes: a two-way relationship, *Diabetologia* 55:21, 2012.
8. Mealey BL: The interactions between physicians and dentists in managing the care of patients with diabetes mellitus, *J Am Dent Assoc* 139(Suppl):4S–7S, 2008.
9. Campbell PR, Shuman D, Bauman DB: ADHA Graduate Student/Faculty Research Project: health history, *J Dent Hyg* 67:378, 1993.
10. Engebretson SP, Hey-Hadavi J, Ehrhardt FJ, et al: Gingival crevicular fluid levels of interleukin-1β and glycemic control in patients with chronic periodontitis and type 2 diabetes, *J Periodontol* 75:1203, 2004.
11. Rhodus NL, Vibeto B, Hamamoto DT: Glycemic control in patients with diabetes mellitus upon admission to a dental clinic: considerations for dental management, *Quintessence Int* 36:474, 2005.
12. Little JW, Falace DA, Miller CS, et al: *Dental management of the medically compromised patient*, ed 8, St Louis, 2013, Elsevier.
13. Gurenlian JR, Ball WL, LaFontaine J: Diabetes mellitus: promoting collaboration among health care professionals, *J Dent Hyg* 83(Suppl):3, 2008.
14. Lalla E, Kunzel C, Burkett S, et al: Identification of unrecognized diabetes and pre-diabetes in a dental setting, *J Dent Res* 90:855, 2011.
15. Gilowski L, Kondzielnik P, Wiench R, et al: Efficacy of short-term adjunctive subantimicrobial dose doxycycline in diabetic patients—randomized study, *Oral Dis* 18:763, 2012.

EVOLVE RESOURCES

Please visit http://evolve.elsevier.com/Darby/hygiene for additional practice and study support tools.

Cancer

Joan M. Davis

CHAPTER 45

COMPETENCIES

1. **Explain terms related to cancer, cancer therapies, and oral healthcare for the cancer patient.**
2. **Discuss the incidence and risk factors associated with cancer and oral cancer.**
3. **Describe the modes of cancer and oral cancer therapy.**
4. **Describe oral considerations of general cancer therapy and oral complication management.**
5. **Discuss oral cancer–specific therapies, including the rationale for bisphosphonate use and the potential for osteonecrosis.**
6. **Explain the dental hygiene process of care for clients with cancer, including development of a dental hygiene care plan for clients before, during, and after cancer therapy.**

Today clients who are in need of oral care are living longer and may very well have survived—or may be currently coping with—a life-threatening disease such as cancer. The dental hygienist will need to understand the oral, physical, and psychologic issues surrounding a client who is currently battling or who has survived cancer. Cancer is not a single disease but rather a broad classification of more than 100 types of diseases. The common element in cancer is the abnormal and unrestricted growth of cells that can invade and destroy surrounding normal body tissues, sometimes spreading to other parts of the body. The difference between a malignant and a benign neoplasm is that a benign tumor is usually circumscribed and encapsulated; it usually grows slowly, and it is composed of cells that resemble the tissue from which it arises. A malignant neoplasm or cancer not only infiltrates locally but also has the potential to metastasize or spread to distant sites. The cells are usually atypical or dysplastic, and they may not resemble the parent tissue. The branch of medicine that studies and treats cancer is called oncology, and the physician specialist is an oncologist.

Cancer

Incidence

To many people, a cancer diagnosis evokes immediate fear of suffering and death. Fortunately there has been a significant decline in cancer deaths during recent years, primarily as a result of a decrease in tobacco use and an increase in cancer screening, early detection, and effective treatment.[1] Figure 45-1 lists the leading types of new cancer cases and deaths according to the American Cancer Society 2012 estimates.[2] Of the estimated 577,190 deaths annually from cancer, 173,200 deaths are caused by tobacco use; another 190,472 deaths are caused by obesity, poor nutrition, and inactivity; and many of the remaining deaths are caused by infectious agents and sun exposure. Although anyone could potentially develop cancer, approximately 77% of newly diagnosed cancer cases occur among people who are 55 years old and older. When cancers are left untreated, they result in significant morbidity and death. In the United States, only heart disease causes more deaths in adults.[2]

Risk Factors

Carcinogenic or cancer-causing influences may be environmental, behavioral, viral, or genetic, thus resulting in potential genetic damage. The National Cancer Institute implicates tobacco use as the single major cause of preventable cancer deaths. Other environmental carcinogenic agents include alcohol, chemical exposure, radon, radiation, sunlight, hormones, and asbestos. Behavioral factors that could lead to the development of cancer include tobacco use, alcohol abuse, an overweight or obese condition, poor nutrition, and inactivity. There is also evidence that certain viruses (e.g., hepatitis B virus, human immunodeficiency virus, human papillomavirus, *Helicobacter pylori*) may be linked to the development of cancers, especially cancers of the liver, nasopharynx, cervix, and lymphatic system.[2] Many of these risk factors could be minimized through behavioral changes as well as the use of vaccines and antibiotics.

Common Signs and Symptoms

During the early stages, most cancers exhibit no symptoms. Box 45-1 lists the most common presenting signs and symptoms of early cancer, which vary depending on cancer type. Pain is not often a symptom during the early stages of cancer. A person who has one of the seven common signs of cancer for more than 2 weeks should see a doctor promptly.

Oral Cancer Incidence and Risk Factors

In 2012 the American Cancer Society estimated that approximately 40,250 new cases (28,540 men and 11,710 women) of oral or pharyngeal cancer would be diagnosed in the United States. Oral cancer incidence rates declined 1% for women and remained stable in men between 2004 and 2008, primarily as a result of the decrease in smoking in the United States. Unfortunately, the incidence of human papillomavirus–related cancers has *increased* over the past decade.[3] These cancers are primarily found in the tongue and the oropharyngeal area (i.e., the throat, the back third of the tongue, the soft palate, the side and back walls of the throat, and the tonsils) of adults who are less than 45 years old.[2]

Leading Sites of New Cancer Cases and Deaths – 2008 Estimates

Estimated New Cases*		Estimated Deaths	
Male	**Female**	**Male**	**Female**
Prostate 241,740 (29%)	Breast 226,870 (29%)	Lung and bronchus 87,750 (29%)	Lung and bronchus 72,590 (26%)
Lung and bronchus 116,470 (14%)	Lung and bronchus 109,690 (14%)	Prostate 28,170 (9%)	Breast 39,510 (14%)
Colon and rectum 73,420 (9%)	Colon and rectum 70,040 (9%)	Colon and rectum 26,470 (9%)	Colon and rectum 25,220 (9%)
Urinary bladder 55,600 (7%)	Uterine corpus 47,130 (6%)	Pancreas 18,850 (6%)	Pancreas 18,540 (7%)
Melanoma of the skin 44,250 (5%)	Thyroid 43,210 (5%)	Liver and intrahepatic bile duct 13,980 (5%)	Ovary 15,500 (6%)
Kidney and renal pelvis 40,250 (5%)	Melanoma of the skin 32,000 (4%)	Leukemia 13,500 (4%)	Leukemia 10,040 (4%)
Non-Hodgkin lymphoma 38,160 (4%)	Non-Hodgkin lymphoma 31,970 (4%)	Esophagus 12,040 (4%)	Non-Hodgkin lymphoma 8,620 (3%)
Oral cavity and pharynx 28,540 (3%)	Kidney and renal pelvis 24,520 (3%)	Urinary bladder 10,510 (3%)	Uterine corpus 8,010 (3%)
Leukemia 26,830 (3%)	Ovary 22,280 (3%)	Non-Hodgkin lymphoma 10,320 (3%)	Liver and intrahepatic bile duct 6,570 (2%)
Pancreas 22,090 (3%)	Pancreas 21,830 (3%)	Kidney and renal pelvis 8,650 (3%)	Brain and other nervous system 5,980 (2%)
All sites 848,170 (100%)	All sites 790,740 (100%)	All sites 301,820 (100%)	All sites 275,370 (100%)

*Excludes basal and squamous cell skin cancers and in situ carcinoma except urinary bladder.

Figure 45-1. American Cancer Society incidence and deaths by site and sex, 2012 estimates. (From the American Cancer Society: Cancer facts and figures 2012. Available at: http://www.cancer.org/acs/groups/content/@epidemiologysurveilance/documents/document/acspc-031941.pdf. Accessed November 19, 2012.)

BOX 45-1

Early Signs and Symptoms of Cancer

- Changes in bowel or bladder habits
- A sore that does not heal
- Unusual bleeding or discharge
- A thickening or a lump in the breast or elsewhere
- Indigestion or difficulty swallowing
- Obvious changes in a wart or mole
- A nagging cough or hoarseness

From the American Cancer Society: *Cancer facts and figures 2012.* Available at: http://www.cancer.org/acs/groups/content/@epidemiologysurveilance/documents/document/acspc-031941.pdf. Accessed November 19, 2012.

BOX 45-2

Common Signs of Oral Cancer

- A swelling, lump, growth, or area of induration or hardness anywhere in or about the mouth or neck that is usually painless
- Erythroplakia patch (velvety, deep red)
- Leukoplakia patch (white or red-and-white patch)
- Any sore (ulcer, irritation) that does not heal after 2 weeks
- Repeated bleeding from the mouth or throat
- Difficulty swallowing or persistent hoarseness

Approximately 9 out of every 10 oral malignancies are squamous cell carcinomas, which often manifest as a painless swelling or lump in the oral cavity or the pharynx and larynx area (Box 45-2). The median age of a person with newly diagnosed oral cancer is 62 years.[4] Of the newly diagnosed cases in 2012, 5440 men and 2410 women were expected to die from these cancers. The overall 1-year survival rate for all stages of oral cancer is about 84%, with a 5-year survival rate of 61%.[2] Even though there has been a slight decline in incidence, oral cancer screening remains a very important component of dental hygiene care, as do continued efforts to educate the public about this life-threatening disease.

Specific oral cancer risk factors include the use of all tobacco products (i.e., cigarettes, cigars, pipes, and smokeless tobacco) and alcohol (Box 45-3). Cigarette smokers have an approximately tenfold-increased chance of developing squamous cell carcinoma as compared with people who have never smoked.[5] The risk of developing any cancer increases with both the amount and duration of tobacco product use.

BOX 45-3

Oral Cancer Risk Factors

- Use of tobacco
- Prior oral cancer lesion
- Use of alcohol
- Older age
- Frequent sun exposure
- Low consumption of fruits and vegetables
- Human papillomavirus

From the American Cancer Society: *Cancer facts and figures 2012.* Available at: http://www.cancer.org/acs/groups/content/@epidemiologysurveilance/documents/document/acspc-031941.pdf. Accessed November 19, 2012.

Individuals who smoke and drink alcohol heavily account for approximately 80% to 90% of oral cancer cases in the United States.

The prognosis for a specific oral cancer is highly variable and depends on the stage and location of the disease when it is first diagnosed. National Cancer Institute data collected between the years 2002 and 2008 demonstrated that persons with a small, localized oral squamous cell cancer have an 82% 5-year survival rate as compared with only a 34% rate among those with late-stage oral cancer.[4] Early detection is the key to survival. The most common intraoral sites for squamous cell cancer are the lateral borders and the ventral surfaces of the tongue, the floor of the mouth, and the oropharynx. Any of the signs and symptoms that persist for more than 2 weeks after the removal of potentially irritating factors or the application of therapeutic measures must be considered to result from cancer until the condition is proven benign by biopsy (i.e., the surgical removal of all or part of the lesion) and microscopic evaluation.

Cancer Therapy

Forms of Cancer Therapy

The choice of cancer treatment is dependent on the type and stage of cancer. Therapy may include one or a combination of the following: chemotherapy, bone marrow and blood transplantation, radiation, surgery, hormone therapy, and immunotherapy. Some cancers respond to a single mode of treatment, whereas others require multimodal treatment strategies. The goal of cancer treatment is to remove or totally destroy the malignant cells in the body. Unfortunately, treatments available today are not able to target only the cancer cells, and normal healthy cells must sometimes be destroyed during treatment. This may result in significant psychologic stress as well as physical morbidity (illness) or death.

Chemotherapy

Chemotherapy is the use of drugs for the treatment of cancer. Combinations of chemotherapeutic agents have resulted in significant improvements in the cure rates of some cancers. Other cancers are not cured by chemotherapy alone, so toxic drugs are used in combination with surgery, radiation, or both to destroy rapidly dividing cancer cells that may spread systemically.

The most common complication of chemotherapy is infection. The high risk of infection is a result of myelosuppression, which is the suppression of bone marrow that results in, among other things, the destruction of white blood cells, thereby leading to a decreased immune response. Bacterial, fungal, and viral infections often increase with chemotherapy; these infections affect both local and distant body sites and lead to potential sepsis and death. Oral infections such as periodontal disease, pulpal disease, and pericoronal disease can significantly increase the likelihood of sepsis occurring if they are not treated before chemotherapy begins. Other complications of chemotherapy include electrolyte imbalances, bleeding, hemorrhage, and acute toxicity from the drugs, including nausea and vomiting, photosensitivity, central nervous system dysfunction, alopecia (hair loss), and poor nutritional status.

Chemotherapy is physically demanding, and it also produces a great deal of stress. Individuals who are undergoing cancer therapy need support from family members, friends, and caregivers who are good listeners and who encourage hope.

Bone Marrow and Blood Stem Cell Transplantation

Bone marrow and blood stem cell transplantation (BMT) is a therapeutic procedure that is used to treat a variety of hematologic diseases, including aplastic anemia, leukemias, lymphomas, neuroblastoma, and immunodeficiency diseases. BMT is also used to treat some solid tumors.

BMT begins with the donation of normal bone marrow or peripheral blood stem cells. The individual with cancer then goes through a "conditioning phase" during which superlethal doses of chemotherapy and sometimes total body irradiation are administered. The goal is to destroy all of the malignant cells and to suppress the immune system to permit engraftment of the normal bone marrow. After clients have been conditioned, the marrow or peripheral blood stem cells are intravenously infused into their blood. If engraftment takes place, the cells begin to reproduce new marrow within 2 to 4 weeks.

A significant problem that exists for clients who receive marrow or peripheral blood stem cells from another individual (allogeneic bone marrow transplant) is graft-versus-host disease (GVHD). This disease results from an immunologic reaction during which the donor cells react against the host tissue antigens. If this occurs within the first 100 days after transplant, it is called *acute GVHD*, and it is characterized by dermatitis, enteritis, and hepatitis. If these characteristics occur after the first 100 days, it is called *chronic GVHD*, and it has manifestations similar to those of autoimmune disorders. These may include skin diseases, keratoconjunctivitis, oral mucositis (mucosal edema, inflammation, and ulcerations), salivary gland dysfunction or xerostomia (dry mouth), esophageal and vaginal strictures, pulmonary insufficiency, intestinal problems, and chronic liver disease. Both forms of GVHD can result in fatal infections. To prevent GVHD, various types of immunosuppressive therapy are used.

During the first 30 days after transplantation, the client experiences cytotoxic and immunosuppressive oral manifestations from the chemoradiotherapy conditioning. These may include severe mucositis, ulceration, hemorrhage, infection, and salivary gland dysfunction. Infections during the first 30 days intensify the mucositis and ulcerations, thereby opening a portal of entry for organisms into the blood.

During the next several months, the client's acute manifestations begin to resolve unless GVHD develops. Common complaints with GVHD include xerostomia and mucositis. In addition, there may be evidence of lichen planus–like or lupus-like lesions, and these may sometimes become erosive. Generalized atrophy of the mucosa and changes that are consistent with scleroderma may be seen. Viral infections, including herpes simplex virus and fungal infections, are common.

After the first 100 days after transplantation, persons with no evidence of GVHD usually do not have any oral complaints other than varying degrees of xerostomia. Those persons with persistent xerostomia may develop rapid tooth demineralization and oral infections. Patients who are scheduled for BMT should undergo a thorough oral and dental evaluation and necessary treatment before transplant. All potential sources of infection and irritation should be treated, because chronic asymptomatic oral infections may become acute during immunosuppression or GVHD and may lead to sepsis and even death.

Head and Neck Radiation and Surgical Treatment

Both head and neck radiation and surgical treatment for oral cancer have unique client care issues that differ somewhat from chemotherapy and BMT. These specific issues are addressed later in this chapter. The following section reviews oral side effects that are common to many cancer therapies.

Oral Considerations of General Cancer Therapy

Oral side effects of cancer treatment that result from the unintended disruption and destruction of healthy tissue can be so debilitating that patients may tolerate only lower, less-effective doses of cancer therapy, or they may delay or discontinue scheduled treatments. Preventing and managing oral complications helps to support optimal cancer treatment and enhances patient survival and quality of life. The National Institutes of Health formally recognized the critical role that dentists and dental hygienists play in the overall care of the individual with cancer.[6] Dental hygiene care is critical to the prevention or amelioration of the oral complications associated with all forms of cancer treatment.

All patients receiving radiation for head and neck malignancies, 80% of BMT recipients, and 40% of patients receiving chemotherapy for any malignancy have oral complications. The risks for oral complications vary with the treatment regimen (Box 45-4). Some oral complications occur only during cancer therapy, whereas others, such as xerostomia and salivary gland dysfunction, may be lifelong after radiation therapy. *Before, during, and after radiation therapy and chemotherapy, the dental hygienist plays a key role in helping clients with cancer to understand that good oral hygiene care prevents or reduces oral complications, which in turn improves clients' quality of life and the likelihood that they will be able to tolerate optimal doses of cancer treatment* (Box 45-5). For example, the dental hygienist collaborates with the client to establish an oral self-care regimen to protect the mouth tissues and to minimize oral complications. To that end, the dental hygienist reviews toothbrushing, interdental cleaning techniques, and other approaches (e.g., the use of antimicrobial and fluoride mouth rinses and fluoride gel) to keep the mouth as moist and clean as possible to reduce risk of dental caries, oral infection, and pain (Table 45-1). The importance of the role of the dental hygienist in enhancing the client's quality of life and potential survival cannot be overemphasized.

BOX 45-4

Risk Levels for Oral Complications

Low Risk
- Patients receiving mildly myelosuppressive chemotherapy that mildly decreases the immune system

Moderate Risk
- Patients receiving single-agent or outpatient therapy

High Risk
- Patients undergoing head and neck radiation for oral and pharyngeal cancer
- Patients receiving stomatotoxic chemotherapy that results in prolonged myelosuppression

Adapted from the U.S. Department of Health and Human Services, National Institutes of Health: *Oral complications of chemotherapy and head/neck radiation (PDQ), 2012.* Available at: http://www.cancer.gov/cancertopics/pdq/supportivecare/oralcomplications/HealthProfessional and http://www.cancer.gov/cancertopics/pdq/supportivecare. Accessed November 19, 2012.

BOX 45-5

Benefits of Good Oral Hygiene Care Before and During Cancer Therapy

- Reduces the risk and severity of oral complications
- Improves the likelihood that the client will tolerate optimal doses of cancer treatment
- Prevents oral infections that could lead to potentially fatal systemic infections
- Prevents or minimizes complications that can compromise nutrition
- Prevents or reduces oral pain
- Prevents or reduces the incidence of bone necrosis in clients undergoing radiation
- Preserves oral health
- Improves quality of life

Adapted from the U.S. Department of Health and Human Services, National Institutes of Health: *Oral complications of chemotherapy and head/neck radiation (PDQ), 2012.* Available at: http://www.cancer.gov/cancertopics/pdq/supportivecare/oralcomplications/HealthProfessional and http://www.cancer.gov/cancertopics/pdq/supportivecare. Accessed November 19, 2012.

Oral Complications of Chemotherapy and Bone Marrow and Blood Stem Cell Transplantation

Not all chemotherapy protocols result in oral manifestations, but many have either a direct or indirect effect on the mouth. Oral problems related to myelosuppression may be significantly prevented or diminished through aggressive preventive dental hygiene interventions. The oral manifestations of

TABLE 45-1
Oral Hygiene Products Used During Cancer Therapy

Product	Description	Indication, Rationale, or Use	Precautions
Toothbrushes	Several are available with extra-soft or super-soft bristles: such as Rx Ultra Suave (PHB, Inc, www.phbdirect.com, 1-800-676-4025) and Biotene SuperSoft (Laclede, Inc, www.laclede.com, 1-877-522-5333). A child-size brush may be helpful for clients with limited mouth opening. Some brushes are available with suctioning capabilities.	Plaque biofilm removal should be performed after meals when clients are not severely compromised from surgery, chemotherapy, or bone marrow transplantation. The tongue must also be brushed, especially by clients who are receiving soft or liquid diets.	Beware of inexpensive, hospital-supplied, hard, unpolished, bristled toothbrushes. The benefits versus the risks of brushing may need to be assessed for clients with severely compromised conditions.
Floss	Unwaxed or waxed versions are available.	Flossing is important for plaque biofilm removal at least once per day.	Assess the client's dexterity, and assist if necessary. Discontinue only when the client is at high risk for bleeding and bacteremia.
Dentifrices	Commercial dentifrices without strong flavoring agents can be used. Paste made from baking soda and water is an alternative.	These help with plaque biofilm removal.	Strong flavoring agents may intensify mucositis. Fully rinse baking soda residue from the oral cavity.
Foam or sponge sticks	These are alternatives to toothbrushes that are available from some medical supply companies. Some are impregnated with cleaning agents.	They are used to cleanse the oral cavity only when the client cannot use a manual toothbrush because of pain associated with ulcerated tissues or when the platelet count is $<20{,}000/mm^3$. If foam or a sponge is used, it should be dipped in a chlorhexidine solution for greatest efficacy. These sticks may also be used to apply topical medications.	These sticks do not adequately remove plaque biofilm. Do not soak them in solution; the sponge top may fall off the stick, and the client could aspirate it. These products may abrade friable tissue. Do not use lemon–glycerin swabs, because they are acidic and drying to the tissues.
Gauze	Gauze is another alternative to a toothbrush. Use 2 × 2 or 4 × 4 squares.	Gauze is used to cleanse the oral cavity only when toothbrushing is not possible as a result of pain associated with ulcerated tissues or when toothbrushing precipitates bleeding. Moisten the gauze in water, saline 0.9% (1 tsp of sodium chloride to 16 oz of water), or baking soda solution. Wrap the gauze around the finger and cleanse the teeth, tongue, and tissues.	Gauze does not adequately remove plaque biofilm.
Baking soda and saline rinse	This is a mucolytic cleansing solution made up of ½ tsp of baking soda, ¼ tsp of salt, and 16 oz of water.	An alkaline soothing rinse is used to cleanse the mouth every 2 to 4 hours for clients with mucositis, xerostomia, or thick secretions or after emesis. It may be used in an irrigation bag to assist with the rinsing of a painful mouth. Rinse the mouth with plain water after use.	This mixture has a high sodium content. Instruct the client not to swallow the solution. This is not to be used by clients on sodium-restricted diets.

Continued

TABLE 45-1

Oral Hygiene Products Used During Cancer Therapy—cont'd

Product	Description	Indication, Rationale, or Use	Precautions
Topical anesthetics	These palliative agents include over-the-counter products such as alcohol-free Benadryl mixed in equal parts with a coating agent such as Maalox to create a rinse. Other agents that are helpful are topical Orabase and benzocaine (www.colgateprofessional.com), which are available over the counter at most pharmacies.	They are used to control the pain associated with mucosal ulcerations.	Topical anesthetics may decrease the gag reflex, thereby resulting in the aspiration of food. Over-the-counter agents or rinses may not provide adequate relief from severe oral ulcerations. The client's oncologist may prescribe analgesics or narcotics.
Saliva replacement and xerostomia palliation	Saliva substitutes include over-the-counter rinses and gels such as Oral Balance Gel (Laclede, Inc, www.laclede.com, 1-877-522-5333) and Moi-Stir (Kingswood Labs, www.kingswood-labs.com/moistir.html, 1-800-968-7772). Dietary guidelines should encourage the intake of high-moisture foods, oily foods, and sugar- and acid-free foods. Saliva stimulants include pharmacologic prescription drugs (pilocarpine) for the systemic stimulation of functional salivary gland tissue and mechanical stimulation with xylitol-containing chewing gum or candy.	They are used for the palliation of xerostomia and dysphagia.	Clients may find saliva substitutes to be unacceptable in taste and too expensive. Clients should be discouraged from using tobacco products, consuming excessive alcohol, and using alcohol-containing mouthwash because these products promote dry mouth or may be irritating.
Chlorhexidine gluconate 0.12%	This is a bactericidal mouth rinse.	These are prophylactic or therapeutic mouth rinses that are used to reduce plaque biofilm and oral microbes. Rinse for 30 seconds with 1 capful twice daily.	Products that are available in United States are prepared with alcohol and may be irritating. This agent should be used only when mechanical plaque control is inadequate. It may cause staining of the teeth, which is removable with dental prophylaxis. It may also alter taste perception.
Commercial mouthwashes	These should be heavily diluted with water.	They may serve as mouth fresheners.	Most commercial mouthwashes have a high concentration of alcohol or phenol, which can be very drying and irritating to tissues unless diluted heavily with water. Flavoring agents may intensify mucositis. Alcohol-free mouthwashes are available (i.e., Biotene, Pro-Health, and Clear Choice).

BOX 45-6

Oral Complications of Chemotherapy

- Oral mucositis
- Neurotoxicity
- Infection
- Bleeding or hemorrhage
- Xerostomia or salivary gland dysfunction
- Dental caries or demineralization
- Altered tooth development

Adapted from the U.S. Department of Health and Human Services, National Institutes of Health: *Oral complications of chemotherapy and head/neck radiation (PDQ), 2012.* Available at: http://www.cancer.gov/cancertopics/pdq/supportivecare/oralcomplications/HealthProfessional and http://www.cancer.gov/cancertopics/pdq/supportivecare. Accessed November 19, 2012.

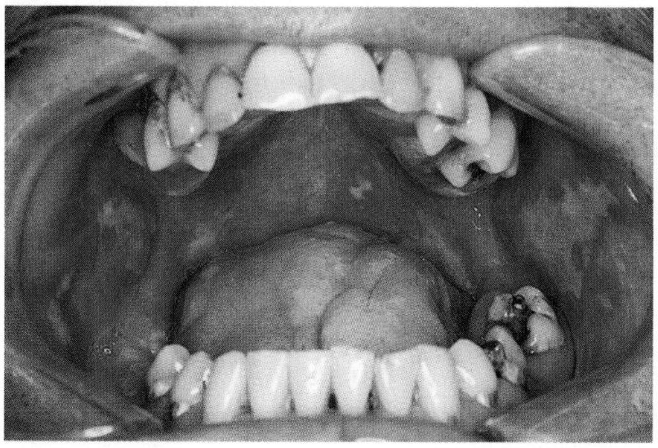

Figure 45-2. Radiation mucositis. (From Regezi JA, Sciubba JJ, Jordan RCK: *Oral pathology for clinical pathologic correlations*, ed 6, St Louis, 2012, Saunders.)

chemotherapy listed in Box 45-6 and described in the following sections are not permanent, but the client will be at risk for these complications throughout the entire period during which the drugs are being administered.

Mucositis

Some chemotherapeutic drugs are toxic to the oral mucosa and cause edema, inflammation, and ulcerations (mucositis) within a few days after the administration of the drug. Ulcerations from chemotherapy and radiation therapy are alike in their clinical presentation, with red, swollen tissue that later develops into a yellowish membrane-covered ulcerated tissue (Figure 45-2). If the tissues do not become secondarily infected, the ulcerated tissue will heal within a few weeks of the drug delivery or radiation therapy. Clients with mucositis report burning, pain, and general discomfort, which can interfere with talking, swallowing, and obtaining proper nutrition.

Management

Mucositis may be prevented or lessened in severity by dental hygiene interventions that create a clean and well-hydrated oral environment, good nutritional status, and control of secondary infection (Box 45-7). The client should be encouraged to rinse frequently with sodium bicarbonate and saline water rinses and with alcohol-free mouth rinses (see Table 45-1).

BOX 45-7

Management of Mouth Pain from Mucositis

- Early detection and treatment of oral infection
- Good oral hygiene, including tongue brushing, to prevent further infection
- Frequent irrigation with 1 tsp of baking soda, ½ tsp of salt, and 32 oz of water
- Frequent rinsing with sodium bicarbonate mouth rinses and nonalcoholic mouth rinses (e.g., Biotene, Clear Choice)
- Daily cleaning of dentures and changing of soaking solution; removal of dentures while sleeping
- Use of prescribed topical anesthetics with caution to avoid anesthetizing the soft palate, which could cause food aspiration; excessive use may potentiate mucositis
- Use of over-the-counter or prescribed systemic analgesics if necessary
- Avoidance of irritating or rough-textured foods
- Use of perioral moisturizers as directed by the radiation oncologist

Adapted from the U.S. Department of Health and Human Services, National Institutes of Health: *Oral complications of chemotherapy and head/neck radiation (PDQ), 2012.* Available at: http://www.cancer.gov/cancertopics/pdq/supportivecare/oralcomplications/HealthProfessional and http://www.cancer.gov/cancertopics/pdq/supportivecare. Accessed November 19, 2012.

These rinses soothe and hydrate the inflamed tissues, help with bacterial plaque biofilm removal, and neutralize pH if the client is vomiting. Pain management begins with mild topical anesthetics and may progress to systemic analgesics and even narcotics.

Neurotoxicity

Some chemotherapeutic agents that are derived from plant alkaloids (e.g., vincristine) are toxic to nerve tissue and may cause severe, deep, and often bilateral odontogenic-like pain known as **neurotoxicity**. When no dental pathology can be found, the drug may be implicated. The pain subsides within a few days after the administration of the drug.

Infection

Some chemotherapeutic agents suppress the bone marrow, thereby resulting in **immunosuppression** (decreased immune response) and bleeding problems. During these periods, the client will be at risk for developing oral infections (fungal, viral, and bacterial) that may increase the risk for a systemic infection, especially if there is a break in mucosal integrity that allows organisms to enter the blood. Oral infections can result in significant morbidity for the client who is undergoing chemotherapy. Oral infections intensify mucositis, and, with a breach in the oral mucosa, such infections may lead to septicemia and death in clients with profound immunosuppression.[5] Inappropriately timed dental and dental hygiene procedures can result in bacteremia, thereby causing sepsis and death.

Management

The final decision regarding the safest time to schedule oral healthcare appointments is made by the oncologist. If necessary, the oncologist may recommend antibiotic prophylaxis before dental and dental hygiene care.

A potential rationale for antibiotic prophylaxis before dental treatment exists when the client has an indwelling central venous catheter for chemotherapy delivery. Some individuals begin chemotherapy without a central venous catheter but have one placed later during therapy. Therefore each time a client is seen it is necessary to ask if a catheter has been placed since the last appointment, because it may become colonized with oral organisms after a dental or dental hygiene procedure. Although no data are currently available to document the absolute need for prophylactic antibiotics in this patient population before dental procedures, the oncologist should be consulted regarding what antibiotics may be necessary (see Chapter 14 for a discussion of antibiotic premedication).

Some cancer centers have clients discontinue toothbrushing and flossing during severe myelosuppression. This practice is controversial, however, because there is evidence that toothbrushing and flossing during immunosuppression are not detrimental, and a decrease in plaque biofilm and local infection reduces the risk for potentially life-threatening systemic infection.

Clients with dentures should be evaluated frequently and encouraged to call the dental office whenever necessary to seek early intervention for an oral complication or dental-related sources of pain, irritation, or dental trauma. Oral tissues may change significantly during chemotherapy as a result of edema, inflammation, ulceration, or weight loss. Clients should understand that, when denture irritation occurs, the prosthesis should be removed from the mouth to avoid further trauma. Persons with oral infections may reinfect their mouths with poorly cleansed dentures. It is important for the client to clean and disinfect the dentures daily and to keep them out of the mouth while sleeping. Denture-soaking solutions must be changed daily, and the soaking container must be cleansed and rinsed thoroughly (see Chapter 56).

Hemorrhage

Myelosuppression from chemotherapy may result in thrombocytopenia (the reduction of clotting factors). Clients with platelet counts of less than 50,000/mm^3 may experience oral hemorrhaging (bleeding) during invasive dental and dental hygiene procedures.[5] The occurrence of spontaneous gingival bleeding increases with a platelet count of less than 20,000/mm^3.[5] When there is a disruption of the mucosal integrity or the presence of periodontal disease, clients are at greater risk for bleeding. This fact emphasizes the need for early debridement and periodontal maintenance care.

Management

When scheduling a client who is undergoing chemotherapy for a dental hygiene appointment, it is imperative to consult the oncologist regarding the status of the client's blood counts and clotting factors to avoid potential bleeding problems associated with chemotherapy. Generally a platelet count of at least 50,000/mm^3 is recommended before invasive dental or dental hygiene procedures occur.[6] If a dental or dental hygiene procedure is absolutely necessary during periods of thrombocytopenia, platelet support therapy may be given by the oncologist. Adequate bleeding times are dependent on the extent of the oral procedure. The client should also be warned that trauma from improper toothbrushing or a poorly fitting dental prosthesis may initiate bleeding when platelet levels are low.

Salivary Gland Dysfunction

Not all persons who are undergoing chemotherapy experience xerostomia or ropy saliva. However, some clients complain of a dry mouth, thickened secretions, or excessive drooling during chemotherapy. Studies are inconclusive regarding the drugs' effects on the salivary glands; however, persons who complain about salivary dysfunction should be offered palliative measures such as adequate hydration (Table 45-2) to help manage this debilitating and uncomfortable side effect and to prevent the further exacerbation of other oral complications.

Dental Caries

Rampant tooth decay is not directly caused by the toxicity of chemotherapeutic drugs. However, clients with chronically dry mouths or persons who increase their intake of high-carbohydrate foods in response to eating problems may experience an increase in caries development. For example, children who are chronically ill may be given nighttime bottle feedings or diets that are high in sugar. During periods of stress, parents and caregivers may allow an unbalanced diet to avoid additional stress that may be caused by insisting on a healthy diet. Such eating patterns may increase dental caries risk.

Management

Depending on the severity of the dental caries problem, various preventive regimens may be prescribed. A fluoride rinse or brush-on 1.1% sodium fluoride gel may be adequate. However, if there is evidence of demineralization and if dryness continues for several months, the client may require custom-fit gel trays for daily gel application. In addition, in-office fluoride varnish applications may be beneficial. The dental hygienist educates the client about the importance of daily fluoride application, good nutrition, and oral hygiene. The dental hygienist also counsels clients and primary caregivers about cariogenic foods and behaviors and suggests alternatives (see Chapters 33 and 35).

Altered Tooth Development

Studies have shown that some chemotherapy drugs given before the age of 10 years—and especially before the age of 5 years—may alter root development.

Oral Cancer–Specific Therapy

The choice of treatment for oral squamous cell cancer depends on the stage of disease at the time of diagnosis. A small lesion of less than 1 cm may require only surgery or radiation therapy. Larger cancers and especially those that have spread to the lymph nodes in the neck may require surgery, radiation, and chemotherapy.

Head and Neck Radiation

Radiation therapy employs the use of ionizing radiation, either from external beams or from internally implanted sources. Radiation therapy may be used by itself for the treatment of oral squamous cell carcinoma when the lesion is

TABLE 45-2

Management of Oral Manifestations of Cancer Therapies

Manifestation	Prevention	Palliative Measures and Management	Dental Hygiene Care Guidelines
Mucositis or stomatitis (related to direct effects of radiation therapy and cytotoxic chemotherapy)	These conditions are caused by the toxicity of the cancer therapy Early onset and severity can be minimized by consistent hydration and excellent bacterial plaque control Gentle tooth and gingival brushing with extra-soft toothbrush Discontinue toothpastes with strong, irritating flavoring agents and replace with baking soda and water paste Discontinue alcohol-based rinses, full-strength peroxide, and irritating foods	Increased hydration with water, saliva substitutes, ice chips, or sugar-free popsicles Cool-mist humidifiers may be helpful, especially in dry environments Baking soda and water solutions (1 tsp of baking soda, ½ tsp of salt, and 16 oz of water) may be used as rinses or placed in a disposable irrigation bag (let the solution flow through the mouth to gently rinse) Topical anesthetics (see Table 45-1)	Do not schedule dental hygiene procedures while the client is experiencing oral ulcerations and pain.
Salivary gland dysfunction or xerostomia (related to direct radiation damage to salivary gland tissue and possible indirect effect of chemotherapeutic agents) Salivary gland dysfunction is permanent after radiation therapy, whereas function usually returns after chemotherapy.	Eliminate use of products with alcohol and irritating agents Diminish caffeine intake Discontinue tobacco use Humidify air with cool-mist humidifier Consult with oncologist for salivary gland stimulant prescription	Suggest over-the-counter saliva substitutes (see recommendations for clients with xerostomia) Stimulate functional salivary gland tissue by chewing xylitol gum or a wax bolus Consult physician for salivary gland stimulant prescription Lubricate the lips with balm or cream (not pure petrolatum) Increase hydration with water, ice chips, and high-moisture foods Thin foods with liquids Recommend the use of a cool-mist humidifier, especially while client is sleeping Suggest baking soda and water rinsing for ropy saliva (see recommendations for clients with mucositis)	To prevent rampant caries, encourage improved oral hygiene measures, a diet low in sucrose, and fluoride supplementation (e.g., the daily use of 1.1% neutral-pH sodium fluoride gels for 5 to 10 minutes in customized fluoride trays for home use).
Infection: fungal, viral, and bacterial (related to chemotherapy-induced immunosuppression) Oral infections may not cause typical signs and symptoms. Candidiasis is common during radiation therapy.	Frequent and consistent oral hydration with water, ices, and saliva substitutes Increase bacterial plaque control Oral infections may be unrelenting when the client is severely immunosuppressed during chemotherapy	Oral microbiologic culturing and assessment Alert oncologist at first signs of oral infection Encourage use of antifungals that are sugar-free	Do not proceed with dental hygiene procedures while a client has an acute oral infection. Schedule dental hygiene procedures when the client's absolute neutrophil count is $>1000/mm^3$. If the client has a central venous catheter, the American Heart Association antibiotic prophylactic protocol should be followed for invasive dental hygiene procedures, including dental prophylaxis.
Bleeding (related to chemotherapy-induced myelosuppression)	Bleeding not preventable but bacterial plaque can exacerbate the complication if not consistently removed	Refer to oncologist for management	Dental hygiene procedures should be delayed until the client has a platelet count of $>50{,}000/mm^3$ or a blood transfusion.

Continued

TABLE 45-2

Management of Oral Manifestations of Cancer Therapies—cont'd

Manifestation	Prevention	Palliative Measures and Management	Dental Hygiene Care Guidelines
Rampant dental caries or demineralization (related to therapy-induced salivary gland dysfunction)	Bacterial plaque control Frequent oral hydration with water, ices, and saliva substitutes Daily 5- to 10-minute application of 1.1% sodium fluoride gel in custom gel carriers (soft vinyl trays adapted to extend beyond the cervical line of the teeth) or topical fluoride In-office application of fluoride varnish to exposed cementum Dietary guidelines to discourage frequent snacking on cariogenic foods, sugared beverages, or acidic beverages (i.e., diet sodas with citric or phosphoric acid) If there is evidence of dental decay despite daily fluoride application, place client on 2-week chlorhexidine regimen and in-office fluoride varnish application	Same as prevention measures	Encourage the participation of client when planning oral hygiene homecare, and ensure strict adherence by frequent monitoring. Establish a 2- to 3-month continued-care interval until the client demonstrates the ability to care for his or her teeth and the acute side effects of therapy have resolved.
Trismus or temporomandibular disorder (related to the direct effect of radiation on the muscles of mastication or the temporomandibular joint)	Daily exercise for muscles of mastication: instruct the client to open and close the mouth 20 times without causing pain to the temporomandibular joint; this should be repeated three times a day	Same as prevention measures Instruct client to encourage further opening of the mouth by placing increasing numbers of tongue blades between posterior teeth for several minutes a day	Dental hygiene procedures may need to be altered for clients with trismus to avoid exacerbating the associated pain (e.g., shortened appointments or sedation).
Soft-tissue necrosis and osteoradionecrosis (related to the direct effect of radiation on tissue and bone) Tissue becomes hypovascular, hypoxic, and hypocellular; damage to the bone and soft tissue is permanent.	All teeth within the field of radiation that have a poor lifelong prognosis should be extracted 14 to 21 days before the initiation of radiation therapy Avoid all surgical insult to irradiated bone throughout the client's lifetime	Referral to an oral surgeon for possible hyperbaric oxygen therapy and surgical management of the necrotic tissue and bone	Establish a frequent and regular dental hygiene continued-care interval to ensure the prevention of periodontal disease and adherence to the oral hygiene homecare protocol.

small and superficial and when a surgical procedure would result in significant functional or cosmetic damage. Radiation may also be used in combination with chemotherapy to enhance the chemotherapy's ability to reduce the tumor or with surgery postoperatively to eliminate residual disease or preoperatively to reduce the size of the tumor. Radiation therapy may also be used for the treatment of other head and neck cancers, including lymphomas and salivary gland tumors.

Radiation damage to some normal cells (e.g., taste buds) may be acute and may resolve after therapy completion. Other normal cells that can be affected (e.g., salivary gland cells) may not have the capacity to repair themselves, thereby resulting in long-term complications. After the first week of radiation, the client will begin to experience some of the acute side effects (e.g., loss of taste, dry mouth), whereas other complications may not become evident until later in the course of radiation therapy.

Oral Side Effects or Complications of Radiation Therapy

The complications associated with head and neck radiation will vary among clients, depending on the field of treatment and the total dose of radiation required. Only the tissues in the direct field or location of radiation are affected. For example, a client undergoing lymphoma treatment may receive only 20 radiation treatments that involve only a portion of the salivary glands and cervical lymph nodes and will therefore experience fewer complications than a client who is undergoing treatment for a squamous cell carcinoma in the oral cavity. To avoid unnecessarily alarming the client and to be able to offer sound advice, the dental professional must establish good communication with the radiation oncologist to understand the anticipated radiation side effects.

The client who is undergoing radiation therapy to the oral cavity and the salivary glands begins to experience some side effects after the first week of therapy. Throughout therapy, it is important to support the client with suggestions to prevent and reduce side effects or complications of radiation therapy. These complications are summarized in Box 45-8 and are described in the following paragraphs.

Xerostomia and Salivary Gland Dysfunction

Salivary gland exposure to radiation is unavoidable during treatment for oral cavity and neck tumors, because the glands are in close proximity to the lymphatic system and cannot be shielded. Ionizing radiation induces fibrosis and atrophy of the salivary gland tissue. Clients begin to experience a change in their saliva after the first week of radiation. They first complain of a thickened and ropy saliva, and, as the treatments progress, their mouths become drier. The degree of dryness is dependent on the radiation dose and the extent of salivary tissue within the radiation field. One study at MD Anderson Cancer Center demonstrated that persons undergoing high doses of radiation therapy to all of the major salivary glands experienced a 67% decrease in saliva after 1 week of radiation, a 76% loss after 6 weeks, and a 95% loss 3 years after the completion of radiation.

Xerostomia as a result of thickened, reduced, or absent salivary flow compromises speaking, chewing, and swallowing and increases the risk of impaired nutrition by causing an inability to eat all foods. Persistent dry mouth also increases the risk of dental caries and other oral infections. Because the irradiated salivary glands are permanently damaged, the change in both the quality and the quantity of saliva remains. Clients often complain bitterly about the complications associated with xerostomia and require ongoing assistance from the dental team to control symptoms.

Management

Clients who undergo radiation therapy to the neck involving the submandibular and sublingual salivary glands with only partial inclusion of the parotid glands complain mostly of a thick, ropy saliva. These clients benefit greatly from baking soda and saline water rinses. A baking soda solution is mucolytic, which aids in the cleansing and refreshing of the mouth. A prescribed medication such as pilocarpine can be provided by the oncologist or dentist to help stimulate residual salivary gland tissue to produce saliva. In addition, commercial saliva substitutes are available as over-the-counter products. Although they be palliative, saliva substitutes do not contain the protective proteins and mucoproteins found in saliva, and some clients do not feel the cost is justified for the limited relief. In addition, the lips should be lubricated with a moisturizing lip balm or cream recommended by the radiation oncologist and not with pure petrolatum, which provides only an occlusive agent and does not moisturize the perioral tissues. These and other suggestions for the management of a dry mouth are listed in Box 45-9.

Alteration of Taste

When the tongue is in the field of radiation, the client experiences partial or full taste loss. Loss of taste is an acute effect, and it usually occurs after the first few treatments. Taste returns a few months after the completion of radiation therapy, but it may be altered from its preradiation status. Taste loss is a significant side effect that makes radiation therapy almost intolerable. Eating becomes a chore; clients complain that all food tastes like mush or straw. Eating ceases to be a pleasurable activity, and clients must force themselves to eat to maintain their nutritional status.

Management

Clients are helped by having someone to listen to their complaints. These individuals should be assured that taste dysfunction is a normal radiation side effect and that taste will return several months after treatment. In addition, clients should be encouraged to continue eating. The use of nutritional liquid substitutes or referral for nutritional counseling

BOX 45-8

Potential Complications of Radiation to the Head and Neck Area

Acute

- Xerostomia
- Loss of taste
- Mucositis
- Dysphagia
- Secondary infection
- Trismus
- Impaired nutrition (from xerostomia, pain, and dysphagia)
- Hearing loss
- Fatigue

Chronic

- Xerostomia or salivary gland dysfunction
- Alterations in sense of taste as compared with preradiation status
- Telangiectasia and friable mucosa
- Continued fungal infections caused by the lack of saliva
- Osteoradionecrosis or soft-tissue necrosis
- Rampant caries
- Muscle fibrosis, temporomandibular disorder, and trismus
- Altered tooth and jaw development in children

Adapted from the U.S. Department of Health and Human Services, National Institutes of Health: *Oral complications of chemotherapy and head/neck radiation (PDQ), 2012.* Available at: http://www.cancer.gov/cancertopics/pdq/supportivecare/oralcomplications/HealthProfessional and http://www.cancer.gov/cancertopics/pdq/supportivecare. Accessed November 19, 2012.

BOX 45-9

Recommendations for Clients with Xerostomia

- Carry bottled water, and sip it often.
- Use liquids to soften or thin foods.
- Use xylitol gum or xylitol hard candies to help stimulate saliva flow.
- Use over-the-counter saliva substitutes (see Table 45-1).
- Rinse frequently with ¼ tsp of baking soda, ⅛ tsp of salt, and 8 oz of water.
- Let ice chips melt in the mouth.
- Suck on sugar-free popsicles.
- Humidify rooms with cool-mist humidifiers.
- Avoid highly seasoned foods, tobacco, and the drying effects of alcohol and alcohol-containing products.
- Ask the dentist or oncologist to prescribe a saliva stimulant.
- Lubricate lips with a moisturizing lip balm or cream rather than with pure petrolatum.

Adapted from the U.S. Department of Health and Human Services, National Institutes of Health: *Oral complications of chemotherapy and head/neck radiation (PDQ), 2012.* Available at: http://www.cancer.gov/cancertopics/pdq/supportivecare/oralcomplications/HealthProfessional and http://www.cancer.gov/cancertopics/pdq/supportivecare. Accessed November 19, 2012.

may be necessary to avoid weight loss and medical complications. If patients do not maintain adequate nutrition during the treatment process, then a stomach tube is surgically placed for liquid feeding at home.

Mucositis, Stomatitis, and Infection

If all nonsurgical dental and dental hygiene procedures have not been accomplished before initiation of radiation, they should be done within the first 2 weeks of therapy, before the onset of mucositis. Usually by the third week of radiation the client begins to experience mucosal inflammation and pain. Like chemotherapy mucositis, the mucosa first becomes edematous and inflamed, and then the tissue becomes thinned; pseudomembranes form, and the tissue becomes denuded (see Figure 45-2). As the treatments progress, small ulcerations may enlarge to become a confluent and pseudomembranous mucositis. Oncologists sometimes schedule a short interruption of therapy to allow for the regeneration of normal cells. Mucositis can increase the risk of severe pain, oral and systemic infection, unpleasant odors, difficulty with talking, and nutritional compromise. A lack of saliva increases ulceration and bleeding risk. In addition, the patient may experience **dysphagia** (the inability to swallow) as a result of salivary gland dysfunction and painful ulcerated tissue within the radiation field.

As a result of the mucositis, secondary oral mucosal infections are common and may intensify the mucosal irritation. The fungal organism *Candida albicans* is most often implicated, but any organism may be responsible for infection when the tissues are severely compromised by xerostomia, mucositis, altered nutrition, and inadequate oral hygiene. Early detection and the treatment of any oral infection are imperative to prevent the exacerbation of mucositis that may require the interruption of cancer therapy. After all radiation treatments have been completed, gradual resolution of the mucositis can be expected; however, the epithelium undergoes permanent fibrosis, and the tissue may be thin and fragile and show evidence of **telangiectasia** (a vascular lesion of dilated small blood vessels).

Management

Box 45-9 summarizes ways to help clients with mouth pain caused by mucositis. A clean, well-hydrated mouth during radiation therapy reduces the severity of mucosal ulceration and the risk for oral infection. Toothbrushes are available that are extra soft and nonabrasive. When the client begins to experience mucositis, it is necessary to modify oral hygiene procedures to be nonirritating and atraumatic but still adequate to remove plaque biofilm and thickened saliva. Toothbrushes should be extra soft, and they may be further softened in hot water. The use of commercial toothpastes with strong flavoring agents may have to be temporarily discontinued and replaced with the use of a paste made from baking soda and water. If toothbrushing becomes impossible as a result of painful tissues, the teeth, gingiva, and tongue may be swabbed with gauze that has been moistened in warm water. Dental flossing should be continued as long as possible and resumed as soon as the mucositis resolves.

Sponge-tipped swabs are supplied for oral care to hospitals through medical supply companies, but they are not effective for plaque biofilm removal. If their use is necessary because of the presence of ulcerated tissue, they should be dipped in a nonalcoholic antimicrobial solution for greatest efficacy.

All commercial mouthwashes with alcohol or phenol should be avoided because of their drying and irritating effects. Although half-strength peroxide and water solutions are sometimes used in hospitals to remove encrusted secretions or for acute infections, they are not recommended for long-term use, because they are acidic and may alter the normal oral flora. Frequent mouth rinses with baking soda and saline water should be suggested. When the mouth is too sore to swish the mouth rinse, gentle irrigation of the mouth with a solution of 1 tsp of baking soda, 1 to 2 tsp of salt, and 32 oz of water can be recommended.

Chlorhexidine gluconate mouth rinse has not been conclusively shown to be beneficial for reducing oral infections and mucositis severity during cancer therapy. Such a rinse, when prepared with alcohol, should be evaluated for its antimicrobial benefit versus the irritating effect of the alcohol. Topical anesthetics and coating agents in addition to the soothing bland rinses (see Table 45-1) give temporary relief. All clients—especially children and their parents—need to be cautioned that topical anesthetic agents may anesthetize the soft palate and the epiglottis, potentially causing the aspiration of food. Excessive use also may increase the mucositis symptoms. Some clients may require systemic analgesics and sometimes even narcotics to control mucositis pain.

During radiation therapy, skin care around the mouth is directed by the radiation oncologist. Some lip lubricants can increase the effects of the radiation and cause significant radiation dermatitis. Physicians may order specific skin care products during therapy for the relief of symptoms.

Clients whose conditions are not compromised are to be scheduled for regular preventive oral healthcare. The role of the dental hygienist in providing professional mechanical oral hygiene care and supportive patient education is

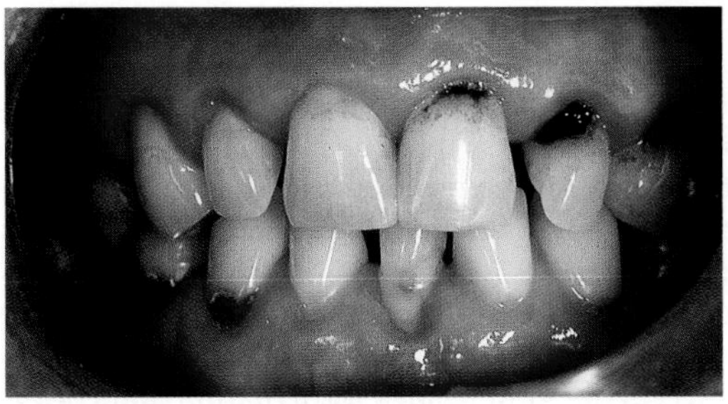

Figure 45-3. Clinical appearance of radiation caries. (Courtesy Dr. Jonathan A. Ship.)

important to prevent mucositis and oral infection. Clients with dentures should be instructed to leave the dentures out of their mouths as often as possible. If the field of radiation encompasses all of the oral tissues, it may be impossible for the client to wear dentures because of significant oral tissue changes from edema and inflammation. The client needs to keep the dentures as clean as possible and to store them in a soaking solution that is changed daily to avoid microbial contamination. These clients often eat a soft or liquid diet, and the tongue becomes coated and infected. Therefore, keeping the mouth well cleansed and the tongue brushed are extremely important.

Trismus, Tissue Fibrosis, and Temporomandibular Joint Dysfunction

The limited ability to open the mouth known as trismus may result from a loss of elasticity of the masticatory muscles or the temporomandibular joint ligaments after a high dose of radiation. Trismus usually occurs within 3 months after therapy, and it remains a lifelong problem. It can result in significant discomfort, and it can interfere with eating, talking, and post-treatment examination.

Management

The client who is receiving radiation therapy to the mastication muscles should be placed on an exercise program to prevent trismus. The jaw should be exercised three times a day by opening and closing the mouth 20 times as wide as possible without causing pain.

Radiation Caries and Demineralization

Rampant caries and tooth demineralization usually begin within the first year after radiation therapy unless intensive oral hygiene and preventive measures are instituted. Figure 45-3 shows the typical clinical appearance of radiation-related caries. Enamel demineralization (the loss of minerals without decay) or rapid decay is a result of changes in both the quality and the quantity of saliva after cancer treatment. The decreased salivary flow limits the availability of calcium and phosphate in the saliva to prevent the natural remineralization of the tooth structure and to buffer the acids produced by cariogenic bacteria in the plaque biofilm. With dry and friable (crumbly) tissues, these clients may change to a soft, high-carbohydrate diet, thereby adding to the lifelong risk of rampant dental decay.

Management

All clients who are receiving cancericidal doses of radiation therapy to any of the salivary glands must have custom fluoride trays made for the daily application of a 1.1% neutral-pH sodium fluoride gel to aid in the prevention of rampant tooth demineralization. The dental hygienist may be responsible for making impressions for study models to fabricate the custom tray. Impressions may be sent to a dental laboratory, or the trays may be made in the dental clinic using a vacuum unit. The fluoride trays are made from a soft vinyl mouth guard material. They should be adapted to extend slightly above the cervical line of the teeth to include full coverage of all teeth. The tray edges must be absolutely smooth and nonirritating to the client's oral tissues to prevent soft-tissue breakdown.

The client should begin use of the fluoride trays at the initiation of therapy. Clients are instructed to first brush and floss their teeth and then to place a thin ribbon of the 1.1% neutral-pH sodium fluoride gel in each of the trays. They place the trays on their teeth and leave them in place for 5 to 10 minutes. After removal, clients rinse the trays well with water but do not rinse the mouth or eat anything for 30 minutes. This fluoride therapy must be done once each day. Many clients feel that it is easiest to use the trays when they are bathing or showering. In this way, the procedure is incorporated into a regular daily routine.

There may be a period of time during therapy when severe mucositis prevents fluoride application with trays. During this time, the client is encouraged to use nonalcoholic and bland fluoride rinses, to increase the hydration of tissues, and to resume the daily fluoride gel application as soon as the mucositis resolves.

In addition, dietary habits and daily food consumption should be discussed to assess the intake of sugar, acidic juice, or soda pop (diet soda included). The dental hygienist plays a critical role in helping clients to prevent radiation caries by educating them about the importance of daily fluoride application, good nutrition, and oral hygiene.

Altered Tooth and Jaw Development

The latent effects of therapeutic radiation therapy on children with cancers of the oral cavity and associated structures vary with the radiation dose and field and the child's stage of growth and development. Radiation has the potential to alter or arrest craniofacial growth and tooth development. Older children who receive minimal doses may experience only slightly altered root development, whereas younger children who are treated at an age when their jaws and teeth are under development may experience gross malformation of the dentition and may suffer significant skeletal deformities.

Soft-Tissue Necrosis and Osteoradionecrosis

Radiation therapy may irreversibly injure the vascularity of soft tissue and bone, result in the decreased ability to heal if traumatized, and increase the susceptibility to infection.[6] Osteoradionecrosis is defined as exposed bone that does not respond to treatment over a 6-month period of time as a result of radiation treatment. There is a higher risk of osteoradionecrosis as the dose of radiation and the volume of irradiated bone and tissue increase. Nonhealing soft tissue or bone may become secondarily infected, and the client may eventually experience intolerable pain and jaw fracture. The mandible appears to be more susceptible than the maxilla because of its dense bone and limited blood supply. Clients who are at the greatest risk are those who have surgery or trauma to irradiated tissue and bone and those who have dental infection in close proximity to bone that has been compromised by radiation. The prevention of osteoradionecrosis by undergoing dental evaluation and treatment before radiation therapy is mandatory. After radiation, the teeth and the periodontium must be professionally managed at intervals to ensure excellent oral hygiene, early intervention, and minimal disease. The dental hygienist is an extremely important member of the professional team that manages this potentially very serious problem.

Hearing Loss and Fatigue

As treatment progresses, the client becomes more easily fatigued and may require daytime naps. In addition, the client may report a partial or total loss of hearing in the ear on the side of the head being irradiated.

Management

As a result of fatigue, clients may need to cut back on their work schedule and obtain plenty of rest. After radiation therapy is completed, hearing and physical energy usually return.

Surgical Treatment of Oral Cancer

Surgery is chosen as the primary treatment when oral cancer is small; when the cancer is completely excisable without complication; when the cancer is not sensitive to radiation therapy; when the lymph nodes, salivary glands, or bones are involved; or when there is a recurrence of tumor in an area that has already received a therapeutic dose of radiation. The disadvantage of surgery is the sacrifice of important functional oral structures.

Potential Complications

Physical

Acute physical complications after head and neck surgery may include infection; airway obstruction; fistula formation; necrosis in the surgical site; impairment of swallowing, hearing, vision, smell, and speech; and compromised nutritional status. Long-term complications include speech impairment, malnutrition from the inability to swallow foods, drooling, malocclusion, temporomandibular disorders, facial deformity, and chronic pain in the shoulder muscles.

Psychosocial

There may be significant psychosocial problems associated with head and neck surgery because the results of the cancer and its treatment are often visible and humiliating and can be psychologically devastating. Physical impairments cannot be completely disguised by clothing, prostheses, or cosmetics. These surgical defects may result in long-term disability, but such problems may be short-term when reconstructive surgery and rehabilitation are available. In today's society, self-image is often equated with body image. As a result, some individuals experience depression, withdrawal and social death, anger, and stigmatization. Some who are heavy smokers and drinkers experience guilt because of the association of these addictions with oral cancer.

Management

The person who has surgery for oral cancer often requires a long postoperative hospital stay. To assist with postoperative management, a dental hygienist who is working in a hospital can do the following:

- Provide in-service programs for nursing staff about oral assessment and oral hygiene care during cancer therapy.
- Act as a liaison between the surgical and dental teams.
- Facilitate ongoing prosthodontic and oral surgery consultations.
- Teach clients to insert, remove, and clean the surgical prosthesis.
- Assess clients' oral tissues for irritation and comfort.
- Teach clients to maintain the oral cavity and all remaining teeth in optimal condition with frequent gentle cleansing and hydration. Cleansing and hydration are usually accomplished with an irrigation bag or bulb syringe, saline rinses, and gentle debridement with large cotton-tipped applicators, sponge swabs, or gauze. Care must be taken when cleansing and suctioning so that new granulation tissue is not disrupted.
- Encourage clients who have been cleared by the surgeon to take food by mouth to use a spoon to place small bites of food on the unaffected side of the mouth and as far back as possible. Forks should be avoided until incisions heal. (Immediately after surgery, a client may not be able to take food and drink by mouth, at which time a tube is placed in the stomach for liquid nutritional supplementation.)

A client who has had a recent head and neck surgical procedure may be in the process of accepting the associated facial deformities and functional alterations. Encouragement to talk about these issues helps the client to move toward acceptance of his or her new body image. It is important for the dental hygienist to listen empathetically to the client's concerns and fears. Taking time to do so decreases client stress and promotes cooperation with recommendations. It is important to remember that, although the surgical treatment may have removed head and neck tissue, it did not remove the person of the client. The client, as a whole person, has human needs related to oral health and disease. It is very important to actively listen to the client, to communicate respectfully and with good eye contact, and to interact directly about ways to promote oral health and cope with the challenges that the surgery has presented.

Prosthetic Rehabilitation

Planning for the rehabilitation of the person with head and neck cancer by the dentist begins at the time of medical diagnosis. When a surgical resection creates facial defects and oral dysfunction, the client must be assured that there is a plan to restore at least partial function and improve cosmetic appearance. The oral and maxillofacial surgeon, the maxillofacial prosthodontist, the general dentist, and the dental hygienist all may play roles in the initial care planning.

Maxillary defects result in unintelligible speech as a result of nasal voice quality, difficulty eating, thickened nasal and sinus secretions, and facial disfigurement. Optimal management begins at the time of surgery, when the prosthodontist may place a surgical obturator (a temporary prosthetic device) to help correct these problems. Approximately 3 to 4 months after surgery, if no complications arise, a permanent prosthesis is fabricated. This prosthesis usually allows for the most effective restoration for the client, because speech, swallowing, mastication, and facial contour all can effectively be

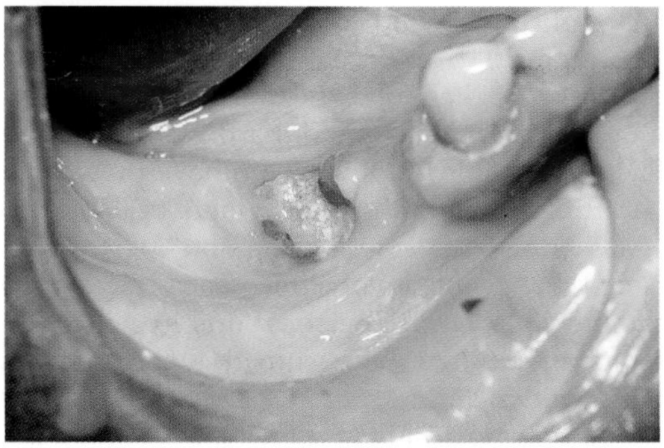

Figure 45-4. Osteonecrosis of the right mandible in a client with metastatic prostate cancer after receiving intravenous bisphosphonate treatment. (Courtesy Dr. Salvatore Ruggiero.)

restored with a prosthesis instead of reconstructed with plastic surgery.

Mandibular defects are often created during oral cancer surgery. Immediate reconstruction is sometimes possible. After extensive intraoral surgery, the client may need additional surgical procedures to release the tongue from the floor of the mouth, to graft skin, to create a vestibule for saliva pooling, and to allow for the extension of denture flanges. These procedures also help with speech, mastication, and swallowing.

After surgical and radiation therapy to the oral cavity, clients who are partially or fully edentulous require conservative prosthetic management. The thinned and friable tissue, the scarring and fibrosis from surgery, and the lack of lubrication and protective qualities of the saliva from radiation treatment make denture placement difficult and place the client at risk for soft-tissue breakdown and osteoradionecrosis. Some clients are never able to wear dentures. Detailed education, close professional supervision, and client acceptance of recommendations are necessary for successful prosthetic rehabilitation.

Bisphosphonates and Osteonecrosis

A potentially painful oral lesion related to a bone-strengthening drug has become an additional concern for clients who have been diagnosed with multiple myeloma or breast, thyroid, lung, or prostate cancer. These individuals may experience metastatic lesions or tumors that spread to the bones. The cancerous bone lesions can lead to **hypercalcemia** (excess calcium in the blood as a result of malignancy) and extreme pain, and they can heighten the potential for bone fractures. To diminish these conditions, oncologists often intravenously administer a class of medications called **bisphosphonates** (e.g., pamidronate [Aredia], zoledronic acid [Zometa], clodronate [Bonefos]). These drugs alter or inhibit the ability of osteoclasts to resorb, thereby suppressing bone turnover. As a result, bisphosphonates stabilize the skeletal matrix and reduce the formation of solid cancerous tumors that are attempting to spread from distant sites such as the lungs.[7] Bisphosphonates are also prescribed in pill form (e.g., alendronate [Fosamax], risedronate [Actonel], ibandronate [Boniva]) to treat osteoporosis and Paget's disease of the bone; they act by increasing bone density.

A potential side effect of intravenously administered bisphosphonate is a condition called **bisphosphonate-related osteonecrosis of the jaw** (BRONJ). This often painful oral or extraoral lesion may resemble an osteoradionecrosis lesion, and it presents as an irregular ulceration with exposed necrotic bone (Figure 45-4). Bisphosphonate-related bone death in the mandible and maxilla is believed to occur as a result of the unique conditions to which the oral cavity is subjected. The mouth, unlike the rest of the body, is constantly being assaulted with small traumas through mastication or poorly fitting dentures as well as oral infection (e.g., periodontitis, apical abscesses). When bisphosphonates are administered, they attach to the bone matrix, and they may remain in the bone for several years. The presence of this drug in the skeletal system prevents the jaw bones from undergoing the forming and reforming that are necessary for normal healing. If traumatized, the bone may then become necrotic and form subsequent lesions. Typical symptoms include loose teeth, pain, drainage, swelling, a heavy feeling, and numbness.

Approximately 0.8% to 12% of patients who are receiving intravenously administered bisphosphonates (and a much smaller number who are using oral bisphosphonates) develop BRONJ. Lesion development risk increases with the form, amount, and duration of bisphosphonate use.[7] The majority of BRONJ lesions are reported to follow invasive dental procedures such as an extraction or implant placement, but BRONJ has also been reported to develop spontaneously in limited cases. Unfortunately, other than palliative care, there currently exists no effective way to treat BRONJ after it has formed.

Management

As with other aspects of cancer treatment, the dental hygienist remains an important treatment team member. In general, the guidelines developed for the oral and dental care of patients who are about to receive head and neck radiation therapy should be followed. Meticulous oral hygiene homecare and professional maintenance during cancer and bisphosphonate therapy can reduce the number of bacteria-induced pathologies in the oral cavity, thereby lowering the risk of developing BRONJ. In addition, the dental hygienist must carefully review the client's health history and explore any medications used during or after cancer treatment. Vigilance must be exercised during intraoral and extraoral examinations for evidence of BRONJ ulcers if an intravenous or oral form of bisphosphonates has ever been used. The patient must also be informed of the risks associated with the use of both oral and intravenous bisphosphonates.

Dental Hygiene Process of Care

The dental hygienist—either as a member of a hospital oncology team (see Web Resources) or as a clinician in consultation with the oncologist—has the opportunity to prevent or ameliorate many of the oral and systemic complications associated with cancer treatment by designing a dental hygiene care plan that promotes a clean and healthy oral cavity. Before the initial dental hygiene care appointment, consultation must be sought with other oncology team members involved in the care of the person with cancer. Open and continuous communication with physicians and nurses reduces the risk of providing care that compromises the client's condition.

Assessment

The dental hygienist collaborates with the dentist to identify sources of infection that may delay postoperative healing for a client who is scheduled for surgery of the oral cavity. In addition, the pretherapy assessment is also critical for a client who is scheduled for intravenous bisphosphonate therapy or radiation therapy of the oral cavity or the salivary glands. Any part of the maxilla or mandible that will be irradiated is at lifelong risk for the development of osteoradionecrosis. Therefore all infections and teeth that cannot be maintained for the client's lifetime should be identified for removal. Teeth to be extracted include not only those with gross caries and refractory periodontal disease but also those that potentially may not be maintained because of the client's lack of personal motivation, physical or mental ability, or financial resources.

Because intraoral infection may spread through the bloodstream and result in sepsis and possibly death during immunosuppression, all potential sources of irritation that may potentiate mucositis must also be identified and eliminated. The assessment of a potential BMT recipient should identify any oral problems that may arise within the first year after the transplant, when the client is in an immunosuppressed condition.

Client Interview

The client interview provides critical information that influences future oral hygiene care and dental treatment. Taking time to listen to the client's perceptions decreases client and family stress, promotes consistency, encourages cooperation among members of the oncology team, and assists the dental hygienist with assessing the client's human needs that will shape the dental hygiene process of care.

The client's current oral status and health and dental histories are reviewed, including frequency of care, dental experiences that were unpleasant or painful, oral self-care habits, and current attitude and knowledge about the teeth and mouth. This information assists the dental hygienist with the planning of dental hygiene care. The interview also reveals the client's socioeconomic status and any cultural and ethnic influences that may affect his or her perceptions of cancer, health beliefs, coping strategies, social support system, dietary habits, and ability to adhere to the supportive care.

Diagnosis

Dental hygiene diagnoses identify human needs related to direct dental hygiene care before the initiation of cancer therapy, during therapy, and after the client has completed all proposed therapy. As therapy progresses and the client moves through various physical changes and psychosocial stages related to the cancer, the dental hygiene diagnoses change, and the care plan is continually revised.

Planning

The client who is undergoing cancer therapy or who is experiencing end-stage disease requires a care plan that is directed toward meeting actual or potential needs associated with the oral and systemic complications of cancer therapies.

Initially, when clients are faced with a life-threatening cancer diagnosis, they are unable to conceptualize the importance of care beyond their most basic physiologic and survival needs. As these needs appear to be no longer at imminent risk, the client often begins to accept the diagnosis, and he or she may be capable of participating in supportive care. Clients in the dental office who have previously had a positive attitude about their teeth and oral hygiene may reveal totally different values during times of stress. It cannot be assumed that clients involved in cancer therapy will continue the previous level of personal oral hygiene care. Alternatively, it should not be assumed that persons with a seemingly overwhelming cancer diagnosis do not have the ability to participate in successful rehabilitation. At appropriate times, a clear understanding of the oral problems associated with cancer therapy must be effectively communicated and trust established by mutual participation in the development of oral health goals.

Oral and Dental Management Before Cancer Therapy

Referral to a Dentist

Conditions found by the dental hygienist that require diagnosis by a dentist should be referred immediately for evaluation and treatment. Before chemotherapy begins, clients need to have all surgical procedures performed at least 7 days before periods of immunosuppression, all sources of infection and irritation removed, and all projected dental needs met. For clients who are scheduled for surgery, all oral surgical procedures need to be scheduled 14 to 21 days before the initiation of radiation therapy involving the oral cavity and the salivary glands. Restorative needs should be cared for before the onset of painful mucositis. Fabrication of new dental prostheses is delayed until several months after radiation therapy ends, when all acute side effects of radiation have been resolved (Box 45-10).

BOX 45-10

Reasons for an Oral Evaluation Before Cancer Treatment

- The identification and treatment of existing infections and problem teeth
- The elimination of potential sites of infection and trauma (e.g., exfoliating teeth in children, partially erupted third molars, orthodontic bands, ill-fitting dentures, fractured teeth or restorations)
- The construction of oral stents to be worn during radiation therapy of the head and neck area
- For clients who are scheduled for head and neck radiation, the extraction of teeth that may pose a future problem (i.e., for the prevention of post-therapy osteoradionecrosis)
- The construction of custom fluoride gel trays and instructions regarding their use
- Instructions regarding oral hygiene, nutrition, and tobacco treatment
- The provision of professional mechanical dental hygiene care (i.e., oral prophylaxis, periodontal maintenance, or nonsurgical periodontal therapy) to reduce periodontal infection and to promote periodontal health

Psychosocial Issues

The initial client appointment is an important time when trust and assurance are established. Clients must feel acceptance in a nonjudgmental environment and sense that their self-esteem will be preserved. The client is a "person living with cancer," not a "cancer case." Additional time is necessary to allow the client to express feelings. All feelings should be acknowledged, and anger should not be mitigated too quickly. The dental hygienist encourages the client to participate in care planning, which provides an opportunity for that client to regain some of the sense of control that was lost to the cancer.

Education

Adequate time must be allotted for education, because the stress related to a cancer diagnosis can easily impede the normal learning process. It is important to engage in the teaching process with full regard for the client's psychologic human need status. Clients in a state of denial are not able to comprehend the importance of preventive oral healthcare until they begin to accept their cancer and therapy plan. Others, stressed by the financial burden of medical treatments, may not place a priority on dental and dental hygiene treatment when it is compared with their impending life-saving cancer therapy. Those who are depressed and who see their prognosis as grave do not value the importance of long-term dental hygiene care until they begin to see cause for hope.

Oral Hygiene Instruction and Self-Care

Oral hygiene self-care assistance is important before cancer therapy initiation to establish good oral hygiene before the oral tissues are compromised. Disclosing agent use helps with instruction and helps the client to identify areas that require closer attention during self-care procedures. This educational approach also provides an opportunity for the dental hygienist to explain the composition of plaque biofilm and the risk of oral and systemic infections during cancer therapy. Oral hygiene technique should be assessed, if possible, and the client should be assisted with establishing plaque-removal techniques that will be useful before and during therapy. If a client is scheduled for therapy that will significantly compromise the oral tissues, initial instruction is given verbally and in print regarding methods for cleansing the mouth in addition to any preventive and palliative products recommended (see Table 45-1). These methods are then elaborated on during therapy. Gentle tooth and gingival brushing can continue during cancer therapy.

Tobacco and Alcohol Cessation Counseling

Usually the oncologist strongly urges the client to stop using tobacco products and to limit excessive alcohol intake during cancer therapy. Tobacco treatment and assistance from the dental hygienist are important (see Chapter 36). Referral to the national tobacco cessation quitline (1-800-QUITNOW or http://www.cdc.gov/tobacco/quit_smoking/index.htmhttp://www.cdc.gov/tobacco/), a local tobacco treatment program, or a support group may be necessary and desired by the client.

Nutritional Counseling

A client's nutritional status affects his or her overall response to cancer therapy and his or her psychologic well-being. The nutritionist on the oncology team assumes primary responsibility for monitoring the client's nutritional status and providing counseling regarding diet selection. The dental hygienist consults with the nutritionist and educates the client about diet selection and dietary habits to promote a clean and healthy oral environment and to reduce caries development. It is important for the dental hygienist to determine the client's understanding of the relationship of a well-balanced diet to dental caries, periodontal disease, and infection. When the client is ready psychologically to assimilate preventive behaviors, the client and the dental hygienist choose foods that are desirable to the client and that are low in sugar, acid, and oral retention qualities. The client needs to understand, however, that it is often difficult during therapy to eat a well-balanced diet that also contains foods that promote oral health.

Dental Hygiene Instrumentation

Dental hygiene instrumentation may need to be altered to accommodate the client's physical condition related to recent surgery, disease manifestations, and the status of the client's blood counts and clotting factors. The oncologist is consulted regarding the safest time to schedule an appointment and the need for antibiotic prophylaxis before dental hygiene instrumentation. Overall, dental hygiene care promotes a clean and well-hydrated oral environment and control of periodontal disease to reduce the risk of oral infection and bacteremia.

Fluoride Therapy

When the client is scheduled for radiation therapy to the salivary glands or total body irradiation for BMT, custom fluoride gel trays are fabricated for daily application of a 1.1% neutral-pH sodium fluoride gel to prevent rampant dental caries. Clients who complain of a dry mouth during chemotherapy require at least a daily fluoride rinse and possibly a 1.1% sodium fluoride toothpaste or gel.

Oral and Dental Care During Cancer Therapy

After therapy is initiated, it is important to continue to support the client and to understand that most cancer therapy is physically and psychologically demanding. With each appointment, the dental hygienist repeats the oral assessment of the client, updates the client's health history, and assesses the client's level of disease acceptance and readiness for new interventions. Clients' anger and bargaining may be signs of acceptance of the diagnosis and an attempt by clients to regain control of their own lives. These times offer the dental hygienist an opportunity to direct the client's interest to positive involvement in oral self-care and dietary planning. Education during care is centered on the immediate real and impending complications of therapy.

Management of Oral Complications

Table 45-2 summarizes dental hygiene interventions that may prevent or ameliorate the oral complications associated with radiation therapy and chemotherapy.

After a client who is scheduled to undergo BMT enters the transplant center, the client is not allowed to leave the unit until the bone marrow has engrafted and blood counts have returned to a normal range. Therefore all dental treatment must be accomplished before the transplant.

Nutritional Counseling During Cancer Therapy

The side effects of cancer therapy often result in a high risk for dental caries. Clients may be placed on a soft and bland diet or a high-carbohydrate liquid diet as a result of recent oral surgery or mucositis from therapy. They may also be encouraged to eat small, frequent meals and snacks to increase their caloric intake and to counteract nausea and vomiting. Additional complications arise from a dry mouth or thickened saliva, taste dysfunction, the inability to practice good oral hygiene because of an oral surgical procedure, or a lack of interest in eating in response to depression and stress. A severely malnourished client may be placed on parenteral nutrition, thereby completely eliminating the mechanical oral cleansing action of foods.

The diets of children who are undergoing cancer therapy are often a problem because there are so many times when they are too sick to eat that parents allow them to eat anything they want when they are feeling well. When working with the nutritionist, the dental hygienist continues to emphasize the importance of a well-balanced, low-sugar diet for the prevention of infection and the promotion of healing after the insult of therapy.

Clients with mouth pain may be helped by hygienists suggesting the use of topical anesthetic or coating agents before eating (see Table 45-1). In addition, clients with oral ulcerations or dry mouth may find it helpful to eat foods that are high in moisture, or they may thin their food with liquids and take frequent sips of water while eating. Irritating, hot, spicy, or acidic foods should be avoided.

Oral and Dental Care After Cancer Therapy

After any kind of cancer therapy, the dental hygienist continues to have an important role in client care. At each client appointment, the dental hygienist reassesses the client's human needs related to oral health. Even when clients have been reassured that their cancer has successfully responded to therapy, they continue to experience stress, anxiety, and concern about the possible recurrence of the cancer. Continued education and frequent contact and support are essential. The dental hygienist tailors the client's oral self-care to the individual's status and human needs and places as much responsibility on the client as possible.

After Chemotherapy

After a client has completed the required rounds of chemotherapy, most of the associated oral manifestations completely resolve. With full bone marrow recovery, all problems associated with acute cytotoxicity, immunosuppression, and thrombocytopenia disappear. After long and intensive chemotherapy, some clients take months to recover fully and experience chronic oral infections such as candidiasis and herpetic infections. Continual assistance with oral hygiene is required to prevent unnecessary infections. The assessment of clients' nutritional intake is important to determine if they have resumed a noncariogenic and normal diet.

After Bone Marrow or Blood Stem Cell Transplantation

After clients are released from a transplant unit, they may have residual effects of the conditioning phase of treatment, and they may remain susceptible to infections for several months as a result of immunosuppressive therapy. Some continue to experience xerostomia, which predisposes them to an altered oral flora and infections, trauma, and rampant dental caries. Clients with GVHD may experience additional complications that involve thinned and friable mucosa and mucosal lesions.

The dental hygienist assists the client with establishing consistent and effective oral hygiene methods that do not create additional trauma and irritation. Bland rinses, gentle but thorough and consistent cleansing of the teeth and tissues, and saliva substitutes are important.

Dental procedures that are deemed necessary are performed only after consultation with the oncologist to assess the client's immune status and his or her need for antibiotic prophylaxis or platelet support. Elective dental procedures are delayed until the client has full hematologic function, which is sometimes up to a year or more after the completion of cancer treatment. Rampant dental caries from xerostomia are prevented with the daily application of fluoride gel in custom fluoride trays.

After Radiation Therapy

Client care after radiation therapy specific to the oral cavity and salivary glands requires lifelong frequent dental and dental hygiene maintenance care. Because damage to the salivary glands and the jaw bones from cancer radiation therapy is permanent, clients are at permanent risk for the development of rampant "radiation caries," tooth demineralization, and osteoradionecrosis. Continued-care appointments are scheduled at intervals to ensure excellent oral hygiene, sound tooth structure maintenance, and the avoidance of soft-tissue irritation. The daily use of the custom fluoride trays with 1.1% neutral-pH sodium fluoride gel for 5 to 10 minutes followed by 30 minutes of abstinence from food and water must continue for the rest of the client's life. If there is evidence of dental decay despite compliance with daily fluoride applications, the client should be placed on a 2-week chlorhexidine regimen to decrease cariogenic bacteria and then scheduled for in-office fluoride varnish applications. A daily remineralizing gel application may also be necessary in addition to the daily fluoride gel application.

With each appointment, the dental hygienist assesses the client's nutritional status and dietary intake. Adjustments are made to return the client to a normal and noncariogenic diet as the acute radiation therapy side effects resolve. Referral for nutritional counseling may be necessary.

A thorough head and neck assessment for oral cancer and for the function of the muscles of mastication, the temporomandibular joint, and any prosthetic appliances is done at each appointment. Deficits in the needs for integrity of the skin and mucous membrane of the head and neck and for a biologically sound and functional dentition require immediate referral to the dentist. Dental disease in an area of irradiated bone is managed as conservatively and as atraumatically as possible by the dentist; management sometimes includes antibiotic prophylaxis. If trismus occurs, treatment consists of introducing tongue blades between the teeth for several minutes each day and gradually increasing the number of blades until adequate opening is achieved. This strategy may be painful, and it requires patience and perseverance. The dental treatment of osteoradionecrosis is conservative but generally requires the conservative surgical removal of necrotic tissue, antibiotics to prevent infection, and, ideally, hyperbaric oxygen therapy to stimulate visualization and new bone growth. When conservative measures fail, surgical resection is usually indicated.

Clients with End-Stage Disease (see Chapter 61)

Evaluation

Client goals that are planned for dental hygiene care vary tremendously, depending on the client's human needs assessment, disease stage, treatment, and psychologic status. Goals and outcomes of care are evaluated repeatedly by assessing clients' responses as they move through the various treatment phases and make psychologic adjustments to their disease. Outcomes of care are evaluated on the basis of whether the planned goals are met, partially met, or unmet.

CLIENT EDUCATION TIPS

- Inform clients about the risk factors for cancer and oral cancer.
- Assist clients with tobacco use cessation (see Chapter 36).
- Educate clients about the potential oral complications associated with the type of cancer therapy that they will undergo and about ways in which such conditions can be prevented or ameliorated.
- Emphasize the importance of excellent oral hygiene during cancer therapy. Individualize self-care plans on the basis of the proposed cancer therapy and the client's needs.
- Ensure that the client has full knowledge of the long-term complications associated with oral cancer radiation therapy and the need to continue preventive measures for the rest of the client's life.
- Ensure that the client has full knowledge of the long-term complications associated with the use of oral and intravenous bisphosphonate therapy and the need for meticulous oral care to prevent trauma to the bone.

LEGAL, ETHICAL, AND SAFETY ISSUES

- Always perform a thorough head and neck examination to screen for oral cancer.
- Inform clients about the potential side effects and complications of various cancer therapies and strategies to prevent and manage them.
- Coordinate clients' oral healthcare before, during, and after their cancer therapy.
- Never abandon clients with end-stage cancer. Good oral health is critical at this time to encourage good oral intake and to improve quality of life.

KEY CONCEPTS

- *Cancer* is a term that defines a wide variety of malignant processes that are usually treated with surgery, chemotherapy, radiation therapy, or bone marrow or blood stem cell transplantation.
- Approximately 40% to 80% of persons treated for non–head and neck malignancies experience oral complications.
- Pre-existing oral or dental pathology can adversely affect the individual who is undergoing cancer therapy.
- The dental hygiene care plan plays a critical role in the care of individuals who are undergoing cancer therapy.
- Head and neck cancer radiation treatment results in some permanent oral complications.
- Complications associated with radiation to the head and neck area, systemic chemotherapy, and bone marrow and blood stem cell transplantation may be prevented or ameliorated by oral hygiene interventions.

CRITICAL THINKING EXERCISES

CLIENT 1: Mrs. G.

Profile: Mrs. G. is a 45-year-old woman with a soft-palate lesion and a large mass in the right side of her neck. A biopsy reveals squamous cell carcinoma. She is scheduled for surgery followed by unilateral radiation therapy to the right posterior mandible and maxilla and the lateral neck.

Chief Complaint: "I need a dental evaluation and dental hygiene care before starting my cancer therapy."

Dental History: Her pretherapy radiographic and clinical oral and dental evaluation reveals no dental caries, generalized gingivitis, and moderate plaque, calculus, and tobacco staining.

Social History: The client is single and lives with her parents.

Health History: The client has been diagnosed with squamous cell carcinoma of the soft palate. She currently takes no medications, and her blood pressure is within normal limits.

Oral Health Behavior Assessment: Mrs. G. states that she brushes her teeth once a day, that she does not use floss, and that she visits her dentist every year. She takes over-the-counter antacids, chewable vitamin C, and Aspergum for her sore throat. She has smoked one or two packs per day for 25 years.

Supplemental Notes: She has dental insurance, she demonstrates sincere interest in and motivation to maintain her teeth, and she is very interested in tobacco cessation interventions.

1. What procedures will be included in the dental treatment plan before radiation therapy?
2. Develop a dental hygiene care plan to be implemented before radiation therapy.
3. What measures do you suggest to relieve this client's xerostomia and the pain associated with mucositis?
4. What dental hygiene interventions and recall schedule are appropriate for this woman after radiation therapy?
5. What are the signs and symptoms of osteoradionecrosis?

CLIENT 2: Mrs. H.

Profile: Mrs. H. is a 23-year-old woman who has been undergoing radiation for Hodgkin's disease.

Chief Complaint: "I need a dental evaluation and necessary treatment before the next phase of my cancer therapy."

Social History: She is single and lives alone.

Health History: She is scheduled for an allogeneic bone marrow transplant for which she will receive total body irradiation and chemotherapy. She will enter the bone marrow transplant unit in 3 weeks.

Dental History: She had no dental support during her previous cancer treatment. Her dental evaluation reveals a sensitive maxillary premolar with a large carious lesion and a radiolucent periapical lesion, several areas of mild demineralization, moderate plaque and calculus, and chapped lips. No other gross caries or periodontal disease is evident. There are no impacted teeth or bony lesions detected by radiographs.

Oral Health Behavior Assessment: The client reports that she brushes her teeth once a day but that she does not use any interdental cleaning devices.

Supplemental Notes: She has dental insurance, and she appears motivated to improve her oral hygiene care.

1. What dental treatment and dental hygiene care would be appropriate for this client before her transplant?
2. Develop a dental hygiene care plan to be implemented before the bone marrow transplant.

REFERENCES

1. Eheman C, Henley J, Ballard-Barbash R, et al: Annual report to the nation on the status of cancer, 1975-2008, featuring cancer in associated with excess weight and lack of sufficient physical activity, *Cancer* 118:2338, 2012.
2. American Cancer Society: *Cancer facts and figures 2012*. Available at: http://www.cancer.org/acs/groups/content/@epidemiology surveilance/documents/document/acspc-031941.pdf. Accessed November 19, 2012.
3. Simard EP, Ward EM, Siegel R, et al: Cancers with increasing incidence trends in the United States: 1999 through 2008, *CA Cancer J Clin* 62:118, 2012.
4. Howlander N, Noone AM, Krapcho M, et al, eds: *SEER cancer statistics review, 1975–2009*. Available at: http://seer.cancer.gov/csr/1975_2009_pops09/ Accessed November 19, 2012.
5. Sturgis EM, Cinciripini PM: Trends in head and neck cancer incidence in relation to smoking prevalence: an emerging epidemic of human papillomavirus–associated cancers, *Cancer* 110:1, 2007.
6. Adapted from the U.S. Department of Health and Human Services, National Institutes of Health: *Oral complications of chemotherapy and head/neck radiation (PDQ), 2012*. Available at: http://www.cancer.gov/cancertopics/pdq/supportivecare/oralcomplications/HealthProfessional and http://www.cancer.gov/cancertopics/pdq/supportivecare. Accessed November 19, 2012.
7. Ruggiero SL, Dodson TB, Assael LA, et al: *American Association of Oral and Maxillofacial Surgeons position paper on bisphosphonate-related osteonecrosis of the jaws—2009 update*. Available at: http://exodontia.info/files/J_Oral_Maxillofac_Surg_2009._American_Association_of_Oral_Maxillofacial_Surgeons_Position_Paper_on_BONJ._Update.pdf. Accessed November 18, 2012.

ACKNOWLEDGMENT

The author acknowledges Gerry J. Barker for her past contributions to this chapter.

EVOLVE RESOURCES

Please visit http://evolve.elsevier.com/Darby/hygiene for additional practice and study support tools.

Human Immunodeficiency Virus Infection

CHAPTER 46

Devan Leonardi Darby, Michele Leonardi Darby

COMPETENCIES

1. Explain the beginnings of the epidemic of human immunodeficiency virus (HIV).
2. Describe the pathogenesis of HIV.
3. Discuss HIV exposure and infection, including transmission routes for HIV.
4. Explain drug therapy used to control HIV.
5. Explain the epidemiology of HIV and acquired immunodeficiency syndrome (AIDS).
6. Describe the risk of HIV infection among healthcare workers.
7. Explain the relationship between HIV and periodontal status.
8. Recognize specific oral conditions related to HIV/AIDS.
9. Describe how to treat patients with HIV infection or AIDS using a healthcare team approach.

The human immunodeficiency virus (HIV) causes acquired immunodeficiency syndrome (AIDS), one of the largest public health challenges facing the world. HIV/AIDS causes gradual impairment of the host's immune system so that the disease is accompanied by other chronic health problems. Knowledge of the continuum of immunodeficiency—from infection with HIV on one end to debilitating disease associated with AIDS on the other—has heightened public awareness of, and concern for, individuals with HIV/AIDS. Although it is still not curable, HIV/AIDS is now a treatable chronic medical condition as a result of the many scientific advances that have been made toward understanding the virus since it was first identified in 1983.

The dental hygiene practitioner must be aware of conditions that commonly accompany HIV/AIDS, knowledgeable about patient care, and comfortable treating clients with HIV/AIDS. Although the knowledge base regarding HIV/AIDS is vast, it is far from complete. The HIV/AIDS epidemic serves as a potent reminder that infectious diseases have not been conquered and that epidemics are not events of the past.

Beginnings of the Epidemic

Immunosuppression is the decreased ability of the body to mount natural immune defenses against disease-causing agents. Unusual opportunistic infections or illnesses associated with severe immunosuppression were first identified in several young, previously healthy homosexual males who were found to have a rare and aggressive pneumonia usually associated only with severe immunodeficiency. These first documented cases of AIDS in the United States were reported in June 1981 by the Centers for Disease Control and Prevention (CDC), but the disease was not given a name until considerably later. HIV was identified and associated with these unusual conditions in 1983. Subsequently, multiple cases of oral Kaposi sarcoma were identified in the homosexual population. Previously Kaposi sarcoma—a rare cancer of the blood vessels characterized by dark red or purple papular lesions—had been found only in elderly men of Mediterranean heritage and then only on the legs.

After these peculiar epidemiologic findings, several deaths in the United States and abroad in the 1970s were suspected of being caused by the same agent. In a retrospective analysis, frozen serum samples from those cases revealed the presence of HIV antibodies. During the early 1980s, similar occurrences of immunodeficiency-related deaths—which would later be identified as early AIDS cases—were also reported in Haiti, in several countries in Africa, and in populations that required routine blood transfusions (e.g., individuals with hemophilia).

Although the disease was first recognized among men who have sex with men, from the early days, HIV/AIDS has also been observed in heterosexual populations, especially in Africa where the epidemic is particularly severe. Today, HIV/AIDS has become a worldwide epidemic. Globally, it has been estimated that 33.4 million people (31.1 million to 35.8 million)* are infected; most of them live in sub-Saharan Africa.[1]

HIV includes two closely related viruses, HIV-1 and HIV-2. HIV-1 is the more common of the two viruses, and it is predominant in most of the world, including the United States. HIV-2 is primarily found in West Africa, and it is more closely related to the simian immunodeficiency virus that has been isolated from sooty mangabey monkeys. HIV-1 is known to have at least nine subtypes or clades that have been identified on the basis of genetic sequencing.[2]

Pathogenesis of Human Immunodeficiency Virus

The HIV virion or virus particle is composed of a core of ribonucleic acid (RNA) encapsulated within a lipid coating. A serologic marker on the coating binds to receptor sites on

*This 2011 UNAIDS global HIV prevalence estimate is higher than the UNAIDS estimate for previous years. This increase in prevalence reflects the combined effects of new HIV infections and increased life expectancy as a result of greater access to antiretroviral medications. Globally, the incidence, or new infection rate, of HIV has declined since 1996.[1]

CD4+ T lymphocytes, a type of white blood cell that is important for cell-mediated immunity. CD4+ T lymphocytes do not have cytotoxicity or the ability to kill a cell, but they do play an important role in activating cytotoxic T lymphocytes. The virus infects by fusing with the cell membrane of the CD4+ T lymphocyte and entering the cell, where it releases its RNA. HIV is called a retrovirus because, once it is within the cell, it uses the enzyme reverse transcriptase to convert viral RNA into deoxyribonucleic acid (DNA). This process is the "reverse" of what typically occurs in animal cells (i.e., the conversion of DNA into RNA).

After the viral RNA is released into the host cell and then changed into DNA, it can integrate into the host cell's genome. This effectively allows HIV to "hijack" the host cell so that it produces more HIV viruses. When activated, the infected cell will synthesize viral protein, create more HIV virions, and kill the host immune cell. The HIV particles produced can then circulate and infect other cells of the immune system.[3] The resultant destruction of immune cells, including CD4+ T lymphocytes and macrophages, weakens the host immune system. The characteristic immunodeficiency occurs when the virus suppresses the immune response, which is the body's natural defense against invasion by an organism.

If left untreated, HIV infection leads to a gradually diminishing immune response as a result of the depletion of CD4+ T lymphocytes. The weakened immune response makes the host susceptible to opportunistic infections and malignancies.[3] This explanation of the disease process is a very simple description of a complex immunologic reaction and is intended to present the general idea of how the virus replicates itself in the human body. For further information, refer to the Suggested Readings section on the website for this textbook.

Human Immunodeficiency Virus Transmission

HIV is transmitted through contact with semen, vaginal secretions, breast milk, and infected blood or platelets. Sexual contact is the primary source of infection among men who have sex with men, whereas intravenous drug users are at high risk as a result of sharing blood-contaminated needles. HIV-positive mothers may transmit the virus to their fetuses during pregnancy, at birth, or when breast-feeding the infant.

Acute Human Immunodeficiency Virus Infection

Acute HIV infection syndrome occurs 6 to 56 days after exposure. Manifestations of initial infection vary but include some or all of the following signs and symptoms:

- Fever
- Lymphadenopathy (lymph node enlargement)
- Headache
- Rash
- Pharyngitis (sore throat)
- Myalgia (aching muscles)
- Arthralgia (aching joints)

There are considerable variations in the presentation of acute HIV infection, but it has been reported that most persons who are undergoing seroconversion (i.e., the acquisition of the antibodies in the blood serum) are ill enough to seek medical attention. Acute HIV infection is also characterized by primary viremia or the initial spike in the viral levels in the bloodstream. Oral manifestations can include erythematous (red) round patches on the hard and soft palate, angular cheilitis, exudative tonsillitis, hairy leukoplakia on the lateral borders of the tongue, and oral ulcers that look similar to aphthous ulcers but that may appear anywhere in the mouth or on the lips.

Human Immunodeficiency Virus Latency and Immune Status

When primary viremia is suppressed by the body's initial immune response, an asymptomatic period follows that may last for a variable period of time that ranges from months to years. Even though symptoms are not present during this latency period, the virus is present and replicating. On average, this asymptomatic period has been reported to lead to the loss of approximately 10% of CD4+ T lymphocytes per year in infected individuals.[3]

Depending on the health status of the human host, HIV infection can remain latent for several years. Only when certain conditions or clinical indicators called *AIDS-defining illnesses* become apparent is the HIV-infected individual classified as having AIDS. The CDC classifies HIV-infected persons according to their immune status. The current system includes categories for asymptomatic infection, symptomatic infection, and AIDS-indicator conditions.[4] The classification system and case definitions are presented in Table 46-1, and the AIDS-defining conditions are listed in Table 46-2. The CDC also performs annual surveillance studies to document the prevalence of HIV/AIDS in the United States on the basis of these classification criteria.

Women with HIV infection or AIDS may have gynecologic manifestations such as vaginal yeast infections, cervical lesions, and cervical cancer. However, there is no general agreement that other HIV-associated conditions behave the same way in both men and women. Drug protocols have been studied much more extensively in men, so the modification of those protocols when applied to women may become part of treatment in the future.

Drug Therapy

The first drugs that were used to control HIV infection were developed in the 1980s. These drugs targeted the reverse transcriptase enzyme that facilitates virus replication in the cells. They inhibited viral replication but were given as

TABLE 46-1

Classification System by Clinical Categories (A to C) and Levels of CD4+ T Cells for HIV Infection and AIDS in Adults[4]

	CLINICAL CATEGORIES		
CD4+ T Cell Categories	A: Asymptomatic Acute (Primary) HIV	B: Symptomatic (No C Conditions) HIV	C: AIDS Indicator
500 cells/mm^3	A1	B1	C1
200 to 499 cells/mm^3	A2	B2	C2
<200 cells/mm^3	A3	B3	C3

TABLE 46-2

AIDS-Defining Conditions and Diagnostic Criteria[4]

Candidiasis of the bronchi, trachea, lungs, or esophagus
Invasive cervical cancer
Disseminated or extrapulmonary coccidioidomycosis
Extrapulmonary cryptococcosis
Chronic intestinal cryptosporidiosis (>1 month in duration)
Cytomegalovirus disease other than of the liver, spleen, or nodes
Cytomegalovirus retinitis with loss of vision
HIV-related encephalopathy
Herpes simplex with chronic ulcer(s) (>1 month in duration) or bronchitis, pneumonitis, or esophagitis
Disseminated or extrapulmonary histoplasmosis
Chronic intestinal isosporiasis (>1 month in duration)
Kaposi sarcoma, either intraoral or extraoral
Lymphoma (Burkitt, immunoblastic, or primary brain)
Mycobacterium avium complex or *Mycobacterium kansasii* (disseminated or extrapulmonary)
Mycobacterium tuberculosis (pulmonary or extrapulmonary)
Pneumocystis jirovecii (formerly *Pneumocystis carinii*) pneumonia
Recurrent pneumonia
Progressive multifocal leukoencephalopathy
Recurrent salmonella septicemia
Toxoplasmosis involving the brain
HIV-related wasting syndrome

TABLE 46-3

Estimated New HIV Infections by Transmission Category, 2009[8]

Transmission Category	Total Cases	Percent of Total
Men who have sex with men	29,300	61%
Heterosexual contact	12,900	27%
Injection drug use	4,500	9%
Homosexual contact and injection drug use	1,400	3%

Adapted from Centers for Disease Control and Prevention: *CDC Fact Sheet. Estimates of new HIV infections in the United States, 2006-2009.* Available at: http://www.cdc.gov/nchhstp/newsroom/docs/HIV-Infections-2006-2009.pdf. Accessed September 8, 2013.

monotherapy (i.e., treatment with just one drug). Monotherapy resulted in resistance mutations and eventually made the drugs ineffective for the suppression of viral replication. During the 1990s other drugs were identified that targeted the enzyme in a variety of ways at different stages of retrovirus development. These have been found to be effective and have led to the use of multiple drugs—the so-called "HIV cocktails"—by individuals with HIV. Treatment with at least three drugs, known as **highly active antiretroviral therapy (HAART)**, is now considered the standard of care.

The process for determining the correct dosages of multiple drugs is extremely complex. It requires close monitoring, clinical testing, and evaluation by a physician. The potent antiretroviral drug cocktails can have potentially serious adverse effects that range from headache and nausea to lactic acidosis, severe skin reactions, lipid abnormalities, and organ failure. While this strategy poses adherence challenges, simultaneous treatment with multiple drugs disrupts viral replication at various stages, thus slowing the development of resistance. When administered and monitored properly, the correct combination will interact beneficially to control the infection, to prevent the development of drug resistance, and to prolong the lives of individuals with HIV.[5]

Epidemiology of Human Immunodeficiency Virus Infection and Acquired Immunodeficiency Syndrome

As of 2008, all 50 states, the District of Columbia, and six U.S.-dependent areas had instituted the confidential name-based reporting of HIV. For these reporting areas, the CDC estimates that, by the end of 2009, the total number of people who were more than 13 years old living with HIV/AIDS was approximately 1,148,200.[6] Precise estimates of HIV incidence are not known because the new infection rate is difficult to track. However, the CDC estimates that approximately 50,000 new HIV infections occur in the United States each year.[7] Overall the infection rate has been decreasing since 1997, but the absolute number of cases or prevalence continues to increase.

Multiple factors play a role in determining one's risk of acquiring HIV in the United States. Men who have sex with men continue to be the most likely to contract HIV due to the high risk associated with male homosexual contact. Although they constituted approximately 2% of the population, men who have sex with men were estimated to account for between 56% and 61% of all new HIV infections between 2006 and 2009. During recent years, young black men who have sex with men have experienced a surge in HIV incidence; they made up 27% of all new infections (12,900) in 2009. Black women are also at particularly high risk, although they are more likely to contract HIV via heterosexual contact.[8] Table 46-3 summarizes new HIV cases in 2009 by transmission category.

Racial and ethnic minorities make up a disproportionately large percentage of the population of people living with HIV/AIDS. On the basis of the ongoing racial disparities seen in the HIV incidence rate, these prevalence trends are likely to continue. Black men are six times more likely than white men to contract HIV, and black women are 15 times more likely than white women to contract HIV.[8] It is thought that multiple factors contribute to these racial disparities, including same-race partner selection, limited access to HIV testing and care services, stigma, sexual power imbalances, and the social disruption caused by poverty. The disproportionate burden of HIV in black and Hispanics is shown in Table 46-4. Current data are available online regarding the prevalence of HIV/AIDS cases among high-risk groups; these are updated regularly.

TABLE 46-4

Diagnoses of HIV Infection by Race or Ethnicity,* 2010

Race/Ethnicity	Cases	Rate†
White	11,821	7.3
Black/African American	18,527	62.0
Hispanic/Latino	8,052	20.4
Asian	668	6.5
American Indian/Alaska Native	201	9.7
Native Hawaiian/other Pacific Islander	51	19.3
Multiple races	547	15.4
Total	37,163	23.9

*In 46 states with confidential name-based HIV infection reporting.

†Rate per 100,000 persons. Adapted from Centers for Disease Control and Prevention: HIV Surveillance Report, 2010; vol. 22. http://www.cdc.gov/hiv/surveillance/resources/reports/2010report/pdf/2010_HIV_Surveillance_Report_vol_22.pdf. Accessed November 11, 2013.

Risk of Human Immunodeficiency Virus Infection Among Healthcare Workers

Healthcare workers are at risk for occupational exposure to HIV infection (as well as the viruses hepatitis B and hepatitis C) as a result of their work-related contact with contaminated blood and bodily fluids. Each year thousands of healthcare workers experience **percutaneous blood exposure**, which is an exposure to contaminated blood through a needle stick or a cut from another sharp instrument. Because accidents can and do occur, it is important for the dental hygiene practitioner to understand the relative risk of contracting HIV from an occupational exposure.

The CDC reports that, as of 2011, there were 57 confirmed seroconversions that resulted from occupational HIV exposure.[9] All documented transmissions were related to blood, visibly bloody fluids, or concentrated laboratory preparations. Needle penetrations accounted for 86% of the transmissions. None of the transmissions occurred in dentists or dental workers. Prospective studies of healthcare workers have estimated the risk of acquiring HIV infection from occupational exposure to be approximately 0.3%; in other words, the vast majority of exposures do not result in HIV infection.[10] The risk of transmission by other routes (e.g., exposure through the eye, nose, or mouth) is even lower at approximately 0.1%.[10]

In 2001 a survey of more than 18,600 dental hygiene students attending 143 U.S. dental hygiene programs sought to determine rates of occupational exposure to blood and body fluids. A total of 687 student exposures were reported between 1996 and 1998. Most exposures occurred during the second year of training, and about 80% of exposures were instrument punctures. Nine contaminated splashes and two bites were also reported.[11] These data emphasize the need for caution and the inclusive application of prevention protocols.

To reduce the risk of contracting HIV from an infected patient, dental hygiene practitioners must follow best practices for infection control to minimize the risk of percutaneous exposure, particularly by needle sticks.[11] The use of adequate sterilization and barrier infection-control procedures (see Chapter 7) are important best practices. It is also important to have an action plan in the event that an occupational exposure does occur. This plan should include the identification and testing of the source individual for blood-borne diseases, the proper reporting of the exposure incident to the CDC, and the initiation of a postexposure antiviral drug regimen if indicated. Table 46-5 shows the indications for HIV postexposure prophylaxis in the case of percutaneous exposures.

Human Immunodeficiency Virus Infection and Its Relation to Periodontal Status

Periodontal disease is commonly seen in clients with HIV/AIDS. There is evidence that HIV-positive individuals have an increased risk for certain types of periodontal disease, especially linear gingival erythema and necrotizing periodontal disease.[13] In the pre-HAART era, it was even hypothesized that necrotizing periodontal disease—along with other oral lesions such as Kaposi sarcoma, oral candidiasis, and hairy leukoplakia—could serve as markers of disease progression in known HIV-positive clients due to their association with low CD4+ lymphocyte counts.[14] Since the advent of widespread HAART, the connection between markers of HIV disease severity (i.e., CD4+ cell count and viral load) and periodontal disease risk has been less clear.

One study comparing the periodontal disease progression of both HIV-positive and HIV-negative clients revealed no significant differences between bleeding on probing, pocket formation, or attachment loss related to HIV status.[15] Likewise, studies of HIV-positive men and women in Western countries indicate that attachment loss was similar for both HIV-positive and HIV-negative groups, and bone loss measured radiographically over time has been shown to be unaffected by HIV status.[16,17] These data suggest that HIV may not be a risk factor for the progression of periodontal diseases; however, given the high prevalence of "conventional" periodontal disease in the HIV-positive population, preventive and restorative oral care is still imperative.

Oral Manifestations Associated with Human Immunodeficiency Virus and Acquired Immunodeficiency Syndrome

The oral manifestations of HIV/AIDS-related immunosuppression are amazingly complex. Considerable investigation has been conducted into the oral lesions associated with HIV infection because of their high incidence among HIV-infected individuals. It is important to recognize HIV-associated oral lesions, because they are often among the first signs to be manifested by the HIV-positive individual.

Oral Candidiasis

Candida is a genus of fungi that is found in the normal oral flora; however, *Candida* can proliferate in immunocompromised, malnourished, or debilitated persons. **Candidiasis**, the disease caused by *Candida*, is the most common HIV-associated oral lesion. Pseudomembranous candidiasis, atrophic or erythematous candidiasis, hyperplastic candidiasis, and angular cheilitis are all common oral lesions in HIV-positive persons caused by the strain *Candida albicans*. Candidiasis is by no means unique to the HIV-infected population, and its presence is not necessarily indicative of HIV/AIDS.

- **Pseudomembranous candidiasis (thrush)** (Figure 46-1) appears as soft, yellow-white, curdlike plaques on the oral

TABLE 46-5

Recommended HIV Postexposure Prophylaxis for Percutaneous Injuries[12]

	INFECTION STATUS OF SOURCE				
Exposure Type	**HIV-Positive Class 1***	**HIV-Positive Class 2***	**Source of Unknown HIV Status†**	**Unknown Source‡**	**HIV-Negative**
Less severe§	Recommend basic two-drug PEP	Recommend expanded three-drug PEP	Generally, no PEP warranted; however, consider basic two-drug PEP‖ for source with HIV risk factors¶	Generally, no PEP warranted; however, consider basic two-drug PEP‖ in settings where exposure to HIV-infected persons is likely	No PEP warranted
More severe**	Recommend expanded three-drug PEP	Recommend expanded three-drug PEP	Generally, no PEP warranted; however, consider basic two-drug PEP‖ for source with HIV risk factors¶	Generally, no PEP warranted; however, consider basic two-drug PEP‖ in settings where exposure to HIV-infected persons is likely	No PEP warranted

PEP, Postexposure prophylaxis.

*HIV-Positive, Class 1—asymptomatic HIV infection or known low viral load (e.g., <1500 RNA copies/mL). HIV-Positive, Class 2—symptomatic HIV infection, AIDS, acute seroconversion, or known high viral load. If drug resistance is a concern, obtain expert consultation. Initiation of postexposure prophylaxis should not be delayed pending expert consultation, and, because expert consultation alone cannot substitute for face-to-face counseling, resources should be available to provide immediate evaluation and follow-up care for all exposures.

†Source of unknown HIV status (e.g., deceased source person with no samples available for HIV testing).

‡Unknown source (e.g., a needle from a sharps disposal container).

§Less severe (e.g., solid needle and superficial injury).

‖The designation "consider PEP" indicates that PEP is optional and should be based on an individualized decision between the exposed person and the treating clinician.

¶If PEP is offered and taken and the source is later determined to be HIV-negative, PEP should be discontinued.

**More severe (e.g., large-bore hollow needle, deep puncture, visible blood on device, or needle used in patient's artery or vein).

Reproduced from Centers for Disease Control and Prevention: *Updated U.S. Public Heath Service guidelines for the management of occupational exposures to HBV, HCV, and HIV and recommendations for postexposure prophylaxis.* Available at: www.cdc.gov/mmwr/preview/mmwrhtml/rr5011a1.htm#box2. Accessed March 1, 2013.

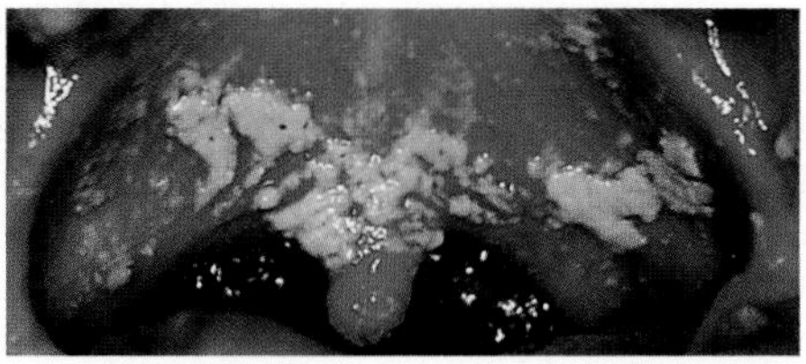

Figure 46-1. Pseudomembranous candidiasis in an individual with AIDS, manifested as white-yellow curdlike plaques on the palate. (Courtesy Dr. James R. Winkler, Marquette University, Minneapolis, Minnesota.)

tissues that, when wiped away, leave red, tender, and bleeding patches of mucosa. These plaques occur most frequently on the hard and soft palate and the labial and buccal mucosa, and they contain desquamated epithelial cells, fibrin, and the fungus.

- **Erythematous or atrophic candidiasis** (Figure 46-2) manifests as smooth, red, denuded patches on the tongue; red patches on the buccal or palatal mucosa; or desquamative gingivitis. These conditions usually result from the persistence of pseudomembranous candidiasis with a loss of the pseudomembrane. They are less obvious and more easily missed than white patches.
- **Hyperplastic candidiasis** (Figure 46-3) manifests as speckled, homogeneous white lesions that appear on the lateral borders of the tongue or the buccal mucosa and that may be associated with oral leukoplakia.

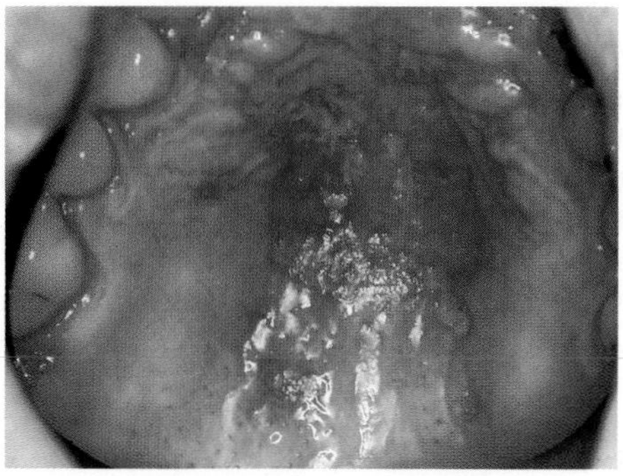

Figure 46-2. Mixed erythematous and pseudomembranous candidiasis of the palate.

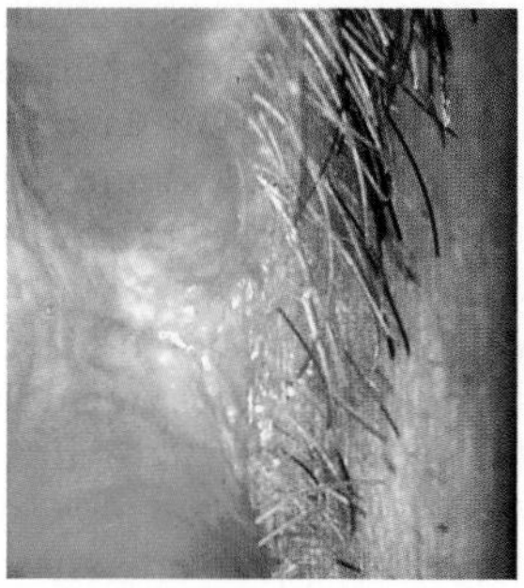

Figure 46-3. Hyperplastic candidiasis at the corner of the mouth. The lesion has persisted despite the use of systemic antifungal drugs.

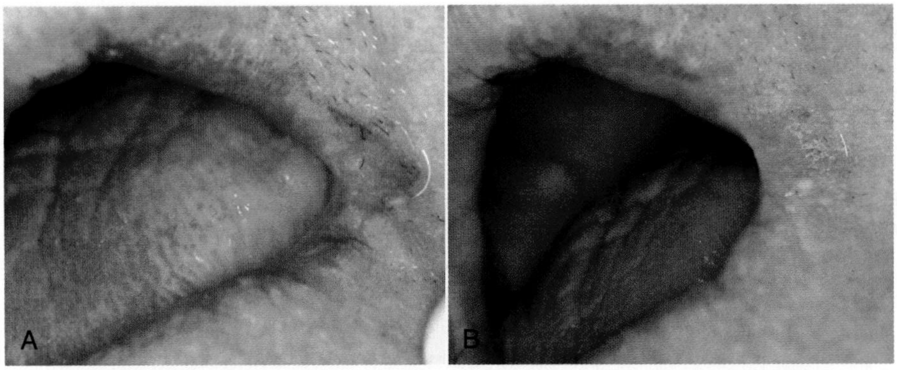

Figure 46-4. **A,** Severe angular cheilitis. **B,** After treatment with systemic fluconazole.

- Angular cheilitis appears as redness, cracks, crusting, or fissures at the commissures of the lips (Figure 46-4). The lesions are moderately painful and eroded. Medical treatment of angular cheilitis that results from *Candida* infection involves a variety of topical or systemic antifungal drugs.

Topical applications of nystatin or clotrimazole are commonly used to treat *Candida* infections. Usually immunocompromised clients require the systemic administration of antifungal medications, such as amphotericin B, ketoconazole, fluconazole, or itraconazole. Please refer to a current dental drug manual for further information about how these drugs are prescribed.

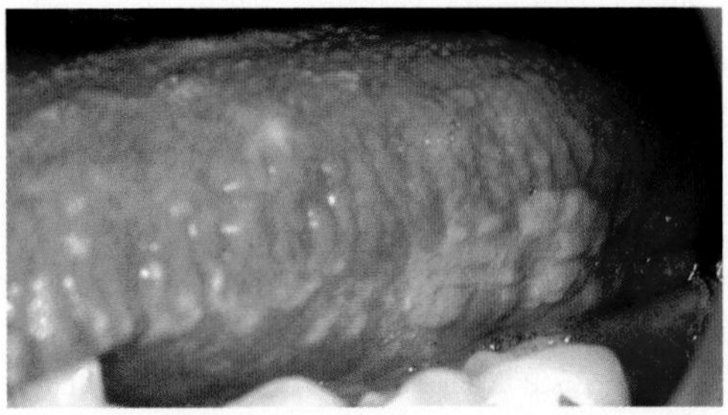

Figure 46-5. Oral hairy leukoplakia of tongue before the initiation of highly active antiretroviral therapy.

Hairy Leukoplakia

Oral hairy leukoplakia (OHL) is a collection of thick, asymptomatic white lesions associated with the Epstein-Barr virus and usually seen on the lateral borders of the tongue (Figure 46-5). The lesions can be unilateral or bilateral with long, fingerlike projections, or they may have a corrugated appearance. OHL is found almost exclusively in persons with HIV/AIDS; prevalence is approximately 20% among HIV-infected persons and up to 80% among those with AIDS.

Treatment for OHL is usually not indicated, but the lesions respond to HAART. Accurate diagnosis of the lesion is imperative as a result of its very high association with HIV infection. OHL is predictive of AIDS, with as many as 80% of individuals with a confirmed diagnosis progressing to the diagnosis of AIDS within 31 months.

Kaposi Sarcoma

Kaposi sarcoma is a malignant, slow-growing, endothelial cell neoplasm that is seen in some persons with AIDS. It has several associated causative factors, including genetic predisposition, viral infection with human herpesvirus-8, environmental influences, and alterations in the immune system. Kaposi sarcoma appears as painless purplish or brownish-red nodules primarily on the skin of the extremities, but it can often occur intraorally. Oral Kaposi sarcoma may present as small innocuous-looking flat reddish, bluish, purplish, or brown lesions of varying sizes, including large nodular lesions (Figure 46-6). Approximately 10% to 15% of HIV-positive clients with Kaposi sarcoma develop intraoral lesions. These lesions may appear anywhere in the oral cavity and, depending on their position, they may cause problems with phonation, swallowing, or breathing.

Oral Kaposi sarcoma lesions often appear on the gingiva associated with the teeth. In these cases, the tumors may be significantly enlarged by the presence of oral biofilm and calculus. Kaposi lesions on the gingiva associated with the teeth require excision or systemic therapy, as do Kaposi sarcomas located further from the teeth. Localized Kaposi lesions tend to respond to a myriad of treatment modalities, including surgical excision, laser excision, antiretroviral agents, cryotherapy, low-dose radiation treatment, intralesional injection with vinblastine, interferon-α, sclerosing agents, and antitumor chemotherapy.

Dental hygiene practitioners and dentists are sometimes hesitant to manipulate gingival tissue for fear of harming nearby Kaposi lesions or causing significant bleeding. However, periodontal care must be provided; in some cases tumor reduction is achieved with nonsurgical periodontal care. Oral biofilm removal, scaling, and root planing are essential to maximizing the effects of periodontal therapy and may help to reduce the size of the tumor before tumor-specific therapy.

Lesions of the Periodontium

As discussed previously, aggressive necrotizing forms of periodontitis have been reported in clients with HIV/AIDS. One form that is not specific to clients with HIV/AIDS is necrotizing ulcerative gingivitis (NUG), a bacterial infection of the gingiva that is characterized by inflammation, bleeding, pain, fever, and halitosis (Figure 46-7). Its treatment will be the same as it is for HIV-negative clients, and it includes the following: (1) cleaning and debriding the areas with cotton or gauze soaked in hydrogen peroxide and a topical anesthetic

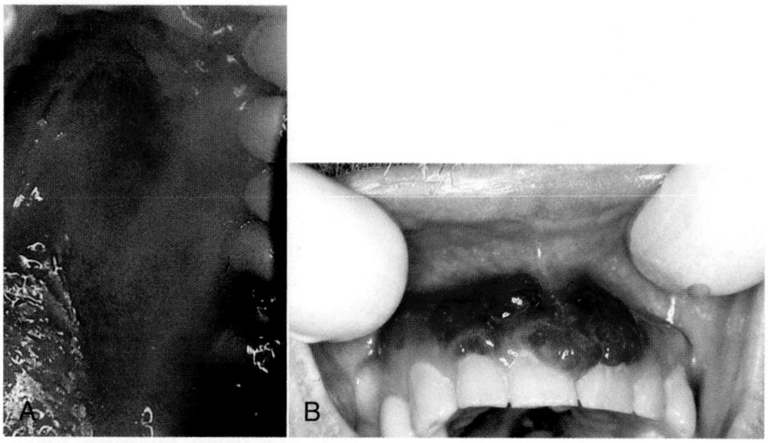

Figure 46-6. **A,** Oral Kaposi sarcoma lesions on the palate of an individual with AIDS. **B,** Oral Kaposi sarcoma on the gingiva. (**A,** Courtesy Dr. James R. Winkler, Marquette University, Minneapolis, Minnesota.)

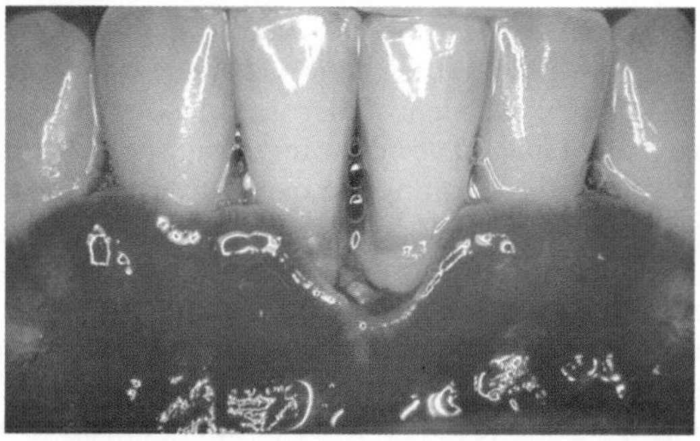

Figure 46-7. Linear gingival erythema and necrotizing ulcerative gingivitis in a client with AIDS.

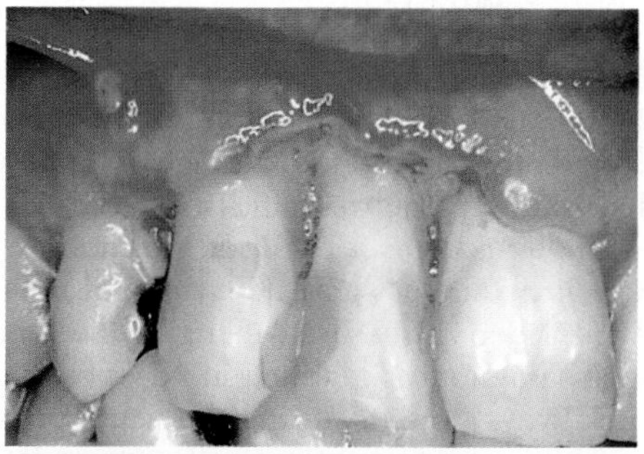

Figure 46-8. Necrotizing ulcerative periodontitis in an individual with AIDS showing color change, necrosis, and sloughing of the periodontal tissues. (Courtesy Dr. James R. Winkler, Marquette University, Minneapolis, Minnesota.)

agent daily or every other day for about 1 week; (2) twice-daily rinses for 30 seconds with 0.12% chlorhexidine gluconate mouth rinse; (3) the introduction of meticulous oral biofilm control as soon as the patient can tolerate it; and, finally, (4) definitive scaling and root planing after the patient has had some improvement in disease symptoms and healing. In the presence of lymphadenopathy, systemic symptoms, and moderate to severe oral tissue destruction, the dentist may initially prescribe an oral antibiotic and prophylactic antifungal medication. The patient should be advised to avoid alcohol and tobacco products and to eat a nutritious diet. Note that hydrogen peroxide mouth rinses are contraindicated in immunocompromised individuals. It is important to note that NUG appears without evidence of attachment loss.

NUG in the presence of rapid attachment and interproximal bone loss, no matter how extensive, is more properly diagnosed as **necrotizing ulcerative periodontitis (NUP)** (Figure 46-8). NUP is very painful, and sequestra or areas of dead bone can occur. Extreme cases of exposed bone and sloughing tissue are sometimes referred to as **necrotizing ulcerative stomatitis**, a condition that is also known as *cancrum oris (noma)*. Treatment is similar to that for NUG. The dentist may need to remove affected bone for healing to occur. See Treatment of Necrotizing Ulcerative Periodontitis later in this chapter.

The examination of the periodontium of a patient with HIV/AIDS may reveal a very red gingiva. This fiery-red soft tissue may sometimes appear as a line that is either localized or generalized along the gingival margin called **linear gingival erythema** (see Figure 46-7). The gingival changes that extend partly toward or directly onto the alveolar mucosa may have the more typical appearance of necrotizing ulcerative disease. In addition, the alveolar mucosa also may be bright red or have red petechiae-like patches.

The subgingival oral biofilm of HIV-positive persons has been shown to harbor high proportions of the same periodontal pathogens found in HIV-negative persons with periodontal lesions along with *Candida* and herpesviruses. More subgingival yeasts have been identified in HIV-positive adults with periodontal disease than in HIV-negative people with periodontal disease.[18] *C. albicans* may play a causative role in these exaggerated cases of gingival and periodontal diseases. These cases are typically unresponsive to the simple mechanical removal of the oral biofilm and calculus. Additional therapeutic agents are often required to control the pathogens that cause the infection.

The precise mechanisms of the severe form of periodontal destruction sometimes seen in HIV-positive individuals are not clearly understood. The relationship among the presence of increased amounts of *Candida,* herpesviruses, xerostomia, altered lymphocyte action, and potentially poor nutrition

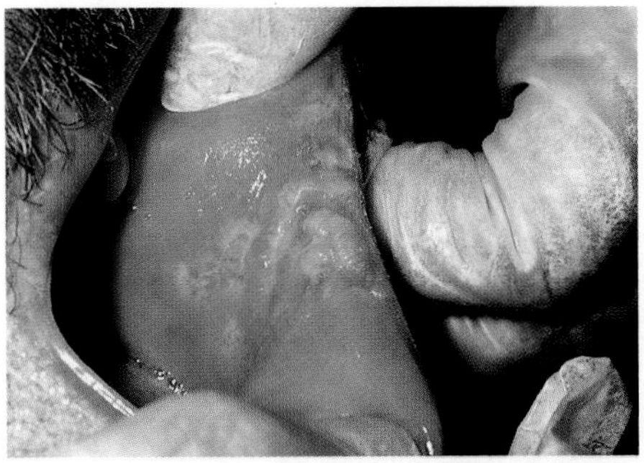

Figure 46-9. Oral warts on the interior of the corner of the mouth. (Courtesy Dr. Deborah Greenspan, University of California–San Francisco.)

remains to be studied in this extremely destructive periodontal disease process. The patient may have gingivitis that extends into the alveolar mucosa, NUG, or NUP with exposed bone. The achievement of successful clinical oral outcomes requires consultation with the dentist and physician.

Lymphadenopathy

Lymphadenopathy or swollen lymph nodes is a nonspecific sign that frequently accompanies a range of human illnesses. Lymphadenopathy typically signifies increased cellular activity in the lymph nodes as a result of infection, malignancy, autoimmune infection, or some other type of inflammation. Cervical lymphadenopathy or swelling of the lymph nodes of the neck is commonly identified in HIV-positive persons. It is almost always present during the acute phase of HIV infection, and it is also found frequently during later disease stages.

Oral Warts

Human papillomavirus is commonly found in HIV-infected individuals. This virus has many subtypes, one of which is associated with the formation of oral warts (Figure 46-9). Although oral warts can occur in any individual regardless of HIV status, recurrence after treatment is uncommon except in the case of HIV-infected individuals. HIV-associated oral warts can be large and multifocal, and they may present aesthetic and functional problems. Among HIV-positive individuals who are receiving antiretroviral therapy, an increase in oral warts with a concurrent decrease in oral hairy leukoplakia and oral candidiasis has been reported.

Recurrent Herpes Simplex Virus Infection

Most individuals have been exposed to primary herpetic infections that are either clinical or subclinical in nature at some time during their lives. Recurrent herpes simplex virus infection can occur in up to 40% of the HIV-positive population, and it is the usual manifestation of herpesvirus infection in individuals with HIV/AIDS. The recurrence of herpes appears to be related to the breakdown in local immune activity or alterations in local inflammatory mediators that allow the herpesvirus to become active again. In general, recurrent herpetic lesions heal within 1 to 2 weeks and are not related to secondary infections. However, when they occur in the HIV-infected population, they can be more severe and persistent. Herpetic lesions can also become secondarily infected with bacteria or fungi. The pain associated with oropharyngeal herpes lesions can significantly restrict the HIV-positive individual's intake of food, thereby compromising adequate nutrition.

Less-Common Lesions

A variety of infections, neoplasms, and other oral lesions have been described in HIV-positive clients. Although rare, they should be recognized and treated. The dental hygiene practitioner plays a role in performing oral evaluations and informing clients of the presence of lesions so that referral for diagnosis and treatment may be encouraged. It is always important to be attentive to changes in the client's health and to encourage him or her to seek additional care immediately.

The Dental Hygiene Process of Care in Clients with Human Immunodeficiency Virus

The dental hygiene practitioner should be sensitive to the many challenges faced by HIV-positive clients. HIV-positive clients are commonly prescribed complex, demanding drug regimens to control the disease process. They may be struggling to live with HIV while striving to maintain a healthy lifestyle. In addition to the medical challenges, people living with HIV/AIDS also encounter social stigma. The HIV-positive patient may have been previously shunned and may fear the same when visiting the dental hygiene practitioner. This may cause the HIV-positive patient to be reluctant or fearful of the clinician's response to knowledge of his or her HIV infection, even though the patient may be eager, cooperative, and happy to comply with recommendations for professional care. One effective way to initiate a professional relationship and to restore a sense of safety to both the client and the dental hygiene practitioner is to shake hands on introduction. The courtesy of this polite touch infuses the professional relationship with confidence and defuses unwarranted fear and alienation.

Patient Interview and Examination

When conducting the patient interview, the dental hygiene practitioner must be particularly sensitive to clues from the patient's health history and pharmacologic history as well as observations of clinical conditions associated with HIV infection. Specific questions on the health assessment form should address the following:

- "Do you have any disease or condition that could impair your immune system?"
- "Have you ever been tested for HIV?"
- "When was the last time you were tested for HIV?"
- "Are you sexually active? With men, women, or both?"
- "Have you ever used injection drugs?"

The dental hygiene practitioner discusses these issues frankly and considers the patient's answers in a nonjudgmental way to stimulate dialogue. When clients indicate that they have been tested for HIV, the dental hygiene practitioner should explicitly ask if they are HIV-positive or HIV-negative. If HIV infection is revealed, the dental hygiene practitioner should assess the patient's support systems, such as family members and partners. The patient's current medication regimen, including antiretroviral drugs and any prophylactic antimicrobials, should also be noted. While validating the health history and during the interview, the patient may report recent hospital stays for conditions associated with HIV status, as listed in Table 46-2. The patient may also report high-risk sexual behavior or intravenous drug use. Throughout the assessment, it is imperative to build trust with the patient by reaffirming professional confidentiality, explaining the medical importance of gathering this sensitive personal information, and showing a supportive attitude.

Medications that an HIV-positive person may be taking include combinations of the following antiviral drugs:

- Nucleoside reverse transcriptase inhibitors (NRTIs), such as abacavir (ABC), zidovudine (AZT), and lamivudine (3TC)
- Nonnucleoside reverse transcriptase inhibitors (NNRTIs), such as efavirenz (Sustiva or Stocrin) and nevirapine (Viramune)
- Protease inhibitors (PIs), such as fosamprenavir (Lexiva) and lopinavir boosted with ritonavir
- Integrase inhibitors (IIs), such as raltegravir

Extraoral assessment may reveal purplish-red nodules on the skin that are indicative of Kaposi sarcoma. Intraoral conditions may include the signs and symptoms associated with candidiasis, OHL, Kaposi sarcoma lesions, or necrotizing forms of periodontal disease. There may also be unusual lesions. Such clients should always be referred to a dentist or a physician for evaluation.

Dental Hygiene Diagnosis

Several of the human needs described in Chapter 2 are relevant to the care of the HIV-infected individual. For example, clients may be extremely anxious about having acquired HIV. The dental hygiene practitioner can help to alleviate this anxiety by focusing the patient on aspects of health that he or she can control. Educating clients about how HIV infection affects the oral structures and how to prevent or lessen the severity of these oral problems may empower the patient to feel some control over the disease. This feeling of empowerment enhances the patient's sense of control. Dental hygiene care for HIV-infected individuals encourages clients to take responsibility for oral health and to understand oral and systemic health-related issues.

Planning Dental Hygiene Care

The dental hygiene care plan must include patient education, therapeutic scaling and root planing, oral biofilm control, the provision of post-treatment instructions, the evaluation of care, and frequent continued care. Dental hygiene care must be integrated with the overall dental treatment plan in consultation with the physician. For example, prescription medication for oral candidiasis, oral biofilm control, or gingival inflammation may be needed.

In the case of more severe forms of NUG and NUP and of oral lesions such as those associated with Kaposi sarcoma, dental hygiene care must always occur in collaboration with the dentist and physician. Sometimes, as in the case of clients with NUP, the need for surgical treatment is so urgent that periodontal surgical intervention may be performed at the same appointment as the dental hygiene care.

HIV-positive clients can be very health-conscious and embrace preventive procedures such as brushing, interdental cleaning, and daily mouth rinsing with an effective antimicrobial agent. This focus on self-care can be a great advantage for the dental hygiene practitioner when designing and implementing a preventive program. The dental hygiene practitioner needs to evaluate the patient's knowledge of oral biofilm and oral disease processes as well as the person's dexterity level before selecting strategies that will lead the patient to optimal oral health. Should deficits in skin and mucous membrane integrity be identified, this interest in prevention can be an asset for motivating the patient to improve his or her oral self-care. An over-the-counter American Dental Association–accepted antibacterial mouth rinse or a prescribed 0.12% chlorhexidine mouth rinse may be recommended to assist with the control of supragingival bacterial plaque and gingivitis. Nutritional counseling may also be helpful to encourage a diet that is conducive to healing and oral maintenance. The patient may also be consulting or may need to consult a nutritionist; therefore the dental hygiene practitioner may be sharing responsibilities with this member of the healthcare team.

Implementation

After it has been formulated, the plan of care is implemented in accordance with the goals and priorities established by the patient and the oral healthcare team.

Infection Control

Some HIV-infected individuals do not reveal their status to healthcare workers. This lack of disclosure may be either because the client has privacy concerns or because the patient is not yet aware of the diagnosis. Standard precautions for infection control are essential for all clients and can be relied on to protect both the client and the dental hygiene practitioner from cross-contamination.

Scaling and Root Planing

Some opinions suggest that scaling and root planing should be performed on HIV-positive clients using only hand-activated instruments because power scaling devices generate an aerosol. To date, there have been no documented cases of HIV infection through an aerosol exposure, so this proposed mechanism of aerosol transmission is not supported by the evidence. In fact, the dental hygiene practitioner may prefer to perform therapeutic scaling and root planing procedures using ultrasonic instrumentation because there is generally less treatment time and because the procedures can often be performed without using injected local anesthetic agents, thereby reducing the possibility of needle sticks.

Generally clients with HIV/AIDS present with oral needs that are similar to those of the HIV-negative population. They can have gingivitis, periodontitis, xerostomia, dental caries, and so on, and they can also have healthy, well-maintained oral tissues. They require meticulous oral biofilm control and periodontal debridement, and they are maintained at regular intervals of 2 to 3 months.

Treatment of Necrotizing Ulcerative Periodontitis

The treatment of NUP consists of the aggressive control of the microbial challenge and local irritants. In addition, periodontal surgery may be required to remove necrosed tissues, including bone. Local irrigation of the gingiva and affected tissues with 0.12% chlorhexidine gluconate or povidone–iodine (Betadine) has also been recommended. Disposable syringes with blunt needles or cotton swabs are required to adequately flush the affected tissues. Persons who are being treated for NUP require frequent monitoring and evaluation. Postoperative care requires good mechanical oral biofilm

Procedure 46-1 Dental Hygiene Care for the Patient with Human Immunodeficiency Virus

EQUIPMENT

Personal protective equipment
Mouth mirror
Explorer
Periodontal probe
Scalers
2 × 2 gauze
Saliva ejector
Disposable syringe with blunt needle
0.12% Chlorhexidine gluconate
Ultrasonic scaling device (power scaler)
Syringe
Oral local and topical anesthetic agents
Cotton swabs

STEPS

1. Assess the client's needs.
2. Establish the dental hygiene care plan with the client; determine the need for consultation with other healthcare professionals.
3. Provide oral disease control instructions.
4. Provide a preprocedural oral rinse of 0.12% chlorhexidine gluconate.
5. Perform debridement procedures as needed. (Note that this may need to be done repeatedly for several consecutive appointments within a week.)
6. Irrigate subgingivally with 0.12% chlorhexidine gluconate after scaling procedures.
7. Postoperative recommendations include oral biofilm control and twice-daily use for 30 seconds of 0.12% chlorhexidine as an antibacterial mouth rinse. Slowly introduce mechanical daily oral care as pain subsides and healing occurs.
8. Establish 2- to 3-month continued-care interval.

Patient with Unexpectedly Severe Periodontal Signs and Symptoms or Oral Lesions

1. Consult with team members. The dentist may need to remove necrotic bone and prescribe medications.
2. Refer the client for lesion evaluation, dental diagnosis, and periodontal consultation.
3. Periodontal care requires irrigating tissues with an effective antimicrobial agent.
4. Debride with the use of hand-activated or ultrasonic instruments and topical or local anesthetic agents as needed.
5. Use postoperative antibiotics or antifungal agents as needed.
6. The client should be monitored every 2 to 3 months by the healthcare team.

Case Documentation

1. Record the services rendered and the client's response to care at each treatment appointment in ink.

control and twice-daily 0.12% chlorhexidine rinses for chemical oral biofilm control throughout the mouth. Clients must be informed about the possible side effects of chlorhexidine, including staining of the teeth, discoloration of the oral mucosa, calculus accumulation, and altered taste sensation. Antibiotics such as metronidazole to control oral anaerobic pathogens must be used with caution and in consultation with the treatment team. HIV-positive clients may experience the overgrowth of other opportunistic organisms when some bacteria are suppressed, including *Candida*. The sequence of procedures for treating NUP in an HIV-positive patient is presented in Procedure 46-1 and the corresponding Competency Form.

Evaluation

After comprehensive dental hygiene care has been completed, the dental hygiene practitioner should evaluate the patient to ensure that the established goals have been met. Evaluation should take place at the expected intervals. After initial therapy, reevaluation should occur in about 4 weeks. This allows time for the healing of the connective tissue so that the patient can be probed and assessed accurately. Continued-care intervals thereafter should be 2 to 3 months. Frequent care intervals provide opportunities to assess the patient's oral health, self-care practices, and nutrition for a good long-term outcome. The evaluation phase of the dental hygiene process also provides the opportunity to identify other human needs related to oral health and disease that may require attention. As with all clients, the process of care for clients with HIV occurs on a continuum.

CLIENT EDUCATION TIPS

- Explain the link between oral and systemic health.
- Explain that periodontal health and oral conditions require frequent evaluation and maintenance (commonly every 2 to 3 months) to maintain and monitor the client's oral health status.
- Remind immunosuppressed clients to avoid hydrogen peroxide rinses that can increase their risk of candidiasis.
- Identify evidence-based oral health products that have a therapeutic effect.

LEGAL, ETHICAL, AND SAFETY ISSUES

- The dental hygiene practitioner has an ethical and legal responsibility to care for individuals with HIV/AIDS.
- Treatment is necessary and effective for persons with HIV/AIDS.
- Standard precautions for infection control must be practiced; accidental exposures are minimized through standard precautions.
- An action plan should be in place in case an occupational exposure to contaminated blood occurs.

KEY CONCEPTS

- HIV infection is a disease that severely suppresses the host's immune response.
- HIV is a chronic, treatable condition.

- The risk of acquiring HIV infection from providing dental hygiene care to infected individuals is extremely low when infection control protocols are followed.
- Standard precautions and efforts to eliminate the risk of percutaneous exposure must always be undertaken.
- Most periodontal disease in HIV-positive individuals is indistinguishable from the disease patterns seen in HIV-negative clients.
- Hydrogen peroxide mouth rinses are contraindicated among immunocompromised individuals.
- Intraoral or perioral lesions observed in HIV-infected persons or persons who are not known to be HIV-positive should be evaluated immediately.
- Healthcare for HIV-infected individuals requires the efforts of a healthcare team.

CRITICAL THINKING EXERCISES

1. Discuss the following issues related to treating a pregnant woman who has HIV: (1) the possible transmission routes of the virus to the fetus; (2) the mother's fears and concerns about taking medications; and (3) the potential for developing aggressive periodontitis and hormone-influenced gingivitis.
2. Discuss the issue of personal safety when treating HIV-infected clients, and review standard precautions. This discussion should include a thoughtful analysis that addresses how many people do not know or may not reveal their HIV status, how individuals' periodontal conditions probably will not provide clues to their HIV status, and how power scaling and polishing devices can be used.

REFERENCES

1. Joint United Nations Programme on HIV/AIDS (UNAIDS): *Global report: UNAIDS Report on the Global AIDS Epidemic, 2012*. Geneva, 2012.
2. Kandathil AJ, Ramalingam S, Kannangai R, et al: Molecular epidemiology of HIV, *Indian J Med Res* 121:333, 2005.
3. Boswell SL, Fuller JD: Pathogenesis and natural history. In Libman H, Makadon HJ, editors: *HIV*, Philadelphia, 2000, American College of Physicians, American Society of Internal Medicine.
4. Centers for Disease Control and Prevention: *1993 revised classification system for HIV infection and expanded surveillance case for AIDS among adolescents and adults*. Available at: http://www.cdc.gov/mmwr/preview/mmwrhtml/00018871.htm. Accessed February 26, 2013.
5. Jacoby HM, Currier JS: Prevention of opportunistic infections. In Libman H, Makadon HJ, editors: *HIV*, Philadelphia, 2000, American College of Physicians, American Society of Internal Medicine.
6. Centers for Disease Control and Prevention: *Monitoring selected national HIV prevention and care objectives by using HIV surveillance data—United States and 6 U.S. dependent areas—2010*. Available at: http://www.cdc.gov/hiv/library/reports/surveillance/2010/surveillance_Report_vol_17_no_3.html. Accessed September 8, 2013.
7. Centers for Disease Control and Prevention: *Estimated HIV incidence in the United States, 2007–2010. HIV Surveillance Supplemental Report 2012;17(No. 4)*. http://www.cdc.gov/hiv/topics/surveillance/resources/reports/#supplemental. Published December 2012. Accessed October 29, 2013.
8. Centers for Disease Control and Prevention: *CDC Fact Sheet. Estimates of new HIV infections in the United States, 2006–2009*. Available at: http://www.cdc.gov/nchhstp/newsroom/docs/HIV-Infections-2006-2009.pdf. Accessed September 8, 2013.
9. Centers for Disease Control and Prevention: *Occupational HIV transmission and prevention among health care workers*. Available at: http://www.cdc.gov/hiv/resources/factsheets/PDF/hcw.pdf. Accessed September 8, 2013.
10. Bell DM: Occupational risk of human immunodeficiency virus infection in healthcare workers: an overview, *Am J Med* 102(Suppl 5B):9, 1997.
11. Tolle-Watts L, Saisbury M: Incidence of student exposures to blood and body fluids and postexposure management protocols in dental hygiene programs, *J Dent Hygiene* 75:214, 2001.
12. Centers for Disease Control and Prevention: *Updated U.S. Public Heath Service guidelines for the management of occupational exposures to HBV, HCV, and HIV and recommendations for postexposure prophylaxis*. Available at: www.cdc.gov/mmwr/preview/mmwrhtml/rr5011a1.htm#box2. Accessed March 1, 2013.
13. Ryder MI, Nittayananta W, Coogan M, et al: Periodontal disease in HIV/AIDS, *Periodontology 2000* 60:78, 2012.
14. Coogan M, Greenspan J, Challacombe SJ: Oral lesions in infection with human immunodeficiency virus, *Bull World Health Organ* 83:700, 2005.
15. Scheutz F, Matee MI, Andsager L, et al: Is there an association between periodontal condition and HIV infection? *J Clin Periodontol* 24:580, 1997.
16. Robinson PG, Boulter A, Birnbaum W, et al: A controlled study of relative periodontal attachment loss in people with HIV infection, *J Clin Periodontol* 27:273, 2000.
17. Perrson RE, Hollender LG, Perrson GR: Alveolar bone levels in AIDS and HIV seropositive patients and in control subjects, *J Periodontol* 69:1056, 1998.
18. Zambon JJ, Reynolds H, Smutko J, et al: Are unique bacterial pathogens involved in HIV-associated periodontal diseases? In Greenspan JS, Greenspan D, editors: *Oral manifestations of HIV infection*, Chicago, 1995, Quintessence.

ACKNOWLEDGMENT

The authors acknowledge Dorothy A. Perry for her past contributions to this chapter.

EVOLVE RESOURCES

Please visit http://evolve.elsevier.com/Darby/hygiene for additional practice and study support tools.

CHAPTER 47

Persons with Neurologic and Sensory Deficits

Dorothy J. Rowe, Brenda S. Kunz

COMPETENCIES

1. Provide general descriptions of dental hygiene care for persons with neurologic and sensory deficits.
2. Discuss dysfunctions of the motor system, including characteristics, treatment and prognosis, oral clinical findings, special considerations, and oral self-care instructions.
3. Discuss peripheral neuropathies, including characteristics, treatment and prognosis, oral clinical findings, special considerations, and oral self-care instructions.
4. Discuss spinal cord dysfunction, including characteristics, treatment and prognosis, oral clinical findings, special considerations, and oral self-care instructions.
5. Discuss seizures, including characteristics, treatment and prognosis, oral clinical findings, special considerations, and oral self-care instructions.
6. Discuss disorders of higher cortical function, including characteristics, treatment and prognosis, oral clinical findings, special considerations, and oral self-care instructions.
7. Discuss cerebrovascular disease, including characteristics, treatment and prognosis, oral clinical findings, special considerations, and oral self-care instructions.
8. Discuss sensory disorders, including characteristics, treatment and prognosis, oral clinical findings, special considerations, communication techniques, and oral self-care instructions.

The nervous system makes each individual unique. It senses and evaluates the internal and external environment, controls one's body, and is responsible for a person's abilities, intellect, and personality. These characteristics are the result of complex interactions within the nervous system, and any structural damage or physiologic change to a component of this system may cause functional loss and a variety of neurologic deficits. Persons with neurologic disorders present unique challenges for the clinician to deliver comprehensive dental hygiene care. The dental hygienist must be knowledgeable about the specific condition, its oral clinical findings, special considerations for dental hygiene care, and oral self-care instructions. Decision making about client care must be based on the best available scientific evidence in conjunction with the clinical expertise of the practitioner and input from the client and/or caregiver (see Chapter 3).

The incidence and prevalence of some of the more common neurologic diseases or conditions are listed in Table 47-1.

General Descriptions of Dental Hygiene Care

Although each neurologic deficit has a unique cause and pathology, the clinical manifestations may be similar. In these situations the oral clinical findings, special considerations for dental hygiene care, and oral self-care instructions also would be similar and therefore are described first in general terms. More specific descriptions, unique to particular neurologic disorders, are reserved for the section on that disorder.

Oral Clinical Findings

Because dental caries and periodontal diseases are frequent oral clinical findings in clients with neurologic deficits, assessing the client's risk for these diseases is essential. Caries risk assessment is the initial step in Caries Management by Risk Assessment (CAMBRA) protocol, which is described in Chapter 18. Risk factors influencing a client's susceptibility to periodontal diseases are described in Chapter 19. Based on the results of these risk assessments, an evidence-based dental hygiene care plan can be developed to manage the client's oral diseases.

Many clients exhibit extensive plaque biofilm accumulations, food debris, supragingival and subgingival calculus, dental caries, and gingival inflammation, possibly extending to the periodontal attachment. The major factor contributing to this poor oral health is the client's inability to perform adequate self-care because of impaired motor coordination, inadequate sensation, or generalized muscle weakness and fatigue. Further debilitation may necessitate dependence on the caregiver, who may be overwhelmed with numerous responsibilities. Access to care may be an additional problem because of limited finances, problems with mobility or transportation to dental care, and the attitudes of oral healthcare practitioners (see Chapter 42). Because of the neurologic deficit, the client may be receiving constant medical attention involving multiple medical appointments. With so many healthcare appointments, professional oral health maintenance may be less of a priority.

Moreover, oral musculature disturbances, observed in many of these clients, interfere with the self-cleansing mechanisms of the tongue, cheek, and lip and consequently the oral clearance of plaque biofilm and food debris. In addition, the client may have lost sensation and may not be aware of the debris collecting in the vestibule. Biofilm and food debris retention around the teeth and oral mucosa is accentuated by the consumption of a soft, carbohydrate-rich diet, which the client chooses because of problems with mastication and swallowing.

TABLE 47-1

Epidemiology of the Common Neurologic Disorders (Median Estimates)

		ANNUAL INCIDENCE		PREVALENCE			
Disorder	**Range of Ages Included**	**Rate per 100,000***	**Number**	**Rate per 1000**	**Number**	**Rate Ratio, M/F†**	**Age(s) of Peak Incidence**
Cerebral palsy	3-13	—	—	2.4	207,000‡	1.3	—
Epilepsy	All	48	142,000	7.1	2,098,000	1.0	<1, ≥80
Multiple sclerosis	All	4.2	12,000	0.9	266,000	0.5	30
Spinal cord injury	All	4.5	13,000	—	—	4.2	20
Stroke	All	183	541,000	10.0	2,956,000	1.1	≥80
	≥65	1093	401,000	—	—	—	
Alzheimer's disease	≥65	1275	468,000	67.0	2,459,000	0.5	≥80
Parkinson's disease	≥65	160	59,000	9.5	349,000	1.8	≥70

*Estimated number of cases in United States in 2005, rounded to nearest 1000.
†Ratio of rates among males to rates among females.
‡Estimated number of cases among children younger than 21 years of age only.
Adapted from Hirtz D, Thurman DJ, Gwinn-Hardy K, et al: How common are the "common" neurologic disorders? *Neurology* 68:326, 2007.

Client medications also may cause oral effects, the most common being xerostomia or dry mouth. Xerostomia in turn causes susceptibility to oral infections such as candidiasis, taste dysfunction, difficulty in swallowing, and dental caries.

Special Considerations for Dental Hygiene Care

Dental hygiene care for clients with neurologic and sensory deficits often requires an interprofessional team approach because of the complex medical conditions. Collaborative actions among healthcare providers offer benefits in terms of patient safety and improved health outcomes. A thorough review of the client's written health and pharmacologic history is mandatory. A consultation with the client's physician may be needed if the client reveals a condition that may jeopardize safety during care, for example, if the condition precludes dental hygiene care or if the client needs urgent medical attention. Further details of physician consultations are discussed in Chapters 10 and 12.

Frequent dental hygiene care appointments usually are needed to achieve and maintain optimal oral health, especially in clients whose neurologic deficit may limit their ability to perform oral self-care. Frequent dental hygiene visits are useful to monitor oral health and hygiene and to reinforce preventive self-care procedures for client and caregiver. Weakness and fatigue increase during the day, so appointments usually are best scheduled early in the morning. Sufficient appointment time must be allowed so that the client does not feel rushed, in terms of communication and physical movements. Also, the dental hygienist may have to provide the client with breaks from treatment.

Clients may be ambulatory but using assistive walking devices or may be confined to a wheelchair. Their need for assistance varies. Certain clients do better without assistance because they have developed their own coping mechanisms; others need aid in seating and rising from the dental chair or in being transferred to and from the wheelchair. Wheelchair transfer techniques are described in Chapter 42. Depending on the client's condition, some may be treated more easily in the wheelchair.

During the appointment, clients with swallowing difficulty and a diminished gag reflex may need to be seated in a more upright position to avoid choking and aspiration of water and foreign substances. Optimal suctioning and limiting the amount of water also help prevent airway obstruction. Mouth props or bite blocks may be useful for clients with impaired oral reflexes, muscle weakness, and tremors and for those easily fatigued; however, extended use of these devices may create problems with the temporomandibular joint. Instrument fulcrums may need additional stabilization. To prevent clinician injury from the client's mouth closing without warning, a finger guard, such as a metal tailor's thimble secured with floss, may be helpful.

In many clients, body stability maintenance is a great concern. The client may need to be secured in the dental chair with restraint or support devices, such as soft ties, belts, or pillows. Moreover, the use of the client's caregiver to hold the client often is the best, least restrictive means. The dental hygienist explains the use of assistance to the client and/or caregiver as being facilitative for treatment, rather than restraint. The client's head can be supported by the clinician sitting or standing at the 12-o'clock position and cradling the client's head with the clinician's nondominant arm. Further suggestions for stabilization are described in Chapter 42.

Oral Self-Care Instructions

Instructions for individualized self-care depend on the client's level of energy and motor coordination (i.e., hand strength, abilities to grasp and to manipulate a toothbrush). It is important to encourage all clients to be as self-sufficient as possible in maintaining their own oral health. The client's motor capabilities are assessed so that devices may be recommended or created to compensate for physical limitations. For example, toothbrush handles with a larger diameter are easier to grip. Toothbrush handles can be enlarged with a bicycle grip, rubber or sponge ball, or modeling clay (see Chapter 42). Power toothbrushes usually have larger handles and do not require the client to produce a brushing stroke; however, supporting and controlling the weight of a power brush may be more difficult than holding a manual toothbrush with both hands. Clients may need to prop their elbows and arms during brushing to maintain motor control and minimize fatigue. For the client who wears dentures, a denture brush secured to the sink by suction would facilitate cleaning the prosthesis with one hand (see Chapter 56).

Other adaptations to assist with plaque control are pump dispensers for toothpaste, toothpaste tubes with flip-top caps, and floss holders. Dental floss use may be too difficult to master, so another interdental aid may be more appropriate (see Chapter 24). Respiratory problems may contraindicate foamy toothpaste, so a brand without the detergent sodium lauryl sulfate may be suggested. Only clients with adequate ability to control gagging and swallowing can use fluoride and chlorhexidine rinses safely at home. Those with severe oral motor dysfunction may be harmed by ingesting those products, so alternate preventive procedures, such as brush-on fluoride gels and fluoride trays, may be suggested.

Clients with mastication and swallowing difficulties may be consuming soft, carbohydrate-rich foods, so noncariogenic and nutritious foods must be recommended. Xylitol products also could be suggested to minimize caries risk (see Chapters 18 and 33). The discomforts from xerostomia may be alleviated by the use of saliva substitutes (see Chapter 55). Fluoride mouth rinses and brush-on gels also may be recommended to xerostomic clients to prevent dental caries, especially root caries, which are prevalent in this population. Because alcohol may dry out the oral mucosa, alcohol-containing mouth rinses are relative contraindications for clients with low saliva production.

For clients requiring assistance with their self-care, their caregivers must be instructed in effective plaque-control procedures (see Chapters 23, 24, 42), as well as the disease process and the importance of daily oral hygiene measures. Written as well as oral instructions should be provided to the caregiver and client so that the information can be reviewed at home. Caregivers also should be instructed in client positioning. For maximal stability and access the caregiver may need to sit or stand behind the person or wheelchair. For the client with uncontrollable movements, a second person may be needed to stabilize the client.

Power toothbrushes may be easier for caregivers to use. Also, the use of a floss holder allows one hand of the caregiver to prop the mouth open while the other hand is grasping the floss holder. If a mouth prop is necessary to keep the mouth open, an inexpensive one can be made by securing five or six tongue depressors together with adhesive tape.

Dysfunctions of the Motor System

Motor actions require the integration of several central nervous system (CNS) and peripheral nervous system (PNS) components. The CNS is composed of the brain and the spinal cord (Table 47-2), and the PNS is composed of the spinal, cranial, and autonomic nerves and ganglia. Several brain regions are involved in voluntary movement control and in motor responses to sensory stimuli, particularly the motor region (frontal lobe) of the cerebral cortex, the cerebellum, and the basal ganglia.[1] The outline of the CNS in Table 47-2 and the diagram of the brain in Figure 47-1 demonstrate the relationship of these specific regions to other components of the CNS. The basal ganglia are clusters of neuron cell bodies (gray matter) embedded deep within the CNS forebrain and midbrain. Although not evident in Figure 47-1, the basal ganglia are represented diagrammatically in Figure 47-2.

Disorders affecting cells of the cerebellum and basal ganglia, which project to the motor regions of the cerebral cortex, disturb movements and produce abnormalities of muscle tone, abnormal posturing, and tremors. There may be hyperkinesis (increase in movement), hypokinesis (lessening of muscular movement), a decrease in associated movements (e.g., arm swing when walking), or abnormal involuntary movements. Degenerative, metabolic, or vascular diseases; toxins; infections; trauma; or neoplasms may cause these abnormalities.

TABLE 47-2

Overview of the Major Subdivisions of the Central Nervous System

Structure ***Brain***	**Primary Function(s)**
Cerebral Hemispheres	
Lobes	
Frontal lobe	Voluntary motor control, including speech
Parietal lobe	Somatic sensations
Occipital lobe	Vision
Temporal lobe	Hearing, memory
Limbic lobe	Drives, emotions, memory
Basal ganglia	Motor control
Diencephalon	
Thalamus	Reciprocal connections with cerebral cortex
Hypothalamus	Integrative control of autonomic functions
Subthalamus	Motor control
Cerebellum	Control of range and force of movement and acquisition of motor skills
Brainstem	
Midbrain	Control of motor and sensory functions; substantia nigra
Pons	Motor relay from hemispheres to cerebellum
Medulla	Control of vital autonomic functions
Spinal cord	Integration of sensory and motor information from body and control of body movements

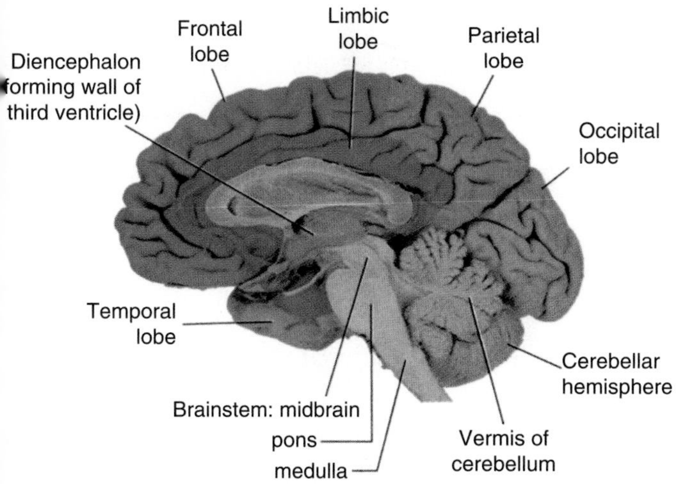

Figure 47-1. Major regions of the brain, as observed in a midsagittal view. Lobes of the cerebral cortex, diencephalon, brainstem, and cerebellum are illustrated; the regions of the basal ganglia are not evident in this view. (Adapted from Nolte J: *The human brain,* ed 6, Philadelphia, 2009, Mosby.)

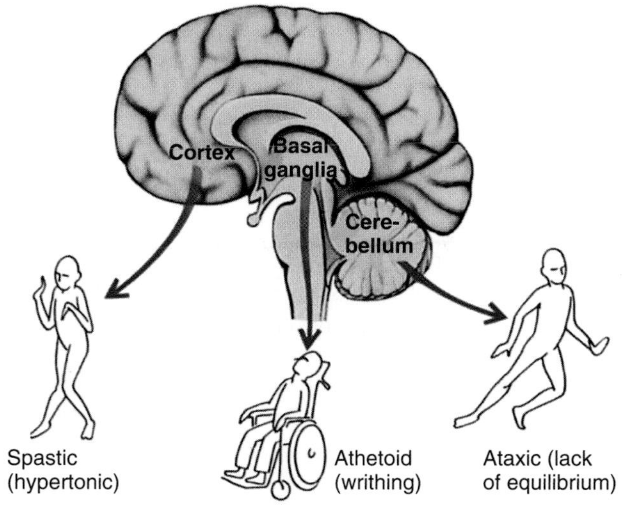

Figure 47-2. Parts of the brain affected in the major types of cerebral palsy. The types of the movement disorders depend on the part of the brain that has been damaged. (Adapted from Nowak AJ: *Dentistry for the handicapped patient,* St Louis, 1976, Mosby.)

Tremors

Tremors are involuntary rhythmic repetitions or oscillations of movement at regular intervals. They may be physiologic, postural, static (resting), or intentional, and there are multiple causes. **Intentional tremor** is the most common tremor and the most common movement abnormality. It may start at any age but most commonly begins in the third or fourth decade. The cause and pathology are unknown. The tremor is most prominent during volitional movements, particularly skilled movements such as writing, and is aggravated when the individual is tense or after caffeine use. Head and voice tremor is common and often is confused with Parkinson's disease tremor; however, essential tremor is faster, is not present during rest, and is not accompanied by other neurologic symptoms or signs. Alcohol, phenobarbital, and diazepam are effective in suppressing the tremor temporarily.

Parkinson's Disease

Parkinson's disease (Parkinson's syndrome, paralysis agitans) is a chronic progressive disorder of the motor system, resulting from the loss of dopamine-producing neurons. It is rather common in middle and old age, with the peak of onset in the sixth decade. The incidence is higher among men than women.[2,3]

Etiology and Risk Factors

Age is a definite risk factor, although an early-onset form of the disease begins before the age of 50. A specific cause for the death of dopamine-producing neurons has not been determined. Many researchers believe that the disease results from a combination of genetic susceptibility and exposure to one or more environmental factors that trigger the disease.[4] The same genes that are altered in inherited cases may be altered in sporadic cases by environmental toxins or other factors, such as viruses.[4]

Pathologic Characteristics

Pathologically the disorder is characterized by the progressive loss of dopamine-synthesizing neurons in the substantia nigra of the midbrain of the brainstem (see Figure 47-1). Dopamine is released from axons that originate from the cell bodies in the substantia nigra and terminate in the basal ganglia, where it serves as a neurotransmitter. A deficiency of dopamine at this site interferes with the conduction of nerve impulses related to muscle activity.

Clinical Symptoms

The cardinal manifestations of Parkinson's disease are rigidity, akinesia (impaired muscle movement), and tremor, although tremor absence does not exclude the diagnosis of the disease. Muscle rigidity is felt in all passive movements. Akinesia or bradykinesia (movement slowness) leads to an expressionless face, infrequent blinking, and posture and gait disturbances, such as the characteristic rapid, short, shuffling steps (Figure 47-3). Other symptoms include a soft, barely audible voice, pitch monotony, and progressive difficulty with writing, which is often extremely small. The tremor is rhythmic, is seen at rest, usually involves primarily the hands, and has been given the name **pill-rolling tremor**. The tremor usually stops during intended movements.

Clients with Parkinson's disease often have great difficulty rising from a sitting position and trying to turn from one side to the other in the recumbent position. They usually stand in a slightly stooped posture with the arms flexed. When attempting to walk, they may have great difficulty getting started, and when they finally succeed, steps are short and arm swing is decreased or absent. When these clients turn, the normal fluid movements become replaced by turning the body as a whole, and they may have difficulty stopping immediately. Depression is common, and dementia is sometimes present.

Treatment and Prognosis

Usually clients with Parkinson's disease progressively deteriorate over the course of the disease. The most efficacious treatment is dopamine replacement in the CNS through the use of levodopa, which is converted to dopamine. Most significantly improve on levodopa therapy, although there is some debate over when to use it. Because of its unpleasant

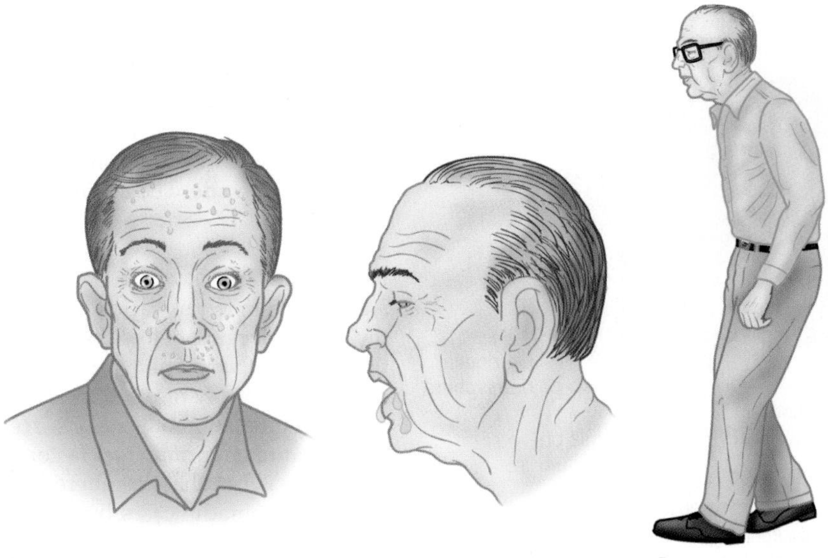

Figure 47-3. Characteristic features of Parkinson's disease. **A**, Expressionless face. **B**, Drooling. **C**, Stooped posture and gait with short, shuffling steps. (From Little JW, Falace DA, Miller CS, et al: *Dental management of the medically compromised patient,* ed 8, St Louis, 2013, Mosby.)

peripheral side effects (e.g., nausea, vomiting, low blood pressure), other medications also are prescribed.

Oral Clinical Findings

One of the first noticeable signs of Parkinson's disease is a lack of facial expression and animation, also known as "masked face." The characteristic tremors also occur in the tongue, lips, and neck. Common manifestations are the "flycatcher" tongue, tongue thrusting, and lip pursing. In the later stages of the disease, the muscles used in swallowing may work less efficiently, causing dysphagia (impaired swallowing) and drooling. Food and saliva may collect in the mouth and the back of the throat, which can cause choking and drooling. On the other hand, xerostomia often results from medications. Some clients experience a pulsating, burning pain involving the anterior tongue, hard palate, lip, and alveolar ridge, termed burning mouth syndrome.

Special Considerations for Dental Hygiene Care

The client's involuntary muscle movements create a safety concern for the clinician, and methods to address this problem were discussed previously. In severe cases it may be necessary to refer the client to be treated under general anesthesia. In addition, the client may be susceptible to orthostatic hypotension and dizziness caused by low blood pressure induced by the medications. Therefore the clinician should be cautious when adjusting the dental chair.

Oral Self-Care Instructions

In the early disease stages, individuals may be able to maintain their own oral hygiene, but the dexterity level must be assessed continually. As tremors and postural instability become more pronounced, they have more difficulty performing their own oral hygiene care and become more dependent on their caregivers (see Chapter 42). Caregivers may find that brushing the teeth with a specially adapted manual or power toothbrush may be helpful. Because xerostomia is a common side effect of the medications, a saliva substitute can be recommended. It can enhance the comfort of wearing prosthetic appliances.

Cerebral Palsy

Cerebral palsy (CP) is a chronic, nonprogressive neuromuscular disorder caused by damage to motor areas of the immature brain, affecting primarily the ability to control posture and movement. It is the second most common neurologic impairment in childhood, intellectual and developmental disability (formerly known as mental retardation) being the first.

Etiology and Risk Factors

Although CP affects muscle movement, it is not caused by problems in muscles or nerves, but by abnormalities inside the brain that disrupt the brain's ability to control movement and posture. Most congenital cases are caused by brain damage occurring during pregnancy or delivery. Risk factors include premature birth, multiple births, maternal infections or exposure to toxic substances, and blood type incompatibility.[5] Acquired cerebral cases arise from brain damage in the first few months or years of life (e.g., brain infections, such as meningitis, or head injury from a motor vehicle accident, fall, or child abuse).[5]

Pathologic Characteristics and Clinical Symptoms

The symptoms of CP vary from mild, with only an awkwardness of movement or difficulty with fine motor skills, to severe, which may incapacitate the child completely. There may be associated conditions such as hearing and vision problems, communication problems, impairment of other senses, epilepsy, and intellectual and developmental challenges. CP is classified into four broad categories according to the type of movement disorder and subdivided based on the number of limbs involved: monoplegia affects one limb; diplegia, two limbs and usually both legs; triplegia, three limbs; and quadriplegia, four limbs. Hemiplegia affects both

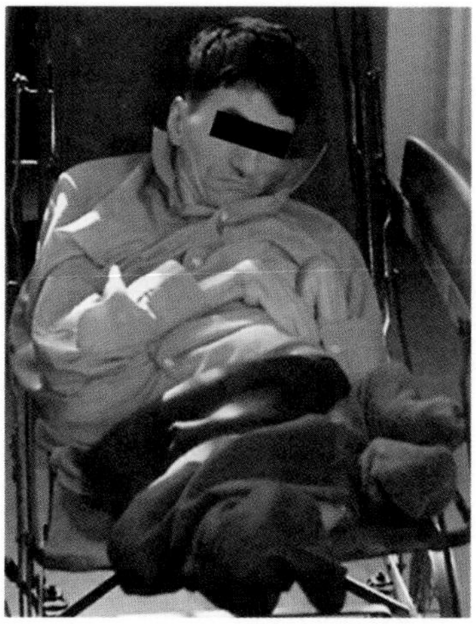

Figure 47-4. A man with the spastic type of cerebral palsy. The spasticity of his antigravity muscles has caused his limbs to assume a severe flexed posture. (From Porter SR, Scully C, Gleeson P: *Medicine and surgery for dentistry*, ed 2, Oxford, England, 1999, Churchill Livingstone.)

limbs on one side of the body. The types of movement disorder are classified on the basis of motor activity and the brain part that was damaged (see Figure 47-2).[5]

- Most CP patients are of the spastic type, characterized by spasticity in the muscles leading to stiffness, resistance to movement, and contractures (Figure 47-4). The sudden, involuntary muscle contractions or spasms result from damage to the motor area (frontal lobe) of the cerebral cortex (see Figure 47-2).
- Athetoid or dyskinetic CP is characterized by slow, writhing, uncontrolled movements that usually affect the hands, feet, arms, or legs and sometimes the face, causing drooling and grimacing. The movements may increase with emotional stress and disappear during sleep. Children with CP may have dysarthria (difficulties with articulation) caused by problems in speech muscle coordination. People often think that children with CP have a mental or emotional problem because of their awkward movements, although this form of CP usually involves only the motor centers, resulting from damage to the basal ganglia (see Figure 47-2).
- Ataxic CP is associated with problems in balance, coordination, and depth perception, caused by damage to the cerebellum (see Figure 47-2). The affected patients have poor coordination, walk with a wide-based gait, and may have difficulty with quick or precise movements.
- Mixed forms of CP, such as spastic-athetoid, have a combination of symptoms.

Treatment and Prognosis

Many types of therapy are used to help each child reach his or her optimum capabilities: physical and occupational therapy, speech and language therapy, biofeedback, orthopedic devices, and medications. Some children die in infancy, but most grow to adulthood. The main causes of death are respiratory and heart diseases.

Oral Clinical Findings

Most oral clinical findings in CP clients are related to disturbances of the oral musculature. Abnormal functioning of the tongue, lips, and cheeks can make oral clearance of food difficult, which is accentuated by the consumption of a soft, carbohydrate-rich diet. Those who have an associated convulsive disorder may be being treated with phenytoin and therefore are susceptible to gingival overgrowth, which are discussed later in this chapter.

Fractures of the maxillary anterior teeth are common because of the uncoordinated ambulation and seizures that lead to frequent falls and the lack of lip protection to the protrusive teeth. Signs of attrition and bruxism result from severe involuntary grinding of the teeth. The teeth of children who are born with CP may exhibit enamel hypoplasia. This enamel defect may be related to the time of cerebral injury. Malocclusion commonly results from the abnormal functioning of the facial, masticatory, and lingual musculature, in conjunction with oral habits, such as tongue thrusting, mouth breathing, and faulty swallowing. Drooling, caused by impaired swallowing and hypotonic lip muscles, frequently is observed.

Special Considerations for Dental Hygiene Care

The client's involuntary muscle movements create a safety concern for the clinician, and methods to address this problem were discussed previously. Abnormal muscle responses or reflexes often are triggered by changing the client's head or neck position in the dental chair. The clinician can control the tonic labyrinthine and asymmetric tonic reflexes, as indicated in Table 47-3. Informing the client when lowering, raising, or tilting the dental chair also may prevent a startle reflex.

Oral Self-Care Instructions

The client's dexterity level must be assessed to develop an oral self-care plan. A specially adapted or power toothbrush, as well as a floss holder, may be needed. Fluoride or chlorhexidine rinses may be recommended, but rinsing probably

TABLE 47-3

Reflex Responses of Cerebral Palsy Conditions and Their Management

Condition	Tonic Labyrinthine Reflex	Asymmetric Tonic Neck Reflex
Stimuli	Tilting head backward, so neck loses support	Turning head to one side, away from midline
Response	Body into full extension Arms and legs extend and stiffen	Arm and leg on face side extend Opposite arm and leg flex
Prevention	Keep head supported and flexed Maintain chair in upright position Hands folded at midline	Use rear operating position Stabilize head in midline position
Management	Bring arms forward Separate legs Massage shoulders	Place face in midline Help flex extended arm and leg

Adapted from DeBiase CB: Treating the patient with cerebral palsy, *Dent Hyg News* 5:13, 1987.

would have to be monitored by a caregiver. Saliva substitutes can be recommended if medications have caused dry mouth. Written instructions should be given to clients and/or caregivers for them to refer to at home.

Multiple Sclerosis

Multiple sclerosis (MS) is an autoimmune CNS disorder in which there is myelin sheath destruction of specific axons causing multiple neurologic symptoms that accrue over time. MS is the most common progressive and disabling neurologic condition affecting young adults. It typically begins in early adulthood, with a mean onset age of 33 years. Caucasian women are affected more frequently, as common with most autoimmune disorders.[6] MS generally has been considered to be more common in the cold and temperate climates of the higher latitudes, predominantly affecting individuals of northern European ancestry. However, current research suggests that the uneven geographic distribution may be attributable to differences in genes and the environment and their interactions.[7]

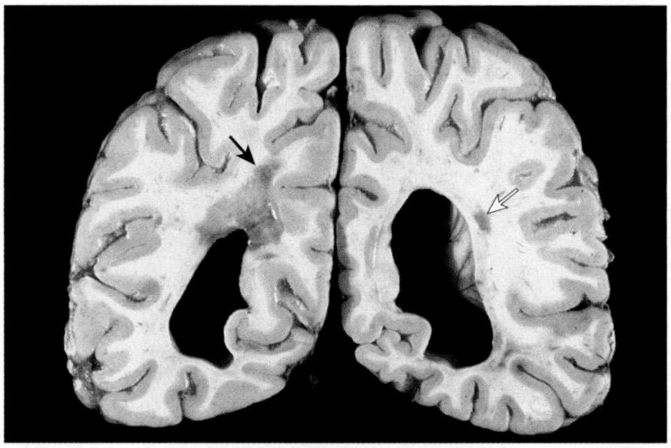

Figure 47-5. Coronal section of the brain of a patient who had multiple sclerosis. Note the large demyelinated plaque over the left ventricle *(black arrow)* and a smaller demyelinated plaque lateral to the right ventricle *(white arrow)*. (From Little JW, Falace DA, Miller CS, et al: *Dental management of the medically compromised patient*, ed 8, St Louis, 2013, Mosby.)

Etiology and Risk Factors

Evidence suggests that MS is caused by a combination of genetic and environmental factors. Susceptibility to MS may be inherited, and all of the identified genes have been associated with immune functions. Deficiency of vitamin D is now known to be a risk factor, possibly because of the vitamin's immunomodulatory effects.[8] MS frequency is correlated strongly with duration and intensity of ultraviolet B radiation from sunlight and serum vitamin D concentrations, as well as low consumption of vitamin D–rich fatty fish.[8] Other environmental risk factors include Epstein-Barr virus infection and cigarette smoking.

Pathologic Characteristics

The main disease characteristic is the presence of numerous demyelinated nerve axons in the brain and spinal cord. The myelin sheath's lipid composition provides axon insulation, so the sheath degeneration interferes with nerve impulse transmission. Current theories favor an immunologic pathogenesis of MS, with or without the presence of a triggering infectious agent. Demyelination results from autoimmune-related inflammation, involving the action of macrophages, lymphocytes, cytokines, antimyelin antibodies, or a combination of these agents. No two individuals with MS are exactly alike, and the clinical manifestations in a particular individual are related to the lesion distribution within the CNS. Lesions may be found virtually anywhere within the white matter regions, which is so called because of the white appearance of the myelinated axons located there. The cerebral hemispheres, brainstem, cerebellum, and spinal cord are particularly vulnerable (see Figure 47-1 and Table 47-2). The affected areas consist of discrete demyelinated plaques that range in size from a few millimeters to several centimeters and are often around the lateral brain ventricles (Figure 47-5).

Clinical Symptoms

Motor symptoms are common and include muscular weakness and spasticity caused by lesions of nerve fibers from the cerebral motor cortex to the spinal cord motor neurons. Lesions in the cerebellar white matter or cerebellar pathways may produce prominent gait and extremity incoordination (ataxia) and a halting or scanning quality of speech. Severe upper-extremity intention tremor may make the simplest self-care tasks impossible, and severe gait ataxia may prevent effective ambulation even when muscular strength is adequate.

Visual disturbances (e.g., impaired visual acuity, impaired color vision, visual field deficits, double vision, optic neuritis, and pain in or behind the eye) are common and may be the first symptom. Other sensory symptoms include numbness, tingling, impairment of temperature sensation, abnormal sense of limb position, and pain. Bladder, bowel, and sexual dysfunction also result from the nerve conduction disturbance. Severe fatigue complaints are common, and exhaustion after an ordinary day's activities may be disabling.

Treatment and Prognosis

The natural progression of MS is unpredictable. Trauma, infection, and surgery have been associated with worsening of MS. Fever, heavy physical exertion, hot weather, a hot shower or bath, and exposure to sunlight may cause a transient and reversible worsening of existing symptoms. In most MS patients the disease is initially exacerbating-remitting, and after several years there is a transition to a slow and relentless chronic progression. In some patients the disease maintains an exacerbating-remitting course, and in others the course is benign, with the patient having only one or two mild exacerbations and no permanent functional disability.

The management of MS includes treating the acute exacerbation with medications, such as steroids, and preventing and treating associated medical and psychologic complications with medications appropriate for the symptoms.

Oral Clinical Findings

Clients with MS exhibit extraoral complications. They often experience facial pain and temporomandibular joint and muscle dysfunction, and sometimes trigeminal neuralgia (see discussion in this chapter). With progression of MS, as the client loses muscular coordination, oral hygiene care is difficult, and the involvement of the tongue and facial muscles interferes with the self-cleansing mechanisms in the oral cavity. Medications may induce xerostomia or gingival enlargement.

Special Considerations for Dental Hygiene Care

Relapses in disease symptoms may be stimulated by various types of infections. Frequent dental hygiene appointments help prevent oral infections and thus prevent exacerbations of the disease process. Short appointments scheduled in the morning may minimize fatigue, and a comfortable, quiet, relaxed environment may reduce stress. The client may be sensitive to heat, so the room temperature must be kept cool. Clients may have incontinence problems, so frequent bathroom breaks may be needed.

Oral Self-Care Instructions

Adaptations for problems in ambulation, muscle weakness, and tremors were discussed at the beginning of the chapter. Disturbances in the MS client's visual acuity must be considered in discussions of oral health maintenance (see discussion of visual deficits). Because of the client's limited dexterity, power or modified toothbrushes may be easier for the client to use. Saliva substitutes and xylitol-containing gum and mints are indicated for dry mouth. Clients may have a slow response to instructions, so visual aids in the office and pamphlets for home are appropriate.

Peripheral Neuropathies

Peripheral neuropathies are abnormalities that affect the PNS. Normally the dendrites of peripheral sensory cranial and spinal nerves receive input (i.e., pain, temperature, touch, pressure, vision, hearing) from the body or external environment, and the axon transmits this information to cells in the CNS. Cells in the CNS process this information and respond via motor nerves to the muscle or internal organs. Interference at any stage impairs the conduction of nerve impulses.

Pain is the most upsetting symptom to the client and the hardest to treat. It can be described in several ways, including burning, constant pain; short jabbing pain; tight or bandlike pressure pain; cold, frostbite-like pain; and painful, sunburn-like hypersensitivity to touch. Other symptoms include paresthesias (prickles or "pins and needles"), sensation loss, unstable balance, sensory loss, or weakness, especially in the lower extremities.

Specific neuropathic conditions are associated with alcoholism (Chapter 52), diabetes (Chapter 44), and human immunodeficiency virus (HIV) infection (Chapter 46). See specific chapters for details.

Facial Neuropathy or Bell's Palsy

Bell's palsy is one of the most common neurologic disorders affecting the cranial nerves and is the most common cause of an acute facial paralysis. The facial nerve (cranial nerve VII) becomes swollen, inflamed, or compressed, which interrupts communication between the brain and facial muscles and leads to facial weakness or paralysis. This disorder can occur at any age, but it is less common before age 15. Pregnant women and individuals with diabetes or upper respiratory ailments are affected disproportionately.[9]

Etiology and Risk Factors

Although the cause is generally unknown, research supports a viral cause. It is thought that the virus triggers edema and inflammation in the facial nerve, leading to infarction and nerve damage. Herpes simplex virus is believed to be the most likely causative virus.[9] Temporary or permanent facial paralysis also may be iatrogenically caused from damage to nerves during intraoral local anesthetic injection or during oral surgery procedures.

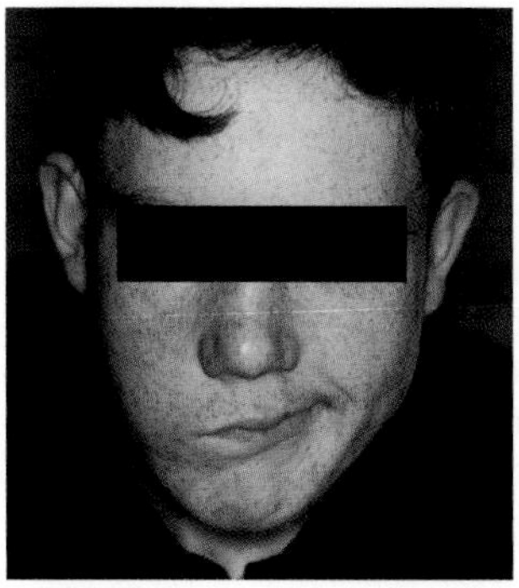

Figure 47-6. Unilateral facial paralysis in a patient with Bell's palsy. On the man's attempt to smile there is a lack of movement of the entire right face and forehead muscles. (From Little JW, Falace DA, Miller CS, et al: *Dental management of the medically compromised patient,* ed 8, St Louis, 2013, Mosby.)

Clinical Symptoms

Patients may describe an abrupt functional impairment. Their face becomes distorted, and they think they have had a stroke (Figure 47-6). Other common signs and symptoms include pain behind the ears, drooling, altered taste, tearing from the eyes, numbness or paralysis on the affected side of the face, and a recent viral syndrome and/or upper respiratory infection.

Treatment and Prognosis

Treatment includes steroids and sometimes antiviral agents, and eye protection with lubricants, artificial tears, and protective eyewear. Other treatments include seventh nerve surgical decompression and galvanic stimulation of paralyzed facial muscles. Most patients recover without cosmetically obvious deformities. With incomplete motor regeneration, patients may have nasal obstruction, excessive tearing, or problems with oral musculature. Incomplete sensory regeneration may result in taste loss or impairment and disagreeable or impaired sensations.

Oral Clinical Findings

Oral musculature numbness affects the ability to chew and to maintain a self-cleansing environment. This numbness could lead to oral trauma, such as cheek biting, and to increased debris on the side of the mouth that is affected. The retention of debris in turn may cause gingivitis and caries. Other common effects are dry mouth, glossitis, and candidiasis.

Special Considerations for Dental Hygiene Care

Adaptations for impaired oral musculature were discussed previously. In addition, the client should wear protective eyewear to prevent foreign material, such as prophylaxis paste, from entering the eye, because the client's eyelids may not close on the affected side of the face.

Oral Self-Care Instructions

Sensation loss impedes the individuals' ability to feel what they are doing during brushing. Establishing a brushing pattern helps the client avoid missing areas. Rinsing with water after eating helps reduce trapped food, which the client may not feel. Use of an oral irrigator also is beneficial.

Trigeminal Neuralgia

Trigeminal neuralgia or tic douloureux is a mononeuropathy of the trigeminal nerve (cranial nerve V) that results in severe pain. The condition is seen more often in females, and most cases occur over the age of 40.[10] It also is observed commonly in clients with multiple sclerosis.[3,10] Some evidence suggests a familial history because of inherited vascular anomalies.[10]

Etiology

Trigeminal neuralgia usually is caused by nerve compression from crossing arteries, benign tumors, or vascular malformations. This pressure can cause wear of the protective myelin sheath around the nerve, leading to abnormal signals to the brain, resulting in pain.

Clinical Symptoms

Trigeminal neuralgia is characterized by sudden, brief, severe lancinating (shooting or sharp stabbing) pains occurring in the distribution of one or more of the branches of the trigeminal nerve. The symptoms are usually unilateral, occur most often in the third or mandibular division, and occur more often on the right side of the face. The pain usually lasts less than a minute and can be triggered by speaking, eating, cold temperatures, or touching the face at specific sites. Pain remission may last months or years, but pain eventually becomes chronic. The condition can be physically and mentally debilitating.

Neurologic examination is usually normal; however, there may be areas of hypesthesia (impaired sensation) in some patients.

Treatment and Prognosis

The first treatment of choice is drug therapy. Anticonvulsant and tricyclic antidepressants commonly are prescribed. Surgical procedures are tried if drug treatment is not tolerated or is ineffective.

Oral Clinical Findings

No significant oral findings are due to the disease alone. Oral ulcerations and xerostomia could result from medications. The patient may avoid oral hygiene owing to the fear that it may trigger pain, therefore increasing the likelihood of plaque-related diseases.

Special Considerations for Dental Hygiene Care

The clinician must be empathetic: to support these clients emotionally as they express their feelings about their pain. Because the pain mimics that of a toothache, a definitive diagnosis can take time and be frustrating to the client and the clinician. Full supine position may relieve pressure on the nerve. Local anesthetic administration may be necessary to relieve tissue pain resulting from manipulation during treatment. Short appointments are recommended to prevent client fatigue. Referral to a pain management physician or support group also is recommended.

Oral Self-Care Instructions

Oral hygiene instruction is individualized to prevent triggering pain.

Spinal Cord Dysfunction

The spinal cord lies within the vertebral column and is the lowest level in the hierarchy of complexity in the CNS. It receives sensory impulses brought in from the periphery, integrates reflex activity, sends motor impulses out to the viscera and skeletal muscles, and/or passes information on to higher CNS structures for synthesis and integration. Connected to the spinal cord are 31 pairs of nerves, which are numbered according to the spinal column level at which they emerge from the spinal cavity. There are eight cervical, 12 thoracic, five lumbar, five sacral, and one coccygeal nerve pairs. All spinal nerves are both sensory and motor.

Spinal Cord Injury

Spinal cord injury (myelopathy) (SCI) may occur from trauma or from diseases such as spina bifida, polio, MS, and cancer. The major causes of SCI are motor vehicle accidents, acts of violence, falls, and sports, especially diving. Most victims are males between the ages of 16 and 30.[11] Injuries result in some function loss in arms and legs (quadriplegia) more commonly than in only trunk and legs (paraplegia). Most victims have some other systemic or head injury.

Clinical Symptoms

The effects of SCI depend on the level and type of injury. The extent of motor function at various levels and the person's potential for independence are indicated in Table 47-4. Clients with SCI also may have problems with temperature and/or blood pressure control, chronic pain, and inability to sweat below the level of the injury.

Treatment and Prognosis

Rehabilitation programs combine physical therapies with skill-building activities and counseling to provide social and emotional support. Even though the spinal cord remains intact, most people with SCI have a loss of function. Only in rare cases do individuals with SCI recover all functioning. The Americans with Disabilities Act (ADA) has promoted mainstreaming people with SCI, but most still are not employed.

People who use ventilators are at risk for respiratory infections and pneumonia. Cutaneous pressure sores (decubitus) are a major concern and if not properly treated can lead to death.

Special Considerations for Dental Hygiene Care

The oral clinical findings and subsequent special considerations for dental hygiene care and oral self-care instructions all depend on the level and type of SCI. Adaptations for specific problems were described previously in this chapter and in Chapter 42. Wheelchair-bound patients may be treated more easily in their wheelchair, either in a reclined or upright position; transferring clients from their wheelchair may risk serious complications (see Chapter 42).

Oral Self-Care Instructions

For clients without the use of their hands, the mouth and teeth play a critical role in performing a variety of tasks. The use of mouth-held appliances assists the client in grasping, stabilizing, and opening objects and contributes to the client's maintenance of independence. A mouthstick for use by quadriplegic persons is illustrated and described in Chapter 42.

TABLE 47-4

Functional Significance of Spinal Cord Lesions

Level	Intact Sensation and Motor Ability	Deficit*	Functional Potential and Independence	Required Aids
C4	Head and upper neck	1, 2, 3, 4	None	WC, ventilator, tracheotomy
C5	Lateral upper arm†	1, 2, 3, 4	Minimal	Electric WC
C6	Lateral forearm and hand†	1, 2, 3, 4	Sitting, eating with devices	Manual WC, hand splints
C7	Middle finger†	1, 2, 3, 4	Personal self-care with devices	Manual WC
C8-T1	Medial hand and forearm†	1, 2, 3, 4	Personal self-care, WC self-transfers	Manual WC
T1-T6	Upper trunk†	2, 3, 4, 5	Complete, WC self-transfers	Manual WC, leg braces
T11-L2	Torso, anterior thigh†	3, 5	Complete, limited walking	Manual WC, leg braces
L4-L5	Medial and lateral leg, dorsal foot†	3, 5	Complete	Foot braces, crutches
S2-S4	Posterior thigh, calf, lateral foot†	4, 6	Complete	Catheter
S5	Complete except ring around anus	None	Complete	None

WC, Wheelchair.
**1,* Quadriplegia; *2,* impaired respiration; *3,* some reflex control of pelvic organs (bowel, bladder), sexual function; *4,* impaired autonomic reflexes, poor thermoregulation, orthostatic hypotension; *5,* paraplegia; *6,* lack of control of pelvic organs.
†Plus regions at preceding levels.

Cleaning the appliance's mouthpiece must be an integral part of the oral self-care regimen. Compliance with procedures to prevent oral disease and subsequent tooth loss is important because edentulousness severely affects the use of these appliances.

Seizures

A **seizure** is a brief (less than 2 minutes) disturbance of cerebral function caused by excessive abnormal neuronal discharge. Seizures are common, and during one's lifetime there is a 10% chance of having one and a 2% to 4% chance of having more than one.[3] About 1% of children have at least one seizure, usually associated with a high fever, during the first 15 years of life.[3] Seizures in the elderly commonly are related to cerebrovascular disease.[3]

Etiology and Risk Factors

Seizures result from primary CNS dysfunction, an underlying systemic or metabolic disorder, or may be clearly linked to infection or trauma (Box 47-1). The specific cause is unknown in most cases. During a seizure there may be a loss or altered state of consciousness, abnormal or cessation of motor activity, abnormal sensory perceptions, and/or loss of bowel and bladder control.

Epilepsy

Epilepsy is a seizure disorder in which the excessive abnormal neuronal discharges from cerebral function disturbances are recurrent. The specific underlying brain dysfunction causing the seizure disorder can be identified only in approximately half of childhood-onset and adult-onset seizures.

Pathologic Characteristics and Clinical Symptoms

There are many types of seizures. Only three of the common ones are described here.[3]

BOX 47-1

Causes of Seizures

Genetic: Inborn errors of metabolism
Congenital abnormalities: Maldevelopment of brain
Perinatal: Anoxia, ischemia, hemorrhage
Central nervous system infections: Encephalitis, meningitis, abscess
Trauma: Penetrating wound, closed head injury, surgery
Neoplastic: Primary gliomas, metastatic
Vascular: Infarction, hemorrhage, arteriovenous malformations
Toxic: Alcohol or cocaine use, alcohol and sedative drug withdrawal
Metabolic: Hypoglycemia, hypocalcemia, high fever
Degenerative: Alzheimer's disease, Creutzfeldt-Jakob disease

Adapted from Collins R: *Neurology,* Philadelphia, 1997, Saunders.

- **Tonic-clonic seizures (grand mal)** are the most common type and can be divided into several phases, beginning with vague prodromal symptoms (aura) that occur hours to days before the convulsion. A series of brief, bilateral muscle contractions may precede the tonic phase. Tonic (stiffening) contractions begin in the trunk and progress, including contraction of abdominal muscles, producing forced expiration across the spasmodic glottis and causing the characteristic vocalization (Figure 47-7). The clonic (convulsion) phase begins after generalized extension, with tonic contractions alternating with loss of muscle tone, causing rhythmic jerking of all four extremities, until contractions cease (Figure 47-8). Autonomic dysfunction (loss of bowel and bladder control) often occurs during the tonic and clonic phases. Persons experiencing seizures may bite the tongue or break bones as a result of the violence of the jerking during the clonic phase. Afterward the

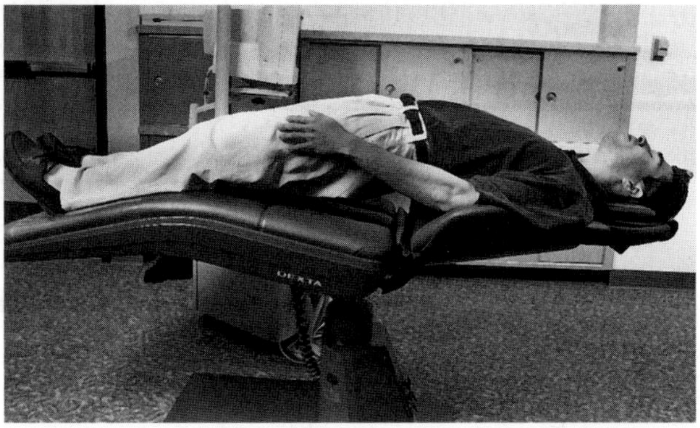

Figure 47-7. A patient during the tonic phase of a generalized tonic-clonic seizure (grand mal). Note the extensor rigidity of the extremities and trunk. (Adapted from Malamed SF: *Medical emergencies in the dental office,* ed 6, St Louis, 2007, Mosby.)

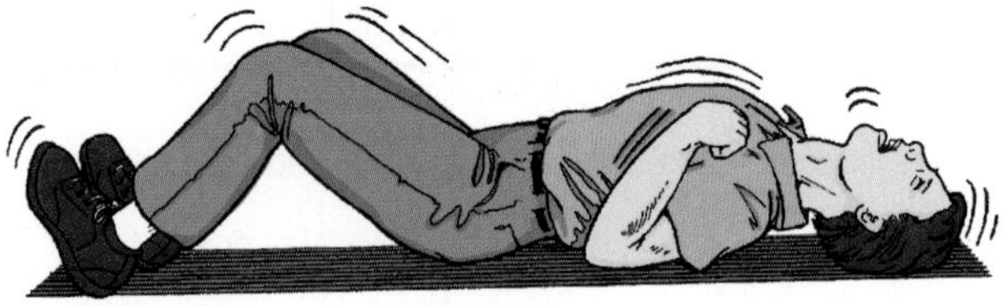

Figure 47-8. Diagrammatic representation of the violent flexor contractions of the clonic phase of a generalized tonic-clonic seizure (grand mal). (Adapted from Malamed SF: *Medical emergencies in the dental office,* ed 6, St Louis, 2007, Mosby.)

individual may enter a deep sleep or experience headaches, muscle aches, and stiffness.

- Typical **absence (petit mal) seizures** are familial and occur almost exclusively in childhood between the ages of 3 and 12 years. The seizures consist of brief (10 to 30 seconds) episodes of altered states of consciousness during which the child has a vacant stare and sometimes eyelid blinking or lip smacking. Muscle tone is maintained. After the seizure the child goes on with normal activities and has no recollection of the seizure.
- **Status epilepticus** is defined as a single seizure lasting for at least 20 minutes or recurrent generalized seizures without regaining of consciousness between the seizure episodes. This is a life-threatening medical emergency and requires prompt and intensive therapy.

Treatment and Prognosis

Anticonvulsant medications, such as phenytoin (Dilantin), are effective in preventing most seizures, and several are available. Sometimes the side effects are worse than the disorder (e.g., when a person has one seizure a year at night), in which case medication is not used.

Oral Clinical Findings

Seizures and epilepsy themselves do not produce oral changes, but the accidents resulting during the seizures and the medications to treat the condition may. Scarring of the lips, buccal mucosa, and especially the tongue may be indicative of past injury to the oral cavity during a seizure. Teeth also may have been injured—fractured from the forceful

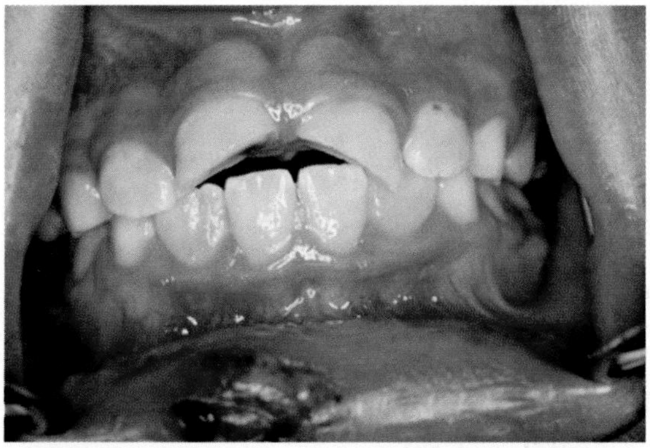

Figure 47-9. Fractured teeth and lacerated lower lip sustained during a grand mal seizure. (From Little JW, Falace DA, Miller CS, et al: *Dental management of the medically compromised patient,* ed 8, St Louis, 2013, Mosby.)

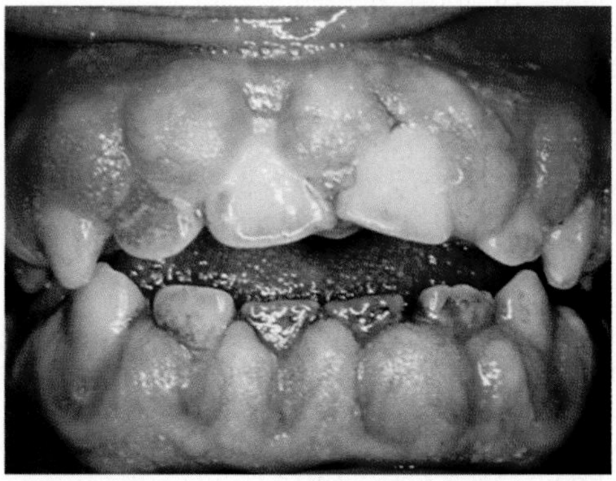

Figure 47-10. Phenytoin-induced gingival enlargement. (From Little JW, Falace DA, Miller CS, et al: *Dental management of the medically compromised patient,* ed 8, St Louis, 2013, Mosby.)

biting that frequently occurs during a grand mal seizure (Figure 47-9). Phenytoin, a common medication to control seizures, may cause severe gingival enlargement or overgrowth (Figure 47-10). The drug alters the metabolism of the gingival fibroblasts so that the cells produce excessive amounts of collagen. This drug-influenced gingival enlargement, which occurs in approximately half of these clients, may be disfiguring and may interfere with mastication and speech.

Special Considerations for Dental Hygiene Care

Major considerations in epileptic client management are prevention of seizures in the dental chair and preparation for managing seizures if they occur. When a client responds positively to seizures on a health history form, further information should be obtained. Examples of questions one could ask are listed in Chapter 12. Based on the client's responses, one may choose to postpone treatment for fear of triggering a seizure in the dental chair. Nitrous oxide and oxygen sedation is known to elicit seizures in epileptics, so it is not recommended for them. Likewise, fatigue can induce seizures, so appointments should be made early in the day. Despite all preventive measures, seizures may still occur. Management focuses on preventing injury and maintaining adequate ventilation. (See Chapter 10.)

Dental hygiene maintenance appointments should be established based on the presence or severity of gingival enlargement induced by phenytoin.

Oral Self-Care Instructions

Frequent maintenance visits, along with immaculate self-care, have been shown to diminish the drug-induced gingival changes, so it is imperative that oral hygiene instruction be stressed at every appointment.

Disorders of Higher Cortical Function

Dementia

Dementia is characterized by a progressive intellectual decline that eventually leads to deterioration of occupational, social, and interpersonal functions Onset is usually insidious, with memory disturbances frequently attributed to the normal aging process. Even though dementia may occur at all ages, the incidence of most dementias, including Alzheimer's disease (AD), rises substantially with increasing age. Dementia differs from the decline of physiologic processes during aging. In old age mental processes become slowed, but the older healthy person still retains a firm grasp on reality, is oriented, can reason, has good judgment, and can continue to lead an active and self-supporting life. Further characteristics of the normal elderly client are described in Chapter 55.

Etiology and Risk Factors

All forms of dementia result from the death of nerve cells and/or the loss of communication among these cells. Although genes play a role, a single abnormal gene has not been associated with the condition.[12] Major risk factors are age and genetics/family history,[12] but risk factors also may include metabolic disorders, anemia, hypoxia and anoxia, brain tumor, trauma, infections, deficiency diseases, toxins, and medications.

Clinical Symptoms

In early stages individuals often complain of diminished energy and enthusiasm, show less interest in subjects they previously cherished, and may show emotional instability and heightened anxiety levels because of the awareness of failing mental functions. As the disease progresses, other areas of cognition become impaired: orientation, language, perceptions, ability to learn new skills, calculation, abstraction, and judgment. The patient becomes increasingly self-absorbed, anxiety increases, and the recognition of personal failure may lead to depression. At this stage there may be pronounced mood swings and poor judgment, followed by diminished drive and feeling. As the mental deterioration progresses, anxiety and depression disappear and are replaced by complete flatness of mood. Personal cleanliness deteriorates and patients will do little, if anything, spontaneously. At this stage, other neurologic dysfunctions, such as hemiparesis (one-sided weakness) and seizures, may develop. Once the patient has reached the point of complete flatness of mood, inability to communicate, and total dependence on others, even treatable dementias are usually irreversible. Consciousness is preserved until terminal stages.

Alzheimer's Disease

Alzheimer's disease (AD) is a brain degenerative disorder that gradually destroys the ability to remember, reason, learn, and imagine. It is the most common form of dementia, affecting 10% or more of those older than 65 years and approximately 50% of those older than age 85.[3]

Etiology and Risk Factors

The etiology of Alzheimer's disease is similar to that described for dementia, with age as a significant risk factor. Researchers have identified several genes, which influence susceptibility to AD, so genetics and family history also are associated with the development of the disease.[12] Other risk factors include smoking and alcohol use, atherosclerosis, and Down syndrome.

Pathologic Characteristics

The brain lesions of AD are characterized by amyloid plaques, which are abnormal clumps of beta-amyloid protein and degenerating neurons and other cells, and neurofibrillary tangles, which are irregular knots of cytoskeletal intermediate filaments found within neurons. Both contribute to the progressive destruction of neurons and atrophy of the cerebral cortex, the area of the brain associated with intellectual functions (Figure 47-11).

Clinical Symptoms

In the early and middle stages of AD, affected individuals may be painfully aware of their intellectual decline, and it is important to support their emotional and mental health with affection and warmth. In the beginning there is simple forgetfulness, especially of directions to familiar places or recent events. There also may be personality changes such as restlessness, increased stubbornness, distrust, poor judgment and impulse control, and increased difficulty with activities requiring planning and decision making. Affected individuals may begin to withdraw socially. As the disease progresses, the ability to perform daily living tasks is lost, and there may be trouble recognizing everyone except the person's closest daily companions. Communication becomes difficult as written and spoken language decline. In the last stages of the disease, patients with AD become bedridden, unable to recognize themselves or their closest family members.

Treatment and Prognosis

Because there is no cure for AD, treatment is aimed at prevention, slowing progression of the disease, and improving quality

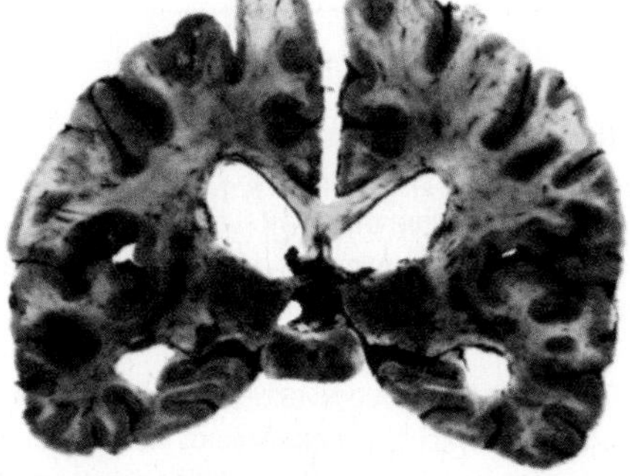

Figure 47-11. Coronal section of the brain from a patient with Alzheimer's disease. The degeneration of the cerebral cortex neurons leads to the thinning of the cortex and secondary enlargement of the lateral ventricles. (From Perkin G: *Mosby's color atlas and text of neurology*, London, 1998, Mosby-Wolfe.)

of life for the patients. Some of the dying neurons use acetylcholine for a neurotransmitter, so acetylcholine drugs are used to improve cognition, although the effects are not permanent. The period from the earliest symptoms to death has an average duration of 8 years. Death usually results from a secondary illness such as urinary tract infection or pneumonia.

Oral Clinical Findings

Clients with AD have more gingival disease and caries than the normal elderly population, mainly because of poor oral hygiene from significant neglect. Clients forget to brush, forget how to brush, may not want to brush, or may be resistant to a caregiver brushing their teeth. Medications, such as phenytoin to control seizures, may cause gingival enlargement (see Figure 47-10), and many induce salivary gland dysfunction.

An association of AD with periodontal disease has been suggested by the observation of components of oral microorganisms in brain tissue of AD patients (see Chapter 20).

Special Considerations for Dental Hygiene Care

A frightened and frustrated client may demonstrate uncooperative, even combative, behavior, so clients with AD are managed best with a caring and understanding approach (Box 47-2). Appointments should be scheduled early in the day and preferably when the office is not busy. The office environment should be as free of unnecessary noise, people, and physical clutter as possible. The caregiver should accompany the client to discuss special client management issues as well as oral care procedures.

Oral Self-Care Instructions

In the early stages of AD the client should be encouraged to be self-sufficient. Toothbrushing instructions should be given slowly, step by step, in simple, concrete language. As the disease progresses, the client becomes more dependent on his or her caregiver for oral homecare, so the caregiver needs to be familiar with these procedures. Although a power toothbrush may be easier for a caregiver to use on the client, electrical appliances are known to disturb or be a safety concern to some individuals with AD. Mouth rinses are not usually recommended because the client may not understand that it would be harmful to swallow.

BOX 47-2

Techniques for Communicating with Clients with Alzheimer's Disease

- Use a calm, soft voice pattern.
- Be cheerful and reassuring.
- Speak slowly and clearly, in short sentences.
- Allow ample time for comprehension.
- Explain procedures before treatment.
- Repeat instructions and explanations in exactly the same words.
- Tell clients what you need them to do instead of giving them a choice.
- Distract clients who are uncooperative or argumentative by changing the activity, or take advantage of their forgetfulness by leaving the room for a few minutes and then returning and cheerfully trying the same activity again.
- Use supportive body posture and facial motion, such as direct eye contact and smiling.

Cerebrovascular Disease

Cerebrovascular Accident or Stroke

Cerebrovascular accident (CVA) or stroke is an abrupt onset of neurologic deficits caused by an interruption of oxygenated blood to the brain, as a result of either ischemia or hemorrhage. It is the fourth most frequent cause of death in the United States, following heart disease, cancer, and chronic lower respiratory diseases.[13] Approximately one-half million people per year in the United States are expected to experience strokes of all causes.[2] It is the major cause of serious, long-term disability in adults.

Etiology and Risk Factors

Risk factors for stroke are listed in Box 47-3. The major factor is hypertension because of its relationship to atherosclerosis or narrowing of the arteries. Hypertension is in most instances a treatable condition, so the single most important measure in preventing strokes is detection and treatment of hypertension.

Pathologic Characteristics

The most common type of CVA, ischemic stroke, results from a lack of oxygen supply to the brain resulting from an occlusion of blood supply. The diminished or lack of blood flow into the brain tissues results from embolism (occlusion of an artery), atherothrombosis (fatty clot within a blood vessel), or systemic hypoperfusion (e.g., from cardiac pump failure).[3] The ischemia leads to infarction (necrosis or death) of brain tissue supplied by the affected artery or arteries. The other type of CVA, hemorrhagic stroke, results from hemorrhage or

BOX 47-3

Risk Factors for Stroke

Common Risk Factors
- Transient ischemic attack
- Recent stroke
- Hypertension
- Cigarette smoking
- Cardiac diseases
- Diabetes mellitus

Uncommon Risk Factors
- Inflammatory disorders
- Hematologic disorders
- Coagulation disorders
- Drug abuse

Possible Risk Factors
- Oral contraceptives
- Obesity
- Physical inactivity
- Alcohol
- Pregnancy

Adapted from Collins R: *Neurology*, Philadelphia, 1997, Saunders.

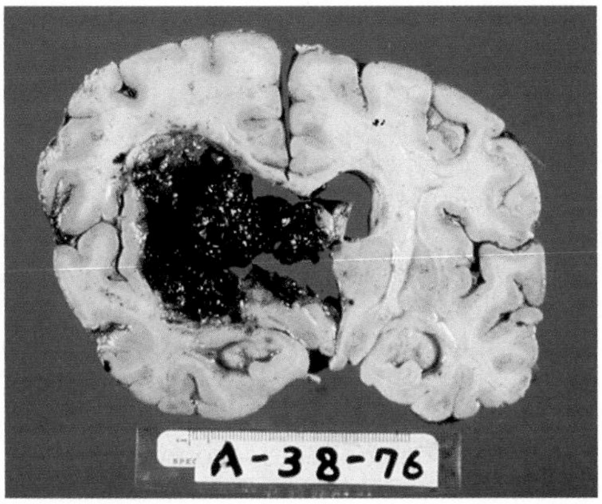

Figure 47-12. Cerebral infarction in an individual who had chronic hypertension. The blood from the intracerebral hemorrhage has displaced the brain tissue. (From Little JW, Falace DA, Miller CS, et al: *Dental management of the medically compromised patient,* ed 8, St Louis, 2013, Mosby.)

BOX 47-4

Differences Between Right-Sided Brain Damage and Left-Sided Brain Damage

RIGHT-SIDED BRAIN DAMAGE	LEFT-SIDED BRAIN DAMAGE
Paralyzed left side	Paralyzed right side
Spatial or perceptual deficits	Language and speech problems
Impaired thought	Decreased auditory memory (cannot remember long instructions)
Quick, impulsive behavior	Slow, cautious, disorganized behavior
Patient cannot use mirror	Memory deficits—language-based
Difficulty performing tasks (toothbrushing)	Anxiety
Neglect of left side	

Adapted from Little JW, Falace DA, Miller CS, et al: *Dental management of the medically compromised patient,* ed 7, St Louis, 2008, Mosby.

rupture of a brain vessel, which causes leakage of blood into the brain tissue, the ventricles, or the space between the brain and skull. The resultant hematoma exerts pressure on brain tissue, causing infarction of adjacent tissue (Figure 47-12).

Regardless of the underlying cause of a stroke, a certain part of the brain does not receive an adequate blood supply for a period of time. If brain tissue is deprived of blood supply for 10 to 20 minutes, infarction will occur. Occlusion of a given artery does not necessarily imply brain tissue infarction in the perfusion territory of that blood vessel because adequate collateral circulation may exist. If adequate blood supply is restored to the brain within time, there will be total resolution of the neurologic deficit. A transient ischemic attack (TIA) is a transient focal neurologic deficit that persists for less than 24 hours and is followed by complete clinical recovery. Most TIAs do not last longer than 10 to 20 minutes.

The right and left hemispheres specialize in different functions, and the two sides of the brain are interconnected. Sensory and motor axons cross on their way to or from the cerebral cortex, so the left side of the brain controls motor and sensory input for the right side of the body and vice versa. Therefore the side of the face and body affected is opposite that of the brain injury. Box 47-4 illustrates the differences between right-sided and left-sided brain damage.[3]

Clinical Symptoms

Stroke can cause various health complications. Signs and symptoms depend on the brain sites affected, but the following are the more common ones:

- Motor impairments. These are the most common deficits and usually involve face, arm, and leg, alone or in combination on the same side. Motor functions affected include cranial nerve functions to muscles of the head and neck, reflexes, gait, balance, and coordination. Often there is apraxia (the inability to perform purposeful movements), although no muscular paralysis or sensory disturbance is present.
- Sensory deficits. Impairments range from loss of primary senses (e.g., vision, pain, temperature, touch) to more complex losses of perception.
- Language and cognition. There is often dysphasia after a stroke, manifested by disturbances in comprehension, repetition, naming, fluency, reading, or writing. Strokes can cause deficits in memory, calculation abilities, attention, and orientation.
- Depression. This is the most common affective disturbance after a stroke. Symptoms of depression include lack of interests, energy loss, insomnia, and appetite loss. Stroke patients also may display emotional instability.

Treatment and Prognosis

Treatment for stroke survivors primarily involves reducing the risk factors, as listed in Box 47-3, and prescribing anticoagulants to prevent clot formation, antihypertensive agents to reduce blood pressure, and aspirin to thin blood. Occupational and physical therapy can help the stroke survivor learn new ways of performing activities of daily living, sometimes with the aid of assistive devices such as braces, wheelchairs, and special utensils.

Oral Clinical Findings

The specific oral findings of a CVA survivor depend on the areas of the brain affected and the type of CVA, as well as the resultant dysfunction. Motor dysfunction effects and xerostomic effects of prescribed medications have been described previously. Dental caries and periodontal diseases are prevalent because of poor oral hygiene. Periodontal disease is associated with the risk of stroke, as well as heart disease (see Chapter 20). Although periodontal pathogen invasion into the periodontium induces bacteremia and a systemic inflammatory response, a causal relationship has not been established.

Special Considerations for Dental Hygiene Care

It is recommended that the stroke survivor not undergo any elective dental care within 6 months of the episode. A positive response to stroke on the health history form should elicit several follow-up questions, which are listed in Chapter 12. This information determines the need for treatment modifications. A client who has had a stroke or TIA is at a greater risk for having another one, so prevention of a recurrence is of utmost concern. Factors such as pain and anxiety add to the risk and so must be managed by creating a safe and comfortable environment. Efforts should be made to minimize fatigue and optimize energy and patience for clinician and client.

Adaptations for these clients' problems in ambulation and muscle weakness were described previously.

Blood pressure should be monitored carefully because marked deviations in blood pressure increase the risk for recurrent CVAs. Blood pressure of 200 mg systolic and/or 115 mg diastolic or higher warrants immediate medical consultation before dental treatment is initiated. Many CVA and TIA survivors receive anticoagulant therapy, which predisposes them to excessive bleeding. Physician consultation is needed to determine whether the therapy should be altered. The physician also must be consulted regarding prophylactic premedication necessity. Oral infection presence may cause changes in blood coagulation factors, which may trigger a repeat CVA. The minimum amount of a local anesthetic with vasoconstrictor is recommended.

Oral Self-Care Instructions

During the immediate poststroke phase, caregivers perform all the daily hygiene functions; therefore they need proper toothbrushing demonstrations and instructions and/or information about maintenance of any dental prosthesis so that they can perform these tasks until the client has relearned them. Even during the rehabilitation phase, clients with residual physical deficits may need assistance performing oral hygiene procedures. Special adaptations that foster the stroke survivor's self-sufficiency were described previously and in Chapter 42.

The discomfort from xerostomia can be alleviated by saliva substitutes and associated dry mouth products (see Chapter 55). Fluoride therapy and xylitol gum and mints are beneficial to prevent root caries (see Chapter 33).

Sensory Disorders

Deficits in Hearing

Hearing loss is the third most common chronic condition in the older population. Approximately 17% (36 million) of American adults report some degree of hearing loss, and 47% of adults 75 years old or older have a deficit.[14] About 2 to 3 out of every 1000 children in the United States are born deaf or hard of hearing.[14] This loss can cause developmental delays of speech and language. Language deficits lead to learning problems, which cause decreased academic achievement. Communication problems also can lead to poor self-concept and social isolation.

Etiology and Clinical Symptoms

Hearing loss is classified based on what part or where in the auditory system there is damage.

- Sensorineural hearing loss occurs when there is damage to the inner ear (cochlea) or to nerve pathways in the auditory nerve (cranial nerve VIII) between the cochlea and the brainstem. This type of loss can be caused by drugs that are toxic to the auditory system (aspirin), viruses, diseases, birth injury, noise exposure, head trauma, tumors, genetic syndromes, and aging. In addition to loss of volume, nerve damage is associated with high-frequency loss, and there are deficits in hearing clearly or understanding speech. Sensorineural hearing loss is a permanent loss.
- Central auditory processing disorders occur when the central auditory processing center (the temporal lobe of the cerebral hemisphere) (see Figure 47-1) is damaged by tumors, diseases, infarcts, heredity, or unknown causes. This type of loss involves problems with sound localization, auditory discrimination, temporal aspects of sound, auditory pattern recognition, and the ability to hear decreasing or competing acoustic signals.

Exposure time length and noise intensity determine effects on hearing loss. The severity of hearing loss is described as the lowest value (decibels or dB) of sound heard at three different frequencies. The normal range is 10 to 15 dB, and values progressively increase with greater impairment. For example, 71 to 90 dB is the severe loss range. Sounds greater than 80 dB are potentially dangerous. Hair cells of the inner ear can be damaged by brief intense sounds, such as an explosion, or by continuous or repeated noise exposure.

Oral Clinical Findings

No specific oral clinical findings are associated with hearing deficits; however, the overall oral health of clients who are deaf or hearing impaired may be compromised because of their limited access to dental care and information.

Special Considerations for Dental Hygiene Care

Communication is the major challenge in achieving and maintaining optimal oral health in clients with hearing deficits. Scheduling and confirming appointments for clients who are deaf or hearing impaired should be conducted by mail, either regular or electronic. Suggestions for facilitating communication with clients with impaired hearing are listed in Box 47-5.

BOX 47-5

Techniques for Communicating with Clients with Impaired Hearing

- Get the client's attention. Do not startle the client when entering the room. Do not approach a client from behind.
- Face the client and stand or sit on the same level. Be sure your face and lips are illuminated to promote lipreading. Keep hands away from mouth. Remove mask.
- If the client wears a hearing aid, make sure it is in place and working before speaking.
- If the client wears glasses, be sure they are on so that your gestures and face can be seen.
- Speak slowly and articulate clearly. Older adults may take longer to process verbal messages.
- Use a normal tone of voice and inflections of speech.
- Do not shout. Loud sounds are usually higher pitched and may impede hearing by accentuating vowel sounds and concealing consonants. If it is necessary to raise your voice, speak in lower tones.
- When you are not understood, rephrase rather than repeat the conversation.
- Use visible expressions. Speak with your hands, your face, and your eyes.
- Talk toward the client's best or normal ear.
- Use written information to enhance the spoken word.

Adapted from Potter PA, Perry AG: *Fundamentals of nursing*, ed 8, St Louis, 2013, Mosby.

Each communication mode has advantages and disadvantages. For each deaf client the preferred mode of communication initially must be established.

- Lipreading or speech reading is difficult to learn and use. Only about 30% of sounds in the English language are visible on the lips. Many sounds appear the same on the lips, and others are not visible at all. Speaking should occur at a natural pace without exaggerated lip movements. Any exaggeration distorts the visible lip pattern for the reader. Although most deaf people can lip-read to some extent, few rely on this method alone.
- American Sign Language (ASL) is the primary means of interpersonal communication for persons who have had a hearing loss since early life. ASL consists of its own vocabulary, idioms, grammar, and syntax, distinct from written and spoken English. Body gestures and facial expressions help convey meaning. The knowledge of a few specific signs may be beneficial for health professionals. ASL classes are widely available, offered at community colleges, universities, and Red Cross chapters.
- Finger spelling (American manual alphabet) is the manual reproduction of English using the hands and fingers. It is tiring and time-consuming; therefore it is used primarily to supplement ASL for proper names and for words that do not have a present sign.
- Interpreter use to translate the spoken words into sign language is costly and limits the client's privacy; however, according to the ADA, the dental office, being a place of public accommodations, must retain and pay for an interpreter if one is needed to achieve equally effective communication. When using an interpreter, practitioners still should focus on the client.
- Writing is probably the best method of communication when the speaker does not know sign language; however, it is time consuming. Some deaf persons do not read or write beyond the fifth-grade level, so your notes must be kept simple and easy to read. Paper and pencil should be located conveniently and disposed of after the visit to prevent cross-contamination. Laminated cards of expressions and phrases commonly used during treatment are also useful.
- Electronic aids are available to facilitate communication. Teletypewriters (TTYs) and telecommunications devices (TDDs), containing an alphanumeric keyboard and an LCD screen, function to send text messages back and forth by telephone; however, both parties must have the equipment. In recent years, electronic mail probably has assumed that function as computers and Internet access are more widely available. Clients with limited hearing also may prefer this mode of communication.

Clients with hearing impairments who wear hearing aids require specific modifications in the dental environment. Although most hearing aids amplify all sounds, some of the newer ones do have a directional microphone to decrease extraneous sounds. In either case, all extrinsic noise should be eliminated or reduced to minimize the client's discomfort. Background music should be turned off, as should the saliva ejector and suction when not in use. Unnecessary instrument rattling should be avoided. The hearing aid should be turned down or removed when ultrasonic scalers or dental handpieces are used but turned on again for oral hygiene instruction.

Oral Self-Care Instructions

Correct brushing and flossing techniques should be demonstrated step by step on clients while they watch in the mirror. Disclosing agents help identify plaque biofilm, and visual aids such as pictures and diagrams are useful to discuss the disease process. Written instructions and pamphlets or brochures on brushing, flossing, and causes of gum disease promote clients' understanding of plaque control and the importance of preventing gingivitis and periodontitis.

Deficits in Vision

Visual deficits can occur anywhere from the eye via the optic nerve (cranial nerve II) to the visual region (occipital lobe) of the cerebral cortex (see Figure 47-1). Terms used to describe common visual deficits are defined in Box 47-6.

In the United States there are approximately 4 million (3%) adults who are blind and visually impaired over the age of 40, of which about 1.3 million (1%) of them are legally blind.[15] Over the age of 80 the percentages increase to about 7% blind and 17% visually impaired.[16]

Etiology and Clinical Symptoms

In general visual impairment can be congenital, perinatal, and postnatal and be caused by trauma, disease, or aging. Age-related loss is the one most commonly observed in the dental office. The following are descriptions of these types of visual deficits:

- Glaucoma is the leading cause of blindness among African Americans and the second most common leading cause of blindness in the United States. It is caused by a buildup of pressure in the eye, with resultant optic nerve damage. Side vision is affected before central vision. It cannot be prevented but usually can be controlled with medication.
- Macular degeneration (age-related macular disease) is the leading cause of vision impairment and legal blindness in individuals 50 years of age and older. There is damage to the central visual area, the macula, which is responsible for the ability to see central vision and detail.

BOX 47-6

Descriptive Terms for Visual Deficits

Low vision: Vision that cannot be improved with corrective aids or surgery

Legal blindness: A field of vision 20 degrees or less in its widest diameter, or central visual acuity for distance 20/200 or less in the better eye with correction

Functional blindness: No useful vision

Myopia (nearsightedness): Blurred vision caused by focusing light in front of the retina, usually because the eyeball is elongated

Hyperopia (farsightedness): Blurred vision caused by focusing light behind the retina, usually because the eyeball is too small or short

Astigmatism: Distortion of the focus of light caused by an irregularly curved cornea

Presbyopia: Loss of accommodation or eye's ability to focus and adjust the eye on the distance between the object and the individual; decreased elasticity of the lens with age, with a progressive loss of focusing ability for near vision

- Diabetic retinopathy is a diabetes complication caused by retinal blood vessel damage. There are effective surgical treatments, so early detection is important to prevent visual loss.
- Cataract is a clouding of the lens preventing light from passing through the lens and thus causing vision to become blurred or hazy. Surgical lens removal and replacement with an intraocular human-made lens is safe and successful.

Oral Clinical Findings

Oral abnormalities would not be expected to occur at a greater rate than in the sighted population, unless a blind or visually impaired person has other medical conditions or disabilities. There may be a greater incidence of poor oral hygiene and the subsequent gingivitis and periodontitis because of the client not being able to see her or his oral hygiene efforts and possibly from not having received effective oral hygiene instructions.

Special Considerations for Dental Hygiene Care

Minor adaptations in client management must be made to accommodate clients with visual impairments effectively, mostly increased verbal descriptions of surroundings and procedures. When a person who is blind or visually impaired arrives in the dental office, he or she should be greeted by someone who acclimates them to the layout of the reception area, especially furniture location and available chairs. When clinicians greet the client in the reception area, they should introduce themselves each time. If at the initial appointment the clinician describes himself or herself, the client is better able to form an image of the clinician as a person. Other office staff should be introduced so that the client can recognize their voices whenever they speak because the client will be hearing the noises, movements, and conversations of others in the background.

Box 47-7 offers suggestions to be used when leading the client to the treatment room. All obstacles should have been cleared away previously. New clients are informed how the operatory is set up, and for returning clients, any changes, especially new furniture arrangements, are described. Guide dogs are permitted to remain in the treatment area so that they can be kept close to their master at all times. The dog should not be distracted or touched but led to a nearby but out-of-the way corner.

For clinical procedures, each step should be described in detail before proceeding, as well as all instruments and materials and their application; for example, the flavor, taste, and feeling of each dental material. Clients can be allowed to handle instruments, but assistance is required when the client explores instruments with sharp ends. A second set of sterilized instruments is used for the actual care. Also, clients can be allowed to feel a moving prophylactic cup on a fingernail. Tapping the mirror and explorer together allows the client to obtain a sense of what these objects sound like when they come in contact with each other. Informing clients first avoids surprising them with sounds, such as from the evacuator, and with movements, such as of the chair, air, water, or power-driven instruments. Maintaining contact of a finger on a tooth or through retraction, while changing instruments, avoids repeated orientation. Clients always should be told when the clinician is leaving and reentering the room to avoid embarrassment.

BOX 47-7

Sighted Guide Techniques to Assist a Person Who Is Blind

- Offer the person who is blind your assistance.
- If assistance is accepted, brush your arm against his or her arm or tap the back of your hand against his or her hand. The person will then grasp your arm just above the elbow. Children will grasp your wrist or hold your hand.
- Walk at a normal pace, staying one step ahead of him or her. Continually describe changes in terrain, as well as stairs, narrow spaces, and so on.
- When approaching a narrow area, such as a doorway, move your forearm and hand so that they rest against the lower portion of your back. The person who is blind will take this cue and move directly behind you at an arm's length.
- To assist seating, guide the patient to the back of the chair. Guide his or her hand over the back, arm, and seat portion of the chair, and then allow the client to seat himself or herself.

Adapted from *Sighted guide techniques*, Braille Institute, 741 N. Vermont Ave., Los Angeles, CA 90029.

Oral Self-Care Instructions

Oral hygiene instruction for clients who are blind can be approached in several ways, all involving clear verbal, step-by-step technique descriptions. One method begins with the client demonstrating current brushing technique in his or her own mouth. Deficiencies can be refined and corrected by the clinician, who places a hand on the client's hand to guide hand position and movements while concurrently verbally describing the technique. Another way of demonstrating proper brushing is for the clinician to perform the task inside the client's mouth. To help children become aware of a clean feeling in the mouth, they can be taught to feel their teeth with the tongue. Flossing is approached in a similar manner. Clients should be told that they should hear the teeth squeak with the floss when the tooth surface is clean. Audiotapes or materials prepared in Braille can be provided to supplement verbal explanations of plaque biofilm and oral disease process.

When oral hygiene instructions are given to clients who are visually impaired, the following factors are considered. Clients should be positioned for the best view and should be wearing their eyeglasses before instructions are started. Clients should not be expected to be able to see fine detail, such as on a radiograph. Written instructions and educational materials in large print must be provided for clients to take home and read at their own pace.

CLIENT EDUCATION TIPS

- Individualize recommendations and expectations for self-care based on evaluating the physical and mental condition of the client.
- Encourage clients to maintain their own oral health for as long as their physical condition allows.
- Facilitate the client's self-sufficiency by modified oral hygiene aids: toothbrushes with adapted handles, power toothbrushes, toothpaste tubes with flip-top caps or pump

dispensers, and floss holders. Twice-daily use of an antimicrobial mouth rinse also is recommended.
- Educate caregivers about the importance of disease prevention as well as plaque control procedures and client positioning for maximal stability and access.
- Provide written and oral instructions to the client and the caregiver so that the information can be reviewed at home.

LEGAL, ETHICAL, AND SAFETY ISSUES

- The dental hygienist should not refuse to care for persons with disabilities because Title III of the Americans with Disabilities Act "makes it illegal to discriminate against persons with disabilities, and those with whom they associate, in the provision of services in places of public accommodation."
- The dental hygienist should obtain informed consent from all clients or their legal caregivers for the performance of all procedures.
- The dental hygienist should be prepared to manage medical emergencies, such as a generalized tonic-clonic seizure, a stroke, or airway obstruction.
- The dental hygienist should be prepared to assist a client in walking safely and in transferring a wheelchair-confined client to the dental chair.
- The dental hygienist should assess carefully vital signs and medications to determine the safety of delivering dental hygiene care to the client.
- The operatory should be clear of all obstacles to prevent accidents from happening to visually or physically impaired clients.

KEY CONCEPTS

- Poor oral hygiene frequently is observed in clients with neurologic deficits because of the following reasons: their poor muscle coordination limits their ability to perform self-care; disturbances in tongue and facial muscles interfere with self-cleaning mechanisms; and when completely debilitated they must depend on caregivers, who may be overwhelmed.
- Xerostomia, which often results from medications, leads to susceptibility to oral infections and root caries, taste dysfunctions, and difficulty in swallowing.
- Malocclusion results from abnormal functioning of the musculature in conjunction with oral habits such as tongue thrusting, mouth breathing, and faulty swallowing.
- Medications, such as phenytoin to control seizures, may cause gingival enlargement. Immaculate self-care and frequent maintenance appointments may diminish this condition.
- Disturbances in musculature cause impaired swallowing and gag reflexes. Good suctioning techniques and possibly an upright position may prevent choking and aspiration of water and foreign substances.
- Stabilizing the client is a concern with clients who have impaired motor control. The head and jaw can be supported by physically cradling the head and using mouth props. Body movements may need to be limited, preferably by the caregiver restraining the client, but physical restraints, such as belts, may be used if necessary.
- Communication with clients with impaired hearing is facilitated by reducing all extraneous noise and articulating clearly. Deaf clients may prefer a specific mode of communication.
- Enhanced verbal descriptions of surroundings and procedures are necessary to care for clients with visual deficits.
- Communicating with clients who have impaired mental function is facilitated by speaking slowly, with direct commands.
- Power toothbrushes or toothbrushes with adapted handles may be easier to maneuver when muscle strength or range of motion is impaired and also when used by a caregiver.
- Caregivers must be educated about the importance of disease prevention as well as plaque control procedures and client positioning for maximal stability and access.

CRITICAL THINKING EXERCISES

Client: Mrs. M.

Profile: Mrs. M., a new client in your dental office, inquires whether you are able and would be willing to deliver dental hygiene care to her 6-year-old daughter, Lisa, who has cerebral palsy.

Chief Complaint: "I recently noticed large amounts of plaque on Lisa's front teeth and am worried about the possibility of dental decay."

Health History: Lisa has been affected by cerebral palsy since birth.

Dental History: Mrs. M. apprehensively explains that she has not previously brought Lisa to a dental office because she assumed that there would be difficulties in caring for Lisa.

Social History: Lisa lives with her parents and is confined to a wheelchair.

Oral Behavior Assessment: Mother reports Lisa uses an electric toothbrush once a day.

Supplemental Notes: Mother reports Lisa has dental insurance and is somewhat fearful of coming to the dental office for care.

1. What questions could you ask Mrs. M. that would help you prepare for Lisa's appointment so that you can deliver optimal dental hygiene care?
2. What factors inherent to cerebral palsy would place Lisa at risk for oral health problems?
3. What barriers to care had Mrs. M. anticipated that would have prevented her daughter from receiving optimal dental and dental hygiene care?

REFERENCES

1. Nolte J: *The human brain*, ed 6, Philadelphia, 2009, Mosby.
2. Hirtz D, Thurman J, Gwinn-Hardy KG, et al: How common are the "common" neurologic disorders? *Neurology* 68:326, 2007.
3. Little JW, Falace DA, Miller CS, et al: *Dental management of the medically compromised patient*, ed 7, St Louis, 2008, Mosby.
4. National Institute of Neurological Disorders and Stroke, National Institutes of Health: *Parkinson's disease*, Bethesda, 2006.
5. National Institute of Neurological Disorders and Stroke, National Institutes of Health: *Cerebral palsy*, Bethesda, 2009.
6. National Institute of Neurological Disorders and Stroke, National Institutes of Health: *Multiple sclerosis*, Bethesda, 2012.
7. Koch-Henriksen N-K, Sorensen PS: The changing demographic pattern of multiple sclerosis epidemiology, *Lancet Neurology* 9:520, 2010.

8. Ascherio A, Munger KL, Simon KC: Vitamin D and multiple sclerosis, *Lancet Neurology* 9:599, 2010.
9. National Institute of Neurological Disorders and Stroke, National Institutes of Health: *Bell's palsy*, Bethesda, 2003.
10. DeLong L, Burkhart NW: *General and oral pathology for the dental hygienist*, Baltimore, 2008, Lippincott Williams & Wilkins.
11. National Institute of Neurological Disorders and Stroke, National Institutes of Health: *Spinal cord injury*, Bethesda, 2003.
12. National Institute of Neurological Disorders and Stroke, National Institutes of Health: *The dementias*, Bethesda, 2004.
13. Mannen J: Oral health and stroke, *Dimens Dent Hyg* 50, 2012.
14. National Institute on Deafness and Other Communication Disorder, National Institutes of Health: *Quick Statistics*. Available at: http://www.nidcd.nih.gov/health/statistics. Accessed December 2012.
15. National Eye Institute, National Institutes of Health: *Statistics and Data*. Available at http://www.nei.nih.gov/eyedata/adultvision_usa.asp. Accessed December 2012.
16. National Eye Institute, National Institutes of Health: *Statistics and Data*. Available at http://www.nei.nih.gov/eyedata/pba_tables.asp. Accessed December 2012.

ACKNOWLEDGMENT

The authors acknowledge Lee E. Wentworth for her past contributions to this chapter.

EVOLVE RESOURCES

Please visit http://evolve.elsevier.com/Darby/hygiene for additional practice and study support tools.

CHAPTER 48

Persons with Autoimmune Diseases

JoAnn R. Gurenlian, Ann Eshenaur Spolarich

COMPETENCIES

1. Explain immune dysfunction.
2. Discuss pathophysiology of autoimmune diseases.
3. Describe pharmacologic considerations for autoimmune diseases.
4. Discuss how autoimmune diseases affect the dental hygiene process of care, including:
   - Recognize the systemic and oral manifestations of common autoimmune diseases covered in this chapter.
   - Identify human needs related to each of the autoimmune diseases listed in this chapter and describe their implications for dental hygiene care.
   - Develop a dental hygiene care plan appropriate for persons with autoimmune disease.

Immune Dysfunction

The human immune system exhibits **self-tolerance**, which is the unique ability to recognize the difference between "self" and "foreign" antigens. This ability to discriminate between one's own antigens and nonself (typically microbial) antigens is known as **immunologic tolerance**. When innate mechanisms that normally prevent the immune system from attacking self-antigens fail, activated T cells and antibodies begin to attack the individual's own tissues, a process known as **autoimmunity**. Conditions associated with autoimmunity collectively are called autoimmune diseases.[1,2]

Understanding how self-antigens induce tolerance is important, because these same mechanisms may be applied to interventions that prevent or control unwanted immune reactions.[3] For example, many of the interventions that have been developed to treat autoimmune diseases target specific cells or mediators that modulate immune function. Other examples include series of injections given to an individual to desensitize the person after exposure to an allergen, or immunosuppressive medications used to prevent organ rejection in transplant recipients.[3]

There are two primary factors necessary for the development of autoimmunity. First, an individual inherits genes that increase susceptibility and contribute to failure of self-tolerance. Multiple genes predispose to autoimmune disease, the most important of which are major histocompatibility complex (MHC) genes that encode cytokines and are recognized by T lymphocytes for antigen processing.[1,3] There is a genetic predisposition for developing an autoimmune disease.

Second, one or more environmental triggers initiate activation of autoantibodies. Triggers may include infection, fever, or severe trauma. The manifestation of many autoimmune diseases is often preceded by an infection.[1,3] An infection triggers a local immune response, causing the release of cytokines and chemical stimulators that activate self-reactive T cells, producing an immune attack against self-antigens. Infections also injure tissues and release antigens that normally are not seen by the immune system or are ignored. The presence of these antigens also can initiate an autoimmune reaction.[1,3]

Pathophysiology of Autoimmune Diseases

Autoantibodies against self-antigens associated with autoimmune diseases bind to self-antigens in tissues, or form immune complexes with circulating self-antigens.[1,3] The tissue destruction observed with autoimmune diseases generally occurs by one of two ways. First, bound antibodies deposit in tissues that express self-antigens, which is usually in a specific tissue or organ. Second, immune complexes deposit in blood vessels, resulting in systemic involvement, manifesting as vasculitis, and joint and kidney damage.[1,3]

However, autoantibodies also can cause disease without directly causing tissue injury. Some autoantibodies inhibit receptor function on cells, as in myasthenia gravis, where acetylcholine receptors are inhibited and neuromuscular transmission fails, causing paralysis of the muscles of the head and neck. Other antibodies stimulate receptors that normally would be stimulated by a hormone. This is evident in hyperthyroidism, where antibodies against the thyroid stimulating receptor stimulate thyroid cells directly.[1,3]

Several common characteristics of autoimmune disease may be observed. Clients often exhibit cluster disorders presenting with more than one autoimmune disease. Because antibodies can travel throughout the body, clients usually experience multisystem organ involvement that may not be explained or diagnosed easily. Signs and symptoms of this involvement are nondescript and often present as fatigue, joint pain, muscle aches, sleep disorders, and anemia. Some clients experience psychiatric difficulties, most commonly depression and frustration, as a consequence of numerous consultations with multiple healthcare providers without receiving definitive diagnosis or treatment recommendations for lengthy periods of time. The result is that clients live with diminished quality of life and ongoing health challenges, including compromised oral health.

There are more than 80 different types of autoimmune diseases.[4] Examples of the more common types of autoimmune diseases appear in Table 48-1.[1,3,5] Omitted from this chapter are specific details concerning three particular autoimmune diseases (immune-mediated diabetes mellitus, rheumatic heart disease, and acquired immunodeficiency

TABLE 48-1
Examples of Autoimmune Diseases[1,3,5]

Autoimmune Disease	Definition
Adrenal insufficiency	Primary condition is known as Addison's disease, which is caused by destruction of the adrenal glands from infections, cancer, or chronic use of steroid hormones Secondary adrenal insufficiency is caused most often by chronic use of steroids Adrenal crisis is a life-threatening condition caused by acute adrenal suppression
Chronic fatigue syndrome	A complex disorder characterized by profound fatigue that is not improved with bed rest and is worsened by physical or mental activity. Blood tests reveal an immune response consistent with viral infection
Cicatricial pemphigoid	A benign chronic blistering disease affecting the oral and genital mucosa, conjunctiva of the eye, skin, characterized by healing of lesions with scarring
Fibromyalgia	A widespread musculoskeletal disorder characterized by pain in the muscles, ligaments, and joints, and fatigue. Has a frequent comorbidity with other autoimmune conditions including chronic fatigue syndrome, rheumatoid arthritis, systemic lupus erythematosus, and hypothyroidism
Hyperthyroidism	Also known as thyrotoxicosis, an excess of thyroxine (T_4) and triiodothyronine (T_3) in the bloodstream, affecting the body's metabolic rate
Hypothyroidism	Characterized by autoimmune thyroiditis, causing progressive gland deterioration, leading to fibrosis and diminished or absent secretion of thyroid hormone
Multiple sclerosis	The most common autoimmune disease affecting the nervous system characterized by demyelination of nerves in the central nervous system because of chronic inflammation
Myasthenia gravis	A chronic autoimmune disease that affects the neuromuscular system representing a decrease in acetylcholine receptors in muscle fibers, resulting in progressive fatigability and abnormality of skeletal muscles
Pemphigus vulgaris	A progressive, severe disease affecting the skin and mucous membranes characterized by bullae that rupture and form painful ulcers
Pernicious anemia	Failure of the stomach to produce intrinsic factor and lack of cobalamin, or vitamin B_{12}
Psoriasis	A common dermatologic condition characterized by well-demarcated erythematous patches with a silver-white scale on the surface of the lesions
Rheumatoid arthritis	A chronic inflammatory condition characterized by pain, swelling, stiffness, and loss of function affecting the joints
Scleroderma	A chronic disease of connective tissue affecting all organ systems secondary to fibrosis and vascular injury. Includes localized and systemic types
Sjögren's syndrome	A triad of keratoconjunctivitis sicca, xerostomia, and connective tissue disorder manifesting as a wide spectrum of severity. Includes primary and secondary forms
Systemic lupus erythematosus	A disease involving multiple organ systems characterized by periods of remissions and exacerbations

syndrome) because these conditions are discussed in other chapters of this text. A description of signs and symptoms reflecting major system involvement of various autoimmune diseases is found in Table 48-2.[2,3]

For more specific details about individual autoimmune diseases, visit the evolve website at http://evolve.elsevier.com/Darby/hygiene.

Pharmacologic Considerations

Management of autoimmune diseases typically includes pharmacotherapy beginning with anti-inflammatory medications and progressing to immunosuppressive drugs. The goals of medication therapy used to treat autoimmune diseases include reduced pain, improved function, slowed rate of disease progression, and limiting tissue destruction.[3] Many autoimmune conditions are treated with drugs that reduce inflammation using corticosteroids and anti-cytokine therapies. Because activated T cells mediate organ-specific autoimmune diseases, immunosuppressive drugs also are used to inhibit T-cell responses. Drugs used to treat rheumatoid arthritis provide a classic model for understanding pharmacologic management of autoimmune diseases, which are described further here. A variety of classes of medications may be indicated for client management, a list of which is found in Box 48-1.

Nonsteroidal anti-inflammatory drugs (NSAIDs) block the synthesis of prostaglandins by inhibiting the enzyme cyclooxygenase, which reduces the formation of inflammatory mediators that create swelling, fever, and pain. NSAIDs are categorized as either salicylates (e.g., aspirin) or nonsalicylates. Aspirin and other salicylates are standard, first-line agents for treatment of rheumatoid arthritis and provide

TABLE 48-2

Signs and Symptoms of Major System Involvement of Autoimmune Diseases[2,3]

System	Features
Constitutional	Fatigue, fever in the absence of infection, weight loss/gain, difficulty sleeping, cold or heat intolerance
Musculoskeletal	Arthralgia, myalgia, arthritis, joint pain and swelling, loss of joint range of motion, carpal tunnel syndrome, flexion contractures, muscle weakness, diaphoresis, tremors, warm/flushed skin
Skin	Photosensitivity, diffuse rash, skin lesions or nodules, mucous membrane lesions, purpura, alopecia, Raynaud's phenomenon, urticaria, vasculitis, skin pigment changes, skin tightness and induration, telangiectasis, calcinosis, edema, alopecia, thin/fine hair, soft or brittle nails
Renal	Hematuria, proteinuria, casts, nephritic syndrome, renal crisis or failure
Gastrointestinal	Nausea, vomiting, gastroparesis, abdominal pain, peritonitis with or without ascites, hepatomegaly, pancreatitis, gastroesophageal reflux disease, dysphagia, dyspepsia, diarrhea alternating with constipation, candidiasis, primary biliary cirrhosis, malabsorption, diverticula
Pulmonary	Pleurisy, pleural effusion, chest pain, shortness of breath, pulmonary parenchyma, pulmonary hypertension, cough from restrictive lung disease
Cardiovascular	Pericarditis, noninfective endocarditis, myocarditis, chest pain, arrhythmia, valve abnormalities, myocardial infarction, congestive heart failure, myocardial fibrosis, palpitations, bradycardia, tachycardia
Reticuloendothelial	Lymphadenopathy, splenomegaly, hepatomegaly
Hematologic/vascular	Anemia, autoimmune thrombocytopenia purpura or thrombocytopenia as a consequence of antiphospholipid antibody syndrome, leukopenia with lymphoma, Raynaud's phenomenon, ulcerations of digits, ischemic resorption of digits, gangrene of digits, lips, nose, and ears
Ocular	Anterior uveitis, iridocyclitis, retinal vasculitis, central retinal artery occlusion, central retinal vein occlusion, ischemic optic neuropathy, xerostomia with keratoconjunctivitis and sicca, retinopathy, blindness, edema of eyelids
Neuropsychiatric	Cerebrovascular accidents, seizure, organic effective disorders, personality disorder, psychosis, coma, vascular or migraine headaches, organic brain syndrome, dementia, cranial neuropathies, peripheral neuropathies, depression, facial pain, nervousness and anxiety, slowed mental acuity
Ear, nose, and throat	Earaches, chronic cough, aberrant voice with nasal tone, dysphagia, gangrene
Oral	Tooth mobility, sicca syndrome, widened periodontal ligaments, microstomia, anterior open bite, resorption of mandible, xerostomia, delayed/early eruption of teeth, salivary gland enlargement, temporomandibular joint swelling, preauricular pain, decreased mobility, locking, crepitus, stomatitis, loss of taste, hyperkeratosis, secondary infection of candidiasis, petechial ecchymosis, bleeding, drug-induced gingival enlargement, gangrene of lips, impaired lip movement, soft palate weakness, tremor of tongue, thickened tongue
Endocrine	Erectile dysfunction, vaginal dryness, dyspareunia, menstrual irregularity, xerostomia, xerophthalmia, miscarriages, goiter, osteoporosis

relief from pain, swelling, and fever. Prevention of joint and tissue damage often necessitates the addition of a DMARD (see later).[6] Large doses of salicylates and NSAIDs often are required for pain relief, which may not be tolerated in some individuals. Although acetaminophen has similar potency and efficacy as aspirin, it has no anti-inflammatory activity, and thus its usefulness is limited.

Disease-modifying antirheumatic drugs (DMARDs) are a wide range of compounds used for the treatment of rheumatoid arthritis and osteoarthritis either in conjunction with NSAIDs, or in clients who have not responded to cyclooxygenase-2 (COX-2) inhibitors. DMARDs slow the course of joint disease and help to prevent further destruction but have a relatively slow onset of action. Clients may need to take these drugs for up to 4 months before seeing an effect.[3,6]

Methotrexate is an immunosuppressant that produces antirheumatic effects within 6 weeks of initiating treatment. It is used alone or in combination with other DMARDs. It is the drug of choice for severe rheumatoid arthritis or psoriatic arthritis and for cases that are unresponsive to NSAIDs. It has a faster onset of action than other DMARDs, often providing relief within 6 weeks after initiating treatment.[3]

Interleukin-1β and tumor necrosis factor-alpha are proinflammatory cytokines that stimulate synovial cells to proliferate and synthesize collagenase, which degrades cartilage, stimulates bone resorption, and inhibits proteoglycan synthesis. Anti-cytokine therapies are used to block these unwanted effects and also provide some anti-inflammatory effects. These drugs are used in clients with severe rheumatoid arthritis who are unresponsive to other DMARDs, and in those

BOX 48-1

Medications Used to Treat Autoimmune Diseases[3,6]

Anti-inflammatory Agents

Salicylates (aspirin)
NSAIDs
COX-2 inhibitors
Corticosteroids:
- Prednisone
- Prednisolone

DMARDs (Disease-Modifying Antirheumatic Drugs)

Immune modulators:
- Methotrexate
- Leflunomide
- Anti-cytokine therapies: etanercept, infliximab, adalimumab, anakinra

Antimalarials: chloroquine, hydroxychloroquine
Penicillamine
Gold compounds: aurothioglucose, auranofin, gold sodium thiomalate
Immunosuppressants:
- Azathioprine
- Cyclophosphamide
- Cyclosporine

BOX 48-2

Complications with Chronic Use of Corticosteroid Medications[3,6]

Insomnia
Peptic ulceration
Osteoporosis
Cataract formation
Glaucoma
Growth suppression
Delayed wound healing
Psychosis
Weight gain

with other autoimmune conditions that affect connective tissue and bones. Examples of these drugs include etanercept, infliximab, adalimumab, and anakinra.[3,6]

Penicillamine depresses circulating immunoglobulin M (IgM) rheumatoid factor and depresses T-cell activity. Antimalarial agents impair complement-dependent antigen-antibody reactions and typically are used in combination with aspirin and steroids, especially for clients with rheumatoid arthritis who are unresponsive to NSAIDs. Antimalarial agents slow the progression of erosive bone lesions and may induce remission. Agents include chloroquine and hydroxychloroquine. Gold compounds inhibit mononuclear phagocyte maturation and function and may suppress cellular immunity.[3,6]

Azathioprine and cyclophosphamide are immunosuppressive drugs used to treat a variety of autoimmune conditions but most often are used for refractory cases of rheumatoid arthritis. Cyclosporine is an immunosuppressant agent that inhibits the production of interleukin-2 by helper T cells and reduces the production and release of other lymphokines in response to an antigenic stimulus.[3,6]

Dental hygienists must be aware that the drugs used to treat autoimmune diseases produce numerous adverse effects, and clients may present with signs and symptoms that reflect their drug treatment and their disease. Each client requires a comprehensive pharmacologic history review to determine the impact of drug therapy on the dental hygiene process of care. Chapter 14 contains detailed information about the pharmacology history review.

Salicylates, NSAIDs, and COX-2 inhibitors are associated with adverse bleeding events, including bruising, gastrointestinal hemorrhage, and gingival bleeding. All of the DMARDs described earlier have many known toxicities, making compliance difficult, and requiring regular monitoring by the physician. Clients often experience general fatigue and malaise, which can be difficult to differentiate from symptoms of the autoimmune disease. Dermatologic problems, including skin lesions, rashes, and hair loss are common, as is delayed wound healing. Lesions may occur on the oral mucosa, including the appearance of bluish-black pigmentation. Clients may experience severe hematologic effects, including alterations in red and white blood cell counts and altered cell function. Because DMARDs alter the immune response, clients become susceptible to infections, such as pneumonia, and may experience a reactivation of latent viruses, leading to diseases such as hepatitis, tuberculosis, and herpetic infections such as shingles. Rarely, immune modulators may promote the development of cancers.[3,6]

Many clients are treated with corticosteroids for their anti-inflammatory effects and for suppression of the immune response. It is this suppressive activity that results in the desired, as well as undesired, effects of corticosteroids. Adverse reactions are proportional to dose, frequency, time of administration, and duration of treatment. Multiple adverse events associated with steroids limit their long-term use. Complications associated with chronic steroid use are listed in Box 48-2.[6]

Clients undergoing chronic corticosteroid therapy are at risk for candidiasis, the most common oral side effect of these medications, which is related directly to their xerostomic effect. They also may exhibit poor wound healing after dental hygiene therapy. Oral infections may be masked because of the anti-inflammatory effects of these medications. Chronic dry mouth increases risks for a variety of oral complications that require dental hygiene interventions (see Table 48-5).

Adrenal Insufficiency and Adrenal Crisis

Regulation of cortisol secretion is controlled by the hypothalamic-pituitary-adrenal axis. Virtually any type of stress, whether physical or psychologic, causes an immediate increase of pituitary secretion of adrenocorticotropic hormone (ACTH), which stimulates the adrenal cortex to produce and secrete cortisol. Surgery is one of the greatest stressors that produces this response.[3,6]

Chronic use of corticosteroids suppresses the body's own production and release of cortisol, resulting in secondary, or medication-induced, **adrenal insufficiency**. The danger is that when the client is physically (infection, surgery) and/or psychologically (fear, anxiety, pain) stressed, the client will not be able to produce an adequate amount of his own cortisol, known as the stress response, placing him at risk for decreased cardiac output, hypoglycemia, and circulatory shock.[3,6] One method used to minimize this suppression is to administer hydrocortisone on alternating days, with higher doses used to maintain adequate serum levels, while still allowing the body to secrete its own cortisone on opposing days.

Dental professionals must determine whether clients on chronic corticosteroid therapy require steroid supplementation before treatment. Other than for major surgical procedures, most clients do not require supplementation for general or routine dental and dental hygiene procedures. Even for minor surgeries, patients taking their medications at their usual dose within 2 hours of the procedure should have enough exogenous and endogenous steroids to handle the procedure. Further, local anesthesia and conscious sedation lower the stress response to pain, which helps to eliminate the need for supplementation.[3,6]

Adrenal crisis is a rare, life-threatening condition caused by acute adrenal suppression. It does not commonly occur with secondary adrenal insufficiency. Four factors contribute to the risk of adrenal crisis during oral surgery: the extent and severity of the surgery, medications used, health status of the client, and the degree of pain control. Adrenal crisis leads to circulatory collapse and death if not treated promptly. Treatment of adrenal crisis requires hospitalization and interventions including intravenous injections of hydrocortisone, glucose, fluids, and electrolyte replacement.[3,6] Dental professionals must recognize the signs and symptoms of adrenal crisis listed in Box 48-3.[3,6] Implementation of a stress reduction protocol in clients with adrenal suppression can minimize the risk for adrenal crisis during dental treatment[3,6] (Procedure 48-1 and the corresponding Competency Form).

Dental Hygiene Process of Care

Autoimmune diseases are multifaceted and present challenges to general and oral healthcare professionals. Given the nature of these diseases, clients may present with multiple human needs that affect dental hygiene care. Using the dental hygiene process of care ensures adequate planning for the delivery of safe and comprehensive oral care.

Assessment

During the assessment phase, it is of utmost importance to obtain a thorough health, oral, and pharmacologic history from the client to identify conditions that warrant referral for medical evaluation. The clinician must be able to determine if the need for medical care supersedes oral care, whether it is safe to provide treatment, and what the client will be able to tolerate in terms of appointment scheduling and procedures. Oral care may have to be deferred until additional medical evaluation and/or treatment is provided.

In some cases, clients report signs and symptoms that may reflect autoimmune disease characteristics without having received a definitive diagnosis. Upon completion of the health history, the dental hygienist can use a risk assessment tool to assist with the identification of autoimmune characteristics, referrals needed, and considerations or modifications necessary to provide dental hygiene treatment. Table 48-3 presents an example of a risk assessment tool for suspected and confirmed autoimmune diseases.[2] This risk assessment tool is to be completed after reviewing the health history when suspecting an autoimmune condition. The clinician should ask all questions of the client and make treatment modifications and referrals based on responses and clinical examination findings.

BOX 48-3

Signs and Symptoms of Adrenal Crisis[6]

Sunken eyes	Myalgias
Profuse sweating	Arthralgias
Hypotension	Hyponatremia
Weak pulse	Eosinophilia
Dyspnea	Hypothermia
Cyanosis	Severe hypotension
Nausea/vomiting	Hypoglycemia
Headache	Circulatory collapse (shock)
Dehydration	Death
Fever	

Procedure 48-1 Implementation of a Stress Reduction Protocol[3,6]

STEPS	RATIONALE
Schedule clients for dental procedures, especially surgical procedures, first thing in the morning.	Cortisol levels are highest in the morning, which helps to ensure client safety by minimizing risks for adrenal crisis.
Use measures to minimize pain and anxiety.	Use of local anesthetics, nitrous oxide sedation, and antianxiety medications helps to minimize exogenous stress from pain and fear associated with dental procedures.
Monitor the client's vital signs before the procedure, during the perioperative period, and before dismissing the client.	Monitoring the client's blood pressure is essential to detect a drop in pressure, an important sign of adrenal crisis. During this crisis, the client may exhibit a weak pulse, temperature changes, and difficulty breathing. Regular monitoring of vital signs helps to ensure early detection of this potential medical emergency so that the client can be treated and maintained safely.
Respond appropriately to a drop in blood pressure.	A blood pressure reading below 100/60 indicates hypotension, and immediate action must be taken to ensure client safety. The patient should be positioned with the feet elevated above the height of the head, with fluid replacement, administration of vasopressors, and treatment of hypoglycemia given as needed. 100 mg of hydrocortisone is administered by IV, and the client then is transported to the hospital.

TABLE 48-3

Risk Assessment Tool for Autoimmune Diseases[2]

Questions	Notes	Dental Hygiene Treatment Modifications and Referrals
How would you describe your overall health?		
Have you had any changes in your health within the last year? (Examples: significant weight loss or gain, chronic or frequent colds, flulike symptoms)		
Have you experienced any of the following: infection, fever, illness, stress, trauma, or motor vehicle accident?		
Have you had any changes to your activities of daily living? (Examples: less active, more difficulty performing routine duties such as laundry, grocery shopping, work, school, sleeping, loss of interest in activities/hobbies, frustration with inability to perform routine tasks, loss of motivation, eating or cooking)		
Have your medications changed since your last visit or are you using your medications differently since last time? (Examples: new medications, increasing frequency of use, taking more NSAIDs, self-medication with drugs and alcohol, use of antidepressants)		
Have you noticed changes in eating behaviors? (Examples: less interested in food, increased eating for comfort, disinterested in or difficulty with eating out with friends)		
Signs and symptoms suggesting autoimmune condition (Examples: fatigue, arthralgia, myalgia, xerostomia, rash, GERD, anemia, shortness of breath, chest pain, lymphadenopathy, arrhythmia, goiter, salivary gland enlargement)		
Assess need for prophylactic antibiotics		
Assess vital signs		
Assess potential for infection		
Assess potential for medical emergency		
Assess need for supportive or assistive devices		

Diagnosis

Human needs assessments differ depending on the client's autoimmune disease(s). The dental hygiene diagnosis depends largely on the signs observed by the clinician and the symptoms reported by the client at the assessment phase. Objective and subjective assessment findings are used to identify key diagnoses and are summarized to support proposed treatment. Figures 48-1 through 48-10 illustrate clinical signs of autoimmune diseases.

Planning

The planning phase may be complicated by the physical demands on the client and medical attention needed at the time of dental hygiene care. Shorter appointments may be necessary to accommodate clients with joint pain, stiffness, swelling, shortness of breath, and other manifestations that may affect their ability to sit for long periods of time. Assistive and supportive devices needed to provide comfort for the client during the dental hygiene appointment should be discussed in advance and included as part of preparation for treatment.

Consultation with the client's physician to establish goals and communication is helpful to determine how to coordinate dental hygiene care with concurrent medical care in a safe manner. Dental hygienists have an opportunity to serve as an advocate for clients who require physical and psychologic support when recognizing that needs are not being met by the current medical system.

In planning for individualized treatment for each client presenting with autoimmune diseases, it is important to consider specific interventions that may be necessary. Clients may have unusual oral complaints or manifestations of autoimmune disease that require attention to comprehensive care. Consultation with the client's physician may be necessary to complete the planning process to ensure client safety. For example, a client who presents with multiple sclerosis should be scheduled for treatment during periods of remission and may need steroid supplementation. Depending on the medications being used to treat rheumatoid arthritis, the dental hygienist may have to evaluate blood work such as bleeding time and platelet function before beginning periodontal debridement. For those individuals who present with systemic lupus erythematosus who have a history of low white blood cell counts from taking immunosuppressants, additional blood assays are needed to determine whether it is safe to proceed with planned treatment and if antibiotic premedication is needed before treatment. Antibiotic premedication also may be indicated for clients with rheumatoid arthritis who have undergone joint replacement surgery. In other instances, depending on the medications used and level of

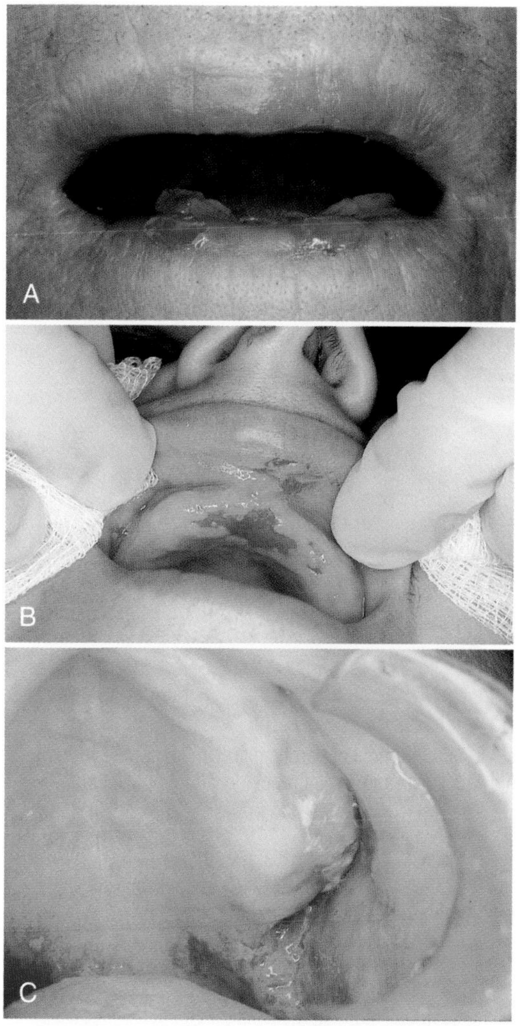

Figure 48-1. **A** through **C,** Examples of oral lesions in pemphigus vulgaris. (*A,* From Ibsen OAC, Phelan JA: *Oral pathology for the dental hygienist,* ed 6, St Louis, 2014, Saunders. *B,* Courtesy Dr. Fariba Younai. *C,* Courtesy Dr. Sidney Eisig.)

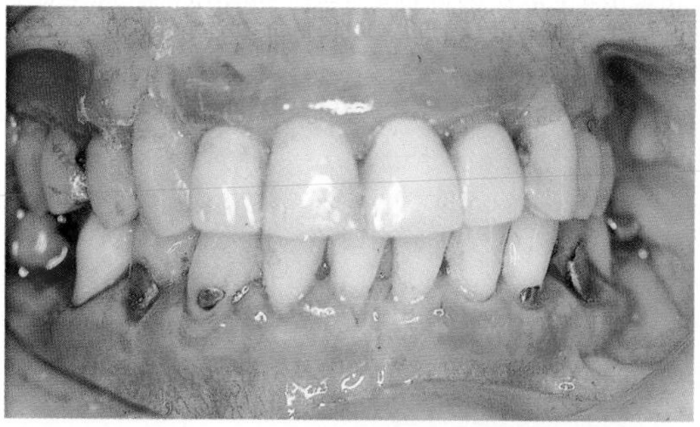

Figure 48-2. Cicatricial pemphigoid (desquamative gingivitis). (Courtesy Dr. Victor M. Sternberg.)

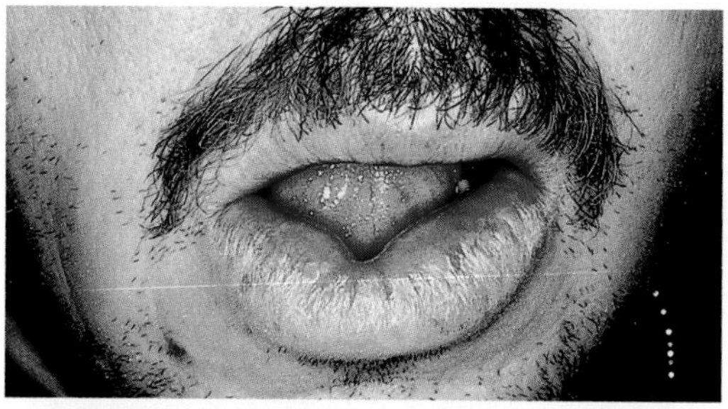

Figure 48-3. Indurated lip lesions characteristic of sarcoidosis. (Courtesy Dr. Donald M. Cohen and Dr. Indraneel Bhattacharyya.)

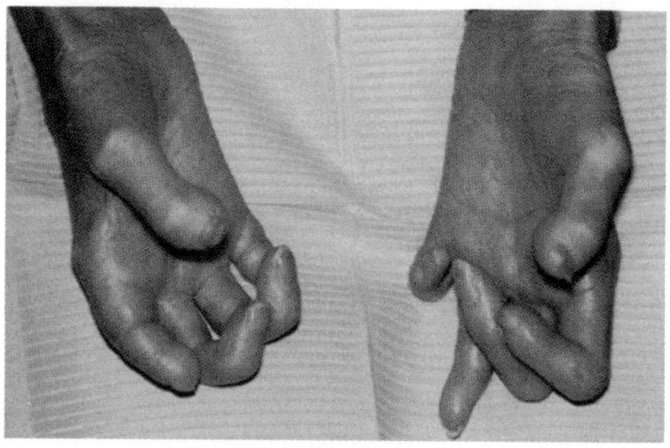

Figure 48-4. Clawlike finger position characteristic of systemic sclerosis.

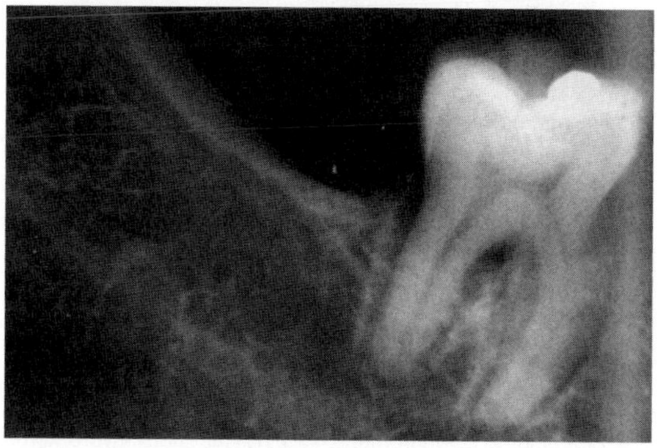

Figure 48-5. Widening of the periodontal ligament space characteristic of systemic sclerosis.

xerostomia, an antifungal therapy for secondary candidiasis may have to be prescribed. Recognizing these special care considerations in the planning process assists the dental hygienist in meeting the multiple needs of the client. Table 48-4 provides an overview of oral manifestations of autoimmune diseases accompanied by respective dental hygiene interventions to facilitate the planning process.

Examples of planning goals may be the following:

- "Client will report a decrease in oral discomfort at next appointment."
- "Client will report greater ability to tolerate time frame of appointment with assistance from use of supportive devices and stabilization techniques."
- "Client will report improved sense of safety maneuvering within the dental hygiene operatory setting."
- "Ease of breathing will be monitored throughout appointment for clients with myasthenia gravis to ensure adequate airway exchange."
- "Avoid administering local anesthesia with epinephrine to clients with uncontrolled hyperthyroidism to minimize risk of thyroid storm."

Further, the clinician should review the potential for a medical emergency to occur given the client's condition and medications taken. Preparing in advance to prevent and/or manage a medical emergency is advised.

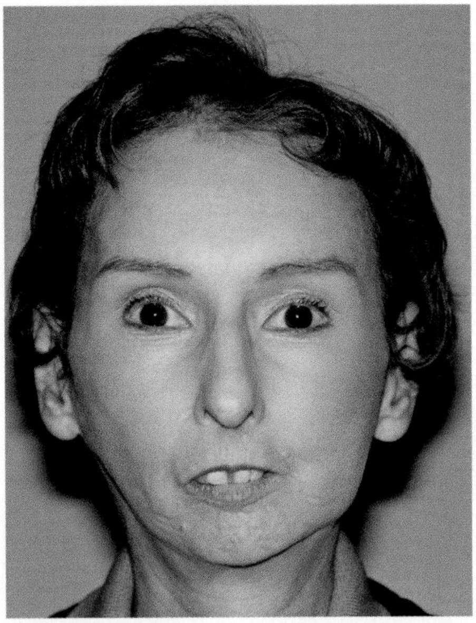

Figure 48-6. Localized scleroderma of the face presenting a scarlike appearance (coup de sabre).

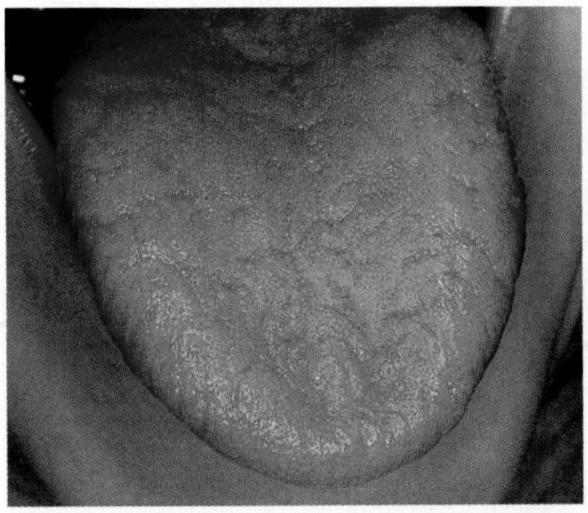

Figure 48-7. Sjögren's syndrome. This individual had severe xerostomia. The filiform papillae are lacking. (From Ibsen OAC, Phelan JA: *Oral pathology for the dental hygienist,* ed 6, St Louis, 2013, Saunders.)

Implementation

Implementation includes the administration of dental hygiene interventions to minimize oral infections and restore oral health, prevent future disease, and client education. It is essential that clients understand the relationship between their autoimmune condition, medical management, and oral care. Some clients may require further care with an oral specialist if mucosal lesions are not responding to initial treatment protocols. Others may need more definitive periodontal treatment. In these instances, referrals to an oral pathologist, oral surgeon, or periodontist are warranted.

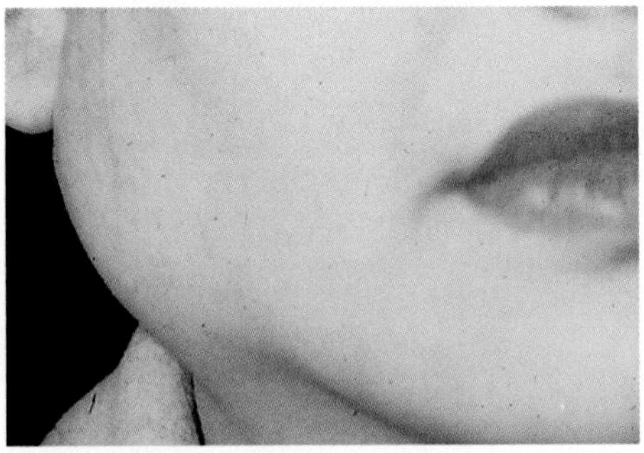

Figure 48-8. Enlargement of parotid gland in Sjögren's syndrome. (Courtesy Dr. Donald M. Cohen and Dr. Indraneel Bhattacharyya.)

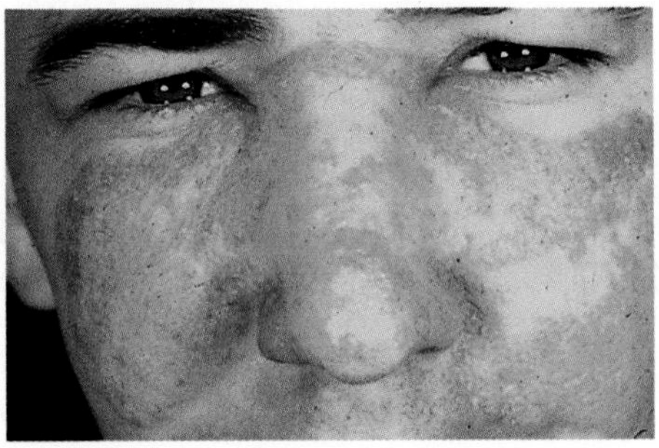

Figure 48-9. Malar rash seen in systemic lupus erythematosus. (Courtesy Dr. Donald M. Cohen and Dr. Indraneel Bhattacharyya.)

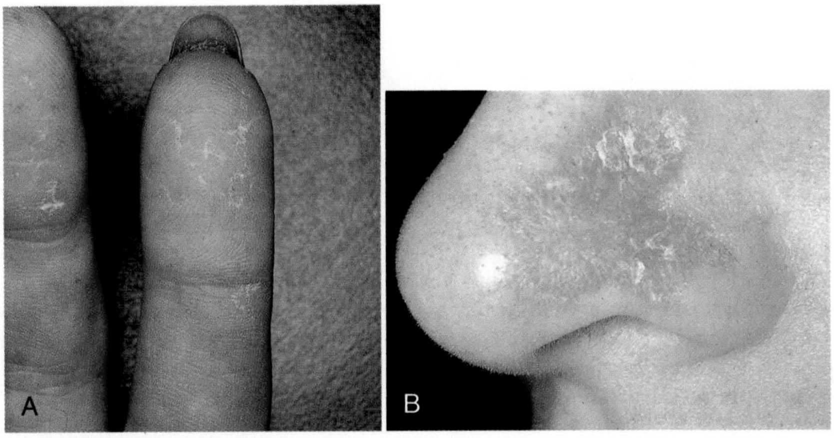

Figure 48-10. **A** and **B,** Two examples of skin lesions in lupus erythematosus. (**A,** From Ibsen OAC, Phelan JA: *Oral pathology for the dental hygienist,* ed 6, St Louis, 2014, Saunders. **B,** Courtesy Dr. Edward V. Zegarelli.)

TABLE 48-4

Oral Manifestations with Dental Hygiene Interventions[2,3,5-7]

Autoimmune Disease	Oral Manifestation(s)	Dental Hygiene Interventions
Chronic fatigue syndrome	Sore throat Tender lymph nodes Headaches Xerostomia Chronic cough Jaw pain	Referral to physician for evaluation Caries risk reduction: fluorides, remineralization therapy, xylitol Salivary replacement therapy Consult for TMJ and jaw pain
Cicatricial pemphigoid	Vesicles or bullae that rupture, leaving large areas of superficial, ulcerated, and denuded mucosa; lesions are painful and may persist for weeks or months if untreated	Physician consult if difficulty with speaking or breathing Treat lesions with topical or systemic corticosteroids Topical pain control for lesions as needed Protect eyes if ocular involvement
Fibromyalgia	TMJ dysfunction Pain in face and head Xerostomia	Referral to physician for evaluation Caries risk reduction: fluorides, remineralization therapy, xylitol Salivary replacement therapy Consult for TMJ and jaw pain
Hyperthyroidism	Mild tremor in tongue Osteoporosis in bones of skull; axial and peripheral skeleton Children: premature loss of deciduous teeth with accelerated tooth eruption and faster development of jaw Adults: marked loss of alveolar process, diffuse demineralization of mandible Rapidly progressive periodontal disease Lingual thyroid tissue appears on posterior dorsal region of tongue, below area of foramen cecum	Inspect thyroid gland carefully: note enlargement, presence of nodules, pain and tenderness on palpation Avoid overpalpation of gland More sensitive to pain: require more anesthesia More sensitive to catecholamines: limit vasoconstrictor: avoid if uncontrolled hyperthyroidism More tolerant to centrally acting drugs: require higher doses of sedatives and analgesics Manage stress, anxiety, and infections to minimize risk of thyroid storm: monitor vital signs
Hypothyroidism	Children: enlarged tongue, delayed eruption patterns, malocclusion Adults: hoarse voice, enlarged tongue, swelling of facial features	More sensitive to central nervous system depressants: lower dose of opiates and sedatives
Multiple sclerosis	Oral manifestations occur in 2% to 3% of population Paresthesia Difficulty with speech Orofacial numbness Trigeminal neuralgia Drug-induced xerostomia	Schedule short morning appointments Treat during periods of remission: avoid treatment during active disease period Steroid supplementation may be needed Provide assistance with ambulation, transfer to dental chair Caries risk reduction: fluorides, remineralization therapy, xylitol Salivary replacement therapy Client education: augmentation of oral hygiene regimen in cases of limited manual dexterity; modify oral hygiene devices or use power devices
Myasthenia gravis	Drooping eyelids and double vision Muscle weakness in face, head, and neck Difficulty chewing, swallowing Difficulty wearing dentures Soft palate weakness Impaired lip movement Altered voice with nasal tone	Client education: assist client with "feel" of oral hygiene aids in mouth if visual impairments Use hands to support lower jaw during mastication Consult with physician for supportive device for lower jaw between meals to prevent spontaneous dropping Consult for implant-supported dentures Schedule short early–morning appointments Use rubber dam, evacuation, and mouth props during appointments Consider nitrous oxide–oxygen sedation to reduce stress and anxiety Consult before prescribing antibiotics and muscle relaxants because some antibiotics have muscle relaxant properties Monitor ease of breathing

Continued

TABLE 48-4
Oral Manifestations with Dental Hygiene Interventions—cont'd

Autoimmune Disease	Oral Manifestation(s)	Dental Hygiene Interventions
Pemphigus vulgaris	Superficial "ragged" erosions and ulcerations, haphazard distribution; most common areas are palate, labial mucosa, buccal mucosa, ventral surface of the tongue, and gingiva	Consultation with physician for early diagnosis Monitor client for long-term effects of treatment with corticosteroids and immunosuppressants
Pernicious anemia	Painful, red, burning tongue with atrophy of papillae Oral ulcerations	Topical pain control for oral lesions and sore tongue
Psoriasis	Oral manifestations are rare Oral lesions appear as white or red plaques, mixed red and white lesions, pustules, vesicles, or ulcerations Geographic tongue may occur	Consult with dermatologist as needed for oral lesions Topical pain control if lesions become symptomatic
Rheumatoid arthritis	Temporomandibular joint (TMJ) involvement (75% of cases) Limited or difficulty opening of the mouth Drug-induced gingival bleeding Drug-induced oral mucosal lesions	Client education: risk of TMJ involvement; regular panoramic radiographs to assess mandibular condylar wear and TMJ Soft diet Moist heat or ice Consultation for occlusal appliance Client education: augmentation of oral hygiene regimen in cases of limited manual dexterity Premedication when indicated before dental services if joint replacement Evaluate bleeding time, platelet function Blood studies if taking immunosuppressants Pain control for drug-induced oral lesions Shorter appointments for comfort if difficulty sitting Use supportive devices to maintain client comfort in the dental chair
Scleroderma	Radiographically: widened periodontal ligament spaces; osseous destruction of TMJ, mandibular angle, coronoid process, or condyle Jaw fractures late in disease process Microstomia Limited opening of the mouth Xerostomia Loss of attached gingival mucosa and generalized recession Firm, hypomobile tongue: difficulty with speech and swallowing Anterior open bite	Client education: augmentation of oral hygiene regimen in cases of limited manual dexterity; modify oral hygiene devices or use power devices Semi-reclined position if gastrointestinal problems Nutritional counseling Caries risk reduction: fluorides, remineralization therapy, xylitol Antimicrobial mouthrinses Salivary replacement therapies Isometric exercises to maintain mobility of muscles of face and neck and to improve mouth opening
Sjögren's syndrome	Erythematous oral mucosa Enlarged salivary glands: especially parotids Severe xerostomia Difficulty swallowing Altered taste Difficulty wearing dentures Fissured tongue; atrophy of papillae Candidasis: often erythematous form Caries: cervical most common Periodontal disease	Referral to physician or ophthalmologist if necessary Client education: daily fluoride application at home to prevent xerostomia-induced dental caries Daily fluoride regimen, remineralization therapy Xylitol gum and candy to stimulate salivary flow and therapeutic doses to interfere with *Streptococcus mutans* Nutritional counseling Use of artificial tears and saliva Salivary stimulants Salivary replacement therapy Antifungal therapy for secondary candidiasis Hydration Avoid spicy or acidic foods

TABLE 48-4

Oral Manifestations with Dental Hygiene Interventions—cont'd

Autoimmune Disease	Oral Manifestation(s)	Dental Hygiene Interventions
Systemic lupus erythematosus (SLE)	Oral lesions (5%-25% of patients) Location of lesions: palate, buccal mucosa, gingiva May appear lichenoid, may look nonspecific or granulomatous Ulceration, pain, erythema, hyperkeratosis Xerostomia Taste alteration Oral mucosal pain Candidiasis Periodontal disease	Referral to physician for consultation because of complex medical history Possible antibiotic premedication if history of pericarditis or noninfective endocarditis, or low white blood cell (WBC) count from immunosuppressants Consult for need for supplemental steroids Antifungal therapy as needed Topical pain control for oral lesions Monitor nutrition if taste alteration Caries prevention: fluorides, remineralization therapy, xylitol Salivary stimulant or replacement therapies Avoid spicy foods Client education: meticulous oral hygiene; avoid excessive sun exposure Schedule shorter appointments
Chronic cutaneous lupus erythematosus (CCLE)	Painful lesions are practically identical to lesions of erosive lichen planus	Referral to dermatologist or physician if necessary Client education: avoid exposure to acidic or salty foods if painful intraoral lesions are present; avoid excessive sun exposure

Client education must include disease pathophysiology, effects on the oral cavity, palliative treatments for oral discomfort, and preventive oral therapies where appropriate. Table 48-4 lists common oral manifestations and dental hygiene interventions for numerous autoimmune conditions.[2,3,5-7] The dental hygienist should consider recommending products and oral devices that will provide the best possible results for biofilm, caries, and xerostomia management.[8,9] Clients presenting with disease- or drug-induced fungal and viral infections require definitive treatment with antifungal and antiviral medications. Clients with medication-induced oral lesions may require agents for topical pain control (Box 48-4). Table 48-5 provides examples of oral health product considerations based on clinical indications.[2,8,9] In addition, clients should be taught to perform an oral self-examination so that they can identify changes that are occurring and seek immediate treatment. Teaching clients to be attentive to their oral health and aggressive in seeking additional evaluation may help avoid long-term adverse effects from their health condition or medication management.

BOX 48-4

Agents for Topical Pain Control

Over-the-Counter Products

- Benzocaine 10% ointment
- Lidocaine 2.5% ointment
- Tetracaine hydrochloride 1% ointment
- Diphenhydramine elixir
- Benzocaine, gelatin, pectin, and sodium carboxymethylcellulose adhesive oral paste

Diphenydramine elixir added in equal amounts to Maalox, Mylanta, or Kaopectate

Prescription Products

- 2% viscous lidocaine mouth rinse
- Sucralfate (Carafate) prepared as a 1 g/15 mL suspension for rinsing

Diphenydramine elixir added in equal amounts to Maalox, Mylanta, or Kaopectate and 2% lidocaine mouth rinse
- Amlexanox oral paste 5%

Evaluation

Clients with autoimmune disease must be placed on 2- to 3-month maintenance intervals because of their compromised immune system. Furthermore, it is important that after initial therapy is completed, an evaluation appointment be scheduled to assess the client's host response to dental hygiene care, determine if additional treatment is needed, and to reinforce self-care.

At each subsequent appointment, the client's overall health, as well as oral health, is reassessed. Continued communication between the dental hygienist, dentist, and physician is extremely important when changes are made in planned professional care.

The dental hygienist relates the client's human needs to the factors that are contributing to the problem(s). The diagnostic statements and goals are used to guide clinical decisions regarding appropriate dental hygiene interventions so that oral health can be achieved. Whether signs and symptoms first documented are still evident at the evaluation appointment determines if the goals were met, partially met, or not met. Further treatment and referral may be necessary, depending on outcomes.

TABLE 48-5

Oral Health Product Considerations[2,8,9]

Product Category	Indications
Fluorides	Caries risk reduction Hypersensitivity
Nonfluoride remineralization therapies	Caries risk reduction Hypersensitivity
Xylitol	Caries risk reduction
Salivary stimulants (pilocarpine, cevimeline)	Oral disease risk reduction Salivary hypofunction and xerostomia Improved comfort and function
Salivary substitutes	Oral disease risk reduction Salivary hypofunction and xerostomia Improved comfort and function
Antimicrobial agents (chlorhexidine, essential oils, triclosan, cetylpyridinium chloride)	Oral disease risk reduction Halitosis
Mechanical devices (power brushes, oral irrigators, interdental aids)	Biofilm removal and oral cleansing Salivary stimulation[8]

Documentation

The final step in the dental hygiene process of care is to document the process and outcomes of each appointment. The practitioner should report the extent to which goals were met and factors influencing outcomes. Proposed future treatment, referrals, and client response to dental hygiene care should be recorded. Any adverse reactions or emergency situations during the provision of care should be noted including details of the event or situation, vital signs, emergency assistance required, treatment provided, and family members and/or healthcare professionals contacted.

CLIENT EDUCATION TIPS

- Explain that daily self-care and 2- to 3-month maintenance care are necessary to control and/or prevent autoimmune disease oral manifestations.
- Explain that regular physician evaluation and reporting of those findings to the oral healthcare team are important to maintain coordinated, comprehensive healthcare.
- Explain that strict adherence to the physician and dental professional recommendations help to ensure that adequate care is rendered. Clients must not self-medicate, stop medications, or ignore preventive practices recommended by the healthcare team.

LEGAL, ETHICAL, AND SAFETY ISSUES

- The dental hygienist thoroughly updates the client's health, dental, and pharmacologic histories and documents any updates or changes in health status at each visit.
- If concern exists that the client is at risk for harm by proceeding with care, the dental hygienist must inform the dentist and client and make a prompt referral to the physician of record.
- The dental hygienist must document any adverse reaction or occurrence during the provision of care. This information must be shared with the dentist and physician of record.

KEY CONCEPTS

- The incidence of encountering individuals with autoimmune diseases in the oral care environment increases as the percentage of aging persons increases.
- The dental hygienist screens for and recognizes typical signs, symptoms, and manifestations of autoimmune diseases.
- Some autoimmune diseases affect the head and neck area only, whereas others can affect multiple organ systems of the body.
- Autoimmune diseases compromise clients' immune systems, which puts them at risk for oral diseases and systemic infections.
- Some autoimmune diseases can be managed effectively with medication.
- Some autoimmune diseases and their treatment effects warrant antibiotic prophylaxis before any invasive care is begun. Consultation with the physician is indicated.
- Scleroderma and rheumatoid arthritis may affect a client's ability to perform adequate oral self-care measures.
- Chronic xerostomia places an individual at extreme risk for dental caries. Professional and daily self-applied topical fluoride applications, use of remineralization therapies, antimicrobials, antiseptics, xylitol, and salivary substitutes may help manage xerostomia and caries risk in those with Sjögren's syndrome and others with chronic dry mouth (see Chapters 16, 18, and 33).
- Referral and consultation with the client's physician are essential to providing optimum dental hygiene care to clients with autoimmune disease.

CRITICAL THINKING EXERCISES

Client: Mrs. M.

Profile: Mrs. M., age 40, who has not been to a dentist for 3 years, was scheduled for care with the dental hygienist.

Chief Complaint: "I have a very dry mouth. Also I cannot eat spicy foods because they irritate the skin inside my mouth. I haven't been able to really taste my food for some time."

Health History: Besides the slight discomfort from her inflamed tissues, she believes her health is satisfactory.

Social History: Married with two children

Dental History: Intraorally, her probing depths range from 4 to 6 mm, with generalized, moderate to severe bleeding on probing. The gingiva and oral mucosa are moderately inflamed and erythematous. The tissues are smooth without stippling, and the tongue is fissured with atrophic papillae. She has Class II periodontitis, with generalized, moderate calculus deposits, and heavy cervical bacterial plaque biofilm. Six Class V carious lesions were identified.

Oral Health Behavior Assessment: She brushes her teeth two times per day but admits that she does not floss.

Supplemental Notes: There is obvious facial swelling bilaterally in the area of the parotid glands; however, she does not report any injury to the head and neck.

1. Use the assessment data to arrive at a dental hygiene diagnosis, set client goals, and plan dental hygiene interventions.
2. What should the dental hygienist do if the client's response to therapy is poor and her periodontal disease continues to progress?

REFERENCES

1. Abbas AK, Lichtman AH: *Basic immunology: functions and disorders of the immune system*, ed 2, Philadelphia, 2004, Elsevier.
2. Gurenlian JR, Spolarich AE: Risk assessment for autoimmune diseases, *Dimensions Dent Hyg* 10(12):18, 21, 2012.
3. Gurenlian JR, Spolarich AE: Immune system dysfunction. In Daniel SJ, Harfst SA, Wilder RS, editors: *Mosby's dental hygiene concepts, cases, and competencies*, ed 2, St Louis, 2008, Mosby Elsevier, p 855.
4. U.S. National Library of Medicine National Institutes of Health: *Autoimmune disorders*. Available at: http://www.nlm.nih.gov/medlineplus/ency/article/000816.hthtm. Accessed August 18, 2012.
5. Walsh MM: Persons with autoimmune diseases. In Darby ML, Walsh MM, eds: *Dental hygiene theory and practice*, ed 3, St Louis, 2010, Saunders Elsevier, pp 919.
6. Little JW, Falace DA, Miller CS, et al: *Dental management of the medically compromised patient*, ed 8, St Louis, 2013, Mosby Elsevier.
7. Ibsen OAC, Phelan JA: *Oral pathology for the dental hygienist*, ed 5, St Louis, 2009, Saunders.
8. Spolarich AE: Xerostomia and oral disease, *Dimens Dent Hygiene* 9(11; Spec Suppl):43, 2011.
9. Papas A, Singh M, Harrington D, et al: Stimulation of salivary flow with a powered toothbrush in a xerostomic population, *Spec Care Dent* 26:241, 2006.

EVOLVE RESOURCES

Please visit http://evolve.elsevier.com/Darby/hygiene for additional practice and study support tools.

CHAPTER 49

Renal Disease and Organ Transplantation

Cheryl Thomas

COMPETENCIES

1. Define solid organ transplant and the United Network for Organ Sharing.
2. Discuss solid organ transplant candidates, including:
   - Determine oral health needs of solid organ transplant candidates, including realistic expectations for persons living with end-stage organ disease.
   - Manage xerostomia as a special consideration in persons living on dialysis.
   - Develop a dental hygiene care plan for the solid organ transplant candidate.
   - Interact with members of the pretransplant and post-transplant healthcare teams.
3. Discuss dental care after solid organ transplantation, including:
   - Determine oral health needs of solid organ transplant recipients.
   - Identify the actions indicated immediately after transplant.
   - Develop a dental hygiene care plan for the solid organ transplant recipient.

End-stage organ disease can occur in persons regardless of socioeconomic status or age, creating a need for organ transplantation to sustain quality of life. **Solid organ transplant** refers to the surgical procedures in which a viable, functioning organ, such as a heart, liver, pancreas, lung, intestine, or kidney, is placed into a patient ailing from end-stage organ disease. The patient's native organs may or may not be removed depending on residual function or medical complications. One commonality of all organ transplant recipients, regardless of etiology, the organ involved, or comorbidities, is infection (sepsis) and organ rejection. Although acute rejection is a relatively rare occurrence in today's world of advanced immunosuppression therapy, sepsis and chronic rejection continue to threaten the medical stability of the organ transplant recipient.

As medical treatment for end-stage organ disease advances, dental hygienists are likely to provide oral healthcare treatment to patients living with dialysis, solid organ transplant candidates, and solid organ transplant recipients. However, dental hygienists often discover variations in patient care and recommendations from hospital to hospital, from organ transplanted to organ transplanted, and the clinician may become confused or frustrated. The National Institutes of Health: National Institute of Dental and Craniofacial Research (NIDCR) now provides dental hygienists with helpful guidelines to patient care (http://www.nidcr.nih.gov/OralHealth/Topics/OrganTransplantationOralHealth/OrganTransplantProf.htm). Because of the complexities and variations of care, however, the importance of understanding the medical complexities of end-stage organ disease and organ transplantation (as well as working closely with the patient's medical team) cannot be overemphasized.

Although no concrete evidence supports a relationship or impact of oral infections on organ transplant recipients, at this time, dental and renal experts consider infections of oral origin as potentially dangerous and preventable to kidney transplant recipients. As a result, several sensible recommendations for providing oral care to the candidate for organ transplantation have been published and include the following[1]:

- Consultation with the patient's physician
- Treatment of active dental disease, including oral debridement
- Postponement of all elective dental treatment
- Removal of all potential sources of dental infection and nonrestorable teeth
- Adjustment of dentures and oral appliances
- Meticulous, daily oral self-care to minimize random bacteremias

United Network for Organ Sharing

The **United Network for Organ Sharing (UNOS)** is a nonprofit, scientific, and educational organization that maintains the nation's only **Organ Procurement and Transplantation Network (OPTN)**. The organ transplant "waiting list" includes persons who have a medical need and qualify medically to benefit from organ transplantation. UNOS manages the OPTN, establishes organ donation policies and procedures, facilitates organ matching and placement, and maintains the national database of organ transplant candidates and donors. Although waiting periods can vary greatly, oral healthcare providers can determine average waiting times for specific hospitals and geographic areas (Figure 49-1). For example, the average renal patient waiting for a deceased donor kidney usually waits at least 2 years before receiving a transplant. Recipients who are fortunate to receive the direct donation from a related or nonrelated living donor can expect to have virtually no waiting time. With this information, a dental hygiene care plan can be developed for the client in the pretransplant waiting phase to avoid postoperative complications from poor oral health and hygiene.

Of the more than 110,000 solid organ transplant candidates listed with UNOS, in 2012 according to UNOS only 23,360 transplants were performed. Of those 23,360 transplants, 13,750 were kidney transplants, by far the largest population

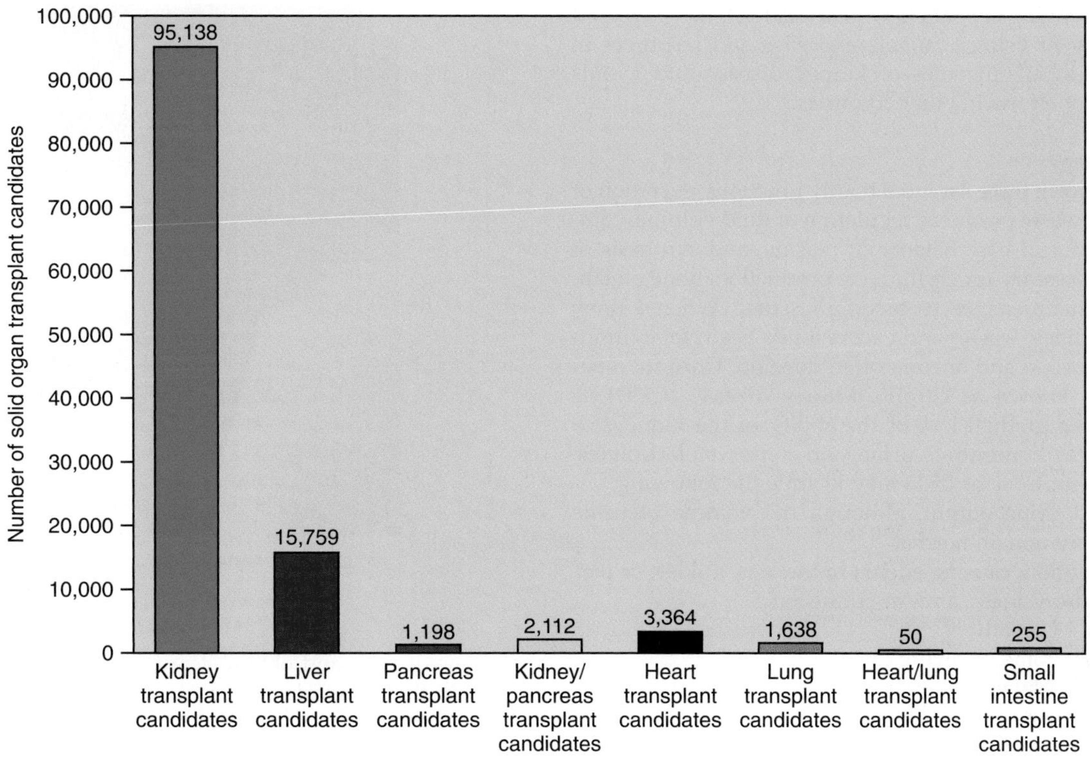

Figure 49-1. Number of persons awaiting organ transplant in 2013. (Data from United Network for Organ Sharing, Richmond Virginia.)

of recipients by organ. Because end-stage renal disease has dialysis to offer patients as a "bridge to transplantation," the fact that kidney transplants can be provided by a living donor (not only by a deceased donor), and deceased kidneys have a 48-hour window (a significantly greater amount of time compared with heart, liver, lung, and other organs), there is an increased number of kidney transplant recipients and candidates, compared with other potential end-stage organ disease candidates.

Solid Organ Transplant Candidates

End-Stage Renal Disease

The National Kidney Foundation (NKF) estimates that 26 million Americans have chronic kidney disease (CKD) and another 20 million are undiagnosed or at higher risk for CKD; these estimates are anticipated to grow as the U.S. population continues to increase. Far more people are awaiting renal solid organ transplant than any other type of solid organ transplant because dialysis is a "bridge" to transplantation.

Dialysis is a treatment method of cleaning and filtering wastes and toxins from the blood when the kidneys lose their function in end-stage renal disease (ESRD). In addition to cleansing wastes from the blood, dialysis:

- Removes salt and extra water to prevent them from building up in the body
- Maintains a safe balance of certain chemicals in the blood, such as potassium, sodium, and bicarbonate
- Helps to control blood pressure

With ESRD, medical treatment modalities include the following:

- In-center hemodialysis
- Home hemodialysis
- Peritoneal dialysis
- Renal transplantation

No dialysis treatment modality is considered medically superior to another; however, the success of treatment is complex and often is geared toward compliance, convenience to the patient, and acceptable clinical outcomes obtained by the treatment modality. For instance, senior citizens living unassisted often are placed in in-center hemodialysis to ensure safety that is required with a home hemodialysis treatment partner (often a spouse, parent, or friend). Furthermore, although renal transplantation is not a cure for ESRD, it provides a less inhibited lifestyle than required with dialysis treatment; therefore many (although not all) patients seek consideration for the National Solid Organ Waiting List.

Kidney Disease Outcomes Quality Initiative

The world-recognized Kidney Disease Outcomes Quality Initiative (K/DOQI) publishes evidence-based practice guidelines for all stages and aspects of kidney disease: anemia and CKD, diabetes and CKD, hemodialysis adequacy, PD, vascular access, anemia management, nutrition, disease classification, dyslipidemia, bone metabolism disorders, and cardiovascular disease in people living with kidney disease.[2]

Kidney Disease: Improving Global Outcomes

Because kidney-related medical outcomes in the United States surpass those in some other countries, the K/DOQI implemented in the United States is part of a larger initiative implemented globally by NKF. This initiative entitled Kidney

Disease: Improving Global Outcomes (KDIGO) has increased the efficiency of using available expertise and resources in improving global outcomes of kidney disease and avoids duplication of efforts in other countries.[3]

Renal Physiology

Kidneys perform three essential bodily functions: excretion of nitrogenous waste products; regulation of fluid volume, composition, and acid-base balance of plasma; and synthesis of hormones necessary for erythrocyte production, bone metabolism, and maintenance of blood pressure.[4] When kidney function declines, wastes and excess fluids begin to accumulate; hypertension and anemia often develop. **Chronic renal failure**, also known as **chronic kidney disease (CKD)**, is defined as the gradual loss of the ability of the kidneys to remove wastes, concentrate urine, and conserve electrolytes. Signs and symptoms of CKD may include the following:

- Decreased urine output, although the volume of urine output may remain normal
- Fluid retention, causing edema in the legs, ankles, or feet
- Fatigue, drowsiness, and/or confusion
- Shortness of breath
- Seizures or coma in severe cases
- Chest pain related to pericarditis

Some people do not notice early signs or symptoms, and many individuals are not diagnosed until there is irreversible, bilateral damage to the kidneys. The most accurate means of measuring renal function is via the **glomerular filtration rate** (GFR), an expression of the quality of glomerular filtrate created each minute in the renal nephrons. The GFR can determine stages of CKD as follows:

- Stage 1: Renal damage with normal GFR (GFR $\geq$ 90). Renal damage may occur before a reduction in GFR. Primary treatment goals are to delay the progression of CKD and reduce risk of cardiovascular disease.
- Stage 2: Renal damage with mild decrease in GFR (GFR 60 to 89). Treatment goals are to delay progression of CKD and reduce risk of cardiovascular disease.
- Stage 3: Moderate decrease in GFR (GFR 30 to 59). Anemia and bone metabolism disorders become more common.
- Stage 4: Severe reduction in GFR (GFR 15 to 29)
- Stage 5: ESRD (GFR less than 15). Patient is unable to maintain essential life functions unless dialysis is initiated.

Preventive treatment to delay (or avoid) ESRD includes the pharmacologic use of angiotensin-converting enzyme (ACE) inhibitors and angiotensin receptor blockers (ARBs).

Dialysis Treatment Modalities

In **hemodialysis** the person's blood (a few ounces at a time) is cleansed with a special filter. The dialysis access (a vascular access, a fistula, or graft) is created surgically by a vascular surgeon, usually in the forearm (Figure 49-2). During each dialysis treatment session a large intravenous cannula is inserted into the vascular access. Hemodialysis treatments may be performed by trained personnel in a dialysis center (typically three times a week for a prescribed period of time for each treatment session) or in the home performed by the patient and a spouse, parent, or friend as a "care partner" with a special home hemodialysis machine and supplies.

Alterations in the dental hygiene care plan for the person receiving hemodialysis treatments are as follows:

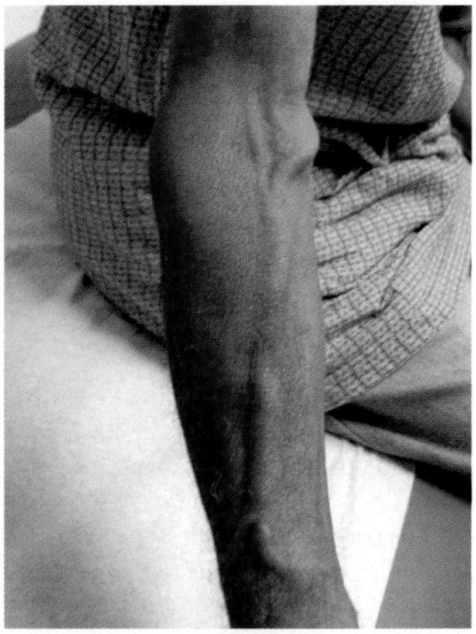

Figure 49-2. Hemodialysis access (fistula).

- Consult with and obtain clearance from the nephrologist to do the following:
  - Confirm that the patient is medically stable to receive dental treatment.
  - Determine if prophylactic antibiotic premedication is indicated to prevent either infection of the dialysis access or infective endocarditis.
- *Do not take blood pressure readings in the dialysis access arm* (this could cause the access to become occluded or infected and may delay or compromise dialysis therapy). The dialysis access is a "life line" and must be protected at all costs.
- Avoid dental treatment *after* dialysis treatment is performed on the same day because of coagulation complications associated with the use of heparin (blood anticoagulant therapy) administered during dialysis therapy.

Peritoneal dialysis (PD), like hemodialysis, filters the blood of the person living with ESRD. However, this treatment modality uses the person's own peritoneal lining to filter the blood. A specialized catheter is placed surgically by a surgeon into the person's abdomen, giving access to the peritoneal lining; the person uses this access to inject a prescribed dialysate solution into the person's peritoneal lining. This fluid contains dextrose, salt, and other minerals dissolved in water. These ingredients create a chemical exchange that allows the person's waste products and extra body fluid to pass from the person's blood, through the peritoneal filter, and into the dialysis solution. After a prescribed period of time, the waste-filled solution is drained from the person's abdomen and immediately replaced with fresh solution, and the dialysis process of filtering the blood begins again.

The two primary forms of PD are as follows:

- **Continual ambulatory peritoneal dialysis (CAPD)**: Dialysate solution is delivered manually to the abdominal catheter for dialysis treatment without the use of a machine. As the word *ambulatory* suggests, the person can walk around freely while the dialysis process is being performed within the peritoneal cavity. Because no equipment is used in the process, there is no need to use electricity. With

CAPD, the solution is removed and replaced during prescribed intervals throughout the day by the patient.

- **Continuous cyclic-assisted peritoneal dialysis (CCPD):** Dialysate solution is delivered to the abdominal catheter via a peritoneal dialysis machine. Unlike CAPD, during CCPD, the solution is removed and replaced during the evening/night during prescribed intervals usually while the patient sleeps at night. Although it does require electricity to operate, it is convenient because it allows a machine to exchange solutions during sleep and frees up valuable time during the day.

PD is offered in-center in select dialysis centers but usually is chosen by patients for its flexibility of self-administered, at-home treatment, and its elimination of an intravenous cannula in a vascular access three times per week in exchange for daily dialysis performed through an abdominal catheter. Neither hemodialysis nor peritoneal dialysis is considered medically "superior"; rather, treatment is prescribed typically based on the patients' needs and abilities and which treatment modality seems to work best for their clinical needs.

Alteration in the dental hygiene care plan for persons living with PD treatments are as follows:

- Consult with and obtain medical clearance from the patient's nephrologist to accomplish the following:
  - Confirm that the patient is medically stable to receive dental treatment. (Oral healthcare appointments may have to be delayed if heparin was used within the last 24-hour period during PD treatment.)
  - Determine if prophylactic antibiotic premedication is indicated to prevent infection of the PD dialysis access, infective endocarditis, or because of other comorbidities.
- Unless patients have comorbidities or evidence-based conditions that indicate antibiotic treatment per the American Heart Association Guidelines or the American Academy of Orthopaedic Surgeons guidelines, PD patients usually do not require prophylactic antibiotic premedication based on PD status alone. However, cardiovascular complications (the most prevalent cause of mortality) are extremely common within the hemodialysis and PD population. With that in mind, all patients should be evaluated individually for antibiotic prophylaxis based on their risk factors.
- Consider the function of compromised organs and how the malfunction of this organ will affect body systems (e.g., secondary hypertension and diabetes).

Etiology

Diabetes mellitus and hypertension are the most prevalent causes of ESRD. Regardless of the cause or treatment modality chosen, ESRD patients are also prone to secondary diabetes and hypertension that may be a complication and also must be considered in the process of care. **Secondary medical conditions** are not part of the original etiology of disease, but rather a complication developed as a result of a disease or condition. For instance, although the primary cause of ESRD in a person living with ESRD being treated with dialysis may be diabetes mellitus, owing to a cascade of complications (e.g., fluid retention, anemia) the person may develop secondary hypertension. Furthermore, a patient living with ESRD with the initial etiology of hypertension also can develop secondary diabetes. In addition to secondary hypertension and secondary diabetes, secondary anemia, hyperparathyroidism, and malnutrition are serious conditions to manage in persons receiving dialysis therapy.

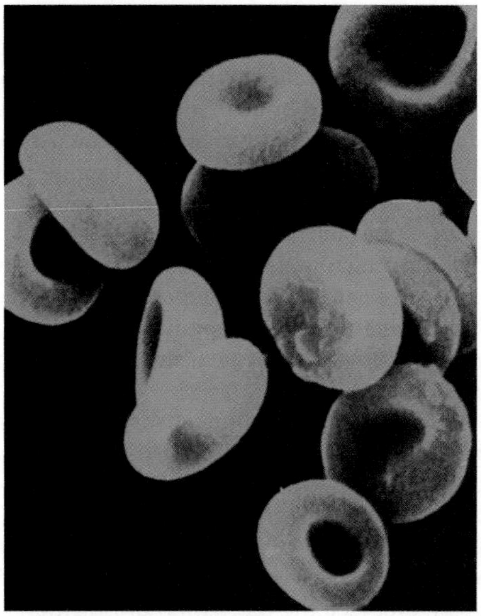

Figure 49-3. Red blood cells. (From Patton KT, Thibodeau GA: *Anatomy and physiology*, ed 8, St Louis, 2013, Mosby.)

Cardiovascular Disease and Inflammation

Persons with renal disease have 10 to 100 times greater risk of cardiovascular disease than persons without renal disease.[5] Regardless of the stage of CKD, inflammation plays an important role in clinical outcomes of medical (and also dental) treatment.

Anemia

With normal, healthy renal function, the kidneys produce the hormone **erythropoietin** (EPO), which stimulates bone marrow to produce red blood cells, essential in delivering oxygen throughout the body. Diseased kidneys fail to make enough EPO, which results in less oxygen distributed throughout the body. **Anemia**, the reduction of the mass of circulating red blood cells, is not a disease but rather a symptom of other illnesses (Figure 49-3). Anemia may be present in the early stages of renal disease and worsens as a renal disease progresses. Nearly all people living with end-stage renal failure (less than 10% renal function) have anemia. Additional factors that contribute to anemia in people with ESRD include iron deficiency, shortened red blood cell life span, hypothyroidism, secondary hyperthyroidism, blood loss, and acute and chronic inflammation. Oral manifestations of anemia include pallor of the oral mucosa, glossitis (an early sign of folate or vitamin B_{12} deficiency), recurrent aphthae, candidiasis, and angular stomatitis (cheilitis). Fatigue and increased risk of infection are common systemic complications of anemia and likely affect a person's ability to perform home oral hygiene. Furthermore, anemia also may contribute to cardiovascular complications.

According to K/DOQI and KDIGO guidelines, persons living with kidney disease are considered anemic when hemoglobin levels are less than 11 g/dL or hematocrit levels fall below 33%. Anemia treatment for those with chronic kidney disease may include a genetically engineered form of the EPO hormone, iron supplements, and/or folate supplements.

Mineral and Bone Disorder

A serious complication of chronic kidney disease characterized by an excessive secretion of parathyroid hormone (PTH) is known as mineral and bone disorder (formerly referred to as secondary hyperparathyroidism). As renal disease progresses, the kidneys lose their ability to excrete phosphorus from the body and produce the active form of vitamin D necessary in bone metabolism. These changes result in decreased serum calcium. In response to reestablish balance, increases in PTH result, causing hypercalcemia. This impediment in bone metabolism is recognized for causing greater potential complications and calcifications within the body's vascular system and organs.

Persons with mineral and bone disorder must limit phosphorus intake. In addition, vitamin D supplements and medications known as *phosphorus binders* may be prescribed to reduce absorption of phosphorus. A renal dietitian (available for consultation at almost all in-center dialysis and transplant centers) works with the nephrologist and patient to plan a renal-friendly diet (see the discussion of nutrition in the following section).

Oral manifestations of mineral and bone disorder may include areas of abnormal calcium leaching from osseous structures and calcium deposits on and in teeth, soft tissues, vasculature, and/or organs. In addition to dental calculus, calcium deposits may be visible on panoramic radiographs as calcifications in the carotid arteries; on periapical radiographs as narrowing of the pulp chamber or abnormal calcifications in soft tissues, or as a radiolucent osseous lesion (also known as a *brown tumor*). Other radiographic manifestations include loss of lamina dura, loss of trabecular pattern, and bone density changes. Early diagnosis and management of mineral and bone metabolism disorders are essential for positive medical outcomes. Dental radiographs may help screen patients with CKD for calcifications because of their high diagnostic potential.[6]

Nutrition

To offset complications associated with chronic kidney disease, patients typically are prescribed a renal diet that restricts fluid and sodium intake (owing to decreased renal output, excess body fluid, and hypertension) and limits dietary phosphorus and potassium. The dental hygienist should reach out to the patient's renal dietitian when counseling the patient for recommended dental products that may be ingested. The dietitian can provide guidance specially designed for the patient's exact needs. The National Kidney Foundation website is a valuable resource for the renal diet. Because diets can vary greatly, however, as a result of such factors as the stage of disease, etiology, compliance of medications and dietary restrictions, and comorbidities, there can be a wide variation in dietary needs. It is always best to consult with the renal dietitian to develop a plan tailored toward specific client dietary needs.

Fluid restrictions result in reduced salivary flow, which interferes with the cleansing role of saliva. Therefore clients receiving dialysis treatment commonly have greater-than-normal deposits of dental calculus and oral candidiasis. Uremia compounds the dental calculus problem.

Because dialysis treatment removes varying amounts of protein during the procedure, dialysis patients routinely have their albumin levels measured and monitored. Albumin is a laboratory test that is an excellent indicator of protein intake. Dietary allowances for dialysis patients may be higher in protein to compensate for protein lost, to aid in tissue healing, and to avoid infection. Patients who have chronic kidney disease stages 1 through 4 are typically on lower amounts of protein and after organ transplantation patients often return to normal dietary intake of protein.

Salivary pH

As kidney disease progresses, nitrogenous materials accumulate in the body, producing a condition known as uremia and altering the pH of blood and saliva. Whether uremia is a protective factor or a risk factor for dental caries remains unclear.[7-9] Dialysis patients often are advised to "suck on lemons" and chew on ice to cope psychologically and physically with chronic xerostomia and strict fluid restrictions. Other alternatives include daily chewing of xylitol gum that contains at least 1.55 g of xylitol as a therapeutic dose, sucking on frozen grapes, and/or sucking on a button tied with a 20-inch string to prevent accidental ingestion. Oral self-care may include use of a power toothbrush, oral irrigation (caution patient about fluid restrictions and ingestion), and sleeping with a humidifier to aid in moisturizing the oral and nasopharyngeal passages. Again, the dental hygienist should consult with the renal dietitian to be sure that all oral self-care recommendations and products are within the client's prescribed renal diet and medical treatment plan.

Periodontal Disease

At best there is a moderate relationship between periodontal disease and renal insufficiency.[10] The evidence-based relationship between periodontal disease and renal disease is the subject of ongoing research.

Communication with Others on the Team

The nephrology team usually includes the following members:

- Nephrologist
- Nephrology nurse
- Renal dietitian
- Nephrology social worker
- Patient care technician
- Pretransplant and post-transplant coordinators

In the pretransplant phase, the dental hygienist likely communicates solely with the pretransplant coordinator on the renal transplant team. In most instances, this is a registered nurse or physician's assistant. The pretransplant coordinator is responsible for coordinating all required preoperative appointments for the transplant candidate.

In the post-transplant phase, the patient receives care at a transplant center or returns to a primary healthcare provider if a transplant center is not located nearby. The dental hygienist should consult with the patient's current healthcare provider to determine the patient's medical stability and precautions during dental hygiene care.

A reliable bridge to transplantation does not yet exist for liver, heart, and lung transplant *candidates*. Therefore they are often in more critical condition and treated in a hospital setting. In this situation, oral healthcare providers consult directly with the patient's medical specialist. These patients should be evaluated carefully before dental hygiene care to determine a safe, effective course of action.

Dental Care After Solid Organ Transplant

Gingival Enlargement

The discovery of the drug cyclosporine provided a breakthrough in solid organ transplantation. Cyclosporine, however, increases risk of nephrotoxicity, the quality or state of being toxic to kidney cells. Most transplant recipients are treated with a trio of immunosuppression medications (e.g., cyclosporine, prednisone, and mycophenolate mofetil). Because even prednisone can cause long-term complications of bone metabolism and adrenal crisis, the pursuit of immunosuppressive therapy with minimal side effects continues. In addition, a wide variety of prescription and common over-the-counter medications are nephrotoxic to transplant recipients. Even common herbs can cause disruption in cyclosporine levels, endangering patient's delicate balance of immunosuppression. Therefore the dental team *always* must consult the medical team to ensure the safety of medications prescribed and over-the-counter medications.

The research literature is replete with instances of drug-influenced gingival enlargement in solid organ transplant recipients. Gingival enlargement, also known as gingival overgrowth, is another adverse side effect associated with immunosuppressive therapy. Gingival enlargement may be due to poor oral hygiene and/or increased sensitivity to cyclosporine. Although modifications in immunosuppressive therapy may be explored when gingival enlargement is a concern, transplant physicians are reluctant to alter the immunosuppressive therapy when the patient's medical condition is medically stable. Drug-influenced gingival enlargement has been associated with the immunosuppressive medication tacrolimus.[11]

Prevention of gingival enlargement is best. Meticulous daily oral self-care should emphasize optimal oral biofilm removal to avoid infection and inflammation, and frequent oral debridement (3- to 4-month continued-care intervals) by the dental hygienist to reduce gingival enlargement risk. The dental hygienist always must be aware that immunosuppressive therapy can mask inflammation.

Infection

Immunosuppressive therapy is at its most aggressive level in transplant recipients immediately after transplant surgery. In the months after surgery, the patient's immunosuppressive therapy gradually is reduced and then maintained at a level that balances the threat of rejection and infection. Any infection (such as vascular or catheter infections, pneumonia, cellulitis, or periodontal abscess) can be reactivated or exacerbated in the immediate postoperative period during the introduction of immunosuppressive therapy or afterward, depending on the overall state of immunosuppression.[12] When providing care, oral healthcare providers should educate patients about the potential risk dental infections play in organ rejection and infection.

Infective Endocarditis and Invasive Dental Procedures

The need for antibiotic prophylaxis for invasive dental procedures in clients who have undergone solid organ transplant remains controversial. Although surveys of transplant survivors demonstrate opposing views, the majority of medical providers recommend antibiotic prophylaxis for invasive dental procedures. The American Heart Association, K/DOQI, nor KDIGO, directly address this issue of care in their guidelines. Extreme variations in variables within the transplant population make blanketed recommendations inappropriate. Therefore organ transplant recipients should be evaluated individually for infectious risk, and necessary medical and dental consultation determine the following:

- If or when the person can receive routine dental care
- Transplant recipient's medical stability
- Comorbidities present (e.g., diabetes, hypertension, cardiovascular disease)
- Medical management of the recipient; concerns during the pretransplant and/or post-transplant phase
- Pharmacologic history

Candidiasis and Viral Infections

Patients taking immunosuppressive therapy often experience candidiasis or recurrence of herpetic infections. The oral healthcare provider works with the transplant team to determine appropriate treatment.

Malignancies

Organ transplant recipients have an increased incidence of squamous and basal cell carcinomas. Therefore frequent screening of the skin and oral pharyngeal area is indicated. Liver transplant recipients with a history of tobacco use and/or alcoholism are at particular risk for oral pharyngeal cancer.

After Solid Organ Transplantation

Immediately after transplantation, only emergency dental care is recommended. During the post-transplant period, a medical consultation is necessary to determine the patient's medical stability and to determine what dental procedures are sensible.

During the stable post-transplant phase, the following actions are indicated:

- Consultation with, and clearance from the physician, for the following:
  - Confirm that the patient is medically stable to receive dental treatment
  - Determine if prophylactic antibiotic premedication is indicated to prevent infection or infective endocarditis
  - Determine if the patient is susceptible to adrenal crisis (a life-threatening condition associated with high doses or long-term use of steroids)
- Meticulous oral-self care including twice-daily antimicrobial mouth rinses and use of xylitol-containing products.
- Necessary professional oral care
  - Frequent oral debridement
  - Frequent oral hygiene counseling
  - Regular screening for oral, head, and neck cancer

CLIENT EDUCATION TIPS

- Explain the reason for pre-solid organ-transplant dental protocols.
- Explain professional dental needs and daily oral self-care needs of the patient living with end-stage renal disease.
- Encourage adherence to recommended daily oral self-care regimen.
- Discuss importance of good oral health to minimizing self-induced bacteremias from eating and oral care.

LEGAL, ETHICAL, AND SAFETY ISSUES

- Medical consultation is required to evaluate the client's medical stability, use of medications, and necessary precautions before invasive dental treatment.
- Document results from the medical consultation, including medical provider's recommendations and conversation with the client or caregiver.
- Use proper standard infection control procedures.
- Obtain and document informed consent from all clients.
- Involve the client in the decision-making process.
- Treat clients with dignity, respect, and empathy.
- Provide oral and written instructions that can be read easily by clients who may have impaired eyesight or hearing.
- Provide definitive instructions and interventions to prevent dental caries, soft-tissue infection, xerostomia, and fungal infections.

KEY CONCEPTS

- Patients awaiting solid organ transplantation outnumber the actual number of transplants performed each year.
- The most common pre–solid-organ transplant recipient is a patient living with end-stage renal disease who is most likely receiving dialysis therapy.
- When assessing a client who is on renal dialysis, do not take blood pressure readings in the dialysis access arm because doing so could cause the access to become occluded or infected.
- Avoid dental treatment *after* dialysis treatment on the same day, because of coagulation complications associated with heparin use (blood anticoagulant therapy) administered during dialysis therapy.
- When treating patients on dialysis, consult with and obtain clearance from the nephrologist to confirm that the patient is medically stable to receive dental treatment and to determine if prophylactic antibiotic premedication is indicated to prevent either infection of the dialysis access or infective endocarditis.
- If the patient received heparin (blood anticoagulant therapy) during peritoneal dialysis therapy within the previous 24-hour period, then professional oral healthcare may have to be delayed.
- Among solid organ transplant centers, K/DOQI, or KDIGO there is no one standard pretransplant or post-transplant dental care protocol. Because of extreme variations in medical conditions and other variables, professional oral healthcare must be tailored to each individual patient.
- The need for antibiotic prophylaxis for invasive dental procedures in clients who have undergone solid organ transplant remains controversial. Clients should be evaluated on an individual basis.
- The Kidney Disease Outcomes Quality Initiative (K/DOQI) and the Kidney Disease: Improving Global Outcomes (KDIGO) Initiative are globally recognized guidelines that address care for medical issues for all stages and aspects of renal disease.
- In persons with mineral and bone disorder, calcium deposits may be visible on panoramic radiographs as calcifications in the carotid arteries, on periapical radiographs as narrowing of the pulp chamber or abnormal calcifications in soft tissues, or as a radiolucent osseous lesion (known as a *brown tumor*). Other radiographic manifestations include loss of the lamina dura, loss of trabecular pattern, and bone density changes.
- Good oral health and effective daily oral biofilm control are important for minimizing the risk of self-induced bacteremias.
- Thorough oral cancer screenings should be performed on a frequent basis.
- The dental hygienist should consult with the client's renal dietitian to be sure that all oral self-care recommendations and products are within the client's prescribed renal diet and medical treatment plan.

CRITICAL THINKING EXERCISES

Activity 1

Client: Mrs. T. is a 60-year-old retired public school teacher with end-stage renal disease. She is on in-center hemodialysis; however, she desires a less-restrictive lifestyle without dialysis.

Chief Complaint: "I would like to get on the waiting list for a new kidney, but I've been told by my dialysis center that I need a dental clearance first."

Social History: Mrs. T. has been on in-center hemodialysis for 3 years. She has a low energy level but does have a daughter and grandchildren who live next door and help her when necessary.

Dental History: Mrs. T. has a history of regular dental visits before she started dialysis but has not had a professional oral debridement since she started dialysis 3 years ago. Her oral hygiene is poor and her gingival tissue bleeds easily upon homecare. Oral assessment findings reveal heavy supragingival oral biofilm and dental calculus deposits, generalized throughout the mouth, spontaneous gingival bleeding, candidiasis, and a uremic mouth odor. Dental examination does not reveal active carious lesions.

Oral Self-Care Assessment: Poor oral hygiene, xerostomia, use of a manual toothbrush once daily, with no interdental or tongue cleaning.

Supplemental Notes: Mrs. T. wants to be listed on the organ transplant waiting list.

1. What are the primary concerns for this patient?
2. If the patient receives an organ transplant, what are the long-term concerns?
3. Develop a dental hygiene care plan including an appointment schedule for this client that includes the dental hygiene diagnoses and client goals.
4. Develop a treatment plan that accommodates a Monday-Wednesday-Friday (afternoons) in-center dialysis schedule.
5. What factors may be contributing to this client's xerostomia and candidiasis? What interventions can be suggested?
6. Identify special precautions and/or care plan modifications for safe, high-quality care.

Activity 2: Learn Empathy, Not Sympathy

This activity asks participants to experience life through the eyes of a dialysis patient and provides insight into the lives of patients living with end-stage renal disease.

1. Avoid or limit fluid intake for a 24-hour period.
2. Sit in a chair for 3 hours (dialysis patients receive treatment over a 3- to 4-hour period three times per week)

during in-center hemodialysis or for over 8 to 10 hours for many types of peritoneal dialysis.

3. Visit or volunteer oral hygiene instruction at a local in-center hemodialysis unit.
4. The renal diet is filled with restrictions of fluids and food groups. Visit the National Kidney Foundation website and make a posterboard or Powerpoint presentation outlining restricted food groups. Discover dental products that are beneficial in the general population but may need to be discouraged with dialysis patients.
5. Explore ways to relieve xerostomia in clients on fluid restrictions.

Activity 3: Critical Thinking Exercise for a Client Who Has Undergone Solid Organ Transplant

Client: Mr. Y. is a 30-year-old accountant. He takes cyclosporine daily as part of his immunosuppressive regimen. He also has type 1 diabetes.

Chief Compliant: "My gums are painful and swollen."

Social History: Mr. Y. received an organ transplant 1 year ago. He has not had a dental visit since before his transplant surgery.

Dental History: Mr. Y. has a history of regular dental visits before he started dialysis but has not had a professional oral debridement since before his transplant surgery 1 year ago. Oral assessment findings reveal gross deposits of moderate supraginginval and subgingival oral biofilms and dental calculus. Dental examination reveals no active carious lesions; however, oral radiographs reveal unusual radiolucent lesions in the soft-tissue areas.

Oral Self-Care Behavior Assessment: Fair oral hygiene, xerostomia, use of manual toothbrush 1 or 2 times per day.

Supplemental Notes: Mr. Y. is an active participant in his medical care but does not quite understand how his oral health can affect other parts of his body.

1. What are the primary healthcare concerns for this client?
2. If the client does receive treatment for drug-influenced gingival enlargement, what are the long-term concerns?
3. Is the client's oral health affecting his diabetes and how can we educate him to understand how his oral health is affecting his general health?
4. Develop a dental hygiene care plan and appointment schedule that includes dental hygiene diagnosis, client goals, education, interventions, and evaluation criteria.
5. What factors are contributing to the client's dry mouth? What interventions can be suggested?
6. Are there any special precautions or considerations that should be considered during this client's care?

Activity 4: Critical Thinking Exercise for Client Who Has Undergone Organ Transplantation

Develop your own case scenario for a patient with liver, heart, heart-lung, lung, or intestinal transplant.

- Investigate available evidence-based research and develop a comprehensive dental care plan.

REFERENCES

1. Guggenheimer J, Egthesad B, Stock DJ: Dental Management of the (solid) organ transplant recipient, *Oral Surg Oral Med Oral Pathol* 95:383, 2003.
2. National Kidney Foundation: *NKF-KDOQI guidelines*. Available at: http://www.kidney.org/professionals/kdoqi/guidelines_commentaries.cfm. Accessed January 30, 2013.
3. *Kidney Disease: Improving Global Outcomes (KDIGO)*. Available at: http://www.kdigo.org/about_us.php. Accessed January 30, 2013.
4. National Kidney Foundation: *How your kidneys work*. Available at: http://www.kidney.org/kidneydisease/howkidneyswrk.cfm. Accessed January 30, 2013.
5. Kuma S: *A double-edged sword in the patient with chronic kidney disease*. Available at: http://www.medscape.com/viewarticle/465461. Accessed January 30, 2013.
6. Antonelli JR, Hottel TL: Oral manifestions of renal osteodystrophy: case report and review of the literature, *Spec Care Dent* 23:28, 2003.
7. Takeuchi Y, Ishikawa H, Inada M, et al: Study of oral microflora in patients with renal disease, *Nephrology (Carlton)* 12:182, 2007.
8. Lucas VS, Roberts GJ: Uremia in a protective role in caries risk, *Pediatr Nephrol* 20, 2005.
9. Lucas VS, Roberts GJ: Oro-dental health in children with chronic renal failure and after renal transplantation: a clinical review. *Pediatr Nephrol* 20:1388, 2005.
10. Kshiragar AV, Moss KI, Elter JR, et al: Periodontal disease is associated with renal insufficiency in the Atherosclerosis Risk in Communities (ARIC) study, *Am J Kidney Dis* 45:650, 2005.
11. Ellis S, Seymour RA, Taylor JJ, et al: Prevalence of gingival overgrowth in transplant patients immunosuppressed with tacrolimus, *J Clin Periodontol* 31:126, 2004.
12. Danovitch GM: *Handbook of kidney transplantion*, Philadelphia, 2001, Lippincott Williams & Wilkins.

EVOLVE RESOURCES

Please visit http://evolve.elsevier.com/Darby/hygiene for additional practice and study support tools.

CHAPTER 50

Respiratory Diseases

Joan Gugino Ellison, Curtis Aumiller

COMPETENCIES

1. **Discuss respiratory diseases, including:**
   - **Identify the risk factors, signs and symptoms, related medications, and dental hygiene care implications for the following respiratory diseases: asthma, chronic obstructive pulmonary disease (chronic bronchitis and emphysema), and tuberculosis.**
   - **Develop a dental hygiene care plan for a person with a respiratory disease.**

Respiratory diseases are common among the general population and can compromise dental and dental hygiene care. To properly manage this group of clients, it is important for the dental hygienist to understand respiratory diseases, medications used in their treatment, their link with periodontal health and oral hygiene, and their implications for dental hygiene care.

The most frequently encountered respiratory diseases are asthma and chronic obstructive pulmonary disease (COPD), including emphysema and chronic bronchitis. In addition, tuberculosis, a disease that has affected mankind for centuries, continues to be a worldwide problem. The emergence of multi–drug-resistant strains of tuberculosis poses yet another infection control and treatment challenge to healthcare providers.[1]

Respiratory Diseases

Asthma

Asthma is a chronic inflammatory respiratory disease characterized by an increased responsiveness of the bronchial airways to various stimuli. Management of the asthma client depends on assessment of the individual's severity level, and degree of control and responsiveness to treatment. Asthma severity is classified as intermittent or persistent (mild, moderate, or severe) based on current impairment of quality of life and risk for future exacerbations and/or lung damage. These classifications are determined by clinical tests as well as the occurrence of airflow obstruction symptoms in relation to environmental factors, exercise, and nighttime sleep disturbances.[2]

Etiology

Various substances or environmental factors can precipitate an asthma attack, including specific antigens such as pollen, ragweed, molds, foods, cockroaches, and house dust mites. Chemical irritants such as tobacco smoke, scents, and house sprays may trigger an asthma attack. Exposure by dental personnel to methacrylates found in dental restorative and sealant materials also has been cited as a possible link with occupational asthma. Adequate ventilation for dental personnel directly exposed to these materials should be ensured to minimize respiratory sensitivity.[3] Other nonallergic stimulators—respiratory infections, environmental pollutants and irritants, exercise, cold air, and emotional stress—also can cause an attack. Generalized narrowing of bronchi and bronchioles caused by mucosal inflammation, increased secretions, and smooth muscle contraction produce asthmatic symptoms[4,5] (Figure 50-1).

Signs and Symptoms

Clinical manifestations of asthma include periodic wheezing, **dyspnea** (difficulty in breathing), coughing, and chest tightness. These and other signs and symptoms are listed in Box 50-1. The onset of an asthma attack usually begins with mild wheezing and coughing, progressing to increased difficulty in breathing. As the attack develops, the individual may experience a sense of pressure or tightness in the chest and a feeling of suffocation. Blood pressure and heart rate may increase slightly during an attack.[4] A severe asthma attack that does not respond to treatment with an adequate dose of commonly used bronchodilators is referred to as **status asthmaticus**. This condition may produce bronchospasms for hours or days without remission and often requires hospitalization.

Implications for Dental Hygiene Care

To prevent an acute asthmatic attack and to address the unique needs of the asthmatic client, the dental hygienist should do the following:

- Assess the frequency, conditions and time of onset, and type—intermittent or persistent (mild, moderate, or severe)—of asthmatic attacks experienced; their management, including the type of medication used and precipitating factors; and whether a previous attack has warranted emergency treatment.[4]
- Seek a medical consultation in cases of persistent severe asthma or when reported symptoms suggest poorly controlled asthma. Document if the client is taking systemic corticosteroids, such as prednisone, for chronic asthma. Assure compliance with the usual regular dose of prednisone on the day of a particularly stressful dental appointment.
- Note the precipitating factors reported by the client, and avoid these factors during professional care.
- Instruct clients to bring the medical inhalers prescribed by the physician to every appointment for use in case of an

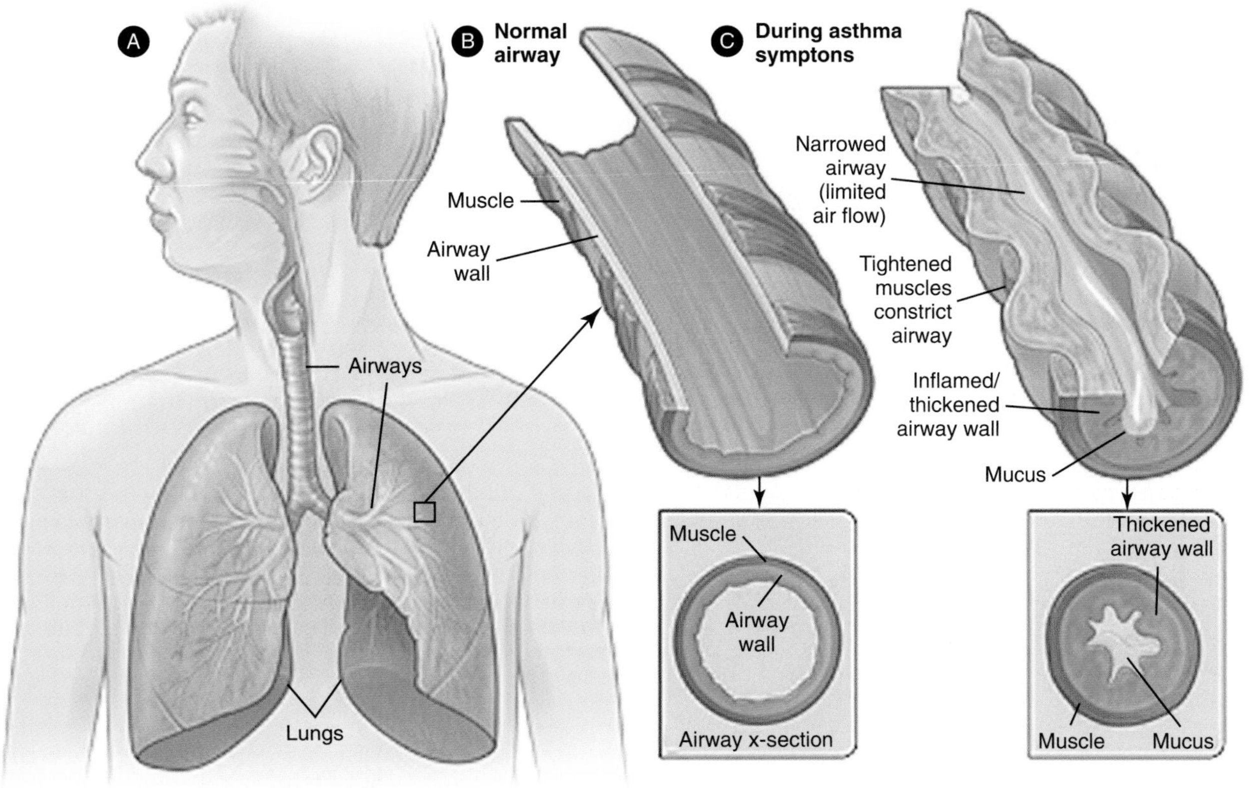

Figure 50-1. **A,** The location of the lungs and airways in the body. **B,** A cross-section of a normal airway. **C,** A cross-section of an airway during asthma symptoms. (From National Heart, Lung, and Blood Institute; National Institutes of Health; U.S. Department of Health and Human Services.)

BOX 50-1

Signs and Symptoms of an Acute Asthmatic Attack

- Wheezing
- Cough
- Nasal flaring
- Dyspnea
- Feeling of pressure or tightness in the chest
- Need to stand, sit upright, or lean forward
- Increased anxiety and apprehension
- Perspiration
- Respiratory rate of more than 30 rpm
- Increased pulse rate of more than 120 bpm
- Rise in blood pressure (particularly in severe attacks)
- Confusion
- Agitation
- Cyanosis

acute attack or prophylactically when chronic moderate to severe disease is present.

- Note that some medications used by clients with asthma cause xerostomia (dry mouth) and unpleasant taste sensation after inhalation use. Consequently the client with asthma may be more prone to dental caries and gingivitis. Children in particular may increase their sucrose intake to combat the unpleasant taste from the inhalant. Table 50-1 describes drugs commonly used in the treatment of asthma.
- Instruct the client to avoid drugs listed in Table 50-2, such as aspirin-containing medications, nonsteroidal anti-inflammatory drugs, barbiturates, and narcotics, because they can precipitate an attack.
- Avoid use of the air polisher or a power-driven polisher (Table 50-3).
- Use preprocedural antimicrobial rinse and high speed suction to reduce contaminated dental aerosols that may be inhaled when using ultrasonic scaler.
- Consider using a local anesthetic agent without epinephrine or levonordefrin because some clients with asthma are sensitive to the sulfite preservatives present in these anesthetic solutions.[4]
- Make the oral care environment as stress-free as possible because anxiety can induce an asthmatic attack in many people, particularly children.
- Use nitrous oxide–oxygen analgesia and/or small doses of diazepam, as prescribed by the dentist, to reduce stress if indicated[4] (see Chapter 41).
- Convey a calm, caring, and compassionate attitude to relax the client and to reduce stress-induced asthmatic attacks.
- Evaluate children carefully for malocclusion; many children with asthma are mouth breathers, and a correlation has been observed between higher palatal vaults, greater

TABLE 50-1
Drugs Commonly Used in the Treatment of Asthma

Action	Indication	Generic Name (Brand Name)	Drug Classification	Adverse Reactions and Dental Drug Implications
Anti-inflammatory agents	Inhibit release of agents that trigger asthma by inflammatory cells; taken on a daily basis to achieve and maintain control of asthma	Beclomethasone dipropionate (Beclovent) Fluticasone (Flovent, Flonase) Flunisolide (Aerobid)	Inhaled synthetic corticosteroids	Cough, hoarseness; oral candidiasis, unpleasant taste, xerostomia
	Used to speed resolution of airway obstruction and reduce rate of recurrence of symptoms	Methylprednisolone, prednisolone (Deltasone, Meticorten) Budesonide (Pulmicort, Rhinocort)	Systemic (oral) corticosteroids	Hyperglycemia, osteoporosis, fluid retention Suppresses adrenal gland; slower healing, infection more likely, symptoms may be masked
Mast cell stabilizers (Antiasthmatics)	To prevent acute bronchospasms	Cromolyn sodium (Intal)	Inhaled antiasthmatic, mast cell stabilizer	Urinary tract infection, nausea, headache, cough; taste perversion, swollen parotid glands, burning mouth/throat, dry throat
Bronchodilators	Temporarily dilate or relax the muscles surrounding the bronchial tubes that tighten during an asthma attack	Albuterol (Ventolin, Proventil) Levalbuterol (Xopenex)	Short-acting inhaled beta$_2$-adrenergic agonists	Nervousness, xerostomia, throat irritation, fast or irregular heartbeat
	Relax bronchial smooth muscles and inhibit release of mast cell inhibitors	Salmeterol (Serevent Diskus) Formoterol (Foradil Aerolizer, Performist) Arformoterol (Brovana)	Long-acting beta$_2$-adrenergic agonists	Nervousness, xerostomia, throat irritation, fast or irregular heartbeat
	Provide maintenance regulation of airway smooth muscle tone; may be used instead of beta$_2$-adrenergic agonists when not well tolerated by patient	Ipratropium bromide (Atrovent) Tiotropium bromide (Spiriva) Aclidinium bromide (Tudorza Pressair)	Anticholinergic, long-acting bronchodilator	Nervousness, xerostomia, headache, cough
Oral sustained-release tablet or capsule	Used as adjunct to inhaled corticosteroids for prevention of nighttime symptoms; relaxes smooth muscles of respiratory system	Theophylline (Theo-Dur, Slo-Bid)	Methylxanthine	Gastric reflux, headache, tachycardia, insomnia, nausea, trembling, nervousness Erythromycin may increase levels of theophylline
Nonsteroidal preventive therapy (leukotriene modifiers)	Long-term control and prevention of symptoms in cases of mild persistent asthma in those 12 years of age or older	Zafirlukast (Accolate) Zileuton (Zyflo) Montelukast (Singulair)	Selective leukotriene receptor antagonist	Nausea, central nervous system depression, increase in liver function test results, myalgia, headache Erythromycin lowers zafirlukast levels; aspirin raises zafirlukast levels
Combined Medications				
Anti-inflammatory agents and bronchodilator		Fluticasone and salmeterol (Advair) Budesonide and formoterol (Symbicort) Mometasone furoate and formoterol (Dulera)		Same possible side effects as each drug individually
Bronchodilators		Albuterol and ipratropium bromide (Combivent)		Same possible side effects as each drug individually

Data from Centerwatch.com. Available at: http://www.centerwatch.com/drug-information/fda-approvals/default.aspx; Haveles EB: *Applied pharmacology for the dental hygienist,* ed 6, St Louis, 2010, Mosby; and Moini J: *Cardiopulmonary pharmacology for respiratory care,* Sudbury, Mass, 2012, Jones & Bartlett.

TABLE 50-2

Contraindicated Drugs for the Individual with Asthma

Drugs	Rationale
Aspirin-containing medications	Ingestion of aspirin is associated with precipitating attacks in some clients
Nonsteroidal anti-inflammatory drugs (NSAIDs)	Ingestion of NSAIDs may precipitate asthma attack in some individuals
Barbiturates and narcotics	Association of these drugs with precipitation of asthma attacks
Erythromycin and ciprofloxacin in clients taking theophylline	May result in toxic blood level of theophylline

TABLE 50-3

Techniques to Be Avoided or Used Cautiously in Individuals with Certain Respiratory Diseases

Disease	Techniques Contraindicated or Used with Precautions	Rationale
Asthma	Use of air polisher Use of power-driven polisher	Aerosols created by air polisher may precipitate asthma attack Polisher may exacerbate existing breathing problems
COPD: chronic bronchitis and emphysema	Avoid use of rubber dam Use of power-driven polisher Nitrous oxide–oxygen analgesia	Rubber dam may cause more breathing difficulties Polisher may exacerbate existing breathing problems May produce cessation of respiration (apnea) if levels are too high
Clinically active tuberculosis	No treatment is provided on an outpatient basis for clients with active tuberculosis	Risk of transmission requires isolation room with special administrative, environmental, and respiratory controls

COPD, Chronic obstructive pulmonary disease.

overjets, posterior crossbite incidence, and mouth breathing in children.[6]

- Observe any asthmatic symptoms during and after dental procedures, because decreased lung function can be triggered by anxiety, supine positioning, tooth enamel dust, and aerosols commonly created by dental procedures.
- Take prompt action to manage symptoms of an acute asthmatic episode (see Procedure 50-1 and the corresponding Competency Form).[4]
- Set goals with the client to achieve meticulous homecare and optimal fluoride benefits to combat negative effects of medication and mouth breathing on oral health.

Chronic Obstructive Pulmonary Disease

Chronic obstructive pulmonary disease is a general term used to describe a spectrum of pulmonary disorders characterized by chronic irreversible obstruction of airflow to and from the lungs.[7] COPD is considered preventable and treatable. However, because many individuals often experience other significant nonpulmonary conditions (weight loss, skeletal muscle wasting, cardiovascular disease, anemia, osteoporosis, and depression) associated with COPD, the severity of the disease may be affected.[8]

When emphysema and chronic bronchitis occur together, the disorder is classified as COPD. **Emphysema** more recently has become a pathologic term to describe the overinflation and irreversible destruction of structures in the lungs known as **alveoli** or *air sacs*. This overinflation is caused by a breakdown of the walls of the alveoli, resulting in decreased respiratory function and often dyspnea.[8] Emphysema describes just one of the structural irregularities characterized by COPD. More prevalent among older men, emphysema is increasing rapidly among women, primarily because of tobacco use.[9] Although chronic bronchitis and emphysema can be described individually, they often coexist and represent the irreversible progression of the disease. Because of the progressive nature of COPD, quality of life is compromised greatly in severe cases.[8]

Bronchitis is an inflammation of the lining of the bronchial tubes. These tubes or bronchi connecting the trachea with the lungs become inflamed and/or infected. As a result, less air is able to flow to and from the lungs, and heavy mucus or phlegm is expectorated.[9] **Chronic bronchitis** is associated with the presence of a mucus-producing cough with expectoration for at least 3 months of the year for more than 2 consecutive years, without other underlying disease to explain the cough.[7] Smokers may dismiss symptoms of chronic bronchitis as a "smoker's cough" and avoid medical care. Consequently the individual may be in danger of developing serious respiratory problems or heart failure. Chronic bronchitis is consistently more prevalent in females than in males and can affect people of all ages but is usually higher in those more than 45 years old.[9] With **spirometry** (common pulmonary test used to measure lung function), COPD can be classified into four levels: stage I, mild; stage II, moderate; stage III, severe; and stage IV, very severe.[7]

Procedure 50-1 Management of an Acute Asthmatic Episode

STEPS

1. Terminate the dental procedure and remove all materials from client's mouth immediately.
2. Place the client in a comfortable position as soon as signs are apparent—usually sitting upright.
3. Remove all dental materials.
4. Try to calm client and allay apprehension.
5. Evaluate ABCs (airway, breathing, circulation), and monitor vital signs.
6. Definitive care:
   a. Administer bronchodilator (client's prescribed medication preferred).
   b. If attack persists, administer oxygen.
   c. Call for emergency assistance if bronchodilators fail to resolve bronchospasm.
   d. Administration of epinephrine by dentist if necessary (available in preloaded syringe).
7. Discharge of the client: alone, escorted, or with emergency personnel, depending on severity of attack.

Adapted from Malamed SF: *Medical emergencies in the dental office*, ed 6, St Louis, 2007, Mosby, and Jennings D, Chernega J: *Emergency guide for dental auxiliaries*, ed 4, Stamford, Conn, 2013, Delmar Cengage.

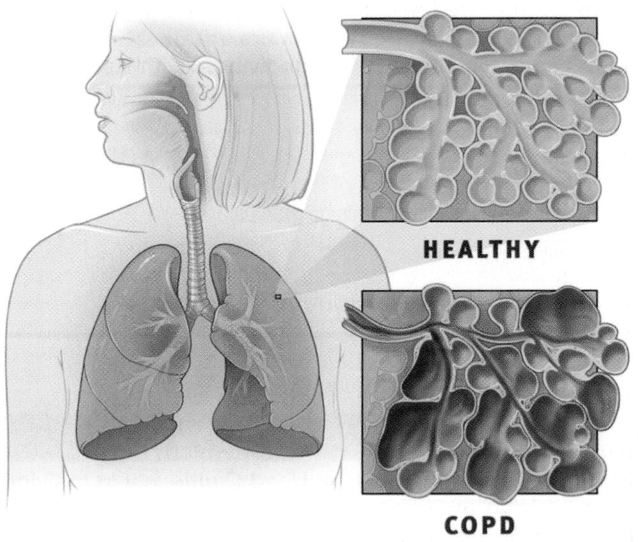

Figure 50-2. Comparing healthy lungs and lungs with chronic obstructive pulmonary disease (COPD). The elasticity of airways and sacs in healthy lungs allows air to move quickly in and out of lungs. The airways and sacs in lungs with COPD lack the elasticity to allow lungs to retain their original shape. These airways lack support and become enlarged and lined with mucus, thereby making breathing more difficult. (From NHLBI Health Information Center. Available at: http://www.LearnAboutCOPD.org.)

Etiology

Cigarette smoking has been identified as the major risk factor in COPD. Air pollutants and industrial dust and fumes may contribute to COPD.[7,8] In some parts of the world air pollutants may be a primary risk factor for COPD.[8] Underlying respiratory disease, severe respiratory infection in early childhood, underdeveloped lungs (during gestation and childhood), and genetic tendencies can be risk factors for COPD.[8]

Emphysema also can have a genetic predisposition known as alpha-1 antitrypsin deficiency or what is commonly called alpha-1. Alpha-1 occurs in about 1 out of every 50 cases of emphysema. **Alpha-1 antitrypsin** is a blood protein produced in the liver that helps to protect the lungs from the enzyme elastase. Elastase is found in white blood cells (WBCs) and helps to kill invading bacteria and neutralize small particles that are inhaled into the lungs. When WBCs are destroyed, the elastase is released into the bloodstream. Alpha-1 antitrypsin inactivates the elastase so that it can be excreted by the body. However, if an individual has low alpha-1 antitrypsin levels, the elastase attacks and destroys the elastic tissues of the lungs, which leads to emphysema. Alpha-1 antitrypsin deficiency can be diagnosed with a blood test, and many patients do not have any other predisposing factors that would lead to such severe emphysema.[7]

Signs and Symptoms of Chronic Obstructive Pulmonary Disease

Chronic bronchitis symptoms appear gradually but intensify in individuals who smoke or when atmospheric concentrations of sulfur dioxide and other air pollutants increase. A cough producing large amounts of sputum may linger for several weeks after a winter cold seems to be cured. With time, upper respiratory infections become more serious, and coughing and expectoration of phlegm continue for longer periods after each episode.[9] Dyspnea (difficulty breathing) initially is mild and is brought on only by exercise or exertion. Eventually, breathing difficulty becomes more frequent and is brought on with less effort. At this point other symptoms of respiratory failure are evident.[4] As the disease progresses and becomes more obstructive, there may be evidence of prolonged expiration and wheezing. Acute attacks of breathing distress with rapid, labored breathing, intensive coughing, and bluish skin can occur; hence the term **blue bloater** has been used to describe an individual with these signs.[7] As seen in Figure 50-2, COPD damages the airways and sacs in the lungs by reducing the elasticity, thereby making breathing more difficult.

Emphysema can be localized or generalized. Individuals with localized emphysema may have no symptoms. At the early stage, symptoms of chronic bronchitis with cough and expectoration predominate. As with chronic bronchitis, dyspnea occurs only with exertion but gradually over time intensifies in severity and frequency. Some individuals may experience rapid progression of dyspnea and disability, and others experience a slower progression. Chronic coughing with expectoration, wheezing, recurrent respiratory infection, and fatigue also may be present. In later stages, severe dyspnea, cyanosis, and other signs of respiratory failure may be evident.[4] As with chronic bronchitis, individuals may experience periods of exacerbation of symptoms usually related to infections or other complications.

Physical findings may be normal in cases of mild or localized emphysema. However, in more advanced cases there is usually weight loss and a "barrel-chest" appearance.[7] The client may appear short of breath and use accessory respiratory muscles. Many may find it easier to breathe in a sitting position, bent over and resting their elbows on their thighs. Usually, the expiration phase of ventilation is prolonged and the client may be breathing against pursed lips. With some individuals, wheezing may be heard on expiration. In advanced stages of emphysema, cyanosis may be evident along with other signs of respiratory failure such as a change in mental state, headache, weakness, and muscle tremor or twitching.[4]

Management of Chronic Obstructive Pulmonary Disease

The management of COPD includes the following components[8]:

1. Assess and monitor disease
2. Reduce risk factors
3. Manage stable COPD
4. Manage exacerbations of COPD

As shown in Figure 50-3, treatment options begin with self-management, education, and avoidance of risk factors, especially smoking. Relieving symptoms and improving overall health through exercise, nutritional counseling, and treatment of complications as part of pulmonary rehabilitation can improve the quality of life greatly for these individuals.[8,10]

Drugs Commonly Used in the Treatment of Chronic Obstructive Pulmonary Disease

Although there is no cure for COPD and medications cannot alter disease progression, they can improve airflow, relieve symptoms, and enhance the quality of life.[8] Antibiotics often are prescribed during the acute attack of symptoms (exacerbation), particularly if there is a bacterial infection present. Bronchodilators, such as those used by people with asthma, have been used commonly as treatment. These drugs, particularly the beta$_2$-agonists, are fast acting and, in addition to relaxing the bronchial tubes, improve mucus clearance.[8]

Advanced cases of COPD often are treated with the addition of more medications as the disease state progresses. Treatment is individualized and monitored based on the response to therapy and side effects reported during treatment. A long-acting beta$_2$-agonist along with an anticholinergic may be followed by a methylxanthine as an add-on therapy for clients who have insufficient relief of symptoms. An inhaled glucocorticosteroid or combinations of medications in one inhaler also may be effective. At this stage many individuals are also on long-term oxygen therapy at home. Surgical removal of one lung may be indicated for some individuals.

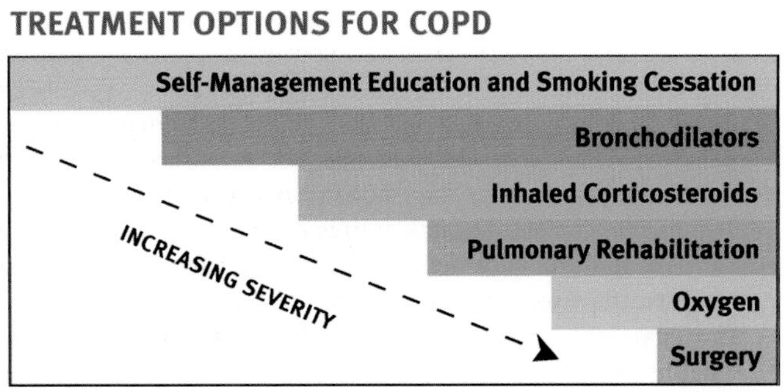

Figure 50-3. Chronic obstructive pulmonary disease (COPD) is a progressive disease but with early diagnosis may progress slowly. Providers must monitor COPD clients carefully, ensuring the treatment is appropriate for the level of disease. (From NHLBI Health Information Center, http://www.LearnAboutCOPD.org.)

Implications for Dental Hygiene Care

To meet the specialized needs of the individual with COPD, the dental hygienist does the following:

- Seat the client in a semi-supine or upright chair position.
- Plan short appointments to decrease stress if the client does not tolerate sitting in a dental chair for long periods of time.
- Assess severity, frequency of symptoms, and conditions that exacerbate symptoms.
- Assess client's signs, symptoms, and self report of acute respiratory infection and reappoint if present.
- Review the health history for evidence of concurrent heart disease; take appropriate precautions if the heart disease is present (see Chapter 43).
- Assess for ineffective salivary flow related to medication-induced xerostomia.
- If applicable, advise client to stop smoking and set goals with the client to initiate a smoking cessation program.
- Monitor periodontal status; the client is at increased risk for disease if he or she is a smoker.
- Be especially observant of the potential for oral lesions if client is a smoker.
- Be especially observant of the potential for oral candidiasis if the patient is on inhaled corticosteroids.
- Avoid use of a rubber dam if possible, because this may further obstruct respiration.
- When needed, cautiously use dental materials with a powder component (alginate or powdered gloves), because they may worsen the client's airway obstruction if inhaled.
- Avoid use of a power-driven polisher (see Table 50-3).
- Use preprocedural antimicrobial rinse and high speed suction to reduce contaminated dental aerosols that may be inhaled when using ultrasonic scaler.
- Offer low-flow (2 to 4 L/min) supplemental oxygen if needed.
- Avoid nitrous oxide–oxygen inhalation sedation with emphysema (see Table 50-3).
- Suggest low-dose oral diazepam or other benzodiazepine, as prescribed by the dentist, if needed to reduce stress.
- Assure that clients taking systemic corticosteroids have taken usual dose on day of appointment, particularly for stressful dental procedures.
- Instruct the client to consult their physician regarding herbal and drug interactions and use of alcohol if the client is taking theophylline.[8]

Tuberculosis

Tuberculosis (TB), an airborne communicable disease, affects primarily the lungs but also can attack other organs and tissues.[9] TB is one of the oldest diseases known to strike humans and still remains one of the most widespread ailments in the world.[1] Although epidemiologic data show a decline in disease incidence among Americans, the worldwide rate continues to increase. The increase in global TB cases has been attributed to adverse social and economic conditions, international travel, and migration of individuals who have TB, and the human immunodeficiency virus (HIV) epidemic. The suppressed immune system of HIV clients and those who are immunosuppressed from use of medications makes these individuals susceptible to opportunistic diseases such as TB, pneumonia, and other fungal, bacterial, and viral lung infections.[1,5]

Etiology

TB is caused by the bacterium *Mycobacterium tuberculosis.* Close contact with persons having TB increases the incidence of disease transmission to others. The following groups are at greatest risk for contracting TB:

- Persons with HIV
- Alcoholics and intravenous drug abusers
- Residents and employees of shared habitation settings: prisons, nursing homes, mental institutions, shelters
- Healthcare workers who care for high-risk individuals
- Immigrants from countries that have a high occurrence of TB
- Medically underserved persons
- High-risk racial or ethnic minority populations
- Persons undergoing immunosuppressive therapy or taking immunosuppressive drugs
- Infants and children under 5 years of age
- Persons with a history of untreated or inadequately treated TB
- Persons with silicosis, diabetes mellitus, chronic renal failure, leukemia, lymphoma, organ transplants, or cancer of the head, neck, and throat
- Persons who are malnourished

Signs and Symptoms

The diagnosis of TB is made via an evaluation of several assessments, including a medical history, physical examination, Mantoux tuberculin skin test, commonly called a TST or *PPD* (purified protein derivative), chest radiograph, sputum culture, and review of clinical symptoms. If TB is diagnosed, testing for drug resistance follows. TB is usually a chronic infection with various clinical manifestations, depending on the stage and duration of the disease.[11] Persons with primary pulmonary TB infection or latent tuberculosis infection (LTBI) often have no clinical evidence of the disease. They test positive on a tuberculin skin test but do not have active TB and are not infectious. When symptoms of active TB infection are present, they are usually mild and include a low-grade fever, listlessness, loss of appetite, malaise, and occasional cough. The most common obvious symptom of active TB is a chronic cough. Other signs of disease progression include fever, night sweats, weight loss, central pulmonary necrosis (death of lung tissue), and cavitation (hollow spaces in the lungs).[7]

Treatment

Treatment of TB depends on whether an individual has active TB or only LTBI. Those persons who test positively for TB but do not have the disease may be treated with a preventive therapy. This treatment usually involves a daily dose of isoniazid (also called INH) or rifampin for 4 to 9 months.[11] Treatment for individuals with active TB may include a short hospital stay along with the concurrent administration of several drugs prescribed for at least 18 months if in the past and at least 9 months if recently treated. Multi–drug-resistant TB is a dangerous form of TB often resulting from low patient compliance or inadequate treatment. A treatment referred to as "directly observed therapy," which involves observing patients as they take each dose of medication, has been successful in some cases to remedy this problem. Patients on a TB drug therapy regimen must be vigilant about taking medication as it has been prescribed even if symptoms have subsided.[11]

Implications for Dental Hygiene Care

When considering treatment options for the individual with a history of TB, the dental professional addresses the major concern: the risk of disease transmission.[1] TB may be transmitted from clients to dental professionals; conversely, if the clinician is infected, clients and other staff members may contract the disease. To prevent disease transmission and meet the needs of the client with a history of TB, the dental hygienist does the following:

- Uses standard infection-control precautions, keeping in mind that many clients with infectious diseases such as TB may not be identified during assessments[12]
- Recognizes signs and symptoms of TB when assessing the client's health history, informs the dentist, and refers for medical evaluation
- Questions clients who report a history of TB, or a positive result from a skin test for TB, concerning dates and results of chest radiographs, sputum cultures, and physical examinations by their physicians, as well as treatment regimens, compliance, and follow-up evaluation
- Determines the type of tuberculosis reported and the current health status of the individual
- Consults with a physician to determine if it is safe to treat the client outside of a hospital setting; a client with active tuberculosis should be treated in a hospital setting under strict infection-control conditions[12]
- Instructs the client with suspected or confirmed TB to observe strict respiratory hygiene and cough etiquette protocols; clients should be kept in the dental setting no longer than is absolutely necessary[12]

CLIENT EDUCATION TIPS

- Explain that rinsing the mouth with water after using an inhaled corticosteroid decreases the risk of oral candidiasis and dental caries.
- Explain that if the client experiences xerostomia and/or an unpleasant taste after inhalant therapy, the use of xylitol-containing chewing gum will increase salivary flow, minimizing the risks of dental caries and gingivitis.
- Explain to clients undergoing drug therapy for tuberculosis (primary or active) the importance of compliance. Inconsistent or incomplete therapy may result in multi–drug-resistant tuberculosis and/or a longer recovery period.
- Explain that smoking cessation is one necessary strategy for managing clients with respiratory diseases.

LEGAL, ETHICAL, AND SAFETY ISSUES

- Acute asthma attacks may occur before, during, and after dental procedures. Dental hygienists must be knowledgeable in the management of such an attack. Avoidance of precipitating factors is the best risk-management strategy.
- Clients reporting a history of asthma must have their bronchodilators at each dental appointment for immediate administration if necessary.
- Clients with active tuberculosis should be treated in a hospital setting to minimize risk of disease transmission to personnel or other clients.

KEY CONCEPTS

- Asthma is a respiratory disease characterized by an increased responsiveness of the airways to various stimuli, which causes periodic wheezing, dyspnea, coughing, and chest tightness.
- An asthma attack may be triggered by allergens, anxiety, cold air, or exercise, or no apparent irritant may be involved.
- Many asthma medications have side effects, including oral candidiasis and xerostomia.
- Two major diseases categorized as chronic obstructive pulmonary disease (COPD) are emphysema and chronic bronchitis.
- COPD is caused most often by cigarette smoking, but the presence of the genetic predisposition of alpha-1 antitrypsin deficiency and chronic exposure to occupational and environmental pollutants are also risk factors associated with COPD.
- The major risk associated with treating clients with active tuberculosis is disease transmission; clients with active tuberculosis should be treated in a hospital setting only for emergency dental care.
- Patient compliance problems during lengthy drug therapy for tuberculosis have contributed to the problem of multi–drug-resistant strains of tuberculosis.

CRITICAL THINKING EXERCISES

Client: Mr. G.

Profile: A 5′10″, 18-year-old white man, weighing 175 lb, arriving for dental hygiene care.

Chief Complaint: "My gums bleed, particularly around my upper front teeth, and I have a dry mouth most of the time, which is very uncomfortable."

Health History: Client's vital signs are as follows: blood pressure of 112/64 mm Hg, pulse rate of 70 bpm, and respiration rate of 14 rpm. Client reports history of asthma for past 10 years, exacerbated by exposure to cats, pollens, and dust. He currently sees physician for acne and a chiropractor for lower back pain. Currently takes doxycycline 100 mg daily for acne and Proventil 90 mcg aerosol inhaler (two puffs as needed for asthma attack).

Social History: Client is single and lives with parents. He appears very quiet and reserved.

Dental History: Suspected carious lesions on occlusal surfaces of teeth 2, 3, 15, and 31.

Gingival evaluation reveals slight gingival enlargement and rolled margins throughout with moderately enlarged, erythematous gingiva and bulbous papillae in the maxillary anterior facial region. Pocket depths 3 mm or less throughout, except in maxillary anterior and posterior molar regions, where some 4- to 5-mm pockets were noted.

Oral Health Behavior Assessment: Client brushes twice daily but does not floss. Moderate plaque biofilm is noted throughout on the gingival third of teeth and interproximal surfaces.

Supplemental Notes: He smokes one pack of cigarettes per week.

1. What are the dental hygiene diagnoses for this client?
2. Develop a dental hygiene care plan for this client that includes goals and interventions.
3. What client education issues should be addressed?
4. What factors could be affecting this client's periodontal health?
5. Are there any contraindications to this client's care?
6. What measures should be taken during treatment to prevent an asthmatic attack?

REFERENCES

1. Centers for Disease Control and Prevention: Trends in tuberculosis incidence—United States, *MMWR Morb Mortal Wkly Rep* 60(11):333, 2010.
2. National Heart, Lung, and Blood Institute, National Asthma Education and Prevention Program Expert Panel: *Expert panel report 3 (EPR3): guidelines for the diagnosis and management of asthma.* Available at: www.nhlbi.nih.gov/guidelines/asthma/asthgdln.htm. Accessed November 11, 2012.
3. Borak J, Fields S, Andrews SA, et al: Methyl methacrylate and respiratory sensitization: a critical review, *Crit Rev Toxicol* 41(3):230, 2011.
4. Malamed SF: *Medical emergencies in the dental office*, ed 6, St Louis, 2007, Mosby.
5. American Lung Association: *Learning about asthma.* Available at: http://www.lung.org/lung-disease/asthma/learning-more-about-asthma/. Accessed November 28, 2012.
6. Tanaka LS, Dezan CC, Fernandes KBP, et al: The influence of asthma onset and severity on malocclusion prevalence in children and adolescents, *Dental Press J Ortho* 17(1):50, e1, 2012.
7. Des Jardins TR: *Clinical manifestations and assessment of respiratory disease*, St Louis, 2011, Mosby.
8. Global Initiative on Chronic Obstructive Lung Disease: *Global strategy for the diagnosis, management and prevention of chronic obstructive pulmonary disease, revised 2011.* Available at: http://www.goldcopd.com. Accessed November 27, 2012.
9. American Lung Association: *Chronic obstructive pulmonary disease (COPD) fact sheet: February 2011.* Available at: http://www.lung.org/lung-disease/copd/resources/facts-figures/COPD-Fact-Sheet.html. Accessed November 27, 2012.
10. National Heart Lung and Blood Institute: *Diseases and conditions index.* Available at: www.nhlbi.nih.gov/health/dci/Diseases/Copd/Copd_WhatIs.html. Accessed November 27, 2012.
11. Centers for Disease Control and Prevention: *TB facts for health care workers.* Available at: www.cdc.gov/tb/pubs/TBfacts_Health Workers/tbfacts_update.pdf. Accessed November 23, 2012.
12. Cleveland JL, Robison VA, Panlilio AL: Tuberculosis epidemiology, diagnosis and infection control recommendations for dental settings: an update on the Centers for Disease Control and Prevention guidelines, *J Am Dent Assoc* 140(9):1092, 2009.

EVOLVE RESOURCES

Please visit http://evolve.elsevier.com/Darby/hygiene for additional practice and study support tools.

CHAPTER 51

Developmentally and Cognitively Challenged

Kelly Marie Schulz, Michele Leonardi Darby

COMPETENCIES

1. Discuss intellectual and developmental disabilities (IDDs), including:
   - Identify causes of IDDs.
   - Describe general characteristics of IDDs.
2. Discuss Down syndrome, including:
   - Explain the cause of Down syndrome.
   - Describe general characteristics of Down syndrome.
   - Describe medical conditions that may accompany Down syndrome and their effect on dental hygiene care.
3. Discuss autism spectrum disorders (ASDs), including:
   - Identify the different types of ASDs.
   - Describe general characteristics of ASDs.
   - Outline instructional strategies to overcome communication barriers with a client who has an autism spectrum disorder.
4. Plan educational interventions for a client with intellectual disabilities, Down syndrome, or autism spectrum disorders.

Intellectual and Developmental Disabilities[1,2]

The American Association on Intellectual and Developmental Disabilities is the overarching organization in support of persons with intellectual disabilities and a leader in innovation and research for persons living with these disabilities.[1]

Developmental disabilities are considered to be lifelong severe chronic disabilities that can be cognitive, physical, or both and that present before the age of 21 years. An intellectual disability (ID) is a type of developmental disability that must occur before the age of 18 years and that is characterized by significantly subaverage general intellectual functioning accompanied by significant limitations in adaptive functioning in at least two of the following skill areas: communication, self-care, home living, social or interpersonal skills, use of community resources, self-direction, functional academic skills, work, leisure, health, and safety. Intellectually and developmentally disabled persons usually have an intelligence quotient (IQ) of less than 70 as well as impairments in their communicative, social, and daily living skills.

Etiology

IDs can stem from genetic biologic factors (e.g., chromosomal and genetic disturbances), nongenetic biologic and nutritional factors (e.g., prenatal, perinatal, or postnatal causes), and psychosocial factors (e.g., inadequate caregiving environment, lack of stimulation). Genetic biologic factors include disorders that are evident at conception. In approximately 15% of affected persons, the ID falls into this category, which includes chromosomal disturbances (10%) such as Down syndrome and metabolic disorders such as in **phenylketonuria** (5%), which causes an abnormal accumulation of phenylalanine that is toxic to the brain.

Nongenetic biologic ID causes are grouped as prenatal, perinatal, and postnatal causes. Approximately 32% of IDs occur during the prenatal period; 11% occur during the perinatal period, and 4% occur during the postnatal period. Prenatal causes include infections such as rubella, toxoplasmosis, syphilis (dental signs: Hutchinsonian incisors, mulberry molars, microdontia), cytomegalovirus infection, and human immunodeficiency virus infection; maternal–fetal blood incompatibilities; drug and alcohol consumption; maternal–fetal irradiation; poor nutrition; and chronic maternal health problems such as hypertension and diabetes. The term *perinatal* refers to the time immediately before, during, and after birth. Premature birth, **hypoxemia** (intracranial hemorrhage), head trauma, infection (e.g., human immunodeficiency virus, herpes), and **kernicterus** (i.e., the toxic accumulation of bilirubin in the brain) are perinatal causes of ID. With advances in medicine, the occurrence of ID as a result of perinatal causes is rare. Postnatal factors include brain infections (encephalitis, meningitis), cerebral trauma (head injury, brain tumor, accident), poison, environmental toxins, and dietary protein deficiency. Psychosocial causes include an environment that is void of sensory and intellectual stimulation during growth and development.

Levels of Intellectual Disabilities

ID is categorized as mild, moderate, severe, or profound as follows:

- *Mild ID (IQ of approximately 50 to 70).* This group represents the largest population with ID (about 85%). These clients are designated as educable and able to acquire some academic skills, and they typically live either independently or in supervised settings. Persons with mild ID can learn simple skills in detail, but their attention spans and memories are short. For clients with mild ID, dental hygienists explain and demonstrate oral hygiene instructions and teach activities instead of concepts. Clients with mild ID require public recognition, praise, and rewards for their progress.
- *Moderate ID (IQ of approximately 35 to 55).* These persons can learn self-care behaviors, social adjustment, and economic usefulness, but they acquire very few academic

skills past the second-grade level. Poor hand and finger coordination may be evident, so clients should be taught only fundamental skills via the show-and-tell method. Additional skills may be taught, depending on client progress. Every successful step performed during therapy and oral hygiene instruction should be rewarded with tangible and verbal praise. Oral hygiene instructions are reviewed at each appointment because of the client's short memory and attention span. Individuals typically live in group settings, where a primary caregiver can supervise the daily regimen to ensure that optimal self-care behaviors are practiced.

- *Severe ID (IQ of approximately 20 to 40).* These individuals can be trained in elementary self-care skills; thus the client can acquire some oral care behaviors with supervision. These clients learn by habit training (i.e., repeating procedures and movements continuously) so that they can grasp the procedures. It is important to set realistic client goals and to include the client's caregiver when teaching oral hygiene behaviors. These individuals typically reside at home with their families or in group homes. Depending on the environment, successfully performed skills should be rewarded by the dental hygienist or the caregiver. See Table 51-1 for suggested awards.
- *Profound ID (IQ of less than 20).* People with this level of ID are incapable of total self-care, social skills, or economic work skills and require continued supervision and care from the primary caregiver. Some self-care may be achievable in a highly structured environment when appropriate training is provided by the caregiver. The caregiver is responsible for the client's general and oral hygiene care, so the caregiver must be educated about the daily oral care regimen and competent with his or her own oral self-care. The caretaker's task is challenging, and oral care may not be a top priority.

General Characteristics of Persons with Intellectual Disabilities

Although common traits are associated with various ID levels, overgeneralization and stereotypic expectations are avoided; instead, individual needs, abilities, and circumstances are assessed.

Health

Persons with ID usually have less physical stamina as compared with the general population. They have delayed physical development and speech in addition to physical challenges such as poor motor coordination, vision, and hearing. Individuals may be overweight or underweight as a result of environmental factors such as inadequate parental or institutional care or genetic and metabolic factors such as phenylketonuria. They may also have poor oral health as a result of nutritional deficiency, limited self-care capabilities, barriers to care, and limited access to care.

Mental and Motor Abilities

Persons with ID usually have short memories, an inability to concentrate or to see differences or likenesses between objects, limited speech, and a lack of adaptive, associative, or organizational skills. Success usually occurs from concrete rather than abstract experiences; therefore these persons are more adept with manual skills than academic skills. Depending on the ID level, clients may be able to render their own oral self-care, and this should be encouraged.

Social and Emotional Abilities

Persons with ID are viewed as followers rather than leaders (i.e., they tend to imitate others). Frequently they have behavioral problems in an effort to gain attention or release emotion. Maladaptive behaviors may be destructive (e.g., aggressiveness directed toward others, property destruction, self-injury). These individuals have an awareness of not fitting in and become discouraged easily. Criticism is not taken positively, and there is an inability to learn through experience.

Self-Injurious Behavior

Persons may exhibit self-injurious behavior (SIB) including head banging, self-biting, self-striking, and bruxism (Figure 51-1). SIB has been viewed as an early developmental stress response that disappears in "normal" children but that remains in clients with ID. Self-injury may be used by a client as positive reinforcement to get something like attention or a favorite food. SIB can also be used to receive negative reinforcement, such as escape from undesired situations (e.g., the dental care experience) or from certain expectations (e.g.,

TABLE 51-1

Rewards That Can Be Used to Reinforce Positive Behavior for Clients with Intellectual Disabilities

Types of Rewards	Examples of Rewards
Social rewards	Attention, smiles, hugs, praise, and other signs of approval and affection
Activity rewards	Any activity that the person enjoys, such as watching television, playing a game, or going to a party
Material rewards	An item that the person can use, play with, wear, or consume, such as toys, money, food, or clothing

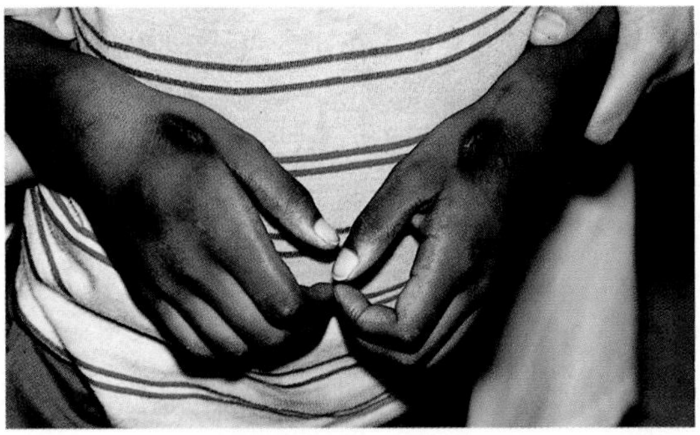

Figure 51-1. Physical outcome of self-injurious behavior in a child with intellectual and developmental disabilities. (Courtesy Dr. F.T. McIver, Department of Pediatric Dentistry, University of North Carolina School of Dentistry.)

daily toothbrushing). These behaviors can intimidate caregivers to the point that the client's demands are met. If the client is allowed this power, he or she becomes difficult to manage.

To prevent SIB, the dental hygienist initiates fact finding with the caregiver to identify SIB triggers and antecedents. The most commonly used behavioral treatment is differential reinforcement of other behavior. The goal of this treatment is to reinforce any behavior other than the SIB. Good results have been shown when differential reinforcement of other behavior and **differential reinforcement of incompatible behavior** are used simultaneously.[3] For example, if the client strikes himself in the mouth, then give the client something to assemble or hold with his hands, or let him hold a cotton roll or mirror until it is needed. Strategies for managing SIB are listed in Table 51-2.

Oral Manifestations

Persons often exhibit specific oral manifestations (e.g., the lips may be larger than those of the general population); tooth anomalies such as microdontia and delayed eruption patterns are usually present as a result of developmental abnormalities (Box 51-1). Tooth surface abrasion from bruxism, which is linked to anxiety and emotional distress, has also been observed.

Consequences of bruxism can include dental attrition, functional problems such as temporomandibular joint disorders, and eventually sensitivity and pain. Wear is usually seen in the incisors and canines and increases with age. By the time these individuals are 30 to 49 years old, wear becomes so significant that restorative measures may be needed. Bruxism may be the result of a lack of personal contact, or it may be a type of self-stimulation. Before treatment can be given for these problems, assessment must be completed to determine the origin and chronicity of the behavior.

Periodontal disease prevalence is attributed to risk factors such as a lack of professional care, a lack of funds to support or to access care, host susceptibility, and poor oral hygiene. These persons usually depend on others to facilitate their access to oral healthcare, and a layperson's assessment of need is likely to differ from that of a dental professional.

Management of Clients with Intellectual Disabilities

Most (89%) individuals with ID who are treated in the oral healthcare environment have mild disabilities. A smaller percentage (6%) have moderate disabilities, and 4.5% have severe or profound disabilities.[4] When developing client oral self-care behaviors, the dental hygienist teaches at a level that is congruent with the client's **mental age** (i.e., the age reflected

BOX 51-1

Some Oral Manifestations Observed in Clients with Intellectual Disabilities

- Self-biting
- Bruxism
- Thick, flaccid lips
- Microdontia
- Malocclusion
- Delayed tooth eruption
- Dental attrition and sensitivity
- Temporomandibular joint disorder
- Periodontal disease
- Heavy oral biofilm accumulation

TABLE 51-2

Strategies for Managing Self-Injurious Behavior in Clients

Strategy	Definition	Examples
Differential reinforcement	Reinforcement of any behavior other than the self-injurious behavior	Draw interest away from the self-injurious behavior (e.g., "Can you sing a song for me about your teeth?")
Positive reinforcement	Used to get a person to repeat a desired behavior	Verbal praise: "You really did well"; "Good job"; "You brush your teeth so well, I want to see you doing this again"
Ignoring unwanted behavior	Refusing to take notice of the self-injurious behavior	Consciously ignoring negative behavior
Positive reinforcement of wanted behavior	Reinforcement when the wanted behavior is directly addressed	"You really cleaned those back teeth well, so I will give you a prize."
Psychoactive medication	Medication that alters one's psychologic state	Neuroleptics, antidepressants, and psychostimulants
Restraint	Physical confinement of a person	Papoose board or Velcro straps
Counseling	Professional guidance of a person using psychologic methods	Offer support, positive reinforcement, and trust
Application of consequences after behavior	Punishment after the unwanted behavior for reinforcement	Time out or not allowing a reward after treatment
Overcorrection	Correction requiring duties above and beyond addressing the specific unwanted behavior	Joe colors on the wall so he should clean more of the wall than where he colored

BOX 51-2

Strategies for Establishing a Trusting Relationship

- Familiarize the client with his or her surroundings, and have the caregiver rehearse the client for the appointment.
- Schedule a time for the healthcare team to meet the client; alleviate anxieties by getting to know the client and by allowing the client to get to know the team.
- Keep the first appointment short, nonthreatening, and fun.
- Give explanations slowly, with one instruction at a time.
- Use a tell-show-do technique when teaching; teach one technique at each appointment to avoid overwhelming the client.
- Validate the client's understanding (e.g., have the client perform the self-care behavior [brushing, interdental cleaning, mouth rinsing, and so on]).
- Reward the client often for positive behavior (e.g., use verbal positive reinforcement such as "Good job"; offer tangible reinforcement such as a toy, a special outing arranged by the caregiver, or public recognition such as a certificate that can be displayed in the client's home or work setting).
- Provide handouts and pictures that have been designed at the appropriate level of reading comprehension for home use.

by the client's level of functioning) rather than his or her chronologic age (i.e., the true age based on the date of birth).

As with any client, a humanistic approach is used, and this is coupled with a care plan designed to address the individual's assessed abilities and dental hygiene–related human needs (see Chapter 2). After the care plan has been designed, the hygienist begins instructions with familiar activities, praises small accomplishments, and uses a gentle but firm demeanor. Extra instructional time may be required for conveying new information. If problems arise (e.g., crying, frustration), the dental hygienist repeats an earlier achievement level to meet the client's need for freedom from fear and stress. Effective communication leads to a trusting relationship, which in turn allows the oral healthcare experience to be successful for both client and the clinician.[4] Approaches to use to form this trusting relationship are listed in Box 51-2.

The process of care increases the likelihood that the visit will be successful. During assessment, the dental hygienist collects data about the client's skills of daily living (e.g., toilet training, oral hygiene regimen, eating habits, dressing). Frequently caregivers are able to suggest behavioral guidance to achieve a pleasant dental experience. Factors to consider include the client's mental age, diet and ability to chew, self-care potential, interests, level of cooperation, and barriers to care as well as the parents' and caregivers' interests, values, and level of cooperation. See Figure 51-2 for a sample dental hygiene care plan.

Down Syndrome[3,4]

Down syndrome, which is the most common and frequently observed chromosomal abnormality in the human race, occurs among individuals of all socioeconomic levels, geographic regions, ethnic groups, and cultures. Down syndrome occurs in 1 out of approximately every 691 live births; therefore approximately 400,000 persons are living with Down syndrome in the United States. These individuals are at increased risk for congenital heart defects, respiratory and hearing problems, Alzheimer's disease, childhood leukemia, and thyroid conditions. Because many of these conditions are treatable, the life expectancy of an individual with Down syndrome is now at about 60 years of age.

Etiology

An abnormality in the number of chromosomes (i.e., three rather than two copies of the 21st chromosome) is responsible for the specific physical characteristics and mental deficiencies observed in persons with Down syndrome. The following three manifestations of chromosomal abnormality can also occur:

1. Trisomy 21, which is the failure of a pair of number 21 chromosomes to segregate (nondisjunction) during the formation of either an egg or sperm before conception, is not inherited. It has no known cause, and it occurs in about 95% of people with Down syndrome. Incidence is correlated with increased maternal age: mothers who are less than 30 years old have a 1 in 900 chance of giving birth to an infant with Down syndrome; those who are 35 years old have a 1 in 350 chance; those who are 40 years old have a 1 in 100 chance; and those who are 45 years old or older have a 1 in 30 chance.
2. Translocation is hereditary and occurs when a piece of chromosome in pair 21 breaks off and attaches to another chromosome, usually chromosome 14, 21, or 22. Translocation occurs in approximately 4% to 5% of children with Down syndrome.
3. Mosaicism occurs in only 1% of children with Down syndrome; it is a result of an error in one of the first cell divisions that occurs shortly after conception.

General Characteristics

Approximately 50 specific physical characteristics have been reported in persons with Down syndrome; however, not every person with Down syndrome manifests all characteristics, and when these characteristics are present, they may occur in various degrees. The most common characteristics follow.

The person's head usually appears small; it is shortened in its anterior-to-posterior diameter (i.e., from the forehead to the crown). The eyes have an upward slant and prominent epicanthal folds, which are the folds of skin that extend from the root of the nose to the median end of the eyebrow. The iris of the eye is speckled with marks called Brushfield spots. The nose is recessed and reduced in size, the nostrils are upturned, and the nasal bridge is depressed. Deviations in the nasal septum also are common. Because of the flat nasal bridge and the underdevelopment of the midfacial region, the face appears flat. This flat facial profile is the most frequently observed characteristic of Down syndrome.

Figure 51-3 depicts the facial features of a person with Down syndrome. The ears may appear small and abnormal in structure and contour, which results in a round or square appearance; the hands may appear short and broad, with nails that are hyperconvex (Figure 51-4). Persons with Down syndrome tend to be short and overweight. Despite IQ limitations in the range of 20 to 85, most children with Down syndrome develop into happy and in some cases self-reliant individuals.

Dental Hygiene Diagnosis	Due to or Related to	As Evidenced by	Client Goal	Evaluative Statements
Biologically Sound and Functional Dentition	Inadequate oral care by caregiver Inadequate self-care Lack of resources	Signs of caries, defective restorations, and missing teeth	Reduce caries index score Seek dental treatment for caries and defective restorations Use 0.12% chlorhexidine mouth rinse to eliminate *Streptococcus mutans* infections	Reduced caries index score at 3-month continued-care interval Completed restorative treatment by 3-month continued-care interval
Skin and Mucous Membrane Integrity of the Head and Neck	Inadequate care by caregiver Inadequate self-care Lack of resources	Presence of numerous gingival bleeding points Attachment loss of 4-7 mm	Decrease gingival bleeding by 50% Stop progression of attachment loss Find additional resources to enable client to receive needed care, e.g., Medicaid program	Decrease gingival bleeding on probing by 50% Attachment loss remains stable Client enrolled in Medicaid program
Freedom from Head and Neck Pain	Inadequate care by caregiver Inadequate self-care	Signs of caries Verbal indicators of pain	Seek dental treatment for pain relief and caries	All carious lesions restored No evidence of oral pain
Responsibility for Oral Health	Impaired mental ability Impaired motor coordination Low value placed on oral health	Presence of plaque, bleeding, and caries Reports no previous dental care and fails to report to appointments	Demonstrate self-care with follow-up by caregiver Seek dental care Verbalizes a commitment to having a healthy mouth	Performs oral hygiene with minimal supervision Reports for scheduled dental visits Verbalizes that she likes the way her teeth feel and look
Conceptualization and Problem Solving	Knowledge deficiency in oral disease risk factors	Inability to verbalize that oral biofilm contributes to bleeding gums and tooth decay	Client and caregiver verbalize the relationship between biofilm, bleeding gums, and caries	Client and caregiver verbalize the role of plaque in oral disease Client and caregiver use disclosing agent to evaluate their oral hygiene

Dental Hygiene Interventions

- Assess Jill's mental level, functional level, and oral health knowledge and skill level.
- Provide education on dental disease.
- Provide education to Jill and the caregiver on toothbrushing (power toothbrush due to limited psychomotor skills) and flossing (by caregiver); power interdental cleaner.
- Communicate importance of at-home fluoride therapy for dental caries control.
- Provide periodontal debridement and prescribe a 0.12% chlorhexidine gluconate antimicrobial rinse to control *Streptococcus mutans* infection (prescription written by dentist).
- Teach Jill and caregiver to evaluate their oral hygiene for progress (i.e., less bleeding points, use of disclosing agent).
- Apply dental sealants.
- Apply fluoride varnish.
- Provide nutritional assessment and counseling including use of xylitol gum and mints to control caries.
- Introduce procedures slowly based on Jill's mental age.
- Provide rewards for oral health and healthy behavior.
- Use techniques for establishing a trusting relationship.
- At 3-month continued-care interval, reevaluate the homecare.
- Refer to dentist for restorative procedures.

Figure 51-2. Sample dental hygiene care plan: client with intellectual and developmental disabilities.

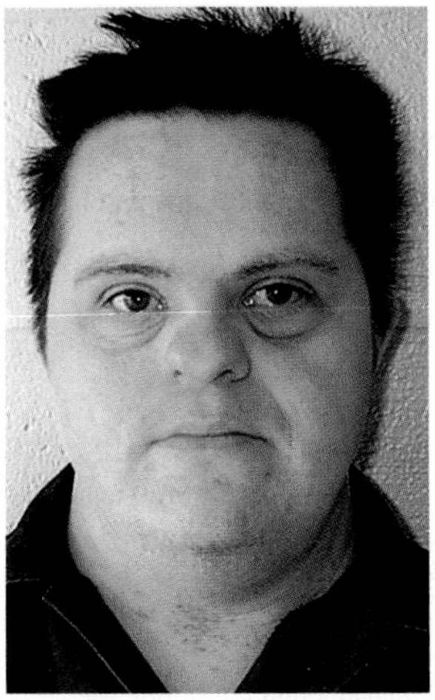

Figure 51-3. Facial characteristics of a person with Down syndrome. (Courtesy Marye J. McClanahan, Gene W. Hirschfield School of Dental Hygiene, Old Dominion University, Norfolk, Virginia.)

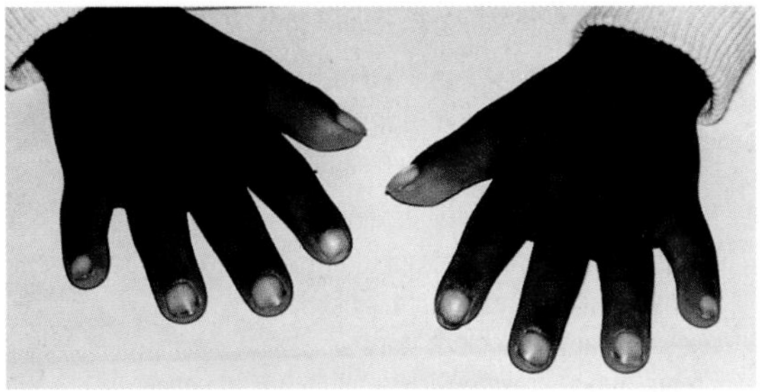

Figure 51-4. Hands of a person with Down syndrome. (Courtesy Dr. F.T. McIver, Department of Pediatric Dentistry, University of North Carolina School of Dentistry.)

Medical Considerations

The life expectancies of persons with Down syndrome can be lengthened by high-quality healthcare, healthy lifestyle behaviors, stimulating home environments, and positive support structures from family, friends, employers, and the community. Individuals with this condition may have various medical conditions that affect the process of care (Table 51-3). Knowledge of potential health problems, care modifications, and available community resources as well as the use of a collaborative approach are required to meet the client's oral health and wellness needs (see the Web Resources section of this book's website). Specific support organizations may not be in the client's immediate geographic location, but they can supply information and referrals. The Internet or a telephone directory (under Social Services, Disabilities, or Intellectual and Developmental Disabilities) can be used to identify local assistance.

Congenital Heart Disease (see Chapter 43)

Congenital heart disease is the most common and serious medical condition among persons with Down syndrome. Most cardiovascular malformations associated with Down syndrome are acutely or chronically life-threatening. Cardiac problems are present in 40% to 60% of newborns with Down syndrome, and heart defects are major causes of high mortality during the first 2 years of the infant's life. In addition, persons with Down syndrome have increased susceptibility to infection, which continues to be a major cause of morbidity and mortality.

Atrioventricular septal defects, ventricular septal defects, atrial septal defects, patent ductus arteriosus, and tetralogy of Fallot are common in the population of clients with Down syndrome with congenital heart disease. The most common congenital heart defects detected by echocardiogram are the

TABLE 51-3

Medical and Dental Hygiene Considerations for Clients with Down Syndrome*

Concern	Clinical Expression	When Seen	Dental Hygiene Care Implications and Management Issues
Congenital heart disease	Septal defects Tetralogy of Fallot Valvular defects Pulmonary arterial hypertension	Newborn through first 6 weeks of life	Increased susceptibility to infection Prevention of infective endocarditis via antibiotic premedication Assess symptoms of secondary concerns before dental hygiene care
Hypotonia	Reduced muscle tone Increased range of joint movement Motor function problems	Throughout life Improvement with maturity	Important to address client's comfort while he or she is in dental chair Limited neck movement and pain Motor function problems that make oral care difficult May exhibit spastic movements Considerations with client positioning Alterations in oral hygiene aids
Delayed growth	Typically at or near the third percentile of the general population	Throughout life	Evaluate mental age Nutrition assessment and counseling During assessment, may see delays in tooth development and facial growth

Continued

TABLE 51-3

Medical and Dental Hygiene Considerations for Clients with Down Syndrome—cont'd

Concern	Clinical Expression	When Seen	Dental Hygiene Care Implications and Management Issues
Intellectual and developmental delays	Some global delay, degree varies Specific processing problems Specific expressive language delay	First year; monitor throughout life	Assess client's mental age to appropriately plan oral care instruction Use caregiver to communicate with client as needed
Hearing deficits	Otitis media Small ear canals Conductive impairment	Assess by 6 months Review annually	May need to speak clearly and use visual aids Obtain a thorough health history to identify hearing problems Involve caregiver to determine what mode of communication would work best with the client
Eye disease	Refractive errors Strabismus Cataracts Tear duct abnormalities Amblyopia Nystagmus	Eye examination during early months of life Regular follow-up	Tactile communication is important Assist client to prevent injury Obtain a thorough health history to identify ocular problems Involve caregiver to determine severity of problem When giving oral care instruction, be in clear view Adjust instruction to client need (e.g., do not expect client to see small anatomy on a radiograph) Avoid glare of dental light in the client's eyes
Cervical spine problems	Atlantoaxial instability Skeletal cervical anomalies Possible spinal cord compression	Radiographic examination by 3 years of age	May require shorter appointments for comfort Help client with walking to treatment area as needed Place client in comfortable position for treatment
Thyroid disease	Hypothyroidism (rarely hyperthyroidism) Decreased growth and activity	Some congenital; most during second decade of life or later Check by age of 1 year, repeat throughout life	Be cognizant of room temperature for client comfort (client may be cold and require a blanket) Assess pharmacologic history Create a low-stress environment Stress good oral hygiene to prevent infection Gingiva may appear spongy; tongue may be swollen
Obesity	Excessive weight gain	Especially when 2 to 3 years old, 12 to 13 years old, and during adult life	May require large blood pressure cuff Offer nutritional counseling If client is in a group home, may consider doing an in-service May have an exaggerated inflammatory response
Seizure disorder	Primarily generalized tonic–clonic (grand mal) seizures Also myoclonic seizures and hypsarrhythmia	Any time	Assess pharmacologic history Minimize stress Avoid flashing dental light into client's eyes Avoid stress-inducing situations Dental sealants and fluoride are beneficial If gingival enlargement present, more frequent continued care may be needed
Emotional problems	Inappropriate behavior Depression	Mid to late childhood and adulthood	Praise client to build self-esteem and cooperation Treat client with respect Assess client's frame of mind (via caregiver or healthcare decision maker) before appointment; validate at appointment Assess pharmacologic history
Premature senescence	Behavioral changes and functional losses	Fifth decade of life and beyond	Evaluate mental age Treat client with respect and concern Assess client's frame of mind with the caregiver before the appointment Assess pharmacologic history

*This information also applies to clients with variable occurrences of congenital gastrointestinal anomalies such as Hirschsprung's disease (an extreme dilation of the colon), imperforate anus, duodenal obstruction, and tracheoesophageal fistula as well as other conditions such as celiac disease, leukemia, Alzheimer's disease, attention-deficit/hyperactivity disorder, autism spectrum disorders, hepatitis B carrier state, keratoconus (conical protrusion of the center of the cornea), dry skin, hip dysplasia, diabetes, and mitral valve prolapse.

atrioventricular septal defects. Endocardial cushions are ridges in the developing fetal heart. These cushions are involved in the formation of the septum that separates the right and left ventricles, the formation of the septum that separates the right and left atria, and the formation of the two valves between the atria and ventricles. Signs of these heart defects are faulty heart valves, severe heart failure, frequent pneumonia, and poor growth. Another condition that is seen in clients with Down syndrome is pulmonary artery hypertension, which is characterized by the constriction of the blood vessels of the lungs; this causes back pressure and right ventricle overload. Pulmonary artery hypertension is often a consequence of the increased flow to the lungs caused by the heart defects.

Multiple cardiac abnormalities exist in approximately 30% of persons with Down syndrome. Medical intervention depends on the severity of symptoms. When providing care, it is imperative to obtain a detailed health and pharmacologic history to determine any cardiac abnormalities that may be present. Prophylactic antibiotic premedication is prescribed when unrepaired congenital heart disease (including palliative shunts and conduits) or repaired congenital heart disease with residual defects at the site or adjacent to the site of a prosthetic patch or device is present because of the highest risk of adverse outcomes from infective endocarditis that could occur after dental hygiene care (see Chapter 12 for a complete discussion of prophylactic antibiotic premedication for cardiac conditions associated with the highest risk of adverse outcomes from endocarditis).

Orthopedic Concerns

Orthopedic problems in these clients are usually a result of hypotonia (low muscle tone).

Atlantoaxial instability, which is found in about 10% to 20% of younger individuals with Down syndrome, is characterized by an abnormal increase in mobility within the joint between the first two cervical (neck) vertebrae, thereby placing the person at risk for spinal cord compression and injury. Most persons with Down syndrome have no symptoms of atlantoaxial instability, but if signs or symptoms are present (e.g., easily fatigued, difficulty walking, neck pain, abnormal gait, extremity weakness, spasticity, limited neck movement, torticollis [head tilt], lack of coordination or clumsiness, sensory deficits, hyperreflexia), they are related to spinal cord compression.

Scoliosis (curvature of the spine), which is frequently detected among individuals with Down syndrome, is usually mild. Persons with Down syndrome usually have excessive external hip rotation and abduction. As a result, a wide-angled gait and widespread legs when sitting are evident. Persons with mild scoliosis may not be aware that they have a spinal problem, but it is still important to ensure client comfort during care.

Other Disorders (see Chapter 48)

Endocrine disorders involving the thyroid, adrenal, or pituitary glands are common among persons with Down syndrome. As many as 50% of older individuals with Down syndrome have thyroid disorders, with hypothyroidism being the most common. Classic symptoms of hypothyroidism include delayed growth, short stature, obesity, lethargy, and dry skin. Evidence suggests that individuals with one endocrine autoimmune disorder (e.g., thyroiditis) are at increased risk for developing a second disorder (e.g., type 1 diabetes mellitus).

As a result of associated anatomic predispositions, ear, nose, and throat problems are common in persons with Down syndrome. Hearing loss that is usually mild to moderate is often caused by persistent fluid in the middle ear and chronic ear infections. Other disorders include chronic rhinitis and sinusitis.

Eye disease affects about 50% of persons with Down syndrome. Cataracts, tear duct abnormalities, strabismus, amblyopia, and nystagmus are known to occur and should be treated by an ophthalmologist.

Seizure activity in infants and young children with Down syndrome occurs at the same rate as it does in the general population; however, at the age of 20 to 30 years, generalized tonic–clonic seizures (i.e., grand mal seizures) are seen more frequently in persons with Down syndrome. Seizures may take the form of staring spells, momentary lapses of attention, jerking of the arms and legs, or loss of consciousness. Gingival enlargement caused by medications that are taken to control seizure activity is of particular significance (Figures 51-5 and 51-6). Effective oral biofilm control reduces the extent of drug-influenced gingival enlargement, so daily self-care must be effective before some seizure-control medications are used.

Adults with Down syndrome often demonstrate neuropathologic changes similar to those of individuals diagnosed with Alzheimer's disease. The anatomic changes of Alzheimer's disease appear to be almost universal among adults with Down syndrome who are more than 40 years old, most of whom do not show behavioral signs of Alzheimer's disease. The relationship between Alzheimer's disease and Down syndrome is under investigation.

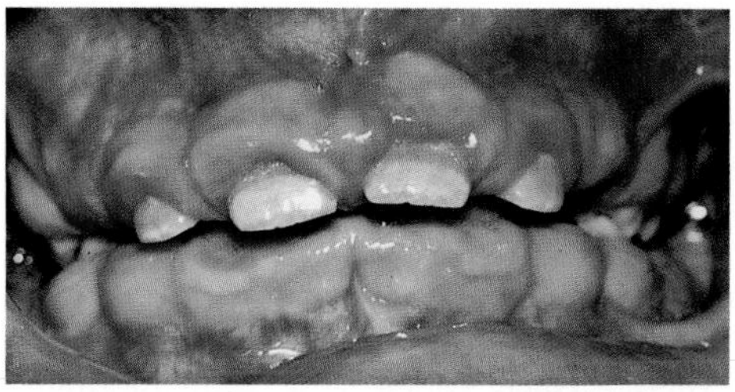

Figure 51-5. Moderate drug-influenced gingivitis associated with Dilantin (phenytoin) therapy for seizure control in a person with Down syndrome. (Courtesy Dr. F.T. McIver, Department of Pediatric Dentistry, University of North Carolina School of Dentistry.)

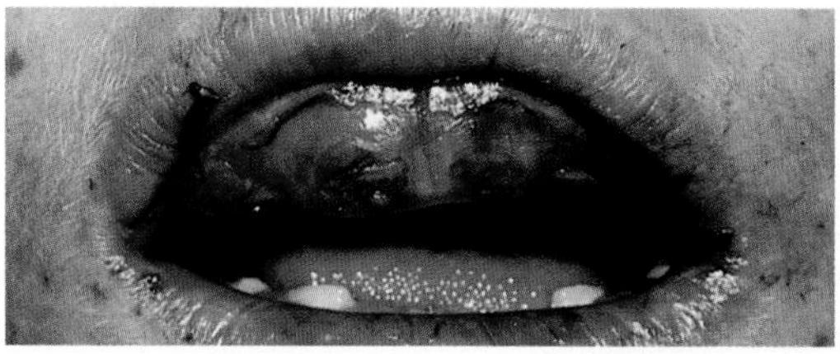

Figure 51-6. Severe drug-influenced gingivitis associated with Dilantin (phenytoin) therapy for seizure control in a person with Down syndrome. (Courtesy Dr. F.T. McIver, Department of Pediatric Dentistry, University of North Carolina School of Dentistry.)

BOX 51-3

Some Oral Manifestations Observed in Persons with Down Syndrome

- Underdeveloped maxilla
- Narrow palate with broadened alveolar ridges
- Congenitally missing teeth
- Malocclusion
- Enamel hypoplasia
- High rate of tooth loss caused by periodontal disease
- Shortened roots
- Enlarged tonsils and adenoids
- Mouth open with protruding tongue
- Fissured tongue
- Enlarged circumvallate papillae on tongue
- Microdontia
- Tetracycline tooth staining
- Periodontal diseases
- Heavy oral biofilm accumulation
- Low caries risk

Oral Manifestations (Box 51-3)

Tongue

A person with Down syndrome often has an open mouth open and a protruding tongue. The tongue seems enlarged as a result of an underdeveloped maxilla, mandibular prognathism, a narrow palate with broadened alveolar ridges, and enlarged tonsils and adenoids, all of which create a small oral cavity space. Tongue fissures and enlarged circumvallate papillae are observed in 37% to 60% of persons with Down syndrome. Therefore good daily oral hygiene—including tongue brushing and the use of an American Dental Association–accepted antimicrobial dentifrice and mouth rinse to reduce oral biofilm, gingivitis, and halitosis—is requisite. The cooperation level of the client must be considered when recommending daily oral care regimens and products.

Sleep Apnea

Approximately 45% of persons with Down syndrome also have obstructive sleep apnea as a result of their flattened midfaces, their narrowed nasopharyngeal areas, the low tone of the muscles of their upper airways, and their enlarged tongues, tonsils, and adenoids. There are many problems associated with obstructive sleep apnea in these clients. It has been shown that, in children with obstructive sleep apnea and heart disease, the low blood oxygenation level causes an increase in the blood pressure of the lungs as the body tries to get more oxygen. This "pulmonary hypertension" can cause the right side of the heart to become enlarged, thereby causing cardiac complications. Children with Down syndrome may also have larger than usual soft palates that usually do not create obstructions but that tend to cause snoring, which is also a problem. When a child sleeps, his or her brain goes to sleep in different stages. A deep sleep is cycled in and out of throughout the night, but this can be disturbed by snoring. The child appears to sleep well, but the brain never actually gets the rest it needs to function at peak performance. A sleep study is required to diagnose obstructive sleep apnea, and treatment ranges from occlusal repositioning appliances to continuous positive airway pressure with or without surgical correction. Adenotonsillectomy in children with Down syndrome and sleep apnea has been helpful in some cases.

Tooth Morphology

The teeth of these clients may be small (microdontia), with maxillary teeth generally more affected in size than mandibular teeth. All teeth except for the maxillary first molars and the mandibular incisors are reduced in size; although the roots are shortened, root formation is complete.[7] The most frequently affected permanent teeth in the maxillary arch are the second molars (52%), the lateral incisors (42%), the canines (41%), the first molars (40%), and the central incisors (35%). In the mandibular arch, the first and second premolars are most commonly affected (63% and 48%, respectively). Tetracycline staining and hypoplastic enamel may be evident as a result of the significant number of early childhood infections requiring antibiotic therapy experienced by persons with Down syndrome.

Missing Teeth and Malocclusion

Congenitally missing teeth and delayed eruption occur in persons with Down syndrome at a much higher rate than in the general population. The increased incidence of congenitally missing permanent teeth (25% to 50%) is probably related to ectodermal dysplasia, local inflammation that damages the tooth germ, or other medical infections. The most frequently missing permanent teeth in persons with Down syndrome are the mandibular second premolar (3.4%) and the lateral incisor (2.2%). Within each quadrant, it is more common to find the most posterior tooth missing than the most anterior tooth. Malocclusion also is seen frequently, with mandibular overjet and posterior crossbite occurring in virtually all persons with Down syndrome. The correction of malocclusion is usually not indicated. If crossbites are corrected, an earlier tissue breakdown may occur as a result of the underdeveloped maxilla and its relation to the basal bone. The lingual movement of the mandibular teeth is difficult because of the tendency of persons with Down syndrome to have large, protruding tongues.

As a result of an increase in the number of persons with Down syndrome working and living in the community, dental professionals have observed an increase in clients with Down syndrome seeking extensive dental care. With most individuals who are working and functioning, there is an increase in self-esteem and self-image. Healthcare professionals assess the client to determine his or her tolerance for extensive treatment. Clients with Down syndrome are given the same treatment options as other clients; treatment objectives should not be limited simply because the client has Down syndrome. Care plans are adapted to the individual's conditions, but overall the goal is to provide comprehensive care.

Periodontal Disease

Individuals with Down syndrome have a high incidence of periodontal disease; this is a function of the associated immunodeficiency and impaired host defense rather than poor oral hygiene alone. Periodontal disease may begin as early as the

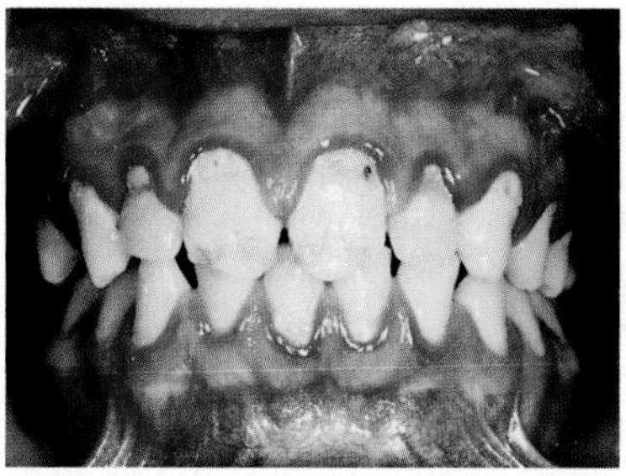

Figure 51-7. Plaque-induced marginal gingivitis and enamel hypoplasia in an individual with Down syndrome. (Courtesy Dr. F.T. McIver, Department of Pediatric Dentistry, University of North Carolina School of Dentistry.)

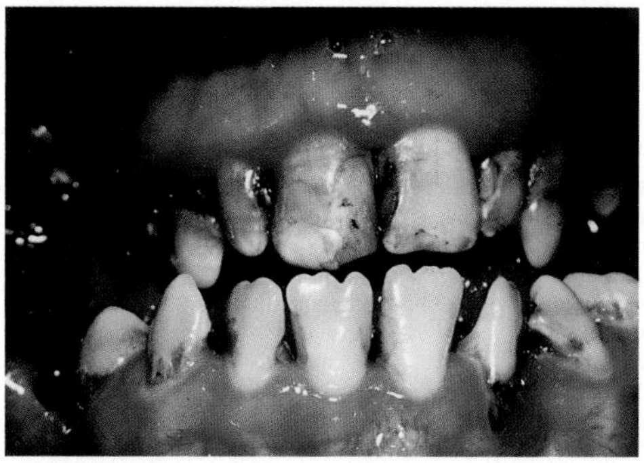

Figure 51-8. Severe chronic periodontal disease in a person with Down syndrome. (Courtesy Dr. F.T. McIver, Department of Pediatric Dentistry, University of North Carolina School of Dentistry.)

age of 6 years in these individuals, and by adulthood nearly all people with Down syndrome are affected. Figure 51-7 depicts a client with Down syndrome with marginal gingivitis and enamel hypoplasia. Figure 51-8 shows more severe periodontal problems in a client with Down syndrome. Periodontal disease is more common among individuals living in institutions as compared with individuals living in the community. This finding may be the result of the lack of education given to the healthcare providers in these institutions, diet, and inadequate daily oral health behavior. In individuals with Down syndrome living in the community, the level of oral hygiene practiced and the extra care given by their caregivers may be sufficient to slow disease progression.

Poor Oral Hygiene

The maintenance of optimal oral hygiene is very difficult for persons with Down syndrome. Therefore dental hygienists educate caregivers and stress the importance of close supervision during oral hygiene procedures and dietary habits that promote health and wellness. If oral healthcare professionals can incorporate effective oral self-care as a part of the client's daily routine, gingival and periodontal conditions may be prevented or controlled. Clear and concise oral hygiene instructions must be presented to the client and the primary caregiver. It is important to communicate directly with the client to build trust. It may be necessary to determine what motivates the client and agree on an award system to augment cooperation.

Persons who are capable of performing their own self-care should do so. Power toothbrushes enable persons with minimal motor control to perform oral self-care independently, thereby facilitating the human need for responsibility for oral health. If persons can perform their own self-care, they own the task and are likely to perform the behavior regularly. Persons with Down syndrome learn better from visual than from auditory teaching; therefore instruction should include pictures, models, and diagrams.

Tooth Loss

Tooth loss occurs in about 50% of individuals with Down syndrome. This tooth loss is attributed to the high prevalence of periodontal disease in this population.

Management of Clients with Down Syndrome

Generally persons with Down syndrome are content and affectionate, but they can become aggressive if they are confused or disoriented. Although their speech patterns are somewhat hindered, most adults with this condition speak intelligently, with a husky quality of voice. It is important to assess the client's intellectual level by observing behavioral patterns, evaluating responses during conversation, and questioning the caregiver. The client may not comprehend the need for care or that it is beneficial. Everything related to care should be introduced slowly, explained, and shown, if possible. Humanistic behavior should be used to calm the client's fears. Some clients with Down syndrome with higher IQs (i.e., those with mild and slightly moderate ID) can participate, and they appreciate the attention given to them during care.

If clients are unmanageable, it is usually because of fear, a previous traumatic dental experience, or mental limitations that do not allow them to comprehend the procedure. Preoperative medications and general anesthesia can be prescribed and administered by the dentist if necessary. When care requires a general anesthetic agent, a thorough health history review is imperative, and all possible needs should be met while the person is anesthetized. A sample dental hygiene care plan for the client with Down syndrome is presented in Figure 51-9.

Autism Spectrum Disorders[5-7]

Autism spectrum disorders (ASDs) cover a wide "spectrum" of neurobiologic disorders that affect how a person interacts, communicates, relates, plays, imagines, and learns. The Centers for Disease Control and Prevention has found that 1 in every 88 children in America has an ASD and estimates that more than 2 million Americans and their families are now affected. ASDs include the following:

- *Autistic disorder (classic autism):* This is the most severe ASD in which the person has difficulty talking and relating to others and the environment; he or she displays compulsive, ritualistic behaviors.
- *Asperger's syndrome:* This is a mild form of autism characterized by impairment in social interactions without significant problems in language, cognitive ability, or age-appropriate developmental skills. Affected individuals are socially awkward; they do not understand the use of gestures, they lack empathy, they avoid eye contact, and they seem unengaged.
- *Rett syndrome:* This rare form of autism, which is found almost exclusively in girls, appears between 6 and 18 months after a period of normal development. It is characterized by poor head growth, a regression of mental and social development, a lack of response to parents, the avoidance of social contact, and excessive hand (e.g., wringing, clapping, washing) and foot activity.

Dental Hygiene Diagnosis	Due to or Related to	As Evidenced by	Client Goal	Evaluative Statements
Biologically Sound and Functional Dentition	Inadequate home-care and diet	Signs of caries at gingival margin	Obtain restorative care Alter diet to exclude cariogenic foods/beverages and include xylitol gum and mints	No evidence of caries activity in 6-month period
Skin and Mucous Membrane Integrity of the Head and Neck	Inadequate daily homecare	Numerous gingival bleeding points	Performance of successful oral hygiene by the caregiver and client (power toothbrush; antimicrobial mouth rinse; tongue brushing	Demonstrates successful oral hygiene at 3-month continued-care interval Decrease gingival bleeding points by 50%
Freedom from Fear and Stress	Fear of dental chair	Client will not sit in the chair while it is moving	Sits in chair without disruptive behavior	Demonstrates comfort level with the dental setting
Responsibility for Oral Health	Lack of caregiver supervision Too much autonomy for self-care by the client Skill deficiency	Biofilm accumulation Signs of caries Coated tongue	Reduce deposit accumulation by next continued-care interval Decrease plaque index score by 1 point by next appointment Client cleans his own teeth then caregiver follows up Both caregiver and client demonstrate effective oral hygiene techniques	Decrease calculus classification from Class III to II Decrease plaque index by 1 point at continued-care interval
Conceptualization and Problem Solving	Oral disease knowledge deficiency of caregiver	Inability to explain disease process and risk factors	Caregiver can explain disease process and risk factors Caregiver can see a difference in James' gingival tissues Caregiver verbalizes the value of oral disease prevention	Client and caregiver report that they evaluate oral hygiene and oral health at least once monthly in the home environment

Dental Hygiene Interventions

- Address concerns with the medication Zyprexa:
  - Monitor vital signs
  - Assess salivary flow
  - Consider semi-supine position
  - Have client sit for 2 minutes before standing
- Conduct nutritional counseling for caries control (include use of xylitol gum and mints).
- Discuss value of daily fluoride for caries control.
- Assess need and apply dental sealants if indicated.
- Instructions for caregiver:
  - Disease risk factors; protective factors
  - Reasoning for plaque index
  - Use of oral hygiene devices
  - Techniques for successful client management
  - How to look for improvements in the tissue
  - Importance of frequent continued-care intervals
- Place dental chair into supine position, then have James get into the chair.
- Introduce procedures slowly based on James' mental age.
- Give client positive reinforcement. Use techniques for forming trusting relationships.
- Complete periodontal debridement and apply fluoride varnish.
- At 3-month continued-care interval, reevaluate the home care.
- Modify plan if needed. Keep open communication between caregiver and healthcare providers.
- Refer to dentist for restorative procedures.

Figure 51-9. Sample dental hygiene care plan: client with Down syndrome.

- *Childhood disintegrative disorder:* This form of autism develops in children who initially seem normal. After at least 2 years of normal development, an affected child exhibits a dramatic loss of vocabulary, language, motor, and social skills. He or she experiences the failure to make friends, a loss of bowel and bladder control, and seizures.
- *Pervasive developmental disorder not otherwise specified:* This is an atypical form of autism in which some but not all classic signs are observed; therefore it does not meet the criteria for a specific diagnosis. This condition is characterized by varying degrees of impairment in communication skills and social interactions, sensitivities to sights and sounds, and restricted, repetitive, and stereotyped behavior patterns.

Given the prevalence of ASDs, dental hygienists are likely to care for individuals with these disorders. Children with ASDs remain in the spectrum as adults and experience problems of independent living and employment. They relate poorly to people and would rather spend high-quality time with objects. For most dental hygienists, care for an autistic person is likely. Men have a four to five times higher incidence of ASDs than women.

Etiology

The cause of ASDs is unknown. Several theories exist, including those related to psychogenic, genetic, biochemical, and neurophysiologic deficits. No single theory has been completely accepted.

Treatment

The care of clients with ASDs is consistent with the theory held by the healthcare provider. Types of treatment include psychotherapy, dietary intervention, educational intervention, music therapy, speech and language therapy, auditory integration therapy, special education, medications, and behavioral therapy. The most commonly prescribed medications include stimulants such as methylphenidate (Ritalin); tranquilizers such as thioridazine or diphenhydramine; anticonvulsants such as phenytoin and carbamazepine; and risperidone, an antipsychotic, to improve behavior.

General Characteristics

From the beginning of life, children with ASDs are unable to relate in an ordinary manner to people and situations. Children with autism are sometimes described as "self-sufficient," "living life in a shell," "happiest when alone," "acting as if people were not there," and "giving the impression of silent wisdom." From the beginning of life, the child desires an extreme autistic aloneness that ignores, disregards, and shuts out anything that comes from outside of him or her. The child has an all-powerful need for being left undisturbed. Everything and anything that changes his or her external environment is looked on as an intrusion. The first characteristic sign of ASD is a lack of posture on being picked up and a failure to adjust the body to that of the person holding the child. Many children with ASD come from highly intelligent families. For a person to be diagnosed with ASD, delays or abnormal functioning must be seen in at least one of the following before the age of 3 years: (1) social interaction, (2) language used for social communication, or (3) symbolic or imaginative play. Approximately 75% of these clients have diagnosed ID, most commonly in the moderate range.

Communication

Children with ASDs are usually devoid of speech or have abnormal language. Their language consists mainly of naming nouns and adjectives that identify objects and indicating colors and numbers that represent nothing specific. This type of language is referred to as *excellent rote memory.* Language becomes a valueless or grossly distorted memory exercise with no use for communication. In other words, autistic children meaninglessly parrot what they hear (**echolalia**). When sentences are formed, they are mostly parrot-like repetitions of word combinations that have been heard. For the autistic child, words become inflexible and cannot be used with any other reference but the original acquired meaning. Autistic children repeat and use personal pronouns just as they are heard. For example, if a child with an ASD desires milk, he may say, "Are you ready for your milk?" Children with ASDs slowly learn to speak of themselves in the first person and of the person addressed in the second person; this occurs around the age of 6 years. It has also been noted that children with autism avoid eye-to-eye contact, facial expressions, and any other form of nonverbal communication.

Behavior

A child with an ASD is controlled by the obsession for sameness that no one can disrupt but the child. Living monotonously repetitious lives makes them feel secure. These clients exhibit restricted, repetitive, and stereotypic patterns of behavior, interests, and activities.

Food is the first intrusion that an ASD infant has to face. Babies with ASD may find eating difficult, and this may result in vomiting. Their unsuccessful struggle against the intrusion of food leads to a limited selection of food choices.[1] If food selection includes regular sucrose intake, dental caries may be a major concern.

An inflexible adherence to specific nonfunctional routines or rituals is evident in these clients. Despair and confusion can be caused by minor changes in routine, everyday tasks, and furniture arrangement. Autistic children also react to loud noises and moving objects with horror. The noise or motion of an object or person is not feared by the child, but rather the disturbance may threaten the child's aloneness. Another characteristic of autism is stereotypic body movements such as rocking, spinning, sniffing, hand clapping, and swaying. A range of behaviors is evident, including hyperactivity, a short attention span, impulsivity, aggressiveness, and SIBs.

Physical Characteristics

Persons with ASD are usually normal physically, although ASD may occur along with other conditions such as metabolic disturbances (e.g., phenylketonuria, Tay-Sachs disease), Down syndrome, and epilepsy. Some individuals with ASD acquire skill in fine muscle coordination, whereas others have a clumsy gait or poor gross motor performance.

Interpersonal Relationships

Children with ASD are more interested in objects than people because objects rarely change in appearance or position. The sameness of objects does not threaten the child, thereby allowing the child to have undisturbed power and control. Children with ASD are not afraid of people but rather of the objects that they acquire. For example, a child with ASD is scared of a pin pricking his body, not of the person doing the pricking. Dental hygienists should try to alleviate a fear of dental instruments by explaining each procedure and the use of each instrument to the client. The children are not interested in surrounding conversation. When addressed, children with ASD respond quickly to "get it over with" so that they can continue their activity, or they may not respond at all. Family members derive the same response as a casual acquaintance. Similarly, children with ASD are very interested in pictures of people but not in people themselves. The pictures of people cannot disturb their environment.

Progress

By the age of 5 or 6 years, language becomes more communicative because the child with ASD has experienced several patterns. Food is accepted, noises and motions are tolerated, and panic tantrums subside. The children also experience increased contact with people, especially people who satisfy their needs, answer their questions, and help them to do things (e.g., reading). By the age of 6 or 8 years, autistic children play alongside other children (this is known as *parallel play*) but never with a group. They also acquire reading skills quickly at this age. As autistic children grow older, several changes begin to occur. They are still in their world of aloneness and sameness, but they emerge from solitude to varying degrees. Some people are accepted into their life because they finally compromise and gradually extend feelers into a world to which they have been total strangers. Other behaviors exhibited by autistic persons at various ages are shown in Table 51-4. Only a small percentage of clients with autism will live and work independently.

Oral Manifestations

Persons with ASD exhibit no specific oral findings, although particular circumstances may increase the risk and prevalence of caries and periodontal disease. Oral care may have been neglected as a result of language difficulties, anxiety, and a lack of social contact. Psychotropic medications may be used as adjuncts to other treatments, thereby causing decreased salivation. The client may benefit from a saliva substitute, daily therapeutic doses of xylitol-containing products, fluoride varnish therapy, and at-home fluoride therapy. Depending on the level of client cooperation, dental sealant therapy should also be considered. Persons with ASD may also have epilepsy, thereby requiring medication that produces drug-influenced gingival enlargement, especially when the individual has poor oral biofilm control.

Individuals with ASD often have nutritional needs as a result of dietary fixation, preferences for soft or sweet foods that require little chewing, a lack of tongue coordination, or pouching their food (i.e., holding food in their cheeks) rather than swallowing. These persons may thus have heavy accumulations of materia alba, food debris, and oral biofilm. Because of these behaviors, nutritional counseling and rigorous plaque-control interventions may be needed.

Management of Clients with Autism Spectrum Disorders

The management of clients with ASD incorporates three approaches: (1) communication techniques, (2) behavioral modification, and (3) pharmacologic therapies. To choose the best approach, the dental hygienist interviews the caregiver to gather information about the client's uniqueness, behaviors, and communication and social skills.

Communication includes the caregiver, the client, and the dental staff. A client with ASD may require conditioning before dental hygiene care. To accomplish this goal, the caregiver is encouraged to bring the client to the office to familiarize the client with upcoming care. Rehearsals at home can be advantageous. The caregiver practices commands that the dental professional may use, such as "Hands down," "Open your mouth," and "Look at me." The reception area should be quiet, with as few people as possible. The client should not wait for extended periods because of the possibility of heightened fear and stress. The dental hygiene procedure is kept short and organized.

A behavioral approach is used to reinforce desired behaviors and to decrease unwanted behaviors. **Behavior modification** techniques that consist of telling, showing, and doing as well as immediate and frequent positive and negative reinforcement are used with short, clear commands (Box 51-4).

Caregivers are encouraged to be present during treatment to provide a familiar face, particularly if immobilization is needed for behavior control. Many methods, including those mentioned earlier, can be used for behavior control (e.g., holding the client's hands down, the use of a papoose board [indicated only when a safe working environment is not attainable] and mouth props). If the client needs to return, the appointments should remain on the same day of the week, at the same time, and with the same dental professionals. The procedure and routine should remain constant as much as possible.

Pharmacologic therapies are needed if all other methods fail. The most commonly prescribed medications include nitrous oxide–oxygen analgesia, diazepam, hydroxyzine, chloral hydrate, meperidine, and promethazine. Pharmacologic therapies may be administered in various combinations and dosages depending on each client's individual needs. See Figure 51-10 for a sample dental hygiene care plan for a client with an ASD.

BOX 51-4

Steps in Behavioral Modification for Individuals with Autism Spectrum Disorders

- Use extensive positive social reinforcement to put the client at ease.
- Use a very simple and suitable reward system, and explain the system to the client (e.g., the client could be given a toy if good behavior is exhibited throughout the appointment). If the client is an adult, a trip to a favorite restaurant may be appropriate.
- Give constant positive social reinforcement throughout each appointment.
- Provide precise verbal praise immediately after each desired behavior.
- Give instructions in a reassuring manner with each desired behavior.
- Do not discuss dental treatment that is needed during dental hygiene care.
- Points earned for desired behavior always entitle the person to a prize at the end.
- Conclude each session with excessive praise.

TABLE 51-4

Possible Behaviors Exhibited by People with Autism Spectrum Disorders

Age Period	Response to Environment	Social and Play Skills	Language Communication Skills	Feeding and Eating	Motor Development
Infancy	Good: Infant is quiet and placid, seldom cries, and is fascinated by lights Irritable: Infant screams and may quiet only with vigorous rocking or car rides Fights washing, dressing, and feedings Stiff, hard to cuddle Body rocks, head bangs	Unresponsive to parents' presence Poor response to social games Little eye contact No reaching or pointing No interest in baby toys May enjoy rough play	Ignores speech Ignores loud sounds Is fascinated with soft sounds Has decreased verbalizations	Poor sucking Refusal to eat lumpy foods Does not cry when hungry	On schedule or uneven May bypass a motor stage, such as creeping
Toddler	Self-stimulating behaviors, rocking, head banging Sleep patterns irregular Resists changes in routine Disturbances in response to stimuli: is fascinated with some sounds Uses touch, taste, and smell to extremes Ignores objects of usual childhood interest Zeros in on details Uses peripheral vision Recognizes parents by outline rather than by features Does not respond to painful stimuli	Inappropriate use of an attachment to objects Stereotypic, repetitive play May be extremely passive May be destructive, aggressive, and self-injurious Difficult to manage Frequent tantrums	Unresponsive to voice, tone, or name Echolalia: delayed or immediate Screams Leads adult by the arm Responds to simple commands	Likes pureed foods Will eat only a limited variety of foods Does not recognize foods in other forms, such as a banana without the peel	Prolonged cruiser Tiptoe walks May be normal May be hyperactive
Preschool	Toddler responses continue	Aloof and expressionless Delayed toilet training More affectionate Socially embarrassing behaviors Tantrums continue Stereotypic, repetitive play continues Passivity may continue	Echolalia may develop Meaningful speech is produced with effort Poor pronunciation and voice control Unable to understand most speech Can understand short, concrete sentences Confusion with pronouns, similar-sounding words, and word order Uses and understands limited gestures	Food jags	May be normal May jump, spin, flap arms and hands May be graceful or clumsy Fine motor ability may differ from gross Difficulty with copying movements May walk with elbows bent, hands together, and wrists dropped Hyperactivity may continue
School years	Behaviors (tantrums) decrease Sleep irregularities may continue Continues to have disturbances in response to stimuli	Increased affection Increased social skills May help with simple household chores	Language skills may increase Same problems seen as preschooler may continue	Food jags continue May begin trying new foods	Increased motor skills Unusual walk Splinter skills may develop May pace, jump, spin
Adulthood	Same as school years	Increased affection Increased social skills	Language skills continue to increase	Diet broadens Food jags continue	Motor skills continue to increase Relatively self-sufficient

Dental Hygiene Diagnosis	Due to or Related to	As Evidenced by	Client Goal	Evaluative Statements
Biologically Sound and Functional Dentition	Inadequate homecare Inadequate diet Harmful toothbrushing technique	Signs of dental caries Signs of cervical abrasion	Obtain restorative treatment Alter diet to exclude cariogenic foods Use a power toothbrush	Decrease plaque index score by 1 point Report ingestion of noncariogenic snacks that include xylitol mints No additional abrasion evident
Skin and Mucous Membrane Integrity of the Head and Neck	Medication (Zoloft) Inadequate homecare	Signs of xerostomia Supragingival soft and hard deposits	Use of saliva substitutes, xylitol gum and mints, and fluoride therapy Caregiver and client to demonstrate use of power toothbrush and moisturizing mouth rinse	Less xerostomia observed and reported Reduction of deposit accumulation at continued-care visit
Freedom from Fear and Stress	Sensitivity to high-pitched noise Client not being sure of his environment	Verbal and nonverbal indicators of stress Tapping Well thought-out (deliberate) walking	Respond positively to the use of equipment that typically causes unpleasant sensation in the ears Decrease behaviors that interfere with treatment	Client appears comfortable and cooperative during care Tapping and deliberate walking behaviors decreased by 50%
Responsibility for Oral Health	Lack of caregiver supervision Too much autonomy for self-care by the client Skill deficiency	Biofilm accumulation Signs of supragingival deposits	Decreased biofilm accumulation by 50% at continued-care appointment Caregiver reports that client cleans his own mouth daily and it is followed up by caregiver Both caregiver and client demonstrate appropriate oral hygiene techniques	Plaque index score decreases by 50%
Conceptualization and Problem Solving	Knowledge deficiency of caregiver and client	Inability to explain disease process and risk factors	Caregiver can explain disease process, risk factors, and protective factors Caregiver can see a difference in client's gingival tissues	Caregiver verbalizes that a difference is observed in Ben's oral health as a result of homecare

Dental Hygiene Interventions

- Addresses concerns with medication Zoloft:
  - Monitor vital signs
  - Assess salivary flow
  - Consider semi-supine position
  - Have client sit for 2 minutes before standing
- Conduct nutritional counseling (include use of xylitol gum and mints).
- Instructions for caregiver:
  - Disease risk factors/protective factors
  - Rationale for plaque index
  - Use of oral hygiene devices
  - Use power toothbrush
  - Techniques for successful client management
  - How to look for improvements in the gum tissue (i.e., bleeding points, tongue cleanliness)
  - Importance of frequent continued-care appointments
- Communicate the value of at-home fluoride therapy for caries control.
- Discuss use of xylitol gum, frequent water, or saliva substitutes for managing xerostomia.
- Avoid equipment with high-pitched noises.
- Give verbal commands for desired behavior. Allow Ben time to process request and wait for response.
- Incorporate behavior modification techniques and techniques for forming a *trusting relationship.*
- Give Ben positive reinforcement for appropriate behavior.
- Complete periodontal debridement and apply fluoride varnish.
- Refer to dentist for restorative procedures.
- After 3 months, re-evaluate home care and oral health status.
- Modify care plan if needed; maintain communication between caregiver and other healthcare providers.

Figure 51-10. Sample dental hygiene care plan: client with an autism spectrum disorder.

Educating Clients with Intellectual Disabilities

Oral hygiene for individuals with ID requires modifications in response to the physical, cognitive, and behavioral challenges that these individuals might have. The client's cognitive and physical limitations and abilities, oral and systemic disease risk, systemic and oral health status, level of deposit accumulation, medications, diet, and ability to cooperate are assessed so that dental hygiene care can meet his or her human needs.

Cognitive Limitations

The client's cognitive level affects his or her oral self-care potential. Wide variations in the ability to learn can exist even within categories of ID. Clients with mild or moderate ID can usually learn to brush their teeth. Successful teaching methods include using pictures, the use of a tell-show-do technique, and modeling. A consistent challenge that these clients face is brushing long enough; therefore an egg timer or a power toothbrush with a built-in timer could be used to lengthen brushing time. Oral irrigators, interdental cleaning aids, and disclosing tablets can be used by clients with mild ID. Clients with moderate ID require repetitive training, but they can usually manipulate a power toothbrush. For clients with severe ID, emphasis is on as much self-care as possible, with the caregiver following up to achieve daily oral biofilm control. Normally these clients are limited to a push–pull stroke, and they often isolate brushing to one side. Clients with profound ID depend on caregivers for oral cleansing. Emphasis is on the acceptance of oral hygiene procedures, which is accomplished through nonverbal communication and desensitization techniques.

Physical Limitations

Communication may be a challenge if the client also has visual or hearing limitations. Visual cues work best for persons with hearing impairments; tactile and auditory cues are used for visually impaired clients. A severe gag reflex may be managed by placing the client in a semi-supine position and eliminating the use of toothpaste to reduce gagging and to provide better visualization for the caregiver. Water, an American Dental Association–accepted antimicrobial mouth rinse, or an ingestible or low-foaming dentifrice can be used in place of toothpaste. Dental professionals and caregivers may need to use a mouth prop to allow for access during oral care. When working with clients with severe and profound ID, the use of a toothbrush designed for a suction attachment can prevent aspiration (see Chapter 42, Figure 42-6).

Selection of Oral Hygiene Aids

As with any client, oral hygiene aids are selected after the assessment of a client with ASD. In general, the brush handle should be longer to facilitate the reaching of posterior areas; the brush head size should be selected on the basis of the client's oral cavity size and his or her ability to open the mouth. Existing toothbrushes can be altered according to client need (e.g., motor ability, grip problems; see Chapter 42, Figure 42-7). Electric toothbrushes are ideal for clients with grip problems and limited fine motor control.

Interdental cleaning may be extremely difficult for clients and caregivers, but some is better than none. Interdental cleaning devices with long handles are recommended to protect fingers from inadvertent or intentional biting and to reach posterior areas. Holders must be easy to thread and to use to ensure compliance. Oral irrigators are not generally recommended for this population except to deliver prescribed antimicrobial agents. The use of 0.12% chlorhexidine gluconate mouth rinse is commonly prescribed for clients with disabilities to help control oral biofilm and gingivitis. It can be administered via an oral irrigator, a spray, or a swab. (Note that chlorhexidine is absorbed through the gastrointestinal system; therefore no harm is caused by swallowing a small amount of the agent.) Other agents may be indicated for these clients, including American Dental Association–accepted antimicrobial mouth rinses, sodium fluoride gels and mouth rinses, povidone–iodine (Betadine) mouth rinses, and similar products. These products are often less expensive and do not stain teeth or alter taste as much as 0.12% chlorhexidine gluconate. The use of an antimicrobial fluoride dentifrice twice daily is also recommended. If cooperation is high, home fluoride application is commonly done with a toothbrush after toothbrushing. Substitute therapeutic doses of xylitol gum and mints for candy and for behavior modification.

CLIENT EDUCATION TIPS

- Teach the caregiver oral self-care behaviors to ensure positive attitudes and habits toward oral health and hygiene.
- Ensure that the caregiver has the knowledge and equipment to perform effective daily oral hygiene with the client.
- Clients with mild intellectual disability are educable, so explain and demonstrate oral hygiene instructions with the use of activities rather than concepts.
- Clients with moderate intellectual disability should be taught fundamental skills by employing the show-and-tell method.
- Discuss preventive therapies (e.g., diet counseling, dental sealants, fluoride therapy, xylitol use, frequent continued-care intervals), their feasibility, and their barriers with the client's caregiver.
- Provide verbal and written instructions so that the caregiver can have a reference if needed.
- Work with the caregiver to overcome barriers to care.

LEGAL, ETHICAL, AND SAFETY ISSUES

- During the provision of health services in places of public accommodation, discrimination against persons with disabilities and those with whom they associate is illegal and unethical.
- Many dental practices do not treat clients with disabilities on the basis of a lack of knowledge and experience, a lack of equipment, and inadequate compensation. Many disabled persons rely on government-funded sources for income and financing healthcare; therefore access to care is a real problem.

- The American Dental Hygienists' Association Code of Ethics states that clients should be treated without discrimination. Dental hygienists who are ill prepared to treat these clients should seek continuing education opportunities or refer these clients so that high-quality care can be rendered.
- Close supervision of disabled clients in the care environment is required.

KEY CONCEPTS

- Causes of intellectual disability (ID) are grouped as prenatal, perinatal, and postnatal causes.
- The level of ID determines if the client is capable of giving informed consent for care. Consultation with the client's physician, social worker, or caregiver (i.e., healthcare decision maker) is necessary.
- When planning oral hygiene interventions for clients with severe or profound ID, the caregiver should be included. Clients with severe ID can learn by habit training but need follow-up by the caregiver.
- Persons with ID may have poor oral health as a result of heightened susceptibility to infection, malnutrition, limited self-care capabilities, economic barriers to care, and limited access to care.
- Oral manifestations observed in clients with ID often coincide with a specific type of syndrome.
- The lips of clients with ID are sometimes larger than those of the general population, and tooth anomalies such as microdontia and delayed eruption patterns are usually present as a result of developmental abnormalities. Tooth surface attrition from bruxism is often seen as a result of anxiety or stress.
- The prevalence of periodontal disease among individuals with ID is attributed to a lack of professional care, a lack of funds to support care, increased susceptibility, and poor oral hygiene.
- When developing oral hygiene skills in a client with ID, teach at a level that is based on the client's mental age rather than his or her chronologic age.
- Down syndrome is the most common and frequently observed chromosomal abnormality in humans.
- Congenital heart disease is the most common and serious medical condition among persons with Down syndrome; therefore the dental hygienist must determine the need for prophylactic antibiotic premedication based on current guidelines.
- Individuals with Down syndrome have a high incidence of periodontal disease.
- Autism spectrum disorders (ASDs) include autistic disorder, Asperger's syndrome, Rett syndrome, and pervasive developmental disorder not otherwise specified, all of which are characterized by varying degrees of impairment in communication skills and social interactions and restricted, repetitive, and stereotyped patterns of behavior.
- Body movements such as rocking are characteristically observed in some persons with an ASD.
- Clients with ASDs may take psychotropic medications that decrease salivation; therefore saliva substitutes and therapeutic doses of xylitol-containing products may be prescribed for daily use.
- Behavior modification is the recommended technique when working with persons with ASDs.
- When educating clients with ID, their cognitive and physical limitations and abilities, level of periodontal health and caries risk, level of deposit accumulation, medications, diet, and ability to cooperate should be assessed.
- When toothbrushes are chosen, the handle should be long, and the brush size should be selected based on the client's ability to open the mouth and the size of the oral cavity. Power toothbrushes are excellent for individuals with limited fine motor control (see Chapters 23 and 42).
- Floss holders are recommended to reach posterior areas and to protect the fingers from inadvertent or intentional biting (see Chapter 24).
- When formulating a care plan for a client with ID, the dental hygienist must be empathetic and realistic, especially if a caregiver is responsible for the client's daily care.

CRITICAL THINKING EXERCISES

1. Visit a sheltered workshop in the community, and invite the workers to receive dental hygiene care. After the completion of treatment, share the challenges that you experienced with your peers. How were you able to overcome the challenges? What strategies were successful or unsuccessful?
2. Visit a school for severely and profoundly intellectually disabled persons. On the basis of your observations and discussions with the teachers, what would you do to improve the oral health status of these students? What recommendations would you have for the teachers?
3. Read each of the dental hygiene care plans (see Figures 51-2, 51-9, and 51-10). Use these to plan a series of appointments to address the diagnosed problems. Are other interventions needed to achieve client goals and therapeutic outcomes? Assuming that the goals are met, what future goals might move these clients to higher levels of oral health and wellness?

REFERENCES

1. American Association of Intellectual and Developmental Disabilities: Available at: www.aaidd.org/about-aaidd#.UmSFWha_Oa4. Accessed August 4, 2012.
2. Schalock RL, Luckasson RA, Shogren KA, et al: The renaming of mental retardation: understanding the change to the term intellectual disability, *Intellect Dev Disabil* 45:116, 2007.
3. National Down Syndrome Society: National Down Syndrome Society Website. Available at: http://www.ndss.org. Accessed October 24, 2012.
4. The National Association for Child Development: *Congenital heart disease in children with Down syndrome*. Available at: http://downsyndrome.nacd.org/heart_disease.php. Accessed October 24, 2012.
5. Centers for Disease Control and Prevention: *About autism*. Available at: www.cdc.gov/ncbddd/autism. Accessed August 4, 2012.
6. *Autism speaks: Autism Speaks Website*. Available at: www.autismspeaks.org. Accessed August 4, 2012.
7. National Institute of Mental Health: *A parent's guide to autism spectrum disorder*. Available at: www.nimh.nih.gov/health/publications/a-parents-guide-to-autism-spectrum-disorder/what-is-autism-spectrum-disorder-asd.shtml. Accessed August 6, 2012.

8. National Institute of Child Health and Human Development: *Autism Spectrum Disorder (ASD) Condition, What is ASD*? Available at: www.nichd.nih.gov/health/topics/autism/conditioninfo/pages/default.aspx. Accessed August 6, 2012.
9. National Institute of Child Health and Human Development: *Intellectual and Developmental Disabilities (IDDs) Overview*. Available at: www.nichd.nih.gov/health/topics/idds/Pages/default.aspx. Accessed August 8, 2012.
10. Raposa KA, Perlman SP: *Treating the dental patient with a developmental disorder*, Ames IA, 2012, Wiley-Blackwell.

ACKNOWLEDGMENT

The authors acknowledge Ginger B. Mann for her past contributions to this chapter.

EVOLVE RESOURCES

Please visit http://evolve.elsevier.com/Darby/hygiene for additional practice and study support tools.

CHAPTER

52

Alcohol and Substance Abuse Problems

Margaret Lemaster

COMPETENCIES

1. Describe alcohol and substance abuse.
2. Describe physiologic, genetic, and environmental causes of substance abuse, including:
   - Identify the action of psychoactive drugs on neurotransmitters.
   - Define the addiction curve and fetal alcohol syndrome.
   - List the risk factors for substance abuse.
3. Compare medical treatment options for substance abuse.
4. Discuss implications for the dental hygiene process of care caused by substance abuse, including:
   - Describe the short-term, long-term, and systemic substance abuse effects.
   - Identify oral signs and symptoms associated with substance abuse.
   - Discuss the dental hygiene process of care related to clients with substance abuse problems and those in recovery.
5. Explain why professionals are at risk for chemical dependence.

Substance abuse is a significant problem in the United States. In 2011 an estimated 22.6 million Americans who were 12 years old or older were current illicit drug users. (Figure 52-1). Although the use of marijuana, psychotherapeutics, inhalants, and hallucinogens among youth between the ages of 12 and 17 years declined from 2002 to 2010 (Figure 52-2), adults between the ages of 50 and 59 showed a staggering increase in illicit drug use from 2002 to 2012[1] (Figure 52-3).

Substance abuse affects the individual, the family, and the community. Alcohol- or drug-impaired drivers cause a significant number of deadly automobile accidents annually. Child abuse and neglect are often directly related to the substance abuse of parents. Because addiction often results in criminal behavior to finance a drug habit, substance abusers are viewed as morally corrupt or weak personalities who willingly engage in self-destructive behaviors that affect themselves and everyone around them. Research has shown that **addiction** is a chronic, cyclic disease; however, unlike other diseases, a social stigma remains.

Clients who are dependent on alcohol or drugs or who are in treatment for substance abuse present the dental hygienist with complex issues related to preventive oral health care. Poor oral health is common among those with substance abuse problems. Risk factors for poor oral health include limited access to care, poor diet, poor oral hygiene, and negative attitudes toward oral health care. Substance abuse directly affects oral health and results in xerostomia, an increased caries rate, enamel erosion, periodontal disease, and poor self-care. Such clients must be identified so that they can be treated safely. To do this, dental hygienists must understand basic concepts associated with substance abuse, its causes, and the associated medical treatment.

Although the scope of dental practice does not include the diagnosis or treatment of alcohol or substance abuse, the dental hygienist must be aware of signs and symptoms of substance abuse and addiction, know an appropriate treatment plan, and implement oral health care appropriately.

According to the Standards for Clinical Dental Hygiene Practice set forth by the American Dental Hygienists' Association, dental hygienists are ethically obligated to take action to promote patient safety and well-being, to assess risk factors that affect oral and general health, and to confer with other health care professionals when appropriate.

Concepts of Alcohol and Substance Abuse

Substances of abuse, which are often referred to as *mood-altering substances,* are those that affect the central nervous system and the perceptions of the environment through chemical changes. Substance abuse includes the use of natural and synthetic substances as well as psychoactive drugs used by those with substance abuse issues.

Alcohol is the most pervasive substance used in the United States, and it is associated with a significant number of health-related diseases and deaths. Nearly 75% of Americans consume alcohol in varying amounts, yet chronic drinkers are often overlooked in the dental setting. Men are more likely than women to be identified, and usually a medical problem caused by alcohol facilitates a medical diagnosis. Self-reporting questionnaires have been shown to be an effective means for identifying alcohol abuse.

There are three main types of alcohol: (1) isopropyl alcohol, (2) methanol, and (3) ethanol. Both isopropyl alcohol and methanol are toxic when ingested, whereas ethanol is the main component of alcoholic beverages. Ethanol is a product manufactured by fermenting simple carbohydrates found in fruit, grains, or vegetables with yeast. The alcohol content of wine, beer, and spirits (hard liquor) differs. On average, beer contains 4.5% alcohol, wine contains 12.9%, and spirits contain 41.1%. A "standard drink" is defined as one that contains approximately 0.5 fluid ounce (12 g) of alcohol. This amount of alcohol is present in 12 fluid ounces of beer, 5 fluid

Figures, tables, and boxes marked as "e" are available as supplemental material on the Evolve site. Visit http://evolve.elsevier.com/Darby/hygiene to access these materials.

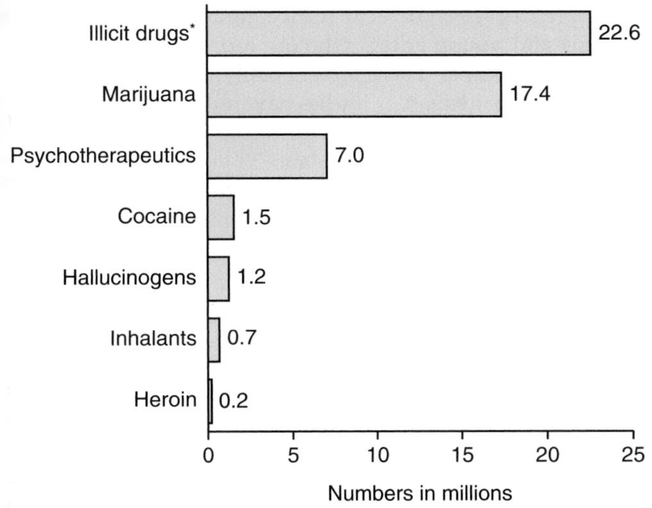

* Illicit drugs include marijuana/hashish, cocaine (including crack), heroin, hallucinogens, inhalants, or prescription-type psychotherapeutics used non-medically

Figure 52-1. Use of specific illicit drugs among persons 12 years old and older.

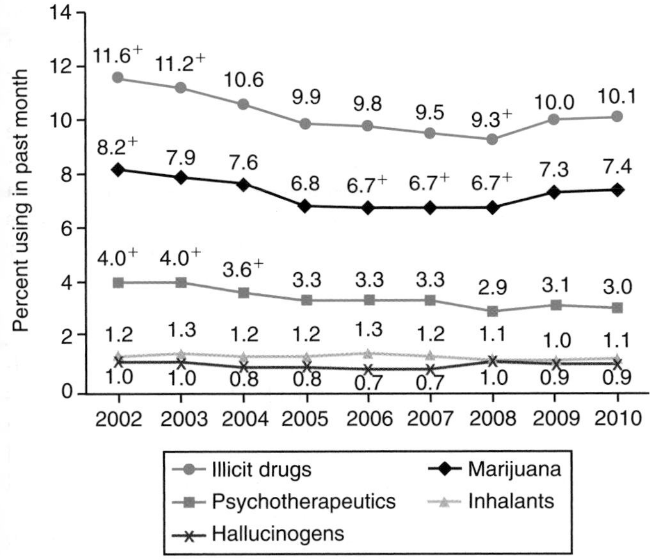

Figure 52-2. Results of the 2011 National Survey on Drug Use and Health. (Prepared for the U.S. Department of Health and Human Services, Substance Abuse and Mental Health Services Administration, Office of Applied Studies, 2010.)

ounces of wine, or 1.5 fluid ounces of 80-proof distilled spirits. **Binge drinking** is defined as drinking five or more standard drinks on the same occasion at least once within a 30-day time frame.

Alcohol reduces anxiety and causes intoxication and sensory alterations. Alcohol enters the blood within 5 minutes of ingestion and remains in the bloodstream for 1 to 4 hours. The liver breaks down alcohol at the rate of one standard drink per hour. Blood alcohol concentration is measured in milligrams per deciliter (mg/dL). In most U.S. jurisdictions, blood alcohol concentrations of more than 100 mg/dL (0.1%) are illegal.

Substance abuse is a pattern of self-administrated drug use that may lead to drug addiction (Table 52-1). **Drug addiction** is a chronic and compulsive need to use drugs despite their causing the user physical harm. **Psychologic dependence** is rooted in the belief that the drug is needed to maintain a state of well-being. **Physiologic dependence** results from a biologic alteration in the user's brain from consistent drug use. A person who has developed physiologic

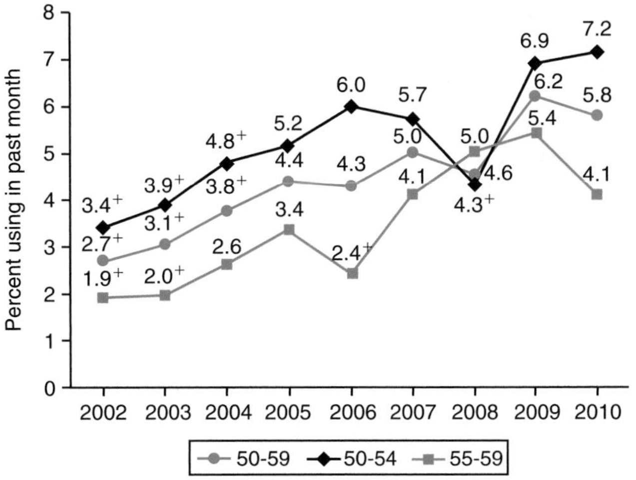

Figure 52-3. Results of the 2011 National Survey on Drug Use and Health. (Prepared for the U.S. Department of Health and Human Services, Substance Abuse and Mental Health Services Administration, Office of Applied Studies, 2010.)

TABLE 52-1

Drug Use Continuum

Classification Based on Use		Behavior
Type 1	Abstainers (about one third of the population)	Never used drugs or alcohol
Type 2	Social drinker or users (majority of population)	Occasional use Able to drink one and stop Does not result in personal problems
Type 3	Drug abusers	Excessive use of substance Binge drinking
Type 4	Physically dependent addicts	Adaptation of the body's chemistry Withdrawal signs and symptoms Not used as a coping device Physician-induced addictions
Type 5	Psychologically dependent addicts	Alcohol or drugs used to cope with life Can never return to social use Tolerance Withdrawal symptoms Compulsive use Loss of control Use despite personal problems Preoccupation Denial

Adapted from Coombs RH: *Drug-impaired professionals,* Cambridge, Mass, 1997, Harvard University Press.

dependence on a drug will go through drug withdrawal when drug use ceases. Withdrawal symptoms may include vomiting, diarrhea, rapid pulse, sweating, anxiety, convulsions, severe cramps, high blood pressure, and severe headaches. People will often continue using drugs because they fear experiencing withdrawal from the drug. Table 52-2 presents the drug categories of abused substances and their effects on the body.

Another aspect of physiologic dependence is the development of drug tolerance whereby an increasingly larger dose is required to produce the same physiologic or psychologic effect obtained earlier with smaller doses. Nicotine, opiates, alcohol, psychedelics, central nervous system (CNS) stimulants, and sedative–hypnotics all require increased doses to establish the same "high" or euphoric feeling that the user experienced with first use. If the drug dosage is not increased, the effects of the drug are diminished, and withdrawal symptoms occur. So-called "club drugs" have joined the list of abused substances in the past 10 years. Methylenedioxymethamphetamine (MDMA, ecstasy), flunitrazepam (Rohypnol), gamma-hydroxybutyric acid (GHB), and ketamine are used by teens and young adults who are a part of the nightclub, bar, and rave scene.[2] These are generally low-cost drugs, and they are readily available. Studies have shown that multidrug use is common among those who misuse stimulants. Young women between the ages of 16 and 25 years are more likely to misuse diet pills or amphetamines, whereas young men of the same age group are more likely to misuse methamphetamine and prescription stimulants such as Benzedrine, Ritalin, and Dexedrine[3] (Table 52-3).

Stages of Change

The stages of change model is an approach to assist clients with changing unwanted behavior.[4] The concept of readiness to change a behavior, such as alcohol or substance abuse, relates to the stages of change theory. For all clients who report some type of substance abuse, the dental hygienist assesses their readiness to quit. To assess readiness to quit, the dental hygienist simply asks clients if they would like to stop their substance use within the next month. The stages of

TABLE 52-2
Effects of Illicit Drug Use

Drug	Short-Term Use	Long-Term Use	Systemic Effects
Hallucinogens			
Cannabinoids Marijuana Hashish Sinsemilla	Relaxation; euphoria; confusion; poor coordination; red, bloodshot eyes; intense hunger or thirst; difficulty with concentration, memory, and learning; distorted perception of sights, sounds, time, and touch; difficulty with problem solving	Leads to use of other addictive substances; increases risk of lung cancer, bronchitis, and emphysema—smoking one joint of marijuana has the same effect as smoking 14 to 16 cigarettes; weakens immune system	Dilated pupils, tachycardia; peripheral vasodilation; bronchial hyperactivity; insomnia; impaired short-term memory; disruption in testosterone secretion Decreases nausea and pressure behind the eyes Sometimes taken by cancer and glaucoma patients to alleviate symptoms Chronic use can result in withdrawal symptoms Can cause thrombocytopenia if injected intravenously
Lysergic acid diethylamide (LSD)	Causes sensory distortions and illusions, extreme emotions from euphoria to panic, and unpredictable reactions	Acute anxiety; fear of loss of control; paranoia; delusions of grandeur	Increased heart rate and blood pressure; hyperthermia; prolonged psychotic reaction or severe depression; mental flashbacks to sensations experienced while taking drug can occur
Phencyclidine (PCP)	Sensory deprivation; reduces inhibitions; deadens pain; mild depression	Combative behavior; inability to speak; confusion, agitation, and paranoia; amnesia	Extremely high blood pressure; cardiovascular instability; respiratory depression; catatonia; coma; convulsions; seizures Retained in fat cells for several months after use and can be released during exercise, fasting, or when under stress, thereby causing flashbacks
Anabolic Steroids			
	Enhanced athletic performance; increased muscle mass; increased aggression; decreased inflammation and swelling of injured tissue; weight gain	Males: shrinking of testicles, reduced sperm count, impotence, baldness, breast development, and enlarged prostate Females: cessation of menses, facial hair growth	Acne; depression; jaundice; tremors; swelling of feet or ankles; halitosis; increased possibility of injury to tendons, ligaments, and muscles; increased blood pressure; liver damage

TABLE 52-2
Effects of Illicit Drug Use—cont'd

Drug	Short-Term Use	Long-Term Use	Systemic Effects
Inhalants			
Volatile solvents Airplane glue Rubber cement Spray paint Hair spray Paint thinner Spot remover Gasoline	Reduced inhibitions; impulsiveness; excitement; irritability; euphoria; dizziness; slurred speech; drowsiness	Confusion; delirium; psychomotor dysfunction; emotional instability; impaired thinking	Brain, liver, kidney, nervous system, bone marrow, and lung disorders as a result of the effect of the solvent or ingredients in the solvent Respiratory arrest; cardiac arrhythmia; asphyxia; suicide
Volatile nitrites Room deodorizers Amyl nitrite	Relaxation of all smooth muscles; altered consciousness; enhanced sexual pleasure (used especially among male homosexuals)	Increased blood flow to the brain resulting in headaches, dizziness, giddiness, vomiting, shock, and loss of consciousness	Nitrite poisoning; damage to the nervous system; impaired perception, reasoning, and memory; dementia; defective muscular coordination
Anesthetics Nitrous oxide	Giddiness; profound laughter; euphoria	Addiction; loss of consciousness; frostbite of the nose and vocal cords from direct inhalation out of a pressurized tank	Peripheral nerve damage; frozen lung tissue; brain cell damage due to oxygen deprivation
Alcohol			
	Feeling of well-being; loss of inhibitions; slowed reactions; intoxication; slurred speech; sedation; unconsciousness; especially dangerous when used with other central nervous system depressants or narcotics	Addiction; increased risk of oral cancer and breast cancer; malnutrition; inflammation of the stomach; hepatitis and other liver damage; alcohol amnestic disorder; dementia	Cognitive impairment; cardiovascular impairment; cirrhosis of the liver; damage to kidneys, central nervous system, and gastrointestinal tract

TABLE 52-3
Drugs That Are Often Abused

Category and Name	Commercial Name	Route of Administration	Drug Effects and Potential Health Consequences
Depressants			
Barbiturates	Amytal, Nembutal, Seconal, Phenobarbital	Injected, swallowed	Reduced pain and anxiety; feeling of well-being; lowered inhibitions; slowed pulse and breathing; lowered blood pressure; poor concentration or confusion; fatigue; impaired coordination, memory, and judgment; slurred speech; dizziness
Benzodiazepines	Ativan, Halcion, Librium, Valium, Xanax	Intravenous, swallowed	
Flunitrazepam	Rohypnol	Intravenous, swallowed, snorted	
Dissociative Anesthetics			
Ketamine	Ketalar SV	Injected, snorted, smoked	Increased heart rate and blood pressure; impaired motor function; memory loss; numbness; nausea and vomiting At high doses: delirium; depression; respiratory depression and arrest

Continued

TABLE 52-3
Drugs That Are Often Abused—cont'd

Category and Name	Commercial Name	Route of Administration	Drug Effects and Potential Health Consequences
Opioids and Morphine Derivatives			
Codeine	Empirin with codeine, Fiorinal with codeine, Tylenol with codeine	Intravenous, injected, swallowed	Pain relief; euphoria; drowsiness; respiratory depression and arrest; nausea; confusion; constipation; sedation; unconsciousness; coma; tolerance; addiction
Fentanyl	Actiq, Duragesic, Sublimaze	Injected, smoked, snorted	
Morphine	Roxanol, Duramorph	Injected, swallowed, smoked	
Opium	Laudanum, Paregoric	Swallowed, smoked	
Opioid pain relievers: oxycodone, meperidine, hydromorphone, hydrocodone	Tylox, OxyContin, Percodan, Percocet, Demerol, Darvon	Swallowed, injected, suppositories, chewed, crushed, snorted	
Stimulants			
Amphetamines	Biphetamine, Dexedrine	Injected, swallowed, smoked, snorted	Increased heart rate, blood pressure, and metabolism; feelings of exhilaration, energy, and increased mental alertness; rapid or irregular heartbeat; reduced appetite; weight loss; heart failure
Cocaine	Cocaine hydrochloride	Injected, smoked, snorted	Increased temperature; chest pain; respiratory failure; nausea; abdominal pain; strokes; seizures; headaches; malnutrition; see also the effects of amphetamines listed previously
Methamphetamine	Desoxyn	Injected, swallowed, smoked, snorted	Aggression; violence; psychotic behavior; memory loss; cardiac and neurologic damage; impaired memory and learning; tolerance; addiction; see also the effects of amphetamines listed previously
Methylphenidate	Ritalin	Injected, swallowed, snorted	Increase or decrease in blood pressure; psychotic episodes; digestive problems; loss of appetite; weight loss; see also the effects of amphetamines listed previously

change theory can be applied to a multitude of behaviors. Because the model is continuous, an individual may enter any stage, relapse to a previous stage, and then restart the change process.

According to this theory, any behavior change involves movement through a series of five stages. These stages are precontemplation, contemplation, preparation, action, and maintenance. **Precontemplation** is the stage of change during which the client has no thought of stopping substance abuse. The substance abuse is not viewed by the client as a problem. Strategies for change initiated by the dental hygienist may be to personalize information about the risks and benefits of the behavior. **Contemplation** is the stage during which clients think that they should stop substance abuse someday, but not within the next month. The dental hygienist may motivate, encourage, and assist the client with specific plans to change. **Preparation** is the stage of change during which clients are willing to set a quit date and to begin changing their behavior and thinking related to substance abuse in preparation for quitting in the next month. The dental hygienist may assist the client with setting attainable goals gradually. **Action** is the stage during which clients have stopped their substance abuse for less than 6 months. The dental hygienist may assist with problem solving, social support, and reinforcement. **Maintenance** is the stage of change during which clients have stopped substance abuse for more than 6 months. The dental hygienist may assist the client with avoiding relapses and by offering continued support. Only when clients perceive that the personal benefits of stopping substance abuse outweigh the benefits of continued use will they make a decision to change their behavior. Nevertheless, personalized advice regarding change that is delivered in a caring and nonjudgmental manner often moves a client who is in the precontemplation stage to the contemplation stage of change. This shift in the stage of change constitutes success, because such movement is in the direction of making a decision to change the behavior someday.

Those individuals in the precontemplation and contemplation stages will have a negative response if the dental hygienist asks or recommends that they change a particular behavior. It is important for the dental hygienist to not take this rejection personally but rather to recognize that the client is not ready to change. Only when the client perceives that the personal benefits of changing a behavior outweigh the benefits of the behavior will they make the decision to change. Client readiness to change will determine the appropriate strategy for assistance by the dental hygienist.

As individuals attempt to stop a behavior such as alcohol abuse, relapse (reverting to regular alcohol use) followed by recycling through the stages of change occurs frequently. When relapse occurs, the client will return to the contemplation or precontemplation stage before attempting to quit again. The dental hygienist encourages clients to view relapse as a learning opportunity: what is learned from relapse can be applied to the next quit attempt.

Helping clients to change a particular behavior is an important role for the dental hygienist, especially when addressing lifestyle adjustments for addictions. Motivation and noncompliance concepts often spotlight failure; however, accepting a client's readiness to change and respecting barriers to change can improve client satisfaction and clinician frustration. By listening to the client and asking nonjudgmental questions about the client's readiness to make a quit attempt, the dental hygienist can respond appropriately for the client's current stage of change. For example, if a client admits to substance abuse but states that he is not ready to stop, providing information about the benefits of stopping would be appropriate to help the client to continue to think about stopping. Asking questions like, "When will you know it is time to quit?" allows the client to think about an answer after the dental hygiene care visit and allows the client more control when making a decision to stop the substance abuse (Figure 52-4).

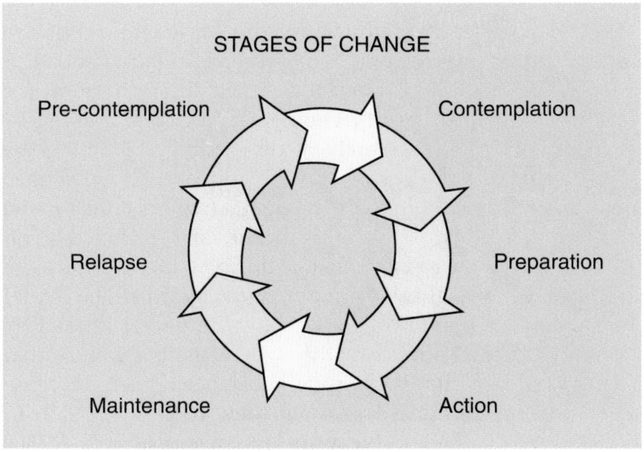

Figure 52-4. Stages of change model.

Whether or not a client is ready to change a behavior, it is critical that the dental hygienist engage him or her by applying patient-centered communication. Characteristics of patient-centered communication include the following:

- *Collaboration, not persuasion:* The dental hygienist–client relationship involves a partnership that honors the client's experience and perspectives. The dental hygienist seeks to create a positive interprofessional atmosphere that is conducive to change but that is not coercive.
- *Eliciting information, not imparting information:* The dental hygienist's tone is not one of imparting information but rather a drawing out of motivation for change from the person. Clients do most of the talking, and dental hygienists listen carefully.
- *Emphasizing the client's autonomy, not the authority of the expert:* The responsibility for change is left with the client.

Causes of Substance Abuse

Physiologic Factors

After a drug enters the body (Box 52-1), it is carried by the bloodstream to the central nervous system (the brain and spinal cord) within 10 to 15 seconds. When a drug crosses the blood–brain barrier, it can affect all parts of the body by interfering with the information sent to the CNS by the autonomic nervous system and the peripheral nervous system. The autonomic nervous system controls involuntary functions such as circulation, digestion, and respiration, and it helps the body to establish a stable internal environment. The peripheral nervous system transmits messages between the external environment and the CNS. The role of the CNS is that of computer and switchboard. As the CNS receives messages from the autonomic nervous system and the peripheral nervous system, it analyzes those messages and sends a response to the correct body system—muscular, skeletal, circulatory, nervous, respiratory, digestive, excretory, endocrine, or reproductive—to react to the stimuli. The CNS is also responsible for reasoning and making judgments. Psychoactive drugs alter the information sent to the brain and disrupt the messages sent back to the body (Figure 52-5). They also disrupt the ability to think and reason.

Neurotransmitters

The three main components of a neuron (nerve cell) are the dendrites, the cell body, and the axons. The dendrites receive signals from other neurons, the cell body nourishes the neuron and keeps it alive, and the axons carry the message

BOX 52-1

How Drugs Enter the Body

- Direct contact with skin or mucous membranes
- Orally, by swallowing
- Snorted through the nose or placed sublingually or against oral mucosa
- Injected either directly into the bloodstream (intravenously), into a muscle mass (muscling), or under the skin (skin popping). All injection methods place the user at risk for hepatitis, septicemia, abscesses, and human immunodeficiency virus infection.

from the dendrites and the cell body to the terminals, which relay the message to the dendrites of the next neuron. Between the neurons lies the synaptic gap, which is the space between the terminal that is sending the message and the dendrite that is receiving the message. This "jump" between neurons is accomplished through biochemicals called *neurotransmitters* that transmit the message from one neuron to the receptors on another. Dopamine, endorphin, enkephalin, serotonin, substance P, epinephrine, and acetylcholine are examples of neurotransmitters. The specific message that is being sent will determine the neurotransmitter that is released from the neuron. For example, substance P is released from neurons if "pain" is the message being transmitted, and dopamine is released if "pleasure" is the message being transmitted.

Psychoactive drugs disrupt the normal functioning of the neurotransmitters. Sometimes this is a desirable effect. **CNS depressants** inhibit the release of substance P, thereby dulling and weakening the pain signal. This effect is desirable if a physician prescribes morphine to alleviate pain in a person with a terminal illness. The illegal CNS depressant heroin also attaches itself to certain receptor sites in the emotional center of the brain and induces a sensation of pleasure or reward; however, it also attaches itself to the area of the brain that controls respiration and can slow it down to a dangerous level. **CNS stimulants** such as cocaine force the release of large amounts of neurotransmitters such as epinephrine and dopamine, which can create, stimulate, and exaggerate messages to and from the CNS (Figure 52-6). Psychedelic drugs will confuse neurotransmitters by exaggerating and distorting messages and by creating visual and auditory images in the brain. Studies show that brain images are altered when methamphetamine, alcohol, nicotine, and cocaine are present in the body. All addictive drugs deplete the brain's receptors for dopamine.[5]

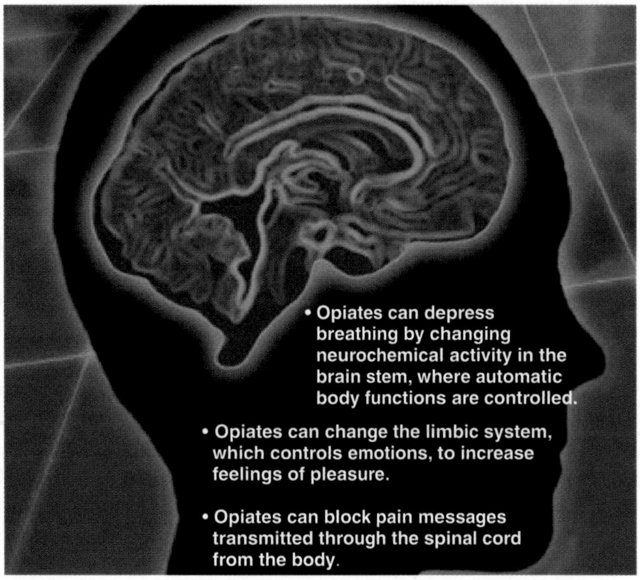

• Opiates can depress breathing by changing neurochemical activity in the brain stem, where automatic body functions are controlled.
• Opiates can change the limbic system, which controls emotions, to increase feelings of pleasure.
• Opiates can block pain messages transmitted through the spinal cord from the body.

Figure 52-5. National Institute on Drug Abuse Research Report Series: heroin abuse and addiction. (From National Institutes of Health, U.S. Department of Health and Human Services, 2006.)

Genetic Factors

Endorphin and enkephalin neurotransmitters have an opiate-like effect on the brain, thereby causing the individual to experience a feeling of well-being. People who are born with the inability to produce sufficient quantities of endorphin and enkephalin have a genetic predisposition toward opiate and alcohol addiction.[6] These are often people who are diagnosed with depression and who look for alternative means to adjust their moods.

Researchers have not yet been able to isolate the specific gene responsible for substance abuse, but it is believed that several modified genes may contribute to addiction. Genes that interfere with serotonin metabolism and that affect the serotonin–dopamine balance in the brain have been implicated in a multitude of psychiatric disorders. Such disorders include alcoholism, drug addiction, depression, suicide, aggressive behaviors, antisocial borderline personality disorder, phobias, panic attacks, eating disorders, and attention-deficit/hyperactivity disorder.

Addiction Dependence, Withdrawal, and Relapse

Because individuals are born with some genetic sensitivity to alcohol and specific drugs, those with a low genetic predisposition for addictive behaviors will take longer to become

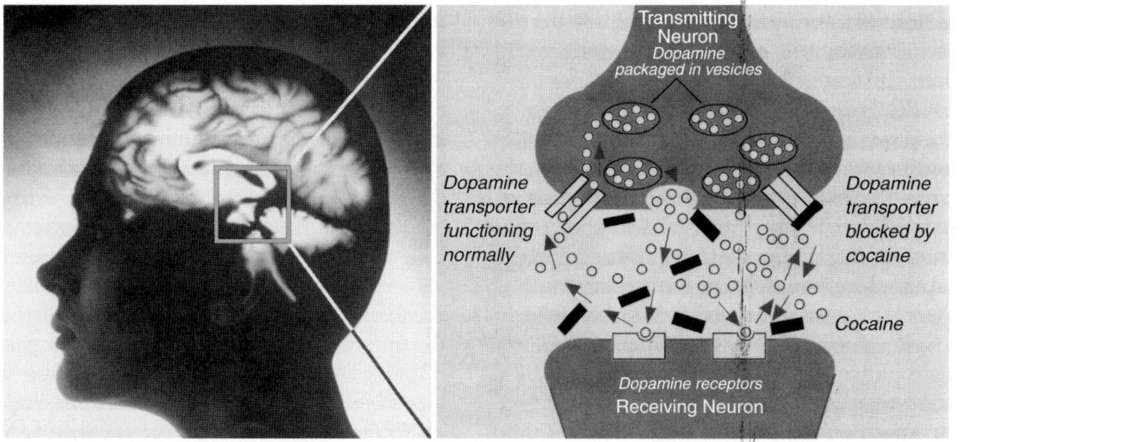

Figure 52-6. Cocaine abuse and addiction. (From the National Institute on Drug Abuse: *Cocaine abuse and addiction.* National Institute on Drug Abuse Research Report Series, National Institutes of Health Publication No. 99-4342, Bethesda, Md, 1999, National Institutes of Health.)

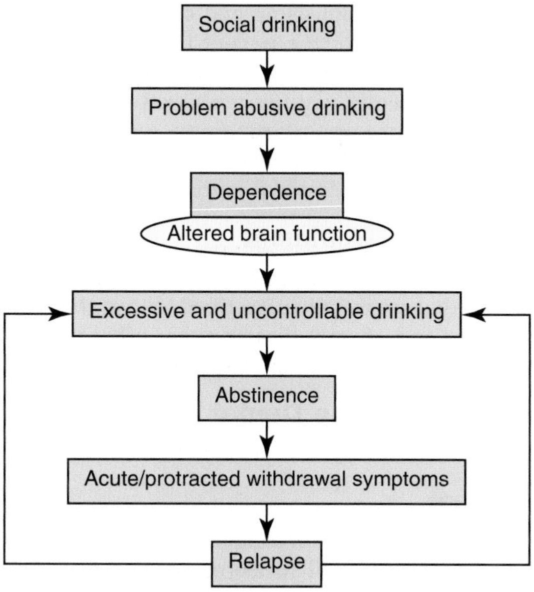

Figure 52-7. Dependence, withdrawal, and relapse. (Adapted from Becker HC: Alcohol dependence, withdrawal and relapse, *Alcohol Res Health* 31:348, 2008.)

addicted or to climb the curve to addiction than those born with a high genetic predisposition. Those with a high predisposition for addictive behaviors start at a point that is closer to addiction on the curve.

Alcohol and drugs are first used experimentally, then socially, and then habitually until addiction is reached. When alcohol and drugs are first used, the predisposition for addictive behaviors increases. Those with a low inherited predisposition for addictive behaviors must use alcohol and drugs over a much longer period of time to become addicted as compared with those with a high inherited predisposition. It may take those with a low predisposition 3 or 4 years of long-term or heavy use to reach the same level of addiction that those with a high predisposition would reach in 2 or 3 months. Predisposition to addiction in the latter group is a result of the deficiency that is already present in their brain chemistry. Evidence suggests that neurotransmitters may rebound back to normal levels in those with short-term, noninherited disruption but not so in those with long-term, inherited imbalance. When the sensitivity does not return to normal, the brain is imprinted and remembers the alcohol and drug-using habits. As a result, if relapse occurs, it will take much less time to reach a level of addiction[6] (Figure 52-7).

Fetal Alcohol Syndrome (see Chapter 51)

A pregnant woman with an active alcohol addiction is at risk for delivering a child with fetal alcohol syndrome. See Box 52-2 for the characteristics of this condition. Intellectual and developmental disabilities, physical impairments, and infant failure to thrive can result.

Environmental Factors

Although substance abuse prevention programs for youth are found in schools, in the media, and in the community, they are insufficient by themselves. Without parental supervision, consistent discipline, and dedicated family relationships, community programs are not as effective. A 2006 study found that nearly 1 in 10 high school seniors abuses a prescription pain reliever each year and that 16% of eighth, tenth, and twelfth graders took cough and cold medications containing dextromethorphan (DXM) to get "high."[7] This abuse of over-the-counter cough and cold medicines has caused many drug manufacturers to change the formulas of their products to eliminate DXM. Many pharmacies have moved products that contain DXM off of store shelves; they must be obtained directly from the pharmacist, and they are out of the easy reach of customers. Stores have also limited the number of DXM-containing products that can be purchased at one time.

Families play an important role in determining how children respond to the temptation to use alcohol, cigarettes, and illegal drugs. Substance abuse by one family member affects all members of the family in some way. Family members feel many of the emotions experienced by the addict, although they tend to suppress their feelings. Often their confidence and self-esteem are diminished, they experience depression, and one third become chemically dependent themselves (Box 52-3).

BOX 52-2

Features Associated with Fetal Alcohol Syndrome

- Abnormal facial characteristics (see Chapter 54, Figure 54-2)
- Intellectual and developmental disabilities
- Learning disabilities
- Hearing, speech, and vision impairments
- Hyperactivity
- Memory and problem-solving deficits
- Poor motor coordination
- Major organ malformations (e.g., heart, liver, kidneys)
- Musculoskeletal system malformations
- Compromised immune system

BOX 52-3

Risk Factors for Substance Abuse

- Children with attention-deficit/hyperactivity disorder
- Children who are alienated, who are rebellious, or who have serious behavioral problems
- Children who experience extreme poverty or peer rejection and who live in areas of high incidence of drug use and crime
- Individuals with a history of child abuse
- Individuals with a genetic sensitivity to specific drugs

Medical Treatment for Substance Abuse

Emergency Treatment

In some instances, substance abuse can be life-threatening. An overdose of an abused substance requires immediate medical attention. Acute alcohol poisoning associated with binge drinking is a condition that has appeared with increasing regularity on college campuses. In addition, alcohol enemas have become an alternative means of consumption; these cause rapid intoxication, severe alcohol toxicity, and death. Symptoms of alcohol poisoning include the following:

- Slow or irregular breathing (<8 breaths per minute)
- Cold, pale, or blue-toned skin
- Rapid pulse
- Vomiting while awake or asleep
- Unresponsive to attempts to awaken
- Semi-consciousness or unconsciousness

Alcohol poisoning is a medical emergency; the contacting of emergency medical services is imperative. While waiting for emergency medical services to arrive, refrain from providing the affected individual food or drink, turn him or her on their side, and monitor his or her vital signs. In the hospital emergency department, the treatment priority is to stabilize the client; this is followed by detoxification by behavioral treatment, pharmacologic treatment, or both. This treatment often is performed on an inpatient basis to limit the individual's access to alcohol or drugs. Clients who have an existing psychiatric problem along with substance abuse are best treated at long-term drug treatment facilities.

Behavioral Treatment

It is often stated that substance abusers must "hit rock bottom" in their lives before they willingly seek help. Reaching rock bottom often means that they are unemployed and lack emotional support from friends and family. The most effective treatments for substance abuse occur when the abuser is motivated to seek medical intervention, behavioral changes, and social reinforcement, although treatment does not need to be voluntary to be effective. Court-appointed treatment and sanctions or enticements provided by family or employers can also result in effective treatment. No single treatment is appropriate for all individuals. Effective treatment attends to the multiple needs of the individual, including medical, psychologic, social, vocational, and legal issues that confront the substance abuser. Remaining in treatment for an adequate amount of time is critical to success. Most patients realize significant improvement by the end of 3 months in treatment. Individual or group counseling and other behavioral therapies are needed to help the patient develop skills to resist drug use. Recovery from drug addiction can be a long-term process and frequently requires multiple treatments. Participation in self-help support programs such as Alcoholics Anonymous or Narcotics Anonymous during and after treatment often helps the individual to maintain abstinence.[8,9]

Pharmacologic Treatment

Treatment for addiction may involve drug therapy (Table 52-4). Drugs that are usually prescribed to treat the symptoms of depression and anxiety disorders are often used to treat clients with addictive behavior disorders.

Implications for the Dental Hygiene Process of Care

Assessment

The problems of the abuse of alcohol, prescribed medications, and illegal drugs affect all socioeconomic groups. However, only about 10% of clients who are alcohol and substance abusers are identified by healthcare providers. Several visits over time for dental hygiene services may reveal behaviors that can be confirmed by a well-focused health history and a thorough extraoral and intraoral examination.

Health History

Chemically dependent clients must be identified so that they may be treated safely. Many will "premedicate" with their drug of choice before coming to a dental appointment. During the health history interview, the dental hygienist identifies all current medications that the client is taking to avoid possible drug interactions between a prescribed or an abused substance and medications offered in the oral health setting. Such interactions may pose a life-threatening situation for the client. The need for prophylactic antibiotic premedication must be considered for the following reasons when treating a client with a history of intravenous drug use:

TABLE 52-4
Pharmacologic Agents Used for the Treatment of Alcoholism

Drug	Purpose	Mechanism of Action	Clinical Effects
Alcohol Sensitizing Agents			
Disulfiram (Antabuse) Citrated calcium carbamide (Temposil)	To cause an aversive reaction when used in the presence of alcohol	Blocks the metabolism of alcohol	If alcohol is ingested while an individual is taking disulfiram, nausea, vomiting, severe stomach pain, and hypotension result. These effects are less severe with citrated calcium carbamide.
Anticraving Agent			
Naltrexone (Trexan)	To reduce or eliminate cravings for alcohol	Antagonizes various opiate receptors	Decreases craving and consumption of alcohol, especially when used as an adjunct to behavioral therapy
Antiemetic Agent			
Ondansetron	Currently used experimentally for the treatment of alcohol addiction	Serotonin antagonism	Decreases nausea and vomiting

- Many intravenous drug users develop venous thrombosis and organic valvular heart disease.
- Damage to the tricuspid valve between the right atrium and the ventricle is often associated with substance abuse.
- Intravenous drug use can result in endocarditis caused by *Staphylococcus aureus* found on nonsterile needles.

Consequently, all clients with a history of intravenous drug abuse should be evaluated by their physician before dental or dental hygiene care to determine if any of these conditions exists, thereby indicating the need for antibiotic premedication (see Chapter 12).

The specific substances being used and how they enter the body influence additional medical conditions that are experienced by chemically dependent clients. For example, clients with a history of intravenous drug use have a higher incidence of human immunodeficiency virus infection and hepatitis B, C, and D infection. Long-term alcohol abuse can result in liver, heart, kidney, and pancreas damage. In addition, damage to the reproductive system, permanent brain damage, and a lack of muscle coordination can result from years of alcohol abuse. The systemic impact of drug addiction can include cardiovascular disease, stroke, cancer, human immunodeficiency virus/acquired immunodeficiency syndrome infection, hepatitis infection, and lung disease, especially after prolonged use.[9]

Questions about substances used and administration routes should appear on dental office health history forms. When reviewing the client's responses and when interacting with the client, the dental hygienist looks for signs of substance abuse. If the dental hygienist suspects that the client may be dependent on a substance, that information should be recorded in the client's dental record (Box 52-4). Specific objective observations, client behavior, and assessment findings such as pupil changes or needle marks should be recorded using objective terminology.

Clients are often reluctant to reveal alcohol or drug use because of the social stigma associated with substance abuse. In addition, many substance abusers are in denial and will not admit to any type of dependence when asked. The astute dental hygienist recognizes signs and symptoms of dependence and discusses the possibility of a substance abuse problem with the client in a nonjudgmental manner.

BOX 52-4

Red Flags for Suspicion of Substance Abuse

- Unreliable; frequently misses appointments
- Careless in appearance and hygiene
- Lapses in memory, concentration, or both
- Alcohol on breath
- Speech is slurred; appears intoxicated
- Needle marks on arm
- Rapid mood swings (within minutes)
- Frequently requests written excuses from work
- Frequently requests specific medication for pain
- Calls the dental office, complains of severe pain, and requests that a prescription for pain medication be given without making an appointment with the dentist
- High tolerance to sedatives and analgesics
- Pupils are abnormally dilated or constricted

eTable 52-5 lists drug categories and the street names of abused substances. The recognition of a drug abuse problem by a healthcare professional may prompt the abuser to seek help. It is essential that clients understand that the reason for obtaining information is to protect them from health risks and that all information will remain confidential.

When abuse is suspected, it is recommended that the dental hygienist ask the following questions:

- Have you ever felt the need to cut down on your drinking or drug use?
- Have you ever felt bad or guilty about your drinking or drug use?
- Have you ever used or had a drink first thing in the morning as an eye opener to steady your nerves or to feel normal?

If the client answers "yes" to two or more of these questions, then the dental hygienist should strongly suspect abuse and consider how to motivate the client to seek treatment. It is necessary to determine if the client "self-medicated" for the dental appointment. If the client used any form of drugs or alcohol before the appointment, then the care plan for that day may need to be modified or canceled to avoid any drug interactions or drug-associated behavioral problems.

The identification of dental hygiene clients who are chemically dependent is important; however, substance abuse treatment is not within the scope of dental hygiene practice. It is helpful if dental offices develop a simple protocol for the referral of clients with substance abuse problems. The oral healthcare setting should have a list of community resources available as a reference for the client. Brochures about specific programs can be provided, or the client can be given the telephone number of the National Council on Alcohol and Drug Dependence.

Extraoral Examination

The general appearance of clients can alert the dental hygienist to the possibility of substance abuse. Do they look substantially older than their stated age, have a disheveled appearance, have poor personal hygiene, insist on wearing sunglasses, and wear long sleeves even in hot weather (perhaps to cover needle marks)? Is alcohol or another odor detected on their breath? Do they appear to be lethargic or intoxicated without the accompanying odor of alcohol? Do they experience tremors? Look at clients' eyes for signs of substance abuse.

Needle marks in the antecubital fossae and forearms or bruises and increased pigmentation over the veins as a result of multiple injections, which may be observed during the taking of a blood pressure reading, may indicate illicit drug use. The subcutaneous "popping" of heroin can cause skin abscesses. Crack abusers will often have burns and scars on the thumb of the dominant hand from the repeated use of a disposable lighter. Multiple healed and healing burns or abrasions may be the result of physical trauma experienced while the client was under the influence of alcohol or drugs. Snorting or inhaling substances can burn nasal passages, cause nosebleeds, and significantly damage nasal structures. Often clients who are substance abusers continually sniff their noses and use handkerchiefs or tissues.

The client's behavior and speech should be watched for signs of confusion, disorientation, lethargy, lack of concentration, or memory impairment. Extreme depression or agitation may indicate a drug overdose.

Tremors of the hands, tongue, and eyelids may be signs of alcohol withdrawal. Other extraoral signs of alcohol abuse include the following:

- Redness of the facial skin and spider petechiae on the nose from dilated blood vessels
- Yellowish facial skin from jaundice caused by liver disease
- Facial trauma as a result of falls when intoxicated
- Angular cheilitis caused by vitamin B deficiency
- Red or swollen eyes

Intraoral Examination

The placement of drugs directly in the vestibule or sublingually may cause localized tissue necrosis. Gingival lesions may be caused by cocaine placement. Alcohol and drug abusers often crave sweets. Consequently, large dark areas of buccal cervical caries from ingesting large quantities of carbohydrates may be present. Other oral manifestations associated with substance abuse include oral candidiasis as a result of immunosuppression and glossodynia (pain in the tongue) as a result of malnutrition and immunosuppression in response to a secondary addiction to alcohol. Cocaine users tend to have severe bruxism, which causes flat cuspal planes on the premolars and molars. Because the substance abuser's body is being taxed by drug use, tissue healing is affected (Box 52-5).

Methamphetamine has recently become the leading drug of abuse: it is easy to produce, it is inexpensive, and it provides extended states of euphoria. Methamphetamine abusers develop "meth mouth," (Figure 52-8), a condition that results in rampant caries, poor oral hygiene, xerostomia, gingival inflammation, and evidence of advanced periodontal disease.[11] Methamphetamine-induced caries has a distinctive pattern of destruction that begins at the gingiva by attacking the buccal smooth surfaces of the posterior teeth and the interproximal spaces of anterior teeth and then progressing to complete destruction of the coronal tooth structure. This severe caries rate may be attributed to decreased salivary flow as a result of the stimulation of inhibitory alpha-2 receptors by methamphetamine use. In addition, methamphetamine users consume high amounts of soft drinks rather than water; they also display poor oral hygiene, poor nutrition, and signs of bruxism.[10] Often the remaining dentition is unsalvageable and extractions are the only option.

BOX 52-5

Oral Manifestations of Alcohol Abuse

- Xerostomia
- Poor oral hygiene
- Gingival bleeding on probing
- Coated tongue
- Glossitis due to nutritional deficiency
- Attrition related to bruxism
- Erosion related to vomiting
- Broken teeth due to accidents related to intoxication
- Buccal cervical caries

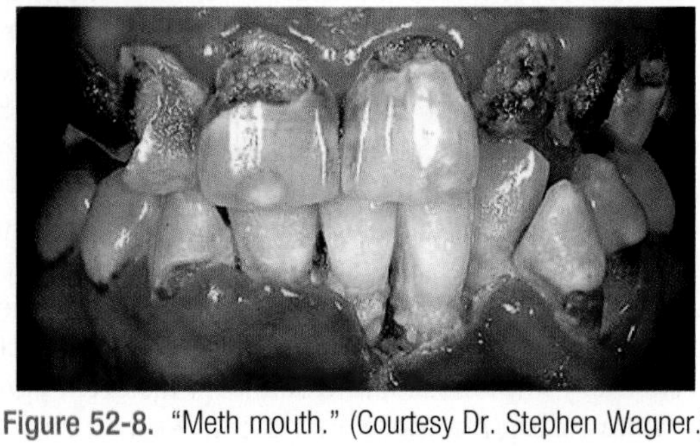

Figure 52-8. "Meth mouth." (Courtesy Dr. Stephen Wagner.)

Dental Hygiene Diagnosis and Care Planning

Substance abuse must be addressed during care planning. People who are deeply immersed in drug abuse will probably seek dental care only when they are in severe pain. Because the pain sensation can be diminished by the use of drugs, the dental problem is usually in an advanced state. Substance-abusing clients may request the use of nitrous oxide sedation for treatment and specific medication for pain. As previously discussed, it is important that oral care professionals have knowledge of the types and amounts of drugs that clients have taken before planning any pain control or other care.

At the same time, clients who are in recovery programs may seek long-neglected dental treatment as part of their attempt to achieve total body health. It is under these circumstances that the dental hygienist will most likely be providing care. Recovering addicts may be extremely cautious or anxious about taking any type of medication, thereby making it difficult to control pain during scaling and root debriding procedures. Some chemically dependent clients may also experience a tolerance to sedatives and analgesics. For clients recovering from substance abuse, pain control should be coordinated with the primary care physician. In addition, chemically dependent clients can experience emotional anxiety or instability and may be able to tolerate only short appointments. For this reason, the use of multiple short (i.e., 20-minute) appointments may be necessary.

After a thorough assessment and consultation with the client's physician, if indicated, complete diagnostic statements are formulated by the dental hygienist on the basis of identified human need deficits. After the diagnostic statements are complete, client goals are set. Care planning priorities include setting realistic goals with the client to improve oral self-care and to enable the client to undergo periodontal scaling and root debridement with a minimum of discomfort. In addition, because malnutrition is clearly associated with substance abuse, dietary analysis and nutritional counseling should be planned. With the permission of clients, consultation with their physicians and counselors may help the dental hygienist to plan effective care.

Implementation

Because good oral health and a pleasant smile add to an individual's self-esteem, receiving necessary dental hygiene care may have a significant positive impact on recovery from substance abuse. A discussion concerning referral for treatment of the substance abuse should be initiated as soon as possible.

Appointments

Chemically dependent clients can experience emotional instability or take little responsibility for their behavior. As a result, they may not keep scheduled appointments. If the client arrives too late for an appointment, the appointment should be canceled. If the client fails to come to an appointment, all remaining appointments should be canceled. Failure to keep appointments should not be reinforced as acceptable behavior. Because of the client's potential unreliability and to provide additional incentive to show up for care, payment should be received in advance of treatment. Aesthetic restorations should be treated last to ensure that clients show up for all necessary treatment. It is unethical to abandon clients after they have been accepted for treatment in a dental practice. If a client continually fails to keep scheduled treatment appointments, the dental office may dismiss the client from the practice by written notification. Legal guidelines dictate that the client must be assured, in writing, that emergency dental treatment will be provided for a length of time sufficient to obtain a new dentist of record; this is usually 30 days or more from the receipt of the dismissal letter. All dental records must be forwarded to the new dentist, along with notification of what services are still needed, when the client makes that request in writing.

Pain and Anxiety Control

Adequate pain control is a necessity for the recovering chemically dependent client, because unrelieved pain can be a relapse trigger. For postoperative pain, nonsteroidal anti-inflammatory medications are recommended, because all other pain medications are potentially addictive. If the dentist feels that narcotic analgesics or sedative–hypnotics for postoperative pain are indicated, substance-abusing clients require a higher dose than non–substance-abusing clients, and a limited number of doses should be prescribed. Analgesic depressants are not contraindicated unless the patient is taking other illicit depressants at the same time. People with methamphetamine addiction rarely seek dental care when under the influence of the drug, but they may seek care between methamphetamine binges.[10] Anesthesia and pain control may be difficult to achieve for heroin-addicted clients who are in a methamphetamine treatment program, because they have developed a tolerance to the analgesic and euphoric effects of their daily methamphetamine dose. Consultation with the client's physician is necessary to determine the best method for alleviating client discomfort.

The control of client anxiety also can help alleviate the client's pain perception. Pain perception has both physical and psychologic components. If the client trusts the clinician, emotional distress can be minimized, thereby reducing the perception of pain. A dental hygienist with excellent communication skills and empathy can help to dispel the client's anxiety. See Table 52-6 for other treatment considerations.

Some substance-abusing clients may see dental treatment as an opportunity to obtain prescriptions for abused substances. Consequently, they often will exaggerate their response to pain in an effort to obtain a prescription for a strong pain control medication. Prescription pads should be kept out of sight and inaccessible to clients. Pain medication in the dental office should be locked in a place that is unknown to clients. Drug-seeking clients often call the dental office, complain that they are in severe pain, and request that a prescription for pain medication be given to them without making an appointment with the doctor. Dental offices should maintain a policy of prescribing medications only after the dentist has evaluated the client.

Dental Hygiene Care

Because short appointments are suggested for these clients, the dental hygienist may be able to complete only limited treatment at each appointment. If there is a need for prophylactic antibiotic premedication, the dental hygienist ensures that the client has taken premedication as directed. General supragingival and subgingival debridement, which will enable the client to initiate adequate homecare, may be all that the client will tolerate during a short appointment. Such treatment would allow the dentist to place needed restorations in a client who is in a state of improved gingival health. This improved tissue response is especially important when cervical restorations are placed, because inflamed gingival margins can interfere with the placement of restorative materials.

The client's response to the initial scaling visit will dictate further appointment planning. The client may be able to tolerate quadrant scaling and root debridement so that optimum treatment for periodontal disease may be provided. Confirmation from the client's physician that there is no immunosuppression or kidney or liver damage should be sought before aggressive nonsurgical or surgical periodontal therapy is undertaken. The use of an ultrasonic scaling instrument and an alcohol-free antimicrobial lavage is indicated to reduce the incidence of a transient bacteremia.

It is best to postpone definitive scaling and root debridement until a later time if the client is unable or unwilling to comply with treatment. In this case, a 2- or 3-month continued-care interval is indicated. When clients have progressed further with their recovery from addiction, they may be more tolerant of dental hygiene care.

Oral Health Instruction

A lack of oral hygiene is common among substance abusers. Oral health instruction should begin with basic toothbrushing instructions and encouragement to practice toothbrushing daily. When daily toothbrushing techniques have been mastered or a power toothbrush has been recommended and demonstrated, interdental oral physiotherapy aids can be introduced. The choice of aid will depend on the client's physical and mental capabilities and the type of embrasures present (see Chapters 23, 24, and 25). If the client does not have the fine motor skills necessary to manipulate dental floss, other aids should be suggested. Interdental wooden stimulators, interproximal brushes, or a power floss aid may be easier for the client to use. If clients are frustrated by an inability to master a technique, they will most likely do nothing. The client in addiction recovery has already been required to make numerous behavioral changes and may see a complex oral hygiene regimen as an additional burden.

Suggesting a daily fluoride rinse regimen is appropriate, especially if the client has a moderate to high caries risk (see Chapters 18 and 33). The use of fluoride therapy is also important for heroin addicts enrolled in a methadone program: the daily methadone dose is administered as a sugary syrup. Antimicrobial rinses to control gingivitis may also be recommended. For alcoholics, it is important to recommend products that do not contain alcohol to avoid supporting their addiction and contributing to the negative health effects that they experience as a result of their alcohol use. Even very small amounts of alcohol ingested by a client who is taking disulfiram or similar alcohol-sensitizing drugs

TABLE 52-6

Assessment Findings Associated with Substance Abuse

Abused Substance	Eye Signs	Oral Findings	Treatment Considerations
Amphetamines	Dilated pupils Slow or no reaction of pupil to light	Xerostomia; increased caries; bruxism (extreme tooth wear seen in ecstasy users) leading to trismus	Can increase bleeding and interfere with coagulation; chronic abusers should have blood tests before surgery or periodontal treatment
Alcohol	Red, puffy	Tooth erosion from sugar in alcohol or regurgitation; sialosis, xerostomia, and glossitis; stomatitis due to nutritional deficiencies and anemia; orofacial injuries from accidents or violence; severe infections due to immunosuppression	Increased dosage of drugs for anesthesia and sedation; increase in bleeding after surgery; increased healing time due to immunosuppression
Cocaine	Dilated pupils Slow or no reaction of pupil to light	Placement of cocaine in maxillary premolar area to test the purity of a drug sample can cause localized gingival and alveolar bone necrosis; increased caries from carbohydrates added to cocaine as filler	Possible spontaneous gingival bleeding from thrombocytopenia; interaction between cocaine and anesthetics that contain epinephrine
Opiates and opioids (heroin, morphine, methadone)	Constricted pupils Nonreactive to light	Methadone is sugary syrup taken orally, which may cause an increase in caries	Increased possibility of hepatitis and human immunodeficiency virus infection from drug injection; poor pain tolerance; increased possibility of bacterial endocarditis with scaling procedures; increased bleeding from thrombocytopenia; interactions between opioids and dentally prescribed medications
Barbiturates and benzodiazepines	Constricted pupils	Xerostomia; lesions on oral mucosa in the area of drug use	Tolerance to sedative drugs
Cannabis (marijuana)	Reddened sclera, swollen eyelids, tears	Leukoplakia and increased incidence of lingual carcinoma; gingival enlargement	Interaction between cannabis and anesthetics that contain epinephrine
Lysergic acid diethylamide (LSD), phencyclidine (PCP)	Dilated pupils Swollen eyelids	Orofacial injuries experienced while "tripping"; bruxism resulting in trismus	Flashbacks that may cause panic attacks can occur in a stressful dental environment; respiratory depression may occur if opioids are prescribed
Inhalants		"Glue-sniffer's rash"; erythema around the labial borders; oral frostbite	Anesthetic toxicity is increased; sensitization to epinephrine can occur; increased risk of seizures
Anabolic steroids		High-carbohydrate diet may cause increased caries	Cardiac dysfunction can result from anesthetics that contain epinephrine; increase in bleeding

can cause an emergency. Nonalcoholic fluoride mouth rinses (e.g., ACT, FluoriGard) and nonalcoholic antimicrobial mouth rinses (e.g., Biotene, Crest Pro-Health) are recommended for homecare and for preprocedural rinses. Xerostomia may be a result of antidepressant medications prescribed for the client. Suggest that the client sip water frequently during the day or use xylitol-containing gums or mints to reduce the effects of dry mouth.

The dental hygienist may also suggest that the client eat a well-balanced diet and limit cariogenic foods to encourage both oral and general health. Positive reinforcement and encouragement should be given to clients for any improvement in their oral hygiene.

Evaluation

The outcomes of dental hygiene care can serve as positive reinforcement for a healthier lifestyle for those clients in recovery. If the evaluation of dental hygiene care occurs 6 to 8 weeks after initial debridement, clients may be further along in their recovery and may be more receptive to additional periodontal therapy, if needed. For those clients who are not in recovery, the evaluation of dental hygiene care provides another opportunity to encourage clients to seek help for their substance abuse. The initial recall or continued-care interval should be 3 months after treatment. This interval is especially important if there was extensive periodontal therapy complicated by immunosuppression.

Dental Professionals and Substance Abuse

Alcohol and drug abuse are widespread in American culture, and dental professionals are not exempt from addiction. In fact, the prevalence of drug and alcohol abuse among professionals may be the same as or higher than it is in the general population.[11] Dental personnel can self-prescribe medications; they have the opportunity for easy access to abuse drugs. Many states have begun monitoring dentists' prescription-writing habits.

Why Professionals Are at Risk for Chemical Dependence

Healthcare professionals are usually required to have high academic grades to be admitted to a professional educational program. Once accepted, the professional education requires hours of instruction to reach competence. Students enrolled in healthcare educational programs are usually competitive, overworked, narrowly specialized, self-sacrificing, and grade conscious.

Dental and dental hygiene students have their work continually criticized by faculty. Trying to prove one's competence can easily lead to little sleep, an unbalanced and emotionally unrewarding lifestyle, physical and emotional exhaustion, stress and anxiety, irritability, and depression.[11] The completion of a professional program often requires students to become "self-denying," and their personal lives become of secondary importance to their education. This situation can lead to emotional conflicts within themselves and their families. Often students will use stimulants to enhance their performance at school, or they may use alcohol on the weekend to relieve stress. This cycle often continues once the student has become a practicing professional.

Although they have been taught to recognize symptoms of chemical dependence in clients, health professionals rarely recognize addiction in themselves. Most are convinced that they are in control of their substance abuse and that they can stop whenever they choose. Chemical dependence may be the underlying cause of licensure suspension or malpractice (Box 52-6).

BOX 52-6

American Dental Association Policy Statement About Chemical Dependency

- The American Dental Association (ADA) recognizes that chemical dependency is a disease entity that affects all of society.
- The ADA is committed to assisting the chemically dependent member of the dental family (including dental hygienists) toward recovery by education, information, and referral.
- The ADA encourages those institutions responsible for dental education to provide an adequate curriculum that addresses substance use, misuse, and addiction.
- To meet the needs of the public and the profession, the ADA also encourages ongoing communication between constituent society chemical dependency committees and their state boards of registration.
- The ADA recognizes the need for research in the area of chemical dependency in dentistry.

Many state dental associations sponsor educational programs and workshops about addiction within the profession. Diversion from the court system to a treatment program is available to addicted professionals unless they have engaged in unethical treatment by causing harm to clients or violating major criminal laws. Health and well-being committees of state dental associations help colleagues with addiction problems. Confidentiality is ensured, and referrals may be made anonymously. The committees may contract for services through the state medical society and provide appropriate referrals, post-treatment follow-up, monitoring, and advocacy.

Many professionals decide that it is time to stop drug abuse when they are faced with the loss of their professional licenses. Some seek help through residential or outpatient formal recovery programs, and others seek help through self-help programs. Dental support groups at Caduceus meetings, which are modeled on the principles of Alcoholics Anonymous, may also provide psychologic support for professionals who are in recovery.

CLIENT EDUCATION TIPS

- Determine at which stage of change a client is before encouraging treatment for substance abuse.
- Discuss the risks of negative interactions between local anesthetics or nitrous oxide–oxygen analgesia and the abused substance.
- Describe how the abused substance affects oral and general health. Inform clients that antibiotic premedication before dental hygiene care may be necessary to prevent infective endocarditis or to manage an immunocompromised status.
- Stress the need for routine professional care, optimal self-care, and proper nutrition. Identify oral manifestations of substance abuse and malnutrition in the client's own mouth.
- Tailor biofilm removal techniques specific to the client's abilities.
- Recommend nonalcoholic antimicrobial mouth rinses and fluoride rinses for alcoholics.
- Positively reinforce and encourage clients for improvements in their oral self-care and movement through the stages of change model.
- Inform clients that alcohol is a risk factor for oral cancer.
- Inform clients with a history of alcohol abuse or those who are taking Antabuse that over-the-counter and prescription mouth rinses (antibacterial and fluoride) may contain up to 30% alcohol and should be avoided.
- Educate women of childbearing age about fetal alcohol syndrome, and inform them that alcohol is transmitted via the breast milk to nursing infants.

LEGAL, ETHICAL, AND SAFETY ISSUES

- Clients' personal, social, and health history forms must be kept confidential.
- Client behavior, assessment findings, professional recommendations, referrals, and treatment should be recorded in the client's permanent record. Personal opinions and judgmental statements are inappropriate.

- Some states have parental notification laws that direct healthcare professionals to reveal knowledge of any medical or psychologic conditions found during an examination to a minor's parent or legal guardian.[10] Knowledge of the statutes in the legal jurisdiction is important so that confidential information about minors is managed correctly.
- Keep prescription pads out of sight and medications locked in a place that is unknown to clients.
- Dentists should never write a prescription for a pain medication without knowing the client's history or without first examining the client.
- With approval from clients being treated for substance abuse, contact their physicians and mental health professionals when planning oral care.
- Reduce the client's anxiety level by keeping appointments short and comfortable.
- Perform only those procedures that the client can easily tolerate.
- Keep oral care products that contain alcohol in a secure place away from persons with alcoholism.
- Do not render treatment that may cause an interaction between an abused substance and dental anesthetics or other drugs offered as part of healthcare.
- Continue to encourage clients to seek help for substance abuse if they have been through a treatment program and have relapsed.
- Identifying dental clients who are chemically dependent is important; however, substance abuse treatment is not within the scope of dental hygiene practice.

KEY CONCEPTS

- Substance abuse is a chronic cyclic disease that affects 20.4 million people in U.S. society, including oral healthcare professionals.
- Substance addiction is the compulsive use of a substance despite adverse medical and social consequences.
- Psychologic and physical dependence on drugs and the presence of a genetic predisposition are the reasons that people continue substance abuse.
- Tolerance to alcohol and drugs creates the need for continued increases in the amounts used to gain the same effect.
- Dental hygienists need to identify chemically dependent clients for the following reasons:
  - To avoid interactions between drugs offered at the dental office (e.g., local anesthetics, nitrous oxide–oxygen analgesia) and abused substances
  - To determine the need for antibiotic premedication before dental hygiene care
  - To recognize increased risk of immunosuppression, heart disease, liver disease, human immunodeficiency virus, and hepatitis B, C, and D
  - To recognize the drug-seeking behavior of clients with a history of abuse
  - To modify care plans as appropriate
- Addictive behaviors are the result of genetic, environmental, psychologic, and physiologic factors.
- Culture, ethnicity, poverty, behavioral problems, child abuse, peer rejection, and environment can be risk factors for substance abuse.
- Drugs affect the transmission of messages among the central, autonomic, and peripheral nervous systems by interfering with neurotransmission. Key neurotransmitters include dopamine, serotonin, and endorphins.
- A pattern of addictive behavior is influenced by genetic factors.
- Women have specific issues with alcohol and other substance abuse during pregnancy because such abuse can affect the health of the fetus.
- Characteristics of children with fetal alcohol syndrome include poor motor coordination, learning disabilities, hyperactivity, sensory impairment, irritability, microcephaly, abnormal facial features, growth retardation, and mental retardation.
- The modification of addictive behavior goes through the stages of change, some of which may have to be repeated before total abstinence is achieved.
- Specific extraoral and intraoral findings are associated with the specific type of substance that the client abuses.
- The American Dental Association encourages treatment rather than punishment of oral healthcare professionals who seek help for substance abuse.

CRITICAL THINKING EXERCISES

Case Study 1

Client: Mr. Y

Profile: Mr. Y, who is 24 years old, was scheduled for dental hygiene care. This is his first dental appointment for preventive care. His last dental appointment was for the extraction of teeth #2 and #15. He has a history of asthma, he smokes one pack of cigarettes a day, and he is currently taking 5 mg of prednisone twice a day. He reports that he took part in a drug and alcohol rehabilitation program 1 year ago. He states that he has seen several television programs about "germs" in dental unit water lines and is worried about being exposed to disease. His girlfriend has suggested that he "do something about his teeth." His chief complaint is that his teeth are discolored and sensitive to cold; they are "soft" and decay easily. He also states that his mouth feels dry. Intraorally, his clinical gingival attachment loss ranges from 3 to 7 mm, with bleeding on probing in the mandibular anterior teeth. His gingivae are pale, except on the mandibular anterior, where the gingival margins are magenta. The tissues are edematous and have rolled gingival margins. The tissue consistency is spongy, and the interdental papillae are blunted. There is inadequate attached gingiva on the facial and lingual areas of teeth #3 and #14 and the mandibular anterior teeth. He has heavy subgingival and supragingival calculus on the mandibular anterior teeth and generalized interproximal nodules throughout the mouth. He has a Class 2 American Academy of Periodontology periodontal classification. Eight carious lesions are identified. He brushes his teeth once a day using a medium-bristle toothbrush, and he uses no other dental aids. His community water is not fluoridated. His diet includes no milk or vegetables, and he eats two king-size chocolate candy bars daily. He knows that the status of his oral health is poor.

1. What are the dental hygiene diagnoses for this client?
2. Develop a dental hygiene care plan that includes goals and interventions for this client.

3. What client education issues should be addressed?
4. What factors could be contributing to this client's periodontal health?
5. Are there any contraindications to this client's care?

Case Study 2

Client: Ms. B

Profile: Ms. B, who is 20 years old, was a new client for dental hygiene care. She completed the health history form when she arrived for the appointment. After reviewing the health history, the dental hygienist noted that Ms. B answered "yes" to the question regarding drug or alcohol addiction. The dental hygienist asked for further clarification from Ms. B and was told that she had been released from a drug and alcohol addiction program 1 year ago. Ms. B had been sent to the treatment program as an alternative to jail. The dental hygienist asked if Ms. B had been able to abstain from using cocaine since she left the program. She encouraged Ms. B to be totally honest in her response and stressed that, if Ms. B was currently using cocaine, it could cause a life-threatening situation if she were to receive a dental anesthetic. Ms. B confided that dental appointments always caused her great anxiety and that she did self-medicate before coming to her appointment.

1. What may happen as a result of the client's drug use before the dental hygiene appointment?
2. Should the dental hygienist proceed with care? If so, what care should be rendered?
3. What are the moral and ethical issues in this situation?

REFERENCES

1. Substance Abuse and Mental Health Services Administration: *2010 National Survey on Drug Use and Health*. Available at: http://oas.samhsa.gov/nsduhLatest.htm. Accessed November 21, 2012.
2. National Institute on Drug Abuse: *NIDA InfoFacts: Rohypnol and GHB*. Available at: www.drugabuse.gov/Infofacts/Rohypnol GHB.html. Accessed November 21, 2012.
3. Wu LT, Pilowsky DJ, Schlenger WE, et al: Misuse of methamphetamine and prescription stimulants among youths and young adults in the community, *Drug Alcohol Depend* 89:195, 2007.
4. Prochaska JO, Norcross JC, DiClemente CC: *Changing for good: the revolutionary program that explains the six stages of change and teaches you how to free yourself from bad habits*, New York, 1994, William Morrow.
5. Sherman C: Drugs affect men's and women's brains differently, *Natl Inst Drug Abuse Notes* 20:14, 2006.
6. Becker HC: Alcohol dependence, withdrawal and relapse, *Alcohol Res Health* 31:348, 2008.
7. National Institute on Drug Abuse: *NIDA-sponsored survey shows decrease in illicit drug use among nation's teens but prescription drug abuse remains high*. Available at: http://www.nih.gov/news/pr/dec2006/nida-21.htm. Accessed November 21, 2012.
8. National Institute on Drug Abuse: *Commonly abused drugs*. Available at: www.nida.nih.gov/DrugPages/DrugsofAbuse.html. Accessed November 21, 2012.
9. Buck JA: The looming expansion and transformation of public substance abuse treatment under the Affordable Care Act, *Health Aff (Millwood)* 30:8, 2011.
10. Marshall B, Grafstein E, Buxton J, et al: Frequent methamphetamine injection predicts emergency department utilization among street-involved youth, *Public Health* 126:47, 2012.
11. Fung EYK, Lange BM: Impact of drug abuse/dependence on dentists, *Gen Dent* September/October:356–359, 2011.

EVOLVE RESOURCES

Please visit http://evolve.elsevier.com/Darby/hygiene for additional practice and study support tools.

CHAPTER

53

Eating Disorders

Laura Lee MacDonald

COMPETENCIES

1. **Define eating disorders and the dental hygienist's role in recognizing them.**
2. **Describe eating disorders, specifically anorexia nervosa, bulimia nervosa, and binge-eating disorder, based on diagnostic criteria and epidemiology.**
3. **Discuss the psychosocial, physiologic, and oral health effects of anorexia nervosa and bulimia.**
4. **Use the dental hygiene process of care to assess a client with an eating disorder, including:**
   - **Engage the client in dialogue of disclosure of an eating disorder.**
   - **Assess oral health needs.**
   - **Plan for harm reduction and oral health promotion.**
   - **Implement dental hygiene interventions.**
   - **Evaluate outcomes of care.**
5. **Explain the value of the dental hygienist's role in interprofessional collaboration for client-centered care.**
6. **List resources available to help clients with an eating disorder.**

The American Psychiatric Association (APA) classifies eating disorders as mental disorders.[1] The APA published the *Diagnostic and Statistical Manual of Mental Disorders, fourth edition, text revision* (DSM-IV-TR) in 2000; it is digitally available from the APA website. The fifth edition (DSM-V) is scheduled for release in 2013. (Please visit the APA website at www.psychiatry.org for the most up-to-date information about the DSM-V.) In both editions, there are two clearly defined eating disorders—anorexia nervosa and bulimia nervosa—and a third diagnosis of "eating disorder not otherwise specified" (EDO-NOS). EDO-NOS is used as a diagnostic category if the person manifests criteria that are not specific to either anorexia nervosa or bulimia nervosa but has clinically significant disturbances in eating. With advances in research and practice, disorders that were formerly categorized as EDO-NOS are being recognized as distinct eating disorders. For example, binge-eating disorder originally fell into the EDO-NOS category, but in the DSM-V it will be identified as a specific eating disorder.

This chapter focuses on anorexia nervosa and bulimia nervosa with some discussion of binge-eating disorder. The dental hygienist should be aware of other eating disorders that fall under the EDO-NOS umbrella, such as compulsive overeating, compulsive overexercising, night-eating syndrome, and sleep-related eating disorder.

Current theories regarding the cause of anorexia nervosa and bulimia nervosa suggest a complex interrelationship among biologic, genetic, psychodevelopmental, neurochemical, and sociocultural components.[1-5] Practice guidelines in response to the etiology of eating disorders are continually being updated on the basis of the best available evidence. Clinical practice guidelines for eating disorders inform health professionals about best practices, such as those published by the APA[2] and the United Kingdom's National Institute for Clinical Excellence.[3] The APA's most recent update discusses the evidence regarding the choice of treatment settings, nutritional rehabilitation, psychosocial interventions, family therapy, pharmacotherapy, and other interventions.[6] An interprofessional collaborative client-centered approach to care is recognized as important to the treatment of and the client's recovery from an eating disorder.

Although mental health counseling and the treatment of eating disorders are outside the scope of dental hygiene practice, the dental hygienist as a primary healthcare provider is ethically responsible to help the client access healthcare. Eating disorders are a challenge for all: the client, the client's family and friends, healthcare professionals, and society in general. The challenge arises from the very nature of the illness, which includes the following: comorbidity with other mental health and medical conditions; insidious onset; secretive behaviors; and the manipulation of the person's way of thinking about his or her body, eating habits, and personal health and wellness. When a person is diagnosed with an eating disorder, the person can be so deeply engaged in the thinking associated with the disorder and the resultant body and mental dysfunction that the restructuring of thought to healthy habits and mindsets is very difficult to manage, often requiring many years for recovery. When a dental hygienist suspects that a client has an eating disorder, the hygienist must address it and become a person in the client's life who enables recovery from the illness rather than one who hesitates and vacillates, saying "I should have" or "I would have, but … ," as illustrated in Scenario 53-1. The time to take action is now. The longer the eating disorder grips a client, the more difficulty he or she will have fighting the illness and repossessing his or her life.

Dental hygienists serve as client advocates. For example, dental hygienists can enable access to needed healthcare; facilitate honest disclosure about the disorder and the behaviors associated with it; promote healthy thinking and being; and help the client to obtain and maintain good oral and general health. Because eating disorders are complex in terms of both cause and treatment, care is enhanced by a client-centered collaborative practice approach involving many health professionals, such as specially trained psychologists for individual and family therapy; psychiatrists and social workers; physicians and nurses with experience with eating

SCENARIO 53-1

When Phillip, the dental receptionist, comes into Sandra Hamm's dental hygiene room, he says, "Have you noticed how skinny Linda Pham is getting?"

"Yes, she had a very fit body last time she was here a little over 2 months ago when she had her braces removed," replies Sandra. "I did notice her weight loss when I walked by the reception area. It looks like she has lost at least 20 pounds. She's a waif of a figure now." Sandra makes a mental note to ask Linda about her weight loss during her dental hygiene appointment. Sandra suspects a possible eating disorder. Sandra has known Linda for most of Linda's 20 years, but she feels uncomfortable asking Linda such questions. She wonders how to go about asking someone "Are you anorexic?"

Throughout the appointment, it becomes evident to Sandra that Linda is not behaving like herself. She is evasive when answering questions about her health history. By the end of the appointment, Sandra hasn't asked Linda about the weight loss and decides that perhaps it is none of her business.

A few months go by, and Linda's father comes in for his dental hygiene appointment. He discloses to Sandra that Linda has been hospitalized for anorexia nervosa. He apologizes for his own oral health state, saying, "All our attention has been centered on Linda. She nearly died from malnutrition. We've been busy with doctor appointments, family therapy sessions, and group support and just plain occupied with strategizing to provide her with support as she recovers from this illness."

SCENARIO 53-2

"Jennifer, are you ready to have your parents come in the room?" asks Dr. Beckham, Jennifer's psychiatrist.

"Oh, whatever. Let's just get this over with! I'm fine. You all are just overreacting. They're going to freak with your diagnosis of bulimia, and then I'll never be able to live again. I hate this! I wish everyone would just leave me alone. I'm 17 years old!" shouts Jennifer back to Dr. Beckham and her healthcare team, Sally Friesen (social worker), Marlee Ford (nutritionist), and Darcy MacAlroy (nurse and case manager).

After team meetings with Jennifer Black over the course of several appointments, Jennifer has been informed that her behavior is consistent with that of a person with bulimia, a mental illness. Darcy invites Mr. and Mrs. Black into the conference room. Jennifer doesn't even look at them; rather, she noticeably sits with her body in a "closed" position. Dr. Beckham welcomes them and informs them that Jennifer is ready to discuss some behaviors that explain why they brought her to the eating disorder clinic program in the first place a couple of weeks ago.

Jennifer begins to cry. "Mom, Dad, I'm so ashamed. I can barely say it, but for the last 7 months I've forced myself to throw up five times a day. At first I only did it once a day, and then I just kept doing it. Dr. Beckham says I have bulimia. Inside I know I do and it is so freaking embarrassing because I think it's disgusting. I can't seem to stop. I'm ready for help. I can't stop doing this on my own."

Mrs. Black, with tears streaming down her face, replies, "Honey, we're all about helping you fight this illness. We'll fight it with you. You can count on us. Admitting you have bulimia is a great first step."

About 2 months ago, Mrs. Black began suspecting that Jennifer was developing an eating disorder. Mrs. Black noticed food missing from their house; Jennifer was excusing herself from the supper table and disappearing into the downstairs washroom. Mrs. Black gently asked Jennifer if she was experiencing any issues with eating, but Jennifer denied any problem. She did mention that her teeth were sensitive and asked to see Claudette, her dental hygienist. In the end, Mrs. and Mr. Black persuaded Jennifer to see Dr. Beckham, which she did, but she was initially very reluctant and dismissive of the idea. Her appointment with Claudette is booked for next week.

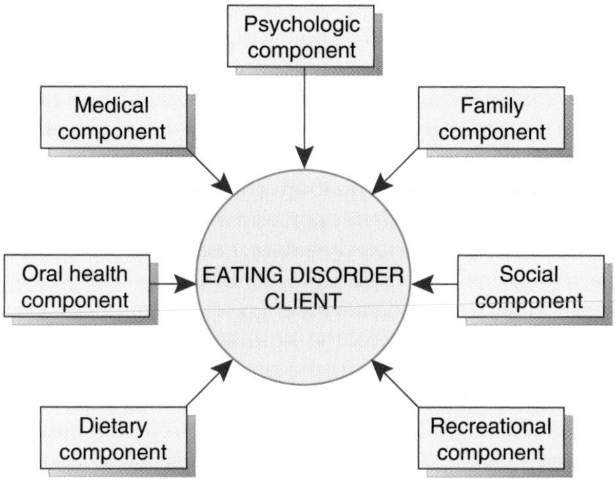

Figure 53-1. An interprofessional collaboration approach to providing care to individuals with eating disorders.

disorders; nutritionists and exercise therapists for education and the reorientation of eating and exercise habits; and the oral health team for the support and treatment of oral manifestations of the illnesses (Figure 53-1). The dental hygienist's collaboration with other health professionals as part of the client's healthcare team is vital. For example, the dental hygienist informs the healthcare team about oral conditions; manages oral health risk and harm reduction; reinforces consistent messages regarding recovery from the illness; and participates in a team approach to care. Scenario 53-2 provides an example of the dental hygienist's role in helping a client to overcome an eating disorder.

Persons with an eating disorder such as bulimia nervosa are likely to eventually seek oral care because of the changing appearance of their teeth or complaints of oral or dental discomfort. Scenario 53-3 illustrates this. Keep in mind that an individual with an eating disorder, due to the nature of the illness, is reluctant to acknowledge the gravity of the eating disorder and carefully protects the disorder as if it is a secret.

SCENARIO 53-3

"My dental hygienist was the first person to help me disclose that I had bulimia nervosa. When she looked in my mouth she saw signs of erosion and asked me about them. It was how she asked me, her tone of voice—calm, kind, empathetic—that enabled me to be truthful to her. I had never ever spoken the words aloud before when I said them to her: 'I throw up. I throw up many times a day and have been doing this for a couple of years. I think I have bulimia.' My dental hygienist helped me to access an eating disorder clinic, and I am now on my way to recovery."

Dental hygienists may be the first health professional to identify the oral and physical manifestations characteristic of these disorders.

Anorexia Nervosa[1]

Anorexia nervosa is a mental illness that affects adolescent girls and young women, although boys and men are not immune to the condition. It is the least common eating disorder, but it has a high profile in society because of publicity related to many public figures who have either died as a result of the illness or who have made public their diagnosis. The term *anorexia* is a misnomer, because it literally means "loss of appetite"; rather, the client with anorexia nervosa suppresses and denies the sensation of hunger. It is suspected that some people have a brief episode of the disorder and recover on their own, but people in whom the course of illness is severe will need help to recover from it.

Diagnosis

There are four key diagnostic criteria for anorexia nervosa, with two specified types: restricting type or binge-eating and purging type (Box 53-1). During an anorexia nervosa episode, persons with the restricting type achieve weight loss through dieting, fasting, or excessive exercise. By comparison, persons with the binge-eating and purging type may engage in purging behaviors such as self-induced vomiting or the misuse of laxatives, diuretics, or enemas in addition to binge eating. These behaviors are seen at least weekly during an anorectic episode. The stereotypic image of the extremely emaciated person may or may not be accurate in clients with anorexia nervosa. The distortion of the body image may be demonstrated by clients with anorexia nervosa through verbalization of how they feel or think about appearance in relation to "being fat" when they are observably thin or underweight.

Epidemiology

Anorexia nervosa affects girls and women, although one tenth of persons with anorexia are male. The lifetime prevalence of strictly defined anorexia nervosa among females is 0.5% to 1%. The onset of the illness primarily occurs before puberty, during adolescence, and during young adulthood. It is a relatively rare eating disorder, but it has the highest morbidity rate of any psychiatric diagnosis; it also has a poor response rate and a protracted course of illness. The incidence appears to be rising.

BOX 53-1

DSM-IV-TR Diagnostic Criteria for 307.1, Anorexia Nervosa

A. Refusal to maintain body weight at or above a minimally normal weight for age and height (e.g., weight loss leading to maintenance of body weight less than 85% of that expected; or failure to make expected weight gain during period of growth, leading to body weight less than 85% of that expected).
B. Intense fear of gaining weight or becoming fat, even though underweight.
C. Disturbance in the way in which one's body weight or shape is experienced, undue influence of body weight or shape on self-evaluation, or denial of the seriousness of the current low body weight.
D. In postmenarcheal females, amenorrhea, i.e., the absence of at least three consecutive menstrual cycles. (A woman is considered to have amenorrhea if her periods occur only following hormone administration [e.g., estrogen].)

Specify Type

- Restricting type: During the current episode of anorexia nervosa the person has not regularly engaged in binge eating or purging behavior (i.e., self-induced vomiting or the misuse of laxatives, diuretics, or enemas).
- Binge-eating and purging type: During the current episode of anorexia nervosa the person has regularly engaged in binge eating or purging behavior (i.e., self-induced vomiting or the misuse of laxatives, diuretics, or enemas).

Data from the *Diagnostic and Statistical Manual of Mental Disorders, Fourth Edition, Text Revision* (Copyright © 2000). American Psychiatric Association.

The course of anorexia nervosa is variable but appears marked by chronicity and relapse. Table 53-1 outlines primary symptoms of anorexia nervosa. Psychologic, emotional, and mental health challenges that are comorbid with eating disorders include major depression and anxiety disorders, substance abuse, self-injurious behavior, and restricted affect and capacity for insight. Table 53-2 identifies medical problems associated with anorexia nervosa. The cardiovascular system, the hematopoietic system, the fluid and electrolyte balance, the gastrointestinal system, the endocrine system, and the bone become medically compromised for persons with anorexia nervosa. Scenario 53-4 shows the role that the dental hygienist may be asked to play with respect to an eating disorder and a comorbid condition, in this case the use of "street drugs." The dental hygienist's holistic approach to oral health recognizes the oral health–systemic health link and understands that upset in one body system affects whole-body wellness.

Bulimia Nervosa[1]

Bulimia nervosa is a mental health illness that affects a person's quality of life and that has the potential to be life-threatening. Unlike people with anorexia nervosa, those with bulimia nervosa are able to maintain a body weight within a normal range for their body type; however, they are unduly

TABLE 53-1
Primary Symptoms of Anorexia Nervosa and Bulimia Nervosa

Anorexia Nervosa	Bulimia Nervosa
• Resistance or refusal to maintain body weight at or above a minimally normal weight for age and height • Weight loss primarily due to reductions in food consumption; even with significant weight loss, reduction continues • Intense fear of weight gain or being "fat" even though underweight • Weight loss viewed as evidence of self-control • Denial of seriousness of medical implications; lack of insight • Loss of menstrual periods in girls and women after puberty	• Regular intake of large amounts of food accompanied by a sense of loss of control over eating behavior • Regular use of inappropriate compensatory behaviors such as self-induced vomiting, laxative or diuretic abuse, fasting, or obsessive or compulsive exercise • Extreme concern with body weight and shape

Data from the *Diagnostic and Statistical Manual of Mental Disorders, Fourth Edition, Text Revision* (Copyright © 2000). American Psychiatric Association.

TABLE 53-2
Examples of Medical and Health Consequences of Anorexia and Bulimia

Anorexia Nervosa	Bulimia Nervosa
• Association with depressive symptoms and social dysfunction • Leukopenia and mild anemia common; other metabolite disturbances • Dehydration and its results (e.g., renal failure) • Signs and symptoms of starvation; emaciation • Amenorrhea • Constipation, cold intolerance, lethargy, and excessive energy • Hypotension, hypertension, bradycardia • Dry skin, hair loss • Lanugo (growth of a downy layer of hair)	• Increased frequency of depressive symptoms and mood disorders • Association with use of stimulants and alcohol is associated • Fluid and electrolyte imbalances, which can lead to serious medical problems • Dental decay and eroded enamel • Salivary gland enlargement • Calloused fingers (from digitally inducing purge) • Dependency on laxatives if used on chronic basis • Esophageal tears, gastric rupture, and cardiac arrhythmias are rare but potentially fatal

Data from the *Diagnostic and Statistical Manual of Mental Disorders, Fourth Edition, Text Revision* (Copyright © 2000). American Psychiatric Association.

SCENARIO 53-4

"Hi, Lynne. Can I have a moment with you before you see Ben for his dental hygiene appointment? We just celebrated his fifteenth birthday," stated Mrs. Friesen, Ben's mother. "I need your help. I suspect Ben has an eating disorder. He's lost a lot of weight in the last few months, he exercises every night at home even though he plays high school volleyball, he swims with the community club team, and he's always out front kicking a soccer ball around. Ben hasn't said he has a problem, and every time I try to bring it up he gets really upset with me. Lately I've noticed him tapping his teeth together. Ben has never done that before. I'm really frightened. I was watching a documentary the other night on TV about teens and street drugs. Tooth tapping is a symptom of that drug ecstasy. The host of the show said sometimes kids will use street drugs like ecstasy and crystal meth to lose weight. When you see him, will you ask him about the tooth tapping? Can you say something to him? The way I look at it, it takes a community to care for our children. I need help getting him help."

focused on body shape and weight and express a general dissatisfaction with their body image. The term *bulimia* literally means "ox hunger," and it accurately describes this abnormal craving for food.

Diagnosis

Bulimia nervosa is characterized by repeated binge eating (i.e., eating significantly more food than what would be considered normal amounts and doing so without control over eating) followed by purging behaviors to offset the binge, such as self-induced vomiting, the use of laxatives or diuretics, excessive exercising, fasting, and enemas. There are two specific types: purging type and non-purging type. The difference between the two is how and what the person does to offset the binge. If the individual engages in self-induced vomiting or the misuse of laxatives, diuretics, or enemas, the condition is the purging type. If he or she uses another type of inappropriate compensatory behavior to prevent weight gain (e.g., excessive exercise, fasting) but does not regularly vomit or misuse laxatives, the condition is the non-purging type. The most common reported means of preventing weight gain is purging by vomiting; 80% to 90% of persons with

BOX 53-2

DSM-IV-TR Diagnostic Criteria for 307.51, Bulimia Nervosa

A. Recurrent episodes of binge eating. An episode of binge eating is characterized by both of the following:
   (1) eating, in a discrete period of time (e.g., within any 2-hour period), an amount of food that is definitely larger than most people would eat during a similar period of time and under similar circumstances
   (2) a sense of lack of control over eating during the episode (e.g., a feeling that one cannot stop eating or control what or how much one is eating)
B. Recurrent inappropriate compensatory behavior in order to prevent weight gain, such as self-induced vomiting; misuse of laxatives, diuretics, enemas, or other medications; fasting; or excessive exercise.
C. The binge eating and inappropriate compensatory behaviors both occur, on average, at least twice a week for 3 months.
D. Self-evaluation is unduly influenced by body shape and weight.
E. The disturbance does not occur exclusively during episodes of anorexia nervosa.

Specify Type

- Purging type: During the current episode of bulimia nervosa the person has regularly engaged in self-induced vomiting or the misuse of laxatives, diuretics, or enemas.
- Non-purging type: During the current episode of bulimia nervosa the person has used other inappropriate compensatory behaviors such as fasting or excessive exercise but has not regularly engaged in self-induced vomiting or the misuse of laxatives, diuretics, or enemas.

Data from the *Diagnostic and Statistical Manual of Mental Disorders, Fourth Edition, Text Revision* (Copyright © 2000). American Psychiatric Association.

bulimia nervosa who report for treatment use this means. See Box 53-2 for the DSM-IV-TR diagnostic criteria for bulimia nervosa.

Epidemiology

Bulimia nervosa is more common than anorexia nervosa. Estimated rates are 1% to 3% of the population, and they are higher for college-aged women. Prevalence is more significant among women than men with a ratio of 10:1. The onset generally occurs during the later teenage years and young adulthood. High-risk populations are those in which weight and appearance are considered to be important to a certain activity, such as ballet, wrestling, long-distance running, and modeling. It appears that industrialized countries support the role of sociocultural factors in the development of bulimia nervosa.

The course and outcome of bulimia nervosa are variable, but the condition tends to be chronic and relapsing. Unlike anorexia nervosa, it does not have a high mortality rate, but it has a comorbid association with other mental health conditions. Scenario 53-5 illustrates a mother's response to her son's relapse with bulimia nervosa and the value that she places on his oral health. On the basis of those persons who have sought help, it seems that the condition is of long-term duration, with recovery requiring diligence, professional assistance, and, at times, pharmaceutical interventions (e.g., antidepressants). Because bulimia nervosa is a secretive illness and the affected person can maintain a normal body weight, it can go on for a very long time without ever being disclosed or diagnosed.

SCENARIO 53-5

Frank's mother was straightforward and kind when she confronted him with her discovery of his relapse back to bulimia nervosa behaviors. She said, "I found Ziploc bags in your closet today when I was picking up your laundry from your room. Dear, I see you are purging again. Please do it in the toilet rather than in these bags. The dog might find these and eat them, which won't do him any good. You'll beat this disorder. Let's book an appointment with your nurse therapist for tomorrow rather than wait until next week's scheduled one. Do you think it would be good to see your dental hygienist this week? It's getting time for another fluoride application, isn't it?"

Some medical complications associated with bulimia nervosa are identified in Table 53-2. Table 53-1 lists the primary symptoms. Persons may develop cardiac problems such as arrhythmias, gastrointestinal problems (e.g., gastroesophageal reflux disease), esophagitis, irritable bowel syndrome, and fluid and electrolyte abnormalities. It is rare to develop gastrointestinal abnormalities, although esophageal tears or gastric ruptures can occur and are potentially life-threatening. Bulimia nervosa is associated with anxiety and mood disorders, particularly major depressive disorders, dysthymic disorder, self-injurious behavior, substance abuse, and personality disorders. Because of the repeated vomiting, some clients will experience dental erosion that results in tooth sensitivity. Professional help may be sought by the person as a result of the discomfort of the dentition, so the dental hygienist may be the first health professional to help the client begin his or her recovery journey.

Binge-Eating Disorder[1]

Binge-eating disorder (BED), according to the DSM-IV-TR is an EDO-NOS. For a diagnosis of EDO-NOS, the person must present with behavior patterns that are not consistent with either anorexia nervosa or bulimia nervosa but have thinking and behavior around food and the body image that are not within normal limits. BED is described as repeated binge eating without compensatory behaviors such as vomiting but associated with shame, guilt, and lack of control. Box 53-3 outlines the research criteria for this disorder. Obesity is associated with BED. Persons with BED have difficulty sustaining attempted weight loss. The disorder appears to be a chronic one. Women are estimated to experience BED 1.5 times more frequently than men, with an overall prevalence of 15% to 50% (mean, 30%) among people surveyed who were accessing weight-loss programs. The onset of the disorder appears during late adolescence and early adulthood. The course and outcome of BED are not known; however, recovery is

BOX 53-3

DSM-IV-TR Research Criteria for Binge-Eating Disorder

A. Recurrent episodes of binge eating. An episode of binge eating is characterized by both of the following:
  (1) eating, in a discrete period of time (e.g., within any 2-hour period), an amount of food that is definitely larger than most people would eat in a similar period of time under similar circumstances
  (2) a sense of lack of control over eating during the episode (e.g., a feeling that one cannot stop eating or control what or how much one is eating)
B. The binge-eating episodes are associated with three (or more) of the following:
  (1) eating much more rapidly than normal
  (2) eating until feeling uncomfortably full
  (3) eating large amounts of food when not feeling physically hungry
  (4) eating alone because of being embarrassed by how much one is eating
  (5) feeling disgusted with oneself, depressed, or very guilty after overeating
C. Marked distress regarding binge eating is present.
D. The binge eating occurs, on average, at least 2 days a week for 6 months.

Note: The method of determining frequency differs from that used for bulimia nervosa; future research should address whether the preferred method of setting a frequency threshold is counting the number of days on which binges occur or counting the number of episodes of binge eating.

E. The binge eating is not associated with the regular use of inappropriate compensatory behaviors (e.g., purging, fasting, excessive exercise) and does not occur exclusively during the course of anorexia nervosa or bulimia nervosa.

Data from the *Diagnostic and Statistical Manual of Mental Disorders, Fourth Edition, Text Revision* (Copyright © 2000). American Psychiatric Association.

SCENARIO 53-6

Clare, a 22-year-old female patient, said the following to Dianne, her dental hygienist: "Annie (anorexia nervosa) was my best friend. Annie and I saw Nurse Joan as an enemy. During my initial days in treatment for anorexia nervosa, she was always telling me Annie was lying to me, that her voice telling me 'I am so fat and I must not eat' was all based on the deceitful nature of the illness. It wasn't until I began to hear Annie's voice as separate from my own that I started to believe what Nurse Joan and my health care team were saying to me: Annie was my enemy, not them." Clare told Dianne that she learned through treatment to call her anorexia nervosa "Annie." Personifying anorexia nervosa enabled her to find her own identity as separate from the illness. When she was able to do this, her recovery from the condition began. It was a long, hard, and intense journey that consumed 7 years of her life.

SCENARIO 53-7

"When I was 21, I discovered by chance that I could throw up all I had eaten and I wouldn't gain weight," said Amanda, a 23-year-old client, to Janet, a dental hygienist. Amanda added, "I was an active university student with good friends, okay grades, and this ever-present worry about weight gain."

Janet asked, "Amanda, do you still throw up? Your teeth are showing very slight erosion. Do they hurt you? Are they sensitive? Sometimes a person who vomits regularly develops enamel erosion. I'm just seeing some slight evidence of this on your teeth."

Amanda replied, "Well, this is so embarrassing, I do feel, oh what's the word—ashamed, mortified—that I even got into this, but I did, and to answer your question, not for awhile, and when I do it's just when I feel too full. I'm better about not eating until I feel too full."

Janet nodded and said, "I'm glad you told me this. It is important to know for your oral health. Let's work on a plan. Have you sought help for this behavior?"

apparently good for those who receive treatment, with less likelihood for relapse than that seen among clients with anorexia nervosa and bulimia nervosa.

Health Effects of Anorexia Nervosa and Bulimia Nervosa

The effects of anorexia nervosa and bulimia nervosa on the psychosocial and physiologic well-being of an individual are significant.[1-6] From a client-centered approach, anorexia nervosa can be thought of as an eclipsing of the person's thinking by the eating disorder; in other words, the person's identity is centered on the eating disorder.[7] Recovery or fighting against the condition is like fighting against one's sense of self or identity. Scenario 53-6 illustrates the possessiveness of anorexia nervosa over the individual. People with bulimia nervosa report an overwhelming sense of lack of control with food; they are driven to consume and purge food as described in Scenario 53-7. For both anorexia nervosa and bulimia nervosa, the treatment is challenging and the recovery period lengthy. Throughout this time period, the dental hygienist must be vigilant to support recovery; he or she must be empathetic to prevent oral implications and deterioration and to enable oral rehabilitation and reconstruction.

Psychosocial Dimension

In the individual with anorexia nervosa, body image distortion and obsession with food restriction results in self-starvation. Keep in mind that the "self" aspect of "self-starvation" is an illness in thinking and not truly self-guidance. Clients with anorexia nervosa report that control of food and perfectionist behavior bring feelings of being more competent and more in control of their lives.

In bulimia nervosa, low self-esteem and subsequent feelings of inadequacy are reinforced by the guilt and embarrassment associated with binge-and-purge behavior. The behavior itself becomes self-reinforcing, because the achievement and maintenance of a lower weight are perceived as bringing increased attractiveness and more friends; hence the eclipsing analogy. Persons with bulimia nervosa do obsess about body image. They may appear quite successful in the management of their lives. Affective expression may appear gregarious to the casual observer; however, underlying the facade is a flattened affect that results from the associated anxiety, guilt, and dysphoria.

Impaired psychologic development and the concomitant distortion of attitudes in the client with an eating disorder provide the foundation for continued dysfunction and the progression of the disorder. Persons with eating disorders rarely seek professional assistance on their own and may resist recommendations and offers of help from family members and friends. Those with bulimia nervosa may eventually seek help as a result of tooth sensitivity or a change in the appearance of their teeth.

Physiologic Responses

Many body systems are at risk for disruption as a result of an eating disorder. The body as a systemic whole is affected, thereby requiring the dental hygienist to consider the oral systemic outcomes of eating disorders. In anorexia nervosa, restricted food intake and resulting undernutrition impair the individual's overall functioning and health. A common physiologic effect of anorexia nervosa behavior is hormonal abnormalities. Among women, a prolonged decrease in estrogen along with a decreased body fat level may contribute to amenorrhea and decreased bone density (i.e., osteoporosis). Osteoporosis may be evident in the jaw and facial bones. The cardiovascular, gastrointestinal, renal, and hematologic systems may be compromised in clients with anorexia nervosa. Vital statistics in the client will likely reveal low pulse rates, decreased blood pressure, and reduced left ventricular output. The client may not openly complain about physiologic symptoms such as constipation; however, a comprehensive health history may identify abnormal function such as this gastrointestinal disturbance. If a person is constipated, he or she may be dehydrated; dehydration is evident in salivary flow and quality, which affects oral health. A person with pale skin or general fatigue may be experiencing hematologic changes and electrolyte imbalances that result in the immune system not functioning optimally. This affects the body's ability to prevent and withstand infection (e.g., oral candidiasis). Conducting a health history is about differentiating normal from abnormal and then following through to improve the diagnosis and resulting care.

The repeated binge-and-purge cycle in the client with bulimia nervosa and the purge subtype of anorexia nervosa may result in dangerous complications, which when left untreated can become life-threatening. Excessive vomiting and diuretic and laxative abuse lead to dehydration and electrolyte imbalance. The loss of potassium is a particular threat, because the resulting hypokalemia and metabolic alkalosis may result in cardiac or renal failure. Ipecac syrup used by some to induce vomiting after binge periods is particularly dangerous. Ipecac syrup contains emetine, which can destroy heart muscle fibers. Chronic ipecac ingestion and absorption can lead to fatal myocardial dysfunction. In addition, repeated binge eating and vomiting can cause gastric dilation, esophagitis, esophageal tears, or rupture. Although not common, these are life-threatening.

Other General Physical Findings

As an eating disorder progresses, general physical characteristics become evident as a result of the disorder. The dental hygienist must be aware to look for these signs during the assessment phase. Two common physical findings for persons with anorexia nervosa during more developed stages of the disorder are lanugo and "feeling cold." Lanugo is a fine downy hair that is usually found on the lower half of the face and the upper body. Dry skin and hair as well as decreased scalp hair are predictable findings as the eating disorder progresses. Clients might even report losing hair or that they no longer brush the hair because it is "falling out." Hypothermia and increased sensitivity to cold may be evidenced by the client wearing inappropriately warm clothing when environmental temperatures are moderate. The dental hygienist needs to be aware of these presentations and gently engage the client in a discussion about them.

The dental hygienist may suspect that a client is engaging in oral purging if they notice callused knuckles. Persons who orally purge using their fingers may have calloused knuckles from the repetitive friction of the teeth riding over the finger during the digital stimulation used to induce vomiting. Although it is common to use one's own fingers to create the urge to vomit, other objects are used as well (e.g., spoons). These objects, in addition to the fingers, can traumatize the palate and other soft tissues of the mouth. During the intraoral examination, the dental hygienist needs to look for lesions and bruises, because these may be cues that a person is orally purging. Additional intraoral and extraoral findings are discussed in the next section.

Oral Health Implications

Intraoral and extraoral manifestations of eating disorders occur, particularly with bulimia and the binge-and-purge subtype of anorexia (Table 53-3).[8-11] The client with an eating disorder may exhibit one or more of these manifestations; some may experience none of them. Many of these signs are seen only after the person has had the disorder for some time. Early identification and prompt intervention for an eating disorder are not likely to occur in the dental hygiene practice given the secretive and nondisclosing nature of a client with an eating disorder. It is more likely that the dental hygienist will notice oral changes in the client who has an established eating disorder and then look to employ tertiary prevention interventions. After conducting a comprehensive health history and oral assessment in a nonjudgmental, respectful environment, the dental hygienist acts to promote prompt intervention to lessen the disorder's effect on the oral cavity and on the person's overall health and wellness.

Parotid Enlargement

Extraorally, parotid enlargement has been observed with both anorexia nervosa and bulimia nervosa. This enlargement is noninflammatory in nature. It gives the jaw an enlarged appearance that subsides with abstinence from self-induced vomiting. Palpation will reveal the enlargement to be soft and generally painless. Clients with parotid gland enlargement may express concern about the unesthetic appearance of the enlargement. If the individual understands that the enlargement usually decreases when the eating disorder behaviors are brought under control, this may increase their

TABLE 53-3
Potential Effects of Eating Disorders on the Oral and Perioral Tissues

Effects on Oral and Perioral Tissues*	Anorexia Nervosa Restricting Type	Bulimia Nervosa and Binge-and-Purge Anorexia Nervosa
Parotid enlargement	Yes	Yes
Diminished taste acuity	Yes	Yes
Dehydration and xerostomia or reduced salivary flow	Yes	Yes
Enamel erosion (perimylolysis)	No	Yes
Intraoral trauma (e.g., palatal abrasion, palatal hematoma)	No	Yes
Increased risk of dental caries (given xerostomia and/or exposed dentin)	?*	?*
Periodontal disease	?*	?*
Other comorbid disorders (e.g., self-injurious behavior)	Yes	Yes
Oral side effects of medications (e.g., antidepressants)	Yes	Yes
Oral health–systemic health issues (e.g., esophageal reflux disease, yeast infection)	Yes	Yes

*Evidence in the literature is not conclusive regarding dental caries and periodontal disease in direct relationship with eating disorders. Both may occur as a result of xerostomia, exposed dentin, poor oral hygiene, and other known risk factors that are general to these two dental diseases.

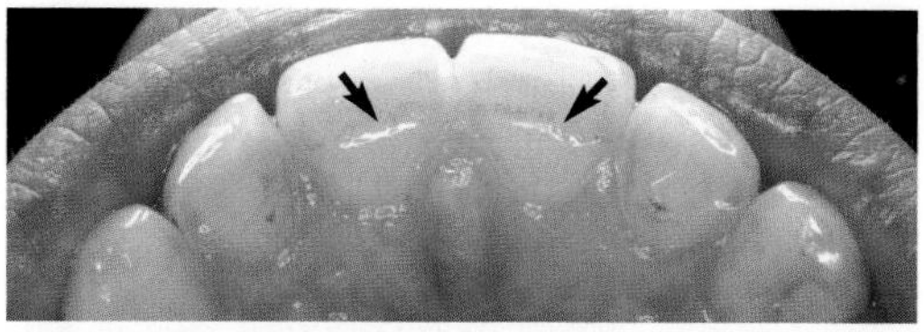

Figure 53-2. Perimylolysis on the maxillary incisors as a result of the habitual vomiting associated with bulimia nervosa. (Courtesy J. Charbonneau, 2008.)

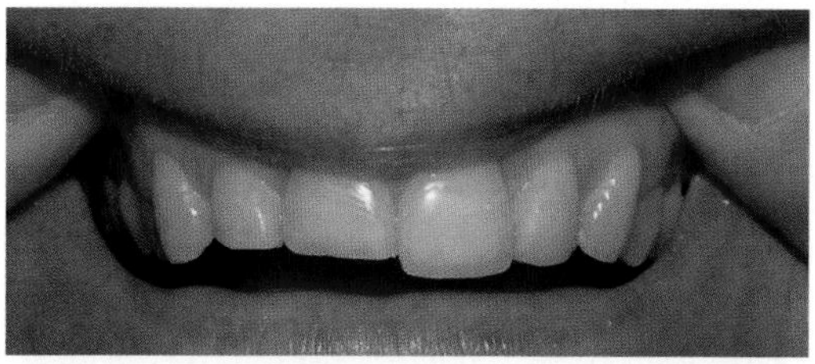

Figure 53-3. Comparison of loss of vertical height of teeth #11 and #12 versus teeth #21 and #22. Vertical height is restored with resin restorations. Height loss was due to the regular vomiting of a client with bulimia nervosa. (Courtesy J. Charbonneau, 2008.)

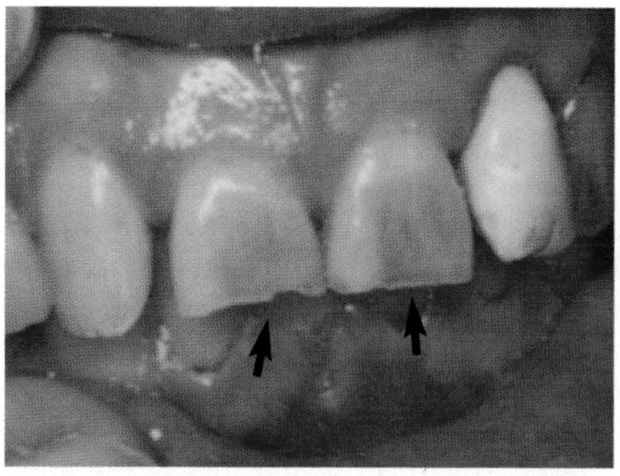

Figure 53-4. Thinning and chipping of incisal third of teeth #11 and #21 in a person with bulimia nervosa. (Courtesy S. Issac, 2008.)

motivation for following through with psychologic and medical care.

Diminished Taste Acuity
Although it will not be obvious from the intraoral examination, diminished taste acuity has been reported by clients with eating disorders. This alteration in taste sensation is thought to be a result of malnutrition (specifically trace metal deficiency) or hormonal abnormalities. Changes in hormonal levels have been shown to decrease sensations of taste and smell.

Dehydration and Xerostomia
Xerostomia, dry chapped lips, and commissure lesions resembling angular cheilitis may occur if the client is dehydrated from vomiting, diuretic or laxative abuse, or antidepressant medications used to treat eating disorders. Little is known about the salivary factors for persons with eating disorders, but it appears that salivary differences exist, such as lower salivary pH, different proteolytic enzymes, and lessened salivary flow rates for persons with bulimia nervosa as compared with healthy individuals.[12-14] Further investigation is needed to understand the cause and effect relationships of these salivary differences. Clients should be informed about the role of saliva in oral health.

Perimylolysis or Enamel Erosion
Perimylolysis (also spelled as *perimylosis*) or enamel erosion is the most common dental finding in the client who orally purges (Figures 53-2 through 53-6). The gastric acids are thought to result in the erosion of tooth surfaces. Initially the maxillary anterior teeth are involved, but, over time, the posterior teeth experience the same erosion. Subsequent mechanical erosion then occurs when the tongue or toothbrush moves against the teeth. Slight pitting is evident on the incisal surfaces of the anterior teeth, and a cupping appearance may be present on the cusps of the posterior teeth. This dished-out appearance should be differentiated from the

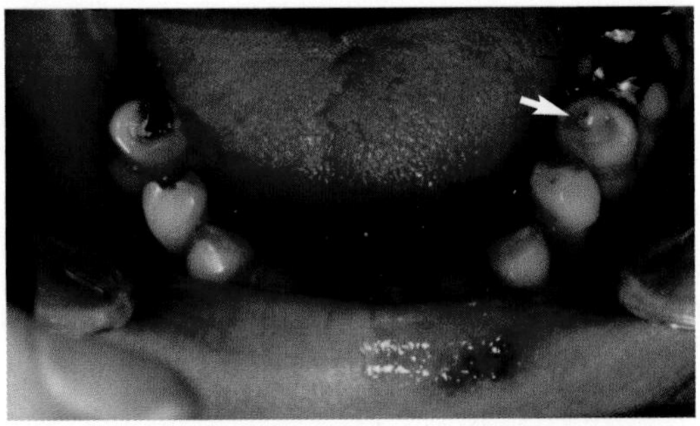

Figure 53-5. Perimylolysis and resin loss on tooth #28; lip lesions caused by oral purging. (Courtesy S. Issac, 2008.)

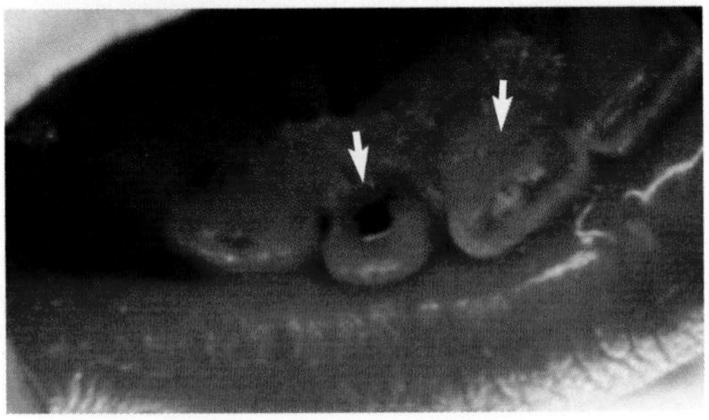

Figure 53-6. Perimylolysis on tooth #12 involving amalgam and on tooth #11 lingual surface. (Courtesy S. Issac, 2008.)

typical flattened appearance that occurs with abrasion. As perimylolysis progresses, the teeth exhibit a loss of normal anatomic features, such as developmental grooves and pits, and they develop a mat-like surface with rounded margins. Enamel loss occurs both vertically and horizontally and may become so extensive that complete enamel loss is evident with dentinal exposure. A loss of lingual and incisal enamel on the anterior teeth weakens the tooth structure, thereby making these teeth susceptible to chipping. An open bite may form as a result of vertical height loss of the anterior teeth. The teeth can appear translucent and "moth-eaten." Enamel loss around amalgam restorations results in a raised-island appearance of the amalgam. Unless the vertical and horizontal dimensions of the teeth are measured and documented via use of dental erosion indices or study casts as part of a routine clinical examination, early perimylolysis is difficult for practitioners to identify, because tooth structure loss usually is subtle. The longer the duration of the illness, the more damage is done to the dentition.

Dentinal Hypersensitivity

Perimylolysis may eventually result in dentinal exposure and associated tooth sensitivity. Clients who purge their food may complain of tooth sensitivity; often this is their chief reason for seeking dental care.

Dental Caries

Decreased salivary flow along with disturbed dietary patterns may predispose the client to an increased dental caries rate. Not all studies support the theory that individuals with eating disorders have an increased dental caries prevalence. However, evidence suggests that persons with bulimia nervosa may be prone to caries as a result of their high carbohydrate intake, changes in their oral pH levels, decreased saliva quantity and quality, and the use of antidepressants or other medications associated with a diminished salivary flow rate. Xerostomia can also result from illicit drug use, which is a potential coexisting condition among clients with eating disorders.

CONSENT FORM

I hereby give consent for my dentist and dental hygienist to contact all healthcare providers and therapists involved in the treatment of my eating disorder. I understand that coordination of care among these health professionals is in my best interests. In addition, I understand that all consultation and discussion among these individuals will be held in strict confidence.

____
Client Signature Date

____
Witness Date

Figure 53-7. Sample client consent form.

Periodontal Disease

Persons who are nutritionally deprived are at risk for periodontal disease. Thus clients with an eating disorder may be at risk for periodontal disease. Moreover, the body is a system; if at a cellular level the nutrients for efficient body function are lacking, then the body is unable to properly maintain itself not only in the oral cavity but also in the heart and other body organs. The client who is taking antidepressants or other medications, including street drugs, may experience dry mouth, which exacerbates dental plaque biofilm growth. Having depression comorbid with an eating disorder may result in apathy toward oral hygiene habits, thus increasing periodontal disease risk.

Intraoral Trauma

Intraoral trauma may be evident in the client who orally purges or regurgitates the stomach contents. In addition, the oral soft tissues may be fragile because of nutritional deficiencies. Findings may include the presence of traumatic lesions such as ulcerations or hematomas on the hard and soft palates as well as cheek and lip bites.

Dental Hygiene Process of Care for Clients with Eating Disorders

The nature of eating disorders and the secrecy and shame associated with them tend to result in clients with eating disorders not seeking dental care until oral manifestations appear. These oral manifestations result in the dental hygienist's involvement in care at a secondary prevention level (Figure 53-7; see Chapter 4). From a primary prevention and health promotion perspective, the dental hygienist and the oral healthcare team can ensure that the practice promotes healthy lifestyle messaging and establishes an environment in which all clients feel safe to disclose their health and lifestyle information. The secondary prevention measures would include screening for eating disorders or for the client's susceptibility to one, harm reduction by preventing further damage to the oral structures, and referring clients for care and interprofessional collaborative practice. All of these measures are aimed at prompt intervention to address the eating disorder to lessen disability. Tertiary prevention measures take place during and after recovery as continued eating disorder behaviors destroy reconstructed dentition, which is very costly for the client. An open dialogue regarding dental rehabilitation or reconstruction during active illness must take place between the dental provider and the client to ensure informed consent.

For individuals with eating disorders who have not been medically diagnosed, the dental hygienist may be the health professional who identifies the need for referral to the healthcare team. A working knowledge of organizations and individuals within the client's community who specialize in caring for individuals with eating disorders allows the dental hygienist to guide the client to appropriate care. This knowledge can be obtained by contacting credible national mental health organizations or eating disorder treatment facilities within the community. The national organizations may not be in the immediate geographic locale, but they are generally knowledgeable about available support throughout the area. Creating a formal referral protocol with eating disorder treatment centers or with healthcare professionals and eating disorder specialists is important for the dental team. Health professionals who are actively treating clients with eating disorders often need oral healthcare professionals to whom they can refer clients who are experiencing oral problems. A liaison between the oral health team and other members of the healthcare team will open the door for comprehensive client care through referrals and interprofessional collaboration.

Evidence that oral health professionals have a low comfort level when dealing with sensitive issues such as addressing or asking a client about an eating disorder led to the development of a framework to better enable oral health clinician communication with clients pertaining to eating disorders.[15] The "Evaluate, Assess, Treat" framework is based on motivational interviewing, and it has been proposed as a means for engaging in the active secondary prevention of eating disorders.

BOX 53-4

Possible Causes for Oral Findings Commonly Associated with Clients Who Have Eating Disorders

Perimylolysis and Erosion

- Gastric or physical disturbances with associated vomiting (e.g., previous pregnancies, chemotherapy, hiatal hernia, duodenal or peptic ulcers, cancer-related therapy)
- High citric acid fruit or fruit juice intake
- Antabuse therapy for alcoholism
- Habitual eating of or sucking on vitamin C tablets or sweet-and-sour candies
- Intake of medications that contain hydrochloric acid
- Exposure to industrial acids

Parotid Enlargement

- Salivary neoplasms
- Inflammatory diseases (e.g., mumps, infectious mononucleosis, tuberculosis, sarcoidosis, histoplasmosis)
- Metabolic disturbances (e.g., malnutrition, alcoholic cirrhosis, diabetes mellitus)
- Autoimmune diseases (e.g., Sjögren's syndrome)
- Parotid duct obstruction
- Acquired immunodeficiency syndrome

Xerostomia

- Medications (e.g., antihypertensives, antidepressants, antipsychotics, antihistamines)
- Systemic diseases (e.g., diabetes, Sjögren's syndrome)
- Side effect of radiation therapy for cancer of the head and neck area
- Dehydration from recent flulike illnesses or high fever

Commissure Lesions

- Loss of vertical dimension or overclosure
- Vitamin B deficiency
- Yeast infection

Dental Hygiene Assessment

The assessment of all dental hygiene clients involves data collection regarding the client's comprehensive health history, intraoral and extraoral statuses, and physical status (Table 53-4). Intraoral photographs, the use of dental erosion indices, and study models are helpful for establishing baseline and follow-up objective clinical observations of enamel erosion. When the clinician observes deviations from normal in a client assessment that are suggestive of an eating disorder, follow-up questions are needed. There are other possible explanations for dental erosion other than an eating disorder (Box 53-4). Possible causes for some observed oral manifestations are as follows:

- Commissure lesions and dry, chapped lips, which are findings typical of an eating disorder, may also be a result of the presence of other illnesses that cause dehydration or undernutrition. Usually, however, clients who have been ill and who subsequently have dehydration willingly convey this information on questioning.
- Dental erosion, which is the most common oral finding in clients with bulimia and the binge-and-purge subtype of anorexia, has also been associated with vomiting as a result of gastric disturbances (e.g., gastroesophageal reflux disease) and other conditions.
- Intraoral trauma may result from an accident, or it may be evidence of self-mutilation that is indicative of psychologic problems other than eating disorders.

During the assessment of a client with a suspected eating disorder, it is imperative that the dental hygienist gather specific information in a professional and nonjudgmental manner. An assessment tool to consider using is the validated SCOFF questionnaire (Box 53-5).[16] Concluding the presence of an eating disorder without adequate assessment is to be avoided. Concluding prematurely that a client has an eating disorder puts the client and the clinician in an unnecessary and uncomfortable position.

TABLE 53-4

Assessment of Client with a Suspected or Previously Diagnosed Eating Disorder

Component	Assessment Technique
Health History	
Physical appearance and gait: skin, build, hair, pallor	Observation
Vital signs: blood pressure, heart rate, body temperature	Objective measurement
Systemic disease: current and past status	Interview, collaborative consultation
Systems review (e.g., bowel movements, postural hypertension)	Interview, collaborative consultation
Medications: drug names, dosage, duration, purpose	Interview, collaborative consultation
Substance abuse: alcohol, nonprescription medications, street drugs	Interview
Physical activity: frequency and duration	Interview
Dietary habits: cariogenicity of diet, general healthy eating habits	Interview, dietary analysis for dental caries control and general healthy eating habits
Oral homecare: routine, products, techniques	Interview, observation
Extraoral Assessment	
Salivary and lymph glands	Palpation
Temporomandibular joint	Palpation, auscultation
Skin: color, moisture, facial hair (lanugo), lesions	Observation
Perioral structures: commissure lesions, lip integrity, trauma	Observation
Hands (knuckles calloused)	Observation
Intraoral Assessment	
Soft-tissue: mucous membranes, palatal tissue, tongue, floor of mouth, throat	Observation and palpation
Salivary flow rate and pH	Observation, salivary flow rate measure, pH test
Dental caries and tooth color	Observation, radiographic assessment, manual assessment
Tooth wear: presence or absence, location, appearance (moth-eaten, cupped, thinned, abraded), open bite	Observation, comparative study model
Periodontal tissues	Observation, radiographic assessment, manual assessment
Oral hygiene	Observation and manual dexterity assessment

BOX 53-5

SCOFF Questionnaire* for Screening for Eating Disorders

1. Do you make yourself **s**ick because you feel uncomfortably full?
2. Do you worry you have lost **c**ontrol over how much you eat?
3. Have you recently lost more than **o**ne stone (14 pounds) in a 3-month period?
4. Do you believe yourself to be **f**at when others say you are too thin?
5. Would you say that **f**ood dominates your life?

*One point for every "yes"; a score of two indicates a likely case of anorexia nervosa or bulimia.

Reprinted with permission from Hill LS, Reid F, Morgan JF, Lacey JH. SCOFF, the development of an eating disorder screening questionnaire, *Int J Eat Disord* 43:344, 2010.

Assessment of the client who reports a history of bulimia nervosa or anorexia nervosa involves several important components. In the client with a diagnosed eating disorder, historic information regarding the course and treatment of the eating disorder, past medical and dental care and treatment interventions, and the current status of the oral environment is necessary to provide appropriate client care. This evaluation should provide a clear depiction of the extent to which the eating disorder relates to associated behaviors, the client's current status regarding psychotherapy or other supportive care, and the current physical and oral findings.

Dental Hygiene Diagnosis

Dental hygiene diagnoses can be accomplished using objective and subjective findings to determine deficits in the human needs related to dental hygiene care. The actual diagnosis of the eating disorder is not a function of members of the oral health team, because this can be determined only through a thorough psychologic evaluation. A client usually manifests several human need deficits that arise directly or indirectly from the eating disorder. For example, the repeated binge eating of carbohydrates followed by vomiting may result in a deficit related to a biologically sound dentition as evidenced by enamel erosion (perimylolysis) and increased signs of dental caries. Dehydration from vomiting or diuretic or laxative abuse may also result in a deficit relating to the integrity of the skin and mucous membranes as evidenced by dry chapped lips and commissure lesions similar to angular cheilitis. It is essential that the dental hygienist consider all possible reasons for these deficits so that appropriate care may follow. Examples of dental hygiene diagnoses for eating disorders are presented in Table 53-5.

Planning

The planning phase for the client who is suspected of having an eating disorder includes the following:

- Phase 1: Referral of the client to medical and psychologic treatment providers
- Phase 2: Establishment of the dental–eating disorder team for interprofessional collaboration
- Phase 3: Support of the client's human needs, specifically the management and support of oral health during and after eating disorder treatment

Planning for the client with a previously diagnosed eating disorder includes phases 2 and 3. Oral healthcare team members must recognize their limitations when treating clients with these disorders. Either palliative or definitive oral and dental treatment may be necessary, but the primary role of the oral healthcare team treating the client with a suspected eating disorder is to refer the client to eating disorder specialists. Such specialists can help clients with the psychologic and medical aspects of their eating disorders. The establishment of a caring and nonjudgmental environment that is based on mutual trust is necessary to successfully achieve a referral. Attention to the client's need for freedom from pain through palliative oral care initially is recommended if the client is experiencing discomfort (see Chapter 61).

Client involvement in the setting of goals is essential. Goals must be set with the following characteristics:

- Specific and measurable outcomes, including target dates for achievement
- Based on the dental hygiene diagnoses
- Realistic
- Measurable by both the client and the healthcare professional

A sample dental hygiene care plan for a client with an eating disorder is shown in Table 53-6.

Implementation

Confirming the presence of an eating disorder with a client may be uncomfortable for the dental hygienist given the sensitivity of the illness itself. Setting the stage and employing an empathetic caring approach, as suggested in Box 53-6, facilitates the dialogue between the client and the dental hygienist.

TABLE 53-5

Example of Dental Hygiene Human Needs Diagnoses for Clients with Eating Disorders

Dental Hygiene Diagnosis Deficit	Due or Related To	As Evidenced By
Wholesome facial image	Self-induced vomiting Excessive diet soda intake Bruxing habits Salivary gland hypertrophy from binge-purge behavior	Client expression of dissatisfaction with tooth discoloration, loss of tooth structure, open bite, visible dental caries, parotid gland enlargement
Freedom from pain	Frequent vomiting Diminished saliva flow rate from diuretic or laxative abuse	Oral discomfort from exposed dentin from enamel erosion, dental caries, and dehydration of oral tissues
Integrity of skin and mucous membranes	Laxative or diuretic abuse and vomiting Use of fingers and other objects to orally purge	Dehydration of oral environment Self-induced trauma during purging and self-abusive behavior Dry skin or hair
Protection from health risks	Self-starvation Anemia or alteration in body metabolism Decreased cardiac function	Dry skin or hair Enlarged parotid glands Bradycardia, low blood pressure, low body temperature, thin, pale
Freedom from fear and stress	Low or endangered self-esteem Need for acceptance by others Feelings of guilt Fear of being found out	Lack of willingness to communicate fully, denial of or providing false explanations for oral manifestations; fatigued
Responsibility for oral health	Lack of self-control Feelings of unworthiness	Lack of ownership of problems, impaired self-care, self-inflicted oral trauma

TABLE 53-6

Example Items for Dental Hygiene Human Needs Care Plan for Client with Bulimia Nervosa*

Human Need Deficit	Dental Hygiene Goal	Dental Hygiene Intervention	Evaluative Statement
Freedom from pain	By 2/28/15, client will have oral function with no discomfort.	Emphasize abstinence from oral purging. Use a professional (fluoride varnish) and offer a home fluoride therapy regimen (neutral sodium fluoride gel or rinse; dentifrice). Use a nonabrasive desensitizing dentifrice. Advise client to avoid toothbrushing for at least half an hour after purging.	Client follows professional and home fluoride therapy program and uses desensitizing dentifrice. Client reports abstinence or attempted abstinence from oral purging. Client avoids toothbrushing after oral purging.
Sound dentition	By 8/1/14, client will have reduced risk of further loss of tooth structure. By 7/7/14, client will not present with further loss of tooth structure.	Use of professional and home fluoride therapy Demonstrate dental plaque-control measures. Refer to dentist for palliative or dental reconstruction and rehabilitation of damaged teeth.	See above, in addition to the following: Client complies with recommended oral hygiene regimen; there is no evidence of progressive enamel loss (perimylolysis). Client is in care of dentist regarding dental palliative care, rehabilitation, and reconstruction needs.
Responsibility for oral health	By 8/1/14, client will participate in treatment of bulimia by attending all health professional appointments, including oral health appointments. By 8/1/14, client will communicate openly with dental hygienist and participate in management of oral conditions.	Consult with the healthcare team or refer the client for care (e.g., eating disorder program, physician, psychologist, dietitian). Recommend that the client consent to collaboration between the oral healthcare team and the eating disorder program or healthcare team. Explain the risks of vomiting to the hard oral tissues (e.g., removal of tooth structure, sensitivity, risk of trauma) Schedule frequent dental hygiene and dental appointments during active bulimia periods.	Client complies with eating disorder healthcare team or program recommendations. Client provides written consent for interprofessional health collaboration for client-centered care. (Liaise with healthcare team after dental or dental hygiene appointments and vice versa when appropriate [e.g., if client is experiencing a period of bulimic activity].) Client states risks of vomiting to oral health. Client self-initiates dental hygiene or dental appointments during active bulimia periods and attends scheduled appointments.
	By 2/2/14, client will participate in management of oral conditions by using oral self-care skills. By 11/10/14, client will self-monitor oral health.	Involve the client in the design of oral self-care skills and monitoring that coordinate with a concomitant eating disorder therapeutic program.	Client demonstrates successful use of oral self-care skills; there is no evidence of perimylolysis, palatal trauma, or dental disease.
Wholesome facial image	By 11/15/14, Client will participate in an active eating disorder program for 2 years.	Collaborate with the client's healthcare team, which includes the oral healthcare team. Refer the client to a dentist for rehabilitation and reconstruction of the dentition.	Client is compliant with oral and healthcare team treatment recommendations and therapeutic program.
	By 12/30/14, client will verbalize that the mouth looks and feels better.	Provide education regarding the client's expressed dissatisfaction with the oral condition.	Client has realistic expectations of dental treatment outcomes. Client states that the mouth looks and feels better.

*Respect and honor each client as an individual with personal needs.

BOX 53-6

Suggestions for Confronting a Person with a Suspected Eating Disorder

Setting
- Use a private setting to ensure client confidentiality.
- Be proactive. Establish an interprofessional collaborative practice for client-centered care.
- Create a climate of calmness, acceptance, and nonjudgment.
- Ensure confidentiality within the collaborative healthcare team.

Approach
- Do no harm. Know your limitations; professionally refer and collaborate with others for client-centered care.
- Focus on the illness rather than the person. Remember that the illness possesses the person's thinking. Separate the disorder from the person.
- Be firm, formal, objective, and concerned. Keep in mind that eating disorder behavior is associated with low self-esteem, depression, and emotional problems.
- Anticipate client resistance and defensiveness. Recognize client sympathy-evoking tactics or manipulation; these are part of the illness.
- Focus on observed signs and symptoms and concern for the client's health.
- Ask if the client engages in specific behaviors associated with the disorder (e.g., "Do you vomit after eating sometimes?" "Do you restrict the amount of food that you usually eat?" "Have you ever heard of bulimia and anorexia?").
- Empower the client to seek help and, if he or she is already engaged in an eating disorder program, to comply with it. Instill hope.
- Gain client consent for interprofessional collaboration.
- Be informed about issues that the client is experiencing that may have an impact on oral health, and likewise keep the healthcare team apprised of oral issues that have an impact on health and recovery.
- Know that eating disorders are complex mental disorders that are often comorbid with other psychiatric disorders such as substance abuse, self-injurious behaviors, anxiety, and depression. Know to look for signs and symptoms of these as well as those of an eating disorder.
- Tell the client that you are ethically obligated to intervene if you believe the client may harm himself or herself or others.
- Value harm reduction, knowing that clients with eating disorders can have a long road to recovery.

The discussion needs to occur in a confidential setting. If dental erosion is the most obvious oral finding, asking questions that eliminate other reasons for erosion allows the clinician to gain valuable information while desensitizing the client to the more direct questions to follow. The discussion should be conducted by asking direct questions while maintaining eye contact. The client's body language may provide clues about whether the suspicion of an eating disorder is accurate. Few clients openly admit having an eating disorder when they are questioned about it. Many have become quite accomplished at denial and can maintain that position in the dental environment. However, most clients with eating disorders experience discomfort when being confronted with objective information that they have attempted to hide. The dental hygienist should be aware of nonverbal cues, such as the avoidance of eye contact by the client or the dropping of the head with a look of embarrassment. These clues are usually an indication that the clinician is on the right track with the questions, even if the client verbally responds negatively.

Individuals with eating disorders commonly react to initial discussions with various emotions. Two common responses are denial accompanied by tears and outright anger. It is important for the dental hygienist to maintain a professional demeanor during emotional outbursts and to reinforce the observation that the client's oral, physical, or health history findings are consistent with an eating disorder and have no other causative explanation. Some clients are relieved at being discovered and are receptive to suggestions for referral to an eating disorder specialist.

Phase 1: Referral of the Client to Medical and Psychologic Treatment Providers

Suggesting that the client make an appointment with an identified eating disorder specialist or treatment center for an evaluation is a less-threatening approach than making a definitive statement that the client has an eating disorder. Many clients are receptive to having the dental hygienist initiate a consultation appointment for them at an eating disorder treatment center (see Box 53-7 for referral suggestions). Others prefer to take the referral information with them to initiate the consultation appointment on their own. Either way, it is important that the client assume personal responsibility for attending a consultation appointment. Follow-up contact is necessary to promote the client's taking action.

The dental hygienist must thoroughly document discussions and decisions regarding referral for evaluation in the client's permanent dental record. This documentation permits subsequent client evaluation and monitoring at future appointments. In addition, it legally documents that the discussion took place and that the oral health team is offering help to the client.

Persistence on the part of the oral health team when no other explanations can be identified for the oral findings of a client who is unable to disclose an eating disorder is crucial, because untreated eating disorders can be life-threatening. Ethically the failure to refer a client who has the signs and symptoms of an eating disorder to an eating disorder specialist or another appropriate healthcare professional is neglecting one's professional responsibility as a healthcare provider.

Phase 2: Establishment of the Dental–Eating Disorder Team for Interprofessional Collaboration

Recovery from an eating disorder and the success of oral healthcare interventions to lessen resultant oral disabilities and to rehabilitate the dentition is largely determined by the client's ability to learn through psychologic therapy to

BOX 53-7

Referring a Person with a Suspected Eating Disorder

Refer the Individual

- Have an established collaboration with an eating disorder program or healthcare professional.
- Meet the client's human need for conceptualization and problem solving. Give specific information about resources for professional evaluation, and offer support.
- Enable and empower the client to access eating disorder programming or help.

Collaborate with the Professional Person to Whom You Are Referring the Client

- Inform the counselor or therapist of the referral.
- Discuss the symptoms and signs of concern, including the oral ones.
- Discuss areas of difficulty with confrontation and referral as well as the appropriateness of the referral.

Follow-up and Support

- Recognize that seemingly small accomplishments may be major to the client.
- Expect periods of recurrence of eating disorder behaviors. Harm reduction is paramount.
- Support recovery, not the illnesses.

manage the thinking and behaviors associated with the eating disorder. For this reason, open dialogue among all health providers prevents segmented care planning and permits an integrated approach to client care. Many persons with bulimia nervosa and binge-and-purge anorexia nervosa have extensive erosion that requires significant dental reconstruction. A lack of coordination among healthcare providers may mean dental failure if the reconstruction is completed before the client has made adequate progress with the eating disorder. The use of a signed release form allows oral health professionals to contact and collaborate with the eating disorder healthcare providers and is recommended when a client with an eating disorder is in active care. A sample release form is shown in Figure 53-7.

Professional collaboration between the oral healthcare team and the eating disorder team permits the oral healthcare team to have a better understanding of the client's specific psychologic issues and increases the success rate of all dental hygiene and dental interventions. The client is often confronting significant personal issues during psychologic therapy; these may influence the timing and ultimate success of definitive oral care. Without dialogue between the oral health team and the eating disorder team, oral health professionals may make care decisions that fail to address the comprehensive needs of the client. If clients are aware that all health providers are working together for their care, then they are less likely to claim that "all is well" to have their short-term desires met. It is not uncommon for clients with eating disorders, given the nature of these conditions, to attempt to manipulate healthcare providers during the course of therapy.

BOX 53-8

Example of Oral Health Education Issues for the Client with an Eating Disorder

- Cause of observed oral signs and symptoms of eating disorder behaviors
- Effect of eating disorder behaviors on oral health
- Connect oral health with systemic health
- Discuss client-specific current oral status
- Inform client of potential progression of oral problems
- Discuss oral health harm-reduction strategies:
  - Abstinence from oral purging
  - Effect of diet/nutrients on dental and oral health
    - Frequency of ingestion
    - Types of foods and drinks consumed
  - Toothbrush abrasion on teeth with perimylolysis
  - Neutralizing oral pH immediately after an oral purge
  - Benefits of fluoride therapy
  - Benefits of dental sensitivity therapy
  - Role of saliva in oral health

Dental hygienists and dentists must maintain a collaborative interprofessional approach to healthcare for maximal success with the client with eating disorders.

Phase 3: Support of the Client's Human Needs, Specifically the Management and Support of Oral Health During and After Eating Disorder Treatment

The implementation of individualized education and preventive strategies to support a healthy oral environment is a primary focus of this phase of the dental hygiene process. To meet the client's human need for conceptualization and understanding, oral health education assists the client with understanding the effects of eating disorder behaviors on oral health and provides self-care strategies to lessen associated problems. There is a paucity of evidence regarding exactly how eating disorders affect oral health and what interventions are effective for lessening the adverse oral health effects. Available literature about oral health and eating disorders is limited to case and case-control reports, literature reviews, practice experiences, and descriptive studies.[8-11] From an evidence-based practice perspective, much of eating disorder care is based on tradition and shared experience. It is from this body of knowledge that the dental hygienist provides the client with information to promote client knowledge and decision making during and after eating disorder care. Sample oral health education strategies for clients with eating disorders are provided in Box 53-8. These strategies may not be relevant for all clients, but an overview of general concepts is included with each educational program.

The dental hygienist is well positioned to educate the client about the following oral health issues related to eating disorders: (1) perimylolysis, (2) the effect of diet on oral health, (3) oral self-care, and (4) pain management during and after periodontal debridement and instrumentation.

Perimylolysis

Education for clients with perimylolysis is aimed at eliminating pain, maintaining and fortifying existing tooth structure, and preventing further erosion. The following have been suggested as oral harm reduction interventions: having an awareness that the low pH of stomach contents is associated with the chemical dissolution of tooth enamel and of the importance of saliva in oral health; rinsing immediately after an oral purge with a pH neutralizing solution; self-applied daily fluoride therapy; desensitization of dentinal hypersensitivity with either professionally applied or over-the-counter agents; waiting 30 to 40 minutes after oral purging before toothbrushing to lessen the mechanical abrasion of an eroded tooth surface; and avoiding abrasive prophylaxis. One suggestion with no evidence of effectiveness is mouth guard fabrication to provide tooth coverage during vomiting episodes.

Effect of Diet on Oral Health

Individuals with eating disorders commonly have eating behaviors that are not conducive to oral health. For example, foods that contain simple carbohydrates such as cookies, cake, and other sweets are common binge foods. It is important for the dental hygienist to counsel the client about the effects of repeated binge eating, frequent sucrose intake, and the extreme intake of dietary carbonated drinks and sports drinks due to their low pH. The continual consumption of low-pH diet beverages in the presence of diminished salivary flow enhances dental erosion and accompanying dentinal hypersensitivity. By adequately assessing eating habits in relation to oral health, the dental hygienist can provide appropriate preventive education and treatment. The dental hygienist, as part of the eating disorder healthcare team, promotes healthy eating and lifestyle; this message never waivers.

Oral Self-Care

Dental hygiene client education is specific to oral care, but, in general, dental hygiene recommendations are to lessen the acidity of the oral cavity; to maintain a wet mouth; to effectively remove dental plaque biofilm without damage to the tooth and surrounding tissues; to remineralize the dentition to protect and restore it; to prevent soft-tissue lesions; and to comply with dental and dental hygiene appointments. Clients need to be informed about the following ways that they can reduce harm to their oral cavities:

- *Rehydrating the mouth with salivary substitutes, frequent sips of water, ice chips, and sugar-free gum.* For the person with an eating disorder such as anorexia nervosa, this may be a formidable expectation during acute phases, because the person is supersensitized to calories and the prospect of water retention and hence "feeling fat." Ice chips may not be tolerable for a person with dentinal sensitivity.
- *Not toothbrushing after a purge owing to the mechanical abrasion of the already chemically assaulted tooth structure.* The client should instead neutralize the acidity in the mouth by promptly rinsing with a neutralizing solution such as sodium bicarbonate (1 tsp in 8 oz of water), slightly alkaline mineral water, or magnesium hydroxide (milk of magnesia) solutions. The toothbrush itself should be soft and used with gentle touch so as to not further destroy enamel crystals.
- *Using desensitizing fluoridated dentifrices and mouth rinses to provide additional benefit for exposed dentin from erosion.*
- *Employing a home fluoride therapy regimen in addition to professional fluoride therapies to remineralize fragile dentition.* The daily use of neutral sodium fluoride gel (administered either with a custom-fabricated tray or by brushing) or a sodium fluoride mouth rinse provides protection while strengthening enamel to prevent additional erosion. Critical to the oral cavity integrity is the reestablishment of normal pH; therefore the fluoride product must have a low pH.
- *Using a fabricated mouth guard for home fluoride application.*
- *Realizing the staining potential of certain agents, such as coffee, red wine, and tobacco products.*

These strategies are aimed at meeting the client's human needs for integrity of the skin and mucous membranes of the head and neck and for a biologically sound and functional dentition.

Pain Management During and After Periodontal Debridement and Instrumentation

During periodontal debridement and instrumentation, appropriate pain management techniques are used to protect sensitive hard and soft tissues. Maintaining a moist, clean environment by frequent rinsing of the oral cavity during instrumentation increases comfort, especially if the individual has xerostomia. Consider the effect of rubber-cup prophylaxis on eroded dentition and if it should be done at all given the damaged tooth structure. Many polishing pastes are abrasive to dentin and should be avoided. Avoid polishing the teeth if the individual does not have extrinsic stains or if the dental hypersensitivity impedes client comfort during stain removal. Dental hygiene care and necessary palliative treatment of discomfort (e.g., the use of desensitization treatments) must be scheduled for both periods of quiescence and those of activity of the eating disorder.

Evaluation

The evaluation of dental hygiene care for the client with an eating disorder consists of the following two parts:

- An objective evaluation that is based on mutual goals previously established by the dental hygienist and the client to determine whether the goals have been met, partially met, or unmet
- A subjective report by the client

Objective Evaluation

For an objective evaluation, the dental hygienist compares baseline findings involving plaque biofilm accumulation, periodontal status, dental caries, enamel erosion, salivary flow rate and quality, dentinal hypersensitivity, and oral tissues obtained at each subsequent appointment in terms of established goals. Many changes that occur over time are subtle and defy detection unless accurate measures are taken for comparison. It is important for the dental hygienist to use objective measurements to monitor the oral impact of the disorder and its associated comorbidities. The comparison of objective measures (e.g., oral dental erosion indices, photographs, study models, salivary flow and quality data) inform the dental hygiene continued-care plan.

Subjective Evaluation

The client's subjective evaluation provides additional information for the dental hygiene continued-care plan. A caring and professional environment ensures that client confidentiality is maintained while oral health human needs are met. The successful treatment of eating disorders requires intensive therapy followed by many years of maintenance. It is common for clients who have successfully controlled eating disorder behaviors for several weeks or months to relapse during the recovery phase. Awareness and verbal acknowledgment of this during the dental hygiene care plan evaluation permits clients to share honestly about areas of progress as well as areas of distress. The oral health findings can then be used in conjunction with observations from other attending health professionals to guide subsequent care.

On occasion, objective and subjective evaluations conflict with each other. A client with previously documented dental erosion may report that binge-and-purge episodes have been under control for 6 months and seemingly want to opt out of continued eating disorder care. The dental hygienist should consider the nature of eating disorders and question whether the client's statement is a reflection of the thinking influenced by the eating disorder. The comparison of the current dental status with intraoral photographs and diagnostic models obtained 6 months previously may indicate that the erosion is progressive. The dental hygienist becomes instrumental in encouraging the client to continue with eating disorder therapy by acknowledging the relapse period as being consistent with recovery. Interprofessional client-centered collaboration is of great value to understanding what dental interventions may be of benefit to recovery and which ones may inhibit it. Explain the need to coordinate nonemergency restorative and prosthetic dental care with psychologic therapy. For example, reconstructing the client's dentition may be viewed by the healthcare team as enabling the continuation of oral purging because the dental concerns of the client have been temporarily addressed while the eating disorder is still possessing the client.

Continual evaluation of the client's oral health status as well as of the status of psychologic therapy is one of the most critical functions of the dental hygienist when managing an individual with an eating disorder. At several points during the dental hygiene process of care, the clinician may need to reassess the client's condition, revise care goals, plan alternative strategies, implement these strategies, and reevaluate the outcome. The dynamic nature of the dental hygiene process of care for clients with an eating disorder creates a challenge for the professional dental hygienist.

Eating Disorder Treatment: Interprofessional Collaboration

The treatment involved for a person with an eating disorder involves many health professionals and interventions in addition to family and social support.[3] With informed consent from the client, health professionals can collaborate with each other for client-centered care to learn about perspectives of care and needs of the client that are outside of the individual health professional's scope of practice. Such collaboration enhances the quality of care and improves client outcomes. An interprofessional health care plan for a person with an eating disorder may be as follows:

- *Inpatient, outpatient, day program, and hospitalization treatment settings.* These settings are determined based on the severity of the client's eating disorder and his or her responsiveness to recommendations.
- *Psychotherapy such as cognitive behavioral therapy, interpersonal psychotherapy, group therapy, and family/caregiver therapy.* Given that the eating disorder is a disorder related to thinking, value is placed on helping the client to think about the eating disorder as a separate entity from his or her own self.
- *Nutritional treatment planning by dietitians with the client and, if applicable, the client's family.* Nutritional treatment is aimed at weight restoration and an understanding of what constitutes a balanced healthy dietary lifestyle. By restoring weight, the mind is better able to respond to cognitive therapy; a starved or nutritionally deprived brain does not function optimally.
- *A physical education therapist.* After a healthy weight is achieved, a physical education therapist may begin discussions with the individual to help establish a healthy approach to physical fitness. Persons with anorexia nervosa often overexercise to burn calories, so the reintroduction of physical activity occurs later during the recovery plan.
- *Possible psychopharmacologic treatment determined by the team and the client.* Appropriate medications may include antidepressants and antianxiolytics. Little evidence exists to support medication use as a single treatment for eating disorders; usually medication is for the treatment of comorbid conditions associated with the eating disorder. These medications do have the potential side effect of dry mouth. Supplemental drug treatment may be provided (e.g., hormone and nutrient replacement).
- *Prevention of oral health risks, particularly with bulimia nervosa and purging-type anorexia nervosa.* Preventing dental erosion and treating dentition with erosion is essential for oral health.

Eating Disorder Resources

There are many myths and misunderstandings that surround eating disorders. Dental hygienists as critical thinkers and client advocates follow an evidence-based, best-practice philosophy that guides dental hygiene practice. Valuable information about eating disorders is available online through credible organizations and associations such as the National Eating Disorders Association (NEDA, United States), the National Eating Disorder Information Centre (NEDIC, Canada), the National Association of Anorexia Nervosa and Associated Disorders (ANAD, United States), the Kings College/London Institute of Psychiatry (IoP, England), and Beating Eating Disorders (beat, United Kingdom). Each association has resource listings for professional and personal help that the dental hygienist can share with clients.

CLIENT EDUCATION TIPS

- Inform the client that help is available and that harm reduction and recovery are possible.
- Explain the need for referral and for the interprofessional collaboration of the healthcare team for comprehensive care.
- Ensure that the client knows about health resources that are available for people with eating disorders.
- Explain the effect of the eating disorder on the oral tissues.
- Promote self-care strategies to prevent or control oral manifestations associated with the eating disorder.
- At a community level, provide educational materials that address oral health and eating disorders both in the practice and in other healthcare settings.

LEGAL, ETHICAL, AND SAFETY ISSUES

- Oral healthcare team members must recognize their limitations with regard to treating clients with eating disorders. The primary role of the oral health team is to refer the client with a suspected eating disorder to specialists who treat the psychologic and medical aspects of eating disorders.
- The documentation of objective and subjective findings and recommendations as well as decisions regarding referral for evaluation in the client's permanent dental record are part of the client's confidential healthcare record.
- Failure to refer a client who has an eating disorder for subsequent psychologic evaluation is neglecting one's professional responsibility as a healthcare provider. Keep in mind that comorbid conditions may necessitate referral as well. Following up after the referral is also important.
- All information related to a client's eating disorder is confidential. The dental practitioner requires the client's consent to refer the client into medical and psychologic therapy systems.
- The use of a signed release form allows oral health professionals to contact and collaborate with the eating disorder treatment team.

KEY CONCEPTS

- Eating disorders are complex mental health illnesses with comorbid associations with other mental health conditions. The impact of eating disorders on the health and wellness of the individual is significant and life-threatening.
- Eating disorders affect oral health and can result in the destruction of the dentition.
- The dental hygienist practices in a professional and nonjudgmental manner that enables client disclosure of an eating disorder
- Dental hygienists must be proactive and have eating disorder information readily available.
- Dental hygienists must have the courage and integrity to openly dialogue with a client regarding objective and subjective observations of an eating disorder.
- Screening for signs of eating disorders and employing evidence-based dental hygiene interventions are part of the professional role of the dental hygiene clinician.
- It is critical to promote health and wellness through interprofessional collaborative practice for the treatment of eating disorders.

CRITICAL THINKING EXERCISES

1. Invite other healthcare professionals to join an interprofessional collaborative forum on eating disorders. Use a client case to learn about, from, and with each other about eating disorders from profession-specific perspectives. Focus on client-centered care.
2. Access a client's story from a credible resource. Discuss empathy as a practice concept in relation to the client's story.
3. Look for evidence-based information about dental hygiene interventions for eating disorders. Discuss practice decisions when an evidence base is lacking.
4. Imagine that the person with an eating disorder being told, "The pizza is in the fridge. I don't get why you won't just eat it." or "You are so beautiful. What do you have to worry about?" or "Did you see that girl, she's so anorexic!" Discuss why these statements are examples of naïveté with regard to eating disorders as complex mental health illnesses.
5. Respond to the following case study:
   Client: Ms. Amanda Telforn
   Profile: A 19-year-old white woman comes to the dental clinic. She attends college and is thin.
   Chief Complaint: "My mouth is always dry, and I need my teeth cleaned."
   Dental History: Client has dental prophylaxis routinely every 6 months. On intraoral examination, you note hematomas on the hard and soft palates and slight gingivitis. She has lingual erosion on teeth #6 through #11. In addition, there is slight pitting on the incisal surfaces of the anterior teeth and a cupping appearance on the cusps of the posterior teeth. Extraorally, there is fine downy hair on the lower half of her face, commissure lesions that resemble angular cheilitis, and enlargement of the parotid gland.
   Social History: The client lives with her parents and appears to be shy and socially introverted. She reports that she works out every day and sometimes twice a day.
   Health History: Client reports no use of medications or systemic disease.
   Oral Health Behaviors Assessment: The client reports brushing and flossing three times per day. She uses a soft toothbrush. She does not use a fluoride mouth rinse.
   Supplemental Notes: Client says that she feels fat but is obviously thin.

Discuss responses to the following questions about the Ms. Amanda Telforn case:

1. How should the dental hygienist proceed with confirming her suspicions that the client may have an eating disorder?
2. What are the dental hygiene diagnoses for this client?
3. What might be goals and interventions for this client?
4. What client education issues should be addressed? How?
5. Are there any contraindications to this client's care?

REFERENCES

1. American Psychiatric Association: *Diagnostic and statistical manual of mental disorders, fourth edition, text revision*, Washington, DC, 2000, American Psychiatric Association.
2. American Psychiatric Association: *Treatment of patients with eating disorders*. Available at: http://psychiatryonline.org/content.aspx?bookid=28&sectionid=1671334. Accessed January 9, 2012.
3. National Institute for Clinical Excellence. National Collaborating Centre for Mental Health. National Clinical Practice Guideline: *Eating disorders: core interventions in the treatment and management of anorexia nervosa, bulimia nervosa, and related eating disorders*, London, UK, 2004, National Institute for Clinical Excellence.
4. National Eating Disorders Association: National Eating Disorders Association Website. Available at: www.nationaleatingdisorders.org. Accessed January 9, 2012.
5. Lask B, Frampton I, eds: *Eating disorders and the brain*, West Sussex, UK, 2011, Wiley-Blackwell. John Wiley & Sons Ltd.
6. Yager J, Devlin M, Halmi K, et al: *Guideline watch (August 2012) practice guideline for the treatment of patients with eating disorders,*

ed 3. Available at: http://www.psychiatry.org/practice/clinical-practice-guidelines. Accessed January 6, 2013.
7. Espindola C, Blay S: Anorexia nervosa treatment from the patient perspective: a metasynthesis of qualitative studies, *Ann Clin Psychiatry* 21:38, 2009.
8. Back-Brito GN, da Mota AJ, de Souza Bernardes LÂ, et al: Effects of eating disorders on oral fungal diversity, *Oral Surg Oral Med Oral Pathol Oral Radiol* 113:512, 2012.
9. Romanos GE, Javed F, Romanos EB, et al: Oro-facial manifestations in patients with eating disorders, *Appetite* 59:499, 2012.
10. Johansson AK, Norring C, Unell L, et al: Eating disorders and oral health: a matched case-control study, *Eur J Oral Sci* 120:61, 2012.
11. Lo Russo L, Campisi G, Di Fede O, et al: Oral manifestations of eating disorders: a critical review, *Oral Dis* 14:479, 2008.
12. Schlueter N, Ganss C, Pötschke S, et al: Enzyme activities in the oral fluids of patients suffering from bulimia: a controlled clinical trial, *Caries Res* 46:130-139, 2012.
13. Aframian DJ, Ofir M, Benoliel R: Comparison of oral mucosal pH values in bulimia nervosa, GERD, BMS patients and healthy population, *Oral Dis* 16:807, 2010.
14. Dynesen AW, Bardow A, Petersson B, et al: Salivary changes and dental erosion in bulimia nervosa, *Oral Surg Oral Med Oral Pathol Oral Radiol Endod* 106:696, 2008.
15. DeBate RD, Cragun D, Gallentine AA, et al: Evaluate, assess, treat: development and evaluation of the EAT framework to increase effective communication regarding sensitive oral-systemic health issues, *Eur J Dent Educ* 16:232, 2012.
16. Hill LS, Reid F, Morgan JF, et al: SCOFF, the development of an eating disorder screening questionnaire, *Int J Eat Disord* 43:344, 2010.

ACKNOWLEDGEMENT

The author acknowledges Karen B. Williams for her past contributions to this chapter.

EVOLVE RESOURCES

Please visit http://evolve.elsevier.com/Darby/hygiene for additional practice and study support tools.

Women's Health and the Health of Their Children

CHAPTER 54

Leslie Ann Wilkerson Mallory

COMPETENCIES

1. Discuss the links between oral and systemic health, including health screening guidelines specific for women.
2. Discuss significant life events of women, including:
   - Explain the relationship between hormonal changes and periodontal diseases.
   - Explain the relationship between periodontal disease status in pregnant women and preterm, low-birthweight infants.
   - Recognize oral manifestations of conditions and diseases prevalent in women.
   - Plan dental hygiene care for the life span of women.
3. Describe the dental care of infants and children, including the planning of their dental hygiene care.

Gender bias, preference given to members of one gender over another, is evident in the history of medicine and healthcare. Research on drugs and diseases has been performed primarily on middle-aged white men, even though sex, age, race, and ethnicity profoundly influence life span, drug efficacy, and risk of disease. For example, little is known about why women live longer than men, are more likely to develop autoimmune diseases, metabolize drugs differently, and manifest brain tissue variation that may influence mood, healing, and disease susceptibility. Scientists have long known of the anatomic differences between the sexes but have just begun to uncover significant biologic and physiologic differences. Sex-based biology is the study of biologic and physiologic differences between men and women. Sex differences are apparent in the composition of bone matter, the experience of pain, the metabolism of certain drugs, and the rate of neurotransmitter synthesis in the brain.

Some women lack the education and self-esteem necessary to advocate for their own healthcare. Limited access to healthcare results in suffering and premature loss of life, especially among women of color and the poor. In the United States, more than 80% of heads of one-parent households are women responsible for securing healthcare for themselves and their children. Even with these constraints, women access the healthcare system more than twice as often as men.

Links Between Oral and Systemic Health

Research evidence links periodontal disease with cardiovascular disease (CVD), valvular heart disease, preterm low-birthweight (PLBW) babies, and pulmonary diseases such as aspiration and ventilator-associated pneumonia and chronic obstructive pulmonary disease (COPD) (see Chapter 20). Moreover, several conditions are risk factors or risk indicators for periodontal disease: type 1 and type 2 diabetes mellitus, tobacco use, stress, depression, financial difficulties, social isolation, and other distress-related, psychosocial factors. Visit http://www.womenshealth.gov/screening-tests-and-vaccines/screening-tests-for-women/index.html for a guide for counseling women on comprehensive healthcare and download the file outlining screening tests for women from http://www.womenshealth.gov/publications/our-publications/screening-tests-for-women.pdf as a reference. Nutrition information for women's health is discussed in Chapter 35.

Women and Heart Disease

Although young women get heart disease less frequently than women over 60 years of age, heart disease is the number one killer of women. Under age 60, one in three men develop heart disease as compared with one in 10 women. A woman's risk rises at menopause but does not equal a man's until about 10 years later. It is surprising to note that heart disease is more severe among women over 60 than among men of the same age; women are twice as likely as men to die within 60 days of having a heart attack and are less likely to survive coronary bypass surgery. It appears that high levels of triglycerides may elevate a woman's risk of heart disease, but there is no evidence that triglycerides have the same effect in men. Increased risks of venous thromboembolism (VTE) are present with postmenopausal hormone therapy (HT), specifically oral estrogen therapy.[1] Postmenopausal hormone treatments may double the risk of developing VTE, and hormone prescriptions, partly as a result of this finding, have declined.

Women may not exhibit the typical signs of a heart attack. In a woman a heart attack may be signaled by indigestion, nausea, vomiting, dizziness, breathlessness, back pain, or deep throbbing in the left or right bicep or forearm, rather than the chest pain frequently observed in men experiencing a cardiac arrest (see Chapter 43).[2]

Significant Life Events

Women need health information on the following:

- Puberty and menses
- Oral contraceptives
- Childbearing years and pregnancy
- Perimenopause, menopause, and postmenopause
- Osteoporosis and osteopenia

Women may need tobacco cessation and nutritional counseling; blood pressure and cholesterol level screening; promotion of exercise for at least 10 minutes three times daily or 30 minutes three times a week; weight control; and stress reduction. Other significant women's health issues include eating disorders, autoimmune diseases, hormone replacement therapy (HRT) and estrogen replacement therapy (ERT), incontinence, and domestic violence.

Puberty and Menses

Puberty and menses are marked by the development of secondary sex characteristics throughout the body and increased estrogen level. The bacteria associated with increased estrogen levels (*Prevotella* species and *Tannerella forsythensis*) have been implicated in periodontal disease. Irregular ovulations usually occur for the first 1 to 2 years before the start of menstruation. Endogenous sex steroid hormone gingival disease, which includes puberty-associated gingivitis and menstrual cycle gingivitis, may occur as estrogen and progesterone levels rise. These gingival diseases are classified as plaque-induced gingival diseases modified by systemic factors (see Chapter 19, Box 19-4). The body reacts to bacterial challenges differently, depending on the integrity of the immune system. The host response appears to be altered in the presence of increased sex steroid hormones, suggesting an effect of these hormones on the immune system.

Swollen, erythematous gingival tissues may be present, as well as herpes labialis and aphthous ulcers, prolonged hemorrhage after oral surgery, and swollen salivary glands. Minor increases in tooth mobility may be seen, along with an increase in gingival exudate. These transient changes are attributed to peak levels of estrogen and progesterone (Figure 54-1).

Although sex steroid hormone effects may be transient, irreversible oral damage could result if proper self-care is lacking. Dental hygiene preventive strategies during puberty and menses include stressing optimal oral hygiene via increased frequency and duration of toothbrushing with an extra soft toothbrush or a power toothbrush and meticulous interdental cleaning (see Chapters 23 and 24). Therapeutic modalities include topical corticosteroids; frequent periodontal debridement, scaling, and root planing; antimicrobial mouth rinses; fluoride rinses, gels, and varnish; and use of xylitol products. Painful oral manifestations of puberty and menses, although disconcerting and uncomfortable, can be managed with topical viscous lidocaine, Orahesive, or Zilactin-B, and over-the-counter systemic analgesics such as aspirin, ibuprofen, or acetaminophen.

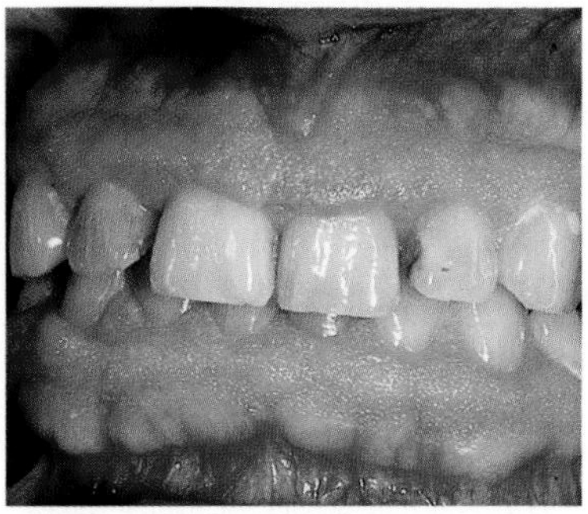

Figure 54-1. Endogenous sex steroid hormone gingival disease. (Courtesy Dr. Jon B. Suzuki.)

Oral Contraceptives

Oral contraceptives are used widely by women of childbearing age. Oral considerations and risks associated with oral contraceptives include gingival inflammation, exaggerated gingival inflammatory response to local irritants, increase in bacterial pathogens, and spotty melanotic pigmentation of the skin and gingiva. Periodontal pathogens (*Prevotella* and *Tannerella* species) increase, fed by estrogen and progesterone from oral contraceptives circulating in the blood. Oral contraceptives induce folate deficiency, which inhibits oral tissue repair and decreases blood clotting, especially in women over the age of 35 who smoke. Some other serious side effects may include the following:

- Vision disturbance (blurred, double, or partial loss of vision; flashing lights; bulging eyes)
- Headaches (severe)
- Unusual leg pain (calf or thigh)
- Chest pain (severe), shortness of breath, or coughing up blood
- Abdominal pain (severe)
- Loss of appetite
- Speech problems
- Depression
- Unusually long menstrual bleeding
- Swelling of hands, feet, ankles, or lower legs

Statistically significant findings suggest an increased risk of venous thromboembolism among current users of combined oral contraceptives compared to nonusers.[3] It is important to encourage clients to discuss the risks and benefits of oral contraceptive options with their doctor if side effects are apparent. In light of the effects and concerns, women may consider using other methods of birth control for a specific time period.

Oral antibiotics can potentially decrease the effectiveness of birth control pills (estrogen-containing oral contraceptives). This occurs because, in addition to killing the bacteria responsible for causing the current illness or infection, oral antibiotics also kill the normal stomach flora responsible for activating the birth control pill. If antibiotics are needed for treatment of oral infection or periodontal therapy, the dental hygienist may recommend women use a back-up method of birth control in addition to remaining on birth control pills to help women avoid pregnancy while taking an antibiotic, and for at least 1 week afterward.

Childbearing Years and Pregnancy

All women of childbearing age should be informed of the critical importance of preventive care so that they may attain optimal oral health before pregnancy and maintain that level of oral health throughout their lives (Box 54-1). A prenatal oral disease prevention program may include increased frequency of periodontal debridement; effective brushing and interdental cleaning (see Chapters 23 and 24), at-home fluoride and nonfluoride caries preventive agents (see Chapter 33), twice-daily antimicrobial rinses (see Chapter 31), use of xylitol-containing products (see Chapter 18), nutritional counseling (see Chapter 35), tobacco cessation (see Chapter 36), and infant oral care to prevent early childhood caries (ECC) (see Chapters 18 and 33). ECC is prevented by inhibiting *Streptococcus mutans* infection of the infant's oral flora in conjunction with avoiding prolonged exposure of the primary teeth to fluids or foods containing carbohydrates. (See section on infant and child care later in this chapter.)

BOX 54-1

Advice to Female Clients of Childbearing Age

- Get early prenatal care, even before pregnancy.
- Eat a well-balanced diet, including a vitamin supplement with vitamins A, C, and D, calcium, phosphorus, and folic acid.
- Select nutritious snacks and avoid those that increase caries risk (sugary foods and drinks).
- Adapt the proper weight for your pregnancy whether that be to gain, lose, or maintain weight.
- Exercise regularly, with doctor's permission.
- Avoid alcohol, cigarettes, illicit drugs, and limit caffeine.
- Avoid hot tubs and saunas.
- Avoid infections (including periodontal disease and dental caries).
- Maintain meticulous oral hygiene by toothbrushing, interdental cleaning, tongue brushing, use of effective antimicrobial and fluoride mouth rinses, as well as use of xylitol products.

During the first trimester of pregnancy (period of organogenesis, when vital organs form), the fetus is most susceptible to **teratogens**. Teratogens are harmful environmental risk factors that include various drugs, chemicals, infections, and/or radiation. Ideally no drug or illegal substances should be used during pregnancy, especially during the first trimester, when the fetus is at greatest risk. There are situations, however, in which drugs are necessary and appropriate to maintain the mother's health under the care of a physician. In those situations drugs classified as category A or B by the U.S. Food and Drug Administration (FDA) are preferred (Table 54-1). The dental hygienist should avoid using or recommending drugs (e.g., some local anesthetics, analgesics, and antibiotics) listed as category C, D, or X. Drugs taken during pregnancy and lactation should be used at the lowest effective dose and shortest duration to minimize harmful effects on the fetus or infant. When pregnant women are treated, if any doubt about any drug, procedure, or client condition is present, the obstetrician of record is consulted.

In the last half of the third trimester, the uterus is very sensitive to external stimuli, and the hazard of premature delivery exists. In a semi-reclined or supine position, the enlarged uterus compresses the inferior vena cava. This interferes with venous return, causing **postural hypotension**, also known as supine hypotensive syndrome. Symptoms may

TABLE 54-1

U.S. Food and Drug Administration Categories of Drugs and Their Implication for Use During Pregnancy*

Category	Description	Examples
A	Adequate studies have failed to demonstrate a risk to fetus (in first trimester) and no evidence of risk in later trimesters; possibility of fetal harm appears remote.	Thyroid supplements (levothyroxine), vitamins (folic acid, riboflavin; vitamins A, D, and C†), potassium chloride
B	Animal studies have failed to demonstrate a risk to the fetus, and there are no adequate studies in pregnant women; or animal studies show an adverse effect on the fetus but well-controlled studies in pregnant women have failed to demonstrate a risk to the fetus.	Acetaminophen, acyclovir, opioids,‡ penicillins, cephalosporins, erythromycin,§ caffeine, cimetidine, insulin, NSAIDs‖
C	Animal studies have shown an adverse effect on the fetus and there are no adequate studies in humans, or no studies are available in either animals or women. Potential benefits may warrant its use.	Epinephrine, phenylpropanolamine, trimethobenzamide, aspirin,‖ atropine, promethazine, theophylline, lisinopril, disulfiram, propranolol, fluoxetine, amitriptyline, sulfonamides,¶ prednisone
D	Positive evidence of human fetal risk based on adverse reaction data, but potential benefits in serious situations may warrant its use.	Warfarin, tetracycline, phenytoin, diazepam, trimethadione, lorazepam
X	Studies in animals or humans have demonstrated fetal abnormalities and/or there is positive evidence of human fetal risk, and the risks clearly outweigh any potential benefits.	Isotretinoin, diethylstilbestrol, phencyclidine (PCP), triazolam

Data from Haveles EB: *Applied pharmacology for the dental hygienist,* ed 6, St Louis, 2011, Mosby.
NSAIDs, nonsteroidal antiinflammatory drugs.
*Any unnecessary medication should be avoided in pregnant women.
†When used at recommended daily allowance (RDA) levels.
‡In usual therapeutic doses.
§Except erythromycin estolate.
‖Except near term, when dystocia and delayed parturition can be produced and then categorized as D.
¶Except near term, when kernicterus can be produced.

include an abrupt fall in blood pressure, bradycardia, sweating, nausea, weakness, or air hunger. A decrease in cardiac output may occur, and if prolonged, could cause a loss in consciousness (fainting). Placing the pregnant woman on her left side and in a supine or semi-supine position while she receives dental hygiene care relieves pressure on the inferior vena cava, which allows blood to return from the lower extremities and pelvic area.

Nitrous Oxide–Oxygen Analgesia Use During Pregnancy[4]

An anxiolytic agent is a drug used to reduce anxiety. Use of the anxiolytic nitrous oxide–oxygen (N_2O-O_2) analgesia in pregnancy has not been assigned a rating by the FDA, but studies demonstrate increased congenital anomalies, altered immune responses, spontaneous abortion, and increased birth defects with prolonged exposure during pregnancy, making the use of N_2O-O_2 a potential occupational hazard for members of the dental team. Scavenging systems, when properly installed and maintained, are effective in reducing ambient N_2O concentration in the oral care environment, a significant improvement for pregnant members of the dental team. Exposure should be no longer than 50 ppm N_2O in the air for longer than 8 hours per week.

Few anxiolytics are safe during pregnancy; however, a single low-dose exposure to N_2O-O_2 analgesia for no more than 30 minutes is considered to be safe.[4] The use of any drugs unless essential during the first trimester is not recommended; therefore, the second or third trimesters are recommended if indicated for anxiety during dental hygiene care that is not elective. An obstetrician should be consulted before this analgesic is administered to a pregnant client and if complications are evident during or following administration (see Chapter 41).

Drug Intake During Lactation

Little conclusive evidence exists about drug dosage during lactation and its effects on the nursing infant because so few studies involve pregnant or lactating women. The amount of drug excreted in breast milk is usually 1% to 2% of the maternal dose. Therefore it is unlikely that most drugs taken by the lactating mother have any pharmacologic significance for the infant. It is prudent for the mother to take the drug just after breast-feeding and then avoid nursing for the required number of hours based on the drug's half-life. To prevent the passage of drugs from mother to infant, lactating mothers should avoid epinephrine, aspirin and other NSAIDs, tetracycline, ciprofloxacin (Cipro), metronidazole (Flagyl), gentamicin, vancomycin, benzodiazepines, barbiturates, and benzodiazepines (diazepam [Valium] and lorazipam). Epinephrine is contraindicated in lactating women because it is excreted in breast milk. If a local anesthetic with epinephrine must be used, the woman should wait 9 hours before breast-feeding her baby. Because of its rapid diffusion from the body, N_2O-O_2 analgesia is considered safe for lactating women and therefore their nursing infants.

Alcohol Intake During Pregnancy

All clients, especially those who are pregnant, should be asked about drug, alcohol, and tobacco habits and educated about cessation options (see Chapters 36 and 52). Pregnant women should be cautioned about alcohol use because their babies could be born with fetal alcohol syndrome (FAS), characterized by damage to the offspring's central nervous system that affects motor skills, skin and muscle innervation, and behavior aspects of the personality. The risk of FAS in babies of women who drink heavily (five or more drinks a day) is high. The risk to women who drink one drink per day, or on occasion, is low. There is evidence that some damage, not full FAS, can occur with a single binge (five or more drinks at one sitting). Characteristics of persons with FAS include short palpebral fissures, a flat midface, an indistinct philtrum, and a thin upper lip. Other less-frequent characteristics may include epicanthal fold, a low nasal bridge, a short nose, ear anomalies, and microdontia (Figure 54-2).

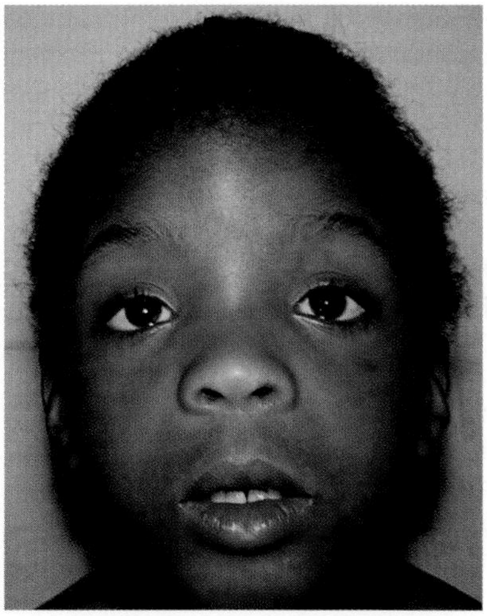

Figure 54-2. Fetal alcohol syndrome. Note distinct facial characteristics such as a flat philtrum, low nasal bridge, short eyelid fissures, thin upper lip, and incomplete development of midface. (From Bird DL, Robinson DS: *Modern dental assisting*, ed 11, St Louis, 2015, Saunders.)

Radiographic Exposure During Pregnancy

The developing fetus is especially susceptible to the effects of radiation, particularly during the first 2 to 18 weeks of development. However, safety features in use such as high-speed film, filtration, long cone rectangular collimation, lead aprons, and thyroid collars significantly decrease radiation exposure. For this reason, the current recommendation that no radiographs be exposed in the absence of clinical signs and symptoms is particularly important when treating the pregnant client. If diagnostic radiographs are needed for the pregnant woman, she must be protected properly by a protective apron and a thyroid collar, and current standards for radiation safety must be maintained to minimize harm to the fetus. Digital radiography may decrease any potential risk even further, because this system uses less radiation than traditional film.

Pregnant dental personnel must use the usual necessary precautions when taking radiographs, that is, wear a lead apron, stand more than 6 feet from the tube head, stand at 90 to 130 degrees to the beam (preferably behind a protective wall), and monitor exposure by wearing a radiation exposure badge (dosimeter). Pregnant dental personnel should receive no greater than 0.5 rem during the gestation period.[5,6]

Oral Manifestations During Pregnancy

Erosion of the lingual, occlusal, incisal, or facial surfaces of the teeth occurs when the enamel is decalcified and softened by gastric acids (see Chapter 53). Perimylolysis, acid erosion of teeth, is rare in pregnancy but may occur if a woman vomits repeatedly from severe morning sickness. Subsequent mechanical abrasion may occur when the tongue or toothbrush moves against the teeth. Clients at risk for tooth erosion should be advised to rinse with water immediately after vomiting and before brushing teeth. An acid-neutralizing preparation of one quart of water mixed with one teaspoon of baking soda is recommended for mouth rinsing after vomiting. At-home daily-use fluoride rinses or gels, xylitol-containing gums or mints, amorphous calcium phosphate–containing products, or other remineralizing products also may be recommended to prevent demineralization of tooth structure.

Pregnancy-associated gingivitis, a sex steroid hormone gingival disease most common in the second trimester of pregnancy, is characterized by an exaggerated host response to oral biofilm. The gingiva may appear fiery red and edematous at the marginal gingiva and interdental papillae, with loss of tissue resiliency. Tissues may be smooth and shiny, bleed easily, and display increased probing depths. These gingival changes occur earlier and more frequently in the anterior than in the posterior areas (see Figure 54-1 and Chapter 19, Box 19-4). Pregnancy-associated gingivitis usually reaches maximum severity during the eighth month and is less severe after childbirth. The tissue, however, may not return to a state of health.

As the most prevalent oral manifestation of pregnancy, pregnancy-associated gingivitis is due to poor oral hygiene, high plasma hormone levels, and an increase in bacteria associated with periodontal disease. The inflammatory response is exacerbated by hormonal and vascular changes and the presence of increased anaerobic bacteria that proliferate in the high-progesterone environment during pregnancy. The marked increase in *Tannerella* species during pregnancy seems to be associated with increased serum levels of the circulating sex steroid hormones estrogen and progesterone. Estrogen and progesterone serve as bacterial nutrients and increase gingivitis during pregnancy. Both hormones have been shown to substitute for naphthoquinone, an essential growth factor for *Tannerella* species and *Prevotella intermedia.* Because bacteria can metabolize estrogen or progesterone as a nutrient, pregnancy favors the colonization of anaerobic bacteria in the gingival sulcus.

When plasma levels of estrogen and progesterone increase, progesterone and estrogen accumulate in gingival tissues. Human gingiva has receptors for progesterone and estrogen. Progesterone causes a dilation of the gingival capillaries, increasing their permeability and thus increasing gingival exudate, edema, and accumulation of inflammatory cells. Estrogens are primarily responsible for vascular changes in other target tissues such as the uterus, yet increased vascular permeability and exudate in the gingiva are essentially the result of progesterone. Tooth mobility is sometimes present in pregnant women and may be related to disturbances in the attachment apparatus. One theory contends that mobility may be related to mineral changes in the lamina dura and not the result of alteration of the alveolar bone.

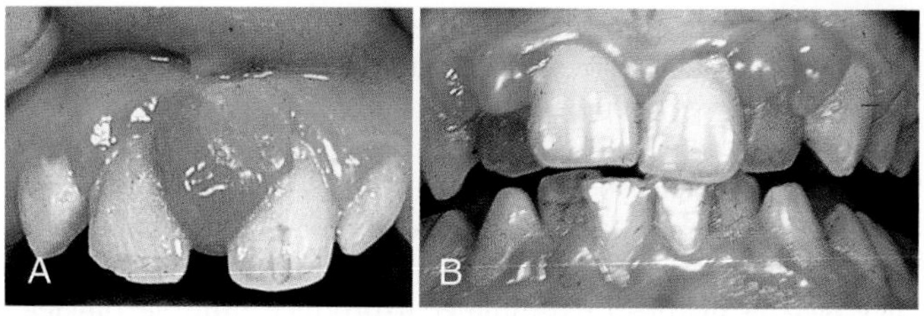

Figure 54-3. Pregnancy granuloma. **A,** Granuloma between the maxillary central incisors. **B,** Granulomas in the maxillary lateral incisor areas. (Courtesy Maria Perno Goldie.)

Tooth mobility usually reverses or declines after the birth of the baby.

Pregnancy granulomas (pyogenic granulomas) are single, tumor-like, soft-tissue growths, typically on the interdental papilla, most often on the labial aspect of the maxillary anterior gingiva; however, bone destruction is rare (Figure 54-3). These granulomas are pedunculated (attached via a stem), with intense red to deep-purple color, depending on the vascularity of the lesion and the degree of blood stagnation. Usually no larger than 2 cm, the granulomas are painless and may bleed readily if disturbed. Occurring in less than 10% of all pregnancies, usually abating after delivery, the lesions often are related to poor oral hygiene and the general effects of progesterone and estrogen on the host immune system. These progesterone-influenced effects inhibit collagenase, the enzyme that breaks down collagen, resulting in the accumulation of collagen within the connective tissue. Typically, surgical or laser excision of the granuloma is performed after delivery; however, situations may dictate immediate removal when the granuloma is painful to the client or when it disturbs tooth alignment, is cosmetically unacceptable, or bleeds easily. If excision is necessary, the second trimester is optimal because of low risk to the fetus during this time. If excised during pregnancy, the granuloma may recur; therefore clients should be advised that an additional procedure may be needed postpartum.

Sex Steroid Hormones and the Inflammatory Process

Prostaglandins, mediators (facilitators) of the inflammatory process, have been shown to increase significantly in the presence of high concentrations of estrogens and progesterones, such as during pregnancy. In addition to stimulating bacterial growth, sex steroid hormones stimulate key factors in the inflammatory response.

Depressed immune function occurs during pregnancy. The maternal immune mechanism is weakened to protect the fetus from rejection; the mother's host resistance to certain diseases, including inflammatory periodontal disease, is also altered. Progesterone and estrogen have been shown to affect the immune system. Neutrophil chemotaxis and phagocytosis and antibody and T-cell responses are depressed in the presence of high levels of sex hormones during a normal pregnancy. Pregnancy also inhibits the migration of inflammatory cells and fibroblasts to the site of injury or insult.

Progesterone functions as an immunosuppressant in the gingival tissues of pregnant women, resulting clinically in an exaggerated appearance of inflammation. As a result, this immunosuppression prevents the rapid, acute inflammatory reaction against oral biofilm and allows for increased chronic inflammation to occur.

Infertility Treatment

Infertility treatment also may affect the oral cavity. Ovulation induction is the most common method of infertility treatment, in which the ovaries are stimulated to produce multiple follicles. One study assessed the effects of three ovulation induction drug protocols on the gingival tissues of women who were undergoing infertility treatment[7]: clomiphene citrate (CC) alone, CC combined with follicle-stimulating hormone, and CC combined with human menopausal gonadotropin. The researchers concluded that ovulation induction exacerbates gingival inflammation, gingival bleeding, and gingival crevicular fluid (GCF) volume and that the duration of the use of these drugs is associated strongly with gingival inflammation severity. Another study suggests there may be an association between periodontal disease and an increased time to conceive. This study found that, on average, a woman with periodontal disease took an extra 2 months to conceive compared with women who did not have periodontal disease. The study also confirmed that other negative influences including an age more than 35 years, being overweight or obese, and being a smoker contribute negatively to conception.[8] Educating clients who are experiencing infertility and those who are seeking treatment about these findings protects the creation of new life and helps to maintain optimal oral and systemic health. Assisting women who are undergoing fertility treatments to achieve optimal oral health prevents associated risks and contributes to lower caries risk in the infant.

Preterm, Low-Birthweight Infants and Periodontal Status

Research has indicated that periodontal infection may be a possible risk factor for preterm, low-birthweight (PLBW) babies (see Chapter 20). Studies demonstrate an association between infection and PLBW babies, specifically genitourinary infections. Infections cause a faster-than-normal increase in the levels of prostaglandin E_2 (PGE_2) and tumor necrosis factor (TNF)–α, molecules that induce labor. PGE_2 is similar in chemical structure to Pitocin (oxytocin), a drug used to induce labor. Other risk factors for PLBW babies include maternal age, cigarette smoking, alcohol use, and drug abuse; multifetal pregnancies; medical problems of the mother such as hypertension; diabetes mellitus; infections; heart, kidney, or lung problems; and an abnormal placenta, uterus, or cervix. With proper precautions, dental care and nonsurgical periodontal therapy is safe and effective during pregnancy, especially during the second trimester.

This topic is currently under debate because of the fact that studies conclude insufficient evidence to indicate that treatment of periodontitis reduces the risk of preterm birth. Treatment may decrease the risk of preterm birth for women at risk of PLBW including women who have previously experienced it or miscarried. Future research is needed to determine the population where risk reduction may be possible.[9]

Menopause

Menopause begins 10 years before the cessation of the menses (menstruation) and continues for about 10 years after. **Perimenopause** consists of the years immediately preceding menopause; **postmenopause** consists of the years after menopause. Most investigators believe that the physical changes accompanying menopause are primarily a result of decreased estrogen production by the ovaries and possibly an increased secretion of gonadotropins, the hormones of the anterior pituitary gland that stimulate the gonads. After menopause, estradiol, the most potent naturally occurring estrogen, ceases to be the major circulating estrogen and is replaced by estrone, which is less potent and demonstrates no cyclic changes. Menopause is accompanied by a number of changes attributed to a variety of geriatric, hormonal, and psychosomatic factors. Estrogens promote maturation and keratinization of vaginal mucosa. In menopause there is a decrease in keratinization and vaginal mucosa atrophy associated with a decline in estrogen level.

Oral Manifestations of Menopause

Thinning of the oral epithelial lining and decreased keratinization, oral discomfort such as burning sensations of the tongue (glossodynia), altered taste perception (salty, peppery, sour), xerostomia, and alveolar bone loss associated with osteoporosis are some of the oral changes observed in climacteric women. Most menopausal women with oral discomfort are relieved by systemic or topical estrogen. Oral mucosae, like vaginal mucosae, are stratified squamous epithelium, and similar desquamative patterns are observed. Human gingiva has specific protein receptors for estrogen; therefore estrogens may stimulate the proliferation of gingival fibroblasts and maturation of connective tissue, mainly through their influence on collagen production. Studies have been unable to demonstrate a correlation between ovarian hormone levels and changes in the oral mucosa during menopause.[10]

Although oral healthcare providers may have clients whose chief complaint is burning and painful sensations in the oral cavity, known as **burning mouth syndrome** (BMS),[11] the diagnostic criteria include (1) pain in the mouth that is present daily and persists for most of the day; (2) oral mucosa is of normal appearance; and (3) local and systemic diseases have been excluded. BMS has many synonyms, including sore mouth, sore tongue, glossodynia, stomatodynia, glossopyrosis, stomatopyrosis, or oral dysesthesia. BMS is not the temporary discomfort that many people experience after eating irritating or acidic foods. BMS is characterized by a burning sensation in the oral cavity even though the oral mucosae appear clinically normal. Establishing a prevalence of BMS in the population is challenging because of the difficulty in establishing whether the disease is primary or secondary. In women, BMS is more frequent during menopause, with a peak incidence in the sixth decade of life. BMS appears to affect women more than men, but evidence of BMS in men has been apparent around 30 years of age. The most prevalent site with burning sensations is the lips and anterior two thirds of the tongue. The pain is chronic (at least 6 months), continuous, and progressive throughout the day, with no apparent cause. Temporomandibular joint (TMJ) pain, facial pain, oral sores, and burning mouth are associated with this syndrome.[11]

Nutritional deficiencies, such as deficiencies of iron, zinc, folate (vitamin B_9), thiamine (vitamin B_1), riboflavin (vitamin B_2), pyridoxine (vitamin B_6) and cobalamin (vitamin B_{12}), may affect oral tissues and cause BMS. These nutritional deficiencies also can lead to vitamin deficiency anemia. BMS also could be due to allergies or reactions to foods, food flavorings, other food additives, fragrances, dyes, or other substances.

Middle-aged women are particularly affected by the condition and are diagnosed with symptoms seven times more frequently than males. Various local, systemic, and psychologic factors may be associated with BMS, but its cause is not understood fully. Identification of symptoms, rather than objective clinical or laboratory findings, often is used to assess this condition. Therefore treatment addressing these factors has had limited success.

Treatment for BMS usually is directed at correction of detected organic causes or involves the use of tricyclic antidepressants, such as chlorpromazine. Interventions may include instruction in proper oral hygiene, saliva-stimulating agents such as pilocarpine, over-the-counter (OTC) xylitol-containing gum or mints, or OTC saliva substitutes depending on the salivary dysfunction severity. Antifungal therapy is necessary if candidiasis is diagnosed. In severely distressed persons, local or systemic corticosteroids may be indicated. Lifestyle changes such as refraining from tobacco and alcohol use, dietary modifications, and avoiding toothpastes containing sodium lauryl sulfate should be initiated. BMS remains an enigmatic disease, and there is insufficient evidence to show the effect of any effective treatment.[11] Future treatment may include agents combining antibacterial and anti-inflammatory actions that show promising effects in clients with oral mucosal diseases secondary to salivary hypofunction.

Hormone Replacement Therapy

Hormone replacement therapy, also known as menopausal hormone therapy (MHT), is the replacement of the female hormone estrogen or progesterone, or occasionally testosterone, to control the negative effects of menopause. This therapy once was considered to decrease the chances of developing heart disease, osteoporosis, and cancer while improving women's lives, but controversy surrounds the risks and benefits of HRT, and individual characteristics and preferences may influence decisions to use this therapy. Estrogen replacement therapy is estrogen alone, used by women who have had the uterus removed. Estrogen's effects on bone health and mental well-being are recognized.[12-15]

A Women's Health Initiative (WHI) study examined a large group of women on combination HRT (estrogen 0.625 mg/day plus progestin 2.5 mg/day) compared with a matched group of women on placebo. However, at about the same time that the Heart and Estrogen/Progestin Replacement Study (HERS I and II) reported no increased risk of CVD-related events for women on HRT, the HRT component of the WHI was halted because of the increased incidence of CVD (22%) and breast cancer (26%) in women treated with combination HRT compared with placebo. The risk of stroke was also significantly higher in the HRT group, accounting for a 41% increase.[16]

The WHI trials found no benefit in the use of HRT as a means of primary or secondary prevention of future CVD events.[17] Results of HERS II and the halting of the HRT component of the WHI all point to the same conclusion: HRT is not beneficial in preventing heart disease or stroke and should not be used in postmenopausal women for the sole purpose of heart disease prevention. Moreover, this conclusion is endorsed officially by the American Heart Association. Increased risks linked with HRT relate to 5 or more years of use.

Oral Effects of Hormone Replacement Therapy

Menopausal or postmenopausal women may experience changes in their mouths that may include the following:

- Xerostomia
- Burning mouth syndrome (BMS)
- Dysguesia (altered taste)
- Periodontal disease (estrogen supplementation in women within 5 years of menopause may slow progression of periodontal disease)
- Gingivostomatitis (may affect a small percentage of women; gingivae appear dry or shiny, bleed easily, and range from abnormally pale to deep red; HRT relieves these signs)

HRT is associated with reduced gingival inflammation and a reduced frequency of clinical attachment loss in osteopenic and osteoporotic women in early menopause. HRT may help protect teeth and does not place women at increased risk of developing TMJ disorders.

Osteoporosis

Bone loss is associated with periodontal disease, menopause, and osteoporosis. **Osteoporosis** is a loss of bone mass affecting 25 million Americans; more than 1.3 million fractures that occur each year in men and women are attributed to osteoporosis. With osteoporosis, more bone is being resorbed than formed. Age is the strongest correlate to bone loss, and menopause is the second strongest correlate. Osteoporosis is more prevalent among white and Asian women and those with early menopause, fair complexions, or small frames. Often osteoporosis may not be detected until a fracture occurs. By this time, significant loss of bone mass has placed the client at risk for future fractures, despite the fact that the original fracture will heal.[19]

Fast and painless tests can diagnose osteoporosis in its early stages: dual-energy x-ray absorptiometry (DEXA or DXA), quantitative computed tomography (QCT), and radiographic absorptiometry (RA). The common x-ray film cannot be used to diagnose osteoporosis early because bone loss must reach at least a 30% level before it is detected radiographically.

The National Osteoporosis Foundation's *Clinician's Guide to Prevention and Treatment of Osteoporosis* represents a major breakthrough in the way healthcare providers evaluate and treat people with low bone mass, osteoporosis, or fracture risks. These guidelines go beyond Caucasian postmenopausal women to include African American, Asian, Latina, and other postmenopausal women and address men age 50 and older for the first time. The *Guide* applies the algorithm on absolute fracture risk called FRAX. Also referred to as a 10-year fracture-risk model and 10-year fracture probability, FRAX estimates the likelihood of a person to break a bone because of low bone mass or osteoporosis over a period of 10 years.[19]

Management of Osteoporosis

Treatment for osteoporosis includes decreasing risk factors and maximizing protective factors, that is, via a calcium- and vitamin D–rich diet plus supplementation (see Chapter 35), weight-bearing exercises, HRT, and drug therapy such as raloxifene (Evista), calcitonin, and sodium fluoride. Evista, a monaminobisphosphonate, inhibits bone breakdown and has been approved by the FDA for prevention and treatment of postmenopausal osteoporosis. Calcitonin, FDA approved in injectable and nasal forms, slows bone breakdown and reduces pain of fractures. Sodium fluoride has been used to stimulate bone formation in the vertebrae, to treat osteoporotic spine fractures, and to prevent fractures at that site.

ERT can decrease the rate of bone resorption, but it cannot replace lost bone. Estrogens affect bone indirectly by interacting with the hormones that control calcium metabolism. HRT has been shown to be beneficial for bone density and architecture. It retards bone loss in postmenopausal women, making bone fractures less likely. All risks and benefits must be evaluated before a woman starts any HRT.

New Risks with Osteoporosis Treatment

Bisphosphonates are a class of synthetic antiresorptive medication given orally or parenterally to clients who exhibit increased bone resorption and are used primarily to increase bone mass and reduce the risk for fracture in persons with osteoporosis. Bisphosphonates also are used to slow bone turnover in individuals with Paget's disease of the bone and to treat bone metastases and lower elevated levels of blood calcium in patients with cancer. Seven FDA-approved bisphosphonates are aminobisphosphonates (nitrogen-containing): alendronate (Fosamax, Fosamax Plus D), etidronate (Didronel), ibandronate (Boniva), pamidronate (Aredia), risedronate (Actonel, Actonel with Calcium), tiludronate (Skelid), and zoledronic acid (Reclast, Zometa).

Significant concern exists in dentistry about the risk of bisphosphonates in the development of osteonecrosis of the jaw (ONJ). Bone necrosis of the jaw, resulting from bisphosphonate therapy, is referred to in a variety of different terms. The American Association of Oral and Maxillofacial Surgeons (AAOMS) refers to the disorder as *bisphosphonate-related osteonecrosis of the jaw* (BRONJ), whereas the most recent November 2011 guidelines from the American Dental Association (ADA) Council on Scientific Affairs adopted the term *antiresorptive agent-induced ONJ* (ARONJ).[20] Although severe musculoskeletal pain is mentioned in the prescribing information for all bisphosphonates, the association between bisphosphonates and severe musculoskeletal pain may be overlooked by healthcare professionals, delaying diagnosis, prolonging pain and/or impairment, and necessitating the use of analgesics. ARONJ may include numbness, tooth mobility, soft-tissue swelling, and sequestra of bones and lesions of exposed bone in the mylohyoid ridge that do not heal. Evidence on the risk of ARONJ is compelling for clients on intravenous bisphosphonate therapy. The long half-life of bisphosphonate in bones justifies the need for long-term studies on its safety. Some physicians recommend using raloxifine hydrochloride (Evista), because these have not been associated with ARONJ and have been approved to prevent and treat osteoporosis. For individuals receiving oral bisphosphonates, care should include the following:

- Eliminating disease (caries, gingival, and periodontal disease) to reduce the need for future extractions or dental implants
- Education about risk for ARONJ and signs of the disease
- Oral health promotion
- Obtain informed consent for all dental procedures
- Delay bisphosphonate therapy until 3 months after dental surgery

Practitioners should keep in mind that ARONJ can develop in an "at-risk" client after routine dental care.

The FDA is investigating reports of increased rates of atrial fibrillation that is life-threatening or results in hospitalization or disability. Researchers in two different studies of older women with osteoporosis treated with the bisphosphonate Reclast or Fosamax have raised questions about the association of atrial fibrillation with bisphosphonate use.[21] In both studies the following occurred:

- More women who received one of the bisphosphonates (Reclast, 1.3%; Fosamax, 1.5%) reportedly developed serious atrial fibrillation as compared with women who received placebo (Reclast study, 0.5%; Fosamax study, 1.0%).
- The rates of all atrial fibrillation (serious plus nonserious) were not significantly different between groups treated with bisphosphonates versus placebo.

The FDA has reviewed some safety data and requested additional data to further evaluate the risk of atrial fibrillation in patients who take bisphosphonates.

Antiresorptive Agent-Induced Osteonecrosis of the Jaw

As mentioned, bisphosphonates are a class of agents used to treat osteoporosis, Paget's disease, and malignant bone metastases. The efficacy of these agents in treating and preventing the significant skeletal complications associated with these conditions has had a major positive impact for patients and is responsible for the widespread use of the agents in medicine. Despite this benefit, antiresorptive agent-induced ONJ (ARONJ) has emerged as a significant complication in a subset of patients receiving these drugs. The most current position paper from the AAOMS delineates three characteristics that must be present to meet the definition of antiresorptive osteonecrosis of the jaw (ARONJ): (1) current or previous treatment with a bisphosphonate, (2) exposed bone in the maxillofacial region that has persisted for more than 8 weeks, and (3) no history of radiation therapy to the jaws.[20] ARONJ looks very much like osteoradionecrosis (ORN); however, involvement of the mandible is extremely rare in ORN but is more common in ARONJ. Based on a growing number of case reports and institutional reviews, bisphosphonate therapy may cause exposed and necrotic bone that is isolated to the jaw with the most common site being the mandibular posterior lingual region close to the mylohyoid ridge. As ARONJ progresses, exposed bone with smooth or ragged borders becomes apparent clinically.[20] Bone lesions vary in color from yellow to grayish-tan and often present with fragmented friable soft tissue. With progression, pain may increase because of inflammation and secondary infection.[20] This complication usually arises after simple dentoalveolar surgery and significantly affects quality of life for most patients. This complication appears to be related to the long half-life of bisphosphonates, the profound inhibition of osteoclast function (prolonged reduction in bone turnover and bone remodeling), and reduced bone quality and strength.[20] Conversely, studies reveal that intravenous bisphosphonate therapy strongly increases the risk of adverse jaw outcomes but that oral bisphosphonates tend to decrease the risk. Intravenous bisphosphonate usually is used to treat bone cancer or severe cases of osteoarthritis. The clinical implications seem to suggest a low incidence of ARONJ, which should be assessed in the context of the clinical benefit of zoledronic acid therapy in reducing hip, vertebral, and nonvertebral fractures in an at-risk population.[22] There is no evidence to suggest that healthy patients with osteoporosis who are receiving bisphosphonate require any special treatment beyond routine dental care or to support altering standard treatment practices, but the clinician must be aware of potential complications. A complete dental assessment (including dentures to ensure proper fit) and elimination of dental disease should be performed before initiation of bisphosphonate therapy; the dentist, dental hygienist, and physician should work collaboratively to ensure that benefits and risks are considered for each client. Currently there is no well-defined effective therapy for treating ARONJ, and more research is needed to determine if treatments given have been beneficial. The ADA recommends that a national registry be created to allow for the study of ARONJ cases.[21]

Dental Implants and Osteoporosis

Some research suggests implants increase risk, whereas other research suggests there is minimal concern. Osteoporosis is not a likely risk factor for failure of osseointegrated dental implants. In fact, the placement of dental implants could aid in maintaining the height and density of alveolar bone. The act of chewing leads to more pressure on the alveolar bone, causing bone remodeling that minimizes or counteracts physiologic age-related bone loss. Osteoporotic bone does not heal differently than bone with more density (see Chapter 58).

Osteoporosis and Periodontal Bone Loss

Loss of teeth and residual ridge resorption are problems associated with oral bone loss. Several studies have linked oral bone loss with systemic bone loss; therefore osteoporosis may affect periodontal bone loss. For example, generalized bone loss from systemic osteoporosis may render jaws susceptible to accelerated alveolar bone resorption. Although osteoporosis is not a causative factor in periodontitis, it may affect the severity of the disease in pre-existing periodontitis and is probably important in the creation of a susceptible host.

HRT and ERT protect against osteoporosis.[15] The Nurses' Health Study examined risk of tooth loss in relation to hormone use in 42,171 postmenopausal women and found that the risk of tooth loss was lower in women taking HRT or ERT. The risk of tooth loss was lower among postmenopausal hormone users, with the most substantial decrease occurring among current users; risk of tooth loss did not appear to change with duration of current or past estrogen use. In addition, greater periodontal attachment loss is found in women with osteoporotic fractures than in normal women. As healthcare professionals, dental hygienists are alert to any rapid changes in alveolar bone, periodontal attachment level, and/or tooth mobility in postmenopausal women and make appropriate referrals for a medical diagnosis.

Domestic Violence

See Chapter 60.

Infant and Child Care

The American Academy of Pediatric Dentistry recommends that a child's first dental examination occur when the first tooth appears or no later than the first birthday.[23] Recent studies note that a majority of pediatricians and general dentists are not advising patients to see a dentist by 1 year of age, which points to the need for increased infant oral healthcare education in the medical and dental communities. To ensure that a child does not experience dental caries or gingivitis, effective oral hygiene routines should be established in infancy and continued throughout life. When a woman is pregnant, she is receptive to advice on the care of her unborn child. New mothers are also receptive in most cases and should be informed of the potential vertical transmission of oral microorganisms from themselves to their infants. Dental neglect can lead to pain, infection, loss of function, and even death. These undesirable outcomes can adversely affect learning, communication, nutrition, and other activities necessary for normal growth and development. The information in Box 54-2 can be shared with pregnant clients, parents, and caregivers of small children.

Early Childhood Caries

Early childhood caries (ECC) is a preventable dental condition that can destroy the teeth of an infant or young child, can cause pain and disfigurement, and, if left to progress, is expensive to treat. ECC is caused by prolonged and repeated exposure of a tooth to fermentable carbohydrates, such as those contained in infant formula, milk, and fruit juice, which ferment in contact with *S. mutans.* The maxillary anterior teeth are the most susceptible to damage, but other teeth also may be affected. Long-term effects of ECC include a higher incidence of orthodontic problems and possible psychologic and social problems that affect children who suffer embarrassment over their appearance (see Box 54-2).

Herpetic Infections

An infection prevalent in infants and young children is primary herpetic gingivostomatitis (herpes simplex virus [HSV]–1). Some of the symptoms of HSV-1 in infants include fever, crying, oral pain, and an unwillingness to eat or drink. Gingivae appear intensely red and painful, with blisters on the tongue and lips. Children can be infected with this herpesvirus by sharing toys, washcloths, towels, or toothbrushes with others who may be infected (home or daycare setting).

Parents with herpetic lip sores can infect their babies by mouth kissing. If a child is in daycare, toys, rattles, and sleeping mats should be wiped and cleaned at least twice a day with a diluted bleach solution to prevent transfer of pathogenic microorganisms.

For other women's healthcare issues, see Chapters 48 and 53 on autoimmune diseases and eating disorders, respectively.

CLIENT EDUCATION TIPS

- Reassure client that information will be kept confidential, but that it is important to identify products used, including over-the-counter and prescription medications,

BOX 54-2

Strategies to Decrease Incidence of Early Childhood Caries and to Promote Healthy Oral Care for Life

Infants (Birth to 1 Year of Age)

- Determine if the water supply that serves the client's home is fluoridated accurately.
  - If there is an inadequate amount resulting from filtration or lack of fluoride in the water, then discuss supplemental options with the parent. Fluoride also is found in over-the-counter mouth rinses, some bottled waters, foods, and beverages (see Chapter 35).
  - Also determine if there is too much fluoride serving the home.
- Establish a dental home before 12 months of age.
- Put babies to bed without a bottle or with a bottle containing only water; do not let babies fall asleep with a bottle containing formula, milk, fruit juice, or other carbohydrate-dense liquid in the mouth. This is especially important because of decreased saliva flow during sleep and an opportunity for disease-causing bacteria to grow.
- Encourage children to drink from a cup as they approach their first birthday; wean children from bottle at 12 to 14 months of age.
- Instead of pacifying a baby with a bottle, rely on strategies such as cuddling, patting, talking, singing, reading, or playing.
- Give babies a clean pacifier. Do not give them pacifiers that have been dipped in sugar, honey, syrup, juice, soda, or other sugary substances or that have been "cleaned" in the mother's or father's mouth.
- Never "clean off" a pacifier in another person's mouth. This practice can infect a baby's mouth with bacterial pathogens that cause dental caries and periodontal disease (vertical transmission of disease from parent or caregiver to infant).
- Never share eating utensils with an infant. Infectious *Streptococcus mutans,* the initiators of the caries disease process, can be transferred from the parent's mouth to the baby's mouth. Caries can develop as early as 11 months of age. The danger of infecting an infant's teeth is increased when the mother already has dental caries herself (vertical transmission of disease).
- Cleaning a child's teeth after ingestion of sugar-containing medication can prevent caries formation. Many over-the-counter medications and prescription drugs such as oral antibiotic liquid formulations contain up to 50% sucrose.
- Consult with a dentist and pediatrician about the need for fluoride supplementation and/or home-use fluoride gels if the fluoride history reveals a fluoride deficiency (see Chapter 12, section on dental history, and Chapter 33).
- Even before teeth begin to erupt, thoroughly clean the infant's gums after each feeding with a water-soaked infant washcloth or gauze pad to stimulate the gum tissue and remove food. When the baby's teeth begin to erupt, brush them gently with a small, soft-bristled toothbrush.
- Schedule regular oral health appointments starting around child's first birthday. The oral health professional checks for cavities in the primary teeth and watches for developmental problems, as well as helps to create a positive experience that may alleviate fear at future visits.
- Fluoride varnish can be used on very young children who are at moderate to high risk of early childhood caries.
- The use of 0.12% chlorhexidine gel or rinse is an intervention for early childhood caries because it inhibits growth of *S. mutans.*
- Thumbsucking should be discouraged after age 4; most children stop by age 2.

Children (2 to 8 Years of Age)

- Do not use fluoridated toothpaste until age 2 to 3 years (unless at a moderate to high risk of caries); fluoride is also found in some over-the-counter mouth rinses, community water supplies, some bottled waters, and some foods.
- Begin teaching the child to expectorate (spit out) the toothpaste and do not use fluoridated toothpaste until the child can accomplish the task successfully.
- Using a small amount (size of a small pea or a smear) of fluoridated toothpaste inhibits decay and minimizes the chance of developing fluorosis when used after 2 to 3 years of age.
- When child is 2 or 3 years old, begin to teach child proper brushing techniques. But remember, parents or caregivers need to follow up with brushing and gentle flossing until age 7 or 8, when the child has the dexterity to do it alone.
- Children should be supervised when using fluoridated toothpaste and oral rinses. If not monitored, they may swallow over four times the recommended daily amount of fluoride.
- Keep dentifrices and oral rinses away from children to avoid accidental ingestion.
- Xylitol-containing gum and mints (1.55 g therapeutic dose at least four to five times daily throughout the day) is used as a healthy treat to inhibit growth of *S. mutans.*
  - Candies and gums should be given only to children who can manage these supplements properly and should be supervised by an adult to avoid choking hazards.
- Sealant applications are used to protect the chewing surfaces of children's teeth.
- Educate the child on limiting use of highly refined carbohydrates (especially sodas, fruit juices, and sports drinks) from vending machines.
- Promote prevention of dental and orofacial athletic injuries in children's sports.
- Encourage the child to discuss any fears about oral health visits; do not mention the word *hurt* or *pain.* Saying "it won't hurt" instills the possibility of pain in the child's thought process.

vitamins, herbs, supplements, and alcohol, to ensure proper care.

- Maintenance of oral health by thorough daily toothbrushing, interdental cleaning, tongue cleaning, and use of an antimicrobial mouth rinse and xylitol products translates to a healthier mouth and body.
- Inform clients about warning signs of heart disease: shortness of breath, nausea, major fatigue, chest pain, mandibular pain, back pain, fainting spells, or gas-like discomfort.
- Inform clients that the American Dental Association and American Academy of Pediatric Dentistry recommend

that a child's first dental examination occur when the first tooth appears or no later than the child's first birthday.

- Explain that the developing fetus is especially susceptible to the effects of radiation, particularly during the first 2 to 18 weeks of development. However, safety features in use such as high-speed film, filtration, long cone rectangular collimation, lead aprons, and thyroid collars significantly decrease radiation exposure. The current recommendation is that no radiographs be exposed in the absence of clinical signs and symptoms. However, if diagnostic radiographs are needed for the pregnant woman, she must be protected properly by a protective apron and a thyroid collar and current standards for radiation safety must be maintained to minimize harm to the fetus.

LEGAL, ETHICAL, AND SAFETY ISSUES

- Respect client confidentiality regarding issues such as oral contraceptives, reproductive health, and domestic abuse.
- Advise clients that systemic antibiotic use can render oral contraceptives ineffective and that an alternative contraceptive method should be considered when antibiotics are taken.
- Consult with obstetrician of record when planning dental hygiene care for pregnant women.
- Report suspected abuse to the proper authorities: child protective services within a Department of Social Services, Department of Human Resources, or Division of Family and Children Services. In some states, police departments also may receive reports of child abuse or neglect. Call Childhelp, 800-4-A-Child (800-422-4453), or the local Child Protection Agency. Take a complete health history, and ask specific questions about drugs, herbs, vitamins, fluoride, and other supplements. The safety of most natural or herbal remedies is unknown because they are not controlled by the U.S. Food and Drug Administration (FDA).
- Ask clients if they have ever taken Phen/Fen, and advise them of the FDA reports of valvular heart disease in women treated for obesity with a combination of fenfluramine and phentermine.
- Make appropriate referrals and initiate consultations with other healthcare professionals as needed.

KEY CONCEPTS

- Women may have different risks for, and symptoms of, heart disease. Heart disease is more severe among women over age 60 than among men of the same age, and women are twice as likely as men to die within 60 days of suffering a heart attack.
- Women are the fastest-growing population of those infected with human immunodeficiency virus (HIV) and acquired immunodeficiency syndrome (AIDS).
- Women live longer and have more chronic disabilities than men.
- Cancer, menopause, cardiovascular disease, diabetes, osteoporosis, autoimmune diseases, and domestic abuse are important issues in women's health and have systemic and oral implications.
- Female dental personnel and the unexposed partners of male dental personnel have cause for concern about regular nitrous oxide–oxygen (N_2O-O_2) analgesia during pregnancy. Difficulty conceiving and birth defects have been documented to occur with its regular use.
- Mechanized instruments are safe to use for clinicians and clients who are pregnant.
- The current recommendation that no radiographs be exposed in the absence of clinical signs and symptoms is particularly important when treating the pregnant client. If diagnostic radiographs are needed, the pregnant woman must be protected properly by a protective apron and a thyroid collar, and current standards for radiation safety must be maintained to minimize harm to the fetus.
- N_2O-O_2 analgesia is safe for use by lactating women; its use is limited to one 30-minute exposure for pregnant women because of risk of birth defects and spontaneous abortion.
- Pregnancy-associated gingivitis is the most prevalent oral manifestation of pregnancy. It often is due to poor oral hygiene, local irritants, sex steroid hormones that serve as bacterial nutrients, and increases in *Tannerella* species and *Prevotella intermedia.*
- As estrogen levels increase, so does the prevalence of *Tannerella* species, *P. intermedia,* and gingivitis. Bacteria associated with increased estrogen levels have been implicated in periodontal disease.
- Sex steroid hormones (estrogen and progesterone) appear to stimulate key factors in the inflammatory response.
- The connection between periodontal infections and adverse pregnancy outcomes is supported by epidemiologic studies. The association is even stronger in women whose periodontal disease is progressing or getting worse.
- Early childhood caries (ECC) is a preventable dental disease that can destroy the teeth of an infant or young child, can cause pain and disfigurement, and, if left to progress, is expensive to treat.
- A prenatal oral prevention program for pregnant women could include increased frequency of periodontal debridement, effective brushing and interdental cleaning, use of xylitol-containing gum and mints, at-home fluoride rinses or gels, antimicrobial rinses, nutritional counseling, infant oral care, and prevention of ECC in preparation for the baby's arrival. Evidence supports the use of 0.12% chlorhexidine mouth rinse and xylitol-containing gum (1.55 g therapeutic dose) during the last 3 months of pregnancy and for 6 months after birth to decrease risk of *Streptococcus mutans* transmission from mother to infant.
- Osteoporosis is not a causative factor in periodontitis but may affect the severity of the disease in pre-existing periodontitis and is probably important in the creation of a susceptible host. Loss of teeth and residual ridge resorption are associated with oral bone loss.
- Osteoporosis is not a risk factor for failure of osseointegrated dental implants. Placement of dental implants may aid in maintaining height and density of alveolar bone.
- Dental hygiene care should include counseling clients about prevention of disease and the oral health–systemic health link, referring to other healthcare providers for assessment and care, and providing tobacco cessation counseling.

- Rapid oral bone loss can indicate systemic osteoporosis. Dental hygienists should be alert to rapid changes in alveolar bone, periodontal attachment level, and/or tooth mobility in postmenopausal women and make appropriate referral to a physician for a medical examination.
- Healthcare professionals, in collaboration with clients, should make treatment decisions. Although a part of the decision-making process, insurance company coverage should not dictate treatment decisions.

CRITICAL THINKING EXERCISES

Scenario 1: Amy, a 16-year-old female client, arrives for her continued-care appointment 2 months late, although she is scheduled every 6 months. After a review of her health, dental, and pharmacologic history, a clinical examination is performed to reveal plaque-induced gingivitis throughout with moderate to heavy bleeding (GI score, 2.0). No periodontal pockets are noted, and her self-care appears adequate. Because of her heavy gingival bleeding, the health history is reviewed again. Amy reiterates that she is not taking any medication, nor has she been diagnosed with any illnesses in the last 8 months.

1. What specific questions could be asked to elicit needed information?
2. Is there concern about client confidentiality?
3. Should Amy's parents be consulted?

Scenario 2: Margie Alexander, a 25-year-old female client, arrives for her 6-month periodontal maintenance appointment. Ms. Alexander's health history is noncontributory, other than that she is in her eleventh week of pregnancy. She had a full-mouth series of radiographs 1 year ago, and her chief complaint is pain in tooth 30. Clinical examination reveals 3- to 4-mm probing depths throughout and bleeding on probing in tooth 14-M (4 mm) and 2-D.

1. What radiographs, if any, should be advised and why? Is it safe to expose radiographs during pregnancy?
2. What discussion should take place between the dental hygienist and the client?
3. Should any other healthcare provider be consulted?

Scenario 3: The practicing dental hygienist is pregnant and concerned about her time in the oral care environment. The dental hygienist heard that exposure to radiation, chemicals in the office, N_2O-O_2, and ultrasonic scaling units may cause birth defects or spontaneous abortion.

1. Are the above concerns substantiated by research evidence in the literature?
2. What precautions, if any, should the dental hygienist take to manage client risks?

Scenario 4: Rose Oliveri, a 50-year-old female client, visited the office after a 1-year hiatus. Her chief complaint is, "My teeth seem to be moving and I don't like it." Her health history reveals that she is taking hormone replacement therapy (estrogen and progestin), a multivitamin, and numerous herbal supplements. Her oral examination reveals probing depths from 3 to 6 mm, with a GI score of 1.0. Her self-care appears to be adequate, with a PI score of 1.

1. Based on the assessment data given, what other diagnostic and therapeutic procedures should be undertaken?
2. What additional questions should be asked regarding her health history, and what recommendations should be offered to the client?
3. What referrals should be made?

REFERENCES

1. Olie V, Plu-Bureau G, Conrad J, et al: Hormone therapy and recurrence of venous thromboembolism among postmenopausal women, *Menopause* 18:488, 2011.
2. Mosca L, Benjamin EJ, Berra K, et al: Effectiveness-based guidelines for the prevention of cardiovascular disease in women: 2011 update, *J Am Coll Cardiol* 57:1404, 2011.
3. Hannaford PC: Epidemiology of the contraceptive pill and venous thromboembolism, *Thromb Res* 127:S30, 2011.
4. Little JW, Falace DA, Miller CS, et al: *Dental management of the medically compromised patient*, ed 8, St Louis, 2012, Mosby.
5. The Centers for Disease Control and Prevention (CDC). *Radiation and pregnancy: a fact sheet for the public*. Available at: www.cdc.gov/netinfo.htm. Accessed on April 12, 2013.
6. American Dental Association Council on Scientific Affairs and U.S. Department of Health and Human Services, Public Health Service, Food and Drug Administration: *Dental radiographic examinations: recommendations for patient selection and limiting radiation exposure*, 2012.
7. Haytaç MC, Cetin T, Seydaoglu G: The effects of ovulation induction during fertility treatment on gingival inflammation, *J Periodontol* 75:805, 2004.
8. Hart R, Doherty DA, Pennell CE, et al: Periodontal disease: a potential modifiable risk factor limiting conception, *Hum Reprod* 27:1332, 2012.
9. Kim AJ, Lo AJ, Pullin DA, et al: Scaling and root planing treatment for periodontitis to reduce preterm birth and low birth weight: a systematic review and meta-analysis of randomized controlled trials, *J Periodontol*, 2012.
10. Meurman JH, Tarkkila L, Tiitinen A: The menopause and oral health, *Maturitas* 63:56, 2009.
11. Torgerson RR: Burning mouth syndrome, *Derm Therapy* 23:291, 2010.
12. Rossouw JE, Anderson GL, Prentice RL, et al: Risks and benefits of estrogen plus progestin in healthy postmenopausal women: principal results from the Women's Health Initiative randomized controlled trial, *JAMA* 288:321, 2002.
13. Hully S, Grady D, Bush T, et al: Randomized trial of estrogen plus progestin for secondary prevention of coronary heart disease in postmenopausal women: Heart and Estrogen/Progestin Replacement Study (HERS) Research Group, *JAMA* 280:605, 1998.
14. Grady D, Herrington D, Bittner V, et al: Cardiovascular disease outcomes during 6.8 years of hormone therapy: Heart and Estrogen/Progestin Replacement Study Follow-up (HERS II), *JAMA* 288:49, 2002.
15. Prentice RL, Chlebowski RT, Stefanick ML, et al: Estrogen plus progestin therapy and breast cancer in recently postmenopausal women, *JAMA* 289:3243, 2003.
16. Wassertheil-Smoller S: Effect of estrogen plus progestin on stroke in postmenopausal women—the Women's Health Initiative: a randomized trial, *JAMA* 289:2673, 2003.
17. Nelson HD, Humphrey LL, Nygren P, et al: Postmenopausal hormone replacement therapy: scientific review, *JAMA* 288:872, 2002.
18. Hammond C, Wild R, Fiorica R: *Straight talk on HRT: benefits and limitations*. Available at: http://www.medscape.com/viewprogram/271. Accessed October 31, 2012.
19. National Osteoporosis Foundation: *Disease statistics "fast facts."* Available at: http://medschool.creighton.edu/fileadmin/user/medicine/images/Creighton_FIRST/Osteo_Spotlight/Fast_Facts.pdf. Accessed October 21, 2012.

20. Ruggiero SL, Dodson TB, Assael LA, et al: American Association of Oral and Maxillofacial Surgeons. Position paper on bisphosphonate-related osteonecrosis of the jaw—2009 update, *J Oral Maxillofac Surg* 67(suppl 1):2, 2009.
21. Hellstein JW, Adler RA, Edwards B, et al: American Dental Association Council on Scientific Affairs Expert Panel on Antiresorptive Agents: Managing the care of patients receiving antiresorptive therapy for prevention and treatment of osteoporosis: executive summary of recommendations from the American Dental Association Council on Scientific Affairs, *J Am Dent Assoc* 142(11):1243, 2011.
22. Eriksen EF, Díez-Pérez A, Boonen S: Update on long-term treatment with bisphosphonates for postmenopausal osteoporosis: a systematic review, *Bone* Oct. 9, 2013. [Epub ahead of print]. Accessed October, 24, 2013.
23. American Academy of Pediatric Dentistry. Guideline on Periodicity of Examination, Preventive Dental Services, Anticipatory Guidance/Counseling, and Oral Treatment for Infants, Children, and Adolescents. http://www.aapd.org/media/Policies_Guidelines/G_Periodicity.pdf. Accessed October 25, 2012.

ACKNOWLEDGEMENT

The author acknowledges Maria Perno Goldie for her past contributions to this chapter.

EVOLVE RESOURCES

Please visit http://evolve.elsevier.com/Darby/hygiene for additional practice and study support tools.

CHAPTER 55

The Older Adult

Joan I. Gluch

COMPETENCIES

1. Explain demographic characteristics and their implications for older adult care.
2. Define the following: geriatrics, gerontology, chronologic age, and functional age.
3. Describe the different theories on why and how people age.
4. Explain general and oral health assessment procedures and findings for the older adult.
5. Explain the importance of health promotion for the aging client.
6. Discuss oral conditions in the aged, including:
   - Differentiate age-related changes from those that occur as a result of diseases or medications.
   - Explain chronic diseases associated with aging and their implications for dental hygiene care.
7. Explain how the five phases of dental hygiene care—assessment, diagnosis, planning, implementation, and evaluation—are customized for care of the older adult.
8. Discuss community health services.

Dental hygienists face many challenges when they provide care for older adults because of the many biologic, psychologic, and social variations within this population. Older adults are a heterogeneous group owing to their lifetime of unique experiences. Life at any given moment is the result of physiologic capabilities, environmental variables, psychosocial factors, and a sense of one's own skills and alternatives. Therefore the human needs of each older adult must be assessed individually, without prior assumptions based on preconceived stereotypes or myths. The healthcare needs of older adults represent the entire continuum of healthy to severely ill individuals. Dental hygienists are challenged to provide care that often involves complex and multiple medical, social, and psychologic needs and the coordination of multiple levels of healthcare.

Demographic Aspects of Aging

Between 2000 and 2010, the group of individuals 65 years old and older increased at a rate faster than the total population.[1] The population of adults 65 years old and older increased by 15.1% as compared with the total population growth rate of 9.7%, and in 2010, those adults over 65 years of age represented 13% of the total U.S. population.[1] The population of adults age 85 to 94 years has grown the fastest, increasing at a rate of 29.9% from 3.9 million individuals in 2000 to 5.1 million in 2010.[1] This substantial rise in the proportion of adults 65 years and older in the population is projected to continue to increase by 36% to 55 million in 2020 and to 72.1 million by 2030, with older adults projected to make up 19.3% of the population in 2030 (Figure 55-1).[2]

This significant demographic increase is caused primarily by increases in life expectancy rather than an increase in the overall life span. **Life span** is the maximal length of life potentially possible in a species—the age beyond which no one can expect to live. For humans, this number is approximately 110 to 120 years. **Life expectancy** is the average number of years lived by any group of individuals born in the same period and is computed at birth or a specific time point. Individuals born in 1900 had a life expectancy of 47.3 years, which increased to 76.8 years for those born in 2000. For those born in 2009, life expectancy is 80.9 years for women and 76 years for men.[2] Life expectancy at ages 65 and 75 also have increased. In 2009 those individuals who survived to 65 can expect to live an average of 19.2 more years, and those individuals who survived to 75 can expect to live an average of at least 12.9 more years.[2]

The increase in life expectancy is explained by the facts that more people are surviving young life (infant and childhood mortality have declined), fertility rates have decreased, and medical care and technology have improved. In addition, the number of people who reach age 65 years in a given year depends heavily on the number of births 65 years earlier. By 2030, all of the "baby boomers" will be 65 years and over, so there will be a "boom" of older adults increasing at a rate greater than the total population. For example, between 2010 and 2030, the population age 65 and over will increase from 13% to 19.3% of the total population.[2]

Other demographic changes in the older adult population that affect healthcare include the following:

- The older adult population is becoming more racially and ethnically diverse. In 2000 older individuals from minority groups made up 16.3% of the elderly, in 2010 increased to 20%, and the minority older adult group is projected to increase to 24% of elderly over the age of 65 in 2020.[3]
- Elderly women outnumber men, and women are more likely to be widowed at each age group. In 2010 women accounted for 58% of the population age 65 and older and 70% of the population age 85 and older. Women age 65 and older were three times as likely as men of the same age to be widowed—44% as compared with 14% of the men. At age 85 and older the differences increase, because 78% of women at this age group are widows as compared with 42% of men.[3]

Figures, tables, and boxes marked as "e" are available as supplemental material on the Evolve site. Visit http://evolve.elsevier.com/Darby/hygiene to access these materials.

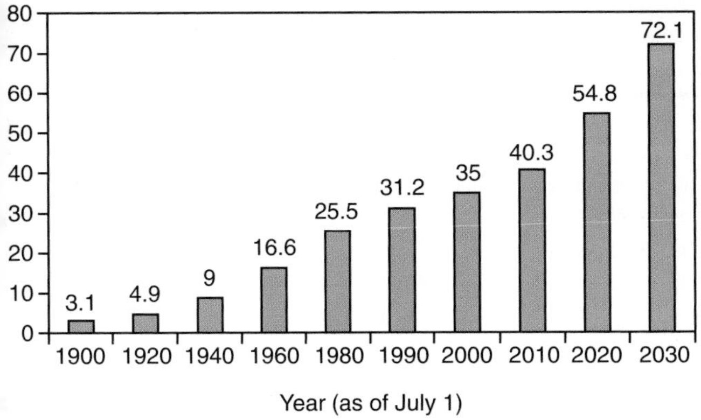

Figure 55-1. Number of older Americans. (From Greenberg S: *A Profile of Older Americans: 2011*. Administration on Aging, U.S. Department of Health and Human Services. Available at: http://www.aoa.gov/aoaroot/aging_statistics/Profile/2011/docs/2011profile.pdf. Accessed March 18, 2013.)

- The older adult population is concentrated in metropolitan areas (78.9%) and in key states. In 2010, 56.5% of the elderly were concentrated in the following 11 states, each with more than 1 million people age 65 and older: California, Florida, New York, Texas, Pennsylvania, Ohio, Illinois, Michigan, North Carolina, New Jersey, and Georgia. In 2010 Florida had the largest proportion of residents aged 65-plus years in the total population (17.3%). Although Alaska was the state with the lowest proportion of elderly residents (7.7%), it also has the largest growth rate for the elderly, growing by 53.9% from 2000 to 2010.[1] As the older population grows in number and age, demands for housing, healthcare, and protective services will increase, particularly in the heavily proportioned states.

These demographic changes in the numbers, composition, and proportion of older adults within the population have a major impact on our society, on healthcare, and on policy implications for federal, state, and local governments.[1] The increase in the population over age 75, in particular, will affect planning for the needs of the aged population, not only for extended care but also for chronic debilitating conditions. Already the increasing number of frail elderly has created changes for nursing home residents. For example, nursing home facilities must ensure that all residents be provided with emergency oral care, be furnished with a referral list of dentists, and have dental care—preventive and therapeutic—as promulgated by the State Medicaid Act.

Healthcare for Older Adults

The terms *geriatrics* and *gerontology* often are used synonymously in discussions of healthcare for older adults, although there is a difference in their implications. Geriatrics is the branch of medicine concerned with the illnesses of old age and their treatment. Gerontology is the scientific study of the factors affecting the normal aging process and the effects of aging. These terms are not interchangeable. A gerontologist is an individual who investigates numerous factors that affect the aging person and the aging process. Gerontologists have divided study of the older population into several categories based on age: young-old (65 to 74 years), middle-old (75 to 84 years), and old-old (85-plus years). Some sociologists have classified those between the ages of 55 and 64 years as the "new-old" and those older than 95 years as the "very old." Whatever terms are used, two important facts exist: (1) characterizations of age should be based on functional ability, not chronologic age, and (2) the majority of older adults perform at a relative level of independent function. Chronologic age refers to age as measured by calendar time since birth, whereas functional age is based on performance capacities. Although a calendar may signify a particular age, functional ability should be the standard that differentiates a person's capability to maintain activity.[4]

Why and How People Age

No single theory can explain why and how people age. Rather, an intermingling of social, psychologic, biologic, environmental, physiologic, and lifestyle factors contributes to the aging process, either in accelerating or in retarding its progress, and produces a different course for each individual.[4] Aging is a progressive yet fluid process, with each factor affecting the others. Understanding the theories of aging—those that have validity and those that contribute to stereotypes—enables the dental hygienist to facilitate human need fulfillment in the older adult through the dental hygiene process of care.

Social Theories of Aging

Social science researchers looking at aging use an interdisciplinary perspective to focus on social, psychologic, and environmental factors that affect the lives of older persons.[4] Dental hygienists, when planning care, must be aware of and consider the dynamic processes that influence each older client. Table 55-1 provides a summary of the three major theories that explain social aspects of aging: disengagement, continuity, and activity theories.[4] Implications for dental hygiene are included within this table to show the application of each of the theories to actions taken during dental hygiene care.

Physiologic Aspects of Aging

Senescence is the term that describes the normal physiologic process of growing old.[4] The fact that everyone, given time, eventually experiences physical changes in all of the body systems makes aging universal. Physical changes that occur are normal for all people, but they take place at various rates and depend on accompanying circumstances (e.g., environmental, psychosocial, lifestyle, and biologic factors) in an individual's life. Typically, normal age changes have been studied in collaboration with pathologic or disease conditions, leading to the misconception that age changes indicate illness or disease. Research continues to uncover evidence that many changes thought to be directly related to the aging process are actually a result of disease or lifestyle influences. For example, a decrease in salivary production was previously thought to be a normal aging feature; however, within the last decade, research has shown that no decrease in salivary production occurs in healthy older adults. Diminished salivary flow is, instead, a by-product of medications or disease.

Biologic Theories of Aging

See the Evolve site at http://evolve.elsevier.com/Darby/hygiene for material on the biologic theories of aging, including eTable 55-2.

TABLE 55-1
Social Theories of Aging

Theory	Hypothesis	Limitation	Dental Hygiene Implication
Disengagement theory	Aging individuals and society gradually withdraw from each other for mutual benefit.	Theory is undermined by the recognition that each individual has a different aging process and that the process often damages the aged and society.	Understand how one's withdrawal from society can affect one's self-concept and motivate behavior. Facilitate human needs for responsibility for oral health and a wholesome facial image.
Activity theory	Aging individuals should be expected to maintain norms of middle-aged: employment, activity, replacement of lost relationships.	Age-related physical, mental, and socioeconomic losses may present barriers to maintaining activity.	Encourage client to seek other support systems to share or continue activities. Discuss appropriate bacterial plaque-control measures and self-examinations.
Continuity theory	Aging depends on a person's psychologic makeup and habitual methods of coping.	Ability to continue in valued social roles depends on an individual's social resources and the opportunities afforded by the social system.	Encourage client to maintain oral wellness. Facilitate human needs for freedom from fear and stress, and responsibility for oral health.

Adapted from Touhy TA, Jett KF: *Ebersole and Hess' gerontological nursing and healthy aging*, ed 8, St Louis, 2012, Mosby.

Health Status and Assessment

Health assessment of older persons always must include a functional appraisal in addition to a review of health, dental, and personal histories.[4] The items generally included within a functional assessment are divided into **activities of daily living** (ADLs) and **instrumental activities of daily living** (IADLs). ADLs are those abilities fundamental to independent living, such as bathing, dressing, toileting, transferring from bed or chair, feeding, and continence. More-complex daily activities, such as using the telephone, preparing meals, and managing money, are examples of IADLs. In 2010 23% of individuals 65 years and over reported limitations in at least one basic action or limitation in complex daily activities.[3] Knowledge of a client's functional abilities helps the dental hygienist customize dental hygiene care, especially in recommending appropriate and realistic preventive homecare routines. In addition, knowledge of functional abilities allows the dental team to identify resources and supports necessary to ensure that the most appropriate level of dental care is provided for the client.

Functional assessment becomes important because the pattern of illness and disease has changed over the past century.[4] Acute conditions were predominant during the early 1900s, whereas chronic conditions present more-prevalent health problems for older adults today. About 80% of seniors have at least one chronic health condition, and 50% have at least two. Five of the six leading causes of death in older adults are chronic diseases. The leading chronic conditions in older adults are arthritis, hypertension and heart disease, cancer, diabetes, and respiratory disorders.[2]

Although the majority of older adults have one or more chronic conditions, most older adults view their health positively. Approximately 72% of older adults living in the community describe their general health as excellent, very good, or good.[2] Little difference exists in perception of health between men and women; however, positive health evaluations decline with age.[2]

Health Promotion and Aging

The increase in numbers and proportion of older adults within the population has coincided with a shifting of priorities to a wellness perspective in health for both consumers and professionals.[4] For the past two decades, efforts to increase the overall health of the nation have been addressed through the ***Healthy People 2020*** initiatives.[5] The health status indicators and focus areas in the *Healthy People 2020* report provide a concrete baseline from which to plan programs, set priorities, and evaluate progress in meeting health objectives and increasing health status.

On the positive side, research indicates that older adults, on average, take better care of their health than does the general population. Individuals of 65-plus years are less likely than younger adults to drink alcohol, be overweight, smoke, or report that stress has affected their health adversely.[4] The lower rates of drinking alcohol and smoking can be attributed to the tendency toward discontinuing these habits in older age, whether done spontaneously or in response to a medical condition or advice, and to the higher mortality rates of those who were drinkers or smokers at younger ages.[4]

Older adults, however, are less likely to engage in regular physical exercise. Inactivity poses serious health hazards to young and old. Lack of exercise can lead to coronary artery disease, hypertension, obesity, tension, chronic fatigue, premature aging, poor musculature, osteoporosis, and inadequate flexibility. Many older adults, and younger adults also, believe that aged individuals are too old to begin or participate in a fitness program; however, research indicates that even those with chronic conditions can benefit from an appropriately designed fitness program.[4]

The dental hygienist as an educator and health promoter can provide appropriate wellness information and reinforce positive lifestyle habits of older clients, thus facilitating the human need for responsibility for oral health, prevention of health risks, and a wholesome facial image.

Oral Conditions in the Aged

As with other physiologic alterations in the body, the distinction between age-related oral changes and those that are disease induced is not always clear or conclusive.[6,7] Disease, consequences of disease, and use of medications often manifest oral changes and pathology independent of the aging process. In the last century, perhaps the most significant change in older adults' oral status is the decline in **edentulousness** (total tooth loss).[6] National data show that in the 65- to 74-year-old age group, edentulousness declined from approximately 50% in 1960 to 24% in 2002, a 50% decrease in prevalence of edentulousness.[6] Changes in treatment philosophies (restore rather than extract), improved treatment modalities, and advances in prevention have played a significant role in reducing tooth loss among older adults, especially the young-old, although significant disparities exist among the current group of older adults, with higher rates of edentulousness (45.3%) seen in low-income individuals with incomes below the poverty level.[6] It is expected that the rate of edentulousness will continue to decline for future cohorts of older adults. Within the focus area of oral health, the *Healthy People 2020* document has identified the target goal of reducing the rate of edentulous older adults to 21.6% of the population.[5]

Dental Changes

Age-Related Changes

With age, teeth undergo several changes, including alterations in the enamel, cementum, dentin, and pulp. Enamel becomes darker in color because of lifetime consumption of stain-producing foods and drink and the formation of secondary dentin. The enamel surface develops numerous cracks (acquired lamellae) and obtains a translucent appearance. The enamel surface has calcium and phosphate constantly demineralized and remineralized during the caries process. During demineralization, the surface appears clinically dull, with slight exploration revealing a chalky surface. Arrested dental caries in older adults often appears as a brownish-black discoloration because of lifelong uptake of stain in enamel lamellae.[7]

Cementum undergoes compositional changes, including an increased fluoride and magnesium content, as individuals age. Abrasion of the crowns of teeth is compensated for by deposition of cementum at the apical end and bifurcated areas of the roots. This secondary cementum normally is deposited slowly and continuously throughout life.[7]

Two independent changes are found within the dentin: secondary dentin formation and obturation of dentinal tubules (dentin sclerosis). As a result, the vitality of the dentin is decreased greatly, and aged dentin may become entirely insensitive and impermeable.[7]

The pulp undergoes the same changes that occur in similar tissues elsewhere in the body: pulpal blood supply decreases, the number of cells decreases, and the number of fibers increases in aged adults. Because pulp calcifications increase with advancing age, the size of the pulp chamber is reduced. Pulp calcifications appear to form in erupted and unerupted teeth.

Attrition is common along the incisal and occlusal surfaces as a result of a lifetime of wear, habits, and dietary factors. Occlusal attrition often smooths the occlusal area, which reduces microbial accumulation in the fissure. These fissures may appear slightly sticky on probing, but they may not need restoring. Therefore vigorous exploring must be avoided in order not to mechanically damage the porous part of the fissure enamel. The attrition present in older individuals is often so severe that dentin is exposed on the incisal and occlusal surfaces.

Many of today's older adults may have used a stiff toothbrush and abrasive toothpaste in the past. Consequently, tooth abrasion, especially in the cervical area and on root surfaces, may be evident.[7] Abrasion, although common among older adults, is the result of a physiochemical process rather than a result of aging. Although modern dentifrices are not sufficiently abrasive to severely damage intact enamel, they can cause remarkable wear of cementum and dentin if the toothbrush is used in a horizontal rather than vertical direction.[7] Dental hygienists can assist individuals in maintaining a biologically sound dentition and freedom from pain through appropriate oral hygiene educational instructions.

Pathology-Induced Changes

Coronal and root caries are active in the older adult population.[6,8] Dental caries once were considered primarily a childhood phenomenon, but research suggests that older adults are more likely to develop new coronal and root caries at a greater rate than the younger population.[8] For example, although 30% of adults ages 18 to 64 had at least one area of untreated decay, 37% of dentate older adults aged 65 to 74 had at least one area of root decay, and 49% of adults 75 years of age or older had at least one area of root decay.[8]

Root caries are most prevalent among older populations because of local oral factors and factors related to aging. Local factors include exposed root surfaces and tooth longevity, and factors related to aging include changes in salivary quantity and composition and inability to complete thorough oral hygiene because of disabilities and chronic conditions. The presence of root caries often indicates disruptions in multiple systems rather than just local factors and requires a multidisciplinary perspective by oral healthcare providers.[8,9] Predictors of caries include the presence of elevated amounts of caries-related bacteria (i.e., *Streptococcus mutans* and lactobacilli), presence of plaque biofilm, presence of restored coronal and root decay, xerostomia, and gingival recession.[9] Root caries can develop rapidly in the absence of inadequate oral hygiene and in the presence of xerostomia, suboptimal periodontal health, and ingestion of fermentable carbohydrates.[10]

Caries control and prevention activities must address three interrelated factors: (1) use of topical fluoride, amorphous calcium phosphate, antibacterial agents, and/or salivary replacement therapy, (2) mechanical removal and chemical control of plaque biofilm, and (3) reduction of refined carbohydrates.[9] Oral hygiene activities often are compromised in older adults because of sensory and neuromuscular changes as a result of aging and/or disease. Use of adaptive devices, such as power toothbrushes and modifications in toothbrush handle size, width, and grip, provides assistance for older adults in thorough plaque removal. Poor dietary practices involving the overconsumption of soft, retentive refined carbohydrates and frequent snacking are often common among older adults and are complicated by salivary changes that promote dental decay.[9,10]

Aggressive caries prevention and management must include risk assessment and frequent and liberal use of topical fluoride products for home use and professional application. In addition to the use of a fluoridated toothpaste, many older adults find 0.05% sodium fluoride rinses easy to use and helpful in caries reduction. Many older adults have difficulty swallowing, however, and prefer the use of the 1.1% sodium or 0.4% stannous fluoride gel, which can be applied directly to the root surfaces and adapted into the proximal surfaces with a toothbrush or small interproximal brush. Professionally applied sodium fluoride in either the 2.0% gel or 5.0% varnish has been shown to be an effective caries-preventive agent for coronal and root caries[9,10] (see Chapters 18 and 33).

Periodontal Changes

Age-Related Changes

There is an increase in alveolar bone porosity and a decrease in cortical width with aging, but this increased porosity has been found to be unrelated to the presence of teeth and does not lead to crestal resorption. Research shows that crestal bone loss with aging is minimal in healthy persons.[7,11] Osteoporosis primarily effects decreases in bone mass and increases in porosity.[11] Also, a reduction in metabolism and reduced healing capacities can influence the quality of bone. Alveolar bone quality can affect significantly the older adult's ability to wear oral prosthetics and achieve proper mastication.

Gingival epithelium reportedly shows no significant morphologic changes with age, although there is evidence of a thinning of the epithelium, diminished keratinization, and increased cellular density. A reduction in cellular elements and an increase in fibrous intercellular substance have been noted in gingival connective tissue. A reduced number of nerves in the gingiva and increased evidence of nerve degeneration with increasing age have been found, along with arteriosclerotic changes in gingival vessels. An increase in gingival width seen with aging has been attributed to growth of the alveolar process, along with eruptive movements of the teeth and supporting tissue.[7]

Alteration in periodontal ligament cellular function, increases in calcification, and arteriosclerosis are seen with advancing age. Numerous morphologic, biochemical, and metabolic changes can be observed in the periodontium with aging, but the overall significance of these factors as they affect susceptibility and periodontal disease progression is unclear. It appears, however, that in the absence of disease the clinical changes in the periodontal structures attributable to aging alone are therapeutically insignificant.[7,9]

Pathology-Induced Changes

Advanced stages of periodontal disease are seen more commonly in people 45 years of age or older; age often is thought erroneously to cause the disease. Research indicates that the effect of age on the progression of periodontitis is negligible when good oral hygiene is maintained and risk factors are decreased. Nevertheless, studies confirm an association between increased age and increased recession, loss of attachment, and higher prevalence of gingival inflammation.[7,11]

The level of periodontal health in middle age can be used as a predictor of periodontal disease in later life.[7,11] Data suggest that the prevalence and severity of periodontal diseases likely will decrease within a few decades as the present younger age groups, with better oral hygiene and less periodontal disease, move into their sixties and seventies.[9]

Dental hygienists should provide aggressive treatment to prevent and control periodontal diseases in older adults. More-frequent dental hygiene care visits provide the opportunity to instruct the older adult in proper oral hygiene, especially in the use of powered toothbrushes, and also in the use of chemotherapeutic agents to control gingivitis, such as triclosan dentifrice and/or essential oil mouth rinse. Prescription of 0.12% chlorhexidine gluconate also may be indicated for older clients who need an additional level of microbial control.[9]

Oral Mucosal Changes

Age-Related Changes

In the absence of disease the oral mucosal status of older adults is comparable to that of younger adults, suggesting that aging alone does not lead to changes in the oral mucosa.[7]

Pathology-Induced Changes

Some mucosal alterations are a result of systemic factors (e.g., xerostomia) and are not related to aging. Systemic disease and medication use cause some older adults to have changes in their oral mucosa, including atrophy of epithelium and connective tissues with a decrease in vascularity. Clinically the oral mucosa appears dry, smooth, and thin. Fungal infections (candidiasis) may result from use of broad-spectrum antibiotics, such as amoxicillin, and xerostomia-causing medications.[10,11]

Lips may appear dry and drawn as a result of dehydration and loss of elasticity within the tissues. Angular cheilitis, commonly evidenced among the aged, clinically appears as fissuring at the angles of the mouth, with cracks, erythema, and ulcerations. Moistness from drooling, deficiency of vitamin B_2 (riboflavin), and infection with *Candida albicans* are the causative factors associated with this condition[8-10] (Figure 55-2).

Ill-fitting dentures or poor denture hygiene also can result in mucosal irritation and infection, including denture stomatitis or candidiasis and denture-induced fibrous hyperplasia. Denture "sore mouth" reflects a commonly seen condition also known as *chronic atrophic candidiasis,* present in as many

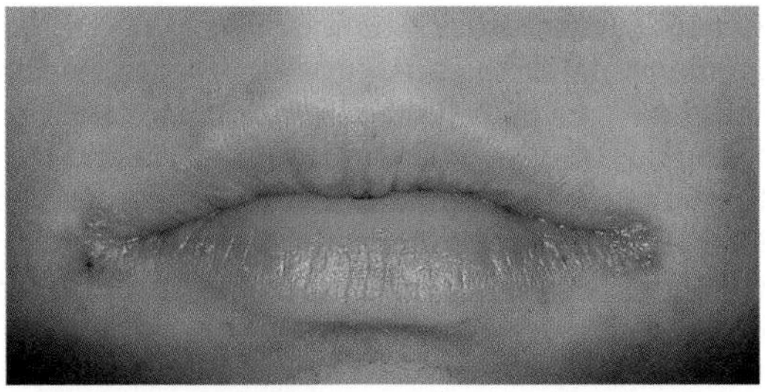

Figure 55-2. Angular cheilitis. (From Ibsen OAC, Phelan JA: *Oral pathology for the dental hygienist,* ed 6, St Louis, 2014, Saunders.)

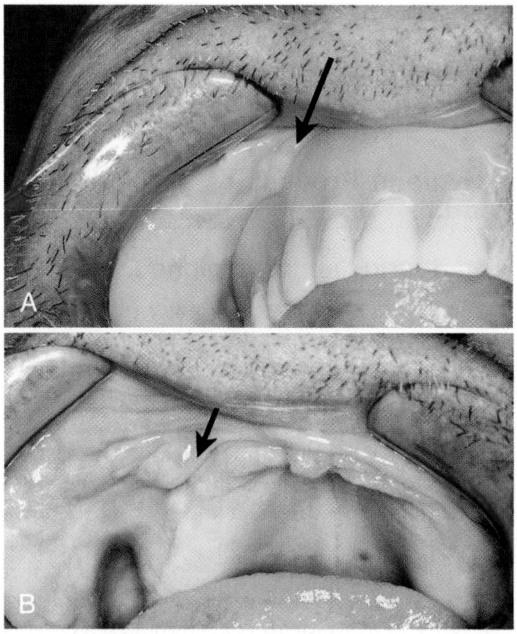

Figure 55-3. Denture-induced fibrous hyperplasia. **A,** With denture. **B,** Without denture. (From Ibsen OAC, Phelan JA: *Oral pathology for the dental hygienist,* ed 6, St Louis, 2014, Saunders.)

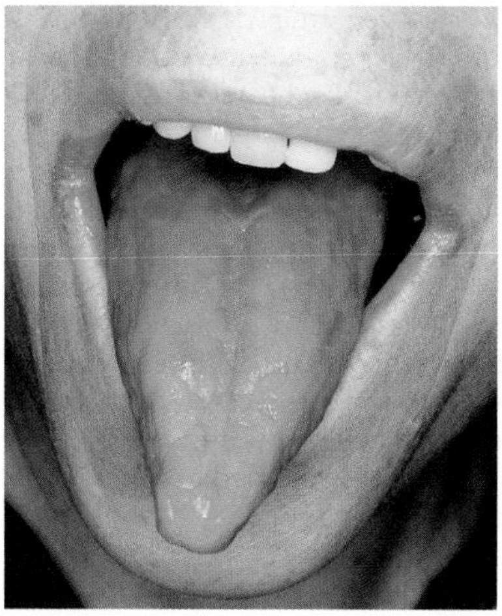

Figure 55-4. Pernicious anemia. The tongue is devoid of filiform papillae. Angular cheilitis is also present. (From Ibsen OAC, Phelan JA: *Oral pathology for the dental hygienist,* ed 6, St Louis, 2014, Saunders.)

as 65% of older individuals who wear dentures. Chronic atrophic candidiasis is associated with poor prosthesis fit, which leads to chronic trauma, and retention of the denture during sleeping hours, which promotes bacterial and fungal growth. The signs of denture-induced fibrous hyperplasia include single or multiple elongated folds near the border of an ill-fitting denture[9,14,15] (Figure 55-3; see Chapter 56).

The human need for skin and mucous membrane integrity of the head and neck necessitates that the dental hygienist provide palliative treatment and refer the individual to the dentist for further evaluation.

Oral cancer continues to be a particular problem for older adults because the average age of diagnosis is 60 years. Oral cancer is more common in men than in women and represents about 2.5% of the total cancers diagnosed each year.[14,15] All older adults should receive a thorough soft-tissue oral examination at each visit so that the dental hygienist can evaluate carefully any early mucosal changes that may indicate precancerous or cancerous lesions and provide early referrals for prompt evaluation and treatment.

Tongue Changes

Age-Related Changes

Changes in the tongue may include a decrease in the number and sensitivity of papillae. Combined with a decline in the sense of smell, some foods have less appeal, and nutritional needs may not be met. Sublingual varicosities are customary findings among the aged; however, they are not problematic. Clinically they appear as deep red or bluish-black dilated vessels on either side of the midline on the ventral surface of the tongue.

Pathology-Induced Changes

Because of nutritional factors, older adults frequently have anemia as a result of iron deficiencies. Atrophic glossitis is a symptom of this condition, and the tongue appears smooth, shiny, and denuded. Often, individuals complain of a burning sensation. In addition, the tongue often increases in size in edentulous mouths or as a result of disease (e.g., pernicious anemia)[8-10] (Figure 55-4). The dental hygienist can assist the individual by recommending an oral lubricant to reduce discomfort and by providing dietary counseling.

Salivary Gland Changes

Research has shown that reductions in salivary flow are not a result of the normal aging process. Rather, decreases in salivary flow usually are attributed to systemic disease, radiation therapy, tumors, or medications that cause temporary or permanent xerostomia.[9,10,12] Signs and symptoms of salivary reduction should be evaluated carefully to determine the cause. In the absence of medications, possible underlying diseases and salivary gland tumors should be investigated.

Sjögren's Syndrome

Sjögren's syndrome is an autoimmune disorder of the salivary glands occurring most frequently in postmenopausal women. Approximately 60% of people with this disorder are older than 50 years. Clinically the oral mucosa is extremely dry and saliva is ropy. Initially the tongue shows marked atrophy of the papillae, and later the surface becomes smooth and lobulated[14,15] (see Chapter 48, Figure 48-7). To meet the need for mucous membrane integrity, persons with Sjögren's syndrome should be instructed to use saliva substitutes and products for dry mouth. For dentate individuals, fluoride therapies (rinses or daily gels) may be recommended to help meet the need for a sound dentition.[12,14,15]

Drug-Induced Oral Changes

Approximately one third of all prescription and over-the-counter drugs are used by older adults, even though these individuals account for only 13% of the population. **Polypharmacy** is the term to describe the common practice of prescribing multiple drugs to clients to manage their many medical conditions.[16] On average, most older adults take more than three therapeutic agents, and the institutionalized elderly use five to seven drugs at the same time. Older clients are more likely to experience adverse reactions because of physiologic changes in the heart, liver, and kidney and also because of the increased exposure and potential for interaction of prescription and over-the-counter medications. Medications most frequently used by older adults include analgesics, diuretics, oral hypoglycemics, antihypertensives, antidepressants, and sedatives. Multiple medical problems, along with multiple drug use, can lead to a high rate of adverse drug reactions. Many drugs produce oral changes in the mouth because of side effects or as a consequence of the actions of the drug.[9,10,16] Dental hygienists play an especially important role in identifying medication usage and potential side effects (see Chapter 14).

Xerostomia

Xerostomia is a common side effect of many prescription and over-the-counter medications, such as antihypertensives, antipsychotics, antidepressives, muscle relaxants, antihistamines, and laxatives. Saliva plays an important role in proper function of the oral cavity because it lubricates the oral mucosa, assisting speech and swallowing, facilitates the retention of oral appliances, and provides a source of minerals for enamel remineralization.[10,12,15] Diminished salivary flow can alter taste, contribute to plaque formation and dental caries, and cause the oral mucosa to appear dry and inflamed. For edentulous persons, denture retention, comfort, and ability to chew and speak may become difficult when less saliva is present.

Management of xerostomia should include palliative care through the use of saliva substitutes, oral lubricants, mouth rinses, and frequent water intake. Attempts to stimulate salivary flow can include the use of xylitol-containing oral care products, candies, or gum, and medications such as the cholinergic agents pilocarpine and bethanechol. Also, consultation with the physician and clinical pharmacist may reveal a substitute medication that may reduce saliva in a less-severe way for the client.[10,12,15]

Clients with xerostomia should return for frequent recall and assessment of caries status. Aggressive caries-prevention efforts should be recommended because the presence of xerostomia places the client in an extreme risk category for caries (see Chapter 18). All of the following caries-prevention efforts are essential for the older adult to control root and coronal caries associated with xerostomia[9,10,12]:

- Daily and thorough brushing with fluoride dentifrice and either high-dose 2.0% sodium or 1.1% stannous fluoride home-use gel and thorough interproximal plaque removal through flossing and/or interproximal brushing
- Frequent use of salivary substitute and dry mouth products
- Nutritional counseling
- Antimicrobial use (e.g., 0.12% chlorhexidine mouth rinses)
- Use of amorphous calcium and phosphate pastes
- Frequent professional debridement
- Frequent professional application of topical fluoride
- Use of xylitol-containing products

Drug-Induced Gingival Enlargement

Persons taking anticonvulsants such as phenytoin may exhibit gingival hyperplasia as a side effect.[15,16] Adequate plaque control, particularly if started before the administration of phenytoin, may reduce the magnitude of gingival enlargement. Also, clients with prescribed cardiovascular drugs (nifedipine) and immunosuppressants (cyclosporine) may exhibit gingival enlargement.[13,14,16]

Dental Hygiene Process of Care with Older Adults

Assessment and Dental Hygiene Diagnoses

Dental hygienists begin their assessment of overall physical factors by observing the older adult in the reception area.[9,13] It is important to observe gait and balance because some elderly persons may require assistance to the treatment area. An arm should be extended for clients who appear unsteady or who have severe visual impairments. The dental chair should be positioned at the level of the knees or higher if the person has difficulty bending the knees. Also, the arm of the chair should be placed back as far as possible. If the client uses a wheelchair, transfer to the dental chair is necessary. The client should be asked if assistance is needed or which method of wheelchair transfer is preferred (see Chapter 42).

Impairments in vision and hearing commonly seen in older adults may necessitate providing assistance in completing any written forms in the office.[9] A health history form in large print allows visually impaired clients to complete the form themselves. At times it may be more effective and efficient to interview older clients. The person should be addressed in a low pitch with the face mask removed. Shouting is unnecessary and ineffective. Background noises such as music should be eliminated if possible. Individuals with hearing aids should be requested to keep them on while the client history is reviewed or oral hygiene methods are discussed; however, the volume should be reduced when a rotary handpiece is used. Older adults accompanied by others should be addressed directly, not the family member or caregiver. By speaking directly to the elderly client, dental hygienists create a respectful, independent environment.[9]

The health history should include the client's personal, medical, and dental background. Personal history, for example, may show that clients are widowed (may live alone, may have reduced income), which could affect their ability to receive dental care. The health history should include previous and past medical conditions. Prescription and over-the-counter medications currently being used must be reviewed for oral implications. Dental hygienists should have readily available a current source for information on medications, such as a reference program, book, or credible website to investigate medications that are unfamiliar or not prescribed as the common drug of choice. Some individuals with more than one disease may experience adverse effects from multiple drug use. The practitioner must consult with the client's physician if there is doubt regarding treatment. Vital signs, including respiration, pulse, blood pressure, and temperature (if indicated), should be evaluated and recorded. In addition to completing a thorough health history, the practitioner should be patient and listen to information that the client shares.

The extraoral examination can reveal abnormalities in the skin of the face and neck, lymph nodes, salivary glands, and underlying muscles.[9,15] The mandible is examined for movement, and the temporomandibular joint should be palpated for crepitation, tenderness, or limitations in movement. A client with arthritis may not be able to open his or her mouth fully.

Lips are evaluated for signs of angular cheilitis, muscle inelasticity, and presence of lesions. A complete dental charting and periodontal assessment are part of every dental history to provide documentation for reevaluation. The saliva quantity and quality are assessed to ascertain if saliva substitutes should be recommended (see Chapter 18).

Radiographs and other diagnostic aids such as study models are used as indicated and appropriate. Referral for biopsy may be indicated for suspicious lesions.

Oral hygiene status including plaque biofilm distribution, calculus, and stains is assessed. Assessment of the client's ability to perform oral hygiene practices is essential. The older person's homecare practices generally should be modified rather than attempts made to change long-term habits completely. Physical changes such as arthritis and impaired vision may affect the client's ability to carry out oral hygiene recommendations.

If the client's vision and dexterity permit, he or she is instructed to perform self-assessments of plaque-control methods and oral soft-tissue examination. Periodic evaluation of bacterial plaque-control measures can be accomplished by using disclosing solution or gingival and plaque indices. Individuals are advised to conduct an oral self-examination monthly to look for lesions that are painless and do not heal within 2 weeks.

The older client's nutritional status should be evaluated because of the many physiologic and psychosocial complexities that have been documented regarding dietary patterns for the elderly[16] (see Chapter 35). Dental hygienists can use the brief nutritional screening questionnaire "Mini Nutritional Assessment" (eFigure 55-5) as part of the health history information; this questionnaire alerts oral healthcare providers to any deficiencies in food intake and related patterns that affect oral health and nutrition. For example, older adults may avoid eating nutritious foods because of decreased oral function or because they are unable or unwilling to cook a full meal because they live alone or cannot shop at the usual location. Merely asking an older adult to describe his or her typical diet often sheds light on multiple issues that affect nutrition and health.[16]

Dental hygienists plan and implement care based on the dental hygiene diagnosis, type and severity of chronic conditions, cognitive abilities and attitudes of the older adult, level of self-care, expectations, and financial ability. Table 55-3 is a presentation of dental hygiene diagnoses related to the older adult. Short morning appointments are recommended because many older adults have a lower stress tolerance and tire more easily than younger people. A written note of date and time of each appointment should be provided to help remind the client and assist caregivers when necessary.

TABLE 55-3

Sample Dental Hygiene Diagnoses Related to the Older Adult

Deficit in the Following Human Need	Cause	Evidence
Wholesome facial image	Ill-fitting dentures	Client's self-report of dissatisfaction with appearance of face and dentures
Freedom from fear and stress	Previous negative dental experiences	Client's report of fear of dentist
Freedom from head and neck pain	Chronic atrophic candidiasis	Client's report of mouth soreness
Protection from health risks	Type 2 diabetes	Client's report of type 2 diabetes
Responsibility for oral health	Inadequate care of mouth and dentures	Stained dentures Chronic atrophic candidiasis Infrequent dental visits
Conceptualization and problem solving	Lack of proper denture and mouth care	Inability to describe appropriate care for mouth and dentures

Planning

Dental hygiene care planning for older adults is often more complex than for younger persons because the vast majority have at least one chronic condition, and many have complex dental and periodontal conditions.[9,11] Also, normal aging alterations may create a compromised oral situation. Treatment modalities must be developed based on individual considerations among the client, dental hygienist, dentist, and at times, the physician and physical and occupational therapists. Table 55-4 provides a general summary of alterations often required in dental hygiene care of older individuals based on common medical conditions.[9,14,15] This summary table will help dental hygienists consider and adapt care customized for the client's medical, dental, and psychosocial needs.

The individual's and his or her family's attitudes toward oral health affects care planning and outcomes. Many older adults view oral problems as an inevitable part of aging. Also, research suggests that older people perceive a lower need for dental care than what actually is required. In addition, cost of care for many is a barrier. Therefore some older adults do not use dental services as frequently as recommended or do so only when dental emergencies occur.[6,9]

Implementation

During instrumentation, as little trauma as possible to the gingiva is required because of reduction in healing capabilities. Loss of elasticity of lips and oral mucosa and xerostomia may make retraction of oral tissues uncomfortable. Older adults with a history of periodontal disease need to be seen for more-frequent periodontal maintenance therapy. Depending on the periodontal classification, scaling should be completed by quadrants to allow for short appointment times.

Text continued on p. 1001

TABLE 55-4
Alterations in Dental Hygiene Care of the Older Adult

Condition	Potential Risk Relating to Dental Hygiene Care	Prevention of Medical Complications	Dental Hygiene Care Plan Modification	Oral Complications
Angina pectoris	Stress and anxiety related to oral healthcare visit may precipitate angina attack in the oral healthcare setting Myocardial infarction may occur when older adult is in the oral healthcare setting Sudden death caused by disruption of cardiac rhythm or cardiac arrest without acute myocardial infarction may occur in the oral healthcare setting	**1.** Detect older adult with history of angina pectoris. **2.** Refer older adult thought to have untreated or unstable angina based on health history for medical evaluation and treatment. **3.** Older adult under medical treatment for angina; during oral healthcare visit, every attempt should be made to reduce stress: a. Concern and warm approach from oral healthcare professionals b. Make older adult feel free to talk about fears c. Morning appointments; however, some evidence supports early afternoon appointments as possibly better. d. Short appointments e. Premedication—diazepam (Valium), 5-10 mg; one tablet preoperatively and/or night before; consider prophylactic nitroglycerin. f. Nitrous oxide–oxygen analgesia or low-flow oxygen via nasal cannula may be beneficial. g. Effective local anesthetic—maximum dose of epinephrine 0.036 mg or levonordefrin 0.20 mg can and should be used; aspirate; inject slowly (do not use vasoconstrictors in patients with a serious arrhythmia). h. Avoid epinephrine-impregnated retraction cords. i. Avoid anticholinergic drugs. j. Daily aspirin or other antiplatelet aggregation drugs do not usually cause clinically significant bleeding. **4.** Reinforce importance of risk factors that can be influenced by older adults. **5.** Terminate appointment if patient becomes fatigued or develops change in pulse rate or volume. **6.** If older adult develops chest pain during hygiene care, stop procedure and give nitroglycerin tablet sublingually. a. If pain is relieved, let older adult rest and then continue with appointment or terminate appointment and reschedule for another day. b. If pain continues longer than 5 minutes, monitor vital signs and give up to two nitroglycerin tablets one at a time during the next 10 minutes; if after three nitroglycerin tablets within a 15-minute time period pain persists and older adult's condition is stable, transport to hospital emergency room and call physician; if patient is unstable, call for medical aid and be prepared to render cardiopulmonary resuscitation.	Older adults with stable form of angina, any routine oral healthcare Older adults with unstable form of angina, only care needed to deal with oral pain and/ or infection	Usually none; however, on rare occasions older adults may have lower jaw pain of cardiac origin (referral pain); history of what initiates the pain and how it is relieved should provide clue to its cardiac origin

TABLE 55-4

Alterations in Dental Hygiene Care of the Older Adult—cont'd

Condition	Potential Risk Relating to Dental Hygiene Care	Prevention of Medical Complications	Dental Hygiene Care Plan Modification	Oral Complications
Congestive heart failure	Sudden death resulting from cardiac arrest or arrhythmia Myocardial infarction Cerebrovascular accident Infection Infective endocarditis (see Chapter 10) Shortness of breath Drug side effects Orthostatic hypotension (diuretics, vasodilators) Arrhythmias (digoxin, overdosage) Nausea, vomiting (digoxin, vasodilators) Palpitations (vasodilators)	**1.** Detect and refer to physician. **2.** No routine dental care until under good medical management. **3.** In older adults under good medical management with no complications, any indicated dental care can be performed. Cause of heart failure and any other complications must be considered in the dental hygiene care plan. a. Hypertension b. Prosthetic cardiac valve, prosthetic cardiac material used for cardiac valve repair, cardiac valvulopathy c. Congenital heart disease d. Myocardial infarction e. Renal failure f. Thyrotoxicosis g. Chronic obstructive lung disease **4.** For older adults in the less-severe stages, Class I and II, use maximum dose of 0.036 mg epinephrine or 0.20 mg levonordefrin; avoid vasoconstrictors in Class III and IV older adults. **5.** Older adults should be in the semi-supine or upright position during care to decrease collection of fluid in lung. **6.** Terminate appointment if older adult becomes fatigued. **7.** Drug considerations: a. Digitalis—older adult more prone to nausea and vomiting b. Anticoagulants—dosage should be reduced so that prothrombin time is two times normal value or less (takes 3 to 4 days) c. Antidysrhythmic drugs (see cardiac arrhythmias) d. Antihypertensive agents (hypertension) e. Avoidance of outpatient general anesthesia	In older adults under good medical management with no complications, any indicated dental care can be performed.	Infection Bleeding Petechiae Ecchymoses Drug-related a. Xerostomia b. Lichenoid mucosal lesions
Hypertensive disease	Stress and anxiety related to oral healthcare visit may cause increase in blood pressure; in older adult with already elevated blood pressure as a result of hypertensive disease, myocardial infarction or cerebrovascular accident may be precipitated. Older adults being treated with antihypertensive agents may become nauseated or hypotensive or may develop postural hypotension.	**1.** Detect and refer older adults with marked elevation of blood pressure and those with moderate prolonged elevation of blood pressure for medical evaluation and treatment. For older adults with blood pressure higher than 180/110, delay elective care and refer to a physician. **2.** Older adults being treated with antihypertensive agents. a. Reduce stress and anxiety of oral healthcare visit by premedication, short appointments, morning appointments, and concerned attitude from oral healthcare professionals; let older adult talk about fears and concerns related to oral healthcare visit; nitrous oxide–oxygen analgesia can be used, but hypoxia must be avoided. b. If older adult becomes stressed, terminate appointment. c. Avoid orthostatic hypotension by changing chair positions slowly and supporting client when he or she gets out of chair.	In older adults under good medical management with no complications, such as renal failure, any indicated treatment may be provided. In older adults with complications, refer for evaluation.	Xerostomia secondary to diuretic agents and other antihypertensive medications Mercurial diuretics may cause oral ulceration or stomatitis Lichenoid reactions may be seen with thiazides, methyldopa, propranolol, and labetalol

Continued

TABLE 55-4

Alterations in Dental Hygiene Care of the Older Adult—cont'd

Condition	Potential Risk Relating to Dental Hygiene Care	Prevention of Medical Complications	Dental Hygiene Care Plan Modification	Oral Complications
	Excessive use of vasopressors may cause significant elevation of blood pressure. Sedative medications used in older adults taking certain antihypertensive agents may bring about hypotensive episodes.	d. Avoid stimulating gag reflex. e. Select sedative medication and dosage cautiously. **3.** Drug considerations: a. Use of local anesthetics with small concentration of vasopressor (epinephrine 0.036 mg; levonordefrin 0.20 mg); aspirate before injection and inject slowly. b. Use caution when using vasoconstrictors in older adults taking a nonselective beta blocker. c. Do not use gingival packing material that contains epinephrine. d. Reduce dose of barbiturates and other sedatives whose actions may be enhanced by many antihypertensive agents. e. Avoid use of general anesthesia in the office.		Lupuslike reaction, rarely seen with hydralazine
Myocardial infarction	Cardiac arrest Myocardial infarction Angina pectoris Congestive heart failure Bleeding tendency secondary to anticoagulant Electrical interference with unshielded pacemaker	**1.** No routine oral healthcare until at least 6 months after infarction because of increased risk of new infarction and arrhythmias. **2.** Consultation with older adult's physician before starting routine oral healthcare to confirm older adult's current status. **3.** Morning appointments **4.** Short appointments **5.** Termination of appointment if older adult becomes fatigued or short of breath or develops change in pulse rate or rhythm; inform physician. If older adult develops chest pain during appointment, manage as described for a client with unstable angina. **6.** Use of local anesthetic with maximum epinephrine 0.036 mg and levonordefrin 0.20 mg; aspirate before injecting; inject slowly; avoid use of vasopressors to control local loss of blood; also avoid use of vasopressors in gingival packing material; do not use epinephrine in local anesthetics with severe arrhythmias. **7.** Premedication before appointment and/or the night before to reduce stress associated with oral healthcare visit—diazepam 5-10 mg. **8.** Anticoagulant medication—if surgery or scaling procedures are planned for older adults taking warfarin, physician should be contacted to confirm that PT ratio (prothrombin time) will be two times normal or less, or international normalized ratio (INR) less than 3.0; patients taking aspirin or other antiplatelet aggregation drug may have increased bleeding, but it is not usually clinically significant.	Older adults 6 months or more after infarction with no complication, any routine oral healthcare can be performed. If complications such as congestive heart failure are present, oral healthcare should be limited to immediate needs only.	

TABLE 55-4

Alterations in Dental Hygiene Care of the Older Adult—cont'd

Condition	Potential Risk Relating to Dental Hygiene Care	Prevention of Medical Complications	Dental Hygiene Care Plan Modification	Oral Complications
		9. Digitalis—older adult more prone to nausea and vomiting; avoid stimulating gag reflex. **10.** Antisialagogues—atropine and scopolamine may cause tachycardia; check with older adult's physician before using. **11.** Antiarrhythmic agents—quinidine, procainamide—nausea and vomiting may occur; hypotension may occur; oral ulceration may indicate agranulocytosis. **12.** Antihypertensive agents (refer to hypertensive disease section in table) **13.** Avoid use of instruments such as ultrasonic scaler with older adults who have unshielded pacemaker.		
Asthma	Precipitation of acute asthmatic attack	**1.** Identify asthmatic older adult by health history. **2.** Determine character of asthma: a. Type (allergic or nonallergic) b. Precipitating factors c. Age at onset d. Frequency and severity of attacks e. How usually managed f. Medications being taken g. Necessity for past emergency care **3.** Avoidance of known precipitating factors **4.** Consultation with physician for severe, active asthma **5.** Older adult should bring medication inhaler to each appointment and use before appointment. **6.** Drug considerations—avoid: a. Aspirin b. Nonsteroidal anti-inflammatory drugs (NSAIDs) c. Narcotics and barbiturates d. Macrolide antibiotics (erythromycin) if older adult is taking theophylline **7.** May want to avoid sulfite-containing local anesthetic solution. **8.** Chronic corticosteroid use may necessitate supplementation. **9.** Premedicate anxious older adult (nitrous oxide–oxygen analgesia or diazepam). **10.** Provide stress-free environment.	None required	Oral candidiasis reported with use of inhaler without spacer but is rare

Continued

TABLE 55-4

Alterations in Dental Hygiene Care of the Older Adult—cont'd

Condition	Potential Risk Relating to Dental Hygiene Care	Prevention of Medical Complications	Dental Hygiene Care Plan Modification	Oral Complications
Tuberculosis	Tuberculosis may be contracted by dental hygienist from actively infectious older adult. Older adults can be infected by oral healthcare professionals.	Many older adults with infectious diseases cannot be identified by history or examination; therefore all older adults should be approached using universal precautions. **1.** In older adults with active sputum-positive tuberculosis: a. Consultation with physician before dental hygiene care b. Care limited to emergency care only c. Care in hospital setting with proper isolation, sterilization, mask, gloves, gown, ventilation d. When older adult produces consistently negative sputum and remains in chemotherapy, is provided same care as normal patient **2.** In older adults with past history of tuberculosis: a. Approach with caution; obtain good history of disease and its treatment (treatment of at least 6 to 18 months' duration); appropriate review of systems is mandatory b. Should give history of periodic chest x-ray films and examination to rule out reactivation c. Consult with physician and postpone care if: 1) Questionable history of proper care 2) Lack of appropriate medical supervision since recovery 3) Signs or symptoms of relapse If present status "free of active disease," care provided is same as for normal older adult. **3.** In older adults with recent conversion to positive skin test (PPD): a. Should have been evaluated by physician to rule out active disease b. May be receiving isoniazid (INH) for 1 year prophylactically c. Care provided same as for normal patient when physician authorizes care **4.** In older adults with signs or symptoms of tuberculosis: a. Refer to physician and postpone treatment. b. If treatment necessary, care provided as in category 1 above.	None required	Oral ulceration (rare), tongue most common Tuberculosis involvement of cervical and submandibular lymph nodes (scrofula)
Joint disease: osteoarthritis	Joint pain, stiffness, and loss of mobility Increased bleeding from aspirin or NSAIDs	**1.** Short appointments **2.** Ensure physical comfort: a. Position changes b. Comfortable chair position c. Physical supports **3.** Aspirin or NSAIDs may result in increased bleeding but it usually is not clinically significant. **4.** If client has joint prosthesis, antibiotics not necessary unless "high risk" (rheumatoid arthritis, diabetic, immunosuppressed or previous infection).	Dictated by severity of disability; if severe, extensive care not indicated; encourage and facilitate oral health–promoting behaviors	Temporomandibular joint involvement

TABLE 55-4

Alterations in Dental Hygiene Care of the Older Adult—cont'd

Condition	Potential Risk Relating to Dental Hygiene Care	Prevention of Medical Complications	Dental Hygiene Care Plan Modification	Oral Complications
Joint disease: rheumatoid arthritis	Joint pain and immobility Increased bleeding secondary to aspirin and NSAIDs Bone marrow suppression from immunosuppressives resulting in anemia, agranulocytosis, thrombocytopenia, and/or increased vulnerability to infection	**1.** Short appointments **2.** Physical comfort: a. Position changes b. Comfortable chair position c. Physical supports **3.** Management of drug complications: a. Aspirin or NSAIDs may result in increased bleeding but it is not usually clinically significant. b. Gold salts, penicillamine, sulfasalazine, corticosteriods, immunosuppressives, or biologic agents; obtain complete blood count with differential and bleeding time. **4.** If joint prosthesis within 2 years of placement, prophylactic antibiotics recommended.	Dictated by severity of disability and temporomandibular joint involvement; if severe, extensive care not indicated; temporomandibular joint surgery may be helpful; encourage oral health–promoting behaviors	Temporomandibular joint involvement; anterior open bite possible Stomatitis secondary to gold salts, penicillamine, and immunosuppressives
Joint prosthesis		**1.** Deep infection around joint prosthesis secondary to bacteremia caused by acute infection elsewhere in body; there is no evidence that transient bacteremias caused by invasive dental procedures can infect these prostheses after 2 years since placement. **2.** Several authors have suggested that patients with active rheumatoid arthritis, severe type 1 diabetes mellitus, congenital or acquired immunodeficiency, hemophilia, loose prostheses, or history of infection of prostheses may be at risk, but there again are few data to support this concept.	Obtain good health history. Few data support use of antibiotic prophylaxis. In contrast, most orthopedic surgeons still recommend prophylaxis. Obtain medical consultation regarding need for prophylaxis. If orthopedic consultant does not recommend prophylaxis, proceed without it. If orthopedic consultant recommends prophylaxis, consult with dentist and patient to determine best course of action.	None

Continued

TABLE 55-4

Alterations in Dental Hygiene Care of the Older Adult—cont'd

Condition	Potential Risk Relating to Dental Hygiene Care	Prevention of Medical Complications	Dental Hygiene Care Plan Modification	Oral Complications
Stroke	Dental hygiene care could precipitate stroke. Bleeding secondary to drug therapy	**1.** Identify stroke-prone older adult from health history (hypertension, smoking, transient ischemic attacks). **2.** Reduce older adult's risk factors for stroke. **3.** For past history of stroke: a. For current transient ischemic attacks (TIAs)—no elective care b. Drug considerations—aspirin and dipyridamole (Persantine), obtain pretreatment bleeding time (less than 20 minutes); warfarin (Coumadin), obtain prothrombin time, which should be <20 seconds on the day of the scheduled procedure c. Short morning appointments d. Monitor blood pressure e. Use minimum amount of vasoconstrictor in local anesthetic f. No epinephrine in retraction cord	Dependent on physical impairment All restorations should be readily cleansable; avoid porcelain occlusals. Modified oral hygiene aids may be needed.	None
Diabetes	In uncontrolled diabetes: a. Infection b. Poor wound healing In older adult treated with insulin, insulin reaction In older clients with diabetes, early onset of complications relating to cardiovascular system, eyes, kidneys, and nervous system (angina, myocardial infarction, cerebrovascular accident, renal failure, peripheral neuropathy, blindness, hypertension, congestive heart failure)	**1.** Detect by: a. Health history b. Clinical findings c. Screening blood glucose level **2.** Refer for medical diagnosis and treatment. **3.** Monitor and control hyperglycemia. **4.** Older adult receiving insulin—prevent insulin reaction. a. Advise older adult to eat normal meals before appointments. b. Schedule appointments in morning or midmorning. c. Advise older adult to inform you of any symptoms of insulin reaction when they first occur. d. Have sugar in some form to give in case of insulin reaction. **5.** Older adults with diabetes being treated with insulin who develop oral infection may require increase in insulin dosage; consult with physician in addition to performing aggressive local and systemic management of infection (including antibiotic sensitivity testing). **6.** Drug considerations: a. Insulin reaction b. Hypoglycemic agents, on rare occasions aplastic anemia, and so on c. In clients with severe diabetes, avoid general anesthesia.	In well-controlled diabetes, no alteration of dental hygiene care plan is indicated unless complications of diabetes present, such as the following: Hypertension Congestive heart failure Myocardial infarction Angina Renal failure	Accelerated periodontal disease Periodontal abscesses Xerostomia Poor healing Infection Oral ulcerations Mucormycosis Numbness, burning, or pain in oral tissues

TABLE 55-4

Alterations in Dental Hygiene Care of the Older Adult—cont'd

Condition	Potential Risk Relating to Dental Hygiene Care	Prevention of Medical Complications	Dental Hygiene Care Plan Modification	Oral Complications
Cirrhosis	Bleeding tendencies; unpredictable drug metabolism	**1.** Identify alcoholic older adult: a. Health history b. Clinical examination c. Repeated detection of odor on breath d. Information from friends or relatives **2.** Consult with physician to verify current status. **3.** Attempt to direct older adult into treatment. **4.** Laboratory screening: a. Complete blood count with differential b. Aspartate aminotransferase (AST), alanine aminotransferase (ALT) c. Bleeding time d. Thrombin time e. Prothrombin time **5.** Minimize drugs metabolized by liver. **6.** If screening test results abnormal, consult physician.	Because oral neglect is seen commonly in alcoholics, older adults should demonstrate interest in and ability to care for dentition before any significant dental hygiene care is performed.	Neglect Bleeding Ecchymoses Petechiae Glossitis Angular cheilosis Impaired healing Parotid enlargement Candidiasis Oral cancer Alcohol breath odor Bruxism Dental attrition Xerostomia

Adapted from Little JW, Falace DA, Miller CS, et al: *Dental management of the medically compromised patient,* ed 8, St Louis, 2013, Mosby.
See Chapter 10 for prophylactic antibiotic premedication guidelines.

Individuals who receive antibiotic premedication need to have as much care as possible at one time; however, the person's medical condition may make lengthy appointments difficult.

Specific and customized oral hygiene instruction is provided to older adults to ensure that they have the knowledge and skills necessary to removal plaque biofilm thoroughly. Chemotherapeutic products, such as triclosan dentifrice, essential oil mouth rinse, or 0.12% chlorhexidine mouth rinse, should be recommended when necessary to supplement mechanical plaque biofilm removal.[8,9] Recommendations for improving the adequacy of the diet with regard to food choices are provided, with specific directions for limiting refined carbohydrate foods and limiting cariogenic snacking.[8,9]

Home use of topical fluoride products has been advocated for all older individuals with teeth. In addition to using a fluoride dentifrice, clients can use a daily nonprescription 0.05% sodium fluoride rinse, especially if they notice decreased quality and quantity of saliva. Many older clients have difficulty rinsing their mouths, however, and a 1.1% sodium fluoride or 0.4% stannous fluoride gel, which is applied by a toothbrush, may be easier to use and may reach susceptible proximal and root surfaces. Clients who have undergone head and neck radiation therapy, who have severe xerostomia, or who have rampant caries can use the tray method to apply the 1.1% sodium fluoride or 0.4% stannous gel in a tray for 5 minutes twice a day. The tray method of application is best completed with an unflavored fluoride product because of the frequency and intensity of the application.[8,9]

For individuals with xerostomia, calcium and phosphate products (e.g., MI Paste, NovaMin) along with self-applied and professionally applied topical fluoride are recommended to promote remineralization. Saliva substitutes that coat the mucosa and teeth to keep them moist are recommended to reduce enamel solubility and the accumulation of plaque biofilm. Saliva substitutes can be used without limit on the frequency of use and come in liquid, gel, or spray formulations that are distributed through the mouth with the tongue. Several over-the-counter products are available, with many containing fluoride and xylitol.[10,12]

Exposed root surfaces are susceptible to dental caries, and professionally applied and home-applied topical fluoride products are recommended to help meet the need for a biologically sound dentition. The role of plaque biofilm and diet in relation to dental caries formation must be stressed. A desensitization treatment and dentifrice also may be recommended to help ensure freedom from pain if root surfaces are sensitive.[9,15]

At the completion of the appointment, dental hygienists should return the dental chair to an upright position slowly. It is important to allow the client to sit up for a short time before dismissal to avoid any problems with postural hypotension. The dental hygienist should pay close attention to see if the client needs assistance out of the chair. Postoperative instructions are reviewed and a written copy provided as indicated.

Evaluation

After care has been completed, older clients need to be reevaluated more frequently and more carefully because of the many physiologic changes, chronic conditions, and pathologic changes frequently seen in this age group. Dental hygienists must be aware that health status can change quickly with an older client, and even small changes may be significant, especially in relation to cardiovascular and cognitive changes. Often a dental hygienist may be the first to notice cognitive declines over a series of appointments or at the recall visit. These qualitative perceptions that "something is not quite right" about the older client should be discussed with the client, relatives, and/or caregivers, and referrals for further medical evaluation provided.[9]

Dental hygienists should allow a longer time to assess results of soft-tissue debridement because of a slower and decreased potential for tissue healing, and provide additional care when necessary. Quantitative evaluation of health status through bleeding and plaque indices and pocket depth recording is essential to document healing and plan new interventions with older clients.

More-frequent maintenance intervals are recommended for older clients to evaluate any changes in functional abilities to complete oral hygiene, any nutritional changes, and the occurrence of new disease. Dental hygienists should not assume that older adults continue to have the same functional abilities, even after a 3-month period. For example, clients with musculoskeletal disorders frequently note varying functional abilities and may need more assistance with oral hygiene at times. In addition, clients may be taking new medications and may alter their nutritional patterns because of the unpleasant taste or increased xerostomia experienced with a different medication. These older adults are at extreme risk for caries and need more aggressive caries management (see Chapter 18). More-frequent visits for dental hygiene care provide opportunity for assessment and to recommend preventive and therapeutic interventions specific to the client's needs.[9,15,16]

Documentation

All components of the process of care are interrelated and depend upon ongoing assessments and evaluation of treatment outcomes to determine the need for change in the dental hygiene care plan. Thus it is critical to document ongoing client progress in the client record to provide documentation for reevaluation. Documenting the client's health status during active therapy and over a lifetime of regular maintenance care is the best defense against a client's accusation of negligence. It is important to provide and document informed consent with all older clients. When necessary, discuss and document treatment with family and/or caregivers.

Community Health Services

Institutionalized elderly make up approximately 4.4% of the elderly population. Homebound, semidependent elderly account for another 5% to 6%. The numbers may be small, but these groups of elderly have the greatest oral needs and the most difficulty reaching dental services.[1,2,17] Individuals who are functionally dependent are more likely to be edentulous and may not have used dental services for several years. Furthermore, research suggests that more than 80% have dental needs, with nearly 40% requiring immediate attention.[1,2,17] Among dentate individuals, three fourths need scaling and selective polishing and have other problems including root caries and poor oral hygiene.[6]

Several factors can be identified that have created this neglect. First, individuals who are in a long-term care facility (LTCF) or are homebound may not be able to care for themselves. They may have numerous complicated and interrelated problems, and dental care may not be a priority. In addition, dental professionals have not been active in providing services because of their own attitudes toward treating the frail elderly, low financial return, and state practice acts that limit dental hygienists' ability to work unsupervised in LTCFs or with the homebound.[17]

The homebound elderly have additional health problems that complicate their care. Some have malnutrition, withdraw socially, or perceive that their speech is affected adversely. These factors can elicit low self-esteem, leading to depression. Problems of not eating and withdrawal can be exacerbated as a result.[9,16]

For older adults, provision of routine dental services is not included under Medicare (federal) benefits. Medicaid (state) dental benefits and eligibility vary by state; however, preventive dental care for elderly is usually not a priority. Given the high dental needs of homebound or institutionalized elderly, systems to provide care must be advocated for and established.[6]

Traditional Dental Office

When dental hygienists treat frail elderly persons, care is complicated by a variety of factors as follows[9]:

- *Appointment time.* Short morning appointments should be scheduled. Most elderly are physically strongest in the morning. Because many cannot sit for long periods, however, 2 hours should be the limit, including transportation time.
- *Accessibility of the dental office.* Parking lots, ramps, and doorways must accommodate wheelchairs. Legally, the Americans with Disabilities Act of 1993 mandates access to all public facilities.
- *Communication with the LTCF.* Most facilities require that services provided and instructions be in writing.
- *Legal considerations.* The elderly client may not be capable of providing informed consent. In such cases the practitioner must have written permission from the individual's physician, family, or facility.
- *Multiple health conditions and drug therapies.* Many elderly individuals have a multitude of chronic health conditions. Consultation with the physician may be necessary.

On-Site Dental Programs

Providing care in a LTCF or client's home has several advantages over the traditional dental office, as follows:

- Frail elderly do not favorably withstand the disruption of being transported.
- Incontinent or catheterized individuals are best treated at their place of residence.
- It is less disruptive to the facility.
- A familiar environment reduces anxiety.

There are three options that dental professionals can use when providing care in an LTCF or to homebound clients. Many facilities have space to build dental operatories, which may be more common in a larger LTCF and provides a more-comfortable permanent arrangement for dental professionals and clients. However, for smaller LTCFs, dedicated permanent space may not be available. Portable dental equipment, including dental chairs, delivery systems, and x-ray equipment, can be transported readily and set up in a conference room or other space so that dental care can be provided as needed for clients. Alternatively, mobile dental vehicles can be deployed when space in the facility cannot be provided.

Mobile vehicles are "dental offices on wheels" and can be customized with dental laboratories and other amenities to customize care with older adults. However the care is provided, it is important to educate the family and/or caregivers about appropriate follow-up care to dental treatment and also about daily, routine oral hygiene care for the client.[17]

Role of the Dental Hygienist

Dental hygienists serve in an important capacity with the institutionalized and homebound elderly in the following activities:

- Providing clinical dental hygiene care either at the LTCF or when the client is transported to the dental office
- Providing in-service education programs for staff and/or family members
- Marking dentures for identification
- Giving fluoride applications
- Developing individual care plans
- Modifying oral hygiene aids

Nursing staff and aides are important intermediaries for oral healthcare professionals.[12] Staff members should be encouraged to refer elderly individuals to the dental office or consulting dentist if they detect unusual signs, such as swelling or discoloration, or if they hear a verbal complaint. The Brief Oral Health Status Examination (BOHSE) can be used by nursing staff members to evaluate oral health of clients systematically at the entrance to the care facility and routinely during care.[17] Dental hygienists can develop and implement in-service education programs to ensure that staff members have the knowledge and skill necessary to complete thorough oral assessments and oral hygiene care.

For homebound individuals, establishment of a prevention program using visiting nurses or home healthcare workers is needed when family members are not available. Some states have developed dental programs that use mobile vans, with professionals and students providing services for homebound elderly. Dental hygienists can collaborate with local agencies, dental and dental hygiene associations, and dental hygiene educational institutions to develop oral screening, referral, and preventive programs for homebound elderly.

CLIENT EDUCATION TIPS

- Explain the differences between normal, physiologic changes seen in aging and pathologic changes.
- Communicate a wellness philosophy of care to maximize health in light of chronic conditions.
- Select and explain health promotion strategies based on older adults' needs.
- Encourage compliance with all medication and medical regimens.
- Relate client's health status to any modifications necessary for dental hygiene care.
- Adapt oral hygiene instructions to any functional limitations and oral health conditions.
- Explain the development and prevention of dental caries and periodontal diseases.
- Provide nutritional counseling regarding the reduction of refined carbohydrates, limitation of cariogenic snacking, and adequacy of dietary intake.
- Recommend the use of topical and professional fluorides to prevent dental decay.
- Recommend the use of oral hygiene products and chemotherapeutic agents by the client to prevent and control periodontal diseases.
- Assist with tobacco cessation efforts.
- Explain the importance of oral cancer prevention and early detection.
- Provide education regarding drug-induced changes in the oral cavity.
- Explain methods to identify and manage xerostomia.
- Instruct family caregivers regarding appropriate oral assessment and oral hygiene care.

LEGAL, ETHICAL, AND SAFETY ISSUES

- Complete and document a thorough medical, personal, and dental history and oral examination with each client.
- Refer older adults for consultation with the physician before dental hygiene care when indicated.
- Evaluate the client's use of medications, and refer client to the physician for consultation when indicated.
- Explain the results of consultation with the older adult, and document conversations and the physician's recommendations in the client's chart.
- Provide and document informed consent with all older clients. When necessary, discuss and document treatment with family and/or caregivers.
- Involve older adults in treatment decisions.
- Treat older adults with dignity and respect.
- Provide written instruction that can be read easily by older clients and/or caregivers, and reinforce instructions verbally.
- Provide aggressive oral health and prevention programs for caries and periodontal diseases.
- Ensure that the dental office facility is wheelchair accessible based on guidelines from the Americans with Disabilities Act.
- Provide care without discrimination.

KEY CONCEPTS

- Older adults are a heterogeneous group, and there is tremendous variability in the physical, psychosocial, and environmental issues within this age group. Functional age, rather than chronologic age, is the best measure to use when providing care to older adults.
- Current demographic reports and projections indicate a significant rise in the number and the proportion of older adults in the United States.
- The older adult population is becoming more racially and ethnically diverse. Elderly women outnumber elderly men. Older adults are concentrated in certain states and are not distributed evenly in the population.
- There is not one accepted theory to explain how and why we age. Multiple social and biologic theories of aging have been proposed and complement each other to shed light on the aging process.
- There are normal, physiologic changes in most body systems that occur as individuals age. These normal changes should not be confused with pathologic changes caused by disease; however, distinctions between normal

aging and pathologic conditions are sometimes difficult to discern.
- Most older adults have at least one chronic condition, and the most common chronic conditions are arthritis, hypertension and heart disease, cancer, diabetes, and stroke.
- Older adults develop coronal and root caries at a rate higher than the adult population; however, the rate of edentulousness (total tooth loss) among elderly is estimated at 15% and is projected to continue to decrease in future years.
- Caries prevention and control strategies for older adults must stress daily removal of plaque biofilm, reduction of refined carbohydrates, and daily use of topical fluorides, salivary substitutes, and calcium and phosphate products, especially when xerostomia is present.
- A small but significant number of older adults have advanced periodontitis, and there is a higher degree of loss of attachment and prevalence of gingivitis among older adults.
- Prevention and control of periodontal diseases should include daily removal of plaque biofilm, use of chemotherapeutic agents, and more-frequent visits for professional debridement and evaluation.
- A small percentage of older adults (6%) reside in long-term care facilities, and a similar percentage (5%) are confined to their homes. These individuals have a higher prevalence of dental disease and a lower usage rate of dental care than the adult population.
- Dental hygienists can work with nursing staff in long-term care facilities, with caregivers, and with homebound individuals in a variety of roles to improve the oral health status.

CRITICAL THINKING EXERCISES

Dental Hygiene Care for an Older Client

Profile: Mrs. F., age 77, returns for a dental hygiene visit on her regular 6-month maintenance schedule.

Chief Complaint: "I have a removable partial denture to replace my lower back teeth that I don't wear because it makes my mouth feel dry and taste bad. Also, I have a large freckle on my left cheek that has grown in the past several months."

Social History: Mrs. F. has been widowed for 3 years and is active with her church and the families of her two daughters who live nearby.

Health History: Mrs. F. has a history of angina for the past 6 years and takes 50 mg atenolol (Tenormin) once a day to prevent angina attacks.

Dental History: Mrs. F. has a history of regular dental visits and has all of her teeth, with the exception of the four mandibular molars. Oral examination reveals a flat, brown, elongated lesion approximately 10 mm long and 6 mm wide on the center of her left cheek. Mrs. F. denies any pain or exudate from this lesion. Dental examination reveals no areas of decay and recession with no evidence of periodontal disease.

Oral Health Behavior Assessment: Good oral hygiene. Uses a power toothbrush and flosses daily.

Supplemental Notes: During dental hygiene care, Mrs. F. states that she thinks her teeth are too short and ugly and asks you if she is too old to get "caps" on her teeth to improve her appearance.

1. What are the dental hygiene diagnoses for this client?
2. Develop a dental hygiene care plan for this client that includes goals and interventions.
3. What client education issues should be addressed?
4. What factors could be contributing to this client's dry mouth?
5. Are there any contraindications to this client's care?
6. What measures should be taken during treatment to prevent an angina attack?

Instant Aging as a Dental Client

This activity asks participants to simulate what it is like to be an older dental client in their office. This exercise provides a good opportunity to learn what older clients may be experiencing and provides insight for participants regarding sensory changes in aging. Students should work in groups of two, alternating the role of client and dental hygienist. Partners are asked to complete tasks while they have simulated several sensory deprivations that older individuals may experience.

Task A: Partner 1 wears glasses with a thin film of oil or lubricant to inhibit clear vision. In addition, partner 1 tapes the fingers of both hands to make fine motor tasks difficult. Partner 1 completes a health history form and/or other office forms for a new client. After the forms are completed (a brief time limit should be imposed), partner 1 walks unassisted back to the treatment room and fills out additional forms in the dental chair.

Task B: Partner 2 wears earplugs or uses cotton or wax ear protectors to limit hearing. In addition, this partner uses an Ace bandage or shoulder harness to restrict shoulder movement. Partner 2 walks unassisted to the treatment room and completes a brief written form in the dental chair. Partner 2 demonstrates brushing and flossing technique and should be asked to describe the technique and answer questions about the performance.

Debriefing Discussion: After the simulated dental appointments are completed, participants discuss their experiences in completing routine dental tasks with some sensory impairments. Although this is only a simulation, partners are encouraged to discuss how this simulation is related to the experiences of their older clients. Partners should complete an "environmental audit" of their dental offices to assess how difficult their office environment is for the older individual to negotiate, based on the environmental considerations discussed in this chapter. Hearing, vision, and motor skill impairments pose significant obstacles even when the environment is optimal for older adults. By adopting the perspective of the client with some sensorimotor deficits, partners may be able to identify difficulties for older clients and make changes to provide care in a more sensitive, appropriate manner.

Visit a Senior Community Center

Most communities provide a variety of services to older adults who currently are living in the community but who may need some assistance with meals, social activities, healthcare, or housing to function in an independent manner for as long as possible.

In this learning activity, readers should contact the director of a local senior center and request to visit and/or volunteer at the center at least twice. Visits to these senior centers provide an interesting window on the daily life of older adults, especially if participants have little experience with older individuals. The centers generally emphasize a philosophy of wellness and provide a wide range of activities to encourage participation by members, such as arts and craft projects, discussion groups, and scheduled trips to social and cultural events.

Students who visit a senior center should keep a diary regarding the activities the seniors completed on the days on which they visited and should participate actively in the events scheduled for the day. For example, learners may wish to volunteer to share a craft activity with the older adults, lead an exercise or dance class, or call bingo for the session. During the visits, the participants should speak with as many seniors as possible to learn of their daily activities, why they participate in the center activities, and which activities and functions of the center they use most frequently. These informal discussions generally are welcomed by the older adults, who view these sessions as a chance to advise and guide younger individuals about the needs of older adults. In addition, these visits provide participants with the opportunity to understand the wide range of abilities these older individuals possess, even in light of chronic and disabling conditions. By observing and sharing activities, participants can view the active and varied nature of the seniors in their daily activities and gain an understanding of the challenges older adults face each day.

REFERENCES

1. Weiner CA: *The Older Population: 2010.* 2010 Census Bureau Briefs, November, 2011 #C2010BR-09, US Census Bureau, US Department of Commerce. Available at: http://www.census.gov/prod/cen2010/briefs/c2010br-09.pdf. Accessed March 18, 2013.
2. National Center for Health Statistics: *Health, United States, 2011, with special feature on socioeconomic status and health*, Hyattsville, Md. Available at: http://www.cdc.gov/nchs/data/hus/hus11.pdf#001. Accessed March 18, 2013.
3. Greenberg SA: *Profile of Older Americans: 2011.* Administration on Aging, U.S. Department of Health and Human Services. Available at: http://www.aoa.gov/aoaroot/aging_statistics/Profile/2011/docs/2011profile.pdf. Accessed March 18, 2013.
4. Touhy TA, Jett KF: *Ebersole and Hess' gerontological nursing and healthy aging*, ed 8, St Louis, 2012, Mosby.
5. U.S. Department of Health and Human Services: *Healthy people 2020: healthy people in healthy communities*. Available at: http://www.healthypeople.gov/2020/topicsobjectives2020/overview.aspx?topicid=31. Accessed March 18, 2013.
6. Brown LJ: Dental services among elderly Americans: utilization, expenditures, and their determinants. In Lamster I, Northridge M, eds: *Improving oral health for the elderly*, New York, 2008, Springer.
7. Russell SL, Ship JA: Normal oral mucosal, dental, periodontal and alveolar bone changes associated with aging. In Lamster I, Northridge M, eds: *Improving oral health for the elderly*, New York, 2008, Springer.
8. Budtz-Jorgensen E, Muller F: Caries, tooth loss and conventional tooth replacement for older patients. In Lamster I, Northridge M, eds: *Improving oral health for the elderly*, New York, 2008, Springer.
9. Ettinger RL: Oral health and the aging population, *J Am Dent Assoc* 138(suppl 1):5S, 2007.
10. Turner MD, Ship JA: Dry mouth and its effects on the oral health of elderly people, *J Am Dent Assoc* 138(suppl 1):15S, 2007.
11. Wolf DL, Papapanou PN: The relationship between periodontal disease and systemic disease in the elderly. In Lamster I, Northridge M, eds: *Improving oral health for the elderly*, New York, 2008, Springer.
12. Mandel L: Saliva and salivary glands in the elderly. In Lamster I, Northridge M, eds: *Improving oral health for the elderly*, New York, 2008, Springer.
13. Little JW, Falace DA, Miller CS, et al: *Dental management of the medically compromised patient*, ed 8, St Louis, 2013, Mosby.
14. Regezi JA, Sciubba JJ, Jordan R: *Oral pathology*, ed 6, Philadelphia, 2011, Saunders.
15. Zegarelli DJ, Woo VL, Yoon AJ: Oral pathology affecting older adults. In Lamster I, Northridge M, eds: *Improving oral health for the elderly*, New York, 2008, Springer.
16. Walls AWG: Mastication, nutrition, oral health and health in older patients. In Lamster I, Northridge M, eds: *Improving oral health for the elderly*, New York, 2008, Springer.
17. O'Connor LJ: Oral health care. In Capezuti E, Zwicker D, Mezey M, et al, eds: *Evidence-based geriatric nursing protocols for best practice*, ed 3, New York, 2008, Springer.

ⓔ EVOLVE RESOURCES

Please visit http://evolve.elsevier.com/Darby/hygiene for additional practice and study support tools.

CHAPTER 56

Persons with Fixed and Removable Dental Prostheses

Leeann R. Donnelly

COMPETENCIES

1. Discuss tooth loss, including:
   - Describe demographics, risk factors, psychologic factors, and disease patterns associated with tooth loss.
   - Describe oral physiologic changes of the edentulous and partially edentulous client.
2. Explain appliances used in fixed and removable prosthodontic therapy.
3. Describe the challenges associated with the replacement of missing teeth.
4. Discuss factors that may affect the oral mucosa of prosthesis-wearing individuals.
5. Discuss the implications for dental hygiene care with removable prostheses, including occlusion and fit, irritations, and lesions that can occur.
6. Explain the importance of regular professional care.
7. Discuss dental hygiene care for individuals with fixed or removable prosthesis, including:
   - Educate prosthesis-wearing clients about expectations, personal responsibility for oral health, importance of oral hygiene measures, regular professional care, and nutrition to maintain oral health.
   - Plan and evaluate dental hygiene care for clients with fixed and removable prostheses.
   - List the types of common prosthesis cleansers available.

Normally, individuals are not conscious of the critical daily functions of teeth: eating, speaking, facial expression, and appearance. Once the teeth are lost, the person quickly realizes that eating becomes more difficult, speech is not as distinct, and facial tissues lose support, which ultimately impairs appearance and other people's perceptions of the person.

The term **edentulous**, derived from the Latin word *edentatus,* means being without teeth or lacking teeth. Although the percentage of persons with tooth loss increases with age, it is not uncommon to find clients in their second through fifth decades of life with prostheses. A **prosthesis** is a fixed or removable appliance that is designed functionally and cosmetically to replace a missing natural tooth or teeth. Although maintaining the oral health of clients with tooth loss entails the same basic preventive and therapeutic care elements as for clients with a complete dentition, those with missing teeth have specialized needs. Dental hygienists must be knowledgeable about how to meet the specialized needs of clients with prostheses.

Demographics of Tooth Loss

Changing patterns in oral disease, professional care, and attitudes toward healthcare have decreased the number of completely edentulous individuals. Nevertheless, surveys indicate that the total number of edentulous individuals is between 20 and 25 million, suggesting that the provision of complete dental prostheses is common in the oral healthcare environment and may remain so given longer life spans and the growing elderly population.[1] At present, approximately one in five adults aged 65 or older in the United States and Canada are edentulous.[2,3] Although edentulous rates have been dropping, these figures suggest that dental hygienists are likely to encounter edentulous clients within any dental hygiene practice setting.

Risk Factors for Tooth Loss

Major risk factors that contribute to a person's edentulous status are as follows:

- Dental caries
- Periodontal diseases
- Low socioeconomic status
- Inadequate access to professional oral care
- Low frequency of professional oral care
- Poor daily oral hygiene

The primary reason for tooth loss before age 35 years is dental caries, whereas periodontal diseases also contribute to tooth loss during the third through the fifth decades of life. Oral cancer, and the corresponding treatment for oral cancer, and oral injury also contribute to tooth loss. In addition, tooth loss is influenced by a client's socioeconomic status, access to professional oral care, frequency of professional oral care, and daily oral hygiene.

Other Factors Associated with Tooth Loss

Psychologic Factors

Client attitude and values influence the success of care, and the edentulous or the partially edentulous person is no exception. Wholesome facial image often is in deficit because of tooth loss, fear of aging, decreased sexuality, feelings of insecurity, fear of rejection, loss of self-esteem, and unrealistic expectations for tooth replacement. Loss of self-esteem is especially related to clients in whom tooth loss is attributed to oral cancer and oral cancer treatment. Human responses associated with tooth loss include the five stages of bereavement, behavioral changes, embarrassment, and loss of dignity. These responses must be considered when providing care for edentulous or partially edentulous clients.[4]

Physiologic Factors

Although prostheses can restore many oral functions when a person experiences tooth loss, remodeling of the orofacial tissues invariably is encountered. Prostheses placement introduces unfamiliar forces that contribute to the following:

- Residual ridge and alveolar bone resorption
- Oral mucous membrane remodeling
- Loss of orofacial muscle tone

Residual Ridge and Alveolar Bone Resorption

After tooth extraction, major bony changes, such as residual alveolar ridge resorption, occur within the first year and continue throughout life. Correlation between degree of alveolar bone resorption and the duration of being edentulous is well documented. Metabolic bone disease, postmenopausal osteoporosis, and a calcium-poor diet also contribute to severe mandibular atrophy in edentulous individuals.[5]

Generally, older individuals resorb bone at faster rates than younger individuals because of anatomic, metabolic, functional, and prosthetic factors. Problems that arise as a result of residual bone resorption are magnified as the person ages. For example, severe mandibular alveolar ridge resorption may expose the contents of the mandibular canal and cause extreme discomfort from the prosthesis. In addition, compression of an exposed mental nerve at or near the crest of the alveolar ridge with only a thin layer of oral mucosa overlying it may cause pain and paresthesia of the lower lip and chin. During assessment, if the dental hygienist finds unmet needs for a biologically sound and functional dentition or freedom from fear and stress, immediate dental referral is indicated.

Resorption of alveolar ridges diminishes stability and retention of the prosthesis as the bony ridges continue to flatten with time. Generally, bony changes observed in the mandibular arch differ significantly from those in the maxilla. The resorption rate is four times greater in the mandible than in the maxilla. Occasionally, irregular patterns of alveolar ridge resorption create numerous sharp spikes, especially in the mylohyoid ridge. Considerable pain can develop as the mucous membrane covering becomes trapped between the hard prosthesis base and sharp bone.[5]

Other bony contours from either growth abnormalities or alveolar resorption may create undesirable consequences and should be noted. **Exostoses**, benign bony outgrowths, frequently occur on the hard palate and lingual aspect of the mandibular alveolar ridge and are known as **palatal tori** and **mandibular tori**, respectively. Their surgical removal, before prosthesis construction, prevents the possibility of irritation of the overlying oral mucosa by the tori. Similarly, large maxillary tuberosities can lead to an unsatisfactory fit of the prosthetic appliance.

Types of Prosthodontic Prostheses

Individuals can have missing teeth replaced by dental implants (see Chapter 58) or by fixed and removable dental prostheses. Transition from a natural dentition to a completely or partially artificial dentition is a major life event that most individuals find challenging. This situation can affect client needs for wholesome facial image, freedom from anxiety and stress, and a biologically sound and functional dentition. If needs are not met, or if clients believe that their needs cannot be met, successful prosthodontic therapy may be jeopardized.

Several types of prostheses ranging from partial to complete can be fabricated to meet clients' needs. The **partial dental prosthesis** is used to replace some, but not all, of the natural teeth (Figure 56-1, *A*). Partial dental prostheses may be fixed or removable. A **fixed partial dental prosthesis** is cemented permanently to natural teeth and commonly is called a *bridge* (Figure 56-1, *B*); it cannot be removed by the client.

Components of fixed partial dental prostheses include the following:

- **Abutment**: the tooth or teeth used to anchor the prosthesis and support the pontic(s)
- **Pontic**: the artificial tooth or teeth that occupy the edentulous space and replace the missing tooth or teeth

Removable partial dental prostheses, commonly called a *partial denture* (Figure 56-2) can be removed and replaced by

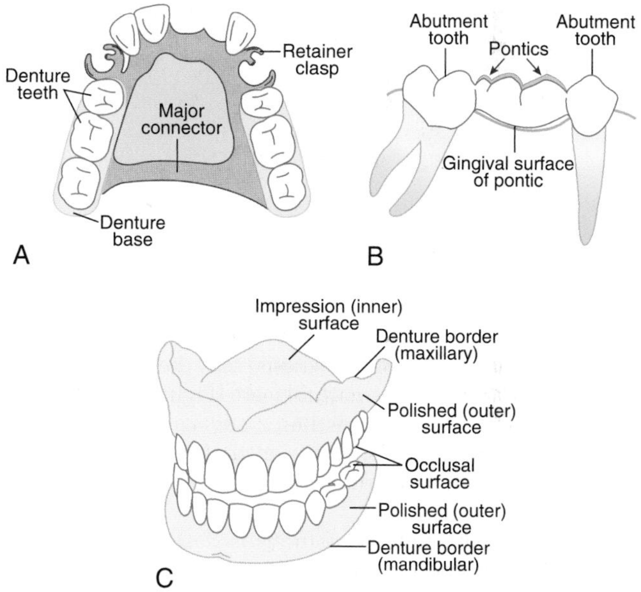

Figure 56-1. Types of prostheses. **A,** Removable partial denture. **B,** Fixed partial denture. **C,** Complete denture.

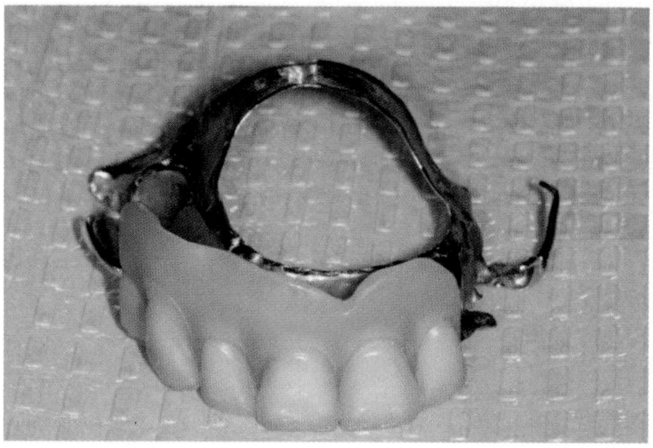

Figure 56-2. Maxillary removable partial denture. (Courtesy Dr. Michael MacEntee, Prosthodontist, Faculty of Dentistry, University of British Columbia, Vancouver, Canada.)

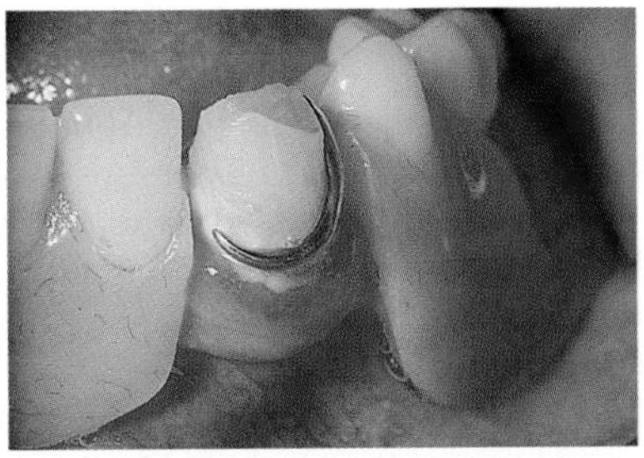

Figure 56-3. Removable partial denture clasp. Note retained plaque biofilm under the clasp in the gingival third of the abutment tooth.

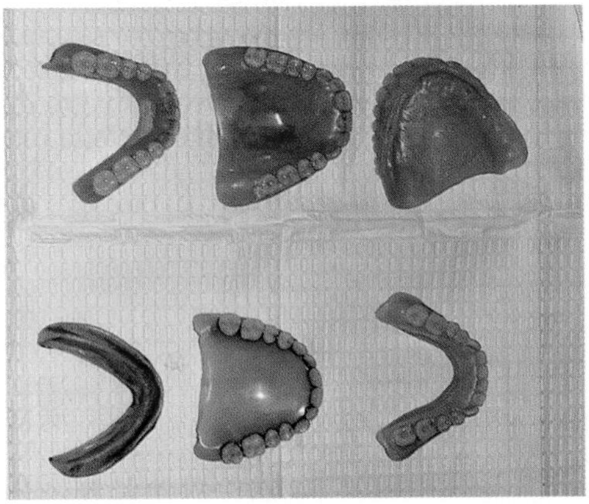

Figure 56-4. Complete (full) dentures. (Courtesy Ivoclar Williams, Amherst, New York.)

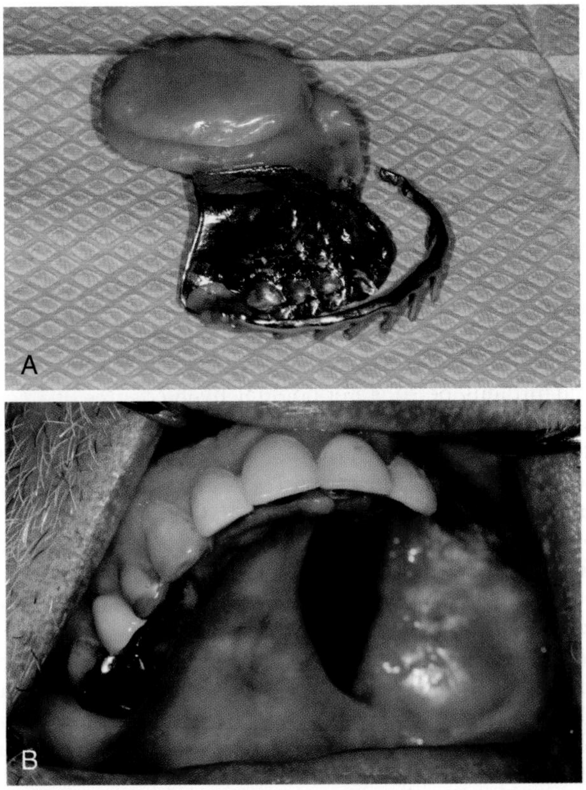

Figure 56-5. **A,** Obturator. **B,** Corresponding oral defect. (Courtesy Dr. Caroline Nguyen, Prosthodontist, Faculty of Dentistry, University of British Columbia, Vancouver, Canada.)

the client. This type of prosthesis may be supported by retainer clasps around the natural teeth (Figure 56-3). Removable complete dental prostheses, or ***complete dentures*** (Figure 56-4; see Figure 56-1, *C*) replace either the maxillary or the mandibular arch or the entire dentition and associated structures.

If a removable dental prosthesis is designed for a client who has undergone oral cancer surgery, it also may need to function as an obturator. An obturator (Figure 56-5, *A*) is a prosthesis that closes an opening or orifice (Figure 56-5, *B*) that may have been created by an accident, that may be a congenital cleft, or that may have been caused by the removal of a cancerous tumor. An obturator is designed to cover an orifice, and in such cases aids in retaining foods and fluids in the mouth and keeping them out of the nasal passage.

Implant dentures are designed to fit over implant fixtures that are inserted partially or entirely into living bone. The increased stability and retention derived from this type of prosthetic appliance has renewed the hopes of the edentulous population for an acceptable alternative to natural teeth (see Chapter 58).

Challenges Associated with Replacement of Missing Teeth

Although prosthodontic therapy can give the edentulous or partially edentulous individual a biologically sound and functional dentition, success depends on the client's attitude and commitment. At the outset, the client must understand the limitations of tooth replacements and their effectiveness as substitutes for natural teeth. Clients need to be informed about the physical manifestations of bone resorption related to facial appearance, potential speech difficulties, and the effects of tooth replacement on masticatory efficiency. If realistic expectations and goals for care of prostheses are outlined early, the client can adapt successfully to the artificial dentition.

Physical Appearance

Alveolar bone resorption dramatically affects physical appearance and facial image. Modifications in appearance often are visible after extensive alveolar bone resorption, such as loss of facial height (vertical dimension), reduced lip support, a sunken maxillary appearance, and increased chin prominence. The effects of physical alterations attributed to bone resorption include decreased stability, unbalanced occlusion, temporomandibular joint (TMJ) disorders, and dissatisfaction with appearance.[6] Usually appearance is judged critically by clients themselves; however, the astute dental hygienist who focuses clients on their positive attributes increases their self-esteem and reduces their anxiety and stress.

Speech Disturbances

Speech patterns are affected by loss of teeth, loss of associated periodontal structures, and the acquisition of prostheses. Transient speech articulation difficulties and oral resonance problems are expected, but soon disappear. To facilitate speaking with a new dental prosthesis, clients need to be instructed to read aloud and to speak in front of a mirror. If a speech disturbance persists longer than a few days, the prosthesis may be ill-fitting and reevaluation by a dentist warranted. A speech deficit also can arise in conjunction with bone resorption because a loosely fitting prosthesis is difficult to control.

Masticatory Efficiency

Masticatory efficiency with prostheses is estimated to be 20% of that of individuals who have a natural dentition.[6] Two primary reasons for reduction in masticatory abilities are loss of periodontal support and stability and periodontal proprioception.

The periodontal ligament support area is critical to the stability of a prosthesis confined to one arch only. However, in edentulous persons periodontal ligament support is one fourth to one half of the support of the natural dentition. Furthermore, proprioception is a major component of the body's reception and interpretation of sensation. Without this feedback regarding movement and position from the pressoreceptors in the periodontal ligaments, chewing ability declines significantly.

Biting and chewing forces also decrease significantly and can be nearly six times less in persons who wear complete dentures. Although the mastication muscles are adequate, the mucous membrane covering the edentulous ridge cannot withstand the pressures exerted. The clients have greater success with a new prosthesis if they are taught to avoid repeated incision using anterior teeth, gum chewing, and sticky foods. Clients also need to be instructed to consume food in smaller pieces, lengthen chewing time, and evenly distribute food to both the left and right sides of the mouth while chewing.[7] Practicing these behaviors is critical to masticatory efficiency and prosthesis stability.

Factors Affecting the Oral Mucosa of Denture-Wearing Individuals

Systemic Diseases and Conditions

Poor general health results in denture problems, such as friable denture-bearing mucosa. For example, a person with kidney dysfunction may have dehydrated mucosal tissues because of a water imbalance, and thus the mucosa becomes vulnerable to trauma. Decreased tolerance to stress, impaired healing, emotional strain, and medications related to poor systemic health adversely affect oral soft tissues. Systemic conditions that may require modification of dental hygiene care include cardiovascular diseases, hypertension, allergies, psychologic problems, and chronic diseases such as diabetes, anemia, and postmenopausal osteoporosis.[7]

Medications taken for systemic diseases or conditions can affect a client's oral condition and must be assessed and documented during each appointment (see Chapter 14). Hormones, digitalis, nitroglycerin, diazepam (Valium), and chlordiazepoxide (Librium) are among the many medications that can affect the oral environment of the edentulous client. Xerostomia, a common side effect of diuretic, antihypertensive, and antidepressive drugs, interferes with complete denture retention and stability as a result of a loss of mucosal lubrication. Uncontrollable tongue and facial movements may develop with psychotropic medications. Drugs such as cortisone, thyroid hormone, and estrogen may perpetuate a chronic mucosal tissue soreness.[7]

Xerostomia (Dry Mouth)

Extreme difficulties experienced by the edentulous client with dry mouth warrant an understanding of the critical role of saliva in the oral health maintenance. Normal salivary flow aids in denture retention and function. A thin film of saliva provides adhesive action as well as lubrication and cushioning effects. When the mouth becomes dry, movement of the denture can cause frictional irritation of the denture-bearing mucosa. Other symptoms may arise as a result of oral dryness, including altered taste perceptions, cracked lips, a fissured tongue, and burning mouth syndrome.[7]Although the exact cause of xerostomia may be difficult to identify, the most common factors associated with it are as follows:

- Sjögren's syndrome
- Emotional and anxiety states
- Negative fluid balance
- Selected nutritional and hormonal deficiencies
- Acquired immunodeficiency syndrome (AIDS)
- Anemia
- Polyuric states
- Drugs or medications
- Therapeutic radiation

Diminished salivary output is not associated directly with increased age; therefore other factors must be considered if xerostomia is observed in older adult clients who wear dentures.

Xerostomia Management

Professional care for the denture client with xerostomia can be challenging because most remedies provide only temporary relief (see Chapter 61, Box 61-12). The dental hygienist may recommend saliva substitutes and frequent mouth rinsing, especially during meals, to keep the mouth lubricated and to provide temporary symptomatic relief. Also, coating the tissue surface of dentures with silicone fluid, or denture adhesive material, and sucking on ice chips and using xylitol or sugarless mints are recommended for the management of soft-tissue dryness. Moisturizing products to recommend include oral lubricants, mouth rinses, toothpastes, sprays, and lozenges.[7]

Pharmacologic management to decrease symptoms associated with xerostomia by increasing salivary flow can be accomplished with cholinergic drugs such as oral pilocarpine. This prescriptive medication is effective in clients who have undergone head and neck radiation therapy or who have Sjogren's syndrome and can experience a severe dry mouth. Although oral pilocarpine has not been tested extensively in denture-wearing populations, it may be of value for those individuals with dry mouth.[7] This treatment option may be discussed with the client's dentist or physician and then presented to the client.

Removable Dental Prostheses Occlusion and Fit

The state of the oral mucosa overlying the ridges directly affects the comfort of removable partial and complete dentures. A thicker mucosal covering is more resilient and provides more padding than a thin mucosa. Unfortunately, dental interventions for minimizing discomfort associated with friable mucosa are limited. Soft lining materials such as tissue conditioners and resilient liners may alleviate discomfort for some individuals. Tissue conditioners and resilient liners, composed of soft, flexible elastomer polymers, palliatively treat chronic soreness and protect supporting tissues from functional and parafunctional occlusal stresses. Dentures with a flexible elastomer require special care because these soft materials cannot be cleaned effectively, and debris can accumulate and support halitosis, a disagreeable taste, and the growth of *Candida albicans.* Most professionals recommend use of a soft brush with soap and water or a nonabrasive denture cleanser (see Chapter 61, Box 61-2 on standard denture care). Oxygenating and hypochlorite-type denture cleansers can damage resilient liners and tissue conditioners and therefore clients must be cautioned about their use.[7]

Oral Hygiene

The client's oral mucosa reveals information about daily self-care. Accumulation of biofilm, stain, and calculus on the denture and oral mucosa leads to offensive odors and mucosal irritations, such as the following:

- **Denture stomatitis**: inflammation of the oral mucosa underlying the denture, characterized by redness, pain, and swelling
- **Papillary hyperplasia:** abnormal increase in the volume of tissue as a result of irritation
- **Chronic candidiasis**: a long-standing *C. albicans* infection (see Box 61-9 on the prevention and treatment of oral candidiasis).

Presence of any of these conditions mandates that the client be educated about oral hygiene interventions to maintain the health of mucosal tissues. (See Chapter 61, Box 61-2.) Specific oral hygiene techniques and products are presented in Chapters 23, 24, 25, 31, and 61.

Continuous Wear of Removable Dental Prostheses

Masticatory stress exerted by dentures may compromise residual alveolar ridges and oral mucosa. In addition, the risk for an inflammatory condition increases if the tissues are not allowed to rest. Therefore clients are advised to remove their dentures overnight or for several hours during each 24-hour period. While out of the mouth, dentures must be cleaned thoroughly and placed in a container either dry or submerged in a cleansing solution.[8] Storing dentures dry is an effective method to prevent the growth of bacteria and fungi with no clinically significant change to denture fit.[9,10]

Removable Dental Prostheses-Induced Oral Lesions

Understanding the soft-tissue response to removable prostheses enables the dental hygienist to assess the client's skin and mucous membrane integrity of the head and neck. The soft tissues associated primarily with dentures are the tongue, floor of the mouth, cheeks, lips, and mucosa overlying the edentulous ridge.

Denture-bearing tissues react differently from individual to individual. For example, differences in the mucosa thickness in conjunction with varying degrees of keratinization can be expected in the mouth of the denture-wearing client. Some edentulous persons develop a denture-induced fibrous hyperplasia as a result of fibrous tissue proliferation after alveolar bone resorption under an ill-fitting prosthesis

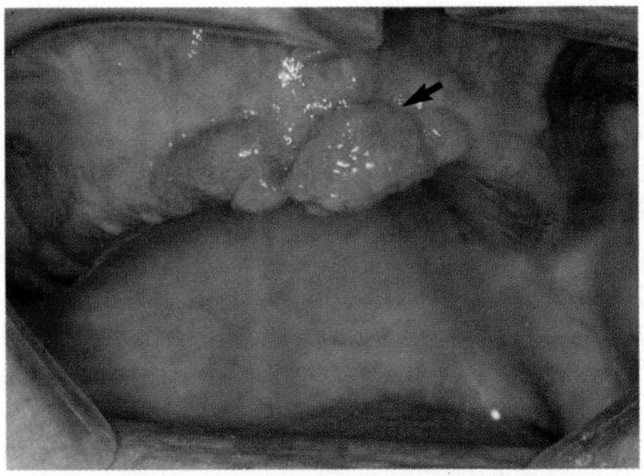

Figure 56-6. Prosthesis-induced fibrous hyperplasia. Chronic denture-induced trauma or irritation has resulted in an overgrowth *(arrow)* of soft tissue. The chief complaint from the patient was an ill-fitting denture. (Courtesy Dr. Catherine Poh, Oral Pathologist, Faculty of Dentistry, University of British Columbia, Vancouver, Canada.)

(Figure 56-6). Although detection is sometimes difficult because of nearly normal color and texture, this flabby hyperplastic tissue is identified by palpating freely movable tissue over edentulous ridges or on the vestibular mucosa.[11]

If fibrous tissue proliferation is observed, the dental hygienist refers the client to the dentist for evaluation and treatment. Depending on the severity of hypermobile tissue, treatment may involve a period of tissue rest, prosthesis adjustment, and/or surgical excision to reduce the excess tissue. Keratinization of edentulous alveolar ridges may be completely absent or may progress to a hyperkeratinized state. This **focal (frictional) hyperkeratosis**, classified as a hyperkeratotic white lesion of the oral mucosa, usually resolves with time on discontinuation of the underlying trauma.[11]

Although it is highly unlikely that chronic irritation resulting from ill-fitting prostheses causes oral carcinoma, trauma induced by dentures and other mechanical irritations probably accelerates the disease progression. The dental hygienist must be especially attentive to oral cancer signs and symptoms: ulceration or erosion, induration, fixation, chronicity, lymphadenopathy, leukoplakia, and erythroplakia (see Chapter 45).

Many oral mucosal conditions in denture wearers are associated with improper oral hygiene care, extended denture wear, or poor prosthesis fit. More specifically, denture-induced lesions are subdivided into the following three categories according to causative factors and clinical features[11] (Table 56-1):

- Reactive or traumatic (Figure 56-7)
- Infectious (Figures 56-8, *A,* and 56-9)
- Mixed reactive and infectious (Figure 56-10)

Reactive or Traumatic Lesions

Reactive or traumatic lesions commonly are secondary to either acute or chronic injury. Lesions in this category are ulcers (see Figure 56-7), focal (frictional) hyperkeratosis, and denture-induced papillary hyperplasia (see Figure 56-10). Figure 56-11 shows an overexuberant repair response that produces hyperplastic tissue. This condition often is painless, but pain may develop if the fibrous lesion is traumatized or ulcerated. Surgical excision and removal of the irritating

TABLE 56-1

Dental Hygiene Diagnoses Related to Deficits in the Need for Skin and Mucous Membrane Integrity of the Head and Neck in Dental Prosthesis–Wearing Clients

Oral Soft Tissue Lesion	Causes	Evidence (Signs and Symptoms)
Reactive Lesions		
Acute ulcers	Ill-fitting prosthesis Chemical agent irritation: Denture adhesive Denture cleanser Self-medication	Yellow-white exudates Red halo Varying pain and tenderness
Chronic ulcers	Same as above	Yellow membrane Elevated margin Little or no pain
Focal (frictional) hyperkeratosis	Chronic rubbing or friction of prosthesis	White patch Asymptomatic
Denture-induced fibrous hyperplasia (epulis fissurata, denture hyperplasia)	Ill-fitting prosthesis	Folds of fibrous connective tissue Varying color Asymptomatic Typical on vestibular mucosa at denture flange contact
Infectious Lesions		
Denture stomatitis (denture sore mouth)	Chronic *Candida albicans* infection Poor oral hygiene care Continuous wear of prosthesis Ill-fitting prosthesis Systemic factors: anemia, diabetes, immunosuppression, menopause Systemic antibiotics Chemical agent irritation: Denture adhesive Denture cleanser Self-medication Denture base allergy	Generalized redness of mucosa Velvet-like appearance Pain and burning sensations Typical under maxillary denture
Angular cheilitis	Chronic *C. albicans* infection Pooling of saliva in commissural folds Riboflavin deficiency	Fissured at angles of mouth Eroded Encrusted Moderate pain
Mixed Lesions		
Papillary hyperplasia	Chronic *C. albicans* infection Chronic low-grade denture trauma	Multiple round to ovoid nodules: "cobblestone" appearance Generalized red mucosa background Rarely ulcerated Typical under maxillary denture

factor are effective methods of treating reactive lesions.[11] Palliative treatment can include over-the-counter products such as Rincinol and Ameseal.

Infectious Lesions

The most common inflammation of the removable dental prosthesis-bearing mucosa is **denture stomatitis** (see Figure 56-8). Despite minimal pain associated with this condition, it often is referred to inappropriately as "denture sore mouth." With a predilection for women, the condition has an incidence of 20% to 40% of the edentulous population and occurs in up to 65% of older adults who wear complete maxillary dentures.[11]

Angular cheilitis is a mixed bacterial and fungal infection typically caused by *Staphylococcus aureus* and *C. albicans* (see Figure 56-9, *A* and *B*). The condition results from small amounts of saliva accumulating at the commissural angles, which promotes the colonization of yeast. Clinically, angular cheilitis appears as cracked, eroded, and encrusted commissural folds and may cause moderate pain. Often it is secondary to overclosure resulting from a reduction in the client's vertical dimension. Vitamin B (riboflavin) deficiency resulting from inadequate nutrition also can cause angular cheilitis.[11]

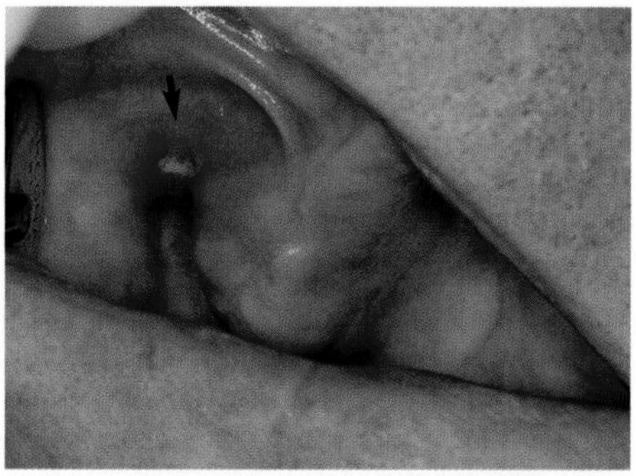

Figure 56-7. Reactive/traumatic lesion. A traumatic ulcer *(arrow)* resulting from elongated buccal flange of the upper complete denture. (Courtesy Dr. Catherine Poh, Oral Pathologist, Faculty of Dentistry, University of British Columbia, Vancouver, Canada.)

Dental treatment requires correcting the prosthesis to eliminate trauma and prescribing antifungal drugs to eliminate the *Candida* infection. Dental hygiene care to prevent recurrence includes client instruction in thorough daily mechanical cleansing of the infected prosthesis as well as chemical immersion in chlorhexidine, or a weak sodium hypochlorite solution (Box 56-1). Sodium hypochlorite damages metal and never should be used when metal is part of any oral appliance. Moreover, if the sodium hypochlorite

BOX 56-1

Inexpensive, Safe, and Effective Cleaning Solution for Removable Dental Prosthesis Devoid of Metal

- 1 tablespoon (15 mL) sodium hypochlorite (household bleach)
- 1 teaspoon (4 mL) detergent (e.g., Calgon)
- 4 ounces (114 mL) water

After soaking, the oral appliance must be rinsed thoroughly with water before reinsertion into the oral cavity.

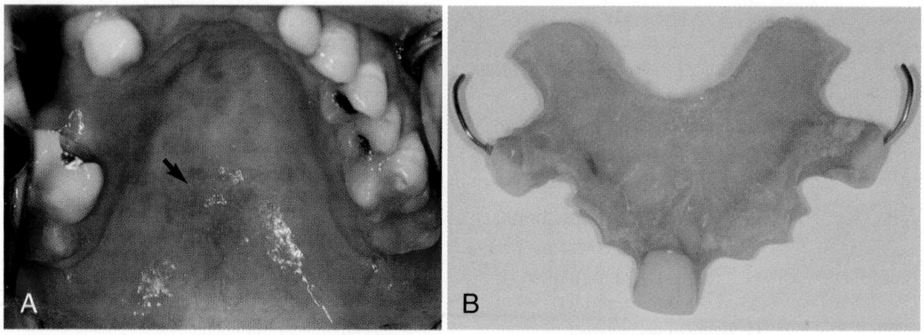

Figure 56-8. **A,** Infectious lesions. *Arrow* points to chronic candidiasis on upper palate (erythematous area). **B,** Upper partial denture worn by client. (Courtesy Dr. Catherine Poh, Oral Pathologist, Faculty of Dentistry, University of British Columbia, Vancouver, Canada.)

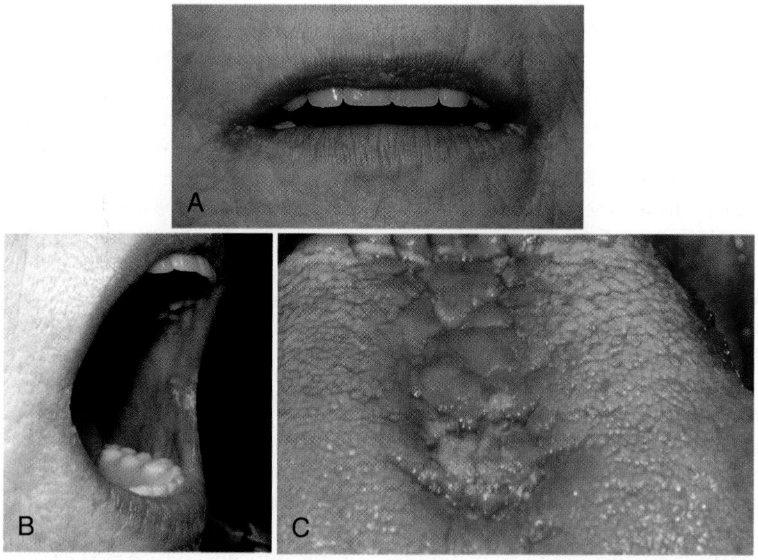

Figure 56-9. Oral candidiasis. **A** and **B,** Angular cheilitis. Note on mouth commissures there are bilateral irregular white plaques on an erythematous base. **C,** Candidiasis on dorsum of tongue (erythematous and de-papillated area at the center). (Courtesy Dr. Eli Whitney, Certified Specialist in Oral Medicine and Oral Pathology, Faculty of Dentistry, University of British Columbia, Vancouver, Canada.)

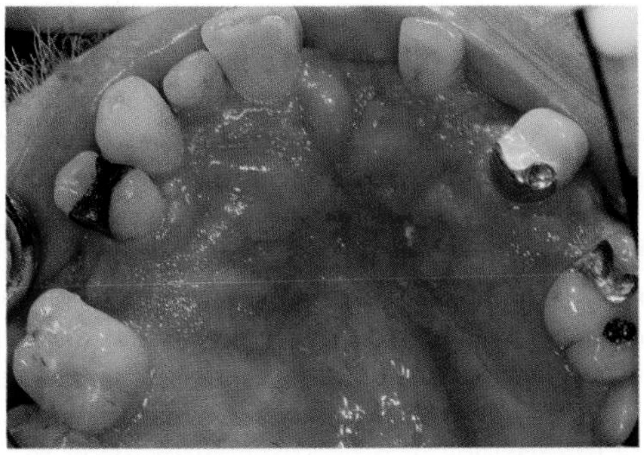

Figure 56-10. Mixed reactive and infectious lesions. Palatal papillary hyperplasia associated with candidiasis. Note that the generalized granular erythematous change of the palatal mucosa matches the shape of a repeatedly relined removable partial denture. Also note denture-induced papillary hyperplasia of the palate. (Courtesy Dr. Catherine Poh, Oral Pathologist, Faculty of Dentistry, University of British Columbia, Vancouver, Canada.)

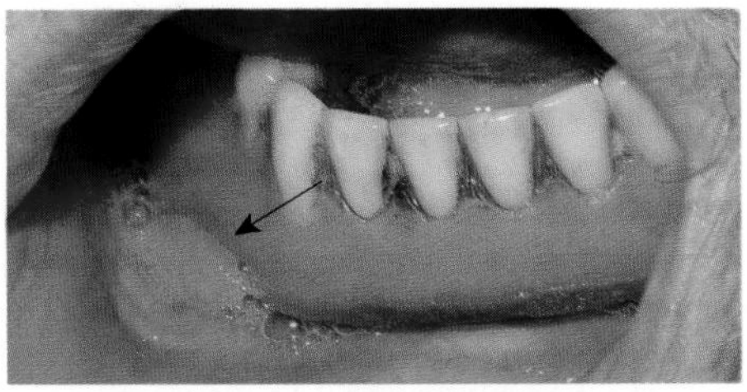

Figure 56-11. Prosthesis-induced fibrous hyperplasia (epulis fissuratum). Chronic denture-induced trauma has resulted in leaflike masses *(arrow)* of soft tissue that overgrow the denture flange. (Courtesy Dr. Catherine Poh, Oral Pathologist, Faculty of Dentistry, University of British Columbia, Vancouver, Canada.)

is too concentrated, or if the denture is soaked for more than 10 minutes, it can bleach the colored portion of the resin base and discolor soft reline materials. Other denture cleansers include nonabrasive denture pastes, commercial denture cleansers, and vinegar. Household cleaners other than a weak sodium hypochlorite solution never should be used to clean oral appliances[8] (see the section on cleansers for removable dental prostheses).

Most removable dental prosthesis-related infections, including denture stomatitis, are caused by a chronic candidiasis infection and are treated using a topical antifungal agent such as Nystatin. Prescribed by the dentist for use at home, Nystatin cream is applied to affected tissues and the dentures to eliminate the fungi. To be effective, topical antifungal agents must be used by the client for approximately 1 week after the disappearance of clinical symptoms.

A chronic *Candida* infection is primarily responsible for the development of denture stomatitis, although recent studies implicate bacteria as the causative agent: gram-positive *Streptococcus* species and *Lactobacillus, Bacteroides,* and *Actinomyces* species. Other contributing factors include biofilm accumulation on dentures; chronic, low-grade soft-tissue trauma resulting from ill-fitting dentures; an unbalanced occlusal relationship; and continuous wearing of the denture at night. In some circumstances systemic conditions such as diabetes, anemia, menopause, malnutrition, and nutrient malabsorption in the digestive tract can predispose an individual to a *Candida* infection.

Chronic candidiasis appears more often on the palatal mucosa rather than on the mandibular alveolar mucosa (see Figure 56-8). Clinical features demonstrate variations in surface texture ranging from a smooth, velvety appearance to a more nodular or hyperplastic form. With severe infections, surfaces may appear eroded, with small confluent vesicles. Characteristically the bright-red color of the denture-supporting mucosa is confined within a well-defined denture border.[11]

Mixed Reactive and Infectious Lesions

Trauma and infection are causative factors contributing to mixed reactive and infectious lesions, such as papillary hyperplasia (see Figure 56-10). A "cobblestone" appearance describes the granular papillary projections that result from a hyperplastic tissue response. This condition can predispose or potentiate the growth of *C. albicans* under the prosthesis and further complicate the problem. Multiple dental therapies to resolve the lesions include surgical excision, antifungal agents, soft-tissue conditioners and liners, and strict oral hygiene measures.[7]

Importance of Regular Professional Care

Findings from a national study reported that only 13% of edentulous seniors had seen a dentist within the previous 12 months, and 67% of them had not visited the dentist within the previous 3 years.[1] These findings underscore a critical role for the dental hygienist in encouraging regular maintenance care and in recognizing oral changes that often go unnoticed by the client.

Periodic maintenance care provides an excellent opportunity to identify denture-related tissue lesions and refer clients for dental evaluation and treatment. Although studies have demonstrated no correlation between cancer at specific sites and the wearing of dentures, denture irritation may be a co-carcinogenic factor in predisposed individuals.

Some clients erroneously perceive that prostheses last a lifetime without further modifications; however, in reality new dentures are needed every 4 to 8 years. Hence education is a priority for the denture-wearing individual.

Dental Hygiene Care for Individuals with Fixed and Removable Dental Prostheses

From the outset, the client must be educated regarding expectations, oral hygiene practices, prosthesis use and care, and regular periodic maintenance appointments. Also, the dental hygienist educates the client about the causes of bone resorption and suggests methods of minimizing the rate of resorption, including removal of dentures at night, regular evaluation to ensure well-fitting dentures, and a calcium-rich diet. Resorption rates vary enormously among individuals, and well-fitting prostheses decrease the rate of resorption. Local factors including trauma can affect the resorption rate so that the denture becomes ill-fitting.

Successful prosthodontic therapy also greatly depends on clients who possess a sense of responsibility regarding their oral health status. The dental hygienist encourages clients to set personal goals for oral health and suggests behavior patterns and techniques that are compatible with their lifestyle, cultural customs, values, and physical capabilities.

The edentulous person's ability to adapt to a denture greatly influences eating pleasure, eating proficiency, and overall health. The quality and quantity of nutritional intake are not necessarily modified in the edentulous individual. Nonetheless, if the prosthesis is ill-fitting, nutritional status may suffer. Eating becomes a chore and less pleasurable. The dental hygienist facilitates success of prosthodontic therapy by assessing the client's nutritional status and providing dietary counseling to ensure that nutritionally rich foods, such as vegetables, meats, beans, fish, and fruits, are not ignored (see Chapter 35).

The dental hygienist assesses loss of retention, stability, and support of the denture and calls problems to the dentist's attention (see Procedure 56-1 and the corresponding Competency Form). The dental hygienist also documents unmet human needs, informs the client and the dentist, and recommends daily self-care to prevent further tissue destruction.

The newly edentulous person commonly requires a denture adjustment within the first 6 to 12 months. Thereafter, annual continued care is essential to denture longevity and meets the need for denture duplication, rebasing, or replacement. Individuals with poor oral hygiene may require more frequent visits.

Clients need to be advised of the importance of daily care of their dentures and the associated soft tissues. Procedure 56-2 and the corresponding Competency Form provides instructions for daily oral care for individuals with removable prostheses. Procedure 56-3 and the corresponding Competency Form provides an overview of instructions for daily oral care for individuals with fixed prostheses. Verbal and written instructions reinforce the homecare regimen, especially for the elderly. A simple reminder to rinse the dentures and mouth after each meal helps reduce accumulation of food debris and biofilm. Written instructions or other formal educational materials that include proper denture hygiene and cleansing of the oral tissues provide specific, tangible recommendations for maintaining oral health. Pertinent information to teach the client is presented in the section on client education issues. At continued-care visits, the dental hygienist assesses the client's ability to perform meticulous oral hygiene care at home.

Removable Dental Prosthesis Cleansers

Maintaining denture hygiene is essential to promote esthetics, control malodor, as well as prevent and treat oral infections in the client. Proper hygienic care can be confusing for the client because of the many products available for home use as well as the various in-office procedures used to maintain hygiene. Commonly available denture cleansers include the following:

- Chemical soak cleansers
- Antimicrobials
- Ultrasonic cleaning devices

Table 56-2 describes common cleansers available. When selecting a cleanser, the client and prosthesis safety are paramount. Abrasive powders and pastes are not recommended for cleaning dentures because of the potential for the client to use these products incorrectly, thus damaging the prosthesis. Denture acrylic can become abraded, and this abrasion may alter the denture fit if a hard-bristle brush or extreme vigor is used when the prosthesis is cleaned.

Prosthesis cleanser efficacy depends partially on the client's dexterity. Brushing with a nonabrasive paste is suitable for the client who is motivated and has the dexterity to clean all denture surfaces thoroughly; however, this cleansing method is the most difficult, especially for the physically challenged or older adult client. Chemical soak cleansers can be alternatives to mechanical cleansing. Alkaline peroxide and hypochlorite solutions can be recommended for dentures with and without metal components, respectively.

Procedure 56-1 Professional Care for Clients with Removable Dental Prostheses

EQUIPMENT

Protective barriers
Prophy cup and bristled brush
Low-speed handpiece
Antimicrobial mouth rinse
Tin oxide
Mouth mirror
Hand mirror
Gauze
Disclosing solution
Tongue blades
Small plastic bag
Stain and calculus remover solution
Ultrasonic cleaning unit

STEPS

Assessment

1. Update client's health history to identify systemic disorders, current medications, and conditions that may affect care and ability to wear the prostheses.
2. Review client's personal history records; note details such as age, occupation, and culture.
3. Review client's dental history.
4. Ask client to explain prostheses problems experienced; listen attentively to complaints.
5. Perform comprehensive assessment of head and neck.
6. Assess the temporomandibular joint (TMJ) and associated musculature as client opens and closes mouth and slides jaw from side to side.
7. Assess extraoral soft tissues.
8. Assess intraoral soft tissues for evidence of local denture trauma or systemic diseases, and record lesion color, texture, size, and contour, and presence of pain.
9. Visually inspect the prosthesis for cleanliness and palpate prosthesis-bearing mucosa with prosthesis out of the mouth.
10. Assess the structure and form of the alveolar ridges.
11. Document changes in associated structures, including the tongue, floor of the mouth, and oropharynx.
12. Assess oral hygiene status.
13. Ask client to displace the prosthesis away from supporting tissues. The posterior border seal of the maxillary denture is checked by attempting to pull the anterior teeth forward.

Procedure 56-1 Professional Care for Clients with Removable Dental Prostheses—cont'd

14. Assess stability of the prosthesis with respect to its position during normal oral functions.
15. Indicate changes in occlusion and articulation.

Dental Hygiene Diagnosis

16. Analyze objective and subjective assessment data; identify unmet human needs.
17. Present significant findings to client and dentist.

Planning

18. Determine a dental hygiene care plan and goals to be achieved in consultation with client and dentist.

Implementation

19. Review self-care and dental care; suggest methods for improvement.
20. Use disclosing solution to stain biofilm on the prosthesis (when appropriate).
21. Counsel client on adequate nutrition.
22. Fill a small plastic bag with cleaning solution, label with client's name, submerge the prosthesis in it, and place the bag in an ultrasonic cleaning unit (Figure 56-12).
23. Lightly polish the prosthesis with an extremely fine polishing agent (tin oxide) *on external surfaces only,* and thoroughly rinse under warm water (when appropriate).

Evaluation

24. Discuss continued-care interval. Emphasize the importance of regular professional care.
25. Measure the achievement of goals established at the previous dental hygiene care appointment.
26. Formulate an evaluative statement regarding the level of goal attainment.
27. Document service in client's record under "Services Rendered," and date entry.

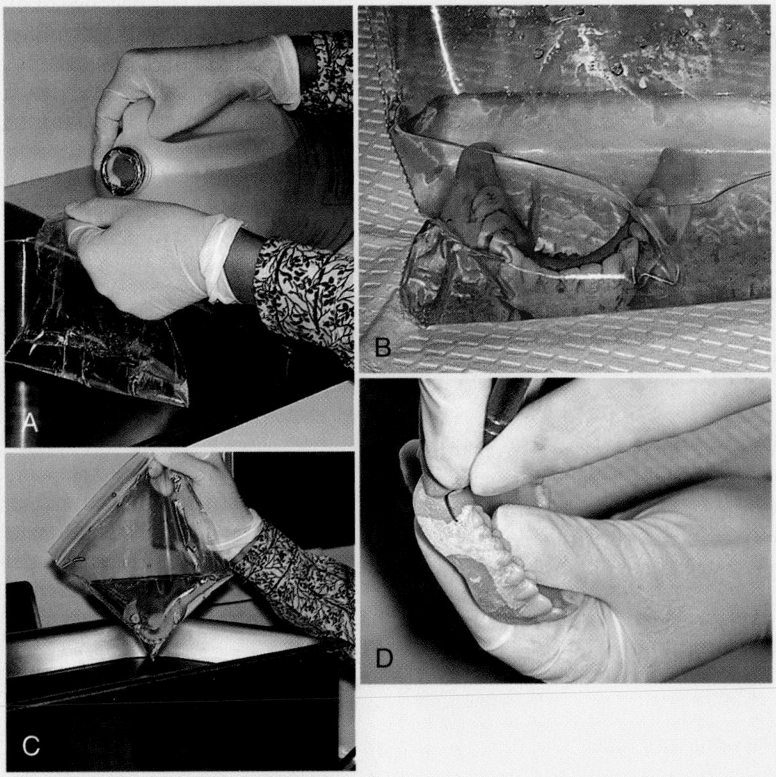

Figure 56-12. Ultrasonic cleaning of denture. **A,** Fill plastic bag with stain and calculus remover solution. **B,** Place denture in bag with solution. **C,** Place bag in ultrasonic cleaner chamber and set for 10 to 14 minutes. **D,** Some dentures may require manual scaling to remove deposits; however, the inner impression is avoided. (Courtesy Bertha Chan.)

The majority of clinical studies report hypochlorites to be an efficacious soaking method for dentures constructed with only acrylic materials. Caution, however, must be taken to avoid use of hypochlorites on any metal-containing prostheses.[8] If an offensive taste and odor linger after the hypochlorite soak, alkaline peroxide may be used subsequently. (See Box 56-1 for how to make an effective denture cleaner.) Table 56-3 presents the variety of oral appliances and dental prostheses that also can be cleaned by these denture-cleaning methods.

Nutritional Considerations for Individuals with Fixed and Removable Dental Prostheses

Many of the lesions associated with prosthesis wearing are a result of ill-fitting dentures, poor denture and oral hygiene care, and prolonged wearing of the prosthesis. Nutritional

Procedure 56-2 Daily Oral and Denture Hygiene Care for Individuals with Removable Prostheses

EQUIPMENT

Soft denture brush, soft intraoral toothbrush, antimicrobial mouth rinse
Basin
Denture cup
Towel
Dilute sodium hypochlorite solution (complete dentures) or commercial denture cleanser (partial dentures)
Warm water
Wall-mounted mirror
Soft nylon toothbrush

STEPS

1. Explain the importance of daily care for both dentures and soft tissues.
2. Describe the consequences of oral and denture hygiene neglect.
3. Summarize the client's responsibilities in monitoring oral function and health status.
4. Advise against the use of denture home-repair kits and encourage the client to return to the dentist for proper care.
5. Discourage use of denture adhesives with a stable and retentive prosthesis. Under dentist supervision, a small amount of adhesive (3-4 pea-sized drops) may be applied to the inner surface that directly contacts the oral mucosa. Denture adhesives are not normally used with partial removable dentures.
6. Remind the client to brush denture after each meal and before retiring or, at the very least, to rinse it under running water.
7. Teach self-examination of denture for proper fit, denture deposits, and abraded inner and outer surfaces.
8. Teach client that some commercially available denture powders and pastes are too abrasive for dentures and are not recommended for use.
9. Suggest daily use of fresh denture immersion cleansers. Recommend a dilute sodium hypochlorite solution as a cleanser for complete dentures (Figure 56-13; see Box 56-1). Soak complete dentures for 5 to 10 minutes, and rinse thoroughly. Partial dentures benefit from alkaline peroxide solutions found in many denture-cleansing products, usually in the form of a tablet. Soak partial denture for 15 minutes or overnight, and rinse thoroughly. Change solutions daily.
10. Teach the client to remove denture when possible and at night while at rest.
11. Assemble supplies.
12. Fill basin with water, and line with a small towel.
13. Gently remove denture, and rinse away saliva and loose debris. In the case of complete dentures, remove any denture adhesive material.
14. Firmly grasp denture in palm of one hand, and hold over water-filled basin.
15. Demonstrate use of a denture brush with a mild soap solution or nonabrasive denture paste to remove accumulations on the inner impression and outer polished surfaces, and adapt brush as necessary (Figure 56-14).
16. Rinse denture and brush under running water to completely remove all denture cleanser.
17. Inspect denture for any remaining biofilm, food debris, or cleanser by visual and tactile examination.
18. Place prosthesis in a denture cup.
19. On removal of denture, rinse mouth with warm water, antimicrobial mouth rinse, or saline solution.
20. Teach client to use a soft toothbrush or soft cloth daily to clean edentulous mucosa and tongue by employing long strokes in a posterior-to-anterior direction.
21. Teach client to use thumb and index finger to massage edentulous tissues daily by applying pressure and then releasing it continually along the ridge. Mechanical, vibratory stimulation with the sides of multitufted soft toothbrush filaments can provide similar results.

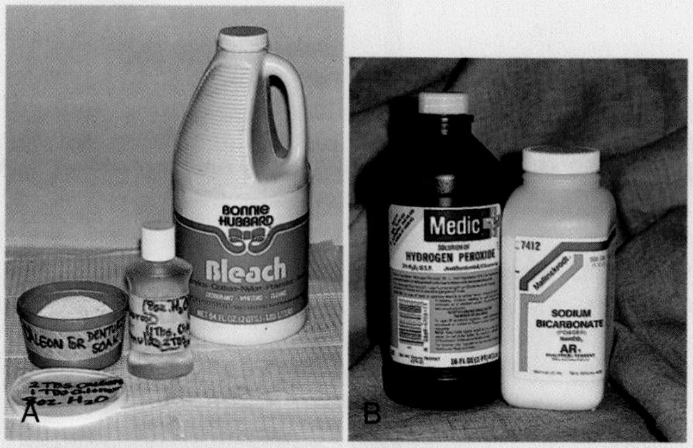

Figure 56-13. Inexpensive denture cleaners. **A,** Combination of sodium hypochlorite, Calgon, and water for denture without metal. **B,** Combination of hydrogen peroxide and sodium bicarbonate forms an alkaline peroxide solution for dentures with metal. (Courtesy Bertha Chan.)

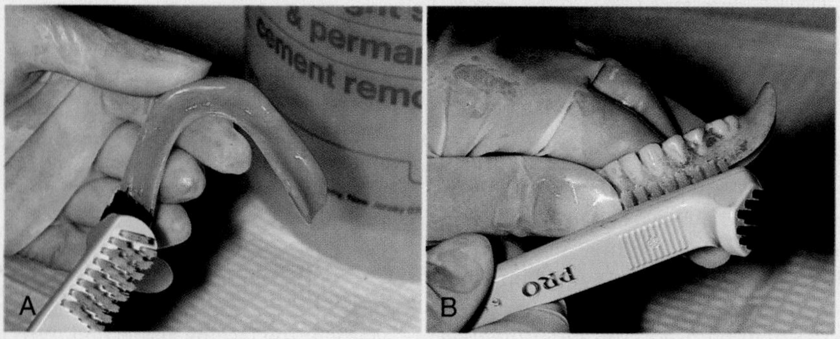

Figure 56-14. **A,** Adaptation of denture brush on inner surface of denture. **B,** Adaptation of denture brush on outer surface of denture. (Courtesy Bertha Chan.)

Procedure 56-3 Daily Oral Care for Individuals with Fixed Dental Prostheses

EQUIPMENT

Soft toothbrush
Interdental cleaners such as variable-diameter floss, dental floss, dental yarn, floss threaders
Antimicrobial mouth rinse
Wall-mounted mirror

STEPS

1. Assemble supplies.
2. Explain the importance of daily self-care for fixed dental prostheses, remaining natural teeth, and periodontal tissues.
3. Describe the consequences of oral and prosthesis hygiene neglect.
4. Summarize the client's responsibilities in monitoring oral function and health status.
5. Teach the client to brush natural teeth and fixed prosthesis after each meal and before retiring. Clients benefit from flossing remaining natural teeth and fixed prosthesis and using an antimicrobial mouth rinse daily.
6. Demonstrate use of a soft toothbrush to remove biofilm and gross debris from fixed prosthesis and remaining natural teeth (see Chapter 23).
7. Demonstrate use of suitable interdental aid to cleanse under the pontic and around abutments and natural teeth (Figure 56-15) (see Chapter 24).

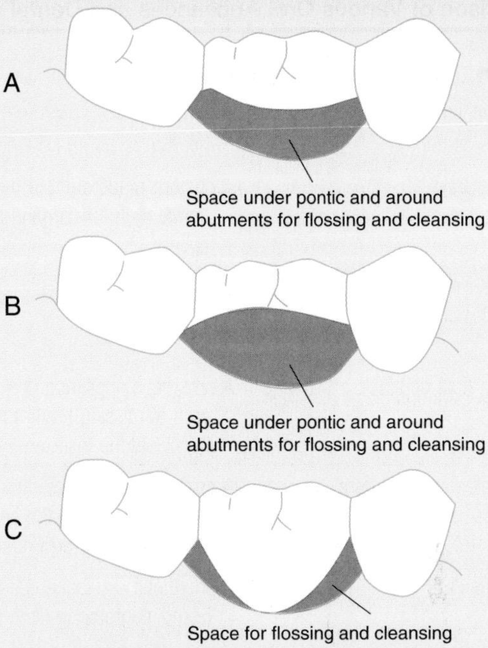

Figure 56-15. Fixed partial denture pontics. **A,** Conventional. **B,** Modified. **C,** Conical (bullet). (Courtesy Dr. Joanne Walton, Prosthodontist, Faculty of Dentistry, University of British Columbia, Vancouver, Canada.)

TABLE 56-2
Removable Dental Prostheses Cleansing Products

Product	Mechanism of Action	Advantages	Disadvantages
Chemical Cleansers			
Alkaline hypochlorite	Dissolves mucins and organic substances of prosthesis biofilm matrix	Bactericidal Fungicidal Bleaches stains May inhibit calculus formation	Corrodes metals Odor and taste may be unacceptable May bleach acrylic if used in high concentration or for prolonged periods
Alkaline peroxide	Mechanical cleansing effect caused by the release of oxygen (bubbling)	Some antibacterial effect Removes stain	Harmful to soft liners Not very effective in removing calculus
Antimicrobial Cleansers			
Chlorhexidine gluconate solution	Antimicrobial action by chemical agent	Antibacterial Antifungal	Temporary relief of denture stomatitis symptoms Stains denture teeth
Ultrasonic cleaning devices	Ultrasonic sound wave action creates vibrating/bubbling effect	Removes biofilm Enhances effectiveness of chemical cleansers	Commonly an in-office procedure Uncertain efficacy of ultrasonic action
Microwave radiation (in-office use only)	Electromagnetic waves kill microorganisms	Bactericidal Minimal negative effect on resilient liners	High temperatures can affect dimensional stability of a denture

TABLE 56-3

Comparison of Various Oral Appliances and Dental Prosthesis*

Appliance	Definition	Purpose
Athletic mouth guard (mouth protector)	An oral appliance designed to protect the teeth and head from trauma during contact sports	Prevents oral and facial injury
Bleaching trays	A custom-made stent in the shape of the teeth and dental arch for carrying the bleaching or whitening agents	Holds the whitening agent against the tooth surfaces
Removable dental prostheses (dentures)		Replaces teeth (form, function, and appearance) in edentulous or partially edentulous dental arches
Complete (full) denture	A prosthetic appliance designed to replace an entire arch of missing teeth and the surrounding alveolar bone; can be inserted and removed by the client	Same as for dentures above
Removable partial denture	A prosthetic appliance designed to replace several missing teeth and the surrounding alveolar bone; can be inserted and removed by the client	Same as for dentures above
Implant denture	A prosthetic appliance designed to fit over osseointegrated implant fixtures	Same as for dentures above
Immediate denture	A prosthetic appliance placed immediately after remaining teeth are extracted from a partially edentulous arch	Same as for dentures above
Fixed partial dental prosthesis (bridge)	A prosthetic appliance designed to replace several missing teeth; permanently cemented in place and removed only by the dentist	Same as for dentures above
Fluoride tray (custom)	A custom-made stent in the shape of the teeth and dental arch for carrying the fluoride agent to the tooth structure	Holds the prescription agent against the tooth surface to decrease caries risk
Bruxing guard (night guard and day guard)	A hard acrylic appliance that fits over all or just several of the maxillary or mandibular teeth to create a functional occlusion or to relax the muscles; may be worn at night or during the day	Controls tooth attrition Eases muscle hyperactivity and pressure on temporomandibular joint
Oral habit appliance	An oral appliance used to interfere with habits such as thumbsucking, tongue sucking, or tongue thrusting	Prevents the habitual behavior from occurring
Orthodontic appliance or repositioner	An oral appliance used for tooth movement and the treatment of malocclusion	Provides tooth movement and stabilization
Stent	A device used after periodontal surgery to support and protect the oral tissues and/or to hold a medicinal or other desired agent in a particular area	Stabilizes general tissue during periodontal surgery Holds anesthetic or antiseptic agents in the area of the surgical site
Sleep apnea or snoring appliance	A flexible, custom-made device that positions the jaw forward during sleep	Opens the airway during sleep Prevents snoring
Space maintainer	A fixed or removable oral appliance to maintain a space created by premature tooth loss	Maintains an open space in the dental arch caused by premature tooth loss until the permanent tooth can erupt

*See also Chapter 37.

deficiencies are seldom noticed and therefore infrequently corrected. For example, a client deficient in B-complex vitamins may have symptoms of atrophic glossitis; angular cheilitis; or cracking, fissuring, or ulceration of the lips. These clinical signs may be interpreted as a chronic *C. albicans* infection rather than a nutritional deficiency. Although nutritional deficiencies are difficult to identify, the dental hygienist must be cognizant of changes related to them in some denture wearers. After assessment the dental hygienist informs the dentist of potential nutritional problems and either recommends dietary measures to the client that may improve oral health or refers the client to a dietitian.

Nutritional Factors

Key nutritional factors for clients include the following (see Chapter 35):

- Negative water balance and its effect on oral structures
- Negative calcium balance and its effect on alveolar bone
- Nitrogen-protein imbalance and resulting muscle weakness and oral tissue fragility

Water is an essential nutrient for all body functions. Therefore evidence of tissue dehydration can be recognized throughout the body, especially in elderly individuals, as wrinkled skin, loss of muscle mass, decreased sweat and sebaceous gland secretions, dry eyes, xerostomia, and a smooth, atrophic tongue. The best dietary recommendation for dehydrated clients is to consume vegetable soup because water and nutrients are retained more effectively in this form.

A negative calcium balance results in osteoporosis, which can precipitate rapid and extensive resorption of the alveolar ridges. A deficit in calcium intake, absorption, or transport may be responsible for the bony changes. Low-fat milk and milk products are good dietary sources of calcium (see Chapter 35 for food sources of calcium).

Protein depletion not only affects muscle mass but also may increase tissue fragility and lip cracking. A decrease in muscle mastication mass and strength is especially evident in the older adult and can be monitored by placing the finger in the vestibule of the mouth and asking clients to clench their teeth. Clients are encouraged to maintain a high-protein diet (e.g., meat, fish, beans, tofu, and legumes) to maintain muscle mass.

Undoubtedly, food nutritional quality depends on the preparation method. Variations in food preparation result from the client's physical capabilities, living conditions, and cultural preferences. Therefore dietary advice should include cooking instructions that maximize the nutrient value of the diet with consideration of individual circumstances and preferences. For example, meat and fish are most nutritious when broiled or boiled rather than fried. In addition to limiting saturated fat intake, boiling foods breaks down complex proteins into more easily digestible components. On the other hand, fried protein-rich foods lose some nutritional value because the protein coagulates and becomes more difficult to digest.

Nutrition and the Edentulous Older Adult

For the edentulous older adult, diet is of great concern. (See Chapters 35 and 55.) Essential nutrient deficiency magnifies the tissue friability and diminishes repair potential observed in geriatric clients. Older adults may have low incomes, inadequate kitchen facilities, loneliness, poor physical health, and other conditions that predispose them to poor nutritional habits. A lack of knowledge and interest in proper nutrition also contributes to malnutrition. The older adult's dietary intake often is affected by wearing dentures, and deficiencies in protein, calcium, and B-complex vitamins may be present. Normally these nutrients are essential in the maintenance and repair of oral tissues and bone. Many older adults have a limited ability to digest and absorb food. This problem can be exacerbated by ill-fitting prostheses, which may result in chewing difficulties and diminish consumption of fibrous foods. Therefore digestion, absorption, and use of nutrients are impaired. Two common dietary tendencies of the aged edentulous person are the following:

- Preference for a soft diet high in carbohydrate and refined sugar
- Consumption of fewer protein-rich and high-fiber foods

For these reasons the dental hygienist routinely assesses nutritional habits and suggests healthy food alternatives to promote weight control and a nutritionally balanced diet (Table 56-4). This assessment and counseling can be accomplished effectively if simple, well-defined, concise guidelines are constructed so that no major changes in food habits and preferences are made. The client and the dental hygienist can set nutritional goals, taking into account lifestyle, financial resources, and cultural preferences. With the edentulous client, nutritional deficits should always be considered during determination of factors that contribute to a denture-related problem.

CLIENT EDUCATION TIPS

- Explain the options available for tooth replacement (e.g., fixed versus removable prostheses).
- Explain the types of chemical cleansing agents, frequency and duration of their application, and other instructions for their use (see Table 56-2).
- Demonstrate techniques for mechanical cleansing of the prosthesis and cleansing and massage of the oral tissues (see Procedures 56-1 through 56-3).
- Provide special instructions for gentle cleansing of soft lining materials if necessary.
- Reinforce the need for regular professional care for denture-wearing individuals that includes intraoral and extraoral assessment and examination of the prosthesis.
- Explain the potentially harmful effects of improper prosthesis care and oral hygiene neglect.
- Emphasize self-care strategies including daily oral hygiene, adequate nutrition, oral tissue self-examination, and resting denture-bearing surfaces.
- Recommend techniques and products for denture use, care, and cleaning. Avoid oxygenating and hypochlorite-type denture cleaners in the presence of resilient liners and tissue conditioners.
- Instruct client to consume foods in smaller pieces, lengthen chewing time, evenly distribute food to both the left and the right sides of the mouth while chewing, and avoid repeated incision with anterior denture teeth.
- Instruct the prosthodontic client to avoid chewing gum and sticky foods.
- Emphasize the value of replacing missing teeth in restoring function; preventing drifting of remaining natural teeth; instructions for use, care, and cleaning of the prosthesis; and importance of regular professional evaluations.

TABLE 56-4

Nutritional Guidelines for Maintenance of Oral Health in Edentulous and Partially Edentulous Clients

Nutritional Goal	Rationale
Eat a variety of foods.	Essential for repair and maintenance of structurally and functionally competent body parts; increases likelihood of getting necessary nutrients
Select foods high in complex carbohydrates: fruits, vegetables, whole-grain bread, and cereals.	Blood glucose levels rise less if complex carbohydrates are consumed rather than simple sugars. Also, fiber in these foods promotes normal bowel function and may reduce serum cholesterol.
Protein-rich foods including lean meat, poultry, fish, dried peas, and beans are required daily.	Maintains strength and integrity of tissues, especially when exposed to physiologic stress
Obtain calcium from dairy products; some nondairy foods also contain substantial amounts of calcium.	Calcium intake is critical to maintain bone mass. Alveolar bone is an early site of calcium withdrawal if dietary calcium intake is low.
Consume fruit juices containing vitamin C and citrus fruit daily.	Essential for repair and healing of wounds and for absorption of other vitamins and minerals
Limit intake of processed foods high in saturated and hydrogenated fats and sodium.	Evidence links high fat intake to heart disease, certain cancers, and obesity. High sodium intake may cause hypertension.
Limit intake of bakery products high in fat and simple sugars.	Bakery products are often high in calories and/or low in nutrients.
Drink eight glasses of water daily.	Essential nutrient for all body functions

Adapted from Zarb GA, Hobkirk JA, Eckert SE, et al: *Prosthodontic treatment for edentulous patients*, ed 13, St Louis, 2013, Mosby.
See also Chapter 35.

- Explain the value of denture marking to prevent loss during short-term or long-term care.

LEGAL, ETHICAL, AND SAFETY ISSUES

- Provide services within the scope of dental hygiene practice as stipulated by the regulatory body of each province or state.
- Maintain written and dated records (in ink) of the status of the client's oral condition, condition of dental appliances, the treatment provided, recommended treatment, recommended referrals, client's refusal or acceptance of treatment, and any pertinent information regarding care.
- Have client remove and reinsert the denture; if the client is unable to do so, the dental hygienist should request that the dentist, accompanying family member, or client's caregiver remove and reinsert the denture.
- Provide a discreet location for the client to remove the denture; this ensures that the client's dignity is respected.
- Have clients maintain control of their own dentures to avoid damage.

KEY CONCEPTS

- A prosthesis is a fixed or removable appliance that is functionally and cosmetically designed to replace a missing tooth or teeth.
- Persons who wear dental prostheses receive an oral examination periodically to monitor the health of hard and soft tissues, the functional integrity of the prosthesis, and changes that may be warranted. Frequency should be based on the client's risk factors for disease.
- A removable dental prosthesis should be marked with the wearer's name or identification number, especially if the person lives in an institutional setting.
- Just like natural oral structures, the dental prosthesis and oral cavity of the wearer must be cleansed thoroughly daily.
- Risk factors for edentulism include caries, periodontal disease, low socioeconomic status, inadequate access to professional care, low frequency of care, and poor daily oral hygiene.
- Loss of natural teeth is associated with fear of aging, decreased sexuality, feelings of insecurity, fear of rejection, loss of self-esteem, and unrealistic expectations for tooth replacement.
- Oral changes related to tooth loss include resorption of the residual ridge and alveolar bone, oral mucous membrane remodeling, and loss of orofacial muscle tone.
- Clients who lose teeth face challenges in their physical appearance, speech, and masticatory efficiency.
- Removable dental prosthesis-induced oral lesions include fibrous hyperplasia, focal hyperkeratosis, denture stomatitis, chronic candidiasis, angular cheilitis, and papillary hyperplasia.
- Client education is a priority for clients wearing prostheses and oral appliances. Clients must know how to clean the mouth and prosthesis or oral appliance to maintain their oral health.

CRITICAL THINKING EXERCISES

In each case, develop a dental hygiene diagnosis, client goals, and a dental hygiene care plan.

1. Jeremy Myers, age 67, is a new client at a dental hygiene care center. Recently widowed, Mr. Myers lives alone in a complex for retired individuals and relies solely on social security payments for living expenses. The client wears a complete maxillary denture and has his natural mandibular dentition remaining. After a review of the client's health, dental, and dental hygiene histories, the dental hygienist identifies unmet human needs experienced by the client that relate to dental hygiene care. The client complains of a sore palate and "loose denture that hurts especially while eating." On intraoral examination the dental hygienist notices a generalized redness on the palatal mucosa. The denture is easily displaced when retention is evaluated. Furthermore, periodontal assessment of the natural dentition reveals a generalized 4- to 5-mm loss of attachment and bleeding on probing. Moderate biofilm and subgingival calculus are present throughout the mandible.
2. Andrea Smith, an 84-year-old widow, visits the dental office twice a year for regular dental and dental hygiene assessments and care. She has a maxillary partial removable denture that replaces her lost molar teeth on both the right and left side of the arch as well as replacing her two maxillary central incisors. Mrs. Smith has retained most of her mandibular teeth except her left second premolar and left first molar. These teeth have been replaced with a fixed partial dental prosthesis or bridge. She is in relatively good health and takes no medications.

   At her current continued-care appointment she has heavy biofilm deposits around her bridge but light to moderate deposits around her remaining natural teeth. She has light calculus deposits localized to the mandibular anterior teeth. On assessment the hygienist finds periodontal probing depths ranging from 3 to 4 mm, with a 6-mm pocket on the mesial surface of the second molar, which serves as an abutment for her bridge. There is 2 mm of recession generalized. Mrs. Smith states that her removable partial denture fits well and that she rarely removes the denture. Mrs. Smith is reluctant to remove the denture.
3. Maxwell Green is a 59-year-old new client. He has had complete removable maxillary and mandibular dentures for 15 years. Since becoming edentulous, Mr. Green has not had new dentures fabricated, nor has he had the existing dentures relined. Mr. Green reports that he is in relatively good health, but on his health history form he has noted that he smokes and avoids regular checkups with his family physician. He states, "The only reason I am here is because my wife is retiring soon and we will lose our dental insurance." Mrs. Green is concerned that Mr. Green's dentures must be replaced, and she wants to ensure that her dental insurance will cover the cost of new dentures.

   On assessment the hygienist notices that the denture teeth are severely worn and covered with heavy accumulations of stain, calculus, and biofilm. The gingival portions of the acrylic dentures are scratched. Mr. Green has stated that the dentures "have never fit right" and that "I often cannot eat with the dentures in my mouth." He also complains of frequent sore spots under the denture when he eats certain foods, such as grains and nuts. Mr. Green's denture care includes soaking the denture in household bleach occasionally and leaving the dentures on the kitchen counter at night before retiring to bed.
4. Judith King, age 75, lives with her 80-year-old husband in a senior citizens' complex close to the dental office. She usually schedules continued-care appointments annually, but it has been 2 years since her last visit. On the health history Mrs. King reports that she missed last year's visit because of a stroke. She is partially paralyzed on the right side, which is her dominant side. Mrs. King also has experienced some facial paralysis as a result of the stroke. Her current medications include a blood thinner and a diuretic. Mrs. King wears a complete maxillary removable denture and a partial removable mandibular denture. She has retained her mandibular anterior teeth from canine to canine. During assessment the hygienist finds moderate to heavy biofilm and food accumulations. Mrs. King has light to moderate calculus accumulations on the remaining natural teeth. Periodontal probing depths are 3 mm or less with bleeding on probing and no gingival recession. The maxillary denture appears to fit well, but the mandibular denture appears to be loose and has a broken supporting clasp.

REFERENCES

1. U.S. Department of Health and Human Services: *Oral health in America: a report of the Surgeon General*, Rockville, Md, 2000, U.S. Department of Health and Human Services, National Institute of Dental and Craniofacial Research, National Institutes of Health.
2. Dye BA, Li X, Beltrán-Aguilar ED: *Selected oral health indicators in the United States, 2005–2008*, NCHS data brief, no 96, Hyattsville, Md, 2012, National Center for Health Statistics.
3. *Statistics Canada: Canada year book 2010*, 2010. Available at: http://www.statcan.gc.ca/pub/11-402-x/2010000/pdf/seniors-aines-eng.pdf. Accessed August 4, 2012.
4. Fiske J, Davis DM, Frances C, Gelbier S: The emotional effects of tooth loss in edentulous people, *Br Dent J* 184:90, 1998.
5. Carlsson GE, Persson G: Morphological changes of the mandible after extraction and wearing of dentures: a longitudinal, clinical, and x-ray cephalometric study covering five years, *Odontol Revy* 18:27, 1967.
6. Allen PF, McMillan AS: A review of the functional and psychosocial outcomes of edentulousness treated with complete replacement dentures, *J Can Dent Assoc* 69:662, 2003.
7. Zarb GA, Hobkirk JA, Eckert SE, et al: *Prosthodontic treatment for edentulous patients*, ed 13, St Louis, 2013, Mosby.
8. Felton D, Cooper L, Duqum I, et al: Evidence-based guidelines for the care and maintenance of complete dentures: a publication of the American College of Prosthodontics, *J Prosthodont* 20:S1, 2011.
9. Abd Shukor SS, Juszczyk AS, Clark RKF, et al: The effect of cyclic drying on dimensional changes of acrylic resin maxillary complete dentures, *J Oral Rehabil* 33:654, 2006.
10. Stafford GD, Arendorf T, Hugget R: The effect of overnight drying and water immersion on *Candida* colonization and properties of complete dentures, *J Dent* 14:52, 1986.
11. Regezi JA, Sciubba JJ, Jordan R: *Oral pathology: clinical pathologic correlations*, ed 6, St Louis, 2011, Saunders.

EVOLVE RESOURCES

Please visit http://evolve.elsevier.com/Darby/hygiene for additional practice and study support tools.

CHAPTER 57

Orofacial Clefts and Fractured Jaw

Joanna L. Harris-Worelds

COMPETENCIES

1. Discuss orofacial clefts, including:
   - Discuss their incidence, prevalence, and etiology.
   - Differentiate between the types of lip and palatal clefts.
   - Educate caregivers about complications and hygiene care associated with orofacial clefts.
2. Discuss jaw fractures, including:
   - Discuss the incidence, prevalence, etiology, and types of fractures.
   - Recognize signs and symptoms of a fractured jaw.
   - Plan dental hygiene care for a client undergoing maxillomandibular fixation.
   - Educate clients about the prevention of jaw fractures.

Orofacial Clefts

The failure of lip and palate tissues to close during embryonic development creates **orofacial clefts**. Orofacial clefts are one of the most common craniofacial anomalies and congenital (birth) defects, and they have the following characteristics:

- They result from a malformation, a deformation, or a disruption in one or more parts of the body.
- They are present at birth.
- They have serious adverse effects on health, development, or functional ability.[1]

These congenital anomalies are categorized into two groups: cleft palate only and cleft lip with or without cleft palate.

Incidence and Prevalence

Orofacial clefts are the most prevalent birth defects in the United States, affecting approximately 6800 to 8000 infants annually.[1,2] One in 600 infants is affected by an orofacial cleft; clefts affecting either the lip, the palate, or both are less common (1 in 1574 infants) than only cleft palate without cleft lip (1 in 940 infants).[2,3] The condition is most common among Asians or individuals with Asian ancestry, such as North American Indians.[3-6] Non-Hispanic whites are five to seven times more likely to have an orofacial cleft than African Americans, who have the lowest prevalence among all ethnic groups.[4,5] Orofacial clefts are more predominant among boys than girls by a ratio of 3:2.[7] Regarding the type of orofacial cleft, boys are more likely to exhibit an orofacial cleft involving both the lip and the palate. There is a female predominance for only cleft palate without cleft lip.[7,8]

Etiology

Orofacial clefts are divided into two etiologic groups: isolated clefts (the client has no other related health problems) and clefts associated with other birth defects or syndromes.[9] A **syndrome** is a set of symptoms that characterize a disease, disorder, or condition. Clefts are associated with more than 300 syndromes, but most of these syndromes are rare.[9] Syndromes commonly associated with orofacial clefts include Van der Woude, Treacher Collins, Crouzon, Apert, and DiGeorge syndromes. Orofacial clefts can be associated with Pierre Robin sequence, which is not a syndrome but a specific presentation of three distinct characteristics: cleft palate, **micrognathia** (small mandible), and **glossoptosis** (airway obstruction caused by tongue displacement).[10]

The cause of nonsyndromic orofacial clefts is not completely understood. Several factors such as maternal smoking, lack of folic acid, nutritional deficiencies, and family history seem to have a strong association with the occurrence of nonsyndromic orofacial clefts.[3,5,9,10] Although a daily vitamin supplement may not completely prevent the occurrence of an orofacial cleft, it is recommended to women of childbearing age to reduce the occurrences of neural tube defects.[5] In addition, isolated clefts may be caused by an interaction between an individual's genetic predisposition and environmental factors.[3,5,9] Risks for orofacial clefts are found within a particular family; however, this is dependent on how many family members have clefts, how closely they are related, the race and sex of the affected individuals, and the type of cleft.[9] Another environmental factor that may contribute to a higher risk of an infant developing an orofacial cleft is the ingestion of drugs by the mother during pregnancy, especially vasoactive or anticonvulsant medications.[5] Palatal clefts without a corresponding lip cleft can be associated with a developmental cause.

Types of Orofacial Clefts

Embryology

Development of the lip and palate occurs during the early to middle portion of the first trimester of pregnancy. A cleft of the upper lip occurs during the fifth week of fetal development. At this time, fusion of the medial nasal and maxillary processes (prominences) forms the philtrum (eFigure 57-1). The primary or anterior palate develops separately from the

Figures, tables, and boxes marked as "e" are available as supplemental material on the Evolve site. Visit http://evolve.elsevier.com/Darby/hygiene to access these materials.

secondary or posterior palate. A cleft of the palate may occur at any time during development of the palate and at different locations and in different structures of the palate. A primary palatal cleft occurs when the cells do not penetrate the grooves between the medial nasal and maxillary processes.

The palate begins to form at the end of the fifth week and is complete by the twelfth week of fetal development. Formation of the secondary palate involves the fusion of the median palatine process with the lateral palatine processes or shelves. The median palatine process is composed of the median nasal process and the maxillary processes. The lateral palatine processes or shelves are the internal aspects of the maxillary processes. During palatal development, these shelves are initially positioned downward and then elevated horizontally for fusion with each other. Failure of fusion might be attributed to late horizontal movement of the shelves, rupture after fusion, or other factors, such as **macroglossia** (enlarged tongue) and micrognathia, which can block or affect the movement of the shelves.[6] Palatal development progresses from the anterior to the posterior or from the primary palate to the uvula (eFigure 57-2).[6,8] Visit http://evolve.elsevier.com/Darby/hygiene for figures illustrating stages of human palatal development.

Location of Clefts

Orofacial clefts may or may not involve both the lip and the palate simultaneously. The severity of the cleft will vary depending on the extent of the lack of fusion between the hard and the soft structures. Severity ranges from least severe, which is an incomplete unilateral cleft lip, to most severe, which is a complete bilateral cleft lip and cleft palate. Table 57-1 provides orofacial cleft types, locations, and illustrations.

Treatment

Cleft lip and cleft palate are treatable birth defects; however, the extent of treatment varies with the type and severity of the cleft. Lip clefts are corrected as early as medically

TABLE 57-1

Orofacial Cleft Embryology

Type of Cleft and Location	Figure
Unilateral or bilateral cleft lip—Lack of fusion of the median nasal process and the maxillary process	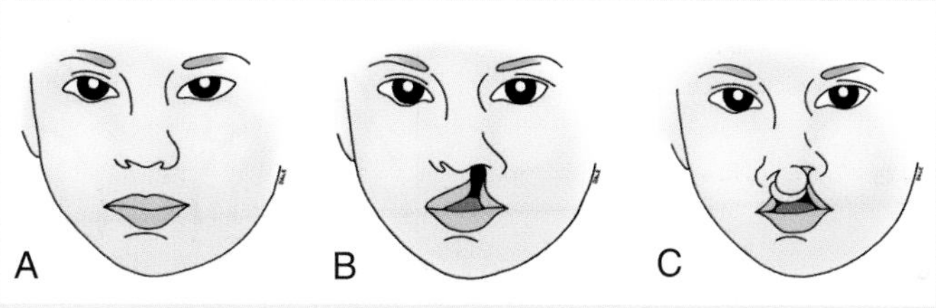 Figure 57-3. Types of facial clefts (frontal view). **A,** Normal. **B,** Unilateral cleft lip. **C,** Bilateral cleft lip. (From Nanci A: *Ten Cate's oral histology,* ed 8, St Louis, 2013, Mosby.)
Complete cleft lip—Involves the alveolar bone and the primary palate; extends into the nostrils	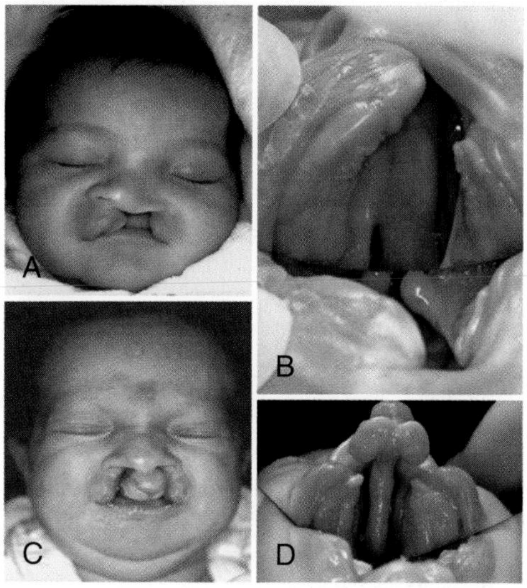 Figure 57-4. Congenital anomalies of the lip and palate. **A,** Newborn male infant with unilateral complete cleft lip and palate. **B,** Intraoral photograph (taken with mirror) showing left unilateral complete cleft of the primary and secondary parts of palate. **C,** Newborn female infant with bilateral complete cleft lip and palate. **D,** Intraoral photograph showing bilateral complete cleft palate. Note the maxillary protrusion and the natal tooth at the gingival apex in each lesser segment. (Courtesy Dr. John B. Mulliken, Children's Hospital Boston, Harvard Medical School, Boston, Massachusetts.)

Continued

TABLE 57-1
Orofacial Cleft Embryology—cont'd

Type of Cleft and Location	Figure
Incomplete cleft lip—Notch of any depth involving the philtrum; does not invade hard structures or the nostrils	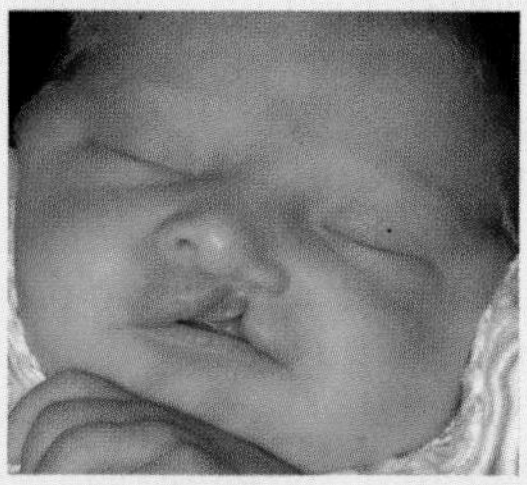 **Figure 57-5.** Incomplete unilateral cleft lip. (From Fonseca RJ, Marciani RD, Turvey TA: *Oral and maxillofacial surgery,* ed 2, St Louis, 2009, Saunders.) 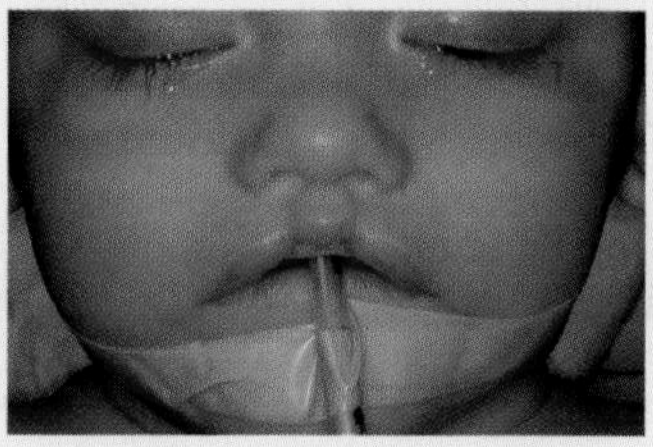 **Figure 57-6.** Incomplete bilateral cleft lip. (From Fonseca RJ, Marciani RD, Turvey TA: *Oral and maxillofacial surgery,* ed 2, St Louis, 2009, Saunders.)
Palatal clefts—Involves anterior (primary palate), posterior (secondary palate), or both	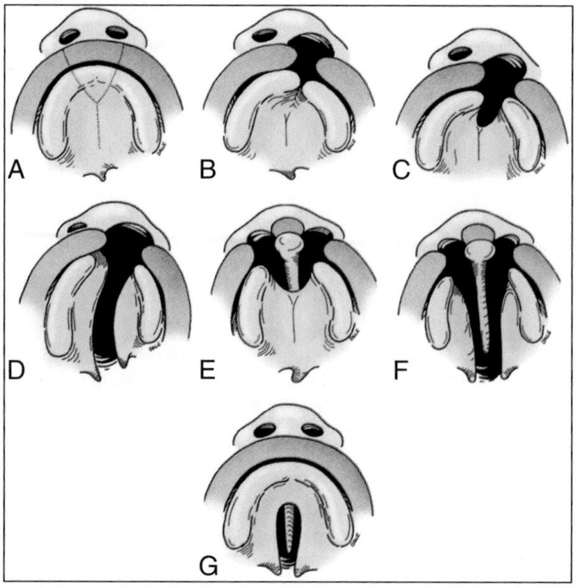 **Figure 57-7.** Palatal clefts (ventral view). **A,** Normal. **B,** Cleft of lip and alveolus. **C,** Cleft of lip and primary palate. **D,** Unilateral cleft lip and palate. **E,** Bilateral cleft lip and primary palate. **F,** Bilateral cleft lip and palate. **G,** Cleft palate only. (From Nanci A: *Ten Cate's oral histology,* ed 8, St Louis, 2013, Mosby.)
Unilateral complete cleft palate—Lack of fusion between one of the two lateral palatine processes and the nasal septum	See Figure 57-4, *A* and *B:* Unilateral complete cleft lip and palate

TABLE 57-1

Orofacial Cleft Embryology—cont'd

Type of Cleft and Location	Figure
Bilateral complete cleft palate—Lack of fusion of either lateral palatine process with the nasal septum	See Figure 57-4, *C* and *D:* Bilateral complete cleft lip and palate
Complete cleft palate: Posterior (secondary) palate: extends posterior to the incisive foramen and involves the hard and soft palate; Anterior (primary) palate: only involved	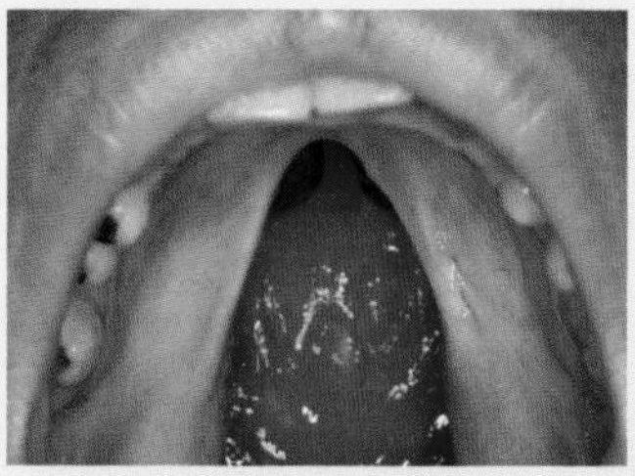 **Figure 57-8.** Palatal view of isolated cleft palate. (From Hupp JR, Ellis E, Tucker MR: *Contemporary oral and maxillofacial surgery,* ed 6, St Louis, 2014, Mosby.)
Incomplete cleft palate—Cleft of the uvula; Submucosal cleft—Lacks muscle or bone fusion yet soft tissue is present	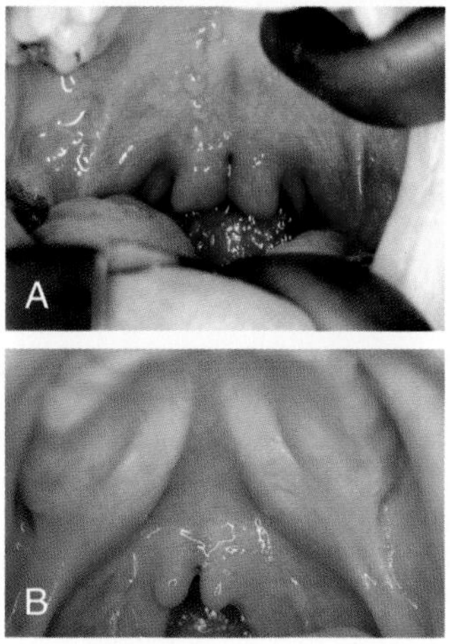 **Figure 57-9.** **A,** Bifid uvula. **B,** Submucosal palatal cleft. (From Hupp JR, Ellis E, Tucker MR: *Contemporary oral and maxillofacial surgery,* ed 6, St Louis, 2014, Mosby; and Neville BW, Damm DD, Allen CM, et al: *Oral and maxillofacial pathology,* ed 3, St Louis, 2009, Saunders.)

possible; however, soft palatal clefts are repaired at 6 to 18 months of age.[3,7] Surgeons adhere to the "rule of 10" to determine when a healthy baby can undergo surgery for an elective procedure (i.e., 10 weeks of age, 10 lb in body weight, and at least 10 g of hemoglobin per deciliter of blood).[7] Closure of the hard palatal cleft is prolonged to allow unimpeded maxillary growth. The majority of maxillary growth occurs by 4 or 5 years of age, and closure of the hard palate often occurs at this time.[7] These primary surgeries can affect facial growth and development. **Orthognathic surgery**—which involves corrective surgery of the jaw and face to alter the relationship of the teeth and supporting bones, sometimes in conjunction with orthodontic treatment—is indicated as a secondary surgery after the primary orofacial cleft surgery if maxillary deficiency, malocclusion, and lip and nasal deformities result.[7,11] Specific treatments for orofacial clefts can be found in textbooks about oral and maxillofacial surgery.

A multidisciplinary or interprofessional team works to manage an orofacial cleft: a plastic surgeon, a pediatrician, a pedodontist, an orthodontist, a speech pathologist, a psychologist, an otolaryngologist, a social worker, an oral and maxillofacial surgeon, a geneticist, an audiologist, a prosthodontist, and a sociologist.[7,11] Table 57-2 explains the problems associated with a facial cleft, the corrective therapy, the specialists involved, and the rationale for specialist involvement. Dental hygienists also participate in interprofessional collaborations for clients with cleft palates.

Complications

Individuals with orofacial clefts can experience feeding difficulties as infants, malocclusion, nasal deformities, and problems with hearing and speech. Feeding problems are associated most often with a cleft palate.[12] Infants with a cleft palate have difficulty producing the negative pressure needed

TABLE 57-2

Multidisciplinary Team Approach

Problem	Therapy	Specialist	Reason
Orofacial cleft	Surgery	Oral and maxillofacial surgeon Plastic surgeon	Perform lip and palatal repair and closure
	Screening and evaluation	Geneticist or genetic counselor	Diagnose a syndrome Establish risk for future pregnancies
Feeding	Squeeze bottles rather than rigid bottles Nipples: soft, elongated, cross-cut opening	Pediatrician	Promote easier feeding for the infant Ensure adequate nourishment
Ears or hearing	Antibiotics Pressure equalization tube placement	Otolaryngologist	Reduce ear infections (otitis media) Address lack of fluid drainage
	Hearing aid	Audiologist	Perform hearing tests to determine hearing impairments
Speech	Surgery	Oral and maxillofacial surgeon	Correct velopharyngeal dysfunction Reduce hypernasal speech
	Speech therapy	Speech pathologist	Retrain or develop articulation skills
	Nonsurgical appliances	Prosthodontist	Fabricate prostheses (obturators): speech bulb or palatal lift

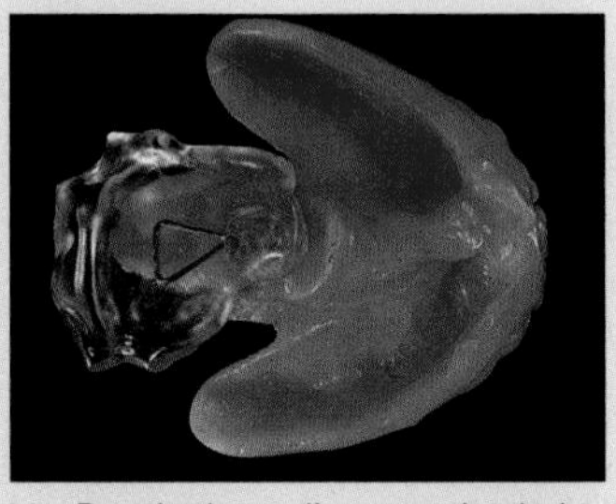

Figure 57-11. Prosthetic appliance: palatal obturator (extraoral view). (Courtesy Dr. Charles Babbush.)

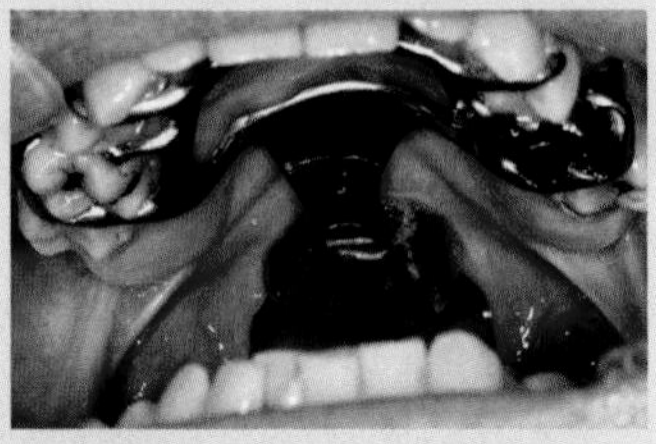

Figure 57-12. Prosthetic appliance: speech bulb (intraoral view). (From Hupp JR, Ellis E, Tucker MR: *Contemporary oral and maxillofacial surgery,* ed 6, St Louis, 2014, Mosby.)

Problem	Therapy	Specialist	Reason
Malocclusion	Orthognathic surgery Orthodontic treatment	Oral and maxillofacial surgeon Orthodontist	Correct function and appearance of jaws Align dentition
Missing teeth	Fixed bridge Denture or partial denture Implants	General dentist or pedodontist Prosthodontist	Improve aesthetics Maximize functionality of dentition
Supernumerary teeth	Retention or extraction	General dentist or pedodontist	Assist or interfere with prostheses Existence aids in maintaining alveolar bone
Nasal deformity	Surgery	Oral and maxillofacial surgeon Plastic surgeon	Modify aesthetics to obtain symmetry Refine nasal breathing
Learning, emotional, or behavioral disorders	Screening and evaluation	Psychologist Sociologist	Counseling and guidance for specific problems Improve performance

Data from Hupp JR, Ellis E, Tucker M: *Contemporary oral and maxillofacial surgery,* ed 6, St Louis, 2013, Mosby; American Cleft Palate-Craniofacial Association: *Parameters for evaluation and treatment of patients with cleft lip/palate or other craniofacial anomalies,* Chapel Hill, NC, 2009, Cleft Palate Foundation; Cleft Palate Foundation: *Your baby's first year,* Chapel Hill, NC, 2010, Cleft Palate Foundation; and Cleft Palate Foundation: *Treatment options for better speech,* Chapel Hill, NC, 2008, Cleft Palate Foundation.

to suck milk from a bottle or breast. The infant's sucking and swallowing reflexes are normal; however, the musculature is underdeveloped or not properly oriented to allow for effective sucking.[7] Nasal regurgitation, long feeding times, and difficulty coordinating swallowing and breathing occur. The excessive inhalation of air necessitates frequent burping. Even with these difficulties, there is no indication that interventions such as spoon-feeding or palate occluding devices will improve feeding.[12]

In children with orofacial clefts, the most common problem is middle ear infection from a lack of ventilation from the Eustachian tubes. Palatal muscles control the opening of these tubes. Without ventilation, fluid accumulates in the middle ear, and bacteria from the nasopharynx multiply to cause acute infections. Hearing impairments are common among persons with cleft palate owing to these chronic infections. However, if the problem is not addressed, permanent damage to the auditory sensory nerves can result.[3,7]

Hearing problems contribute significantly to the speech disorders that are common in persons with orofacial clefts.[7] Individuals with an isolated cleft lip have normal or close to normal speech, and approximately 80% of those with a cleft palate will develop normal speech after closure.[3] Speech is affected by a palatal cleft due to the function of the soft palate, which is to prevent air from escaping through the nose.[7] During speech, the muscles of the soft palate elevate and draw it posteriorly to the pharyngeal wall for closure (eFigure 57-10).[7] If closure does not occur, it is called **velopharyngeal dysfunction** (VPD).[13] VPD, which allows air to escape into the nasal cavity, may cause a client to have hypernasal speech.[7] Cleft palate closure surgery does not prevent VPD from occurring; children may develop VPD after palate repair.[13]

Clients affected by orofacial clefts may experience malocclusion; this is especially likely among those with cleft palates. Class III malocclusion is most common. **Malocclusion**, which is the improper alignment of the upper and lower teeth, can result from missing teeth or stunted maxillary growth. Maxillary growth is constricted as a result of scar tissue formation after primary surgeries to correct orofacial clefts. Other dental problems that may be present are congenitally missing teeth and supernumerary teeth. Because of the location of the cleft, the lateral incisor and the canine may be absent or severely displaced. Teeth may also be morphologically deformed, hypoplastic, or hypomineralized. Nasal architecture can also be deformed if a cleft involving the lip extends into the floor of the nose.[7]

Dental Hygienists' Role

Oral Hygiene Care

Hygiene care for a client with cleft lip, cleft palate, or both is crucial during childhood, because caries risk is high. Children with orofacial clefts have 3.5 times more decayed surfaces than children without clefts, and the prevalence of caries is more evident in the primary dentition among clients with orofacial clefts, particularly the maxillary incisors, the teeth adjacent to the cleft, and the molars. Clients with a cleft palate have a higher prevalence of caries because of a longer oral clearance time for foods, a higher generation of fermentable sugars from starches, and the tenacious nature of nasal fluid, which promotes the adherence of oral biofilm. Other factors include insufficient parental dietary counseling, insufficient education about a toothbrushing technique specific to babies and toddlers, the trauma of coping with a baby with a cleft, and the poor accessibility of the toothbrush around the cleft area.[14]

Soft-food consumption increases caries risk owing to the retention of these substrates, thereby allowing for increased acid production. With orthodontic appliances, more surface irregularities retain food and biofilm; this also increases caries risk. Children with orofacial clefts who are treated with an intraoral appliance (obturator) have a 7.6 times higher chance of exhibiting dental caries at the age of 2.5 years than those without intraoral appliances.[14] With the risk of demineralization, systemic and topical fluoride therapy, dental sealants, and the use of therapeutic doses of xylitol-containing products daily are indicated (see Chapters 33 and 34).

The Fones technique of toothbrushing and the sulcular toothbrushing technique are most appropriate for children (see Chapter 23). A power toothbrush and a small brush head size may be indicated, because toothbrushing may be inadequate or tooth inaccessibility may interfere with biofilm removal as a result of the loss of elasticity of the surgically repaired lip, the anatomy of the cleft, and the fear of brushing around the cleft area.[14] In addition, crowding of the dentition restricts the toothbrush and the self-cleaning ability of the mouth.[14] Clients with orofacial clefts also need to clean interdentally daily to remove biofilm and food debris. Caregivers who are responsible for oral hygiene of children need to be educated about the importance of daily food debris and oral biofilm removal.

Oral hygiene instructions also need to address the care of intraoral speech prostheses and **obturators**, which are removable acrylic prostheses fabricated to close an opening of a cleft palate (Figures 57-11 and 57-12). These appliances can also retain replacement teeth. Daily care for these appliances is similar to the care of partial and full dentures (see Chapter 56).

Fractured Jaw

Although the mandible is the largest and strongest facial bone, it is the second most commonly fractured facial bone after the nasal bone. There are no specified patterns of mandibular fractures.[15]

Incidence and Prevalence

The age groups that most commonly experience mandibular fractures range from the late teens to the early thirties followed by the early thirties to the late forties.[15-17] Males incur fractured mandibles two to six times more often than females for all age groups; however, the rate can be higher depending on the population and age studied.[15,16] Fractures involving the mandible as compared with the other facial bones occur less frequently in children than in adults.[17]

Etiology

Fractures of facial bones generally result from direct force or trauma (e.g., motor vehicle accidents, assault and battery, occupational injuries, falls, recreational accidents). Midfacial fractures are usually the result of high-impact forces. The causes of maxillofacial fractures vary by the population, its characteristics, and its geographic region.[16] Among adults, the most common causes of mandibular fractures are interpersonal violence (e.g., physical assaults and battery) and motor vehicle accidents.[15,18] In addition, the use of illicit substances correlates with the incidence of interpersonal violence.[15,16] In children, the causes of most facial fractures are falls, motor vehicle accidents, and road traffic accidents (e.g., pedestrian and bicyclist incidents).[16,17]

Types of Fractures

The type and location of a fracture, which is a partial or complete break in the bone, is dependent on the source, size, and direction of the traumatizing force. Trauma distributed to a larger surface area may cause several fractures as a result of the distribution of the force throughout the mandible. The direction of the force can help with the diagnosis of concomitant fractures.

Fracture types that reflect the severity of the break are *greenstick, multiple,* and *comminuted.* The terms *simple, compound,* and *complex* relate to injury of the adjacent soft tissue.[19] eFigure 57-13 illustrates these types of fractures. eTable 57-3 describes the classification of fractures and the potential causes of facial fractures. See Evolve website for illustrations of types of fractures and a table describing the classification of fractures and the potential causes of facial fractures.

Signs and Symptoms of a Fractured Jaw

Emergency Care

Contact with a physician or dentist is needed if the client has sustained a blow to the mandible and has any of the following conditions:

- Deformed, crooked, or shifted mandible
- Painful lump in the mandible or below the ear
- Malocclusion of the dentition
- Loose, broken, or missing teeth
- Painful swelling or bruised gingival tissue at the site of injury
- Difficulty opening or pain in the temporomandibular joint
- Numbness in the chin and lower lip[20,21]

If a client has sustained a mandibular bone injury, the healthcare professional may need to maintain the client's airway, breathing, and circulation until emergency medical service providers arrive (see Chapter 10). Attention to the mandibular injury is secondary to securing and maintaining the vital body functions. When the jaw has sustained a fracture or dislocation, a client can have increased bleeding or a breathing problem. Treatment of the fracture occurs immediately, as long as the client's condition is stable and there are no neck fractures or other life-threatening injuries.[7] While the client travels to the healthcare facility, the mandible should be supported in place with the client's hands, or a bandage may be wrapped over the top of the client's head and under his or her jaw. The bandage should be easily removable in case the client needs to vomit. eFigure 57-14 illustrates one method of temporary jaw stabilization and immobilization.

Physical and Clinical Examination of a Suspected Jaw Fracture

A client with a possibly fractured jaw should be examined for signs of injury such as facial lacerations, swelling, and hematomas. The location of the injury can correlate with the location of the fracture. To help with the detection of a jaw fracture, do the following:

- Examine extraorally the inferior border of the mandible from the symphysis to the angle from behind the supinely positioned or seated client for the detection of deformity, tenderness, or numbness.
- Examine the condyle and the function of the temporomandibular joint while standing in front of the client.
- Examine intraorally for malocclusion, fractured or loose teeth, mucosal or gingival lacerations, and ecchymosis on the floor of the mouth.
- Assess mobility of the mandible through gentle bimanual manipulation.[19]

eTable 57-4 lists the signs and symptoms, the location of injury or trauma, and the potential anatomic location of a suspected jaw facture. eBox 57-1 compares the symptoms of a dislocated jaw and a fractured jaw.

Treatment

Before treatment, the healthcare provider must determine if the injury has resulted in a dislocation or fracture of the jaw. Treatment should be rendered in a hospital or emergency department. The treatment goal for a fractured jaw is rapid bone healing; normal ocular, masticatory, nasal, and speaking function; and an acceptable orofacial appearance.[7]

Dislocated Jaw

If the mandible is dislocated, the healthcare professional may be able to return it to its correct position by using the thumbs placed intraorally on the occlusal plane with the other digits cupping the inferior border of the mandible. An anesthetic may be needed to control pain or to relax the jaw muscles. Stabilization of the jaw is indicated to prevent repeated dislocation when opening widely, yawning, or sneezing. Rarely is surgery indicated for the treatment of a dislocated jaw.[21]

Fractured Jaw

Basic procedural treatment follows these steps: (1) restoration of proper occlusion (fixation); (2) repair of bony fractures (reduction); and (3) soft-tissue repair.[7] Fixation can be either maxillomandibular or intermaxillary and involves wiring teeth together. Elastics attached to arch bars are used to pull the jaws together into their proper positions before wiring (Figure 57-15). Closed reduction does not involve direct opening, exposure, or manipulation of the fracture area; open reduction requires surgical exposure of the bone for fixation.

If elastics are removed in the event of nausea or vomiting, replacement is needed to continue appropriate treatment. Wiring of the maxillary and mandibular arches immobilizes

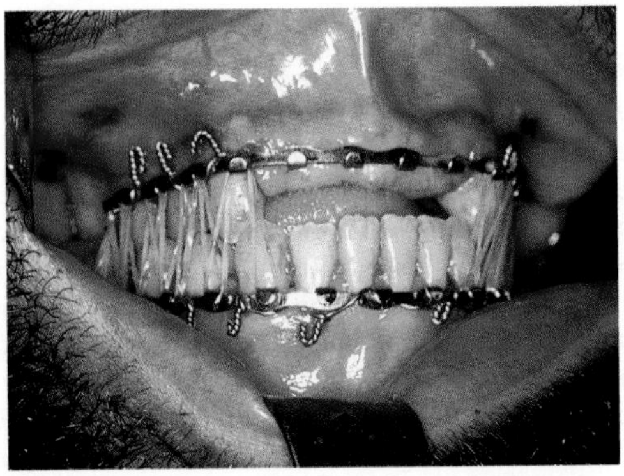

Figure 57-15. Arch bars and heavy interarch elastics. (From Hupp JR, Ellis E, Tucker MR: *Contemporary oral and maxillofacial surgery,* ed 6, St Louis 2014, Mosby.)

the fracture for usually 4 to 8 weeks to allow for the maximum healing of the fracture.[7,21] Specific treatments for mandibular and maxillary fractures can be found in textbooks about oral and maxillofacial surgery.

Complications

Infection, which is the main complication of a mandibular fracture, occurs when oral bacteria enter the open wound caused by the fracture.[19,22] No evidence supports a specific causal relationship to the development of infection; however, risk factors include the treatment modality (i.e., open versus closed reduction), a lack of compliance with the postoperative regimen, the duration of antibiotic use, the severity and number of fractures, inadequate nutrition, the client's age, and the client's inability to resist infection.[22,23] There is inconclusive evidence that suggests that teeth in the line of the fracture contribute to a higher risk of infection.[23] Systemic and behavioral factors (e.g., immunosuppression, such as from human immunodeficiency virus infection; diabetes mellitus; chronic infections; alcoholism; intravenous drug abuse) can delay the healing process and contribute to postoperative infection.[22,23]

Other complications besides infection are **malunion** (misalignment during healing) or **nonunion** (failure to heal) of the fracture, **osteomyelitis** (inflammation of the bone and bone marrow), wound dehiscence (opening), malocclusion, mobile teeth at the fracture site, and facial nerve injury.[19,23] A rare complication that mainly affects mandibular fracture in children is **ankylosis**, a disturbance or underdevelopment of the bone on the affected side of the fracture. The prevention of ankylosis can be achieved with a short immobilization period and consecutive active mobilization of the temporomandibular joint.[19]

Although harmful effects involving the teeth or the periodontium seldom occur during maxillomandibular fixation of a jaw fracture, this topic needs more research. Periodontal complications can include increased tooth mobility, periodontal pockets, tooth sensitivity, caries, root resorption, or dentoalveolar ankylosis. A Swedish study reported that no permanent changes occurred in the tissues surrounding the teeth after wiring fixation was used for jaw fractures. The study noted that changes in the periodontium were temporary and resolved completely after fixation.[24] A periodontal condition expected during immobilization is gingivitis, which should resolve when the client resumes normal oral hygiene care.

Dental Hygienists' Role

Oral Hygiene Care

Daily oral self-care is essential while the maxillary and mandibular jaws are immobilized with wires and elastics during the 4- to 8-week healing period. During immobilization, only facial and buccal tooth surfaces can be accessed with a toothbrush. However, brushing may not be allowed for a specified time period after surgery, or it may be impossible for the client immediately after surgery. A cotton or sponge swab moistened with water or 0.12% chlorhexidine gluconate should be used on the gingival and tooth surfaces until brushing can be performed. Oral cleaning needs to occur after every meal or snack with a soft-bristled toothbrush. Lingual surfaces are debrided and the gingiva massaged with normal tongue movements.

Thorough removal of the oral biofilm and food debris will decrease the risk of infection and enamel demineralization. Dentifrices recommended should contain fluoride to minimize enamel demineralization and antiplaque and antigingivitis ingredients to decrease gingival inflammation. Desensitizing dentifrices should be considered to help with tooth sensitivity when necessary. Oral rinsing or oral irrigation with an over-the-counter American Dental Association–approved or Canadian Dental Association–accepted antimicrobial or fluoridated mouth rinse should also be performed after every meal or snack. (See Chapters 25, 31, and 33.)

Care of the skin and the mucous membranes is essential for the prevention of infection, for healing, and for the minimization of scarring. Wires can irritate the mucosal membranes during fixation. Warmed beeswax or orthodontic wax can be applied to the ends of wires to limit mucosal irritation. The client also needs to care for the lips and the wounds associated with the jaw injury or surgery. Under fixation, the client no longer has the ability to moisten the lips with the tongue. For the prevention of dry, cracked lips, Aquaphor, Blistex, Carmex, vitamin E ointment, or mineral oil is recommended. The client can use soap and water, hydrogen peroxide diluted 1:1 with water, and topical antibiotic ointment as wound care. Most importantly, the client should follow care instructions given by the oral surgeon and should refrain from the behaviors associated with delayed healing, such as smoking and alcohol consumption.

Diet and Nutrition

A client who has had a fractured jaw and subsequent jaw surgery will experience a loss of approximately 10% of the body weight. The oral surgeon may recommend a high-protein, high-calorie blenderized liquid diet for the duration of treatment to maintain the body's immune and protective systems and to build healthy tissue. Calorie and protein supplements such as Ensure, Boost, Carnation Instant Breakfast, and other protein powders are encouraged. In addition, the client will need to reduce the risk of dehydration by drinking plenty of water and other fluids daily.

Additional Care Instructions

Postoperative instructions should address communication, pain control, precautions during healing, physical activity, and other expectations of jaw immobilization that the client may experience. The client should limit verbal communication and use a dry-erase board, a pad and pen, email, or text messaging for easy communication. The client should be encouraged to create and maintain a nonstrenuous daily routine during healing. Prescription pain medications and antibiotics should be taken as prescribed. Acetaminophen or ibuprofen can be taken for mild pain or discomfort.

Prevention

The prevention of a mandibular fracture relates to causes of such fractures (e.g., refrain from altercations or situations that involve the potential for assault). Motor vehicle accidents are more difficult to avoid. However, preventive laws that focus on speed limits, alcohol, cell phone use restrictions, shoulder restraints and seatbelts, and vehicle safety modifications have led to a decrease in maxillofacial injuries.[16] The use of seatbelts and shoulder restraints will prevent facial bones from contacting the dashboard or windshield in the event of a motor vehicle accident.[16,20] For children, proper child safety restraints should be used to prevent facial and bodily injuries. Prevention during contact sports should include the wearing of headgear or a helmet, a mouth guard, and other protective equipment.[16,20] Education about safety guidelines is the best preventive measure for facial and bodily injuries.

CLIENT EDUCATION TIPS

- Explain the contributory factors of nonsyndromic clefts.
- Discuss the role of embryology in the development of facial clefts.
- Explain the roles of specialists for addressing orofacial cleft complications.
- Individualize oral hygiene instructions for orofacial clefts, malocclusion, missing teeth, and prostheses.
- Provide nutritional counseling to reduce caries risk.
- Educate clients about the prevention of facial fractures specific to adults and children.
- Inform clients about the signs and symptoms of a fractured jaw or a dislocated jaw.
- Explain the potential complications of a fractured jaw.
- Explain the development and prevention of demineralization and caries during immobilization.
- Recommend appropriate nutritional foods and liquids that can be used by a postsurgical client or a person who has immobilized jaws.

LEGAL, ETHICAL, AND SAFETY ISSUES

- Dental hygienists should recognize symptoms of a fractured and dislocated jaw and refer clients to emergency personnel.
- The dental hygienist should not abandon the client throughout treatment, particularly after surgery.

KEY CONCEPTS

- Orofacial clefts are a common birth defect that the dental hygienist will encounter during practice; corrective cleft treatment is likely to be completed in industrialized nations.
- Syndromes are rarely associated with orofacial clefts; several factors can contribute to the occurrence of a cleft lip, a cleft palate, or both, and clients need to be educated before pregnancy about possible preventive measures.
- Embryology plays a vital role in the development of orofacial clefts.
- Caregivers must be educated about cleft complications, the specialists involved in their management, and the importance of oral hygiene care for the prevention of dental caries.
- Facial fractures result from direct force or trauma.
- The assessment of a client's signs and symptoms in conjunction with the dentist and the physician is essential to provide appropriate care for a suspected fractured jaw.
- Minimize periodontal complications during immobilization through appropriate diet and nutrition, oral hygiene instruction, and professional care and self-care.
- Emphasize client adherence to the oral surgeon's instructions for jaw fracture treatment.
- The use of preventive safety measures is the best approach for avoiding facial fractures.

CRITICAL THINKING EXERCISES

CLIENT 1: A 33-year-old female client of record arrives for her 6-month dental hygiene appointment. She has her 2-month-old infant son in a car carrier and a light blanket draped over the child. As you bring the client and her infant into the treatment area, you inquire about seeing the child. The mother becomes visibly upset, and she states that her son has a birth defect: a cleft lip and palate. How would you react to the situation? What questions would you ask the mother to determine her current knowledge about her son's birth defect? What resources and dental hygiene information could you give the mother?

CLIENT 2: A 4-year-old girl arrives with her mother for her first dental appointment in your office. The health history interview reveals a history of ear infections, hearing problems, and speech difficulties. During follow-up questioning, the mother states that these problems are associated with the child's having been born with a cleft palate. The mother indicates that the child will have corrective surgery next year and is currently wearing an obturator. What instructions would you give the caregiver about obturator cleaning and care? What oral hygiene instructions are appropriate for the client and caregiver? About what other complications involving cleft palates would you educate the caregiver?

CLIENT 3: Mr. S.

Profile: The client is a 26-year-old man who called this morning for an emergency visit.

Chief Complaint: "My jaw is swollen on the left side, and my teeth feel funny when I bite. I can't open my mouth very wide because it hurts."

Health History: Mr. S.'s last physical examination was 2 years ago, and he uses two cans of spit tobacco a week. He reports that he recently began attending Alcoholics Anonymous meetings for alcohol dependency.

Social History: The client is single and lives with a roommate.

Dental History: Mr. S. has a history of infrequent dental visits and has several two- and three-surface amalgam restorations on teeth #2, #3, #14, #19, #30, and #31. His previous charting and bitewing radiographs reveal that teeth #17 and #32 are impacted. His record and treatment plan from 8 months ago indicate that carious lesions are present on tooth #15 mesial and tooth #18 occlusal. His gingival tissue margins are erythemic, edemic, and rolled. The tissue consistency is spongy, and the interdental papillae are blunted. He has heavy oral biofilm accumulation in the swollen area and on the tongue and generalized moderate interproximal biofilm.

Oral Health Behavior Assessment: He reports brushing twice daily, but he does not floss or clean his tongue.

Supplemental Notes: Mr. S. knows that his oral health is poor. He has no dental insurance, and he wants to be relieved from the sudden onset of pain. Visually, you observe on Mr. S.'s left side a swelling and a faint hematoma on his left cheek apical to the zygoma.

1. What are the dental hygiene diagnoses and possible differential dental diagnoses for Mr. S.?
2. What follow-up questions would you ask Mr. S. about his pain?

3. What types of radiographs could help the dentist determine the course of treatment?
4. Develop a dental hygiene care plan for this client. Develop a homecare plan for oral disease prevention that also includes nutritional counseling.

REFERENCES

1. Centers for Disease Control and Prevention: Improved national prevalence estimated for 19 selected major birth defects—United States, 1999-2001, *MMWR Morb Mortal Wkly Rep* 54:1301, 2006.
2. Parker SE, Mai CT, Canfield MA, et al: Updated national birth prevalence estimates for selected birth defects in the United States, 2004–2006, *Birth Defects Res A Clin Mol Teratol* 88:1008, 2010.
3. Cleft Palate Foundation: *Your baby's first year*, Chapel Hill, NC, 2010, CPF Publications Committee. Available at: www.cleftline.org/docs/Booklets/FYL-01.pdf. Accessed on November 3, 2013.
4. Canfield MA, Honein MA, Yuskiv N, et al: National estimates and race/ethnic-specific variation of selected birth defects in the United States, 1999-2001, *Birth Defects Res A Clin Mol Teratol* 76:747, 2006.
5. Texas Department of State Health Services: *Birth defect risk factor series: oral clefts*. Available at: www.dshs.state.tx.us/birthdefects/risk/risk-oralclefts.shtm. Accessed November 4, 2012.
6. Nanci A: *Ten Cate's oral histology: development, structure, and function*, ed 8, St Louis, 2013, Mosby.
7. Hupp JR, Ellis E, Tucker M: *Contemporary oral and maxillofacial surgery*, ed 6, St Louis, 2013, Mosby.
8. Moore KL, Persaud TVN, Torchia MG: *The developing human: clinically oriented embryology*, ed 9, Philadelphia, 2013, Saunders.
9. Cleft Palate Foundation: *Genetics and you*, ed 2, Chapel Hill, NC, 2008, Cleft Palate Foundation. Available at: www.cleftline.org/docs/Booklets/GEN-01.pdf. Accessed on November 3, 2013.
10. Hoeein MA, Rasmussen SA, Reefhuis J, et al: Maternal smoking and environmental tobacco smoke exposure and the risk of orofacial clefts, *Epidemiology* 18:226, 2007.
11. American Cleft Palate-Craniofacial Association: *Parameters for evaluation and treatment o patients with cleft lip/palate or other craniofacial anomalies*, Chapel Hill, NC, 2009, American Cleft Palate-Craniofacial Association. Available at: www.acpa-cpf.org/uploads/site/Parameters_Rev_2009.pdf. Accessed on November 13, 2013.
12. Bessell A, Hooper L, Shaw WC, et al: Feeding interventions for growth and development in infants with cleft lip, cleft palate or cleft lip and cleft palate, *Cochrane Database Syst Rev* (2):CD003315, 2011.
13. Cleft Palate Foundation: *Treatment options for better speech*, Chapel Hill, NC, 2008, Cleft Palate Foundation. Available at cleftline.org/docs/Booklets/SPE-01.pdf.
14. Cheng LL, Moor SL, Ho CTC: Predisposing factors to dental caries in children with cleft lip and palate: a review and strategies for early prevention, *Cleft Palate Craniofac J* 44:67, 2007.
15. Ogundare BO, Bonnick A, Bayley N: Pattern of mandibular fractures in an urban major trauma center, *J Oral Maxillofac Surg* 61:713, 2003.
16. Chrcanovic BR: Factors influencing the incidence of maxillofacial fractures, *Oral Maxillofac Surg* 16:3, 2012.
17. Imahara SD, Hopper RA, Wang J, et al: Patterns and outcomes of pediatric facial fractures in the United States: a survey of the national trauma data bank, *J Am Coll Surg* 207:710, 2008.
18. Allareddy V, Allareddy V, Nalliah RP: Epidemiology of facial fracture injuries, *J Oral Maxillofac Surg* 69:2613, 2011.
19. Laub DR: *Mandibular fractures*. Available at: emedicine.medscape.com/article/1283150-overview. Accessed November 23, 2012.
20. Aetna InteliHealth: *Broken jaw*. Available at: www.intelihealth.com/IH/ihtIH/WSIHW000/7165/32146/211418.html?d=dmtHealthAZ. Accessed November 23, 2012.
21. Vorvick LJ: *Jaw—broken or dislocated*. Available at: www.nlm.nih.gov/medlineplus/ency/article/000019.htm. Accessed November 23, 2012.
22. Senel FC, Jessen GS, Melo MD, et al: Infection following treatment of mandible fractures: the role of immunosuppression and polysubstance abuse, *Oral Surg Oral Med Oral Pathol Oral Radiol Endod* 103:38, 2007.
23. Malanchuk VO, Kopchak AV: Risk factors for development of infection in patients with mandibular fractures located in the tooth-bearing area, *J Craniomaxillofac Surg* 35:57, 2007.
24. Thor A, Andersson L: Interdental wiring in jaw fractures: effects on teeth and surrounding tissues after a one-year follow-up, *Br J Oral Maxillofac Surg* 39:398, 2001.

EVOLVE RESOURCES

Please visit http://evolve.elsevier.com/Darby/hygiene for additional practice and study support tools.

CHAPTER 58

Osseointegrated Dental Implants

Mehran Hossaini-Zadeh

COMPETENCIES

1. Discuss osseointegrated dental implants, including:
   - Define basic components of a dental implant.
   - Define the steps of dental implant treatment planning, implementation, and maintenance.
   - Discuss dental implant indications, contraindications, benefits, and risks.
2. Discuss the diagnosis and planning of dental hygiene care, including peri-implantitis and its management.
3. Identify recommended devices and strategies for cleaning dental implants.
4. List the professional armamentarium used in conjunction with oral self-care aids for patients with dental implants.
5. Define a failed implant.

Dental implants, a proven and established method of tooth replacement, offer an alternative to the use of conventional removable and fixed dental prostheses. Dental implants are considered the standard of care and a required part of the informed consent process when discussing tooth replacement. In edentulous clients, dental implants provide a unique opportunity for the management of clients who are physically or psychologically unable to tolerate a removable prosthesis. For example, without the use of dental implants, there are no realistic treatment options available for individuals with severely atrophic mandibles (Figure 58-1). In partially dentate clients, preparing otherwise healthy teeth for the fabrication of a fixed bridge creates a dilemma that renders dental implants as a viable and predictable alternative for the replacement of single and multiple teeth.

Dental hygienists must be experts at dental implant hygiene maintenance so that they can educate clients throughout and after dental implant therapy.

Osseointegrated Dental Implants

Natural tooth function describes the security of having a sound foundation on which to bite, chew, and grind. Tooth loss attributed to periodontal disease, dental caries, or trauma prevents many individuals from experiencing natural tooth function. Although conventional restorative and prosthetic dental care assists individuals with adapting to their lost dentition through fixed and removable prosthetic appliances, dental implants clearly provide a chance to regain natural tooth function.

Dental implants provide a method for stabilizing or anchoring a dental prosthesis to the supporting hard and soft tissue. Despite the variation in terminology, generally this stabilization is achieved by three main components: the implanted device, the abutment, and the prosthesis (Figure 58-2. The **implanted device** (i.e., the root form dental implant) must rely on a predictable, stable, and long-term connection to the supporting bone. This connection is defined as **osseointegration**, which is the functionally stable interface between the bone and an implanted device without the presence of any connective tissue. This interface must remain stable with functional loading and throughout the life of the implant. The **abutment**, which is an intermediate connector, allows for the connection of the prosthesis to the dental implant that has osseointegrated to the supporting bone. This abutment may be integrated into the prosthesis, such as in a single crown, or separated from the prosthesis, such as in a multiunit fixed or removable prosthesis. This abutment also creates a soft-tissue interface for a healthy transition between the oral environment and the dental implant.

The final **prosthesis** can be completely supported by the implant, as in the case of a single or multiunit fixed prosthesis, or it may be retained by the implant and supported by the soft tissue, as in the case of a removable prosthesis (Figure 58-3). There are many different forms of tooth replacement that involve the use of dental implants; some examples can be seen throughout this chapter (Figure 58-4; see also Figures 58-5 and 58-6 in Scenario 58-1 and Figures 58-7 and 58-8 in Scenario 58-2).

Historically, various metals including Vitallium, cobalt alloys, ceramic, aluminum, and vanadium have been used for dental implant manufacturing. Contemporary dental implants, however, are made from titanium or titanium alloys. Extensive biomaterial research has provided various surface modifications to improve the interface between the implant, the bone, the soft tissue, and the prosthesis.

The soft-tissue interface with different parts of the implant is critical to the overall health and longevity of the dental implant. Oral biofilm control must be achieved to maintain the health of the soft-tissue interface. With oral biofilm present and host susceptibility, the peri-implant tissue is at risk for inflammation and infection (i.e., **peri-implantitis**).

Indications, Contraindications, and Client Selection

Regardless of the cause of the tooth loss, the replacement of a tooth with a dental implant can certainly be considered a viable option. However, functional or aesthetic deficits rather

Figures, tables, and boxes marked as "e" are available as supplemental material on the Evolve site. Visit http://evolve.elsevier.com/Darby/hygiene to access these materials.

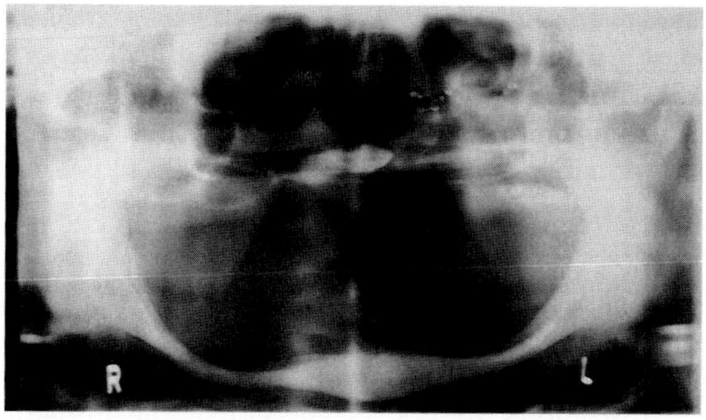

Figure 58-1. Radiograph of an atrophic mandible. (Courtesy A.K. Lakha.)

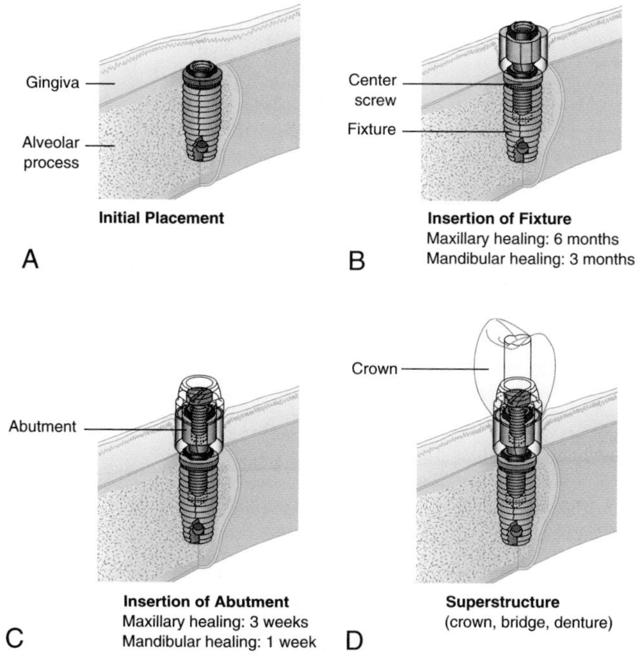

Figure 58-2. **A** through **D,** The sequence of treatment with osseointegrated dental implants. (Courtesy Nobel Biocare, Yorba Linda, California.)

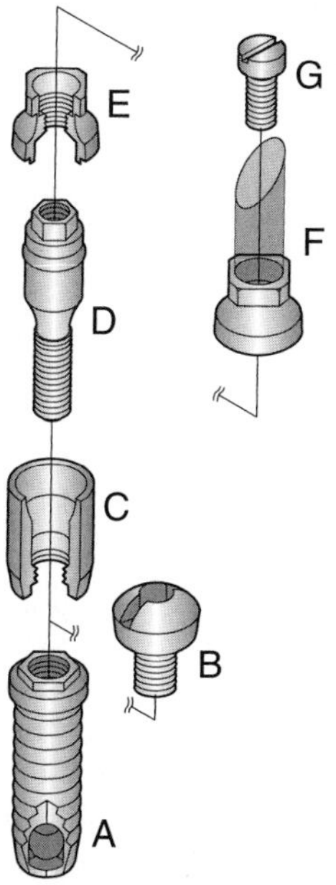

Figure 58-3. Brånemark system components. **A,** Implant. **B,** Cover screw. **C,** Abutment. **D,** Abutment screw. **E,** Cylinder. **F,** Cylinder. **G,** Gold screw. (From Worthington P, Lang BR, Rubenstein JE: *Osseointegration in dentistry: an overview,* Carol Stream, Ill, 2003, Quintessence.)

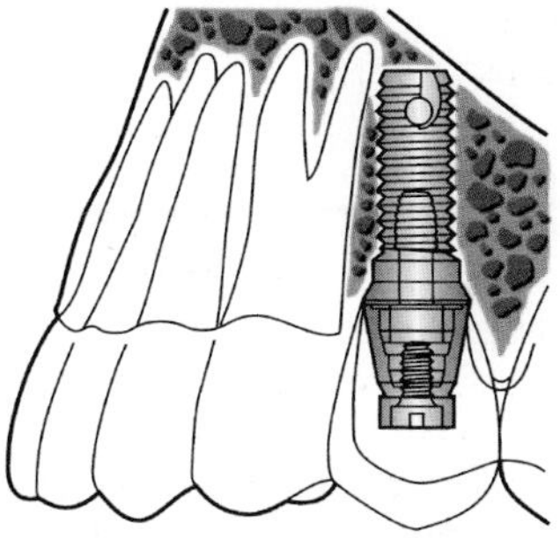

Figure 58-4. The cast crown is attached to the endosteal implant abutment by a gold screw. (From Worthington P, Lang BR, Rubenstein JE: *Osseointegration in dentistry: an overview,* Carol Stream, Ill, 2003, Quintessence.)

than indiscriminate tooth replacement should be analyzed critically and considered as an indication for dental implant use. Although there are no specific absolute contraindications for the use of dental implants, other contraindications for oral surgical procedures do apply. These contraindications include—but are not limited to—a history of head and neck radiation therapy, prolonged bisphosphonate use, and poor control of systemic conditions such as diabetes mellitus. When including a dental implant as a possible treatment option, factors such as the client's expectations, his or her willingness to participate in the treatment plan, and his or her compliance with oral hygiene must be taken under consideration.

Stages of Treatment

For the most successful dental implant outcomes, a restoratively driven team approach to treatment planning and the sequential implementation of the treatment is necessary. In general, the treatment team consists of the client, the surgeon, and the restorative team. The restorative team, which includes a dental hygienist, is responsible not only for the prosthesis fabrication but also for the maintenance and long-term dental implant evaluation (eFigure 58-9). In general, the treatment sequence can be summarized as follows: (1) the extraction of the tooth and a healing period of 3 to 6 months; (2) the surgical placement of the implant (stage 1 surgery) and a healing period of 3 to 6 months; and (3) the uncovering of the implant (stage 2 surgery) and a healing period of a few days, followed by the restorative process. Admittedly there may be significant variations in this generalized summary on the basis of such factors as the individual's specific condition, the implant location, the bone quality, and the practitioner's expertise. After the completion of the implant restoration procedures, it is critical to initiate well-planned oral hygiene and maintenance protocols.

Presurgical Workup

After a thorough evaluation of the client's general and oral health, all of the active dental disease should be addressed or treatment planned in an appropriate sequence with the

SCENARIO 58-1

A CLIP AND HADER BAR IMPLANT WITH A REMOVABLE PROSTHETIC APPLIANCE OR DENTURE (FIGURES 58-5 AND 58-6)

A 70-year-old client has developed severe aggressive periodontal disease. Her facial contours have collapsed from extensive bone resorption. The general dentist and the dental hygienist have discussed the diagnosis and care options with the client and have referred her to an oral surgeon for the extraction of her remaining teeth. In consultation with the client, the general dentist and the oral surgeon plan treatment to include a full removable upper denture and a lower endosteal implant system. The endosteal implant will consist of a two-implant system with a bar between the implants and a full lower removable denture with a clip to hold it in place. With this dental implant approach, the client can readily remove the full lower denture. The client's ability to remove the prosthetic appliance promotes long-term success of the implant by allowing daily access to oral biofilm accumulation. The maxillary removable prosthetic appliance adds rounded facial contours and alleviates deep furrows.

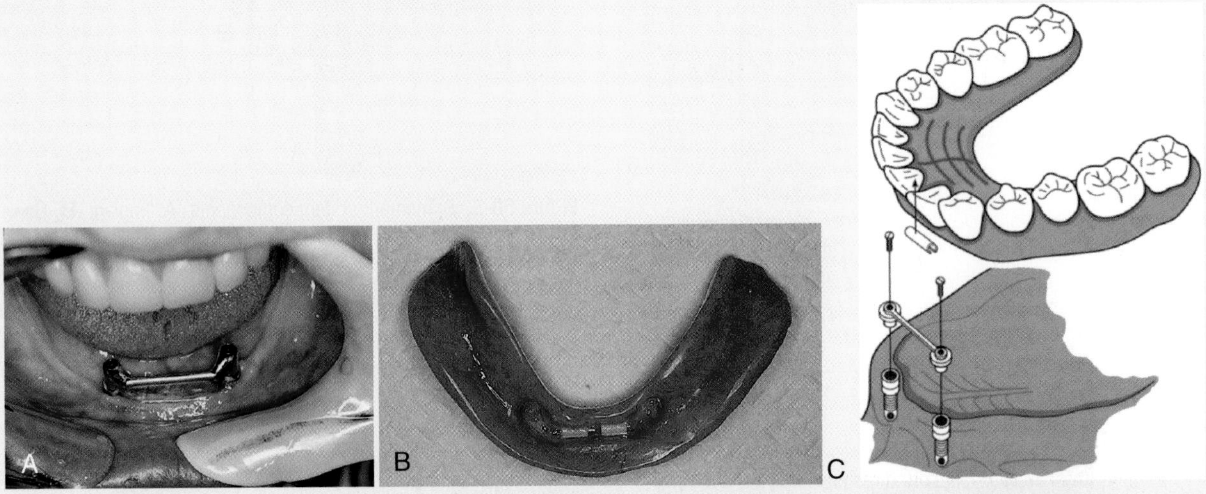

Figure 58-5. A, Crossbar endosteal implant. **B,** Clip-on type of overdenture. **C,** Components of the attachment. (*B,* Courtesy M.A. Conover. **C,** From Worthington P, Lang BR, Rubenstein JE: *Osseointegration in dentistry: an overview,* Carol Stream, Ill, 2003, Quintessence.)

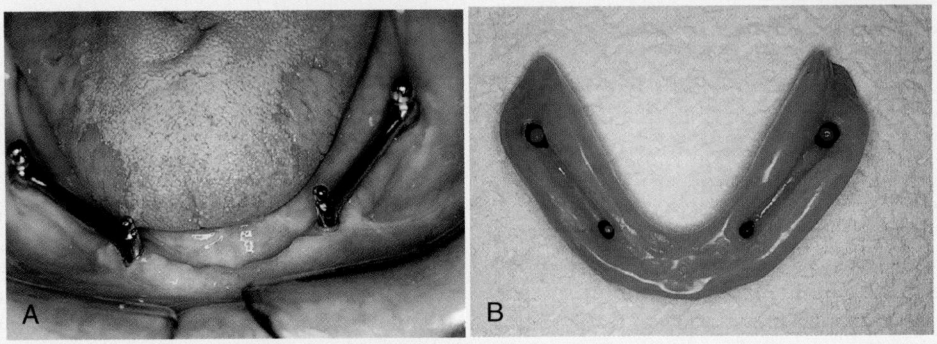

Figure 58-6. A, Ball and crossbar endosteal implant. **B,** Socket-type overdenture. (Courtesy M.A. Conover.)

SCENARIO 58-2

A TWO-IMPLANT SYSTEM WITH A TWO-UNIT RESTORATION AND A CANTILEVER BRIDGE (FIGURES 58-7 AND 58-8)

A client developed a benign tumor within the lower right mandible. The oral surgeon extracted two molars, removed the tumor, and inserted synthetic bone to promote bone growth. A few months later, two implants were placed in the mandibular right premolar area. The oral surgeon is hesitant to place another implant in the mandibular right molar region out of fear of disturbing the inferior alveolar nerve. Therefore a two-unit crown restoration with a cantilever bridge is fabricated. A cantilever bridge allows for a posterior occluding surface area without the placement of a third implant.

SCENARIO 58-2

A TWO-IMPLANT SYSTEM WITH A TWO-UNIT RESTORATION AND A CANTILEVER BRIDGE (FIGURES 58-7 AND 58-8)—cont'd

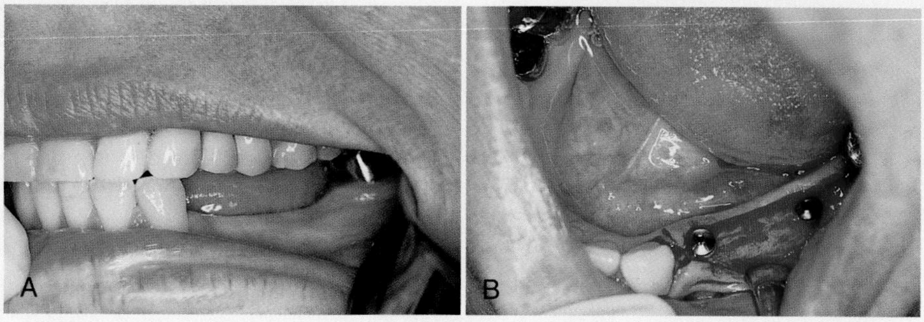

Figure 58-7. **A,** Partial edentulism. **B,** Two endosteal implants surgically placed in an edentulous area. (Courtesy M.A. Conover.)

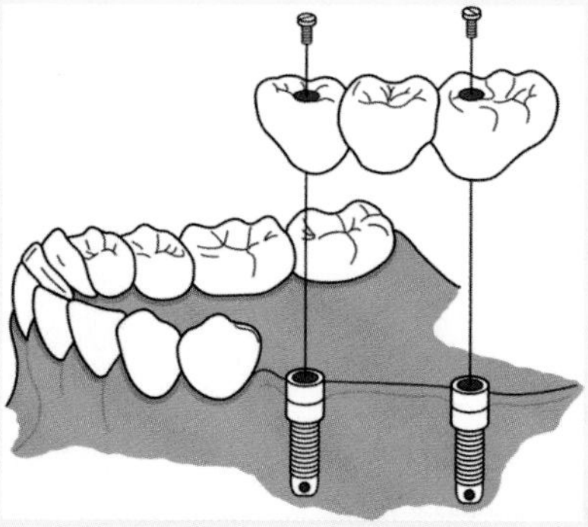

Figure 58-8. Endosteal implant–supported restoration in a partially edentulous mandible is not attached to the adjoining natural tooth. (From Worthington P, Lang BR, Rubenstein JE: *Osseointegration in dentistry: an overview*, Carol Stream, Ill, 2003, Quintessence.)

planned dental implants. The presurgical workup usually includes diagnostic study models, radiographic imaging, and a wax-up followed by the fabrication of the surgical guide and, at times, the fabrication of a temporary or final prosthesis. In addition to bitewing and periapical films, a panoramic radiograph or a cone-beam computed tomography scan is required for better visualization of the anatomic landmarks and assessment of the available bone for implant placement. Much of the diagnostic workup and treatment planning can be done virtually. The objective of this workup is to determine the implant position in relation to the planned prosthesis, the anatomic landmarks, and the available bone volume. Some of the critical anatomic landmarks include the maxillary sinus, the nasal cavity, the inferior alveolar nerve, the mental foramen, and the roots of the adjacent teeth. At least 2 mm of healthy and viable bone is required between the implant and the adjacent anatomic structures (Figures 58-10, 58-11, and 58-12).

Virtual Treatment Planning (Scenario 58-3)

Three-dimensional or virtual implant treatment planning allows the surgeon to better visualize a client's bony anatomy in three dimensions for dental implant placement by using computed tomography via medical grade computed tomography scanning or in-office cone-beam computed tomography scanning. Various software can be used to view these images and to virtually place implants in relation to all pertinent vital structures, including nerves, sinuses, soft-tissue thicknesses, and the available bone volume. In addition, the implant-to-restoration relationship, distances, and angulations can be visualized and planned before the surgery. From the virtual treatment plan, surgical drilling guides can be fabricated to help the surgeon with accurate implant placement in relation to the preplanned prosthesis.

Virtual planning helps the surgical and restorative teams to plan implant cases more accurately and efficiently.

Stage One: The First Surgical Procedure

Using the surgical guide fabricated by either conventional or virtual planning, osteotomy (bone removal) sites are created for the implant placement. The implants are placed and stabilized within the osteotomy sites at a preplanned location and angulation that is suitable for the final prosthesis. The primary stabilization of the implant at the time of placement is one of the main markers for the success of a dental implant. At this time, the implant is left in place for a period of 3 to 6 months and allowed to undergo the physiologic healing processing needed for osseointegration with the surrounding bone (Figures 58-13 and 58-14). The healing period is determined by a number of factors, such as the initial stabilization of the implant, the quality and quantity of bone, and the need for any concurrent bone grafting at the time of implant placement.

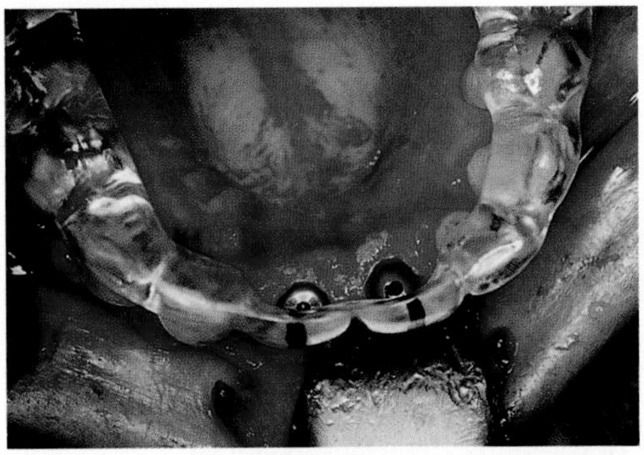

Figure 58-10. Surgical guide stent used to confirm the positioning of the intended restoration.

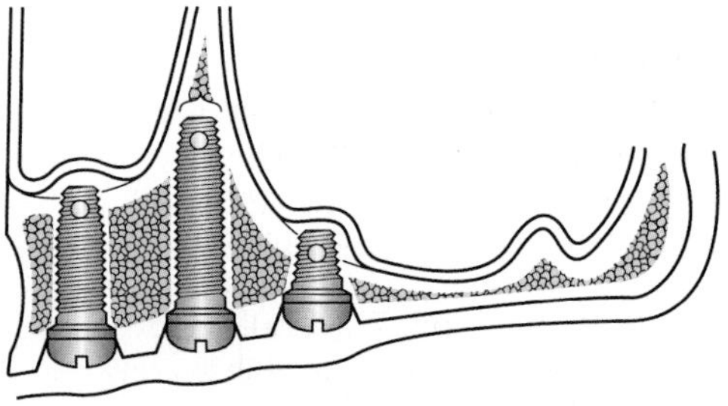

Figure 58-12. Amount of bone relative to the length of the endosteal implant from the anterior to the posterior maxilla. (From Worthington P, Lang BR, Rubenstein JE: *Osseointegration in dentistry: an overview,* Carol Stream, Ill, 2003, Quintessence.)

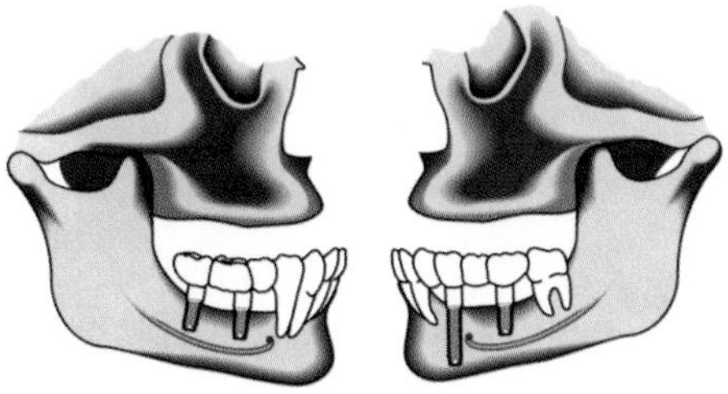

Figure 58-11. Placement of implants with respect to the mandibular nerve and canal. (From Worthington P, Lang BR, Rubenstein JE: *Osseointegration in dentistry: an overview,* Carol Stream, Ill, 2003, Quintessence.)

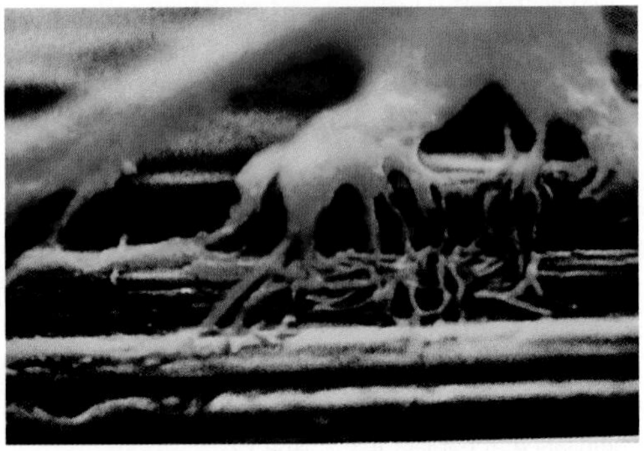

Figure 58-13. Bone cells fusing to a titanium implant, which is termed *osseointegration.* (Courtesy Professor Per-Ingvar Brånemark, Institute for Applied Biotechnology, Gothenburg, Sweden.)

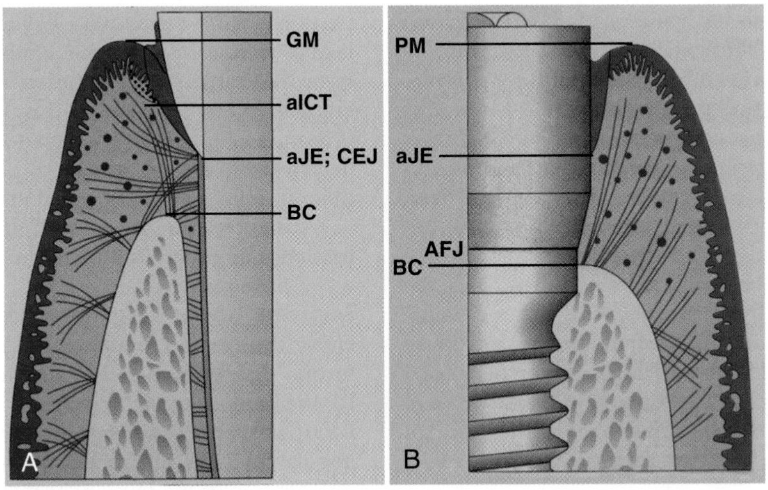

Figure 58-14. **A,** The sulcular tissue around a tooth is similar to an implant, and so is the junctional epithelial zone. The connective tissue zone, which attaches to the cementum on a natural tooth, is completely different around the implant. **B,** The peri-implant tissues exhibit histologic sulcular and junctional epithelial zones that are similar to those of a natural tooth. The primary difference is the lack of connective tissue attachment and the presence of primarily two fiber groups (rather than the 11 seen with a natural tooth). (From Misch CE: *Dental implant prosthetics,* St Louis, 2005, Mosby.)

Stage Two: The Second Surgical Procedure

Traditionally implants are left buried under the mucosa during the initial healing period of 3 to 6 months. However, some surgical protocols accommodate one-stage implant placement and leave the implant exposed into the oral cavity with a healing abutment, which appears as a cap during the healing period. Wound care and oral hygiene are critical during this healing period. The healing abutment protrudes through the mucosa and allows for the healing and formation of a mucosal collar around the implant, which creates access for the connection of the prosthetic parts to the implant (Figures 58-15 through 58-18).

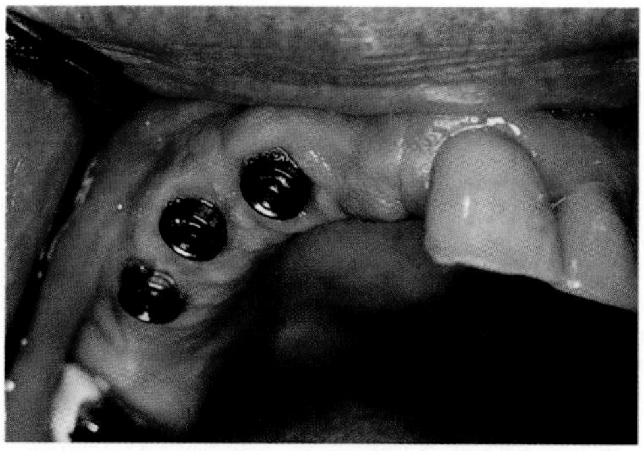

Figure 58-15. This client has healthy peri-implant tissue and good oral hygiene compliance. (Courtesy A.K. Lakha.)

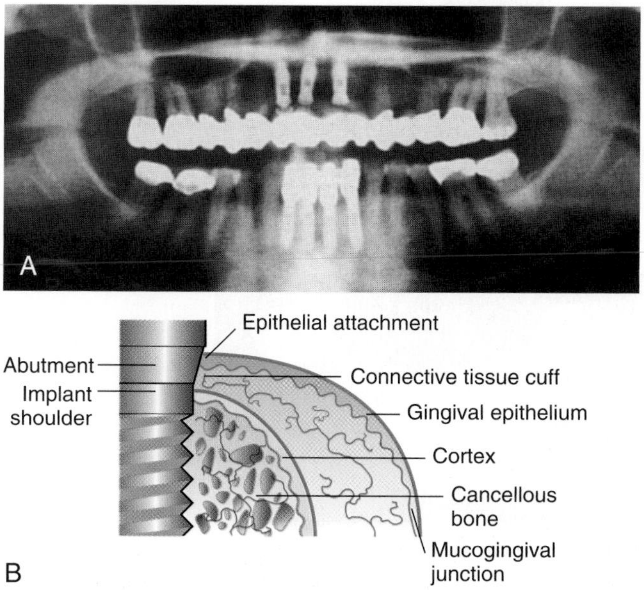

Figure 58-16. **A,** Radiograph of endosseous implants used for clinical follow-up. **B,** Blood supply of the connective tissue cuff surrounding the implant or abutment is scarcer than in the gingival complex around the teeth because none of it originates from the periodontal ligament. (**A,** From Babbush CA: *Dental implants: the art and science,* Philadelphia, 2001, Saunders. **B,** From Newman MG, Takei HH, Klokkevold PR, et al, eds: *Carranza's clinical perodontology,* ed 11, St Louis, 2012, Saunders.)

Stage Three: The Fabrication of the Prosthetic Appliance or the Restorative Crown

Fabricating the prosthetic appliance may require several appointments to achieve a desirable fit. The prosthetic appliance design should ensure a wide interproximal space for access during daily oral biofilm control. Oral self-care education is provided 1 to 2 weeks after the prosthetic appliance placement. Within a few months, natural tooth function should be restored (Figure 58-19).

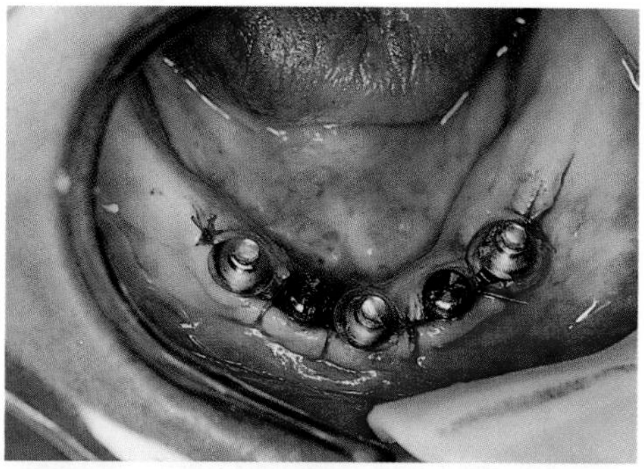

Figure 58-17. Stage two: endosseous implants with healing caps. (Courtesy M.A. Conover.)

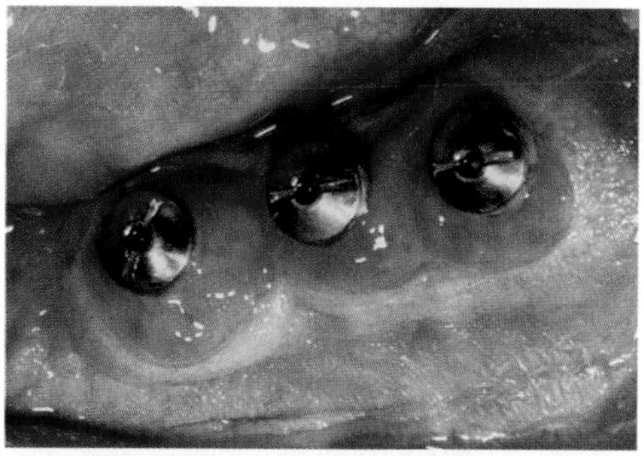

Figure 58-18. Implant fixtures uncovered 6 weeks after stage two. Note the tissue hyperplasia at the soft-tissue–titanium interface. The implant fixtures are uncovered. (From Babbush CA: *Dental implants: the art and science,* Philadelphia, 2001, Saunders.)

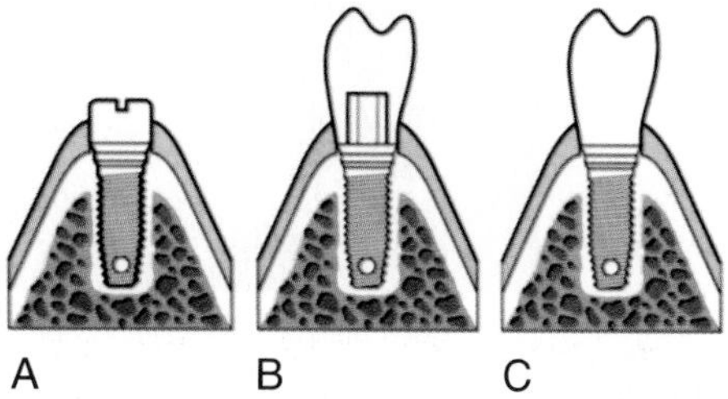

Figure 58-19. Stage two surgery for two-stage endosseous implant systems. **A,** The cover screws are located, removed, and replaced by an abutment cylinder that penetrates the mucosa into the mouth. **B,** The prosthetic component is then mounted on the abutment. **C,** The final stage-three restoration is attached with a screw or cement. (From Worthington P, Lang BR, Rubenstein JE: *Osseointegration in dentistry: an overview,* Carol Stream, Ill, 2003, Quintessence.)

SCENARIO 58-3

VIRTUAL DENTAL IMPLANT PATIENT

A 75-year-old woman had severe atrophy of her maxillary and mandibular ridges from long-term denture wear (Figure 58-20). She was unhappy with her inability to retain her dentures and function normally; an implant-stabilized overdenture was her best option. Given the severe atrophy of her maxillary and mandibular ridges, it was impossible to determine the anatomy of the underlying bone for the evaluation and placement of dental implants. Barium upper and lower dentures were fabricated (Figure 58-21) with the use of the SimPlant protocol. While the client was wearing these barium dentures, computed tomography scans were taken (Figure 58-22). After the evaluation of the scans and after a determination of the full extent of the atrophy of the ridges was made, the client underwent virtual treatment planning for five Endopore implants (Sybron Implant Solutions, Orange, California) in the maxilla and six Nobel Biocare implants in the mandible. Bone-borne SurgiGuides (Materialise Dental, Leuven, Belgium) were ordered on the basis of the virtual treatment plan (Figure 58-23).

Through use of the SurgiGuides, all of the implants were successfully placed during one visit (Figures 58-24 through Figure 58-27). After 4 months of osseointegration, a framework and overdenture were successfully fabricated and inserted into each arch (Figure 58-28).

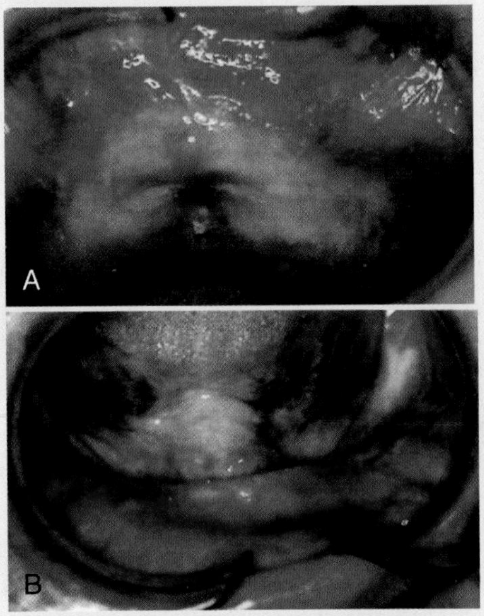

Figure 58-20. Virtual dental implant treatment plan. **A,** Maxilla and **(B)** mandible preoperative views.

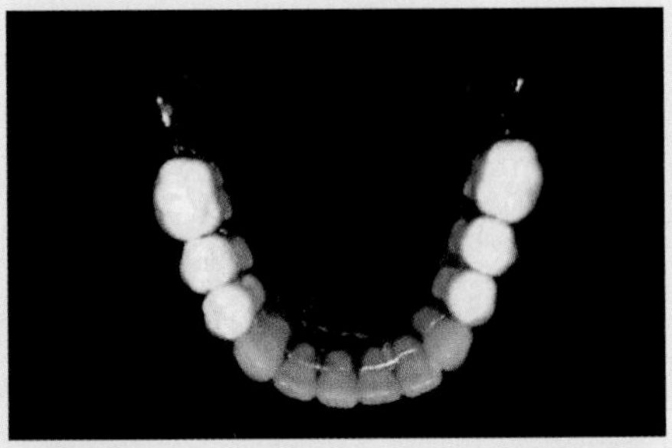

Figure 58-21. Barium scan prosthesis, mandible.

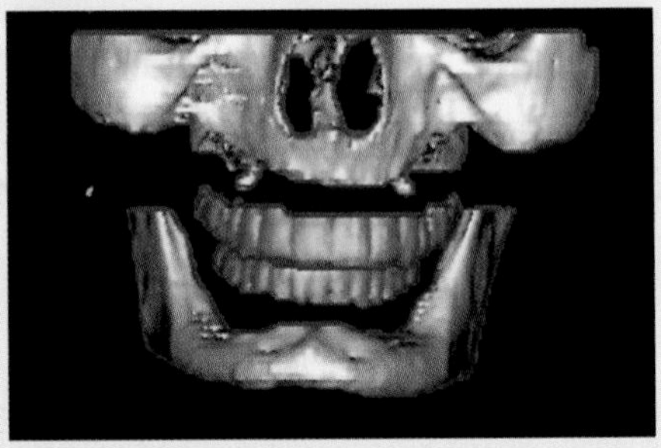

Figure 58-22. Preoperative computed tomography scan, maxilla and mandible, while scanning prosthesis is worn.

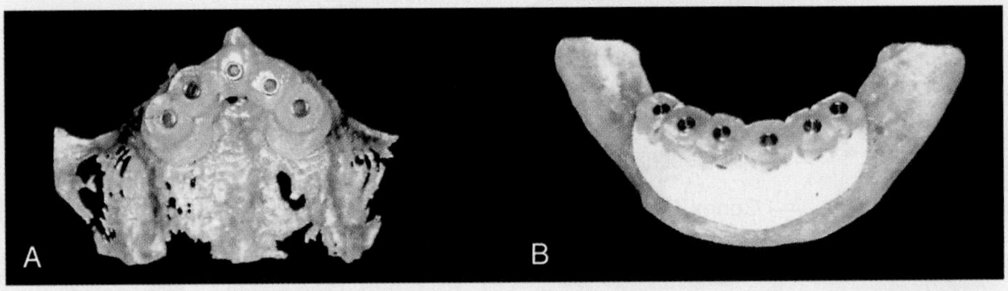

Figure 58-23. Stereolithographic model and bone-borne SurgiGuides. **A,** Maxilla. **B,** Mandible.

SCENARIO 58-3

VIRTUAL DENTAL IMPLANT PATIENT—cont'd

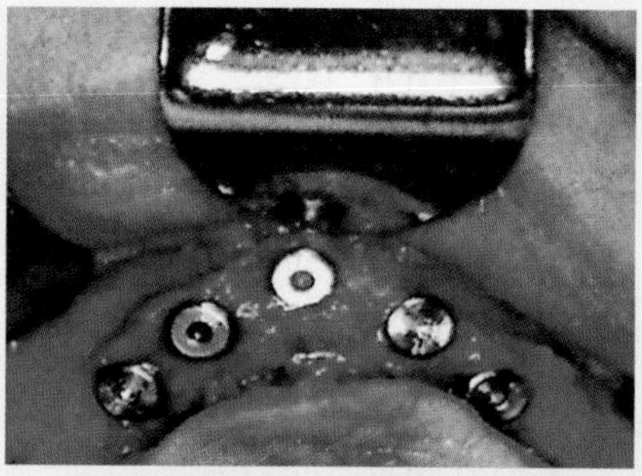

Figure 58-24. Implant placement, maxilla. SurgiGuide was used.

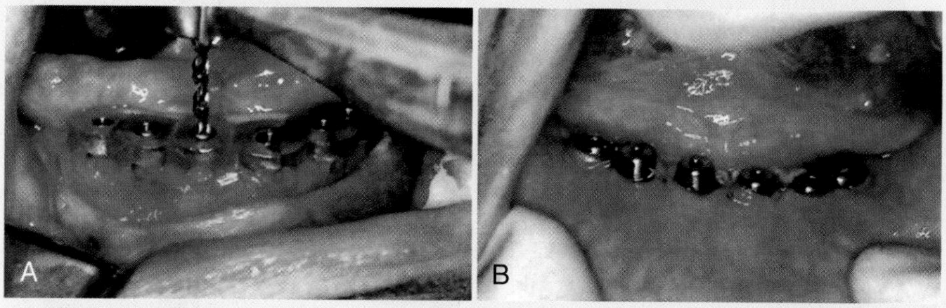

Figure 58-25. A, Implant placement, mandible, using implant-specific drilling instruction and SurgiGuide. **B,** Final implant placement with healing abutments.

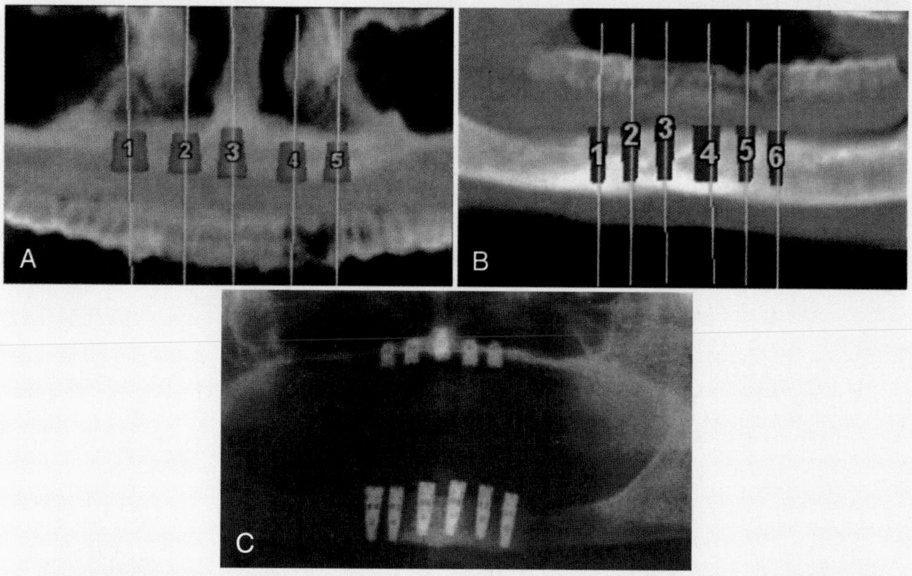

Figure 58-26. Virtual treatment plan. **A,** Maxilla. **B,** Mandible. **C,** Postoperative panograph.

Continued

SCENARIO 58-3

VIRTUAL DENTAL IMPLANT PATIENT—cont'd

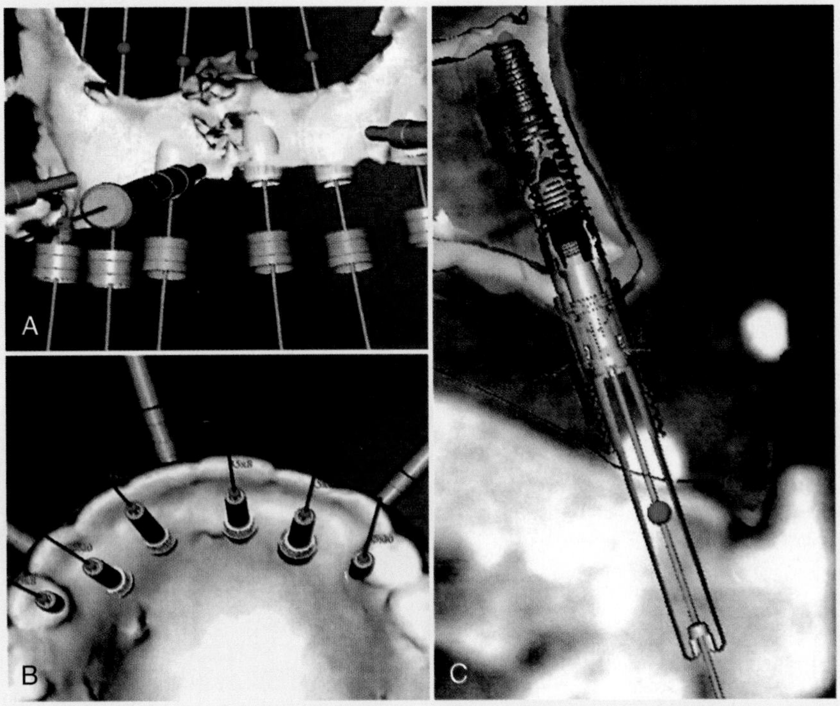

Figure 58-27. **A** and **B,** Computer models of the maxilla and **(C)** palatal view of the proposed implants' emergence. The images resemble a traditional radiograph.

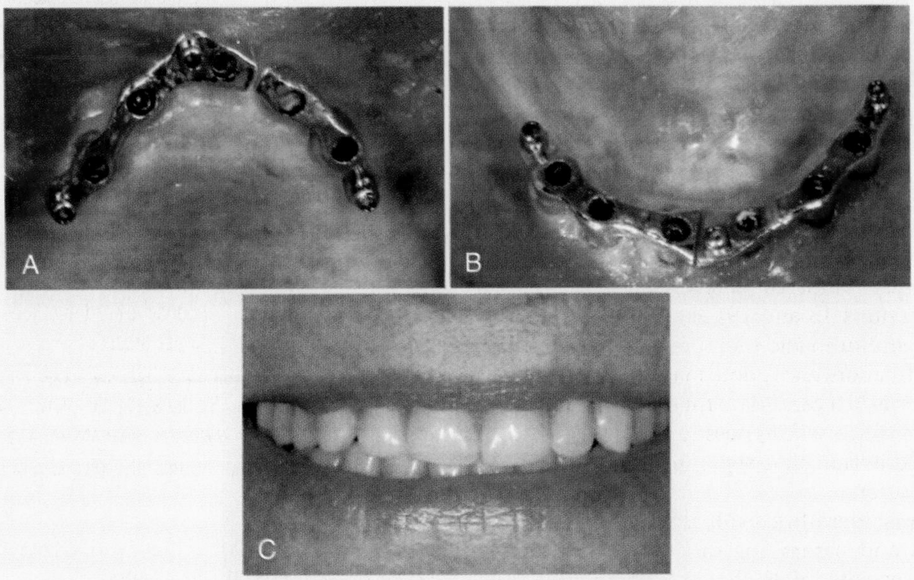

Figure 58-28. Overdenture framework. **A,** Maxilla. **B,** Mandible. **C,** Final overdenture fabrication.

Maintenance and the Role of the Dental Hygienist

During the initial planning stages and throughout treatment (eFigure 58-29), the need for compliance with oral self-care recommendations should be emphasized. Unfortunately, many clients view the dental implant as a new tooth that will tolerate mistreatment better than a natural tooth. This myth must be dispelled, and the client must realize that the gingival tissue around the dental implant needs more daily oral care to control plaque biofilm than the gingival tissue around a natural tooth.

Some dental implant candidates have lost their natural teeth as a result of significant oral risk factors for periodontal

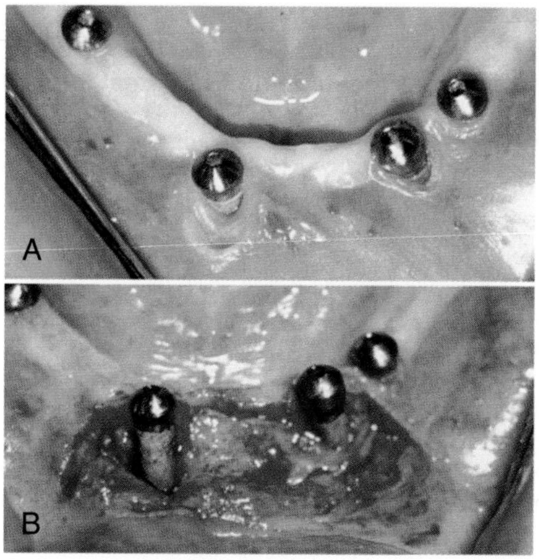

Figure 58-30. **A,** Clinical appearance of peri-implantitis. **B,** Soft tissue is reflected to reveal a loss of osseous support in areas #22 and #27. (From Babbush CA: *Dental implants: the art and science,* Philadelphia, 2001, Saunders.)

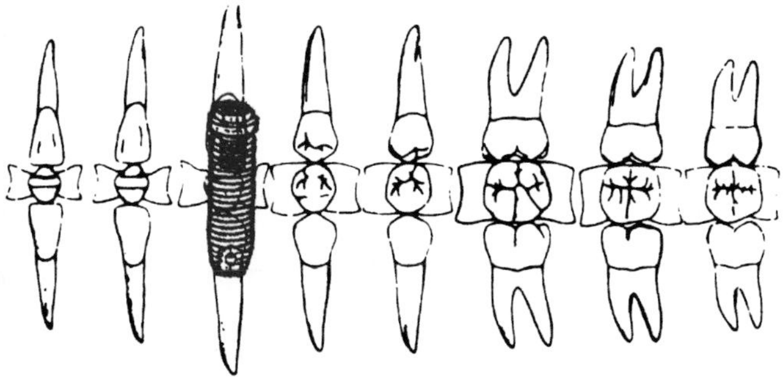

Figure 58-31. Dental implant stamp used to show the location of the dental implant for documentation in the client record.

disease. These individuals may also be at risk for failure of the dental implant (Figure 58-30).

The dental hygienist evaluates the client's risk factors for oral disease (see Chapters 18 and 19) and the client's value system regarding their mouth and their oral health behaviors. A high level of motivation and good manual dexterity are important requirements in a candidate for dental implants for long-term success. In fact, a willingness to perform daily oral biofilm control is a criterion that separates a good implant candidate from a poor one.

The dental hygienist identifies, evaluates, and documents[1] the following signs and symptoms of oral problems, risk factors, and issues associated with the dental implant:

- Changes in the health history
- Location of implants using the implant stamp (Figure 58-31)
- Diagnostic record evaluations
- Oral mucosa conditions
- Discomfort, pain, or infection related to the implant
- Color, texture, and overall condition of the gingival peri-implant tissues, as measured by the following:
  - Attached peri-implant tissue index (Table 58-1)
  - Peri-implant tissue bleeding index (Table 58-2)

TABLE 58-1

Attached Peri-Implant Tissue Index

Grade*	Clinical Impression
0	No keratinized epithelium
1	≤1 mm keratinized epithelium
2	≤2 mm and >1 mm keratinized epithelium
3	>2 mm keratinized epithelium

From Koth D, McKinney RV Jr, Steflik D: *Clinical dentistry: evaluation of the implant-gingival tissue interface,* Hagerstown, Md, 1984, Harper and Row.

*Create tension by retracting the lips laterally to form the mucoperi-implant tissue junction. Use a probe to measure the external surface of the attached peri-implant tissue (note that this measurement uses the tissue that is outside of the sulcus); measure from the mucoperi-implant tissue line to the peri-implant tissue margin to determine width.

TABLE 58-2

Peri-Implant Tissue Bleeding Index

Grade*	Clinical Impression
0	No inflammation Peri-implant tissue of normal color and stippling No bleeding on probing
1	Mild inflammation Peri-implant tissue with slight change in color and stippling with slight hyperemia No bleeding on probing
2	Moderate inflammation Peri-implant tissue hyperemic with redness, edema, glazing, and loss of stippling Bleeding on probing
3	Severe inflammation Peri-implant tissue markedly red, edematous, and ulcerated Tendency toward spontaneous bleeding with finger pressure

From Koth D, McKinney RV Jr, Steflik D: *Clinical dentistry: evaluation of the implant-gingival tissue interface,* Hagerstown, Md, 1984, Harper and Row.

*Visual assessment and the use of a plastic probe determine the grade of the peri-implant tissue.

- Periodontal probing depths
- Bleeding on probing
- Presence of exudate in sulci around abutments
- Amount of oral biofilm and calculus formation as measured by disclosing solution and the plaque and calculus index (Table 58-3)
- Visualization of salivary percolation when applying pressure to the implant crown. (The formation of bubbles at the sulcus indicates a breakdown of the biologic seal.)
- Bridgework mobility as measured by the mobility index (Tables 58-4 and 58-5)

TABLE 58-3

Plaque and Calculus Index for Dental Implants

Grade*	Clinical Impression
0	No plaque in the peri-implant tissue area The amount of plaque is determined by running a pointed plastic probe across the implant surface at the entrance of the peri-implant crevice No calculus
1	A film of plaque can be removed but is not visible to the clinician or supragingival calculus extending no more than 1 mm below the peri-implant tissue margin and adjacent area of the implant The plaque may be recognized only by running a probe across the implant surface
2	Visible plaque within the peri-implant crevice or on the implant and peri-implant tissue margin and adjacent peri-implant tissue surface; moderate accumulation of soft debris; or subgingival calculus extending more than 1 mm into the crevice or moderate amounts of supra–peri-implant and sub–peri-implant calculus can be seen visually
3	Heavy accumulation of plaque within the crevice or on the implant surface and peri-implant tissue margin and adjacent implant surface; an abundance of soft matter or heavy accumulation of supra–peri-implant and sub–peri-implant calculus

From Koth D, McKinney RV Jr, Steflik D: *Clinical dentistry: evaluation of the implant-gingival tissue interface,* Hagerstown, Md, 1984, Harper and Row.

*Visual assessment and the use of a plastic probe determine the grade of plaque and calculus.

TABLE 58-4

Mobility Evaluation Scale

Grade	Clinical Impression
0	Absence of clinical mobility with 500 g in any direction
1	Slight detectable horizontal movement
2	Severe horizontal movement >0.5 mm
3	Moderate visible horizontal mobility ≤0.5 mm
4	Visible moderate to severe horizontal and any visible vertical movement or apical migration of crestal bone with accompanying severe mobility

From Misch CE: *Contemporary implant dentistry,* ed 3, St Louis, 2007, Mosby.

- Microbiologic monitoring test results
- Marginal bone height surrounding the fixture as indicated on radiographs
- Score on the implant quality scale (Table 58-6)
- Oral hygiene knowledge, beliefs, and behaviors

TABLE 58-5

Mobility Index for Freestanding Endosteal Implants and Attached Prostheses

Grade*	Clinical Impression
0	No mobility
1	Slight buccolingual mobility, <0.5 mm
2	Slight buccolingual mobility, >0.5 mm but <1.0 mm
3	Mobility >0.5 mm in buccolingual and mesiodistal directions
4	Depressible, salivary percolation (bubbling around implant)

From Koth D, McKinney RV Jr, Steflik D: *Clinical dentistry: evaluation of the implant-gingival tissue interface,* Hagerstown, Md, 1984, Harper and Row.

*Use of two single-ended metal instruments to determine mobility. Rock the implant to test horizontal mobility. Test vertical mobility by applying pressure occlusally.

eFigure 58-32 provides a sample assessment form for establishing the client's baseline status maintenance record. This form can be used in conjunction with the human needs assessment form found in Figure 21-3 of Chapter 21.

Diagnosis and Planning of Dental Hygiene Care

Depending on the client's diagnosed unmet needs, the dental hygienist sets goals and develops a dental hygiene care plan in conjunction with the client. Client preferences significantly affect the client's acceptance of oral hygiene recommendations and should be incorporated into the care plan. The dental hygienist works collaboratively with the client to ensure that the proposed dental hygiene care plan is understood and accepted.

Personal Oral Hygiene Care

Ongoing oral self-care education should be customized on the basis of client preferences and in collaboration with the dentist with regard to abutment length and position; the prosthetic design and the ease of biofilm removal between the appliance and gingival tissue; client motivation, compliance, and manual dexterity; and peri-implant tissue health. Clients who have lost their teeth because of periodontal risk factors need education about the modification and control of those risk factors (see the discussion of periodontal risk factors in Chapter 19). The hygienist impresses on clients the idea that implants also are vulnerable to periodontal risk factors that can cause peri-implantitis.

The dental hygienist monitors the oral tissues to ensure that the client is not causing trauma with an oral hygiene aid. As clients' oral conditions change, so do their dental hygiene needs. For example, if a client has an increased amount of gingival bleeding, the dental hygienist may need to modify homecare to include the daily application of 0.12% chlorhexidine gluconate or a new implant cleaning strategy.

Peri-implantitis

Peri-implant inflammation can occur around the implant abutment if biofilm and calculus continue to accumulate

TABLE 58-6

Implant Quality Scale

Group	Management	Clinical Conditions
I. Success (optimum health)	Normal maintenance	No pain or tenderness on function 0 mobility <2 mm radiographic bone loss from initial surgery Probing depth <5 mm No exudate history
II. Survival (satisfactory health)	Reduction of stresses Shorter intervals between hygiene appointments Gingivoplasty Yearly radiographs	No pain 0 mobility 2 to 4 mm of radiographic bone loss Probing depth of 5 to 7 mm No exudate history
III. Survival (compromised health)	Reduction of stresses Drug therapy (antibiotics, chlorhexidine) Surgical reentry and revision Change in prosthesis or implants	No pain on probing 0 mobility Radiographic bone loss of >4 mm Probing depth of >7 mm May have exudate history
IV. Failure (clinical or absolute failure)	Removal of implant	Any of the following: Pain on function Mobility Radiographic bone loss of less than one half of length of implant Uncontrolled exudate No longer in mouth

From Misch CE, Perel ML, Wang H, et al: Implant success, survival, and failure: the International Congress of Oral Implantologists (ICOI) Pisa Consensus Conference, *Implant Dent* 17:5, 2008.

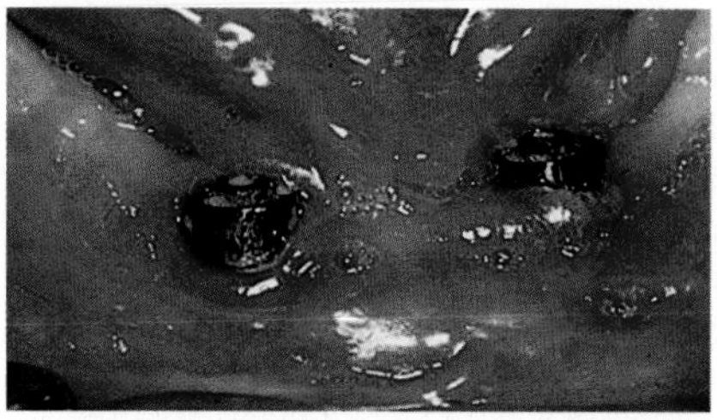

Figure 58-33. Peri-implantitis, an infectious disease around an implant. Note the amount of plaque and the changes in the tissue's color, size, contour, and consistency. (Courtesy A.K. Lakha.)

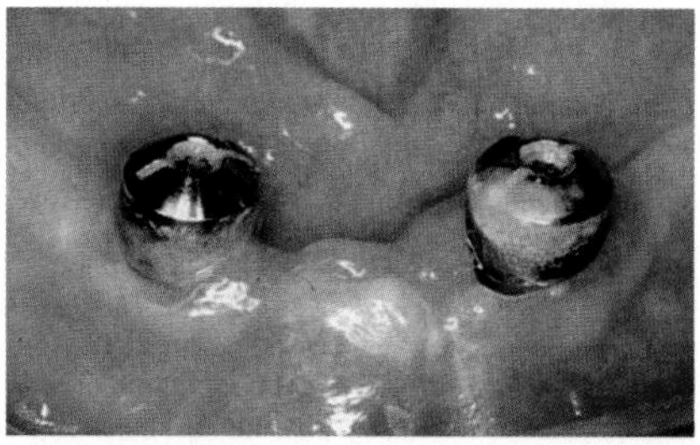

Figure 58-34. Heavy plaque and calculus accumulation around these healing heads have caused a breakdown of the perimucosal seal. The implants are at risk for failure. (From Babbush CA: *Dental implants: the art and science,* Philadelphia, 2001, Saunders.)

(Figures 58-33 and 58-34). A widely used definition of **peri-implantitis** is the loss of crestal peri-implant bone in conjunction with bleeding on probing.[2] This definition implies that the initial dental implant healing was uneventful and that osseointegration was achieved as anticipated. It is important to note that bony destruction can progress without any notable impact on osseointegration and implant mobility.

The inflammation causes bleeding and/or suppuration upon gentle probing with a blunt instrument. The marginal tissue may be swollen or red; however, these characteristics are not always clearly visible. Unless the lesion access is obstructed, a periodontal probe can be advanced 4 mm or more into the peri-implant sulcus; pain is usually not recorded. Since osseointegration is generally maintained apically to the peri-implantitis defect, bone destruction can progress without any signs of implant mobility. Mobility indicates the complete loss of osseointegration and total implant failure.

Depending on the criteria that are used to define peri-implantitis, it has been reported in as many as 20% of research subjects and in 10% of implants with 5 to 10 years of functional loading (i.e., the pressure brought to bear on the implant by occlusion over time). The differences in the defining criteria are due to the use of different thresholds in research studies for bone loss and inflammatory parameters such as bleeding on probing or probing depth. The lack of standardized criteria to define peri-implantitis, in addition to other factors such as early bone remodeling around the implants unrelated to inflammatory processes, can result in variability in diagnosis and the inconsistent reporting of peri-implantitis. For example, bleeding on probing has been reported in as many as 80% of cases in some studies.[3-7] Nevertheless, bleeding on probing alone tends to overestimate gingival inflammation, even in periodontally healthy subjects.[8] Due to the discrepancy between the bleeding on probing and the clinical manifestations of peri-implantitis, it may be a poor prognostic marker for future periodontal attachment loss.

It is difficult to define the continuum between inflammatory changes of the mucosa or mucositis surrounding the implant and peri-implantitis. Therefore, peri-implantitis management may be equally challenging. Peri-implant mucositis may respond well to nonsurgical treatment modalities such as mechanical debridement, whereas there is a limited response to nonsurgical mechanical debridement alone in peri-implantitis cases.

The first step in the management of peri-implantitis is to identify and remedy the local factors and the etiology, such as retained dental cement, poor contours of the prosthesis, and poor personal oral hygiene. Nonsurgical debridement in conjunction with the medical management of peri-implant inflammation should then follow. Surgical therapy may ultimately be required. Surgical therapy includes granulation tissue removal and thorough cleaning of the contaminated surface.

Recommended Devices and Strategies for Cleaning Dental Implants (eBox 58-2)

Disclosants (see Chapter 17)

Disclosing agents for professional and home use are applied to teeth and dental implants for oral biofilm visualization. For example, the client may not see biofilm on the lingual aspect of abutments or on the posterior portion of a bridge without a disclosant. These agents are used as a monitoring strategy after effective self-care behaviors are confirmed.

Intraoral Mirror and Penlight

A magnifying intraoral mirror and penlight can be used by the client in conjunction with disclosants for an adequate visual examination of oral biofilm accumulation and color changes in the soft tissue.

Toothbrushes (see Chapter 23)

Clients should clean their implants, teeth, and gums two to three times daily with a toothbrush directed at a 45-degree angle toward the soft tissues. Because titanium is less rigid than a natural tooth, the abutment surface can be damaged with hard-bristled toothbrushes, thereby facilitating oral biofilm accumulation and gingival or peri-implant recession (i.e., the loss of gingival tissue around the implant). Therefore soft-bristled brushes are recommended. To prevent trauma to the delicate mucosa that surrounds the abutment, the soft-bristled brush should have a small, compact head for reaching the facial, lingual, and occlusal surfaces and for tongue brushing. The toothbrush can be dipped into a 0.12% chlorhexidine gluconate solution to enhance oral biofilm and gingivitis control. Clients also should invest adequate time into brushing their prosthetic appliances.

Unituft Interspace Brushes: Tapered or Flat (see Chapter 24)

The unique design of the unituft interspace brush allows the client to focus on one implant or tooth at a time (Figure 58-35). The brush has soft-bristled nylon fibers that do not damage the peri-implant tissue. The facial and lingual surfaces of dental implants can be reached with the unituft interspace brush with either the tapered or flat design. The plastic handle can be placed under hot water and bent for greater access to hard-to-reach areas. The unituft toothbrush is recommended for use two or three times daily to remove oral biofilm and to strengthen the peri-implant and gingival tissue. The unituft brush can be dipped into a 0.12% chlorhexidine gluconate solution to enhance biofilm and gingivitis control.

Power Brushes (see Chapter 23)

Power brushes may be prescribed for clients so that they may thoroughly clean around the abutments and the interproximal areas under the prosthetic tooth or appliance (Figures 58-36 and 58-37). Brushes can be dipped into 0.12% chlorhexidine gluconate and then used. The brush motion should follow the curvature of the dental implant along the gingiva. Power brushing is recommended one or two times daily.

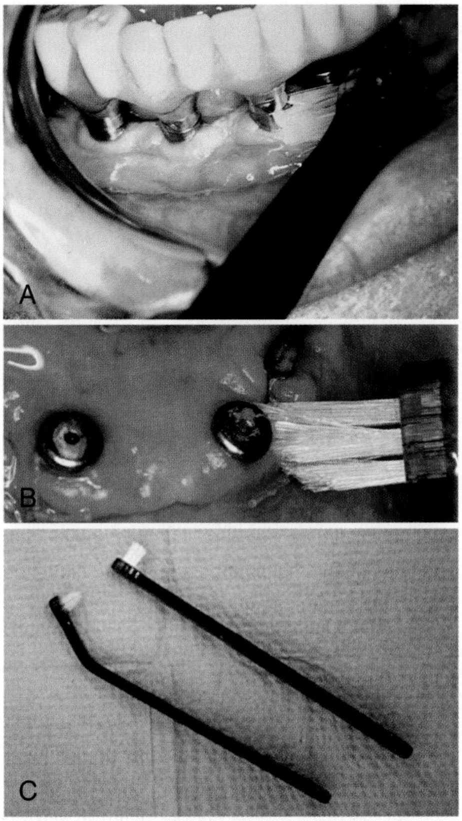

Figure 58-35. **A,** The application of an end-tuft toothbrush to an endosseous implant. **B,** The application of a tapered end-tuft toothbrush to healing surgical sites. **C,** Tapered and flat end-tuft toothbrush design. The plastic handle can be bent to a position for use in the lingual areas. (**A,** Courtesy J. Kleinman. **B** and **C,** From Babbush CA: *Dental implants: the art and science*, Philadelphia, 2001, Saunders.)

Plastic Nylon-Coated Interdental Brush and Foam Pads: Tapered or Cylindric (see Chapter 24)

The interproximal areas of dental implants can be reached with a cone-shaped or cylindric interdental brush, foam tip, or Proxi-Tip (Figures 58-38 and 58-39). To avoid alteration of the abutment surface, nylon-coated wires are required rather than the conventional metal-wired brushes. Interdental brushes should be discarded when the nylon coating has worn down to the metal wire. The interdental brush can be used from the facial or lingual areas and interproximally. Interdental brushes are recommended for use at least one time daily. The interdental brush also may be used with 0.12% chlorhexidine gluconate for target delivery of the antimicrobial agent.

Rubber Tip

The rubber tip may be used to remove debris accumulation from all surfaces, including the gingival sulcus toward the coronal and abutment surface. The rubber tip may also stimulate and massage the peri-implant tissue. Performance of this procedure is recommended once daily (Figure 58-40).

Dentifrice (see Chapter 25)

Abrasive dentifrice can alter the abutment surface; therefore clients should use a low-abrasive toothpaste, which is defined as one that has a radioactive dentin abrasion score of 130 or less. Toothpastes that carry the American Dental Association Seal of Acceptance or the Canadian Dental Association Seal of Recognition meet this criterion for low abrasiveness. For example, a low-abrasive dentifrice such as Crest Pro-Health or Colgate Total could be safely recommended for implant clients to use twice daily in conjunction with an oral hygiene aid. Baking soda (sodium bicarbonate) toothpastes also have a low level of abrasiveness.

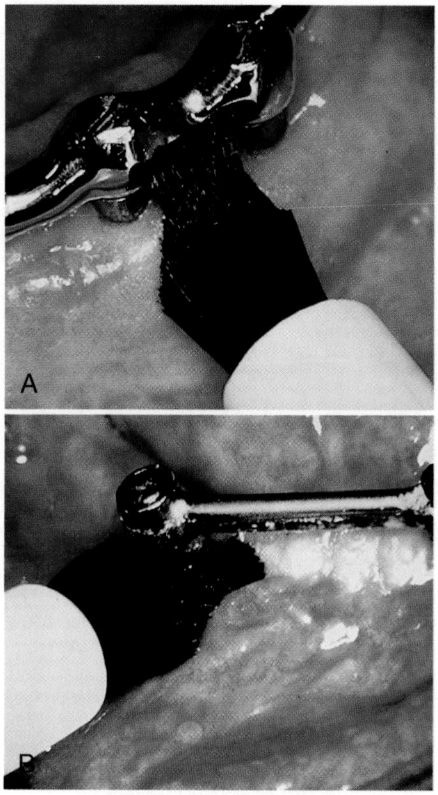

Figure 58-36. **A,** Application of a Rota-dent (Pro-Dentec) power rotary long-tip brush to clean the crossbar of an endosseous implant. **B,** Application of Rota-dent (Pro-Dentec) power rotary brush to an endosseous implant. (Courtesy J. Kleinman.)

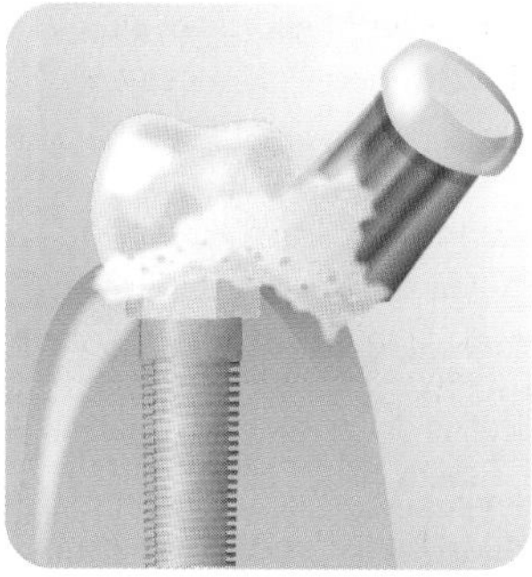

Figure 58-37. Sonicare power brush. (Courtesy Philips Oral Healthcare, Stamford, Connecticut.)

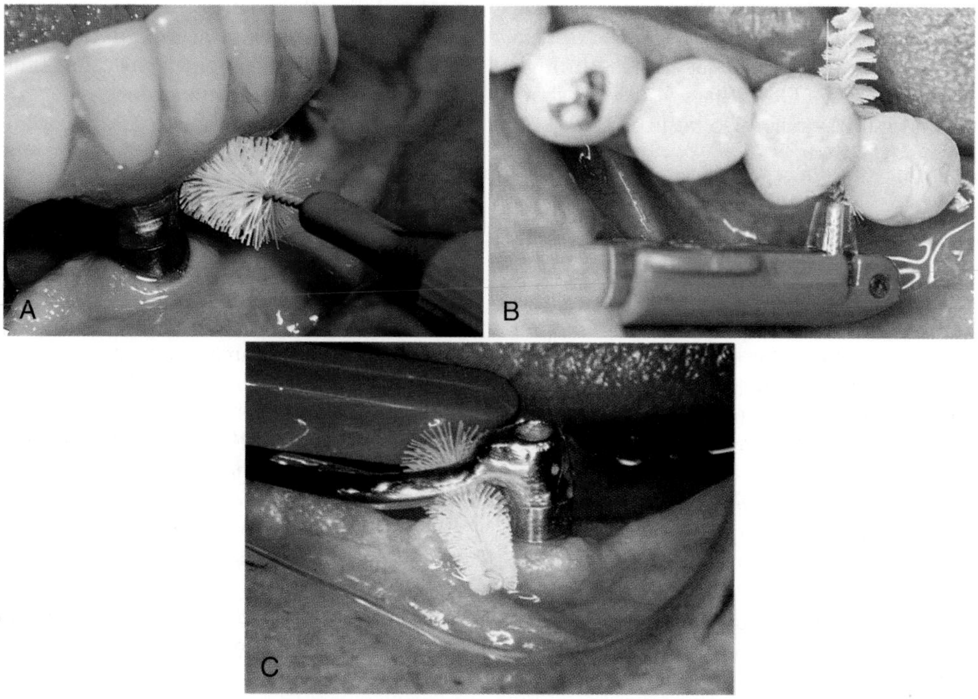

Figure 58-38. **A,** Application of a John O. Butler nylon-coated Proxabrush to an endosseous implant. **B,** A coated interproximal brush is used when embrasure space allows for easy insertion and removal. **C,** Connector bars can usually accommodate interproximal brushes for ease of use and effective self-care. (**A,** Courtesy J. Kleinman. **B,** Courtesy Procter & Gamble, Professional and Scientific Relations, Cincinnati, Ohio. **C,** From Babbush CA: *Dental implants: the art and science,* Philadelphia, 2001, Saunders.)

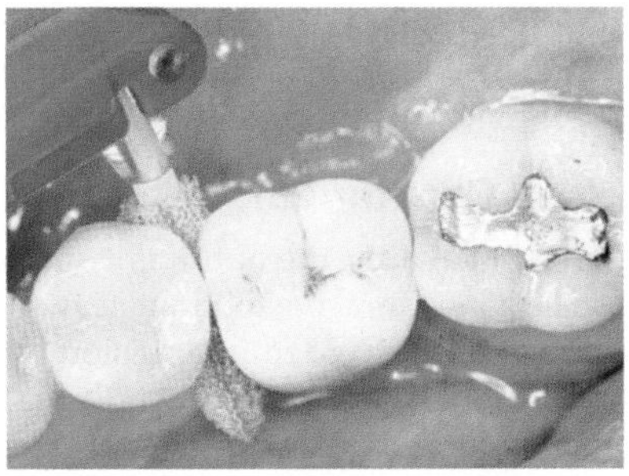

Figure 58-39. Application of an Oral-B Foam Tip device to an endosseous implant interdentally. This product can be used to target-deliver chemotherapeutic agents while reducing the amount of tooth staining. (Courtesy Oral-B, Belmont, California.)

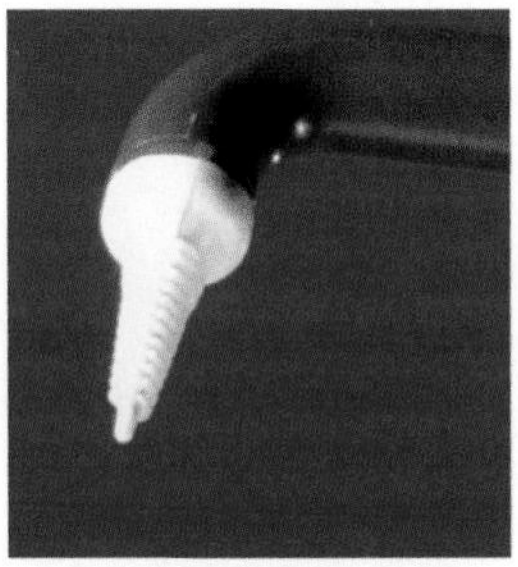

Figure 58-40. Application of the Advanced Implant Technologies Proxi-Tip. (Courtesy AIT Dental, Beverly Hills, California.)

Dental Floss and Dental Tape (see Chapter 24)

If abutments are spaced close to each other, dental floss or tape should be used to clean their proximal surfaces at least once daily (Figures 58-41, 58-42, and 58-43). The floss is placed around the implant, crisscrossed, and pulled in a shoe-shining motion to clean the abutment. Floss or tape can be used in conjunction with a floss threader to allow easy access through the embrasure or limited areas. Other aids—such as shoelaces, ribbon, yarn, and gauze—may also be used if embrasure space permits.

Oral Irrigation

An oral irrigator (Figure 58-44) may be indicated for use in limited access areas where there is evidence of soft-tissue inflammation surrounding the abutment cylinder. The flow rate of the unit should be set at the lowest force (see Chapter 24). Solutions used in the oral irrigator may include water, an American Dental Association–accepted antimicrobial mouth rinse, or a 0.12% chlorhexidine gluconate mouth rinse (see the discussion of oral antimicrobial agents in Chapter 31).

Antimicrobial Agents (see Chapter 31)

For approximately 5 to 7 days after the abutment connection surgery, the use of a capful of the antimicrobial 0.12% chlorhexidine gluconate solution as a 30-second rinse is recommended twice daily to control plaque formation. A cotton swab, a soft toothbrush, a unituft interspace brush, a power rotary brush, an interdental brush, or a subgingival irrigator (Figure 58-45) may be used for the target delivery of an agent to a site. Rinsing with 0.12% chlorhexidine gluconate reduces both gram-positive and gram-negative oral bacteria by 100% for up to 5 hours after use with the 30-seconds-twice-a-day

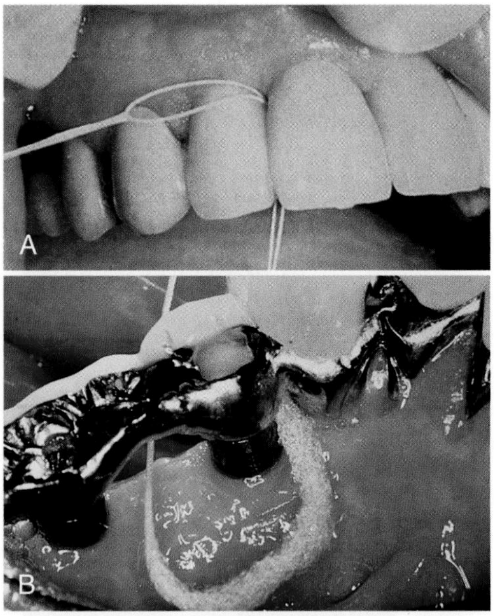

Figure 58-41. **A,** Application of floss threaders for challenging areas. **B,** Application of Oral-B Super Floss to an implant. (**A,** From Babbush CA: *Dental implants: the art and science,* Philadelphia, 2001, Saunders. **B,** Courtesy Procter & Gamble, Professional and Scientific Relations, Cincinnati, Ohio.)

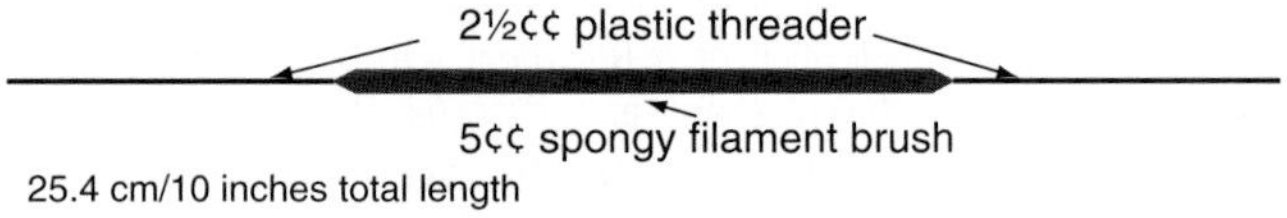

Figure 58-42. Characteristics of the Thornton Bridge and Implant interdental cleaner.

protocol, thereby resulting in less peri-implant gingivitis and bleeding; however, the use of chlorhexidine gluconate as a rinse for more than a month may cause staining of the natural teeth or the prosthetic appliance.

Cervitec Plus varnish with chlorhexidine gluconate can be used to protect at-risk, exposed, and sensitive implant tissue areas. The combination of 1% chlorhexidine and 1% thymol firmly adheres to the implant surfaces, thus creating a shield of long-lasting protection. A heavy metal salt agent, hyaluronic acid, can be placed in the implant area with the solution in a syringe. It reduces bacterial colonization and bleeding within the first 2 months and has tissue-healing properties.

Professional Care and Maintenance of Dental Implants (Box 58-1 and eBox 58-2)

Armamentarium

The clinical armamentarium (Table 58-7) needed to provide professional dental hygiene implant care includes the following:

- Antimicrobial agent such as 0.12% chlorhexidine gluconate
- Plastic disposable syringe or gingival irrigation unit
- Periodontal probe; preferably a flexible plastic probe (Figure 58-46; see also Figure 19-6 in Chapter 19)
- Set of plastic Teflon-coated scalers (Figures 58-47 and 58-48)

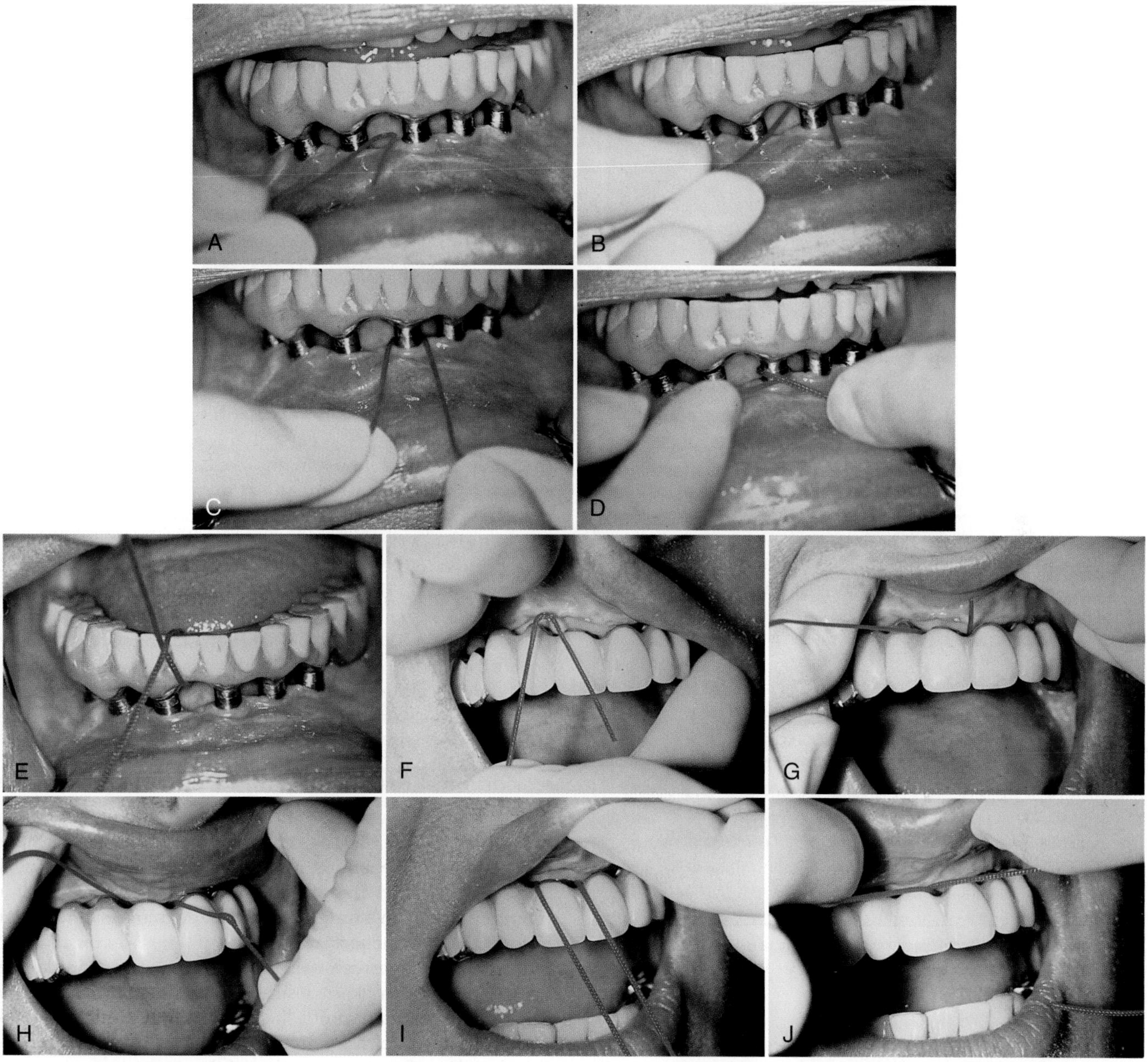

Figure 58-43. **A** through **J,** Systematic demonstration of how to use the John O. Butler Postcare Implant Flossing Cord. (Courtesy J. Kleinman.)

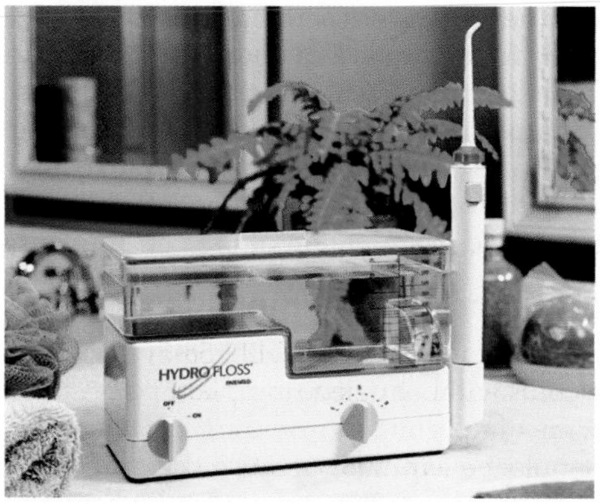

Figure 58-44. Hydro Floss oral irrigator. (Courtesy Oral Care Technologies, Inc., Birmingham, Alabama.)

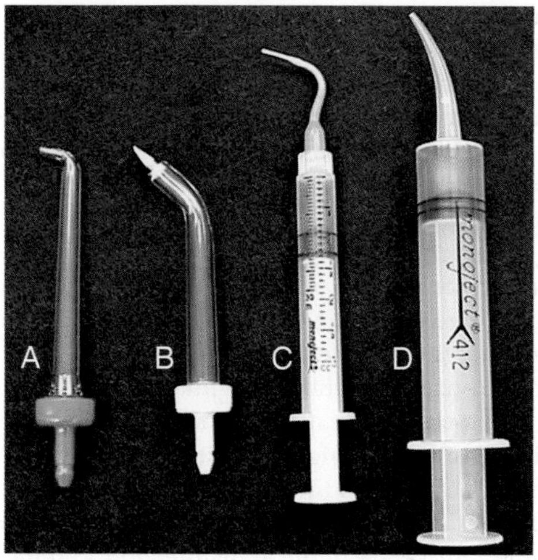

Figure 58-45. Irrigation tip styles. **A,** Supragingival and **B,** marginal tips are designed to attach to a power irrigator. The two tips on the right are attached to simple syringes. **C,** Marginal irrigator tip. **D,** This tip has the most difficult fit because it becomes progressively wider. (Courtesy Dr. W.B. Stilley II.)

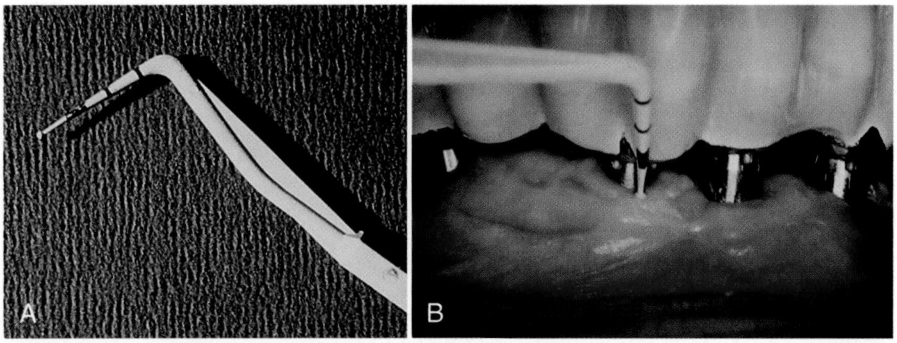

Figure 58-46. **A,** Plastic flexible probe (Pro-Dentec) that can be used to measure sulcus, if absolutely necessary; it does not alter the abutment surface. **B,** Plastic flexible probe measuring sulcus. (Courtesy J. Kleinman.)

BOX 58-1

The Role of the Dental Hygienist in Implant Maintenance

- Identification of potential implant clients
- Provision of education and motivation throughout treatment
- Development, continual assessment, and modification of client-specific oral hygiene procedures
- Evaluation of prosthesis (components, attachments, mobility, and retention)
- Evaluation of peri-implant tissue
- Probing when necessary
- Exposure of clinically acceptable radiographs
- Removal of oral biofilms as well as soft and hard accretions
- Recommendation of oral hygiene products and devices; providing instruction
- Determination of a client-specific continued-care interval
- Co-therapists to identify potential problems or complications
- Documentation of implant status

Adapted from Misch CE: *Contemporary implant dentistry,* ed 3, St Louis, 2007, Mosby.

- Set of gold-tipped Gracey scalers, such as an 11/12 or 13/14 set
- Set of gold-tipped titanium-covered implant hygiene scalers (all types of tips available) (Figure 58-49)
- Set of graphite-reinforced nylon scalers (Figure 58-50) or high-tech plastic scalers (Figure 58-51)
- Wood-tipped porte polisher
- Ultrasonic scaler with a disposable polysulfone plastic tip (Figure 58-52)
- Implant ultrasonic scaler (Figure 58-53)
- Strip of 2-inch × 2-inch gauze
- Thick (red) and thin (green) implant floss
- Gel dentifrice, tin oxide, or nonabrasive prophylaxis paste
- Rubber cup and pointed polisher
- Soft, multi-tufted toothbrush with a compact head design and other appropriate aids for self-care instruction

Peri-implant tissue irrigation with an antimicrobial agent such as 0.12% chlorhexidine gluconate, before instrumentation, reduces the pathogenicity of bacterial colonies and the risk of local infection. Chemical disinfection to remove endotoxins with agents such as chlorhexidine, citric acid, hydrogen peroxide, stannous fluoride, and tetracycline is under investigation. The clinical efficacy of these agents for total mouth disinfection remains unclear. A plastic disposable syringe or a power oral irrigation unit may be used to accomplish this irrigation procedure, because both techniques allow access to the peri-implant sulcus and deliver the antimicrobial solution to the peri-implant sulcus easily and effectively. A solution of 0.12% chlorhexidine gluconate is an excellent antimicrobial agent for peri-implant tissue irrigation. To minimize generalized staining, the solution may be applied locally with a cotton applicator rather than rinsing. An American Dental Association–accepted antimicrobial mouth rinse is acceptable if a client cannot tolerate the stain or taste of some antimicrobial solutions.

Periodontal Probing Around Dental Implants

Periodontal probing around the peri-implant tissue continues to be controversial. This controversy stems from the concerns that periodontal probing can break down the fragile epithelial attachment around the dental implants or scratch the titanium surface. The available research does not suggest any harm to the implant surfaces or to the prognosis of the implant with careful and proper periodontal probing. In addition, it appears that the soft-tissue health and function is based on its close adaptation around the implant rather than any histologic attachment to the implant surfaces. Despite the controversy, periodontal probe use in the evaluation of dental implants is widely used as a diagnostic tool and reported throughout the literature. Therefore it seems quite reasonable to use a periodontal probe as a diagnostic tool to evaluate the health of the dental implant and the surrounding soft tissue. The use of a plastic disposable probe or a single-use plastic probe that connects to a fiberoptic light source has been suggested. The fiberoptic light gives good visibility during the measurement and examination of the peri-implant sulcus.

Scaling Around Dental Implants

Several types of instruments will remove oral biofilm and dental calculus without damaging the implant surface (Figure 58-54). Scratching, gouging, or contaminating the titanium surface should be avoided, because this will create an area that becomes more retentive to biofilm accumulation and its bacterial by-products. Instrument rigidity and design, prosthetic appliance design, biofilm location, and calculus tenacity should be carefully assessed before instrumentation. Because the titanium abutment surface can be easily abraded

TABLE 58-7

Clinical Implant Hygiene and Maintenance Armamentarium

Company	Product	Features
Advanced Implant Technologies	Implant-Prophy+	Standard instrument designs and blade angles Sharpenable Autoclavable High-performance plastic Exceptional strength Certified as U.S. Food and Drug Administration Class 3 device in full compliance with regulatory protocol
Brevet	Implant Cleaning Kit	Six instrument designs Composite resin material Sterilizable
Quixonic SofTip	Plastic Prophy Tips for Quixonic Sonic Scaler	Three sonic tip designs, fully autoclavable Disposable plastic sheaths
Hu-Friedy	Implacare	Disposable Mirror paired tips Three standard instrument designs Plasteel (high-grade resin)
Pro-Dentec	Sensor Probe	Thermoplastic Maintains consistency of probing pressure Autoclavable
Pro-Dentec	Mandrels	Soft-bristle brushes that can attach to slow-speed handpieces for polishing Flat and tapered shapes available
Premier	Implant Scalers Implant Cleanic Paste Periowise Plastic Probe	Universal and facial designs High-carbon plastic Autoclavable Sharpenable
Straumann (ITI)	Light Curet	Universal design Sterilizable Resharpenable
Steri-Oss	Scaler System	Standard instrument designs Graphite reinforced nylon Packaged sterile and sterilizable Exceptional strength Sharpenable

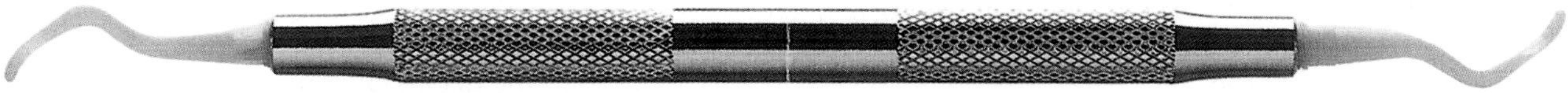

Figure 58-47. Hu-Friedy Implacare Maintenance Instrument with disposable Plasteel (high-grade resin) tips that screw into the handle. (Courtesy Hu-Friedy, Chicago, Illinois; photography by Dr. Roland Meffert.)

by metal scalers, sonic instruments, and abrasive agents, the following are strongly contraindicated for use on dental implants: metal curets and scalers, metal tip inserts of sonic and ultrasonic scaling instruments, air polishing devices, air abrasive systems, and rubber cup polishing with flour of pumice or abrasive paste (Figures 58-55 and 58-56). A polysulfone disposable tip may be used with a sonic scaler to remove tenacious calculus deposits.

Plastic, Teflon-coated, graphite, wood-tipped, and gold-tipped Gracey instruments have been developed for use when scaling dental implants (see Figures 58-47 through 58-51). The plastic and Teflon-coated instruments are designed to prevent abrasion to the titanium implants and tend to be preferred. The wood-tipped instrument or porte polisher is designed to prevent scratches on the implant surface. Half of a round, pointed toothpick inserted through the end of an interdental brush handle is considered a very safe and effective scaler for use around dental implants. Wood-tipped instruments are used only once, however, and then thrown away to prevent splintering and damage to the peri-implant tissue.

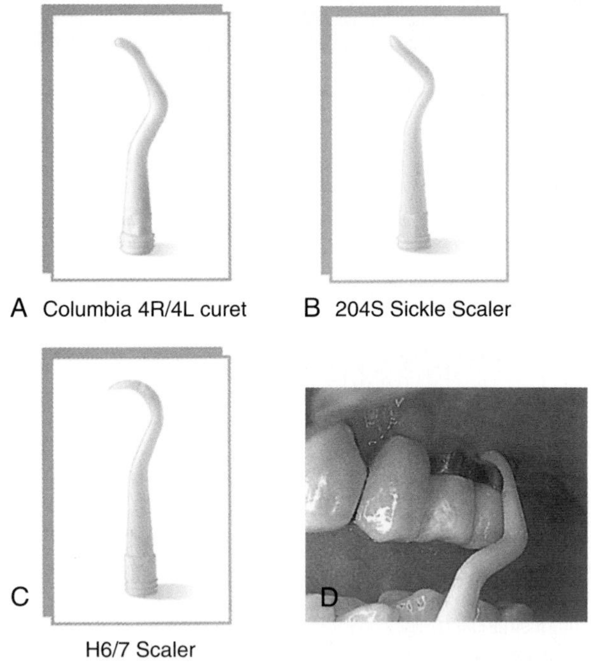

Figure 58-48. **A, B,** and **C,** Close-up of working ends of scalers. **D,** Clinical application of the universal scaler. (Courtesy Hu-Friedy, Chicago, Illinois.)

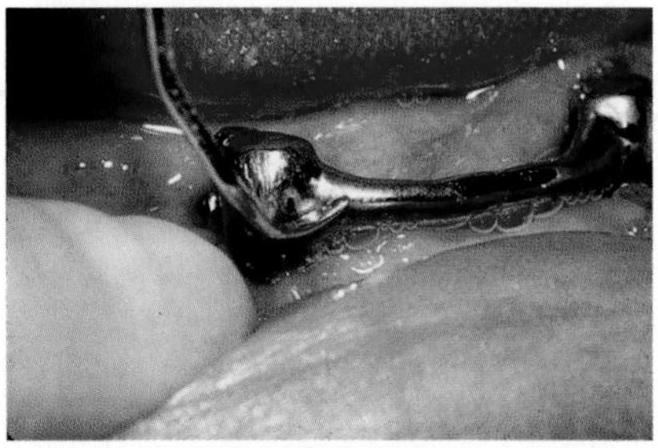

Figure 58-49. Gold-tipped titanium-covered dental hygiene implant scalers are available with all types of tips. (Courtesy Denise O'Connor Lirette.)

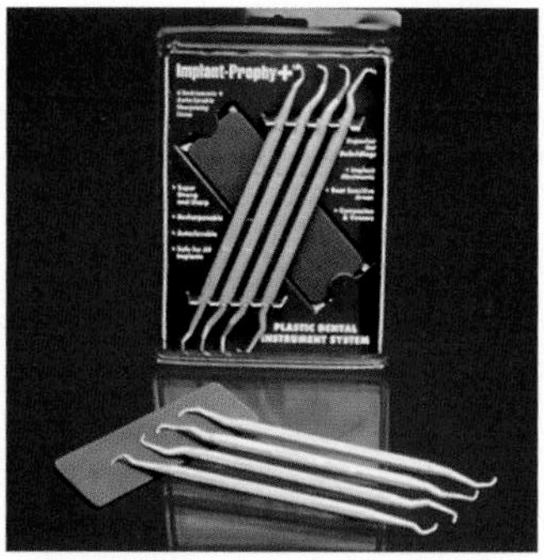

Figure 58-51. Implant-Prophy+ instrument system. (Courtesy Advanced Implant Technologies, Beverly Hills, California.)

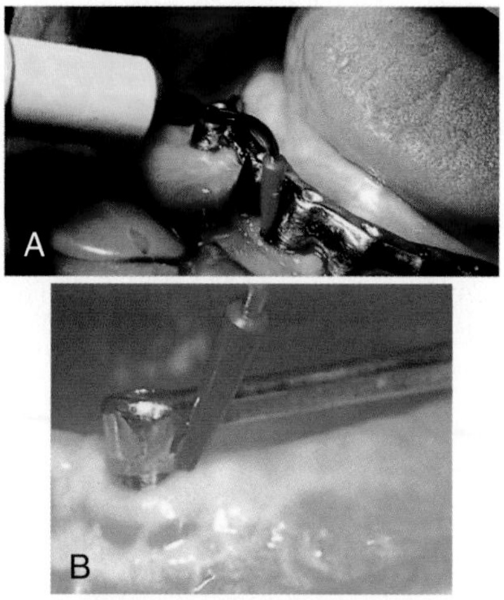

Figure 58-52. **A,** Disposable polysulfone plastic Cavitron SofTip for Ultrasonic scaling of implants. **B,** Ultrasonic scaler insert for scaling titanium implants. (**A,** Courtesy DENTSPLY, York, Pennsylvania. **B,** Courtesy Tony Riso Company, North Miami Beach, Florida.)

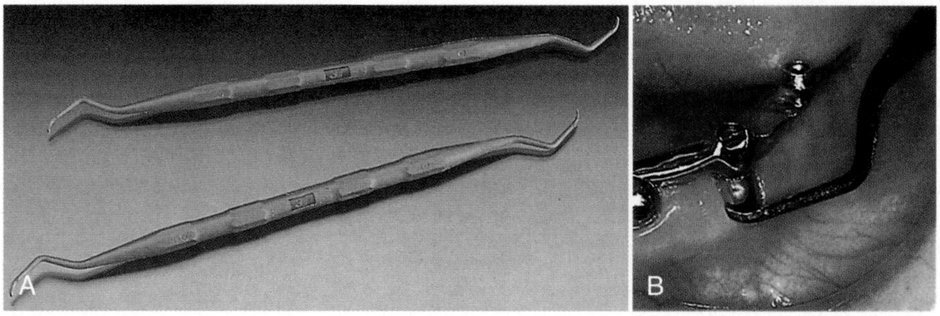

Figure 58-50. **A,** Graphite-reinforced nylon scalers. **B,** Application of graphite-reinforced nylon scaler to the dental implant. (Courtesy Steri-Oss, Yorba Linda, California.)

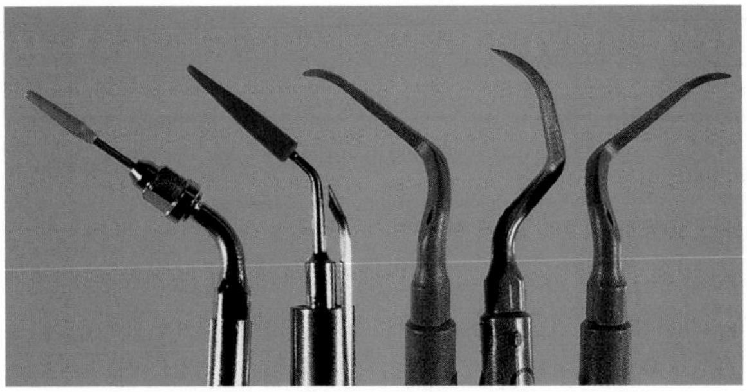

Figure 58-53. Ultrasonic tips for implants. **A,** Plastic Piezo implant insert (EMS). **B,** Blue plastic magnetostrictive insert. **C, D,** and **E,** Carbon composite piezoelectric inserts: PH1, PH2R, PH2L (Satelec). (**B,** Courtesy Tony Riso Company, North Miami Beach, Florida. **C, D,** and **E,** From Newman MG, Takei HH, Klokkevold PR, et al, eds: *Carranza's clinical periodontology,* ed 10, St Louis, 2006, Saunders.)

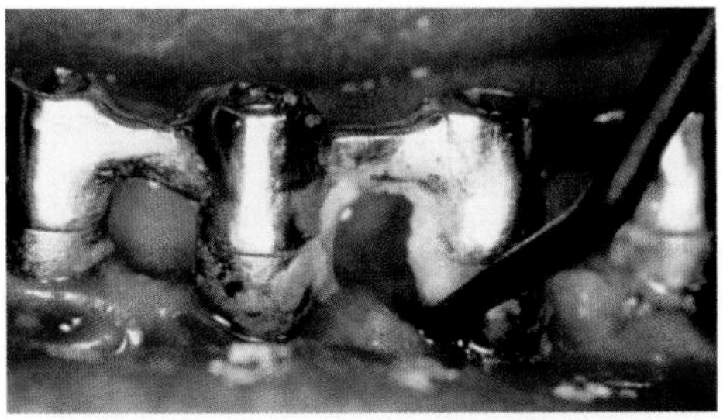

Figure 58-54. Tenacious calculus needs to be removed by a plastic scaler. (From Babbush CA: *Dental implants: the art and science,* Philadelphia, 2001, Saunders.)

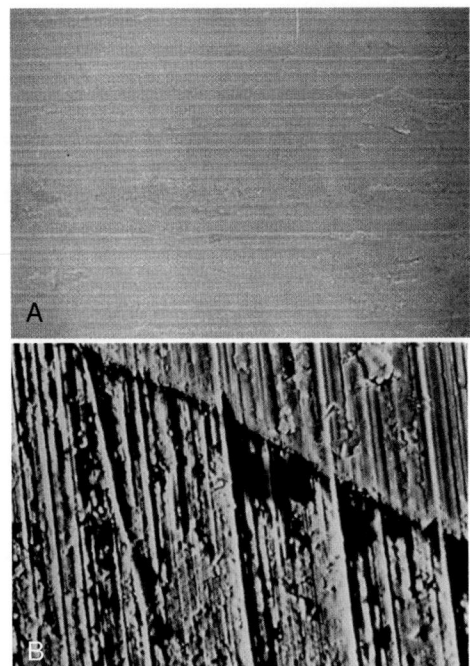

Figure 58-55. **A,** A smooth titanium implant surface. **B,** Effects of air abrasion use. Note the roughened implant surface. (From Babbush CA: *Dental implants: the art and science,* Philadelphia, 2001, Saunders.)

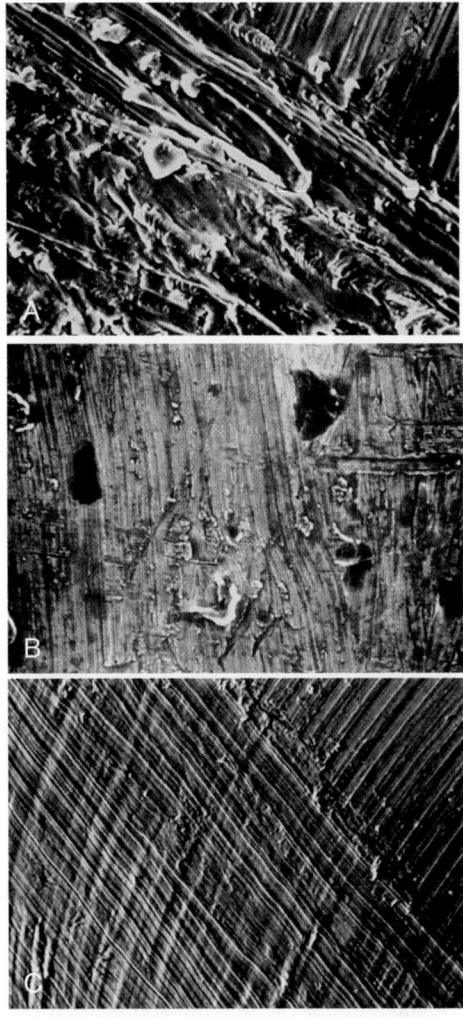

Figure 58-56. **A,** Effects of ultrasonic scaler use. Note the roughened implant surface. **B** and **C,** Effects of metallic scaler use. Note the roughened implant surface. (From Babbush CA: *Dental implants: the art and science,* Philadelphia, 2001, Saunders.)

The gold-tipped Gracey instruments are fabricated from a special gold alloy that is softer than titanium and therefore does not roughen the abutment surface or cause the retention of acquired deposits. Gold-tipped Gracey scalers should not be sharpened, because the gold is then removed, thereby exposing the underlying metal. Some believe that graphite and gold-tipped scalers may change the implant surface topography and should thus be avoided. Polishing with a gel dentifrice or tin oxide in a rubber cup or with a rubber point is recommended. Buffing the abutments "shoeshine style" with long gauze strips or floss is effective for biofilm removal. An ordinary cotton shoestring can help to remove biofilm from underneath the prosthetic appliance.

The dental hygienist continually assesses whether the client has problems associated with the dental implant that are related to oral hygiene or to the peri-implant tissue. For example, the dental hygienist can monitor the peri-implant tissue; remove acquired deposits from natural teeth and implants; discuss oral hygiene needs; provide customized instructions (Box 58-3); review self-care recommendations; evaluate the client's acceptance of and ability to perform the oral self-care regimens; encourage client compliance with

TABLE 58-8

Continued-Care Schedule for Clients with Dental Implants*

Care	Care Schedule
After implant is placed	Oral hygiene education and instruction
Radiographic evaluation of bone and periodontal structures	Every 3 months for first year and annually thereafter, unless necessary earlier
Continued-care appointment	Every 3 months for first year; thereafter evaluate for 4-month continued-care appointments
Removal and cleaning of implant superstructure	Annually, during continued-care appointment
Any signs of infection	Return to general dentist within 10 to 14 days or refer to specialist

*Be sure to commit client to the next continued-care appointment before the current appointment ends.

BOX 58-3

Oral Self-Care Guidelines for Dental Implant Clients

- Clean implants and bridges at least twice daily, preferably after breakfast and after the last food intake before going to sleep. This is especially important because the flow of saliva decreases during sleep.
- Clean thoroughly but not too aggressively. Avoid any materials or behaviors that might damage the implant surface.
- Use a systematic regimen so that all areas are cleaned.
- Clean the neck of the implant.

BOX 58-4

Criteria for Implant Success

- An individual unattached implant is immobile when tested clinically.
- A radiograph does not demonstrate any evidence of peri-implant radiolucency.
- Vertical bone loss is less than 0.2 mm annually after the first year of service of the implant.
- Individual implant performance is characterized by an absence of persistent or irreversible signs and symptoms such as pain, infections, neuropathies, paresthesia, or violation of the mandibular canal in the context of the foregoing; success rates of 85% at the end of a 5-year observation period and 80% at the end of a 10-year period are the minimum criteria for success.

From Misch CE: *Contemporary implant dentistry,* ed 3, St Louis, 2007, Mosby.

implant examinations; take necessary radiographs; and facilitate caries prevention in the existing natural dentition via fluoride and amorphous calcium phosphate therapy, sealants, xylitol use, and nutritional counseling.

Clients with dental implants should maintain a 3- to 4-month (or as needed) continued-care schedule (Table 58-8). The biofilm and dental calculus accumulated on the appliance also should be removed using the same procedures that are used with conventional dentures.

Failed Implants[9] (Box 58-4; see eFigures 58-29, 58-33, and 58-34)

A failed implant is one that has lost its integration. Unfortunately, the removal of the entire dental implant is the only option. Clients may elect to have another implant in this site, but further augmentation or bone grafting may be necessary. It is important to make an attempt to identify the cause of the implant failure; causes may range from surgical failure due to infection or poor bone healing at the time of implant placement to peri-implantitis and client noncompliance. Other factors that may result in failure include insufficient client maintenance, poor initial implant stabilization, insufficient bone, premature loading, prosthodontic difficulties, illness or systemic disease, and the need for bone augmentation that is not initially provided.

CLIENT EDUCATION TIPS

- Explain the cause and pathogenesis of periodontal disease and the importance of oral biofilm control in the prevention of oral diseases and the maintenance of oral health.
- Emphasize client responsibility for daily maintenance care to sustain the health of peri-implant tissues and to prevent periodontal disease and dental caries in existing natural dentition.
- Instruct the client to never use a rigid toothbrush, an abrasive dentifrice, safety pins, paper clips, or metal objects to self-clean the implants or abutments.
- Encourage clients to access professional oral hygiene maintenance care regularly.
- Educate clients about the risk factors for implant periodontitis and dental implant failures.
- Educate clients about the benefits of dental implant reconstruction, and assist them with the determination of whether they are candidates for dental implants.
- Encourage clients to maintain a daily self-care regimen by developing an individual implant hygiene care package that includes a written daily plan and the oral hygiene tools needed for daily care.
- Demonstrate the recommended daily strategies for cleaning dental implants.
- Recommend evidence-based oral care products, and provide instructions regarding their use.

LEGAL, ETHICAL, AND SAFETY ISSUES

- Dental hygienists must assess for possible peri-implantitis at each professional dental implant care session. The sulcular area around the implant or insert is the primary area of concern.
- Clients should be referred to a general dentist, a periodontist, or an oral and maxillofacial surgeon for the informed consent, implant surgery, and placement.
- Dental hygienists discuss the risks and benefits of dental implant placement with potential candidates.
- Never provide periodontal debridement around implants with the use of metal scalers or sonic and ultrasonic scalers (unless the ultrasonic or sonic tip is specially designed for implants).
- Implant mobility and signs of inflammation and exudate around the implant sulcus should be recognized, documented, and called to the attention of both the client and the dentist.
- Peri-implantitis and poor client adherence with oral self-care are the leading causes of dental implant failure. Signs of peri-implantitis or client nonadherence must be recognized, documented, and called to the attention of both the client and the dentist.
- Each year the superstructure of the implant should be removed for evaluation and cleaning. Many insurance plans now cover this service.

KEY CONCEPTS

- Dental implants provide an alternative to missing dentition. Dental hygienists must be able to recognize good candidates who will benefit from this investment.
- Dental implants need more maintenance than natural teeth. The dental hygienist emphasizes and describes the importance of daily oral self-care and professional dental hygiene care to dental implant clients.
- Osseointegration is a unique biologic phenomenon in which living bone cells fuse to the metal titanium.
- The benefits and risks of dental implants should be explained to the client.
- Recommend strategies for cleaning dental implants with appropriate oral hygiene aids.
- Air abrasion, metal instruments, or metal ultrasonic and sonic instruments are not recommended for dental implants. Abrasives and metal instruments may cause scratches and irregularities on the implant, thereby leading to oral biofilm accumulation and inflammation. If metal instruments are used, they should be made of metals as pliable as or more pliable than titanium. Plastic, gold-tipped, Teflon-coated, graphite, or wooden instruments may be used for scaling dental implants. The dental hygienist must know which instruments are safe for titanium metal. Some mechanized instrument manufacturers market plastic tips that can be used with dental implants.
- The plastic periodontal probe may disturb the biologic seal between the healthy peri-implant tissue and the titanium abutment. Caution is indicated during the rare times that a plastic periodontal probe is used.

CRITICAL THINKING EXERCISES

1. Place artificial calculus on an implant typodont or model. Use a sonic or ultrasonic scaler with a polysulfone plastic tip and plastic scaling instruments to remove the calculus.
2. With colleagues, discuss the characteristics of current edentulous and partially edentulous clients. Which clients would be good candidates for dental implants and why? Which clients are poor candidates and why?
3. Read the cases presented in Scenarios 58-1 and 58-2. Develop an oral self-care plan for each of the clients, and justify your clinical decisions.

REFERENCES

1. Daniels A: The importance of accurate charting for maintaining dental implants. *J Pract Hyg* 2:9, 1993.
2. Lang and Berglundh in 2011.
3. Rutar et al, 2001.
4. Baelum and Ellegaard, 2004.
5. Roos-Jansaker et al, 2006b.
6. Koldsland et al, 2010.
7. Dierens et al, 2012.
8. Lang et al, 1991.
9. Meffert RM: How to treat ailing and failing implants. *Implant Dent* 1:25, 1992.

ACKNOWLEDGMENT

The author acknowledges Vivian L. Young-McDonald, RDH, for her past contributions to this chapter.

EVOLVE RESOURCES

Please visit http://evolve.elsevier.com/Darby/hygiene for additional practice and study support tools.

CHAPTER

59

Orthodontic Care

Margaret M. Walsh, Denise M. Bowen

COMPETENCIES

1. **Discuss classification of occlusion in the permanent dentition, including:**
   - **Classify malocclusions in the horizontal, vertical, and transverse planes of space.**
   - **Describe the clinical characteristics indicating abnormal development of the permanent dentition.**
2. **Discuss the primary dentition, including:**
   - **Explain the classification of the primary dentition.**
   - **List the sequence of tooth eruption.**
3. **Discuss transitional dentition.**
4. **Define skeletal, dental, and chronologic age.**
5. **Explain the equilibrium theory.**
6. **List the baseline factors to be assessed for orthodontic care, as well as the components of diagnostic records.**
7. **Discuss treatment planning.**
8. **Explain the biologic mechanism for orthodontic tooth movement.**
9. **Describe the effects of orthodontic force on the teeth and periodontium.**
10. **Compare the types of orthodontic appliances, including advantages and disadvantages.**
11. **Discuss orthodontics in the preadolescent child, including the three stages of comprehensive orthodontic treatment.**
12. **Discuss periodontal aspects of adult orthodontic treatment.**
13. **Discuss dental hygiene maintenance, including:**
    - **Describe mechanical plaque control aids as well as the use of fluorides and antimicrobial agents for the orthodontic client.**
    - **Identify special oral hygiene considerations in managing the client who has undergone orthognathic surgery.**

Orthodontics is a dental specialty that deals with the recognition, prevention, and treatment of conditions involving irregularities of the teeth, jaws, and face and their influence on the physical and mental health of the individual. The goals of orthodontics are as follows:
- Establish or maintain a normal functioning occlusion
- Improve facial aesthetics or maintain good facial aesthetics
- Promote long-term stability
- Establish the best physiologic position of the condyle in the temporomandibular joint
- Establish periodontal health

Any deviation from the normal relationship of the maxillary arch or teeth to the mandibular arch or teeth is called a *malocclusion.* The problems that can arise from an untreated malocclusion include the following:
- Psychosocial problems caused by poor facial aesthetics, poor word enunciation, and increased plaque biofilm, debris, and stain retention
- Oral function problems, such as difficulties with chewing, swallowing, and speech, as well as temporomandibular dysfunction, a chronic impairment of the function of the temporomandibular joint
- Injury caused by trauma to, and breakage of, protruding teeth
- Parafunction (i.e., clenching, grinding, and other habits outside of the range of normal)
- Periodontal involvement (i.e., gingival recession and discrepancies, mucogingival problems, alveolar defects

The dental hygienist plays a key role in identifying malocclusions that can be corrected orthodontically, preparing the client to begin orthodontic therapy, and maintaining the client's dental and periodontal health during and after orthodontic treatment. This chapter provides an overview of the basic concepts involved in orthodontics and of specific techniques for oral health self-care for persons undergoing orthodontic treatment.

Classification of Occlusion in the Permanent Dentition

The first guidelines to clearly describe the normal and abnormal relationships of the teeth were developed during the 1890s by Edward H. Angle. Angle's method of malocclusion classification was based on the principle that the maxillary first molars are the keys to occlusion. Applying the system to the permanent dentition only, Angle classified the occlusion based on the relationship of the mandibular first molars to the maxillary first molars as Class I, Class II, or Class III (see Chapter 16).

Although Angle's classification system is simple to use, it describes malocclusion only in terms of teeth and dental discrepancies (i.e., poor tooth position). In addition, it considers only the anteroposterior plane of space. However, malocclusions must be assessed further to determine if a skeletal discrepancy exists. A **skeletal discrepancy** exists when the problem is caused by the position of the jaws relative to one another. For the classification of skeletal malocclusions, there are three basic spatial planes involved: the sagittal (vertical),

Figures, tables, and boxes marked as "e" are available as supplemental material on the Evolve site. Visit http://evolve.elsevier.com/Darby/hygiene to access these materials.

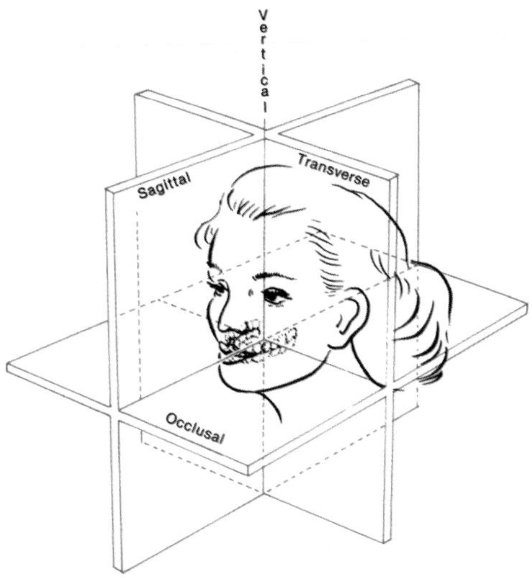

Figure 59-1. Perspective view of the planes of reference normally employed for orthodontic examination. The alignment of teeth and the asymmetry of the dental arches are best seen in projection against the occlusal plane; profile and facial aesthetics along with anteroposterior and vertical relationships are best studied in projection against the sagittal plane; and transverse dentofacial relationships are best evaluated in projection against the transverse plane. (From Graber LW, Vanarsdall, Jr. RL, Vig KWL: *Orthodontics: current principles and techniques,* ed 5, Philadelphia, 1994, Mosby.)

transverse (horizontal), and occlusal planes (Figure 59-1). Horizontal malocclusions are classified as Class II or Class III malocclusions that are similar to Angle's classification system. Vertical malocclusions include open bites and severe overbites (also called *deep bites* or *deep overbites*). Transverse or horizontal malocclusions also include crossbites (see Chapter 16).

In most cases, a malocclusion is caused by a combination of skeletal and dental discrepancies. Nevertheless, it is possible that an anterior open bite could occur if the posterior teeth erupt too far or if the anterior teeth erupt too little. Thus an anterior open bite could be the result of a dental malocclusion (Figure 59-2, *A*). An anterior open bite, however, is not usually caused by a malocclusion of the teeth alone. Called the "long face syndrome," an anterior open bite typically involves a skeletal problem in which the mandible is positioned too far downward and backward and the posterior teeth are overerupted (Figure 59-2, *B*). In adolescents, an anterior open bite is most likely caused by skeletal malrelationships, and it is complex to treat.

Conversely, a skeletal "short face" with insufficient eruption of the posterior teeth (Figure 59-3, *A*) would result in a mandibular plane that is too flat, thus predisposing the client to a severe anterior overbite (Figure 59-3, *B*). Although the condition is often seen clinically as a problem with the relationship of the anterior teeth, it is important to understand that the treatment of an open bite or a severe overbite requires the correction of eruption problems of the posterior teeth, thereby allowing the mandible to assume a more ideal relationship with the maxilla.

A posterior crossbite is a malocclusion in the transverse plane of space that exists when the buccal cusps of the maxillary teeth are lingual to their normal relationship with the mandibular teeth (Figure 59-4). The presence of a posterior

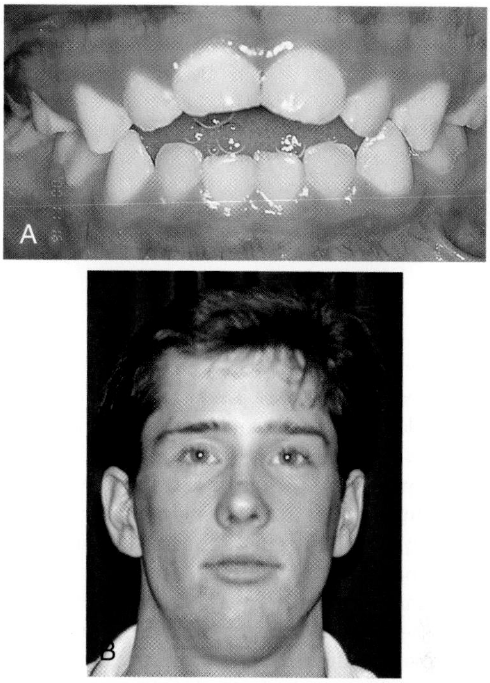

Figure 59-2. **A,** An anterior open bite, which is a malocclusion in the vertical dimension. **B,** Long face syndrome. (**B,** From Graber KW, Vanarsdall RL Jr, Vig KWL: *Orthodontics: current principles and techniques,* ed 5, Philadelphia, 2012, Mosby.)

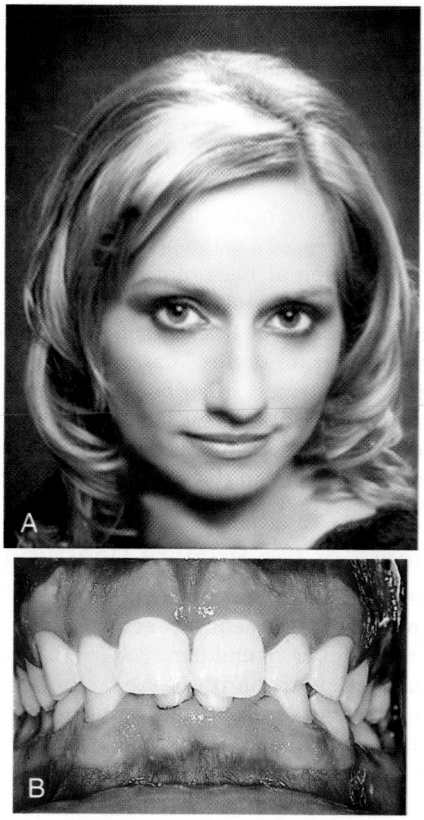

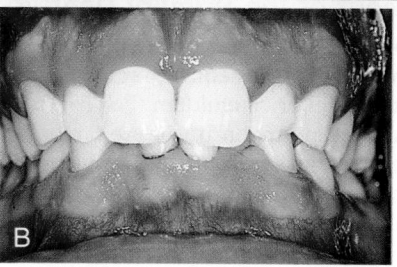

Figure 59-3. **A,** Short face syndrome. **B,** A severe overbite, which is a malocclusion in the vertical dimension. (**A,** From Graber KW, Vanarsdall RL Jr, Vig KWL: *Orthodontics: current principles and techniques,* ed 5, Philadelphia, 2012, Mosby.)

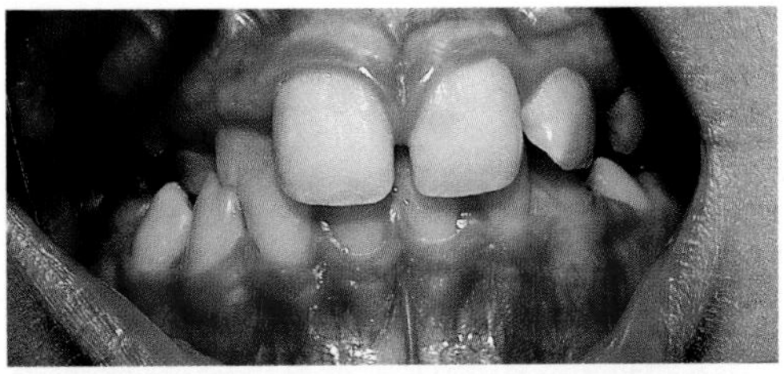

Figure 59-4. A posterior crossbite, which is a malocclusion in the transverse plane.

crossbite can be studied to determine if it is related to skeletal or dental causes. If the palate is too narrow or the mandible is too wide and if the teeth are in an appropriate position, the crossbite has a skeletal cause. If the palate is of adequate width but the maxillary posterior teeth incline lingually, the crossbite is dental in origin. The malocclusion is of skeletal and dental origin if both the relationship of the jaws and the alignment of the teeth are involved.

The important point for dental hygienists to appreciate is that the treatment of a Class II or Class III malocclusion that is caused by malpositioned teeth alone (i.e., dental discrepancies) will be very different from the treatment of the same malocclusion caused by skeletal relationships that are not ideal. To determine if skeletal malrelationships of the jaws exist, diagnostic tools other than the clinical assessment of the teeth must be used. Impressions for diagnostic dental casts in addition to a specialized cephalometric radiographs must be taken. As a result, it can be determined whether Class II and III malocclusions involve poor skeletal relationships of the jaws or simply malpositioned teeth. The use of diagnostic dental casts and cephalometric radiographs will be discussed in greater detail later in this chapter.

TABLE 59-1

Occlusion in the Primary Dentition and Its Effect on Occlusion in the Permanent Dentition

Occlusion Classification	Effect
Flush terminal plane 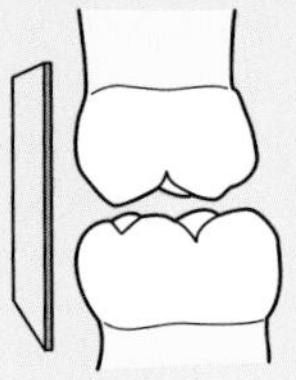	This should develop into a Class I relationship if primate spaces exist between the primary mandibular first molar and canine. If no primate spaces exist, then a Class II relationship will develop. However, a Class I relationship may develop if the permanent mandibular first molars can migrate mesially into the leeway space provided by the mesiodistal dimensions of the exfoliated primary second molars and the permanent second premolar teeth.
Mesial step 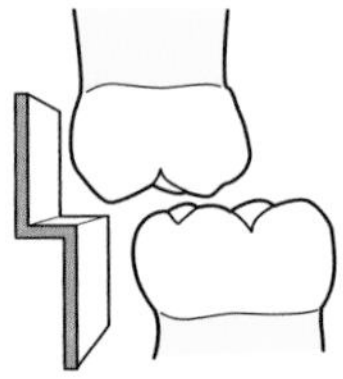	This should develop into a Class I relationship. However, it can also be an indication of excessive development of the mandible and develop into a Class III malocclusion.
Distal step 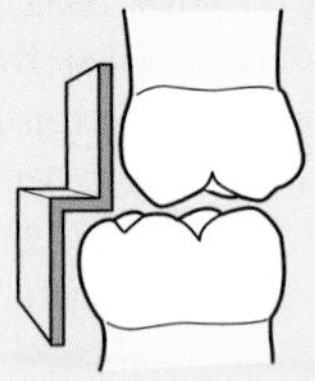	This should develop into a Class II relationship. At best, an end-to-end molar relationship of the molars will be present in the permanent dentition.

Classification of Occlusion in the Primary Dentition

Angle's classification of malocclusion, which was described in Chapter 16, applies only to the permanent dentition. Similarly, the classification of the primary dentition's occlusion uses the distal surfaces of the primary maxillary and mandibular second molars. Both of these systems are only a starting point for occlusal assessment, because other relationships (e.g., transverse, vertical, sagittal) and the functional status must also be evaluated. Table 59-1 reviews these classifications of primary dentition occlusion and summarizes their effects on the occlusion of the permanent dentition.

Development of the Primary Dentition

Although the dates of the eruption of the teeth of the primary dentition are variable, the sequence in which the teeth erupt is usually the same for all children (Box 59-1).[1] The eruption time is considered normal if it is up to 6 months before or 6 months after the age of eruption. The mandibular incisors typically erupt first and are easily visible when a baby smiles. The remaining incisors should erupt thereafter. The next teeth to erupt are the first molars, which are followed by the canines. By 24 to 30 months of age, the primary dentition is completed with the eruption of the second molars.

In a young child, spacing in the primary dentition is normal and desirable (Figure 59-5, *A*). Spacing that occurs predominantly in two locations is referred to as **primate space**, because it exists on a permanent basis in subhuman primate species. Primate space occurs in the maxilla between the lateral incisors and canines and in the mandible between the canines and the first molars. Another type of spacing called **developmental spacing** develops between the incisors, and it is an indication that growth of the alveolar processes is adequate to provide room for the permanent teeth (Figure 59-5, *B*). The permanent incisor teeth are each 2 to 3 mm larger mesiodistally than the primary incisors that they replace. The dental hygienist explains to parents that any spacing in the primary anterior teeth is a positive sign of optimal arch development as long as it is not related to a tongue thrust or congenitally missing incisors. The absence of spacing in this region, however, is a clear sign of crowding in the permanent dentition.

Transitional Dentition

Three dentitions exist over the life span of the natural teeth: the **primary dentition** (before the eruption of the first permanent tooth), the **transitional dentition** (in children after the eruption of the first permanent tooth but before the teeth

BOX 59-1

Sequence and Ages of Eruption

Primary Dentition

Mandibular central incisor (8 months)
Maxillary central incisor (10 months)
Maxillary lateral incisor (11 months)
Mandibular lateral incisor (13 months)
Mandibular first molar (16 months)
Maxillary first molar (16 months)
Maxillary canine (19 months)
Mandibular canine (20 months)
Mandibular second molar (27 months)
Maxillary second molar (29 months)

Permanent Dentition

Mandibular first molars (6 years)
Mandibular central incisor and maxillary first molars (6¼ years)
Maxillary central incisor (7¼ years)
Mandibular lateral incisor (7½ years)
Maxillary lateral incisor (8¼ years)
Maxillary first premolar (10¼ years)
Mandibular canine and first premolar (10½ years)
Maxillary second premolar (11 years)
Mandibular second premolar (11½ years)
Maxillary canine (11½ years)
Mandibular second molar (12 years)
Maxillary second molar (12½ years)
Maxillary and mandibular third molars (20 years)

Adapted from Proffit WR, Fields HW Jr, Sarver DM: *Contemporary orthodontics*, ed 4, St Louis, 2007, Mosby.

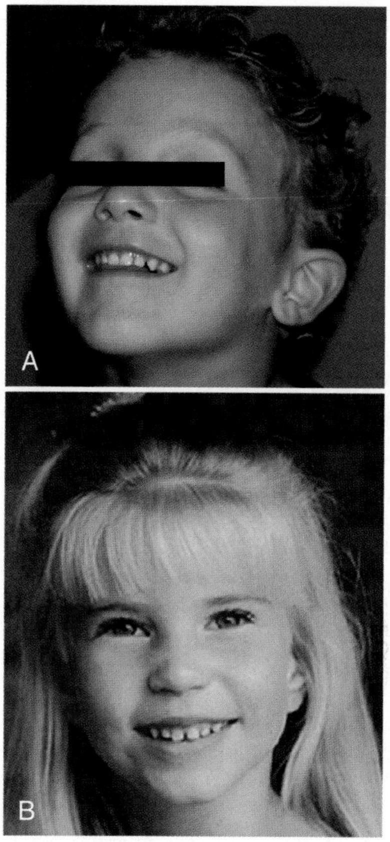

Figure 59-5. A, Primate spaces can be seen in this client's maxillary arch. **B,** Both primate and developmental spaces are present in the primary maxillary anterior teeth of this child.

come into occlusion) and the permanent dentition (before the eruption of the third molars).

Clinically the dental hygienist may notice in the young adolescent that the posterior teeth appear to have short clinical crowns. By the time this vertical growth stops during the late teens, the gingival attachment is located at or near the cementoenamel junction. The slow continued eruption of the posterior teeth in response to the growth in the vertical height of the ramus during later adolescence enables continued eruption, thereby increasing the height of the clinical crowns and placing the gingival attachment at an appropriate level on the root.

The eruption mechanisms remain active throughout adult life. After all of the permanent teeth have erupted and the pubertal growth spurt is completed, the adult occlusal equilibrium phase begins. During this adult phase, eruption continues at a very slow pace that compensates for the normal and slight occlusal wear patterns of the teeth so that the vertical height of the face is maintained. Eruption cannot compensate, however, for extreme occlusal wear, and a reduction in the vertical height of the lower face will be noted in these clients. A relatively more rapid eruption process can occur in an adult when a tooth in an opposing arch is lost. After losing its occlusal contact, a tooth will erupt into the extraction space. At times, teeth will erupt until they contact the gingiva in the opposing arch.

The sequence in which the permanent teeth erupt is a consideration that is more important than the age at which they erupt.[1] A change in the sequence of eruption is a much more reliable sign of a developmental problem than the age at which the teeth erupt. It is within normal limits for a maxillary canine to erupt at the age of 14 years rather than the age of 12 years as long as the eruption of the second premolars is also delayed. If the maxillary second premolars have erupted and the canine has not, a problem with the development of the canines is likely. The eruption sequence of the permanent dentition that produces the most favorable occlusion is shown in Box 59-1. Eruption symmetry is also a consideration. Right and left contralateral pairs normally erupt at the same time. Asymmetric tooth eruption may be a sign of developmental discrepancies.

Diagnostic Records

The diagnosis and treatment planning process in orthodontics follows a problem-oriented approach in which a diagnosis or problem list is formulated from client data. After the problem list is developed, the problems are prioritized so that the most important problem receives the greatest priority in treatment. All possible solutions to each problem are considered, and, from this list, the best possible treatment options for the client in terms of cost, effectiveness, complexity, and risk are presented to the client for consideration.

An objective scientific appraisal of the client's condition must be made on the basis of data obtained from the health history and interview, the clinical examination, and the diagnostic records. Table 59-2 highlights pertinent data collected from the client health history questionnaire and interview and their implication for orthodontic care.

Intraoral Photographs

Intraoral photographs are taken to document the client's status before treatment. A set of photographs should include an anterior view with the teeth in occlusion, right and left buccal views of the posterior sextants with the teeth in occlusion, occlusal views of the maxillary and mandibular arches, and profile views (both smiling and nonsmiling). Additional photographs are taken of any special conditions, such as gingival recession or clefting or enamel anomalies not visible on the standard photographs.

Radiographs

A panoramic radiograph is exposed to examine the perioral structures for the presence of pathology or for supernumerary or impacted teeth (Figure 59-6). The mandibular condyles

TABLE 59-2

Baseline Factors to Be Assessed and Implications for Orthodontic Care

Factors	Implications for Care
Personal Factors	
Chief complaint	Must be a priority in treatment planning
Age of client	May affect client motivation and cooperation (Adults are generally internally motivated, whereas a child may be completing treatment because of a parent's wishes.)
History of previous orthodontic treatment of client or of client's parents or siblings	Provides insight into hereditary factors involved in the orthodontic problems as well as into the client's or parents' understanding of orthodontic treatment and the ability to understand and help a child manage orthodontic discomforts
Health History	
History of trauma to teeth or jaws	Provides insight into cause of an existing skeletal asymmetry Alerts the dental hygienist to the need to study radiographs for the presence of fractures of the teeth or jaws
Osteoarthritis of the temporomandibular joint	Orthodontic treatment will not improve degenerative changes
Nickel or latex allergy	Metal orthodontic appliances contain nickel, and elastics contain latex; alternative materials will need to be planned
Medications	
Pharmacological agents for the management of hypertension, epilepsy, and organ transplants	Risk for gingival enlargement that may lead to increased plaque retention and associated gingival inflammation and dental caries
Osteoporosis and its treatment	Bone remodeling may occur at a slower rate Hormonal management of osteoporosis may be an option
Indomethacin, a potent prostaglandin inhibitor used for the treatment of arthritis	Response of the teeth to orthodontic forces may be reduced
Corticosteroids and nonsteroidal anti-inflammatory agents	Potent medications used on a chronic basis may reduce the response of the teeth to orthodontic forces
Tricyclic antidepressants, antiarrhythmic agents, antimalarial agents, methylxanthines, and some tetracyclines may influence prostaglandin levels	Response of the teeth to orthodontic forces may be reduced
Oral Health and Function	
Dental caries and endodontic pathology	Before orthodontic treatment, clinical and radiographic assessment must be completed, caries must be controlled, and endodontic lesions must be treated
Periodontal health	Before orthodontic treatment, a thorough periodontal assessment must be completed, diseased sites must be controlled, and areas of inadequate attached gingiva must be corrected with gingival grafting
Occlusal function	In children, shifting of the mandible during closure may affect the skeletal development of the mandible

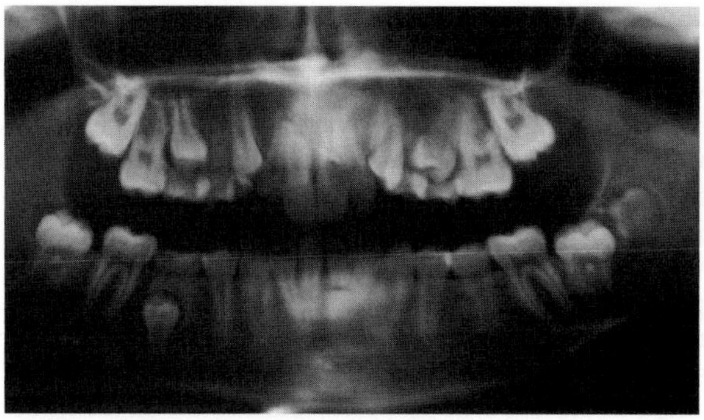

Figure 59-6. A panoramic radiograph is taken to evaluate the dentition for the presence and location of the permanent teeth, pathology, and temporomandibular joint conditions.

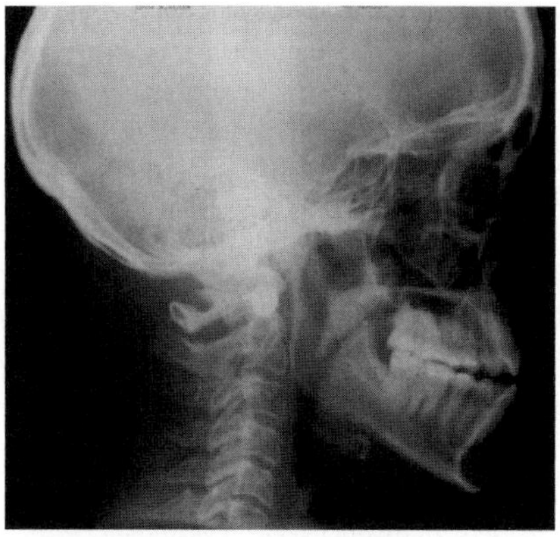

Figure 59-7. A lateral cephalometric radiograph is taken to evaluate the impact of skeletal and dental–skeletal relationships.

are evaluated, and the possible need for additional radiographs of the TMJ is determined by the dentist. If the anterior teeth are not clearly visible, anterior periapical films are taken to evaluate the roots of these teeth for a predisposition to apical resorption.

A lateral cephalograph presents a lateral view of the skull and is always indicated in orthodontics to assess the skeletal relationship of the jaws to each other and to the base of the cranium and to determine the need to reposition the anterior teeth (Figure 59-7). The use of cephalometrics in orthodontics is valuable because, although two cases of malocclusion may appear similar clinically or on a study model, significant differences in the two cases become apparent when the skeletal components of the malocclusion are analyzed. The only instance in which a lateral cephalometric radiograph would not be indicated is when a client presents only minor orthodontic problems. If serious facial asymmetry is present, then a cephalometric radiograph taken from the frontal aspect is also indicated.

Cephalometric analysis is also used to evaluate changes that occur as a result of orthodontic treatment. Taken before, during, and after orthodontic therapy, cephalometric radiographs can be used to assess changes in dental and skeletal relationships. Finally, cephalometric analysis is used to develop a visualized treatment objective; this is a plan that is used to predict treatment results.

Bitewing radiographs are taken to rule out the presence of active caries. An adult with a history of periodontal disease requires a full set of periapical radiographs in addition to the panoramic film.

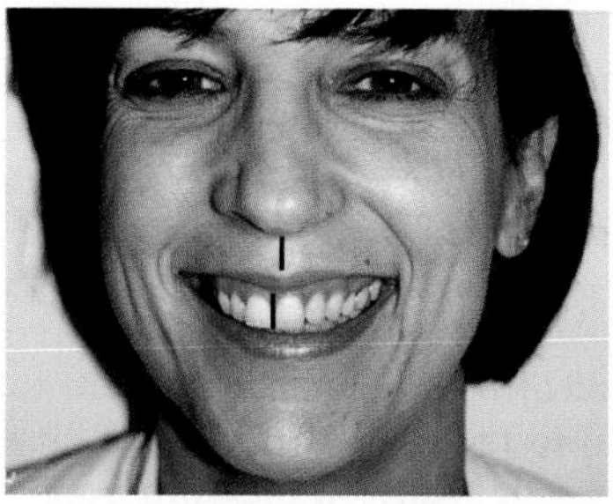

Figure 59-8. The relationship of the midline of the maxilla to the philtrum. In this case, the midline of the maxilla deviates to the client's right.

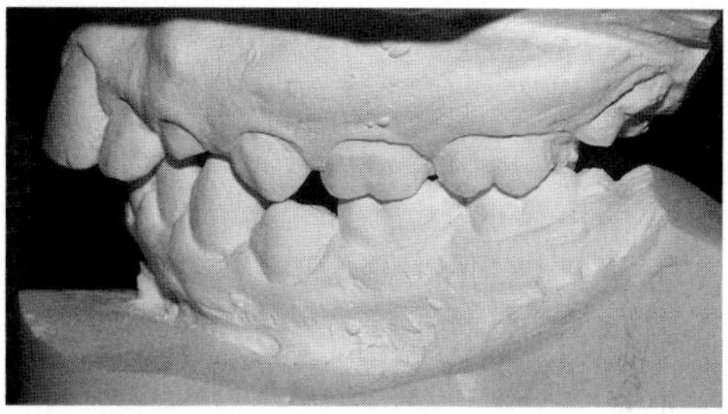

Figure 59-11. Study model of a child with a Class II, division I malocclusion.

Facial Photographs

Although the facial and jaw proportions are assessed clinically and measured on lateral cephalometric radiographs, an analysis of the face and the profile is also made with the use of facial photographs. Viewing the client from the frontal view, the face is evaluated for bilateral symmetry. The midline of the maxilla is also assessed in relation to the philtrum and the nasal columna (Figure 59-8).

At a minimum, four facial photographic views are taken: (1) full face with lips relaxed, (2) full face smiling, (3) a smiling profile, and (4) a nonsmiling profile. The assessment of the profile can be used to differentiate those individuals who have an acceptable or nearly acceptable profile from those with serious skeletal malrelationships. Visit http://evolve.elsevier.com/Darby/hygiene for information on the goals of profile analysis and eFigures 59-9 and 59-10.

Diagnostic Dental Casts or Study Models

Mounted and unmounted diagnostic dental casts or study models are used to assess the occlusion, the symmetry of the form of the dental arches, and the symmetric positioning of the individual teeth within the arches (Figure 59-11). Impressions of the maxillary and mandibular arches must be taken, along with a wax-bite registration, to prepare the models that are used to study the occlusion (see Chapter 37).

Treatment Planning Concepts

The American Association of Orthodontists recommends that a child be examined by an orthodontist by the age of 7 years.[2] The specifics of orthodontic treatment planning are beyond the scope of this chapter; however, certain concepts are important for the dental hygienist to understand. Although the diagnostic phase of treatment is scientific and objective in nature, treatment planning is more subjective and reflects both the experience and judgment of the clinician as well as the priorities of the client. Although client concerns must be given priority, the orthodontist is not obligated to provide treatment that the client requests if the plan requested does not comply with professional standards.

The goals of orthodontic treatment are to achieve ideal occlusion, facial aesthetics, periodontal health, and stability. In clients who present with complex orthodontic problems, it may be impossible to achieve all goals, and a compromise must be made. Efforts to achieve an ideal dental occlusion may, for example, produce a good dental result with poor facial aesthetics. The achievement of ideal aesthetics, on the other hand, may require a compromise in the dental occlusion or the long-term stability of the result. For cases in which all three goals cannot be achieved, priority must be given to the client's chief complaint. If aesthetics are the client's main concern, the client would be unhappy with treatment that did not correct problems of facial aesthetics or that possibly even worsened, even if it resulted in an ideal occlusion with maximum long-term stability. The dental hygienist must recognize this issue when seeing a client for maintenance after the completion of orthodontic therapy. All too frequently the dental occlusion evaluated using Angle's classification is used as a single criterion for assessing the success of treatment. Before seeing orthodontic clients for a maintenance appointment, the dental hygienist reads all written communication from the orthodontist to be aware of treatment results and any compromises required as well as recommendations for maintenance.

Other issues to be considered in treatment planning are the cost, risks, and benefits of various options. Plans that are complex and difficult must be considered in terms of financial expense as well as cost in terms of discomfort and time, and they must also be compared with the expected client benefits. Alternatively, simple treatment plans may not be worth their cost if the benefits achieved are too limited. A more complex plan, such as one that involves **orthognathic surgery** (i.e., surgery that involves the bones of the jaws), may improve treatment results so much more that the benefits achieved far outweigh the costs and risks.

Clients with Skeletal Malocclusions

Three approaches to the treatment of a skeletal malocclusion are as follows:

1. Growth modification of the jaws to correct the problem
2. Camouflage of the jaw discrepancy via tooth movement to correct the dental occlusion within the limits of the existing jaw discrepancy
3. Surgical correction of the jaw discrepancy

Growth modification is the preferred method of treatment; it involves manipulating the growth of the jaws to correct a skeletal malocclusion. Camouflage of the discrepancy by repositioning the teeth is a compromise that is acceptable in mild or even moderate skeletal cases. Surgical correction is limited to severe skeletal malrelationships. Visit http://evolve.elsevier.com/Darby/hygiene for additional information about treatment for skeletal malocclusions.

Monitoring Treatment Response

Despite careful analysis, diagnosis, and treatment planning, it is impossible to predict with complete certainty the result of any treatment plan, especially those that include growth modification for preadolescent and adolescent clients. If growth occurs as expected and if the client cooperates and attends all appointments, a good result is expected. If growth, cooperation, or both fail to meet required expectations, an alternative plan that includes camouflage therapy with extractions may be required. To reduce the amount of uncertainty associated with treatment planning, the client's initial response to treatment is evaluated 6 to 9 months after therapy is initiated. If the client is responding to growth modification as expected at that time, the orthodontist can assume that the planned treatment is appropriate and should be continued. If treatment results are less than expected at this initial assessment, the treatment plan can be changed as indicated. The client's response to treatment must be monitored throughout therapy.

Treatment Planning for Multiple Dental Problems

Treatment planning for children or adult clients with multiple dental problems must follow a specific sequence. First, any active dental disease must be treated or controlled. Carious teeth must be restored, any indicated extractions completed, any endodontic pathology treated, and periodontal disease controlled by aggressive scaling and root debridement with the use of local anesthesia. Mucogingival surgery (e.g., free gingival grafting) is completed, if needed, before orthodontic treatment as well. Orthodontic treatment can then be initiated, including orthognathic surgery, if required. Definitive periodontal therapy (e.g., osseous surgery) is delayed until after orthodontic therapy is completed, because the architecture of the alveolar bone often changes as a result of orthodontic treatment. Finally, definitive restorative procedures are completed, including crowns, bridges, implants, and partial dentures.

Biology of Orthodontic Tooth Movement

Tooth movement occurs when light pressure is exerted on the tooth. This pressure results in bone being resorbed on one side of the tooth and new bone growing in and slowly hardening on the other side of the tooth. This new bone holds each tooth in its new position. The reason this occurs can be described as follows.

The PDL consists of collagenous fibers, undifferentiated mesenchymal cells and the fibroblasts and osteoblasts into which they differentiate, nerve fibers, blood vessels, and tissue fluids. These constituents function together to support the teeth during normal function in addition to making orthodontic tooth movement possible. The PDL space is filled with the same extracellular fluid that is found in all tissues of the body. This fluid allows the PDL to function as a shock absorber during normal function.

When light, sustained force is applied to a tooth, the tooth moves in the socket within seconds, which expresses fluid from the PDL space. The PDL becomes compressed between the tooth and the alveolar wall, and pain is felt. Within a few minutes after pressure is applied, altered blood flow occurs in addition to changes in oxygen levels and the release of cellular mediators such as prostaglandins and cytokines within the PDL. After 6 hours of sustained pressure, cellular activity in the PDL, including differentiation into osteoclasts and osteoblasts, occurs. This needed pressure explains why a force must be applied to a tooth for at least 6 hours per day to result in tooth movement.

Osteoclasts must form within the PDL to remove bone from the area adjacent to the compressed part of the PDL. These osteoclasts attack the lamina dura and remove bone on the pressure side during a process called **frontal resorption**. Osteoblasts are needed to then remodel bone on the pressure side of the tooth as well as to form new bone on the side to which tension is applied. Both osteoclastic and osteoblastic activities are stimulated by prostaglandin E, a chemical mediator that is important to tooth movement.

Forces that are light and continuous and that produce only frontal resorption are ideal. Clinically, however, it is likely that, with even the lightest force, some areas of PDL necrosis and undermining bone resorption are likely to develop, temporarily weakening the base or foundation needed for tooth support. If undermining bone resorption does occur, tooth movement will occur about 10 days after activation. A period of another 10 to 14 days is then needed to allow for repair and regeneration of the PDL before force should be applied again. Based on this process, orthodontic appointments are typically made no more frequently than every 4 weeks to allow healing and to prevent damage to the teeth or bone that could occur.

Effects of Orthodontic Force on the Teeth and the Periodontium

Effects on the Pulp

Properly applied orthodontic forces will, at most, affect the dental pulp minimally. A mild, transient pulpitis may occur and is usually experienced by clients as discomfort during the first few days after appliances are **activated** (i.e., adjusted to apply desired pressures). Occasionally, however, a loss of pulpal vitality may occur during orthodontic treatment. This loss may occur because of a history of trauma to the tooth (and therefore is unrelated to orthodontic treatment) or as a result of the poor control of orthodontic forces.

Effects on Root Structure

As in the PDL and the adjacent bone, the resorption and repair of dentin and cementum occur during orthodontic movement. Cementum and dentin are removed during periods of force application and replaced by cementum during periods of rest. As a result, the tooth root is remodeled during optimal orthodontic tooth movement in the same manner as alveolar bone is remodeled. Remodeling, however, will not occur if more serious damage develops, such as the damage that may occur at the root apex, where portions of cementum or dentin may actually break away from the root. These portions will be resorbed by the body and will not be replaced. The permanent loss of root structure occurs only at the root apex. This **apical root resorption** appears radiographically as a loss in the length and apical blunting of the root (Figure 59-12).

Some loss of root length will occur in almost every individual who is treated orthodontically, and this is usually of little clinical significance. The maxillary and mandibular incisors are the most frequently affected teeth. At times, however, the severe loss of one third to one half of the root length occurs from even routine orthodontic tooth movement. Although the cause of this type of resorption is not clear, some

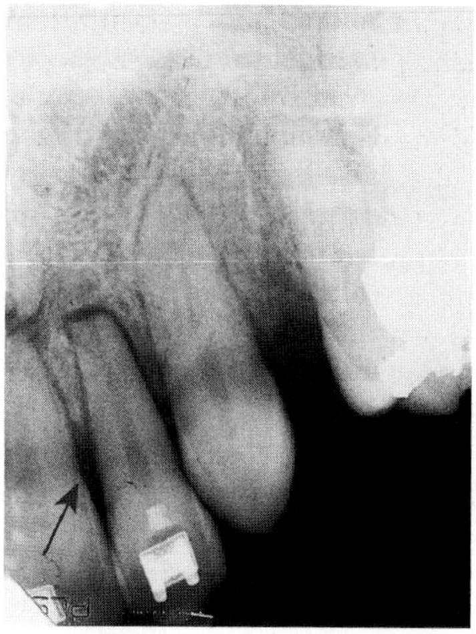

Figure 59-12. Apical root resorption.

individuals are found to be more prone to resorption than others. Treatment factors and characteristics that make the teeth prone to resorption are presented in eBox 59-2. The use of low-force wires has reduced the occurrence of root resorption when they are placed low on the teeth and move the teeth slowly.

Effects on the Height of Alveolar Bone

Orthodontic therapy is not associated with an increase in the loss of alveolar bone. The only situation in which bone loss is exacerbated by orthodontic tooth movement is when teeth are moved in the client who has active periodontal infection. When periodontal disease has been controlled before and during orthodontic treatment, improved tooth position and placement will actually improve the osseous contours as well. This improvement is demonstrated by the uprighting of mesially drifted second molars to allow for the construction of crown and bridge prostheses. As the tooth is uprighted during orthodontic treatment, the osseous contours on the mesial aspect of the tooth are improved because the crestal bone is uprighted along with the tooth (Figure 59-13).

Mobility and Pain

Increased tooth mobility is expected during orthodontic treatment. PDL fibers become disorganized and detached from the bone and the root cementum, and the adjacent bone must remodel. Radiographs taken during treatment will reveal widened PDL spaces. However, excessive mobility may be an indication that too much force is being applied, thereby causing too much undermining bone resorption. If a tooth becomes extremely mobile during therapy, all force should be discontinued until the mobility reduces to moderate levels. Usually this problem can be corrected without causing permanent damage.

Several hours after an appliance is activated during an orthodontic visit, a client may feel a mild aching sensation and sensitivity to pressure so that chewing a hard food is painful. This pain will likely last for 2 to 4 days and then disappear until the appliance is again adjusted. Pain after orthodontic adjustments varies among individuals. One client may experience severe pain after the application of a mild force, whereas another client may not experience any

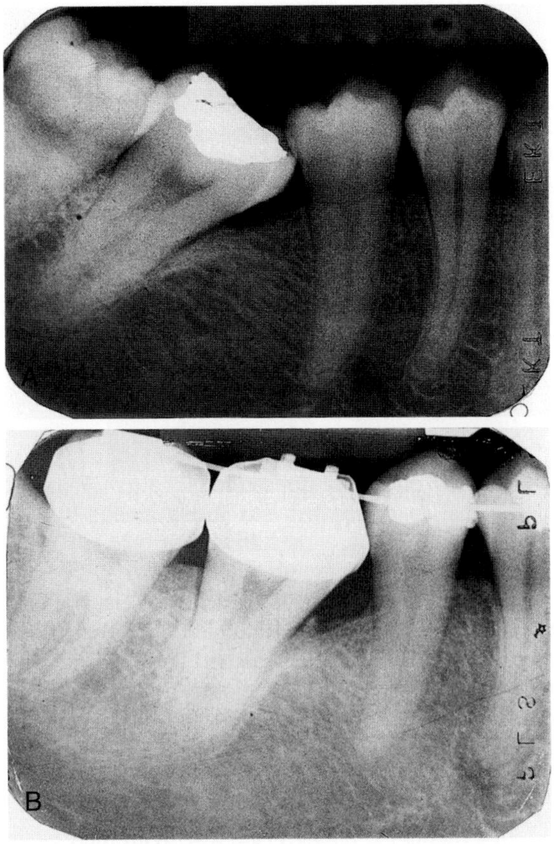

Figure 59-13. **A,** Mesial drifting of tooth #31 into extraction space. Note the bony defect on tooth #31. **B,** Note the improvement in the contour of the alveolar bone near tooth #31 mesial as the tooth is uprighted.

pain at all from the application of a heavier force. When planning dental hygiene appointments with clients who are undergoing orthodontic treatment, it is generally more comfortable for a client to be seen before rather than immediately after orthodontic adjustments. Scaling procedures are particularly uncomfortable for teeth that are already painful as a result of an orthodontic adjustment.

Pain is the result of the development of ischemic areas within the PDL. Tenderness with the chewing of firm foods is caused by the mild pulpitis that occurs and by inflammation at the tooth apex. The greater the force applied to the tooth, the greater the amount of pain expected, because larger areas within the PDL will undergo sterile necrosis. If light forces are applied, painful symptoms can be relieved by having the client chew gum during the first 8 hours after the adjustment. Chewing temporarily displaces the teeth enough to allow some blood flow through the compressed areas of the PDL, thereby preventing the buildup of metabolites that stimulate pain receptors.

Effects of Orthodontic Force on the Maxilla

The sites of maxillary growth where growth modification may be effective are the sutures where the maxilla is attached to the cranium and the mid-palatine suture area. To counter excessive maxillary growth, forces would be applied to oppose the natural soft-tissue forces that place tension on and separate the craniofacial sutures. To treat deficient growth,

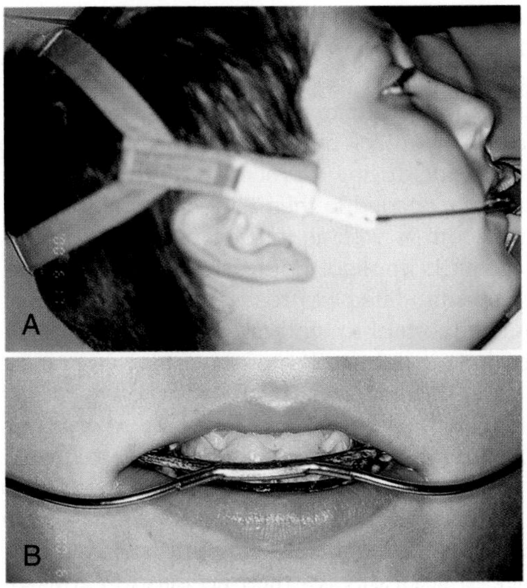

Figure 59-14. **A,** Headgear appliance. **B,** Anterior view of headgear appliance.

forces would be applied to enhance the natural forces that stimulate maxillary growth.

Extraoral headgear appliances are used to restrain maxillary growth (Figure 59-14). The appliance must be worn at least 8 hours per day, and wearing it for 12 to 14 hours per day is preferable. Physiologic reasons exist for wearing headgear at night. More growth hormone is secreted in children during the night than during the day. The growth of the long bones of the body has been found to be greater at night than during the day. Although it is not known if facial bones grow in the same pattern, it is reasonable to expect that they do. As a result, the use of headgear to modify skeletal growth is more effective at night than during the day.

Orthodontic Appliances

Orthodontic appliances can be categorized as removable or fixed.

Removable Appliances

Removable appliances are those that can be removed by the client. They typically consist of various wires attached to an acrylic base that is supported by the teeth or the soft tissues. See Box 59-3 for advantages and disadvantages.

Removable appliances are used for the following:

- Growth modification in adolescents and children with mixed dentition
- Limited movement of the individual teeth
- Retention after treatment completion

Removable appliances that are used during growth modification are referred to as functional appliances. A functional appliance is one that changes the posture of the mandible to a position that is open or both open and forward. These appliances modify the growth of the mandible by stretching the soft tissues that surround the mandible. One example is the twin-block appliance shown in Figure 59-15.

During the late 1990s, a technology with which a series of sequential clear plastic tray aligners could be used to correct

BOX 59-3

Advantages and Disadvantages of Removable Orthodontic Appliances

Advantages

- They can be removed for social functions.
- Less chair time is needed to make removable appliances, because they are fabricated in a laboratory rather than directly in the client's mouth.
- More modification of skeletal growth is possible with removable appliances than with fixed appliances.

Disadvantages

- Treatment response is heavily dependent on client compliance, because treatment progresses only when the client wears the appliance.
- Removable appliances can be accidentally thrown away or lost, thereby causing a setback in treatment and incurring additional financial costs for the client.
- Complex tooth movement cannot be completed with a removable appliance, so the use of a removable appliance in complex cases may require a compromised treatment result.

malalignments was developed.[3] Marketed for adults but appropriate for responsible adolescents who will comply with directions, this system incorporates the use of a three-dimensional digital model of the dental arches on the basis of a computed tomography scan of dental impressions submitted by the dentist. After a plan is approved by the dentist or orthodontist, the digital client information is used to produce a series of as many as several dozen sequential aligners that have been designed to produce the desired tooth movement. Each aligner is worn 22 hours per day for 2 weeks before the next aligner in the sequence is used. These removable appliances may also be used in combination with other therapies (e.g., interproximal enamel reduction, short-term fixed appliance therapy) when conditions are more complex. A second orthodontic tray system, Invisalign, has also been developed recently. This system involves only one or two plastic appliances that can be fabricated and then modified as needed in the dental office to produce the desired tooth movement.[4]

Fixed Appliances

In most cases, fixed appliances are required. In contrast with removable appliances, fixed orthodontic appliances consist of brackets and other attachments that are fixed to the teeth with bonding or attached to bands that are cemented to the teeth (Figure 59-16). See eTable 59-3 for descriptions of components of fixed appliances and their auxiliary attachment purposes.

Separation

Teeth that have tight interproximal contacts must be separated before a band is placed. Various separators are available to wedge the teeth apart. Separators may consist of a brass wire that is twisted tightly around the contact, steel springs to squeeze the contact open, or elastomeric "doughnuts" that are slipped into place around the contact.

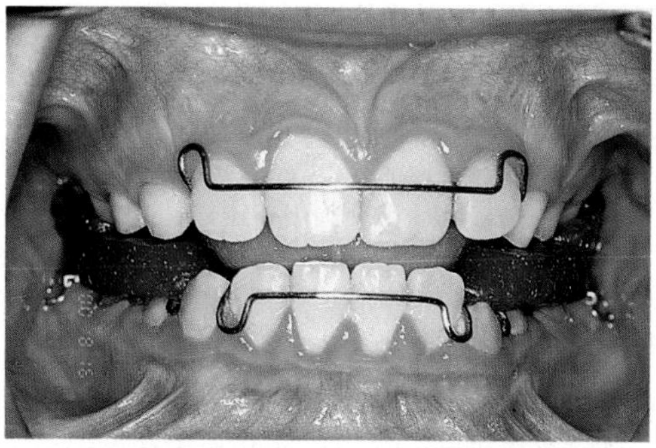

Figure 59-15. Twin-block appliance.

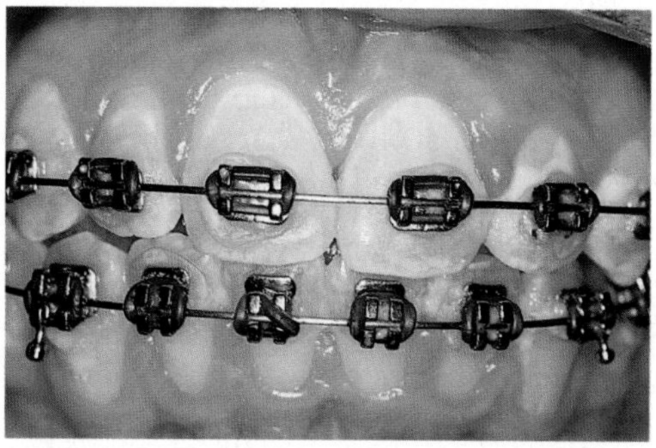

Figure 59-16. Fixed orthodontic appliance. Note the white spot lesions on the anterior teeth.

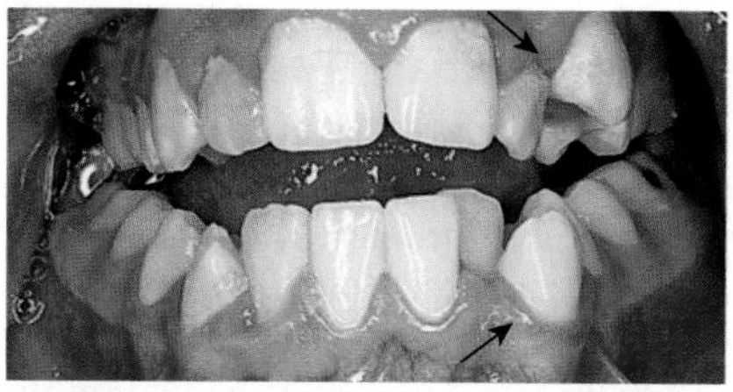

Figure 59-17. Malalignment of the permanent canines caused by a lack of space in the dental arch.

Bonded Attachments

Bonding is an area in orthodontics that is continually changing and improving. Bonding is based on the mechanical locking of an adhesive to irregularities in both the tooth surface and the base of the bracket. Successful bonding requires attention to the tooth surface preparation, the bracket base design, and the bonding material used. Additional information on bonding is presented in eTable 59-4.

Orthodontics in the Preadolescent Child

Early orthodontic treatment initiated during the mixed dentition or even during the primary dentition may be beneficial to improve the orthodontic situation. A second stage of treatment, however, will likely be needed after the permanent teeth have erupted.

Malaligned teeth during the early mixed dentition may be caused by one of the following two basic problems:

- Lack of adequate space in the arch, thereby causing an erupting tooth to be deflected from its normal position (Figure 59-17)

- Interference with or delay in permanent tooth eruption, thereby leading to space problems because the existing adjacent teeth shift into improper positions

The dental hygienist can play a valuable role in the treatment of preadolescent children by recognizing signs that indicate the need for early orthodontic treatment. The following are oral conditions that should alert the dental hygienist to potential problems warranting the dentist's attention and possible referral for treatment.

Altered Sequence of Eruption

The knowledge of eruption patterns that are considered "normal" (Box 59-1) will enable the dental hygienist to recognize any abnormalities that may predispose a child to orthodontic problems. Early detection by the dental hygienist and referral to the orthodontist may prevent the later development of a more complex **malalignment** or malpositioning of the teeth. The following variations in the eruption sequence of the permanent dentition are signs of the need for early orthodontic treatment:

- Mandibular second molars erupt before the mandibular second premolars, thereby reducing the space available for the second premolars.
- Maxillary canines erupt at about the same time as the maxillary premolars, thus causing the canines to be displaced labially.
- The eruption of a permanent tooth on one side without eruption of the same tooth on the other side within a 6-month time frame indicates the need to take a radiograph of the unerupted tooth to determine if some physical obstruction is present.

Overretention of Primary Teeth

The overretention of the primary teeth requires orthodontic consideration (Figure 59-18). A permanent tooth should erupt when three fourths of its root is completed. If the primary tooth still has significant root structure remaining at this time, it should be extracted. This problem typically occurs when the permanent tooth bud develops in a position that is too far lingual to the primary tooth or when a primary molar root is still intact and prevents exfoliation.

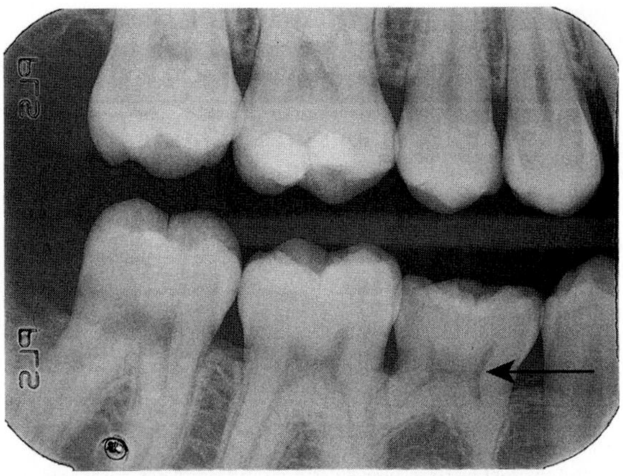

Figure 59-18. Retained primary second molar.

Early Loss of Primary Teeth

Premature primary tooth loss that results from severe caries or trauma will create an alignment problem, because existing other teeth will drift into the space of the missing tooth.

The loss of a tooth is considered premature if it occurs 6 months before the permanent tooth is expected to erupt. If a primary second molar is lost prematurely and the first permanent molar tips mesially, it is possible that the permanent first molar will close all space available for the permanent second premolar. To prevent the loss of space caused by the drifting of adjacent teeth, an appliance to maintain the space of the missing tooth is used (Figure 59-19).

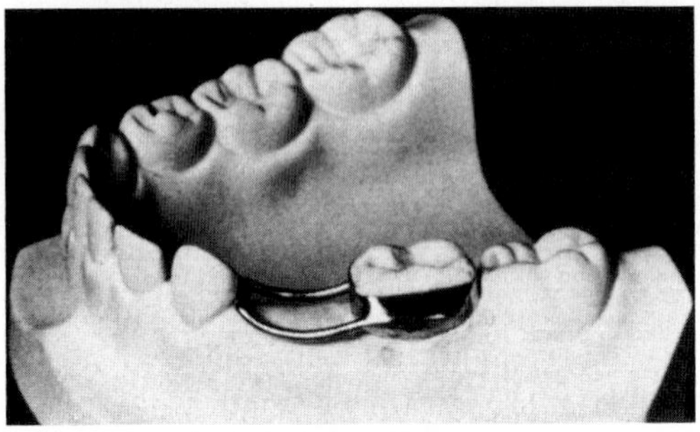

Figure 59-19. A band and loop space maintainer, with the band placed on the second primary molar and the loop extended to maintain the space of the missing primary first molar. (From Proffit WR, Fields HW Jr, Sarver DM: *Contemporary orthodontics,* ed 2, St Louis, 2013, Mosby.)

Early primary tooth loss, however, will delay eruption of the permanent tooth, because a layer of dense bone and tissue forms over the developing tooth. The permanent tooth should be given the chance to erupt on its own and may not do so until after the root is completely formed. The surgical excision of the overlying gingiva or forced eruption by placing an attachment on the permanent tooth may be required if the tooth fails to eventually erupt on its own.

Supernumerary Teeth

Supernumerary teeth are most frequently found in the maxillary anterior area (Figure 59-20). To minimize the displacement of other teeth within the arch, the extraction of a supernumerary tooth should be completed as soon as it can be done without harming the developing permanent tooth. Early detection of the presence of supernumerary teeth by the dental hygienist is very important.

Congenitally Missing Teeth

Congenitally missing teeth are an additional problem seen during the permanent dentition. The teeth most likely to be congenitally missing are the mandibular second premolars and the maxillary lateral incisors. Whether the condition is unilateral or bilateral, a congenitally missing tooth will cause the dental arch to develop asymmetrically, even if the primary tooth remains. Missing permanent teeth can be managed by the orthodontic closure of the space, the replacement of the tooth (or teeth) with a bridge, or the placement of a dental implant.

Crowding of Mandibular Incisors

A slight space deficiency in the arch for the eruption of permanent mandibular incisors will result in mild crowding and malalignment of these teeth. A phase of slight mandibular incisor crowding is considered normal, however, until a child approaches the age of 10 years. Space then becomes available

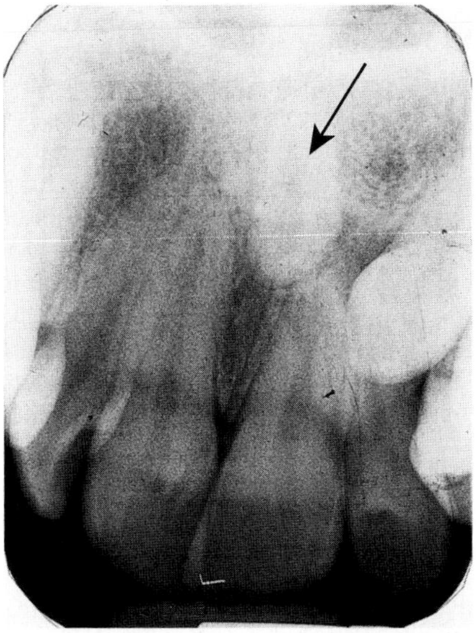

Figure 59-20. Supernumerary tooth (mesiodens) and impacted canine.

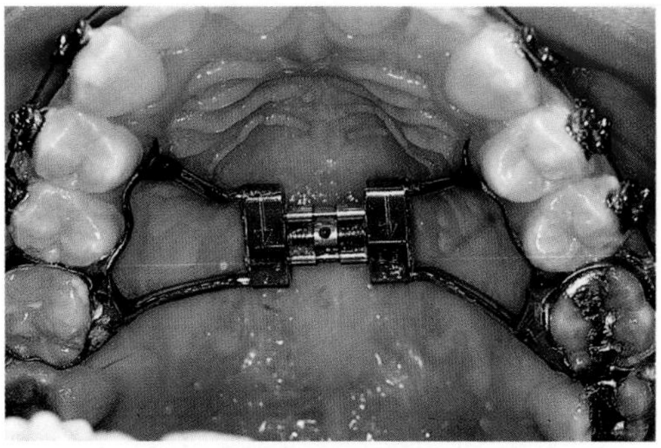

Figure 59-21. Palatal expansion device.

to eliminate this crowding after the mandibular canines erupt, for the following reasons:

- The distance between the canines will increase slightly because the incisors erupt not only incisally but also facially, thereby increasing the length of the arch.
- The mandibular canines move distally into the primate spaces, thus creating more room for the alignment of the incisors.

If crowding of the permanent mandibular incisors is severe, these processes will not create enough space to relieve the crowding. The most common form of malocclusion, in fact, is an Angle Class I malocclusion with crowding of the incisors.

Severe Crowding

Clients with severe crowding during the mixed dentition may experience early loss of the primary canines. The severe crowding and malalignment of the anterior teeth cause the roots of the primary canines to be resorbed by the eruption of the permanent lateral incisors. Affected clients may be treated with expansion of the dental arches or by serial extraction therapy.

Methods for expansion of the dental arches include orthodontic and orthopedic approaches.[3]

The goal of orthodontic expansion is to increase the length of the arch by tipping the crowns of the teeth facially with the use of conventional fixed appliances in addition to removable expansion appliances. Relapse will occur after treatment because forces applied by the cheek musculature can tip the teeth back to their original lingual positions.

Orthopedic expansion is achieved by applying forces so that the underlying skeletal structures are changed rather than by the movement or tipping of teeth within stationary alveolar bone. The goal of orthopedic expansion during the mixed dentition is to reduce the need for the extraction of the permanent teeth by establishing adequate arch length and promoting an optimal skeletal relationship between the maxilla and the mandible. Various types of appliances are used (Figure 59-21).

For children with severely crowded teeth, it may be decided during the early period of mixed dentition that there will not be enough room within the arches for all of the permanent teeth. For clients who have a Class I molar relationship, a normal overbite, and normal skeletal relationships, serial extraction is a treatment option in which select teeth are extracted at planned points in time to reduce crowding during the transition from the primary dentition to the permanent dentition. A second phase of fixed orthodontic therapy must also follow serial extraction. The second phase of fixed orthodontic therapy, however, can be expected to be less complex than it would have been if the extractions had not been completed.

Midline Diastema

In contrast with the crowding of mandibular incisors, spacing typically occurs in the maxillary incisors; this is seen as a slight diastema, or naturally occurring space, between the permanent central incisors. This "ugly duckling" stage occurs because the mesially inclined positions of the unerupted canines displace the roots of the lateral and central incisors mesially, thus flaring their crowns distally. If the midline diastema is 2 mm or less in size, it is likely to close as the maxillary lateral incisors and canines erupt.

Most children with a maxillary midline diastema at age 9 will have complete closure of the diastema by the age of 16 without any orthodontic intervention. If, however, the size of the diastema is initially more than 2 mm, total closure may not occur. A diastema of more than 2 to 3 mm in size may be caused by the following:

- A midline supernumerary tooth
- A midline soft-tissue or intrabony lesion
- Missing lateral incisors
- A tooth-size discrepancy (e.g., peg lateral incisors)

Malposed and Lingual Eruption of the Permanent Anterior Teeth

The permanent maxillary and mandibular incisor tooth buds develop lingual to the existing primary teeth. As a result, the permanent mandibular incisors may erupt malposed and lingual to the primary incisors, even in children with normal spacing (Figure 59-22). The permanent maxillary lateral incisor is also particularly prone to eruption lingual to its ideal position in the arch. The extraction of the primary canines may be needed to allow for labial positioning of the lateral incisors with an orthodontic appliance.

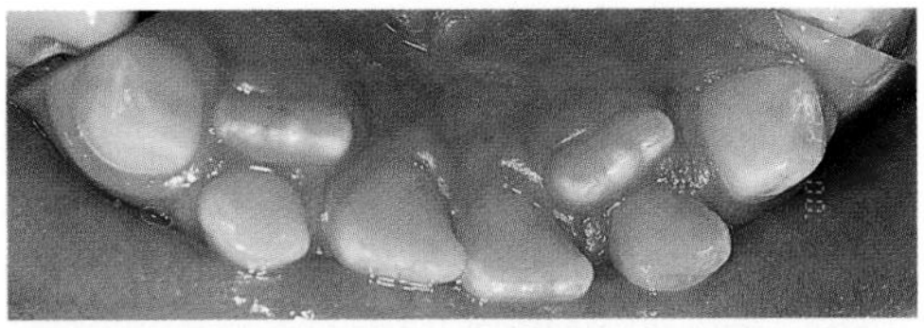

Figure 59-22. Lingual eruption of the mandibular incisors.

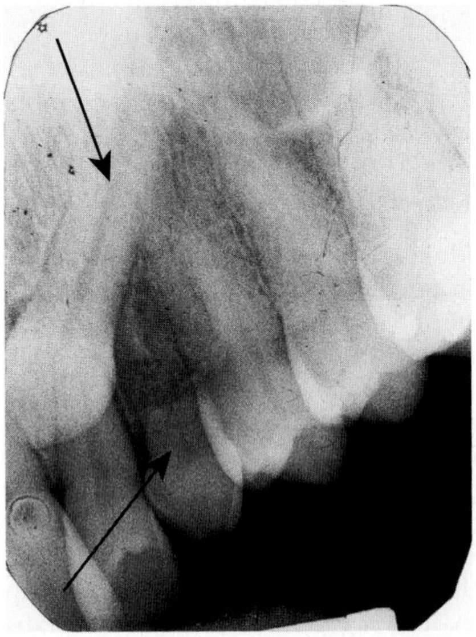

Figure 59-23. Impacted permanent canine and resorption of the primary canine root.

Impacted Canines

The maxillary canine is the most likely tooth to become impacted within the bone (Figure 59-23). Depending on the impaction severity, the canine may erupt normally after the primary canine extraction. If this is not expected to be successful, an impacted canine can be surgically exposed, bracketed, and brought into occlusion orthodontically after space in the arch has been created. The age of the client must also be considered when making the treatment decision. The older the client, the more likely it is that the tooth will be ankylosed (fused to the bone), thus making orthodontic movement impossible.

Lack of Leeway Space for the Eruption of the Permanent Premolars

Exactly opposite to the situation in the permanent anterior teeth, the permanent premolar teeth are smaller than the primary molars that they replace. This additional space, called the *leeway* or *E space,* is on average 5 mm in size in the mandibular arch and 3 mm in size in the maxillary arch. When the primary second molars are lost, the first permanent molars will rapidly shift mesially into this leeway space, thereby contributing to an ideal Class I occlusion in the permanent dentition. If a problem of crowding of the permanent dentition is apparent in the child at this time (i.e., at approximately 11 years of age), the orthodontist may choose to prevent the mesial drifting of the permanent molars by maintaining the leeway space with the use of a space maintainer.

Protruding Maxillary Incisors

The treatment of protruding maxillary incisors is indicated only when the protruding incisors have spaces between them and are esthetically objectionable or in danger of traumatic injury because of their degree of protrusion. This situation, in addition to an open bite, often occurs as a result of prolonged thumbsucking. Thumbsucking is considered prolonged if it is practiced for more than 6 hours per day and into the mixed dentition. The American Academy of Pediatric Dentistry recommends intervention to stop a thumbsucking habit if the habit continues to the age of 4 years.[5] The following types of malocclusion are caused by prolonged thumbsucking:

- Anterior open bite (the thumbsucking interferes with the normal eruption of the incisors and allows for the excessive eruption of the posterior teeth)
- Constricted maxillary arch (the maxilla develops into a V shape rather than a U shape)
- Posterior crossbite

When seeing a child who has a thumbsucking habit, it is important for the dental hygienist to discuss the problems that will result from continuing the habit. Some children will respond to advice from a dental professional rather than a parent. In the case in which the child unconsciously sucks the thumb or finger during sleep or while reading or watching television, a glove can be worn or a bandage applied to the thumb to discourage the habit. For a child who wants to stop the thumbsucking habit but is unable to do so, a wire crib appliance can be cemented onto the maxillary arch to prevent the placement of the thumb onto the palate. It must be explained to children that the purpose of this appliance is not punishment but rather that it has been placed to help them stop the thumbsucking habit. After the habit has been stopped, the appliance should remain in place for an additional 3 months to ensure that the habit has truly been broken.

Considerations in the Final Phases of Orthodontics

At the completion of the correction of Class II or Class III malocclusion, some rebound of the teeth back toward their initial positions can be expected. Because of this reaction, the malocclusions may be slightly overcorrected during treatment. For example, when a Class II malocclusion with a deep overbite is treated, the teeth may be overcorrected to an end-to-end incisor relationship before forces are removed. Because the teeth will rebound after the orthodontic forces are removed, the incisors should shift into an ideal relationship in which the maxillary incisors overlap the mandibular incisors to a slight degree. A period of 4 to 8 weeks is allowed for this rebound to occur before the fixed bands and brackets are removed.

Rebound is also an issue during palatal expansion procedures. The maxilla is overexpanded to enable the teeth to come into an ideal transverse occlusion as the expected rebound occurs.

A tooth positioner is a clear plastic or rubber appliance that covers the teeth and the gingiva. The inherent elasticity of the plastic or rubber allows for the settling of the teeth into their final occlusion. A tooth positioner may be delivered to the client immediately after the fixed appliances are removed. It should be worn full time during the first 2 days, because the most tooth movement occurs during this time. Thereafter the positioner is worn during the night as well as for a 4-hour period during the day. The full effects of the positioner are achieved in 3 weeks. After that, the positioner no longer provides a finishing function.[1]

It is important for the dental hygienist to understand these final procedures of orthodontic treatment, because it is common for the client to be anxious to have the appliances removed at this point. As far as the client is concerned, the teeth look as though they are fully corrected and treatment is finished. This concern is especially an issue for adolescent clients, who will often express a strong desire to have the appliances removed to the dental hygienist when they are seen at the continued-care appointment. The dental hygienist can be of great service to clients by helping them understand the importance of this finishing phase to the development of a solid occlusion that will have long-term stability.

Fluoride Therapy to Treat Decalcification

The presence of fixed orthodontic appliances places clients in a moderate to high caries risk category (see Chapter 16). The client is considered to be at moderate risk for dental caries as the result of the presence of fixed orthodontic appliances alone, even if the client has had neither incipient nor cavitated caries during the past 3 years. The presence of dental caries in the orthodontic client who also has additional risk factors such as poor oral hygiene or xerostomia places the client at high risk for experiencing further dental caries.[6] The development of "white spot" lesions on the teeth is a significant problem for the client who is undergoing orthodontic therapy. Occurring under and adjacent to orthodontic bands and brackets, the white spot lesion is early caries (see Figure 59-15). If the lesion is visible only when the tooth is dried, it likely involves the enamel only. If the white spot lesion is visible without drying, demineralization has progressed deeper within the enamel, although a relatively intact outer enamel surface remains. A sharp explorer should not be used to probe the intact surface of a white spot lesion, because the intact outer surface may be broken by the explorer, thereby requiring restoration of the lesion. If the lesion continues to progress, the outer surface will break down and form an open carious lesion.

The dental hygienist must help orthodontic clients to understand their responsibility for preventing enamel decalcification by completing optimal homecare, including daily rinsing with a 0.05% sodium fluoride mouth rinse or the application of a brush-on 5000 ppm fluoride gel or paste in addition to the daily use of an over-the-counter fluoride dentifrice.

The white spot lesion may be reversible after appliances are removed, especially if the lesion has a smooth surface. The regimen recommended is based on the premise that areas of softened enamel surface remineralize faster than subsurface areas. Because the entire remineralization process occurs from the surface only, the use of fluoride rinses immediately after debonding would remineralize the enamel surface lesion; however, doing so would block access to remineralization by the subsurface lesion and prevent complete repair. It is therefore recommended that topical fluoride supplementation be delayed until 2 to 3 months after debonding to allow for the remineralization of areas of the subsurface lesion to occur naturally.[3]

During this period, good oral hygiene is essential to increase the rate of natural remineralization. After this initial period, fluoride is recommended to treat the lesion surface, because fluoride ions greatly enhance remineralization. With remineralization, the lesion should reduce in size and develop a shiny surface similar to that of healthy enamel.[3]

Retention

Retention of the teeth after orthodontic treatment is necessary for the following reasons:

- Gingival and periodontal tissues need time to reorganize after the appliances are removed.
- Soft-tissue pressures from the tongue, lips, and cheeks may contribute to relapse if the musculature has not had time to adapt to the new occlusion and if tooth position is unstable.
- Skeletal growth can continue to affect the occlusion as it did before treatment, depending on the age of the client.

Time for the reorganization of the gingival and periodontal tissues is necessary because orthodontic tooth movement causes widening of the PDL and the disruption of the supporting collagen fibers. This is evident clinically by the mobility of the teeth that are present when appliances are removed. The teeth are not only mobile at treatment completion but also susceptible to displacement as a result of forces applied by the surrounding soft tissues and the occlusion. Reorganization of the periodontium takes 3 to 4 months and can occur only when each tooth is able to respond individually to the forces of mastication. Although retainers should be worn full time for the first 3 to 4 months after treatment, they should be removed during eating. The natural flexion of the individual teeth during eating will encourage periodontal tissue remodeling and a reduction in tooth mobility. If a fixed retainer is placed, it should not be so rigid that the natural flexion of teeth within the alveolar process cannot occur.

Retention after the correction of severe malalignments should be continued for at least 12 months because of the slow remodeling of the gingival fibers. After 3 to 4 months, however, removable retainers are not required on a full-time basis. Permanent retention may be required for teeth that are not able to tolerate the forces of the lips, cheeks, and tongue. For clients who are still growing, retention should be maintained until growth has stopped. The dental hygienist must encourage the client to strictly follow the orthodontist's recommendations for the use of retainers. If any indication of relapse is noted, the client must be referred to the orthodontist.

Removable Retainer Appliances

The most common type of retainer is the Hawley appliance, which is worn on the maxillary arch. This appliance consists of an acrylic palatal component with clasps on the molar teeth and a labial bow with adjustment loops at the canines (Figure 59-24, *A*). The labial bow can function to retain the position of the maxillary anterior teeth, or it can be adjusted to close spaces between anterior teeth that were banded. A clear plastic tooth positioner (Figure 59-24, *B*) may also be used for the first 3 weeks following removal of fixed appliances.

Fixed Retainers

Fixed retainers are bonded to the teeth and used for the long-term control of orthodontic alignment. Specifically, these

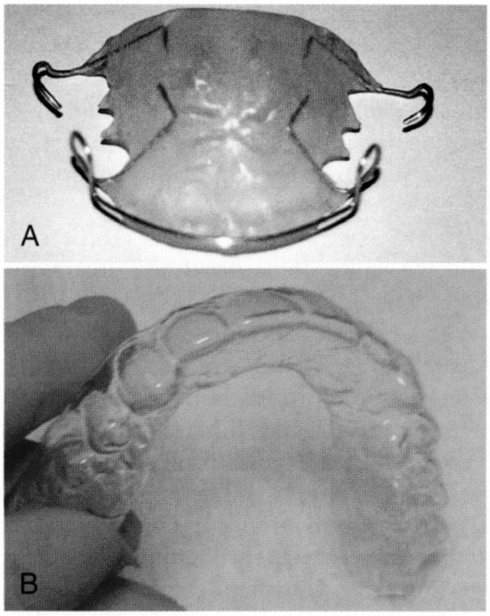

Figure 59-24. **A,** The Hawley appliance is commonly used as a removable retainer on the maxillary arch. **B,** The tooth positioner may also be used as a removable retainer.

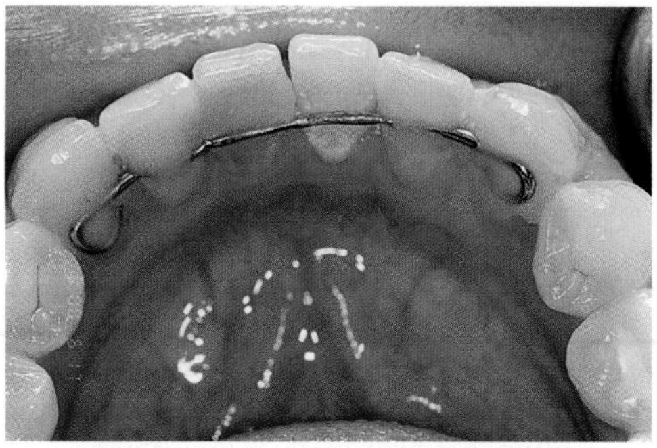

Figure 59-25. Bonded canine-to-canine (3-3) lingual retainer bonded to all incisors.

retainers are used to retain alignment of the mandibular incisors during the late growth that occurs between the ages of 16 and 20, for maintaining diastema closure, and for maintaining pontic space before crown and bridge restoration to replace a missing posterior tooth or teeth.

Bonded lingual canine-to-canine retainers, which are also referred to as *3-3 retainers,* are used most frequently in the mandibular anterior teeth to prevent relapse of crowding and malalignment of the incisors (Figure 59-25). Typically a round stainless steel wire that extends across the anterior teeth from the right to the left canine is bonded to the lingual surfaces of the canine teeth with restorative composite material. When seeing a client with a bonded retainer for continued-care appointments, the dental hygienist checks the appliance for breakdown of the bonding material. Bond failure can be detected by gently rocking each tooth with the blunt handle ends of two instruments and by observing the teeth for mobility when pressure is applied during scaling. The dental hygienist also ensures that the client understands how to clean around the appliance (see the interdental cleaning section later in this chapter).

Periodontal Aspects of Adult Orthodontic Treatment

Treatment of the adult with a history of periodontal disease must be planned carefully and must include the opinions of all dentists involved in the treatment of the client (e.g., orthodontist, periodontist, prosthodontist, endodontist). The primary form of periodontal treatment completed before orthodontics is that completed by the dental hygienist: periodontal scaling and root planing. Dental hygiene care is considered complete only when the inflammatory conditions are controlled well enough for the client to safely begin orthodontic tooth movement.

The control of plaque biofilm, which is described later in this chapter, is key to managing the adult with periodontal disease. A client's ability to remove plaque is complicated by the presence of orthodontic bands and brackets. The most difficult areas for the adult client to keep clean are the tooth surfaces between and subgingival to the brackets.

The width and thickness of the attached gingiva must be assessed carefully in the adult client. When the arch is expanded by labial movement of the teeth to relieve crowding problems, the risk of gingival recession is increased. Labial movement of the teeth may result in the development of a dehiscence in the bone. The labial gingiva becomes thin, and recession begins. Recession can progress rapidly if the labial keratinized gingiva is thin or nonexistent. It is preferable to prevent gingival recession rather than to correct it after it has occurred. A gingival graft procedure should be considered for many adult clients, especially those with keratinized gingiva that is thin in width and thickness and those who will be undergoing arch expansion to align the incisors.

Clients with previously treated periodontal disease must be seen for professional supportive periodontal maintenance every 2 to 3 months.

Dental Hygiene Care for the Orthodontic Client

The dental hygienist plays a critical role in maintaining oral health during and after treatment. In addition to providing professional mechanical dental hygiene care to promote the client's periodontal health, the dental hygienist provides ongoing instruction and feedback with regard to personal oral self-care. It is often beneficial to have written directions regarding various aspects of dental hygiene care recommendations. These directions, which should be given to clients as they leave the dental office, will enable them to better understand and remember specific directions given to them. Parents should always be included when youth are informed of the risks and necessary preventive home measures, but it is important that young clients be in agreement with recommended programs. The dental hygienist must work with the individual to design a regimen that is acceptable and effective.

Oral Biofilm Control

Plaque biofilm removal for the orthodontic client presents a special challenge. The accumulation of plaque biofilm around dental brackets and marginal gingivae may lead to enamel decalcification, which can be seen as white spot lesions and gingival disease (Figure 59-26).

The key is to find approaches that clients are able to use effectively and incorporate into their lifestyle. However, it is

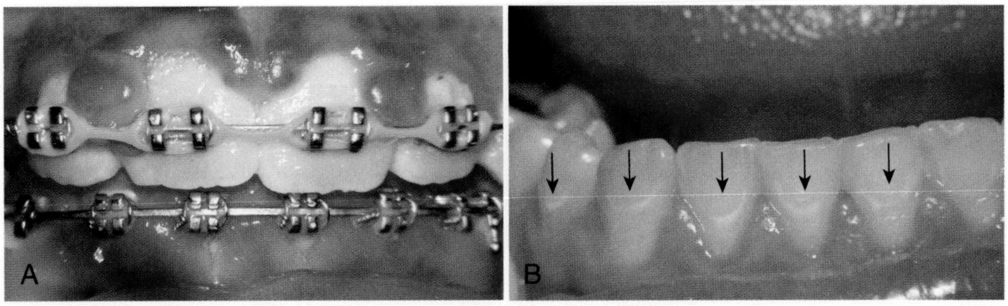

Figure 59-26. **A,** Enlarged papillae with the development of clefts in the mandibular incisor region as a result of prolonged poor oral hygiene in an adolescent client with fixed orthodontic appliances. **B,** White spot lesions as seen after the removal of bonded brackets.

BOX 59-4

Oral Hygiene Recommendations for Clients with Fixed Appliances

- Brush three times a day with fluoride dentifrice (0.22% sodium fluoride).
- Aim toothbrush bristles at the gingival margin to stimulate and debride the gingival margin area.
- Brush around brackets, first placing the bristles above and aiming them down toward the brackets and then placing the bristles below and aiming them up toward the brackets.
- Consider using specialized orthodontic brushes.
- Consider using power toothbrushes.
- Use a floss threader or super floss to clean subgingivally on the proximal surfaces.
- Use an interdental brush or wooden wedge (e.g., Proxabrush or a Stim-U-Dent) to get under the archwire and between teeth if the space is wide enough.
- Use the oral irrigator on low power at least once a day. Aim it perpendicularly to tooth contacts just above the papilla.
- Use disclosing tablets to check for plaque removal.
- Use 0.05% sodium fluoride rinse or 1.1% sodium fluoride gel/paste once daily.
- Use chlorhexidine 0.12% to 0.2% if prescribed for short periods (i.e., a few weeks); however, separate chlorhexidine from fluoride use by 60 minutes for the effective use of each.

important to not overload the client with too many adjuncts (Box 59-4).

Toothbrushing

Various toothbrush designs are now available. Styles include two-row sulcular brushes that can be placed gingival and coronal to the brackets, brushes with middle rows of bristles that are shorter to facilitate their use over brackets, end-tufted brushes to remove plaque biofilm around brackets, and brushes with bristles of various lengths. Clients' plaque removal efforts should be directed to the gingival margin using the modified Bass technique and to the cervical and incisal or occlusal aspects of the brackets (Figure 59-27). Powered toothbrushes may help the client with plaque biofilm removal, especially those brushes that have timers incorporated into them to ensure that the client uses the brush for a long enough period.

Interdental Cleaning

Interproximal plaque removal presents a particular challenge for the client. Various plaque removal aids, which were detailed in Chapter 22, include interdental brushes, rubber-tip stimulators, toothpicks, wooden wedges, and floss and floss threaders (Figure 59-28) or water floss.

For clients with fixed appliances, floss threaders must be used to place the floss interproximally. For young clients, teaching the parents to floss around their child's appliances is an option that should be considered.

For clients with fixed retainers to use floss, floss threaders must also be used to place floss interproximally. If the retainer is bonded to the canines only, the floss threader needs to be used only once, and floss can be pulled under the wire to floss each contact area without rethreading it between each tooth. If the client has large cervical embrasures as a result of a history of periodontal disease, interproximal brushes may be more effective for plaque biofilm removal. Triangular wooden wedges are also an alternative aid for interproximal plaque removal.

When orthodontic treatment is planned so that a bridge will be fabricated, it is often necessary to place a fixed retainer between abutments to maintain the pontic space. The same aids that are used for plaque biofilm removal around fixed retainers on the anterior teeth can be used around the wires that retain the pontic space.

Clients with fixed orthodontics, implants, bridges, and gingivitis and for those in a periodontal maintenance program can also clean the interdental areas by irrigating them with a dental water jet, or water flosser, that produces pulsating streams of fluid. Water flossing has been reported to reduce plaque biofilm, bleeding, gingivitis, probing depth, pathogenic microorganisms, and calculus at least as effectively as dental floss in orthodontic care. Orthodontic clients might prefer water floss for daily use over flossing with a floss threader because of the difficulty of threading the floss under the orthodontic wire to access each interdental space. A low-power or orthodontic tip should be used, and the irrigating stream should be directed perpendicularly to the long axis of the tooth rather than into the gingival sulcus. Antimicrobial agents may be added to the irrigator reservoir or used as a mouth rinse when indicated to reduce gingival inflammation.

Chlorhexidine Mouth Rinse

The use of a prescription rinse that contains chlorhexidine should also be considered for the client who has difficulty controlling gingival inflammation or dental caries. The rinse

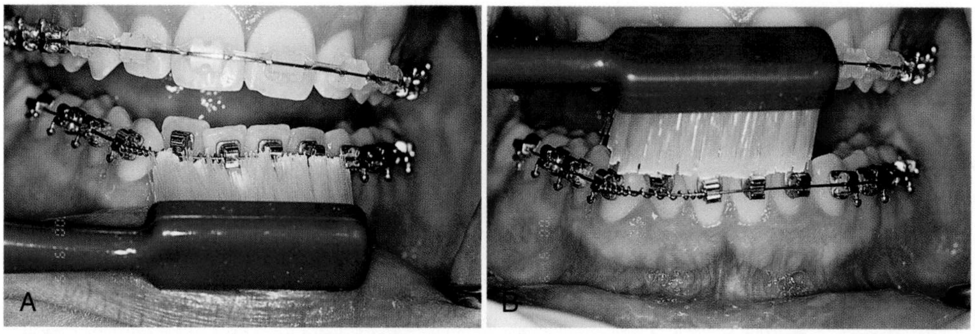

Figure 59-27. **A,** Placement of the toothbrush for the removal of plaque from the cervical aspect of brackets. **B,** Placement of the toothbrush for the removal of plaque from the incisal aspect of brackets.

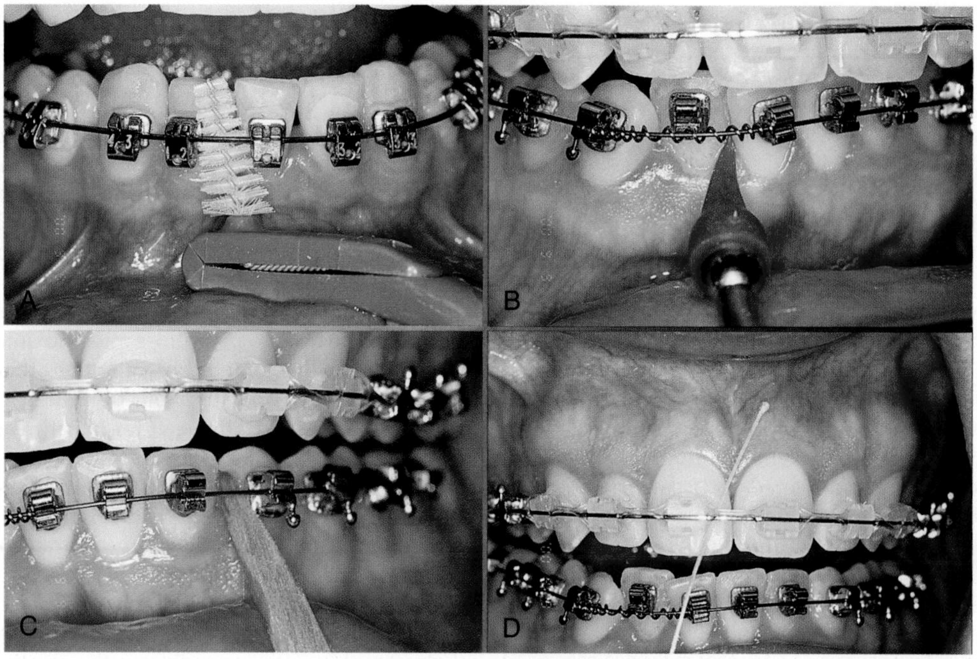

Figure 59-28. **A,** Use of an interdental brush to clean around brackets. **B,** Use of a rubber-tip stimulator to disrupt plaque and to massage the papillae. **C,** Use of a wooden wedge to remove plaque. **D,** Use of a floss threader to place floss under the archwire.

can be applied locally with an interproximal brush to treat a local area of gingival inflammation and to minimize brown staining that may occur as a side effect.

Fluoride Therapy

The presence of orthodontic appliances is a risk factor for dental caries. Daily fluoride therapy is essential preventive care for the orthodontic client to prevent enamel demineralization and tooth decay. The use of home fluoride therapies is as important in the adult client as it is in the child. Adult clients may be even more susceptible to tooth decay than children if they have poorly contoured margins on restorations, root exposure caused by gingival recession, or reduced salivary flow or gingival enlargement as a result of prescription medication.

In addition to a standard fluoride toothpaste, an over-the counter sodium fluoride rinse or 5000 ppm sodium fluoride dentifrice or gel should be used daily at home, depending on caries risk assessment (see Chapter 18). Numerous products that contain neutral and acidulated fluorides have been recommended as safe and effective for preventing white spot lesions and promoting enamel remineralization in the orthodontic client. However, the effectiveness of these products relies on client compliance.

Dietary Counseling

Because plaque control is more difficult for the client who wears fixed orthodontic appliances, sugar intake should be minimized during the period of active treatment. If sweets are eaten, they should be eaten as part of a meal to limit the number of acid attacks throughout the day. The dental hygienist informs the client that foods that cannot be cleaned off of the fixed orthodontic appliances may lead to dental caries, white spots, and unattractive food debris accumulation. Moreover, even though orthodontic bands and wires are made of metal or porcelain, they can be fragile and damaged by eating the wrong foods, thereby delaying the completion of orthodontic treatment (Box 59-5).

BOX 59-5

Foods to Avoid and to Include When Wearing Fixed Orthodontic Appliances

Foods to Avoid
- Chewing gum, sugarless or otherwise
- Sticky foods (e.g., peanut butter; sticky candies such as caramels, Sugar Daddies, and Tootsie Rolls)
- Hard foods (e.g., nuts, corn on the cob, popcorn, hard candy, bagels, apples, whole carrots, hard pretzels, hard chips, jerky)
- Ice

Foods to Include
- Foods low in sugar
- Fresh fruits and vegetables cut in pieces
- Applesauce
- Yogurt
- Pasta
- Representatives from all areas of the food pyramid, cut in pieces if needed (see Chapter 33)

Frequent Professional Dental Hygiene Maintenance Care

For the client who, despite all efforts, has limited plaque-control abilities, continued-care appointments every 3 to 4 months may be required. Clients who are undergoing active orthodontic treatment are considered to be at moderate to high risk for the development of dental caries.[6] As a result, topical treatments that involve applying a fluoride varnish, 2% sodium fluoride, or 1.23% acidulated phosphate fluoride or fluoride varnish should be applied at 3- to 6-month intervals, depending on client need. Dental hygiene care of the orthodontic client includes procedures performed during the dental hygiene appointment, such as client assessment, deposit removal, self-care recommendations, and communication with other dental offices involved in the client's care.

Client assessment consists of the same procedures used for a client without orthodontic appliances. The hard and soft tissues are evaluated clinically and supported with periodontal probing and radiographs when indicated. The soft tissues are examined for trauma caused by sharp appliances. Trauma can result in areas of abrasion or laceration. Warm salt water rinses (i.e., 1 tsp of salt added to an 8-oz glass of water) and the use of utility wax to cover sharp appliance surfaces can relieve discomfort from the offending wire until it can be remedied. Soft wax should be offered to all orthodontic clients to prevent mucosal injury and to control pain. Common oral manifestations observed in clients who are undergoing orthodontic treatment include the following:

- Gingival inflammation caused by plaque biofilm accumulation around brackets or contact hypersensitivity to the nickel titanium wires and plastic brackets
- Gingival hyperplasia caused by plaque biofilm accumulation
- Decalcification of enamel around brackets (white spot lesions)
- Dental caries around brackets
- Canker sores or other soft-tissue lesions from the friction of the braces rubbing against the soft tissue of the mouth
- Root resorption

The removal of plaque biofilm and calculus requires the patient and skillful application of the instruments and materials used for the maintenance of any client. An ultrasonic or air-powder device may be especially effective for removing the stains that develop under archwires and between brackets. Cone-shaped prophylaxis cups may also be applied for better access to these areas.

Communication with the orthodontist and any other office involved in the treatment of the client is an essential duty of the dental hygienist. Whenever a client is seen for dental hygiene, the dental hygienist sends a written note to the involved dentists informing them of the client's appointment outcomes; any changes in his or her general, dental, or periodontal health; and recommendations for homecare. Any additional concerns or questions—as well as the date of the client's next dental hygiene visit and duplicates of exposed radiographs—are included. In addition, before treating a client who is seeing numerous dentists, the dental hygienist reads any communication from those dentists to be aware of the client's status. Comprehensive and professional communication is appreciated by all involved, including the client.

Oral Hygiene Care for the Surgical Orthodontic Client

While the client is in the hospital, oral hygiene care consists of frequent saline irrigation with a 30-mL syringe and a blunt needle and, if available, with special brushes that can be placed on the end of a suction unit. Thorough oral debridement is essential for preventing infection of the surgical incisions, gingival inflammation, and dental decalcification (Box 59-6).

For the first 2 weeks after surgery, clients continue to irrigate with the use of saline and a syringe several times daily, especially after eating. The oral and maxillofacial surgeon must be consulted regarding postoperative hygiene, especially that involving the use of mouth rinses and powered irrigators.

If the client has been placed in maxillomandibular fixation for 6 to 8 weeks, a small, soft-bristled brush; a modified sulcular technique; and any aids for cleaning interproximally as best as possible are beneficial. Dietary recommendations are especially important for helping the client to heal and maintain his or her overall health after surgery. Caloric requirements increase after surgery, which is also when the client will have the most difficulty ingesting foods. All foods must be prepared to a thin consistency in a blender. Water, nutritious drinks, and high-caloric nutrition supplementation liquids are encouraged. Carbonated beverages are to be avoided.

After fixation is removed, clients require instruction in physical therapy techniques to restore the function of the lips and the ability to open and close the jaws. The final postsurgical phase of orthodontic treatment is completed to allow the teeth to settle into better intercuspation. Elastics are used to guide the occlusion. Settling generally takes 2 months to complete. Retention of the surgically treated case is no different than retention for any adult orthodontic case. Definitive periodontal surgery and prosthetic treatment can be completed after the final occlusion is established.

BOX 59-6

Postsurgical Plaque-Control Procedures During Maxillomandibular Fixation

First 2 Weeks After Surgery

- Frequent saline rinses (especially after eating) are performed with a 30-mL syringe with a blunt needle.
- If available, use special brushes that can be placed on the end of a suction unit to remove plaque biofilm and debris from the labial surfaces of the teeth; the lingual surfaces will not be accessible.
- After the surgical incisions have healed, a diluted (1 : 1 ratio) antimicrobial mouth rinse may be applied with the use of a powered irrigator. The irrigator must be set on a low setting and directed perpendicularly to the tooth at the gingival margin. Chlorhexidine is a recommended antimicrobial agent because of its effectiveness and low alcohol content.
- The surgeon is consulted regarding postoperative hygiene procedures.

2 to 8 Weeks After Surgery

- Modified sulcular brushing may be started with the use of a small, soft-bristled brush.
- Interproximal aids such as Stim-U-Dents, toothpicks, a rubber-tip stimulator, and an interproximal brush may be used.
- Fluoride rinses that are low in alcohol content and gels and toothpastes are used to prevent decalcification.
- Dietary recommendations for the ingestion of water, nutritious drinks, and high-caloric supplementation liquids should be provided. Carbonated beverages are to be avoided.

CLIENT EDUCATION TIPS

- Explain the dental and skeletal conditions that warrant orthodontic treatment.
- Explain changes that are occurring during treatment and the importance of retention after treatment.
- Explain the need for further periodontal and prosthodontic procedures.
- Work carefully with clients to develop a plaque-control regimen that is acceptable and effective; to limit dietary sugars; to use home fluoride rinses, gels, and dentifrices; and to clean removable appliances.
- Reinforce the importance of following procedures and attending orthodontic appointments as recommended by the orthodontist.

LEGAL, ETHICAL, AND SAFETY ISSUES

- The dental hygienist maintains written communication with the orthodontic office regarding mutual clients. In this communication, the orthodontist is advised of the date of the last maintenance appointment with the dental hygienist, any changes in the client's health history or oral health, recommendations provided for plaque control or home fluoride, and any problems with the orthodontic appliances noted (e.g., loose brackets or bands, wires impinging on tissues). Any radiographs that have been taken also need to be enclosed.
- Before seating the client, the dental hygienist reads any letters sent by the orthodontist since the last visit. This routine keeps the dental hygienist up to date on the progress of the client's treatment and allows him or her to follow up with any concerns expressed by the orthodontist.
- The dental hygienist carefully evaluates young clients to identify malocclusions that may benefit from early orthodontic intervention and brings any findings to the attention of the dentist and the parents. Failure to note such malocclusions could result in the need for more lengthy orthodontic treatment with less favorable results.
- When seeing a client for continued-care visits after orthodontic therapy has been completed, the dental hygienist continually evaluates the dentition for relapse. If any areas of relapse in the malocclusion are noted, the dentist must be advised and the client referred back to the orthodontist for evaluation.

KEY CONCEPTS

- Evaluation of the occlusion includes not only the relationship of the teeth to one another as categorized by Angle I, II, and III classifications but also the skeletal relationship of the maxilla and mandible to each other.
- Children's skeletal development and their chronologic age must be determined to take appropriate advantage of growth modification procedures. Such procedures are most effective when applied during the preadolescent growth spurt. Growth modification can be used to restrain maxillary growth, to enhance mandibular growth, and to expand the palate to correct transverse discrepancies and to create more space within the arch.
- The sequence of tooth eruption is more important than the date of eruption. During the primary dentition, spacing is preferred. Primate and developmental spaces provide room for the developing permanent teeth. A lack of space in the primary dentition indicates that the permanent dentition will be crowded.
- Eruption of the permanent teeth occurs as a result of cellular activities within the periodontal ligament. Eruption is a process that continues at various rates throughout life. The primary dentition plays a critical role in the optimal eruption of the permanent teeth.
- Light, sustained orthodontic forces result in optimal tooth movement through a process of frontal resorption.
- Orthodontic treatment planning is a complex process that must take into consideration a client's chief complaint. It also is based on the clinical judgment and experience of the orthodontist. It may be impossible to achieve all orthodontic goals. The dental hygienist must be aware of this when seeing a client for maintenance after treatment has been completed.
- Properly applied orthodontic forces will affect the dental pulp, cementum, and dentin to a minimal degree. Apical root resorption occurs in almost all orthodontic cases, but it is usually not clinically significant.
- Orthodontic brackets are made of metal, ceramic, or plastic material and attached directly to the teeth through bonding or to stainless steel bands that are cemented around the teeth.
- Client education is particularly important during orthodontic therapy. The dental hygienist must help the client

to develop skill in removing plaque biofilm from around the orthodontic appliances as well as in understanding the treatment procedures that are needed to ensure an optimal result.

- The dental hygienist plays a key role in preparing the client for orthodontic treatment as well as maintaining the client's oral health during and after orthodontic treatment. The dental hygienist may complete data collection procedures, including taking the medical and personal histories, completing periodontal and dental chartings, taking radiographs, and preparing study models.
- For the client with active periodontal disease, the dental hygienist must complete periodontal debridement and client education to eliminate infection.
- During treatment, the client must be seen regularly by the dental hygienist for clinical maintenance procedures and follow-up regarding homecare recommendations.

CRITICAL THINKING EXERCISES

Client: T.J. Langer

Profile: T.J. is a 5-year-old boy who has come with his mother to have his teeth cleaned.

Chief Complaint: T.J.'s mother is concerned that there is spacing between T.J.'s upper front teeth and between some of his lower teeth. She asks you if he will need braces to close these spaces.

Social History: The client lives with both parents.

Medical History: Noncontributory.

Dental History: On inspection, you notice that the primary spaces are between the maxillary lateral incisors and the canines and between the mandibular canines and the first molars. You also notice that the primary second molars are in an end-to-end relationship.

Supplemental Notes: The client lives in a fluoridated community.

1. What would you say to T.J.'s mother about his potential need for orthodontic treatment?

REFERENCES

1. Proffit WR, Fields HW Jr, Sarver DM: *Contemporary orthodontics*, ed 4, St Louis, 2007, Mosby.
2. Rinchuse DJ, Rinchuse DJ: Developmental occlusion, orthodontic interventions, and orthognathic surgery for adolescents, *Dent Clin North Am* 50:69, 2006.
3. Graber TM, Vanarsdall RL Jr, Vig KWL, eds: *Orthodontics: current principles and techniques*, ed 4, St Louis, 2005, Mosby.
4. Wong BH: Invisalign A to Z, *Am J Orthod Dentofacial Orthop* 121:540, 2002.
5. American Academy of Pediatric Dentistry: Oral health policies, guidelines, and quality assurance policies, *Pediatr Dent* 23:1, 2002.
6. American Dental Association Council on Scientific Affairs: Professionally applied topical fluoride: evidence-based clinical recommendations, *J Am Dent Assoc* 137:1151, 2006.

ACKNOWLEDGEMENT

The authors wish to acknowledge the former chapter author, Leeann Branscome Simmons, BSDH, MS, and the review provided by orthodontist, Dr. Rufus Van Dyke.

EVOLVE RESOURCES

Please visit http://evolve.elsevier.com/Darby/hygiene for additional practice and study support tools.

CHAPTER 60

Abuse and Neglect

Sheryl L. Ernest Syme, Susan Camardese

COMPETENCIES

1. Define the following terms: maltreatment, abuse, neglect, and P.A.N.D.A.
2. Discuss child maltreatment, including how to distinguish the physical findings that may be mistaken for abuse including injuries occurring from accidents, genetic and acquired conditions, infections, and cultural practices.
3. Discuss family violence, including bullying and domestic violence.
4. Discuss the abuse and neglect of the elderly and other vulnerable adults.
5. Explain human trafficking and list indicators of possible victims.
6. Discuss the disclosure and reporting of abuse, including:
   - Explain the oral health professionals' ethical and legal responsibilities regarding reporting abuse and neglect, implement appropriate screening questions, and eliminate reporting barriers.
   - Identify appropriate local and national agencies to report abuse and neglect.

Oral health professionals are positioned uniquely to identify signs and symptoms of all manifestations of abuse and neglect and can play an important role in early recognition of related oral manifestations. The frequency of dental hygiene care visits provides the opportunity to develop close and trusting client-provider relationships and to obtain detailed medical and dental histories and extra- and intraoral clinical assessments, key factors in early recognition of signs of abuse and neglect. Abusers often avoid the same physician but return to the same dental office.[1] **Maltreatment** is the term used to define abuse and neglect of victims. Legislation in all 50 states, the District of Columbia, and the U.S. territories mandates the reporting of suspected child maltreatment to child protective services agencies. Many states also mandate the reporting of suspected intimate partner violence and elder abuse to social or law enforcement agencies. Oral health professionals, however, make very few reports. This chapter provides information on how to recognize and report abuse and neglect to increase the frequency of these early recognition and reporting behaviors by dental hygienists in the dental hygiene care setting. Dental hygienists should be familiar with their state's definitions of abuse and neglect along with reporting requirements.

Abuse and Neglect

The public health approach to abuse and neglect prevention seeks to improve the health and safety of all individuals by addressing underlying **risk factors** that increase the likelihood that an individual will become a victim or a perpetrator of violence. The World Health Organization defines risk factor identification and the need to provide important information about populations requiring preventive interventions, as criteria of the public health model.[2] Oral health professionals are vital to identifying risk factors of abuse and neglect.

Abuse is a public health problem that can be physical, sexual, emotional, and verbal, or a combination of any or all of these victimizing social issues that include child maltreatment, spousal or intimate partner violence, elder abuse, and human trafficking. **Neglect** refers to acts of omission by parents or caretakers, which may include failure to provide adequate care, support, nutrition, health or surgical care; failure to follow through with recommended healthcare; and in the case of children, failure to provide for their educational needs as required by law (Table 60-1).

Because the majority of abuse and neglect occurs within the head and neck region, oral health providers are often the first to render care to victims, yet they infrequently recognize risk factors and make timely reports or referrals to the proper authorities.[3-5] The need for increased abuse and neglect education for dental professionals has been well established in past literature. **Prevent Abuse and Neglect through Dental Awareness (P.A.N.D.A.)** is an educational and awareness program created to promote an atmosphere of understanding in dentistry and other professional communities to increase the prevention of abuse and neglect through early identification and appropriate intervention for victims. Nevertheless, research continues to show the need for abuse and neglect education among all oral health professionals.[6,7]

Child Maltreatment

Historical U.S. Perspective

Although child abuse and neglect have occurred throughout the ages and worldwide, child maltreatment was not identified as a public health issue among the medical community until the early 1960s. Before the 1960s, physicians attempted to submit research identifying suspicious physical findings and medical history inconsistencies among emergency room child patients but the medical community refused to publish this information. At the time it was determined to be a "family problem," not a medical issue. In addition to the lack of

TABLE 60-1
Types of Abuse

Category	Description
Neglect	Deprivation of adequate food, water, clothing, shelter, medical care, or supervision; also includes failure to educate a child as required by law
Physical abuse	Nonaccidental injury or threatened injury (e.g., kicking, biting, hitting, pushing, choking, assault with weapons)
Sexual abuse	Use of sex to hurt, degrade, dominate, humiliate, and gain power over the victim. As a violent act of aggression, forced sexual activity, marital rape, and sexual sadism are forms of sexual domestic violence and often accompany physical abuse.
Emotional and/or psychologic abuse	Intimidation with gestures, yelling, smashing things, or destroying the victim's property; threats to harm a child or children or keep them from the victim; isolating the victim from family and friends; and economic domination. Destroys the victim's self-esteem; includes verbal abuse, excessive demands on the child's performance, and withholding love and affection. Scars of emotional and/or psychologic abuse are traumatic and long term.

recognition by the medical community, there were no laws protecting children from maltreatment in and outside of the home. It was not until 1938 that a law was enacted stating the minimum ages of employment and allowable hours of work for children. Up until that time children could be removed from school to work as laborers. The first child in the United States to be removed from the home as a result of family violence occurred in New York City in 1874. At that time, animals had more protection from cruelty than children with the establishment of the American Society for the Prevention of Cruelty to Animals (ASPCA). However, no such organizations or laws existed protecting children.

In 1974 the federal government established the Child Abuse Prevention and Treatment Act (CAPTA: P.L. 93-247) to define broadly abuse and neglect. The Child Abuse Prevention and Treatment Act (CAPTA; 42 U.S.C. §5101) as amended by the CAPTA Reauthorization Act of 2010, retained the existing definition of child abuse and neglect as follows:

- Any recent act or failure to act on the part of a parent or caretaker that results in death, serious physical or emotional harm, sexual abuse, or exploitation, or
- An act or failure to act that presents an imminent risk of serious harm

Each state is then responsible for establishing its own definitions within the minimum standards set by federal legislation.

In 1980 CAPTA began the use of the term *child maltreatment* for abuse and neglect. In 1988 the Child Maltreatment Report Series was established to collect and publish the child maltreatment information/statistics for each state and the District of Columbia.

Current Prevalence

Child maltreatment occurs in families from all socioeconomic strata and geographic areas spanning all ethnicities. The U.S. Department of Health and Human Services reports that more than 695,000 children were victims of maltreatment in 2010, and victims in the age group of birth to 1 year had the highest victimization.[8] Many of the reported children suffered from multiple forms of maltreatment, and many were subjects of repeated reports, indicating that abuse and neglect are not isolated episodes. In many cases, the abuse and neglect escalates in violence and trauma to victims. It is estimated that 1560 children died from abuse and neglect in 2010. The Centers for Disease Control and Prevention identifies child maltreatment as a public health problem[9] and the Child Welfare League of America categorizes child abuse as a rising epidemic.[10]

Child Maltreatment Defined

Child maltreatment includes all types of abuse and neglect of a child under the age of 18 by a parent or caregiver, or another person in a custodial role (e.g., clergy, coach, teacher). The four types of child maltreatment are physical abuse, sexual abuse, emotional abuse, and neglect (see Table 60-1). Physical abuse is the use of physical force, such as hitting, kicking, burning, or another show of force against the victim. Sexual abuse is unwanted sexual activity, with perpetrators (abusers) using force, making threats, or taking advantage of victims not able to give consent. Most victims and perpetrators know each other. Immediate reactions to sexual abuse include shock, fear, or disbelief. Long-term symptoms include anxiety, fear, or post-traumatic stress disorder. Emotional abuse is a pattern of behavior that retards a child's development and self-esteem, such as constant criticizing or belittling or not providing love or guidance. Neglect may include deprivation of adequate food, clothing, shelter, healthcare, psychologic support, and other needs or supervision, and in some legal jurisdictions, failure to educate a child as required by law.

Neglect accounts for more than 78% of all reported cases of abuse, followed by reports of physical, sexual, and emotional abuse (Figure 60-1). Children with special needs have a higher victimization risk for maltreatment than children not reported to have special needs.[7] Common indicators of abuse and neglect are found in Table 60-2.

Physical Maltreatment

Physical maltreatment is the use of physical force, such as hitting, kicking, burning, or another show of force against the victim.[8] Signs of physical abuse may include imprints or marks made by objects used by the perpetrators of abuse that

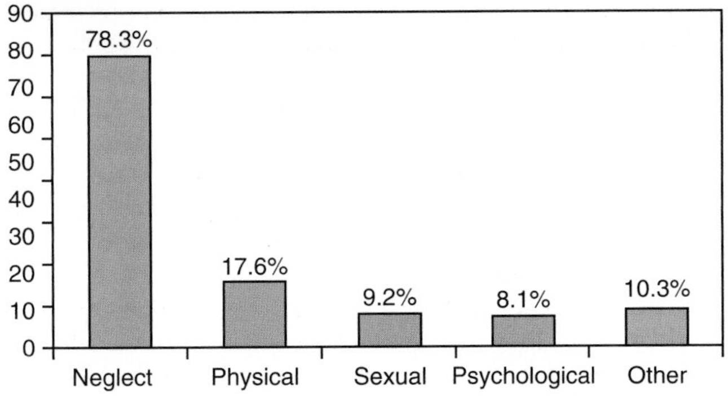

Figure 60-1. Types of reported cases of abuse and neglect. (From U.S. Department of Health and Human Services, Administration on Children, Youth and Families, Children's Bureau: *Child maltreatment 2010,* Washington, DC, 2011. Available at: http://www.acf.hhs.gov/programs/cb/stats_research/index.htm#can.)

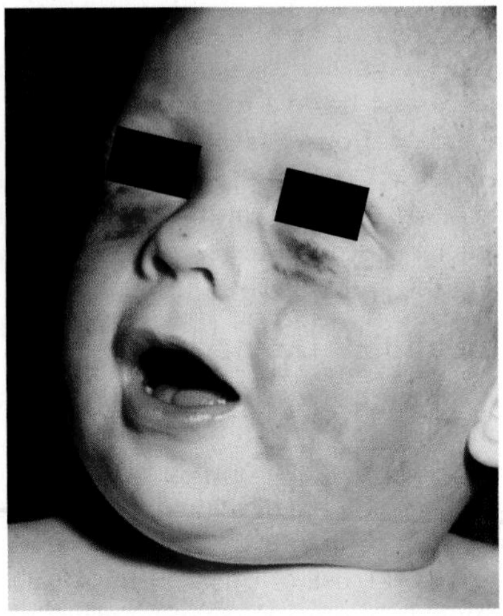

Figure 60-2. Infant with bilateral facial bruises from multiple beatings. (Courtesy Dr. Lynn Douglas Mouden, cofounder of P.A.N.D.A. [Prevention of Abuse and Neglect through Dental Awareness].)

may leave "tattoo" effects on the victim's skin. The victim's skin can reveal tell-tale imprints left by belt buckles, ropes, and looped cords, as well as linear markings from skin compressed between the perpetrator's fingers during an open-handed slap or strike.

Other indicators of abuse include bruises, welts, bite marks, burns, fractures, lacerations, abrasions, head injuries (Figure 60-2), and delay of treatment. Typical sites for inflicted injuries of abuse are the buttocks and lower back, genitals and inner thighs, cheeks, ears, lip and labial frenum, neck, arms, and hands. Because head and neck injuries are common in abuse victims, the dental professional should be knowledgeable of dentofacial trauma associated with abuse. Notably, tongue, lip, gingiva, and frenum lacerations; jaw fractures; tooth fractures; avulsed teeth (Figure 60-3); and nonvital teeth warrant further assessment of suspected abuse. Aside from blows to the face, forced feeding with utensils, bottles, cups, or fingers or scalding liquids or caustic substances cause many oral injuries associated with abuse.

TABLE 60-2

Indicators of Abuse and Neglect in Clients

Type of Abuse	Indicators
Physical abuse	Unexplained bruises in various stages of healing Multiple bruises on face, lips, arms, legs Bruising on nonbony protrusions* Shaped or patterned injuries or bruises such as belt or belt buckle marks, iron burns, hand slap or finger markings, rope burns Cigarette burns Scalding injuries (glovelike immersion burns) Broken nose Black eyes Inappropriate seasonal dress (long sleeves in the summer to cover bruises) Cuts or lacerations especially on the face or neck Oral trauma including the following: Torn frenum Avulsed teeth Discolored teeth (resulting from pulpal necrosis), indicator of past traumatic injury Fractured teeth Gingival abrasions Burns from scalding liquids or hot utensils Oral lacerations resulting from forced feeding Trauma to the corners of the mouth (may indicate the use of gags) Gingival contusions Petechiae or bruising (may indicate forced oral sex) Palatal lesions and scars
Neglect	Poor hygiene Rampant caries, early childhood caries Unmet medical or dental needs Lack of regularity of dental hygiene appointments Poor or no parental supervision
Sexual abuse	Petechiae on soft palate (may be a sign of forced oral sex) Venereal warts (condyloma acuminatum) on lips, tongue, palate, or gingivae Venereal disease (in prepuberty) Itching of genitalia Difficulty in walking or sitting
Emotional maltreatment	Withdrawn or fatigued Record of suicide attempts Parent or caregiver: Constantly blames or berates child Is unconcerned about child Overtly rejects child

*Normal childhood injuries tend to occur on bony protrusion (e.g., knees and elbows). Bruises caused by abuse often are found on nonbony areas (e.g., arms, legs, and neck).

Inappropriate seasonal clothing worn to cover injuries to the arms and legs, unlikely stories about how the injuries occurred, and evidence of repeated injuries or multiple bruises in various stages of healing may indicate frequent violent abuse.

Sexual Abuse

Sexual abuse is unwanted sexual activity, with perpetrators using force, making threats, or taking advantage of victims not able to give consent. Most victims and perpetrators know each other. Immediate reactions to sexual abuse include shock, fear, or disbelief. Long-term symptoms include anxiety, fear, or post-traumatic stress disorder.

The identification of sexually transmitted disease in children beyond the perinatal period suggests sexual abuse. Postnatally acquired gonorrhea, syphilis, and nontransfusion, nonperinatally acquired HIV are usually diagnostic of sexual abuse. Signs of sexual abuse often present in a child's oral cavity. Some oral indicators of sexual abuse include condyloma acuminatum (venereal warts), which appear as a cauliflower-like growth on lips, palate, gingiva, or tongue (Figure 60-4). Syphilis may emerge as an ulcerated chancre or mucous patch (Figure 60-5). Gonorrhea may appear as pharyngitis, tonsillitis, or gingivitis. Herpes can manifest as gingivostomatitis (Figure 60-6). Human papillomavirus (HPV), an emerging sexually transmitted disease, is recognized as yet another indicator in child sexual abuse associated with the formation of oral warts.

Palatal petechiae could be a sign of forced oral sex (Figure 60-7). After documenting all observations and obtaining a complete client history, the dental hygienist should report suspicions to a child protective services (CPS) agency immediately.

Emotional Maltreatment

Emotional maltreatment is a pattern of behavior that retards a child's development and self-esteem such as constant criticizing or belittling or not providing love or guidance. Behavioral and emotional signs of maltreatment include expressions of aggression, disruptive behavior, or anger, rage, or unusual anxiety or fear.

Neglect

Neglect is typically a failure by the parent, caregiver, or guardian to provide for basic physical, educational, or emotional needs. It may include deprivation of adequate food, clothing, shelter, healthcare, psychologic support, and other needs or supervision.

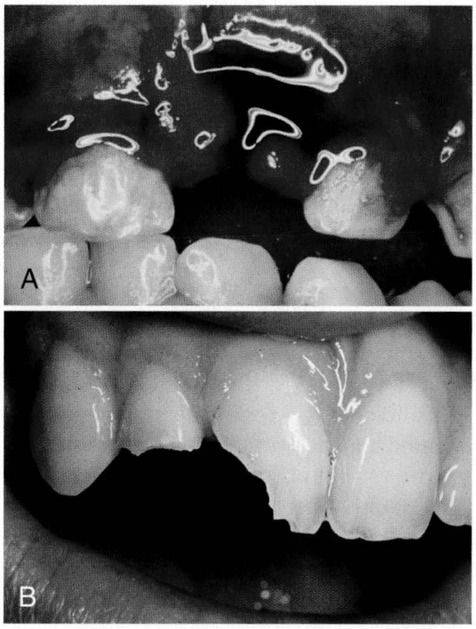

Figure 60-3. **A,** Tooth avulsion in a child as a consequence of being punched in the mouth. **B,** Tooth fracture of central and lateral incisors consequent to a beating when child landed against a chest of drawers. (Courtesy Dr. Lynn Douglas Mouden, cofounder of P.A.N.D.A. [Prevention of Abuse and Neglect through Dental Awareness].)

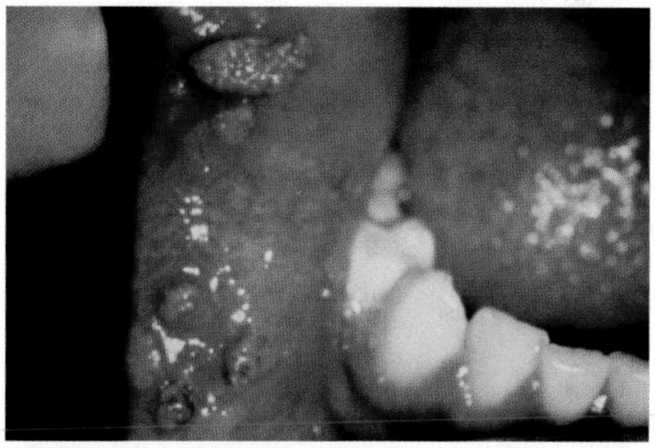

Figure 60-4. Indicator of oral sexual abuse. Condylomas. Venereal warts transmitted to the oral cavity through sexual abuse. (Courtesy Dr. Lynn Douglas Mouden, cofounder of P.A.N.D.A. [Prevention of Abuse and Neglect through Dental Awareness].)

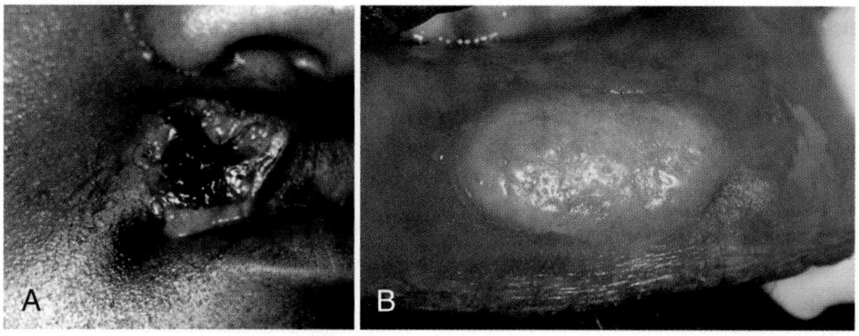

Figure 60-5. **A,** Indicators of oral sexual abuse. Syphilis emerging as an ulcerated chancre on lip. **B,** Syphilis emerging as a mucous patch on lip.

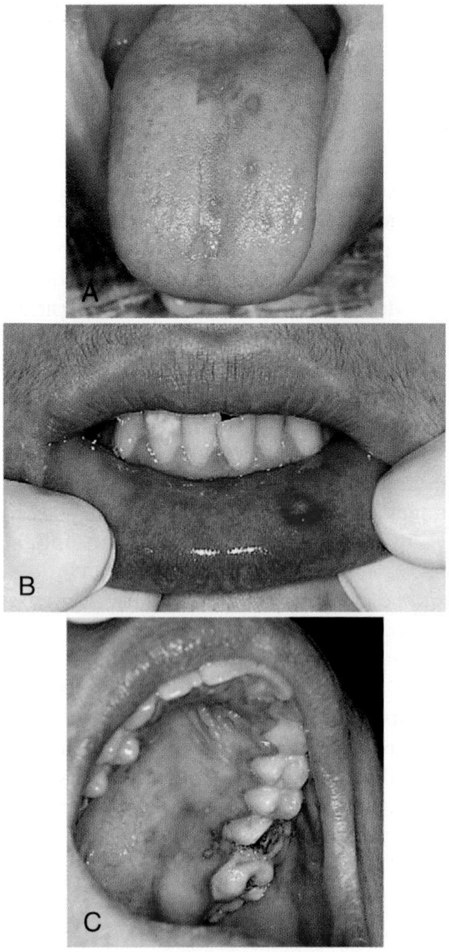

Figure 60-6. **A,** Indicators of oral sexual abuse. Herpetic gingivostomatitis in a child. **B** and **C,** Herpetic gingivostomatitis in an adolescent.

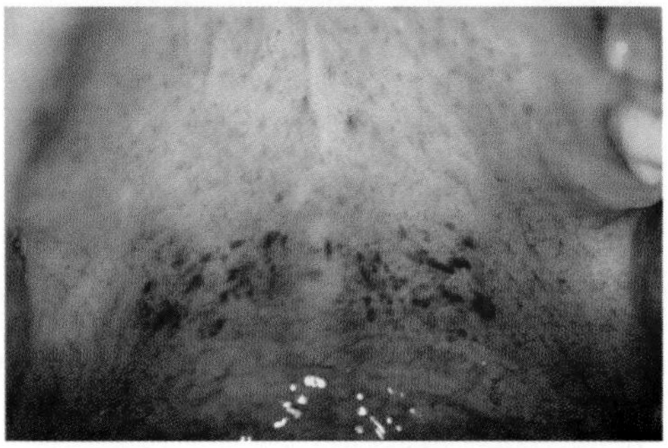

Figure 60-7. Indicator of oral sexual abuse. Palatal petechiae may indicate forced oral sex.

Dental neglect manifests as poor oral hygiene, untreated dental disease (rampant dental caries, pain, infection, bleeding, trauma), and lack of continuity of care once informed (Figure 60-8). The American Academy of Pediatric Dentistry defines dental neglect as the willful failure to seek and follow through with treatment to ensure oral health. Poor oral health literacy and/or lack of access to oral healthcare may contribute to dental neglect, presenting a conundrum for oral health

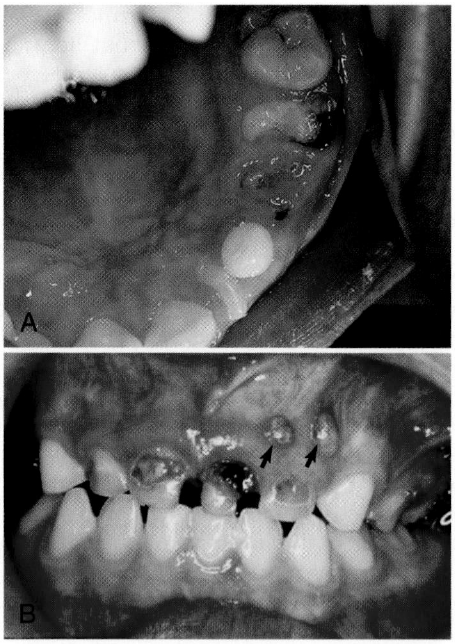

Figure 60-8. **A,** Dental neglect. Rampant dental caries destroyed primary maxillary molar to the root. **B,** Dental neglect. Multiple paruli caused by rampant tooth decay. (Courtesy Dr. Lynn Douglas Mouden, cofounder of P.A.N.D.A. [Prevention of Abuse and Neglect through Dental Awareness].)

professionals. Even with improved oral health literacy, inability to obtain care may continue as a result of barriers such as financial limitations, lack of providers, and geographic constraints.

Indicators of Maltreatment

The abused child may present with warning signs of abuse, such as repeated injuries (multiple bruises in different stage of healing) and/or inappropriate behaviors or a neglected appearance. The client may confide in the caregiver, complain of hunger or thirst, or display a lack of interest in the surroundings. Abuse victims may exhibit passive or withdrawn behavior, poor self-image, sexual acting out, depression, anxiety disorders, substance and alcohol abuse, eating disorders, hostility, lack of cooperation, self-destructive or self-abusive behavior, suicidal thoughts, social or academic problems, and/or reluctance to return to a waiting adult. The victim's abuser may monitor interactions, answer questions directed to the client, seem overly solicitous, refuse to leave the treatment area, or display hostility.

The goal of good parenting is enabling a child to grow up with feelings of satisfaction, security, and self-respect. An abused child may not experience these positive feelings because they are growing up in non-nurturing environments. Overly critical or strict parents and extremely isolated families are other warning signs of non-nurturing environments.

Nurturing caretakers would not hesitate to seek immediate medical or dental treatment for an injured child. Perpetrators, on the other hand, are typically less forthcoming about the nature of nonaccidental injuries and more likely to delay seeking treatment intentionally for the child because they fear discovery.

Abuse versus Findings Mistaken for Abuse

Physical findings mistaken for abuse may be of accidental, genetic, acquired, infectious, or cultural origin. Healthcare providers use their professional judgment and clinical skill to assess the location, size, shape, and mode of injuries. Accidental injuries normally heal at the same time, whereas injuries from abuse are in various stages of healing. Accidental injuries also normally occur over bony prominences such as knees and elbows, whereas injuries from abuse often occur on surfaces away from bony prominences such as the neck, head, trunk, buttocks, hands, and upper arms.[5]

Children are typically forward moving during activities, and therefore an accidental childhood injury would occur in areas of bony protuberances, such as knees, elbows, chin, and hands. In addition, several genetic conditions have manifestations that mimic the signs of physical abuse such as the following:

- Sturge-Weber syndrome (encephalotrigeminal angiomatosis) is a rare disorder that is present at birth. A child with this condition has a port-wine stain birthmark (usually on the face) and nervous system problems.
- Ehlers-Danlos syndrome (EDS) is a group of inherited connective tissue disorders marked by extremely loose joints, hyperelastic skin that bruises easily, and easily damaged blood vessels. Symptoms of EDS include fragile and stretchy skin and easy scarring and poor wound healing.
- Idiopathic thrombocytopenic purpura (ITP) (immune thrombocytopenic purpura) is a bleeding disorder in which the immune system destroys platelets, which are necessary for normal blood clotting. Persons with the disease have too few platelets in the blood. Symptoms include abnormally heavy menstruation; bleeding into the skin, which causes a characteristic skin rash that looks like pinpoint red spots (petechial rash): easy bruising, nosebleeds, or bleeding in the mouth.

HIV and hemophilia are acquired medical conditions that have indicators that mimic physical abuse. Infectious skin conditions such as eczema, dermatitis, or impetigo may be mistaken as abuse. Cultural practices such as cupping, coining, or scraping (gua sha) used in some families to alleviate illness may cause unintentional injuries to the child. In some cultures it is believed that use of cups warmed by a flame placed on the back of a child with respiratory illness will draw out the infections. The suction created by the cup-to-skin contact on the back leaves markings appearing to be the result of inflicted child abuse. In addition, copper is believed to be a healing metal. In some cultures, a copper coin is rubbed in various directions on the back of a sick child to help draw out illness. The rubbing produces various red markings on the child's back resembling abuse. Scraping, performed with a kitchen spoon rubbed over the back for up to 30 minutes, is an East Asian home remedy for respiratory problems. The scraped skin may look alarming but is reported to be not painful.

Assessment

All clients are assessed for health history and physical, behavioral, and oral findings. Documentation procedures are consistent among all dental hygiene clients. Consultation with other providers such as physicians, social workers, and other interdisciplinary professionals may be needed for the best client care.

Suspected cases of child maltreatment may warrant taking separate child and adult patient histories (stories) to elicit the nature of the observed injury.

- Do the child and adult histories match?
- Is there consistency with the injury, timeline, and explanation?
- Have other similar injuries occurred with the client and/or other household members?

Determine whether to discuss your suspicions with the adult based on the child's safety. Parents and caregivers should be approached separately, always in private, without the child or others present. Because there may be a suspicion of child maltreatment, there may be a lack of awareness by the adult who brought the child. Do not accuse or use judgmental language. Remind the adult that you are concerned about the welfare of the child and the well-being of all your clients. Effective statements if you decide to talk with the adult include the following:

- "Because I care about children and I care about your child…"
- "I am concerned about your situation…"
- "In my practice I care about my clients' overall health and well-being…"

Based on the interviewed adult's response:

- If the adult's response or attitude seems suspicious and you are not sure, you may consult with other health care providers or contact Child Protective Services (CPS).
- If you feel the child may be in danger…contact CPS.
- If the histories (stories) match…all is fine.

Documentation

Documentation includes text, photographs, and other pertinent information or data that serve as an official and legal record of present and past dental or dental hygiene care. Separate fact from opinion.

If child maltreatment is suspected, the following documentation should be included:

- All clinical and behavioral findings in the client record
- Conversations that transpired during the appointment
  - Full names should be used
  - Use quotes for verbal statements associated with the person
- Record reason for seeking treatment (or reason for delay in treatment)
- Obtain usual consent for clinical photographic and or radiographic needs
- Document report made to CPS

Family Violence

More than 3 million children are victims of family violence[8]:

- 87% are aware of domestic violence
- 69% have witnessed domestic violence
- More than 60% are also victims
- 90% are under age 10
- 64% under age 2

Long-range health implications in children have been attributed to domestic violence exposure. The Adverse Childhood Experiences Study (ACES) is the largest public health study that assessed associations between childhood maltreatment and later-life health and well-being.[11] Ten categories of

BOX 60-1

Childhood Risk Factors Leading to Chronic Health, Psychologic, and Social Problems in Adulthood

Recurrent emotional abuse
Sexual abuse
Recurrent physical abuse
Alcohol and/or drug abuser in household
Incarcerated household member
Presence of a chronically depressed household member
Mentally ill, institutionalized, or suicidal household member
Mother is treated violently
One or no parents in the household
Emotional or physical neglect

childhood experiences (Box 60-1) were identified that are major risk factors for the leading causes of illness and death as well as poor quality of life in the United States. For those children who have been victims of abuse and/or neglect or witnessed domestic violence in the home or who have experienced any combination of adverse childhood situations are at a greater risk for chronic health, psychologic, and social dysfunction throughout adulthood. Clearly, abuse and neglect have far-reaching negative risks for the health, well-being, and longevity of its traumatized victims.

Bullying

Bullying is the use of force or coercion to abuse or intimidate others. The behavior can be habitual and involve an imbalance of social or physical power. It can include verbal harassment or threat, or physical assault directed repeatedly toward particular victims, perhaps on the grounds of race, religion, gender, sexuality, or ability. It may be in person or electronic.

In addition, bullies, victims of bullying, and bully-victims were more likely to be exposed to violence at home.[12] Bullying is an extremely prevalent public health problem, and it does not happen in isolation. Bullying continues in a variety of settings, including in schools; cyberspace via computers, cell phones, and other devices; and the workplace.

Domestic Violence

Domestic violence and bullying are similar forms of abuse with the power and control behaviors of one person dominating another. Domestic violence/intimate partner violence (IPV) is a pattern of abusive behavior in any relationship that is used by one partner to gain or maintain power and control over another intimate partner occurring in heterosexual and homosexual partnerships and dating relationships. IPV crosses all barriers including age, race, economic level, educational level, and ethnic groups. IPV victims are primarily women, but men are also victims. Sexual violence, stalking, and intimate partner violence are major public health problems in the United States. More than one in three women and more than one in four men in the United States have experienced rape, physical violence, and/or stalking by an intimate partner in their lifetime.[13] Ninety-four percent of high school students report being hit, slapped, or physically hurt on purpose by their boyfriend or girlfriend.[14]

Routinely ask about IPV always in private and document disclosures. Always assess the safety of the client and refer to local resources for assistance in leaving the abusive relationship. Examples of screening questions are the following:

- "Do you feel safe at home?"
- "Because domestic violence is so common, we are asking all our clients, because we know health is affected by this."
- "Has your partner ever threatened you?"

If adults deny any issues, you may jeopardize their safety if you pursue the line of questioning. If a client discloses information, the oral health professional should assure the client by using such phrases as, "It is not your fault, help is available, and I can give you information if you like." If client denies abuse, but you suspect IPV, your response may be, "I'm concerned. There is help available for you. I have information if you would like." You should never put yourself or the client in jeopardy by forcing the issue if the client does not feel safe pursuing or receiving further information at the time.

Domestic violence is rampant, yet not all states have mandatory reporting requirements for IPV. Many states do, however, encompass domestic violence reporting requirements under laws requiring the reporting of injuries resulting from violent criminal acts, deadly weapons, or moving vessels. Oral health professionals should check their state's legislative policies for reporting responsibilities.

Elderly and Vulnerable Adults

Definitions in state laws vary for elder and vulnerable adult maltreatment Generally, however, **elder and vulnerable adult maltreatment** is a term referring to any knowing, intentional, or negligent act by a caregiver or any other person that causes harm or a serious risk of harm to a vulnerable adult, which occurs in three different areas: domestic, institutional, and self-neglect or self-inflicted.

Domestic elder abuse generally refers to any form of maltreatment of an older person by someone who has a relationship with them (a spouse, a sibling, a child, a friend, or a caregiver), which occurs in the home. **Institutional abuse** occurs in residential facilities (e.g., nursing homes, foster homes, group homes, **board** and **care facilities**). Perpetrators of institutional abuse usually are staff, professionals, or caregivers who are paid to provide care and protection.

Elder maltreatment and self-neglect are separate yet related sets of behaviors and interactions. **Self-neglect** is the harm or the potential for harm created by one's own behaviors rather than resulting from others' actions. Self-neglect occurs when vulnerable adults fail or refuse to address their own basic physical, emotional, or social needs.

Elder maltreatment includes the following:

- Physical abuse
- Financial exploitation
- Emotional abuse
- Sexual abuse
- Neglect

Most reports of elder maltreatment involve neglect. Elder neglect includes failure of caregivers to provide (1) protection from health and safety hazards such as withholding medical devices and medications and (2) basic needs such as personal hygiene, clothing, shelter, or nutrition, and failure to follow up with medical/dental care.

Elder abuse is expected to rise as the number of older Americans increases. Any person can be mistreated, but it is more likely to occur in an individual who is frail because of a disabling chronic condition or who suffers from a cognitive disorder such as dementia. However, not all elderly adults are vulnerable. Conversely, not all vulnerable adults are elderly. Often, because of social isolation and limited mobility, visits to medical or dental professionals are the only contact that elderly or vulnerable adults have outside the home. This places the burden of identifying maltreatment in the hands of healthcare professionals.

Human Trafficking

Human trafficking is a form of modern-day slavery, in which people profit from the control and exploitation of others. As defined under U.S. federal law, victims of human trafficking include children involved in the sex trade, adults age 18 or over who are coerced or deceived into commercial sex acts, and anyone forced into different forms of "labor or services," such as domestic workers held in a home or farm workers forced to labor against their will. The common factors among each of these situations include elements of force, fraud, or coercion that are used to control people.

Human trafficking is a crime against humanity. Thousands of men, women, and children are victims of human trafficking in their own countries and abroad. Trafficking includes recruiting, transporting, transferring, harboring, or receiving a person through use of force or coercion to exploit them. Every country holds responsibility for trafficking, whether as country of origin, transit, or destination for victims.

Human trafficking is the fastest growing and second largest criminal industry in the world. Over the last 10 years there has been a significant awareness of the criminality of human trafficking, yet health consequences for the victims are now just surfacing. Given the prevalence and migratory nature of trafficking, public health implications indicate the need for healthcare providers to be trained adequately to provide appropriate and safe care for trafficked victims. Many victims encounter a healthcare professional, and these individuals may not be recognized as victims by the untrained healthcare provider. Most victims suffer from malnutrition and therefore are subject to severe dental decay and pain. Many of the victims are children. Potential health consequences of human trafficking include mental health issues, effects of physical violence and sexual abuse, and risks associated with unhygienic and overcrowded working and living conditions, which may result in infectious illnesses.

Traffickers control victims using financial tactics such as debt bondage and economic control. Other means of control include social restriction (isolating victims and restricting contact and movement) and legal insecurity (including threat of deportation or reporting immigration violation). Traffickers are family members, community members, neighborhood or nationally known gangs, international criminal syndicates, or small-scale, "mom and pop" organizations.

Indicators of trafficked victims may include the following:

- Victim is brought to the office by someone and is not allowed to come alone.
- Client may be shy.
- Another is "in charge" of them.
- Trafficker dictates the dental treatment.
- Victims have no form of identification.
- They do not speak or understand English.
- The trafficker wants the best dental work; cost is no object.
- Esthetics is the reason for the visit, not the victim's health.
- Victim will be taken to more than one office and will not have a dental "home."

Because human trafficking is a federal crime, dental hygienists should report all victims to the Federal Bureau of Investigation (FBI), Department of Homeland Security.

Disclosures of Abuse

Given a relationship of trust and rapport, clients may disclose personal information or confide in the dental hygienist. Dental hygienists who suspect abuse can create an opportunity for the client to mention an abuse problem by saying something like the following:

- "Now that violence against women is so common, and there is help available for those who suffer from abuse, I am asking all clients routinely about violence in their lives."
- "Are you in a relationship that threatens or hurts you?"
- "Is someone hurting you?"

Although maintaining confidentiality is important, allegations or reports of abuse must be reported as required by law and ethics (referred to as **disclosure**). When a client reports abuse, the hygienist must document that disclosure in the client record and report the disclosure to the proper authorities. It is not the responsibility of the dental professional to diagnose or investigate suspected abuse; rather, law enforcement and CPS agencies have the expertise and resources to investigate such reports.

Reporting Abuse

Persons required by state statutes to report suspected abuse and neglect to the proper agency are **mandated reporters for child and vulnerable adult victims**. Dental hygienists and dentists are mandated reporters for child abuse/neglect, vulnerable adults, and victims of human trafficking. State-established **immunity** laws protect reporters from civil law or criminal penalties resulting from filing a confidential report of suspected abuse and/or neglect.

Each state has its own reporting mechanisms for suspected abuse and/or neglect. For example, suspected child abuse or neglect can be reported to CPS, but the mechanisms for reporting suspected IPV, domestic violence, and elder or vulnerable adult abuse can vary. Some states have dedicated family violence or adult protective services, but regardless of the state or type of abuse suspected, oral health professionals always may report suspected abuse as an emergency by dialing 911.

Oral healthcare professionals do not gather evidence to build an abuse or neglect case if they suspect abuse; rather, their duty is to report their suspicions to the appropriate authority and document their observations in the client record. As a legal document, the treatment record must document objectively all findings and disclosures made by the client.

For a complete list of definitions and reporting hotlines, go to the website for U.S. Department of Health & Human Services, Administration for Children & Families, http://www.childwelfare.gov/responding/reporting.cfm. Other

BOX 60-2

Abuse and Neglect Resources

- Family Violence Prevention Fund, (800) 595-4889
- National Health Resource Center on Domestic Violence, (888) 792-2873
- National Committee for the Prevention of Elder Abuse, (646) 462-3603
- National Coalition Against Domestic Violence, (303) 839-1852
- National Human Trafficking Resource Center, (888) 373-7888

abuse and neglect resources are listed in Box 60-2 and the Web resources section of the Evolve website.

Reporting is not an accusation; it is a cry for help. Painful physical, cognitive, and emotional effects may result from not reporting; of course, the worst consequence is death. Victims often become adult offenders.

Child Protective Services (CPS) and law enforcement have the expertise and resources to investigate such reports. CPS is the designated agency that receives child maltreatment reports, investigates cases, and provides intervention and treatment services to children and families when child maltreatment has occurred. Frequently, this agency is located within governmental social service agencies, such as the Department of Social Services.

Adult Protective Services are those services provided to older people and people with disabilities who are in danger of being mistreated or neglected, are unable to protect themselves, and have no one to assist them. Mandated reporting by oral health professionals varies among states for the elderly and victims of domestic violence. Refer to your state licensing board for reporting requirements. A complete state-by-state list of toll-free elder reporting and adult protective services can be found in the Web resources section of the Evolve website related to Chapter 60.

Legal and Liability Issues

Failure to report suspected neglect and/or abuse by a mandated reporter can carry harsh penalties, including fines and prison times. Penalties for failing to report neglect or abuse can range from 10 days' to 5 years' imprisonment and fines ranging from $100 to $5000. Although penalties vary, most states classify a first failure to report as a misdemeanor; however, several states upgrade a second failure to report to a felony. Failure to report suspected abuse jeopardizes the dental professional's license, but even worse, a victim may be harmed further or die.

Why Dental Health Professionals Fail to Report

The American Dental Association's Principles of Ethics and Code of Professional Conduct states that its members "shall be obliged to become familiar with the signs of abuse and neglect and to report suspected cases to the proper authorities." Nonetheless, lack of reports of suspected abuse and neglect by oral healthcare providers stems from lack of knowledge of requirements and procedures. Dental hygienists and dentists must be aware of reporting requirements and know the signs and symptoms of abuse and neglect.

CLIENT EDUCATION TIPS

- Provide community-based domestic violence resources in dental office restrooms or inconspicuous places where the victim can get away from the perpetrator, read, and memorize helpline phone numbers.
- Encourage client–dental hygienist communication without being judgmental.
- Ask clients about physical findings and observations related to suspected abuse or accidental injuries.
- Let client know that help is available to escape an abusive relationship.

LEGAL, ETHICAL, AND SAFETY ISSUES

- The law provides protection for mandated reporters who make their report in good faith.
- Given certain state requirements and the litigation protection provided to mandated reporters, failure to report suspected neglect and/or abuse by a mandated reporter can carry harsh penalties, including fines and prison time.
- Failure of a mandated reporter to report suspected abuse is a misdemeanor in most states.
- All states have enacted legislation for prosecution of persons who falsely report abuse cases (reports made without having a reasonable belief that the report is true).
- Visit the state's child protective services website, and contact the state bar association for specific information about child, domestic, and elder abuse.

KEY CONCEPTS

- Dental hygienists should be especially cognizant of physical abuse, because the majority of all physical signs of abuse occur on the neck and craniofacial regions.
- Legislation in all 50 states mandates that dentists and dental hygienists report suspicions of child abuse and neglect, vulnerable adult abuse and neglect, and victims of human trafficking to appropriate agencies and provides protection from retaliatory litigation from perpetrators.
- Failure of a mandated reporter to report suspected child abuse or neglect is a misdemeanor in most states, punishable by fine and/or imprisonment.
- Parents or guardians of abused children often change physicians, but they are more likely to continue to visit their child's dentist.
- Neglect accounts for most of all reported cases of abuse in the United States.
- Each state establishes its own definitions for abuse within the minimum standards set by federal legislation.
- The American Academy of Pediatrics reports that lips are the most common site of injuries associated with child abuse.
- Oral indicators of abuse include a wide range of oral injuries that are evident during an oral examination.
- Because the client's dental hygiene care record is a legal document, the dental hygienist should record all indicators of abuse or neglect accurately and clearly.
- Given a relationship of trust and rapport, clients may disclose information to dental hygienists pertaining to abuse.
- Oral healthcare professionals do not diagnose or investigate incidents of suspected abuse and neglect. Rather, they

report suspected cases of abuse or neglect to the proper authorities.

CRITICAL THINKING EXERCISES

Consider these questions when analyzing the following cases:

1. Do you recognize any signs or symptoms of abuse and neglect?
2. Is the client in a dangerous situation?
3. Is there a risk to the client's safety if you approach the caregiver or the person accompanying the client to the appointment to seek additional information?
4. Is this incident reportable by mandate? Why?
5. What actions should be initiated by an oral healthcare professional?
6. Given the legal jurisdiction of licensure, what agency is contacted to report a case of suspected abuse or neglect?

Case Study 1: You are the dental hygienist treating a 12-year-old girl whose parents are going through a divorce. The girl lives with her mother, and her parents are working out custody arrangements through the judicial system. During the past 4 months, the girl failed to show up for two of three previously scheduled restorative appointments. On examination you find very poor plaque control and the same unrestored carious lesions noted from the last visit. The girl now complains of tooth sensitivity when drinking cold beverages, which prompted the father to make today's appointment. On review of the girl's record, you note that the caries and poor oral hygiene were discussed with the mother and the girl and also documented during her initial examination and the one restorative visit that was attended. During today's appointment, you speak with the girl's father, explain the importance of good oral hygiene and the need to control the progression of the caries, and recommend that the carious teeth be restored as soon as possible. The girl's father makes the recommended restorative appointments to address his daughter's unrestored caries and painful oral symptoms. The father schedules the recommended restorative appointments and seems concerned about his daughter's oral health. He states that the girl's mother will hear about this in court.

Discussion of Case 1: Initially, this scenario may appear to be a case of neglect given that the client has several untreated carious lesions and the mother failed to keep two of the previous three restorative appointments despite being fully informed of the caries. According to the CAPTA definition of abuse, because the client was not in pain at prior appointments and there was no evidence of impaired function or quality of life until today, this scenario, although sad that some of the caries have progressed, most likely does not qualify as a case of neglect. There is no indication that the mother or the father willfully failed to ensure a level of oral health essential for adequate function and freedom from pain and infection. Because the dad secured a dental appointment as soon as his daughter complained of cold sensitivity, brought her in for her visit today, and was compliant with making the recommended restorative appointments, he appears to demonstrate the behaviors of a concerned, nurturing parent. Because he is not living with his daughter and he has a strained relationship with the girl's mother, he may have been unaware of the missed visits and the unrestored caries. He appears to want to rectify the missed appointment and seems committed to improving his daughter's oral health. He and his daughter appear to have a positive father-daughter relationship. The daughter spoke fondly of time she gets to spend with her father. Given the extensive education that you provided to the father and the daughter and the father's follow-through with recommended treatment, it is likely he will be more proactive and alert to his daughter's oral health in the future. Although there is no indication that the mother willfully failed to ensure a level of oral health essential for adequate function and freedom from pain and infection, you nonetheless will be cognizant of the social and family situation of your client and alert to enhanced need for follow-through with recommended treatment should the mother present with the daughter for future dental visits. It is also important not to take sides when there is a family conflict. The priority and concern is the child's oral health and well-being and not the conflict between the mother and the father.

The dental hygienist is expected to document clinical findings, note to whom oral health information and recommendations are provided when treating minor children, report suspicions of dental neglect when signs and symptoms are present, and consult with CPS agencies when in doubt.

Case Study 2: You are the dental hygienist treating an 8-year-old boy who has been a client in your practice for several years. The child appears withdrawn and won't make eye contact when you speak to him. The boy winces when you ask him to lay back in your dental chair. Your extraoral palpation exam of the boy's head and neck is physically uncomfortable for the boy who expresses his neck and throat hurt. Your oral assessment reveals a torn maxillary frenum and cuts and bruising of the maxillary gingivae and alveolar mucosa. When asked how the injuries occurred, the child says that he fell off his swing set. Suspicious, you review the client's record to see if there are any past references to oral injuries and discover that the boy had similar injuries several visits ago, reportedly from falling off his scooter. You look carefully at the client's face, neck, and arms for any other signs, and you notice faint bruising on all sides of the boy's neck and on both of his upper arms. The marks on his upper arms look like marks that thumbs and fingers would leave if both arms are grabbed and squeezed at the same time. When you ask the child's mother about the injuries, she pauses and then says that she thinks it happened when he tripped down the stairs last week. Suddenly she becomes concerned about what her son has told you, says that he lies a lot, and abruptly ends the appointment stating she has another appointment to get to, and doesn't allow his treatment to be completed.

Discussion of Case 2: Although the child's oral injuries could occur from a fall, the bruises on the back and both sides of his neck, as well as bilaterally on both arms are not likely to have occurred from a fall off a swing nor from falling down stairs. Accidental falls would likely result in asymmetric injuries on the upper and lower portions of the body, as well as to hands and fingers from the child trying to stop his fall. The combination of the oral and upper body injuries, delay in seeking treatment, and the inconsistent history of the injuries reported by the child and mother are signs of nonaccidental trauma. The oral injuries are more consistent with trauma from being slapped or force-fed, for example, having a cup or utensil forced into the mouth. When someone is grabbed forcefully by the upper arms by another person, the thumbs of the perpetrator could leave a thumb-bruise print along with the prints of fingers that are wrapped around the back of the upper arm. Similar "tattoo" markings from the thumbs and fingers of the perpetrator would be evident on the child's neck when strangled. When the mother's sudden change in behavior and the child's withdrawn demeanor are considered along with a documented history of the same type of injury, there is most likely enough information to arouse suspicion. If you suspect abuse, as an oral healthcare professional you have a legal and moral obligation to report your suspicions immediately to Child Protective Services.

REFERENCES

1. Mouden LD: Dentistry addressing family violence, *Missouri Dent J* 76(6):21, 24, 27, 1996.
2. World Health Organization: *Global health risks: mortality and burden of disease attributable to selected major risks*, Geneva, Switzerland, 2009, World Health Organization Press. Available at: http://www.who.int/healthinfo/global_burden_disease/GlobalHealthRisks_report_full.pdf. Accessed November 27, 2012.
3. Mouden LD, Bross DC: Legal issues affecting dentistry's role in preventing child abuse and neglect, *J Am Dent Assoc* 126(8):1173, 1995. Available at: http://jada.ada.org/content/126/8/1173.full.pdf+html. Accessed November 15, 2012.
4. American Academy of Pediatric Dentistry: *Guideline on oral and dental aspects of child abuse and neglect*. Reference Manual. Clinical Guidelines, Adopted 1999, Revised 2005, Reaffirmed 2010. 34(6):158-161. Available at: http://www.aapd.org/policies/. Accessed November 7, 2012.
5. Kellogg N: Oral and dental aspects of child abuse and neglect, *Pediatrics* 116(6):1565, 2005. Available at: http://pediatrics.aappublications.org/content/116/6/1565.full.pdf. Accessed November 15, 2012.
6. Gutmann ME, Solomon ES: Family violence content in dental hygiene curricula: a national survey, *J Dent Educ* 66(9):999, 2002.
7. Nelms AP, Gutmann ME, Solomon ES, et al: What victims of domestic violence need from the dental profession, *J Dent Educ* 73(4):490, 2009.
8. U.S. Department of Health and Human Services, Administration on Children, Youth and Families, Children's Bureau: *Child maltreatment 2009, 2010*, 2011. Available at: http://www.acf.hhs.gov/programs/cb/stats_research/index.htm#can. Accessed November 25, 2012.
9. Centers for Disease Control and Prevention, National Center for Injury Prevention and Control, Division of Violence Prevention: *The public health approach to violence prevention*. Available at: http://www.cdc.gov/ViolencePrevention/overview/publichealthapproach.html. Accessed November 26, 2012.
10. Child Welfare League of America, Practice Areas: *Child protection*. Available at: http://www.cwla.org/programs/childprotection/default.htm. Accessed November 26, 2012.
11. Corso PS, Edwards VJ, Fang X, et al: Health-related quality of life among adults who experienced maltreatment during childhood, *Am J Public Health* 98(6):1094, 2008. Available at: http://www.ncbi.nlm.nih.gov/pmc/articles/PMC2377283/. Accessed November 26, 2012.
12. Centers for Disease Control: Bullying among middle school and high school students—Massachusetts, 2009, *MMWR Morb Mortal Wkly Rep* 60(15):465, 2011. Available at: http://www.cdc.gov/mmwr/preview/mmwrhtml/mm6015a1.htm?s_cid=mm6015a1_w. Accessed November 27, 2012.
13. Black MC, Basile KC, Breiding MJ, et al: *The National Intimate Partner and Sexual Violence Survey (NISVS): 2010 Summary report.* Atlanta, 2011, National Center for Injury Prevention and Control, Centers for Disease Control and Prevention. Available at: http://www.cdc.gov/violenceprevention/pdf/nisvs_report2010-a.pdf. Accessed November 28, 2012.
14. Centers for Disease Control and Prevention: *Youth risk behavior surveillance—United States, 2011, MMWR Morb Mortal Wkly Rep* 61(4):1, 2012.

EVOLVE RESOURCES

Please visit http://evolve.elsevier.com/Darby/hygiene for additional practice and study support tools.

CHAPTER 61

Palliative Oral Care

Elizabeth T. Couch, Margaret M. Walsh

COMPETENCIES:

1. **Define palliative care, including:**
   - **Discuss the purpose of palliative care and its goals based on the World Health Organization.**
   - **Explain the importance of palliative oral care at end of life.**
2. **Discuss palliative oral care, including:**
   - **Explain standard oral hygiene care.**
   - **Assess signs and symptoms of oral complications commonly found among palliative care patients and intervene appropriately to maximize comfort using oral care.**
3. **Describe the role of the dental hygienist as part of the palliative care team.**
4. **Explain the steps of the dental hygiene process of care.**

Any form of care that focuses on decreasing disease symptom severity in individuals with life-limiting illnesses rather than trying to delay or reverse disease progression is called palliative care.[1]

Traditionally, palliative care includes an interdisciplinary team of physicians, social workers, pharmacists, nurses, and chaplains. The importance of oral care often is overlooked in palliative care settings because of the absence of dental professionals, such as dental hygienists, as members of the palliative care team.[2,3] **Palliative Oral Care** is the management and prevention of oral problems caused by a patient's disease or from treatments received. Palliative oral care focuses on the patient's immediate quality of life. This chapter focuses on palliative care, palliative oral care, oral complications commonly found among patients with life-limiting illness, and evidence-based dental hygiene interventions aimed at maximizing comfort and quality of life in individuals with life-limiting illnesses. In addition, the role of the dental hygienist as part of the palliative care team is addressed.

Palliative Care

According to the World Health Organization (WHO), palliative care is "a healthcare approach that improves the quality of life of patients and their families who face problems associated with life-limiting illnesses. Palliative care aims to prevent and relieve suffering by early identification, assessment, and treatment of pain and other types of physical, psychologic, emotional, and spiritual distresses."[4] Specific goals of palliative care are listed in Box 61-1.

Although the term *palliative care* initially referred to end-of-life palliative care, the scope of palliative care has expanded to include maintaining and improving quality of life for all patients and their families during any stage of a life-limiting illness, whether acute, chronic, or terminal.

Palliative care often is initiated after a person receives a diagnosis of a life-limiting illness. It can be delivered in the home as well as in long-term and acute care facilities. Palliative care often includes hospice care before or at the end of life. End of life has been defined by the Institute of Medicine as "the period of time during which an individual copes with declining health from a terminal illness or from the frailties associated with advanced age, even if death is not clearly imminent."[1] Hospice is not a place, but a concept of care that provides compassion, support, and care for persons in the last phases of terminal illness so that they may live as fully and comfortably as possible.[1] Palliative care extends into the end-of-life period, the final phase of one's illness, as well as the bereavement period after the patient's death. Communication among the patient, the family, and the palliative healthcare team is important to provide optimal care.

Palliative Oral Care

Oral care is important in all phases of palliative care (Figure 61-1). A mouth free of discomfort and bad odors helps to maintain self-esteem and aids in social communication, preventing some of the loneliness experienced at the end stage of life. During this time, the mouth often becomes the center of existence because it maintains nutritional status and is used to communicate needs and emotions to loved ones.

A consistent oral assessment is needed to evaluate oral mucosal changes and other oral complications from medical treatment. Based on this assessment, evidence-based interventions are implemented to improve patient comfort and quality of life. Oral problems are frequent in patients receiving palliative care. Evidence suggests that meticulous oral hygiene care often can prevent the onset of such problems and dramatically improves the patient's quality of life.[5] Therefore it is important to ensure that standard oral hygiene care is implemented for every patient receiving palliative care.

Standard Oral Hygiene Care

If the mouth is determined to be healthy, then standard oral hygiene care is prescribed for the patient to perform on a daily basis (Box 61-2). Standard oral hygiene care includes brushing all teeth and cleaning the tongue twice daily, and lubricating the lips with gauze moistened with water-based products, such as Oral Balance gel (Laclede Professional

Figures, tables, and boxes marked as "e" are available as supplemental material on the Evolve site. Visit http://evolve.elsevier.com/Darby/hygiene to access these materials.

BOX 61-1

Goals of Palliative Care

- Provide relief from symptoms, especially pain.
- Support holistic patient care and enhance quality of life.
- Offer support to patients to live as actively as possible until death.
- Affirm life and neither hasten nor postpone death.
- Regard dying as a normal process.
- Offer support to family during the patient's illness and in their own bereavement.

Adapted from World Health Organization. Available at: http://www.who.int/cancer/palliative/definition/en.

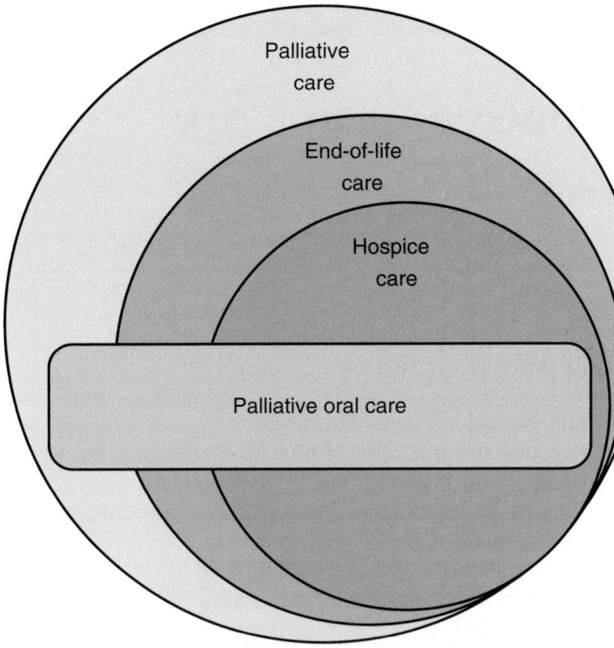

Figure 61-1. Palliative oral care as it relates to palliative care, end-of-life care, and hospice care. (Adapted from Heitkemper M: Palliative care at end-of-life. In Lewis SL: *Medical-surgical nursing*, ed 8, St Louis, 2011, Elsevier, pp 153.)

BOX 61-2

Standard Oral Hygiene Care

NO DENTURES

- Brush teeth twice daily with a soft toothbrush.
- Electric toothbrushes with a small head are easier to use on patients.
- Toothbrushes should be changed every 3 months or more frequently if there has been a fungal infection.
- If the mouth is sore, use an extra-soft brush (e.g., Colgate 360° Sensitive Pro-Relief).
- Toothpaste with 1000 ppm fluoride should ideally be used.
- If patients cannot tolerate toothpaste, then fluoride mouth rinse or water is sufficient.
- Clean tongue using soft toothbrush or tongue scraper.
- Lubricate lips with gauze moistened with water-based product.
- Refer to dentist when needed.

DENTURES

- Take lower denture out first and put upper in first.
- Rinse mouth and dentures with water after meals.
- Remove dentures at night.
- Clean with soap and water using a soft denture brush twice daily; rinse over a partially filled bowl.
- Soak overnight in dilute sodium hypochlorite (1:9 parts water).
- Soak those with metal clasps in 0.12% chlorhexidine solution or alkaline peroxide, found in many denture-cleansing products.

Adapted from the National Health Service. Oral Care Guidelines for Publicly Funded Healthcare Systems in the United Kingdom. Reference number C028. 2010, Herefordshire Primary Care Trust.

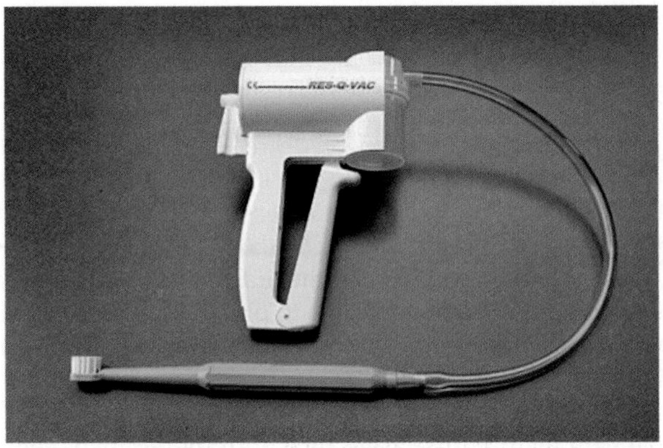

Figure 61-2. Plak-Vac/Res-Q-Vac Combination suction toothbrush. (Copyright 2010 Trademark Medical.)

Products, Gardena, CA). Toothbrushing techniques differ depending on the patients' ability to swallow or spit. For those who have no difficulty swallowing or spitting, a small smear of fluoride toothpaste can be used. For patients with xerostomia, a small smear of no-foaming toothpaste (e.g., Biotene) is recommended. For those who have difficulty swallowing and spitting, a suction toothbrush (Figure 61-2), dipped in a nonalcohol fluoride rinse with concurrent suction use is needed.[6]

Standard oral hygiene care also includes denture care for patients with removable prosthetics (see Chapter 56). Patients with ill-fitting dentures must be referred to the dentist for denture adjustment to avoid the onset of denture sores or ulcers (Figure 61-3). Dentures must be removed at night and cleaned with soap and water using a soft denture brush twice daily and soaked overnight in a labeled container of liquid solution such as water or dilute sodium hypochlorite (1:9 parts water). Appliances with metal clasps, however, must be soaked in 0.12% chlorhexidine gluconate or alkaline peroxide solution found in many denture-cleansing products to avoid corrosion of the metal. Dentures should be rinsed well before use. They are not left out to dry, because they will warp and change form. Modifications to standard oral hygiene care are done on a case-by-case basis, depending on the individual needs of each patient.[6]

Standard oral hygiene care also may include the use of mouth rinses to promote patient comfort because they can leave a fresh and pleasant taste in the mouth. A mouth rinse should be used in conjunction with good oral care.

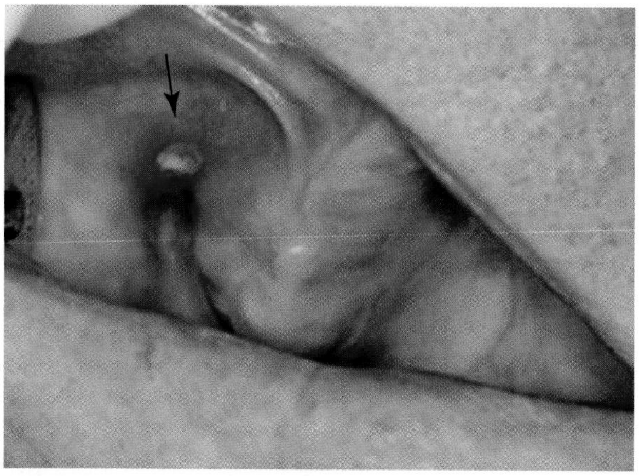

Figure 61-3. Ulcer from ill-fitting denture. (Courtesy Margaret Walsh.)

BOX 61-3

Recommended Mouth Rinses to Promote Oral Health and Comfort

- Water or sodium chloride 0.9% solution given warm or cold, as needed
- 0.12% chlorhexidine solution (alcohol-free) can be used for patients with or at risk of bacterial infection but should not be used more than twice daily
- 0.05% fluoride mouth rinse is nontraumatic, pleasant tasting, prevents dental caries, and helps relieve the pain of sensitive teeth

Data from Sweeney P: Oral hygiene. In Davies A, Finlay I: *Oral care in advanced disease*, 2005, Oxford University Press.

Alcohol-containing mouth rinses are to be used with caution because of their drying effect on the oral tissues. Box 61-3 lists some recommended mouth rinses to promote oral health and enhance patient comfort.

Patients Who Need Assistance with Standard Oral Hygiene Care

For patients who require assistance with the performance of standard mouth care, the dental hygienist educates the primary caregiver or family member on how to perform daily standard mouth care, which may include denture care (see Box 61-2).

Intubated Patients

For intubated and semi-conscious or unconscious patients, Box 61-4 describes the recommended standard oral care procedure to be followed. A suction toothbrush (see Figure 61-2) and disposable mouth prop are used when performing oral care on persons with a decreased level of consciousness to avoid aspiration or injury.[7,8] For additional information on patient positioning and stabilization see Chapter 41.

Oral Complications

If pain is reported and signs of oral complications are observed, then appropriate evidence-based interventions must be implemented immediately to ensure the patient's comfort and quality of life. Common oral complications observed or reported in palliative care patients are mucositis, ulcers, oral candidiasis, and xerostomia.

BOX 61-4

Treatment for Patients Requiring Assistance and Intubated Patients

- Gather supplies.
- Don mask and gloves.
- Position for comfort and control.
- Use disposable mouth prop.
- Lubricate lips with water-based product.
- Clean teeth, gingiva, tongue with soft toothbrush or gauze moistened with fluoride or chlorhexidine mouth rinse 2 to 3 times daily.
- Suction to remove excess secretions.
- Power or suction toothbrush may be needed, especially with intubated patients.

Data from Wiseman M: The treatment of oral problems in the palliative patient, *J Can Dent Assoc* 72(5):453, 2006; Feider L, Mitchell P, Bridges E: Oral care practices for orally intubated critically ill adults, *Am J Critical Care* 19(2):175, 2010.

Mucositis and Ulcerations

Mucositis is a condition that commonly occurs in patients receiving palliative care, especially those undergoing cancer chemotherapy and radiation treatment (see Figure 61-4). Chemotherapy affects the oral cavity by reducing the mitosis rate in the oral tissues.[8] A reduction in mitosis predominantly causes atrophy in the tissues of the floor of the mouth, buccal mucosa, and soft palate. In the chronic presence of plaque biofilm, tissue atrophy soon leads to erythema and edema, which often progresses into painful ulcerations (Figure 61-4). These oral ulcerations not only cause discomfort but also create a portal for oral flora to cause systemic infections. Chemotherapy drugs such as 5-fluorouracil and methotrexate cause mucositis within 5 to 7 days of treatment, lasting a few weeks if no secondary infection occurs.[9] Moreover, radiation therapy acts on salivary glands, causing xerostomia, creating a more susceptible environment for pathogen invasion and onset of painful ulcerations.[8]

Chemotherapy and radiation-induced mucositis often presents clinically as red, edematous tissue with a yellow membrane covering the ulcerations. Individuals with mucositis often report a burning, tingling sensation followed by generalized pain and discomfort, often hindering the patient's ability to talk, eat, and swallow (see Chapter 45).

Management

Mucositis and ulcer management involves primarily prevention and relief from pain and discomfort (see Table 61-1 and eBox 61-5). Keeping the client's mouth clean and hydrated is key to preventing mucositis onset. Warm baking soda, saline, and water rinses every 1 to 3 hours for 7 days helps soothe the ulcerated tissue while hydrating and neutralizing the pH in the mouth (Box 61-6). Clients with mucositis also need to rinse with 10 mL of 0.12% chlorhexidine solution (alcohol free) twice daily to reduce the oral bacterial load and help prevent the onset of secondary infections. Topical corticosteroids also may be used with caution to reduce oral discomfort because they may decrease the gag reflex, increasing the risk of aspiration pneumonia (Box 61-6), the leading cause of

TABLE 61-1
Common Oral Complications: Signs and Symptoms, Prevention, and Treatment

Manifestation	Signs and Symptoms	Prevention	Treatment
Mucositis and Ulcerations 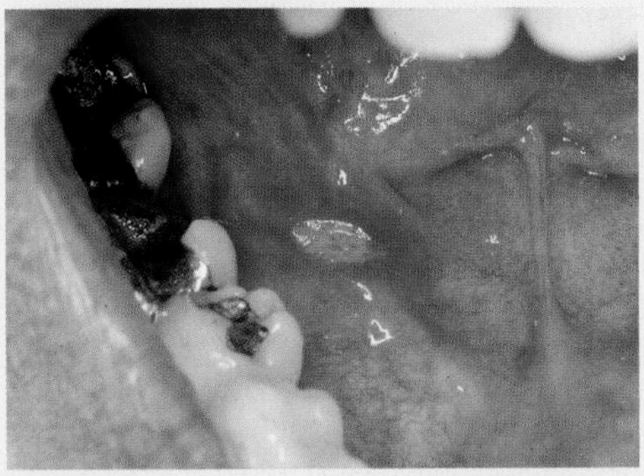 **Figure 61-4.** Oral ulceration from cancer treatment. (From Ibsen OAC, Phelan JA: *Oral pathology for the dental hygienist,* ed 6, St Louis, 2013, Saunders.)	• Red, swollen tissue • Yellow membrane-covered • Burning, pain, and general discomfort reported by client	• Consistent hydration • Standard oral care • Avoid milk of magnesia because it will dry the mouth • Avoid spicy foods, smoking, and alcohol	• Soothing baking soda, saline, and water rinse (eBox 61-5) • Topical lidocaine 2% • Dyclonine hydrochloride 0.5% or 1% • Diphenhydramine hydrochloride 5% (Benadryl, Pfizer Inc., New York) and loperamide (Kaopectate, Pfizer Inc., New York; Maalox, Novartis Consumer Health Canada Inc., Mississauga, Ont.) equal parts as a rinse • Sucralfate suspension, 10 mL 4 times/day, swish and swallowed or expectorated • Benzydamine, 15 mL 3-4 times/day, rinse and expectorate (Tantum, 3M Pharmaceuticals, London, Ont.) • "Magic Mouthwash": often prescribed by oncologists with varied ingredients such as antihistamines, anti-fungals, topical anesthetics, and antibiotics • Morphine 2% solution for preselected patients

Oral candidiasis
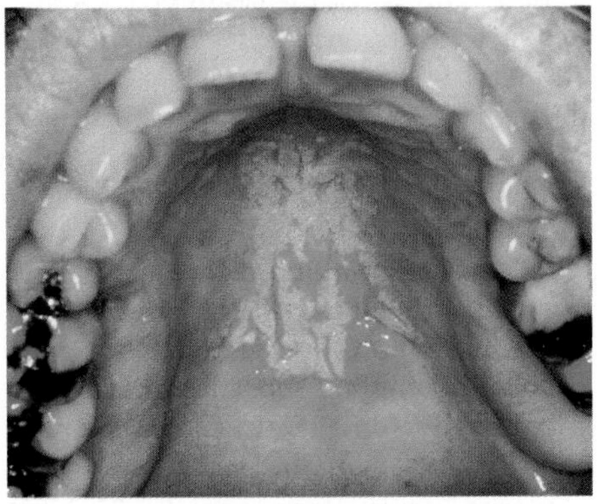
Figure 61-5. Oral candidiasis. (From Ibsen OAC, Phelan JA: *Oral pathology for the dental hygienist,* ed 6, St Louis, 2013, Saunders.)
	• **Pseudomembranous candidiasis**
	  • White cottage cheese–like mass that wipes off with red inflamed and bleeding tissue underneath
	• **Erythematous candidiasis**
	  • Red lesions, usually on the hard palate and dorsal surface of the tongue
	• **Hyperplastic candidiasis**
	  • Elevated white-yellow patches that cannot be wiped off
	• **Angular cheilitis**
	  • White and red fissures at the corners of the mouth
		• Routine oral care
		• Daily denture care
		• Dentures out overnight
		• Saline rinses (½ tsp of salt in 1 qt water)
		• Mouth moisturizer
			• **FIRST ROUTE:**
			  • Topical antifungal medication:
			    ■ Nystatin oral suspension 200,000-500,000 IU, swished and swallowed 3-5 times/day
			    ■ Nystatin suspension frozen (200,000-500,000 IU) in sugarless fruit juice
			    ■ Clotrimazole troche, 10 mg, 5 times/day for 14 days
			    ■ Angular Cheilitis can be treated with 0.5% triamcinolone and 2% ketoconazole cream
			  • Do not eat/drink for 20 minutes after treatment
			  • New denture container and toothbrush
			  • Remove denture and treat denture every day
			• **SECOND ROUTE:**
			  • Systemic medication:
			    ■ Fluconazole, 100-200 mg orally stat, then 50-100 mg/day for 7-14 days
			    ■ Ketoconazole, 200-400 mg orally for 7-14 days
			    ■ Itraconazole, 100-200 mg/day orally for 7-14 days

TABLE 61-1

Common Oral Complications: Signs and Symptoms, Prevention, and Treatment—cont'd

Manifestation	Signs and Symptoms	Prevention	Treatment
	• Symptoms: pain, bleeding, burning mouth, inability to taste food, malnutrition, and impaired quality of life		■ Amphotericin B, 0.25-1.5 mg/kg a day intravenously • Continue with denture treatment and new oral care products • May need further lab test (cytologic smear, culture, biopsy) if not responding to treatment
Xerostomia (dry mouth) 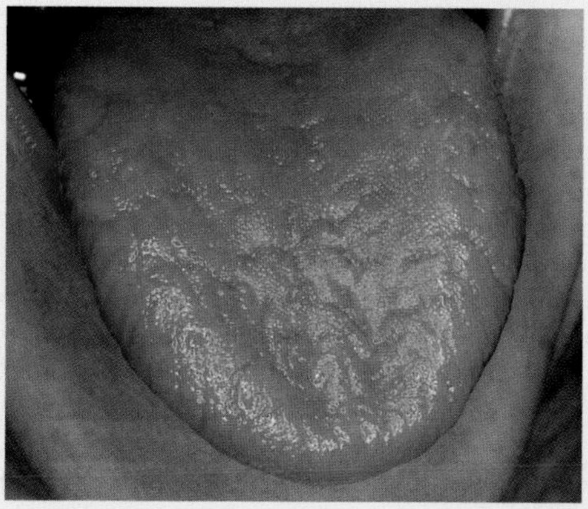 **Figure 61-6.** This patient has severe xerostomia. The tongue filiform papillae are lacking. (From Ibsen OAC, Phelan JA: *Oral pathology for the dental hygienist,* ed 6, St Louis, 2013, Saunders.)	• Dryness of mucous membranes • Dryness of lips • No "pool" of saliva at floor of mouth • Difficulty chewing and swallowing • Difficulty speaking • Fissured tongue	• Routine oral hygiene • Maintain hydration • Avoid use of products containing alcohol, lemon, and glycerin, and petroleum-based products • Review medications and consult with physician about modifications to prescriptions • Non-alcohol fluoride mouthwash	• Swab water-soluble lubricants throughout mouth: ○ Oral Balance gel (Laclede Professional Products, Gardena, CA) • Baking soda and saline rinse every 1-3 hours for 7 days (see Box 61-6) • Increase hydration by having client: ○ Suck on ice chips and/or sugar-free popsicles ○ Chew on sugar-free gum ○ Suck on partly frozen melon ○ Thin foods with liquids ○ Take frequent sips of water or water sprayed from pump dispenser • Saliva substitutes: ○ Carboxymethylcellulose (CMC) or mucin-containing lozenges ○ Moi-Stir (Kingswood Lab, Indianapolis, IN) ○ Lactoperoxidase containing toothpaste ○ Polyglycerylmethacrylate and glucose oxidase (Oral Balance) • Consult with physician or dentist about pilocarpine prescription • Water-based products for lips: ○ Aquagel, KY Jelly, Oral Balance

Adapted from National Health Service: Oral Care Guidelines for Publicly Funded Healthcare Systems in the United Kingdom. Reference number C028, 2010, Herefordshire Primary Care Trust; Wiseman M: The treatment of oral problems in the palliative patient, *J Can Dent Assoc* 72(5): 453, 2006; Hospice and Palliative Care Association Clinical Guidelines for Mouth Care in Palliative Care Patients. 1, 2008.

death in personal care homes (Box 61-7).[10,11] In severe cases patients may be prescribed systemic analgesics and narcotics for pain management (see Table 61-1 and eBox 61-5).

Oral Candidiasis

Oral candidiasis is the most common fungal infection in humans and has a 70% to 85% incidence among clients in palliative care (Figure 61-5).[8] **Candida albicans**, a natural oral cavity inhabitant, is the organism responsible for most cases of candidiasis. Although there are many causes of oral candidiasis (Box 61-8), the main cause can be attributed to an imbalance in oral flora and host immunity.

Oral candidiasis can be classified into four clinical types: pseudomembranous (thrush), erythematous, hyperplastic candidiasis, and angular cheilitis.[12] **Pseudomembranous candidiasis** is present clinically as a white cottage cheese–like mass that wipes off with red, inflamed, and bleeding tissue underneath. **Erythematous candidiasis** appears as red lesions, usually on the hard palate and dorsal surface of the tongue. **Hyperplastic candidiasis** presents as elevated white

BOX 61-6

Soothing Baking Soda, Saline, and Water Rinse

- ¼ tsp. baking soda, ¼ tsp. salt, and 16 oz water
- Used to cleanse mouth every 1-3 hours for 7 days
- May be used in disposable irrigation bag to assist in rinsing painful mouth
- Rinse with plain water after use
- High sodium content (not to swallow)
- Not for patients with sodium-restricted diet

BOX 61-7

Aspiration Pneumonia

- Aspiration of oral and throat secretions are the main cause of pneumonia.
- Pneumonia is the leading cause of death in personal care homes.
- A correlation has been shown between aspiration pneumonia and the following:
  - Swallowing disorders
  - Impaired cough reflex sensitivity
  - Compromised health
  - Poor management of oral secretions
  - Dependent in feeding
  - Recent antibiotic therapy
  - Periodontal disease
  - Poor dental plaque control
  - Dry mouth
  - Having natural teeth, especially with untreated dental caries
  - Uncooperative behavior during oral hygiene care

Data from Munro CL, Grap MJ, Elswick RK Jr, et al: Oral health status and development of ventilator-associated pneumonia: a descriptive study, *Am J Crit Care* 15(5):453, 2006.

BOX 61-8

Predisposing Factors for Oral Candidiasis

LOCAL FACTORS	MEDICAL FACTORS
• Poor oral hygiene	• Immunosuppression
• Xerostomia	• Corticosteriods, including inhalers
• Wearing dentures	• Broad-spectrum antibiotics
• Overclosure of mouth, drooling	• Obesity/diabetes
• Tissue trauma	• HIV/AIDS
• Smoking tobacco	• Cancer chemotherapy
	• Head and neck radiation
	• Poor nutritional status

Data from Bertone M, Wener ME: There is a FUNGUS Among Us! Oral Care in Palliative Care. Hospice and Palliative Care. Presentation at 19th Annual Provincial Conference, 2010, Manitoba.

yellow patches, similar to pseudomembranous candidiasis, only it cannot be wiped off. **Angular cheilitis** occurs as white and red fissures at the commissures of the mouth. Each clinical type can occur in combination or independently of one another.[12] Oral candidiasis symptoms include pain, bleeding,

BOX 61-10

Denture Treatment for Oral Candidiasis

- Thoroughly clean with brush and liquid soap
- Heavy deposits:
  - Ultrasonic cleaning
  - Full-strength vinegar for 10 minutes (no metal)
- Disinfect each day along with treatment
- Change solution daily
- Store in well identified container overnight in solutions of the following:
  - Water
  - Mouth rinse
  - 0.12% chlorhexidine
  - Listerine antiseptic (Pfizer Canada, Toronto, Ont.)
  - Water + 5 mL of nystatin for 2 weeks
  - Dilute sodium hypochlorite (1:9 parts water)

Data from Bertone M, Wener ME: *There is a FUNGUS among us! Oral care in palliative care: hospice and palliative care.* Presentation at 19th Annual Provincial Conference, 2010, Manitoba; Wiseman M: The treatment of oral problems in the palliative patient, *J Can Dent Assoc* 72(5):453, 2006.

burning mouth, inability to taste food, malnutrition, and impaired quality of life. If left untreated, oral candidiasis can progress systemically, increasing mortality. Systemic candidiasis has a mortality rate of 70%.

Management

Oral candidiasis can be treated locally (route 1) or systemically (route 2) depending on the severity of the infection (see Table 61-1 and eBox 61-9). Route 1 begins with meticulous oral hygiene care. The main topical treatment is nystatin (200 to 500,000 IU) or Clotrimazole (10 mg, five times a day, for 14 days), which are available in many forms, including troches, oral suspensions, creams, and ointments. If using an oral suspension, clients rinse with 5 mL of nystatin for 5 minutes, three to five times a day, for 2 weeks. Oral suspensions are contraindicated in patients with difficulty swallowing, because the medication is expectorated. When using an oral suspension, patients should not eat or drink for 20 minutes after application.

Salivary *Candida* levels have been reported to be higher in denture wearers than dentate individuals.[8] Therefore it is imperative that patients and their caregivers regularly treat dentures to avoid fungal infections (see Box 61-2 for details about standard denture care). (See Box 61-10 for information on the treatment of dentures for oral candidiasis.)

The second route of candidiasis treatment involves the use of prescribed systemic medications. This type of treatment is reserved for cases in which the first route of treatment was ineffective. Fluconazole is the most frequently used systemic medication. When taking fluconazole, patients take two tablets (100 mg) immediately, followed by one tablet daily for 7 to 14 days.[8,9,12] Denture care and routine oral hygiene care are continued throughout the treatment.

Xerostomia

Xerostomia (dry mouth) is the subjective feeling of oral dryness that is a common symptom affecting palliative care

BOX 61-11

Causes of Xerostomia

Normal Salivary Flow
- Anxiety

Drug-Induced
- Anticholinergic drugs such as Cogentin to treat Parkinson's disease and Atrovent to treat chronic obstructive pulmonary disease (COPD) and acute asthma
- Antihistamines
- Antihypertensives

Dehydration
- Diabetes mellitus
- Diarrhea, vomiting, hemorrhage
- Reduced fluid intake

Salivary Gland Disease
- Radiation therapy
- Sjögren's syndrome
- Calculi (mineral deposits that block the salivary glands)
- Mumps
- Sarcoidosis
- Parotid agenesis

From Sweeney MP, Bagg J: The mouth and palliative care, *Am J Hosp Palliat Care* 17(2):118, 2000.

patients.[8,12] Many factors cause xerostomia onset (Box 61-11), but medications and drug therapies are the most important (see Chapter 14, Box 14-5). Drug-induced xerostomia (see Figure 61-6) occurs from a change in the nature and quality of the saliva as well as the overall flow rate. This change in consistency and volume of saliva facilitates the adherence of food and oral biofilm to the oral tissues, tooth surfaces, dentures, and appliances. This oral debris increases a client's risk of developing tooth decay, periodontal disease, and mouth infections. It also leads to difficulty eating, tasting, chewing, swallowing, speaking, and denture discomfort and retention.[13]

Management

Xerostomia treatment (see Table 61-1 and eBox 61-12) includes frequent hydration with sips of water, saliva substitutes, ice chips, or sugar-free popsicles. A soothing baking soda, saline, water rinse (see eBox 61-5) is recommended to cleanse the mouth every 1 to 3 hours for 7 days. This rinse should not be swallowed or used by clients on a sodium-restricted diet. Products containing lemon, glycerin, or alcohol are contraindicated for clients with xerostomia because of their acidic and drying effect. Instead, lips should be lubricated with water-based products such as Aquagel, KY Jelly, or Oral Balance. Use of a nonfoaming toothpaste and a humidifier also helps to prevent dehydration.[6,8,12]

The Role of the Dental Hygienist

Dental hygienists have the educational background and expertise needed to contribute greatly to the palliative care team. Within the palliative care team, dental hygienists provide education and in-service training, conduct client assessments, and plan and evaluate care. It is the responsibility of the dental hygienist to either directly perform the dental hygiene process of oral palliative care or train palliative health professionals to perform the process of oral palliative care for their patients.

The Dental Hygiene Process of Care

Oral Health Assessment

Routine oral health assessment and standard oral hygiene care reduce the risk of oral problems developing, are pivotal to planning quality care, and are required for assessment, diagnosis, and evaluation of any oral problems.[12] The oral health assessment consists of (1) interviewing patients (or their caregivers) to ask questions about the patient's oral health and (2) performing an extraoral and intraoral evaluation to determine oral health and hygiene status. A family member or primary caregiver should be present at the assessment to discuss any concerns regarding the patient's oral care needs and to ask any questions regarding palliative oral care.

Interview

During the patient and caregiver interview the following relevant questions should be asked:
- Does the patient wear dentures?
- Is the patient's mouth painful?
- Is the patient able to eat and drink?
- Is the patient's mouth dry?

In addition, the patient's chart is reviewed to determine drug history, medical problems, diet, and prior treatment that would have implications on the patient's oral health. Relevant issues are clarified and discussed with the patient and caregiver.

Oral Health Screening Evaluation

An evaluation of the extraoral and intraoral structures of the head and neck is done to determine the integrity of the face, head, neck, lips, buccal mucosa, tongue, palate, floor of mouth, and gingiva. (See Chapter 15, Procedures 15-1 and 15-2, on conducting extraoral and intraoral assessments.) This evaluation is done with the use of proper protective equipment (gloves, mask, protective lenses), a tongue depressor, light source, water-based ointment, and gauze. Figure 61-7 presents an algorithm of questions and appropriate interventions the dental hygienist, or other healthcare professionals, can use as a guide when conducting oral health screening evaluations. When conducting the intraoral evaluation, clinicians ask themselves the following:
- Is the mouth healthy?
- Are mucositis or ulcers present?
- Is oral candidiasis present?
- Is the mouth dry?
- Overall, what specific human needs related to palliative oral care are in deficit?

Dental Hygiene Diagnosis

Based on information gathered during the assessment phase, the dental hygienist identifies the human need deficits related to the patient's palliative oral care. The diagnosis phase is ongoing and ever-changing, depending on the patient's

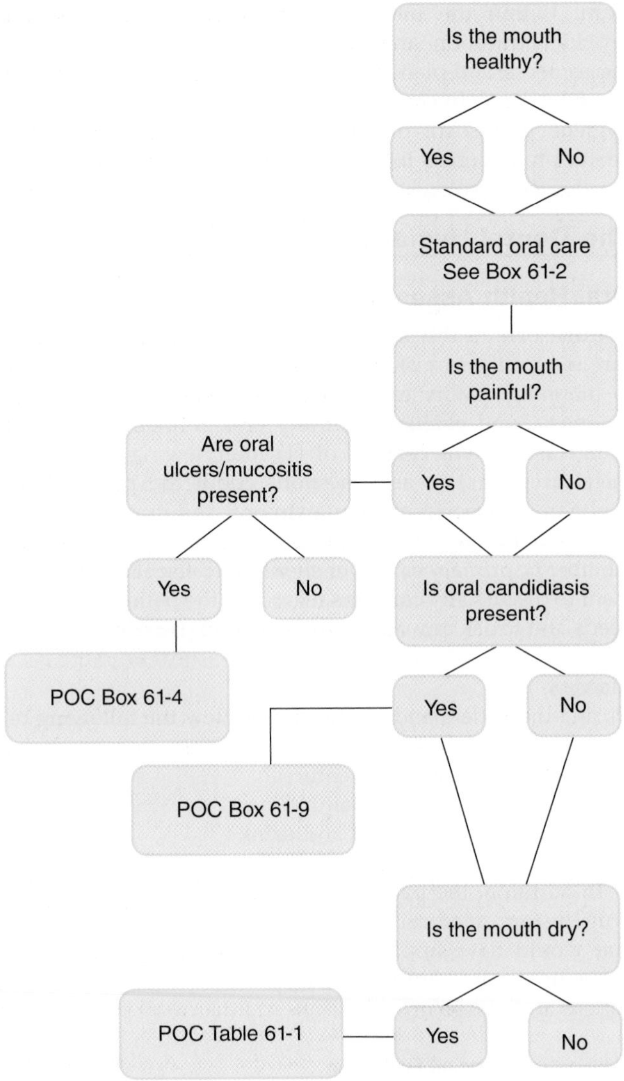

Figure 61-7. Guide to conducting oral health assessments on palliative care patients.

current human need deficits identified at the time of each assessment. This deficit identification is critical to determine the best palliative oral care plan to maintain oral comfort and quality of life.

Planning Palliative Oral Care

The palliative oral care plan focuses on maintaining oral comfort to improve the patient's quality of life. Palliative oral care plans include setting goals for standard oral hygiene care along with the prevention and management of oral complications if indicated (Box 61-2, Table 61-1). Pain management and maintenance of hydration are top priorities when setting goals for palliative oral care. In addition, the plan addresses concerns perceived by the patient, family, caregiver, nurse, dental hygienist, or other members of the palliative care team. The dental hygienist presents the palliative oral care plan to the palliative care team for feedback and integrates the plan goals into the patient's overall treatment regimen. If restorative treatment is needed, a goal is set to refer the patient to a dentist for further evaluation.

Implementation of Care

Depending on the dental hygienist's assessment, diagnoses, and palliative oral care plan, dental hygiene interventions are introduced to meet the patient's human need deficits.

Evaluation of Care

The physical and psychologic needs of patients in palliative care are continually changing; therefore it is imperative that goals and outcomes of palliative oral care are evaluated continuously. Proper evaluation is based on whether the goals are met, partially met, or unmet. See the Critical Thinking Exercises for an example of the dental hygiene process of care.

Conclusion

The dental hygienist as a member of the palliative care team provides in-service training on palliative oral care for nursing staff and other healthcare professionals. Applying the human needs conceptual model to the dental hygiene process of care ensures a comprehensive and humanistic approach to developing a palliative oral care plan that enhances the person's dignity and quality of life. Facilitating personal comfort, hydration, normal eating, and social communication is of critical importance. Many people do not realize how important the mouth becomes to the dying individual. Simple explanations and procedures related to oral hygiene can help to reduce the stress related to this time. Such explanations provide a significant opportunity for family members to assist in the care of their loved one, because oral hygiene care aids so much in their overall comfort. This assistance with care may be especially important for parents of dying children. Many medical procedures must be performed by nurses or physicians, but oral care procedures are simple and provide an opportunity for the family to participate with tender care.

CLIENT EDUCATION TIPS

- Explain to patients, families, and other caregivers the potential oral complications associated with medications and medical treatment and strategies to prevent them.
- Explain to family and palliative care team members the importance of oral care as a component of palliative care.
- Identify oral health products that will ensure that the oral cavity remains moist and clean to promote quality of life.
- Educate caregivers on how to deliver oral care properly to patients who require assistance, especially those who are intubated.

LEGAL, ETHICAL, AND SAFETY ISSUES

- Legally, patients are considered competent to make decisions when they are informed and able to understand the facts, are able to make rational treatment decisions and understand their implications, and can communicate their choices.
- Clinicians must respect and not pressure patients when they request withholding or withdrawing treatment.
- When the patient is not competent, the patient's best interest then must be considered by clinicians and the patient's loved ones; they are challenged to balance potential benefits with previously expressed wishes, if known.

- Do not abandon oral care for patients during the end stage of life. Good oral care helps improve the quality of life during this important and limited time.

KEY CONCEPTS

- Palliative care is any form of care that focuses on decreasing disease symptom severity in individuals with life-limiting illnesses, rather than trying to delay or reverse disease progression.
- The importance of oral care often is overlooked in palliative care settings because of the absence of dental professionals, such as dental hygienists, as members of the palliative care team.
- Oral hygiene care is important in promoting comfort by maintaining moist oral tissues and self-esteem as well as by preventing bad odors and the loneliness experienced at the end stage of life among palliative care patients.
- Consistent, ongoing oral health assessment is needed to evaluate oral mucosal changes and other oral complications from medical treatment. Based on this assessment, evidence-based interventions are implemented to improve patient comfort and quality of life.
- If the mouth is determined to be healthy, then standard oral hygiene care is prescribed for the patient to perform on a daily basis.
- For patients who require assistance with the performance of standard mouth care, the dental hygienist educates the primary caregiver or family member on how to perform daily standard oral hygiene care, which may include denture care.
- If pain is reported and oral complications are observed, then appropriate evidence-based interventions must be implemented immediately to ensure the patient's comfort and quality of life.
- Common oral complications observed in or reported by palliative care patients are mucositis, ulcers, oral candidiasis, and xerostomia.
- Within the palliative care team, dental hygienists provide oral health education and in-service training on conducting oral health assessments, using evidence-based interventions to promote oral comfort, and evaluating outcomes of oral palliative care.
- The dental hygienist is responsible for either directly performing the dental hygiene process of care related to palliative oral care or training other palliative care team members to conduct oral assessments, and implement and evaluate outcomes of evidence-based interventions to improve the comfort and quality of life of their palliative care patients. The process of care for a palliative care patient includes conducting oral health assessments (client interview and oral health screening evaluation), formulating dental hygiene diagnoses, and planning, implementing, and evaluating care outcomes.

CRITICAL THINKING EXERCISES

Profile: Mrs. D., age 78, is a hospice resident.

Chief Complaint: "I have a removable partial denture to replace my upper back teeth that I don't wear because it makes my mouth feel dry and taste bad. Also, I have a sore on the roof of my mouth from the denture sliding back and forth when I talk or eat."

Social History: Mrs. D. has been widowed for 3 years. Her two daughters live nearby.

Health History: Mrs. D. has a history of angina for the past 6 years and takes 50 mg atenolol (Tenormin) once a day to prevent angina attacks. She is in congestive heart failure and expected to live less than 6 months.

Dental History: Mrs. D. has a history of regular dental visits and has all of her teeth, with the exception of the four maxillary molars. Oral examination reveals a maxillary ulcer and a warped denture resulting from sitting out in the air overnight. Mrs. D. reports pain on her palate and dry mouth. Dental examination reveals no signs of decay and some evidence of gingival inflammation, food debris, and plaque biofilm.

Oral Health Behavior Assessment: Poor oral hygiene. Uses a manual toothbrush once a day.

1. What are the dental hygiene diagnoses for this patient?
2. Develop a dental hygiene care plan for this patient that includes goals and interventions.
3. What patient education issues should be addressed?
4. What factors could be contributing to this patient's dry mouth?
5. Are there any contraindications to this patient's care?
6. What is the main palliative oral care priority for this patient?

REFERENCES

1. Heitkemper M: Palliative care at end-of-life. In Lewis SL, Dirksen SR, Heitkemper MM, et al: *Medical-surgical nursing*, ed 8, St Louis, 2011, Elsevier, pp 153.
2. Ettinger RL: The role of the dentist in geriatric palliative care, *J Am Geriatr Soc* 60(2):367, 2012.
3. Brown J, Hoffman L: The dental hygienist as a hospice care provider, *Am J Hosp Palliative Care* 7:31, 1990.
4. World Health Organization: *Palliative care.* Available at: http://www.who.int/hiv/top-topics/palliative/palliative care. Accessed November 14, 2012.
5. Wiseman M: Palliative care dentistry, *Gerodontology* 17(1):49, 2000.
6. National Health Service: *Oral care cuidelines for publicly funded healthcare systems in the United Kingdom.* Reference number C028. 2010, Herefordshire Primary Care Trust.
7. Feider L, Mitchell P, Bridges E: Oral care practices for orally intubated critically ill adults, *Am J Crit Care* 19(2):175, 2010.
8. Wiseman M: The treatment of oral problems in the palliative patient, *J Can Dent Assoc* 72(5):453, 2006.
9. Thanvi J, Ashok KP, Thanvi R: Oral care in palliative patients, *Dental Impact* 4(1):9, 2012.
10. Bertone M, Wener ME: *There is a FUNGUS among us! Oral care in palliative care: hospice and palliative care.* Presentation at 19th Annual Provincial Conference, 2010, Manitoba.
11. Munro CL, Grap MJ, Elswick RK Jr, et al: Oral health status and development of ventilator-associated pneumonia: a descriptive study, *Am J Crit Care* 15(5):453, 2006.
12. Sweeney MP, Bagg J: The mouth and palliative care, *Am J Hosp Palliat Care* 17(2):118, 2000.
13. Rydholm M, Strang P: Physical and psychosocial impact of xerostomia in palliative care: a qualitative interview study, *Int J Palliat Nurs* 8:318, 2002.

EVOLVE RESOURCES

Please visit http://evolve.elsevier.com/Darby/hygiene for additional practice and study support tools.

CHAPTER 62

Practice Management

Michelle Sirois

COMPETENCIES

1. Describe techniques used for successful practice management.
2. Discuss techniques used for successful client and record management, including:
   - List the elements of a complete case presentation.
   - Describe the advantages and disadvantages of electronic health or dental records.
3. Discuss time management and scheduling, including the types of appointment book management systems.
4. Explain economic considerations for a profitable practice, including office overhead, production, and collection.
5. Discuss the marketing of dentistry and dental hygiene, including:
   - List the four Ps of marketing.
   - Compare and contrast types of social media used for marketing.
6. Discuss quality assurance and the auditing of client records.

Practice Management

Participation in management of the dental and dental hygiene practice adds a dimension of administrative responsibilities and decision making to the dental hygienist's daily routine and affords professional growth opportunities. Such participation increases the value of the dental hygienist as a team member and enhances job satisfaction.

Practice management can be defined as the organization, administration, and direction of the professional practice in a style that facilitates high-quality client care, efficient use of time and personnel, reduced stress for staff members and clients, enhanced professional and personal satisfaction for staff, and financial profitability.[1] Those who strive to manage a successful practice must be prepared, organized, and able to act upon the goals established for the organization. The practice owner(s) must devise a list of these goals and objectives, often as a part of the **mission statement** or **vision**. This visionary statement should be realistic about the current state of the practice, where the owners and providers want the practice to be in the future, and the strategies that will allow the practice to achieve those goals.[2] For this mission statement to be operational, it must be accompanied with specific measurable objectives, a plan for how the vision for the office goals will be achieved, and specification of what each team member can contribute toward achieving these goals.

The first step is to identify and prioritize the essence of what makes the practice exceptional and unique. Emphasis on the specialties of the clinicians along with key elements such as providing quality dentistry, excellent client service, employee satisfaction, and effective team communication contributes to a successful dental or dental hygiene practice. Consider how all of these elements can be managed successfully. The leader must start with understanding good leadership skills and implementing them into the practice. Management styles vary from person to person; effective leadership begins with a talented person to lead a group effectively. Good leaders motivate and inspire co-workers to become involved in the practice. Team members need to be appreciated and praised, a benefit that can be viewed as a bigger motivator than financial compensation to many employees.[3]

Micromanagement takes valuable time away from client care and focuses on every detail no matter how minor. *Micromanagement often is viewed as "over-managing."* It creates fatigue for the leaders as well as counterproductive employees, loss of team unity, loss of confidence among staff members, increased staff turnover, and increased stress for all involved. Clients sense a stressful work environment, which may lead to increased anxiety, frustration, and decreased confidence in the team or leader. These negative effects may decrease the practice's positive financial growth. An effective leader must understand how to recognize the pitfalls of micromanagement and consistently employ self-management skills to prevent these scenarios.

Undermanaged staff can be just as counterproductive as micromanaged practices. Poor organization, deficient communication, ineffective leadership, and/or insufficient guidance may encourage employees to take on a withdrawn, "it's not my job" approach. Poorly managed practices often suffer from inconsistency in client care and record keeping because of high employee and client turnover, decreased employee satisfaction, increased client and staff frustration, and loss of financial profitability.

A **shared management** style is the best method to approach team leadership for success. This style involves team empowerment, shared responsibility, frequent and constructive communication and, most importantly, flexibility. Shared

Figures, tables, and boxes marked as "e" are available as supplemental material on the Evolve site. Visit http://evolve.elsevier.com/Darby/hygiene to access these materials.

management increases job productivity, reduces stress for team members and clients, improves team morale, and maximizes practice profitability. To develop a shared management approach, the team must start by developing shared goals, answering questions such as, "What is desired for the future of the practice?" and "How will client care be enhanced when changes are made?" Encouragement of all team members' equal contributions to the office goals helps personnel to become more vested, responsible, and dedicated to carrying out the objectives. Developing shared goals and standards for the practice inspires teamwork, self-delegation, and personal accountability. Goals may include professional development for employees. They also may focus on scheduling pitfalls and successes, productive time utilization, client needs, current technologies, and treatment modalities. Shared management style is founded on using personnel's individual talents for the betterment of the group and practice. Offices that follow this approach tend to have high financial profitability and client satisfaction. Clients often refer friends and family to the practice, which allows for continual improvements, growth, and cutting-edge, comprehensive client-centered care.

Practice management styles vary; however, a successful practice requires a dedicated leader. An effective leader understands the importance of flexibility and mentorship. As the practice and number of employees continue to grow, so must the goals, strategies, and standards of the practice. Flexibility and good listening skills during communication help to avoid dictatorship and contribute to successful relationships. Frequent communication and appropriate amendments to the office's mission, goals, and objectives for the practice and client care also can enhance greatly colleagues' feelings of inclusion and appreciation. Successes must be rewarded and acknowledged as well as personnel awareness of shortcomings or deficiencies. The mission is the framework for success and must be revisited often for effective growth of the practice. Each practice requires different emphasis areas, depending on where the practice wants to position itself in the future. Successful leaders mentor, inspire, and applaud good performance and also promote integrity, accountability, and a positive outlook. Leadership is less about power and more about empowerment. There is nothing more dynamic than an empowered team.[2]

Standards for Clinical Dental Hygiene Practice

Management styles aside, when devising a framework for quality dental hygiene care provided by the practice, dental professionals should begin with the American Dental Hygienists' Association's Standards for Clinical Dental Hygiene Practice.[3] (See Chapter 1.) It is imperative that practices consistently revisit similar documents and standards to ensure quality oral healthcare is being delivered and practitioners continue to maintain competence.

Effective Office Collaboration Through Frequent Communication

Collaboration can be defined as working jointly with others in an intellectual endeavor. The importance of collaboration in dental and dental hygiene practice is vital to success for all members of the team and the client group. Collaboration on the part of each professional in the office fosters high-quality client care. For collaborative care to exist in a practice, all practitioners must be able to support the diagnoses and deliver the suggested treatment in a respectful manner for the benefit of the client. Using a collaborative approach requires identifying each individual's knowledge, personal skills, or qualities and using those attributes to their fullest potential. Fundamental elements to creative and productive collaboration and communication are team meetings, which often occur in the form of morning huddles as well as weekly or monthly lunch gatherings.

For a meeting to be productive, it must be well defined, organized, and constructive. Leadership of the individual(s) planning the meeting requires advanced preparation, an outline of areas of weakness or change that must be addressed, and active involvement of others to share solutions or concerns as well as instill confidence in one another. Morning huddles and regular team meetings are most productive when the approach includes shared responsibility, clear standards of client care, brainstorming, action plans, constructive feedback, empowerment, and praise. Poor meeting planning and communication create frustration for employees. Preparing an effective outline for morning huddles or meetings includes the following three considerations:

1. What is the key motivating issue(s) that should be discussed?
2. What are the topics or issues identified and prioritized by the group?
3. How can successful problem solving strategies be used during the meeting?

Answering these questions in advance helps meetings flow productively. Some groups find it helpful to assign a member of the team a specific time and topic to prevent deviation or over-discussion on any matter. If the team cannot come to a conclusion on one issue, the leader considers follow-up assignments and allots a more appropriate amount of time for consideration at a later date. A team member not leading the discussion should be assigned to take notes for documentation of the discussion and decisions made. Notes ensure that any employees that could not attend will be able to review all information and decisions and feel included. Posting these notes in a central employee area such as the breakroom or an online discussion forum encourages access by all team members. If all team members are allowed to speak freely about concerns in the practice without fear of penalty, the team can gain insight into deficiencies and brainstorm ways to circumvent these issues in the future.

A practice manager should allot approximately 15 minutes before the start of each workday to discuss any successes or pitfalls of the previous day as well as solutions to how those pitfalls can be avoided in the future. Morning huddles are short, so they are intended to identify individual client needs on a daily basis, resolve scheduling concerns, and enhance management and coordination of client services planned for that day. These huddles allow little or no time for practice or team development. Because of the ever-changing demands of the profession and clients, a practice manager should schedule different meetings or gatherings to discuss current topics and needs of the practice (Table 62-1). A creative leader should vary the discussion topics often to avoid monotony and evoke motivation. Open discussions and communication are key to a successful and dynamic practice. The leader can never forget or disregard the education and experience of each individual team member.

TABLE 62-1

Suggested Meeting Topics

1. FYI	Share data, facts, and practice policies or logistics
2. Planning	Create long-range action plans usually mission oriented
3. Problem solving	Deal with immediate issues related to day-to-day business
4. Decision making	Finalize a process and gain commitment to decisions
5. Monitors	Review progress of practice or assess team accomplishments
6. Evaluating	Assess the performance of an individual or project
7. Training	Develop skills or knowledge of the team
8. Celebrating	Provide social opportunities and reward team performance
9. Marketing	Brainstorm ideas and/or update team on status and successes
10. Client services	Debrief client visits and/or plan for future visits or services
11. Team building	Develop a cohesive, congruent, and collaborative team
12. Leadership	Revisit vision, mission, direction, and goals
13. Daily huddle	Review schedule and ensure exceptional client care
14. Learning moments	Coach and debrief with individuals in training
15. Improving care	Share new educational theories and behaviors that can enhance the client care experience

TABLE 62-2

Steps for Conflict Resolution

1. Explain the current situation as you perceive it. Be brief and to the point without including your own judgments or feelings.
2. Show that you understand how the other person is feeling and then express your own feelings in regard to the matter.
3. Be respectful of others' opinions and beliefs.
4. Offer a compromise to allow both sides to feel heard and validated.
5. Explain what the outcome is likely to be if you both can agree to the compromise proposed.
6. Walk away from the discussion if it escalates to shouting or anger. Collect thoughts, calm down, and appoint another time to meet to discuss the issue.
7. Ask a neutral party to mediate a solution if needed.
8. Be willing to accept the final decision of the situation whatever it may be. Be able to back down from the situation and let it go.

Employing a teamwork attitude in the dental office is not a new concept; however, it has been adopted slowly among healthcare providers, possibly because of a lack of understanding of one another's roles and educational backgrounds, as well as limited time interaction between co-workers. Dental hygienists are trained to be critical thinkers through their rigorous dental hygiene educational experiences. At times employers or practice managers are unfamiliar with their expertise; therefore the autonomy to use those skills is limited once in a private dental practice or alternative practice setting. It is the role of the dental hygienist to educate other healthcare professionals about preventive oral hygiene care and their vital role in delivering quality oral health services.

Conflict Resolution in the Dental and Dental Hygiene Practice

Not all communication among employees is productive and without conflict. A professional can mediate feelings effectively between employees by following the steps of conflict resolution. Dental professionals often find themselves practicing in tight quarters with various individuals and personalities and sometimes experience differences or disagreement with one another. The challenge is to identify approaches to work through differences, areas of compromise, and challenging work environments. Learning and practicing effective communication skills assist team members in the workplace when faced with conflict.

The first rule of conflict resolution is to understand that a person cannot change anyone else but oneself. If a team member desires a change in a relationship with someone else, that individual must understand clearly his or her own goals, beliefs, and motivations first. It may be impractical to think that one co-worker can work harmoniously with a challenging co-worker. Nonetheless differences do not have to result in constant disagreement and antagonism. Changing reactions to one another can change the interactions shared between co-workers. All communication consists of *reaction* and *counter-reaction*.[4] If co-worker "A" changes reaction(s) to co-worker "B," that difference in response may evoke a different reaction from co-worker "B." Co-worker "A" should take a moment to reflect upon a typical reaction experienced in the past when dealing with co-worker "B" and determine, "Did the interaction involve disrespect, shouting, silence, gossiping with others, or swallowing down anger?" Exploring how to identify and cope with one's own reactions should preclude any expectation of change in the interactions of the other person. Some individuals find it difficult to identify objectively their true feelings or beliefs when reflecting on a situation. It may be helpful for them to use personality tests such as Myers Briggs or DiSC to identify their personality traits and reactions from a more scientific standpoint. Discovering a person's character strengths and weaknesses can assist in pinpointing why conflict may be arising with another person and how to use certain strengths to resolve it. Negotiation and communication among co-workers is the best way to reshape a relationship. When conflict arises, dental professionals first must be introspective and then follow conflict resolution steps to change the situation (Table 62-2).

Respectful behavior among co-workers contributes to a more pleasant workplace for everyone.

Personnel Management

A practice that has defined the specific job descriptions for each professional and support staff member in the office provides a foundation for an organized collaborative team framework. Well-defined job descriptions allow the employer and employee(s) to recognize and communicate easily what is expected of both parties and lead to reduced workplace stress as well as increased productivity and job satisfaction. Job descriptions help to establish the role each team member plays and how he or she completes an integral part of the bigger picture. Encouraging a flexible discussion about what responsibilities each employee would like to accept or oversee results in each contributing team member feeling as though he or she brings something unique and valued to the team. A large part of productivity and proficiency in the workplace comes from job satisfaction and a perception of being an appreciated team member. A happy member of the team tends to be the person whose day-to-day task suits his or her personality.[5] The key to creating a productive and effective team is having the right person for each job. Various personalities in the office can either increase or decrease office morale; for example, an optimistic team member faces each challenge as an opportunity, whereas the pessimist views the challenge as an obstacle or hinderance.[5] Some employers use personality tests previously mentioned for self-assessment, such as DiSC or Myers Briggs, to understand each team member better, align responsibilities around their characteristics, and foster productivity. Once a personality type is identified, a discussion with that individual employee about his or her roles, responsibilities, and visions can be used as a means of producing a more tailored job description and evoking a feeling of acceptance and flexibility.

Brainstorming about how to address challenges, development of problem-solving strategies, and clear measures of accountability help prepare staff members to respond appropriately to issues as they arise. Finally, developing measures to gauge success[2] and allow for revisiting of ineffective actions encourages movement in a positive direction and ongoing change as the needs of the practice evolve. This process is accomplished by individual and team meetings and frequent discussions. Employees who perceive that they are included, valued, and validated become essential employees. Allowing experienced members of the team the autonomy to practice using evidence-based decision making as well as their critical thinking skills also brings about a feeling of importance and appreciation, which is vital to the success of a healthcare team. When every employee in the practice is part of idea generation, each member also is more responsive to participating in solutions. Change is difficult for some, but clear job descriptions, frequent discussions, practice guidelines and policies, and employer and employee accountability reduce apprehension of everyone involved.

Office Policies

Office policies should address all areas that are viewed as important to the practice's efficient operation. Office policies should be comprehensive and address a variety of topics essential to management of the practice. They often include information about employee benefits, attendance, hours, office attire, professional expectations and behavior, morning huddles and meetings, inexcusable conduct, and penalties for unprofessional actions. Examples of office policies related to client care include infection control, current CPR/AED certification, current licensure, continuing education units (CEUs), medical emergency protocols, and client care approaches. Office policies often fail to address pressing matters such as conflict resolution among co-workers. It is important to make each employee aware of the steps to resolve an issue with a fellow co-worker and how the office prefers conflicts be handled. Informing employees that there are steps to be taken to resolve conflict in the office can alleviate employee frustrations and lead to quicker resolutions. As the practice evolves, so should the office policies. A yearly or bi-yearly review of office policies should be incorporated into a team meeting and reviewed with all team members for clarity.

A practice that uses clearly defined practice policies, standards, and job descriptions informs employees of practice expectations to achieve the ultimate goal of providing quality client care services. Periodic performance reviews enhance performance and lower stress levels of the employees because they understand what is expected of them. Job satisfaction results when each team member knows what is expected and when consistent performance evaluation is based objectively on those expectations.

Accountability is the obligation of an individual to account for activities, accept responsibility for them, and report the results in a transparent and honest manner. Strategies for accountability must be developed to ensure everyone is acting responsibly and working toward the same goals. Accountability can be just as important as the goal itself. If not enforced, it may encourage laziness, ineffectiveness, and decreased job satisfaction resulting from lack of action on the manager's part. Discussion of circumstances and consequences for failing to perform job responsibilities, collaborate effectively for the achievement of the established goals of the practice, or exhibit productive behaviors and actions is the responsibility of the practice manager. In addition to defining the rights and responsibilities of all office employees, an office manager must define rights and responsibilities of the client and ensure they are available in writing for all clients and team members.

Client Management and Records

The client is the most important member of the oral healthcare team; without clients there would be no practice. A healthy functional relationship with the client must be established early and reinforced often through effective communication regarding treatment needs, individual progress, and education. To be effective at establishing this relationship, the clinician must understand that each client has his or her own physical, psychologic, spiritual, and emotional needs. Human needs are influenced by many factors, such as current and previous experiences and socioethnocultural factors.[1] A clinician who appreciates and understands these needs will be successful at gaining the client's trust and nurturing the client-provider bond.

Establishing a healthy relationship starts when the client makes initial contact with a front desk employee seeking information or requesting an appointment. Front desk employees are the first to establish a relationship with the client and establish the foundation for a successful client-provider relationship. This interaction provides an opportunity to showcase the unique qualities of the practice, philosophies, office polices, and/or office expectations for the client. If front desk personnel are not welcoming and forthright about office policies and expectations, or if they are abrupt or unfriendly, it may diminish or prevent a successful relationship with the client. When office policies change, continuing clients should receive those changes in writing. Some practices ask clients to sign a statement indicating they have been informed and understand the new policies.

Client motivation is achieved when clients have autonomy and are involved actively in their oral healthcare options, decisions, and treatment. Fulfillment of this obligation requires providers to deliver understandable information to the clients about their needs, treatments, options, and costs. It also may require the provider to offer written/printed information the client can read over, review, and reflect on before scheduling recommended treatment. Strategies providers can use to motivate clients to accept recommendations for comprehensive care include the following:

- Making the information relevant and meaningful to the clients by using their culture, beliefs, attitudes, and values
- Relating information by building on the client's existing knowledge, experiences, and feelings
- Using success and rewards to promote learning and encouragement rather than criticism to gain acceptance of treatment

Case Presentation

A case presentation is the process of explaining and educating clients on all assessment findings identified during the dental hygiene care appointment (Box 62-1). Case presentations should include why the client is experiencing the change or issue, intervention or treatment options, risks of proceeding or not proceeding with recommendations, and associated costs. Case presentations and the client's response should be documented in the client record. The dental hygienist is often responsible for presenting a case presentation about dental hygiene care plans, or reinforcing information in the dental care plan and referrals, to clients within a general dental or dental hygiene practice. To meet the client's human needs for freedom from fear and stress and for conceptualization and problem solving, it is important that the discussion be held in a manner that is informative and nonthreatening to the client, using terminology that is easily understandable. Written documentation during case presentation also may aid in client understanding and comprehension. Treatment acceptance depends on how the information is received and understood by the client.

Client nonadherence or noncompliance is a lack of client action after the suggested intervention has been suggested and discussed with the client. Client noncompliance may lead to disease progression, tooth/bone loss, and an increase in systemic health concerns. Noncompliance also results in compromised care, unsatisfactory outcomes for the client and practitioner, and possibly litigation. In the event of a lawsuit, the judicial decision, outcome, or amount of settlement may be altered based on negligence of the practitioner if nonadherence was ignored or not properly documented in the client's record. The following are examples of noncompliance that may occur during dental hygiene care:

BOX 62-1

Elements of a Complete Case Presentation to a Client

Information
Data collected and assessment findings are shared with the client, using visual aids such as radiographs, photographs, models, or a periodontal chart when appropriate.

Education
An explanation of the significance of the assessment findings is given to the client, including short- and long-range possibilities and consequences of the condition present. At the same time the practitioner asks questions and initiates discussion to bring the client into the conversation so that a determination of the client's level of understanding, priorities, and interest in pursuing care can be made. Media, research evidence, and other instructional strategies should supplement client education.

Options
A list of alternative methods of care is given to the client, including benefits, time involved, treatment risks, risks of not completing treatment, and the cost of each option.

Choice
An informed decision is made by clients based on their understanding of the information presented, priorities, desire for treatment, values, and perceived needs.

Agreement
The client and professional concur on a course to follow, including sequencing of care and assignment of responsibilities. The dental hygienist, as an advocate, supports the informed decision made by the client. A written summary of the case presentation should be composed during the discussion and agreement of care and a copy given to the client for personal records.

- Routinely tardy for scheduled appointments or necessity for an early departure
- Repeated postponement or cancellations
- Failure to appear for scheduled appointments
- Unwillingness to provide consent for diagnostic tests (e.g., radiographs, saliva testing)
- Unwillingness or inability to accept recommended specific procedures or care plans
- Unwillingness or inability to follow referrals to specialists
- Failure to use medications as prescribed
- Failure to follow oral hygiene recommendations

The management of client nonadherence begins with recognizing when it occurs and documenting it each and every time. The following list describes the process of documenting client nonadherence to prescribed care:

- Record recommended care as given to the client. (Written directions should be provided to the client each time suggestions are made and scanned into the record for documentation purposes.)

- Describe all instructions that have not been followed when seeing the client for a re-care visit. If a client has partially met the agreed on goal(s), the partial adherence should be documented as well as the client's statement about why the goal was not achieved.
- Describe the client's nonverbal response when questioned about nonadherence, if noted.
- Record in quotations the client's verbalizations about nonadherence, including reasons for inability or choice.
- Document modifications made to recommendations.
- Note any discussion of the consequences of not following recommendations or instructions that occurs between office personnel and the client.

Client Records

A complete client record consists of a signed HIPAA form; current and past health histories; intraoral, extraoral, dental, and periodontal charting findings; radiographs and findings of other diagnostic tests with corresponding dental and dental hygiene diagnoses; informed consents and informed treatment refusals; copies of prescriptions, photographs, and study models; documented conversations with clients regarding appointments, treatment, and oral hygiene suggestions; a record of services including all treatment delivered with dates; and any correspondence with other dental specialists and/or medical providers.

Client records serve as a client's treatment timeline by documenting the client's history with the practice. This record also can serve as legal documentation if needed. Client records serve as an accurate verification of all experiences shared between office personnel and the client. Maintaining an accurate client record is a vital component of thorough client care and also can enhance practice procedures and future appointments. Maintaining detailed records for each client achieves the following:

- Organize all treatment procedures performed
- Record each client's oral and health goals related to their beliefs, attitudes, and habits
- Provide the basis for correlating dental hygiene care with other components of comprehensive care
- Aid in evaluating dental hygiene and dental diagnoses as well as effective care planning
- Serve as a communication tool between all team members and the client
- Guide consistent, individualized preventive care
- Provide documentation of necessary treatment needs to third-party insurers
- Demonstrate accountability for responsible quality care
- Provide legal protection for oral healthcare providers and serve as documentary evidence for defense, if needed

To maintain proper records management, treatment entries should be made promptly after the procedure, discussion, and/or treatment is performed using clear, concise statements describing the appointment and signed by the treating clinician. Clinicians must ensure a complete and legible name is documented in the chart; initials are not acceptable for legal documentation. Illegible written client records are to blame for numerous incorrect prescriptions, treatments, or diagnoses. It is imperative to have decipherable writing if paper charting still is being used for proper client treatment and follow-up. Written client charts are becoming obsolete in the wake of electronic dental records.

Electronic Software and Dental Records

Dental practice software packages offer a variety of features from day-to-day activities to monthly or yearly productivity and losses. Software programs offer practice management features such as word processing; spreadsheet programs with automated accounting functions; data management for entering, storing, sorting, and retrieving data; graphic programs; desktop publishing; scheduling formats; payroll functions; e-billing and accounts payable functions; intraoffice communication; and client education functions. Computers are stationed in each treatment room as well as at the front desk areas so that client information can be accessed from every area. Networked systems allow for this smooth communication to occur in the office. Software functions also can create office letterhead, pamphlets, fliers, and all other necessary marketing tools needed for business advertising.

Electronic dental programs offer assistance to clinicians through voice-activated programs that record periodontal chartings, dental charting, soft tissue assessments, risk factors, oral care services, and treatment record notes. These features enhance the clinician's ability to document clinical findings and record notes quickly and easily to ensure information is not missed or left out. Once client information is recorded, it then can be compared to past documentation and used for client educational purposes. Photographs, illustrations, graphs, or spreadsheets illustrate tissue or bone loss for the client to visualize and enhance communication between the provider and client.

Computerized client records and software allow client records to be uniform, understandable, and transferable between providers. Electronic health records (EHR) are an online combination of information such as health histories for medical, dental, pharmacy, vision, lab tests, medical alerts, radiographic documentation, appointment scheduling, current and future treatment plans, financial aspects, and various other medical records (Box 62-2). Electronic client records allow multiple clinicians to view the same records simultaneously, which leads to increased communication and quality care for the client. This transferability allows for confidential and efficient sharing of general and oral health information among healthcare providers addressing interrelated client needs, according to the Health Insurance Portability and Accountability Act (HIPAA).[6] HIPAA is a federal law that protects the privacy of health information that can be identified with an individual client; the HIPAA Security Rule sets national standards for the security of electronic protected health information; the confidentiality provisions of the Patient Safety Rule protects individually identifiable information from being used to analyze patient safety events. In other words, individual information is shared only as the client directs it or as needed by the client's healthcare providers for diagnoses and treatment. Dental and dental hygiene professionals have been striving to connect with other healthcare professionals on a greater level based on the established link between oral and systemic health, and shared electronic client records improve communication between various health entities while protecting client privacy.

In 2009 President Obama signed into law the American Recovery and Reinvestment Act, which has aided in the expansion of wireless services and transportability of health records. By 2015, all medical records including dental records

BOX 62-2

Definitions of Electronic Record Acronyms

EMR	Electronic medical record	• Legal medical record used within one organization • Nontransferable
EHR	Electronic health record	• Information that conforms to interoperability standards • Used across more than one healthcare organization component
PHR	Personal health record	• Electronic data that provide clients with their personal health information • Conforms to nationally recognized interoperability standards • Readily shared with healthcare providers with client-controlled access
PHI	Protected health information	• Individual identifiable health information that can be linked to a specific client. • HIPAA defines the type of information and circumstances in which PHI can be used and disclosed
HIE	Health information exchange	• A system that enables the exchange of EHR information between hospitals and regions with nationally recognized standards, facilitating the coordination of care
HIT	Health information technology	• Application of information processing involving computer hardware and software that deals with storage, retrieval, sharing, and use of healthcare information, data, and knowledge for communication and decision making
EDR	Electronic dental record	• Proposed name for legal dental records

must be converted to an EHR. A task force has been established by the American Dental Association (ADA) to put together a dental online database system to allow providers to communicate client's information to their EHR using a universal method. The ADA task force created Systematized Nomenclature of Dentistry (SNODENT) for this purpose. As of 2012, several dental practice software companies such as Dentrix, PracticeWorks, and EagleSoft had launched usable EHR programs. Not all dental software packages available on the market are truly transferable EHRs; thus research is recommended before investing in a software system appropriate for each practice. Government incentives have been made available to dental providers who adopt EHRs and treat a high percentage of underserved clients, especially children. All dental providers are expected to integrate EHRs into their practices by 2015, although most will not benefit from the financial incentives because their client population is not composed of a majority of underserved clients. Nonetheless, if the transition from paper to EHRs is handled properly, the practice can reap significant advantages.

Advantages of Electronic Health and Dental Records and Dental Software

Electronic health and dental record software has allowed clinicians to truly use the totality of a client's record in an easily accessible way. Electronic records offer many advantages over standard paper files. Electronic files can send alert prompts to remind the provider of clients' needs, such as diagnostic tests, updates on the medical history, follow-up visits, and medication refills. Electronic software can assist clinicians in clinical decision making and treatment planning of client conditions by supporting access to online scientific literature. Software features can differ from practice to practice depending on the needs of the staff and clients. Other features offered by dental software can provide alerts for chronic conditions, client trend trackers, client treatment preferences, appropriate re-care interval reminders, pending treatment, past referrals, radiographic needs, allergies, and redundant or inconsistent procedures. Dental software also serves as a safety barrier for the client and provider by linking with pharmacies to list all current medications or recently filled medications to indicate potential drug interactions or repeat medication prescriptions such as painkillers. These electronic reminders can reduce errors in treatment especially during busy or stressful times. Using technologic assistance enhances treatment through feedback.

Almost every client at one time or another moves between healthcare settings or experiences out-of-town emergencies, and networked electronic data transfer allows the smooth transition of information from setting to setting while eliminating time spent faxing, scanning, or copying radiographs. Secure Internet networks encrypt client information for safe transfer. **Data encryption** is the process of transforming data to make them unreadable to anyone except those possessing special knowledge in computer formats. Encryption is a risky undertaking because the loss of the password results in loss of data; however, it is necessary whenever data exist where the security of physical media cannot be ensured. In practice terms, before electronic data are backed up and moved offsite (which all practices should be doing), the data first must be encrypted. Once appropriate, strong encryptions have occurred, the information is sent to an offsite server for safe storage. Cloud-based software stores data in servers offsite and providers can access programs through a Web browser on the Internet. All that is needed is a secure Internet connection from a remote access away from the office or clinic. Information is backed up to the minute, and memory and hardware requirements are less because of "outside storage." Time-consuming backups and external hard drives are no longer necessary. If a power surge or fire destroyed a computer or software, the practice's information would be untouched. Upgrading software is easy with Web-based systems because it is completed remotely and the server operates continuously. Failures are possible just as with every other technology, but failures are far less than most other systems. Security is better on electronic/digital records/files than paper. **Date stamping** features also add to the level of protection with all electronic files. Each entry is date stamped, documenting when the entry was placed. If changes are made to a previous entry, date stamping documents the newer entry. This feature provides legal protection of all parties involved. Databases can be linked between dental labs and offices or clinics to check the status on cases and communicate questions between the lab clinician and the provider via the Internet. These systems also can track supplies and alert staff of reordering needs.

Electronic software increases intraoffice communication. With a click of the mouse staff members can inform others that the client is in the chair, ready for an exam, running late, or has canceled the appointment. Networked programs can be established in a practice for smooth communication between treatment rooms and providers. Dropdown features can be used and added to clinical entry notes for consistent verbiage and decreased time spent on entry notes. Electronic software eases day-to-day front desk operations by sending appointment reminders via email regarding upcoming appointments, decreasing time spent scheduling over the phone, returning missed calls, or confirming appointments. Clients can schedule or reschedule appointments online and receive online prompts when needed to update their personal medical history in advance, saving time in the office. Insurance coverage also can be auto-checked when the client schedules online to assess or confirm coverage.

Electronic billing is emailed automatically to third-party providers when the clinician submits client notes and confirms treatments completed during the procedure. All of these features reduce the number of staff needed. Because of reduced paperwork and data entry requirements, front desk personnel have more time for client education and interaction, allowing for better rapport with office staff. Continued-care prompts can be programmed to appear according to the client's periodontal status and scheduled while clinicians are entering clinical data. Tracking of office productivity opportunities in dental software allows for discussion and treatment improvement. These programs allow the practice to operate in a more environmentally friendly capacity.

Some healthcare professions have not only adopted EHRs for client care and documentation but also are employing a tablet. Because of their size and portability, tablets are ideal for clinical workflow tasks such as entering handwritten notes into electronic records, generating accurate prescriptions, and sharing information such as radiographic records or intraoral photographs with clients for educational purposes. With the advent of teledentistry the need for EHRs increased. Teledentistry has been using EHRs, programs and technologies such as intraoral cameras, digital radiography, and high-speed Internet to diagnose client needs successfully in remote areas or across the globe. Clinicians placed in remote sites also have access to vital information.

Electronic files increase communication in the office and between the provider and client. Some databases allow client access to their personal records to support the concept that body and oral conditions are linked and affect overall health. Most programs offer features such as "ask a nurse" or "email your provider" to build the relationship between parties. At times, these features also decrease the need for an appointment saving chair-time and the client's time. Providers may not lose revenue because these discussions may be eligible for billing as consultation time. These software programs feature client-assisted preventive and disease management services where available. Online multimedia oral health education programs can provide clients with valuable information from demonstrations on basic oral hygiene care to detailed explanations of complex dental procedures. Care planning formats as well as informed consents can be created while entering data regarding each client. At the same time clients have an opportunity to increase their awareness; clients tend to become more involved and motivated in their personal care.

Disadvantages of Electronic Health and Dental Records

Electronic databases have many advantages that are revolutionizing the practice management and client assessment; however, there are disadvantages with all technologies. Currently, there is not one secure system in which all healthcare entities can share client records. To this point, there are still no answers to the questions: "Where will this information be stored?" or "Which organization will oversee its security and management?" Governmental policymakers have not been able to address these concerns.

Small businesses may find the costs of implementing EHRs daunting. These costs include equipment and technology, startup, converting historical medical/dental records to EHRs, ongoing technology upgrades, and ongoing technical support. Practices must comply with laws such as HIPAA and revise systems as needed. Those who do not may suffer loss of accreditation and licensure. There also may be technical limitations that have to be addressed to adapt existing EHR systems in individual practices, adding additional fees.

Time Management and Scheduling

Appointment scheduling is essential for controlling the flow of an office by allocating appropriate time increments for appointments, lunch breaks, staff meetings, holidays, vacations, and professional conferences. Dental software scheduling templates offer a variety of features to a dental or dental hygiene practice to track such matters as daily, monthly, or yearly office production; pending client treatment; individual provider productivity; overhead versus production costs; and accounts payable/receivable. Each practice requires and uses various functions so that unique features can be developed. Popular scheduling templates used by the majority of practices include the following:

- Unlimited future booking. This approach allows appointments to be scheduled as far in advance as necessary to accommodate all clients. Most offices use this feature to book the next appointment for clients before they leave the current appointment. Clients appreciate being able to secure a preferred appointment time in advance to best fit their personal schedule. This format has some disadvantages. For example, lost may be the flexibility to schedule new clients in a timely fashion or the ability to accommodate longer appointments for clients needing periodontal maintenance or root planing and scaling. Unlimited future booking also requires careful advanced planning by the dental hygienist for time away from the practice.
- Restricted appointment booking. This approach limits scheduling to a specific period of time such as 1 to 3 months ahead. Clients who need an appointment but are not scheduled to return in that time frame are listed on a waiting list. Clients who need a continued-care appointment in 4, 6, or 12 months are called or asked to call closer to that date. Often a phone call, card, or email is sent to

scheduled clients reminding them of the upcoming appointment. This reminder is helpful for clients who travel frequently or have a fluctuating schedule. This restricted format requires less advanced planning for needed time off but can influence how full the schedule is at any given time.

- Computer and telephone contact files. This approach uses a waiting list of clients in need of appointments and their preferred time. Clients who are available on short notice to fill changed or canceled appointments benefit most from these lists. If an office does not participate in this type of booking, it is best to have a list of clients who can be available on short notice and those who need special treatments to be able to fill cancellations. To best use this approach, the ongoing list must include the client's full name, cell or work telephone number, treatment and time needed, and availability of the client to allow for easy scheduling.
- Production-based booking. This approach is used to schedule clients based on the type of production or procedure being performed. To use this format the office first must establish daily production goals. Based on those goals a format can be tailored to the practice needs. Procedure time blocks are established daily and clients are scheduled according to the specific procedure block needed.

Dental Hygiene Scheduling

A dental hygienist can provide a variety of services to each and every client seen in the practice. Full time dental hygiene work typically involves 32 or more hours a week. Dental hygienists should refrain from working more than 4 days a week in clinical practice, if possible, to allow their bodies time to rest. Time away from clinical dental hygiene helps to avoid repetitive motion injuries that plague dental and dental hygiene professionals. Two typical scheduling approaches for dental hygienists in a general dental practice follow:

- Traditional dental hygiene booking. A dental hygienist delivering comprehensive dental hygiene care completes certain procedures at each new series of visits such as health history review, blood pressure monitoring, preprocedural rinsing, extra and intraoral screenings, risk assessments, periodontal charting, dental charting, client education, exposing and interpreting radiographs or other diagnostic tests as needed, scaling and root planing, coronal polishing, pit and fissure sealants, fluoride therapy, and providing recommendations for follow-up care. For a clinician to provide quality care and comprehensive services for adult clients, a minimum of 1 hour should be allocated per appointment. New clients or periodontal therapy may require a longer appointment. For children, less time may be needed because of reduced charting and treatment requirements. A dental hygiene schedule using a traditional booking format allows the hygienist to treat approximately seven clients per day.
- Assisted dental hygiene booking. Some practices use the support of a hygiene assistant. A dental hygienist and a hygiene assistant work together to increase the number of clients on a given day. This **accelerated dental hygiene practice** allows the dental hygienist to work at a faster pace increasing production and productivity by 50% or more. Hygiene assistants are used at the maximum capacity permitted by law to aid in this fast-tracked pace. eFigure 62-1 illustrates the tasks of the hygiene assistant and dental hygienist in a sample daily schedule. When the daily production for this team increases it also must lead to an increased salary for the dental hygienist and hygiene assistant. This scheduling format may become increasingly popular in community clinics as a way to increase client access to care using dental hygienists and advanced dental hygiene practitioners.

Continued-Care Systems

Also referred to as **re-care** or **recall system**; **continued-care systems** are designed to organize and maintain an appropriate schedule for each client to be seen in the practice based on their individual needs. When applied to patients with periodontitis who have completed active nonsurgical or surgical periodontal therapy, the term used may be *periodontal maintenance care*. In some practices, the dental hygienist is responsible for establishing and managing the continued care or periodontal maintenance schedule for each client. The dental hygienist(s) and dentist(s) must define and establish office policies and parameters for how continued-care intervals are determined for each client. Tracking formats provided by dental software programs allow front desk personnel or the dental hygienist to schedule clients easily according to their re-care timeline. Online technologies have allowed clients to schedule or reschedule their own continued-care appointments via the Internet. Confirmation of these appointments also can be handled through email or text.

Reclamation is a process of electronic periodic purging of all files to identify clients whose care is not complete, who have missed appointments, or who have been absent from the practice and are in need of care. Once identified, clients can be called, emailed, texted, or mailed notification of needed treatment and their last appointment at the office. The dental hygienist may be responsible for reviewing charts and managing reclamation protocols. Most electronic software programs easily can complete this task for clinician viewing and documentation.

Economic Overhead

Practice Overhead

The financial considerations of a practice require determining income and expenditures (e.g., productivity, overhead expenses, collections, and profit). Expenses include the following:

- Employee salaries and fringe benefits
- Rent, lease, and utility expenditures
- Equipment and maintenance
- Lease-hold improvements
- Supplies
- Marketing and advertising
- Accounting and payroll expenses
- Insurance policy payments for the building or personnel

The **office overhead**, based on these expenses, is a determination of the dollar amount it costs per hour to run the office. **Office production** is the total fees billed for services performed. **Collection and income** comprise the amount of money paid to the office from clients, dental insurance companies, and health agencies. **Profit** is the amount remaining after all practice operating costs have been paid. **Cash flow** is the balance between the rate at which money flows into the practice and the rate at which it flows out. Equity is a combination of the practice assets, such as equipment, fittings, and fixtures and the practice's goodwill. Assuming a professional reputation and current practices, goodwill is valued at about five times earnings before interest, tax, depreciation, and amortization.

Financial arrangements must be confirmed with each client before oral healthcare is performed. The practice's policy statement presented in writing to new clients should summarize the financial arrangement options and client's responsibilities. Financial discussions involving treatment with the client may involve the dental hygienist, dental assistant, front desk, dentist, or a combination. To encourage prompt fee collections, some practices offer a small discount to clients who make payments in full at the time the service is rendered. If the office requires a down payment before extensive services are performed or if a fee is charged when a client carries a balance over 30, 60, or 90 days, the clients need to be informed of these policies and made aware that these fees may be added to their account balance. Special long-term financial arrangements also may be offered to some clients to assist in paying for care provided. Dental insurance assists many clients including those who otherwise may not be able to afford oral healthcare. Misunderstandings occur when clients do not fully understand their policies and benefit limits or are unfamiliar with how dental insurance coverage is determined. Dental insurance coverage varies from company to company and policy to policy. It is important to educate clients on their financial responsibilities for services not covered by their dental insurance. Even with the help of the office staff in completing and submitting insurance claims to maximize allowable benefits, it is the clients' responsibility to investigate and understand their individual policy and coverage. Many insurance policies pay a percentage of the "usual and customary" fee for services and require that regular visits be maintained to receive a larger percentage of the service fee. Having a basic understanding regarding insurance policies and coverage is beneficial for the dental hygienist because many clients will ask the hygienist about dental insurance coverage when specific treatment is recommended.

At the present time it is illegal for a dental hygienist to own and operate a dental practice in most states and jurisdictions; however, it is legal in some (e.g., Colorado). In several states (e.g., Montana, Oregon, California, Connecticut, and Washington) an independent practice or limited access permit dental hygienist may own a dental hygiene practice. For dental hygienists who choose to own and operate practices, partnerships are made with dental practices to provide clients with dental care as needed. These arrangements are unique in that hygienists with a collaborative practice or limited access permits are able to work under general supervision or no supervision other than according to a prescription or authorization to provide care. Therefore the dental hygienist must optimize knowledge of practice management principles and practices, the leadership and managerial roles, and the opportunities to enjoy the rewards of a financially successful practice.

Facility Management

Dental hygiene care rooms and equipment must be cleaned and maintained carefully to ensure the maximum life span of these costly items. To keep overhead costs to a minimum, dental hygienists are expected to perform daily, weekly, or semi-annual maintenance (as recommended by manufacturer specifications) to ensure proper equipment function and longevity. Written guidelines are useful to direct personnel in the care of all items. Such guidelines include the following:

- Information on special cleansing and lubricating repairs
- Specially trained personnel to contact when in need of specialty repair
- Intervals of cleaning and oiling
- Schedules for changing of o-rings, drains, filters
- Assignment of personnel responsible for equipment resource management

A materials resource inventory file including MSDSs is needed for all dental hygiene equipment, products, and services. Standards of work allow all team members in the dental office the information needed to maintain all equipment and products.

Adequate stock should be available, but an excess accumulation of items should be avoided because of shelf life and storage problems. Dental supply companies always can supply lists of previous orders, prices, and new items available for purchase; however, if a practice orders from multiple suppliers, a master list should be compiled. An inventory control system consists of the following:

- A list of supplies and materials used
- The manufacturer or distributor
- Cost of item
- Quantity and frequency of ordering

Offices should assign one person as responsible for ordering supplies and maintaining material and supplies in stock to avoid repeat orders or confusion. Dental hygienists often control and manage dental hygiene supplies and client samples for the hygiene operatory, whereas dental assistants oversee other materials and supplies needed for the practice. A specialized budget should be allocated for the dental hygiene department to allow for the purchase of new instruments, ultrasonic inserts, and equipment in addition to any needed repairs.

Dental Hygiene Revenues

The dental hygiene department is a vital, consistent income source for an oral healthcare practice. Without a healthy dental hygiene department, many offices fail to be or stay profitable or to maximize profitability. Some dentists provide preventive oral health or nonsurgical periodontal therapy services; however, this choice can be counterproductive and costly to production. Dental hygienists providing comprehensive care, and especially those with an awareness of practice management, increase the productivity and profits of a practice.

Preventive oral health service fees should be set at a level that validates the education and training of the professional providing the service, and with suitable compensation for the time spent rendering the service. Clients value quality preventive oral healthcare and education and nonsurgical periodontal care provided by the dental hygienist. Additional benefits to the practice are realized when dental hygienists motivate clients to proceed with long-term, comprehensive reconstructive and cosmetic dental treatment, which increases overall profits for the practice.

Some procedures provided directly by the dental hygienist are more productive for the practice, for instance, radiographs, continued-care and periodontal maintenance appointments, active nonsurgical periodontal therapy, chemotherapeutic drug therapy, periodontal supportive services, dental implant maintenance, emergency periodontal treatment, placement of dental sealants, and cosmetic tooth whitening. Protocols and fee structures must be established in the office regarding approaches for each stage of periodontal health and disease. Monitoring of periodontal status is needed at every visit along with altering or adjusting care plans to address the current status of the client.

For all providers, guidelines for professionalism also may contribute to the success of the practice. Displaying a positive professional image and attitude, staying on schedule, adhering to office policies, and always building upon positive provider-client relationships always reflect confidence on the dental hygiene department and the practice. Maintaining current knowledge about oral health conditions, oral hygiene aids and products, clinical and didactic skills, and therapies also increases a client's confidence in the quality of care.

Integral Contributions of the Dental Hygienist

The dental hygienist is a valuable member of the oral healthcare team. Most dental hygienists monitor the health status of clients; educate clients about oral and systemic health, risk factors, and diseases; generate revenues for the practice; attract clients; and maintain client satisfaction through good communication and quality care. The valuable contributions made each day by the dental hygienist are not measured easily. Dental hygienists are recognized best for such roles or actions as the following:

- Providing client education, motivation, and encouragement regarding personal oral and systemic care
- Performing multiple roles as a clinician, researcher, client advocate, oral health educator, and practice manager
- Providing thorough intraoral and extraoral examinations as well as client information on recommended treatment
- Providing answers to client questions and directing clients to additional resources related to recommended dental care and presenting practice philosophies
- Providing a supporting clinical and professional partnership with others in the office, offering a collaborative relationship through communication
- Performing and documenting multiple assessments with expertise (e.g., vital signs, medical history review, premedication validation, extraoral and intraoral examinations, evaluations of outcomes of surgical and nonsurgical periodontal therapies) and monitoring and communicating those findings to the client
- Functioning as a practice builder, interacting with clients as a professional relationships specialist, client confidant, practice ambassador, and friend. Dental hygienists who speak highly of the practice and the quality of work offered in the practice build confidence in clients that leads to client-to-client referrals.
- Filling leadership roles as well as team member roles are two of the many hats worn by the dental hygienist. The dental hygienist has the background and knowledge to educate others in the practice.
- Being responsible for the evaluation of client care in the prevention portion of the practice; therefore the role of practice analysis, recommendations for revisions, and implementation of changes are responsibilities often fulfilled by the dental hygienist.

A dental hygienist always should record and monitor the changes he or she has implemented in the office. Building a portfolio of contributions to the office, client outcomes and overall productivity is a great resource to use when negotiating salary or practice revisions (see Chapter 7). At times the assets a dental hygienist brings to an office are overlooked and become expected, instead of rewarded. It is the duty of the dental hygienist to record these contributions in measurable terms, using portfolios to highlight these talents.

Marketing Dentistry and Dental Hygiene

Marketing is the act of developing, communicating, delivering, and exchanging services in a structured, researched, and organized approach that offers value to the public. Marketing satisfies the needs and wants of the public through exchanging services for currency while building a long-term trusting relationship. The purpose of marketing dental and dental hygiene services is to obtain and maintain the needed share of the client population to keep the practice productive as desired and inform society of the benefits of the practice. The **marketing plan** of a practice should include the four Ps of marketing:

- Product (or service)
- Price
- Place
- Promotion

Product includes the services provided by the practice as well as the philosophies, objectives, and quality of care provided. **Price** involves the cost of the service, which is based on healthcare financing mechanisms, such as reasonable and customary fees and practice expenses such as materials and staffing. **Place** encompasses the entire location and environment of the practice. **Promotion** includes strategies that communicate with target markets and external public groups, such as advertising with newsletters, television, and social media, and all other advertising.

Brainstorming discussions occur between staff members on promotional ideas and select services that should be showcased and how they could be advertised effectively. Some practices appoint outside marketing groups to handle all forms of marketing; however, small practices may find these resources unapproachable because of high costs. In a traditional setting the practice manager is responsible for the marketing relations of the practice. The marketing plan must contain the desired target audience, allotted budget, mode(s) of advertising selected, as well as evaluation measures, which determine if the marketing is successful for the practice. Within the oral healthcare setting, the dentist(s), dental hygienist(s), dental assistant(s), front desk staff, practice manager, and dental laboratory technician(s) should be aware of the marketing plan and incorporate it into daily practice. The most effective marketing is generated from the clients. Satisfied customers who believe their needs have been met with high-quality oral health services at a reasonable fee in a caring environment recommend the practice to friends, family, and business associates. Table 62-3 represents marketing strategies that can promote the providers and the practice and its staff. **Practice promotion** occurs when all team members project the desired professional image and gain public exposure on behalf of the practice. **Internal marketing** reaps the best results often in the form of client referrals.

TABLE 62-3

Marketing Strategies for Practice Promotion

1.	Write articles for local newspapers, town websites, area health magazines, Twitter, Facebook, blogs, YouTube/videos, professional affiliation websites on oral disease, dental service updates, dental emergency care, and evaluation of over-the-counter products.
2.	Participate in community wellness fairs that advocate for overall wellness, health, and disease understanding.
3.	Sponsor free oral cancer screening days for oral health awareness. Perform oral health screenings at schools, senior centers, health fairs, career days, community and athletic programs, civic groups, and special events.
4.	Give lectures to community members regarding oral health and dental diseases to increase awareness.
5.	Invite local newspaper reports or use social media sites to feature an article on the practice, new technology used, new staff members, new degrees or certification obtained.
6.	Participate in broadcast media programming, local radio station and television with special interests information, talk shows, and community service announcements.
7.	Participate in health coalitions, civic, religious, and fraternal group activities in which the practice professionals meet new people and share common interests, providing business cards and referral slips.
8.	Participate in community, cultural, and recreational events in town, state, or region.
9.	Teach health information and cardiopulmonary resuscitation workshops to consumers and other professionals.
10.	Teach dental health to local children by sponsoring a "dental hygienist day" for oral health month(s).
11.	Sponsor an open house event to welcome neighbors to meet the dental office staff members and learn about services offered.
12.	Buy advertising space or time in telephone book or website, local paper, radio stations, Internet sites, in other community media.
13.	Use direct mail methods to distribute oral health education materials, practice brochures, or a newsletter to client's population or local community. Welcome letters for new member to community are also effective.
14.	Design a website for the dental practice that can be accessed by the dental consumer through popular search engines.

Table 62-4 outlines steps that should be taken for productive internal marketing.[7]

Social media is defined as online technologies and practices that people use to share opinions, insights, experiences, and perspectives with friends, family, strangers, or customers. Social media is the newest form of effective advertising and communication; it has revolutionized the marketing world. Social media best lends itself to practice updates, customer service, building relationships, feature articles, practice promotion, client referrals, online practice and clinician credibility, advertising, and even treatment acceptance. Using social networking shows clients a modern edge to the practice, accessibility to clinicians, and approachability. Social media alone cannot replace all forms of advertising but complements current forms of advertising because large portions of the population use some form of social media on a regular basis. Effective websites can showcase a practice or providers' unique talents to set the practice apart. Website designers have to update links constantly, which assist search engines in the finding of the practice website and increase viewing. Keyword-rich content is essential for building credibility with customers and search engines. To keep readers stimulated it is imperative that beneficial and enlightening articles be posted on a regular basis along with ongoing management of Web-based activity and communication. Social media is an effective tool for a practice and works in a budget-friendly manner because most forms are free or very inexpensive. Costs for media sites are associated with Web design, technologic support, and maintenance.

Facebook, Myspace, and other such social networking services can feature a practice page, which shows client cases, staff, office locations, and amenities, as well as lists and describes all services available. This form of social media allows the client to gain confidence in the practice and feel a sense of comfort from already knowing staff and services before ever setting foot in the practice. Facebook also can be used to engage clients by posing questions that require input such as, "What do you like about our office?" Advertising through this type of social networking requires considering a targeted ad campaign based on location, age, gender, education, and interests. These services offer effective and low-cost features that allow communication with existing clients who have the option of encouraging their friends to use the office as well. Twitter is a real-time information network that allows members to connect with one another and to receive information of interest in small bursts. Twitter provides for ongoing conversation and can be used to build a trusting relationship through posts to those with whom one wishes to communicate on a regular basis. This network can be used to engage clients with individual interests and to post short feature articles about new treatments or medication. Twitter requires time on the part of the "tweeter" to post thoughts or ideas on a regular basis.

A Weblog, most often referred to as a blog, is a personal online journal meant to be updated frequently and intended for general public use. Personal or practice blog sites are easy to implement and can be linked into the practice website. Blogs are great for search engine marketing, engaging clients

TABLE 62-4

Successful Internal Marketing Tools

1.	Train staff to ask clients in good standing for referrals.
2.	Remind clients how much your practice appreciates referrals. Place sign(s) in easily seen areas to encourage practice referrals.
3.	Use incentives to build a referral system. Examples include tooth whitening, power toothbrushes, or a reduced treatment fee.
4.	Display posters and/or brochures promoting the dental services offered in the practice.
5.	Ask for client testimonials; encourage letters and emails to your office with positive feedback about treatments received from current clients.
6.	Build strong practice website with links to other social media, such as Facebook, Twitter, Blogs, YouTube, MySpace.
7.	Establish a practice e-newsletter highlighting promotional offerings, events, services, and updates.
8.	Consistently survey clients, asking for feedback on how to improve the office.
9.	Always provide the best customer service. This always leads to satisfied clients, which then lead to client referrals.
10.	Send thank-you notes to clients after each visit, expressing your appreciation for their patronage.
11.	Offer various ways to accommodate your clients (e.g., booking an appointment online even if the office is closed).

in conversations, putting a human voice to the practice, building brand awareness, and generating interest in the practice. Interesting blog posts keep the reader coming back for more, so the topics should be exciting, evoke curiosity, and involve opinions.

YouTube is a form of video marketing that allows a practice or provider to upload and share video advertisements, treatment procedures, and/or educational videos to promote the practice. YouTube allows for great exposure of the upload materials and can expand the practice exponentially. It is important to tag the video or upload with an exciting or descriptive caption for increased interest and viewing. Uploading videos onto YouTube is easy and, best of all, free.

No matter which type of social media the practice decides to use it is imperative that personal drama and negative opinions be left out at all costs. It is also understandable that sometimes less than flattering reviews may be posted from time to time by an unhappy client. It is best to address any negative reviews openly as soon as possible with intentions of presenting accurate information for the client.

Client Satisfaction

To appeal to a broad-based population, the practice must offer a comprehensive spectrum of oral health services including state-of-the-art preventive, therapeutic, maintenance, restorative, cosmetic, counseling, and reconstruction services, or referrals must be made to specialists who offer such treatments. High-quality care is the key to obtaining client satisfaction. Clients recognize dentists and dental hygienists who are sensitive to human needs; provide consistent, technical expertise with an attitude of caring and gentleness; and are respectful of team members and clients.

Correct pronunciation of clients' names can be facilitated by writing them phonetically in the chart. Giving personalized attention, respecting each client as an individual, listening carefully, thoroughly discussing reported symptoms, and being responsive are methods that help develop special relationships that are appreciated by the client. As a consumer advocate, the dental hygienist stays abreast of consumer trends and educates clients about oral healthcare changes as new services and products become available. When care plans are explained, alternatives are offered, including explanations of all options and the costs of each, with clear recommendations given. Clients need to understand the difference between what treatment is necessary and what treatment is ideal. The client's informed decision then is supported fully.

Written, emailed, texted, and/or telephone communications further enhance client satisfaction. A practice website and brochure should be developed and distributed to describe the philosophy of care, introduce the providers and staff, describe services offered, and list office hours plus emergency arrangements, and note special features about the practice for client convenience. Outlines of assessed needs and sequencing of appointments help clients to stay involved with their personal treatment. Sending copies of letters to or from other healthcare professionals concerning needed or ongoing treatment informs the client of the shared interest in his or her oral health. Mailing or emailing clients brief personalized notes of appreciation, congratulations, well wishes, and sympathy communicates appreciation and caring. Telephone contact between the dental hygienist and client should occur after lengthy or complex treatment to check on the client's comfort or healing.

Client satisfaction leads to team member satisfaction. The dentist and dental hygienist should recognize one another and all staff members by expressing appreciation for daily cooperation and team spirit, offering congratulations for tasks well done, noting client loyalty, and recognizing referrals received from staff members' marketing efforts.

Quality Assurance and Auditing of Client Records

All healthcare providers, including dental and dental hygiene practices, must have a formal written patient care quality assurance plan that includes the following:

- Standards of care that are patient centered, focused on comprehensive care, and written in a format that facilitates assessment with measurable criteria
- An ongoing review of a representative sample of patients and patient records to assess the appropriateness, necessity, and quality of the care provided
- Mechanisms to determine the cause of treatment deficiencies
- Client care review policies, procedure, outcomes, and corrective measures

The practice should have a system in place for continuous review of established standards of care. This review requires that objective, measurable criteria be established to review client records with the goal of determining the extent to which the standards of practice have been met. The practice manager should have a written system and process for regular chart auditing. Charts may be selected randomly or auditing of a particular area of concern may be reviewed. A checklist with standards and expectations is helpful for audits. It should have a place to note when policies have not been followed, standards have not been achieved, or treatment deficiencies existed. The record should reflect some commentary or explanation for the deviation. If not, the provider should be asked to comment and to provide needed documentation in the record. Appropriate follow-up with the client also should be noted. If not, actions to correct deficiencies are taken. If multiple providers or team members are responsible for the client care being audited, a record of standards met and standards not met for clients of each provider or each procedure being performed should be recorded. As such, quality assurance involves concurrent review as well as retrospective review of client records. Records also can be flagged for certain areas of interest and reviewed accordingly. A valid method of sampling should be created and documented. The review must be consistent and unbiased. For example, a goal of 1% of all monthly records may be the number of records set for the practice and every tenth chart may be reviewed until that goal is reached.

Other information examined during record audits as a part of quality assurance includes the distribution and honoring of patient rights. The statement should be delivered to all patients and that fact is recorded in all records. The practice manager or designee determines if those rights have been granted to all clients and, if not, addresses that concern.

The Association for Healthcare Documentation Integrity has identified best practices for Quality Assessment and Management.[7] They indicate that three types of error can be detected during audits: critical, noncritical, and feedback errors (or educational opportunities). Critical errors affect client rights, safety, care, or treatment (Box 62-3). Noncritical errors are related to document integrity. Feedback errors do not affect client care but are minor areas in the system or process needing improvement, commonly typographic or spelling errors that do not affect quality of care.

Some dental software programs can perform client record audits systematically. The data produced then can be reviewed by the practice manager or designee. Figure 62-2 presents a sample form used for dental hygiene client record audits.

Please visit the website http://evolve.elsevier.com/Darby/hygiene for additional resources on practice management and quality assurance.

BOX 62-3

Example Client Rights Statement

Client Treatment Rights

- Your right to privacy and confidentiality is important to us and will be protected according to all legal and ethical standards.
- After an assessment has been completed, an explanation of recommended treatment, treatment alternatives, expected outcomes of various treatments, and the risk of no treatment will be explained.
- Once you understand the information about each procedure, consent for care will be requested. You also have the right to refuse treatment at any time. Before initiating your care, costs will be explained. The provider will strive to complete all treatment that has been discussed and accepted.
- When treatment is completed, referrals will be made as needed for specialty care that is beyond the scope of practice here.
- If at any time during or after treatment you wish complete and current information about your care, please contact the front desk and request copies. We also can send information to your other healthcare providers according to the HIPAA statement you signed about privacy of your protected health information.
- This practice uses strict infection-control practices as recommended by the Centers for Disease Control and Prevention and the Occupational Safety and Health Administration. These practices are incorporated to protect you as well as the individuals providing your care.
- You have the right and are encouraged to be an active participant in your oral healthcare decisions, and your right to individual decisions will be respected. Your treatment outcomes largely depend on your adherence with preventive, self-care, treatment, and follow up.
- We strive to adhere to current standards of care and honor your right to receive such care.
- We encourage you to inform the practice manager or your care provider if you have any comments, questions, or concerns. They will be addressed to the best of our ability.

CLIENT EDUCATION TIPS

- Provide clients with written documentation and practice information through social media stating the philosophy of care, introducing the staff, describing services offered, listing office hours, and providing suggested websites for continued education, emergency arrangements, and special features of the practice.
- Provide clients with office expectations and policies (e.g., arriving promptly for scheduled appointments, timely notice if an appointment must be changed).
- Provide practice information about office policies with regard to medical precautions and the need for oral radiographs and collaboration with other health professionals.
- Provide written outlines to clients of their assessed needs and sequencing of appointments to help the client to review and recall verbal case presentations.
- Send clients copies of letters to or from health professionals concerning needed or ongoing care to inform the client of the shared interest in his or her oral health.
- Provide clients with a patient bill of rights and assure them they will be respected.

LEGAL, ETHICAL, AND SAFETY ISSUES

- Client autonomy is an important right and ethical principle; therefore it is important to ensure patients are given options and a thorough informed consent process is followed.
- Client nonadherence to recommended oral healthcare regimens is significant because it can result in compromised care, unsatisfactory care outcomes, client and practitioner dissatisfaction, and possible litigation. In the event of a lawsuit, the judicial decision, outcome, or amount of

Chart Audit Form

Dental Hygiene Client Chart Audit #: ________________ **Date:** ____________

Reviewer: ______________________________ **Provider:** ____________

Note: For each area listed, note yes (Y) or no (N). If no (N) is selected, please give explanation for the deviation in comment section.

Y N (a) Health history completed, updated, and signed
Y N (b) Extra-oral and intraoral examinations completed
Y N (c) Periodontal examination completed
Y N (d) Dental charting completed
Y N (e) Oral hygiene status/self-care assessed and recorded
Y N (f) Radiographic surveys and other diagnostic tests completed and evaluated PRN
Y N (g) Dental hygiene diagnosis including caries risk assessment and periodontal disease classification completed
Y N (h) Consultations with other health professionals for diagnoses and care plan, PRN
Y N (i) Care plan is comprehensive and meets standards
Y N (j) Consent forms completed and signed, PRN
Y N (k) Comprehensive care delivered or recommended as appropriate
Y N (l) Fee payment schedule accurately reflects services provided
Y N (m) Reevaluation completed or planned appropriately
Y N (n) Referrals to dentist, specialist, or other healthcare provider, PRN
Y N (o) Client treatment completed with continued care or periodontal maintenance interval recorded
Y N (p) Record of services follows documentation guidelines in policy manual
Y N (q) Other ______________________________

Comments: ______________________________

Follow up required: ______________________________

Figure 62-2. Sample form used for dental hygiene client record audits.

settlement may be altered based on negligence of the practitioner if nonadherence was ignored.

- Client adherence or nonadherence must be documented carefully, including recommended care and instructions not followed, the client's specific behavior and verbalizations about nonadherence, and any discussions of the consequences of not following recommendations.
- Accurate records provide legal protection by providing documentary evidence if necessary.
- Regular record audits as part of quality assurance measures are needed to determine if practice standards and standards of care are being met by all providers and documentation is accurate and complete.

KEY CONCEPTS

- Practice management is the organization, administration, and direction of the professional practice to produce high-quality care, effective use of time and personnel, stress reduction, and satisfaction enhancement.
- The team concept in dental and dental hygiene practice is the interaction and independence of all staff members to promote the unity and efficiency of the group.
- High-quality care and good communication are the keys to client satisfaction.
- Office policies are established to guide expectations and establish consistency.
- Case presentations for dental hygiene therapy explain the examination findings, discuss the treatment options, explain risks and benefits of proposed procedures and not accepting treatment, present an estimate of costs, and make recommendations to guide and motivate the client in settings goals and choosing a care plan.
- Dental and dental hygiene records serve as a communication, education, assessment, and legal documentation and therefore must be accurate, concise, clear, and thorough.
- Continuing-care and periodontal health maintenance systems are established within dental and dental hygiene practices to ensure regular scheduling of appointments for health maintenance for established clients.

- Economic considerations within a dental and dental hygiene practice include office expenses, production, collection, and profit.
- Marketing a dental and dental hygiene practice involves the planning and management of services that benefit clients at a profit to the practice and involves the participation of all team members.
- Client satisfaction will do more for practice promotion than any other strategy for marketing.
- Social media should be used to introduce potential clients to the practice as well as showcase the uniqueness of the practice, office philosophy, staff, education, services offered, and fees.

CRITICAL THINKING EXERCISES

1. Case presentation: Find an example of a client case with localized severe periodontitis, including a sample periodontal chart demonstrating deep probing depths. Assure the practice client case selected has full-mouth radiographs with evidence of subgingival calculus. One resource for finding cases is www.dentalcare.com.
   a. Role-play the case presentation of the dental hygienist presenting findings to the dentist to reach a collaborative dental hygiene care plan.
   b. Role-play the case presentation of the dental hygienist presenting findings and the recommended dental hygiene treatment plan to the client. Be certain that the discussion contains all elements, including information about findings, education regarding significance of findings, options for care, choice by the client, agreement by the client, and recording of the case presentation in the treatment record.
2. Develop a marketing plan to promote the dental hygiene portion of a dental practice.
   a. The plan should include specific activities or behaviors the team members intend to initiate and what each task is intended to accomplish.
   b. Include an overall timeline to complete the project, time frame for each task, labor division outline, outcome evaluation, and budget.
3. Interview a dental hygienist about the office management of a local dental and dental hygiene practice. Report on the "recall" or continued-care system, the management of supplies and equipment, use of electronic dental records systems, the mission and goals for the practice, HIPAA and OSHA compliance, and the hygienists' role in practice management.
4. Visit a local dental and dental hygiene practice to observe the various uses of a client's electronic record. Report on how each team member (e.g., dentist, dental hygienist, dental assistant, laboratory technician, front desk, and office manager) uses the numerous features of the electronic client record differently and describe the role each team member plays in ensuring accuracy and documentation in the client's electronic record.

REFERENCES

1. Henson H: Practice management. In Darby ML, Walsh NN, eds: *Dental hygiene theory and practice*, Philadelphia, 2010, Saunders.
2. Sharma S: Leadership and management: get organized, get started, *Dent Nurs* 6:9, 2010.
3. American Dental Hygienists' Association: *Standards for clinical dental hygiene practice*. Available at: http://www.adha.org/downloads/adha_standards08.pdf. Accessed August 13, 2012.
4. Sharma S: Personnel management: ergonomics and teamwork in dental practice, *Dent Nurs* 6:12, 2010.
5. Gross T: Creating the authentic practice, *Dent Econ* 8, 2009.
6. Health Insurance Portability and Accountability Act of 1996 (HIPAA): *Privacy and Security Measures*. US Department of Health and Human Services. Available at: http://www.hhs.gov/ocr/privacy/. Accessed March 30, 2013.
7. Association of Healthcare Documentation Integrity (AHDI): *Healthcare documentation quality assessment and management best practices*. 2010. Available at: http://www.ahdionline.org. Accessed March 30, 2013.

ACKNOWLEDGEMENT

The author and editors wish to acknowledge Harold Henson for his former contribution to this chapter.

The author and editors wish to acknowledge Angie Bailey, RDH, MS candidate for her review of this chapter for the fourth edition.

EVOLVE RESOURCES

Please visit http://evolve.elsevier.com/Darby/hygiene for additional practice and study support tools.

CHAPTER 63

Career Planning and Job Searching

Jennifer L. Brame

COMPETENCIES

1. Discuss career development in dental hygiene, including:
   - Identify the steps to career development.
   - Select one or more individuals that may serve as a mentor and/or reference, and serve as a networking source for your career.
   - Write a personal career plan including short-term and long-term goals and objectives for career development in dental hygiene.
2. Discuss the opportunities within dental hygiene as a career.
3. Discuss the job search and interview process, including:
   - Describe how to search for a job in dental hygiene.
   - Develop a résumé or curriculum vitae that highlights professional expertise and accomplishments and a cover letter to obtain an interview for a desired dental hygiene position.
   - Create a list of questions and considerations that may be used during a job interview.
4. Describe additional employment factors, including:
   - Types of possible compensation within the dental hygiene field.
   - Employment rights and the performance evaluation process.
   - Job exiting, including sources of burnout or stress in dental hygiene.
5. Describe the expanding scope of dental hygiene.
6. Explain the significance of career satisfaction.

Career Development in Dental Hygiene

Dental hygiene is a unique and exciting profession that provides opportunities for lifelong learning through continuing education, maturation of professional skills, participation in the growth of the profession, research, education, organizational leadership, and contributions to community service. Career development in dental hygiene should be a continual process that professionals assess throughout their career to adapt to ever-evolving personal characteristics and life changes, as well as the changing face of the profession. Analyzing oneself, cultivating and exploring personal and professional interests, building a team of mentors, creating professional and personal goals, and organizing those goals in a plan empower a person to navigate the profession and offer a path to career satisfaction.

Steps to Career Development

Self-Assessment

Self-assessment enables oneself to discover particular interests, abilities, and environments conducive for success. This knowledge may affect one's desire for career choices and job selection and is also a strong educational tool in developing critical thinking and problem-solving skills.[1]

Self-assessment may be completed using various tools. Performance evaluation and personal observation are means of self-assessing skills and job performance. Assessment instruments also may be used, for example, the personality assessment examination, such as the Meyers-Briggs Type Indicator (MBTI), which includes more than 90 questions to reveal overall trends in a person's personality type and preferences. Expansion in self-awareness is a lifelong process that can lead to broadening functions, relationships, and responsibilities within career activities and events that may enhance career development and satisfaction.

Building a Relationship with a Mentor

Whether beginning a career in dental hygiene or practicing for many years, dental hygienists find it rewarding, personally and professionally, to have one or more mentors. A mentor is a trusted advisor who can evaluate a person's professional strengths and serve as a resource. Mentorship can provide support and guidance during the transition from student to clinician, reducing anxiety and improving confidence in clinical practice. Powerful mentors also can provide positive differences in mentees' careers and help them to grow professionally. Good candidates for a mentor include a former professor, a past or present employer or supervisor, close colleagues, or others knowledgeable in a specific area of interest. Dental hygienists may consider seeking mentors by enrolling in advanced education programs or volunteering for professional activities of the American Dental Hygienists' Association (ADHA), their constituent (state) organization, or local component (area in which the dental hygienist resides), alumni associations, or by collaborating with dental hygienists who have become known in an area of expertise in dental hygiene.

Figures, tables, and boxes marked as "e" are available as supplemental material on the Evolve site. Visit http://evolve.elsevier.com/Darby/hygiene to access these materials.

Networks for Professional Enhancement

Networks in dental hygiene are professional friendships and business relationships designed to exchange knowledge and develop a support system for achievement of professional goals. Positive networks in dental hygiene may be found via membership in professional associations and community organizations. Additional sources include online networks such as DHNet, LinkedIn, and Facebook.

Dental professionals must seek out opportunities to meet new people and build professional networks. Once established, a professional network can serve as a career-long resource for job openings, continuing education, leadership opportunities, development of relationships with mentors, and references.

Career Goals

The road to a successful and fulfilling career begins with self-assessment and the development of career goals and a career plan. A career plan is developed by creating a list of personal goals one hopes to attain within his or her career. These career goals should include short- and long-term goals, such as 2- and 5-year goals to consider when developing a career plan. Next strategies for attaining these goals and specific actions needed are listed for each goal identified. A timeline sometimes is helpful as a means of assessing progress. The plan should be realistic and feasible but not restricted to safe boundaries. Dental hygienists should update their career plans and self-assess routinely, as changes in life occur, to ensure job satisfaction throughout the span of their career.

Dental Hygiene as a Career

Although most dental hygienists work in private dental practices, there are a variety of career opportunities.[2] Dental hygienists may choose to work clinically in privately owned dental offices, school-based dental clinics, military dental clinics, managed care organizations, health departments, community health dental clinics, hospitals, state and federal correctional institutions, and long-term care facilities. Other nonclinical career opportunities include public health and government positions, sales or marketing positions, education, research, administration roles, consulting, consumer advocacy, and in healthcare policymaking.[2]

According to the Bureau of Labor Statistics, employment of dental hygienists is expected to grow 38% from 2010 to 2020, which is faster than the average for all occupations.[3] This projection is based on population growth, aging of our current population, growing emphasis on preventive dental care, and research linking oral health and general health.[3,4] As a result of these projections and other factors outside of the discipline, dental hygiene education programs have been expanded in number and the unmet need is being fulfilled for basic, entry-level practice positions.

The Job Search

Researching Employment Opportunities

Resources for job searching include professional networks; online job search engines; social media websites, such as LinkedIn, Facebook, and Twitter; and online classifieds, such as Craig's List. Consider online resources for employment searching and as tools to locate potential employers' website to learn more about the organization, its clients, and its staff as well as the typical services delivered there. For positions in education, the applicant should visit educational institutions' websites, public health organizations within the state or province of the job seeker's preference, and research facilities or other institutions where research is being conducted. For dental hygiene positions abroad, visit the International Federation of Dental Hygienists (IFDH) (http://www.ifdh.org) or the specific country's dental hygiene association's website. Remember that word-of-mouth is also a valuable tool for learning about job opportunities, thus reinforcing the power and necessity for strong professional networks. Box 63-1 identifies sources for locating dental hygiene employment.

BOX 63-1

Sources for Locating Dental Hygiene Employment

- Professional networks (e.g., local professional association, alumni associations, and study clubs)
- Verbal or printed announcements at dental hygiene meetings and continuing education courses
- Public or county health departments
- Dental hygiene school employment opportunities bulletin boards
- Dental hygiene and dental association newsletters and journals
- Professional journals and magazines
- Public employment agencies
- ADHA website: http://www.adha.org/career-center
- Social media websites such as LinkedIn, Facebook, and Twitter
- Newspaper and web-based classified advertisements
- Websites for employment opportunities

Additional Internet sites may be found on the textbook resources page.

Writing a Résumé

The **résumé** is a document that highlights achievements, experience, skill sets, and education. There are various styles that may be used when tailoring a résumé. Websites such as how-to-write-a-résumé.org can serve as a guide for development and format. The functional résumé lists primary skill sets and accomplishments that support a specific job position and reflect ability in individual areas of expertise. Box 63-2 describes the contents of a high-quality résumé.

Honesty and accuracy are the most important elements of résumé writing. It is important to highlight skills necessary for the desired job, and those of a new graduate such as familiarity with new technologies and treatment modalities. The résumé format is brief; one to two pages is preferred. A high-quality document on medium-weight white or ivory paper is most appropriate and professional. The résumé must appear polished, neat, accurate, and letter-perfect with correct spelling and grammar. Sample résumés appear in Figures 63-1 and 63-2.

Curriculum Vitae

A **curriculum vitae** (CV) is a comprehensive résumé used typically for individuals seeking an academic position. The CV format is more complex than the résumé and is not limited to one to two pages. A CV should include information such as educational background, licensure, continuing education,

BOX 63-2

Components of a High-Quality Résumé

Personal Identification
- Name
- Address
- Telephone number and email address

Job Objective (Optional)
- Statement of the exact job being sought, giving résumé focus
- Professional goals

Career Summary
- Skills
- Strengths

Professional Employment Experience
- Summary of any responsibilities not generally encompassed by the normal dental hygiene job description, noting any special awards received; for new licentiates, list of special skills or interests from school, jobs in related fields, or academic honors and awards
- Students should document professional experiences with diverse client populations treated in rotations during school.
- Private practice
- Teaching
- Administrative experience
- Research
- Government

Professional Data (Optional)
- Professional affiliations
- Community and professional services
- Publications
- Presentations given
- Continuing education courses attended
- Professional projects

References (Optional)
- "Available on request"

professional employment, teaching experience, professional membership, leadership roles, community service, publications, and research involvement.

Electronic Portfolio

An electronic portfolio, also known as an e-portfolio or digital portfolio, is a digital collection of material that provides evidence supporting your efforts, achievements, and progress gained from education, work, and life experiences (see Chapter 7). A personal website can provide an alternative web presence to social networks, helping build a positive digital identity.[5]

Maintaining Professionalism on Social Media Websites

Although participation in social media (e.g., Facebook, Twitter) is the norm, remember that these media may play a role in determining whether one is hired or not. Keep these postings professional; remove any potential image-damaging posts and pictures before the job search. Keep in mind that potential employers have the ability to view these sites and may glean a perception that is misinterpreted or negative.[6] Social media sites never should be used as a means to complain about professional issues or work-related events. Never comment on clients, client care, or practice-related issues. Maintaining client privacy and abiding by HIPAA laws is vital for a dental hygiene professional.

References and Recommendations

References are personal testimonies to the job candidate's competence and character. When identifying potential references, a person should ask if they would be willing to serve as a reference, and if they can provide a favorable recommendation. Job seekers with many years of experience want to touch base with anyone listed on their reference list before distributing it. A friendly phone call periodically keeps the connection current, offers a networking opportunity, and may be a source of job leads. References should be selected and contacted before résumé distribution.

Cover Letter

A cover letter is an introductory letter, accompanying the résumé, designed to introduce the job candidate to a potential employer. The cover letter is the applicant's first contact with a prospective employer and provides a succinct introduction and marketing opportunity spotlighting skills and qualifications. Cover letters should accompany résumés when distributing to potential employers.

Unless the employer is requesting an electronic submission, the résumé and cover letter should be typed and printed on high-quality paper. Applicants should either hand-deliver or mail résumés and cover letters when inquiring about a position. Job ads typically indicate the method of delivery preferred. Figure 63-3 illustrates a sample cover letter.

Response and Follow-up Before the Interview

A follow-up letter should be sent at least 1 to 3 weeks after the résumé is sent, if no reply has come from the prospective employer. Following up avoids any implication of disinterest or lack of desire for the position and may clarify the status of an application. In addition, good business etiquette requires a prompt response to all calls, emails, and interviews. Figure 63-4 presents an example of a follow-up letter.

Preparing for the Job Interview

The job interview is the employer and applicant's opportunity to determine if the position is a good fit for him or her. The initial impression that an applicant makes on the employer may have long-standing implications and may determine whether one is hired. Before the interview, job applicants should locate important information regarding the practice, university, company, agency, or organization with which they will be interviewing. Complete an online search to learn about such issues as the setting, types of clients seen, and mission of the office. Equally important, make sure that you know where the office is located and how to locate it before the scheduled interview.

For a university position, determine the university's mission; the administrative department that houses the position; job responsibilities; and salary scales and benefits. For

Jill Thompson, RDH, BSDH, BS
123 New Way
Anytown, ST 60123

Objective	To utilize my educational and clinical expertise to work as a dental hygiene educator in an oral care company.
Professional Experience	**Dental Hygienist** **2007-Present** **Tom Levine, DMD, General Dentist, Berkeley, California** Responsibilities included medical history assessment, intra/extra oral examination, vital signs, full mouth and bitewing digital radiography, oral cancer screening, oral caries detection, professional prophylaxis, fluoride application, and review of oral hygiene techniques. • Led the development and implementation of eco-friendly practices in the office to incur a 30% profit in the purchasing of products and tools to carry out dental and dental hygiene procedures. • Developed the dental health product store in our office to sell oral care products and systems to patients to use at home, which resulted in a 45% profit to the practice and increased patient compliance by 20%. **Children's Author** **2001-2003** **Hoobey Publishing, Los Angeles, California** Wrote three children's books on learning experiences for 4-5 year olds and assisted in selling these books with parents to target educational skills and opportunities. • Fifteen percent of the proceeds from the sale of the books went to the St. Jude's Children's Foundation. **Kindergarten Teacher** **1996-2003** **Berkeley Elementary School, Berkeley, California** Responsibilities included educating 20 kindergarteners on vocabulary, spelling, reading, and math for a 10-month period of time. Exercises included fun and exciting programs to gain the students' interest.
Education	**Bachelor of Science Degree in Dental Hygiene** **2007** University of Pacific School of Dentistry, San Francisco, California **Bachelor Degree in Education** **1996** University of California, San Francisco, California
Volunteer Experience	**Newbawn Nursing Home, Alamo, California** **2008-Present** Worked with geriatric patients to provide medical history assessment, intra/extra oral examination, vital signs, oral prophylaxis, fluoride application, review of oral hygiene techniques, and education of the staff at the nursing home.
Global Community Activities	**Honduras Children's Foundation, July 2006; Mexico Operation Blessings** **2009**
Professional Licensure	**Dental Hygiene License in the states of:** — California — Arizona
Professional Organizations	American Dental Hygienists' Association, California Dental Hygienists' Association, Arizona Dental Hygienists' Association, American Academy of Dental Hygiene, American Teacher's Organization
Professional Honors	2007 Sigma Phi Alpha, 1998 and 2002 Teacher of the Year Award
References	Available on request

Figure 63-1. Example of an experienced professional résumé.

an interview in a corporate setting, determine the philosophy, mission, and goals of the company; new developments and products; sales and revenue; the number of employees; dental professionals who work in the company; job responsibilities of the dental hygienist; person(s) to whom the dental hygienist reports; colleagues who assist or work with the dental hygienist; travel requirements and meetings to attend; questions about salary and benefits for possible discussion; and whether the position is new, is existing, or has been modified for this search.

The applicant should prepare questions before the interview regarding the position, job description, practice management, salary, and benefits (vacation time, sick days, holidays, medical and dental insurance, stock options, professional development opportunities, retirement plan), depending on the setting. Refer to Box 63-3 for questions and considerations for job interviews.

The Interview

During the interview, employers frequently outline or discuss the job description, responsibilities, and expectations. Compatibility is established by linking the candidate's skills and strengths with the job description and needs of the practice. Depending on the time and depth of conversation, some

Jill Thompson, RDH, BSDH
123 New Way
Anytown, ST 60123

Objective	**To work in a state-of-the-art dental/cosmetic dental practice in Berkeley, California.**	
Education	**Bachelor of Science Degree in Dental Hygiene** University of Pacific School of Dentistry, San Francisco, California	**2013**
Professional Experience	**Dental Assistant** **Tom Levine, DMD, General Dentist, Berkeley, California** Responsibilities include full-mouth and bitewing radiographs, assist the dentist in dental procedures (i.e., restorations, aesthetics, prosthodontics), clean and sterilize instruments, provide infection control procedures between patients, set room up for patients being treated including tray set-up, and perform patient education when needed.	**2012-Present**
	Student Dental Hygienist **University of Pacific School of Dentistry, Department of Dental Hygiene, San Francisco, California** Responsibilities included medical history assessment, intra/extra oral examination, vital signs, full-mouth and bitewing radiographs, prophylaxis, fluoride application, and review of oral hygiene techniques.	**2009-2013**
	Student Dental Hygienist **Home Health Nursing Home, Berkeley, California** Responsibilities included medical history assessment, intra/extra oral examination, vital signs, full-mouth and bitewing radiographs, oral health education to patients and nursing home healthcare team, patients.	**2011-2013**
Volunteer Experience	**Miles for Smiles Organization, California** Worked with nondisabled children and disabled children in oral health education, and took bite registrations to be used in the case of missing children.	**2012-Present**
Professional Licensure	**Dental Hygiene License in the state of:** — California	
Professional Organizations	American Dental Hygienists' Association California Dental Hygienists' Association	
References	Available on request	

Figure 63-2. Example of a student résumé.

employers may request a second interview. This should include a thorough discussion of job description, office policies and procedures, work schedule, compensation package of starting wage and benefits, performance evaluation, fringe benefits, and frequency and basis of raises. Please note that not all employers use multiple interviews and may discuss these specifics during one interview. Some employees or employers also propose a working interview in which the dental hygienist works in the potential job setting for a half-day or day to evaluate the fit.

Professional appearance makes a long-standing impression. Consider your appearance as you would want to be perceived: professional, organized, neat, and clean. Interview attire should include wearing a business suit (pants or skirt) with short, groomed nails with clear or neutral polish and a clean and neat hairstyle. Avoid excessive jewelry, makeup, and perfume. Keep in mind that the position is one of a healthcare provider, so it is essential to project professionalism, integrity, and critical thinking skills.

Interview Communication

Professional behavior and effective communication are keys to conducting a successful interview. The applicant should listen to each question thoroughly and provide open and honest answers that impart a sense of integrity and self-esteem during the interview. Likewise, it is vital that the applicant take time to ask questions of the employer. The applicant should take notes during the interview to reference after the interview. Other recommendations for successful job interviews are as follows:

- Turn off all cell phones and other electronics.
- Be prompt. Arrive 10 minutes early.
- When applicants enter a room, they should shake the interviewer's hand as well as anyone else's hand on the team.
- Make eye contact during communication.
- Listen carefully to each question and answer the actual question asked, responding with direct, thoughtful, concise answers.

May 1, 2013

Lucy Smith
111 Drive Way
Chapel Hill, NC 27514
lucysmith@emailaddress.com

Dr. Alicia Brown
222 Dental Road
Durham, NC 27713

Dear Dr. Brown,

I saw your advertisement on LinkedIn for a full-time dental hygienist stating that you wanted a sincere, dedicated, and patient-centered hygienist. I feel that I meet all of those qualifications and am very interested inapplying for the position. I have enclosed a résumé, and would appreciate your consideration for this position.

During my education in the dental hygiene program, I had many opportunities to develop skills necessary to become a competent and successful hygienist. I am a dedicated clinician, compassionate and caring to each patient, and thorough in my care. As a dental hygiene student, I had the opportunity to provide care to patients in various settings including rotation sites at hospital dental clinics and community dental clinics. I have excellent interpersonal and communication skills, and am confident working with a variety of patient types. I feel confident in my skills as a developing dental hygiene clinician and am excited about the opportunity to continue learning.

Thank you for your consideration of me for this position. I look forward to hearing from you and welcome the opportunity to meet and further discuss.

Sincerely,
Lucy Smith

Figure 63-3. Example of a cover letter.

Jill Thompson, RDH, BSDH, BS
123 New Way
Anytown, ST 60123

March 1, 2010

Dr. Larry Birkshire
Birkshire Dental Associates
XYZ Lane
Anytown, ST 60123

Dear Dr. Birkshire:

I sent my cover letter and résumé to you on February 18 for the dental hygiene position in your dental and cosmetic practice in Berkeley, California. I am excited to learn more about this computer-driven dental practice and the dental hygiene position within it, which was highlighted in the *Berkeley Tribune*.

My experience working with many diverse patient populations (i.e., children, adolescents, teenager, adults, and geriatric) at the University of Pacific School of Dentistry provided me the opportunity to utilize my Spanish language skills in treating many Hispanic patients. My rotations in clinic and public health, as well as working with special-needs patients utilizing a computerized software program, have improved my dental technology skills, which include digital radiography.

Please call me during the day at 555-123-1234. I look forward to speaking with you in the next week. Thank you for your assistance.

Sincerely,
Jill Thompson, RDH, BSDH, BS

Figure 63-4. Example of a follow-up before-an-interview letter.

BOX 63-3

Questions and Considerations for Job Interviews

Practice Team and Practice Management

- What types of clients and treatment services are provided?
- What is the management style?
- Are there staff meetings? If so, how often are staff meetings held?

Health Maintenance, Disease Prevention, and Health Promotion

- How often are the health history questionnaire and vital signs completed?
- Under what circumstances is a client's physician consulted for advice regarding oral healthcare?
- What is the practice protocol for antibiotic premedication and restrictions on treating clients with elevated blood pressure?

Job Description and Client Care

- What is the job description?
- What are the expectations for the person in this position?
- How many days per week are available for work? Which days?
- What are the work hours?
- What is the daily schedule for dental hygiene clients?
- Are there variable appointment lengths for healthy adults, active periodontal therapy care, periodontal maintenance care, new client care, and/or children?
- Is there an assistant for the dental hygienist?
- What is the protocol for both planned time off and unexpected time off?
- Are there days or hours when the dental hygienist will provide client care in the absence of a dentist (if state supervision laws permit)?
- Are there opportunities for professional growth?
- What are radiographic exposure recommendations?
- Do the dentist and dental hygienist work collaboratively to determine a care plan for periodontal needs?
- What are the elements of nonsurgical periodontal therapy that the practice supports and performs?
- What is the level of client compliance with prevention and periodontal health maintenance efforts?
- How are continued-care intervals established for clients?
- What is the percentage of cancellations and broken appointments?
- Who discusses risks, benefits, and alternatives to the recommended treatment with the client?
- Who discusses fees and dental insurance with the client?
- What products (e.g., antimicrobials, anesthetics, fluorides, and desensitizing agents) are available for client treatment?
- What products (e.g., toothbrushes, floss, toothpick holders, interproximal devices, fluorides) are available for distribution as samples to clients? If you have preferences that are not available, will the practice purchase them?
- What methods of pain or dental anxiety control are used and how often?

Office Observation

- Ask to see the dental hygiene treatment room, sterilization, and radiographic facilities.
- Is there adequate space in the room to move around the dental chair?
- Is the space adequate and accommodating for left-handed operators, if applicable?
- What types of instruments are available?
- What is the instrument maintenance policy? How and when are new instruments ordered?

Other Work Responsibilities

- What are the record-keeping and documentation requirements for dental hygiene services?
- Are there dental hygienist responsibilities elsewhere?
- Does the practice adhere to OSHA guidelines and standards?
- What is the practice attire? Is protective clothing provided?
- How are instruments sterilized? Are the sterilization units monitored?
- Where and how are biohazards disposed of?

Medical Emergencies

- Does the office provide CPR recertification for the practice team?
- Does the staff have a practice plan in case of medical emergency?
- Where is the emergency medical kit and oxygen tank located? How frequently are they checked, and by whom?

- Ask for clarification if a question is not clearly understood. If there is an unanswerable question, say so; do not pretend you have an answer.
- Be articulate, and answer with details to establish a memorable impression; give examples of proven ability and professionalism but keep responses brief.
- Establish credibility and trust; above all, be honest and do not misrepresent yourself.
- Do not offer information about your personal life.
- Ask specific, intelligent questions that provide the information needed to determine if this is the position sought. Asking questions shows the employer a genuine interest in the job.
- Be cautious to contain nervous habits (e.g., inappropriate laughter, chattiness); do not fidget or chew gum.
- Project confidence during the interview, and do not be afraid to discuss limitations and potential weaknesses. The key to discussing limitations is knowing how to spin them into a positive opportunity. (For example, a new graduate may point out that time management is a short-term weakness; however, it is also an opportunity to learn and grow.)
- Make sure to highlight the special skills that you have, setting you apart from other applicants. This may include familiarity with new technologies and treatments, computer skills, and experience with intraoral photography.
- Demonstrate that the primary reason for the interview is to gain information about the position and resist the temptation to ask about money. Although there may be brief mention of the wage or salary range during the interview, any salary negotiations should occur after a job offer is received.

Working Interview

Dental hygienists may be asked to or may request a working interview, in which they actually perform the job within the work environment with staff members before being offered the position. This is an excellent opportunity for the applicant and office members to examine their potential working relationship. It also gives the dental hygienist a firsthand view of the interoffice working specificities and their potential to succeed in the environment.

Office Observation

Applicants should ask for the opportunity to observe the office. It provides the dental hygienist an opportunity to view a typical workday in an office setting, therefore giving insight on the interoffice dynamics, including communication between the staff members, management styles, flow of schedule, atmosphere of working environment, efficiency, teamwork among peers, and client relations. Other important observations may include safety, sanitation, and sterilization methods, equipment and instrument quality, and the overall reality of how the office functions.

Follow-up Communications

After the interview, candidates should thank the interviewers in person and in writing. A post-interview thank-you letter (Figure 63-5) should be mailed the day after the interview. The letter should be typed and signed by the applicant and sent via mail. The letter does not have to be long or detailed, but it does show a potential employer a genuine interest and level of respect, making the candidate more memorable to a potential employer.

Job Selection Considerations

When considering which job to select, the dental hygienist should compare career needs and desires with what is being offered by the potential employer. Although sometimes challenging, patience and careful selection of a job is important in helping to identify the best fit. It is important to determine which of the following details are of greatest importance personally:

- Overall practice ambiance and atmosphere
- Practice philosophy, goals, and values
- Personal harmony felt with the office atmosphere and staff members
- Practice standards and quality of care provided
- General job description, including the specific responsibilities and the scope of dental hygiene care provided
- General work conditions (e.g., workload, scheduling, pace, hours, equipment, supplies, instruments)
- Compensation package consisting of salary, fringe benefits, opportunity for bonuses, schedule, and basis for remuneration increases
- Opportunity for professional growth, continuing education, and personal satisfaction
- Job security with an assured client load plus established record of employee longevity
- Location of employment setting, commuting, and parking situation

Jill Thompson, RDH, BSDH, BS
123 New Way
Anytown, ST 60123

March 1, 2010

Ms. Sarah Jameson
OnHealth Pharmaceuticals, Inc.
XYZ Lane
Anytown, ST 60123

Dear Ms. Jameson:

Thank you for the opportunity to interview for the position of dental hygiene educator and exhibit specialist with OnHealth Pharmaceuticals, Inc. I am impressed with the detailed training your organization provides to dental hygiene educators. I know I will be confident and prepared to demonstrate the company's new line of oral care products to the dental and dental hygiene communities.

I look forward to an opportunity to return to the trade show environment and exercise my sales skills again. I am certain other dental hygienists will be as excited as I was to learn more about the flexibility of this new product line and how it will help their patients improve their oral health. My experience in education and private practice will provide a distinct advantage for this position.

Please contact me during normal business hours at 555-123-1234. I hope to become a part of your professional team and look forward to hearing from you shortly. Thank you for this opportunity.

Sincerely,
Jill Thompson, RDH, BSDH, BS

Figure 63-5. Example of a post-interview thank-you letter.

- Practice well established, new and growing, stable, or restructuring and in transition; staff large or small

Compensation

The methods of compensation for dental hygiene employment are varied and determined by agreement between the employee and employer. Dental hygienists may be paid on an hourly, daily, salary, or commission basis. Methods of compensation include the following:

- Fixed salary: A guaranteed fixed wage is paid for hourly, daily, weekly, or monthly employment.
- Salary plus commission: A base salary is paid, plus an additional percentage of fees charged for dental hygiene services.
- Salary plus fringe benefits: Fringe benefits or "perks" are special services and items offered in addition to salary. The most common fringe benefits that dental hygienists receive are continuing education, free or discounted dental care, and paid vacations or holidays (Box 63-4).
- Commission with guaranteed minimum salary: A percentage of fees charged for dental hygiene services is paid, with an assured minimum wage per day regardless of daily gross production.
- Commission: Earnings are based on a percentage of fees charged for dental hygiene services.
- Independent contractor: In some states a dental hygienist may work as an independent contractor with a supervising dentist to provide services to the clients of that dentist by referral prescription while adhering to the state dental practice act. The dental hygienist sets and collects all fees and pays overhead costs with the profit fluctuation based on production, collection, and expenses.
- Profit-sharing bonus: A work incentive is awarded to employees after profit goals are achieved for a specified period; may be calculated monthly, quarterly, or annually.
- Fringe benefits: Paid services in addition to regular wages. Some benefits are required by law, and some are optional services offered by the employer or requested by the dental hygienist. Fringe benefits paid for by the employer are tax deductible to the employer.

Salary Ranges

To find general statistics on dental hygiene pay, the job seeker may visit a few helpful websites, including the U.S. Department of Labor's Bureau of Labor Statistics or sites such as http://www.payscale.com, to compare the prospective employer's salary with national standards. The dental hygienist also may contact other dental hygienists working in the area, contact the component dental hygienists' association employment chairperson, or contact a local employment

BOX 63-4

Optional Fringe Benefits

- Paid absences
- *Sick leave.* Salary paid during occasional short-term illnesses; sometimes, sick days are allowed to accumulate if not used, or unused days are paid at the end of the year as a bonus
- *Holidays.* Salary paid for usual, nationally observed holidays
- *Vacation.* Salary paid for vacation time often varies according to the length of service with the employer. Vacation pay may be cumulative; for part-time employees, vacation days are prorated
- *Educational leave.* Salary paid for time off to attend educational programs that are work related
- *Emergency personal leave.* Paid time off for unexpected events such as a family illness, death, or funeral; jury duty, legal depositions, or court appearances; or extreme weather conditions
- *Maternity leave.* Time off, usually without pay but with the guarantee of job protection on return from leave; reasonable time limits usually apply
- *Extended leave.* Leave without pay for a few weeks to several months for the purpose of travel, family, or personal needs. The position is held during the absence with an agreed-on time of return
- *Sabbatical, developmental, or research leave.* Usually involves leave without pay or reduced pay for a few weeks to several months for the purpose of education or research. The position is held during the absence with an agreed-on time of return

Employee Assistance Program

- Provides confidential and professional assistance for employees and their family members experiencing problems affecting their job or overall quality of life.

Retirement

- Employer contributes entire sum or employer matching contribution combined with employee contribution or pension plans

Insurance Benefits

- Health insurance
- Dental insurance
- Vision insurance
- Liability (malpractice) insurance
- Long-term permanent disability insurance
- Life insurance

Professional Expenses

- Professional license renewal
- Uniform allowance
- Professional equipment expenses
- Professional education assistance
- Professional activities
- Professional journals or texts
- Transportation expenses
- Expense account

agency, if possible specializing in dental office employment, to learn about average salary ranges.

Employment and Evaluation

Employment Rights

Dental hygiene employment falls under the Nondiscrimination Act, Title VII of the Civil Rights Act of 1964. The law establishes equal employment opportunity for all during the hiring process and throughout the course of employment.

Minimal standards for working conditions are set by each state and include guidelines pertaining to hours and days of work, minimum wage and reports for pay, employee records, uniforms and equipment, meal periods and eating area, rest periods and rest facilities, and environmental temperature. The Occupational Safety and Health Administration (OSHA) sets minimum federal requirements for industrial safety.

Employment Contracts

An employment contract may be used to describe the terms of employment agreed on by the dental hygienist and the dentist (eFigure 63-6). The contents may include administrative terms of the agreement, settings and terms of employment, job description, compensation, probationary period, performance evaluation, and termination procedures (Box 63-5). An employment contract is not a required document and therefore may not be completed.

Performance Evaluation

The dental hygienist should be given the opportunity for evaluation on a periodic and consistent basis via **performance evaluation**. The performance evaluation is a valuable tool that provides a progress report for the employee, recognizes and supports desired behavior, develops strengths, pinpoints weaknesses, and gives specific direction for change. The performance evaluation may assist in determining a salary increase or can be used as a legal supporting document for employee dismissal. A job evaluation should be performed at the completion of the probationary period if the employee is new, then once or twice a year for the duration of employment. Figure 63-7 provides an example of an employee performance evaluation.

BOX 63-5

Terms of Employment

- *Permanent.* The employee's service with the employer is relatively secure and of unlimited duration.
- *Temporary.* The employee's service is known to be of limited duration.
- *Probationary.* A service trial period, usually 1 to 3 months, for employee and employer to work together, followed by evaluation of each other. During this period the employee may resign or be dismissed immediately for any reason.
- *Full time.* The employee works solely in one office, or for one employer in multiple offices, for a customary number of hours. Normally, 32 to 40 hours per week constitutes full-time employment.
- *Part time.* The employee works less than full, customary hours of the facility's operation, usually fewer than 30 hours per week.
- *Job sharing.* Two or more people share one full-time job by the day, week, month, or year. The time can be split in any fashion agreeable to the job sharers and the employer. The salary and benefits are divided proportionally with the time worked.

Job Exiting

Job Termination

Job termination may occur through dismissal by the employer or resignation by the employee. In the event of dismissal, the dental hygienist should make all attempts to understand the reasoning and clarification.

When the dental hygienist decides to resign from a job, notice of intentions should be given to the employer as soon as possible, before any of the office co-workers are told. A minimum of a 2-week notice should be given to the employer; however, resignation should allow the employer an adequate and appropriate amount of time to fill the position before departure. Maintaining a positive relationship with the employer is an essential component to assist your career by expanding your professional network and potential list of references. Remember that dentistry is a community; burning professional bridges can have a negative impact on your career.

Stress and Burnout Among Dental Hygienists

Dental hygienists may experience work-related stress and burnout. Becoming complacent with client care and losing motivation in one's efficiency are signs of fatigue and burnout. Spark a new interest in dental hygiene by attending continuing education courses, joining a dental hygiene study club, or becoming active in local and/or state organizations. Network contacts and mentors also may be a positive influence and resource to assist in identifying what may assist in overcoming the burnout. Sources of stress and burnout in a dental hygiene career may include the following:

- Intense interpersonal relations with clients and staff members
- Development or persistence of chronic work-related pain or physical symptoms
- Monotonous tasks, giving a lack of intellectual stimulation
- Lack of feeling appreciated, which leads to reduced self-esteem and motivation
- Sensing a lack of accomplishment of personal and/or professional goals
- Generalized lack of change of responsibilities

Dental Hygiene's Expanding Scope

Changes in the Profession

The dental hygiene profession constantly is evolving and advancing to accommodate changes in the population needs and practice environment.[7,8] The development of new technologies, changes in policy at the state and federal levels to address access to care issues, workforce trends, and the professional interests of dental hygienists are factors that have been the drive for advancement within the profession[7] (see Chapter 1).

In addition, clinical practice standards are changing to allow more direct access to dental hygiene services with

Employee Name: ______________________ Date: ________

(Registered Dental Hygienist)

Evaluation completed by: ______________________

	EXCELLENT	ACCEPTABLE	NEEDS IMPROVEMENT
PROFESSIONAL BEHAVIOR:			
1. Attitude	___	___	___
2. Cooperation	___	___	___
3. Responsibility	___	___	___
4. Initiative	___	___	___
5. Communications	___	___	___
6. Contributions to Office	___	___	___
CLIENT MANAGEMENT:			
1. Information and Instruction	___	___	___
2. Assistance in Decision Making	___	___	___
3. Respectful	___	___	___
4. Contribution to Comfort	___	___	___
5. Client Acceptance	___	___	___
RISK MANAGEMENT:			
1. Infection Control	___	___	___
2. Protect Self/Client from Injury	___	___	___
PROCESS OF CARE:			
1. Systematic Approach	___	___	___
2. Performs All Necessary Care	___	___	___
3. Care Procedures (List specific concerns)			
______________________			
______________________			
______________________			
______________________			
4. Documentation Skills	___	___	___
5. Evaluation Skills	___	___	___
6. Modification of Care	___	___	___
7. Coordination with Other Care	___	___	___

CHANGES/GROWTH SINCE LAST EVALUATION:

____

____

GOALS FOR CHANGE/GROWTH:

____

____

COMMENTS:

____

____

SIGNED:

______________________________ Date: ________

Supervisor

______________________________ Date: ________

Employee

Figure 63-7. Example of an employee performance evaluation.

declining supervision levels, thus enabling dental hygienists more opportunities to provide care to those in need. Collaborative practice agreements (Minnesota, New Mexico), limited access permits (Oregon), and public health endorsements (Nevada, Maine) are examples of legislative means to provide more access to care using dental hygienists.[9]

California licenses registered dental hygienists in alternative practice (RDHAPs) who may provide direct services for clients via prescription from a dentist or physician in residences of the homebound, schools, residential facilities, institutions, and dental health professional shortage areas. Special education is required for this licensure. Moreover, in 2012, nearly half of the states in the country allow dental hygienists meeting specific experience and training requirements to provide preventive services via **direct access** to care. Direct access to care means that dental hygienists are able to initiate treatment based on their assessment of clients' needs without the specific authorization or presence of a dentist. The administration of local anesthetics by dental hygienists is another area where the profession has advanced greatly in the past decade. In 2012, there were 44 states including the District of Columbia that permitted dental hygienists to administer local anesthesia.

Expanding Educational Opportunities

As the opportunities for employment expand, so too does the prospect for advanced education. Positions in education, research, and corporate settings many times require educational degrees beyond an associate's degree. To accommodate this need, schools have created **degree completion programs**, designed to allow a licensed dental hygienist with an associate's degree advanced education and earning a baccalaureate degree. As of 2012, there were 58 degree completion programs, many of which offer online coursework and distance education, allowing greater flexibility for completion. Furthermore, as of 2012, there were 20 master of science programs designed to prepare students to become educators, administrators, and researchers.[10,11]

Beyond traditional education, establishment of a new mid-level oral healthcare provider has a greater impact on access to care and dental hygienists' scope of practice. The **Advanced Dental Hygiene Practitioner (ADHP)** is based on a concept passed by the 2004 ADHA's House of Delegates. The ADHP works as a part of healthcare teams to improve access to oral healthcare for underserved populations through the provision of preventive services currently under the purview of dental hygienists.[12] ADHPs earn a master's degree and serve in a capacity similar to that of the nurse practitioner in the medical field. Minnesota was the first state to implement education for licensure of a mid-level provider via the **dental therapist (DT)** and **advanced dental therapist (ADT)**. The DT may administer services including extractions and restorative procedures with the supervision of a dentist. ADTs may practice as a DT but have a more expanded scope of practice with less limiting restrictions allowing for evaluation, assessment and treatment plan development, and nonsurgical extractions of permanent teeth.[9]

Career Satisfaction

To excel in dental hygiene is to create a plan that offers security and confidence for self and adapts to conform to life changes and personal goals and interests. Many leave the profession because of stress and burnout, family responsibilities, and changing interests. Continually learning about new advancements in research and treatment modalities helps keep the profession interesting. Discover opportunities for personal and professional growth, which may include furthering education, changing job setting, or expanding one's professional responsibilities and practices. Other means to enhance career satisfaction include the following:

- Hold membership and/or leadership role in professional organizations.
- Contribute to the oral healthcare team. The dental hygienist must be willing to step in and pick up tasks for other team members and collaborate with those team members to offer superior client care.
- Continue to develop lifelong learning and use evidence-based decision making in practice. Dental hygienists must keep abreast of the published research on dental hygiene and dentistry to make relevant evidence-based decisions regarding products, tools, technology, and procedures in practice. One way of achieving this goal is to join a study club that can serve as a means for keeping up with research and can act as a vehicle for professional networking.

Oral healthcare is a diverse, dynamic profession. Finding one's role within it is vital to developing career satisfaction and contributing to the profession as a whole. The dental hygienist must seize the opportunity to determine how best to meet both of these criteria.

CLIENT EDUCATION TIPS

- When legally working in alternative settings without dental supervision, the dental hygienist informs the client that the dentist must review the client records annually when it is required by law that he or she do so (e.g., in New Hampshire).
- When legally working in alternative practice settings without dental supervision, the dental hygienist informs clients that they must be referred annually to a licensed dentist for treatment evaluation and planning when it is required by law that the dental hygienist do so (e.g., in Oregon and Washington).
- It is important to educate clients on the scope of dental hygiene practice and licensure, especially for the newer expanding roles including DT, ADT, and ADHP.

LEGAL, ETHICAL, AND SAFETY ISSUES

- Honesty (veracity) and accuracy are the most important elements of résumé writing.
- The dental hygienist can provide services in certain settings without direct supervision when allowed by law.
- Dental hygiene employment falls under the Non-Discrimination Act, Title VII of the Civil Rights Act of 1964. The law establishes equal employment opportunity for all during the hiring process and throughout the course of employment.
- Dental practice acts are legislative laws that define whether a dental hygienist works under general or direct supervision. These acts do not apply to the business association between the dentist and the dental hygienist.
- Minimal standards for working conditions are set by each state.

- The Occupational Safety and Health Administration (OSHA) sets minimum federal requirements for workplace health and safety.
- Employment contracts may or may not be legally binding.
- The performance evaluation can be used as a legal supporting document for employee dismissal.
- In the event of dismissal, the dental hygienist must (1) make all attempts to understand clearly the grounds and (2) clarify the severance arrangements.
- Financial arrangements between the dentist and the dental hygienist are solely the concern of those two individuals.
- An independent contractor dental hygienist may hire employees and function as an employer.

KEY CONCEPTS

- A career is a lifelong journey that may change to adjust to changes in life.
- The elements of career development include self-assessment, seeking employment, professional development, and career mobility, requiring the dental hygienist's ongoing thoughtful and active participation.
- Searching for a dental hygiene position begins with writing a résumé, composing a cover letter, preparing a list of questions for an interview, and rehearsing for the event.
- Dental hygienists must identify resources, such as mentors and references, for career development and networking.
- Various employment arrangements, terms of employment, and compensation packages are available, depending on the employer and dental hygienist's ability to negotiate an agreement with the employer.
- Job performance is determined by a combination of factors, including evaluation of dental hygiene skills and production, adherence to the job description, and contribution to the practice.
- The performance evaluation is a communication tool based on the agreed-on performance plan and includes compliments and criticisms plus an outline for specific recommended changes.
- Career satisfaction may be met through continuous self-assessment and adaptation to one's needs and desires.
- The dental hygiene profession is constantly expanding, providing more job opportunities as well as better access to care.

CRITICAL THINKING EXERCISES

1. Answer the following questions based on introspection and reflection:
   - What do you value about yourself as a person?
   - What values are important to you in your career and position at work?
   - What skills and expertise do you have that you can use in your position?
   - Are there skill areas in which you need further development?
2. Write two or three professional goals that you would like to obtain in the next 2 years and 5 years. How do you plan on meeting these goals? What steps will you need to take to achieve these goals? Who can help you obtain these goals?
3. Create a cover letter, résumé, and follow-up communication letter(s) for your job search. You may design something for yourself, have a friend with a creative eye do it for you, or use a computer template.
4. Write a job placement advertisement for what you would consider to be your dream job. Then write a specialty cover letter to answer the advertisement.
5. Develop your own interview questions using the interview styles discussed in this chapter. Pair up with a partner and pose the questions to each other. Evaluate your answers, body language, and delivery.

REFERENCES

1. Mould MR, Bray KK, Gadbury-Amyot CC: Student self-assessment in dental hygiene education: a cornerstone of critical thinking and problem-solving, *J Dent Educ* 75(8):1061, 2011.
2. American Dental Hygienists' Association: *Survey of dental hygienists in the United States*. Executive Summary 2007. Available at: http://www.adha.org. Accessed October 2012.
3. Bureau of Labor Statistics, U.S. Department of Labor: Dental hygienists. In *Occupational outlook handbook*, 2012-13 edition, Dental Hygienists. Available at: http://www.bls.gov/ooh/healthcare/dental-hygienists.htm. Accessed October 23, 2012.
4. American Dental Hygienists' Association (ADHA): *Employment trends and wages*. 2012. Available at: http://www.adha.org/careerinfo/wages_and_trends.htm. Accessed October 9, 2012.
5. Parsons KM, Holt ER: Shape your future with an e-portfolio, *Access* 19, 2012.
6. Henry RK: Maintaining professionalism in a digital age, *Dimen Dent Hyg* 10(10):28, 32, 2012.
7. Rhea M, Bettles C, American Dental Hygienists' Association (ADHA): *Dental hygiene at the crossroads of change*. 2011. Available at: http://www.adha.org/downloads/ADHA_Environmental_Scan.pdf. Accessed November 8, 2012.
8. Albino JE, Inglehart MR, Tedesco LA: Dental education and changing oral health care needs: disparities and demands, *J Dent Educ* 76(1):75, 2012.
9. American Dental Hygienist's Association (ADHA): *ADHP Fact Sheet*. 2012. Available at: http://www.adha.org/adhp/index.html. Accessed October 23, 2012.
10. American Dental Hygienist's Association (ADHA): *2012 Dental hygiene education curricula, program, enrollment, and graduate information*. 2012. Available at: http://www.adha.org/downloads/edu/dh_ed_fact_sheet.pdf. Accessed October 1, 2012.
11. American Dental Hygienist's Association (ADHA): *2006 Dental Hygiene Education Program Director Survey*, 2008. Available at: http://www.adha.org/downloads/AD-exec_report-2008.pdf. Accessed October 23, 2012.
12. Stolbert RL, Brickle CM, Darby MM: Development and status of the advanced dental hygiene practitioner, *J Dent Hyg* 85(2):83, 2011.

ACKNOWLEDGMENT

The author acknowledges Christine Hovliaras for her past contributions to this chapter.

EVOLVE RESOURCES

Please visit http://evolve.elsevier.com/Darby/hygiene for additional practice and study support tools.

Legal and Ethical Decision Making

Pamela Zarkowski

CHAPTER 64

COMPETENCIES

1. **Describe the foundations of ethical decision making, including:**
   - **Describe key ethical principles and philosophies affecting healthcare.**
   - **Identify responsibilities and themes in the dental hygiene code of ethics.**
2. **Apply the ethical decision-making framework to resolve ethical dilemmas encountered in practice.**
3. **Recognize and define basic legal concepts.**
4. **Explain the legal concepts of the dental hygienist–client relationship.**
5. **Explain the legal concepts of the dental hygienist–dental hygienist relationship.**
6. **Describe risk management strategies to reduce legal risks and liabilities associated with dental hygiene practice.**
7. **Define the various roles of the dental hygienist.**

Foundations of Ethical Decision Making

Ethics Defined

Ethics is a branch of philosophy that deals with thinking about morality, moral problems, and moral judgments. Ethics is a concern for everyone because it forces the question of what one should do and why.[1] A discussion of professional ethics relates to what is professionally right or conforms to professional standards of conduct. This definition reflects the traditional view of a profession as a group that determines its own standards, writes its own code of ethics, and disciplines its own members. This traditional view is undergoing change to include a broader perspective that argues professional ethics involves not merely what practitioners regard as custom but rather what the profession and society agree are appropriate rules of conduct. eBox 64-1 provides the executive summary of the American Dental Hygienists' Association (ADHA) Code of Ethics. For example, the ADHA Code of Ethics points out that a dental hygienist should not discuss a client's medical condition with anyone without the individual's authorization. Another example found within the ADHA Code of Ethics is a statement that the dental hygienist should inform the client of proposed care and allow the person to become involved in treatment decisions.

A code of ethics recognizes the following three relationships:

- Professional and client
- Professional and professional
- Professional and society

In dental hygiene, ethics focuses on moral duties and obligations of the professional to clients, colleagues, and society. Although it is not specifically stated, there is also a critical element of trust as an ethical obligation in the three relationships. The influence of society in evaluating professionals and their ethical conduct is increasingly evident. If a health professional is reported in a local newspaper as having unprofessional conduct, letters or emails to the editor or blogs suggest improved monitoring of health professionals. The public has strong expectations for appropriate professional behavior.

Historically the health professions were viewed as groups that followed codes of ethics and monitored their members; however, recurring charges of malpractice, impropriety, and fraud and the scrutiny of various public and private agencies have projected the health professions into the arena of public concern and criticism. Consumers who are aware of inappropriate or perceived unethical behaviors contact professional organizations and peer review groups to express their concerns. Professional conferences and publications now address issues such as ethics, ethical decision making, peer review, quality improvement, and related issues. Professional groups meet to form alliances among state boards, academics, publishers, manufacturers, and military and public health services, leading to a common code of ethics.[2]

Legal obligations and ethical obligations are distinct. Rules of conduct, promulgated by state or federal statutes, are by their nature obligatory customs or practices of a community (legal obligation). A dental hygienist must follow legal obligations or face the consequences. For example, a hygienist is obligated by both federal and state statutes not to discriminate against individuals belonging to certain classes or to sexually harass another person. Such behaviors may result in legal action against the dental hygienist. Consequences for violating statutory laws include fines or imprisonment or both, depending on the severity of the violation.

Rules of conduct promulgated by the ADHA or the Canadian Dental Hygienists Association (CDHA) serve as guidelines for conduct or ethical obligations. A professional who violates an ethical code may frustrate a client or lose the respect of professional colleagues, but there may or may not be legal consequences to an ethical violation. For example, the

Figures, tables, and boxes marked as "e" are available as supplemental material on the Evolve site. Visit http://evolve.elsevier.com/Darby/hygiene to access these materials.

BOX 64-2

How to Maintain Professional Accountability

Self
- Report any conduct or conditions that endanger clients.
- Stay informed and practice current dental hygiene theory.
- Make judgments and evaluate based on evidence.
- Maintain current licensure and continuing education requirements

Client
- Provide clients with thorough and accurate information about care.
- Conduct dental hygiene care in a manner that ensures client safety and well-being.
- Encourage communicating within a professional client-provider relationship.

Profession
- Maintain ethical standards in practice.
- Encourage professional colleagues to follow the same ethical standards.
- Report colleagues' unethical behavior to appropriate peer review entities.

Employment Situation
- Remain current regarding state rules and regulations governing dental and dental hygiene practice.
- Follow appropriate policy and procedures.

Society
- Maintain ethical conduct in care of all clients in all settings.

dental hygienist who refuses to provide care to individuals on Medicaid is violating the ethical standard that suggests dental hygienists should not discriminate, but there are no legal consequences.

Accountability and Responsibility

Accountability refers to the ability to answer for one's actions. Dental hygienists provide client care and are accountable for their actions to themselves, their clients, the profession, employers, and society (Box 64-2).

The purposes of professional accountability are as follows:
- Evaluate new professional practices and reassess existing ones
- Maintain standards of care
- Facilitate personal reflection, ethical thought, and personal growth on the part of health professionals
- Provide a basis for ethical decision making
- Demonstrate qualities important to professional status

Dental hygienists are accountable for dental hygiene care and do not rely on others to assume this responsibility. (Visit http://evolve.elsevier.com/Darby/hygiene for eBox 64-3 and historical background on major ethical perspectives.)

Fundamental Ethical Principles

The ethical principles that underlie healthcare are:
- Autonomy
- Beneficence
- Nonmaleficence
- Justice
- Veracity
- Fidelity

Autonomy is based on the principle of respect for persons. Individuals have a right to self-determination, that is, freedom to make their own judgments based on their own evaluations. It is the belief that independent actions and choices of an individual should not be constrained by others. Recognizing autonomy occurs when the dental hygienist involves the client in decision making and obtains informed consent. The caregiver provides clients with enough information to make judgments about their care. All clients should be provided with understandable information about their oral health status and treatment options. To meet this obligation a dental hygienist uses communication that is appropriate for the client's comprehension and competence level.

Beneficence is the provision of benefit, preventing evil or harm, removing evil or harm, or promoting good. A professional has a duty to help others by doing what is best for them. Acting on this principle, a professional is responsible for contributing to the health and welfare of others. Examples of beneficent actions include taking only necessary radiographs and maintaining equipment to prevent client injury, such as replacing worn instruments so that instrument tips do not break in a client's mouth. A dental hygienist participating in a community-based oral cancer screening and referral program is another example of promoting good.

Nonmaleficence is summarized by "above all, do no harm." A dental hygienist seeks to never harm a client. An example of potential harm is when a dental hygienist is asked to provide treatment in which she is not qualified. A dental office, as part of its treatment options, begins using the dental hygiene staff to provide tooth-bleaching treatments for clients. A dental hygienist, although not appropriately trained, provides the treatment to clients. Her actions may be viewed as having the potential to inflict harm and violate the principle of nonmaleficence.

Justice relies on fairness and equality. A person is treated justly when given what he or she is due, owed, deserves, or can legitimately claim. All clients receiving care should be treated equally. A dental hygienist who provides substandard care to persons in a nursing home because they are institutionalized is not treating all clients equally.

Veracity, truth telling or integrity, is critical to meaningful communication and therefore to relationships between individuals. Dental hygienists are obligated to be truthful with clients and associates. For example, a dental hygienist fails to tell a client that during sealant application to tooth 19, the primary tooth anterior to tooth 19 fractured. A dental hygienist employed on a commission basis erroneously codes a procedure for insurance reimbursement to receive higher financial reimbursement. The dishonest behavior is apparent in these aforementioned situations.

Fidelity is the obligation to keep implied or explicit promises. A dental hygienist who says that she is going to call the client with some additional information about dental implants and then follows through with her promise is demonstrating fidelity.

Other core principles suggested in ethics forums warrant a brief review. *Societal trust* is an obligation to follow the highest ideals and standards of a health profession and the belief that all members of the profession strive to achieve the standards outlined by their profession. Other ethical principles include *reparation,* which suggests that a practitioner responsible for an injury to others must make amends. In *confidentiality,* when information is divulged by one person to another, there is an implicit promise that the information will not be revealed to a third person.

Codes of Ethics

The ADHA Code of Ethics assists dental hygienists in achieving high levels of ethical consciousness, decision making, and practice. The Code describes the basic beliefs on the importance of oral health and the role of dental hygienists in preventing and treating oral diseases. The Code contains categories of Standards of Professional Responsibilities, a key section to the code (see eBox 64-1). The categories begin by explaining the dental hygienists' responsibility to maintain personal health and well-being, competence, and a collaborative and safe work environment. Also highlighted are responsibilities to clients, colleagues, employees and employers, the dental hygiene profession, the community, society, and scientific investigation.

The responsibilities within each category reflect themes, including professional obligations to contribute to society and the profession, communication with clients and colleagues, professional collaboration, and participation to advance the profession. The responsibilities under each category provide a framework for reflection and guide the identification of a potential ethical concern or resolution of an ethical dilemma. Codes of ethics serve as a component of the self-policing responsibility of a profession. Code of Ethics documents can be obtained from the ADHA and the CDHA websites.

Ethical Problems in Dental Hygiene

Ethical, moral, and legal issues intertwine in the many dilemmas faced by dental hygienists. An **ethical dilemma** is a situation in which two ethical principles are in conflict. Regardless of the decision made or actions taken by the dental hygienist, an ethical principle will be violated. In this section, examples of ethical dilemmas in different career situations are presented, followed by a decision-making framework for resolving the dilemmas.

Clinical Practice

Dental hygienists report ethical problems such as unprofessional behavior on the part of the dental team, inappropriate client treatment decisions, providing unnecessary dental treatment, delegation to unqualified personnel, insurance fraud, harassment or disrespectful behavior, and substandard care. ADHA members identified three commonly encountered ethical dilemmas in dental hygiene practice[3]:

- Observation of behavior in conflict with standard infection-control procedures
- Failure to refer clients to a specialist
- Nondiagnosis of dental disease

Examples are the colleague who uses a chemical disinfectant rather than properly sterilizing instruments; the staff person who recycles disposable items, such as saliva ejectors or rubber cups; use of instruments "sterilized" in malfunctioning equipment; the new dental assistant who is unfamiliar with standard barrier techniques.

Failure to refer a client to a periodontist occurs in dental hygiene care situations. For example, the dental hygienist responsible for client assessment observes a client's deteriorating periodontal status. The dental hygienist's employer, a general dentist, chooses not to refer; however, the dental hygienist recognizes that the skill level of the dental staff cannot meet the client's periodontal needs. The failure to inform the client of the need for a referral to a periodontist, depending on the facts, may constitute an ethical dilemma as well as malpractice. The ADHA Code of Ethics speaks specifically to the responsibility to refer clients to other healthcare providers when the client's needs are beyond the dental hygienist's ability or scope of practice. The standard to provide optimum oral healthcare using professional knowledge, judgment, and ability must be considered. Another ethical obligation is to serve as an advocate for the welfare of clients; however, in some states the dental hygienist cannot legally refer. Alternatives for solving the dilemma may include working to change office policy, educating colleagues about current referring guidelines, informing clients of their need to seek care in another office, or seeking another position. Each solution carries consequences such as upsetting the employer, frightening the client, performing an activity outside the scope of dental hygiene practice, or losing a valued position.

Consider the scenario when the dental hygienist–dentist team fails to detect dental disease. Perhaps thorough client assessment does not occur. The dental hygienist has the skills to assess the client and record findings but is not given adequate time to fulfill those responsibilities. The dentist conducts a cursory dental caries examination, but other conditions such as periodontal disease, cancer, malocclusion, or temporomandibular joint dysfunction are ignored. Violation of the Code includes failing to provide optimal oral healthcare, compromising the public's confidence in members of the dental health profession, and failing to educate clients about high-quality oral healthcare. The failure to assess the client who then experiences a medical emergency also is an example of malpractice because a systemic condition requiring medical evaluation was not detected. The dental professional is skilled to detect possible systemic diseases based on oral manifestations and health history assessment.

The legal obligations include completing appropriate clinical examinations and following consistent referral protocols. It is suggested that dental offices have a standard protocol for dealing with clients with medical conditions that require evaluation and treatment beyond the scope of dental practice. Adherence to the protocol may protect the practitioner from malpractice. The office protocol should comply with the Americans with Disabilities Act, ensure that the client is counseled and referred to an appropriate healthcare agency or provider, and ensure that consultations and referrals are documented in the services rendered section of the dental chart.[4] The protocol should be used consistently with all clients.

Public Health

Public health hygienists frequently face ethical problems because their decisions concern allocating limited resources and maximizing benefits for a large population. A dental hygienist must implement a dental sealant program for elementary school children. Funding is limited, and therefore all students are not able to participate. How are the recipients selected? Should children receiving the benefits of water fluoridation also have the benefit of a dental sealant program? Or should children without access to water fluoridation or other fluoride therapies participate in the sealant program? With knowledge that sealants are useful in preventing occlusal caries, children without the benefit of fluoridation are at a higher risk for developing smooth-surface dental caries. Does socioeconomic status play a role in access to dental services? In this situation, the ethical standard of providing optimal oral healthcare using sound professional judgment to meet the oral health needs of the public guide decision making. An additional ethical responsibility is access to oral health services for all, supporting justice and fairness in the distribution of healthcare resources. The dental hygienist may choose to maximize the preventive potential by using the funding for a sealant program in the fluoridated community. One outcome may reduce the incidence of caries in children living in the fluoridated community. Another outcome may be that the children at risk for caries without access to fluoride or dental sealants continue to be at risk.

Consider the situation of a dental hygienist employed by the state department of public health. The responsibilities of the position include monitoring quality and quantity of oral health services provided by different public health clinics throughout the state. State law does not allow dental hygienists to practice unless a dentist is on the premises. The dental hygienist responsible is aware that although dental hygienists are providing care in settings where a dentist is not always present, high-quality care, within the dental hygienist's scope of practice, is being provided to individuals in need. A legal and ethical dilemma exists. Should the dental hygienist at the local clinic continue care? Is it fair to discontinue services to particular groups because a local clinic cannot afford to employ a dentist full-time? To whom is the dental hygienist ethically responsible—the citizens of the state, the profession, or the state board? From a legal perspective, the dental hygienist is violating the law. The standard advocating provision of care and prevention of dental disease can be used to argue that ethically the dental hygienist is meeting the obligation; however, ethical codes also direct dental hygienists to uphold the laws and regulations governing the profession. Thus this is a difficult dilemma. Unethical and illegal behavior cannot be justified. The dental hygienist coordinating the clinics should seek to remedy the situation legislatively or through creative strategies such as staffing alternatives and affiliation agreements with local dentists or clinics.

In another situation the dental hygienist travels with a mobile dental clinic program throughout a metropolitan area providing oral health education and preventive services to city residents. The program receives funding from the state to provide care for underserved populations. The dental hygienist begins receiving telephone calls reporting that the dentist staffing the mobile clinic, deluged by the large number of clients, is providing substandard care. The dental hygienist has been a strong advocate of the program, a pilot project that was to be a model for other regions. The dental hygienist knows that reporting the dentist may result in discontinuing services to a population in need. At the same time, the dental hygienist is obligated to document and report inadequate or substandard care. The dental hygienist must protect the clients and stop the inadequate care. Solutions to the dilemma may include working with a local dental society or dental school to assist in staffing the clinic until a replacement dentist is identified.

Other examples of ethical problems in public health may include:

- misuse of funds supporting items other than client care
- non dental personnel making treatment decisions
- compromising or alternating client care or populations served due to local or state politics

Administration

Administrators, whether in educational or business-based institutions, face ethical dilemmas. A client visits a dental hygiene clinic for care. The client refuses to be treated by a specific student and makes unpleasant comments about the student's ethnic background. The administrator must protect the student from the client and provide a comfortable and safe learning environment free of harassment. At the same time, the reputation of the dental hygiene program to willingly treat all persons in the community must be maintained. The administrator may educate the client about his rights and responsibilities or dismiss the client and refer him to another provider for care. In some instances, institutional protocol guides the administrator in choosing a particular option; however, this situation addresses the standard of managing conflicts constructively and promoting human relationships that are mutually beneficial.

In another example, students in a dental hygiene program are assigned to provide nonsurgical periodontal therapy at an urban, hospital-based clinic. The clients treated at the clinic are high risk for acquired immunodeficiency syndrome (AIDS). The dental hygiene program director is aware that there is always the possibility of a puncture wound occurring, with the result that a dental hygiene student may be injured by a contaminated instrument. Does the director choose not to have students assigned to the clinic? Should students and their families be informed of the risk? The situation may create a dilemma in some settings, but using the principle that all individuals should be treated without discrimination, as well as the knowledge that students are using the appropriate standard of care, all students should be assigned.

An administrator also deals with ethical problems among colleagues. The administrator is asked to evaluate the faculty for merit salary raises. Not all faculty members contribute equally to the department. One tenured faculty member fulfills the minimum responsibilities; however, if that faculty person's raise is not comparable to others' raises, she may contribute even less and accuse the administrator of discrimination. Some less-productive faculty members may decide to quit, leaving those remaining with the burden of heavier workloads, especially because the college is experiencing a hiring freeze. Does the administrator recognize all the faculty members as equally meritorious? Is there an obligation to report weaker faculty contributions to the administration? What obligation exists to those who are most productive? The administrator must identify the specific problem and, with the questions previously raised, consider the alternatives. One solution is to suggest a merit raise for the weak faculty person, then structure that faculty member's obligations to improve her productivity. The consequences include other faculty members' lowered morale when all faculty members receive merit raises, although not all are justified.

Research

Informal research occurs in practice when a dental hygienist surveys clients' attitudes, evaluates their acceptance of products and procedures, or compiles salary survey data. Dental hygienists also are involved in research conducted at educational institutions or in association with the manufacturing of oral- or health-related products.

Perhaps a dental hygienist is conducting research to evaluate the effectiveness of a chemotherapeutic agent on selective pathogenic and nonpathogenic microorganisms. The manufacturer is providing funding for the research. The dental hygienist discovers that although the research design is valid, her co-investigator is allowing personal bias to influence observations and interpretations. Both are aware that if the research establishes the chemotherapeutic agent as effective, the pharmaceutical company that produces the agent will provide generous funding in the future. Should the dental hygienist confront the co-investigator? Should the dental hygienist ignore the unethical and illegal behavior of the co-investigator? Knowing that research is replicated, should the dental hygienist ignore what has occurred and assume that follow-up research will reveal the flaws of the current research?

Other examples of ethical problems in research include:

- Individuals who steal another's idea or concept
- Individuals who take credit for a colleague's success in research
- Manipulation of data
- Intentional bias in sampling and failure to report research that does not support or confirm a hypothesis
- Misuse of funds or resources

Dental Hygienist–Dentist-Client Relationships

One of the most difficult and common problems is when the dental hygienist and dentist do not agree on the type of oral healthcare required by a client. A dental hygienist observes signs of cancerlike soft-tissue changes during the client's assessment. The dental hygienist suggests that the lesion be biopsied. The dentist disagrees. The dental hygienist feels a responsibility to the client that conflicts with that of the dentist. Does the dental hygienist express concern to the client? Should the dental hygienist identify another dentist in the office for a second opinion? Should the dentist's decision stand? The dental hygienist considers all the alternatives and chooses one that supports ethical principles. If the dental hygienist seeks another dentist in the office to evaluate the client, the dental hygienist may be satisfied with a second opinion. The consequences can include an unhappy dentist and frightened client; however, if a biopsy is performed, the personal and professional satisfaction gained by the dental hygienist and effects of the biopsy on the client's health outweigh the other consequences. Conflicts between the dental hygienist and dentist are not easily solved.

Dental hygienists may be employed where they work under the policies and procedures outlined by the dentist-employer(s). When policies and procedures dictate that the dental hygienist is allowed 45 minutes for all clients, that care must be completed in one appointment, or that everyone gets a "routine oral prophylaxis," the dental hygienist is being forced to provide substandard care. Should the dental hygienist work within the policies, ignoring the quality-of-care standard? Does the dental hygienist terminate the position? It may be difficult to leave a position because of location, salary, and benefits. Does the dental hygienist inform the client that care is limited and recommend referral for a second opinion? Or does the dental hygienist attempt to provide optimal care and work more diligently? Issues about client care, length of time allotted for care, referral protocols, and other work expectations should be addressed in the preemployment interview process. If issues arise after employment, the dental hygienist may resolve the concerns by scheduling an appointment with the employer or as part of an employee evaluation process, whichever occurs earliest.

Conflicts arise when a client refuses specific treatment, decides to ignore a referral, or continues an unhealthy practice. What ethical obligations does the dental hygienist have to the client and the employer?

A client makes a decision based on information. Some ethical dilemmas created by client actions, or failure to act, could be eliminated if the client were given an appropriate amount of information. With overly brief appointments, ill-informed or uncommunicative staff members are unable to adequately educate clients. Client education and service should remain priorities and should guide office practice and policies.

Other examples of ethical problems in dental hygienist–dentist-client relationship may include:

- Ethnic, gender, or racial harassment of staff, vendors, or clients
- Office staff practicing outside the defined scope of practice
- Inappropriate use of social media
- Violation of appropriate business practices (i.e., denying a patient a copy of their dental record)

Dental Hygienist–Dental Hygienist Relationships

It is difficult to work in an environment in which the care provided by a colleague is below the acceptable standard. For example, the dental hygienist colleague may be compromising client care by not thoroughly assessing the client or may be performing services beyond the scope of dental hygiene care. Situations that may affect the client's care or health status create an immediate dilemma. Does one report the activity to the employer, regulatory boards, or the ethics board of the professional association? Does one attempt to educate or update the colleague? Or does one ignore the situation, assuming it is the employer's responsibility?

In situations like these, talking with the dental hygienist in question may be the best alternative. The dental hygienist may be unaware of the quality-of-care issues or illegal activities. Respectfully confronting individuals while offering solutions to the problem is a step toward resolution. Other solutions may include an office in-service session, attending a continuing education class, or developing a dental hygiene office manual outlining specific roles and responsibilities.

Employer-Employee Relationships

In a dental or dental hygiene practice or other work environment, various professional, personal, and business relationships coexist. As an employee, one may be asked to function in a role that creates ethical problems. Perhaps a dental hygienist suspects that an employer is sexually harassing an employee, that insurance fraud is occurring during billing procedures, or that a colleague has a substance abuse problem. One may immediately determine that the dental hygienist has an obligation to act on the situations observed. Is it the dental hygienist's responsibility to act, or is it the employer's? Should the dental hygienist be concerned about the ethical and legal issues? Does one address the issue with the offending practitioner? What if after the problem is addressed no change occurs? It is especially exasperating when one recognizes that the dental hygienist is expected to practice within the ADHA or CDHA Code of Ethics but is not in control of the work environment.

The ADHA Code of Ethics says to participate in the development and advancement of the profession. Many dental hygienists are not members of their professional association. Are the dental hygienists who are not members of the association aware of the Code of Ethics? Is it the ethical obligation of a dental hygienist who is a member to encourage nonmembers to join the professional association? As a member of a professional association, a dental hygienist has access to scientific literature, continuing education courses, and other resources. Should these items be shared with nonmember dental hygiene colleagues? Each question raises multiple ethical dilemmas. The Code of Ethics encourages a work environment that promotes individual growth and development. Educating nonmember dental hygienists about the association or sharing new knowledge or expertise supports the professional development philosophy.

Ethical Decision-Making Framework[5]

Define the Problem or Conflict

The problem may be defined by personal criteria, such as one's feelings, sense of professionalism, or moral code. Ethical or legal standards or a combination of ethical and legal principles also may define the problem. In some instances the conflict arises from a difference in philosophy, management style, or professional priorities. It is advisable to define precisely the problem or conflict creating the dilemma. It is vague to state, for example, that a conflict has arisen because of different educational backgrounds. It is more precise to identify the conflict as lack of consistency in referring for biopsy or client assessment techniques.

Identify the Ethical Issues

What are the issues? Can one major issue be defined? For example, when a conflict exists between the dental hygienist's suggestion to refer to a specialist versus the dentist's refusal to support the suggestion, the dilemma occurs between a professional obligation to follow the dentist's diagnosis and the dental hygienist's obligation to assess the client's needs and provide high-quality care. From the client's point of view, the referral may satisfy the client's need for a specialist's evaluation and possible treatment; however, if the dental hygienist's recommendation is incorrect or based on some misconceptions, the second opinion creates an additional expense in time and money for the client, resulting in conflict within the employment setting and a frustrated client.

Gather Relevant Information

When faced with an ethical dilemma, the dental hygienist must gather all relevant information (e.g., personal data such as family status, age, lifestyle, habits, medical and dental facts, and the professional and personal values involved). Subjective and objective information is included to evaluate the evidence-based and human-based elements. As part of information gathering, one may want to reevaluate a client, research the evidence, investigate a diagnosis, or obtain a third opinion. If the dilemma is focused on an office protocol or policy, the dental hygienist may want to contact other healthcare providers, a lawyer, or a professional association representative for verification of standard practices.

Identify the Ethical Alternatives

To answer the question, the dental hygienist should list possible courses of action. For example, in one situation alternatives may include resigning from a position, confronting an employer, or calling the client to express a concern or suggest a course of action. Each alternative may carry serious personal, financial, and professional implications.

In most situations the list of alternatives takes into consideration the parties involved—the client, dentist, dental hygienist, and co-workers. When listing the alternatives, consider the following:

- Obligation(s) to the client (legal, professional, and ethical)
- Obligation(s) to others involved (client's family, employer, colleagues)
- Personal beliefs and values
- Client's legal rights, responsibilities, values, and interests
- Alternatives that protect the client's best interests
- Alternatives that protect the professional's best interests
- Alternatives that do the least amount of harm
- Practical constraints
- Professional judgment

Establish an Ethical Position

Once alternatives are delineated, the dental hygienist must make a choice. In establishing an ethical position, there may be ethical conflicts. For example, a client refuses to be premedicated with an antibiotic before an appointment. If the dental hygienist honors the client's request, the ethical principle of autonomy is followed; however, ethically, the dental hygienist who treats a client without appropriate premedication would potentially harm the client, violating the ethical principles of nonmaleficence. In selecting the course of action, one may weigh which action promotes the best balance between the negative and positive aspects of the situation.

Or one may evaluate the alternatives and choose the least negative alternative. For example, a dental hygienist chooses, in order to balance her recommendations versus the dentist's decision not to refer a client for biopsy of a lesion, to reschedule the client in 2 weeks and reevaluate the lesion. The consequences may include a harmonious working relationship, an opportunity to further study the pathology, and the ability to keep open the possibility that in 2 weeks both the dental hygienist and dentist can conduct a more informed assessment. The conflict may be internal, within the work environment, or with the parties involved, such as the dentist-employer. If one is resolved that the ethical choice is the correct one, however, identifying the consequences assists the decision maker in anticipating and preparing for implementing or acting on the choice.

Select, Justify, and Defend the Alternatives

Once the consequences of a choice have been evaluated, and before the choice is acted on, one should review the decision. What are the supporting ethical principles? Does the ADHA code address the issue or offer guidance? What might be a strong argument against the position? Identifying an argument, aside from an ethical position, that supports the decision is helpful. Evaluation at this stage assists the decision maker before the choice is implemented or acted on. Individuals need to evaluate their decisions. It may be that the consequences are so negative that another alternative or compromise might need to be considered (Box 64-4).

Dental Ethics Committee

The dental team must use ethical principles and codes for resolving an ethical dilemma. Establishing a dental ethics committee (DEC) for the office is one action to facilitate ethical decision making.[6] The DEC could identify dilemmas, use the ethical decision-making model and existing codes of ethics for in-service and discussion to address concerns, and create a team approach for resolving difficult issues. Guidelines could be developed for the DEC, outlining its purposes, functions, and membership. Staff meetings could periodically include the DEC as one of the agenda items. A committee approach assists in raising issues of concern to all office members and educates staff members about ethical decision making. This approach encourages an ethics-based office philosophy.

Jurisprudence

Oral Health Professionals at Risk

Clients have become sophisticated consumers of high-quality healthcare that is accessible and reasonably priced. Therefore an individual who is dissatisfied with oral healthcare frequently looks to the legal system for assistance. Malpractice suits against dental professionals have consistently become more prevalent (Box 64-5).

Common malpractice litigation includes accusations of the following:

- Violation of standard of care, negligence
- Failure to treat problems related to temporomandibular joint disease
- Failure to diagnose, refer, or treat periodontal disease
- Failure to obtain informed consent
- Use of defective products
- Abandonment of the client
- Failure to identify and protect a person with a medically compromising condition, such as a heart murmur or drug allergy
- Failure to maintain proper records
- Incorrect medical or dental history taking
- Failure to meet the standard of care, administering incorrect treatment

Oral health professionals are governed by statutory laws enacted by legislators, administrative laws (regulations) promulgated by regulatory boards, and common law or case law determined by judicial decisions in court cases (Figure 64-1). Each governing body affects the practice of dental hygiene. The professional is presumed to be aware of all the rules and regulations influencing practice and cannot claim ignorance of the law. Sanctions for violations exist, and a practitioner who violates a particular rule may be adjudicated under multiple governing bodies.

For example, a dental hygienist who administers nitrous oxide–oxygen analgesia in a state that restricts dental hygiene to traditional practice has violated the rules and regulations outlined by the state regulatory board and may, based on a review of the board, have his or her license revoked or suspended. If harm occurs as a result of the administration of the nitrous oxide, the individual may be charged with a civil violation, such as negligence. In addition there may be allegations of a criminal violation, specifically administering drugs without a license, depending on state and local statutes, resulting in court action or fines. A dental hygienist must be aware of the rules and regulations governing the practice of dental hygiene in the jurisdiction where licensing is maintained.

Basic Legal Concepts

The **law** is divided into civil and criminal categories. Although these categories are separate, one can be accused of both a civil and a criminal violation simultaneously.

- **Civil law** includes offenses for violating private or contractual rights or, in simpler terms, a breach of legal duty against a person. In a civil lawsuit, a violation against a person is purported to have occurred. The remedy that person seeks is to be "whole" because some type of "damage" has occurred, and the manner in which one is made "whole" is to receive monetary damages.
- **Criminal law** is that law established for preventing harm against society and describes a criminal act as well as the appropriate punishment. In a criminal lawsuit, the individual found guilty is punished based on society's rules and regulations. Fines, prison terms, or other punishments are based on the specific criminal violation.

Two distinctly different levels of proof are used to determine innocence or guilt:

- For a criminal act, the level of proof required is that **beyond a reasonable doubt.** To meet the level of proof, a jury or judge must be absolutely convinced that the criminal act occurred to establish guilt. If one is not absolutely convinced, an individual must be found innocent.
- A civil action requires a less-strict level of proof, called a **preponderance of evidence.** This level requires that the jury or judge, based on the evidence presented, must be 51% certain that someone is guilty or innocent. For example, a dental hygienist committed an error during client care. If the jury or judge is 51% sure that error caused a harm to the client, the dental hygienist will be found liable.

The requirement of a preponderance of evidence to prove guilt or innocence is weaker than a requirement of proof beyond a reasonable doubt. Professional malpractice suits filed against oral health professionals are usually in the civil arena; therefore the level of proof required is a preponderance of evidence. Understanding the level of proof required for civil lawsuits assists in explaining how dental hygienists or dentists are found guilty or innocent when charges are filed against them.

Parties in a lawsuit include the plaintiff(s) and the defendant(s). In a legal dispute, the **plaintiff** is the person who brings the action or files the suit; the **defendant** is the person defending himself or denying the action charged.

BOX 64-4

Example of the Ethical Decision-Making Process

Scenario

A recent dental hygiene graduate takes a position in an office with a staff consisting of two dentists, two dental hygienists, and three dental assistants. The dental hygienist works late one evening a week with a dentist. The dental hygienist notices that after dinner, and throughout the evening, the dentist steps into the laboratory and drinks from a bottle in a paper bag that he hides in the laboratory. He then gargles with mouthwash and returns to client care. His care of clients does not appear compromised. He treats clients and staff with respect, completes care as planned, and manages the office. He meets all the requests of the dental hygienist, and the evening office hours run smoothly; however, the dental hygienist notes that the dentist's drinking behavior is repeated week after week. The dental hygienist questions the staff about the drinking. The staff indicates that they find him a great dentist, the office environment is a good one, and they really like the job. They imply that they hope that the dental hygienist will ignore the situation so that everything will remain the same. Using the framework for ethical decision making, how would the dental hygienist use the model to assist in evaluating the decision?

Define the Problem

The dental hygienist may find it personally offensive that a person is drinking on the job and providing client care. The dental hygienist may feel that the quality of care provided by the dentist is compromised by the drinking, thus violating the ethical mandate of providing the most comprehensive care available. There may be legal issues such as negligent behavior on the part of the dentist. There are also interpersonal issues with the staff members who are ignoring the situation and pressuring the dental hygienist to do the same. The problem is that the dentist is drinking, providing client care, and compromising client safety and staff interaction.

Identify the Ethical Issue

A professional is responsible for protecting clients' well-being (nonmaleficence, beneficence). This responsibility is clearly delineated in the American Dental Hygienists' Association (ADHA) and the Canadian Dental Hygienists Association (CDHA) Codes of Ethics. A dental hygienist must prioritize her responsibilities to the client versus the wishes of the staff to ignore the situation. Working with someone in an alcoholic state may affect client care, decision making, and problem solving by the dentist (confidentiality, veracity).

Gather Relevant Information

Are other staff members noticing the behavior? How long has the pattern existed? Does the drinking occur throughout the whole day? Have there been any untoward incidents identified with the dentist's care or client management? Has the dentist or is the dentist currently participating in alcoholic rehabilitation? Is there a personal crisis in the dentist's life? The dental hygienist should document her observations and those of others.

The dental hygienist may want to investigate the types of services available to professionals with substance abuse problems. Perhaps a protocol is in place within the state dental society to work with the dentist to overcome his problem and maintain his professional status, or Alcoholics Anonymous may have information about programs. The dental hygienist may want to research alcoholism and the characteristics of an alcoholic to assist in confirming that a problem exists.

Identify the Alternatives

In this situation, alternatives may include the following:

- Discussing observations with the dentist involved
- Discussing and confirming observations with co-workers
- Confronting a single staff member to get additional support
- Discussing observations with others
- Ignoring the situation
- Contacting appropriate agencies, such as the dental association or state board
- Quitting the employment situation
- Refusing to work with the dentist
- Contacting the local dental hygiene or dental component for guidelines or advice
- Talking to peers to get ideas or solutions
- Consulting the Code of Ethics and the state statutes that govern practice

The dental hygienist is required by the Code to follow the rules and regulations governing the practice of dental hygiene. Thus if a mandate exists requiring the dental hygienist to report situations when client care may be compromised, the alternative of choice is clearly delineated. In most dilemmas the ethical code is useful to generate alternatives for consideration.

Establish an Ethical Position

As part of the decision-making process, the dental hygienist chooses to confront the dentist and offer information about counseling services available to persons with a drinking problem.

Select, Justify, and Defend the Alternatives

One considers the decision in light of supporting ethical principles. In this case the principles include beneficence, nonmaleficence, veracity, and confidentiality. One may also consider a strong argument against the position, such as the dentist's possible denial or a consequence such as the dentist terminating the dental hygienist's employment rather than admitting a substance abuse problem. Evaluation of the alternatives is an ongoing part of the process. As each alternative is identified, its advantages, disadvantages, and consequences are reviewed. The mental exercise of justifying and defending assists the dental hygienist in the decision-making process and helps generate additional alternatives. The dental hygienist goes through a process of "what if" and finishes the sentence.

Act on the Ethical Choice

The most difficult part is acting on the choice. In the best scenario the dentist welcomes the identification of a problem and seeks counseling to overcome it. The worst scenario may be denial and an effort on the part of the dentist to dismiss the dental hygienist; however, the guiding ethical principle of nonmaleficence, the ADHA Code of Ethics, and genuine concern for fellow employees should strengthen the dental hygienist, whatever the consequences.

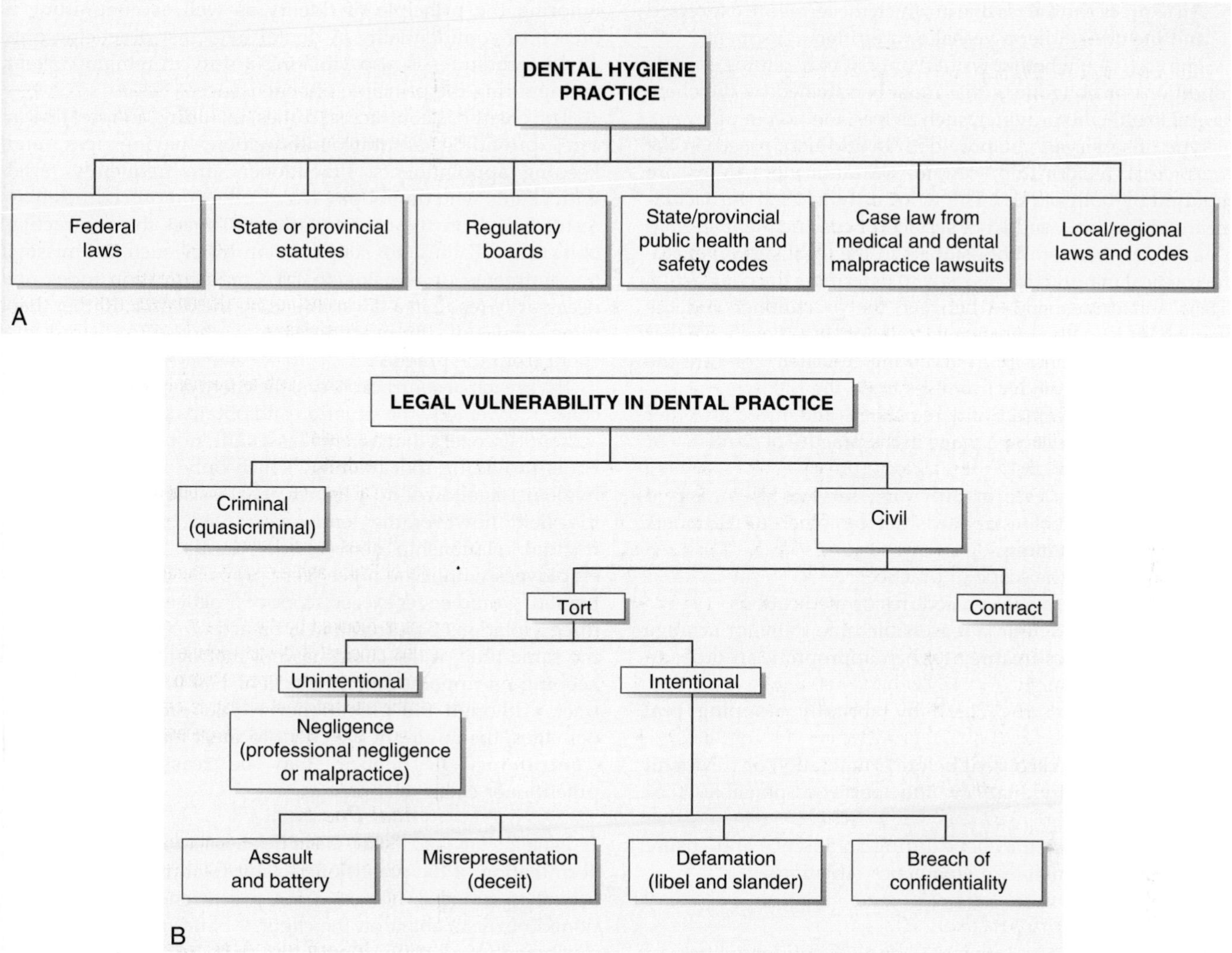

Figure 64-1. A, Diagram of governing bodies affecting the practice of dental hygiene. **B,** Diagram of legal vulnerability in dental practice. (**B,** Redrawn from Pollack B: *Risk management manual,* Fort Lauderdale, Fla, 1986, National Society of Dental Practitioners.)

BOX 64-5

Are You Contributing to Potential Malpractice Situations or Illegal Dental Hygiene Practice?

It is not my responsibility to report violators of the dental practice act. I assume that it is someone else's responsibility.
I sometimes treat clients with severe periodontal disease for years rather than refer them.
If I am running late on my schedule, I may not update a client's health history.
There is probably a procedure or two that a dental assistant performs in my office that is not allowed under state law.
Before treating a client, I rarely explain the reason for the procedure or the risks involved because it takes too much time.
If a client insists, we do not always premedicate an individual who should have appropriate antibiotics before treatment.
If a dentist asks me to do something that I know is illegal, I should do it because the dentist will get sued, not me.
If I do not like a client, I may eliminate the name from my continued-care list.
If you checked any of these statements, you or your clients are at risk.

Contract Principles and Relationships

Malpractice lawsuits are civil in nature. A common concept of liability used in dental malpractice lawsuits is **breach of contract** (i.e., failure to perform a promise). When one thinks of a contract violation, business transactions come to mind, rather than oral healthcare. Applications of the breach of contract concept were originally limited to business transactions; however, society has become more consumer-oriented, and the courts now recognize the dentist-client relationship as a contract. A legal definition states that a contract is an agreement between two or more consenting and competent parties to do or not to do a legal act for which there is sufficient consideration. **Consideration** is an exchange of something of value, such as money, between two people.[7] The contractual relationship between the oral health practitioner and the client is one of the following two types:

- An **implied contract** can begin in a number of situations, including the performance of a professional act, such as taking radiographs or expressing a professional opinion. Although there is no written document of agreement in an implied contract, a contractual relationship exists.

- An express contract is one in which the terms are expressed and includes either a verbal or a written agreement.

The contract, whether written or oral, may outline specific conditions or obligations that must be satisfied by the client or oral healthcare provider, such as fees, method of payment, or type of services to be provided. In addition, based on the contractual relationship, certain warranties or duties are required by both parties. The word duty in legal vernacular means obligatory conduct or service, or conducting oneself in a particular manner. Professionals in the legal system evaluate medical malpractice case law to determine the contractual rights and duties shared between the practitioner and the client based on the contractual relationship. Based on that contractual relationship, in accepting the client for care the oral healthcare provider promises to do the following[8]:

- Be properly licensed and registered and meet all other legal requirements to engage in the practice of dentistry or dental hygiene
- Use reasonable care in providing services as measured against acceptable standards set by other practitioners with similar training
- Never exceed the scope of practice
- Not use experimental procedures or medications
- Complete care within a reasonable time frame or arrange other sources of treatment when appropriate in order to complete treatment
- Never abandon the client by abruptly stopping oral healthcare
- Obtain informed consent before examination or treatment from the individual or the party responsible (i.e., guardian)
- Arrange care for the client during an absence and ensure that care is available in emergency situations
- Make appropriate referrals and request necessary consultations
- Maintain client privacy and confidentiality of information
- Maintain a level of knowledge in keeping with current advances in the profession
- Keep clients informed of their treatment progress and health status
- Inform the client of unanticipated occurrences
- Never exceed the scope of practice authorized by the license; never permit any person acting under another's direction to engage in unlawful acts
- Keep accurate records of the care provided to the client
- Comply with all laws regulating the practice of dentistry and dental hygiene
- Practice in a manner consistent with the code of ethics of the profession
- Charge a reasonable fee for services based on community standards
- Not attempt a procedure for which the practitioner is unqualified

The duties or warranties listed are enforceable, although not written or stated in any document given to the client. A dental hygienist who uses an experimental periodontal therapy rather than evidence-based procedures may be violating a contractual responsibility to use only standard procedures. A dental hygienist who casually discusses confidential information obtained from a client during the health history interview is violating a contractual obligation, ignoring the principle of fidelity as well as committing a breach of confidentiality. A dental hygienist practicing outdated techniques is also violating a duty to remain current and ignoring the principle of beneficence.

The client has contractual duties, including cooperating in care, providing accurate information, paying fees, and keeping appointments. Practitioners are frequently faced with clients who do not pay fees. Collection procedures may result based on the client's failure to meet the contractual obligation. Failing to cooperate in care, such as missing appointments or refusing to take premedication, does not necessarily result in a lawsuit filed by the dentist. Rather than filing a lawsuit, the practitioner may choose to dismiss the client from the practice.

If a breach of contract occurs, the client can use the contract concept to remedy the situation and obtain damages. Perhaps a client discovers that a dental assistant, not a dental hygienist, is providing root planing, which only a licensed dental hygienist is allowed to perform. The assistant did not harm the client; however, the dentist warranted, based on the contractual relationship between the dentist and client, that employees within the office were properly licensed and that the staff would never exceed scope of practice. In this example, three violations occurred and a breach of contract exists. At the same time, if the client has not met obligations, such as keeping an appointment, that client has breached the contract. Although the practitioner would probably not seek damages, the failure of the client to meet his responsibilities (contributory negligence) may be reason to end the practitioner-client relationship.

Terminating the Practitioner-Client Relationship

Termination of the practitioner-client relationship frequently occurs in practice; however, the practitioner must be cautioned never to abandon the client. Abandonment is a relinquishment of all connection with the client. The relationship between professional and client may end without charges of abandonment if the following conditions are met:

- Both parties agree to end it.
- The death of the client or oral health practitioner occurs.
- The client ends the relationship by act or statement.
- The client is cured, or treatment completed, as with a specialist.
- The practitioner unilaterally decides to terminate care.

If the practitioner seeks to end the relationship, the following specific steps are necessary:

- The client should receive written notification of termination and the reasons (e.g., lack of payment for services rendered or nonadherence to recommended care).
- Reason for termination should be provided in objective language. If a client is being terminated because of harassing behaviors, the letter does not have to describe the specific behaviors. Instead, the letter can indicate that the dentist is terminating the relationship because of "disrespectful attitudes and behaviors toward staff." Another reason may be noncompliance impacting the prognosis.
- The letter should state that the individual will remain a client of the practice for a certain length of time, the date services will be terminated, and that, if necessary, emergency care will be provided for a designated time period.
- The letter must suggest that the client seek another dental care provider and state that copies of the client's records

September 27, 2013

Mr. Daniel Powers
12214 Harvard Road
Point Park, MI 48000

Dear Mr. Powers:

Our records indicate that you have failed to respond to six notices for periodontal maintenance care, sent over the 4-year period from 2009-2013 requesting that you make an appointment for an examination and oral maintenance. Your lack of response to both mail and telephone messages suggests that you do not agree with our preventive philosophy. Thus, effective October 27, 2013, your relationship with this office is terminated. You will remain a patient in the practice for the next 30 days. Emergency treatment only will be provided during that 30-day period. I strongly suggest that you identify another oral healthcare provider. I shall be happy to forward a copy of your records once that practitioner is identified. Enclosed is a permission slip to transfer your records. Please sign the transfer slip and return to the office.

Mary L. Mesial, RDH, BS, MSDH

Figure 64-2. Letter of protection, terminating dental hygienist–client relationship.

I, ____________, hereby grant permission
(Print Name)
to ____________
(Print Name of Doctor or Hospital)

to release information related to my health history, status, and care, and copies of my health record, radiographs, and any test results to:

____
at ____________
____________.

Signature: ____________
Date
(If a Minor, Parent or Guardian Must Sign)

Figure 64-3. Request for release of information (Waiver of confidentiality.)

will be forwarded to the new provider. It is advisable to include a permission slip for transfer of records that the client can sign and return to expedite the process (Figures 64-2 and 64-3).

- The letter should be sent by certified or registered mail with return receipt requested. The termination process is done carefully to ensure continuity of care and diminish the possibility of charges of abandonment. A copy of the termination letter and returned receipt should be kept in the client's file.

Avoiding charges of abandonment becomes an issue in dental hygiene care when clients of record do not respond to a continued-care notice. Although office procedures may not require that an individual receive notification that he or she is no longer a client of record, actions such as the written notification should be taken.

Another example of a situation that may require termination of the practitioner-client relationship is when the client refuses necessary oral radiographs or prophylactic antibiotic premedication for the prevention of infective endocarditis. Rather than jeopardize quality of care, the dental hygienist may dismiss the client of record from the practice. Again, written notification of termination is necessary to protect the dental hygienist and the employer from charges of abandonment.

Related Responsibilities

The law states that a practitioner may refuse to treat an individual for any reason except race, creed, color, national origin, or certain condition, such as a disability. For example, a practice specializing in prosthodontic care may refuse to accept children as clients. As long as there is not a discriminatory reason such as ethnic origin, not accepting children as clients is legal. An office that fails to schedule individuals with Hispanic-sounding surnames, however, is discriminating based on national origin.

Dental hygienists should obtain information about the rules and regulations governing the care of clients within their state to avoid charges of discrimination. Different jurisdictions (states, commonwealths, provinces) have defined special groups with certain statutory implications relating to civil rights and discrimination. For example, in some states, statutes related to the rights of the disabled protect persons with human immunodeficiency virus (HIV) infection.

One can refuse to treat a client of record and not violate a contract obligation. A practitioner should refuse to treat a client if the practitioner does not have the competence to provide the appropriate standard of care. The practitioner without the necessary skills is expected to refer the client to the appropriate oral health provider. Lawsuits have resulted from practitioners attempting to provide care that is beyond the practitioner's level of competence. Perhaps a dental hygienist evaluates the client's periodontal health and, although referral is indicated by the condition presented, the dentist chooses to provide treatment. If a certain skill level is required to provide the appropriate treatment (e.g., root planing and periodontal surgery) and those skills are not present in the personnel of that practice, the practitioner has failed to meet the obligation to refer. The referral is not viewed as a discriminatory practice, but rather is the appropriate action under contract principles.

Tort Principles

The legal basis most commonly used by clients to file suit against healthcare providers is the negligence principle. Negligence falls within the category of law known as *torts*. A tort is an interference with another's right to enjoy person, property, or privacy.[7] Categories of torts are as follows:

- Intentional torts
- Unintentional torts

Intentional Torts

Intentional torts are committed with intent on the part of the person. Intentional torts include battery, assault, false imprisonment, mental distress, breach of confidentiality, interference with property (e.g., trespassing on private property), and misrepresentation or deceit. Professional liability insurance frequently covers only the unintentional tort of negligence. Intentional torts require that the person accused of the tort intended the harm that occurred. An intentional tort is a serious offense. Some intentional torts of interest to dental hygienists are discussed in the following paragraphs.

An assault[7] occurs when one intends to cause apprehension in someone without touching him or her. An example of an assault may be threatening someone with a raised hand. A practitioner that threatens to harm someone or causes fear may be guilty of assault, as in the example, "If you do not sit still, I am going to stick you with the needle."

A battery[7] is a harmful or offensive contact with someone—touching someone without their permission (e.g., restraining a child without parental permission). A technical battery[7] is when a dental hygienist, in the course of treatment, exceeds the consent given by the client. Examples of technical battery include placing dental sealants on teeth when consent was not obtained or giving a fluoride treatment without the client's consent. In such cases, the person bringing the charges (plaintiff) argues that the contact was offensive, and the dental hygienist (defendant) could be charged with both assault and battery. Assault and battery are considered intentional torts, and professional liability insurance may not provide coverage for charges filed under these categories. The dental hygienist should obtain informed consent to prevent charges of assault and battery. (Informed consent is discussed later in the section.)

Deceit or misrepresentation can occur in the provision of oral healthcare. A failure to inform a client that an instrument tip has broken and is lodged in the sulcus is an example of deceit. A practitioner must always keep the client informed of his or her oral healthcare status and not misrepresent personnel or services rendered. If a dental hygienist is ill and a dental assistant substitutes, there is an intent to misrepresent the dental assistant as a dental hygienist, and the employer is guilty of an intentional tort.

Another tort that could be classified as intentional is breach of confidentiality. A dental hygienist who violates the confidential relationship between the dental hygienist and the client is committing a tort. Discussing a specific client's history over lunch with a friend is a violation of confidentiality between the practitioner and client. If a dental hygienist responds to a request for client information without obtaining the client's permission, the confidential relationship is violated.

Unintentional Torts and Negligence

Unintentional torts are not intended by the person accused of committing the tort. Negligence and dental malpractice are used synonymously. Negligence[7] is a failure of one owing a duty to another to do what a reasonable and prudent person would ordinarily have done under the circumstances. The defining characteristics of negligence are the following:

- A duty or standard exists (e.g., health history taking, assessing blood pressure levels, assessing periodontal health, recording oral health status, referral).
- A breach or failure to exercise requisite care occurs (e.g., failing to assess the client, treat the client; failing to meet the standard of care for the practice of dental hygiene; incorrectly using anesthesia).
- A harm results (e.g., medical emergency occurs; periodontal status declines; paresthesia develops).
- The harm is directly caused by the breach of duty.

The plaintiff's responsibility is to prove that the defendant was negligent. The plaintiff must prove, by a preponderance of the evidence, all of the elements listed previously. For example, a dental hygienist is placing dental sealants on a child's teeth. The treatment area is a typical environment, with the operator's supplies on the dental bracket tray. The supplies include a receptacle with acid-etch material. The dental hygienist is etching the teeth while holding the acid-etch–filled receptacle. The child suddenly moves, the acid etch spills on the child, and a chemical burn occurs on the side of the child's face. Has negligent behavior occurred? One would need to evaluate the elements of negligence to answer the question. The dental hygienist did not intend to burn the child; however, a duty existed to be careful while applying the acid-etch solution. For the most part the dental hygienist was practicing cautiously; however, evidence may indicate that keeping the acid-etch solution away from the child is recommended to avoid spilling. The dental hygienist failed to use certain precautionary measures (reasonably prudent man rule) and harm resulted. The harm was proximately caused by the dental hygienist's actions, and thus the hygienist is found negligent by a judge or a jury. Again, the jury or judge would have to be only 51% sure that the dental hygienist's actions caused the harm. The jury or judge may recognize that the child's actions influenced what occurred but may still find the dental hygienist negligent.

Another example of negligent behavior is if a dental hygienist leaves infection-control chemicals (like those used to clean out suction units) in a cup on a counter. If, when the dental hygienist is away from the treatment room, a client mistakes the liquid for water or mouth rinse and drinks it, harm occurs although there was no intent to harm the client.

Standard of Care

Standard of care[7] is the degree of care a reasonably prudent professional would exercise under the same or similar circumstances. The standard of care is not defined by the courts, but rather is determined by members of the profession. In negligence actions, in order to define the standard of care and determine if the defendant is guilty or innocent, expert witnesses are called to testify. (A lawyer may seek information from a professional association, such as the ADHA or CDHA, professional literature, or a nationally recognized group, such as the Centers for Disease Control and Prevention, as a source of acceptable standards.)

An expert witness is a member of the defendant's professional group with a similar background (e.g., in a periodontal malpractice lawsuit, a dental hygienist working in a periodontal practice). Lawyers for both the plaintiff and defendant may call into court expert witnesses that best satisfy their arguments. Therefore the dental hygienist, who may be defending specific actions, may identify an expert witness to support the standard of care demonstrated by that dental hygienist's practices. The plaintiff, on the other hand, has an expert witness testify that the dental hygienist did not meet the acceptable standard of care. The decision of liability is left to the jurors and judge. Jurors, it should be noted, are primarily composed of non–healthcare providers. As indicated earlier, the level of proof required in civil actions is a preponderance of the evidence.

After listening to the testimony of both the expert witnesses, jurors decide whether the plaintiff was negligent. If there is a failure to meet that standard, as determined by the jurors or a judge, the dental hygienist may be found negligent. For example, a dental hygienist fails to monitor and record a client's blood pressure before care. During treatment the client experiences a cardiac arrest related to high blood pressure. The standard of care for dental hygiene includes taking and recording blood pressure as part of client assessment. The dental hygienist failed to meet the standard.

The failure to meet the standard of care can include the following:

- An act of omission (i.e., not doing something)
- An act of commission (i.e., performing an act inappropriately)

Omitting a procedure or step because one is unaware that it is the current standard is not an acceptable excuse in a court of law.

Dental hygienists are obligated to practice the concepts and techniques currently accepted (i.e., to meet the standard of care). Although the dentist is ultimately responsible for the actions of the dental hygienist, the dental hygienist still may be found negligent in a court of law if a required duty is not met. Typically, dental practitioners may be found negligent when harm is caused to the client as a result of failure to stay current. It is difficult for any dental professional to accept a verdict of guilty of negligence because, as was noted earlier, there is no intent on the professional's part to provide inadequate care; however, members of the legal system attempt to evaluate the facts objectively. They evaluate the actions of the practitioners and then assess the impact of those actions on the client. If harm occurs, the legal system decides who is at fault and awards damages, if appropriate.

Informed Consent

Another legal argument that falls within the negligence theory used in lawsuits against practitioners is lack of informed consent. Informed consent is a person's agreement to allow something to happen based on full disclosure of facts required to make an intelligent decision; consent is the individual's right to self-determination. As part of the consent process, clients must be informed of the material risks involved in care. Obtaining informed consent cannot be delegated to an assistant; it is the professional's responsibility to obtain consent.

A material risk is one that a "reasonable person" would consider in determining whether to proceed with the proposed treatment. Court decisions have determined that the client has the final say in his or her care, the client must be of sound mind when giving consent, and the consent must be informed to be valid.[7]

To achieve informed consent, clients must be told, in a language that they understand, the following information:

- Diagnosis of the condition
- Recommended procedure
- Nature and reasons for the procedure
- Benefits of the procedure
- Material risks in performing the procedure
- Prognosis if the procedure is performed or not performed
- Alternatives to the recommended procedure
- Risks and benefits to the alternative procedures
- Potential consequences if client does not choose the recommended procedure

In lawsuits that focus on informed consent, clients claim a lack of understanding of the risks involved in care, or that alternatives to treatment were not presented. The dental hygienist should explain any technical terms and make sure that the client comprehends the information; a linguistic interpreter may be necessary. Consent must be obtained for minors from parents or guardians. It is important to obtain consent from the parent(s) legally allowed to provide consent for medical and dental treatment. Issues of consent for minors with divorced or separated parents must be carefully monitored so that legal consent is obtained. If a client is legally incompetent, consent must be obtained from a guardian. Consent can be documented using a standardized form that allows portions to be completed on a case-by-case basis (see Chapter 22, Figure 22-4).

Clients should sign the consent form. If care is modified or if additional invasive procedures are performed, consent should be obtained again. Dental hygienists must take the time to obtain informed consent and allow the client an opportunity to ask questions. This opportunity to ask and have questions answered also must be documented in the client's record. Informed consent should be obtained for all surgical and invasive procedures as well as fluoride therapy, radiographs, and similar services. It is suggested that office policy be developed so that informed consent is obtained in a consistent manner from all clients.

Informed Refusal (Figure 64-4; see Chapter 22, Figure 22-5 and Box 22-6)

A risk of a lawsuit occurs when the client refuses to follow the advice of the treating dentist or dental hygienist. The lawsuit may occur if a client experiences serious injury or consequences after refusing care and claims he or she did not fully understand the consequences of refusing a recommendation or treatment. A basic rule to follow when a client refuses advice is to inform the client of possible consequences.

Date	Progress Notes
11-5-10	Care plan suggests periodontal surgery. Explained justification for surgery, risks, and alternative of three-month maintenance care, with reevaluation of need for surgery; client opted for three-month maintenance care. Client states that she understands three-month regimen must be strictly followed. Explained limitations of maintenance care versus surgery. Client asked questions about procedures at maintenance appointment.
	I, Mary Gorski, refuse periodontal surgery as recommended by M. Mesial. I opt to cooperate in a three-month maintenance care appointment program for a nine-month period. The risks, benefits, and reasons for both treatment alternatives have been adequately explained, and my questions answered.

Figure 64-4. Informed refusal.

This rule is known as informed refusal. The rules for informed refusal follow those for obtaining informed consent to care. They include that the client be told in understandable language the following information:

- The diagnosis and recommendation for treatment or referral
- The reasons for the recommendation
- Risks and possible consequences to client's oral and general health

There must be discussion about the refusal and the effects as well as an opportunity to discuss the recommendation. During the discussion, if it appears that the client refused care because of lack of understanding, the dental hygienist reexplains the recommendation. The client's refusal can be documented on an informed refusal form that includes the following:

- Recommendation
- List of the consequences of refusal
- Documentation that the client understood the risks of refusing care
- The date
- Signatures of the dentist, client, and a witness

If the client refuses to sign the informed refusal, this should be noted and the form signed by the provider and the witness. A copy of the form should be given to the client and another copy kept in the chart.

Statute of Limitations

The statute of limitations is the length of time an aggrieved person has to enter lawsuits against another for an alleged injury.[7] A statute of limitations places a time limit on a contract or tort action. Once the time period has ended, the lawsuit cannot be filed. For example, the statute of limitations for a contract action may be 6 years and for a tort action 3 years. In some states the statute of limitations starts either at the time an injury occurs or at the time the plaintiff discovers the injury or reasonably should have discovered the injury. This ability to sue when an injury is discovered expands the length of time in which someone can file a lawsuit. Perhaps a client is diagnosed with severe periodontal diseases 5 years after ending a client-provider relationship. The client still may be allowed to file a lawsuit. Risk constantly exists for a lawsuit to be filed. Practitioners must be aware of the statute of limitations and rules within their state to assist in planning for record keeping and record storage.

Legal Concepts and the Dental Hygienist–Client Relationship

Confidentiality

The dental hygienist–client relationship raises additional areas of concern that extend the legal duties and obligations outlined. Confidentiality means that information about a client's care is not to be shared without the client's permission. To release confidential information without the client's permission is an invasion of privacy. Invasion of privacy includes releasing client information to an unauthorized person, such as a spouse, or discussing a client's health history outside the scope of treatment. In large, open clinics, discussions with clients may appear less private. It is important that the practitioner maintains confidentiality of information in all settings and takes steps to protect client privacy and confidentiality.

A person can waive confidentiality through words or actions. For example, an individual who is referred to a specialist waives confidentiality. The referring practitioner is expected to inform the specialist of the client's status. Confidentiality can be waived by action of law, such as a requirement to report specific communicable diseases or the suspicion of child abuse to a state or provincial agency. A client's waiver of confidentiality should be documented in a progress note or separate form titled Waiver of Confidentiality (see Figure 64-3).

Defamation

Defamation is a communication that injures an individual's reputation. Defamation may be:

- Libel (written defamation)
- Slander (verbal defamation)

To be libelous or slanderous, the defamatory comment must be false. If an individual's reputation is not harmed by the defamatory comment, there is no libel or slander. In certain defamation cases, malice (intent to inflict an injury) must be shown. If a lawsuit is filed, the plaintiff must show actual damages to property, business, trade, profession, or occupation, or diminish the esteem, respect, or confidence in which the person is held. Thus an informal comment to one person about an "incompetent dentist" by a recently fired dental hygienist would not be considered slander. The dentist's reputation was not harmed and those listening would consider the source and not necessarily believe the comment. Repeated comments by a dental hygienist in a periodontal practice stating that one periodontist is more skilled than another may result in a lawsuit if the comments harm the dentist's reputation or influence clients' return to the practice.

Legal Concepts and the Dental Hygienist–Dentist Relationship

Discrimination in Employment

In seeking employment, an individual is protected against unlawful discriminatory practices. Federal and state labor laws exist to protect both employers and employees. State laws protecting against discrimination may be more inclusive than federal laws. If an employee believes they have been the subject of discrimination, consulting with an attorney familiar with state law is advised. A federal statute, Title VII of the Civil Rights Act of 1964, prohibits discrimination based on race, color, religion, gender, or national origin as it relates to hiring, firing, and terms, conditions, or privileges of employment. Gender discrimination includes discrimination based on pregnancy, childbirth, and related medical conditions such as gynecologic or gender-related problems. Title VII applies to employers with 15 or more employees; however, human rights acts enacted in almost all states outlaw the same type of discriminatory activity and may affect employers with as few as one employee. State laws may also expand the types of discrimination banned (e.g., discrimination based on marital status, physical handicap, or sexual orientation). The Age Discrimination in Employment Act of 1967 (ADEA) is a federal law that affects employers with 20 or more employees. The act prohibits discrimination on the basis of age between 40 and 70 years.

The Equal Employment Opportunity Commission (EEOC) deals with discrimination on any of the federally prohibited grounds. The EEOC assists by investigating or advising on appropriate agencies to contact. There are strict guidelines on the timeliness of the complaint, such as a requirement to bring a complaint within 180 days. If the EEOC is unable to obtain a solution, an individual may have the right to file a lawsuit. The EEOC has local offices that will answer questions or direct an individual to appropriate sources to resolve issues. Federal laws prohibiting employment discrimination are available from the EEOC website. Dental hygienists who believe they have been discriminated against in the employment setting should contact their state civil rights agency.

Americans with Disabilities Act

The Americans with Disabilities Act (ADA) prohibits employment discrimination against qualified individuals with disabilities. The law applies to employers with 15 or more employees. An individual qualifies for protection under this act if he or she has a physical or mental impairment that substantially limits one or more major life activities. Major life activities include walking, breathing, seeing, hearing, speaking, learning, and working. If an individual satisfies the position requirements, the employer is required to provide reasonable accommodations such as modifying equipment, facilities, schedules, or job routine. For example, an office receptionist with a hearing impairment may require telephone amplification in order to meet the job requirements.

Equal Pay Act

The Equal Pay Act of 1962 protects men and women who perform substantially equal work in the same establishment from gender-based wage discrimination. The law would not allow an employer to reduce the wages of either a man or a woman to equalize inequities in pay.

Pregnancy and Employment Status

A significant percentage of dental hygienists are female; therefore discrimination based on pregnancy is an important issue. Federal law prohibits an employer from terminating or refusing to hire or promote a woman because of childbirth, pregnancy, or related medical conditions, such as abortion. The EEOC is the agency that administers Title VII provisions. Guidelines distributed by the EEOC state that disabilities caused or contributed to by pregnancy or childbirth must be treated like any other disability. Mandatory leave arbitrarily set at a specific time for pregnant women without regard to their ability to work is also prohibited, as well as a policy that prohibits an employee from returning to work for a predetermined length of time after childbirth. Pregnancy benefits cannot be limited to married women only. Dental hygienists, in order to be informed and to assist their employers, should obtain information from a local department of human rights if a maternity leave is anticipated.

Employer-Employee Relationships

Seeking employment is a common occurrence. An employment application can include the following:

- Identification of the applicant (e.g., name, address, telephone number)
- Applicant's interests (jobs, salary levels)
- Summary of applicant's background including education, employment history, and skills

Unlawful pre-employment inquiries include the following:

- Applicant's maiden name
- Birthplace of applicant
- Religious denomination or affiliation
- Complexion or skin color
- Disability status
- Requirement of a photograph
- Height, weight
- Marital status or children
- Arrest record
- National origin, ancestry, or descent
- Society or club memberships or affiliations

Applicants need not provide the information that falls within the unlawful category. Individual states have legislation that regulates employment. An excellent resource is a state department of civil rights or a related agency.

Unlike some employer-employee relationships, the dental hygienist rarely has a written employment contract. Traditionally, responsibilities of employment, financial arrangements, benefits, and length of employment are verbally agreed on. Lack of a written agreement may leave the dental hygienist in a precarious situation. The contract is written documentation that clearly outlines the rights and responsibilities of the parties involved (see Chapter 63, eFigure 63-6). The ADHA provides a sample employment contract template to its members. A dental hygienist–employee needs to assist an employer so that a complete and fair contract is drafted, addressing the following issues:

- Position title and responsibilities
- Scheduled days and hours of the week
- Remuneration:
    - Amount
    - Pay period schedule
    - Benefits to be deducted
    - How remuneration will be calculated—commission, hourly, daily
- Schedules of review or evaluation:
    - Influence on remuneration
    - Method of evaluation: formal or informal

- Fringe benefits
- Notification requirements for contract severance
- Specific expectations

In most jurisdictions the dental hygienist works as an employee of the dentist. The law views this as a basic employer-employee relationship where there is direct control and supervision of the employee by the employer. The doctrine governing the relationship is **respondeat superior**,[7] Latin for "let the superior [master] answer." Based on the traditional structure of most state dental practice acts, the dentist-employer answers for the actions of the dental hygienist. The dental hygienist, as a licensed professional, is legally accountable and can be sued. Because of the doctrine of respondeat superior, however, dentists are also named in lawsuits filed against dental hygienists. Including the dentist as one of the parties of a lawsuit is a reflection of the "deep pocket" theory. That is, the monetary damages sought can be increased because of the larger malpractice insurance coverage of the dentist-employer.

Another business relationship with the dentist-employer that may exist for the dental hygienist is that of an independent contractor. As an independent contractor, the dental hygienist is under contract to fulfill certain responsibilities but has little guidance from the contracting party. The Internal Revenue Service (IRS) distinguishes whether a person is an independent contractor or employee as related to federal taxes (Box 64-6). The criteria include 20 different points to consider in determining the status of a worker. The key in reviewing the points is the control by the respective parties in the relationship and the substance of the relationship over form.

The independent contractor is self-employed. With the increased freedom of independent contracting, there is also an increased liability and total responsibility for income and Social Security taxes. An individual interested in an independent contracting agreement should investigate the area within the jurisdiction and seek legal advice. A comparison of an employee's role vs. that of an independent contractor is available at http://www.texasworkforce.org/ui/tax/forms/c8.pdf.

Sexual Harassment

Federal guidelines classify sexual harassment as a form of sexual discrimination. **Sexual harassment** is defined as sexual discrimination because it forces a female or male to work under adverse employment conditions. The EEOC defines sexual harassment as follows:

> *Unwelcome sexual advances, requests for sexual favors and other verbal or physical conduct of a sexual nature when submission to or rejection of this conduct is made either explicitly or implicitly a term or condition of an individual's employment; submission to or rejection of such conduct by an individual is used as the basis for employment decisions affecting the individual; or such conduct has the purpose or effect of unreasonably interfering with an individual's work performance or creating an intimidating, hostile or offensive working environment.*[8]

BOX 64-6

Internal Revenue Service Guideposts for Independent Contractors

As an aid to determining whether an individual is an employee under the common law rules, 20 factors are identified as indicating whether sufficient control is present to establish an employer-employee relationships.

Instructions—when, where, and how work is performed

Training—requiring the worker to work with experienced employees, corresponding with the worker, requiring the worker to attend meetings or use other methods

Integration—refers to integration of the worker's services into business operations

Services rendered personally—if services must be rendered personally, it is presumed the persons for whom services are performed are interested in methods used

Hiring, supervising, and paying assistants—if the persons for whom services are performed hire assistants, that generally shows control; the reverse is also true

Continuing relationship

Set hours of work

Full-time standard—worker performs full-time and is restricted from performing other work

Doing work on the employer's premises—suggests control over the worker, especially if the work could be done elsewhere

Order of sequence set—if the worker must follow a sequence set out by the entity for whom he or she is performing the services, this would indicate an employer-employee relationship

Oral or written reports—written reports indicate control

Payment by hour, week, month—indicates employer-employee relationship; payment by job indicates independent contractor relationship

Payment of business and/or travel expenses—if the person for whom services are performed pays for travel expenses, this generally indicates employer-employee relationship

Furnishing of tools or material—furnishing of tools by person for whom work is performed indicates employer-employee relationship

Significant investment—lack of investment in the facilities indicates employer-employee relationship

Realization of profit or loss—realization of profit or loss by worker would indicate independent contractor; but the worker who cannot realize profit or loss is generally considered an employee

Working for more than one firm—if the worker performs work for more than one unrelated firm, it generally indicates the worker is an independent contractor

Making service available to the general public—making service available to the general public on a regular basis indicates an independent contractor

Right to discharge—indicates employer-employee relationship

Right to terminate—right to terminate by the employee without incurring liability indicates employer-employee relationship

Data from Texas Workforce Commission: *Employment status—a comparative approach.*

Two types of sexual harassment occur, as follows:

- **Quid pro quo**, which means something for something, involves a superior-subordinate relationship in which the offender has control over the working conditions of the victim. Examples of sexual harassment include demands for sexual favors in exchange for better working conditions or reviews, raises, or promotions.
- **Hostile environment** includes unwelcome, demeaning verbal or physical conduct of a sexual nature that creates a hostile, intimidating, or offensive work environment. Behaviors that may create a hostile work environment include conversation with sexual content, telling sexually explicit jokes, displaying sexually suggestive objects or pictures, sending inappropriate texts or email messages, and using names such as "honey," "sweetie," or "blondie." The environment may interfere with the ability of the harassed employee to do the job; however, there is no tangible employment loss evident. Supervisors, co-workers, or nonemployees may be involved.

Sexual harassment occurs in the dental environment.[9] A dental hygienist reported that every time she asked for a dentist "to check" a client after a dental hygiene appointment, the dentist asked the dental hygienist to perform a sexual act. The dental hygienist, flustered and embarrassed, did not want to work alone with the dentist. Although the request for sexual favors was not related to salary or employee evaluation, it easily could have developed into that type of situation. The dentist's actions constitute sexual harassment. A second example may be a client who makes inappropriate remarks or gestures of a sexual nature. Clients, who are considered nonemployees, influence the environment in which a dental hygienist is employed. A dental hygienist should report the behavior of the client to the employer. The employer is obligated to make the working environment nonthreatening.

An employer is required to maintain a professional, businesslike relationship among employees and prevent or stop all situations considered harassment in the workplace. Prevention is the best strategy. Employers should communicate to all employees that sexual harassment will not be tolerated. If an individual has been the victim of sexual harassment, immediate action is necessary. An employee's response to either physical or verbal harassment must be prompt, serious, specific, and assertive. If faced with sexual harassment, one should do the following:

- Directly inform the harasser that the conduct is unwelcome, and specifically identify the conduct.
- Directly inform the harasser that the conduct is to stop.
- Review office policies and protocol and/or notify an employer or supervisor of the incident.
- Talk to co-workers; determine whether there have been similar experiences shared by others or if others have witnessed harassing behaviors.
- If a refusal may affect the job, report the incident to a co-owner of the practice or appropriate supervisory personnel.
- Document the harassment and keep accurate notes of what was said and done, the date, the time, the place, and the names of any witnesses.

If the situation is not remedied, options exist. In settings that employ 15 or more employees, the district office of the EEOC is contacted. The EEOC will guide an individual through the process of filing a complaint against the harasser. If there are fewer than 15 employees, assistance may be available from a state agency such as the State Department of Civil Rights. Although hiring a lawyer may not be necessary, legal representation is helpful to guide the victim and represent the victim if the case progresses. The district EEOC office is a resource.

Termination of Employment

Dental hygienists may have their employment terminated for little or no reason, defined as "at will." The small business atmosphere of dental practice allows the "at will termination" by either party to exist. Some states have developed legal remedies for individuals wrongfully terminated. Some jurisdictions, for example, have laws that allow employers to terminate employees for good cause (i.e., someone can lose his or her position with a documented cause such as failure to meet performance standards). A dental hygienist should be familiar with the state's policy on termination. Various states have developed criteria that must be met to prove either appropriate or inappropriate employer behavior if an employee is terminated. The termination process can also be outlined in a contract (e.g., termination requiring 2-week written notice). Given the "at will" termination process, notice of termination is a courtesy but not a requirement to end employment.

Risk Management[10]

A risk management program is recommended to identify potential risks in the delivery of oral care. After risk is identified and measured, efforts can be made by the office staff to minimize or eliminate the risk. Potential areas of risk exposure include the following:

- Liability associated with professional actions of employers or employees
- General liability exposures for injuries to clients, vendors, and others
- Property and casualty exposures associated with the office, building, or surrounding area (e.g., parking lot)
- Exposure to defamation actions among staff, office managers, and other personnel
- Exposure to financial losses such as fraud, embezzlement, or theft
- Exposure to contracts, warranties, and similar entities associated with the purchase and use of goods and services
- Fraud and abuse exposure associated with federal and state third-party reimbursement programs
- Exposure to losses associated with staff hiring, promotions, and termination practices
- Inappropriate or incorrect use of dental equipment or dental materials
- Violation of privacy or confidentiality requirements

Box 64-7 provides sample questions that can be considered when assessing the potential risks in an employment setting.

Communication as a Risk Management Tool

Dental Hygienist–Client

Open communication between the dental hygienist and client minimizes misunderstandings, reducing the likelihood of lawsuits and allowing for direct, timely resolution of problems. A dental hygienist who spends 45 to 60 minutes in a one-on-one relationship with a client can reduce the potential

BOX 64-7

Sample Checklist for Assessing Litigation Risk in a Dental Employment Setting

Is the staff properly licensed and practicing within the appropriate scope of practice?
Is the dental equipment properly maintained and monitored?
Are there procedures for educating and updating staff concerning the components of the dental record and record-keeping techniques?
Do the staff members use appropriate verbal and nonverbal communication techniques?
Are the health and dental histories updated at every appointment?
Are appropriate intraoral and extraoral data collected and recorded?
Do the staff members comprehensively document crucial data or conversations?
Are referrals (to dentists, physicians or other healthcare providers) documented?
Is informed consent or informed refusal documented?
Does the office have a medical emergency protocol, and has the procedure been rehearsed?
Are the staff members qualified in cardiopulmonary resuscitation (CPR) and first aid?
Is there a medical emergency kit available, and are the drugs in it kept current? Is someone in the office capable of administering the medications in the emergency kit?
Is there an office manual that outlines protocols for client care, referral, and termination?
Is office protocol or documentation available to all staff outlining roles and responsibilities and important policies, such as sexual/ethnic harassment prevention guidelines?
Are the staff members practicing the latest infection-control procedures according to Occupational Safety and Health Administration (OSHA) and Centers for Disease Control and Prevention (CDC) guidelines?
Are the staff members familiar with the uses of major equipment in the office (e.g., automatic processor, panoramic radiology, dental handpieces, sedation equipment, and autoclaves)?
Are broken toys or sharp objects removed promptly from the reception area?
Are the sidewalks, parking lots, and driveways clear of any debris (e.g., nails, glass, ice)?
Are the handicapped ramps operable?
Is signage clear and understandable?

for negligent actions. The one-on-one relationship with a client gives the dental hygienist an opportunity to explain the care that will occur and answer client questions. Concepts must be presented clearly, with appropriate use of professional jargon. A client who senses professional interest and expertise on the part of the dental hygienist may not be as prone to file a lawsuit if a procedure is unsuccessful. A diverse clientele may require that an office employ bilingual staff to assist in improving communication.

Dental Hygienist–Employer

The dental hygienist plays a key role in educating employers about potential liabilities for dental hygienists and their prevention. Written standards for office protocol can be developed and coordinated by the dental hygienist in conjunction with the employer. A resource library that includes updated website addresses, literature, textbooks, and other related material, such as a current copy of the rules and regulations outlining the rights and responsibilities of licensed office staff, provides a quick resource if questions arise. The use of Web-based resources allows for a large array of resources to be available quickly to respond to questions, clarify information, or identify potential risks. If a risk management philosophy is practiced and reinforced by the employees and the employer, legal risks are reduced for the entire staff.

Dental Hygienist–Colleagues

The best resources for the development of a risk management philosophy are the personnel within the employment setting. Consistent criteria for record keeping and referral can be developed; specific evidence-based literature to support particular treatment modalities can be shared; and office protocols and handbooks can be developed. Each activity contributes to improved practice habits. Persons employed in similar roles should meet for a risk management day to identify areas of potential risk and develop mechanisms to reduce that risk. Suggested activities are the following:

- Brainstorm to identify risks in the practice; these can include treatment techniques, client management, record keeping, communication, and preventive practices.
- Have each person review the plan of care for a client; write down the key steps followed.
- Sample client records and review record-keeping styles, abbreviations, charting records, informed consent and refusal, and other written aspects of care.
- Discuss risky practices that have become apparent.
- Develop a consensus that focuses on reducing risky behaviors that can be comfortably incorporated by all on a consistent basis (e.g., procedures for client care, charting techniques, abbreviations, referral guidelines, periodontal and other preventive therapies).
- Develop a dental hygiene office manual, which can be a separate manual or incorporated as a component of a larger manual. It can focus on the dental hygiene staff, client assessment, treatment and evaluation, insurance information, risk management suggestions, record keeping protocol, standardized periodontal assessment and charting guidelines, and premedication information. Once consensus occurs, chapters can be delegated and written. The manual serves as a guidebook to assist current and future employees. The manual is also helpful to other office staff and dentists.
- Propose and/or conduct a similar risk management workshop for the dentists and assistants on staff.

Client Record

The client record can be a provider's best defense or worst enemy in a malpractice action. The record provides the following information:

- Complete record of both the health and dental status at the time of the initial examination, including the pharmacologic and fluoride history
- Comprehensive and chronologic documentation of treatment provided

- Potential legal document on the client's behalf (e.g., use in corpse identification or insurance claims or fraud)
- Legal document for the defense of litigious claims against a dental practitioner
- Records as required in some states as part of the laws regulating professional practice
- Tool for quality assessment and assurance
- Communication mechanism among health professionals involved in the client's care

Documentation begins with initial client contact and continues throughout the relationship between the provider and the client, including reasons for termination of the relationship, if that occurs.

Client Identification Data

Client identification data are standard pieces of information such as name, address, telephone number for home and work, best time to call, emergency contact person, legal guardian, physician of record, and insurance-related information such as a Social Security number. Practices have grown larger, client numbers have increased, and client populations reflect multicultural backgrounds. Inaccurate client data make it difficult to identify a record that may be critical in a lawsuit. Poor documentation reflects on the oral healthcare provider. There may be an assumption that sloppy records reflect sloppy care.

Information about a client may change frequently, so periodic updating should be routine. Updated material should be dated. A client's photograph, as part of the record, has been recommended for identification purposes.

Health and Dental History (see Chapter 12)

All health and dental history information should be pursued and answered. If an item on the history form is not appropriate, it should be indicated "NA" (not applicable). If the condition is normal, a notation such as "WNL" (within normal limits) is appropriate. The oral healthcare provider should review the history to make sure every question has been answered. A client history should be obtained at every visit. After a review is complete, notations should be made and dated in the progress notes or on the health history, noting changes.

One needs to document the individuals involved in each step of the history-taking process. For example, names of those who completed the health history with the client, names of those who reviewed the history with the client (if not the dentist or dental hygienist), and dates and signatures for each step should be recorded.

Assessment data should be recorded consistently. For example, a client initially comes to the office with moderate periodontitis. If the condition does not improve, the practitioner has a record of the condition from the moment care began. Therefore the dentist or dental hygienist cannot be accused of contributing to the client's condition.

Clinical Assessment and Diagnosis

A protocol should be established for the initial clinical assessment and subsequent visits. A diagnosis should be documented in order to justify treatment. The plaintiff's attorney frequently suggests that malpractice occurred because there was no clear diagnosis documented in the dental chart that would guide treatment.

Treatment Information

Concise, accurate, clear, and comprehensive records of care should include the following:

- Nature of the care or treatments provided
- Area in the mouth where care is provided
- Use of special dental equipment, such as an ultrasonic scaler
- Type and dose of anesthetic agent and/or analgesia used
- Details about conditions presented, gingival health, oral hygiene status, specific areas of change
- Language that is specific (e.g., a notation such as "some deep pockets in the posterior" provides little definitive information)
- Details of conditions noted during or as the result of treatment, such as hematomas, excessive bleeding
- Specific recommendations for postoperative instructions and whether written postoperative instructions were provided to the client
- Medication prescribed or administered and dosages
- Unexpected occurrences or reactions, such as fractured restorations
- Client education conducted, as well as client's response
- Continued-care interval or maintenance schedule

All procedures must be documented. Each client has one dental hygienist and remembers each visit. Each dental hygienist has a large clientele and needs to record information that may be required in future litigation. Cancellations, late arrivals, changes of appointments, and conversations with front desk personnel are documented.

The record should reflect objective information; subjective information is included only if it affects client care (e.g., writing "Client was very apprehensive and asked many questions during the procedure," rather than "Client was a bother and questioned everything"). A record must be maintained in a professional manner. It is advisable not to comment on client or guardian personalities or characteristics, such as "Mom is very protective."

The record assists in the defense against a charge of breach of contract, negligence, or lack of informed consent. The lawyer for the plaintiff who reviews a thorough, complete record may determine that there is no reason to pursue a lawsuit. The record may clearly indicate that the practitioner has met all obligations and caused no harm. An incomplete or inaccurate record under close scrutiny provides multiple opportunities for the plaintiff's lawyer to prove inadequate or negligent care (Box 64-8).

Legal Issues and Roles of the Dental Hygienist

Dependent Practitioner

The status of a dependent practitioner may be somewhat misleading. An individual is dependent as a result of the licensing and regulation laws of the state; however, the individual is not dependent on the employer to assume legal responsibility for one's actions. The dependent practitioner is providing client care. Based on the educational background and licensed status, the dental hygienist has professional obligations and legal duties that must be fulfilled. Failure to fulfill specific legal duties may result in charges of negligence (malpractice).

BOX 64-8

Suggestions for Managing Client Records

Entries should be legible, written in black ink or ballpoint pen.

When there is more than one person making entries, entries should be signed or initialed.

When errors occur, they should not be blocked out so that they cannot be read. Instead, a single line should be drawn through the entry, and a note made above it stating "error in entry, see correction below." The correction should be dated at the time it is made.

Electronic records should never be altered.

Financial information should not be kept on the treatment record.

Entries should be uniformly spaced on the form. There should be no unusual or irregular blank spaces.

On health information forms, there should be no blank spaces in the answers to health questions. If the question is inappropriate, a single line is drawn through the question, or "not applicable" (NA) is recorded in the box. If the response is normal, a "within normal limits" (WNL) notation is made.

All cancellations, late arrivals, and changes of appointments are recorded.

Consents are documented, including all risks and alternative treatments presented to the client and remarks made by the client.

The client is informed of any adverse occurrences or untoward events that take place during the course of care; a note on the record that the client was informed is necessary.

All requests for consultations and responses are recorded.

All conversations held with other health practitioners relating to the care of the client are documented.

All client records should be retained for at least the period of the statute of limitations equal to that of contract actions. In most jurisdictions it is 6 years; however it can be longer. In the case of minors, it is until the person reaches the age of 24 years. However, a case of alleged negligence involving a very young patient may arise 16-18 years after treatment. Check for special laws in your local jurisdiction. A dental office may consider additional record retention options that may include record storage facilities, microfilm, and/or imaging to allow retrieval at a later date. If at all possible, keep records forever.

Electronic dental records continue to become more popular. There should be a standardized protocol that includes daily backup of records and weekly transfer of records. Software programs allow transfer of information. Security measures may be integral to the system. Health Insurance Portability and Accountability Act (HIPAA) security regulations should be followed.

No subjective evaluations, such as an opinion about the client's mental health, should be recorded on the treatment record unless the writer is qualified and licensed to make such evaluations.

Confidentiality of information contained on the record should be guarded. Staff should be trained to follow HIPAA guidelines.

The original record should not be surrendered to anyone, except by order of a court.

A record should never be altered once there is some indication that legal action is contemplated by the client.

Staff are instructed that they must retain the records of clients and comply with any written request for a copy.

Adapted from Pollack BR: *Dentist's risk management guide,* Fort Lauderdale, Fla, 1990, National Society of Dental Practitioners.

A dental hygienist may be charged with **negligence** if a breach of duty occurs and harm results. One can omit a service, resulting in negligence, such as assessing a client's blood pressure. A practitioner can also commit a negligent act, such as harming a client with an instrument or using hand-over-mouth technique practices to discourage inappropriate behavior in children. In any situation the duty or standard of care expected is evaluated. A conflict arises when the dental hygienist cannot provide care at an acceptable standard. For example, an individual has a periodontal condition that requires four 1-hour appointments to adequately root plane and scale, followed by an appointment for reevaluation. The care planning philosophy of the dentist is to allow two appointments. The dental hygienist may fail to adequately treat the client in two appointments and may contribute to a declining periodontal status. The issue of the standard of care for the dental hygienist is addressed during the lawsuit. Thus the dental hygienist is liable for professional actions taken or omitted.

Independent Practitioner

As an independent practitioner a hygienist is responsible for all the legal principles that influence client care, including negligence, referral, abandonment, informed refusal, and informed consent. An independent practitioner also is an employer and is responsible for knowledge of labor and employment laws, discrimination issues, tax laws, and related business obligations. Assessing and minimizing risks contributes to long-term success in practice.

An independent practitioner is advised to seek legal and business assistance for some of the following items. Contracts and other related agreements are necessary to a business owner and must be drafted, negotiated, and signed. Employer-employee relationships and office protocols must be developed, and guidelines established. An independent practitioner is the owner of a business, and functioning as such requires managerial skills outside the realm of client care (e.g., building and equipment maintenance, material and human resources management, and strategic planning). State and federal laws affect many aspects of the business, including hiring, firing, and evaluating personnel. Other laws affect the physical plant, such as incorporating barrier-free access or selecting and maintaining equipment according to Occupational Safety and Health Administration (OSHA) guidelines.

The financial commitment to the practice is a significant one. Therefore protecting personal assets, as well as keeping personal and professional expenses separate, is essential. Separate accounts are advisable for ease of bookkeeping. In addition, separation of personal and professional assets is important so personal assets cannot be taken if the business is affected by either financial or legal problems. An independent practitioner is responsible for policies and procedures used, quality of care provided, documentation, and the actions of employees. Given the litigious environment affecting dentistry and dental hygiene, the independent practitioner may be scrutinized by those seeking to find errors or illegalities. A clear understanding of the laws governing practice is imperative.

Independent Contractor

The independent contractor must recognize the contractual responsibilities inherent in both business and professional relationships. The dental hygienist is contracting to provide services. Both parties in the relationship, the dental hygienist and the contracting party, have specific rights and responsibilities. For example, the dental hygienist assumes that the contracting party will pay a salary and provide certain facilities and support staff. Failure to fulfill specific obligations of a contract is a breach of contract. Dental hygienists should seek legal counsel before any commitment as an independent contractor. Issues such as labor laws, income tax, and Social Security taxes, as well as liability issues are additional and important considerations. The independent contractor and practitioner must also remain cognizant of the legal issues affecting client care such as negligence, informed consent, referral, abandonment, and record keeping.

The dental hygienist, as an independent contractor, must approach practice with a strong risk management philosophy. A dental hygienist need not be put at risk because of the poor quality of care provided by someone else. Therefore, during the interview process, before establishing a relationship, the dental hygienist should evaluate the employer in terms of potentially negligent activities, referral philosophies, infection control, and record keeping, to name a few considerations. Reviewing client records (with an understanding of HIPAA regulations) to observe how client care is managed may assist a dental hygienist in deciding whether to contract with a specific care provider.

Dissolution of the contract relationship after a preliminary period should be addressed as part of the initial negotiations. Rights and responsibilities of all parties should be clearly outlined so that the working relationship is defined. At the same time the reasons and methods for ending the relationship, such as justifications to dissolve and notice requirements, also must be reviewed and agreed on.

Independent contracting requires careful scrutiny of tax laws and definitions of the independent contracting status. Legal counsel should be sought before committing to any relationship.

Educator

An educator has contact with both colleagues and students. Confidentiality—an obligation not to violate confidences shared—is one aspect of the relationships developed in an educational setting. In today's society, issues that must remain confidential have become more difficult to define. Educators are grappling with issues such as the student who confides a high-risk lifestyle for contracting a sexually transmitted disease or a colleague who has had a positive HIV test result. Institutions of higher education have developed policies to address such situations, but state and local laws may also address topics such as the students' rights and health issues.

Some states have general policies concerning issues such as the infected healthcare worker that can be used by institutions to guide their activities. Discrimination may also be an issue. Educators must be certain that decisions affecting admission, hiring, clinical assignments, workload, promotion, and evaluation are not influenced by actions that are considered discriminatory. Informal comments previously made about an individual or group of individuals may resurface if allegations of discrimination occur. Clearly outlined policies for personnel hiring and management and student admission and continuance assist in decreasing potentially discriminatory practices.

The educator who serves as a clinical instructor must recognize that the legal principles apply to clinical education. Informed consent, standard of care, confidentiality, referral policies, and contract and tort duties must be purposefully applied. Clinical faculty members ultimately are liable for a student's actions. Therefore client interactions and care should be carefully monitored. Client information written by a student and co-signed by a faculty member should be read critically to ensure accuracy and completeness. Student-faculty interactions in a clinical setting must be free of bias or discriminatory practices. Similar issues apply to the educator, who also may provide clinical care as part of an in-house faculty practice. Policies to prevent charges of abandonment must be developed and implemented. Careful documentation of client care, referral, and dismissal with standardized language ensures consistency within the institution.

An educator may be involved in supervision of clerical and clinical staff. Employee rights, contractual responsibilities, employee evaluation, and dismissals involve legal issues. Again, the educator must consider written documentation, discriminatory practices, civil rights issues, and issues within the area of labor law and employer-employee relationships.

The educator also works with administrators. Issues such as the educator's contractual rights, civil rights, and related topics should be understood, and if an issue arises, legal counsel may be sought. Failure on the part of an institution to recognize specific rights may lead to legal resolution. Promotion and tenure, salary issues, and job descriptions and responsibilities have a legal component.

Administrator or Manager

The administrator or manager is involved in hiring, evaluating, and possibly dismissing students, colleagues, or employees. Knowledge of federal and state law affecting civil rights and sexual harassment, and the protection of those rights, is important policy to know and follow. Administrators must recognize that specific questions cannot be asked as part of an employment interview. Evaluation of an employee should be completed carefully and documented. In some instances, dismissal of an employee or student can occur only after a series of evaluations, warnings, and in some instances, counseling, is completed. Again, colleagues who make discriminatory remarks, exhibit sexual misconduct, or conduct themselves inappropriately reflect on the administrator's ability to manage effectively.

Contracts are a common part of an administrator or manager's life. A **contract**, the agreement between two consenting parties, reflects certain rights and responsibilities. All parties involved require a clear understanding of the rights and responsibilities delineated in the contract. Failure to understand the contract may lead to charges of a breach of contract based on the failure to fulfill a responsibility. For example, if a breach of contract occurs, there may be financial ramifications. If an employee is inappropriately dismissed without due process of the law, the court may require that the employer be responsible for fulfilling the salary terms of the contract. In such a situation, although the employee is gone, the employer is still obligated under law to pay salary and benefits.

The administrator or manager may be responsible for ensuring the safety of an employee from the tortious acts of another (e.g., a responsibility to protect an employee from a client or student who may commit an assault or battery). In addition, a responsibility exists to prevent negligence in maintenance of the physical plant, such as faulty steps, icy or wet entrances, or other dangerous situations. The administrator or manager may be responsible for following federal or state mandates in areas such as employment or safety. Adherence to laws, rules, and regulations within the workplace may be the responsibility of the manager.

Labor laws and related legal concepts may dictate what documentation is important and also appropriate. Employees have access to their employment files, and therefore one must be objective and thorough in documenting events and personal interactions. State and federal laws seek to protect the rights of involved individuals.

Consumer Advocate

The consumer rights advocate should be aware of legislation on legal issues, civil rights, healthcare, labor issues in employment of the disabled, geriatrics, and issues regarding children and adolescents. Advocates should focus on areas that best meet personal needs and the needs of the population group(s) they represent. Understanding the political system, how laws are enacted, and lobbying techniques assists the advocate to keep updated by pursuing information and getting on mailing lists. Working with professional groups with similar interests also provides a valuable resource for information or to respond to a situation, such as through a letter-writing campaign.

Contracts and torts are applied in many situations. Did a group promising to provide services breach its contract? Did an agency violate the terms of its contract? Was an individual negligent in his responsibilities? Was informed consent obtained? Is there a duty to an individual or group of individuals based on an interpretation of the law? Can one argue that some have misrepresented themselves or an issue? In most instances a lawyer can assist in defining the legal principles that apply. The code of ethics for lawyers suggests that they perform some legal work pro bono (for free). Therefore an individual working as a consumer advocate may find legal assistance from someone willing to work pro bono and obtain valuable advice and guidance from the legal perspective.

Researcher

Researchers should be familiar with issues such as institutional review boards, confidentiality, rights of human and animal subjects, informed consent, record keeping, data management, and abandonment. For instance, researchers must also consider legal issues not addressed in this chapter, such as product liability, fund management, and tax issues.

CLIENT EDUCATION TIPS

- Educate the client about the legal justification for particular activities (e.g., questions about the use of protective barriers can result in a discussion about Occupational Safety and Health Administration [OSHA] regulations).
- Explain issues of standards of care, scope of practice, and duty to the client.
- As the operator records information, such as periodontal assessment data, the need to keep accurate records to assist in client care and protection from health risks can be described.
- If a client is refusing a particular recommendation for treatment, the ethical principles of autonomy, beneficence, and nonmaleficence can be discussed.
- If a client raises a concern about treating particular clients, such as those with infectious diseases, the legal issues of discrimination and the ethical principle of justice can be discussed.

LEGAL, ETHICAL, AND SAFETY ISSUES

- Before making a legal or ethical decision, the dental hygienist seeks resources that guide the process (e.g., American Dental Hygienists' Association or Canadian Dental Hygienists Association Code of Ethics, American Dental Association Principles of Ethics and Code of Professional Conduct, Standards of Clinical Practice, research evidence, current rules and regulations governing the practice of dental hygiene in the state in which the license is held). Public health statutes may identify responsibilities such as mandatory reporting of child or adult abuse, infectious disease reporting, and record-keeping requirements.
- Written office protocols that reflect evidence-based practice protect the healthcare team from litigation, if these protocols are used and practiced.

KEY CONCEPTS

- Ethics focuses on the moral duties and obligations of the professional to self, the profession, clients, colleagues, employees, employers, family, friends, the community, scientific investigations, and society.
- Dental hygienists are guided by the core ethical principles of autonomy, veracity, justice, beneficence, nonmaleficence, and fidelity.
- Dental hygienists are accountable to clients, colleagues, employers, and society.
- A code of ethics is characteristic of a profession and assists in raising ethical sensitivity and providing a guiding framework for decision making.
- An ethical decision-making model includes identifying the conflict and the ethical principles involved and gathering relevant information in order to identify a list of alternatives from which a dental hygienist can choose one ethically based alternative on which to act.
- Civil law is that branch of law that includes offenses violating private or contractual rights.
- Dental hygienists can have a contractual relationship with a client that requires the dental hygienist to fulfill specific obligations.

- Abandonment results if a relationship between a practitioner and client is severed without appropriate notification and documentation.
- Technical battery occurs if a practitioner performs a procedure on a client without informed consent.
- Negligence is a professional's failure to fulfill a specific duty to a client that results in an injury or harm.
- A dental hygienist must meet the standard of care for the profession (i.e., the degree of care a reasonably prudent professional would exercise under the same or similar circumstances).
- Informed consent allows a client to agree to allow something to happen based on full disclosure of information and is based on the ethical principle of autonomy, recognition of an individual's right to self-determination.
- Informed refusal allows a client to decline dental advice; the refusal should be documented in order to protect the practitioner.
- Confidentiality is an important responsibility that protects a client's privacy.
- Federal and state laws exist to protect dental hygienists from employment discrimination in hiring, firing, compensation, and promotion decisions.
- Dental hygienists may be subject to sexually harassing behaviors and should be familiar with steps to stop or prevent the behavior.
- Risk management involves identifying risks and implementing strategies to reduce or eliminate risks.
- Record keeping is important to protect the practitioner and the client and to assist in client care.

CRITICAL THINKING EXERCISES

1. Obtain a current document from the ADHA or CDHA that provides a synopsis of the supervision requirements for services provided by dental hygienists by state or province. How is the legal doctrine of respondeat superior affected by this variability in supervision requirements in the various legal jurisdictions?
2. Obtain the current Code of Ethics from both the ADHA and the CDHA. Read both. How are they similar? How do they differ?
3. Answer the questions in Scenarios 64-1 to 64-4 and eScenario 64-5 for analysis and discussion.

SCENARIO 64-1

Ivy Smith has been a licensed dental hygienist for 8 years. She is not active in the dental hygiene professional association and looks to her employer to keep her "updated." She relies on her employer, Dr. Albert Brady, to tell her what is "legal" or "illegal" in dental hygiene. She rarely attends professional meetings or reads scientific publications. She discusses with you, a dental hygiene colleague, some of the things that she is doing in her private practice. Her employer has told her that under his direction she can perform some expanded duties, so she has cemented some crowns and used nitrous oxide–oxygen analgesia during client care activities (both of which are illegal for dental hygienists in the state/province). She was also told by her employer not to spend time reviewing health or dental histories or using other client assessment methods, such as evaluating periodontal disease status, in order to save time. According to her employer, when it comes to history review and assessment, "Once is enough" and her job is to "clean teeth." She has raised a concern about potential malpractice liability, but her employer told her not to worry because he is responsible under the doctrine of respondeat superior.

1. Which sections of the ADHA or CDHA Code of Ethics apply to this case?
2. Is Ivy Smith meeting the standard of care for dental hygiene?
3. What strategies would you use to encourage Ivy to join the ADHA or CDHA?
4. Does the concept of respondeat superior excuse Ivy Smith from her legal and ethical responsibilities?
5. Assume Ivy Smith schedules a meeting to discuss her concerns with Dr. Brady. What legal and ethical issues should she raise with her employer?

SCENARIO 64-2

You have been working in a practice for 3 years and have developed a close friendship with Alice Gunn. Alice moved from Georgia 3 years ago, is a single parent, and is a technically proficient dental hygienist. Her dental hygiene skills and communication skills with clients and staff have impressed you. One night after work you and Alice go out for dinner, and she confides in you that she is not licensed in the state. Alice admits that because of the job opportunity that occurred in the office, the great health benefits, the hours, and the employer and employees, she could not wait to get a license and took the job. Your employer never asked for proof of licensure, and so she never had to admit or deny that she wasn't licensed. She asks you not to mention the situation because she really can't afford to stop practicing until she gets a license. She also does not want to be exposed because she is active in the local dental hygiene association and it would be embarrassing. She promises to try to get a license but doesn't want anyone to know that she isn't currently licensed.

1. Use the ethical decision-making model to resolve the dilemma presented.
2. How would a copy of the dental practice act assist the dental hygienist?
3. How could the employer have prevented this situation?
4. What aspects of the ADHA or CDHA Code of Ethics apply to this situation?

SCENARIO 64-3

Andrew Pierce is a second-year dental hygiene student who has been described as client centered. Andrew works diligently and carefully to make sure that his clients receive outstanding dental hygiene care. Many of the clients who visit the dental hygiene clinic are on limited incomes and do not have dental insurance. Andrew knows the importance of fluoride therapy for his child and adult clients. He tries to give fluoride treatments, when appropriate, to all clients. He knows that preventive therapies are important and feels he is serving the needs of the clients; however, he knows that some of his clients cannot afford the fluoride fee and would decline the treatment if given a choice. Andrew gives a fluoride treatment to clients who cannot afford the treatment or do not have insurance coverage. In order for them not to be charged, he does not record the fluoride treatment in the progress notes and does not indicate the fluoride treatment on the charge slip given to the cashier. The dental hygiene faculty members often do not notice that the fluoride treatment is not documented because they are busy with many students.

1. Which ethical principles apply to this case?
2. Identify some of the risks to the client, student, faculty, and dental hygiene program.
3. Take the part of the dental hygiene program director. What steps would you take with the student and with the dental hygiene faculty to address the problem?
4. Take the role of a student colleague of Andrew Pierce who is aware of the situation. Based on your program's academic and professional decorum policies, what would you do?

SCENARIO 64-4

An assistant, your best friend, is employed in the office where you practice dental hygiene and is pregnant. The doctor has been very understanding about her condition; however, she is scheduling her physician visits during the workday. Your employer "gently" asks her to schedule the doctor appointments toward the end of the day, when the office is closed. She becomes very offended and quits. She calls you the evening she quits and tells you that she is going to call the state OSHA office and report some violations related to the standards. You think this is unfair because the office is in compliance and she is creating issues where none exist. She also starts saying unkind things about the employer and suggests to you that she is also considering contacting the EEOC concerning possible sexual harassment.

1. Accusations of sexually harassing behaviors are serious. Discuss the types of sexual harassment that can occur in a dental office. If the dentist had been sexually harassing the assistant, what steps should she have taken?
2. If the employer had not been supportive of the pregnant assistant, what steps could the assistant have taken to resolve the conflict?
3. Use the ethical decision-making model to resolve the dilemmas presented.
4. What aspects of the ADHA or CDHA Code of Ethics apply to this situation?

REFERENCES

1. Nash DA: Ethics and the quest for excellence in the profession. *J Dent Educ* 49:198, 1985.
2. Peltier B, Hasegawa TK, Ozar DT, et al: Ethics Summit. II: Creating a sustaining structure for an ethic alliance of oral health organizations. *J Am Coll Dent* 67:4, 2000.
3. Gaston MA, Brown DM, Waring MB: Survey of ethical issues in dental hygiene. *J Dent Hyg* 64:217, 1990.
4. Grimes RM, Richards E, Flaitz CM: Avoiding malpractice for nondental conditions: the example of human immunodeficiency virus. *J Am Dent Assoc* 132:499, 2001.
5. Gairola G, Skaff KO: Ethical reasoning in dental hygiene. *Dent Hyg* 57:16, 1983.
6. Homenko DF: A committee's morals. *RDH* 19:32, 1999.
7. Garner BS, ed: *Black's law dictionary*, ed 7, St Paul, Minn, 1999, West.
8. Title VII of the Civil Rights Act, Part 1604.11 Code of Federal Regulations [Title 29, Vol 4, Parts 900 to 1899] [Revised July 1, 1997], Washington, DC, US Government Printing Office.
9. Pennington A, Darby M, Bauman D, et al: Sexual harassment in dentistry: experiences of Virginia dental hygienists. *J Dent Hyg* 74:288, 2000.
10. Pollack BR: *Dentist's risk management guide*, Fort Lauderdale, Fla, 1990, National Society of Dental Practitioners.

EVOLVE RESOURCES

Please visit http://evolve.elsevier.com/Darby/hygiene for additional practice and study support tools.

GLOSSARY

A

Abrasion Pathologic tooth wear caused by a foreign substance.

Abutment Tooth, tooth root, or dental implant that anchors a fixed or removable prosthetic appliance.

Acquired pellicle Thin, clear, unstructured organic membrane that forms over exposed tooth surfaces and restorations within minutes after removal by professional and self-polishing techniques.

Acute periapical abscess Localized inflammation that occurs when bacteria or toxins rapidly enter the periradicular tissues, usually from the tooth pulp chamber.

Acute pericoronitis Abscess associated with a partially erupted tooth or fully erupted tooth that is covered completely or partially by a flap of tissue (operculum).

Acute periodontal abscess Exacerbated inflammatory reaction occurring usually in a periodontally involved area and caused by a blockage of the area by some foreign body.

Aerosols Artificially generated solid or liquid airborne particles less than 50 microns in size.

Alginate Irreversible, flexible hydrocolloid impression material used primarily for making study casts of a client's dentition.

Alveolar bone Bone composed of compact or cortical bone and spongy bone that is marked by trabecular spaces seen on radiographs.

Alveolar mucosa Nonkeratinized epithelium characterized by a smooth and shiny surface that covers the vestibule and floor of the mouth and becomes the buccal and labial mucosa.

Amalgam Alloy of mercury with silver, copper, and tin; used to restore form and function of teeth.

Amide local anesthetics Agents that undergo biotransformation in the liver by microsomal enzymes; metabolic products of amide local anesthetic agents are almost entirely excreted by the kidneys.

Amorphous calcium phosphate (ACP) Substance containing the same minerals as the hydroxyapatite crystals of tooth enamel; calcium and phosphate ions in ACP seek out areas of demineralization to prevent caries progression, enhance enamel remineralization, and occlude dentinal tubules.

Anaerobic Occurring or existing in the absence of free oxygen.

Ankylosis A disturbance or underdevelopment of the bone on the affected side of a fracture; immobility of a joint resulting from infection, injury, surgery, or disease; fusion of bone to bone or tooth to bone.

Anodontia Congenital absence of teeth. Defects of ectodermal structures are causative effects; also known as *edentia.*

Apical third The third of the tooth involving the tip or apex of the root.

Approximal (proximal) caries Dental caries between teeth at the point of their proximal contact.

Area-specific curets Curets designed for use in specific locations, usually slightly narrower in blade width and longer in terminal shank length than are universal designs (e.g., Gracey curet series).

Assessment instruments Instruments, such as the periodontal probe, dental explorer, and mouth mirror, used for taking measurements and for detecting tooth irregularities, restorations, probe depths, soft-tissue changes, clinical parameters of oral disease, acquired deposits, and other intraoral manifestations.

Attached gingiva Portion of the gingiva that is connected firmly to the alveolar bone.

Attrition Tooth-to-tooth wear from opposing tooth contact.

Auscultation Physical assessment technique that uses the clinician's sense of hearing to determine an abnormality; act of listening to and detecting body sounds to determine variations from normal (e.g., listening for clicking sounds in the temporomandibular joint).

Autoclave Most common method of heat sterilization in the dental care setting. Uses moist-heat and pressure to sterilize instruments and materials that are not moist-heat sensitive.

B

Bacteremia Presence of microorganisms in the bloodstream.

Bacterial plaque biofilm See *Dental plaque; Oral biofilm.*

Behavior modification Technique used to reinforce desired behaviors and extinguish behaviors considered detrimental via the consistent application of rewards and punishment.

Beneficence Ethical principle that endorses the promotion of benefit, goodness, kindness, and charity and removal of harm.

Biofilm A complex, three-dimensional arrangement of bacteria living together as a self-sufficient, secure, self-sustaining community that is resistant to conventional antibiotics and antimicrobial agents. Dental plaque is a biofilm; therefore the term *oral biofilm* is used.

Bitewing radiographs Radiographs that include images of the crown and some of the roots of several teeth in both arches. Bitewing radiographs are standard diagnostic tools for posterior teeth, producing the best image of the tooth crowns, the main area of concern for dental caries and tooth restoration.

Bone loss (horizontal and vertical) Loss of alveolar bone that normally supports the teeth; the pattern of bone loss may be horizontal when the bone loss is parallel to the cementoenamel junction (CEJ) of adjacent teeth or vertical when the bone loss is oriented diagonally to the CEJ of adjacent teeth.

Bruxism Stress-induced, involuntary behavior of grinding the teeth together; does not cause bone loss itself but can cause loss of bone secondary to periodontitis, headache, muscle spasm, and facial pain.

Buccal mucosa Tissue that lines the inner cheek; may be glistening pink or pigmented with melanin; frequent areas of cheek-biting lesions.

C

Candidiasis (thrush) Fungal infection of the oral cavity caused by *Candida albicans;* also known as *thrush;* when it occurs under a denture, it is called *denture stomatitis*. Atrophic candidiasis is characterized by erythematous pebbled patches on the hard or soft palate, buccal mucosa, and dorsal surface of the tongue.

Carcinogenic Cancer-causing.

Cardiovascular disease (CVD) Alteration of the heart and/or blood vessels that impairs function.

Caries balance Balance between protective factors and pathologic factors to remineralize early carious lesions and/or prevent future caries.

Caries management Care plan to restore and maintain a balance between protective factors and pathologic factors to remineralize early carious lesions and/or prevent future caries, known as the *caries balance*.

Caries risk assessment Process by which the client is categorized based on the probability of developing dental caries; includes an individual's caries disease indicators, risk factors, and protective factors. The goal of caries risk assessment for clients 6 years old or older is to assign a client to a caries risk level for developing future caries as the first step in managing the disease process. The level of caries risk (low, moderate, high, or extreme) is based on the presence of caries disease indicators and the balance between pathologic and protective factors.

Case presentation Process of explaining assessment findings to a client along with options and recommendations for therapy to reach agreement on a care plan and client goals.

Cementoenamel junction (CEJ) Location on a tooth where the cementum and enamel meet; demarcation between the anatomic crown and the anatomic root of the tooth.

Cementum Mineralized bonelike substance that covers the roots of teeth and provides a surface for attachment and anchorage for the periodontal fibers; may be cellular or acellular.

Centric occlusion Relationship between the maxillary and mandibular occlusal surfaces that provides the maximum contact and/or intercuspation.

Cerebrovascular disease Disease of blood vessels supplying the brain.

Chemotherapeutic agent Chemical agent used to treat a disease or alter host response to the disease.

Chemotherapy Treatment of a disease with a chemical agent that destroys the pathogens causing the disease or alters their ability to replicate; also known as *pharmacotherapy.*

Chief complaint Client's primary reason for seeking the oral healthcare appointment as verbalized by the client. The chief complaint is written in the client's own words.

Chlorhexidine gluconate (CHG) A bis-biguanide used as a disinfectant for skin and mucous membranes; an antiplaque and antigingivitis agent. It is used predominantly in prescription oral rinses, irrigation solutions, and controlled-release products.

Client Biologic, psychologic, spiritual, social, cultural, and intellectual human being whose behavior is motivated by human needs and who has eight human needs related to dental hygiene care; the contemporary healthcare consumer; the term suggests one who is an active participant in oral healthcare and who is responsible for personal choices and the consequences of those choices; may refer to an individual or group.

Clinical crown Portion of the tooth that is exposed above the epithelial attachment.

Conceptual model Set of concepts and propositions integrated into a meaningful configuration within the domain of dental hygiene; school of thought.

Concrescence Fusion of two teeth at the root through the cementum only. Originally teeth are separate but later are joined because of excessive cementum deposition.

Conscious sedation Method of pain control that decreases client's response to pain, anxiety, and stress; client is awake and able to respond, breathe, and cough; also known as *inhalation sedation, nitrous-oxide psychosedation,* and *relative analgesia.*

Consistency Degree of firmness or density of the soft tissue; some terms used to define firmness include *spongy, fibrotic,* and *nodular.*

Continued care Maintenance care or periodontal maintenance therapy that occurs at regular intervals after completion of active therapy. Also known as *re-care* or *recall.*

Cross-arch fulcrum Fulcrum established by holding the working end of the instrument and the index finger of the hand holding the instrument on separate dental arches.

Cross-contamination Transfer of oral fluids and debris from a client to surfaces, equipment, materials, workers' hands, or another client or person (co-worker, family member, or friend).

Curet Subgingival scaling instrument designed to enhance access and adaptation on teeth with periodontal pockets.

D

Dental calculus Oral biofilm that has been mineralized by calcium and phosphate salts within the saliva and can attach to teeth, restorations, and dental appliances; commonly referred to as *tartar;* calcified oral biofilm.

Dental caries An infectious, chronic, bacteria-caused disease characterized by the acid dissolution of enamel and the eventual breakdown of the more organic, inner dental tissues.

Dental impression Negative imprint taken of the teeth and surrounding tissues so that a diagnostic cast (study model) can be made.

Dental index Quantifiable measure of the amount of oral disease or condition in a population or individual.

Dental plaque Dense, nonmineralized mass of bacterial colonies in a gel-like intermicrobial, enclosed matrix (slime layer) that is attached to a moist environmental surface. Also known as *microbial plaque, oral biofilm, dental biofilm, dental plaque biofilm, bacterial plaque biofilm.*

Dentifrice (toothpaste) Substance (gel, paste, or powder) used in conjunction with a toothbrush or interdental cleaner to facilitate bacterial plaque biofilm removal, or as a vehicle for transporting therapeutic or cosmetic agents to the tooth and its environment.

Dentinal hypersensitivity A painful condition that occurs when vital dentinal tubules are exposed to the oral environment; fluid movement within the dentinal tubule, caused by a stimulus (thermal, evaporative, tactile, osmotic, or chemical) initiates a pain sensation in the pulp because of dental attrition, dental erosion, gingival recession, and scaling and root planing. Also referred to as *dental hypersensitivity.*

Disclosing agent (disclosant) Liquid concentrate or tablet containing an ingredient that temporarily stains oral deposits and debris so that the client and clinician can see them.

Dyspnea Difficulty breathing.

E

Early childhood caries (ECC) Severe decay caused by *Streptococcus mutans* and by sugars and acids in a bottle of milk or juice left in contact with a child's primary teeth; causes rapid demineralization of hard tooth structure; affects children ages 0 to 2.

Edentulous Lacking or being without teeth.

Embrasure space The area immediately under the contact point of adjacent teeth. Size of the embrasure space is important in selecting the correct interdental cleaning aids.

Ergonomics Study of human performance and workplace design to maximize health, comfort, and efficiency.

Erythema A red area of variable shape and size reflecting tissue inflammation, thinness, and irregularity. The tissue then may be described as erythematous.

Essential oils Volatile oils derived from plants; contain phenolic compounds (e.g., thymol, eucalyptol, menthol, and methyl salicylate) and are used in some commercial mouth rinses.

Ester anesthetics Ester-type local anesthetics (primarily 20% benzocaine) used as topical anesthetic; injectable ester-type local anesthetics are off the market.

Extraoral fulcrum Fulcrum established outside of the mouth and used predominantly for teeth with deep periodontal pockets; the leverage point may be the client's jaw or side of the face. Also known as an *external fulcrum.*

F

Filled sealant Sealant composed of a mixture of resins, chemicals, and fillers.

Fluoride Most effective agent and nutrient for the prevention and control of dental caries on smooth surfaces of teeth.

Fluoride-releasing sealant Glass ionomer sealant.

Fremitus The vibration or movement of the teeth when in contacting positions from the client's own occlusal forces. Used in part to determine occlusal trauma.

Fulcrum Source of stability or leverage on which the finger rests and against which it pushes for the clinician to hold a dental instrument with control during stroke activation.

Furcation Areas between the branching roots of posterior teeth where the root trunk divides into separate roots.

G

Gingival margin Edge of the marginal gingiva nearest to the incisal or occlusal area of the tooth; marks the opening of the gingival sulcus.

Gingival recession Reduction of the height of the marginal gingiva to a location apical to the cementoenamel junction, resulting in root surface exposure; signifies attachment loss.

Gingival sulcus Space between the marginal gingiva and the tooth. The healthy gingival sulcus measures 0.5 mm to 3 mm from the gingival margin to the base of the sulcus. Also known as a *gingival crevice.*

Gingivitis Inflammation of the gingival tissue with no apical migration of the junctional epithelium beyond the cementoenamel junction; characterized by inflammation and redness of the gingival tissue and bleeding on probing. See also *Periodontitis.*

H

Health history Assessment of a client's health status to identify predisposing conditions, current and past treatment experiences, past responses to healthcare, and risk factors that may affect dental hygiene care and outcomes of care. Also known as *medical history.*

Host defense system A host's natural defense system against invasion by an organism (e.g., the inflammatory process and immune system).

Host immune system Consists of antibodies, lymphocytes, leukocytes, macrophages, and other specialized cells that protect the body from invasion by foreign substances. Specialized cells that fight infectious agents.

Human need Internal tension that results from an alteration in a state of a person's system. Eight human needs related to dental hygiene practice follow:

Biologically sound and functional dentition: The need to have intact teeth and restorations that defend against harmful microbes, provide for adequate function, and reflect appropriate nutrition and diet.

Conceptualization and problem solving: The need to grasp ideas and abstractions in order to make sound decisions about one's oral health.

Freedom from fear and stress: The need to feel safe and to be free from fear and emotional discomfort in the oral healthcare environment.

Freedom from head and neck pain: The need to be exempt from physical discomfort in the head and neck area.

Protection from health risks: The need to avoid medical contraindications to dental hygiene care, including the need to be protected from health risks related to dental hygiene care.

Responsibility for oral health: The need to be accountable for one's health as a result of interaction among one's motivation, physical capability, and environment.

Skin and mucous membrane integrity of the head and neck: The need to have an intact and functioning covering of one's head and neck area, including the oral mucous membranes and periodontium, which defend against harmful microbes, resist injurious substances and trauma, and reflect adequate nutrition.

Wholesome facial image: The need to feel satisfied with one's own oral-facial features and breath.

Human needs conceptual model Conceptual model of dental hygiene that defines the paradigm concepts of client, environment, health and oral health, and dental hygiene actions in terms of human needs theory.

Human needs theory Theory that explains and predicts human behavior by focusing on human need fulfillment and unmet human needs as motivators.

Hypertension Condition characterized by a persistent elevation of the systolic and diastolic blood pressures. Blood pressure ranges are as follows:

Normal: Less than 120/80 mm Hg

Prehypertension: 120-139/80-89 mm Hg

Stage 1 high blood pressure: 140-159/90-99 mm Hg

Stage 2 high blood pressure: 160 and above/100 and above mm Hg

I

Iatrogenic factors Adverse factors caused by the healthcare practitioner that result in a negative outcome for the patient.

Immunity The nonsusceptible state of a host to an infectious agent or antigen. In terms of the law, established to protect persons from civil lawsuits and criminal prosecution resulting from filing a report of child abuse and neglect.

Immunosuppression Suppression of the body's natural immune response, measured by a decrease in certain immune system cells.

Inactive ingredient (nontherapeutic agent) A product additive that is necessary to make the formulation thick, hold together, clean efficiently, or have a particular color or flavor for consumer appeal.

Incipient caries Carious lesions limited to the enamel surface: if in a pit or fissure, it can be treated with a dental sealant.

Inflammatory mediators Soluble, diffusible molecules that promote or enhance the process of inflammation and therefore can cause hard- and soft-tissue destruction observed in periodontal disease. Some examples include endotoxin (LPS), interleukin, tumor necrosis factor-α, and prostaglandins.

Informed consent Written agreement from a mentally competent person that allows an action on the part of the healthcare provider; required before the performance of invasive healthcare procedures or procedures on a minor, and before a person is used as a participant (subject) in research. The agreement may come from a legal guardian or healthcare decision maker in the case of a minor or others who cannot self-determine.

Inhalation sedation Synonym for nitrous oxide and oxygen analgesia; gases are inhaled through the nose, resulting in the reduction in the perception of pain and reduction in anxiety in the client. Also known as *conscious sedation, psychosedation,* and *relaxation sedation.*

Initial therapy Also known as *phase I periodontal therapy* or *anti-infective therapy,* most of which falls within the scope of dental hygiene practice. Includes client education, diet assessment, tobacco cessation, fluoride therapy, dental sealants, debridement, desensitization, antimicrobial therapy, selective polishing, restorative prosthetic treatment, and occlusal therapy.

Interdental papilla Gingival tissue located in the interdental space between two adjacent teeth; the tip and lateral borders are continuous with the marginal gingiva, whereas the center is composed of alveolar gingiva.

Interproximal or interdental area The proximal surfaces of teeth (mesial and distal surfaces) and the embrasure spaces.

Intraoral fulcrum Traditional fulcrum established inside the mouth against tooth structure.

Intrinsic stain Internal discoloration of the tooth that may be caused by taking medication (e.g., tetracycline), excessive fluoride ingestion, or genetics during tooth development.

J

Junctional epithelium (JE) Cufflike band of nonkeratinized squamous epithelium that completely encircles and adheres to the tooth surface at the base of the gingival sulcus via hemidesmosomes; histologically the apex, or base of the sulcus, is formed by the JE.

Justice Ethical and legal principle that relies on fairness and equality; a person is treated justly when given what he or she is due, is owed, deserves, or can claim legitimately.

K

Kaposi's sarcoma Malignant neoplasm associated with HIV infection and manifesting as brown or purplish tumors on the gingiva near the teeth or on the skin.

L

Lateral pressure Force used by a dental hygienist to engage the cutting edge of the periodontal scaling instrument against the tooth.

Lavage Therapeutic washing of the periodontal pockets and root surface to remove endotoxins and loose debris with water under pressure.

Lingual Surface nearest the tongue.

Local anesthesia Loss of sensation in a circumscribed area of the body as a result of the depression of excitation in nerve endings or the inhibition of the conduction process in peripheral nerves; results from use of a local anesthetic agent.

Local delivery Mode of application in which the antimicrobial agent is transported directly to the oral cavity, or a specific location within it, for topical application.

Low-velocity evacuation tubing (LVE) Tubing that facilitates low level of suctioning to rid the oral cavity of saliva and debris during oral care; also facilitates patient rinsing, operator's ability to see, and oral fluid control during care.

M

Malalignment Malposition of the teeth.

Materia alba Loosely attached collection of soft oral debris and bacteria seen as a whitish, curdlike mass on the teeth or overlying oral biofilm.

Meta-analysis A statistical process often used with systematic reviews; involves combining the data analyses of numerous individual studies into one analysis; considered one of the gold standards for evidence because of strict protocols to reduce bias and to include the findings of only the very best studies.

Mobility Property of a lesion; refers to whether the lesion is free or fixed in relationship to the neighboring tissues; also used to describe the degree of movement of a tooth in a socket infected with periodontitis.

Modified pen grasp Standard grasp used for assessment and treatment instruments.

Motivation The incentive or drive to satisfy unmet human needs or human needs in deficit.

Motivational interviewing Form of patient-centered communication to help clients get "unstuck" from the ambivalence that prevents a specific behavior change. The goal is to have the client verbalize arguments for stopping an unhealthy behavior like smoking.

Mucogingival conditions Conditions that occur when the periodontal disease process extends beyond the attached gingiva and into the alveolar mucosa.

Mucogingival junction Demarcation between the alveolar mucosa and the attached gingiva.

N

Nitrous oxide Gas used in combination with oxygen for the control of pain and anxiety during dental and dental hygiene care.

Nodule Elevated solid mass; deeper and firmer than a papule of between 0.5 cm and 2 cm in size.

Nonadherence or noncompliance A lack of client cooperation with recommended oral healthcare.

Nonmaleficence Ethical principle stating that, above all, a health professional should do no harm.

Non–plaque-induced gingivitis Gingival diseases of specific bacterial, viral, or genetic origin; gingival manifestations of systemic conditions such as mucocutaneous disorders and allergic reactions; or traumatic lesions, foreign body reactions, or otherwise nonspecific gingival lesions.

Nonsteroidal anti-inflammatory drugs (NSAIDs) Drugs that block enzymes that promote the inflammatory response, thus reducing inflammation.

Nonsurgical periodontal therapy (NSPT) Periodontal scaling and root planing performed with the aim of increasing connective tissue attachment level. Also includes the use of chemotherapeutic agents to control periodontal pathogens.

Nonverbal communication Interactions between two or more persons using body language to communicate a message.

Nutritional counseling Process used to help clients develop healthful food selection and eating behaviors that promote overall health.

O

Occlusal Biting or chewing surfaces of posterior teeth.

Occlusion Contact relationship between maxillary and mandibular teeth when the jaws are in a fully closed position.

Occupational exposure Exposure to an infectious agent that occurs in the workplace. A percutaneous injury or contact of mucous membrane or nonintact skin with blood, saliva, tissue, or other body fluids that are potentially infectious. Exposure incidents may pose a risk of hepatitis B virus, hepatitis C virus, or HIV infection and are a matter of medical urgency.

Occupational Safety and Health Administration (OSHA) Federal agency responsible for safety in the workplace.

Opposite-arch fulcrum Intraoral fulcrum established on a tooth surface on the opposing arch from the arch being scaled.

Oral biofilm A biofilm that grows on surfaces within the oral cavity; is a necessary condition for initiation and progression of dental caries and periodontal disease, depending on the pathogens present in the biofilm. See also *Biofilm; Dental plaque.*

Oral biofilm control (plaque control) Regular mechanical or chemical removal of dental plaque from the teeth and adjacent oral tissue or the prevention of its growth and maturation.

Oral hygiene Degree to which the oral cavity is kept clean and free of soft and hard deposits by daily oral self-care or, when necessary, oral care provided by a caregiver.

Oral irrigation Method of directing a steady or pulsating stream of water or chemotherapeutic agent over the teeth, over the gingival tissues, or into a periodontal pocket; goal is to remove oral debris, reduce pathogens and their by-products, or deliver an antimicrobial agent.

Oral malodor (halitosis) Offensive breath odor associated with poor oral hygiene, periodontitis, sinus infection, tonsillitis, lung disease, diabetes, or uremia.

Oral rinses Available for both cosmetic and therapeutic use and in prescription and over-the-counter formulations.

Therapeutic uses include plaque and gingivitis reduction and caries prevention; cosmetic uses include breath freshening, tartar control, and tooth whitening. Also known as *mouth rinses* and *mouthwashes.*

Oropharyngeal Referring to an area consisting of the throat, back third of the tongue, soft palate, and side and back walls of the throat and tonsils.

Osteoporosis Condition involving demineralization of the bone and a decrease in bone mass caused by excessive leaching of calcium from the bone matrix.

Over-the-counter (OTC) drugs Medications and healthcare products that can be purchased without a prescription directly off the store shelf. The American Dental Association Seal of Acceptance includes only OTC products and devices. The Seal is no longer given for prescription drugs.

P

Palpation Act of using the sense of touch to collect client data; compressing or moving tissue to check for abnormalities during an intraoral and extraoral examination.

Panoramic radiograph Radiograph in which the entire dentition, in addition to the adjacent osseous structures from the orbits of the eyes to the base of the mandible and the temporomandibular joints, is displayed on one rectangular film.

Peri-implantitis Inflammation affecting the soft and hard tissue around a dental implant.

Periodontal debridement Removal of subgingival calculus and oral biofilm and its by-products while preserving as much tooth surface as possible.

Periodontal maintenance (PM) Supportive phase of care initiated after successful completion of active periodontal treatment; also known as *supportive periodontal therapy.*

Periodontal pocket Pathologic deepening of the gingival sulcus from the apical migration of the junctional epithelium and destruction of the periodontium.

Periodontitis Inflammatory disease of the periodontium that results from progression of gingivitis; caused by specific microorganisms; characterized by progressive destruction of the periodontal ligament and alveolar bone, recession, clinical attachment loss, pocket formation, and possible tooth mobility. The four major types are chronic, aggressive, necrotizing, and systemic. See also *Gingivitis.*

Periodontium Supporting structure of tissues that surrounds the teeth; includes the gingiva, periodontal ligament, root cementum, and alveolar bone.

Piezoelectric Type of ultrasonic scaling device that has a ceramic transducer; alternating currents applied to the transducer create dimensional change that is transmitted to the tip; tip moves in a linear pattern, and only two sides of the tip are activated and applied to the tooth for mechanized instrumentation.

Pit and fissure sealant Thin plastic coating of an organic polymer (resin) placed in the pits and fissures of teeth to act as a physical barrier. Also known as a *dental sealant.*

Preliminary impression Impressions taken to construct study models for diagnosing, documenting clients' dental arches as part of permanent records, and enhancing client education as a visual aid.

Preprocedural rinse A therapeutic oral rinse used before and during professional care to decrease oral microorganisms available to the clinical environment from oral procedures that cause aerosols and spatter.

Preventive sealant Sealant that is placed in caries-free teeth in an effort to prevent dental caries.

Professionally applied fluoride Fluoride therapy administered in an oral healthcare setting by a dental hygienist; high-potency, low-frequency fluoride therapy.

Prophylactic antibiotic premedication Drug therapy administered before invasive dental hygiene instrumentation to clients at the highest risk of a negative outcome from infective endocarditis.

Proximal contact The contact between teeth (mesial to distal and mesial to mesial at the midline) that stabilizes their position in the dental arch and prevents food impaction between the teeth.

Q

Quadrant Any one of the four quarters of the maxillary and mandibular arches.

R

Rampant caries Rapidly progressive decay that requires urgent intervention to gain control, eliminate the disease, and prevent progression.

Recession Reduction of the height of the marginal gingiva to a location apical to the cementoenamel junction, resulting in root surface exposure; signifies clinical attachment loss.

Re-evaluation Appointment that takes place 4 to 6 weeks after completion of nonsurgical periodontal therapy so that a client's response to active therapy can be determined.

Referral To direct to a source of information or care for a suspected problem, disease, or condition such as child abuse or neglect.

Remineralization Deposition of minerals into previously damaged areas of a tooth; process of replenishing calcium, phosphate, and fluoride ions to damaged tooth structure that has lost minerals; facilitated by fluoride therapy and amorphous calcium phosphate therapy.

Removable partial denture Partial denture that can be removed from the mouth by the client.

Restorative therapy Restoration of damaged tooth structure, defective restorations, esthetic inconsistencies, and anatomic and physiologic abnormalities.

Risk assessment Act of determining the likelihood of a disease occurring in the future based on the balance between risk factors and protective factors.

Risk factors Behaviors and conditions present in the client, child, parent, family, or environment that may contribute to future disease, disability, or abuse and neglect. Conditions, behaviors, lifestyles, or genes that if present will increase the likelihood of a disease occurring.

Root planing Definitive procedure to remove cementum or surface dentin that is rough, impregnated with calculus, or contaminated with toxins or microorganisms.

Rubber cup polishing Removal of tooth stains after scaling using a low-speed handpiece, prophylaxis angle with rubber cup, and prophylaxis polishing paste; coronal polishing.

S

Same-arch fulcrum Intraoral fulcrum established by a finger resting on a tooth surface on the same arch near the area being assessed or treated with a dental hygiene instrument.

Scaling Instrumentation of the crown and root surfaces of the teeth to remove oral biofilm, dental calculus, and extrinsic stains from surfaces without the intentional removal of tooth surface.

Self-care (home care) Client's care regimen performed at home daily.

Sign Objective condition that can be observed directly.

Standard precautions Synthesis of the major features of universal precautions and body substance isolation precautions applied to blood; other body fluids, secretions, and excretions except sweat; no-intact skin; and mucous membranes.

Sterilization Destruction of all living organisms, including highly resistant bacterial spores.

Subgingival calculus Calculus located below the gingival margin and attached to cementum or dentin.

Sulcular epithelium Nonkeratinized epithelial lining of the gingival sulcus.

Supragingival calculus Calculus located above the gingival margin; may attach to any hard surface including enamel, restorative materials, prosthetic appliances, or exposed cementum.

Symptom Subjective condition reported by the client.

Systematic reviews Reviews of published research reports that provide a summary of numerous, high-quality research studies that have investigated the same specific question. Systematic reviews use explicit criteria for retrieval of studies, assessment, and synthesis of evidence from individual randomized clinical trials and other well-controlled methods. Many are published by the Cochrane Collaboration.

Systemic delivery system Mode of application in which the agent (drug) is ingested and then delivered via the bloodstream; agents so delivered include products such as fluoride supplements, fluoridated water, and antibiotic medications.

T

Tachycardia Abnormally high heart rate, usually above 150 beats per minute.

Tactile sensitivity Ability to distinguish relative degrees of roughness and smoothness on the tooth surface via the vibrations transferred from the instrument's working end, shank, and handle to the clinician's fingers.

Temporomandibular joint (TMJ) dysfunction (TMD) Impaired function of the joint characterized by pain, headache, tinnitus, impaired hearing, and pain around the tongue; any one or combination of the following maladies: pain in the area of the TMJ and or muscles of mastication, limitation or deviation in the movement of the mandible, and/or detectable sounds during movement of the mandible. Also known as *temporomandibular dysfunction.*

Therapeutic communication Process of sending and receiving messages between a client and a healthcare provider that assists the client to make decisions and reach goals related to comfort and health.

Therapeutic sealant Sealant that is placed in teeth with incipient carious lesions in an effort to stop the decay process.

Tobacco cessation Evidence-based intervention for becoming tobacco free.

Tooth bleaching (whitening) Use of a chemical oxidizing agent, sometimes in combination with heat, to lighten tooth discoloration.

Topical fluoride Products that are self-applied by clients in a nonprescription form, self-applied by clients in a prescription form, or professionally applied prescription products that are delivered for variable amounts of time to exposed crown and root surfaces and then expectorated.

Transient bacteremia Temporary presence of bacteria and other microorganisms in the bloodstream.

Trauma Injury that results when the client inadvertently chews or bites oral tissues while they are still anesthetized. An injury caused by accident or a violent act.

U

Ulceration Loss of skin surface, with a gray to yellow center surrounded by a red halo; results from destruction of epithelial integrity caused by discrepancy in cell maturation, loss of intracellular attachments, and disruption of the basement membrane.

Ultrasonic scaler Mechanized device that produces vibratory motions of the instrument tip from 18,000 to 50,000 cycles per second; removes all types of supragingival and subgingival deposits from tooth surfaces; includes magnetostrictive and piezoelectric mechanized instruments.

Unfilled sealant Sealant that does not contain particles and is therefore less resistant to wear; useful in school-based settings when occlusion cannot be adjusted with a finishing burr and dental handpiece.

Universal curet Curet that has two cutting edges on each working end; designed for use in all areas throughout the mouth.

Unmet human needs (human need deficits) Human needs related to oral health, which are in deficit. See also *Human need.*

W

Working end Part of the instrument attached to the shank that determines the general purpose of the instrument.

X

Xerostomia Dry mouth caused by a variety of conditions such as a salivary gland dysfunction, medications, and radiation therapy to the head and neck.

Y

Yokes Devices to hold gas cylinders in contact with the gas machine.

Z

Zones of territory Appropriate distances, or personal spaces, that are maintained between people in various situations; such zones may be based on the degree of respect, authority, and friendship between the individuals communicating.

Page numbers followed by "f" indicate figures, "t" indicate tables, and "b" indicate boxes.

A

B

M

O

P

S

X

Y

Z